DEDICATION

To the memory of my father and mother, Pietro and Giuliana:
They would have been proud to see the results of my efforts
—*Andrea Gabrielli*

To my best friend and partner Susana E. Picado—who makes me better.
To those who, in service to our people, struggle for justice and peace;
Giuliana and Pietro were two.
—*A. Joseph Layon*

To my dad, General Jae Hung Yu, and the Seventh Division for their sacrifices and
changing history for the better.
To my Mom, the late Esang Yoon who was the wind beneath our wings.
To the late Dr. Thomas J. Whelan Jr. who continues to mentor me in the practice of
Surgery and Code of conduct.
To Joe and Judy Civetta who sparked my continuing love for Critical Care and being the
guiding light for all Peepsters.
And to my late daughter Pearl (and CD) who has the Master Key to All...
—*Mihae Yu*

■ CONTRIBUTING AUTHORS

The authors would like to gratefully acknowledge the efforts of the contributors of the original chapters in *Civetta, Taylor, and Kirby's Critical Care*, Fourth Edition.

Steven G. Achinger, MD

Gareth Adams, MD

Olufemi Akindipe, MD

Serge Alfandari, MD, MSc

Adrian Alvarez, MD

Marcelo Amato, MD

Giuditta Angelini

Djillali Annane, MD, PhD

Massimo Antonelli, MD

Juan Carlos Ayus, MD, FACP, FASN

Keri A. Baacke, MD

Sean M. Bagshaw, MD, MSc, FRCPC

Philip S. Barie, MD, MBS, FCCM, FACS

Claudia L. Barthold, MD

Robert H. Bartlett, MD

Miho K. Bautista, MD

Maher A. Baz, MD

Elizabeth Cordes Behringer, MD

Giuseppe Bello, MD

Rinaldo Bellomo, MBBS, MD, FRACP, FJFICM

Howard Belzberg, MD, FCCM

Ira M. Bernstein, MD

Rebecca J. Beyth, MD

Indermeet S. Bhullar, MD

Luca M. Bigatello, MD

Thomas P. Bleck, MD, FCCM

Ernest F.J. Block, MD, MBA

Eric L. Bloomfield, MD

Karen L. Booth, MD

Karen Bordson, DO

Adrien Bougle, MD

Philip Boysen, MD

James E. Calvin, Jr., MD

William G. Cance, MD

Lawrence J. Caruso, MD

Juan C. Cendan, MD

Cherylee W.J. Chang, MD, FACP

Marianne E. Cinat, MD, FACS

Cornelius J. Clancy, MD

Michael Coburn, MD

Giorgio Conti, MD

Jamie B. Conti, MD, FACC, FHRS

Timothy J. Coons, RRT, MBA

Mark S. Cooper, BM, BCh, PhD

C. Clay Cothren, MD, FACS

Douglas B. Coursin, MD

Claudia Crimi, MD

Kristina Crothers, MD

Gohar H. Dar, MD

Rabih O. Darouiche, MD

Elizabeth Lee Daugherty, MD, MPH

David A. Decker, MD

Leonardo De Luca, MD

Demetrias Demetriades, MD, PhD, FACS

Clifford S. Deutschman, MS, MD, FCCM

Karen E. Doucette, MD, MSc

Quan-Yang Duh, MD

Stephanie H. Dunlap, DO

Herbert L. DuPont, MD

Soumitra R. Eachempati, MD, FACS

Rodney K. Edwards, MD, MS

Elamin M. Elamin, MD, MSc, FACP, FCCP

Timothy C. Fabian, MD, FACS

Samir M. Fakhry, MD, FACS

Kevin J. Farrell, MD

Robert J. Feezor, MD

Niall D. Ferguson, MD, FRCPC, MSc

Sebastian Fernandez-Bussy, MD

Joseph Ferreira, BS, CPTC, CTOP II

Henry E. Fessler, MD

Jay A. Fishman, MD

Timothy C. Flynn, MD

Michael A. Frölich, MD, MS

Brian Fuehrlein, PhD

Andrea Gabrielli, MD, FCCM

Robert Peter Gale, MD

George D. Garcia, MD

Achille Gaspardone, MD, Mphil

Dany E. Ghannum, MD

Lewis R. Goldfrank, MD

Shankar P. Gopinath, MD

Dietrich Gravenstein, MD

J.S. Gravenstein, MD

David M. Greer, MD, MA

Jeffrey S. Groeger, MD

Jonathan Haft, MD

Stephen B. Hanauer, MD

Ikram U. Haque, MD

Cathleen Harris, MD

Kevin W. Hatton, MD

George Hatzakis, MSc, PhD

Steven O. Heard, MD

Alan W. Hemming, MD, MSc

Dean R. Hess, PhD, RRT

Zoltan G. Hevesi, MD

Thomas L. Higgins, MD, MBA

Brian L. Hoh, MD

M. Barbara Honnebier, MD, PhD

Charles W. Hoopes, MD

Ramona O. Hopkins, PhD

David B. Hoyt, MD, FACS

Laurence Huang, MD

Thomas S. Huber, MD, PhD

Ahamed H. Idris, MD

Steven R. Insler, DO

Felicia A. Ivascu, MD

James C. Jackson, PsyD

Sridivya Jaini, MD, MS

Michael A. Jantz, MD, FCCP

Edgar Jimenez, MD, FCCM

Aaron Joffe, MD

Raja Kandaswamy, MD

Scott R. Karlan, MD

Paraskevi A. Katsaounou, MD

Robin D. Kim, MD

Craig S. Kitchens, MD

Charles T. Klodell, MD

Marin H. Kollef, MD

Meghavi S. Kosboth, DO

Andreas H. Kramer, MD, FRCPC

Anand Kumar, MD

Aseem Kumar, PhD

Franco Laghi, MD

A. Joseph Layon, MD, FACP

Marc Leone, MD, PhD

Olivier Y. Leroy, MD

David M. Levi, MD

Lawrence Lottenberg, MD, FACS

Harrinarine Madhosingh, MD

Michael E. Mahla, MD

Patrick T. Mailoux, DO

Daniel R. Margulies, MD, FACS

Paul E. Marik, MD, FCCm, FCCP

Claude Martin, MD

Larry C. Martin, MD

Mali Mathru, MD

S. Anjani D. Mattai, MD

Kristin L. Mekeel, MD

Richard J. Melker, MD, PhD

Scott T. Micek, PharmD

William M. Miles, MD

Taro Mizutani, MD, PhD

Jerome H. Modell, MD

Ernest E. Moore, MD

Frederick A. Moore, MD, FACS

Sharon E. Moran, MD

Jan S. Moreb, MD

Alison Morris, MD, MS

Thomas C. Mort, MD

David W. Mozingo, MD, FACS

Susanne Muehlschlegel, MD

Deane Murfin, MBBCh, DA(SA), FCA(SA)

Michael J. Murray, MD, PhD

Neil A. Mushlin, DO

Ece A. Mutlu, MD, MBA

Gökhan M. Mutlu, MD

Bhiken I. Naik, MBBCh(Wits), DA(SA)

Minh-Hong Nguyen, MD

Minh-Ly Nguyen, MD

Jennifer A. Oakes, MD

Nimisha K. Parekh, MD, MPH

Robert I. Parker, MD

David A. Paulus, MD

V. Ram Peddi, MD

Kevin Y. Pei, MD

Carl W. Peters, MD

Frederic M. Pieracci, MD, MPH

Michael R. Pinsky, MD, CM, Drhc, FCCP, FCCM

F. Elizabeth Poalillo, RN, MSN, ARNP, CCRN

Andrew Pollak, MD

David T. Porembka, DO, FCCM

Raymond O. Powrie, MD, FRCP, FACP

Issam I. Raad, MD

Amin Rahemtulla, PhD, FRCP

S. Sujanthy Rajaram, MD

H. David Reines, MD

Zaccaria Ricci, MD

Winston T. Richards, MD

Claudia S. Robertson, MD

Steven A. Robicsek, MD, PhD

Claudio Ronco, MD

Amy F. Rosenberg, PharmD

Stephen J. Roth, MD, MPH

Daniel T. Ruan, MD

Steven Sandoval, MD

Stephanie A. Savage, MD

Sherry J. Saxonhouse, MD

Thomas M. Scalea, MD

Denise Schain, MD

Carten M. Schmalfuss, MD

Eran Segal, MD

Allen M. Seiden, MD, FACS

Steven A. Seifert, MD, FACMT, FACEP

Hani Seoudi, MD

Christoph N. Seubert, MD, PhD

David Shade, BA, JD

Stephen D. Shafran, MD, FRCPC

Jack D. Shannon, MD

Marc J. Shapiro, MD, MS, FACS, FCCM

Takeru Shimizu, MD, PhD

William C. Shoemaker, MD

Marc A. Simon, MD, MS, FACC

Jennifer A. Sipos, MD

Lee P. Skrupky, PharmD, BCPS

Robert N. Sladen, MBChB, MRCP(UK), FRCP(C), FCCM

Matthew S. Slater, MD

Danny Sleeman, MD, FACS, FRCS

Wendy I. Sligl, MD

Arthur S. Slutsky, MD

Eric S. Sobel, MD, PhD

Howard K. Song, MD, PhD

Edward D. Staples, MD

John K. Stene, MD, PhD

Deborah Stern, MD, MPH

Andrew Stolbach, MD

R. Todd Stravitz, MD, FACP, FACG

Kathirvel Subramaniam, MD

Murat Sungur, MD

David E.R. Sutherland, MD, PhD

Maria Suurna, MD

Sankar Swaminathan, MD

Danny M. Takanashi, Jr., MD, FACS

Christopher D. Tan, PharmD, BCPS

Jamie Taylor, MD

Lisa Thannikary, MD

S. Rob Todd, MD, FACS

Krista L. Turner, MD

Andreas G. Tzakis, MD, PhD

Kimi R. Ueda, PharmD

Kürsat Uzun, MD

Johannes H. van Oostrom, PhD

Thomas C. Vary, PhD

Theordoros Vassilakopoulos, MD

George C. Velmahos, MD, PhD, MSEd

J. Matthias Walz, MD

Hsiu-Po Wang, MD

Michael F. Waters, MD, PhD

Carl P. Weiner, MD, MBA, FACOG

Eelco F.M. Wijdicks, MD

Robert D. Winfield, MD

Charles C.J. Wo, BS

Linda L. Wong, MD

Gregory W. Woo, MD

Kenneth E. Wood, DO

Jean-Pierre Yared, MD

Mihae Yu, MD, FACS

Arno L. Zaritsky, MD

Janice L. Zimmerman, MD

In the Preface to the Fourth Edition of the textbook, we quote Nikos Kazantzakis' *Report to Greco*. Did our attempt succeed? Early reports suggest yes.

However much we have succeeded, the foundation for this was laid by Doctors Civetta, Taylor and Kirby—our teachers and mentors. We truly stand on the shoulders of giants.

We hope you—our readers—will provide us feedback on the quality of this handbook, as you have the textbook. Our desire with the *Manual* was to distill the full textbook into a short, pithy and readable contribution. We are pretty sure the "short" part did not work too well; let us know if we have, however, created something useful for you.

As we noted in the Preface to the textbook, the mistakes of omission or commission found herein are ours and ours alone.

We three editors share a friendship, have given each other guidance and moral support, and will share any failures and successes of our travail.

A. Joseph Layon
(ajlayon@geisinger.edu)
Danville, Pennsylvania

Andrea Gabrielli
(agabrielli@anest.ufl.edu)
Gainesville, Florida

Mihae Yu
(mihaey@hawaii.edu)
Honolulu, Hawaii

■ ACKNOWLEDGMENTS

We thank our colleagues at Lippincott—Nicole Dernoski, Tom Gibbons, and Brian Brown–for their assistance. Indu Jawwad from Aptara did superb work.

Our families are part of this handbook, to them, we bow in thanks and respect.

Andrea Gabrielli
A. Joseph Layon
Mihae Yu

■ CONTENTS

CHAPTER 1 ■ FUNDAMENTALS OF CARDIOPULMONARY RESUSCITATION

MAJOR PROBLEMS

- Cardiopulmonary resuscitation (CPR) is a series of assessments and interventions performed during a variety of acute medical and surgical events wherein death is likely without immediate intervention.
- Sudden cardiac arrest (SCA) is a leading cause of adult death in the United States and Canada.
  - Cardiac arrest (CA) is defined as "cessation of cardiac mechanical activity as confirmed by the absence of signs of circulation."
    - In the prehospital arena, CA is most commonly due to ventricular fibrillation (VF) secondary to ischemic heart disease.
      - Asystole and pulseless electrical activity (PEA) are less common initial rhythms with SCA, although these rhythms may represent the initial identified rhythm in adults who actually experienced an acute VF or ventricular tachycardia (VT) event.
    - Although VF and VT are considered to be the most common out-of-hospital (OOH) arrest rhythms, only 20% to 38% of in-hospital arrest patients have VF or VT as their initial rhythm.
    - Children and young adults require CPR most commonly for respiratory arrest, airway obstruction, or drug toxicity.
      - VF/VT is identified as the initial rhythm in 5% to 15% of OOH arrests in children.
    - Other conditions such as trauma, external or internal hemorrhage, and drowning may call for resuscitation at any age.
- Immediate and effective CPR can save lives.
  - With witnessed VF CA, CPR doubles or triples the rate of survival.
  - Only about 27% of OOH arrest victims receive bystander CPR.
- The primary goal of CPR is to generate sufficient oxygen delivery to the coronary and cerebral circulations to maintain cellular viability while attempting to restore a perfusing cardiac rhythm by defibrillation, pharmacologic intervention, or both.

IMMEDIATE CONCERNS

- Effective CPR can be performed by following a few basic rules.

- Immediately assess the environment for danger and move the patient if necessary. Never assume that an environment is safe.
- Minimize the time from CA recognition to starting effective CPR.
  - For every minute without CPR during witnessed VF CA, survival decreases by 7% to 10%.
  - This is cut in half (3%–4% per minute) when bystander CPR preceded attempted defibrillation.
  - Defibrillate immediately if a defibrillator is rapidly available (less than 3–5 min) in patients with VF.
    - This is the primary treatment focus within the first few minutes of SCA due to VF.
      - For each minute delay in defibrillation, chances of eventual hospital discharge decreased by 8% to 10%.
      - If the time from arrest to emergency medical service (EMS) arrival and initiation of CPR is more than 5 minutes, provision of 2 minutes of CPR before defibrillation is associated with improved outcome.
- "Push hard and fast" during chest compressions and minimize the duration of interruptions to reassess the patient's rhythm.
  - Interrupt chest compressions only briefly, about every 2 minutes, to assess the rhythm, and switch rescuer if feasible.
- While CPR is in progress, attempt to identify the cause of arrest.
  - Other resuscitation interventions may be indicated based on the cause of CA.
  - If no response to standard CPR interventions, think about delayed recognition and recall the H's and T's (Table 1.1).
  - Good teamwork increases the effectiveness of resuscitation when more than one rescuer is available.
- Attention to postresuscitation care is an important element of neurologic outcome.
  - Restore and support adequate cardiac output and tissue perfusion.
  - Monitor and maintain normal blood glucose concentrations.
  - Treat the underlying cause of the arrest.
  - Maintain normothermia.
  - Consider therapeutic hypothermia to maximize survival and cerebral recovery.
- If there is no response to effective CPR, appropriate judgment is needed in determining when to stop resuscitative efforts.

TABLE 1.1

POTENTIAL CORRECTABLE PROBLEMS DURING CARDIAC ARREST: "6 H'S AND 5 T'S"

Hypovolemia
Hypoxia
Hydrogen ion (acidosis)
Hypo-/hyperkalemia
Hypoglycemia
Hypothermia
Toxins
Tamponade, cardiac
Tension pneumothorax
Thrombosis, coronary or pulmonary
Trauma

Adapted from 2005 American Heart Association Guidelines for Cardiopulmonary Resuscitation and Emergency Cardiovascular Care. *Circulation.* 2005;112[24]SIV-1–IV-211.

OUT-OF-HOSPITAL CARDIAC ARREST

- Despite improvement in the scientific basis for resuscitation practices and extensive efforts at CPR training of lay and professional rescuers
  - Outcome of most adult victims of out-of-hospital cardiac arrest (OOHCA) remains poor.
    - Median reported survival to hospital discharge is 6.4%.
    - Adults who had a witnessed CA were more likely to arrive to the hospital alive (39% vs. 31%, $p = 0.049$) and were more likely to have a good neurologic outcome after 6 months (35% vs. 25%, $p = 0.023$) as compared with patients who had a CA in a nonpublic location.
  - In children, epidemiology and physiology of OOHCA are different.
    - Recent systematic review of 41 OOHCA studies, including trauma, revealed a restoration of spontaneous circulation (ROSC) of 30%, with survival to admission of 24% but survival to discharge of 12% and neurologically intact survival of only 4%.
    - Initial cardiac rhythms observed in these children were as follows:
      - Asystole, 78%
      - PEA, 12.8%
      - VF/pulseless VT, 8.1%
      - Bradycardia with a pulse, 1%

IN-HOSPITAL CARDIAC ARREST

- Objective survival rates over the years have hardly changed.
  - Current adult in-hospital cardiac arrest (IHCA) has overall survival of about 18%.
  - Analysis of data from the national CPR registry found
    - Prevalence of VF or pulseless VT as the first documented pulseless rhythm during IHCA was only 23% in adults and 14% in children.
    - Prevalence of asystole as the initial rhythm was 35% in adults and 40% in children.
    - Prevalence of PEA was 32% versus 24% in adults and children, respectively.
  - Survival rate to hospital discharge after pulseless CA

- Higher in children than adults (27% vs. 18%, respectively)
- Of these survivors, 65% of children and 73% of adults had good neurologic outcome.
- After adjusting for known predictors, such as arrest location and monitoring at time of arrest, outcome was surprisingly worse when the rhythm was VF/VT in children compared with asystole and PEA.
  - Further analysis of these data showed that VF/VT occurred during CPR in children more commonly than it occurred as the initial rhythm.
  - Survival to discharge is highest (35%) when VF/VT is the initial rhythm compared with survival of 11% if this rhythm develops during resuscitation.

NEUROLOGIC OUTCOME

- Determined by the following:
  - The cause of arrest (e.g., degree of shock or hypoxemia prior to arrest)
  - The duration of no flow, adequacy of flow during CPR
  - Restoration of adequate flow after ROSC
  - Subsequent injury secondary to postarrest management such as the occurrence of hyperthermia or hypoglycemia
- Survivors who ultimately have a good outcome
  - Generally awaken within 3 days after CA
  - Most patients who remain neurologically unresponsive due to anoxic–ischemic encephalopathy for more than 7 days will fail to survive.
    - Those who do survive often have poor neurologic recovery.
      - Neurocognitive impairment ranges from dependency on others for care to remaining in a minimally conscious or vegetative state.
- Achieving good functional outcome is the ultimate goal for successful CPR.
  - The financial implications of caring for patients with disordered consciousness are substantial.
  - Most studies reporting outcome data have used crude methods to describe neurologic outcome, such as the composite scores from the Glasgow Outcome Scale and Cerebral Performance Category.
    - An important limitation of these scales is the possibility of wide variation of neurologic function for the same score.
    - In children, the Pediatric Cerebral Performance Category and Pediatric Overall Performance Category have been used.
  - 11% to 48% of CA patients admitted to the hospital will be discharged with good neurologic outcome.
    - Recent data from the National Registry for Cardiopulmonary Resuscitation (NRCPR) show that neurologic outcome in discharged adult survivors is generally good, with 73% of patients with Cerebral Performance Category 1.

INITIAL CONSIDERATIONS

- CPR is primarily based on two principles.
  - Providing artificial ventilation and oxygenation through an unobstructed airway
    - Cardiac output is limited; avoid ventilation in excess of that required for adequate ventilation/perfusion matching.

- Delivering chest compressions to maintain threshold blood flow
  - Especially to the heart and brain, while minimizing interruption of compressions

Basic Life Support

- Basic life support (BLS) is the initial "ABCs" phase of CPR.
  - A: airway
  - B: breathing
  - C: circulation
- Effective BLS can provide almost 30% of normal cardiac output with adequate arterial oxygen content.
  - Sufficient to protect the brain for minutes until effective defibrillation or other definitive therapeutic maneuvers are provided Table 1.2.

Advanced Life Support

- Advanced life support (ALS) entails the following:
  - Advanced airway management including use of ancillary equipment to support ventilation and oxygenation

- Prompt recognition and, when appropriate, treatment of life-threatening arrhythmias using electrical therapy including defibrillation, cardioversion, pacemaker insertion, and pharmacologic therapy
- Inclusion of the use of pharmacologic therapy and advanced procedures extending into the postarrest setting such as the use of therapeutic hypothermia

Advanced Airway Management

- Tracheal intubation
  - Endotracheal intubation (ETI) is indicated if unable to adequately ventilate or oxygenate the arrested or unconscious patient with bag-mask ventilation or if prolonged ventilation is required and airway protective reflexes are absent in the patient with a perfusing rhythm
  - A properly placed endotracheal tube (ET) is the gold standard method for securing the airway.
    - Attempted ETI by less skilled rescuers results in a 6% to 14% incidence of misplaced or displaced ETs.
- Confirmation of correct ET placement
  - Clinical signs used to confirm correct ET placement
    - Visualization of bilateral chest rise

TABLE 1.2

SUMMARY OF BASIC LIFE SUPPORT ABCD MANEUVERS FOR INFANTS, CHILDREN, AND ADULTS FOR LAY RESCUERS AND HEALTH CARE PROVIDERS (NEWBORN INFORMATION NOT INCLUDED)

Maneuver	Adult lay rescuer: ≥ 8 y HCPs: Adolescent and older	Child lay rescuers: 1– 8 y HCPs: 1 y to adolescent	Infant ≤ 1 y of age
Airway	Head tilt–chin lift (HCPs: Suspected trauma, use jaw thrust)		
Breathing: Initial	Two breaths at 1 sec/breath	Two breaths at 1 sec/breath	
HCPs: Rescue breathing without chest compressions	10–12 breaths/min (approximate)	12–20 breaths/min (approximate)	
HCPs: Rescue breaths for CPR with advanced airway	8–10 breaths/min (approximately)		
Foreign-body airway obstruction	Abdominal thrusts	Back slaps and chest thrust	
Circulation HCPs: Pulse check (≤10 s)	Carotid	Brachial or femoral	
Compression landmarks	Lower half of sternum, between nipples	Just below nipple line (lower half of sternum)	
Compression method • Push hard and fast • Allow complete recoil	Heel of one hand, other hand on top	Heel of one hand or as for adults	Two or three fingers HCPs (two rescuers): Two thumb–encircling hands
Compression depth	1½–2 inches	Approximately one-third to one-half the depth of the chest	
Compression rate	Approximately 100/min		
Compression:ventilation ratio	30:2 (one or two rescuers)	30:2 (single rescuer) HCPs: 15:2 (two rescuers)	
Defibrillation AED	Use adult pads Do not use child pads	Use AED after five cycles of CPR (out of hospital) Use pediatric system for child 1–8 y if available HCPs: For sudden collapse (out of hospital) or in-hospital arrest use AED as soon as available	No recommendation for infants <1 y of age

AED, automated external defibrillator; CPR, cardiopulmonary resuscitation.
Note: Maneuvers used by only health care providers are indicated by HCPs. AED, automated external defibrillator; CPR, cardiopulmonary resuscitation.
Adapted from 2005 American Heart Association Guidelines for Cardiopulmonary Resuscitation and Emergency Cardiovascular Care. *Circulation.* 2005;112[24]SIV-1–IV-211.

- Bilateral breath sounds over the lateral lung fields
- Absent breath sounds over the epigastrium
- Presence of water vapor/mist in the tube
- None of these signs is confirmatory, and an $ETCO_2$ detector or esophageal detector is indicated to confirm correct tube placement.
  - *$ETCO_2$ detector device* is a disposable colorimetric device that detects $ETCO_2$ has been investigated as a guide to correct ET placement.
    - The device fits on the end of the ET and is normally purple; exhaled CO_2 turns the color to bright yellow, indicating that the ET is in the trachea.
    - The positive predictive value of this device for correct tube placement is close to 100%, but the negative predictive value ranges from 20% to 100% depending on whether the patient has a perfusing rhythm.
      - False-negative results are seen if there is no or very low pulmonary blood flow, such as during CA or with a large pulmonary embolus.
      - False-positive (i.e., the detector remains yellow) results are seen when it is contaminated with an acidic drug (e.g., epinephrine) or gastric contents.
  - *Esophageal detector device* comes in two versions: the bulb and the syringe esophageal detector devices (EDD).
    - Bulb EDD consists of a bulb that is compressed and attached to the ET. When released, if the tube is in the esophagus, the suction collapses the lumen of the esophagus or pulls the esophageal tissue against the tip of the tube, and the bulb will not re-expand (positive result for esophageal placement).
    - Syringe EDD consists of a syringe attached to the ET; the rescuer attempts to pull the plunger of the syringe. If the tube is in the esophagus, it will not be possible to pull out the plunger (i.e., aspirate air) with the syringe.
      - This device has high sensitivity for esophageal placement of ETs in both CA and patients with a perfusing rhythm but poor specificity for tracheal placement.

Electrical Therapy

- One of the mainstays of ALS, especially in adults
  - Electrical energy is used to treat life-threatening cardiac dysrhythmias.
    - Constitute 16% to 85% of OOH and 14% to 56% of in-hospital CAs
      - Recent data suggest that VF and VT are decreasing, with only 24% of the initial rhythms in more than 36,000 adult arrests being VF- or VT-based in a recent analysis from the NRCPR.
      - In hospitalized children with CA, VF is the initial rhythm in approximately 10% of cases and subsequently occurs during 15% of the cases.
- Defibrillation
  - Defined as delivery of electrical energy resulting in termination of VF for at least 5 seconds after the shock
  - The goal is to quickly depolarize the entire myocardium, terminating the rhythm and hoping that a sinus rhythm will start.
  - *Defibrillator device*
    - Manual defibrillator devices require the rescuer to analyze the rhythm and then manually set and determine the electrical energy dose.

- Automatic defibrillator devices analyze the rhythm, determine whether a shock is required, and deliver the shock if needed automatically.
  - Two types of automatic defibrillators: internal implantable cardioverter defibrillator and automated external defibrillator (AED)
- Defibrillators are also characterized by the mode and waveform of electrical current delivered into monophasic and biphasic defibrillators.
  - Animal and human data show that biphasic defibrillators have a higher first-shock success in terminating VF compared with monophasic devices.
- *Defibrillation dose*
  - Optimal initial energy dose for the first shock \ required for effective defibrillation remains unknown despite multiple studies.
    - Reasonable to use selected energies of 150 J to 200 J with a biphasic truncated exponential waveform or 120 J with a rectilinear biphasic waveform for the initial shock
    - For second and subsequent biphasic shocks, the same or higher energy can be given.
      - Most manual defibrillators are set to an initial default of 200 J of energy.
    - If only a monophasic defibrillator is available, an energy dose of 360 J is recommended for all shocks.
  - The optimal dose for effective defibrillation in infants and children
    - Not known
    - Upper limit for safe defibrillation also not known
      - Doses more than 4 J/kg (as high as 9 J/kg) have effectively defibrillated children.
      - Recommended manual defibrillation (monophasic or biphasic) doses for children are 2 J/kg for the first attempt and 4 J/kg for subsequent attempts.
- *Electrode position*
  - Either handheld paddles or self-adhesive pads are used for shocks.
  - Electrodes are applied to the bare chest in the conventional sternal–apical (anterolateral) position.
    - The right (sternal) chest pad is placed on the victim's right superior–anterior (infraclavicular) chest, and the apical (left) pad is placed on the victim's inferior–lateral left chest, lateral to the left breast.
- *Electrode size*
  - The largest pad or paddle that can be placed on the chest while avoiding contact between the pads or paddles should be used. There should be at least 1 inch between the pads.
  - Paddles that are too small increase the risk of skin burn injury.
- Electrical cardioversion
  - Used for some life-threatening arrhythmias causing rapid cardiovascular deterioration
    - Including VT and supraventricular tachycardias (SVTs) such as paroxysmal atrial tachycardia, atrial flutter, or atrial fibrillation with a rapid ventricular response
  - The technique, unlike defibrillation, must be synchronized with the patient's electrocardiogram.
    - Delivery of the energy during the T wave of the QRS may result in VF.
  - *Energy level*
    - The amount of energy recommended for emergency cardioversion varies with the rhythm.

○ 100 J is recommended for atrial fibrillation and 50 J for atrial flutter.

○ Monomorphic VT responds well to cardioversion, and 100 J should be attempted first.

○ Pulseless VT behaves like VF, and 200 J should be used initially.

○ In conscious patients, sedation with intravenous diazepam, midazolam, or methohexital is indicated, and the cardioversion is accomplished with the lowest energy possible (50–200 J).

○ In children, the recommended initial cardioversion dose is 0.5 to 1 J/kg.

- External cardiac pacing
  - External (transcutaneous) pacing is not recommended for patients in asystolic CA, but it should be always considered in the ICU or other critical care areas of the hospital where the device and adequate skill are promptly available.
  - Pacing can be considered in patients with symptomatic bradycardia when a pulse is present.

Pharmacologic Therapy

- Used in CA to increase the rate of ROSC and terminate or limit the risk of recurrent arrhythmias
- Route of administration for resuscitation medications
  - A central venous line may not be available at the time of the arrest and immediate placement is not necessary to ensure survival.
    - Peripheral IV access can be used effectively with the advantage of not interrupting CPR.
      ○ Rapidly follow the medication bolus with a 10- to 20-mL fluid bolus to ensure central delivery.
      ○ Intraosseous cannulation is an effective alternate for drug delivery.
      ○ Instillation can be made through an ET, if available. Lipid-soluble medications that can be delivered via ET are lidocaine, epinephrine, atropine, naloxone, and vasopressin.
      ○ Recommended to administer at least 2 to 2½ times the IV recommended doses.
- *Epinephrine*
  - The most commonly used medication during CPR
    - Primary action in CA is to increase the coronary perfusion pressure through systemic vasoconstriction mediated by its α-adrenergic effects. The β-adrenergic effects are relatively unimportant.
    - Epinephrine is used primarily during CA due to asystole and PEA.
    - A second-line agent used for shock-refractory VF or pulseless VT
    - Little pharmacologic data supporting the currently recommended dose of 1 mg of epinephrine in adult CA and 0.01 mg/kg in children
- *Vasopressin*
  - An endogenous antidiuretic hormone that, when given at high doses, causes vasoconstriction by directly stimulating vascular smooth-muscle V1 receptors.
  - Improves coronary perfusion pressure but, unlike epinephrine, offers theoretical advantages of cerebral vasodilation, possibly improving cerebral perfusion.
    - Lack of β_1-adrenergic activity potentially avoids unnecessary increases of myocardial oxygen consumption, resulting in postresuscitation arrhythmias.

- Half-life of 10 to 20 minutes compared to the 3 to 5 minutes observed with epinephrine
- *Sodium bicarbonate*
  - Metabolic and respiratory acidosis develops during CA resulting from anaerobic metabolism, leading to lactic acid generation and inadequate ventilation along with reduced blood flow during CPR, which leads to inadequate pulmonary delivery of carbon dioxide for elimination.
  - Untreated acidosis suppresses spontaneous cardiac activity, decreases the electrical threshold required for the onset of VF, decreases ventricular contractile force, and decreases cardiac responsiveness to catecholamine such as epinephrine.
    - Elevated PCO_2 tension probably is more detrimental to myocardial function and catecholamine responsiveness than metabolic acidosis.
  - If arterial blood gas and pH measurements not available:
    - Recommended initial dose of sodium bicarbonate is 1 mEq/kg intravenously.
    - Half of this dose may be repeated at 10-minute intervals.
    - In pediatric patients, the 1 mEq/kg dose should be diluted 1:1 with sterile water to reduce the osmolality.
- *Atropine*
  - Used in sinus bradycardia when accompanied by hypotension or frequent premature ventricular contractions (PVCs) secondary to unsuppressed ectopic electrical activity arising in the area of injured tissue during the prolonged period after repolarization
  - Sinus bradycardia after myocardial infarction may predispose the heart to the onset of VF.
    - When profound bradycardia is present, acceleration of the heart rate above 60 bpm may improve cardiac output and reduce the incidence of VF.
  - Dosage of atropine for severe symptomatic bradycardia is 0.5 to 1.0 mg intravenously repeated every 3 to 5 minutes until the desired pulse rate is obtained or a maximum of 0.04 mg/kg has been given.
    - A larger dose has little therapeutic value, and a smaller dose may actually slow the heart rate.
    - Endotracheal dose is 2 to 2.5 mg.
- *Lidocaine*
  - Decreases ectopic electrical myocardial activity by raising the electrical stimulation threshold of the ventricle during diastole
  - In ischemic myocardial tissue after infarction, it may suppress re-entrant arrhythmias such as VT or VF.
    - The 2005 guidelines recommend lidocaine only when amiodarone is not available.
    - Lidocaine may be used in stable monomorphic VT and polymorphic VT with normal or prolonged QT interval if ventricular function is not decreased.
  - Loading dose of lidocaine is approximately 1 to 1.5 mg/kg given as an IV bolus.
  - If needed, repeat 0.5 to 0.75 mg/kg every 5 to 10 minutes, up to a total of 3 mg/kg.
    - Followed by a continuous infusion of 30 to 50 μg/kg/minute (1–4 mg/min in a 70-kg patient)
  - Toxicity may occur in oliguric or anuric patients because renally excreted lidocaine degradation products also have pharmacologic effects and toxic potential.
    - Early signs of lidocaine toxicity are due to central nervous system effects and include anxiety, loquacity, tremors, metallic taste, and tinnitus.

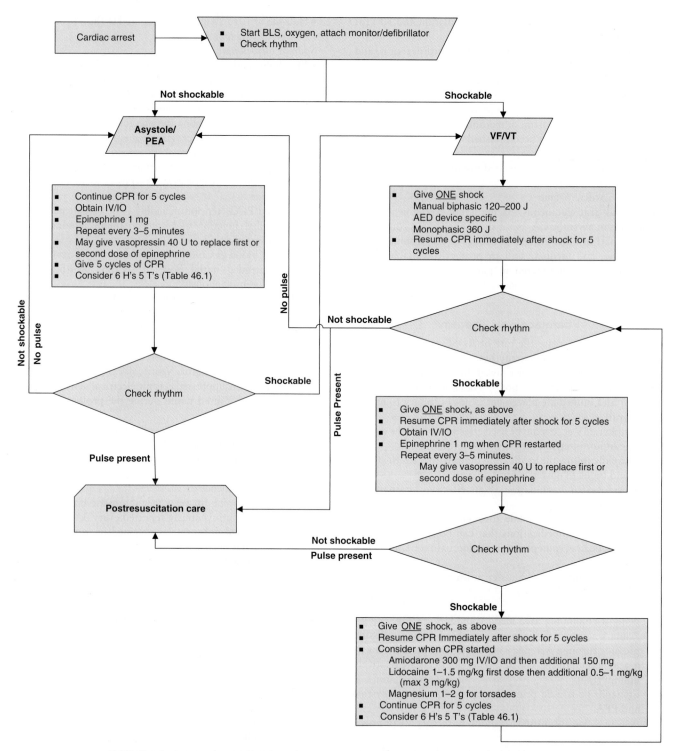

FIGURE 1.1. Suggested treatment algorithm for pulseless cardiac arrest. It is important that resuscitation drugs should be given during the cardiopulmonary resuscitation (CPR) cycles to minimize "no CPR" time. BLS, basic life support; PEA, pulseless electrical activity; VF, ventricular fibrillation; VT, ventricular tachycardia; AED, automated external defibrillator; IO, intraosseous. (Adapted and modified from 2010 American Heart Association Guidelines for Cardiopulmonary Resuscitation and Emergency Cardiovascular Care. *Circulation.* 2010;122:S729–S767).

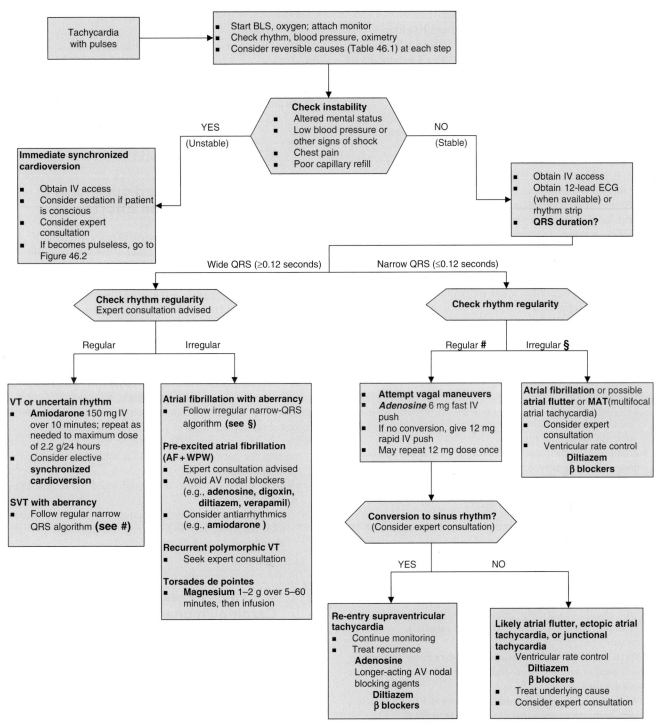

FIGURE 1.2. Suggested treatment algorithm for tachycardia with pulse. BLS, basic life support; ECG, electrocardiogram; VT, ventricular tachycardia; SVT, supraventricular tachycardia; WPW, Wolff-Parkinson-White syndrome. (Adapted and modified from 2005 American Heart Association Guidelines for Cardiopulmonary Resuscitation and Emergency Cardiovascular Care. *Circulation.* 2005;112[24]SIV-1–IV-211.

- • May be followed by somnolence, respiratory depression, apnea and, in severe cases, cardiovascular collapse.
- • *Procainamide*
  - • Suppresses both atrial and ventricular arrhythmias with mechanisms of action similar to those of lidocaine

- • Is used in the management of PVCs, VT, and persistent VF, but amiodarone is usually preferred
- • Incremental bolus injections are slowly infused at 20 mg/minute until
  - • The arrhythmia is controlled.

- Hypotension occurs.
- The QRS complex is widened 50% from baseline.
- A total dose of 17 mg/kg (1.2 g in a 70-kg adult) is given, followed by a continuous infusion of 1 to 4 mg/minute to prevent recurrent arrhythmias.
  ○ Therapeutic plasma level of 4 to 8 μg/mL.
- *Amiodarone*
  - A complex drug with effects on sodium, potassium, and calcium channels on myocardial cells and α- and β-adrenergic blocking properties
  - The 2005 guidelines denote it the preferred agent for both atrial and ventricular arrhythmias, especially in the presence of impaired cardiac function.
    - Amiodarone is recommended for narrow-complex tachycardias that originate from a re-entry mechanism (re-entry SVT); ectopic atrial focus; control of hemodynamically stable VT, polymorphic VT with a normal QT interval, or wide-complex tachycardia of uncertain origin, and control of rapid ventricular rate due to accessory pathway conduction in pre-excited atrial arrhythmias with AV nodal blockade in patients with preserved or impaired ventricular function
  - In treatment of arrhythmias with a pulse, 150 mg amiodarone is given IV over 10 minutes, followed by a 1 mg/minute infusion for 6 hours and then a 0.5 mg/minute maintenance infusion over 18 hours.
    - Supplementary infusions of 150 mg can be repeated every 10 minutes as necessary for recurrent or resistant arrhythmias to a maximum manufacturer-recommended total daily IV dose of 2.2 g.
  - When used in the treatment of VF or pulseless VT, a bolus dose of 300 mg is recommended diluted in 20 to 30 mL of D5W.
    - A single second dose may be given (150 mg) in 3 to 5 minutes for shock-refractory VF or VT.
    - In children, 5 mg/kg is given as a rapid bolus and may be repeated up to 15 mg/kg.
  - Major adverse effects of amiodarone are hypotension and bradycardia.
    - Can be prevented by slowing the rate of drug infusion
    - Amiodarone can increase the QT interval; therefore, its use should be carefully considered when other drugs that can prolong the QT interval are administered.
- *Calcium*
  - Plays a critical role in myocardial contractility and action potential generation, but studies have shown no benefit of calcium in CA
  - When indicated, the recommended dose is 5 to 10 mL of a 10% solution of calcium chloride (8–16 mg/kg).
  - Calcium gluconate is given in a dose of 6 to 8 mL if peripheral IV access is available. Undiluted calcium chloride given through a peripheral vein may cause sclerosis and tissue injury; therefore, if a central site is not available and the patient is not in CA, it either should be diluted or calcium administered in a less irritating form (e.g., calcium gluconate).
  - In children, a dose of 10 to 20 mg/kg of calcium chloride is recommended.
- *Magnesium*
  - Recommended for the treatment of torsades de pointes VT with or without CA

- Given at a dose of 1 to 2 g diluted in D5W over 10 to 60 minutes
- In children, a dose of 25 to 50 mg/kg is used.

Algorithms for Advanced Life Support
- The treatment algorithms of pulseless CA and tachycardia with pulse are summarized in Figures 1.1 and 1.2, respectively

ETHICAL CONSIDERATIONS

Termination of Cardiopulmonary Resuscitation Efforts

- CPR is inappropriate when survival is not expected.
- There are few criteria that can reliably predict the futility of CPR.
- Recommended that all patients with cardiopulmonary arrest receive CPR with the following exceptions:
  - There is a valid Do Not Attempt Resuscitation order, which can be verified
  - Signs of irreversible death are already present (e.g., rigor mortis, decapitation, decomposition, dependent lividity).
  - No physiologic benefit can be expected with further CPR.
  - In newborns, gestational age or congenital abnormality is related to almost certain early death.
- In the ICU, CPR is started without a physician's order, which is based on implied consent for emergency treatment.
  - The decision to stop CPR should be made by a physician treating the patient, ideally familiar with the patient's pre-existing conditions.
    - Rarely good outcome with prolonged CPR has been reported.
    ○ Acceptable to prolong resuscitative efforts in children with recurrent VF or VT, drug toxicity, or a primary hypothermic insult.

Family Presence during Cardiopulmonary Resuscitation

- Has been a common practice to exclude family of the arrest victim during CPR efforts
  - Helping the family of a dying patient is an important part of CPR and should be done in a compassionate manner considering the family's cultural and religious beliefs and practices.
    - Concern that allowing family presence may become disruptive, interfere with resuscitation, cause them to experience syncope, and increase the risk of legal liability were not substantiated by good evidence.
    - Family surveys after CPR suggested that the majority of family members want to be present during CPR.
    - In pediatric arrest, most parents surveyed wanted an option to be present during CPR.
    - The resuscitation team should be sensitive to the family's presence, and a team member should be assigned to comfort the family, answer questions, and clarify the procedures.

CHAPTER 2 ■ AIRWAY MANAGEMENT

GENERAL PRINCIPLES

- You may *not* neglect the "A" of the ABCs and wait for airway management to turn into an emergency.
- Bag-valve-mask should be attempted by application of a mask and initiation of bag ventilation with an increased FiO_2 while equipment for intubation is prepared.
- An appropriate mask provides a tight seal around the nose and mouth, and the colorless plastic with soft and pliable edges allows visualization of the mouth and secretions.
- The mask is attached to the resuscitation (self-inflating or collapsible) bag with a high-flow oxygen source.
- Proper inflation requires two hands
  - One to hold the mask firmly in place against the patient's face
  - The other to compress the bag
  - The mandible must be lifted to create a seal without airway occlusion.
    - An oropharyngeal or nasal airway facilitates oxygen delivery by bypassing or retracting the tongue.
    - Forceful bag compression should be avoided to prevent gastric distention and possible pulmonary aspiration.
    - Gentle insufflation allows assessment of lung compliance and minimizes complications.
- Contraindications to bag-valve-mask ventilation include:
  - Airway obstruction
  - Pooling of blood or secretions in the pharynx
  - Severe facial trauma
- Critically ill patients require tracheal intubation for the reasons listed in Table 2.1.
- Relative or absolute contraindications to **conventional** tracheal intubation
  - Traumatic or severe degenerative disorders of the cervical spine
  - Acute infectious processes such as acute supraglottitis or intrapharyngeal abscess
  - Extensive facial injury and basal skull fracture
- Blind nasal intubation may be contraindicated in the following situation:
  - Upper-airway foreign-body obstruction, because the tube may push the foreign body distally and exacerbate airway compromise

ANATOMIC CONSIDERATIONS

Adult

- Neck flexion aligns the pharyngeal and tracheal axes, whereas head extension on the neck and opening of the mouth align the oral passage with the pharyngeal and tracheal axes.

- This maneuver places the patient in a "sniffing position" (Fig. 2.1).
  - Flexion/extension of the head decreases 20% by 75 years of age.
  - Degenerative arthritis limits cervical spine motion, more with extension than flexion.
  - Spine movement is contraindicated in the presence of potential cervical spine injury.
    - Hence, patient is maintained in a neutral position with in-line stabilization.
    - Barring the edentulous patient, the front component of the hard cervical collar is commonly removed to allow full mandibular movement/optimize mouth opening.
- Knowledge of anatomic landmarks may help during direct laryngoscopy (Fig. 2.2).
  - The cricoid, a circle of cartilage above the first tracheal ring, can be compressed to occlude the esophagus (Sellick maneuver) to prevent passive gastric regurgitation into the trachea.
  - The epiglottis lies in the anterior pharynx.
  - The vallecula, a furrow between the epiglottis and base of the tongue is placement site for the tip of a curved laryngoscope blade.
  - The larynx is located anterior and superior to the trachea and contains the vocal cords.

Pediatric

- Differences exist between the adult and the pediatric airways.
  - Pediatric patients have a relatively large head and flexible neck.

TABLE 2.1

INDICATIONS FOR TRACHEAL INTUBATION

Open an obstructed airway
Provide airway pressure support to treat hypoxemia
PaO_2 <60 mm Hg with an FiO_2 >0.5
Alveolar-to-arterial oxygen gradient 300 mm Hg
Intrapulmonary shunt >15%–20%
Provide mechanical ventilation
Respiratory acidosis
Inadequate respiratory mechanics
Respiratory rate >30 breaths/min
FVC <10 mL/kg
NIF >−20 cm H_2O
V_D/V_T >0.6
Facilitate suctioning, instillation of medications, and bronchoscopy
Prevent aspiration
Gag and swallow reflexes absent

FiO_2, fraction of inspired oxygen; FVC, forced vital capacity; NIF, negative inspiratory force; V_D/V_T, dead space/tidal volume ratio.

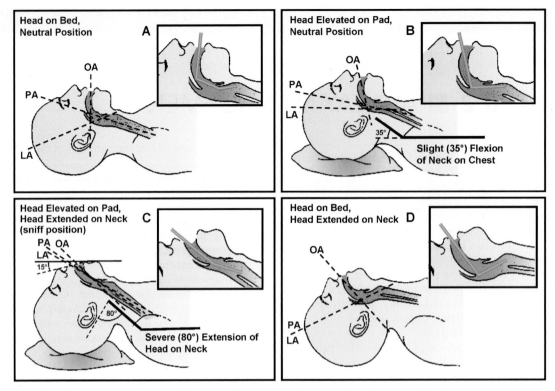

FIGURE 2.1. Demonstration of the "sniffing position" for optimal visualization of the glottic opening.

• The air passages are small.
• The tongue, adenoids, and tonsils are larger than those in adults.
• The epiglottis is floppy.
• The glottis is typically slanted at a 40-degree to 50-degree angle, making intubation more difficult.
• Mucous membranes are softer, looser, and more fragile and readily become edematous when an oversized endotracheal tube is used.
• The epiglottis and larynx of infants lie more cephalad and anterior.

• The cricoid cartilage ring is narrowest portion of the upper airway in children.
  • In the adult, the glottic opening is narrowest.
• The pediatric vocal cords have a shorter distance from the carina.
  • The mainstem bronchus angulates symmetrically at the level of the carina at about 55 degrees.
    • In adults, the right mainstem angulates at about 25 degrees and the left at about 45 degrees.
• The cupulae of the lungs are higher in the infant's neck, increasing the risk of lung trauma.

Intubation

• All anticipated equipment/drugs must be available for the planned intubation technique (Table 2.2).
• A difficult-airway cart or bag with a variety of airway rescue devices—and a bronchoscope and/or fiberoptic laryngoscope—should be readily available.

MEDICATIONS

• Local anesthetics
  • Aerosolized or nebulized 1% to 4% lidocaine can readily achieve nasopharyngeal and oropharyngeal anesthesia if the patient is cooperative and capable of deep inhalation, thus limiting its usefulness in the ICU.
  • Transtracheal (cricothyroid membrane) instillation of 2 to 4 mL of 1% to 4% lidocaine with a 22- to 25-gauge needle causes sufficient coughing-induced reflex to afford ample

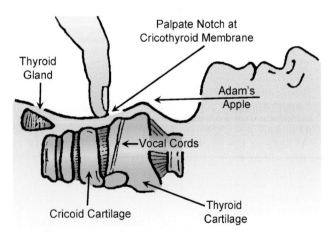

FIGURE 2.2. Laryngoscopic landmarks. Panel shows the cricoid cartilage.

TABLE 2.2

STANDARD EQUIPMENT AND DRUGS FOR TRANSLARYNGEAL INTUBATION

Bag-valve-mask resuscitation bag
LMA-type device
Oxygen source
Suction apparatus
Selection of oral and nasal airways
Magill forceps
Assortment of laryngoscope blades and endotracheal tubes
Tape, stylet, lubricant, syringes, and tongue depressors
Monitors (ECG, blood pressure monitor, pulse oximeter, capnography, or similar device) and defibrillator[a]
Fiberoptic bronchoscope,[a] rigid fiberscope,[a] and specialty blades[a]
A drug tray or cart with vasoconstrictors, topical anesthetics, induction agents, muscle relaxants, and emergency medications
14-Gauge IV, scalpel, assortment of supraglottic airways,[a] bougie,[a] Combitube,[a] ET exchanger,[a] and Melker-type cricothyrotomy kit

[a]Immediately available.
LMA, laryngeal mask airway; ECG, electrocardiograph; ET, endotracheal tube.

distribution to anesthetize the subglottic and supraglottic regions plus the posterior pharynx in 90% of patients.
- Cocaine provides excellent conditions for facilitating intubation through the nasopharynx due to its outstanding topical anesthetic and mucosal and vascular shrinkage capabilities. In-hospital availability may limit its use in favor of phenylephrine or oxymetazoline combined with readily available local anesthetics.
- Lidocaine ointment applied to the base of the tongue with a tongue blade or similar device allows performance of direct laryngoscopy in many patients.
  - If time permits, nasal spraying with a vasoconstrictor followed by passing a progressively larger nasal airway trumpet from 24 French to 32 French that is coated/lubricated with lidocaine gel/ointment provides exceptional coverage of the nasocavity in preparing for a nasal intubation.
- Barbiturates
  - Sodium thiopental, an ultra-short-acting barbiturate, decreases the level of consciousness and provides amnesia without analgesia.
    - Intubation dose in the operating room (OR) of 4 to 7 mg/kg ideal body weight (IBW) (1 to 2 mg/kg in the ICU) dose over 20 to 50 seconds (more rapidly via central venous line (CVL))
      - Duration of action 5 to 10 minutes
      - Lowers cerebral metabolic rate while maintaining cerebral blood flow as long as systemic blood pressure is maintained within an adequate range
      - Thiopental may lead to hypotension in critically ill patients due to its vasodilatation properties, especially with hypovolemia.
- Narcotics
  - Morphine, hydromorphone, fentanyl, and remifentanil reduce pain perception and allay anxiety, making intubation less stressful.

- Fentanyl and the ultra-short-acting remifentanil have a more rapid onset (seconds) and shorter duration of action (about 20 minutes and 5 minutes, respectively) than the conventional narcotics used in the ICU.
- Morphine may lead to histamine release and its potential sequelae.
- Though all narcotics cause respiratory depression, the newer synthetic narcotics may lead to glottic spasm that may hamper ventilation.
- Benzodiazepines
  - Lorazepam and midazolam have excellent amnestic and sedative properties.
    - May be combined with an analgesic agent during intubation
      - Lorazepam use for intubation is possible, but it is hampered by a slower pharmacodynamic onset (2–6 minutes) as compared to midazolam.
      - Hypotension may occur with hypovolemia.
- Neuromuscular blocking agents
  - Administration of a sedative-hypnotic agent with a rapid-acting muscle relaxant, typically succinylcholine, is cited as improving intubation conditions and leading to fewer complications.
    - If one does not fully contemplate the patient's risk for airway management difficulties and does not have access or a good working knowledge of airway rescue devices if conventional laryngoscopy techniques fail, disaster may ensue. Any clinician who administers drugs such as induction agents, including paralytics, must have developed a rescue strategy coupled with the equipment to deploy such a strategy.
  - Indications: include agitation or lack of cooperation not related to inadequate or no sedation
  - Neuromuscular blocking agents may cause depolarization of the motor end-plate (succinylcholine, a depolarizing agent) or prevent depolarization (nondepolarizer: pancuronium, vecuronium, rocuronium).
    - Succinylcholine has a rapid onset and short duration of effect
      - It may raise serum potassium levels by 0.5 to 1.0 mEq/L.
      - It is contraindicated in bedridden patients and in those with pre-existing hyperkalemia, burns, or recent or long-term neurologic deficits.
      - Other side effects are elevation of intragastric and intraocular pressures, muscle fasciculation, myalgia, malignant hyperthermia, cardiac bradyarrhythmias, and myoglobinuria.
      - At a dose of 0.25 mg/kg IBW - the ED95 - succinylcholine has a duration of about 3 minutes. This is our recommendation, despite the commonly-used dose recommended in the literature of 1.0 to 1.5 mg/kg IBW.
    - Nondepolarizing muscle relaxants have a longer time to onset and duration of action as compared to succinylcholine.
      - Rocuronium (typical OR dose, 0.6 mg/kg) can approach succinylcholine in rapid time of onset if dosed at 1.2 mg/kg).
- Ketamine
  - A phencyclidine derivative that provides profound analgesia, amnesia, and dissociative anesthesia
    - Airway reflexes often, but not always, preserved.

- Has a rapid onset and relatively short duration of action
- Its myocardial depressant action is often countered by its sympathomimetic properties, leading to hypertension and tachycardia.
  - Use in the critically ill patient with ongoing activation of his or her sympathetic outflow could lead to profound hemodynamic instability, as the underlying myocardial depression may not be successfully countered.
- Has significant bronchodilatory properties but promotes bronchorrhea, salivation, and a high incidence of dreams, hallucinations, and emergence delirium (at doses well above those noted)
- Dose at 0.5 to 1 mg/kg leads to anesthesia for about 20 minutes and analgesia for about 60 minutes.
- Propofol
  - IV administration of 1 to 3 mg/kg IBW results in unconsciousness within 30 to 60 seconds.
    - Awakening is observed in 4 to 6 minutes.
- Hypotension, cardiovascular collapse, and, rarely, bradycardia may complicate its use.
- Etomidate
  - Considered the preferred induction agent in the critically ill patient due to its favorable hemodynamic profile
    - Role as a single-dose induction agent is in question due to its transient depression of the adrenal axis, and this adrenal suppression may be influential in the outcome of the critically ill.

EQUIPMENT FOR ACCESSING THE AIRWAY

- Esophageal Tracheal Combitube
  - The esophageal tracheal Combitube (ETC) is recommended by the American Heart Association Advanced Cardiovascular Life Support course and other national guidelines as an advanced variant of the older esophageal obturator airway and the pharyngeal tracheal lumen airway.
    - The double lumens with proximal and distal cuffs allow ventilation and oxygenation in a majority of nonawake patients whether placed in the esophagus (95% of all insertions) or the trachea.
    - The proximal cuff is placed between the base of the tongue and the hard palate and the distal cuff within the trachea or upper esophagus.
  - The ETC is inserted blindly, assisted by a jaw thrust or laryngoscopic assistance.
- Laryngoscopes
  - Fiberoptic versus conventional is used to expose the glottis to facilitate passage of the tracheal tube.
  - The utility of the laryngoscope under elective circumstances, with otherwise healthy surgical patients, is essentially limited to individuals with a grade I or II view that can be easily intubated.
    - Difficult view (grade III or IV) has been documented in 14% of patients despite optimizing maneuvers such as the optimal external laryngeal manipulation (OELM) and the backward upward right pressure (BURP) technique (Fig. 2.3).
      - Up to 33% of critically ill patients have a limited view with laryngoscopy (epiglottis only or no view at all).

Determining Optimal External Laryngeal Manipulation with Free (right) Hand

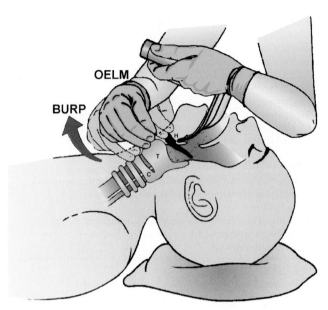

FIGURE 2.3. Diagrammatic representation of the optimal external laryngeal movement (OELM) and backward upward rightward pressure (BURP) maneuvers for optimal visualization of the glottis.

  - Hence, critical care practitioners responsible for airway management must be prepared to embark on a plan B or plan C immediately if conventional direct laryngoscopy fails.
- Blades
  - Laryngoscope blades are of two principal kinds, curved and straight, varying in size for use in infants, children, or adults (Fig. 2.4)
- Endotracheal tubes
  - The tube size used depends on the size of the patient (Table 2.3).
- Malleable stylet
  - A well-lubricated malleable stylet is preferred by many to pre-form the endotracheal tube (ET) into a shape that may expedite passing through the glottis.

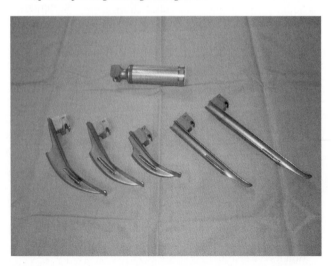

FIGURE 2.4. Various types of laryngoscope blades in common use.

TABLE 2.3

RECOMMENDED SIZES FOR ENDOTRACHEAL TUBES

Patient age	Internal diameter of tube (mm)[a]
Newborn	3.0
6 mo	3.5
18 mo	4.0
3 y	4.5
5 y	5.0
6 y	5.5
8 y	6.0
12 y	6.5
16 y	7.0
Adult female	7.0–7.5
Adult male	8.0–9.0

[a]One size larger and one size smaller should be allowed for individual intra-age variations and shorter-stature individuals. Where possible, the subglottic suction endotracheal tube should be used.

- The stylet is a guide, not a "spear," and its tip should be safely inside the ET, never distal to the ET tip.
- Ideally, the styleted ET tip should be placed at the entrance of the glottis, and then, with stylet removal, the ET will advance into the trachea less traumatically.

HOW MIGHT THE AIRWAY BE ACCESSED?

General Indications and Contraindications

- The oral approach is the standard method for tracheal intubation today unless there is limited access to the oral cavity due to trauma, edema, or anatomic difficulties.
- If the nasal approach is not feasible, a surgical approach via the cricothyroid membrane or a formal tracheostomy would be clinically indicated.

Orotracheal Intubation

- Expediently prepare both the patient and the equipment for the airway management procedure.
  - While bag ventilation (preoxygenation) is being provided, obtain appropriate towels for optimizing head and neck position or blankets for ramping the obese patient and adjusting the bed height and angulation (Fig. 2.5).
    - Assemble the necessary equipment, such as the ET, syringes, suction equipment, lubricant, CO_2 detector, and a stylet, if desired.
  - Obtain a rapid medical–surgical history.
  - Review previous intubation procedures sought.
  - Complete an airway examination.
  - Ensure IV access and develop a primary plan for induction.
  - Place airway rescue devices at the bedside.
  - Insist on clear communication among team members.
- Awake intubation
  - Awake intubation techniques comprise both nasal and oral routes and, most often, involve topically applied local anesthetics or local nerve blocks.
  - Practitioners may prefer to maintain spontaneous ventilation during emergency airway management by avoiding excessive sedative–hypnotic agents and/or muscle relaxants.
    - Light sedation and analgesics, however, are typically administered despite the label of being "awake."
  - After proper preparation, unless the patient is unconscious or has markedly depressed mental status, the "awake look" technique incorporates conventional laryngoscopy to evaluate the patient's airway to gauge the feasibility and ease of intubation.
    - If viewing the airway structures during an "awake look" proves fruitful, intubation should be performed during the same laryngoscopic attempt either directly—grade I or II view—or by bougie assistance—grade I, II, or III—or by other means.
- Rapid sequence intubation (RSI)
  - RSI refers to the administration of an induction agent followed by a neuromuscular blocking agent, with the goal

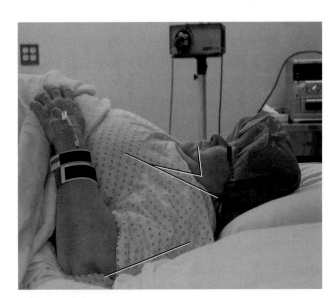

FIGURE 2.5. Ramping of an obese patient's torso to improve glottic visualization is noted on the left panel. The right panel shows the patient position *without* proper ramping.

of hastening the time needed to induce unconsciousness and muscle paralysis and minimizing the time the airway is unprotected with less risk of aspiration.

- Preoxygenation is paramount via a bag-mask.
- Cricoid pressure is applied to reduce the risk of passive regurgitation of any stomach contents.
  ○ Cricoid pressure may sometimes worsen the laryngoscopic view, plus impede mask ventilation; hence, adjustment or release of cricoid pressure should be considered in these circumstances.
- RSI is said to be associated with a lower incidence of complications and higher first-pass intubation success rate as compared to the "sedation only" method.
  - A predetermined induction regimen, such as etomidate and succinylcholine—0.25 mg/kg IBW etomidate and 0.25 mg/kg IBW of succinylcholine—generally works well for most critically ill patients.

Positioning the Patient

- One of the most important factors in improving the success rate of orotracheal intubation is positioning the patient properly (see Fig. 2.1).
  - Classically, the sniffing position, namely cervical flexion combined with atlanto-occipital extension, will assist in improving the "line of sight" of the intubator.
  - Bringing the three axes into alignment (oral, pharyngeal, and laryngeal) is commonly optimized by placing a firm towel or pillow beneath the head (providing mild cervical flexion) combined with physical backward movement of the head at the atlanto-occipital joint via manual extension.
  - This, when combined with oral laryngoscopy, will improve the "line of sight" for the intubator to better visualize the laryngeal structures in most patients.
  - Optimizing the position of the obese patient (see Fig. 2.5, left panel) is an absolute requirement to assist with the following:
    - Spontaneous ventilation and mask ventilation
    - Opening the mouth
    - Gaining access to the neck for cricoid application, manipulation of laryngeal structures, or invasive procedures
    - Improving the "line of sight" with laryngoscopy
    - Prolonging oxygen saturation after induction

Blade Use

- Curved blade
  - After opening of the mouth either by the extraoral technique (finger pressing downward on chin) or the intraoral method (the finger scissor technique to spread the dentition), the laryngoscope blade is introduced at the right side of the mouth and advanced to the midline, displacing the tongue to the left.
    - The epiglottis is seen at the base of the tongue and the tip of the blade inserted into the vallecula.
  - The laryngoscope blade should be lifted toward an imaginary point in the corner of the wall opposite the patient to avoid using the upper teeth as a fulcrum for the laryngoscope blade.
    - A forward and upward lift of the laryngoscope and blade stretches the hyoepiglottic ligament, thus folding the epiglottis upward and further exposing the glottis.
  - With visualization of the glottic structures, the ET is passed to the right of the laryngoscope through the glottis into the

trachea until the cuff passes 2 to 3 cm beyond the vocal cords.
  - A blind guide underneath the epiglottis (tracheal tube introducer, bougie) or a rigid fiberoptic stylet may be incorporated to improve the insertion success rate.
- Straight blade
  - Intubation with a straight blade involves the same maneuvers but with one major difference.
    - The blade is slipped *beneath* the epiglottis, and exposure of the larynx is accomplished by an upward and forward lift at a 45-degree angle toward the corner of the wall opposite the patient.
      ○ Leverage must not be applied against the upper teeth.
- Repetitive laryngoscopies are not in the best interest of patient care and may place the patient at extreme risk for potentially life-threatening airway-related complications.
  - Conventional laryngoscopy should be abandoned in favor of incorporating an airway adjunct to assist the clinician.

Nasotracheal Intubation

- Nasotracheal intubation is still commonly used in oral and maxillofacial operative interventions but less commonly in emergency situations outside the OR.
  - The presence of midfacial or posterior fossa trauma and coagulopathy are absolute contraindications to this technique. It is also contraindicated in the presence of acute sinusitis or mastoiditis and best avoided in patients with a basilar skull fracture, a fractured nose, or nasal obstruction.
  - As the nasal portal dictates a smaller-diameter tracheal tube, the length of the tracheal tube will be shortened; hence, the length must be considered when placing a small-caliber tube (e.g., a 6.0-mm diameter in an individual taller than about 69 inches), as the nasal tracheal tube may end up as an elongated nasal trumpet, without entrance into the trachea.
- The method of intubation via the nasal approach is variable.
  - It may be placed blindly during spontaneous ventilation, combined with oral laryngoscopic assistance to aid with ET advancement utilizing Magill forceps; utilize indirect visualization through the nares via an optical stylet or a flexible or rigid fiberscope; or incorporate a lighted stylet for transillumination of the laryngeal structures.
- Technique
  - The patient is prepared for the nasal approach by pretreatment of the mucosa of both nostrils with a solution of 0.1% phenylephrine and a decongestant spray such as oxymetazoline for 3 to 10 minutes.
  - This is followed by progressive dilation, starting with either a 26 French or 28 French nasal trumpet, and progressing to a No. 30 French to No. 32 French trumpet lubricated with 2% lidocaine jelly. Conversely, placement of cotton pledgets soaked in a mixture of vasoconstrictor agent and local anesthetic is equally effective.
  - Supplemental oxygen may be provided by nasal cannulae placed between the lips or via a face mask.
  - The patient is best intubated with spontaneous ventilation maintained.
    - Incremental sedation/analgesia may be provided. Sitting upright has the advantage of maximizing the oropharyngeal diameter.

- Orientation of the tracheal tube bevel is important for patient comfort and to reduce the risk of epistaxis and tearing or dislocation of the nasal turbinates. On either side of the nose, the bevel should face the turbinate (away from the septum).
- Tube advancement should be slow and gentle, with rotation.
- If advancement is met with resistance from glottic/anterior tissues, helpful maneuvers include sitting the patient upright, flexing the head forward on the neck, and manually pulling the larynx anteriorly.
- Conversely, if advancement is met with posterior displacement into the esophagus, sitting the patient upright, extending the head on the neck, and applying posterior-directed pressure on the thyrocricoid complex may assist in intubation.
  - Rotation of the tube and manual depression or elevation of the larynx may be required to succeed.
  - Voluntary or hypercapnic-induced hyperpnea helps if the patient is awake because maximal abduction of the cords is present during inspiration.
- Entry into the trachea is signified by consistent breath sounds transmitted by the tube and inability to speak, if the patient is breathing, and by lack of resistance, often accompanied by cough. Confirmation with end-tidal CO_2 measurement or fiberoptic viewing is imperative.
- Nasotracheal intubation may also be accomplished with *fiberoptic assistance.*
  - Advancement of the ET into the glottis may be impeded by hang-up on the laryngeal structures: the vocal cord, the posterior glottis or, typically, the right arytenoid.
  - When resistance is met, a helpful tip is as follows: Withdrawing the tube 1 to 2 cm, rotate the tube counterclockwise 90 degrees, and then readvance with the bevel facing posteriorly.
  - Matching the tracheal tube to the fiberscope to minimize the gap between the internal diameter of the tube and the scope may also improve advancement.
  - Tracheal confirmation and tip positioning are added advantages to fiberoptic-assisted intubation.
  - The nasal approach has decreased in popularity due to
  - A restriction of tube size
  - The potential to add epistaxis to an already tenuous airway situation
  - The potential for sinus obstruction and infection beyond 48 hours

CONFIRMATION OF TRACHEAL INTUBATION

Physical Examination

- Confirmation of ET location after intubation is imperative and consists of the following:
  - Observation of the ET passing through the vocal cords
  - Absence of gurgling over the stomach with bag-valve ventilation
  - Chest rise with bag-valve ventilation
  - Presence of condensation upon exhalation
  - Presence of breath sounds over the **lateral** midhemithoraces
  - Presence of CO_2

Capnography

- Identification of exhaled CO_2 measured *via* disposable colorimetric devices or capnography is a standard of practice.
- Capnography may fail due to
  - Low-flow or no-flow cardiac states (no pulmonary blood flow as a source of exhaled carbon dioxide)
  - Soilage from secretions, pulmonary edema fluid, or blood, temperature alterations (outside helicopter rescue), age, lack of maintenance

Other Devices

- Esophageal detector devices
- Syringe or the self-inflating bulb models (Fig. 2.6) assist in the detection of ET location based on the anatomic difference between the trachea (an air-filled column) and the esophagus (a closed and collapsible column).
  - Applying a 60-mL syringe to the ET and withdrawing air should collapse the esophagus, while the trachea should remain patent.
    - False-negative results may still be seen (no reinflation even though the ET is in the trachea) in less than 4% of cases.
    - Technique failures include ET soilage, carinal or bronchial intubation in the obese, and those with severe pulmonary disease (chronic obstructive pulmonary disease, bronchospasm, thick secretions, or aspiration), and gastric insufflation.
- Two infallible or fail-safe techniques when used under optimal conditions
  - Visualizing the ET within the glottis
  - Fiberoptic visualization of tracheal/carinal anatomy

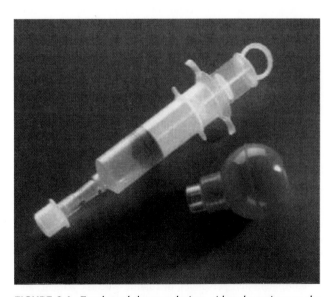

FIGURE 2.6. Esophageal detector devices, either the syringe or the self-inflating bulbs, assist in the detection of endotracheal tube location based on the anatomic difference between the trachea (an air-filled column) and the esophagus (a closed and collapsible column). Note that a 15-mm adaptor inserts onto the tip of the bulb syringe so that the connection may be made.

Cheney Test

- Clinically useful adjunct for assisting in the verification of the ET location
  - Hang-up test
    - Passing a bougie or similar catheter-like device for the purpose of detecting tip impingement on the carinal or bronchial lumen
    - Gently advancing a bougie to 27 to 35 cm depth may allow the practitioner to appreciate hang-up on distal structures.
      - Compared to unrestricted advancement if ET is in esophagus
      - Care must be taken not to perforate the trachea

DEPTH OF ENDOTRACHEAL TUBE INSERTION

- Classic depth of insertion is height and gender based.
  - Also affected by the route of ET placement (i.e., oral vs. nasal)
  - Final tip position is best at about 2 to 4 cm above the carina to limit irritation with head movement and patient repositioning.
    - ET depth in the adult patient less than or equal to 62 inches (157 cm) in height should be approximately 18 to 20 cm.
    - Otherwise, 22 to 26 cm may be the appropriate depth.
    - Chest radiography only determines the tip depth at the time of film exposure.

AMERICAN SOCIETY OF ANESTHESIOLOGISTS PRACTICE GUIDELINES

- Airway management procedures should be accompanied by capnography or similar technology to reduce the incidence of unrecognized esophageal intubation.
- Preintubation evaluation to recognize the potential difficult airway is paramount (Table 2.4)
  - Is there a reasonable expectation for successful mask ventilation?
  - Is intubation of the trachea expected to be problematic?
  - Should the airway approach be nonsurgical or surgical?
  - Should an awake or a sedated/unconsciousness approach be pursued?
  - Should spontaneous ventilation be maintained?
  - Should paralysis be pursued?

Awake Pathway

- If difficulty is recognized, an awake approach may be appropriate.
  - Patient preparation with an antisialagogue, assembling equipment and personnel, discussion with the patient, and optimal positioning should be pursued unless emergent.
  - The awake choices, following optimal preparation,
    - May allow an "awake look" with conventional laryngoscopy
    - May allow bougie-assisted intubation

- May allow laryngeal mask airway (LMA) insertion
- May allow indirect fiberoptic techniques (rigid and flexible) or proceeding with a surgical airway
- Access to the airway via cricothyroid membrane puncture via large-bore catheter insertion with either modified tubing or a jet device to ventilate, or via Melker cricothyrotomy kit, is an option prior to other awake or asleep methods.

Asleep Pathway

- After induction in the patient with a known or suspected difficult airway or in the unrecognized difficult airway (Table 2.5)
  - Ability to adequately mask ventilate will determine direction of management
    - Mask ventilation adequate but conventional intubation is difficult
      - The nonemergency pathway is appropriate, utilizing the bougie, specialty blades, supraglottic airway, flexible or rigid fiberoptic technique, or surgical airway.
      - Mask ventilation is suboptimal or impossible, intubation of the trachea may be attempted, but immediate placement of a supraglottic airway such as the LMA is the treatment of choice.
      - If the supraglottic device fails, an extraglottic device such as the Combitube or similar device can be placed.
        - Otherwise, transtracheal jet ventilation may be used or a surgical airway placed.

COMPLICATIONS RELATED TO ACCESSING THE AIRWAY

- Complications occur in four time periods (Tables 2.6 – 2.9):
  - During intubation
  - After placement
  - During extubation
  - After extubation
- Cuffed tube usage for prolonged intubation and artificial ventilation increases rate of tracheal and laryngeal injury.
  - Cuff pressures above 25 to 35 mm Hg further add to risk by compressing tracheal capillaries.
  - Other factors include the duration of intubation, reintubation, and route of intubation. More complications occur from: nasal intubation versus oral, patient-initiated self-extubation, excessive tracheal tube movement, trauma during procedures, poor tube care.

Failed Intubation

- In the clinical situation of can't ventilate, can't intubate, the practitioner will need to rapidly deploy the rescue plan.
  - After *failure* of conventional mask ventilation (no ventilation or oxygen delivery) or when mask ventilation is *failing (inadequate gas exchange, SpO$_2$ less than 90%, or a falling SpO$_2$).*
    - Supraglottic airway (LMA) should be placed.
    - If unsuccessful, placement of the LMA, the Combitube may serve as a backup for LMA failure.

TABLE 2.4

AMERICAN SOCIETY OF ANESTHESIOLOGISTS DIFFICULT-AIRWAY ALGORITHM

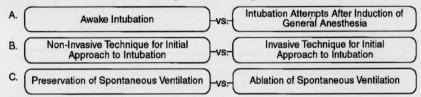

DIFFICULT AIRWAY ALGORITHM

1. Assess the likelihood and clinical impact of basic management problems:
   A. Difficult Ventilation
   B. Difficult Intubation
   C. Difficulty with Patient Cooperation or Consent
   D. Difficult Tracheostomy

2. Actively pursue opportunities to deliver supplemental oxygen throughout the process of difficult airway management

3. Consider the relative merits and feasibility of basic management choices:

   A. Awake Intubation — vs. — Intubation Attempts After Induction of General Anesthesia

   B. Non-Invasive Technique for Initial Approach to Intubation — vs. — Invasive Technique for Initial Approach to Intubation

   C. Preservation of Spontaneous Ventilation — vs. — Ablation of Spontaneous Ventilation

4. Develop primary and alternative strategies:

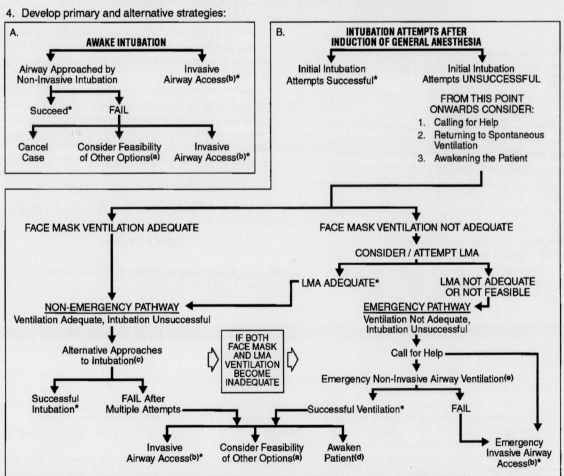

* Confirm ventilation, tracheal intubation, or LMA placement with exhaled CO_2

a. Other options include (but are not limited to): surgery utilizing face mask or LMA anesthesia, local anesthesia infiltration or regional nerve blockade. Pursuit of these options usually implies that mask ventilation will not be problematic. Therefore, these options may be of limited value if this step in the algorithm has been reached via the Emergency Pathway.

b. Invasive airway access includes surgical or percutaneous tracheostomy or cricothyrotomy.

c. Alternative non-invasive approaches to difficult intubation include (but are not limited to): use of different laryngoscope blades, LMA as an intubation conduit (with or without fiberoptic guidance), fiberoptic intubation, intubating stylet or tube changer, light wand, retrograde intubation, and blind oral or nasal intubation.

d. Consider re-preparation of the patient for awake intubation or canceling surgery.

e. Options for emergency non-invasive airway ventilation include (but are not limited to): rigid bronchoscope, esophageal-tracheal combitube ventilation, or transtracheal jet ventilation.

Source: http://www.asahq.org/publicationsAndServices/Difficult%20Airway.pdf.

TABLE 2.5

STRATEGY FOR EMERGENCY AIRWAY
MANAGEMENT OF THE CRITICALLY ILL PATIENT

1. Conventional intubation—grade I or II view
2. Bougie—grade III view
   a. May use for grade I and II if needed
3. LMA/supraglottic device—grade III or IV view
   a. LMA/supraglottic rescue for bougie failure
   b. Or use the LMA/supraglottic device as a primary device
      (i.e., known difficult airway, cervical spine limitations,
      Halo-vest)
4. Combitube—rescue device for any failure or as a primary
   device if clinically appropriate
5. Fiberscope (optical/video-assisted rigid or flexible
   models)—primary mode of intubation, an adjunct for
   intubation via the LMA

LMA, laryngeal mask airway.

○ Both devices have a high rate of success for ventilation,
  are placed rapidly and blindly, and require a relatively
  simple skill set.
• Limiting intubation attempts is a key to successful manage-
  ment.
  • Repeated attempts are probably futile (e.g., a grade IV view
    with conventional methods) and markedly increase the risk
    of hypoxemia and other potentially devastating complica-
    tions.
• Conventional intubation failure should be supplemented by
  an airway adjunct.
  • Bougie, specialty blades, or fiberscopes if immediately avail-
    able
  • Key point: **Use them early and use them often.**
  • More invasively, transtracheal jet ventilation via a large-
    gauge (12- or 14-gauge) IV catheter through the cricothy-
    roid membrane may be an appropriate alternative.

• However, advanced planning with ready access to the proper
  equipment and a sound understanding of "jetting" principles (lowest PSI setting to maintain SpO_2 in the 80%–90%
  range, prolonged inspiration-to-expiration ratio [i.e., 1:5],
  6–12 quick breaths per minute, allowing a path for exhalation, constant catheter stabilization, and barotrauma vigilance) must be followed; otherwise, **the consequences may
  be very serious.**

EXTUBATION OF THE DIFFICULT AIRWAY IN THE INTENSIVE CARE UNIT

• Airway management also constitutes maintaining control of
  the airway into the postextubation period.
• The known or suspected difficult-airway patient should be
  evaluated in regard to factors that may contribute to his or
  her inability to tolerate extubation (Tables 2.10 and 2.11).
  • "Difficult extubation" is defined as the clinical situation
    when a patient presents with known or presumed risk fac-
    tors that may contribute to difficulty re-establishing access
    to the airway.
  • Reintubation, immediately or within 24 hours, may be
    required in up to 25% of intensive care unit patients.
    ○ Measures to avert reintubation such as noninvasive ven-
      tilation may reduce mortality rate if done so upon extu-
      bation.

PARAMETERS OF AIRWAY EVALUATION FOR EXTUBATION

NPO Status

• Although not thoroughly studied, it makes clinical sense to
  consider 2 to 4 hours off of distal enteral feeds prior to

TABLE 2.6

RISKS OF TRACHEAL INTUBATION

Time	Tissue injury	Mechanical problems	Other
Tube placement	Corneal abrasion; nasal polyp dislodgement; bruise/laceration of lips/tongue; tooth extraction; retropharyngeal perforation; vocal cord tear; cervical spine subluxation or fracture; hemorrhage; turbinate bone avulsion	Esophageal/endobronchial intubation; delay in cardiopulmonary resuscitation; ET obstruction; accidental extubation	Dysrhythmia; pulmonary aspiration; hypertension; hypotension; cardiac arrest
Tube in place	Tear/abrasion of larynx, trachea, bronchi	Airway obstruction; proximal or distal migration of ET; complete or partial extubation; cuff leak	Bacterial infection (secondary); gastric aspiration; paranasal sinusitis; problems related to mechanical ventilation (e.g., pulmonary barotrauma)
Extubation	Tear/abrasion of larynx, trachea, bronchi	Difficult extubation; airway obstruction from blood, foreign bodies, dentures, or throat packs	Pulmonary aspiration; laryngeal edema; laryngospasm; tracheomalacia; intolerance of extubated state

ET, endotracheal tube.

TABLE 2.7

AIRWAY COMPLICATIONS CONTRIBUTING TO HYPOXEMIA

Esophageal intubation
Mainstem bronchial intubation
Inadequate or no preoxygenation
Failure to "reoxygenate" between attempts
Tracheal tube occlusion: Biting, angulation
Tracheal tube obstruction after intubation
   Due to:
      Particulate matter
      Blood clots
      Thick, tenacious secretions

Regurgitation/aspiration
Multiple attempts
Duration of laryngoscopy attempt
Airway obstruction, unable to ventilate
Accidental extubation after intubation
Bronchospasm, coughing, bucking

extubation and maintaining the NPO status after extubation until the patient appears at low risk for failing the extubation "trial."

Cuff Leak

- Hypopharyngeal narrowing from edema or redundant tissues, supraglottic edema, vocal cord swelling, and narrowing in the subglottic region of any etiology may contribute to the lack of a cuff leak.
  - Too large a tracheal tube in a small airway should be considered.
  - If airway edema is the culprit
    - Steps to decrease airway edema include elevation of the head, diuresis, steroid administration, minimizing further airway manipulation, and "time."
  - The performance of a cuff leak test varies by institution and protocol.
    - A relatively crude yet effective method of cuff leak test involves auscultation for cuff leak with or without a stethoscope.

- Cuff leak volume (CLV) may be measured as the difference of tidal volume delivered with and without cuff deflation and stated as a percentage of leak or as an absolute volume. An absolute CLV less than 110 to 130 mL or 10% to 24% of delivered tidal volume is helpful in predicting postextubation stridor.
  - Single- or multiple-dose steroids may reduce postextubation airway obstruction in pediatric patients.
  - Steroid use in adults (1–4 mg dexamethasone IV) administered 6 hours prior to extubation—rather than 1 hour prior—may reduce postextubation stridor.

Risk Assessment: Direct Inspection of the Airway

- It is mandatory that the records of the known difficult-airway patient be reviewed.
- Some patients may need evaluation of their hypopharyngeal structures and supraglottic airway to assess airway patency and resolution of edema, swelling, and tissue injury.
  - Conventional laryngoscopy is a standard choice for evaluation but often fails due to a poor "line of sight."
  - Flexible fiberoptic evaluation is useful but may be limited by secretions and edema.
  - Video-laryngoscopy and other indirect visualization techniques that allow one to see "around the corner" are especially helpful.

TABLE 2.8

FACTORS CONTRIBUTING TO POSTINTUBATION HEMODYNAMIC INSTABILITY

Anesthetic medications
Sympathetic surge, vasovagal response
Excessive parasympathetic tone
Loss of spontaneous respirations
Positive pressure ventilation
Positive end-expiratory pressure (PEEP)
Auto- or intrinsic PEEP
Hyperventilation with pre-existing hypercarbia
Decrease in patient work
Underlying disease process (i.e., myocardial insufficiency)
Volume imbalances (sepsis, diuretics, hypovolemia, hemorrhage)
Preload dependent physiology
   Valvular heart disease, congestive heart failure, pulmonary embolus, right ventricular failure, restrictive pericarditis, cardiac tamponade
   Hypoxia-related hemodynamic deterioration
Hyperkalemia-induced deterioration (succinylcholine)

TABLE 2.9

TRACHEAL INTUBATION COMPLICATIONS SEEN AFTER EXTUBATION

Time of occurrence	Complications
Early (0–72 h)	Numbness of tongue Sore throat Laryngitis Glottic edema Vocal cord paralysis
Late (>72 h)	Nostril stricture Laryngeal ulcer, granuloma, or polyp Laryngotracheal webs Laryngeal or tracheal stenosis Vocal cord synechiae

TABLE 2.10

RISK FACTORS FOR DIFFICULT EXTUBATION

Known difficult airway
Suspected difficult airway based on the following factors:
   Restricted access to airway
   Cervical collar, Halo-vest
   Head and neck trauma, procedures, or surgery
   ET size, duration of intubation
Head and neck positioning (i.e., prone *vs.* supine)
Traumatic intubation, self-extubation
Patient bucking or coughing
Drug or systemic reactions
   Angioedema
   Anaphylaxis
   Sepsis-related syndromes
   Excessive volume resuscitation

ET, endotracheal tube.

AMERICAN SOCIETY OF ANESTHESIOLOGISTS PRACTICE GUIDELINES STATEMENT REGARDING EXTUBATION OF THE DIFFICULT AIRWAY

- The American Society of Anesthesiologists guidelines have suggested that a preformulated extubation strategy should include:
  - Consideration of relative merits of awake extubation *versus* extubation before the return of consciousness (clearly more applicable to the OR setting than to the ICU)
  - Consideration of the short-term use of a device that can serve as a guide to facilitate intubation and/or provide a conduit for ventilation/oxygenation

Clinical Decision Plan for the Difficult Extubation

- A variety of methods are available to assist the practitioner's ability to maintain continuous access to the airway after extubation, each with limitations and restrictions.

TABLE 2.11

THE DIFFICULT EXTUBATION: TWO CATEGORIES FOR EVALUATION

1. Evaluate the patient's inability to tolerate extubation
   a. Airway obstruction (partial or complete)
   b. Hypoventilation syndromes
   c. Hypoxemic respiratory failure
   d. Failure of pulmonary toilet
   e. Inability to protect airway
2. Evaluate for potential difficulty re-establishing the airway
   a. Difficult airway
   b. Limited access to the airway
   c. Inexperienced personnel pertaining to airway skills
   d. Airway injury, edema formation

TABLE 2.12

AIRWAY EXCHANGE CATHETER (AEC) – ASSISTED EXTUBATION: TIPS FOR SUCCESS

1. Access to advanced airway equipment
2. Personnel
   a. Respiratory therapist
   b. Individual competent with surgical airway?
3. Prepare circumferential tape to secure the airway catheter after extubation
4. Sit patient upright; discuss with patient
5. Suction ET, nasopharynx, and oropharynx
6. Pass lubricated AEC to 23–26 cm depth
7. Remove the ET while maintaining the AEC in its original position
8. Secure the AEC with the tape (circumferential); mark AEC "airway only"
9. Administer oxygen:
   a. Nasal cannula
   b. Face mask
   c. Humidified O_2 via AEC (1–2 L/min)
10. Maintain NPO
11. Aggressive pulmonary toilet

ET, endotracheal tube.

- The LMA offers the ability for fiberoptic-assisted visualization of the supraglottic structures while serving as a ventilating and reintubating conduit.
- The bronchoscope is useful for periglottic assessment after extubation but requires advanced skills and minimal secretions.
- The airway exchange catheter (AEC) allows continuous control of the airway after extubation, is well tolerated in most patients, and serves as an adjunct for reintubation and oxygen administration. Dislodgment may occur, resultant from an uncooperative patient or a poorly secured catheter. Observation in a monitored environment with experienced personnel is top priority (Table 2.12).
  - Clinical judgment and the patient's cardiopulmonary and other systemic conditions, combined with the airway status, will guide in establishing a reasonable time period for maintaining a state of "reversible extubation" with the indwelling AEC (Table 2.13).

TABLE 2.13

SUGGESTED GUIDELINES FOR MAINTAINING PRESENCE OF AIRWAY EXCHANGE CATHETER

Difficult airway only, no respiratory issues, no anticipated airway swelling	1–2 h
Difficult airway, no direct respiratory issues, **potential** for airway swelling	>2 h
Difficult airway, respiratory issues, multiple extubation failures	>4 h

TABLE 2.14

STRATEGY AND PREPARATION FOR ENDOTRACHEAL TUBE (ET) EXCHANGE

1. Place on 100% oxygen
2. Review patient history, problem list, medications, and level of ventilatory support
3. Assemble conventional and rescue airway equipment including capnography
4. Assemble personnel (nursing, respiratory therapy, surgeon, airway colleagues)
5. Prepare sedation/analgesia ± neuromuscular blocking agents
6. Optimal positioning; consider DL of airway
7. Discuss primary/rescue strategies and role of team members; choose new ET (soften in warm water)
8. Suction airway; advance lubricated large AEC via ET to 22–26 cm depth
9. Elevate airway tissues with laryngoscope/hand, remove old ET, and pass new ET
10. Remove AEC and check ET with capnography/bronchoscope or use a closed system and place small bronchoscope through swivel adapter while at the same time ventilating, checking for CO_2, with the AEC still in place

DL, direct laryngoscopy; AEC, airway exchange catheter.

EXCHANGING AN ENDOTRACHEAL TUBE

- Exchanging an ET due to cuff rupture, occlusion, damage, kinking, a change in surgical or postoperative plans, or self-extubation masquerading as a cuff leak, or when a different size or alteration in location is required, is common.
- Four methods typify the airway manager's armamentarium of exchanging an ET (Table 2.14)
  - Direct laryngoscopy
  - Flexible or rigid fiberscope
  - Airway exchange catheter
  - A combination of these techniques

SUGGESTED READINGS

1. Borasio P, Ardissone F, Chiampo G. Post-intubation tracheal rupture. A report on ten cases. *Eur J Cardiothoracic Surg.* 1997;12:98–100.
2. Massard G, Rouge C, Dabbagh A, et al. Tracheobronchial lacerations after intubation and tracheostomy. *Ann Thorac Surg.* 1996;61:1483.

CHAPTER 3 ■ TEMPORARY CARDIAC PACEMAKERS

INDICATIONS

- Most common indication for temporary pacing is hemodynamically unstable bradycardia
  - May be the result of primary degenerative conduction system disease or secondary causes such as medications, metabolic abnormalities, or acute myocardial infarction (AMI)
  - Medications include antiarrhythmic drugs and β- or calcium channel blockers, in particular diltiazem or verapamil.
  - Hyperkalemia and other electrolyte disturbances cannot only cause bradycardia but also may contribute to high pacing thresholds.
    - Secondary causes of bradycardia must be corrected for pacing to be successful. Table 3.1 lists some indications for temporary cardiac pacing.
- Not all bradycardias in the setting of acute myocardial infarction require temporary pacing (Tables 3.2 and 3.3).
- Atrioventricular (AV) block
  - Occurring during an inferior wall myocardial infarction (MI) from a right coronary artery occlusion may be secondary to ischemia of the region supplied by the AV nodal artery. In this setting, AV block rarely progresses to high-degree AV block, typically resolves within 2 weeks, and probably will not require temporary pacing.
  - AV block in the setting of an anterior wall MI carries a worse prognosis. Anterior wall MIs can be more extensive, and AV block seen in this situation is usually from infarct involvement of the interventricular septum and infranodal conduction system. AV block from an anterior wall MI may rapidly deteriorate to asystole.
    - Temporary pacing in the setting of an anterior wall MI and complete heart block is strongly suggested.
- Other indications for temporary pacemakers are considered prophylactic.
  - There are some procedures performed in the cardiac catheterization or electrophysiology lab in which temporary pacing is strongly considered.

TABLE 3.1

INDICATIONS FOR TEMPORARY CARDIAC PACING

Bradyarrhythmias
Asystole
Any symptomatic or hemodynamically unstable bradycardia
Second-degree Mobitz type II or third-degree heart block
Other conduction abnormalities at high risk for progression
  to complete heart block such as alternating bundle branch
  block or new bifascicular block

Tachyarrhythmias
Bradycardia or pause-dependent polymorphic ventricular
  tachycardia
Ventricular tachycardia that is treatable with overdrive pacing
Atrial tachycardias or atrial flutters that are treatable with
  overdrive pacing

Preventive
Patient undergoing right heart catheterization with a left
  bundle branch block
Cardiac interventions with high risk of bradyarrhythmia such
  as rheolytic thrombectomy (AngioJet), rotational
  atherectomy (Rotoblation), or alcohol septal ablation
Pacemaker generator change in a patient who is pacemaker
  dependent

- A patient undergoing alcohol septal ablation has a risk for needing a pace maker of as high as 55% to 70%, but a much smaller percentage requires permanent cardiac pacing—11% to 17%.
- Other examples include percutaneous coronary rotational atherectomy (Rotoblation), rheolytic thrombectomy (AngioJet), or a generator replacement in a patient who is pacemaker dependent.
- Temporary pacing is also commonly used after cardiac surgery.
  - Incidence of hemodynamically unstable bradycardia after cardiac surgery has been reported to be as high as 4%.

TABLE 3.2

STANDARD AMERICAN COLLEGE OF CARDIOLOGY/ AMERICAN HEART ASSOCIATION CLASSIFICATION FOR RECOMMENDATIONS AND INDICATIONS

Class I	Conditions for which there is evidence and/or general agreement that a given procedure or treatment is beneficial, useful, and effective
Class II	Conditions for which there is conflicting evidence and/or a divergence of opinion about the usefulness/efficacy of a procedure or treatment
Class IIa	Weight of evidence/opinion is in favor of usefulness/efficacy
Class IIb	Usefulness/efficacy is less well established by evidence/opinion
Class III	Conditions for which there is evidence and/or general agreement that a procedure/treatment is not useful/effective and in some cases may be harmful

From Gregoratos G, Abrams J, Epstein AE, et al. ACC/AHA/NASPE 2002 guideline update for implantation of cardiac pacemakers and antiarrhythmia devices—summary article: a report of the American College of Cardiology/American Heart Association Task Force on Practice Guidelines (ACC/AHA/NASPE Committee to Update the 1998 Pacemaker Guidelines). *J Am Coll Cardiol.* 2002;40: 1703–1719.

- AV block is not uncommon after valvular heart surgery and is likely a result of either direct injury to the surrounding conduction system or edema.
- Sinus bradycardia occurs in 64% of postcardiac transplant patients.
  - Though this bradycardia often resolves, temporary pacing may be required to maintain adequate heart rates for optimal cardiac output in the immediate posttransplant recovery period.
  - In addition, temporary atrial pacing may reduce the incidence of postoperative atrial fibrillation.
- Temporary pacemakers may also be used for other reasons besides bradycardia and heart block.

TABLE 3.3

INDICATIONS FOR PACING IN ACUTE MYOCARDIAL INFARCTION

Class I	Class IIb	Class III
Asystole	Persistent second- or third-degree AV block at the AV node level	Transient AV block in the absence of intraventricular conduction defects
Persistent second-degree AV block in the His-Purkinje system with bilateral bundle branch block or third-degree AV block within or below the His-Purkinje system after acute myocardial infarction		Transient AV block in the presence of isolated left anterior fascicular block
Transient advanced (second- or third-degree) infranodal AV block and associated bundle branch block. If the site of block is uncertain, an electrophysiologic study may be necessary		Acquired left anterior fascicular block in the absence of AV block
Persistent and symptomatic second- or third-degree AV block		Persistent first-degree AV block in the presence of bundle branch block that is old or age indeterminate

AV, atrioventricular.
From Gregoratos G, Abrams J, Epstein AE, et al. ACC/AHA/NASPE 2002 guideline update for implantation of cardiac pacemakers and antiarrhythmia devices—summary article: a report of the American College of Cardiology/American Heart Association Task Force on Practice Guidelines (ACC/AHA/NASPE Committee to Update the 1998 Pacemaker Guidelines). *J Am Coll Cardiol.* 2002;40:1703–1719.

- Pause or bradycardia-dependent polymorphic ventricular tachycardia, such as that occurring in the long QT syndrome, can be treated with temporary pacing, which will shorten the QT interval.
- Overdrive or rapid ventricular pacing may also prevent ventricular tachycardias triggered by premature ventricular contractions; some ventricular tachycardias may be terminated by ventricular pacing.
- Certain atrial tachycardias, such as atrial flutter, can be terminated with rapid atrial pacing.

TEMPORARY PACING CATHETERS

Deciding on Atrial, Ventricular, or Dual-Chamber Pacing

- Most ICU pacing needs can be met with single-chamber, right ventricular pacing
  - In some clinical situations, dual-chamber pacing is necessary.
  - Some patients with congestive heart failure, significant diastolic dysfunction, and right ventricular infarction with AV block rely on AV synchrony and atrial contraction to maintain optimal physiologic cardiac contraction for adequate cardiac output.
    - Dual-chamber pacing is most readily available in postcardiac surgical patients, as temporary epicardial wires are routinely placed at the time of surgery.
    - Otherwise, insertion of two separate pacing catheters or a specialized dual-chamber pacing catheter will be necessary.
  - Single-chamber atrial pacing can also be used in many of the aforementioned situations, as long as the only conduction system abnormality is from sinus node dysfunction and not AV block.
  - Single-chamber atrial pacing may be preferred if the patient has a mechanical tricuspid valve to avoid catheter entrapment or tricuspid valve endocarditis to avoid dislodgement of the vegetation.
  - Table 3.4 summarizes the available pacing modes for temporary pacing.

Ventricular

- Most temporary transvenous pacing catheters are designed for placement in the right ventricle (RV).
  - These are constructed of a wire insulated with a polymer such as polyethylene or polyvinyl chloride and are available in various sizes.
  - In general, these catheters should be placed with fluoroscopic guidance.
  - Balloon-tipped catheters are available to allow for flow-assisted placement, which is critical if fluoroscopy is not available (Fig. 3.1).
  - Specialized pulmonary artery catheters that have dedicated pacing ports for the placement of a pacing wire electrode while still allowing for routine hemodynamic monitoring are available

Atrial

- Multiple catheter designs for atrial pacing
  - Some pacing catheters are preformed to facilitate placement into the right atrial appendage or coronary sinus, thus allowing atrial pacing.
  - A new design consists of several electrodes positioned 10 to 20 cm proximal to the distal-tip electrodes. These electrodes are positioned to lie along the lateral right atrial wall, allowing atrial sensing and pacing.
  - The vast majority of temporary pacing catheters are designed to lie against the ventricular myocardium once positioned (passive fix).
    - Newer designs, especially those for right atrial pacing, have a deployable screw that is embedded in the myocardium (active fix) (Fig. 3.2). All leads placed in the heart carry a risk of migration and perforation, but active fix leads may reduce the risk of dislodgement.

EXTERNAL PACEMAKER UNIT

- The external temporary pacemaker unit controls the pacing mode, stimulus output, stimulus frequency, and threshold for sensing intrinsic activity.
  - Pacing modes can be synchronous (demand/inhibited) or asynchronous to pace the atrium, ventricle, or both.

TABLE 3.4

COMMON PACING MODES AVAILABLE FOR TEMPORARY PACING

Mode	Chamber paced	Chamber sensed	Synchronous or asynchronous	Advantages	Disadvantages
VVI	Ventricle	Ventricle	Synchronous	Technically simple	Nonphysiologic; may exacerbate CHF
AAI	Atrium	Atrium	Synchronous	Physiologic (AV node intact)	Technically more difficult; requires intact AV nodal conduction
DDD	Atrium and ventricle	Atrium and ventricle	Synchronous	Physiologic	Technically more difficult; may require two pacing catheters
VOO	Ventricle	n/a	Asynchronous	Same as VVI	Same as VVI
AOO	Atrium	n/a	Asynchronous	Same as AAI	Same as AAI
DOO	Atrium and ventricle	n/a	Asynchronous	Same as DDD	Same as DDD

CHF, congestive heart failure; AV, atrioventricular.

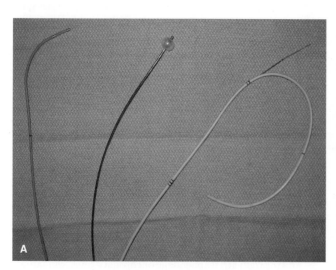
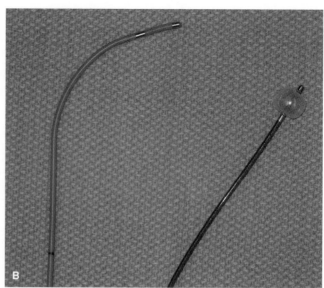

FIGURE 3.1. Close-up view of the tips of the torque-guided and balloon-tipped pacing catheter.

- Range of output varies from 0 to 20 mA.
- Frequency can be adjusted from 30 to 180 beats/minute.
- Sensing threshold can be varied from no sensing (asynchronous) to <1.5 mV.

ASSESSMENT OF THE PATIENT

- A complete patient assessment must be made prior to pacemaker placement.
- Bradycardia alone is not sufficient.

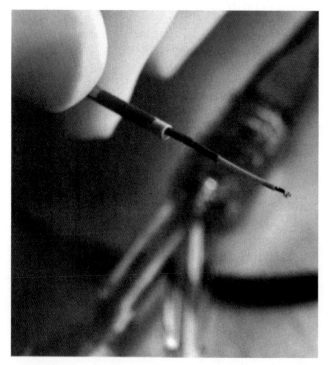

FIGURE 3.2. An example of an active fixation lead with a screw helix. (Compliments of Medtronic, Inc., Minneapolis, MN.)

- Hemodynamic instability, symptoms, or evidence of significant conduction system disease on the electrocardiogram (ECG) (bundle branch block, high-degree heart block) favors therapy.
- Reversible causes, especially medications, should be sought.
  - Glucagon may be effective for β-blocker overdose, calcium for calcium channel overdose, and digoxin immune Fab (Digibind) for digitalis glycoside overdose
  - Some bradycardias can be treated medically with agents such as isoproterenol, a β_1-receptor agonist that increases heart rate.
  - Electrolyte abnormalities such as hyperkalemia and other adverse metabolic states, such as severe acidosis, should be corrected.

PREPARING EQUIPMENT

- All the necessary equipment should be available and inspected.
  - The external pacing unit should be programmed to the desired settings and turned to the "on" position.
  - A new battery should be installed.
  - The lead should be examined for any defects.
  - The connector cables should be inserted into the pacing generator to make sure that they are compatible.
- Continuous ECG monitoring and a defibrillator at the bedside are required.
- Fluoroscopy is preferred but is not mandatory.

VENOUS ACCESS

- Access is obtained using the Seldinger technique.
  - Placing an introducer sheath that is large enough to accommodate the size of the pacing catheter, usually No. 4 to 7 French

TABLE 3.5

COMMON SITES FOR CENTRAL VENOUS ACCESS WHEN PLACING A TEMPORARY PACING CATHETER

Access site	Advantages	Disadvantages
Internal jugular vein	Relatively easy placement; fluoroscopy generally not necessary	Pneumothorax
Subclavian vein	Relatively easy placement; fluoroscopy generally not necessary	Pneumothorax; site commonly used for permanent pacing
Femoral vein	Relatively easy access	Leg immobilization; high risk of infection; fluoroscopy needed for placement

- Common placement sites
  - Internal jugular vein
  - Subclavian vein
  - Femoral vein
- Advantages and disadvantages of various access sites are given in Table 3.5.
- For bedside placement
  - Right internal jugular vein or left subclavian vein is the preferred site.
  - In the cardiac catheterization lab, the femoral vein is commonly used.
    - If the patient is likely to require permanent transvenous pacing, the subclavian vein should be avoided on the side of the planned permanent implantation.
  - Other potential sites
    - The basilic or cephalic veins
    - The downside is that access of these vessels usually requires a surgical cut-down approach.

PLACEMENT OF THE TRANSVENOUS PACING CATHETER

- Once the sheath is in place
  - The pacing catheter is advanced through the sheath into the venous system.
  - The lead is attached to the connector cables, inserted into the pacing unit.
  - The lead is gradually advanced under continuous electrocardiographic monitoring, with care not to use excessive force, as this may lead to perforation.
    - If performed under fluoroscopic guidance, an inferior or septal position in the distal third of the apex is preferred.
      - Apical right ventricular capture is noted by a left bundle branch, superior axis pattern.
    - If no fluoroscopy is available, a balloon-tipped catheter must be used.

- Placement into the right ventricle is confirmed by ventricular capture on the ECG with a left bundle branch block, superior axis pattern.
- Once ventricular capture is obtained, threshold testing is performed.
- The balloon is deflated to avoid advancement into the pulmonary artery.

PACE SENSING AND THRESHOLD DETERMINANTS

- With good anatomic positioning of the pacing catheter, determine a stimulation threshold
- With continuous ECG monitoring
- Begin pacing at a rate at least 10 beats/minute faster than the patient's intrinsic heart rate.
- Output set at 5 mA
  - Pacemaker output is gradually decreased until the stimuli fail to produce ventricular (or atrial) capture (Fig. 3.3).
  - Current setting at which capture fails to occur is the *pacing threshold*
    - Should be less than 1 mA
    - Pacemaker output should be set at three to five times the pacing threshold.
- If pacemaker is to be used in a demand mode
  - It is important that there is adequate sensing of the endocardial electrogram.
    - To ensure good sensing, the pacing rate is set lower than the patient's intrinsic rate.
    - Sensitivity of the pacing unit is set at its most sensitive level (lowest value) and is then decreased (higher values) gradually.
    - Setting at which the pacemaker fails to sense and begins pacing competitively with the patient's intrinsic rhythm is called the *sensing threshold*.

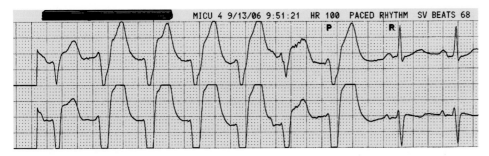

FIGURE 3.3. Loss of capture during threshold testing. Temporary pacing rate was set at 100 beats/min. Loss of capture is obvious with change in QRS morphology. *P* is the last paced ventricular beat. The patient's own rhythm comes through with loss of ventricular pacing. *R* denotes an intrinsic ventricular beat.

○ For demand pacing, the sensitivity should be set at a more sensitive level than the sensing threshold.

POSTINSERTION CARE

- The electrode catheter and its introducer should be secured to the skin under sterile conditions.
- Coiling the proximal electrode catheter around the insertion site and firmly taping to the skin prevents dislodgement of the distal catheter.
- An extension cable should be used to connect the catheter electrode pins to the pulse generator.
  - The pulse generator should be secured to a location where it will unlikely be moved or disconnected inadvertently.
- The plastic shield provided with the pulse generator should be slipped over its controls to prevent accidental control movement
- Obtain a portable chest radiograph to ensure proper positioning of the pacing catheter and assess for complications, particularly pneumothorax.
- A baseline 12-lead ECG should be obtained to document the QRS morphologic features, with the pacing catheter in proper position.
  - A right bundle branch block morphology in lead V_1 with ventricular pacing may indicate pacing of the left ventricle (via an atrial septal defect, ventral septal defect, etc.) and increases the patient's risk of a thromboembolic stroke.
  - A change in the morphology of the paced QRS may be the first sign of electrode displacement.
    - Continuous electrocardiographic monitoring of the patient is imperative.
- Daily evaluation includes:
  - Inspection of the entry site, cardiac auscultation, threshold determinations, and evaluation of intrinsic rhythm
  - Complications of the pacemaker can often be determined by auscultation.
    - Pericardial friction rub may indicate ventricular penetration.
    - A clicking sound may imply intercostal muscle stimulation.
    - Marked changes in thresholds may occur with catheter movement or perforation.
    - The intrinsic rhythm can be evaluated by reducing the rate of the pacemaker until the underlying rhythm emerges.

TROUBLESHOOTING

- A stepwise approach to determine the nature of problems
  - The two most common problems are
    - Failure to capture (pacing artifact without a conducted QRS)
    - Failure to pace (no pacing artifact)
    - Common reasons for noncapture
    - Lead dislodgement
      ○ Lack of apposition of the catheter against tissue or cardiac perforation
    - Change in pacing threshold, or *undersensing*
    - Changes in the patient's clinical status or introduction of new medications can lead to increased pacing thresholds.

○ Electrolyte abnormalities and acidosis may prevent pacing.
○ Antiarrhythmic medications, especially sodium channel blockers such as flecainide or propafenone, may also increase pacing thresholds.
- Failure to pace may occur from
- Loss of output from the pacemaker generator
  ○ Loss of power (low batteries) or disconnection of the pacing catheter from the generator
- Break in the circuit
- *Oversensing*—the inhibition of the pacemaker by events that the pacemaker should ignore
  ○ May be caused by electromagnetic interference in the intensive care unit, T waves, and myopotentials
- Troubleshooting begins with a thorough review of the patient's clinical status and medications.
  - Also includes the following steps:
    - Check labs to evaluate for electrolyte abnormalities such as hyper- or hypokalemia and correct any reversible causes of increased pacing thresholds.
    - Increase the output of the generator to restore capture.
    - Review the settings on the generator box for appropriate programming and to see whether the device has been turned on.
    - Replace the batteries if they are suspected to be depleted.
    - Inspect the box for any obvious abnormalities and examine the connectors from the generator to the pacing catheter for any loose connections, fractures, or insulation breaks.
    - A chest radiograph should be part of any workup for pacing problems; it is useful to evaluate for not only lead dislodgment but also pneumothorax
    - An echocardiogram may help in determining whether there is a new effusion, which may be seen if a perforation has occurred.

COMPLICATIONS

- Although the insertion of a temporary transvenous pacing catheter is generally a safe and well-tolerated procedure, there are potential complications that can occur.
- A complication can occur at any point during the procedure from the time of initial catheter insertion to the time that the catheter is finally removed.
- These include:
  - Vascular injury
  - Inadvertent arterial puncture
  - Bleeding
  - Infection
  - Cardiac tamponade
  - Tricuspid valve injury
  - Pneumothorax
  - Hemothorax
  - Air embolism
  - Phrenic nerve injury
  - Thoracic duct injury
  - Guidewire fracture
  - Thromboembolism
  - Atrial or ventricular arrhythmia
- Insertion of a temporary pacemaker in the setting of an acute MI may increase the risk of certain complications.

- Bleeding risk is increased because the patient is usually anti-coagulated.
- Infarcted myocardium may be soft and necrotic, increasing the risk of cardiac perforation.
- Infarcted tissue may result in high pacing thresholds or inability to capture.
- Myocardium may be irritable, increasing the risk of arrhythmia.
- Metabolic and electrolyte abnormalities may also result in high pacing thresholds or myocardial irritability, and must be corrected.

ALTERNATIVE TEMPORARY PACING METHODS

External Noninvasive (Transcutaneous) Pacing

- External transcutaneous pacing was introduced by Zoll in 1952.
  - Pacing is achieved through two large, self-adhesive electrode pads, usually placed in an anteroposterior position, which are connected to an external pulse generator.
  - Successful pacing with this method has been reported to be as high as 94%
  - However, pectoral muscle stimulation is common and may require sedation.
  - Reliable capture is still not as consistent as with other pacing methods.

Transesophageal Pacing

- Possible because of the posterior position of the esophagus to the left atrium
  - Advantages are that its placement is relatively noninvasive and has minimum complications.
  - The major disadvantage is that ventricular capture is unreliable.

- Therefore, most useful for patients who need atrial pacing only.
- This technique requires a special transesophageal pacing electrode and generator, which provide higher outputs necessary for transesophageal pacing—usually between 2 and 530 mA.
  - The electrode is introduced orally or nasally and is advanced to the proximity of the left atrium.
  - Optimal electrode position occurs at a location with the largest atrial electrograms.

Transthoracic Pacing

- This approach has been used successfully on many occasions, but less invasive temporary pacing techniques have made this procedure quite uncommon.
- Highly invasive technique is performed by direct percutaneous placement of pacing catheters or wires into the right ventricle through a transthoracic needle.
  - Approaching from the precordium or from the subxiphoid region
  - A needle and stylet are introduced into the right ventricle.
  - As needle and stylet are being advanced, they are connected to the V_1 lead of a standard ECG.
    - A current of injury pattern is seen upon penetration of the right ventricular wall, provided that there is no complete ventricular asystole.
    - Removal of the stylet and aspiration of blood verify intracardiac positioning.
    - A pacing catheter is then passed through the needle and the needle is removed.
    - Electrodes are connected to a standard pacing box.
  - Several complications that are potentially severe
  - Pneumothorax
  - Coronary artery perforation
  - Mediastinal bleeding
  - Cardiac tamponade
- Approach should be used **only** when other pacing options are not available.

CHAPTER 4 ■ ALTERED CONSCIOUSNESS AND COMA IN THE INTENSIVE CARE UNIT

MAJOR PROBLEMS

- Impaired consciousness is a very common neurologic problem in the ICU.
- Assessment is a complex undertaking.
- Multiple factors include:

- Prolonged accumulation of sedative agents with impaired renal or hepatic function
  - Allowance of time for metabolism would lead to improvement
- Hypoxic/ischemic injury to the brain more likely than commonly appreciated
- Clinical spectrum of the neurologic aspect of critical illness

ANATOMY OF COMA

- In general, structural lesions interrupt the ascending reticular-activating system.
  - System consists of the reticular formation, neuronal network that signals the thalamus, and cortex.
    - The thalamus participates in arousal.
      - Without this neuronal network, a person cannot be aroused.
    - The thalamus, through the interlaminar nuclei, maintains arousal and relays sensory, motor, and critical cortical circuits.
  - Generally, altered consciousness is caused by lesions that are dorsally located in the pons and thalamus or are bihemispheric.
    - Bilateral lesions of the thalamus, bilateral white-matter lesions, or bilateral cortical lesions necessary to impair consciousness.
    - Alternatively, a hemispheric mass could produce bilateral injury when brain shift occurs or when obstructed ventricular system results in acute hydrocephalus.
- The mechanism of derangement of the brain in acute metabolic abnormalities is not well understood.
  - Not uncommonly, a structural lesion is involved.
  - Examples include:
    - Patients with rapid sodium correction that causes osmotic demyelination, central pontine myelinolysis, or extensive white-matter disease
    - Cerebral edema may also occur in patients with acute ketoacidosis or in those with fulminant hepatic failure.

DEFINITIONS

- Major categories of altered level of consciousness arbitrarily defined for interphysician communication
  - *Acute confusional state*: Impairment of attention, inability to retain memory, and incoherent conversation. Patient not following commands, including tracking a finger
  - *Delirium*: Hallucinations occur and are accompanied by signs of autonomic hyperactivity (tachycardia, hypertension, sweating). Patients may be combative, noisy, and have a markedly abnormal sleep pattern. Hallucinations can be vivid and often visual, particularly in cyclosporin toxicity.
    - Delirium tremens probably more common than appreciated. Warning signs are increased pulse to more than 120 beats/minute, systolic blood pressure more than 160 mm Hg, respiratory rate of more than 30 breaths/minute, fever, new-onset seizures, and a need for incremental doses of lorazepam or other benzodiazepines to control confusion.
  - *Coma*: Unresponsive, eyes closed. Painful stimuli should not produce a localizing response to the pain stimulus, or eye opening, grimacing, or—absent an endotracheal tube—speech. The patient is unable to fixate on an object.
    - With prolonged comatose state, the patient will eventually open eyes, start to fixate on persons around the bedside, and gradually show improvement by following commands and uttering a few words
  - *Persistent vegetative state*: Variation on the comatose state. Patients with pathologic motor responses—extensor (decerebrate) posturing or flexor (decorticate) posturing—who remain comatose may open their eyes, then typically start to develop sleep–wake cycles
    - Periods when patient has eyes open without fixation and periods in which the eyes are closed and the patient in a deep sleep
    - No recognition of external stimuli, no meaningful expression, no visual tracking
    - Brainstem function, including respiration, preserved
    - If vegetative state persists 1 year after traumatic brain injury (TBI) and 3 months after anoxic ischemic injury, it is termed *permanent*.
- Anoxic-ischemic encephalopathy after CPR or asphyxia spares the brainstem but damages cortex; common cause of vegetative state
- After TBI, often some improvement in the level of consciousness
  - Termed *minimally conscious state*
  - Some communication possible, but profound disability
  - *Brain death*: All brain function is lost
    - Occurs in patients with catastrophic neurologic injury, such as a sudden increase in intracranial pressure due to TBI or cerebral hemorrhage
    - Clinical diagnosis can be made, allowing for legal declaration of patient's death.
  - *Locked-in syndrome*: State that mimics coma. Patients have normal consciousness but complete paralysis, except for vertical eye movements. Unable to move limbs, grimace, or swallow but able to look up and down and blink; lesion is typically in base of the pons—often an embolus to the basilar artery—with sparing of the ascending reticular formation, so consciousness unimpaired and patients fully alert

CLINICAL EXAMINATION

- Consists of two parts
  - First to evaluate in a broad manner using coma scales
    - The Glasgow Coma Scale has been used for many years and is a useful means of conducting such an examination.
    - The FOUR (Full Outline of UnResponsiveness) score—devised and validated both in emergency departments, medical, and surgical ICUs
  - Four components, each of which has 4 as the maximal grade Figure 4.1
  - Neurologic examination
    - Brainstem reflexes
- Pupillary responses typically present
  - Bilateral myosis often seen in patients treated with opioids.
  - Unilateral myosis represents Horner syndrome when ptosis is present.
    - Commonly reflects damage to sympathetic pathway after placement of an internal jugular (IJ) vein catheter
    - Extensive thoracic surgery or brachial plexopathies are also causes for unilateral myosis.
  - Bilateral mydriasis with good light responses due to delirium or anxiety
    - Fixed, dilated pupil indicates third cranial nerve involvement.
- Direct compression from herniated brain tissue or due to shift of brainstem in which third nerve is tethered

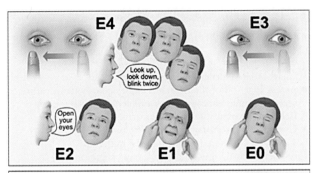

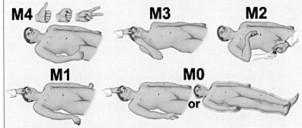

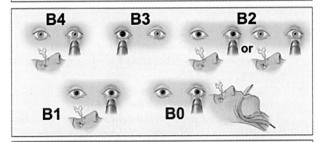

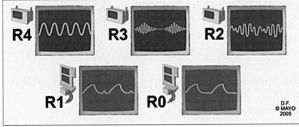

FIGURE 4.1. The FOUR score components are eye response, motor response, brainstem reflexes, and respiration. The eye responses are E0 for eyelids that remain closed with pain; E1 for eyelids closed but open to pain; E2 for eyelids closed but open to loud voice; E3 for eyelids open but not tracking; E4 for eyelids open or open to tracking or blinking to commands. The motor responses are M0 for no response to pain or a generalized myoclonic status epilepticus; M1 for extension response to pain; M2 for flexion response to pain; M3 for localizing to pain; M4 for thumbs up, fist, or peace sign. The brainstem reflexes are B0 for absent pupil, corneal, or cough reflex; B1 for pupil and corneal reflexes absent; B2 for pupil or corneal reflexes absent; B3 for one pupil wide and fixed; B4 for pupil and corneal reflexes present. And finally, respiration responses are R0 for breathes at a ventilator rate or apnea; R1 for breathes above ventilator rate; R2 for not intubated and irregular breathing; R3 for not intubated and Cheyne-Stokes breathing pattern; and R4 for not intubated, regular breathing pattern.

- Important clinical sign indicating brainstem distortion and the presence of a new structural mass
- Major pitfall in ICU is unilateral pupillary dilatation: can be seen with aerosolized anticholinergics and may cause alarm.
  - Mist condenses on eyelids and then touches the cornea, causing a dilated pupil
- Gaze deviation an important clinical sign.
  - Has little localizing value

- May be seen in acute hepatic or renal failure without structural brain lesion
- *Downward gaze* indicates a lesion in the thalamus or dorsal midbrain, frequently seen after hypoxic/ischemic injury
- *Gaze preference* indicates a lesion in one hemisphere, usually a lesion of frontal lobe
  - Eyes turn *toward* abnormality because one eye field is unopposed
    - *Skew deviation*, in which the eyes at rest are not lined up correctly, classic sign of a midbrain or pons lesion
- Spontaneous eye movement abnormalities
  - *Ping pong*: Horizontal conjunctive deviation of the eyes alternating every few seconds
  - *Convergence nystagmus*: Ocular divergence in slow motion followed by rapid convergent jerk
  - *Ocular bobbing*: Rapid downward conjugate movement with slow return to baseline
  - *Ocular dipping*: Slow downward conjunctive movements with rapid return
  - These abnormalities indicative of bihemispheric lesion
    - Rarely observed in toxic encephalopathies
    - Motor tone
- Patient observed for the presence of rigidity or flaccidity
- Marked flaccidity often indicates poisoning or drug intoxication, critical illness polyneuropathy.
- Twitching of the face and mouth may indicate seizures.
  - More often represents myoclonus status epilepticus
    - With repetitive twitching in face, arm, and legs an important clinical sign
    - Seen in drug intoxications, after CPR
    - A poor prognostic sign
    - Localization principles
- Major categories of coma are noted in Table 4.1.
- Table 4.2 shows a systematic diagnostic approach
  - Imaging
    - After the cause of the coma state is localized on examination
- CT or MRI scans, CSF testing, or electrodiagnostic tests may be helpful.
  - MRI may help determine the immediate action to undertake.
  - MRI requires anesthesia support in many patients.
  - Abnormalities seen on neuroimaging studies of comatose patients are shown in Table 4.3
  - The EEG can be performed to detect nonconvulsive status epilepticus.
    - In which the patient has subtle eye blinking or eye movements or gaze preference associated with epileptic discharges
  - Laboratory tests that should be known are shown in Table 4.4

FAILURE TO AWAKEN AFTER SURGERY

- Common problem in general or vascular surgical procedure
  - Vast majority of patients
    - Anoxic/ischemic injury or multiple infarcts are detected
    - May also be due to multiple emboli to the brain
      - Risk of embolization is most significant in patients with severe atherosclerotic disease of the ascending aorta and

TABLE 4.1

CLASSIFICATION AND MAJOR CAUSES OF COMA

Structural brain injury
Hemisphere
Unilateral (with displacement)
  Intraparenchymal hematoma
  Middle cerebral artery occlusion
  Hemorrhagic contusion
  Cerebral abscess
  Brain tumor
Bilateral
  Penetrating traumatic brain injury
  Multiple traumatic brain contusions
  Anoxic-ischemic encephalopathy
  Multiple cerebral infarcts
  Bilateral thalamic infarcts
  Lymphoma
  Meningitis/encephalitis
  Gliomatosis
  Acute disseminated encephalomyelitis
  Cerebral edema
  Multiple brain metastases
  Acute hydrocephalus
  Acute leukoencephalopathy
Brainstem
  Pontine hemorrhage
  Basilar artery occlusion
  Central pontine myelinolysis
  Brainstem hemorrhagic contusion
Cerebellum (with displacement of brainstem)
  Cerebellar infarct
  Cerebellar hematoma
  Cerebellar abscess
  Cerebellar glioma

Acute metabolic-endocrine derangement
Hypoglycemia
Hyperglycemia (nonketotic hyperosmolar)
Hyponatremia
Hypernatremia
Addison disease
Hypercalcemia
Acute hypothyroidism
Acute panhypopituitarism
Acute uremia
Hyperbilirubinemia
Hypercapnia

Diffuse physiologic brain dysfunction
Generalized tonic-clonic seizures
Poisoning, illicit drug use
Hypothermia
Gas inhalation
Basilar migraine
Idiopathic recurrent stupor

Psychogenic unresponsiveness
Acute (lethal) catatonia, malignant
Neuroleptic syndrome
Hysterical coma
Malingering

From Wijdicks EFM. *Catastrophic Neurologic Disorders in the Emergency Department.* 2nd ed. Oxford University Press; 2004, with permission.

TABLE 4.2

DIAGNOSTIC APPROACH TO COMA IN CRITICAL ILLNESS

- Chart sedative drugs and doses
- Assess function of the liver and kidneys, body temperature, serum albumin concentration, and acid-base balance
- Reconstruct plausible drug interactions
- Consider antagonists for benzodiazepines (flumazenil, 1 mg), narcotics (naloxone, 0.1–0.4 mg), and nondepolarizing muscle relaxants (neostigmine, 0.035–0.070 mg/kg, with atropine, 1 mg)
- Localize examination findings to one main category (see Table 22)
- Obtain CT scan of the brain
- Consider MRI (T_2-weighted, fluid attenuation, inversion recovery)
- Obtain electroencephalogram and somatosensory potentials (optional)
- Obtain spinal fluid for cell count, glucose, Gram stain, and cultures (optional)

CT, computed tomography; MRI, magnetic resonance imaging.

thus is applicable to patients with major cardiovascular surgeries.
- Commonly, patients do not awaken because of the accumulation of narcotic and sedative agents.
  - Many of these patients have underlying liver dysfunction that further increases accumulation of these drugs.
- Acute postoperative hyponatremia due to administration of a large volume of hypertonic fluid to patients may be a cause of failure to awaken.

Failure to Awaken after Transplantation

- Vast majority of patients
- Delirium that may evolve to coma due to immunosuppressive toxicity
- Other reasons for loss of consciousness
  - Hypoxic ischemic encephalopathy
  - Central pontine myelinolysis
  - Air embolization
  - Acute uremia
  - Acute graft failure
  - Multiple intracranial abscesses from aspergillosis
  - Immunosuppressive agents—cyclosporin and tacrolimus—can produce a marked neurotoxicity.
    - Patients evolve from rambling speech and visual hallucinations into a stuporous stage that is associated with marked MRI abnormalities.
      - MRI often shows diffuse lesions in the white matter that are fully reversible with discontinuation of the medication.
      - Tacrolimus and cyclosporin are known offenders; sirolimus much less frequently so.
- Central nervous system infections often caused by opportunistic infections.
  - Cytomegalovirus the most common viral infection after organ transplantation.
    - Rarely results in cytomegalovirus encephalitis

TABLE 4.3

FREQUENT ABNORMALITIES ON NEUROIMAGING STUDIES IN COMA

Findings	Suggested disorders
Computed tomography	
Mass lesion (brain shift, herniation)	Hematoma, hemorrhagic contusion, MCA territory infarct
Hemorrhage in basal cisterns	Aneurysmal SAH
Intraventricular hemorrhage	Arteriovenous malformation
Multiple hemorrhagic infarcts	Cerebral venous thrombosis
Multiple cerebral infarcts	Endocarditis, coagulopathy, CNS vasculitis
Diffuse cerebral edema	Cardiac arrest, fulminant meningitis, acute hepatic necrosis, encephalitis
Acute hydrocephalus	Aqueduct obstruction, colloid cyst, pineal region tumor
Pontine or cerebellum hemorrhage	Hypertension, arteriovenous malformation
Shear lesions in the white matter	Head injury
Magnetic resonance imaging	
Bilateral caudate and putaminal lesions	Carbon monoxide poisoning, methanol
Hyperdense signal along sagittal, straight, and transverse sinuses	Cerebral venous thrombosis
Lesions in corpus callosum, white matter	Severe head injury
Diffuse confluent hyperintense lesions in white matter, basal ganglia	Acute disseminated encephalomyelitis immunosuppressive agent, or chemotherapeutic agent toxicity, metabolic leukodystrophies
Pontine trident-shaped lesion	Central pontine myelinolysis
Thalamus, occipital, pontine lesions	Acute basilar artery occlusion
Temporal, frontal lobe hyperintensities	Herpes simplex encephalitis

MCA, middle cerebral artery; SAH, subarachnoid hemorrhage; CNS, central nervous system.
From Wijdicks EFM. Neurologic Complications in Critical Illness. Contemporary Neurology Series 2nd ed. Oxford University Press; 2002.

TABLE 4.4

LABORATORY TESTS IN THE EVALUATION OF COMA

Hematocrit, white blood cell count
Electrolytes (Na, KCl, CO_2, Ca, PO_4)
Glucose
Urea, creatinine
Aspartate transaminase and γ-glutamyltransferase
Osmolality
Arterial blood gases (pH, PCO_2, PO_2, HCO_3, HbCO) (optional)
Platelets, smear, fibrinogen degeneration products, activated partial thromboplastin time, prothrombin time (optional)
Plasma thyrotropin (optional)
Blood and cerebrospinal fluid cultures (optional)
Toxic screen in blood and urine (optional)
Cerebrospinal fluid (protein, cells, glucose, India ink stain, and cryptococcal antigen, viral titers) (optional)
PO_2/PCO_2, partial pressure of O_2/CO_2; HbCO, carbon monoxide hemoglobin.

From: Wijdicks EFM. Neurologic Complications in Critical Illness. Contemporary Neurology Series 64. 2nd ed. Oxford University Press; 2002.

- Infection with *Cryptococcus neoformans* or *Aspergillus fumigatus*
  - Leave multiple brain abscesses and multiple intracranial hemorrhages
  - Outcome from these infections is very poor.
- Sudden loss of consciousness
  - May indicate a new onset of seizures in transplant recipients
    - Incidence in liver transplantation is about 20%.
    - In cardiac transplantation, incidence is between 10% and 15%.
  - Usually an intracranial hemorrhage or bacterial abscess is causative.
  - An acute metabolic derangement—hypernatremia or hyperglycemia—may be implicated.
  - In cardiac transplantations, it is usually associated with an ischemic stroke.

Failure to Awaken in Multisystem Trauma

- Multitrauma patients are at high risk of TBI, so close observation is important.
  - May need intracranial pressure monitoring
    - Particularly if no localization to or eye opening to pain or have brainstem reflex abnormalities
  - Many traumatic parenchymal lesions are localized in the frontal and temporal lobes.

- Significant risk of secondary deterioration from swelling
- Most severe circumstances: Diffuse axonal injury is present.
  ○ Multiple *shear lesions* in the brain
  ○ Typically in the frontal cortex, white matter, basal ganglia, thalamus, and internal capsule
- Rarely failure to awaken after trauma due to fat embolization syndrome
- Patients have large bone fractures.
- Often present 12 to 75 hours after the initial traumatic injury
  ○ Patients often have axillary or subconjunctival petechiae.
  ○ Are markedly hypoxemic
  ○ Frequently have pulmonary edema

Management of Coma

- Initial management is determined by the presence or absence of increased intracranial pressure.
  - Supratentorial mass lesion or diffuse edema (Table 4.5).
  - Placement of an intracranial pressure monitor
  - 20% mannitol solution
    ○ Typically administered at a dose of 0.25 to 1 g/kg
    ○ Goal is to increase plasma osmolality to 310 mOsmol/L.
      – Decreases brain volume by extracting water from brain
      – Generated through an osmotic gradient
      – Important initial intervention and can bridge the patient to neurosurgical evacuation
  - Hypertonic saline (7.5% or 23.4%) may be more effective
    ○ 30-mL bolus through a central line
  - Brief (hours) use of hyperventilation, with target $PaCO_2$ of 30 mm Hg
  - Surgical evacuation of the mass is indicated before further brainstem compression occurs and all brainstem function is lost.

TABLE 4.5

MANAGEMENT OF ACUTE SUPRATENTORIAL MASS WITH BRAIN SHIFT

Stabilizing measures
Protect airway: Intubate
Correct hypoxemia with O_2 nasal cannulae, 3–4 L/min, or face mask
Elevate head to 30 degrees
Treat extreme agitation with lorazepam, 2 mg intravenously, or propofol, 0.3 mg/kg/h
Correct coagulopathy with fresh-frozen plasma, vitamin K (if applicable), consider factor VIIa

Specific medical measures
Hyperventilation: Increase respiratory rate to 20 breaths/min, aim for a $PaCO_2$ of 25–30 mm Hg
Mannitol 20%, 0.25 to 1 g/kg; if no effect, 2 g/kg; aim for a plasma osmolality of 310 mOsm/L
Dexamethasone, 10 mg intravenously (in tumors only)

Specific surgical measures
Evacuation of hematoma
Placement of drain in abscess
Decompressive craniotomy in brain swelling of one hemisphere
$PaCO_2$, arterial partial pressure of CO_2

- Corticosteroids role only for edema surrounding a metastatic lesion or primary brain tumor
  ○ No role in closed-head injury, cerebral infarction, or cerebral abscess

Coma from an Infectious Disease Such as Acute Bacterial Meningitis

- Immediate IV infusion with antibiotics
- Empiric treatment includes:
  - Cefotaxime (2 g IV every 6 h)
  - Vancomycin (2 g IV every 12 h)
  - Corticosteroids
  - If herpes simplex encephalitis considered, acyclovir (10 mg/kg IV every 8 h) is administered.
- In most patients with an infectious cause but no clear etiologic factors, both antibacterial and antiviral treatments initiated until CSF examination reveals the true cause of infection.

Neurosurgeon's Role in the Treatment of Comatose Patients

- Removal of the mass
- Placement of a ventriculostomy, particularly in patients with a subtentorial mass or brainstem lesion
- Craniotomy to remove a bone flap can be performed to allow for swelling
  - This is an option in patients with massive middle-cerebral artery infarction or those with a swollen traumatic contusion.
- For brain abscess in the setting of organ transplantation, a drain can be placed in the abscess. The management of patients in coma from a subtentorial lesion is noted in Table 4.6.

Prognosis

- Prognosis may be determined before hospital admission.
  - Time without circulation and poor airway control may all play an important role in outcome.
  - In TBI, outcome is related to prehospital hypoxemia.

TABLE 4.6

MANAGEMENT OF ACUTE SUBTENTORIAL MASS OR BRAINSTEM LESION

Stabilizing measures
Intubation and mechanical ventilation
Correct hypoxemia with 3 L of O_2/min
Flat body position (in acute basilar artery occlusion)

Specific medical measures
Intra-arterial tpa (in basilar artery occlusion)
Mannitol 20%, 0.25–1 g/kg (in acute cerebellar mass)
Hyperventilation to $PaCO_2$ of 25–50 mm Hg (in acute cerebellar mass)

Specific surgical measures
Ventriculostomy
Suboccipital craniotomy
$PaCO_2$, arterial partial pressure of CO_2

- Certain neurologic conditions may be associated with no hope for good recovery:
  - Patients with myoclonus status epilepticus and brain swelling after cardiac arrest
  - Patients with multiple territorial infarcts and brain swelling after cardiac surgery
  - Occlusion of the basilar artery and coma
  - Multiple intracranial hemorrhages associated with tissue plasminogen activator (tPA)
  - Pontine hemorrhages with hypertension and extension to the midbrain and thalamus
  - Multiple hemorrhagic contusion and associated extradural hematomas
  - Patients with gunshot wounds
  - Intraventricular extension
- In any of these circumstances, outcome is poor, and the level of care should be discussed with family members.

Brain Death

- May occur after traumatic brain injury, severe anoxic/ischemic injury, cardiac resuscitation, catastrophic intracranial hemorrhages, massive hemispheric infarcts, cerebral edema, and fulminant hepatic failure
- Brain death equivalent to death
  - Time of its determination is the time of death
- Definition of brain death implies
  - Documentation of loss of consciousness
  - No motor response to painful stimuli
  - No brainstem reflexes
  - Apnea
- Structural lesion on CT scan is commonly found
- The diagnosis of brain death is made in the following steps:
  - First, the cause has to be identified, and coma has to be irreversible.

- Major confounding factors have to be excluded, and there should be no reversible medical illness.
- Core temperature should be at least 32°C.
- No confounding pharmaceutical agents should have been administered or lingering.
- On examination
  - There is no motor response to pain applied to the face and limbs.
  - Any movement seen must be attributable only to a spinal cord response.
  - There should be:
    - Absent pupil response
    - Absent cold caloric oculovestibular response
    - Absent corneal reflex
    - Absent cough to bronchial suctioning
    - Apnea with a $PaCO_2$ of 60 mm Hg—or a 20 mm Hg increase from pretest baseline
      - Apnea test is done under controlled circumstances using the oxygen diffusion method.
- If patient fulfills all these criteria, brain death can be diagnosed.
  - Useful to have two examinations 6 hours apart; the American Academy of Neurology considers this optional
  - In younger children, electrophysiologic tests are required.

Withdrawal of Care

- Discussion of withdrawal of care must involve senior clinician to explain to the family members the findings and how they play a role in the assessment
- Palliative care includes:
  - Lorazepam and phosphenytoin to prevent seizures
  - Propofol to reduce myoclonus status epilepticus

CHAPTER 5 ■ BIOTERRORISM

IMMEDIATE CONCERNS

- The emergency department (ED) is the key component in protecting the hospital from contamination
  - Isolation/decontamination areas for early suspicious cases must be available to prevent dissemination throughout the facility and community
- Depending on the type of agent released.
  - Affected population may present acutely, with a large number of simultaneous cases.
  - Insidiously over a period of days to weeks.
    - Latter presentation is far more dangerous.

- May not trigger hospital defense systems.
- Resulting in a severe compromise of the facility.

KEY COMPONENTS TO BE ADDRESSED IN ANY PLAN

- Implementation of the Hospital Incident Command System (Fig. 5.1)
- Notification and coordination with public and other authorities (Fig. 5.2)
- Delineation of perimeters and facility access

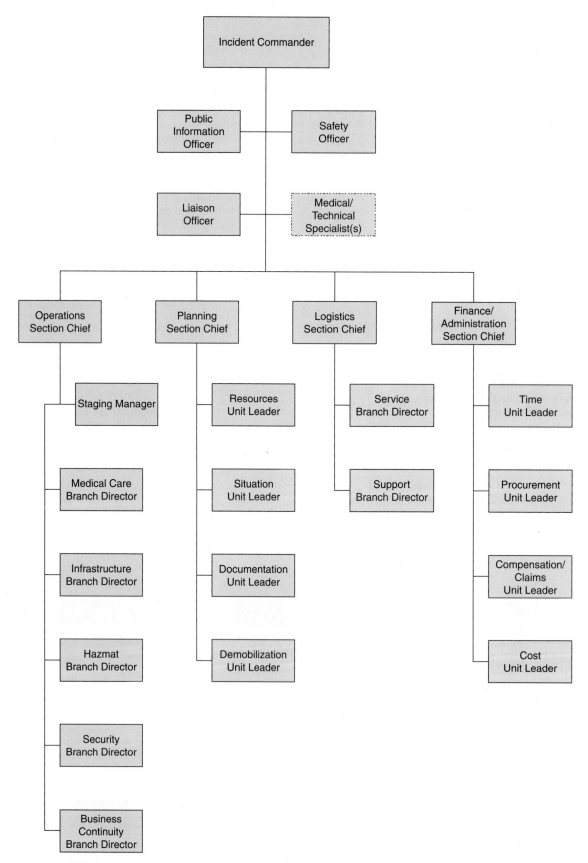

FIGURE 5.1. Basic elements of the Hospital Incident Command System. (From *HICS Guide Book* 2006: 21. http://www.emsa.ca.gov/HICS/files/Guidebook_Glossary.pdf. Accessed October 27, 2008.)

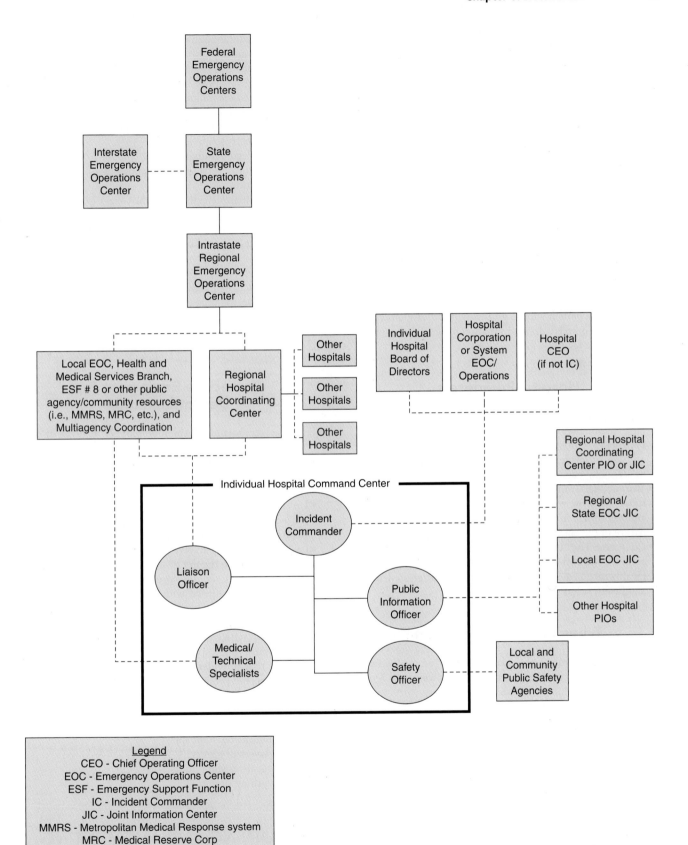

FIGURE 5.2. Diagram illustrating the potential coordination of the Hospital Incident Command System with organizations to the facility. (From *HICS Guidebook* 2006: 21. http://www.emsa.ca.gov/HICS/files/Guidebook_Glossary.pdf. Accessed October 27, 2008).

- Deployment of decontamination equipment, first receivers, and personal protective equipment (PPE)
- Distribution of surge teams, equipment, and medications
- Establishment of patient flows to designated surge areas, including discharge and transfer of patients
- Critical care equipment, designated areas, and personnel: crucial parts of the response
- Large number of these patients require a high level of support.
- Especially airway management, mechanical ventilation, and hemodynamic interventions

DECONTAMINATION AND FIRST RECEIVERS

- Process begins with the designation and enforcement of perimeters around hospital.
  - To ensure that patients flow through a predetermined corridor
  - Usually *any* patient should go through a thorough, supervised, and complete decontamination prior to accessing the inside of the facility.

Hospital Perimeters

- Hospital perimeter is divided into three areas, or zones
  - *Hot zone*: Everything outside the facility's perimeter. Patients have not been through decontamination or triage, and credentials for access have not been verified by security or screening personnel.
  - *Warm zone*: Transition zone, where decontamination and triage happens, where security personnel verify credentials and health-screening clearance for access, depending on the nature of the event
  - *Cold zone*: The "inside" of the hospital. Patients' access this zone only after decontamination is completed and verified. Health care providers are granted access after credentials and health status are corroborated.

Types of Decontamination

- **Primary decontamination:** Occurs when an individual's clothes are removed, in conjunction with showers with a low-pressure, large-volume water delivery system.
  - In colder climates, it is important to ensure warm water delivery systems and to consider of indoor or pool decontamination techniques.
  - Privacy is another major consideration that will help improve compliance by the establishment of corridors and barriers installed to protect patients' dignity after clothing has been removed for decontamination.
- **Secondary decontamination:** Performed by either health care workers following specific guidelines for nonambulatory patients or by the ambulatory patients themselves
  - Recommended that plain water, in conjunction with scrubbing, be used
  - Usually implemented very quickly to expedite the removal of the agent and decrease any possible absorption
  - Mild soapy solutions can be used for oily residues, but decontamination process should not be delayed to add soap.

- **Chemical decontamination:** Begins with the identification of the potential agent
  - Accomplished by evaluation of the clinical presentation
  - Or by using definitive colorimetric chemical identification kits similar to the military type M-8/M-9 paper, or through electrochemical sensors, radiologic detectors, surface acoustic wave technology, infrared mass spectroscopy, and/or ion mobility spectroscopy units
- **Radiologic decontamination:** The presence of radioactive material requires very specific equipment to ensure proper decontamination.
  - Multiparticulate detectors (e.g., the Geiger-Mueller counter) can be used for initial detection and to ensure adequate decontamination.
    - Extreme care should be used to prevent contamination of devices.
    - Scanning should be performed close to but without any skin contact, with a plastic disposable cover.
    - External decontamination is carried out with plain water and scrubbing and should be repeated until the skin shows no evidence of emissions.

Protective Equipment for Decontamination

- First receivers include hospital employees working at a site remote from where the "release" occurred.
  - The primary first receivers have the highest risk and, thus, require a higher level of protection.
- Levels of PPE include class A, B, and C ensembles.
  - Level A ensembles include the highest level of respiratory protection—a self-contained breathing apparatus that is worn inside vapor-protective chemical clothing.
  - Level B ensembles involve heavy-splash chemical protective clothing with the use of self-contained breathing apparatus (some PPE in this level may be encapsulated but should not be confused with the garment rating of vapor protective).
  - Level C ensembles involve light-splash chemical clothing in conjunction with either a filter cartridge face mask or powered air-purifying respirator (PAPR) in which the appropriate filter that provides respiratory protection must be used for the specific product involved within a qualified atmosphere containing an appropriate level of oxygen.
    - Level C ensembles usually suitable for hospital first receivers and consist of:
      - A chemical-resistant suit
      - Two layers of gloves
      - Chemical-resistant boots
      - A breathing device

PLANNING AND AUGMENTING RESPONSES

- In the United States, most medical facilities are functioning at full or near-full capacity during routine operations.
- Recommendations to increase capacity to respond are summarized in Table 5.1.

TABLE 5.1

PLANNING ASSUMPTIONS AND RECOMMENDATIONS FOR MASS CRITICAL CARE

Planning assumptions regarding the current critical care medicine response capacity for bioterrorism
1. Future bioterrorist attacks may be covert and could result in hundreds, thousands, or more critically ill victims.
2. Critical care will play a key role in decreasing morbidity and mortality rates after a bioterrorist attack.
3. Mass critical care could not be provided without substantial planning and new approaches to providing critical care.
4. A hospital would have limited ability to divert or transfer patients to other hospitals in the aftermath of a bioterrorist attack.
5. Currently deployable medical teams of the federal government would have a limited role in increasing a hospital's immediate ability to provide critical care to large numbers of victims of a bioterrorist attack.
6. Hospitals may need to depend on nonfederal sources or reserves of medications and equipment necessary to provide critical care for the first 48 h after discovery of a bioterrorist attack.

Recommendations for hospital planning and response for emergency mass critical care
Modifying usual standards of care
1. Hospitals should develop a set of emergency mass critical care practices that could be implemented in the event critical care capacity of that hospital is exceeded.
Decisions regarding which critical care interventions should be provided: essential elements of critical care
2. To ensure the availability of essential critical care interventions, the Working Group recommends that hospitals give priority to interventions that fulfill the following criteria: (a) interventions that have been shown or are deemed by critical care experts' best professional judgment to improve survival and without which death is likely; (b) interventions that do not require extraordinarily expensive equipment; and (c) interventions that can be implemented without consuming extensive staff or hospital resources.
3. Hospitals should plan to be able to deliver the following during emergency mass critical care: basic modes of mechanical ventilation, hemodynamic support, antibiotic or other disease-specific countermeasure therapy, and a small set of prophylactic interventions that are recognized to reduce the serious adverse consequences of critical illness.
4. Hospitals should plan to be able to administer intravenous fluids resuscitation and vasopressor to large numbers of hemodynamically unstable victims and should stockpile sufficient equipment to do this without relying on external resources for at least the first 48 h of the hospital medical response.
5. Hospitals should plan to provide at least two widely accepted prophylactic interventions that are used every day in critical care: maintaining the head of a mechanically ventilated patient's bed at 45 degrees to prevent ventilator-associated pneumonia and thromboembolism prophylaxis.
Decisions regarding who receives critical care services
6. If there are limited hospital resources and many critically ill patients in need, triage decisions regarding the provision of critical care should be guided by the principle of seeking to help the greatest number of people survive the crisis. This would include patients already receiving ICU care who are not casualties of an attack.
Who should provide emergency mass critical care
7. In the event that critical care needs in a hospital cannot be met by intensivists and critical care nurses, usual ICU staffing should be modified to include non-intensivist clinicians and non–critical care nurses, using a two-tiered staffing model.
8. When there are inadequate numbers of intensivists, hospitals should plan for non-intensivists to manage approximately six critically ill patients and to have intensivists coordinate the efforts of up to four non-intensivists.
9. If a hospital has insufficient numbers of critical care nurses to appropriately manage patients, noncritical care nurses should be assigned primary responsibility for patient assessment, nursing care documentation, administration of medications, and bedside care (e.g., head of bed at 45 degrees, moving patient to prevent pressure ulcers), and critical care nurses should advise non–critical care nurses on critical care issues such as vasopressor and sedation administration.
10. If possible, a non–critical care nurse should be assigned to no more than two critically ill patients, and up to three noncritical care nurses would work in collaboration with one critical care nurse.
11. Bioterrorism training for noncritical care practitioners should include basic principles of critical care management.
Infection control for emergency mass critical care
12. Hospitals should develop pre-event plans to augment usual or modified airborne infection isolation capacity for critically ill victims of a bioattack with a contagious pathogen.
13. Hospitals should stockpile enough PPE to care for mass casualties of a bioterrorist attack for up to 48 h. Also, all hospital clinical staff should receive initial and periodic training on principles of health care delivery using PPE.
Where emergency mass critical care should be located
14. When traditional critical care capacity is full, additional critically ill patients should receive care in non-ICU hospital rooms that are concentrated on specific hospital wards or floors.
15. Hospitals should plan to be able to measure oxygen saturation, temperature, blood pressure, and urine output for the victims of bioattacks in emergency mass critical care conditions.
Learning during emergency mass critical care
16. Hospitals should have information technology capabilities for analyzing clinical data for patients receiving emergency mass critical care and for quickly sharing new observations with a broader clinical community.
Medications for emergency mass critical care
17. Hospitals should develop a list of drugs to stockpile for up to a 48-h response to a mass casualty event using selection criteria that include likelihood the drug would be required for care of most patients, proven or generally accepted efficacy by most practitioners, cost, ease of administration, ability to rotate into the hospital's formulary prior to expiration, and resources required for medication storage.

ICU, intensive care unit; PPE, personal protective equipment.
From Rubinson L, Nuzzo J, Talmor D, et al. Augmentation of hospital critical care capacity after bioterrorist attacks or epidemics: recommendations of the Working Group on Emergency Mass Critical Care. *Crit Care Med.* 2005;33(Suppl.):E2393.

Classification and Initial Treatment for Bioterrorism Agents

- Bioterrorism agents are classified as category A, B, or C based on:
  - Availability
  - Potential for dissemination and infectivity
  - Ability to cause events of large magnitude
    - Category A agents are the most severe

- Early warnings of a bioterrorism event, signs and symptoms of syndromes caused by biologic agents, and initial steps to take if an illness is suspected to be related to a bioterrorism activity are summarized in Table 5.2.
- Tables 5.3 and 5.4 enumerate the clinical presentations, diagnostic tests, and available treatments for category A, and categories B and C, respectively.
- Table 5.5 details dosing of drugs for treatment of potential bioterrorism agents.

TABLE 5.2

GUIDELINES FOR IDENTIFICATION OF A BIOTERRORISM EVENT

- Unusual temporal or geographic clustering of illness
- Unusual age distribution of common disease (e.g., an illness that appears to be chickenpox in adults but is really smallpox)
- Large epidemic, with greater caseloads than expected, especially in a discrete population
- Disease more severe than expected
- Unusual route of exposure
- A disease that is outside its normal transmission season or is impossible to transmit naturally in the absence of its normal vector
- Multiple simultaneous epidemics of different diseases
- A disease outbreak with health consequences to humans and animals
- Unusual strains or variants of organisms or antimicrobial resistance patterns

A. Sentinel clues for a category A biologic agent

Pneumonia or influenzalike syndromes

- Chest pain, dry cough, possible nausea, and abdominal pain, followed by sepsis, shock, widened mediastinum, hemorrhagic pleural effusions, and respiratory failure

Gram-positive bacillus may be isolated.

Consider inhalation anthrax.

- Pneumonia associated with mucopurulent sputum, chest pain, and hemoptysis, particularly in an otherwise normal host

Gram-negative bacillus isolated

Consider pneumonic plague.

- Bronchopneumonia associated with pleuritis and hilar lymphadenopathy, particularly in an otherwise normal host

Gram-negative coccobacillus isolated

Consider tularemia.

Cutaneous ulcer or ulceroglandular syndromes

- Painless ulcer covered by a black eschar, surrounded by extensive nonpitting edema that is out of proportion to the size of the ulcer. Fever and regional lymphadenopathy may be present.

Consider cutaneous anthrax.

Fever and rash syndromes

- An abrupt, influenzalike illness with fever, dizziness, myalgias, headache, nausea, abdominal pain, diarrhea, and prostration. Evidence of "leaky capillary syndrome" with edema or signs of bleeding ranging from conjunctival hemorrhage, mild hypotension, flushing, petechiae, and ecchymoses to shock and generalized mucous membrane hemorrhage and evidence of pulmonary, hematopoietic, renal, and neurologic dysfunction

Consider viral hemorrhagic fevers.

- Febrile illness with myalgias, followed in 2 to 3 d by a generalized macular or papular-vesicular-pustular eruption, with greatest concentration of lesions on the face and distal extremities, including the palms. On any one part of the body (face, arms, chest), all lesions are at the same stage of development (all papules, vesicles, pustules, or scabs).

Consider smallpox.

Paralytic syndromes

- Paralytic illness characterized by symmetric, descending flaccid paralysis of motor and autonomic nerves, usually beginning with the cranial nerves

Consider botulism.

B. Reporting protocols if bioterrorism is suspected as responsible for an illness

- Establish isolation and personnel protection level.
- Contact local public health department immediately.
- Do not wait for confirmation.
- Record data and order tests.
- Alert clinical laboratory.
- Arrange for consultations.
- Follow hospital protocol.
- Notify hospital epidemiologist/infection control specialist.
- Discuss findings with all involved parties.

From *The American College of Physicians Guide to Bioterrorism Identification.*
http://www.acponline.org/bioterro/bio_pocketguide.pdf. Accessed October 27, 2008.

TABLE 5.3

BIOLOGICAL AGENTS CATEGORY A

Entity	Agent	Transmission	When to suspect	Presentation	Diagnosis	Treatment	Alternative treatment	Prophylaxis	Minimum PPE (ideal PPE)	Vaccine
Anthrax	*Bacillus anthracis*	Direct contact: Cutaneous anthrax Airborne: Inhalational anthrax (consider terrorist activity) Ingestion: Gastrointestinal anthrax and Oropharyngeal No person to person	Characteristic skin lesions Rapidly progressive pneumonia CXR: Widened mediastinum (lympha-denopathies) and pleural effusions	Pustule that progresses to a skin ulcer with black necrotic center Respiratory failure Septic shock Diarrhea	Gram stain cultures	Ciprofloxacin (1)	Doxycycline (2) + 1 or 2 additional antimicrobials	Ciprofloxacin (3) or Doxycycline (4) or Amoxicillin (if pregnant and sensitive strain)	Standard precautions	Yes
Botulism	BoNT	Ingestion of toxin (consider terrorist activity: water supply) Inhalation of toxin Infection with toxin production No person to-person	Oculobulbar paralysis	Symmetric descending paralysis	Clinical BoNT detection (days)	Supportive antitoxin (early) (CDC)		Antitoxin monoclonal Ab (limited supply)	Standard precautions (droplet if meningitis suspected)	No
Plague	*Yersinia pestis*	Vector (rodent fleas) (bubonic plague) Inhalation (pneumonic plague) (consider terrorist activity) *Person- to-person*	Large inguinal and axillary lym-phadenopathies (bubonic) Sepsis Unusual number of patients with a fulminant course of productive cough and pneumonia. Sepsis	Buboes DIC, sepsis Respiratory failure Pneumonia, sepsis	Gram stain Cultures Immunofluores-cence	Streptomycin (5) or Gentamicin (6)	Doxycycline (2) or Chloramphenicol (7) or Ciprofloxacin (1)	Doxycycline (4) or Ciprofloxacin (3)	Droplet (airborne)	No

(continued)

39

TABLE 5.3

BIOLOGICAL AGENTS CATEGORY A (CONTINUED)

Entity	Agent	Transmission	Minimum PPE (ideal PPE)	When to suspect	Presentation	Diagnosis	Treatment	Alternative treatment	Prophylaxis	Vaccine
Smallpox	Variola virus	Direct contact Fomites Airborne *Person-to-person*	Airborne (PAPR)	Papulopustular rashes	Progression from: (duration) No symptoms: incubation (7–14 d) Enanthema (2–4 d): contagious Early rash: maculopapular (4 d) Umbilicated centrifugal rash *All lesions at same stage* Scabs (5 d) Pustules (5 d) Scabs resolve: noncontagious	Clinical PCR (CDC)	<3 days of exposure: Vaccinia vaccine Vaccinia immune globulin (VIG) (8) Vaccinia immune globulin IV (VIGIV) (9) Cidofovir (10) 3 days of exposure: supportive		See Treatment	Yes
Tularemia	*Francisella tularensis*	Direct contact with infected animal carcasses (rabbits, hares, rodents) Arthropod bites (tick, deerfly) Ingestion of contaminated food or water Inhalation (consider terrorist activity) *No person-to-person*	Standard precautions	Unusual number of patients with respiratory or systemic illnesses	Ulceroglandular Oculoglandular Oropharyngeal Pneumonic Sepsis	Gram stain Direct fluorescent antibody Culture requires special media Serology only retrospective value	Streptomycin (5) or Gentamicin (6)	Doxycycline (2) or Chloramphenicol (7) or Ciprofloxacin (1)	Doxycycline (4) or Ciprofloxacin (3)	No
Viral hemorrhagic fevers	Ebola Marburg Lassa Machupo Rift Valley	Direct contact Airborne (hypothetical) *Perso-to-person*	Droplet (airborne) (PAPR)	Unusual number of patients with fever, myalgias, conjunctivitis in a severely ill patient with either a purpuric or hemorrhagic maculopapular rash	Maculopapular rash, purpuric or hemorrhagic Bleeding diathesis: epistaxis, hematemesis, hematochezia Pneumonitis	Clinical CDC	Supportive Ribavirin (11) (not effective against Ebola or Marburg) Specific immune globulin (difficult to obtain)		Ribavirin (12) (in needle sticks)	No

PPE, personal protective equipment; CXR, chest x-ray; CDC, Centers for Disease Control and Prevention; DIC, disseminated intravascular coagulation; PCR, polymerase chain reaction; PAPR, powered air-purifying respirator; BoNT, *Clostridium botulinum* neurotoxin.
Adapted from:
1-*Pandemic Point-of-Care Guide*. Joint Commission Resources. 2007.
2-*Fundamentals of Disaster Management*. 2nd Edition. Society of Critical Care Medicine. 2004.
3-Centers for Disease Control and Prevention—*Bioterrorism*, available at: http://www.bt.cdc.gov/agent/agentlist-category.asp (Accessed 1–5-08).

TABLE 5.4

BIOLOGIC AGENTS CATEGORIES B AND C

Entity	Agent	Transmission	Minimum PPE	When to suspect	Presentation	Diagnosis	Treatment	Alternative treatment	Prophylaxis	Vaccine
Brucellosis	Brucella sp.	Direct contact, Ingestion (consider terrorist activity), Person-to-person (extremely rare)	Standard precautions	Unusual number of patients with: fever, myalgias, malaise, sweats, sepsis	Nonspecific	Gram stain, Blood cultures, Anti-O Antibody titer (≥1:160)	Doxycycline (2) plus Rifampin (13)	Trimethoprim/sulfamethoxazole (14, 15) plus Gentamicin (6)	Doxycycline (4) plus Rifampin (13)	No
Ricin toxin	Toxin from castor bean plant Ricinus communis	Direct contact, Ingestion, Inhalation (consider terrorist activity)		Unusual number of patients with nausea, vomiting, abdominal pain, diarrhea, Dyspnea, ALI, ARDS	Gastrointestinal symptoms, Hypovolemic shock, Respiratory failure	Difficult, Urinary ricinine (CDC), Environmental specimens to CDC for immunoassays and PCR				Yes
Cholera	Vibrio cholerae	Ingestion	Standard precautions	Abrupt, copious watery diarrhea	Abrupt, copious watery diarrhea, Very rare abdominal pain or fever		Rehydration, aggressive Doxycycline 300 mg PO, 1 dose or Ciprofloxacin 1 g PO, 1 dose or Azithromycin 1 g PO—1 dose			
Foodborne infections	Escherichia coli (O157:H7, enterotoxigenic), Campylobacter sp., Salmonella typhi & non-typhi, Shigella sp., Giardia lamblia, Listeria monocytogenes, Entamoeba histolytica, Yersinia enterocolitica, S. aureus (enterotoxin B), Others…	Ingestion	Standard precautions	Diarrhea, nausea, vomiting, fever, chills	Diarrhea, nausea, vomiting, fever, chills	Direct smear, Stool cultures, Blood cultures	Azithromycin (16) or Ciprofloxacin (3)	Azithromycin (16), Ciprofloxacin (3), Ciprofloxacin (3), Metronidazole 500–750 mg PO tid, Ampicillin 2 g IV q6h, Metronidazole 500–750 mg PO tid, Trimethoprim/sulfamethoxazole (15), Supportive, Various other antibiotics	Ceftriaxone (16), Azithromycin (16), Paromomycin (16), Paromomycin (16)	No
Glanders	Burkholderia mallei	Direct contact, Ingestion, Inhalation, Person-to-person	Standard precautions, Droplet in pulmonary cases	Massive numbers of patients with similar clinical presentation	Localized infection, Pulmonary infection, Bloodstream infection, Chronic infection (extremities, spleen or liver)	Skin cultures, Sputum cultures, Blood cultures, Urine cultures	Trimethoprim/sulfamethoxazole (14)	Tetracyclines (16), Ciprofloxacin (16), Streptomycin (16), Imipenem (16), Ceftazidime (16)		No
Melioidosis	Burkholderia pseudomallei	Direct contact, Ingestion, Inhalation, Person-to-person	Standard precautions, Droplet in pulmonary cases	Massive numbers of patients with similar clinical presentation	Acute localized infection, Pulmonary infection, Acute bloodstream infection, Chronic suppurative infection	Skin cultures, Sputum cultures, Blood cultures, Urine cultures	Trimethoprim/sulfamethoxazole (14) or Ceftazidime (16)	Imipenem (16), Meropenem (16), Chloramphenicol (16)		No

PPE, personal protective equipment; ALI, acute lung injury; ARDS, adult respiratory distress syndrome; CDC, centers for disease control; PCR, polymerase chain reaction.

Adapted from:

1- *Pandemic Point-of-Care Guide.* Joint Commission Resources. 2007

2- *Fundamentals of Disaster Management. 2nd Edition.* Society of Critical Care Medicine. 2004

3- Centers for Disease Control and Prevention—*Bioterrorism,* available at: http://www.bt.cdc.gov/agent/agentlist-category.asp (Accessed 1–5-08)

TABLE 5.5

TREATING AGENTS

1.	Ciprofloxacin	
	Adults	400 mg IV q12h
	Pregnancy	400 mg IV q12h
2.	Doxycycline	
	Adults	100 mg IV q12h
	Pregnancy	100 mg IV q12h
3.	Ciprofloxacin	
	Adults	500 mg PO bid
	Pregnancy	500 mg PO bid
4.	Doxycycline	
	Adults	100 mg PO bid
	Pregnancy	100 mg PO bid
5.	Streptomycin	
	Adults	1 g IM q12h
6.	Gentamicin	
	Adults	5 mg/kg IM or IV q24h
	Pregnancy	5 mg/kg IM or IV q24h
7.	Chloramphenicol	
	Adults	25 mg/kg IV q6h
8.	VIG	
	Adults	0.6 mL/kg IM
9.	VIGIV	
	Adults	100 mg/kg IV at rate:
		1 mL/kg/h for 30 min, then
		2 mL/kg/h for 30 min, then
		3 mL/kg/h for 30 min
10.	Cidofovir	
	Adults	5 mg/kg IV over 1 h
11.	Ribavirin	
	Adults	30 mg/kg IV loading dose
		16 mg/kg IV q4h for 4 d, then
		8 mg/kg IV q4h for 6 d
12.	Ribavirin	
	Adults	500 mg PO q6h for 7 d

Note: These are starting doses for adults only; for length of therapy, pediatric therapies, and further indications, consult with health authorities or infectious disease specialists.

Classification and Initial Treatment for Chemical Agents

- The chemical agents are divided into five different groups (Table 5.6).
  - Nerve agents: Anticholinesterase activity
  - Asphyxiants or blood agents: cyanide-based
  - Choking or pulmonary-damaging agents: direct airway cytotoxicity
  - Blistering or vesicant agents: direct skin cytotoxicity; may also affect airway
  - Incapacitating agents: for riot control

PERSONAL PROTECTIVE EQUIPMENT IN THE INTENSIVE CARE UNIT

- The Society for Critical Care Medicine (SCCM) and the World Federation of Societies of Intensive and Critical Care Medicine have adopted new recommendations for PPE.

- If possible, the ICU area designated should be turned into a negative-pressure environment.
- Patient rooms should function as negative-pressure areas either by design or by installing portable negative-pressure units.
- Entire ICU is a "warm" zone, where all staff—including medical, nursing, respiratory therapy, secretarial, and housekeeping—wear a basic layer of PPE that includes
  - Scrubs
  - Gown
  - Gloves, with longitudinal taping
  - N-95-type mask
  - Nonabsorbent-material shoes
- Donning and doffing of PPE should follow a checklist (Table 5.7).
- If a patient's room needs to be accessed for routine care **not** resulting in the generation and dispersion of aerosols, a second layer of PPE is recommended.
  - Eye protection (taped goggles)
  - Hair-covering device (hair net or hat)
  - A second gown
  - A second layer of gloves, with longitudinal taping
- If patient's room needs be accessed where there is a **high risk** for aerosolization of secretions (e.g., the use of bag-valve-mask, endotracheal intubation, open-circuit suctioning, bronchoscopy, or disconnection from ventilator), a higher level of PPE should be used.
  - PAPR
  - The second layer noted earlier
  - The PAPR used indoors in the ED or ICU should be of a light material and should not be confused with the PAPR used in decontamination lines at the entrance of the hospital.
- The doffing (removal) of the PPE is probably—and remarkably—the most important phase.
  - The likelihood of contamination increases significantly if procedures are not properly followed (see Table 5.7).

VENTILATOR TRIAGE

- Distribution of mechanical ventilators requires evaluation when demand exceeds availability.
- Well-defined, objective criteria need be used for their assignment (Table 5.8).
- In a major mass casualty incident (MCI), where the number of patients far exceeds the available resources
  - Imperative to utilize a protocol with easy-to-follow tools, with clear definitions based on objective criteria
    - Sequential organ failure assessment (SOFA) may be used as the base for the initial classification of patients.
    - With follow-up at 48 and 120 hours
    - Once a patient has passed the inclusion and exclusion criteria, the SOFA-based initial (Tables 5.9) and 5.10) evaluation is performed.
    - There are repeat evaluations at 48 and 120 hours (Tables 5.11 and 5.12, respectively).

TABLE 5.6

CHEMICAL AGENTS

Type	Acronym	Other name	Military detection	Classic findings	Other signs and symptoms	Decontamination	Treatment	Miscellaneous
Nerve	GA GB GD GF VX	Tabun Sarin Soman Cyclohexyl sarin Methylphosphon-othioic acid	M256A1 CAM M8 paper M9 paper M8A1 alarm M8 alarm	Miosis Sialorrhea Rhinorrhea Fasciculation	Blurred vision Headache Nausea and vomiting Sialorrhea Diaphoresis Diarrhea Seizures Dyspnea	Remove clothing Gently wash skin (avoid abrading skin) Flush eyes with water or saline	Atropine 2 mg IV/IM every 5 min Repeat as needed based on symptoms Pralidoxime 600–1,800 mg IM or 1 g IV (max 2 g/h) MARK-I kit contents: AtroPen—atropine sulfate 2 mg in 0.7 mL ComboPen—pralidoxime chloride (2-PAM) 600 mg in 2 mL Benzodiazepines for seizures Oxygen Ventilatory support	In high exposures: Unconsciousness Flaccid paralysis
Blood/ asphyxiant	AC CK	Arsine Hydrogen cyanide Cyanogen chloride	M256A1 Ticket NOT—M8A1 NOT—CAM	Cherry-red skin or Cyanosis or Frostbite (when applied in liquid form)	Few: Giddiness Palpitations Dizziness Nausea and vomiting Gasping Hyperventilation Drowsiness Seizures (terminal)	Remove clothing (if no frostbite) Gently wash skin (avoid abrading skin) Flush eyes with water or saline	Oxygen *Antidotes:* Amyl nitrate by inhalation 1 amp (0.2 mL) every 5 min Sodium nitrate 300 mg IV over 5–10 min Sodium thiosulfate 12.5 g IV over 10–20 min Repeat sodium nitrate based on patient's weight and hemoglobin level	Metabolic acidosis Venous oximetry above normal Arsine and cyanogen may cause delayed pulmonary edema

(continued)

TABLE 5.6

CHEMICAL AGENTS (CONTINUED)

Type	Acronym	Other name	Military detection	Classic findings	Other signs and symptoms	Decontamination	Treatment	Miscellaneous
Pulmonary/ choking	CL CG DP PS	Chlorine Phosgene Diphosgene Chloropicrin	No detection	Odor of newly mown hay or grass or corn	Eye irritation Airway irritation Dyspnea Wheezing Coughing Laryngeal edema Pulmonary edema ALI and ARDS	Fresh air Oxygen Remove clothing Gently wash skin (avoid abrading skin) Flush eyes with water or saline	Termination of exposure No antidote Supportive treatment	
Blistering/ vesicant	CX H HD HN L	Phosgene oxime Mustard gas Sulfur mustard Nitrogen mustard Lewisite	CX: M256A1 M8 alarm Mustards: M256A1 CAMM8 paper M9 paper M8 alarm NOT – M8A1 alarm L: M256A1 only	CX Odor: Pungent or pepperish HD odor: Garlic or horseradish L odor: Geranium	Eye edema and tearing Skin erythema and blistering Airway sloughing Dyspnea Coughing Pulmonary edema	Remove clothing Gently wash skin (avoid abrading skin) Flush eyes with water or saline	Termination of exposure Supportive treatment Mustards: No antidote Antidote for lewisite: British anti-lewisite (BAL) or Dimercaprol	Bone marrow suppression
Riot control agents	CN or MACE CS	Chloroacetophenone Ortho- chlorobenzylidene malononitrile	No detection	Lacrimation Rhinorrhea Erythema	Dyspnea Tachypnea Wheezing	Flush eyes with water or saline Flush skin with water Decontamination usually is not indicated	Supportive treatment	Usual: self-limiting Unusual: pulmonary edema

ALI, acute lung injury; ARDS, adult respiratory distress syndrome.
Adapted from references 22 and 26.

TABLE 5.7

PERSONAL PROTECTIVE EQUIPMENT (PPE): DONNING AND DOFFING AND ENHANCED AIRBORNE PRECAUTIONS WITH POWERED AIR-PURIFYING RESPIRATOR (PAPR)[a]

Prior to entering the room
(For leaving the room, proceed to step VI)
Step I
The following articles must be put on in the anteroom. If there is no anteroom, they should be donned prior to entering the ICU
1. Properly fitted N-95 mask (minimum)
2. Impervious isolation gown
3. Gloves (place two strips of tape onto the glove and the gown, one anterior and one posterior)

Step II
Routine-care PPE (second layer)
The following articles are to be worn in addition to PPE in step I, prior to entering the patient's room for *routine* patient care
WARNING: If you anticipate aerosolization of secretions (e.g., endotracheal intubation, cardiac arrest, tracheostomy, bronchoscopy, endotracheal tube exchange), skip this section and *proceed to steps III, IV, and V* prior to entering the room
1. Disposable goggles (place a strip of tape onto goggles and forehead)
2. Second impervious isolation gown (see picture 2 on PAPR sheet)
3. Second set of gloves (place two strips of tape onto the glove and the gown, one anterior and one posterior; see picture 3A,B on PAPR sheet)
4. Hair net or hat (optional)
You may now enter the room for routine care

Step III
Testing the HEPA filter and electric pump battery efficiency
1. Attach breathing tube (black) to the air pump/filter/battery (PAPR) assembly box (gray) with a twist-and-lock motion
2. Turn the power switch ON
3. Check airflow by inserting floater cone inside the free end of the black tube. Floater device should remain suspended, with the lower indicator line *not* touching the tube's end. This indicates proper functioning of the unit If cone does not float, *do not use this unit* and send for servicing
4. Turn the power switch OFF and set unit aside.

Step IV
Donning the hood (*requires assistance*)
1. Secure long hair
2. Put on a hair cover (optional)
3. Peel off protective layer from face shield
4. Attach breathing tube to the top of the hood; a snap should be heard
5. Place the pump/filter/battery assembly (gray) (PAPR) box around waist and adjust belt. Leave the box in the back
6. Turn the power switch ON
7. Ensure the breathing tube is free from twists, kinks, or damage
8. With assistance, put hood on, face first. Ensure that the elasticized edge of the face seal is under the chin and along the cheeks. Ensure the N-95 mask remains securely in place (4)
9. Center inner headband around forehead and verify that straps on top of the hood are in contact with the top of the head

Step V
PAPR PPE (second layer)
1. Lift the outer shroud of the hood
2. Put on a second impervious isolation gown, ensuring that it covers the inner shroud *only* (5)
3. Allow the outer shroud to cover the top portion of the isolation gown
4. Apply second pair of gloves (place two strips of tape onto the glove and the gown, one anterior and one posterior)

You may now enter the room to perform procedures where aerosolization of secretions are anticipated.
Prior to leaving the room
Step VI
Removal of routine-care PPE
1. Grasp front of second isolation gown (top layer) with both hands and pull forward to remove from shoulders
2. Remove second isolation gown with taped gloves as one unit, as you roll inside out, prior to discarding
3. Remove disposable goggles, grasping above the ear. *Do not* touch the frame area around the eyes. Discard goggles

Step VII
Removal of PAPR PPE (*requires assistance*)
1. Second person detaches breathing tube from the assembly unit and turns OFF unit
2. From the outside, grasp the hood at the top of the head and under chin simultaneously and remove hood
3. Dispose of hood respirator and breathing tube
4. Second person unties second isolation gown (top layer)
5. Grasp front of second isolation gown with both hands and pull forward to remove from shoulders.
6. Remove second isolation gown with taped gloves as one unit, as you roll inside out, prior to discarding
7. Remove air pump/filter/battery assembly box and place inside double plastic bags while in the room
8. Exit the room, maintaining the first PPE layer (N-95 mask, hair net, goggles, and gown); bring the double-bagged air pump/filter/battery assembly box for processing

ICU, intensive care unit.
[a]The following guidelines are intended to illustrate a suggested donning and doffing sequence for enhanced airborne precautions, using the 3M BE-10 Series PAPR. They are not intended to substitute the recommendations of the Infection Control or Critical Care Groups of your institution. Please refer to the manufacturer's instructions for further details of assembly, handling, and cleaning.

TABLE 5.8

VENTILATOR AND INTENSIVE CARE TRIAGE TOOL

Inclusion criteria
The patient must meet one of either criteria A or B
A. Requirement for invasive ventilatory support
 • Refractory hypoxemia (SpO_2 <90% on nonrebreather mask/FiO_2 >0.85)
 • Respiratory acidosis with pH <7.2
 • Clinical evidence of impending respiratory failure
 • Inability to protect or maintain airway
B. Hypotension
Hypotension (systolic blood pressure [SBP] <90 or relative hypotension) with clinical evidence of shock (altered level of consciousness, decreased urine output, or other end-organ failure) refractory to volume resuscitation requiring vasopressor/inotrope support *that cannot be managed on the ward*

Exclusion criteria
The patient is excluded from admission/transfer to critical care if *any* of the following (*) is present:
*Severe trauma (defined by each center based on their experience with the Injury Severity Score [ISS], Trauma and Injury
  Severity Scoring system [TRISS], or similar)
*Severe burns
A patient with any two of the following:
  i. Age >60 years
  ii. Total body surface area (TBSA) >40%
  iii. Inhalation injury
*Cardiac arrest
  *Unwitnessed cardiac arrest
  *Witnessed cardiac arrest not responsive to electrical therapy (defibrillation, cardioversion, or pacing)
  *Recurrent cardiac arrest
*Severe cognitive impairment
*Advanced untreatable neuromuscular disease
*Metastatic malignancy
*Advanced and irreversible immunocompromise
*Severe and irreversible neurologic event/condition
*End-stage organ failure meeting following criteria:
  *Cardiac:
  i. New York Heart Association (NYHA) class III or IV heart failure
  *Lung:
  i. Chronic obstructive pulmonary disease (COPD) with forced expiratory volume in 1 second (FEV_1) <25% predicted,
    baseline PaO_2 <55 mm Hg, or secondary pulmonary hypertension
  ii. Cystic fibrosis with post-bronchodilator FEV_1 <30% or baseline PaO_2 <55 mm Hg
  iii. Pulmonary fibrosis with vital capacity (VC) or total lung capacity TLC <60% predicted, baseline PaO_2 <55 mm Hg, or
    secondary pulmonary hypertension
  iv. Primary pulmonary hypertension with NYHA class III to IV heart failure, or right atrial pressure >10 mm Hg, or mean
    pulmonary arterial pressure of >50 mm Hg
  *Liver
  i. Child Pugh score >7
*Age >85 years
*Requirement for transfusion of >6 units packed red blood cells within 24-h period
*Elective palliative surgery

Adapted from Christian M, Hawryluck L, Wax R, et al. Development of a triage protocol for critical care during an influenza pandemic. *CMAJ.* 2006;175(11);1377.

TABLE 5.9

THE SOFA SCALE

Variable	Value				
	0	1	2	3	4
PaO$_2$/FiO$_2$, mm Hg	400	≤400	≤300	≤200	≤100
Platelets (×1,000/μL)	150	≤150	≤100	≤50	≤20
Bilirubin, mg/dL (μmol/L)	<1.2 (< 20)	1.2–1.9 (20–32)	2.0–5.9 (33–100)	6.0–11.9 (101–203)	12 (>203)
Hypotension	None Epi ≤0.1[a] Norepi ≤0.1[a]	MAP <70 mm Hg Epi >0.1[a] Norepi >0.1[a]	Dop ≤5[a]	Dop >5[a]	Dop >15[a]
Glasgow coma score	15	13–14	10–12	6–9	<6
Creatinine, mg/dL (μmol/L)	<1.2 (<106)	1.2–1.9 (106–168)	2.0–3.4 (269–300)	3.5–4.9 (301–433)	5 (>434)

Dop, dopamine; Epi, epinephrine; Norepi, norepinephrine.
[a] μg/kg/min.

TABLE 5.10

INITIAL ASSESSMENT

Critical care triage tool (initial assessment)		
Color	Criteria	Priority/action
Blue	Exclusion criteria or SOFA >11	Medical management ± palliate D/C from CC
Red	SOFA ≤7 or Single organ failure	Highest
Yellow	SOFA 8–11	Intermediate
Green	No significant organ failure	Defer or D/C Reassess as needed

SOFA, sequential organ failure assessment; D/C, discharge; CC, critical care.
Adapted from reference 30.

TABLE 5.11

48-HOUR ASSESSMENT

Critical care triage tool (48-hour assessment)		
Color	Criteria	Priority/action
Blue	Exclusion criteria or SOFA >11 or SOFA 8–11 no	Palliate and D/C from CC
Red	SOFA <11 and Decreasing	Highest
Yellow	SOFA <8 no Δ	Intermediate
Green	No longer ventilator dependent	D/C from CC

D/C, discharge; CC, critical care; SOFA, sequential organ failure assessment; Δ, change.
Adapted from reference 30.

TABLE 5.12

120-HOUR ASSESSMENT

Critical care triage tool (120-hour assessment)		
Color	Criteria	Priority/action
Blue	Exclusion criteria or SOFA >11 or SOFA <8 no	Palliate and D/C from CC
Red	SOFA <11 and Decreasing progressively	Highest
Yellow	SOFA <8 minimal decrease (<3 points in past 72 h)	Intermediate
Green	No longer ventilator dependent	D/C from CC

D/C, discharge; CC, critical care; SOFA, sequential organ failure assessment; Δ, change.
Adapted from reference 30.

CHAPTER 6 ■ INVASIVE PRESSURE MONITORING: GENERAL PRINCIPLES

PRINCIPLES OF ARTERIAL WAVE TRANSMISSION

Natural Frequency

- A pressure wave travels down the conducting tubing and deflects the transducer diaphragm, which rebounds and generates a reflected wave. When this reflected wave reaches the tip of the catheter, another reflected wave travels back toward the transducer.
- The *natural frequency* (f_n) of a system is the frequency at which a signal, such as a change in pressure, will oscillate in a uniform, frictionless tube. This frequency is measured in hertz (Hz) cycles per second. Natural frequency decreases with increasing tube length, since at any given wave speed, a round trip in a longer tube simply takes more time.
- Natural frequency increases with wave speed, which in turn increases with tube radius and tube wall stiffness and decreases with the density of the conducting medium. Thus, short, wide, rigid tubing; a stiff transducer; and dense conducting media (e.g., saline rather than air) yield a higher f_n.

Damping

- The friction generated by the movement of the conducting medium decreases the amplitude of the reflected pressure wave, or *damps* it. Stiffer transducer diaphragms and stiffer conducting tubing will result in less damping as smaller volumes are required to displace them. Damping is also influenced by the mass of the conducting medium and tubing resistance, which impedes the minute amount of reciprocative flow needed for pressure wave transmission, causes dissipation of energy from the pressure wave, and increases damping.

TROUBLESHOOTING

- Simplicity and uniformity in transducer and catheter setup are key to minimizing opportunity for errors. Tubing should be stiff tubing designed for pressure monitoring, used with a minimum length and few stopcocks and connectors.

Zeroing

- A common source of error is the zero reference level for pressure measurement. All pressures are measured relative to the horizontal plane at which the transducer is set to zero.

When the transducer is connected to a fluid-filled catheter, any hydrostatic pressure imposed by the catheter will be sensed by the transducer. The recorded pressure will rise as the transducer is lowered, and vice versa. This continues to occur when the catheter is attached to a patient.

- Most agree that vascular pressure should be referenced to the level of the heart; that is, the recording system should read zero pressure when the open end of a transduced fluid-filled tube is held at the horizontal plane of the heart. The optimal external anatomic landmark representing this plane remains a subject of debate. Many suggest the midaxillary line, but others have recommended estimation of the uppermost boundary of the heart. For simplicity and uniformity, the midaxillary line is best for general use.
- This anatomic reference level should be on the same horizontal plane, not of the transducer diaphragm but of the port or stopcock that is opened to atmospheric pressure when the electronics are zeroed. One simple way to provide consistency is to secure the transducer to the patient's arm near the heart and zero it using the port molded into the transducer body. This will allow fewer errors than attaching the transducer to an IV pole, in which case elevating the bed or sitting the patient up will change his or her horizontal relationship to the zero point. However, re-zeroing to the cardiac level will be needed when patient orientation is changed (such as lateral decubitus or prone positions). Care must also be taken that the transducer has not rotated to a dependent position on the arm or slipped to the elbow in a patient who is anything but completely flat.

Testing the Frequency Response

- Intensive care units, operating rooms, and other monitoring settings combine various components from various manufacturers into their systems for vascular pressure measurement. The parts may vary between units or perhaps even from patient to patient or nurse to nurse and will change as suppliers change over time. The performance specifications of individual components such as transducers and amplifiers are provided in their user manuals, but the performance of the integrated system is usually untested.
- Fortunately, the catheter–tubing–transducer system allows simple bedside study. By using the flush device, one can apply a near square-wave pressure signal, and the features of the recorded output can be examined. When the flush device resistor is bypassed, a high-pressure signal is produced, which goes off-scale on the bedside monitor. When the lever is released, however, a square-wave low-pressure signal is

generated, which falls within the range of the display. Proper functioning is indicated when this signal rapidly reverberates a few times and then decays back to the underlying vascular pressure.

Overdamping and Underdamping Errors

- Overdamping is a common problem that causes errors in the measurement of systolic and diastolic pressure. Overdamping is suggested during a bedside flush test by a gradual pressure decay or an undershoot and slow return to baseline without any oscillation. The effect of overdamping on the waveform is to first cause the wave to lose details such as the dicrotic notch and a brisk systolic upstroke, or the a, v, and c waves of a venous pressure. With more damping, the wave will appear sinusoidal, systolic pressure will fall, and diastolic pressure rise toward the mean arterial pressure. Even with extreme overdamping, the mean pressure remains accurate.

- Numerous problems in the catheter–tubing–transducer subsystem can cause overdamping. These include air bubbles, blood clots, or fibrin within the catheter or tubing, catheter tips abutting a vessel wall, or kinks or partially closed stopcocks. Flushing or changing the tubing and obsessively purging air bubbles solves many overdamping problems. If the damped waveform is associated with kinking or thrombosis of the catheter, poor blood return, or sensitivity to minor catheter movement, it may need replacement.

- In tachycardic, hyperdynamic patients, excessive oscillation may be apparent in the pulse recording, especially at peak systole. This problem occurs when important harmonics of the pulse approach the transducer system's f_d. Underdamping causes systolic and diastolic pressure to be over- and underestimated, respectively. The excessive oscillations will also interfere with the algorithms used to calculate a digital display of systolic and diastolic pressure. Even manual estimation of these pressures from the bedside oscilloscope or printed record is inaccurate, since the pulse pressure is exaggerated.

- The characteristics of the transducer system can be studied and optimized to reduce under-damping errors. During observation of a fast flush, oscillations that are widely spaced indicate a low f_d, which may poorly suit a patient whose pulse is dynamic with upper harmonics of high amplitude. Natural frequency is reduced by lengthy or compliant tubing or by bubbles. Removing unneeded tubing extensions and diligently clearing bubbles will bring the flush test oscillations closer together, and the waveform will show more detail with greater accuracy.

- The reverberations in the pulse can be smoothed away by injecting a tiny bubble of air into the transducer or catheter. However, this practice is not recommended. While the air bubble will increase the damping, it also decreases f_d. The waveform will be made to appear more normal but may be no more accurate. If larger bubbles are introduced, the excessive damping causes the pulse pressure to narrow toward the mean arterial pressure. One would like to increase the damping of the system without decreasing its natural frequency. This effect can be achieved by reducing the amplifier high-pass filtration frequency just enough to eliminate the reverberations, as is outlined in most monitoring equipment users' manuals. Too much electronic damping will degrade the waveform just as would excess mechanical damping. Filtering should generally not be reduced below 12 Hz to avoid removing the higher-order harmonics contributing to the systolic waveform. There are also mechanical devices that attach to a stopcock near the transducer and increase damping. These devices are designed to match the transducer impedance to that of the tubing, decreasing wave reflections without altering f_d.

- Artifact that appears similar to under-damping can also occur when long, flexible catheters are vibrated by high-velocity blood flow, termed "catheter whip." This phenomenon should be suspected when long intravascular catheters are used in high-flow vessels of much larger diameter, such as long femoral or pulmonary artery catheters. Contributions of under-damping to the waveform appearance can be ruled out by inspecting the fast flush and optimizing the external tubing system. Artifact due to movement of the catheter tip is difficult to eliminate. In the pulmonary artery, stabilizing the catheter tip by inflating the balloon to measure a pulmonary artery occlusion pressure will remove the "whip." Measurement of mean pressures will also remain accurate.

CHAPTER 7 ■ HEMODYNAMIC MONITORING: ARTERIAL AND PULMONARY ARTERY CATHETERS

CLINICAL USE OF ARTERIAL LINES

Pressure Measurement

- Continuous measures of systolic blood pressure (SBP), diastolic blood pressure (DBP), and mean arterial pressure (MAP) are displayed with invasive arterial catheters.
- Waveform analysis (Fig. 7.1) demonstrates the typical points associated with (a) systolic upstroke, (b) systolic peak, (c) systolic decline, (d) dicrotic notch, (e) diastolic runoff, and (f) end diastole. Examination of the arterial waveform provides useful information regarding a patient's clinical status. Left ventricular ejection produces the first, sharp upstroke at the beginning of aortic valve opening (see Fig. 7.1, points 1 and 2). As the ventricular flow is dispersed peripherally, the waveform declines (point 3); this is also when the heart is in isovolumetric relaxation and diastolic filling. Just prior to closure of the aortic valve and as a result of isovolumetric relaxation, there is a slight drop in pressure known as the incisura (at the aorta) or dicrotic notch (at the periphery; point 4). Further decrease in the pressure waveform reflects the runoff to distal arterioles (points 5 and 6). More peripheral arteries exhibit narrower waveforms and higher systolic pressures and wider pulse pressures, although the MAP remains similar to central vessels. The etiology of varying pulse contours in the periphery is related to the elasticity, amplification, and distortion of smaller arteries.
- Various cardiac conditions produce characteristic arterial waveforms. In aortic stenosis, narrow waveform and loss of the dicrotic notch secondary to diseased valve are seen. Aortic regurgitation may exhibit widened pulse pressures and a sharp upstroke, sometimes accompanied by two peaks.
- Arterial cannulation is relatively safe, with nonocclusive thrombosis and hematoma being the most common complications. Selection of anatomic site is an important consideration; percutaneous arterial catheters can be introduced in the radial, brachial, axillary, femoral, and dorsalis pedis arteries. Placement in brachial arteries is ill advised; it is an end artery, and patients may develop ipsilateral hand ischemia in up to 40% of insertions. The radial artery remains the most popular placement site due to its ease of access and relatively low complication rates. A pre-procedure Allen test assesses the patency of collateral arteries, but this test has poor correlation with distal flow and likelihood of hand ischemia.

Systolic Pressure Variation

- Variations in systolic blood pressure and ventricular stroke volume are of greater magnitude in hypovolemic states. Originally, SPV was described as two components (Fig. 7.2): delta up (Δup) and delta down (Δdown)—while emphasizing the strong correlation between Δdown and hypovolemic states. Δup is the difference between maximum SBP and a reference SBP (usually at expiratory pause during mechanical ventilation). Δdown is similarly the difference between minimum SBP and reference SBP and represents a decrease in stroke volume during expiration. SPV >0 mm Hg indicates hypovolemia and suggests responsiveness to fluid challenge. SPV also has significant correlation with the left ventricular end-diastolic area by echocardiogram and pulmonary artery occlusion pressure (PAOP). Note that SPV, like stroke volume variation, may be sensitive to changes in volume status but may not necessarily equate to actual intravascular blood volume.

STROKE VOLUME VARIATION

- Arterial pressure variation during the respiratory cycle is a well-documented phenomenon. Pulsus paradoxicus describes falls in arterial pressures (>0 mm Hg) during inspiration and rises in pressures during expiration in spontaneously breathing patients. Reverse pulsus paradoxicus occurs in ventilated patients. Stroke volume variation (SVV) is not a measurement of absolute preload; rather, it is an assessment of response to fluid resuscitation. SVV >9.5% to 15% is associated with fluid responsiveness. SVV is approved for use only in sedated, mechanically ventilated patients who are in sinus rhythm

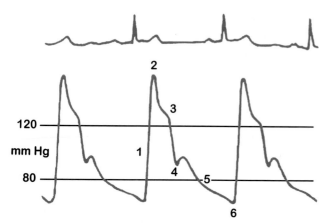

FIGURE 7.1. Arterial waveform analysis (see text for explanation of points 1–6).

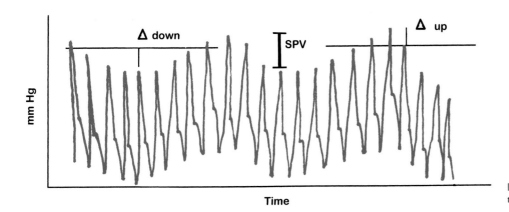

FIGURE 7.2. Systolic pressure variation (SPV) (see text).

(rhythm must be regular or the variation may be due to irregular rate rather than volume status).

$$SVV = (SV\ maximum - SV\ minimum)/[(SV\ maximum + SV\ minimum)/2] \times 100$$

PULMONARY ARTERY CATHETER

- Inherent in the use of the pulmonary artery catheter (PAC) is the assumption that flow-related variables such as cardiac output/cardiac index and oxygen delivery (DO_2) to the tissues are important for survival. The biggest criticism of the supply dependency concept was the mathematical coupling between DO_2 and VO_2 as cardiac output is on both sides of the equation. An easier clinical end point of resuscitation is the central ($Sc\bar{v}O_2$) or mixed venous oxygen saturation (SvO_2) or which reflects the balance between DO_2 and VO_2.
- Review of all the literature studying resuscitation to CI, DO_2, and SvO_2 goals is summarized in the practice guidelines for the PAC. The controversy is not whether DO_2 is important to tissues but rather *how much* is necessary to meet the demands of individual tissues. It is also clear that global values of DO_2 may not translate into transport of oxygen to the individual tissue beds, but until we have a tool to measure all tissue oxygenation states (or one tissue bed that is a surrogate marker for the rest of the body), the amount of oxygen delivery necessary for tissue perfusion will remain controversial.
- Over the decades, clinicians have progressed from treatment of BP, HR, and urine output to markers of anaerobic metabolism such as lactic acid and base deficit and then to flow-related variables such as DO_2, VO_2, and SvO_2.

INDICATIONS FOR PULMONARY ARTERY CATHETER INSERTION

- Indications for PAC insertion have been broadly categorized in Table 7.1.

TABLE 7.1

INDICATIONS FOR PULMONARY ARTERY CATHETER INSERTION

Precautionary reasons
For prevention of multisystem organ failure in high-risk patients (perforated viscus)
For preoperative assessment of high-risk patients with cardiac, pulmonary, and renal dysfunction
For management of high-risk patients postoperatively (major hemorrhage)
For patients with expected large fluid shifts: sepsis, bleeding, multiple trauma, burns, and cirrhosis

Treatment of shock
Hypotension not relieved with fluid
Suspected cardiac event or cardiac compromise contributing to shock
Oliguria not responding to fluid
Patients with multiple organ dysfunction
For continuous SvO_2 monitoring

To guide treatment in pulmonary dysfunction
To differentiate cardiogenic causes of hypoxia from acute respiratory distress syndrome and guide fluid management
For monitoring cardiac output in patients requiring high positive end-expiratory pressure (≥ 15 cm H_2O)

Treatment of cardiac dysfunction
Complicated myocardial infarction
Congestive heart failure with poor response to afterload reduction and diuretic therapy
Suspected tamponade or contusion from blunt chest injury
Pulmonary hypertension with myocardial dysfunction

TABLE 7.2

NORMAL HEMODYNAMIC VALUES

Hemodynamic parameter	Normal range
Systolic blood pressure	100–140 mm Hg
Diastolic blood pressure	60–90 mm Hg
Mean arterial pressure (MAP)	70–105 mm Hg
Heart rate	60–100 beats/min
Right atrial (RA) or central venous pressure (CVP)	0–8 mm Hg
Right ventricle systolic pressure	15–30 mm Hg
Right ventricular diastolic pressure	0–8 mm Hg
Pulmonary artery (PA) systolic pressure	15–30 mm Hg
PA diastolic pressure	4–12 mm Hg
Mean PA	9–16 mm Hg
Pulmonary artery occlusion pressure (PAOP, wedge)	6–12 mm Hg
Left atrial pressure (LAP)	6–12 mm Hg
Cardiac output (L/min)	Varies with patient size
Cardiac index (L/min/m²)	2.8–4.2 L/min/m²
Right ventricular ejection fraction (RVEF)	40%–60%
Right ventricular end-diastolic volume indexed to body surface area (RVEDVI)	60–100 mL/m²
Hemoglobin	12–16 g/dL
Arterial oxygen tension (PaO₂)	70–100 mm Hg
Arterial oxygen saturation	93%–98%
Mixed venous oxygen tension (PvO₂)	36–42 mm Hg
Mixed venous oxygen saturation (SvO₂)	70%–75%

PRESSURE MEASUREMENTS

- Normal hemodynamic values are presented in (Table 7.2).
- While passing from the vena cava to a branch of the pulmonary artery, characteristic waveforms are displayed on the monitor (Figs. 7.3 and 7.4).
- Whether the patient is on mechanical ventilation (positive intrathoracic pressure) or spontaneously breathing (negative intrathoracic pressure), all pressure measurements should occur at end expiration when the intrathoracic pressure is closest to atmospheric pressure (Fig. 7.5) (unless the patient is on higher levels of positive end-expiratory pressure [PEEP]).
- The first characteristic waveform seen when inserting a PAC is the right atrium (RA) tracing (Fig. 7.6). The tracing can be seen while inserting the catheter or by transducing the right atrial pressure once the PAC is in position. There are two main positive pressure deflections, called the a and v waves. The a wave follows the P wave of the electrocardiogram and is due to the pressure increase during atrial systole (Figs. 7.6 and 7.7). The v wave results from atrial filling against a closed tricuspid valve during ventricular systole. Between these two positive deflections is a small c wave due to tricuspid closure. Two negative deflections called the *x* and *y* descents occur when pressure in the atrium decreases. The *x* descent occurs during atrial relaxation. The *y* descent is seen when the tricuspid valve opens and blood flows from the atrium to the ventricle.
- The pressures observed in the RA range from 0 to 8 mm Hg. Higher pressures may not necessarily mean fluid overload but reflect the volume of the right heart and the ability of the

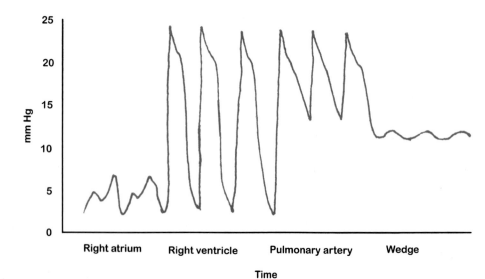

FIGURE 7.3. Waveforms seen during pulmonary artery catheter insertion.

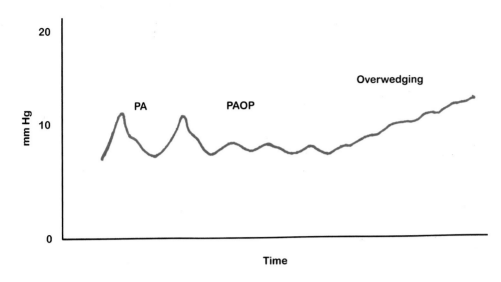

FIGURE 7.4. Over-wedged tracing. PA, pulmonary artery; PAOP, pulmonary artery occlusion pressure.

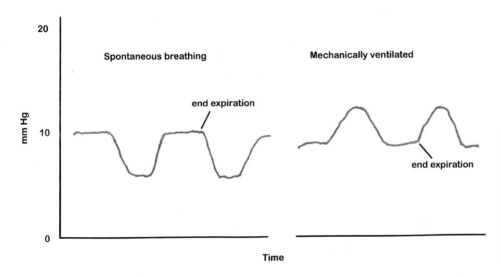

FIGURE 7.5. Reading of pulmonary artery occlusion pressure (PAOP) at end expiration. During spontaneous breaths, PAOP dips down during peak inspiration due to negative intrathoracic pressure. During mechanical ventilation, PAOP goes up during peak inspiration due to positive pressure ventilation and intrathoracic pressure. In both situations, PAOP should be read at end expiration.

A) Atrial Fibrillation

B) Atrial Flutter

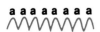

C) Complete AV Block

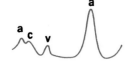

NORMAL

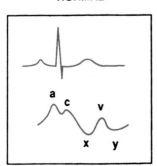

D) Tricuspid Regurgitation

E) Pericardial Tamponade

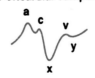

F) Constrictive Pericarditis

FIGURE 7.6. Pressure tracings from the right atrial port in normal and pathologic conditions (refer to text).

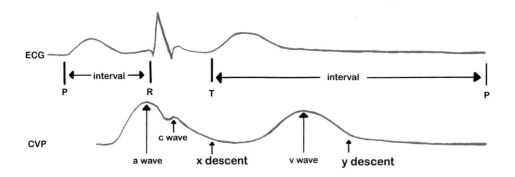

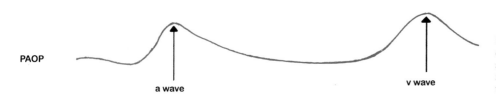

FIGURE 7.7. Reading of central venous pressure (CVP) and pulmonary artery occlusion pressure (PAOP) in relationship to the cardiac cycle (electrocardiogram).

ventricle to eject that volume. There is little relationship between the central venous pressure (CVP) and PAOP or left heart pressures in patients with valvular or coronary artery disease or when pulmonary artery pressures are elevated. It is in these situations of right heart failure, severe pulmonary disease, and in most of the critically ill patients when monitoring the CVP only (and not the PAOP) would be misleading.

• The next waveform seen is that of the right ventricle (see Fig. 7.3). The pressures here are higher with a wider difference between systolic and diastolic. If no RV waveform is seen after inserting the catheter 30 cm from the internal jugular or subclavian vein entry site, the catheter may be curling in the atrium or passing into the inferior vena cava. The catheter should be quickly advanced through the ventricle both to avoid dysrhythmias and to keep the catheter from warming and losing its stiffness. The right ventricular (RV) systolic pressures generally range from 15 to 30 mm Hg and diastolic pressures from 4 to 12 mm Hg. In right heart failure, the RV diastolic pressures may be high enough that the waveform mimics the pulmonary artery (PA). Low RV pressures will be seen in hypovolemic shock and they will also be close to PA pressures. One concern at this point of insertion is causing a right bundle branch block or even complete heart block in patients with pre-existing left bundle branch block. However, the incidence of complete heart block appears to be no greater in patients with left bundle branch block than without.

• Once the catheter enters the pulmonary artery, the waveform shows an increase in diastolic pressure while the systolic pressure remains about the same as in the ventricle, sometimes referred to as the "step up" (see Fig. 7.3). This transition may be difficult to discern when there is hypovolemia, tamponade, RV failure, or catheter whip. If there is no change in waveform after inserting the catheter 50 cm, it may be coiling in the ventricle and is at risk of knotting. A chest radiograph will discern the problem, and fluoroscopy may be used to guide placement. Normal PA pressures range from 15 to 25 mm Hg systolic over 8 to 15 mm Hg diastolic. The beginning of diastole is marked by a dicrotic notch on the PA tracing, corresponding to the closure of the pulmonic valve. This incisura distinguishes the PA from the RV when RV diastolic pressures are elevated. As blood flows through the lungs to

the left atrium, the PA pressure drops until it reaches a nadir at the end of diastole. Since the pulmonary circulation has low resistance, the diastolic pressure is able to decrease until it is just higher than PAOP. The highest PA systolic pressure occurs during the T wave of the corresponding electrocardiogram (ECG). The pulmonary circulation is very dynamic and is affected by acidosis, hypoxia, sepsis, and vasoactive drugs. An increase in cardiac output (CO) may also seemingly paradoxically lower the PA pressures by a reflexive decrease in pulmonary vascular resistance with fluid resuscitation and decreased sympathetic nervous system discharge.

• The transition to the wedge position is noted by a drop in mean pressure from the PA. The PAOP usually ranges from 6 to 12 mm Hg in normal states. PAOP most closely reflects left ventricular end-diastolic volume (LVEDP) after atrial contraction and before ventricular contraction (see Fig. 7.7). There are often no clear a, c, or v waves. When v waves are prominent such as in mitral insufficiency, the bottom of the v wave or the a wave may be used to measure the PAOP (Fig. 7.8). A prominent v wave may fool the novice into thinking that the catheter is not wedging. It is important to note the change in wave form from PA to v wave tracing (although the two waves may look remarkably similar). One way of differentiation is that the v wave occurs later in the ECG cycle after the T wave while the PA wave occurs right after QRS (Fig. 7.8). There may be large a waves secondary to a decrease in left ventricle compliance; the point 0.05 seconds after initiation of QRS again best reflects LVEDP. Even though the measurements are correlated with the ECG and are done during end expiration, the PAOP may be exaggerated by respiratory muscle activity, especially during active or labored exhalation.

Principles of Measuring Pulmonary Artery Occlusion Pressure

• When the balloon is inflated, the blood flow in that segment of the pulmonary artery is occluded, and the PAOP is measured. Since there is no flow, the pressure between the occluded pulmonary artery segment and the left atrium will equalize (Fig. 7.9), analogous to closing off a pipe with pressures

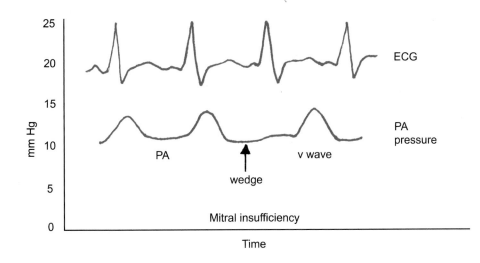

FIGURE 7.8. Regurgitant mitral valve generating a v wave seen during wedging. PA, pulmonary artery.

equalizing between the two ends. With the closed pipe analogy, there is a list of assumptions that may not necessarily hold true in a critically ill patient, regardless if mechanically ventilated or otherwise: PAOP ≅ PcP ≅ LAP ≅ LVEDP ≅ LVEDV, where PcP is pulmonary capillary pressure, LAP is left atrial pressure, and LVEDV is left ventricular end-diastolic volume. As long as there is no obstruction in this conduit, the relationship between PAOP and LVEDP may hold. The final assumption is equating pressure to volume by estimating LVEDV or "preload" with LVEDP. We will now assess the pitfalls with each one of these assumptions.

- PAOP ≅ PcP ≅ LAP occurs only in the dependent areas of the lung, where the pressures from blood flow in the RA and

pulmonary artery are greater than the alveolar pressure, or zone 3 in the West classification. Placement of the catheter in other areas of the lung (zone 1 or 2) may cause errors in estimation of PAOP to LAP due to pulmonary venous obstruction and respiratory variation as well as high ventilator support (PAOP reads higher than LAP).

- Increased intrathoracic pressure secondary to respiratory failure and the addition of PEEP in ventilated patients affects pulmonary vascular pressures. Up to about 15 cm H_2O, PAOP closely correlates with LAP. During higher PEEP states, the PAOP may not reflect the true filling pressure of the heart (i.e., pressure outside minus pressure inside the heart).

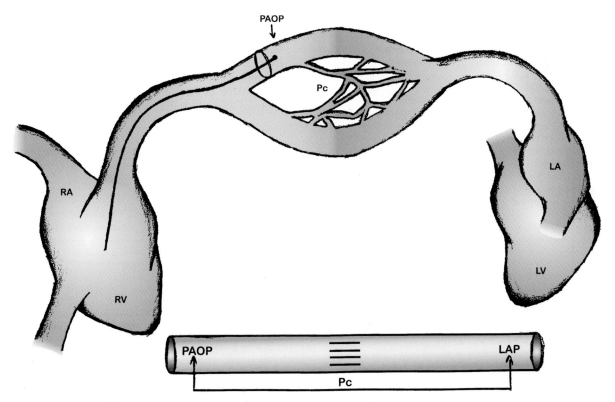

FIGURE 7.9. Closed pipe analogy: blocking of flow by the balloon with theoretical equalization of pressure in the conduit. RA, right hetrium; RV, right ventricle; PAOP, pulmonary artery occlusion pressure; Pc, pulmonary capillary; LAP, left atrial pressure; LV, left ventricle.

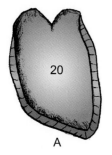 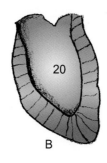 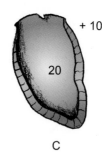

FIGURE 7.10. The same pulmonary artery occlusion pressure of 20 mm Hg reflecting three different clinical conditions. **A:** Distended hypervolemic ventricle in a normal heart. **B:** Normal volume in a noncompliant heart (ventricular hypertrophy). **C:** Low volume in a normal ventricle with high juxtacardiac pressures such as high positive end-expiratory pressure.

- LAP □ LVEDP. LAP (and thus PAOP) will overestimate LVEDP if there is an obstruction between the left atrium and the left ventricle such as a myxoma or mitral stenosis. Mitral valve regurgitation also causes the PAOP to read higher than the true LVEDP because of the additional pressure of the retrograde flow of blood across the valve resulting in a large v wave (see previous). LAP (and thus PAOP) will underestimate LVEDP when severe aortic regurgitation causes premature closure of the mitral valve when the left ventricle is still filling. LAP (and PAOP) is higher when there is a left atrial kick in a failing heart and decreased ventricle compliance such as in ischemic states, left ventricular hypertrophy, and restrictive cardiomyopathies. This is especially true when LVEDP is greater than 25 mm Hg.
- LVEDP □ LVEDV. The pressure–volume relationship depends on the compliance of the ventricle and the transmural ventricular distending force. The compliance of the ventricles will change with ischemia, infarct, and hypertrophy. A stiff heart (myocardial hypertrophy) will need higher pressures to obtain the same amount of volume as a normal heart (Fig. 7.10). The transmural ventricular distending force (intracavitary pressure minus juxtacardiac pressure) will depend on the pressure inside and outside the heart. External forces elevating juxtacardiac pressures may be high ventilator support or pericardial tamponade, which may cause elevation of PAOP but may not reflect ventricular filling pressure.

Clinical Use of the Pulmonary Artery Occlusion Pressure

- As long as the previously mentioned assumptions regarding the relationship between PAOP, LAP, and LVEDP have been evaluated, the PAOP may be used as an estimate of LAP with reasonable correlation. The optimum wedge pressure depends on the patient but has been defined as the pressure where there is minimal increase in stroke volume or left ventricular stroke work. Although the normal PAOP values may be 10 to 14 mm Hg, some patients require a high pressure to reach the optimum stroke volume (Fig. 7.11).
- The Starling curve-plotting stroke volume index to PAOP (as an estimate of LVEDP) may help identify the optimum wedge, but some patients may have a flat curve. If vasoactive agents are started, the heart may now be on a different curve requiring new assessment of the optimum PAOP. The optimum PAOP varies not only from patient to patient but temporally within the same patient as the clinical condition changes (such as vasoactive agents, myocardial compliance, and external forces around the heart). There are no set numbers to treat to, but each patient must be individually assessed and assessed *repeatedly*, making the PAC a highly user-dependent tool.
- Elevated wedge pressures may help differentiate hydrostatic pulmonary edema from that caused by increased permeability. A PAOP of 24 mm Hg or higher is associated with a tendency for hydrostatic edema. Lower pressures may imply

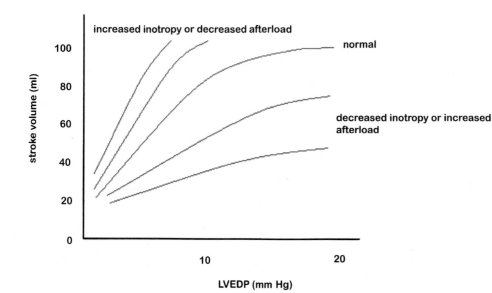

FIGURE 7.11. Frank–Starling curves (family of curves) showing the relationship between left ventricular end-diastolic pressure (LVEDP) to stroke volume (SV, mL/beat). Augmenting preload increases LVEDP with a concomitant increase in SV (up to a certain point). The effects of manipulating preload, afterload, and contractility and shifting to another curve can be seen.

Modified Stewart-Hamilton equation

$$Q = \frac{VI\ (TB - TI) \times SI \times CI \times 60 \times CT \times K}{SB \times CB \quad {_0^\infty}\int \Delta TB\ dt}$$

Q = Cardiac Output
VI = volume of injectate
TI = injectate temperature
TB = blood temperature
CI = specific heat of the injectate (D5W = 0.965, saline = 0.997)
SI = specific gravity of the injectate (D5W = 1.018, saline 1.005)
60 = seconds/minute
CT = correction factor (loss of thermal indicator due to time lost in injecting, catheter length, patient's temperature)
$= \dfrac{TB - \text{mean temperature of the injectate delivered to the right atrium}}{TB - TI\ (\text{pre-injectate temperature})}$
SB = specific gravity of blood (1.045)
CB = specific heat of the blood (0.87)

$_0^\infty\int \Delta TB\ dt$ = integral of blood temperature change

Computation constant (K) $= \dfrac{SI \times CI \times 60 \times CT \times VI}{SB \times CB}$ = changes with VI

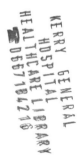

FIGURE 7.12. The modified Stewart–Hamilton equation for estimating cardiac output.

increased capillary permeability and traditionally, a PAOP of <18 mm Hg has implied a pulmonary (or noncardiogenic) cause of lung edema. When there is an increase in PVR, the wedge pressure underestimates Pc, and hydrostatic pulmonary edema may therefore occur at lower wedge pressures.

- Volumetric PACs are designed with the ability to measure right ventricular ejection fraction, from which the right ventricular end-diastolic volume indexed to body surface area is calculated.

Cardiac Output

- The ability of the heart to meet increasing tissue oxygen demand is perhaps the single most important determinant in oxygen delivery and tissue perfusion.
- Crystalloid solution (usually 10 mL, but 5 mL may be used in volume-restricted patients) is injected into the RA port at similar parts of the respiratory cycle (end expiration), within 4 seconds in a smooth manner. The thermistor near the tip of the PAC detects the change in temperature, and the change in blood temperature over time is proportional to the blood flow from the ventricle. Several measurements (three to five) should be taken and the average of the values (within 10% of each other) used. Principles of the modified Stewart-Hamilton equation calculate the cardiac output (Fig. 7.12).
- Falsely low CO will occur if an error in the system increases the change in temperature (which is in the denominator of the Stewart-Hamilton equation): The temperature probe reading the injectate is cooler than the actual injectate (or the solution is warmer than the temperature reading of the injectate), more than allotted "dye" amount is injected (>10 mL fluid), there is too rapid an injection, or the injection occurs during positive pressure ventilation. Falsely high CO may occur if the temperature probe measuring injectate reads warmer than the actual injectate (if the solution is cooler than the tempera-

ture reading of the injectate), less than the allotted amount of "dye" (<10 mL) is used, or the catheter has migrated distally with less change in temperature difference. Most institutions use temperature probes at the site of injection (RA port) so that variations in injectate temperature should not contribute to errors in CO measurements.

- Another development in the evolution of measuring CO is the PAC with continuous cardiac output monitoring.

Starling Curves

- Drs. Frank and Starling described the relationship between myocardial stretch and contractility (see Fig. 7.11). Myocardial stretch is an independent determinant of stroke work, and the actin–myosin interaction has a linear correlation with the strength of systolic contraction up to a certain point. Given the heart's dynamic environment, a family of curves is more representative of the true preload-to-stroke volume relationship. Increasing afterload or decreasing contractility shifts the curve down and to the right (i.e., more stretch is necessary to produce a similar difference in stroke volume). One cannot stress enough the importance of reassessment after each therapy. For example, initiating afterload reduction may put the heart on a different Starling curve (to the left and up; see Fig. 7.11) but may decrease the preload. Unless more fluid is given to optimize the LVEDP (i.e., PAOP), the best stroke volume may not be achieved.

MIXED VENOUS OXYGEN SATURATION

- The SvO_2 value indicates the balance between oxygen delivery to the tissues and the amount consumed by the tissues before returning to the heart.

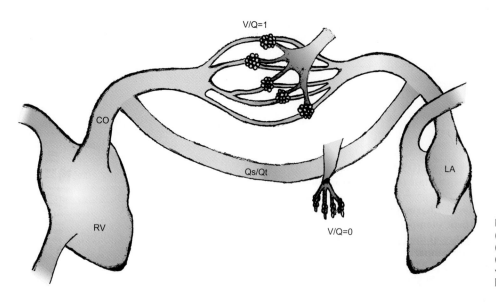

FIGURE 7.13. Intrapulmonary shunt (Qs/Qt) is the percent of cardiac output (CO) not involved with gas exchange (goes through collapsed alveoli), with ventilation/perfusion V/Q = O. LA, left atrium; RV, right ventricle.

Rearranging the Fick Equation

$$SvO_2(\%) = \frac{VO_2}{SaO_2 - CO\ (L/min) \times Hgb\ (g/dL) \times 1.36\ (mLO_2/g\ Hgb) \times 10}$$

Four factors determine the SvO_2 value: three parameters contributing to oxygen delivery (CO, hemoglobin, and SaO_2) and one parameter for O_2 consumption. Low SVO_2 suggests insufficient O_2 delivery or increased O_2 consumption. SVO_2 is also a harbinger of shock and may decrease before overt shock is apparent. Mixed venous oxygen saturation has also regained popularity as an end goal of resuscitation with decreased mortality.

- Inadequate oxygen delivery can be the result of decreased cardiac output, low hemoglobin, or low oxygen saturation. Increased consumption may occur due to activity, fever, hyperthyroid state, or repayment of oxygen debt. High SvO_2 suggests low cellular consumption such as in late sepsis, arteriovenous shunts (cirrhosis), or excessive inotrope use. Hypothermia, sedation, paralysis, anesthesia, hypothyroidism, and cyanide poisoning can also reduce VO_2.
- The catheter should also be checked to ensure that distal migration has not occurred leading to sampling of pulmonary capillary blood that is normally highly saturated (~100%). Inflating the balloon (wedging) should determine that the catheter is in too far if the PAOP tracing is seen with <1.25 mL of air. The oximeter should be calibrated daily in vivo.

INTRAPULMONARY SHUNT

- "Shunt" refers to the portion (in %) of blood that flows (CO) from the right side of the heart to the left completely deoxygenated (Fig. 7.13). Physiologic shunt = anatomic shunt + intrapulmonary shunt. "Anatomic shunt" refers to the direct drainage of the venous system to the left ventricle through the bronchial, thebesian, and pleural veins (~2%–5% of CO).

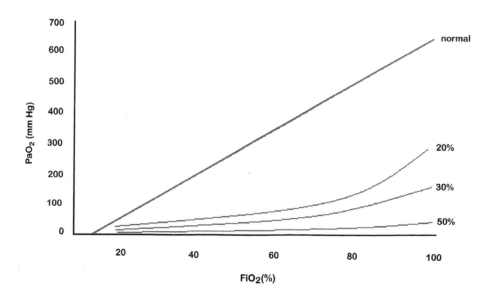

FIGURE 7.14. The effect of FiO_2 on PaO_2 depending on the degree of intrapulmonary shunts of 20%, 30%, and 50%. This assumes that other parameters that affect SvO_2 such as cardiac output, hemoglobin, and oxygen consumption are remaining constant.

Intrapulmonary shunt (Qs/Qt) is expressed as the percentage of cardiac output passing through completely collapsed alveoli with no or little gas exchange so that the ventilation-to-perfusion ratio is zero (i.e., V/Q = 0).

- "Venoarterial admixture" or "shuntlike states" refer to blood flow passing through partially open alveoli (i.e., V/Q <1). Acute shunt will not respond to FiO_2, and the treatment is PEEP to open the alveoli and make them responsive to FiO_2. Venous admixture will demonstrate some response to FiO_2.

If the shunt is minimal (normal condition), there is almost a linear relationship between FiO_2 and PaO_2, but as the shunt increases, FiO_2 no longer affects PaO_2 in a linear fashion (Fig. 7.14). This is an important concept as one cannot improve hypoxemia by increasing FiO_2 alone but needs to open the alveoli with PEEP. If the shunt equation is calculated on a FiO_2 of <1.0, both the shunt and venous admixture will be captured in the equation. Intrapulmonary shunt (Qs/Qt) is calculated as $(CcO_2 - CaO_2)/(CcO_2 - CvO_2)$, where CcO_2 is

TABLE 7.3

DERIVED CALCULATIONS (ALL INDEXED TO BODY SURFACE AREA)

Parameter	Equation	Key	Normal	Units
Stroke volume indexed (SVI)	CI/HR or EDVI – ESVI	Amount of blood ejected with each contraction (per m^2)	30–65	mL/beat/m^2
Left ventricular stroke work index (LVSWI)	SVI × (MAP – PAOP) × 0.0136	External work for the left ventricle in 1 beat	43–61	g · m/m^2
Right ventricular stroke work index (RVSWI)	SVI × (MPAP – CVP) × 0.0136	External work for the right ventricle in 1 beat	7–12	g · m/m^2
Pulmonary vascular resistance indexed (PVRI)	$\dfrac{(MPAP - PAOP) \times 80}{CI}$	Resistance for right ventricle; 80 converts mm Hg/min/L to dynes · sec/cm^5	255–285	dynes · sec/cm^5
Systemic vascular resistance (SVR)	$\dfrac{(MAP - CVP) \times 80}{CI}$	Resistance for left ventricle	1,970–2,390	dynes · sec/cm^5/m^2
Arterial oxygen content of blood (CaO_2)	(Hgb × 1.36 mL O_2/g Hgb × SaO_2) + (0.0031 × PaO_2)	Amount of oxygen in arterial blood, majority is carried by Hgb (1.36 mL of O_2/g of Hgb if blood is 100% saturated), very little is dissolved (0.0031 × PaO_2)	16–22	mL O_2/dL blood
Mixed venous oxygen content of blood (CvO_2)	(Hgb × 1.36 mL O_2/g Hgb × SvO_2) + (0.0031 × PvO_2)	Amount of oxygen in mixed venous blood (sampled at the pulmonary artery)	12–17	mL O_2/dL blood
Arterial-mixed venous oxygen content difference ($AVDO_2$)	CaO_2–CvO_2	How much O_2 was consumed by the tissues before returning to the heart	3–5	mL O_2/dL blood
Delivery of oxygen indexed (DO_2I)	CaO_2 × CI × 10	Primary determinant of organ perfusion	500–600	mL O_2/min/m^2
Oxygen consumption indexed (VO_2I)	(CaO_2 – CvO_2) × CI × 10	Oxygen consumed by the tissues	120–160	mL O_2/min/m^2
Intrapulmonary shunt (Qs/Qt)	$(CcO_2 - CaO_2)/(CcO_2 - CvO_2)$ CcO_2 = (Hgb × 1.36 × 100% saturation) + (0.0031 × PAO_2) PAO_2 = FiO_2 × [(760 mm Hg – 47 mm Hg)] – ($PaCO_2$/RQ)	% of CI that is not involved with gas exchange and goes to the arterial side deoxygenated; >20% usually requires ventilator support. Since pulmonary capillary blood cannot be sampled, 100% saturation is assumed. 760 is atmospheric pressure at sea level; 47 is water vapor pressure	3–5	% of cardiac output
Coronary perfusion pressure (CPP)	CPP = DBP – PAOP	The major determinant of flow in a fixed, diseased conduit is the pressure difference	50–60	mm Hg

CI, cardiac index (mL/min/m^2); HR, heart rate (beats/min); EDVI, end-diastolic volume index (mL/m^2); ESVI, end-systolic volume index (mL/m^2); MAP, mean arterial pressure; DBP, diastolic blood pressure (mm Hg); PAOP, pulmonary artery occlusion pressure (mm Hg); CVP, central venous pressure; Hgb, hemoglobin (g/dL); CcO_2, pulmonary capillary content of oxygen; PAO_2, partial pressure of oxygen in the alveoli; RQ, respiratory quotient VCO_2/VO_2 is 0.8 for a mixed fuel diet.

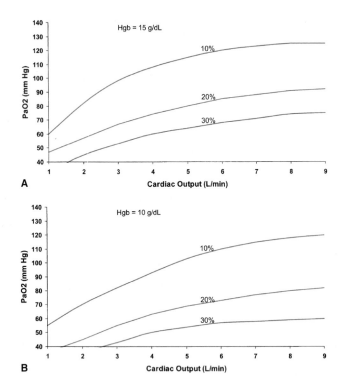

FIGURE 7.15. Relationship between PaO₂, cardiac output, and three different intrapulmonary shunt states (10%, 20%, and 30%) for patients with a hemoglobin of 15 g/dL and 10 g/dL. This graph demonstrates "nonpulmonary" causes for PaO₂ changes where a low cardiac output or low hemoglobin will impact PaO₂ depending on the degree of shunt.

the pulmonary capillary content of O₂, CaO₂ is the arterial content of O₂, and CvO₂ is the mixed venous content of O₂ (Table 7.3).
- Since pulmonary capillary blood cannot be sampled, the saturation is assumed to be 100%, which usually holds true when the FiO₂ is 1.0. It is important to understand the contribution of a low SvO₂ to PaO₂ if there is a moderate shunt (>20%).
- Any decrease in SvO₂ in a patient with >20% shunt will allow more deoxygenated blood to go into the arterial circulation, resulting in a lower PaO₂. This is called nonpulmonary cause

of hypoxia. For example, if a patient with a 20% intrapulmonary shunt and a hemoglobin of 15 g/dL has an acute cardiac event and the CO decreases from 5 to 3 L/minute, the PaO₂ will decrease from ~80 to 65 mm Hg (Fig. 7.15).
- In exactly the same scenario, if the patient's hemoglobin is 10 g/dL, the PaO₂ will decrease from 70 to 55 mm Hg. This demonstrates the importance of low SvO₂ contributing to lower PaO₂. If the PEEP had been increased in this patient to treat a low PaO₂, a further decrease in CO would have resulted in worsening SvO₂ and PaO₂. Treatment in this case is to optimize CO first to see whether PaO₂ improves. Another example: If a patient is agitated and the arterial saturation decreases, this may be due to increased oxygen consumption and low SvO₂ in a patient with a moderate intrapulmonary shunt and not from an acute pulmonary event. Treatment is to decrease agitation and VO₂. There are times when severe cardiorespiratory compromise warrants titration of both cardiac output and PEEP simultaneously in patients with life-threatening hypoxia. It is important to understand the interaction of one organ on the other and the relationship between PaO₂, hemoglobin, and cardiac output (see Fig. 7.15).

DERIVED VARIABLES

- See Table 7.3 for the equations and normal values.

COMPLICATIONS OF PULMONARY ARTERY INSERTION

- PAC insertion is an invasive procedure and carries inherent risks. The overall complication rate associated with PACs can be as high as 25%. The procedural risks are pneumothorax, hemothorax, and knotting of catheters. Multiple prospective and retrospective studies have reported the most common complications including infection, thrombosis, arrhythmias, new bundle branch blocks, and pulmonary artery rupture.
- Serious complications (PA rupture and cardiac perforation with tamponade) are infrequent, but they can be fatal if unrecognized.

CHAPTER 8 ■ NONINVASIVE CARDIOVASCULAR MONITORING

- Recent experiences have demonstrated that early intervention is associated with improved outcome. Identification of the adequacy of perfusion is a function of balancing oxygen delivery with oxygen demand. Invasive monitoring requires time and technology, often leading to delays that reduce the

potential benefit of the information gathered. In addition to the need for rapid monitoring, the challenge of continuous data collection and analysis as opposed to intermittent static observations is of major concern in the selection of monitoring techniques.

- Noninvasive hemodynamic monitoring can be safe for patients and staff, convenient, inexpensive, reasonably accurate, and available anywhere in the hospital, doctors' offices, or prehospital areas. Early recognition of abnormal hemodynamic or respiratory patterns allows therapy to be given earlier, more vigorously, and with greater effectiveness. Timing of treatment is as essential as the therapy itself in achieving good outcome.

TISSUE PERFUSION

Conventional Vital Signs

- Conventional vital signs include heart rate and mean arterial pressure; heart rate may be automatically derived from the electrocardiogram and the systolic, diastolic, and mean arterial pressure measured directly or automated by DynaMAP (Tampa, FL) or from an indwelling arterial catheter if one is already in place.

Arterial Hemoglobin Oxygen Saturation by Pulse Oximeter

- The standard pulse oximeter (Nellcor, Pleasanton, CA) is routinely used for continuous hemoglobin saturation (SpO_2) monitoring. Two different wavelengths of infrared light are reflected from the capillaries to identify and evaluate the oxygen saturation of the arterial component. Sudden changes in the arterial hemoglobin saturation are useful in assessing changes in pulmonary function. This has had a major impact on clinical practicet both inside and outside the operating room. Unfortunately, arterial oxygen saturation by itself does no indicate the oxygen delivery (DO_2) or the oxygen consumption/demand (VO_2) and is not a reliable measure of tissue oxygenation/perfusion or the hemodynamic status.

- Oximetry is based on the Beer–Lambert law of optical wavelength-dependent absorption of light energy. The Beer–Lambert law describes that light intensity (I) decreases exponentially when transmitted through a measurement compartment. The rate of the exponential decrease depends on the concentration of material inside the measurement compartment (C) and a wavelength-dependent absorption coefficient (a). In addition, the decrease depends on the optical pathlength (L) of the compartment: Pulse oximetry fundamentally relies upon adequate perfusion of the vascular bed being monitored. Without sufficient blood flow, oxygen content cannot be adequately analyzed. Decreased perfusion may be caused by a variety of factors including hypotension, medications, ambient temperature, poor circulation, and so forth

- Pulse oximeters are calibrated using saturation curves of healthy adult volunteers. They are, therefore, the most accurate at high saturation levels and less so at low saturation levels. Unfortunately, from the clinical standpoint, the low saturation levels are where they are the most useful to us. Nonetheless, this is rarely of major consequence, as the clinical difference between a saturation of 83% and 80% is usually very minimal.

- Other sources of error include ambient light and motion artifact. Error rates with excess ambient light can be as high as 63% for heart rate and 57% for saturation. Additional sources of error include darkly pigmented skin, nail polish, thermal injuries to fingers and/or toes, and inaccessibility of the extremities.

CHAPTER 9 ■ PULSE OXIMETRY AND PHOTOPLETHYSMOGRAPHY

- Photoplethysmography is the measurement of volume changes with light transmission. The photoplethysmograph (PPG) is displayed on most pulse oximeter devices; however, it is frequently ignored as oxygen saturation and pulse rate are the numbers of interest.

- The pulsatile cardiac component (PCC) of light hitting the photodiode corresponds to changes in the arterial blood volume with each heartbeat. The magnitude of change of the PCC with each heartbeat is related to stroke volume, and the area under the curve of each heartbeat is related to the volume of blood entering the vascular bed with each beat. The PCC is therefore a representation of flow into a vascular bed while the low frequency component (LFC) is a representation of changes in venous volume

TISSUE OXYGEN MONITORS

- Experimental studies have shown that transcutaneous oxygen monitoring is sensitive to arterial oxygen tension during normal cardiac output but is more sensitive to perfusion in low-flow shock. In adult patients, $PtcO_2$ is approximately 80% of the arterial oxygen tension (PaO_2) during normal hemodynamic conditions. However, when blood flow is diminished, $PtcO_2$ also decreases. $PtcO_2$ is therefore related to both perfusion and oxygenation.

- When perfusion is normal, $PtcO_2$ varies with arterial oxygenation. When perfusion is inadequate, $PtcO_2$ varies with cardiac output. Hence, a normal $PtcO_2$ value indicates that both oxygenation and perfusion are relatively normal. A low $PtcO_2$ indicates that either oxygenation and/or cardiac output is inadequate. If arterial oxygenation is normal (as indicated by blood gases or pulse oximetry), low $PtcO_2$ indicates low-flow shock.

- The relationship between $PtcO_2$ and PaO_2 can be quantitated, utilizing the $PtcO_2$ index, which is simply defined as $PaO_2/PtcO_2$. In a study that simultaneously measured cardiac index, $PtcO_2$, and PaO_2 in a large number of critically ill surgical patients, it was found that when cardiac output was relatively normal (cardiac index >2.2 L/min/m²), the $PtcO_2$ index averaged 0.79 ± 0.12. In individual patients with these normal cardiac outputs, $PtcO_2$ varied linearly with PaO_2. When cardiac output decreased, however, the $PtcO_2$ index decreased as well. For patients with a cardiac index between 1.5 and 2.2 L/minute/m², the $PtcO_2$ index averaged 0.48 ± 0.07. For patients with a cardiac index below 1.5 L/minute/m², the $PtcO_2$ index was 0.12 ± 0.12. These data confirm that when blood flow is relatively normal, $PtcO_2$ varies with arterial oxygenation. However, with low-flow shock, $PtcO_2$ becomes very sensitive to changes in cardiac output.

- Clinical studies have demonstrated the usefulness of transcutaneous oxygen monitoring in detecting shock. When $PtcO_2$ monitors are placed during acute emergency resuscitation, low $PtcO_2$ values detect both hypoxemia and hemorrhagic shock. Moreover, the response of $PtcO_2$ during fluid infusion is a sensitive indicator of the efficacy of shock resuscitation.

- Transcutaneous oxygen monitoring thus has benefit both as an early detector of shock and as a monitor to titrate resuscitation to a physiologic end point. It is noninvasive and inexpensive and is therefore widely applicable for patients at risk, such as during emergency resuscitation of trauma and acute surgical emergencies, in the perioperative and postanesthesia period, and in the intensive care unit. However, though end points of successful resuscitation utilizing transcutaneous oxygen monitoring have been suggested, such values have not been validated in large prospective studies. The only risk of transcutaneous oxygen monitoring is minor skin burn beneath the probe if probe temperatures exceed 44°C or if the device is left in place for excessive periods of time.

- Two techniques for direct tissue oxygen monitoring are available. Polarographic electrodes incorporated into needles have been most widely utilized. In addition, a technique utilizing the phenomenon of fluorescence quenching is available. Tissue oxygen probes contain a fluorescent compound that is O_2-sensitive, such that its fluorescent emission is diminished in direct proportion to the amount of O_2 present. Energy from the monitor is transmitted through fiberoptic elements to the florescent compound in the probe, resulting in the emission of light, which is then measured by sensors in the tissue probe. The intensity of the emitted light is inversely proportional to the tissue pO_2.

- Another method of tissue oxygen monitoring is transconjunctival. The conjunctiva of the eye does not have a stratum corneum, so oxygen is freely diffusible. Transconjunctival probes are placed against the eye and allow continuous tissue oxygen monitoring without heating; the technology has been utilized both during anesthesia and shock.

Near-infrared Spectroscopy

- Near-infrared spectroscopy (NIS) has been developed as a noninvasive measure of tissue oxygenation. NIS measures the ratio of oxygenated hemoglobin to total hemoglobin (StO_2) in the microcirculation of the underlying muscle by measuring the absorption and reflectance of light. Using cutaneous probes placed upon the thenar eminence, values of $87\% \pm 6\%$ have been measured in normal volunteers. Early clinical experience suggests that StO_2 values decrease during shock and increase with successful resuscitation. A recent multicenter trial in trauma patients suggested that an StO_2 value of 75% may be a therapeutic goal. Clinical data are limited. Tissue edema may be a confounding factor, as the distance between the probe and the underlying muscle affects measurements. Again, the sensitivity and specificity of this device compared to other tissue oxygen–monitoring devices has not been studied. NIS has been demonstrated to have a close relationship to base deficit in critically injured patients and predicting development of organ failure in traumatic shock patients.

Gastric Tonometry

- The mesenteric circulatory bed, particularly the gut mucosa, is prone to hypoperfusion and ischemia during shock. Tonometry has been developed as a technique to detect adequacy of gastrointestinal mucosal perfusion. The potential usefulness of gastric tonometry has been suggested in clinical studies in which it has been reported to reflect the severity of shock and to increase during successful resuscitation. However, the technique has not gained widespread acceptance, in part because the accuracy of the pHi measurement has been questioned.

Transcutaneous and End-tidal Carbon Dioxide

- In combination with low $PtcO_2$, increased transcutaneous pCO_2 gives additional evidence of circulatory shock. End-tidal CO_2 may also be utilized as a measure of perfusion; end-tidal CO_2 is decreased during low-flow states due to decreased pulmonary flow. Decreased end-tidal CO_2 values in combination with increased transcutaneous pCO_2 and normal arterial pCO_2 values are strong evidence of circulatory shock.

Cardiac Output Monitoring by Thoracic Electric Bioimpedance

- In thoracic electric bioimpedance methods, pairs of noninvasive disposable prewired hydrogel electrodes consisting of an outer injecting electrode and an inner sensing electrode are positioned on the anterior thoracic skin surface at the levels of the lung apex and the base; electrocardiogram leads are also placed on the precordium and shoulders. The outer pairs of electrodes pass a small-amplitude (0.2–5.0 mA) alternating current at 40 to 100 kHz through the patient's thorax to produce an electrical field. The injected electrical signals travel predominantly down the aorta, which has lower electrical resistance than aerated lung. Each ventricular contraction propels the stroke volume down the aorta, increasing aortic blood volume and aortic flow and lowering impedance. The impedance is sensed by the inner recording electrodes that capture the baseline impedance (Zo), the first derivative of the impedance waveform (dZ/dt), and the electrocardiogram. Changes in aortic blood flow throughout the cardiac cycle are quantitatively related to changes in the electrical impedance It has been reported an average difference of 9.7% between thoracic electric bioimpedance and COtd and an average difference of 9.5% between rapidly repeated COtd measurements in the same patient.

- Lithium dilution cardiac output measurements, arterial pressure pulse, contour cardiac output system, and noninvasive partial CO_2 rebreathing cardiac output measurement have been recently introduced as noninvasive alternatives to pulmonary artery catheters. These techniques share the shortcomings of thermodilution with pulmonary artery catheters in that they give only episodic sets of measurements, require critical care conditions, and need frequent recalibration.

CHAPTER 10 ■ CAPNOGRAPHY

- *Capnometry* refers to the measurement of carbon dioxide, regardless of the method used.
- *Capnography* describes the method of obtaining a capnogram: that is, a tracing of carbon dioxide concentration as a function of time or volume.
- With modern methods, continuous readings of exhaled carbon dioxide tensions and volumes can be obtained. We speak of steady state when the tension is exerted by carbon dioxide in different tissue and organ compartments and blood and alveolar gas have reached equilibrium and when the input of carbon dioxide from metabolism equals the output of carbon dioxide via ventilation and, to a small extent, via skin, flatus, feces, and urine.
- A steady state can exist with high, normal, or low arterial, alveolar, or end-tidal carbon dioxide tension ($PaCO_2$, $PACO_2$, or $PETCO_2$). However, all too often, we do not have a steady state: Tissue depleted of carbon dioxide can absorb liters of carbon dioxide from blood until tissue PCO_2 and blood PCO_2 reach equilibrium; conversely, such tissue stores can contribute CO_2 to that generated by metabolism. For example, prolonged hyperventilation can exhaust tissue stores of carbon dioxide and bicarbonate. Under these conditions, the maintenance of a normal $PaCO_2$ requires less than normal ventilation because some of the metabolic carbon dioxide filters back into the tissues instead of being exhaled.
- Conversely, high tissue stores of carbon dioxide (e.g., after a cardiac and respiratory arrest) will call for greater-than-normal ventilation until steady state is once again reached. A depressed respiratory center (e.g., under the influence of an opiate) will lead to an imbalance of input and output as the tissues take up some of the carbon dioxide while the rest leaves the body in the exhaled gas. Once the tissues and blood reach equilibrium, steady state will once again supervene in the presence of elevated levels of $PaCO_2$, $PACO_2$, and $PETCO_2$.
- Renal compensation of metabolic acidosis or alkalosis will also lead to an unsteady state that can last for many hours. The point: Capnograms can hide as much as they reveal, and thus the interpretation of capnograms calls for discerning clinicians.
- Instead of plotting the respired gas as a function of time, we can also plot CO_2 as a function of volume. This calls for a method to measure, breath by breath, the respired volume of gas. Together with an arterial blood gas, the single-breath method enables the clinician to estimate the volume of carbon dioxide in the exhaled breath, the volume of the alveolar dead space, and the volume of the anatomic dead space.

SUMMARY

- Noninvasive systems are able to continuously display variables online in real time throughout the patient's hospital course and with information systems to predict outcome and support therapeutic decision making.
- Because they are simple, safe, easy to use, inexpensive, reasonably accurate, and available anywhere in the hospital, some form of noninvasive hemodynamic monitoring with an appropriate information system will replace invasive monitoring for acutely ill patients.

CHAPTER 11 ■ ECHOCARDIOGRAPHY IN THE ICU

- Two-dimensional Doppler echocardiography maps the anatomic relations of the heart by ultrasonic wave pulses sent out from transducers placed on the chest wall, esophageal tube, or endotracheal tube. The sound waves are bounced off the walls and valves of the heart and are captured by sensors as echoes that are electronically plotted to produce images corresponding to anatomic features of the heart, including the right and left atrium, the atrial septum, valves, pulmonary vessels, and the thoracic duct.

- Transesophageal echocardiography is useful in evaluating heart valve abnormalities, tumors, blood clots, and congenital defects and dissecting aortic aneurysms. Doppler techniques are for diagnostic imaging rather than a continuous hemodynamic assessment tool; the images may be distorted by obesity, chronic obstructive pulmonary disease, hyperinflation of the lungs, chest trauma, and surgical dressings.

- Doppler techniques are able to provide some qualitative information about flow through vessels but are limited by the need for expert interpretation of the images and the need for very sensitive transducer placement. These factors provide for a useful diagnostic tool but limit the reproducibility of the measurements and their use for continuous monitoring.

CHAPTER 12 ■ CLEAN AND ASEPTIC TECHNIQUES AT THE BEDSIDE

CATHETER-RELATED INFECTION

- Although bloodstream infection generally accounts for fewer than 15% of all cases of nosocomial infections, critically ill patients and persons with cancer have disproportionately higher rates of nosocomial bloodstream infections. Not only do bloodstream infections account for 20% of all cases of nosocomial infections among intensive care unit patients, but 87% of bacteremias originate from an infected central vascular catheter.
- Catheter-related bloodstream infection (CRBSI) is defined as the isolation of the same organism (i.e., the same species with identical antimicrobial susceptibility) from the colonized catheter and from peripheral blood in a patient with clinical manifestations of sepsis and no other apparent source of bloodstream infection.
- Until recently, catheter colonization was defined as the growth in cultures from either the tip or subcutaneous segment of the catheter of ≥15 colony-forming units/mL by the semiquantitative roll-plate method or ≥1,000 colony-forming units/mL by the quantitative sonication method.
  - This method of diagnosing CRBSI requires removal and culture of the vascular catheter. Only 15% to 25% of central venous catheters removed because of suspected catheter-related infection yield growth.
- There are two potential methods that could indicate whether the catheter is the source of bloodstream infection *without removing the catheter.* Both methods require concurrent collection of peripheral and central (i.e., through the lumen of the catheter) blood cultures.
  - The first qualitative method—differential time to **positivity**—which relies on the understanding that the culture of a blood sample that contains higher bacterial concentration would become positive, as detected by production of carbon dioxide by multiplying organisms, at least 2 hours before this would occur in a culture from peripheral blood. The supposition is that the bacterial load of the infected catheter is higher than that seen in peripheral blood.
  - The other quantitative method—**paired quantitative blood cultures**—is based on the anticipation that the number of colony-forming units retrieved from a central blood culture would be greater than or equal to fivefold higher than that grown from cultured peripheral blood.
- Because the patient's skin around the catheter insertion site and the hands of medical personnel provide the two most common sources of pathogens, at least two-thirds of cases of catheter-related infection are caused by **staphylococcal organisms (coagulase-negative Staphylococci and *Staphylococcus aureus*).**
- Less common pathogens, including gram-negative bacteria and *Candida* spp., collectively cause about 25% of infection cases.

Approaches that Significantly Reduce Catheter-related Bloodstream Infections

- The most recent Centers for Disease Control and Prevention guidelines include new recommendations for using all of the following clinically protective measures, including cutaneous antisepsis with **chlorhexidine** (category IA), maximal sterile **barriers** (category IA), and catheters coated with the combinations of **chlorhexidine plus silver sulfadiazine**, or *minocycline plus rifampin* (category IB).
- The superiority of *chlorhexidine* over iodophor and alcohol could be predicted by comparing their characteristics. Unlike iodophor and alcohol, chlorhexidine provides a residual and persistent antimicrobial activity that is not impaired by exposure to organic matter such as blood, does not irritate the skin, and has minimal absorption through the skin.
- Although 2% chlorhexidine compounds appear to be optimal in terms of both efficacy and safety, only recently has aqueous chlorhexidine become available in the United States, where the most frequently used form of chlorhexidine is in combination with an alcohol, usually isopropyl alcohol.
- Another important Centers for Disease Control and Prevention guideline is the practice of maximal sterile precautions: the use of gloves, a *large* drape, a cap, a mask, and a gown
- Finally, there are choices of antibiotic coated catheters. Catheters coated with **minocycline and** *rifampin* provide two agents both active against the vast majority of staphylococcal isolates, including methicillin-resistant *S. aureus* and *S. epidermidis*, thereby reducing the likelihood of developing superinfection by Gram-negative bacteria or *Candida* spp.
  - The clinical efficacy of this catheter was confirmed in a **prospective randomized trial** (PRT), with mean placement duration 6 days, where these central venous catheters were significantly less likely than uncoated catheters to become colonized (**8% vs. 26%;** *p* <0.001) with less bloodstream infection (0% vs. 5%; *p* <0.01). In another PRT, minocycline rifampin catheters were more protective than the first-generation chlorhexidine/silver sulfadiazine–coated catheters, with a threefold lower rate of catheter colonization (7.9% vs. 22.8%; *p* <0.001) and a 12-fold lower rate of CRBSI (0.3% vs. 3.4%; *p* <0.002).
  - The second-generation chlorhexidine/silver sulfadiazine–coated catheters have a longer durability of antimicrobial

activity than the first-generation catheters. A PRT demonstrated that second-generation chlorhexidine/silver sulfadiazine–coated central venous catheters were less likely to become colonized than uncoated catheters (9% vs. 16%, p <0.01) but had a statistically insignificant trend for a lower rate of CRBSIs (0.3% vs. 0.8%).

Other Practices

- A controversial practice is **guidewire exchange** of vascular catheters.
  - In hemodynamically stable patients with limited vascular access and in whom catheter-related infection is possible but not very likely, it is reasonable to insert the new catheter over a guidewire as long as the removed catheter is cultured; should culture of the removed catheter yield growth, it is recommended to remove the catheter that was newly inserted over a guidewire and place yet another catheter at a different site.
  - Although it is theoretically plausible that insertion at the same site of a vascular catheter with effective antimicrobial coating along both the external and internal catheter surfaces may obviate the need to manipulate another vascular site, this approach requires clinical investigation.

- Attachment of an **antimicrobial hub** containing iodinated alcohol to central venous catheters is another available tool.
- Because this antimicrobial catheter hub protects only against organisms that migrate through the hub along the internal surface of the catheter but not against skin organisms that advance along the external surface of the catheter, the potential clinical benefit of using this preventive approach in the context of vascular catheters that remain in place for less than or equal to 7 to 10 days is doubtful.
- The relationship between **infection and thrombosis** of vascular catheters prompted numerous investigations of the clinical efficacy of flushing or locking the catheter lumen with various **antibiotic–anticoagulant combinations** that do not result in systemic levels of the antibiotic
  - Because this approach provides antimicrobial activity against only organisms that exist in the catheter lumen, clinical investigations have generally focused on long-term vascular catheters that are frequently infected by such a route. Clinical trials have yielded **discrepant results.**
  - Although there were no observed cases of infection of vancomycin-locked catheters by vancomycin-resistant organisms, the potential emergence of resistance to vancomycin, a drug that is still used to treat most cases of catheter infections, continues to underscore the equivocal role of this strategy.

CHAPTER 13 ■ VASCULAR CANNULATION

VENOUS CANNULATION

- The decision to place a central venous access device should be made after considering the risks and benefits to each patient. Indications include the following:
  - Patients who have **difficult peripheral intravenous (IV) access** such as obese patients or drug abusers
  - Administration of **chemotherapy or caustic drugs** such as amphotericin B, sulfamethoxazole trimethoprim, ciprofloxacin, dobutamine, doxycycline, erythromycin, ganciclovir, lidocaine, penicillins, pentamidine, phenergan, phenytoin, potassium (depending on dilution), ceftriaxone, vancomycin, and tobramycin
  - Infusates with an **osmolality >280 to 300 mOsm** such as parenteral nutrition
  - Performance of **plasmapheresis,** and **hemodialysis**

General Considerations

- **Obtain informed consent:** Informed consent is a process of communication between a patient (or patient's surrogate) and

physician that results in the patient's authorization or agreement to undergo a specific medical intervention.
- **Obtain procedure-directed history and physical exam,** such as
  - Location and number of **previous** central venous catheters **(CVCs)** and ports
  - Location of known **venous thrombi**
  - History of **infected** ports and their sites
  - History of **clavicle fracture** (pertinent for subclavian approach)
  - History of **bleeding** associated with CVC placement
  - History of **pneumothorax** or other complications from previous CVCs
  - History of inferior vena cavae **(IVC) filter** placement
  - Current or recent use of warfarin, aspirin, clopidogrel bisulfate, heparin, low-molecular-weight heparin, or other **anticoagulants**
  - History of **pacemaker** insertion
- Prior to starting the procedure, obtain all necessary items listed below and, using an aseptic technique, open them onto a working table in close proximity to the patient.
  - Sterile **gown** and **gloves**
  - **Hat** and **mask**

- Central line kit with a **large** enough **drape** to cover the insertion area and to prevent contamination of long wires
- 2% **chlorhexidine** or 10% povidone iodine
- Sterile **saline flush**

General Technique for Central Venous Catheters

- Prepare the skin with **2% chlorhexidine** (preferred over povidone due to less infection rate) or **10% povidone iodine** if patient is allergic to chlorhexidine.
  - Ten percent povidone iodine has no immediate effect due to slow release of iodine and takes about 2 minutes to be fully effective. Appropriate time for drying prior to draping should be allowed.
- This gap can be filled as the time to obtain a **maximum sterile barrier.**
  - This includes the placement of a **sterile cap, mask, gown, and gloves** for every single procedure.
  - The use of all four elements consistently along with appropriately prepped skin reduces **catheter-related septicemia by sixfold.**
- The patient's scrub should include a generous area and extend **10 cm** outward in a circular manner from the planned insertion point. If the line is placed in an area with hair, the hair need not be removed.
- **Prepare the CVC kit prior** to starting the line placement as follows:
  - Load the 1% **lidocaine.**
  - Bring the wire onto the sterile field close to the insertion point to minimize movements after cannulation of the vein with the finder needle.
  - Adjust the wire by pulling the **J-curve of the tip into the hub** of the guidewire holder so that it is straightened out and ready for insertion.
  - Remove the distal port cap off the catheter for easier placement over the wire.
  - **Flush the ports** of the catheter with sterile saline to remove air.
  - Next, place the **large sterile drape** over the insertion site. Do not occlude the air supply or field of vision when draping neck areas of conscious patients. An assistant, electronic devices, or both must **monitor** relevant parameters of the patient's well-being continually through the procedure, because the operator may lose valuable clues while concentrating on the procedure and because much of the patient is obscured by drapes.
- Local analgesia may be obtained by injecting 1 to 5 mL of 1% lidocaine without epinephrine subcutaneously so that a 1-cm wheal is raised. Use the **smallest needle** available (preferably 30 gauge) and **inject slowly** to minimize discomfort of tissue distention.
  - Attention should be paid to the **track** of local anesthetic instilled so that subsequent larger needles are not inserted into an area where there is minimum anesthetic.
  - Some operators use the smallest needle to create a skin wheal, leave that needle in the skin after removing the syringe, and then replace the small needle with a longer 21- to 22-gauge needle into the same site to further infiltrate the deeper tissues. This longer needle is then **left in**

the tissues after removing the syringe and serves as a **guide** to insert the final large needle precisely into the tissue that has been well anesthetized.
  - Conscious sedation must be used with great caution in nonintubated patients.
- After accessing the vein, use the **Seldinger technique** for catheter insertion.

Seldinger Technique

- The desired vessel or cavity is punctured with a sharp hollow needle called a trocar.
- A round-tipped (J-tipped) guidewire is then advanced through the lumen of the trocar, and the trocar is withdrawn.
- Any hollow catheter or cannula can now be passed over the guidewire into the cavity or vessel. The guidewire is then withdrawn.
  - **Do not force** the wire through the finder needle; resistance of any type is an indication to stop, remove the needle and guidewire, and hold pressure on the vein.
- Check the **distance of the catheter** inserted from skin entry site (Table 13.1).
- After catheter insertion, verify that **all ports allow aspiration of blood** and can be flushed with saline without resistance.
- Secure the catheter, cover with a **nonocclusive sterile dressing.** Antibiotic ointments (bacitracin, neomycin, and polymyxin) should not be used, as they increase the rate of catheter colonization by fungi, promote the emergence of antibiotic-resistant bacteria, and do not lower the rate of catheter-related bacteremia.
- Obtain a **stat chest radiograph** to verify the position and exclude pneumothorax or other injuries (x-ray not needed with femoral approach).
- **Document** the procedure appropriately in the chart.

Caution: **Excessive dilation** extending beyond the subcutaneous tissue and fat into the vein increases the risk of postprocedure complications (oozing, hematoma formation, arteriovenous fistula formation, and pseudoaneurysm formation).

- **Inadvertent arterial puncture** and subsequent hematoma or pseudoaneurysm formation can be prevented by providing **direct pressure** manually or with a standard device for at least 30 minutes.

TABLE 13.1

DISTANCE FROM SKIN PUNCTURE SITE TO ATRIA-CAVAL JUNCTION

Insertion site	Distance
Right internal jugular vein to atria-caval junction	16.0 cm
Right subclavian vein to atria-caval junction	18.4 cm
Left internal jugular vein to atria-caval junction	19.1 cm
Left subclavian vein to atria-caval junction	21.2 cm

From Tan BK, Hong SW, Huang MH, et al. Anatomic basis of safe percutaneous subclavian venous catheterization. *J Trauma.* 2000;48(1):82–86.

Technique of Central Venous Cannulation

Femoral Vein Cannulation

- The femoral vein is punctured in the femoral triangle (inferior to the inguinal ligament, lateral to the adductor longus, and medial to the sartorius muscles) where it lies medial to the femoral artery (Fig. 13.1).
  - Locate the femoral artery, keep a finger on the artery, and introduce the finder needle attached to a 10-mL syringe at an angle 45 degrees to the skin, about 1 cm medial to the femoral artery pulsation, **2 cm below** the inguinal ligament.
  - Slowly advance the needle **cephalad and posteriorly** while continuously withdrawing the plunger. **Too much suction** applied to the plunger in a hypovolemic patient may lead to vein collapse with minimum blood return. This may mislead the operator into assuming the needle is not in the vessel lumen.
  - Once venous blood is obtained, use the **Seldinger technique** to complete the procedure (see earlier discussion).

Caution: **Stay below the inguinal ligament.** The distal tip of the finder needle should not traverse cephalad to the inguinal ligament to avoid **retroperitoneal hematoma** and/or **intra-abdominal** injuries.

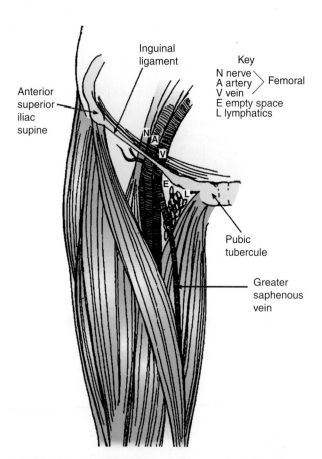

FIGURE 13.1. Anatomy of the femoral artery and vein. Use the pneumonic NAVEL (Nerve, Artery, rein, Empty space, Lymphatics) to recall structures as you move in a lateral to medial direction toward the navel.

Internal Jugular Vein Cannulation

- The anatomic relationship of the internal jugular (IJ) vein to the carotid artery varies. For purposes of IJ vein access, an important anatomic triangle is formed by the two heads of the sternocleidomastoid and the medial one-third of the clavicle. Within this triangle, the carotid artery lies medial and slightly posterior to the IJ vein, decreasing its chances of accidentally being punctured during catheter insertion (Fig. 13.2). **Ultrasonography** (US) lessens the complications of inadvertent puncture and/or cannulation of the carotid artery and is becoming the standard of care.
- Stand at the head of the bed.
- Place the patient in a **Trendelenburg** position, at least 15 degrees head down to distend the neck veins and to reduce the risk of air embolism.
- Slightly turn the head (**no more than 20 degrees**) away from the puncture site. Turning it too far increases the risk of arterial puncture.
- The syringe and needle should be stabilized by resting the hand on the mandible of the patient at its midpoint (Fig. 13.3)
- The vein is usually **within 2 to 3 cm** of the skin. If the vein is not found, redirect the needle more laterally.
- Use the **Seldinger technique** (see earlier discussion).
- If the patient is intubated and on **high positive end-expiratory pressure** (PEEP) settings, holding the inspiratory effort for a few seconds while cannulating the IJ vein may decrease the overinflation of the lung apex and decrease the chances of obtaining a pneumothorax. (This should be performed only if no deleterious effects occur toward the patient's oxygenation, ventilation, alveolar recruitment, or overall status.)

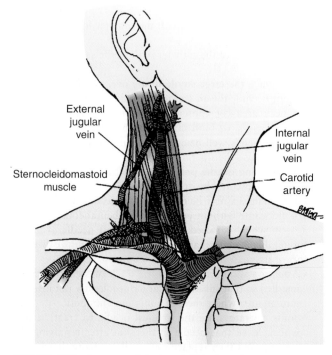

FIGURE 13.2. Anatomy of the internal jugular vein.

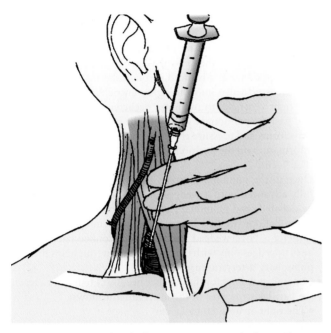

FIGURE 13.3. Attach a fresh 10-mL syringe to the large 18-gauge 2-inch finder needle and, using the previously placed 22-gauge needle as a guide, find the internal jugular vein.

Subclavian Vein Cannulation

- The subclavian vein is a continuation of the axillary vein and runs from the outer border of the first rib to the medial border of anterior scalene muscle where it joins with the IJ vein to form the innominate vein (brachiocephalic vein). The vein is separated posteriorly from the subclavian artery by the insertion of the scalenus anterior and posteromedially from the dome of the pleura by Sibson fascia (suprapleural membrane). The pleura lies only 5 mm posterior to the subclavian vein. Its diameter is approximately that of a man's small finger. The left subclavian vein is the site at which chyle, formed in the intestines from dietary fat and lipids, enters the blood stream via the thoracic duct.
  - The position that provides the **greatest exposure** of the subclavian vein was with the shoulders in the **neutral position and slightly retracted.** However, in the **Trendelenburg** position, the shoulders assume a protracted (shrugging) position secondary to the effects of gravity. This must be actively reversed by **pulling the arm in a caudal direction** while performing the venipuncture to return the shoulder to a neutral position and maximize vein exposure from under the clavicle.
    - This maneuver is extremely helpful even in patients who cannot be in the Trendelenburg position or who are unable to have a roll inserted between the scapulae.
  - Second, a retracted position of the shoulder, as obtained by placing a rolled towel beneath the vertebral column between the scapulae to allow the **shoulders to fall back,** was shown to serve two very important purposes: (a) It prevents the interference between the path of the needle insertion and the humeral head of the shoulder, ensuring that the needle and syringe are always parallel to the coronal plane; and

(b) it brings the subclavian vein into close contact with the undersurface of the clavicle, which is desirable for accurate identification of the vein.
- Place a rolled towel beneath the vertebral column between the scapulae to allow the shoulders to fall back into a slight neutral-retracted position (*contraindicated* in patients with **cervical spine injuries** since elevation of the shoulders may lead to neck flexion and should not be done on trauma victims without spine clearance. Place the patient in a **Trendelenburg** position, at least 15 degrees head down to distend the subclavian veins and to reduce the risk of air embolism).
- Identify the **middle one-third** of the clavicle as it follows a **gentle curve up** toward the shoulder. **Have an assistant pull the arm caudad at the initiation of venipuncture.**
- Enter the skin at the anesthetized point along the upper border of the medial one-third of the clavicle at the junction of the sternocleidomastoid muscle and the clavicular head (Fig. 13.4). While maintaining **constant suction** on the syringe, point the needle tip **toward the suprasternal notch** and a parallel line to the coronal plane and the floor and gently advance the needle tip cephalad until it **hits the clavicle.** The index finger rests on the suprasternal notch and provides the direction toward which the tip of the finder needle is directed.
- **Withdraw the needle and syringe back 2 cm** from the clavicle prior to making an effort to pass under the leading edge. Not withdrawing the needle 2 to 4 cm is a common mistake and makes the maneuvering of the needle tip around the convex leading edge of the clavicle difficult.
- A common mistake, especially in overweight patients or patients with large stature, is to use a puncture site that is **too close to the clavicle.**
- This makes it extremely difficult to pass the finder needle under the clavicle while maintaining the needle and syringe parallel to the coronal plane and the floor.
- As the angle of entry between the patient's chest and the syringe increase in an effort to get under the clavicle, the

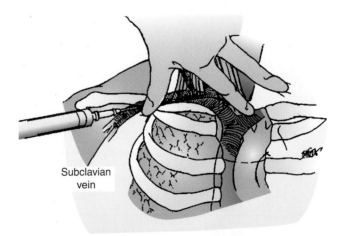

Subclavian vein

FIGURE 13.4. Enter the skin at the anesthetized point and point the needle tip toward the suprasternal notch. While maintaining constant suction on the syringe and a parallel line to the coronal plane and the floor, gently advance the needle tip cephalad until it passes under the clavicle and into the vein.

chances of producing a pneumothorax also increase proportionally.
  • A distance more than **2 cm from the edge of the clavicle** may be necessary in larger patients.
Caution: **At all times maintain the needle and syringe parallel to the coronal plane and floor.**
  • Once the vein is accessed, use the **Seldinger technique (see** earlier discussion).

Pulmonary Artery Catheter Insertion

• Insert the **introducer** for the PAC in similar fashion as the central line (see earlier discussion). Flush the introducer with saline to prevent thrombosis.
• Take great care in maintaining sterile technique at all times while working closely with the nonsterile assistant. Protect the sterile portion of the catheter by resting it on the **large sterile field** while the transducers are attached.
• Have the assistant check the proximal and **distal ports** for patency by **flushing** them with sterile saline. Also have the assistant check the **patency of the balloon** using the syringe provided in the kit.
• Familiarize yourself with the markings on the PAC prior to placing the catheter. **Single thin lines** are used to indicate a distance of **10 cm,** while a **single wide line** indicates a distance of **50 cm** from the tip.
  • These lines are used in combination to indicate the distance from the tip (i.e., two thin lines indicate 20 cm from the tip). The wedge position is achieved in most patients at **45 to 55 cm** from the tip.
• Place the sterile **plastic sleeve** over the catheter after flushing all ports to further protect the catheter in a sterile cover during manipulation (Fig. 13.5).
• The distal end of the PAC is then inserted into the central venous introducer hub and is threaded down the central vein into the superior vena cava.

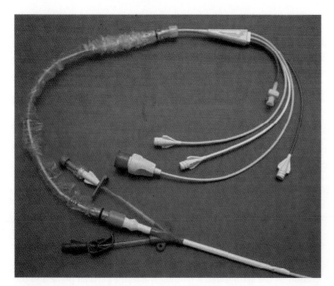

FIGURE 13.5. Place the plastic sleeve cover over the catheter to maintain sterility during placement tend to help secure and lock its final position onto the introducer.

• The PAC must be placed at **least 30 cm** (three thin lines) into the introducer for the **balloon** to clear the distal end of the introducer sheath prior to inflation.
• Once at 30 cm in the central vein, the balloon is inflated, and the catheter is advanced through the right atrium, past the tricuspid valve into the right ventricle, quickly through the right ventricle (to minimize occurrence of arrhythmias), and past the pulmonary valve into the pulmonary artery. The **waveforms and pressure** readings on the monitor provide the information on the position of the catheter in the vasculature (Fig. 13.6).
• Once in the pulmonary artery, the catheter should be carefully advanced until it wedges. At this point, the balloon can be deflated, and pulmonary artery tracings should reappear. If the balloon wedges before maximal reinflation, then the catheter is **"overwedged"** and should be pulled back slightly until it wedges only with maximal inflation (this helps prevent pulmonary artery rupture).
• General guidelines for the distance necessary to travel to reach the various structures of the heart are as follows:
  • The right atrium: 20 to 25 cm
  • The right ventricle: 30 to 35 cm
  • The pulmonary artery: 40 to 45 cm
  • The catheter usually wedges at 50 to 55 cm
• Once the PAC is in the correct position, the balloon should be deflated and the catheter **secured** in place by **locking the plastic sleeve tip** onto the hub of the introducer at two places to avoid movement.
• Correct catheter placement is confirmed with a chest radiograph.
Caution: **AT NO POINT SHOULD THE PAC EVER BE WITHDRAWN WHILE THE BALLOON IS INFLATED! Always verify that the assistant has deflated the balloon prior to withdrawing the PAC. This avoids the complication of rupture of the pulmonary artery, which can lead to massive life-threatening hemorrhage and death.**

Complications of Pulmonary Artery Catheterization

• Overall complication rate is 15%.
• Mechanical complication rate is 5% to 19%.
• Infectious complication rate is 5% to 26%.
• Thrombotic complication rate is 2% to 26%.
• Arrhythmias are the most common complication of PAC insertion and occur secondary to ventricular irritation as the catheter passes to the pulmonary artery (PA). More than 80% of these are premature ventricular contractions or non-sustained ventricular tachycardia. They are self-limiting and resolve with advancement of the catheter from the right ventricle (RV) into the PA or with prompt withdrawal of the catheter back into the right atrium. Significant arrhythmias requiring treatment occur in fewer than 1% of patients, usually those with concurrent cardiac ischemia.
• Right bundle branch block occurs in 5% of PAC insertions and usually is transient after positioning the catheter into the PA. The presence of a pre-existing left bundle branch block puts the patient at risk for complete heart block should sight bundle branch block occur. In these patients, temporary pacing equipment should be kept nearby on standby.

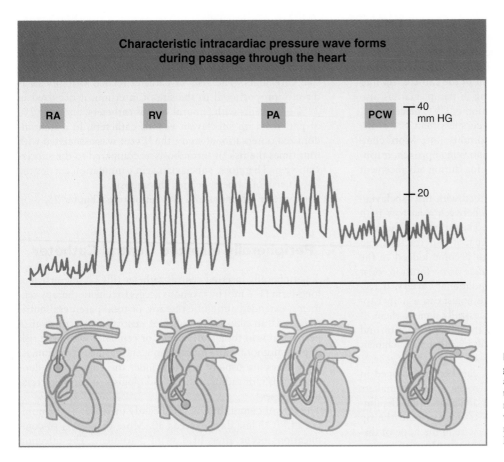

FIGURE 13.6. Use the waveforms to guide the placement of the pulmonary artery catheter from the right atrium, through the right ventricle, to the pulmonary artery, and finally into the wedge position. RA, right atrium; RV, right ventricle; PA, pulmonary artery; PCW, pulmonary capillary wedge.

- The incidence of knotting of the PAC on itself, on intracardiac structures, or on pacing wires is less than 1%. This risk is increased in patients with dilated cardiac chambers. A persistent RV tracing despite advancement of the PAC further than 20 cm into the patient should alert the physician to this possibility.
- Pulmonary artery rupture is the most catastrophic complication of PAC insertion. Although it occurs in fewer than 1% of cases, it carries a mortality rate of 50%. Age over 60 years, anticoagulation therapy, and the presence of pulmonary hypertension increase the risk of rupture. The presence of sudden and large quantities of hemoptysis, especially immediately after PAC balloon inflation, greatly indicates this possibility. Management includes lateral decubitus positioning (bleeding side down), intubation with a double-lumen endotracheal tube, and increasing positive end-expiratory pressure. Embolization via bronchoscopy or angiography or lobectomy may be necessary if bleeding continues or is massive.
- PAC-related infection is a fairly common complication. The incidence of positive catheter tip culture result is 45% in some series. Fortunately, the risk for clinical sepsis is less than 0.5% per day of catheter use.
- The incidence of pulmonary infarction is less than 7%. Unintentional distal migration of the PAC tip is the usual cause. Some evidence indicates that catheter-related thrombi also may be a significant cause. Though postmortem studies have shown that the rate of endocardial lesions (e.g., thrombi, hemorrhage, vegetations) related to PAC use is significant, correlation with clinical events has not been established.

Central Line Complications

- More than 15% of all patients who receive CVCs have complications. At least 52% of the reported complications are related to practitioner **technique** and the level of **experience**. Physicians who have placed >50 CVCs are half as likely to have a mechanical complication as those who have performed <50. The incidence of mechanical complications after three or more **insertion attempts** is six times that after one attempt. An increasingly important tool for improving safe learning curves for CVC placement is the two-dimensional ultrasound imaging and guidance.
- **Mechanical complications** associated with CVC placement include **cardiac tamponade, hemothorax, pneumothorax, carotid artery injury, subclavian artery injury, venous rupture, air embolism, catheter malpositioning, catheter transection, and wire or catheter embolism.** Compared to the subclavian vein cannulation, the IJ route is more likely to be complicated by arterial puncture (3%–4% vs. 6%–9%) and less likely to be complicated by pneumothorax (1%–3% vs. 0.1%–0.2%). The femoral route, in comparison to the other two routes, is associated with a much higher rate of arterial puncture (9%–15%) and hematoma formation (3%–5%) but, in the emergent setting, offers the advantage of avoiding pneumothorax and hemothorax.
- The tip of an intact catheter can **migrate** into the opposite brachiocephalic vein, jugular vein, or azygous veins. Interventional radiology can play an important role in repositioning **misplaced catheters.**

- If a catheter was placed without imaging guidance, it may be placed into an **artery.** Appropriate consultation of the **vascular or cardiothoracic service** should be obtained prior to removing misplaced catheters from the subclavian artery and the carotid artery. Malposition of the catheter tip into the lumbar venous plexus resulting in paraplegia has also been described as a rare complication of CVC placement.
- **Perforation of the great vessels** occurs less than 1% of the time but carries nearly a 40% mortality rate. More commonly seen with the right subclavian vein approach, it usually is the result of guidewire kinking during advancement of the dilator.
- **Pinch-off syndrome** has been described with the subclavian route when the catheter is crushed between a narrow path between the clavicle and the first rib. The catheter can become occluded and, with repeated trauma, it can fracture and embolize distally. The fragment can become lodged in the heart, resulting in cardiac arrhythmias or perforation, or it can be embolized further into the pulmonary artery. If recognized early, the interventional radiologist can usually capture the catheter fragments and successfully remove them. If the fragments remain unrecognized, thrombus formation and fibrosis around the catheter can result in catheter attachment to the vessel wall.
- **Guidewires** used for venous access can become **trapped** in indwelling vena cava filters or electrodes from pacemakers and other implantable devices. Fluoroscopy often demonstrates that the J-wire has become trapped around the tip of an IVC filter. Pulling back on the wire in the hope of dislodging it can have catastrophic results, with migration of the filter, tears in the IVC, hemorrhage, and death. Several techniques are available to the interventional radiologist to remove broken wires or wires trapped in filters. The key is to **stop** if there is resistance or if the wire is trapped and difficult to remove and immediately enlist the assistance of the interventional radiologists.
- **Air embolism** may also occur as a rare complication during CVC placement. It is more common in conditions that diminish the central venous pressure, such as decreased intravascular volume and upright sitting position. Rapid introduction of air into the venous circulation of greater than 300 to 400 mL at a rate of 100 mL/second is considered to be fatal. Clinically, the patient will have immediate **hypoxemia** and/or **cardiovascular collapse.** The hypoxemia is a result of V/Q mismatch (ventilation without perfusion) due to mechanical obstruction of vessels by the air bubbles. The air further has a chemical activation of the pulmonary endothelium resulting in activation of complement, free radicals, and inflammatory mediators, which results in bronchoconstriction and/or noncardiogenic pulmonary edema. The physical exam reveals the wheezing and crackles of **heart failure.** The classic finding of **mill wheel murmur,** a churning sound heard throughout the entire cardiac cycle from air bubbles in the RV, is a relatively specific sign of air embolism but is insensitive and occurs late in the course. Management includes **securing the airway** and placing the patient in the **left lateral decubitus position with right side up,** making it more difficult for the air to enter the right ventricular outflow tract (pulmonary artery) because it is in a dependent position. The best intervention is **prevention;** placing the patient in 15 degrees of Trendelenburg position prior to placing the CVC increases the central

venous pressure and decreases the chance for air embolism to occur.
- **Catheter-related venous thrombosis,** diagnosed with US, occurs in approximately 15% of patients in the medical intensive care units. The risk of catheter-related thrombosis is directly proportional to the site of insertion; it occurred in 22% of patients with femoral venous catheters, and only 2% of patients with subclavian venous catheters. In a nonrandomized observational study, the IJ vein was associated with four times the risk of thrombosis as compared to the subclavian vein. Therefore, subclavian vein cannulation carries the lowest risk of catheter-related thrombosis.
- **For catheter infections and prevention, see Chapter 75.**

Peripherally Inserted Central Catheter

- A peripherally inserted central catheter (PICC) line provides long-term (1–6 mo) intravenous access for chemotherapy regimens, extended antibiotic therapy, or total parenteral nutrition. It is an alternative route of central access through a peripheral vein (brachial, basilic, or cephalic) with little risk of pneumothorax, air embolization, and cardiac arrhythmias. PICC lines are usually inserted under the guidance of fluoroscopy, US, or radiographs by radiologists or certified registered nurses.
- The rate of complications significantly increases as the number of PICC line days exceeds 30. More than 70% of complications occur after 30 days of placement. The infection rate for PICC lines is similar to conventionally placed CVCs; however, they have the added disadvantages of being more vulnerable to thrombosis and dislodgement and less useful for drawing blood specimens.
- Another concern is over usage that potentially exhausts upper-extremity venous access sites. This may have serious implications in chronically ill patients, especially those with renal failure who may eventually require arteriovenous fistulas for dialysis access. Complication rates (infection, sepsis, and thrombosis requiring removal) as high as 40% to 50% have been reported with the use of PICC lines in chemotherapy patients. Based on the foregoing evidence, we recommend strong caution against the routine use of PICC lines.

ARTERIAL CANNULATION

- Continuous blood pressure monitoring is essential for the management of critically ill patients. Significant differences may occur between arterial pressures measured by direct versus indirect invasive methods (see **Chapters 6 and 8**).
- The indications for peripheral arterial cannulation include:
  - **Continuous blood pressure** (BP) monitoring in postoperative and critically ill patients
  - **Hypotension or hypertension** requiring continuous drug infusion
  - Mechanically ventilated patients that require **repeated blood gases**
- Use *caution* in the following circumstances:
  - Extremities with burns or trauma
  - Extremities with carpal tunnel syndrome

- Broken or infected skin
- Coagulopathy
- Raynaud disease
- Near arterio-venous (AV) fistulas and synthetic grafts
- The most frequently used site for direct arterial cannulation and blood pressure measurement is the **radial artery.** Use of the femoral artery, axillary artery, dorsalis pedis artery, and temporal artery has also been described. Utilization of the **brachial artery** is *not* **recommended** due to poor collateral circulation and secondary ischemia to the radial and ulnar artery in the setting of obstruction, due to the potential for **loss of the hand.**
- With regard to radial artery cannulation, the value of the **Allen test** in predicting potential ischemic damage after cannulation is at best **unreliable.** The original test described in 1929 was for the purpose of evaluating palmar collateral circulation in thromboangiitis obliterans. In critically ill patients, the test has poor predictive power.

General Technique

- First **palpate** the artery at **two points** 2 cm apart.
- Using an 18-gauge needle, make a small superficial **break** through the **skin** over the artery. This penetrates the tough skin barrier and prevents shearing and damage of the tip of the catheter during subsequent arterial penetration.
- The catheter cannula is advanced through the puncture site along the course of the artery at a 30- to 45-degree angle to the skin.
- Once the anterior wall of the artery is penetrated, the needle is withdrawn, and the plastic cannula is gently advanced into the arterial vessel at a lower angle (15–30 degrees) to facilitate smooth passage.
- The catheter with the needle may pass though the **anterior and posterior walls** of the artery. In this case, after removing the inner needle, gently withdraw the plastic cannula until pulsatile blood flows freely from the open end. Then advance the plastic cannula at a lesser angle into the arterial lumen.
- The use of a guidewire and the Seldinger technique may be employed to assist with the threading of the cannula into the artery after penetration.
  Caution: **Never try to thread the guidewire against even slight resistance.**
- If *complications* occur, such as distal ischemia, local infection, inability to withdraw blood effectively, or poor waveform, the arterial catheters should be changed to another site. Before removal, pressure should be applied proximally and distally to the insertion site. Attaching a syringe to the catheter and applying suction during extraction (for removal of developed clots) decreases the incidence of arterial thrombotic occlusion. After catheter removal, fingertip pressure should be applied for 10 minutes or as long as necessary to achieve hemostasis and prevent hematoma or aneurysm formation.

Radial Artery

- The radial artery is one of the best cannulation sites due to its accessibility and the safety of extensive collateralization.

- The **nondominant hand** of the patient should be cannulated first. Placing a small rolled towel under the wrist and securing it with tape onto a backboard in a **hyperextended position (about 20 degrees)** diminishes the arterial tortuosity and increases the cannulation success rate.
- The artery should be cannulated 1 to 2 cm proximal to the wrist flexion point where there is a lower risk for digital ischemia because of better collateral circulation.

Femoral Artery

- See the preceding section for identification and cannulation techniques for the femoral vein.
- The femoral artery is **lateral** to the femoral vein. The artery can be easily palpated in most patients.
- It should be punctured **below the inguinal ligament** to prevent intra-abdominal injury and retroperitoneal hematomas. The artery is usually reached 3 to 5 cm from the skin.
- The modified Seldinger technique is usually required for femoral cannulation.
- Consider using a **Doppler US** to guide cannulation in high-risk patients who are anticoagulated or obese.

Axillary Artery

- The axillary artery should be cannulated as **high as possible in the axilla,** close to the thoracic apex, because of a rich anastomotic network surrounding the artery in this region.
- The axillary artery is fraught with a number of complications. Care must be taken with needle punctures high in the apex of the thoracic cavity to avoid **pneumothorax** or hemothorax. Thromboembolism can also occur from the axillary artery down to the radial or ulnar artery. Hematoma from a puncture leak of the artery can fill the axillary sheath around the neurovascular bundle and compress the brachial plexus, resulting in nerve damage and peripheral neuropathy
- Since the risk of **cerebral air embolism** from accidental air injection into the axillary artery is higher with **right-sided catheterization,** placement should be performed preferentially on the left side first.

Dorsalis Pedis Artery

- This small artery is congenitally absent in 3% to 12% of the population and is often difficult to cannulate; furthermore, blood pressure measured in the dorsalis pedis artery may differ significantly from that measured in more central arteries, especially in the presence of vasopressor infusion.

Temporal Artery

- Rich collateral circulation and easy accessibility make the temporal artery an attractive site for cannulation; tortuosity and its location, however, make cannulation and maintenance extremely difficult.

Complications of Arterial Catheters

- The most common complications include local ischemia, infection, hematoma, bleeding, thrombosis, distal embolism, ischemic necrosis, arteriovenous fistula formation, air embo-

lism, and neuropathy. Of these, ischemic necrosis and thrombosis are two of the most concerning complications occurring 1% to 2.5% of the time. The incidence of local infection at the catheter insertion site is reported to be as high as 10% to 15%, whereas the incidence rate of catheter-related sepsis is 0.2% to 5%.

CHAPTER 14 ■ FEEDING TUBE PLACEMENT

For critically ill patients, enteral nutrition is preferable to parenteral whenever feasible. Although parenteral nutrition can effectively deliver protein and calories, it does not prevent intestinal mucosal atrophy. It is now well recognized that the healthy gut mucosal layer provides a barrier to pathogen invasion. Microbial invasion through the gut into the systemic circulation is thought to represent a major cause of the nosocomial sepsis, and possibly the multiple organ dysfunction, seen with critical illness.

- The initial consideration for determining the choice of an enteral access system is the anticipated duration of enteral feeding.

  Short term: Patients predicted to need enteral feeding for **2 weeks or less** are said to have short-term requirements. These patients are best served with bedside placement of a **nasoenteric tube.**

  Long term: Patients thought to need enteral feeding for greater than **6 to 8 weeks** are described as having long-term requirements. **Percutaneous or surgically placed** tubes are most appropriate for this subgroup of patients.

  Intermediate: Patients with the anticipated need for enteral feeding for greater than 2 weeks but less than 6 to 8 weeks are said to have an intermediate requirement. These patients are well served by nasally, percutaneously, or surgically placed feeding tubes.

- Determine whether the patient can tolerate enteral nutrition.
- Based on the patient's overall condition, associated medical conditions, the **functional status of the gastrointestinal tract,** and available hospital resources, the most appropriate type of feeding tube and placement technique can be chosen.
- If the attempted placement technique is unsuccessful, reconsider the foregoing and choose another enteral access option.
- Roughly half of critically ill patients have **gastric emptying dysfunction.**
  - Many underlying conditions such as diabetes mellitus, medication use, gastritis, sepsis, and electrolyte abnormalities also affect gastric emptying. For these patients, enteral tubes may need to be placed beyond the pylorus.
  - Although **postpyloric feedings** are generally favored, postpyloric tube placement should not unduly delay the start

of enteral nutrition as gastric feedings are often well tolerated.
- Though bolus gastric feeding may occasionally be used, continuous infusion of enteral feeds is better tolerated than bolus feeding.

NASOGASTRIC TUBE

- The least complicated and quickest feeding access is the **nasogastric tube.**
  - Although the stiffer, wider tubes used for gastric decompression also can be used for feeding, it may be preferable to replace these tubes with the thin, softer, more flexible tubes.
  - The tube is lubricated and then passed blindly through a nostril. It travels down the posterior pharynx into the esophagus and then into the stomach. Placement is aided by wire stylets or weighted tips.
- **Auscultation of air instilled** into the nasogastric or nasoenteric tube is useful for determining proper tube placement. It is important to confirm that the tube was not inadvertently placed into the bronchial tree.
- **Complications** are similar to those of the sump tube, such as **epistaxis, rhinitis, esophageal perforation or hemorrhage, pneumothorax,** and inadvertent placement into the **trachea or bronchus.**
  - After placement of a nasogastric or nasoenteric feeding tube, an abdominal **radiograph** should be obtained to confirm proper tube location **before infusing the enteral formula**
- If gastric feeding is used, the addition of **promotility agents** may be helpful.
- **Metoclopramide** increases upper gastrointestinal motility by blocking dopamine receptors. Metoclopramide is associated with movement disorders, which may be irreversible.
- **Erythromycin,** a macrolide antibiotic that is also a motilin agonist, increases gastric emptying and tolerance to gastric feeding. The commonly used dose is 200 mg, but **70 mg** may be just as effective.
  - Unfortunately, patients often develop **tachyphylaxis** to the drugs after several days, requiring close monitoring of gastric volumes and feeding tolerance.
- The long-term use of any antibiotic raises concerns about the development of resistance.

POSTPYLORIC TUBES

- A large variety of tube designs are commercially available. For nasal placement, tubes tend to be thin, soft, and flexible.
  - Most are polyvinyl chloride, silicone, or polyurethane.
  - Many are weighted at the tip with mercury, whereas others are unweighted.
  - Most contain a thin metal stylet to assist in placement.
  - All are radiopaque to enable confirmation of position by radiographic study.
  - Their soft, flexible construction and narrow diameter enables these tubes to be well tolerated by the patient. However, these tubes are prone to occlusion, particularly if feeding is interrupted without irrigating the tube free of formula and when the tube is used for the delivery of crushed or dissolved medications.
- Several bedside techniques have been described to aid in achieving **postpyloric placement of tubes** inserted through the nose. These techniques are highly successful in experienced hands.
- Manually passing the soft, thin, flexible tube across the length of the stomach and beyond the pylorus is often challenging (Fig. 14.1). Often, the tube coils back into the fundus or cannot easily be negotiated through the antrum and pylorus. In most cases, the difficulty in tube advancement into the duodenum is related to the blind nature of the passage and to the inability to steer or guide the tube.
- Several techniques have been described to aid in passage. Some authors have reported improved success with simple maneuvers such as placing the patient in **the right lateral decubitus position,** giving the tube a gentle **clockwise twist** as it is being passed, or **bending the tip** of the stylet.
  - House officers who learned the technique were able to achieve placement rates of **70% to 80%.**

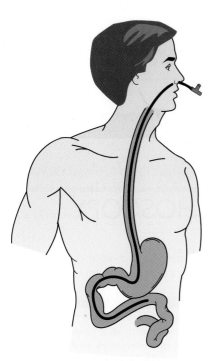

FIGURE 14.1. Nasoenteric feeding tube.

- The use of **ultrasound, electrocardiogram, or electromagnetic transmitter** for **location of the tip** of the tube during insertion have all been described and may decrease the time of insertion and the number of confirmatory radiographs. However, these techniques do not actually guide the tube in its course.
- A technique using an **industrial magnet to guide a magnet-tipped tube** into the duodenum has also been described.
  - All these techniques have reported success rates above 75%, but large trials comparing them to other techniques are lacking.
- **Continuous pH monitoring** using a specially designed tube that has a built-in pH sensor in the tip has been described to facilitate passage by enabling recognition of the tube tip location. Generally, **lower pH** values are found in the **stomach** compared with the duodenum even in patients receiving H_2-receptor antagonists.
  - This device may obviate the need for radiographic confirmation of tube location. Although the need for fewer radiographs may save money, the requirement for specialized tubes and a pH monitor may offset the savings.
    - These tubes are generally two to three times more expensive than traditional tubes, and most pH monitors cost a few hundred dollars.
  - Serial or continuous pH monitoring also can be used to **indicate whether the tube has migrated back into the stomach.** However, the ability to use pH values to determine location may be less accurate in the setting of H_2-blocker administration or with achlorhydria, where the stomach has less acid production and, hence, higher than normal pH readings.
- If there is concern that a nasoenteric tube has migrated back into the stomach, its position must be clarified with a **radiograph.**
- **Fluoroscopic or endoscopic** support may be necessary for passing the tip of the nasoenteric tube beyond the pylorus. Even with the assistance of these modalities, success is not guaranteed.
- **Fluoroscopic guidance** is an excellent method for placing the tip of the feeding tube beyond the pylorus. Because the tubes are **radiopaque,** they are easily seen under fluoroscopy. Tube passage can then be guided by **direct vision.**
  - Though this technique increases the likelihood of success, it has several drawbacks: The critically ill patient must be **transported** to the radiology department or the **radiography equipment** must be brought to the ICU. The technique also exposes the patient to **radiation.**
- **Endoscopy** provides an alternate means of delivering the tube past the pylorus, but it is also the most invasive. After positioning the tube into the stomach, an esophagogastroscopy is performed. The tip of the tube, or a suture secured to the tip, can then be grasped with a biopsy forceps that was passed through the endoscope and **dragged into the duodenum.**
  - Although this technique is effective, the tube may get pulled back into the stomach by the withdrawal of the endoscope, and the procedure places the patient at risk for all of the complications associated with endoscopy, including injury to the esophagus, stomach, or duodenum; perforation; bleeding; and aspiration.
- Nasoenteric tubes also can be placed at the **time of laparotomy** for patients requiring temporary jejunal access. The surgeon will **manually thread** the catheter past the pylorus while the anesthesiologist pushes it in.

- Even after the successful nasoenteric placement, tubes easily can be inadvertently removed or pulled back into the stomach
- No method for **tube immobilization** (i.e., sutures, bridles, or taping) is completely secure.
  - Occasionally, replacement requires considerable effort.
  - **Frequent checks** by nurses on the secure immobilization of the tubes assist with inadvertent dislodgement during turning.

PERCUTANEOUS PLACEMENT

- Percutaneous gastrostomy has been shown to be less costly and less time consuming and has **fewer complications** than surgical gastrostomy.
  - Placement requires **fluoroscopic or endoscopic** assistance to direct the tube into the appropriate lumen after skin puncture.
    - These tubes are less likely to dislodge but can **leak**, cause **pain** at the insertion site, and induce a local soft-tissue **infection**. With long-term use, they also may begin to decay.
    - Some models have separate ports for simultaneous jejunal feeding and gastric decompression.
    - Most are secured from within the lumen of the viscus by a small flange or balloon contained within the tip; removal may require endoscopy.
- **Percutaneous endoscopic gastrostomy** tube placement generally requires one of two techniques, termed "push" and "pull." There are numerous commercially available insertion kits that contain the tube and the equipment necessary for **placement** (see Chapter 16).
- The incidence of **major complications** with this technique is generally described as between **1% and 3%,** and the reported mortality rate is about 0.5%.
- Complications include **colonic injury, gastric perforation, hemorrhage, leakage with peritonitis, necrotizing fasciitis, and skin infection.**
- Conditions that preclude the ability to perform upper endoscopy such as **obstruction, varices, and severe** *Candida*

esophagitis are contraindications to this procedure. Relative contraindications include **ascites** with its attendant risk of **peristomal leakage** and **peritonitis** from gastric leakage. Previous upper-abdominal surgery and adhesions may prevent the stomach from being manipulated up to the abdominal wall. If **transillumination** cannot be achieved, the procedure should be aborted.

- An alternative method for percutaneous gastrostomy is the **radiographic approach.** The stomach is distended with air using a nasogastric tube. Radiopaque contrast is then instilled in the stomach to enable it to be seen with fluoroscopy. The abdominal wall then can be pressed down onto the stomach. A needle is passed into the gastric lumen and a guidewire inserted through the needle. The tract is dilated to the appropriate diameter and the tube is pushed into the lumen.
  - This technique eliminates the need for endoscopy; however, many of the **same contraindications and complications** apply. In addition, this method does not allow inspection of the mucosa before tube placement or direct visualization of tube position after it is in place.

JEJUNOSTOMY

- Surgically placed jejunostomy tubes are excellent for long-term infusion feeding but expose the critically ill patient to the risks and complications of an **operative procedure.**
- In the early 1970s, the **needle catheter jejunostomy** was introduced. Although easy to insert, it is frequently **too narrow** to allow rapid flow of the more viscous feeding solutions, and the small diameter does not allow for medication administration through the tube.
- Other options for jejunostomy placement include soft rubber tubes (**red rubber or Robinson catheters**).
  - Their wider internal diameter improves infusion and decreases the likelihood of occlusion
- These tubes are prone to **dislodgement** and need to be secured diligently. Balloon and mushroom-tipped tubes are less susceptible to inadvertent removal because their tips are wider than their shafts, which help to anchor the tubes in place.

CHAPTER 15 ■ FLEXIBLE BRONCHOSCOPY

INDICATIONS

Potential indications for flexible bronchoscopy in the ICU include the following:
- *Airway management* (intubation, changing of endotracheal tubes [ETs], and extubation)
- Diagnosis and/or management of *respiratory infections, certain parenchymal lung disease,* acute *inhalational injury,*

airway injury from intubation or chest *trauma, hemoptysis, atelectasis, airway obstruction,* and *bronchopleural fistulae*

Both fiberoptic and video bronchoscopes are utilized for flexible bronchoscopy in the ICU. With the *video bronchoscope* and with attachment of a camera head to the fiberoptic bronchoscope, observation by multiple parties is possible, which decreases the possibility of missed findings and facilitates teaching and education.

CONTRAINDICATIONS

Only a few absolute contraindications to flexible bronchoscopy exist in critically ill patients:
- Absence of informed consent
- Unavailability of trained personnel
- Inability to maintain adequate oxygenation during the procedure
- Unstable cardiac conditions
- Uncontrolled bronchospasm
- Inability to correct coagulopathy to safe levels if biopsy or protected specimen brush (PSB) is planned (relative contraindication). A platelet count should be at least 50,000 cells/μL if biopsies are going to be performed.

GENERAL CONSIDERATIONS

- Obtain informed consent.
- Enteral feeding or oral intake should be discontinued for at least 4 hours before and 2 hours after the procedure.
- Patients with asthma should receive bronchodilators prior to bronchoscopy.
- Platelet counts and coagulation studies should be obtained in those patients with risk factors for bleeding if bronchoscopic biopsies are planned.
- Continuous monitoring with electrocardiogram, pulse oximetry, intra-arterial blood pressure, or intermittent cuff blood pressure every 3 to 5 minutes is advised.
- Monitoring intracranial pressure and end-tidal CO_2 is suggested for patients with a serious head injury. Bronchoscopy has been noted to increase intracranial pressure by at least 50%, in 88% of patients with head trauma, despite the use of deep sedation and paralysis.
- Equipment for reintubation and bag-valve-mask ventilation should be readily available, and suctioning equipment, including Yankauer and ETs, should be accessible at the bedside.
- In mechanically ventilated patients, a special swivel adapter with a perforated diaphragm through which the bronchoscope is passed should be used to prevent loss of delivered tidal volumes.
- The lumen of the ET should be 2 mm larger than the external diameter of the bronchoscope. Due to narrowing of the airway, bronchoscopy in the mechanically ventilated patient may cause hypoxemia, hypoventilation, generation of auto–positive end-expiratory pressure (PEEP), and potential barotrauma.
- The fraction of inspired oxygen (FiO_2) should be increased to 1.0 prior to and during the procedure to ensure adequate oxygenation. Exhaled tidal volumes should be monitored during the procedure. The bronchoscope should be withdrawn periodically to allow for adequate ventilation; prolonged suctioning through the bronchoscope can decrease delivered tidal volumes and oxygenation.
- Resuscitation medications, materials for chest thoracostomy should be readily available.

PREMEDICATION

- **Topical anesthesia** (lidocaine jelly and nebulized or sprayed lidocaine) of the nares and oropharynx is used to sup-

press the gag reflex and coughing in non-intubated patients.
- In intubated patients, 1% lidocaine can be administered through the ET or through the working channel of the bronchoscope after insertion into the ET.
- Lidocaine is absorbed through the mucous membranes and achieves peak serum concentrations that are similar to that of intravenous administration. The total dose of lidocaine should not exceed **3 to 4 mg/kg.** Patients with **cardiac or hepatic** insufficiency have reduced clearance of lidocaine, and the dose should not exceed **2 to 3 mg/kg.**
- The use of lidocaine should be kept to a minimum if samples for culture are to be obtained, as bacteriostatic lidocaine preparations may decrease culture yields.
- **Sedation and analgesic agents** are often used to provide anxiolysis, antegrade amnesia, analgesia, and cough suppression. A combination of opiates and benzodiazepines is typically used. Propofol may also be used in intubated patients and patients with adjunctive airway support; advantages include rapid onset and offset of action, with the potential disadvantage of drug-induced hypotension.

DIAGNOSTIC AND THERAPEUTIC FLEXIBLE BRONCHOSCOPY

Bronchoalveolar Lavage

- Bronchoalveolar lavage (BAL) allows for sampling of cellular and non-cellular components from the **lower respiratory tract.**
- The tip of the bronchoscope is wedged into a distal airway, and sterile saline solution (aliquots of 20–60 mL) is instilled through the bronchoscope and then aspirated with the syringe or suctioned into a sterile trap. Infusions of 120 mL to 240 mL are needed to ensure adequate sampling of secretions in the distal respiratory bronchioles.
- The first aliquot of aspirated fluid is likely to contain material from the proximal airways, and some authors recommend discarding this aliquot.
- In patients with emphysema, collapse of the airways with negative pressure during aspiration or suctioning may limit the amount of fluid obtained and give false-negative results.
- Suctioning prior to having the bronchoscope in the appropriate wedged position should be minimized to avoid contamination with upper-airway secretions and potential false-positive results.
- In addition to quantitative bacterial cultures for the diagnosis of ventilator-associated pneumonia, BAL samples may also be sent for **cytology, antigen tests, and polymerase chain reaction tests,** which provide additional information for the diagnosis of noninfectious pulmonary disease.

Protected Specimen Brush

- The protected specimen brush (PSB) is used to obtain a lower–respiratory tract specimen for microbiology that is not contaminated by organisms in the proximal airways.
- A retractable brush within a double-sheathed catheter has a distal dissolvable plug occluding the outer catheter.

- After the tip of the bronchoscope is positioned in the desired area, the catheter is advanced through the working channel and situated 1 to 3 cm beyond the distal end of the bronchoscope to prevent collection of secretions pooled around the distal end of the bronchoscope.
- The inner cannula containing the brush is advanced to eject the distal plug, and the brush is then advanced into the desired subsegment under direct visualization.
- Once the sample is obtained, the brush is retracted into the inner cannula, the inner cannula is then withdrawn into the outer sheath, and the entire catheter is removed from the bronchoscope.
- The distal ends of the outer and inner cannula are wiped with alcohol, cut with sterile scissors, and discarded. The brush is advanced beyond the remaining portion of the inner cannula, cut with sterile scissors, and placed in 1 mL of non-bacteriostatic sterile saline or transport media.

Cultures and Diagnosis of Pneumonia

- Specimens for culture should be rapidly processed within **30 minutes** to prevent a decrease in pathogen viability or contaminant overgrowth.
- A quantitative culture result of more than 10^4 **colony forming units (CFU)/mL** is considered diagnostic for pneumonia with **BAL**, while whereas more than 10^3 **CFU/mL** is considered diagnostic for pneumonia with **PSB**.
- An evidence-based review of 23 prospective studies of BAL in suspected ventilator associated pneumonia (VAP) showed a sensitivity of 42% to 93% with a mean of 73% ± 18%, and a specificity of 45% to 100% with a mean of 82% ± 19%.
- In a review of studies evaluating PSB, the sensitivity ranged from 33% to 100% with a median sensitivity of 67%, whereas the specificity ranged from 50% to 100% with a median specificity of 95%
- It is unclear whether BAL is superior to PSB or vice versa in the diagnosis of VAP. In a meta-analysis of 18 studies on PSB (795 patients) and 11 studies on BAL (435 patients), there was no difference in the accuracy of the two tests.
- Despite studies of BAL and PSB showing a greater accuracy than tracheal aspirates, the routine use of bronchoscopy for establishing the diagnosis of **ventilator-associated pneumonia** remains controversial. This controversy is in part due to critiques in study methodologies and in part due to conflicting results regarding outcomes.
- Performing microbiologic cultures of pulmonary secretions for diagnostic purposes **after initiating new antibiotic therapy** can lead to **false-negative** results. Culture positivity at 24 and 48 hours after the onset of antimicrobial treatment is markedly diminished.
- In an **immunocompromised** patient with pulmonary infiltrates risk for **fungal, viral, protozoal, mycobacterial, and atypical bacterial** pulmonary infections, BAL fluid should be sent for cytopathology to evaluate for viral cytologic changes and Gomori methenamine silver staining to evaluate for fungal organisms and *Pneumocystis jiroveci*. Alternatively, Papanicolaou, Giemsa, toluidine blue O, or direct fluorescent antibody staining may be used for detection of *Pneumocystis*.
- For the diagnosis of pulmonary **fungal infections,** BAL fluid should be sent for fungal stains and cultures in addition to

cytology stains. Some fungi, such as *Mucor* and *Rhizopus*, are difficult to grow on culture, and diagnosis relies on BAL cytology or biopsy specimens. ***Aspergillus*** is the most commonly encountered pulmonary fungal infection. BAL cytology and culture are diagnostic in approximately 50% to 60% of cases of invasive pulmonary aspergillosis. The diagnostic yield from BAL appears to be increased with the use of galactomannan antigen and PCR testing. Antigen testing for **histoplasmosis** and **blastomycosis** on BAL samples is now available.

- To evaluate for **viral infections,** respiratory viral cultures and a respiratory syncytial virus antigen assay should be obtained. BAL cytology may demonstrate characteristic intracytoplasmic inclusions, but sensitivity is lacking. Immunofluorescence and polymerase chain reaction (PCR) for cytomegalovirus may be performed on BAL specimens.
- If there is suspicion for tuberculosis or nontuberculous **mycobacteria,** BAL samples should be sent for acid-fast bacillus stains and mycobacterial culture
- For atypical bacterial infections, additional stains and cultures may be required. *Legionella* requires specific culture media. A direct fluorescence antibody stain is also available for *Legionella*. Some laboratories utilize specific media if *Nocardia* is suspected. *Nocardia* can often be identified with a combination of Gram stain and modified Ziehl–Neelsen stains and are observed as delicately branched, weakly Gram-positive, variably acid-fast bacilli. Methenamine-silver stains may demonstrate the organisms in tissue specimens.

Transbronchial and Endobronchial Biopsies

- Histologic samples of **lung parenchyma** may be obtained with transbronchial lung biopsies and offer a less invasive option to open lung biopsy. However, for some interstitial lung diseases and pulmonary vasculitides, transbronchial biopsy specimens are inadequate to make a definitive diagnosis.
- The major risks of transbronchial biopsies are **bleeding and pneumothorax.** A chest radiograph should be obtained after transbronchial lung biopsy. Rates of pneumothorax after transbronchial lung biopsy in mechanically ventilated patients have been reported up to 7% and 23%, but <5% in nonventilated patients.
- Samples of **bronchial mucosa** and **endobronchial** abnormalities may be obtained with endobronchial biopsies. Transbronchial and endobronchial biopsies may be sent for bacterial, mycobacterial, and fungal cultures as indicated, in addition to histology.
- Transbronchial biopsy may be able to establish other **noninfectious diagnoses of pulmonary infiltrates** in the ICU including idiopathic interstitial pneumonia and graft-versus-host disease in stem cell or bone marrow transplantation patients, leukemic infiltrates, drug-induced pneumonitis, bronchiolitis obliterans organizing pneumonia/cryptogenic organizing pneumonia, bronchoalveolar carcinoma, lymphangitic carcinomatosis, and acute rejection after lung transplantation.
- Transbronchial biopsy is associated with a **2.7% and 0.12%** risk of **morbidity and mortality**
- Transbronchial biopsy should be restricted to nonuremic patients with platelet counts >50,000 cells/μL and prothrombin times and activated partial thromboplastin times less than twice that of controls.

Airway Management

Endotracheal intubation can be technically difficult in select patient groups (Table 15.1).

- *Spontaneous ventilation* keeps the airway open and assists the bronchoscopist in locating the glottis when airway anatomy is distorted.
- Bronchoscopic endotracheal intubation can be performed using either a nasal or oral approach. With the **nasal approach,** after preparation of the nasal mucosa with a local anesthetic such as lidocaine and a mucosal vasoconstrictor such as 1% phenylephrine, the bronchoscope is passed through the nares and situated directly above the glottic opening. It is then passed into the trachea, and the ET is passed over the bronchoscope into the trachea. The major limitation of this approach is epistaxis (especially in coagulopathic patients), potential for sinusitis with prolonged nasal intubation, dislocation of adenoids, and limited diameter of the nares.
- With the **oropharyngeal approach,** topical anesthesia is achieved with spraying of 4% lidocaine. A bite block is placed, and the flexible bronchoscopy is guided past the tongue and directly over the larynx, facilitating endotracheal intubation with the ET passed over the bronchoscope.
- Use of these airways in the completely awake patient with inadequate topical anesthesia may be problematic due to **gagging and vomiting.** This is less of a problem in the sedated or unconscious patient.
- Flexible bronchoscopy allows for **ET changes** in patients with ET cuff leaks, inadequate ET internal diameters, and nasotracheal tube-associated sinusitis.
- Before bronchoscopy, the oropharynx should be suctioned thoroughly. The ET should be advanced over the bronchoscope before its placement in the pharynx. The bronchoscope tip is advanced to the level of the cuff of the existing ET, and secretions are aspirated through the suction channel. If necessary, the cuff is deflated and the bronchoscope advanced into the tracheal lumen. The existing ET is then withdrawn with the cuff fully deflated, the bronchoscope tip advanced to the carina, and the new ET advanced over the bronchoscope into the trachea.
- **Percutaneous dilatational tracheostomy** has become a well-accepted method for performing bedside tracheostomy in the ICU. Bronchoscopic visualization ensures that the guide-wire needle is introduced in the appropriate interspace in a midline position and that the needle does not penetrate the membranous **posterior tracheal wall,** thereby decreasing the risk of misplacement of the tracheostomy tube and creation of a false paratracheal passage. Bronchoscopy also provides feedback to the operator during dilator passage so that pressure on the posterior wall is minimized and the potential for posterior wall tears is reduced.
- Flexible bronchoscopy can be extremely useful in the placement of a **double-lumen ET.** If a right-sided tube is used, adequate positioning of the tube with the tracheal port proximal to the carina and bronchial port proximal to the right upper lobe orifice can be confirmed by using a small-diameter (3.5-mm outer diameter) flexible bronchoscope to inspect the airway through each lumen. Positioning of left-sided tubes is not as problematic given the longer length of the left mainstem bronchus relative to the right mainstem bronchus and less likelihood of obstructing the left upper or left lower lobe.

TABLE 15.1

FACTORS ASSOCIATED WITH DIFFICULT
ENDOTRACHEAL INTUBATIONS

Anatomic
Short muscular neck
Receding mandible
Prominent upper incisors
Microglossia
Limited mandible movement
Large breasts
Cervical rigidity

Congenital abnormalities
Absence of nose
Choanal atresia
Macroglossia

Infectious
Bacterial retropharyngeal abscess
Epiglottitis
Diphtheria
Infectious mononucleosis
Croup
Leprosy

Noninfective inflammation
Rheumatoid arthritis
Instability of cervical spine
Cervical fixation
Temporomandibular disease
Cricoarytenoid disorders
Hypoplastic mandible
Ankylosing spondylitis

Neoplasia
Laryngeal papillomatosis
Stylohyoid ligament calcification
Laryngeal carcinoma
Mediastinal carcinoma

Trauma
Mandibular fracture
Maxillary fracture
Laryngeal and tracheal trauma
Mediastinal carcinoma

Endocrine
Obesity
Acromegaly
Thyromegaly

Atelectasis

- Complete lung atelectasis will produce **opacification** of the hemithorax and usually **ipsilateral mediastinal shift.**
- In patients who do not improve after chest physiotherapy, endobronchial obstruction due to **inspissated mucus, endobronchial tumor, foreign body, or blood clot** should be excluded by bronchoscopy.
- With the exception of large, obstructing central airway mucous plugs, the radiographic response to successful removal of secretions is **delayed from 6 to 24 hours.**

- Instillation of saline or a dilute 10% solution of **acetylcysteine** through the working channel may help to clear thick, tenacious secretions. Acetylcysteine is a bronchial irritant, however, and may exacerbate bronchospasm in patients with reactive airway disease. Typically 10- to 20-mL aliquots of saline are used as the irrigant to facilitate clearing of mucous plugs. If saline irrigation fails, then instillation of acetylcysteine or **rhDNase (Pulmozyme)** may be considered. In some patients, holding continuous suction while withdrawing the bronchoscope through the ET allows removal of large mucous plugs that cannot be suctioned directly through the working channel.

Hemoptysis

- **Early** bronchoscopy should be considered regardless of the degree of hemoptysis, to localize the site of bleeding and attempt to determine the underlying etiology. It is important to guide temporizing therapy such as angiographic embolization and definitive therapy such as surgical resection.
- **Massive hemoptysis** is defined as expectoration of blood exceeding 200 to 1,000 mL over a 24-hour period, with expectoration of >600 mL in 24 hours as the most commonly used definition.
- Only 3% to 5% of patients with hemoptysis have **massive hemoptysis,** with the mortality rates approaching 80% in various case series.
- Causes of massive hemoptysis are presented in (Table 15.2)
- **Airway patency** must be ensured in patients with massive hemoptysis. While preparing for intubation and bronchoscopy, the patient may be positioned in the **lateral decubitus position** with the **bleeding side down.**
- The **largest possible ET** should be inserted to allow for introduction of bronchoscopes with a 2.8- to 3.0-mm working channel for more effective suctioning and to allow for better ventilation with the bronchoscope in the airway for prolonged periods of time. In severe cases, the mainstem bronchus of the nonbleeding lung can be **selectively intubated** under bronchoscopic guidance to preserve oxygenation and ventilation in the normal lung.
- **Endobronchial tamponade** with flexible bronchoscopy can prevent aspiration of blood into the contralateral lung and preserve gas exchange in patients with massive hemoptysis. This can be achieved with a No. **4-French Fogarty balloon-tipped catheter.** The catheter may be passed directly through the working channel of the bronchoscope, or the catheter can be grasped by biopsy forceps placed though the working channel of the bronchoscope prior to introduction into the airway. The bronchoscope and catheter—with the latter held in place adjacent to the bronchoscope by the biopsy forceps—are then inserted as a unit into the airway. Care must be taken not to perforate the catheter or balloon by the forceps. The catheter tip is inserted into the bleeding segmental orifice, and the balloon is inflated. If passed through the suction channel, the proximal end of the catheter is clamped with a hemostat, the hub cut off, and a straight pin inserted into the catheter channel proximal to the hemostat to maintain inflation of the balloon catheter. The clamp is removed, and the bronchoscope is carefully withdrawn from the bronchus with the Fogarty catheter remaining in position, to provide endobronchial hemostasis. The catheter can safely remain in

TABLE 15.2

POTENTIAL CAUSES OF MASSIVE HEMOPTYSIS

Neoplasm
Bronchogenic cancer
Metastasis (parenchymal or endobronchial)
Carcinoid
Leukemia

Infectious
Lung abscess
Bronchiectasis
Tuberculosis
Necrotizing pneumonia
Fungal pneumonia
Septic pulmonary emboli
Mycetoma (aspergilloma)

Pulmonary
Bronchiectasis
Cystic fibrosis
Sarcoidosis (fibrocavitary)
Diffuse alveolar hemorrhage
Airway foreign body

Cardiac/vascular
Mitral stenosis
Pulmonary embolism/infarction
Arteriovenous malformation
Broncho-arterial fistula
Ruptured aortic aneurysm
Congestive heart failure
Pulmonary arteriovenous fistula

Iatrogenic/traumatic
Blunt or penetrating chest trauma
Tracheal/bronchial tear or rupture
Tracheo-innominate artery fistula
Bronchoscopy
Pulmonary artery rupture from Swan-Ganz catheter
Endotracheal tube suctioning trauma

Hematologic
Coagulopathy
Disseminated intravascular coagulation
Thrombocytopenia

Drugs/toxins
Anticoagulants
Antiplatelet agents
Thrombolytic agents
Crack cocaine

position until hemostasis is ensured by surgical resection of the bleeding segment or bronchial artery embolization.
- Additional bronchoscopic techniques may be useful as a **temporizing measure** in patients with massive hemoptysis. Bronchoscopically administered **topical therapies** such as iced sterile saline lavage or topical 1:10,000 or 1:20,000 epinephrine solution may be helpful. Direct application of a solution of thrombin or a fibrinogen–thrombin combination solution and, recently, oxidized regenerated cellulose mesh has recently been described.
- For patients who have hemoptysis due to **endobronchial lesions,** particularly endobronchial **tumors,** hemostasis may be achieved with the use of neodymium-yttrium-aluminum-garnet (Nd:YAG) laser phototherapy, electrocautery, or cryotherapy via the bronchoscope.

Trauma

- The classic signs of tracheobronchial disruption include shortness of breath, **massive subcutaneous emphysema, persistent pneumothorax** despite chest tube insertion, and a large air leak after tube thoracoscopy.
- **Tracheobronchial disruption** rarely occurs as an isolated injury and is associated with fractures of the ribs, clavicle, sternum, and pulmonary contusion. Rapid **deceleration** results in shearing forces, acting predominantly at the distal trachea near the carina where the relatively fixed trachea joins the more mobile distal airways. If the trachea and mainstem bronchi are crushed between the chest wall and vertebral column and the glottis closed, airway pressure suddenly increases, and resultant rupture of the airway may occur.
- **Prompt diagnosis and surgical correction** or tracheobronchial disruption produce a better outcome, and delay in diagnosis is usually detrimental to the patient. Failure to diagnose disruption may result in a delayed stricture formation at the site of injury, resulting in dyspnea, distal atelectasis, and chronic recurrent infections.
- If a persistent **bronchopleural fistula** exists because of proximal airway trauma, the cuff of the ET sometimes can be positioned just distal to the rupture site and inflated, and adequate ventilation can be established before surgical repair.
- **Cervical tracheal rupture** is less common than rupture of the intrathoracic trachea. Cervical tracheal rupture, however, may be more difficult to diagnose once the patient is intubated because of the proximal location of the tear, and may itself be an impediment to intubation.

Bronchopleural Fistula

- In patients who are not candidates for surgical management of a bronchopleural fistula (BPF), flexible bronchoscopic techniques may offer alternative methods for closure of the BPF.
- Detection of a proximal BPF due to stump breakdown after lobectomy or pneumonectomy or a BPF due to bronchial dehiscence is usually relatively straightforward, as these abnormalities can be directly visualized. In the setting of a BPF due to a rent or tear on the lung periphery, locating the bronchial segment that provides ventilation to that area of the lung can be more difficult.
- *Airway stents* may be used to cover and seal the fistula in selected patients, depending on the location of the fistula.
- Successful endobronchial occlusion of BPFs has been reported with **cyanoacrylate-based tissue adhesives** (Histoacryl, Bucrylate), **fibrin sealants** (Tisseel, Hemaseel, thrombin plus fibrinogen or cryoprecipitate), absorbable **gelatin sponge** (Gelfoam), vascular occlusion **coils**, doxycycline and blood, Nd:YAG **laser, silver nitrate,** and lead shot. The agent initially seals the leak by acting as a plug and subsequently induces an inflammatory process with fibrosis and mucosal proliferation permanently sealing the area.

Foreign-body Removal

- Risk factors for foreign-body aspiration include age younger than 3 years, altered consciousness, trauma, and disordered swallowing mechanisms.

- Patients may present **with dyspnea, coughing, wheezing, or stridor.** Foreign-body aspiration may be relatively occult, with no obvious history for aspiration. Radiographically, there may be evidence of atelectasis, bronchiectasis, or recurrent pneumonitis.
- For most situations, the **rigid bronchoscope** remains the instrument of choice in young children and infants. In adults, flexible bronchoscopy has clearly been shown to be an effective diagnostic and therapeutic tool in cases of suspected foreign-body aspiration. Several **extraction devices** are available for use through the flexible bronchoscope. Biopsy forceps, graspers, and foreign-body baskets are most commonly employed.

Upper-airway Obstruction

- Causes of upper-airway obstruction include **epiglottitis, bilateral vocal cord paralysis, laryngeal edema, and foreign body.** In the pediatric patient, **subglottic stenosis** secondary to croup should also be considered.
- The flexible bronchoscope affords immediate direct visualization of the upper airway and, if performed with an ET placed over the bronchoscope, affords visualization and guidance for endotracheal intubation.
- If **epiglottitis** is suspected, it may be prudent to perform bronchoscopy in the **surgical suite,** with the surgical team available for **emergency tracheostomy** in case of failure.
- When performing bronchoscopic intubation in suspected upper-airway obstruction, the **nasotracheal approach** may be preferable because the turbinates offer stabilization and a more controlled approach to the area of acute airway obstruction. Flexible bronchoscopic intubation in upper-airway obstruction may be performed in the **sitting position** with **decreased posterior displacement of the epiglottis** over the compromised upper airway as compared with laryngoscopic examination in the supine position.
- If **foreign-body obstruction** is known or suspected as the cause of the upper-airway obstruction, rigid (not flexible) bronchoscopy may be preferable.
- Central airway obstruction may be from primary lung cancer or metastatic **malignancies.** Treatment for malignant airway obstruction from endoluminal tumor has typically consisted of Nd:YAG **laser photoresection** and metal or silicone **stent** placement, although endobronchial electrocautery or argon plasma coagulation has more recently been used in lieu of the Nd:YAG laser.
- Benign causes of obstruction occur most commonly from previous intubation or tracheostomy tube placement, leading to **cicatricial stenosis** with or without **granulation tissue.** Patients with an indwelling tracheostomy tube may also develop a fibrous stenosis or granulation tissue just beyond the tip of the tracheostomy tube, thereby causing airway obstruction. The granulation tissue may be resected with laser electrocautery therapy. The stenosis may be dilated with a rigid bronchoscope or balloon dilatation catheters.

Inhalation Injury

- Patients with singed nasal hairs, facial burns around the nose or mouth, oral/nasopharyngeal burns, carbonaceous sputum, or hoarseness should be suspected of having an upper-airway injury.

- **Stridor, wheezing,** or other manifestations of upper airway symptomatology may imply **impending ventilatory failure.**
- Flexible bronchoscopy should be performed **early** by an experienced bronchoscopist to identify evidence of thermal airway injury with direct examination of the **supraglottic and infraglottic** areas. The need for intubation should be anticipated and an ET placed over the bronchoscope before examining the airways.
- **Serial examinations** may be necessary in patients with apparent minimal thermal airway injury on initial evaluation.
- Signs indicating impending airway obstruction include **inflammation, edema, ulceration, or hemorrhage** of the upper-airway mucosa.
- In the intubated patient, repeat airway examination by bronchoscopy may be necessary before **extubation** to ensure airway patency and resolution of the supraglottic or laryngeal edema. The endotracheal tube can be withdrawn over the bronchoscope while inspecting the airway mucosa and replaced if the airway is compromised.

COMPLICATIONS

- The incidence rate of major complications ranges from 0.08% to 0.15%, and the mortality rate ranges from 0.01% to 0.04%.
- The characteristics of high-risk patients are summarized in Table 15.3.
- Life-threatening complications including hypoxemia, hypercapnia, barotrauma, cardiac arrhythmias, myocardial ischemia, intracranial hypertension, local anesthetic toxicity, and pulmonary hemorrhage.
- In critically ill patients, the decrement in PaO_2 can exceed 30 to 60 mm Hg and hypoxemia may occur as much as 20% of the time. The greater the amount of normal saline instilled for lavage during bronchoscopy, the more frequent the hypoxemia—seen in as many as 23% of patients—and the longer its duration, up to 8 hours.
- Complications associated with the administration of sedation, analgesia, and topical anesthesia include hypotension and allergic reactions, and hypoventilation and hypoxemia from over-sedation and respiratory depression.
- The overzealous use of local anesthetic agents within the airways has potential for toxicity with the rapid uptake of these agents into the systemic circulation from the bronchial mucosa. Lidocaine in excessive doses can cause sinus arrest

TABLE 15.3

CHARACTERISTICS OF INCREASED-RISK PATIENTS FOR BRONCHOSCOPY ON MECHANICAL VENTILATION

Pulmonary
PaO_2 <70 mm Hg with FiO_2 >0.70
PEEP >10 cm H_2O
Auto-PEEP >15 cm H_2O
Active bronchospasm

Cardiac
Recent myocardial infarction (<48 h)
Unstable dysrhythmia
Mean arterial pressure <65 mm Hg on vasopressor therapy

Coagulopathy
Platelet count <20,000 cells/μL
Increase of prothrombin time or partial thromboplastin time 2.0 times control

Central nervous system
Increased intracranial pressure

FiO_2, fraction of inspired oxygen; PEEP, positive end-expiratory pressure.

and atrial ventricular block, especially in patients with underlying heart disease. Other potential adverse reactions include respiratory arrest, seizures, laryngospasm and, rarely, hypersensitivity reactions. Although not as commonly used for topical anesthesia, benzocaine has been associated with the development of methemoglobinemia.

- The incidence rate of bronchoscopy-related hemorrhage in normal hosts approaches 1.4%. In immunocompromised hosts, the rate of hemorrhage ranges from 25% to 29%, whereas hemorrhage occurs in as many as 45% of uremic patients.
- Postbronchoscopy fever occurs in as many as 16% of patients.
- Bronchoscopy-related pneumonia is rare, occurring in fewer than 5%, and bacteremia is exceedingly rare. In general, endocarditis prophylaxis is not required with flexible bronchoscopy.
- Neurosurgical patients are at risk for intracranial hypertension as a result of bronchoscopy-induced elevation of intrathoracic pressure, arterial hypertension, and hypercapnia. Bronchoscopy-associated cough or retching must therefore be avoided. Deep sedation with or without neuromuscular blockade may be utilized if bronchoscopy is deemed necessary.

CHAPTER 16 ■ OTHER IMPORTANT INTENSIVE CARE PROCEDURES

Invasive procedures are performed at the bedside of critically ill patients with increasing frequency. With the development of safety systems and new techniques, the morbidity of these bedside procedures is not higher than the morbidity of similar procedures performed in the operating room, emergency department, or angiography suite.

TUBE THORACOSTOMY

- Fluid or air that remains undrained into the pleural cavity may cause infection, lung collapse, or entrapment and should be drained.
- A **pneumothorax** is usually drained if it exceeds 15% to 20% of the hemithoracic volume or causes hemodynamic instability.
- A *h*emothorax after blunt trauma is drained if more than 200 mL of blood is in the thoracic cavity as found by blunting of the costodiaphragmatic angle on erect chest radiograph or estimated on computed tomographic (CT) imaging.
- After trauma, a **thoracotomy** may be indicated if the chest tube output is more than 1,500 mL at placement or if output of more than 200 mL/hour persists over 4 to 6 hours after placement. A hemodynamically unstable patient who is bleeding in the chest should be taken to the operating room even with lower than the preceding chest tube outputs.

Percutaneous Technique

- The **percutaneous technique** is safe for patients who do not have risk factors for intrathoracic adhesions (e.g., previous thoracic operation, empyema, clotted hemothorax). A **No. 28 Fr or No. 32 Fr** chest tube is adequate according to the size of the patient and does not cause excessive pain. For the drainage of simple pneumothorax, smaller tubes (*No. 18 Fr or No. 22 Fr*) may be used.
- The most common site is at the intercostal space above the nipple (usually the **fourth intercostal space**) and at the **midaxillary line.** The diaphragm can elevate up to the nipple in expiration and, for this reason, lower placement of chest tubes is not safe and may risk injury to the diaphragm and intra-abdominal organs.
- **Adequate local analgesia** is key because tube thoracostomy is a painful procedure. The entire tract should be infiltrated including the **muscles and the rib periosteum and the superior border of the rib,** not just the subcutaneous tissue.
- A needle covered by a plastic sheath and connected to a fluid-filled syringe is inserted through the skin with the intent to hit the underlying rib. Once the rib is felt, the needle is slightly

withdrawn and then redirected immediately **over the rib** to avoid injury to the **neurovascular intercostals bundle** that travels under each rib. Under continuous suction, the syringe and needle are slowly advanced until bubbles of air are aspirated. This indicates that the needle has entered into the pleural space. The needle and syringe are withdrawn and the plastic sheath left in place. A **guidewire** is inserted into the sheath (Fig. 16.1). If there is any resistance during advancement of the guidewire, the procedure should be repeated from the beginning. With the guidewire in place, the plastic sheath is removed. A 2-cm skin incision is made, and **sequential dilatation** with three consecutive dilators is done over the guidewire. After this, the chest tube, loaded on a plastic guide, is placed over the guidewire into the chest. The plastic guide and guidewire are withdrawn, and the chest tube is left in place.
- **Securing the chest tube** is a very important part of the procedure. The tube is tied to the skin with a 0 nonabsorbable suture. A separate suture should be placed as a purse-string around the tube and left untied. This suture will serve to close the incision once the chest tube is removed. The tube should also be **taped** to the skin. Extra precautions should be taken to have the chest tube and its connection to the drainage bottles **secured** to avoid inadvertent partial or complete removal.

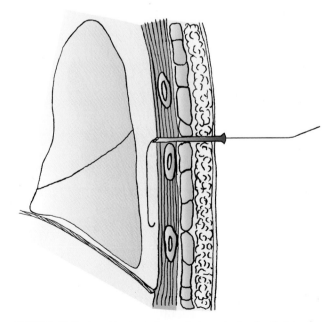

FIGURE 16.1. A guidewire is inserted through the sheath into the pleural space, guiding sequential enlargement of the tract by tapered dilators.

- Usually, **20 cm H$_2$O negative suction** is applied at least for the first 48 hours although there is no evidence that this shortens the period of placement or decreases the rate of residual pneumothorax compared to water seal.

Open Thoracostomy Technique

- The open thoracostomy technique is similar to the percutaneous thoracostomy except the skin incision made parallel to the ribs is slightly larger (**3–4 cm**). Blunt dissection using a sturdy clamp (some use Mayo scissors) is done through the subcutaneous tissue and muscle. It is then opened wide to **spread the muscles and enlarge the tract.** This is an **important step,** as the novice tends to make the skin incision large but the intermuscular tract too small, resulting in difficulty with tube insertion.
- The clamp is finally inserted into the pleural space in a controlled way over the rib underlying the skin incision and spread wide to admit the chest tube (Fig. 16.2). There is no reason to "tunnel" the track to the rib above the skin incision. Tunneling causes more pain, makes the procedure more difficult, and offers no benefit.
- A **finger** is inserted to explore for the presence of adhesions at the site of insertion (Fig. 16.3). Then, the chest tube is guided by a clamp into the opening and toward the superior and posterior hemithorax (Fig. 16.4). The tube is secured as discussed earlier.

Pitfalls and Complications

- A **misplaced chest tube** may not drain adequately.
- Do not assume that air or fluid will be drained because a chest tube is in place.

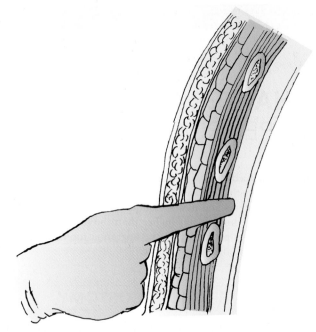

FIGURE 16.3. A finger is inserted into the tract prior to tube insertion to ensure a clear pleural space and absence of adhesions.

- Confirm correct placement with a chest radiograph, and have a low threshold to **replace or add a chest tube,** if the symptoms are not relieved, hemodynamic instability persists, or drain seizes abruptly.
- Injury to the intercostal vessels or lung may cause significant **bleeding.** The chest tube should then be removed and on rare occasions the bleeding site explored if the hemorrhage continues
- **Intraparenchymal placement** may cause a persistent air leak. It is usually diagnosed by CT. The tube should be removed, and the leak usually seals.
- The chest tubes should be **securely tied and taped** to the skin and checked daily. Accidental removal of a tube equals a sloppy technique.

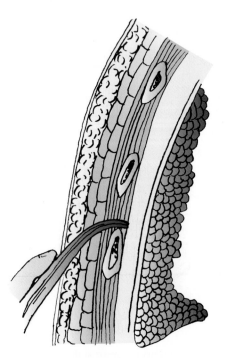

FIGURE 16.2. A sturdy clamp is necessary to spread the muscles wide to allow easy insertion of the chest tube.

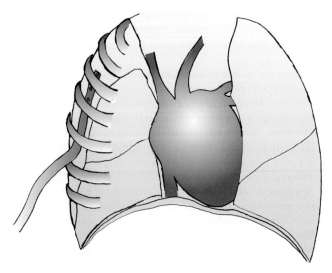

FIGURE 16.4. The final position of the chest tube.

- **Infection** is the most common related complication. Poor aseptic technique, long duration of the tube in the chest, and no antibiotic prophylaxis (one dose before tube placement) are associated with this complication.
- Significant **undrained hemothorax** (estimated at more than 400 mL) should be managed by thoracoscopic evacuation or intrathoracic thrombolysis.

Removal of Chest Tubes

- Removal takes place when there is no air leak and fluid output is <2 mL/kg per 24 hours. The patient is asked to inspire maximally and hold the breath. Warn the patient that the tube must be **pulled quickly** to prevent air entry into the chest. With one hand against the chest wall, the physician pulls abruptly the chest tube with the other hand and immediately ties the purse string to seal the insertion site. The site is dressed. If a purse-string suture is absent, it is important to apply occlusive dressing to prevent air entry into the chest.

DIAGNOSTIC PERITONEAL ASPIRATION AND LAVAGE

The most common reason for a diagnostic peritoneal aspiration and lavage is the diagnosis of **intra-abdominal injury**. Portable ultrasonography and the liberal use of helical CT have limited the usefulness of diagnostic peritoneal aspiration and lavage. Occasionally, aspiration or paracentesis of the abdomen is also performed to diagnose and treat **ascites**.

- Currently, diagnostic peritoneal aspiration (DPA) and diagnostic peritoneal lavage (DPL) are used only on rare occasions due to lack of appropriate technologic resources or due to major physiologic **instability** that precludes patient transport to CT.
- Another indication for DPL may be to detect **bowel injury,** as CT scan may miss intestinal infarction and perforation.
- Once the peritoneal cavity is accessed, **aspiration** is performed first (DPA) and is considered positive if **10 mL** of gross blood is aspirated. If the DPA is negative, 1 L of normal saline is infused (DPL), and the abdomen is gently shaken or "lavaged." By lowering the normal saline bag below the level of the body, the lavage fluid returns into the bag, but not all is retrieved, usually less than half; the fluid is sent for analysis.
- A count of more than **100,000 red blood cells/mm³** indicates bleeding. More than **500 white blood cells/mm³** or the presence of bile, enteric content, or high-amylase in the effluent of the lavage may indicate bowel injury. However, the red cell criteria are oversensitive and frequently lead to unnecessary operations. These cell counts are valid for **blunt** but not for penetrating trauma.

Percutaneous Insertion of Peritoneal Catheter

- Patient must have a Foley catheter placed to **decompress the bladder** to avoid injury to a distended bladder.
- A 0.5-cm skin incision is placed under the umbilicus (or over it in the presence of pregnancy, pelvic hematoma, or a lower

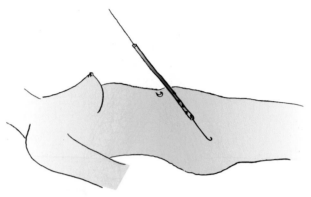

FIGURE 16.5. A peritoneal lavage catheter is placed over the guidewire.

midline operative scar). A sheathed needle is introduced in the direction of the pelvis. The needle is connected to a fluid-filled syringe and advanced slowly. When the flow of fluid becomes unobstructed, the needle is in the peritoneal cavity. Needle and syringe are withdrawn, and the plastic sheath is left in place. A guidewire is introduced through the sheath, which is then removed. A dilator is placed over the guidewire and withdrawn. Then, the DPL catheter is introduced, and the guidewire is removed (Fig. 16.5).
- A simpler DPL system includes only a catheter fed over a trocar. After the skin incision, the **trocar and catheter** are introduced in a controlled and slow fashion into the abdomen in the direction of the pelvis. **Two points of resistance** are felt as the trocar passes through the anterior fascia and the peritoneum. As soon as the tip of the trocar passes the second point of resistance—and is presumably into the abdomen—the catheter is fed over it toward the pelvis, and the trocar is removed. Experience is needed to perform this technique to prevent trocar injury of abdominal contents.

Open Technique for Peritoneal Catheter Insertion

- A 2- to 4-cm skin incision is performed under or over the umbilicus. The **fascia is visualized** and retracted. The fascia is then incised and the peritoneal cavity entered (Fig. 16.6). Under direct observation, a DPL catheter is introduced toward the pelvis (Fig. 16.7). Sometimes, sutures are placed in the fascia to close the perforation.

Pitfalls and Complications

- The introduction of needles and catheters in the abdominal cavity carries the (very low) risk of **injuring the bowel or vessels.** The procedure needs to be performed by physicians experienced with the procedure, which is becoming uncommon as the procedure is not frequently performed.
- Once-useful cell counts need to be viewed with caution, as the indications for surgical exploration after abdominal trauma have changed, and many injuries are managed nonoperatively.

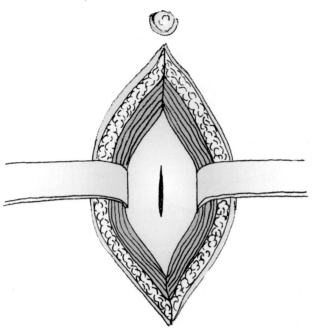

FIGURE 16.6. Open technique for peritoneal lavage catheter insertion with direct visualization and incision of the abdominal fascia.

• Infusing the lavage fluid but being unable to retrieve it is not uncommon. Slight repositioning of the catheter may help.

CRICOTHYROIDOTOMY

Indications

Cricothyroidotomy is a real emergency and reserved for those patients who cannot be intubated orally or nasally or have lost

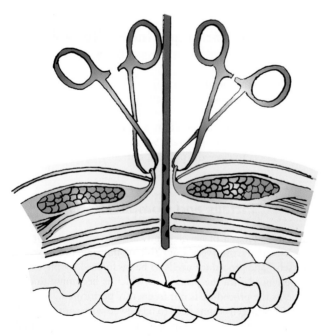

FIGURE 16.7. Insertion of the peritoneal lavage catheter under direct vision.

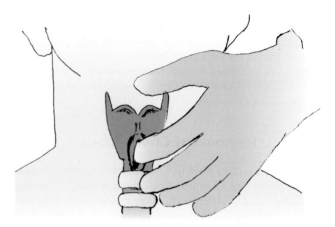

FIGURE 16.8. Digital identification of the cricothyroid space.

a pre-existing oral airway and are desaturating. It would be a mistake to attempt a tracheostomy in such patients, as this consumes considerably more time. Because the cricothyroid space is superficial in relationship to the skin, it should be selected as the easiest point—even if suboptimal—for insertion of a life-saving airway.

Open Cricothyroidotomy

• A **vertical incision** is placed above the cricothyroid space. Compared to a horizontal incision, this incision decreases the likelihood of bleeding from injury to the anterior jugular veins
• After sharp incision of any soft tissue between the skin and cricoid cartilage, the cricothyroid space is identified by **palpation** (Fig. 16.8). Any bleeding at this point is ignored, as the sheer goal is to establish an airway as soon as possible.
• A pointed clamp is introduced through the cricothyroid membrane and opened to dilate the space (Fig. 16.9). Experienced surgeons can use the scalpel to incise the membrane, although the risk exists for injuring the cartilage or posterior wall. The thyroid cartilage is immobilized and pulled upward and anteriorly with a tracheostomy hook. The **tracheostomy hook** is essential for this procedure. A No. 4 tracheostomy tube is introduced. If the space is wide, a No. 6 tube is preferable. The bleeding is controlled by sutures, electrocoagulation, or pressure.

Percutaneous Cricothyroidotomy

• A vertical incision is made. A hollow needle is introduced through the cricothyroid space and a guidewire is introduced through the needle (Figs. 16.10 through 16.12), which is then removed.
• Dilation of the trachea takes place over the guidewire by introducing a dilator (Fig. 16.13). Finally, a No. 4 tracheostomy tube is placed over a guiding dilator and the guidewire. The dilator and guidewire are removed, and the tube is left in place and secured to the skin.

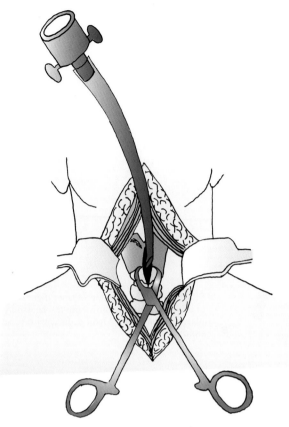

FIGURE 16.9. Dilatation of the cricothyroid membrane and insertion of the tracheostomy tube.

Pitfalls and Complications

- Cricothyroidotomy can become a **challenging procedure**, as the pressure to establish an airway in a dying patient is great. Blood can obscure the field and create additional difficulty.
- **Incorrect identification of the cricothyroid space** and placement of the incision above the thyroid cartilage are possible.
- **Inadequate opening** of the cricothyroid membrane and loss of valuable minutes while trying to insert the tracheostomy tube through a very narrow opening is not uncommon.

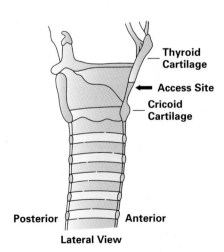

FIGURE 16.10. Access site for cricothyroidotomy (lateral view). (From Cook Medical, Inc., with permission.)

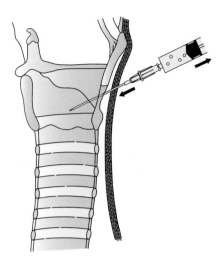

FIGURE 16.11. Localization of the cricothyroid space and placement of catheter (lateral view). (From Cook Medical, Inc., with permission.)

- **Injury** of the thyroid and cricoid cartilage, vocal cords, or posterior tracheal wall and esophagus are additional intraoperative complications.
- There is controversy about the need to **convert** the cricothyroidotomy to a tracheostomy at a later stage. Previous standard teaching recommended that a tracheostomy should be performed because cricothyroidotomy is associated with a higher degree of tracheal stenosis if left in place for a long time, but studies vary in results.

PERCUTANEOUS TRACHEOSTOMY

- The neck is **hyperextended** by placing a pillow under the patient's shoulder (except in patients with spinal precautions).
- After preparation of the neck, the site of incision is selected to be in the middle between the cricoid cartilage and sternal notch, which corresponds to the **second or third tracheal cartilage**.

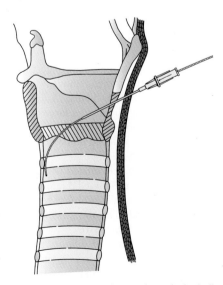

FIGURE 16.12. Insertion of guidewire through the hollow catheter (lateral view). (From Cook Medical, Inc., with permission.)

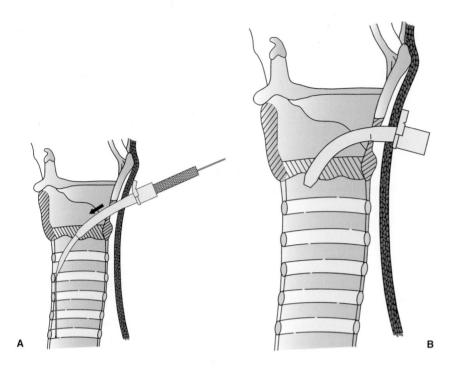

A   **B**

FIGURE 16.13. Dilation of tract (figure A, lateral view). Figure B shows the tracheostomy in place. (From Cook Medical, Inc., with permission.)

- The procedure is performed under **bronchoscopic guidance.** The bronchoscope is introduced through the orotracheal tube, and the tube is pulled to the level immediately below the vocal cords (usually at approximately 16 cm at the lip). A common error is not withdrawing the tube far enough, leading to impalement of the orotracheal tube by the introductory needle.
- A 2- to 3-cm **vertical incision** is placed, and the subcutaneous tissue and pretracheal muscles are bluntly dissected until the trachea is palpated
- A sheathed needle connected to a fluid-filled syringe is introduced. **Aspiration of bubbles into the syringe** indicates entry into the trachea, also confirmed by the bronchoscope. The needle is pushed in 2 mm farther, as the sheath is shorter than the needle. The needle and syringe are removed, and the sheath remains in place. The syringe is placed back on the sheath and **air reaspirated** to confirm that the sheath remains in the airway and has not dislodged during removal of the needle (a **crucial step**).
- A J-tipped **guidewire** is introduced through the sheath into the trachea, and the sheath is then removed (Fig. 16.14). The tract is dilated by a short firm dilator. A thin **guiding tube** is threaded over the guidewire, then a **large curved dilator** is fed over a guiding tube and the guidewire (Fig. 16.15). The large curved dilator has a **mark** to guide how deep it should be inserted into the airway.
- Now the trachea is adequately dilated to accommodate the tracheostomy tube. The large curved dilator is removed, and the tracheostomy tube (usually a Shiley No. 8) is fed over a No. 28 Fr dilator, guided by the guidewire/guiding tube complex into the trachea (Fig. 16.16).
- The kit contains several sizes of dilators to accommodate different-caliber tracheostomy tubes. A **single cannula tracheostomy tube** will have the same internal diameter as a double cannula tube but a smaller external diameter, making it easier for insertion.

- All these steps are visualized through the bronchoscope although during insertion of the main dilator, the force required to push the dilator may temporarily collapse the trachea for several seconds with poor visualization through the bronchoscope.
- Finally, the guidewire, guiding tube, and curved dilator are removed, and the tracheostomy tube is left in place. The bronchoscope is withdrawn from the endotracheal tube (which remains in place) and inserted into the newly placed tracheostomy tube to **confirm correct placement by visualizing** the carina. The cuff of the tracheostomy tube is inflated, and the tube is connected to the ventilatory circuit.

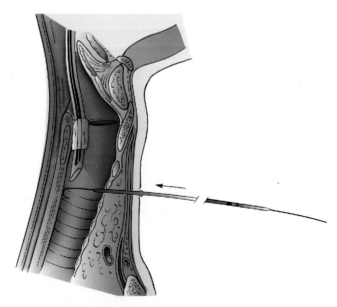

FIGURE 16.14. Insertion of guidewire and guiding catheter.

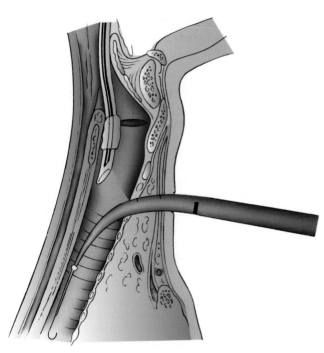

FIGURE 16.15. Dilation with the large progressive curved dilator.

Pitfalls and Complications

- **Loss of airway** is the most important concern. It can occur by unrecognized pretracheal or paratracheal placement of the dilators, which dilate the soft tissues instead of the trachea,

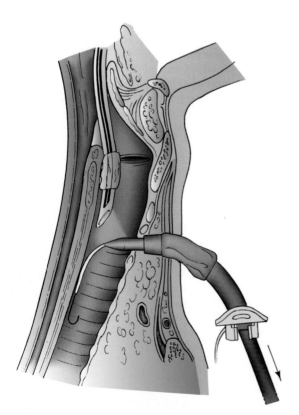

FIGURE 16.16. Insertion of the tracheostomy tube over a guiding dilator.

leading to placement of the tracheostomy tube outside of the trachea (usually the mediastinum).
- **Posterior tear** to the trachea and even the **esophagus** can occur. **Bronchoscopic guidance** is key to avoid placement of the tube in non-tracheal sites.
- **Bleeding** is usually not a problem. On occasion, however, injury to an anterior vessel or the thyroid may cause bleeding through the wound. In most cases, one needs to complete the procedure rapidly to prevent blood from draining into the airway and achieve hemostasis by compression of the tracheostomy tube against the track. It is very rare that bleeding will persist. Anterior veins may easily be suture ligated as well.
- A common error is not withdrawing the endotracheal tube far enough, leading to impalement of the tube/cuff (or even the bronchoscope) with the finder needle (see preceding).

PERCUTANEOUS GASTROSTOMY

A gastrostomy is required for patients who cannot be fed through the mouth because of inability to swallow, prolonged intubation, obstructing lesions of the pharynx or esophagus, or extensive neck operations.
- The procedure starts with an esophagogastroscopy and insufflation of the stomach, so that it opposes the anterior abdominal wall. An appropriate site of placement is selected by applying digital pressure on the skin, which is seen through the gastroscope as an indentation to the stomach. **Transillumination through the abdominal wall** should also be possible at the selected site of placement. This area is infiltrated with local anesthesia.
- A long needle covered by a plastic sheath is introduced through the skin and abdominal muscles into the stomach (Fig. 16.17). The needle is withdrawn and the plastic sheath left in place. A snare is introduced through the appropriate port of the gastroscope. A guidewire is placed in the stomach

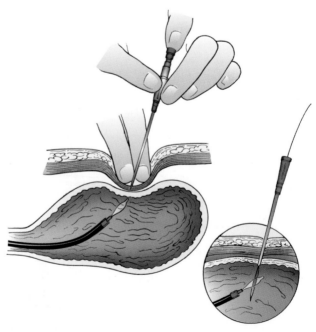

FIGURE 16.17. Insertion of needle into the stomach under endoscopic guidance.

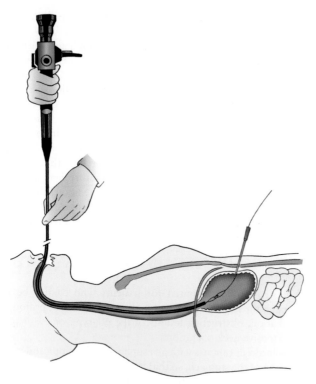

FIGURE 16.18. Guidewire snared and pulled with gastroscope through mouth.

through the plastic sheath and grasped by the snare (Fig. 16.18). The gastroscope, snare, and guidewire are withdrawn out of the mouth.

- The guidewire at the oral end is tied to the tip of a percutaneous gastrostomy tube. A 2-cm incision is made on the skin of the abdomen at the site of guidewire entry, and the guidewire is pulled from the abdominal side. In this way, the gastrostomy tube is pulled back into the mouth and, through the esophagus and stomach, out through the abdominal wall (Fig. 16.19). The gastroscope is reintroduced into the stomach and confirms correct placement of the tube. The tube

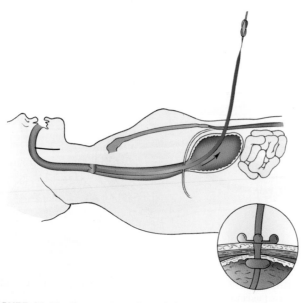

FIGURE 16.19. Gastrostomy tube pulled through stomach.

is secured by placing a flange and suturing it to the skin. It can be used within 6 hours for medication and 12 hours for feeds.

Pitfalls and Complications

- It is necessary to confirm that there are no vessels and no intervening hollow viscera (such as the colon) **between the stomach and anterior abdominal wall.** The indentation created by digital pressure should be clearly evident by the gastroscope, and transillumination at that site should be clear.
- **Infection of the wound** should be recognized early and can be avoided with strict sterile technique. Usually, the tube does not need to be removed. The infection is treated by opening the wound and administering antibiotics.
- **Tube dislodgement** may occur either if the stomach is under tension (e.g., on a patient with hiatal hernia or with adhesions) or because the tube was not secured adequately and was inadvertently pulled. Both complications are usually preventable and should be avoided by recognizing that the anatomy is not favorable for a gastrostomy or suturing the gastrostomy tube adequately to the skin. Early tube dislodgement may lead to extravasation of gastric contents and **peritonitis.**

ABDOMINAL PRESSURE MONITORING

Abdominal hypertension, the elevation of pressure in the abdominal cavity due to bleeding or visceral swelling, leads to compromise of cardiac output, tissue perfusion, and ventilation, all eventually resulting in death if untreated. Intra-abdominal pressures below 10 cm H_2O are considered normal, 10 to 15 acceptable for postoperative patients, 15 to 20 worrisome and possibly in need of action, and more than 20 is cause for decompression in most cases. Bladder pressures are widely used to reflect intra-abdominal pressures, as intraperitoneal pressure is transmitted on the bladder wall.

- Patients must have a Foley catheter decompressing the bladder. With the patient lying flat and under aseptic technique, a three-way stopcock is connected to a syringe and pressure monitor. Fifty to 100 mL of saline are injected into the bladder, and the stopcock is opened toward the pressure monitor. It is important to level the monitor in advance, so that the 0 mark corresponds to the level of the pubic symphysis.
- An easy and simple technique that does not require any instruments is the U-tube technique. The Foley catheter is elevated while allowing a U-loop to form. If there is not enough urine in the tube, saline needs to be injected. The column of urine or injected fluid that forms is measured between the pubic symphysis and meniscus (Fig. 16.20).
- There are several systems on the market that allow continuous measurement of pressures without interrupting the continuity of the Foley circuit and therefore decreasing the risk of urinary infection.

Pitfalls and Complications

- The most dangerous pitfall is the exclusive reliance on bladder pressure measurements. **Clinical examination** should always

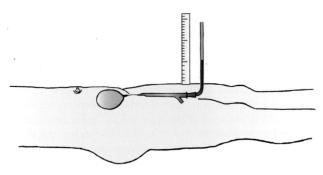

FIGURE 16.20. Measurement of intra-abdominal pressure using column of urine/water in the Foley catheter tubing.

be the principal reason for continued observation or immediate decompression. Bladder pressure measurements should support only the clinical diagnosis.

PERICARDIOCENTESIS

The pericardial space can accommodate large volumes of fluid if accumulation occurs over a long period of time, whereas **cardiac tamponade** develops with even small quantities of fluid if occurring abruptly. Pericardiocentesis is indicated to treat tamponade or diagnose the nature of chronic fluid. The latter is performed under ultrasonographic guidance. The former will be described later, although pericardiocentesis for traumatic tamponade **is rarely useful.** Unless the patient is in a remote area with difficult access to a trauma center, pericardiocentesis is not indicated; rapid **sternotomy** and control of the bleeding is the treatment of choice.

- With the patient supine, a standard pericardiocentesis kit or, in true emergencies, a central line kit can be used. A hollow needle is inserted approximately **1 cm below the costal margin** and slightly to the left of the midline. The direction is **toward the left shoulder.** The needle is advanced slowly under the rib (Fig. 16.21). Electrocardiographic monitoring

is possible by attaching an alligator clip to the needle. **ST-segment elevations** indicate contact of the needle with the epicardium. Aspiration of fluid or blood obviously indicates that the needle is in the pericardial sac. Aspiration of blood relieves the pericardial tamponade, and a guidewire is inserted through the needle. Using a Seldinger technique, a catheter is inserted and used to withdraw further fluid or blood over time, if needed. With wide availability of portable **ultrasound machines,** emergent tapping of pericardial space may be safer than the "blind" technique previously used.

Pitfalls and Complications

- Pericardiocentesis is a potentially **dangerous** technique if performed blindly. When performed under emergency situations for presumed cardiac tamponade, there is risk of **injuring the heart,** particularly if the clinical diagnosis of tamponade is not correct and the space between the pericardium and epicardium is very narrow. Additionally, misplacement of the needle—most typically under the heart—is not unusual. As mentioned previously, blind pericardiocentesis for traumatic injury purposes has been nearly abandoned in urban hospital settings.
- When performed using radiologic guidance for stable conditions, little risk if involved.

PERCUTANEOUS INFERIOR VENA CAVA FILTER PLACEMENT

- **Absolute indications** for filter placement are recurrent pulmonary embolism despite anticoagulation, contraindications to anticoagulation in the presence of pulmonary embolism or proximal deep venous thrombosis, and complications of anticoagulation prompting its cessation.
- **Relative indications** include polytrauma patients at high risk for venous thromboembolism, critically ill patients with

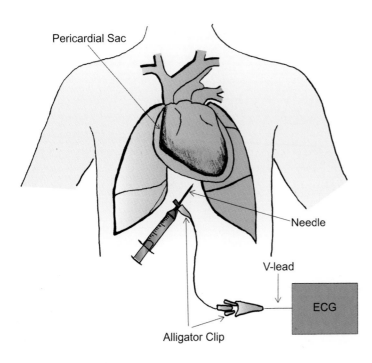

FIGURE 16.21. Technique of pericardiocentesis.

tenuous respiratory status in whom even a small pulmonary embolism may prove detrimental, and large free-floating venous clot.

- Multiple types of permanent filters exist, although **removable filters** are used with increasing frequency. All devices are **magnetic resonance imaging–compatible.** Two techniques are dominant in performing filter insertion at the bedside and will be described further: the fluoroscopy-guided and the endovascular ultrasound-guided techniques.

Fluoroscopy Guided

- After a screening duplex ultrasound is performed to examine for femoral venous clots, portable fluoroscopy is used to define the **L2–4 lumbar** region. The site of venous access is selected—typically the left or right **femoral vein**—and venous cannulation is performed using a Seldinger technique. A No. 4 or No. 5 Fr angiographic catheter is advanced over a guidewire into the inferior vena cava and up to the second lumbar vertebra.
- **Contrast material is injected,** and the cava is imaged to delineate its anatomy and size. In particular, **the renal veins** are defined as the landmark for which the filter should be placed **below.**
- The pigtail catheter is exchanged for the **sheath,** which is inserted over a dilator. The sheath is positioned **caudad to the renal veins,** and the filter carrier system is advanced into the sheath. The filter is then deployed, completion venography is performed, and the sheath is withdrawn

Intravascular Ultrasound Guided

- Insertion is usually performed through a **right femoral vein** approach. A micropuncture is made in the vein using a No. 4 Fr catheter, and a 0.035 wire is introduced.
- A No. 8 Fr sheath is inserted into the inferior vena cava, and the intravascular ultrasonographic (In-Vision Gold, Volcano Corp, Rancho Cordova, CA) is advanced over the wire through the iliac venous system up to the level of the **right**

atrium. Then, it is slowly withdrawn to evaluate the inferior vena cava in a retrograde fashion. The **right renal artery and bilateral veins** are visualized, and the maximum diameter of the vena cava is measured.

- After a **second puncture** in the right common femoral vein, the delivery sheath for a vena cava filter (VCF) is introduced over a 0.035 guidewire. The sheath and then the VCF are advanced to the level of the renal veins. Deployment is performed under **direct** intravascular ultrasonographic **visualization.** Confirmation of correct placement below the renal and above the iliac veins is established ultrasonographically.
- A postinsertion plain radiograph is routinely performed to verify correct placement at the L2–4 level. This technique is valuable in patients at risk for renal failure due to avoidance of radiocontrast dye.

Pitfalls and Complications

- Complications of venous access include bleeding, hematoma, arteriovenous fistula, hemopneumothorax, and cardiac dysrhythmias.
- Misplacement outside the inferior vena cava (IVC) at an incorrect location has been reported to be as high as 4.6%. Locations for filter misplacement include renal veins, gonadal veins, or unintended suprarenal placement.
- Insertion-site venous thrombosis and vena cava occlusion are potential complications of filters. Access via the internal jugular or subclavian vein results in a lower incidence of thrombosis when compared to femoral access. Caval thrombosis rates do not appear to vary significantly among the available filters.
- Pulmonary embolism in the presence of an IVC filter has been reported in 3% to 7% of patients after filter placement.
- Guidewire entrapment may occur during placement of central venous and pulmonary artery catheters and during catheter exchanges. Attempts at removal of an entrapped item can lead to filter displacement and vessel damage when excessive force is applied. Straight guidewires should be used for all new central venous catheters in patients with indwelling IVC filters.

CHAPTER 17 ■ FLUIDS AND ELECTROLYTES

GENERAL COMMENTS

- In an average person without extremes of weight, approximately **60% of total body weight is water.** Of this total body water, two-thirds (40% of total body weight) is in the **intracellular** *fluid* (ICF) space, and one-third (20% of total body weight) is outside the cells (i.e., **extracellular fluid space** [ECF]).
- Extracellular volume is divided into **intravascular space and interstitial fluid** (5% and 15% of total body weight, respectively). The intravascular space contains **plasma volume** that is the most mobile fluid compartment and the first to be released to areas of injury and the first to be repleted through intravenous infusion. Also in the intravascular space are **red cells. Red cell volume plus plasma volume comprise the blood volume (BV),** which is estimated to be 7% of the total body weight. In a 70-kg person, total body water is 42 L (60% × 70 kg), circulating BV is 4.9 L (7% × 70 kg), ICF is 28 L (40% × 70 kg), and ECF is 14 L (20% × 70 kg). The percentage of weight used will vary depending on deviation from ideal body weight and gender.
- Maintaining BV or "**effective circulating** *BV*" is an important part of resuscitation, as BV consists of red cells (carrying O_2) and plasma (carrying glucose), which supply fuel and oxygen to the cells to synthesize adenosine triphosphate **(ATP).**
- Water is **freely permeable** between body compartments and migrates to areas of higher solutes, but this **takes time.** Therefore, **chronic hypotonic losses** with ability to "borrow" from ICF (approximately 28L in a 70-kg person) are better tolerated than **acute isotonic losses,** which have only the ECF (approximately 14 L in a 70-kg person) to borrow from.
- **Osmolality** (tonicity) defined as number of particles in solution is normally 280 to 300 mOsm/L in the serum.
- The **ICF concentration of solutes** is vastly **different from** that of the *ECF,* and approximately 80% of ATP generated is used to maintain this gradient. Some of the ECF cations (in mEq/L) are as follows: sodium (Na^+), 142; potassium (K^+), 4; calcium (Ca^{++}), 5; and magnesium (Mg^{++}), 3. The ICF cations (in mEq/L) are: K^+, 150; Mg^{++}, 40; and Na^+, 10. Some of the ECF anions (in mEq/L) are chloride (Cl^-), 103; and bicarbonate (HCO_3^-), 27. The major ICF anions (in mEq/L) are phosphates, 107; proteins, 40; and sulfates, 43.
- This difference in ICF and ECF electrolyte composition explains the clinical observations regarding electrolyte **shifts between ECF and ICF.** This explains why large amounts of certain electrolytes are needed to replete small deficiencies in the serum (ECF) if the ICF stores are depleted. One of our limitations is the inability to assess ICF electrolyte composition easily at the bedside.

- Because water is freely permeable, the osmolality of all body compartments should be the same but, in reality, the protein concentration in the plasma to interstitial fluid is 16:1, generating an **oncotic pressure difference** between the two compartments.
- **Starling forces** describe **net fluid flux** between **intravascular space** and the **interstitium:**

$$Q = Kf\{(Pc - Pi) - \sigma(\pi c - \pi i)\},$$

where Q is the net fluid flux (mL/min), (Pc – Pt) is hydrostatic pressure difference between capillary (c) and interstitium (i), and ($\pi c - \pi i$) is the oncotic pressure difference between the capillary and interstitium. Kf is the filtration coefficient for that membrane (mL/min/mm Hg), and is the product of capillary surface area and capillary hydraulic conductance, and σ is the permeability factor (i.e. reflection coefficient), with "one" being impermeable and "zero" being completely permeable.

- The **permeability factor** explains why, in times of capillary leak as in shock states, colloids cannot maintain an oncotic pressure difference and tend to leak out into the interstitium.
- The general principle of **fluid resuscitation** is that intravascular hypovolemia should be replaced with **isotonic fluid,** which tends to distribute in the ECF (3:1) intravascular:interstitium. Hypotonic fluid will distribute between all body compartments with only a small amount remaining in the intravascular space (as water is freely permeable).
- Frequently used **isotonic solutions** are 0.9% **normal saline,** which contains 154 mEq/L of Na^+ and Cl^- each, and **lactated Ringer** solution that contains 130 mEq/L Na^+, 109 mEq/L Cl^-, 4 mEq/L K^+, 3 mEq/L Ca^{2+}, 28 mEq/L lactate.
- The **end point of fluid resuscitation** continues to be an area of great debate, as direct measurement of intravascular (plasma) volume is not the norm. Surrogate markers are used to assess adequate fluid resuscitation: blood pressure, heart rate, urine output, and parameters of perfusion and cardiac function. Although every clinician wants to treat patients to "**euvolemia,**" there are only a few centers measuring intravascular volume using **radioisotope studies** and **measuring plasma volume.** Debates will continue on how much fluid to give until an easy method of measuring intravascular volume is available.

REGULATION OF WATER BALANCE

- ECF **tonicity** is generally reflected in the concentration of **sodium** in the serum. The serum sodium (Na_{pl}) is proportional to the total body exchangeable sodium (Na_e) plus the total body exchangeable potassium (K_e): $\{(Na_e + K_e)/(\text{total body water})\} \propto Na_{pl.}$

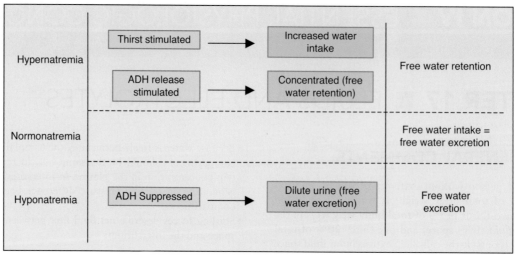

ADH = anti-diuretic hormone

FIGURE 17.1. Water intake and excretion regulation. ADH, antidiuretic hormone.

- This equation illustrates the **relationship** between **total body solutes and total body water.** Decreases in potassium often accompany hyponatremia, and replacement of intracelllular solute losses can also be an important part of treating hyponatremia.
- As water intake and excretion are tightly regulated to maintain near-constant plasma osmolality (Fig. 17.1), disturbances in serum sodium indicate **disorders in water balance, not** gains or loss of **sodium.** This is a **crucial point in understanding dysnatremias**
- The actions of **antidiuretic hormone (ADH),** also called arginine vasopressin, on the kidney tightly regulates water excretion. To maintain water balance, an **intact thirst mechanism** and the ability of the kidneys to **vary urinary concentration** are required.

RENAL WATER HANDLING

- In the absence of ADH activity (as **in diabetes insipidus**), **urine concentration** will remain very low (**50–80 mOsm/kg**). When

TABLE 17.1

STATES OF IMPAIRED WATER EXCRETION IN THE INTENSIVE CARE UNIT RESULTING IN HYPONATREMIA

Volume-depleted states
Volume depletion
Diuretics

Normal-volume states
Syndrome of inappropriate antidiuretic hormone (SIADH)
Pain
Postoperative state
Nausea
Hypothyroidism

Volume-expanded states
Congestive heart failure
Renal failure
Cirrhosis

ADH activity is maximal, urinary concentration can be as high as **1,200 mOsm/kg.** This ability to excrete very dilute or a very concentrated urine allows the body to achieve water balance across a very wide range of water intake (between approximately **0.8 L/day** and **15 L/day**).
- Administration of water to a patient with **impaired water excretion** (Table 17.1) can lead to hyponatremia.

Electrolyte Free Water

- **Electrolyte free water** is a conceptual volume of a body fluid (usually urine) that represents the volume of that fluid that would be required to dilute the electrolytes contained within total volume of the fluid to the same tonicity as plasma electrolytes.
- The remainder of the volume (total volume minus electrolyte free water) can be thought of as containing the **nonelectrolyte osmoles.** This nonelectrolyte water excretion is the amount of water excreted above the excretion of electrolyte solutes, and thus, if it is not replaced, will have an effect on the plasma sodium concentration. In other words, the osmolality of a solution is not important in determining whether it contains "free water"; rather, it is the **concentration of electrolytes that is important.**
- An important concept is **urine electrolytes** and *not* the **urine osmolality** determine the **degree of free water excretion** in the urine. If the concentration of electrolytes in the urine is greater than the concentration of electrolytes in the plasma, free water is not being excreted in the urine. If the concentration of electrolytes in the urine is less than that in the plasma, the patient is excreting free water in the urine. This relationship is illustrated in Figure 17.2.

SODIUM

Hyponatremia

- Hyponatremia commonly occurs in hospital settings. Often the condition is asymptomatic, but **hyponatremic**

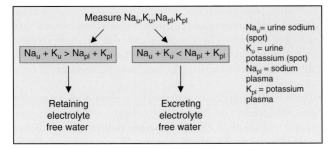

FIGURE 17.2. Relationship of electrolyte concentration in urine and plasma to the amount of free water excreted.

encephalopathy (brain dysfunction due to cerebral edema) can result in a life-threatening emergency.

- Risk factors for life-threatening hyponatremia are **female gender of premenopausal age, children, and hypoxia.**
- Hyponatremia is defined as **serum sodium of <135 mEq/L.** The ability of the kidney to dilute the urine and thus excrete free water is the body's primary defense against the development of hyponatremia.
- **Excess ingestion of water** as the sole cause of hyponatremia is **rare,** as the typical adult with normal renal function can excrete a massive free water load (15 L of free water per day).
- The combination of factors necessary for the development of hyponatremia are **free water intake** in the setting of an underlying condition that impairs free water excretion (see Table 17.1).
- The states that impair water excretion are usually states where **ADH release** is a physiologic response to a stimulus such as **volume depletion, pain, nausea, postoperative state, or congestive heart failure** (due to decreased circulating blood volume). Pathologic release of ADH occurs in syndrome of inappropriate ADH release (syndrome of inappropriate antidiuretic hormone [**SIADH**]) and with certain medications such as **thiazide diuretics and anticonvulsants.**

Clinical Manifestations of Hyponatremia

- **Hyponatremic encephalopathy** is the clinical term for symptomatic cerebral edema secondary to hyponatremia, and this condition can have a fulminant presentation. Early signs are usually nonspecific—**nausea, vomiting, headaches**—often go unrecognized, and are thought to be due to cerebral edema. When pressure is exerted on the skull by the brain, **seizures** may occur and, if uncorrected, brainstem **herniation** with respiratory failure and death will follow.

Risk Factors for Hyponatremic Encephalopathy

- The **time to development** of hyponatremia (i.e., acute versus chronic) has been presumed to be an important risk factor in determining severity of symptoms, but there is disparity in patient outcomes even when the time to development of hyponatremia is similar.
- There are **three major risk factors** for poor outcomes after hyponatremic encephalopathy: **female of premenopausal age, hypoxia** at disease presentation, **younger age,** and **children** (high brain–to–cranial vault ratio).

Approach to a Hyponatremic Patient

- The first step in working up the *hyponatremic* patient is to exclude hyperosmolar hyponatremia (Fig. 17.3). An osmot-

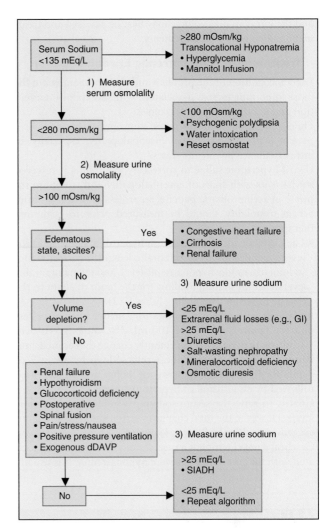

FIGURE 17.3. Diagnostic approach to hyponatremia. DDAVP, desmopressin; GI, gastrointestinal; SIADH, syndrome of inappropriate antidiuretic hormone.

ically active substance that is confined to the extracellular fluid (usually glucose or mannitol) will remove water from the intracellular space and will dilute the serum sodium concentration (**translocational hyponatremia**).

- To correct for hyperglycemia, 1.6 mEq of Na^+/L is added for every 100 mg/dL increase of the serum glucose above 100 mg/dL.
- **Pseudohyponatremia** may occur due to hyperproteinemia and hyperlipidemia when samples are diluted prior to measurement of the serum sodium. If a **potentiometric method** is used, this is not a concern. In pseudohyponatremia, the measured serum osmolality will be normal.
- After assessment of osmolality, the remainder of the diagnostic approach is based on the **history, urinary electrolytes, and clinical assessment** of the patient's **intravascular volume** status.
- Physical examination can be **unreliable** in the clinical assessment of volume status and thus should be interpreted with caution (see Fig. 17.3). A difficult group of patients to assess are those with **total body fluid excess** (with edema, weight gain) due to shock and loss of fluid into the interstitial space but who are **intravascular volume-depleted.** Despite edema, they would be categorized as the "volume depletion" group,

and the intravascular volume may best be assessed and treatment guided by **BV** measurements.

Treatment of Hyponatremic Encephalopathy

- **Early recognition** of the problem and prompt therapy are the most important factors associated with successful intervention and good neurologic outcomes.
- Fluid restriction alone is never appropriate to manage a patient with hyponatremic encephalopathy, **especially in intravascular hypovolemic states.**
- Use of **hypertonic saline** to correct hyponatremia is reserved for patients with signs of encephalopathy and is not appropriate in asymptomatic patients regardless of serum sodium. **Serum osmolality** should be measured prior to beginning therapy.
  - The rationale for treatment with **hypertonic saline** is (a) for severe manifestations of cerebral edema, (b) correct serum sodium to a mildly hyponatremic level, and (c) maintain this level of serum sodium to allow for the brain to adapt to the change in serum osmolality (Table 17.2).
- In patients with severe manifestations (**active seizures or respiratory failure**), a **bolus** of 100 mL 3% saline (given over 10 minutes) can be given to promptly change the serum osmolality. The goal is to raise the serum sodium by about 2 to 4 mEq/L. If symptoms persist, the bolus may be **repeated** followed by an infusion of hypertonic saline.
- Goal is to raise the serum sodium to mildly hyponatremic levels. However, the total change in serum sodium should not exceed **15 to 20 mEq/L over 48 hours.**
- **Cerebral demyelination** is a rare, serious complication associated with the correction of severe hyponatremia. It is usually

a **delayed phenomenon** occurring days to weeks after correction of hyponatremia and can manifest as a **pseudocoma** with a locked-in stare. This condition can also be asymptomatic and **magnetic resonance imaging** (which is sensitive for the detection of demyelinating lesions) may be necessary for the diagnosis.
- The rate of correction of serum sodium alone does not predict the development of cerebral demyelination. What is important is the **absolute change in serum sodium over 48 hours exceeding 15 to 20 mEq/L** and overly aggressive correction to **normonatremic** levels. **Liver disease** and **hypoxia** increase the risk of demyelination, and care must be exercised in these groups.
- The serum sodium should never be corrected to **normonatremic** levels for a **few days** after hyponatremic encephalopathy. This allows the patient to adjust to the new plasma tonicity.
- In patients with **impaired cardiac output** in whom pulmonary edema may develop with vigorous volume expansion, intravenous **furosemide** should be given in addition to hypertonic saline to prevent volume overload.

Hypernatremia

- Hypernatremia, a serum sodium >145 mEq/L is commonly encountered. **Thirst** is a powerful protective mechanism and, therefore, **restricted access to water** is nearly always necessary for the development of hypernatremia.
- In critically ill patients, usually there is a combination of **impaired access to water** and **ongoing free water losses** (Fig. 17.4).
- A detailed history focusing on **fluid intake and losses** and an estimate of the patients intravascular volume is the first step in the evaluation. Sources of water losses are in the **urine**, from the **gastrointestinal tract** (diarrhea and nasogastric suction), and **insensible losses** (fever, sepsis, massive diaphoresis, burns).
- The urine osmolality alone cannot be used to determine whether there is free water loss in the urine. This is because water is excreted with **nonelectrolyte osmoles** (which under physiologic conditions is typically **urea**) and with electrolyte osmoles. Both contribute to the osmolality of the urine but have differential effects on water balance. Water that is excreted with nonelectrolyte osmoles is water that is lost in excess of electrolyte loss. Therefore, **loss of water** with the **nonelectrolyte osmoles will raise the serum sodium.** Water that is excreted with electrolyte osmoles will not affect the serum sodium (as long as the concentration of electrolytes in the urine and serum are similar).
- Failure to concentrate the urine in the face of hypernatremia should raise suspicion of a **urinary concentrating defect.** Renal failure, loop diuretics, tubulointerstitial renal disease, and diabetes insipidus are the main causes of urinary concentrating defects.
- During hypernatremic states, the brain is subject to osmolar stress that favors the movement of water out of the brain and can lead to significant **brain damage.**

Central Diabetes Insipidus

- **Central diabetes insipidus** (CDI) is most commonly in the setting of head injury, pituitary surgery, and cerebral

---

TABLE 17.2

TREATMENT OF HYPONATREMIA

High-risk groups for poor outcomes
Menstruant females
Children
Hypoxic patients

Hyponatremic encephalopathy with evidence of severe cerebral edema (active seizures, respiratory arrest)
- –Bolus, 100 mL of 3% NaCl over 10 min
- –Can repeat bolus 1–2 times with the goal of increasing serum sodium 2–4 mEq/L or until clinical improvement
- –Begin infusion as for hyponatremic encephalopathy

Hyponatremic encephalopathy (seizures, decreased mental status, headache, nausea, vomiting)
- –Infuse 3% NaCl at a rate of 1 mL/kg/h. ICU setting using infusion pump
- –Check serum sodium every 2 hours until symptom-free
- –Stop hypertonic saline when patient is symptom-free or serum sodium has increased by 15–20 mEq/L *in the initial 48 hours of therapy*

Asymptomatic hyponatremia
- –Fluid restriction unless hypovolemia is suspected
- –Demeclocycline
- –Vasopressin V_2 receptor antagonists

From Ayus JC, Krothapalli RK, Arieff AI. Treatment of symptomatic hyponatremia and its relation to brain damage. A prospective study. *N Engl J Med.* 1987;317(19):1190–1195.

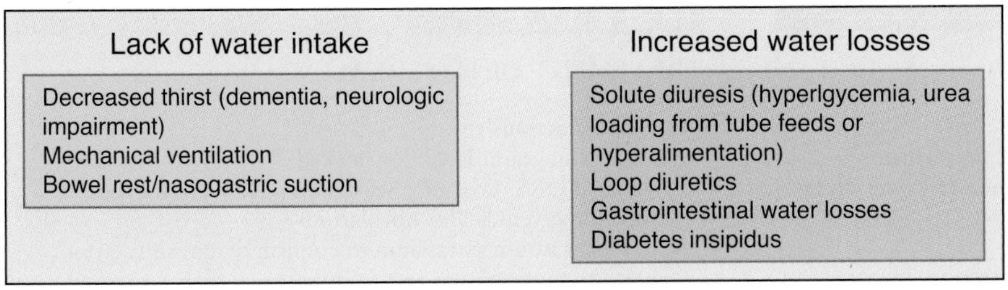

Lack of water intake	Increased water losses
Decreased thirst (dementia, neurologic impairment) Mechanical ventilation Bowel rest/nasogastric suction	Solute diuresis (hyperlgycemia, urea loading from tube feeds or hyperalimentation) Loop diuretics Gastrointestinal water losses Diabetes insipidus

FIGURE 17.4. Common causes of hypernatremia in the intensive care unit.

hemorrhages. Urine is not concentrated in the setting of hypernatremia. In general, the plasma osmolality exceeds the urine osmolality.

- A simple and reliable clinical test that can be used to distinguish **CDI** from **nephrogenic diabetes insipidus** is to administer a V$_2$ receptor agonist, such as DDAVP. A **50% increase in urine osmolality** after DDAVP administration strongly suggests CDI. Once the diagnosis is established, DDAVP can be given either subcutaneously or intranasally with close monitoring of water intake to avoid hyponatremia, and monitoring of electrolytes.

Treatment of Hypernatremia

- The goal of treatment is to achieve **normal circulatory volume** as patients typically have circulatory volume depletion, and then to correct the serum sodium with free water replacement (Table 17.3). **Oral hydration** is preferable to parenteral and should be used in patients with functional gastrointestinal tract.
- It is also possible to be **hypernatremic** and **hypervolemic,** in which case sodium should be withheld and patient allowed to be in negative fluid balance.
- In hypernatremic states, **insulin resistance** has also been observed leading to severe hyperglycemia and potential worsening of hyperosmolality.
- In patients without evidence of hypernatremic encephalopathy, the serum sodium should not be corrected more quickly than **15 mEq/24 hours.** In severe cases (>170 mEq/L), sodium

TABLE 17.3

TREATMENT OF HYPERNATREMIA

1. Replete intravascular volume with colloid solution, isotonic saline, or plasma
2. Estimate water deficit. Deficit should be replaced over 48–72 hours, aiming for a correction of 1 mOsm/L/hour. In severe hypernatremia (>170 mEq/L), serum sodium should not be corrected to below 150 mEq/L in the first 48–72 hours. Replacement of ongoing water losses are given in addition to the deficit
3. Hypotonic fluid should be used. Usual replacement fluid is 77 mEq/L (0.45 N saline). A lower sodium concentration may be needed if there is a renal concentrating defect or sodium overload. Glucose-containing solutions should be avoided, and an oral route of administration should be used
4. Monitor plasma; electrolytes should be monitored every 2 hours until patient is neurologically stable

Reproduced from Medical Knowledge Self-assessment Program (MKSAP) 2006.

should not be corrected to below 150 mEq/L in the first 48 to 72 hours to prevent cerebral edema.

POTASSIUM

- Potassium is present mainly in the **intracellular space** (approximately 4,000 mEq of total body stores) and is sequestered in the intracellular space through the action of the Na$^+$/K$^+$ ATPase pump.
- The serum potassium level is **tightly regulated** so that the potential differences across membranes, especially cardiac, are not affected by alterations in potassium level.
- The major influences that favor potassium movement **into cells** are **insulin and** β_2-adrenergic stimulation.
- Metabolic **acidosis** favors potassium movement **out of cells** as H$^+$ is exchanged for K$^+$ when H$^+$ moves intracellularly. However, this may have less importance in settings where an organic anion is generated as a result of the acidosis (such as lactic acidosis) as the organic ions may also move intracellularly and thus negate the electrogenic stimulus for potassium to move out of the cell.
- There are two main determinants of **potassium excretion** of clinical significance: **flow of tubular filtrate** into the distal nephron and **secretion** of potassium into the electronegative filtrate through epithelial potassium channels.
- The effect of **aldosterone** with sodium retention is the most important influence increasing the action of ENaC and therefore **stimulates potassium excretion.**
- Medications such as **amiloride, triamterene, and trimethoprim** block ENaC and lead to decreased K$^+$ secretion and can lead to clinically important hyperkalemia.
- **Decrease in the rate of tubular flow** into the distal nephron stimulates the renin angiotensin system, which in turn stimulates release of aldosterone with increased **potassium excretion.**

Hyperkalemia

- Hyperkalemia occurs through several mechanisms: **shifting** of potassium from intracellular compartment to the extracellular fluid compartment or through total body excess (either **too much intake or too little excretion** from renal failure) (Table 17.4). Other causes for impaired renal excretion are adrenal insufficiency, type IV renal tubular acidosis (usually seen in diabetics).
- Chronic renal failure alone typically does not lead to hyperkalemia until the glomerular filtration rate (GFR) falls below approximately **15 mL/minute.**
- Medications are a very important risk factor for the development of hyperkalemia (Table 17.5).

TABLE 17.4

CAUSES OF HYPERKALEMIA

Assess for increased potassium intake
Low-sodium salt substitutes and potassium supplements
Assess for shift of potassium intracellular fluid to extracellular fluid
Metabolic acidosis
Tissue necrosis (rhabdomyolysis, bowel infarction, tumor lysis) or depolarization
Insulin deficiency
β_2-Blockade

Assess for reduced potassium excretion in urine
Renal failure
Low aldosterone action (Think drugs: especially heparin, cyclosporine, tacrolimus, ARB, ACE-I)
Decreased distal nephron flow rate

ARB, angiotensin receptor blockers; ACE-I, angiotensin-converting enzyme inhibitor.
From Medical Knowledge Self-assessment Program (MKSAP) 2006.

Management of Hyperkalemia

- The first step is to differentiate **life-threatening hyperkalemia** from less urgent cases and then to identify the diagnosis.
- The absolute levels of the potassium cannot be reliably used to determine if a life-threatening condition exists, and the effect of elevated potassium on the cardiac membrane must be determined through an **electrocardiogram.**
- The management of emergent hyperkalemia is detailed in Table 17.6. As a temporizing measure, **shifting of potassium intracellularly** with insulin or beta-agonists can be used until definitive removal therapy is instituted. If normal renal function is present, diuretics and intravenous saline can be used to remove potassium. Cation exchange resins can be used as an adjunctive therapy.
- In patients with renal failure, especially with oliguria, **emergency dialysis** is often necessary.
- Hyperkalemia not associated with electrocardiographic changes can sometimes be managed with discontinuation of

TABLE 17.5

MEDICATIONS THAT CAUSE HYPERKALEMIA

Drugs that interfere with potassium excretion
Interfere with renin–angiotensin–aldosterone axis:
ACE-I, ARB, aldosterone blockers, heparin (decrease aldosterone synthesis), beta-blockers (decrease renin release)
Interfere with tubular potassium handling
Potassium-sparing diuretics (amiloride, triamterene), trimethoprim, calcineurin inhibitors (cyclosporine, tacrolimus)

Drugs that shift potassium from intracellular fluid to extracellular
β_2-blockers, depolarizing paralytics (e.g., succinylcholine), digitalis

ACE-I, angiotensin-converting enzyme inhibitor; ARB, angiotensin receptor blockers.
From Medical Knowledge Self-assessment Program (MKSAP) 2006.

TABLE 17.6

TREATMENT OF HYPERKALEMIA

Immediate actions
Electrocardiogram: Look for peaked T waves, loss of p waves, widened QRS. Loss of p wave and widened QRS suggest impending ventricular fibrillation
Send repeat serum potassium to confirm diagnosis (do not wait for confirmatory test to initiate emergency therapy)

Hyperkalemia with electrocardiographic (ECG) changes
Stabilize cardiac membrane
—Intravenous (IV) calcium gluconate or chloride to stabilize cardiac membrane, may repeat in 5 min if ECG changes persist
—Place patient on cardiac monitoring
Shift potassium into cells
—IV insulin (with IV dextrose if necessary to prevent hypoglycemia)
—Albuterol, 10–20 mg by nebulization (caution in heart disease)
—IV $NaHCO_3$ may be of benefit

Potassium removal
—Dialysis
—Diuretics (with IV saline if patient is not volume overloaded) if renal function is normal
—Cation exchange resins (caution with decreased gastrointestinal motility as bowel necrosis can occur)

Hyperkalemia without electrocardiographic changes
—Remove offending agents
—Otherwise follow same therapy as above with dialysis, diuretics, and/or cation exchange resins.

the offending agent. Some medications causing hyperkalemia such as spironolactone can have a long half-life, and the effect can last for up to 1 to 2 weeks.

Hypokalemia

- Hypokalemia can occur either through **shifting** from ECF to ICF or through total body potassium **depletion** via gastrointestinal losses (distal to the stomach) or urinary losses (Table 17.7). It should be noted that gastric secretion contains only 10 mEq/L of K^+, but hypovolemia associated with vomiting/nasogastric (NG) suction stimulates aldosterone with sodium retention and potassium excretion.
- **Shifting of K^+** into the **intracellular compartment** is a normal physiologic process in response to **insulin** secretion after a meal. This avoids a dangerously high K^+ level as the total amount of K^+ contained within the extracellular space is quite low. β_2-**adrenergic stimulation** is another avenue for cellular uptake of potassium. This is clinically significant as β_2 agonists can be used to transiently treat hyperkalemia and possibly lead to hypokalemia in certain clinical settings.

Clinical Manifestations of Hypokalemia

- The effects of hypokalemia are related to the effect on **neuromuscular transmission** and **conduction in the heart.** A

COMMON CAUSES OF HYPOKALEMIA

Potassium shift into cells
Alkalosis, recovery from diabetic ketoacidosis, β_2-agonists,
  insulin
Gastrointestinal potassium losses
Vomiting, nasogastric suction, diarrhea
Renal potassium losses
Diuretics, hypomagnesemia, hyperaldosteronism, drugs
  (amphotericin B, cisplatin), proximal (type II) and distal
  (type I) renal tubular acidosis (RTA), Bartter and Gitelman
  syndromes
Decreased potassium intake
Intestinal secretion contains 30–60 mEq/L of potassium
Gastric secretion contains only 10 mEq/L of potassium, and
  hypokalemia may be a result of hypovolemia with
  stimulation of aldosterone. Aldosterone will lead to sodium
  retention and potassium excretion in the kidneys

From Medical Knowledge Self-assessment Program (MKSAP), 2006.

decrease in extracellular potassium makes the **membrane less excitable** and muscle weakness results.
- Hypokalemia can lead to **arrhythmias** (especially in patients on **digitalis** or with heart disease). Other effects include **ileus, muscular cramps, augmented ammonia production in the kidney** (which can potentiate hepatic encephalopathy), and **rhabdomyolysis.**
- Hypokalemia is often associated with **hypomagnesemia,** and serum magnesium status should be assessed in all patients with hypokalemia.

Management of Hypokalemia

- As K^+ is a major intracellular cation, serum levels may not reflect the severity of deficiency. Total body potassium deficits are typically large (**200–300 mmol** for serum potassium of 3.0 mEq/L; i.e., for each **1 mEq below normal**), and repeated replacements may be needed with serial measurements.
- For severe hypokalemia, potassium chloride should be given intravenously (IV) at a rate of **10 to 20 mEq/hour.**
- **Hypomagnesemia** should also be corrected if present.

PHOSPHORUS

Phosphate Homeostasis

- The need for phosphate for proper **cellular energy metabolism** through high-energy phosphate compounds (**ATP**) is among the most important. Phosphate is obtained in the diet primarily through protein intake.
- The typical Western diet contains sufficient phosphate to meet metabolic demands; however, in patients with **poor nutritional** status, often seen in alcoholics, hypophosphatemia may develop.
- The **phosphate excretion in the kidney** is regulated by several factors that favor tubular phosphate **reabsorption** (such as **insulin, prostaglandin E$_2$,** and **thyroid hormone**) and factors that **inhibit phosphate reabsorption** (such as **parathyroid hormone** and the newly characterized phospha-

turic hormone FGF-23 that plays a role in hereditary and acquired **phosphate-wasting disorders**). Phosphate reabsorption is handled principally in the **proximal tubule** through the **NPT2** sodium phosphate cotransporter. Therefore, disorders of the proximal tubule, such as Fanconi syndrome, may lead to renal phosphate wasting.

Hypophosphatemia

- There are three major mechanisms of hypophosphatemia: decreased absorption, increased loss, and ECF to ICF shifts (Table 17.8).
- Phosphate, like potassium and magnesium, is mainly an **intracellular ion,** and low serum phosphate usually represents significant total body phosphate depletion.
- Hypophosphatemia commonly occurs in alcoholics and in hospitalized patients with nasogastric suction, malnutrition, extensive bowel resection, malignancy, low sun exposure, and diuretic use.
- If the cause is in doubt, **renal phosphate losses** can be assessed by calculating the fractional excretion of phosphorus at a time when serum phosphorus is low:

Fractional excretion of phosphorus $= (P_u \times Cr_{pl})/(P_{pl} \times Cr_u)$

where P is phosphorus level, u is urine, pl is plasma, and Cr is creatinine level.

If the value is **below 5%,** the kidney is appropriately conserving phosphate and, therefore, the **losses are extrarenal.**

CAUSES OF HYPOPHOSPHATEMIA

Decreased phosphate absorption, GI phosphate losses
- Alcoholism/poor nutrition
- Diarrhea
- GI tract surgery
- Ingestion of phosphate-binding medications or antacids
- TPN preparations with inadequate phosphorus
- Vitamin D deficiency
- Use of corticosteroids

Shifting of phosphate from extracellular space
- Refeeding syndrome
- Respiratory alkalosis
- Hungry bone syndrome
- High-grade lymphoma, acute leukemia
- Administration of glucagon, epinephrine

Increased renal losses of phosphate
- Hyperparathyroidism
- Fanconi syndrome (proximal tubular dysfunction seen in several diseases especially multiple myeloma)
- Diuretics, especially carbonic anhydrase inhibitors
- Acute volume expansion
- Amphotericin B
- Oncogenic osteomalacia
- Hypophosphatemic rickets (X-linked and AD)

GI, gastrointestinal; TPN, total parenteral nutrition; AD, autosomal dominant.
From Medical Knowledge Self-assessment Program (MKSAP), 2006.

Clinical Manifestations of Hypophosphatemia

- The most life-threatening events are failure of two important muscles leading to cardiac and ventilatory failure.
- In severe depletion, muscular weakness (especially large muscle groups, proximal extremity weakness), arrhythmias, rhabdomyolysis, hypotension, hypoventilation, seizures, coma, and hemolytic anemia may occur.
- Other undesirable effects of hypophosphatemia are the following: shift of oxygen dissociation curve to the left from deficiency of 2,3,DPG; depressed immune function (chemotaxis, phagocytosis, bacteriocidal activity); platelet dysfunction (adhesion and aggregation); metabolic acidosis (impaired bicarbonate resorption and ammonia production); and abnormal glucose metabolism from decreased entry into the cell to make high-energy phosphates.

Treatment of Hypophosphatemia

- Parenteral phosphorus administration should be undertaken in symptomatic patients or in patients with severe depletion (<1.0 mg/dL) or when the oral route is not appropriate. Parenteral phosphate preparations are generally ordered in millimoles. **One millimole (mmol)** of phosphate equals **31 mg of phosphorus.**
- As phosphate is administered as either a sodium salt or a potassium salt, intolerance to either of these should be considered in settings such as renal failure or congestive heart failure.
- Phosphorus replacement in asymptomatic patients should be oral and can be given as a potassium or sodium salt.
- Be careful of the **refeeding syndrome** in total body depleted patients as phosphorus is a major intracellular anion, and sudden decreases in ECF may lead to cardiovascular and respiratory failure.

Hyperphosphatemia

- Occurs primarily in the setting of **impaired renal function**
- Significant **phosphate loading** can occur due to exogenous phosphate administration or as part of the **tumor lysis** syndrome; however, renal insufficiency also commonly complicates this condition. Occult sources of phosphate loading include **sodium phosphate solutions** (either orally or as an **enema**), which can produce significant and, in some rare cases, fatal outcomes.
- In renal failure, elevated serum phosphorus is associated with cardiovascular disease and cardiovascular mortality.

Clinical Manifestations of Hyperphosphatemia

- There are few overt symptoms of hyperphosphatemia, and the syndrome may be insidious. Nephrocalcinosis can complicate hyperphosphatemia and manifest as renal insufficiency.
- On rare occasions, **acute dialysis** may be indicated to treat hyperphosphatemia. Extended dialysis session (>4 hours) may be necessary as phosphorus mobilization is time dependent and phosphorus removal in short dialysis sessions is limited.
- Patients may exhibit **signs of hypocalcemia,** hypotension, and impending cardiovascular collapse that can occur with acute hyperphosphatemia.

CALCIUM

Calcium Homeostasis

- Calcium concentration in plasma is tightly regulated by processes that promote **calcium influx** into the extracellular fluid (mainly intestinal calcium absorption and release of calcium from bone demineralization), and **remove calcium** from the extracellular fluid (urinary calcium excretion and bone formation).
- Intracellular calcium levels are very low, whereas the total body calcium stores in the bone are abundant.
- The hormonal influences that regulate these processes are complex but involve the actions of two principal hormones: **parathyroid hormone and calcitriol.**
- Calcium exists in the plasma as **protein-bound calcium** and **ionized calcium,** usually measured in mmol/L.
- Measurement of the total serum calcium reflects the aggregate amount of these two pools of plasma calcium. **Ionized calcium** is the **active component** and the more important physiologically.
- Albumin is the predominant calcium-binding protein in the circulation. A reduction in plasma **albumin of 1 g/L** will decrease the serum total **calcium by 0.8 mg/dL.** The **validity** of this correction in critical illness has been **questioned,** possibly due to other factors that affect binding of calcium to albumin.
- Therefore, measurement of **ionized calcium** levels in critically ill patients is a good practice, and results may be available within minutes of using point-of-care testing.

Hypocalcemia

- The causes of hypocalcemia can be divided into either efflux of calcium **out of the extracellular space** or by **decreased entry** of calcium into the extracellular space (Table 17.9).
- Normally, homeostatic mechanisms can maintain serum calcium levels despite low intake by increasing mobilization from the bone.
- Hypocalcemia can result from **decreased calcium absorption and mobilization** from bone stores in **hypoparathyroidism** and **vitamin D deficiency.**

TABLE 17.9
CAUSES OF HYPOCALCEMIA
Hypoparathyroidism/pseudohypoparathyroidism Hyperphosphatemia Hypomagnesemia Vitamin D deficiency • Dietary deficit • Reduced sun exposure • Decreased 25-hydroxylation of vitamin D (liver disease, alcoholism) • Decreased vitamin D–sensitive rickets type 1 (1-α-hydroxylase deficiency) and type 2 (receptor deficiency) Renal failure (reduced 1-hydroxylation of vitamin D) Osteoblastic metastases (prostate, breast) Saponification in severe pancreatitis Citrate load (blood transfusion)
From Medical Knowledge Self-assessment Program (MKSAP), 2006.

- Increased calcium removal from the serum occurs in severe pancreatitis through **saponification** of fats and in **osteoblastic metastatic** disease.
- **Ionized calcium** is impacted by conditions that alter **protein binding** of calcium. **Alkalemia** will increase the affinity of albumin for calcium (through altering the net charge of the protein) and will lower the ionized calcium. Acute increases in total albumin may lower ionized calcium.
- **Risk factors** for hypocalcemia include the following: neck irradiation, parathyroid surgery, renal transplantation in patients with tertiary hyperparathyroidism, malignancy, alcoholism, low sun exposure, and malnutrition.

Clinical Manifestations of Hypocalcemia

- Altered **mental status** and **tetany** (Chvostek and Trousseau signs)
- In sepsis, hypocalcemia may be associated with parathyroid hormone (PTH) insufficiency, altered vitamin D metabolism, hypomagnesemia, chelation of calcium by lactate, and calcitonin precursors.
- The association between **hypocalcemia and sepsis** is not well understood although it is now recognized that elevated intracellular calcium levels are a common mechanism for cell death, and low calcium levels may not reflect intracellular concentration of calcium.

Treatment of Hypocalcemia

- The first questions should be to what degree is the ionized calcium altered and why? If the ionized calcium is decreased due to chelation from hyperphosphatemia, treatment of the hypocalcemia can be dangerous, as it can precipitate vascular calcification.
- In **sepsis**, hypocalcemia is common, and treatment is not usually necessary unless cardiovascular collapse with ionized calcium levels of <0.8 mmol/L is present. Data from animal models suggest that it may be harmful to treat hypocalcemia in the setting of sepsis. There are no randomized clinical studies to guide treatment of hypocalcemia in sepsis, and treatment should be reserved for those with symptomatic hypocalcemia such as hemodynamic instability.
- For acute symptomatic hypocalcemia, administer intravenous **calcium chloride** or **calcium gluconate**. Calcium gluconate is advantageous because it is less caustic to veins. Calcium should not be infused more rapidly than **2.5 to 5 mmol in 20 minutes** because of the risk of cardiac abnormalities and asystole. Intravenous calcium will transiently normalize the calcium level, and an infusion should be started after the bolus, especially in settings where there is an ongoing process such as the hungry-bone syndrome after parathyroidectomy.
- **Magnesium deficiency,** by inducing resistance to the actions of parathyroid hormone, can be an important cause of hypocalcemia. If magnesium deficiency is the cause, calcium levels should return to normal once magnesium is replaced.

Hypercalcemia

- Hypercalcemia is caused by entrance of calcium into the intravascular space in excess of renal excretion and calcium incorporation into bone. Two sources of **calcium influx** into the intravascular space are **intestinal absorption** and **bone**

TABLE 17.10

CAUSES OF HYPERCALCEMIA

Excess calcium influx into vascular space
–Primary hyperparathyroidism (usually adenoma, gland hyperplasia; parathyroid malignancy is rare)
–Malignancy (multiple myeloma, carcinomas through production of PTH-related peptide, osteosarcomas)
–Immobilization
–Granulomatous disease (increased vitamin D production?)
–Sarcoidosis
–Tuberculosis
–Paget disease
–Milk-alkali syndrome
–Vitamin D intoxication
–Hyperparathyroidism (stimulation of osteoclasts)

Decreased calcium excretion
–Primary hyperparathyroidism
–Thiazide diuretics
–Familial hypocalciuric hypercalcemia

PTH, parathyroid hormone.
From Medical Knowledge Self-assessment Program (MKSAP), 2006.

---

reabsorption. Decreased renal excretion occurs in primary hyperparathyroidism and with thiazide diuretics.
- Causes are listed in Table 17.10, with the most common causes being primary hyperparathyroidism, malignancy, and granulomatous diseases.
- Total calcium must be corrected for serum albumin because of protein binding, and **ionized calcium** should be measured in hypercalcemic patients.

Clinical Manifestations of Hypercalcemia

- There is a decrease in neuromuscular excitability and decreased muscular tone. Other manifestations include **lethargy, confusion, coma, nausea, constipation, polyuria, and hypertension.** Hypercalcemia can lead to **volume depletion, nephrolithiasis,** and **nephrogenic diabetes insipidus.**

Approach to Diagnosis

- First step is to measure PTH level.
- Failure to suppress PTH secretion in the face of hypercalcemia denotes hyperparathyroidism. Primary hyperparathyroidism typically does not result in severe, symptomatic hypercalcemia.
- In hypercalcemia of malignancy, PTH is usually suppressed (this is the normal response of the parathyroid gland). PTH-related peptide should also be ordered if malignancy is suspected, as many cancers express this protein product that stimulates PTH receptors.
- 1,25-hydroxyvitamin D and 25-hydroxyvitamin D levels can be helpful if abnormal vitamin D metabolism is suspected. Certain granulomatous conditions lead to increased 1,25 vitamin D, and in cases of vitamin D intoxication, high levels of 25-OH vitamin D may be seen.

Management of Hypercalcemia

- In most patients with symptomatic hypercalcemia, **volume depletion** occurs, and one of the first steps is volume repletion with intravenous **saline** (0.9% saline is the treatment of choice). This replacement of the extracellular volume will increase calcium excretion in the urine. Caution is advised in infusing large amounts of saline to an oliguric patient.

- After fluid resuscitation, normal saline should be continued, and **furosemide** can also be given to **increase urinary calcium excretion.** Diuretics should not be given until the patient is completely volume-resuscitated. The action of loop diuretics is distinct from that of thiazide diuretics. Loop diuretics act in the ascending limb of Henle and will promote calcium excretion in the urine. Thiazide diuretics act more distally in the nephron and will decrease calcium excretion.
- **Bisphosphonates** are a good long-term treatment for hypercalcemia of malignancy by **impairing bone reabsorption,** but these agents must be used with caution in patients with renal insufficiency. **Calcitonin** is usually effective in the short term, but tachyphylaxis develops. It is best used early in the management while waiting for diuresis to remove calcium from the body.
- In patients with renal failure, **dialysis** is usually necessary to treat symptomatic hypercalcemia.

MAGNESIUM

Hypomagnesemia

- Magnesium depletion occurs in many conditions (Table 17.11) and is common in critical illness through urinary or gastrointestinal losses with inadequate intake in malnourished patients.
- It is important to identify low magnesium levels, especially in those with known (or at risk for) **cardiac arrhythmias** due to membrane-stabilizing effects on myocardium.
- Magnesium depletion has effects on the homeostasis of other ions and often occurs with **hypokalemia** and **hypocalcemia.** Low magnesium causes a potassium-wasting state, and patients with hypokalemia should be assessed for magnesium depletion. Hypomagnesemia induces a state of **reduced PTH secretion** and **PTH resistance.**
- Tissue magnesium depletion can be present in the absence of decreased serum magnesium levels (as more magnesium is in the **intracellular space**).
- Decreased total serum magnesium levels are often due to a decrease in serum albumin, which is the principal binding

TABLE 17.11

CAUSES OF HYPOMAGNESEMIA

Gastrointestinal losses
- Diarrhea
- Nasogastric suction
- Malabsorption
- Steatorrhea
- Extensive bowel resection
- Acute pancreatitis
- Intestinal fistula

Urinary losses
- Diuretics, aminoglycosides, cisplatin, alcohol
- Pentamidine, foscarnet, cyclosporine, amphotericin B
- Phosphorus depletion
- Metabolic acidosis

From Medical Knowledge Self-assessment Program (MKSAP), 2006.

protein of magnesium, and many of these patients do not have decreased ionized magnesium levels. The correlation of ionized hypomagnesemia and mortality in ICU patients is controversial. Magnesium is not actively mobilized from a body pool (unlike calcium) and, therefore, serum levels are very dependent on intake. If magnesium intake is exceeded by magnesium loss (e.g., urinary losses), the serum magnesium levels will be decreased.

Clinical Manifestations of Hypomagnesemia

- The most serious consequences of hypomagnesemia are its **cardiovascular effects;** it is associated with poor outcomes in acute myocardial infarction and may predispose to arrhythmias. Magnesium treatment may decrease **arrhythmias** after myocardial infarction. Magnesium depletion increases the risk of **torsades des pointes,** a form of polymorphic ventricular tachycardia. Intravenous magnesium is regarded as a treatment for torsades des pointes and refractory ventricular tachycardia, even in the absence of documented hypomagnesemia. Hypomagnesemia may contribute to **atrial arrhythmias** after cardiopulmonary bypass.
- Other manifestations include **altered mental status, seizures, and muscular weakness.**
- Magnesium is an important cofactor for multiple enzyme function (including **ATPase**).

Treatment of Hypomagnesemia

- For acutely symptomatic patients, parenteral administration should be undertaken; **8 to 16 mEq** should be administered intravenously in 5 to 10 minutes followed by 48 mEq over the next 24 hours.
- In asymptomatic patients, the oral route should be used although absorption is variable. Parenterally administered magnesium inhibits magnesium reabsorption in the ascending limb of Henle, and much of a parenterally administered dose may be wasted in the urine.

Hypermagnesemia

- Hypermagnesemia is not a common condition, and it is often **iatrogenic.** Magnesium is readily excreted by the kidney unless overwhelmed by large ingestions (Epsom salt and magnesium-containing cathartics).
- In the presence of peptic ulcer disease, **magnesium absorption** can be enhanced, and magnesium-containing antacids in this setting can lead to toxic hypermagnesemia.
- Patients with **renal failure** are at highest risk for developing hypermagnesemia, and the administration of magnesium-containing cathartics to these patients can be fatal.
- **Clinical manifestations** of hypermagnesemia include **hypotension, bradycardia, respiratory depression, decreased mental status, and ECG abnormalities.**

Treatment of Hypermagnesemia

- **Removal of the offending agent** may be sufficient in mild cases with normal renal function.
- In symptomatic hypermagnesemia, the neuromuscular membrane can be stabilized by administration of **1 g of calcium chloride** intravenously over 5 to 10 minutes. **Dialysis** is usually necessary in the setting of renal insufficiency or severe toxicity.

CHAPTER 18 ■ BLOOD GAS ANALYSIS AND ACID-BASE DISORDERS

Acid-base physiology is among the most complex topics in clinical medicine. Disturbances of this system are common in the critically ill, and important clinical decisions based on measured acid-base parameters occur on a daily, even hourly basis. The purpose of this chapter is to provide a conceptual introduction to the current approach to acid-base physiology, while de-emphasizing calculations and formulas.

MAINTENANCE OF THE ARTERIAL pH AND ACID-BASE BALANCE: BUFFERING AND ACID EXCRETION

- Buffering of acids is the first line of defense against perturbations in systemic pH.
- pH is a logarithmic scale that is a function of the concentration of H_3O^+ species in solution (H^+ will be used interchangeably with H_3O^+ in this chapter).
- A **buffer** can be thought of as a substance that, when present in solution, **takes up [H^+] and therefore resists change in pH when [H^+] is added.**
- The overall **buffering system** of the body is complex and includes several components. These are listed in Table 18.1.
- The most important system is the **carbon dioxide–bicarbonate system,** which is the principal buffer in the extracellular fluid. It is the only buffering system where the **two components (acid and conjugate base) are readily measurable** in the extracellular fluid.
- Buffers work by **binding the free H^+ as the conjugate base,** which is a weak acid.
- Buffering capacity will be depleted if acid is continually added. In humans, the net fixed acid production is approximately 70 to 100 mmol/day. The excretion of the daily acid load occurs through two distinct mechanisms: (a) the **renal excretion of fixed acid** and (b) the **respiratory excretion of volatile acid** (i.e., carbon dioxide).
- Through the interconversion of **bicarbonate, carbonic acid, and carbon dioxide,** fixed and volatile acids can be buffered

until they can be excreted through the urine or respiration (Fig. 18.1).
- In the lung, CO_2 **is released,** which ultimately leads to **more H^+ reacting with HCO_3^- to generate water and more CO_2.**

URINARY EXCRETION OF FIXED ACIDS

- In the kidneys, the **entire filtered load of bicarbonate is**—to avoid losing base—**reabsorbed.** When the kidney excretes one H^+ in the urine, one "new" HCO_3^- is generated.
- Most **bicarbonate reabsorption** occurs in the **proximal tubule,** the renal secretion of H^+ is ten times greater in the proximal tubule—approximately 4,000 mmol/day—as compared with the distal tubule—approximately 400 mmol/day. However, in the **distal tubule,** there is a much **higher luminal–intracellular H^+ gradient** than that seen in the proximal tubule—a ratio of approximately 500:1, due to **active secretion of H^+ into the tubule.**
- In the absence of buffers, the ability to excrete acid in the urine would be limited. Through the use of **buffers in the urine** with modestly acidic pH (approximately 5.5 under maximal conditions), the excretion of H^+ in the urine occurs with different conjugate bases, which are grouped as **titratable acids—mostly phosphates, and nontitratable acids—ammonium.**
- The excretion of **titratable acid** has a **limit,** as it is dependent on the filtered load of phosphate and makes up a relatively small proportion of the acid excreted.
- However, the kidney can generate its **own buffer—ammonia** in substantial amounts, which can be up-regulated in the face of systemic acidosis. Ammonia is produced in the kidney, traverses the plasma membrane, and is "trapped" in the tubular

TABLE 18.1

BLOOD AND EXTRACELLULAR FLUID BUFFERS

Acid	Conjugate base
H_2CO_3	HCO_3^-
Albumin-H	Albumin$^-$
H_2PO_4	HPO_4^-
Hgb-H	Hgb$^-$

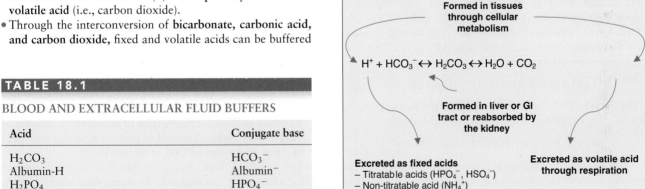

FIGURE 18.1. Normal acid-base homeostasis.

lumen because the low pH drives the following reaction to the right, as the plasma membrane is much less permeable to the charged species ammonium.

$$NH_3 + H^+ \Leftrightarrow NH_4^+$$

Therefore, **ammonia–ammonium** acts as a urinary buffer system, allowing the elimination of one H^+ for nearly every ammonia produced.

- Through **active secretion of H^+** in the distal tubule, the H^+ concentration gradient can be maintained approximately 100:1 between the urine and the intracellular space of the tubular epithelial cells. This corresponds to the maximally acidic urine of approximately pH 5.
- In the presence of systemic acidosis, the kidney will compensate by increasing the excretion of fixed acids, mainly in the non-titratable form (i.e., ammonium), which exists in the NH_4^+ form at a pH of 7 or below.
- This manifests as a change in the **urine anion gap** where ammonium is the **unmeasured cation**. The urinary anion gap is a useful clinical test that can be used to answer the question, "Are the kidneys excreting the acid load appropriately, or are the kidneys part of the acid-base problem?"

$$\text{Urinary anion gap} = [Na^+] + [K^+] - [Cl^+]$$

- Because ammonium is not a measured cation, the presence of significant amounts of ammonium causes an abundance of chloride relative to the measured cationic constituents of the urine (sodium and potassium).
- If there is a high level of ammonium in the urine, the **urine anion gap** will be **negative**, suggesting nonrenal causes of metabolic acidosis. If the **urinary anion gap is zero or positive**, this suggests **inability of the kidney** to excrete acid.
- A caveat that is often clinically important is that the presence of unmeasured anions in the urine (such as β-hydroxybutyrate) may falsely depress the urinary anion gap, and therefore this test does have some limitations, such as during ketonuria.

RELATIONSHIP BETWEEN SYSTEMIC pH AND BUFFER CONCENTRATIONS: AN EVOLVING CONCEPT

Traditional Paradigm

- One of the earliest observations by Hendersen was that the concentration of H^+ in the blood was dependent upon the concentration of CO_2, H_2CO_3, and HCO_3^-. The **Henderson–Hasselbalch equation** was later derived by using the **Sorenson** convention of expressing $[H^+]$ as pH. This relationship is usually expressed as follows:

$$pH = 6.1 + \log[HCO_3^-]/[H_2CO_3]$$

As the $[H_2CO_3]$ in plasma is related to the partial pressure of CO_2, this relationship can be rewritten as follows:

$$pH = 6.1 + \log([HCO_3^-]/0.03 \times PCO_2)$$

This relationship became very meaningful clinically as the methodologies to measure the key variables pH, HCO_3^-, and PCO_2 were developed.

- However, the relationship between pH, HCO_3^-, and PCO_2 failed to completely describe the **relative contributions of fixed acids and volatile acids** (the respiratory component) to acidosis. This is because PCO_2 and HCO_3^- are not truly independent of each other, as changes in one will lead to changes in the other, as seen in this relationship: $CO_2 + H_2O \Leftrightarrow H_2CO_3 \Leftrightarrow H^+ + HCO_3^-$
- Additionally, no single value accurately **quantifies** the degree of fixed acids present during metabolic acidosis or alkalosis. The degree of acidemia could be considered as simply the pH, as the **pH is ultimately a composite of the net respiratory and metabolic components of the acid-base disturbance.**
- Historically, several theoretical frameworks have been developed in an attempt to overcome this lack of exactitude in the concepts of **quantification** and etiology. The first is that the **HCO_3^- system** was **not the only quantitatively important buffering system** to be considered. The erythrocyte membrane is permeable to H^+, and, therefore, H^+ can diffuse inside the cell, and **hemoglobin** can act as an intracellular buffer. Other buffering systems, such as **phosphate** and circulating **proteins**, can act as clinically relevant buffers as well (see Table 18.1).
- By quantitative chemistry, the **pH** of a system is dependent on the relative concentrations of the acids and conjugate bases of **all of the buffering systems** present. Clinically, we measure accurately the concentration of the acid (CO_2) and conjugate base (HCO_3^-) of **only one buffering system** while perturbations in the other buffering systems are not accounted for.
- Another major complicating factor is the fact that the human body is **not a closed system**. CO_2 is both continually being generated in the tissues and continually excreted through the respiratory system. Changes in CO_2 can occur very rapidly in humans as the respiratory rate increases or decreases. Additionally, the kidney can modulate the production of HCO_3^- to adjust the HCO_3^- concentration and the pH, albeit at a much slower pace than respiratory effects
- This means that the **concentration of the measured parameters** (HCO_3^- and PCO_2) are not just **dependent on the inciting insult**—the disease process—that caused them to change but on the body's response to that change (i.e., **compensation**).

Base Excess and Standard Base Excess

- The change in pH of a system is dependent on both the amount of acid (or base) added to the system and the buffering capacity present in the system. As acid is added to a buffered solution, for every H^+ that is buffered, one molecule of conjugate base of the buffer is consumed.
- Therefore, assessing **changes in concentrations of the conjugate base** is more helpful than the degree of change in the pH in **quantifying** the degree of fixed acids present.
- The difficulty in describing the buffering system of a patient is the **inaccessibility** for measurement of a fair proportion of the buffers (see Table 18.1), especially **intracellular buffers.**
- **Base excess** has been proposed to quantify the degree of acid loading based on the change in body buffers. Siggaard–Andersen defined the **base excess** of blood as the **number of mEq of acid (or base) needed to titrate 1 L of blood to a pH of 7.4 at 37°C with a PCO_2 of 40 mm Hg.**
- The **standard base excess** is the base excess corrected for changes in hemoglobin, recalling that hemoglobin is an important intracellular buffer. The base excess can be

considered as a **measurement of the "metabolic portion"** of an acid-base disturbance as the concentration of CO_2 is being held constant at a normal level.

The Anion Gap

- The anion gap is calculated by taking the difference between the concentrations of the measured cations and the measured anion; it takes on a value of approximately **8 to 12 mEq/L** in healthy individuals.
- The anion gap is an indirect estimation of the amount of **"extra anions"** in the circulation. The anion gap reflects the serum albumin (negatively charged), phosphates, and other minor anions. The gain of acid is usually associated with the presence of an unmeasured anion. The **extra base** present leads to a greater difference between the measured anions and cations and, therefore, a **greater anion gap.**
- The anion gap is calculated using the following formula:

$$[Na^+] - ([Cl^-] + [HCO_3^-])$$

- There is a wide range for the normal anion gap. When interpreting the anion gap, caution must be exercised, as it can be influenced by many conditions other than metabolic acidosis
- **Hypoalbuminemia** is the most common condition that affects the normal anion gap, as albumin normally contributes to the net negative charge of the blood. For every **1 mg/dL** fall in the plasma albumin concentration, the anion gap should decrease by approximately **3 mEq/L.**
- In plasma cell dyscrasias, such as **multiple myeloma,** the presence of cationic proteins (immunoglobulins) in the serum is a cause for falsely depressing the anion gap.
- Other conditions that decrease anion gap are **hypercalcemia** and **hyponatremia.**
- Conditions that have been noted to **increase the anion gap** in the absence of metabolic acidosis are renal failure, volume depletion, metabolic alkalosis, and some penicillins.
- Because of the wide variation in the anion gap and the variety of conditions that can affect it, it is best to **directly measure** "unmeasured anions" such as lactate or ketones whenever feasible
- Metabolic acidosis is subdivided into **anion gap** and **non–anion gap** metabolic acidosis based on the value of the anion gap and to guide with the differential diagnosis.

Newer Models of Acid-base Quantification: Stewart Approach

- In the traditional model, acids behave as Brønsted/Lowry acids (i.e., proton donors), which causes a decrease in buffers. This is best approximated by the decrease in serum bicarbonate, but other unmeasured buffers, such as Hgb-H, are also decreased during acidosis.
- A nontraditional approach is the **Stewart model** that defines acids and bases differently. An acid is defined as any substance that **raises the [H⁺]** of a solution, not necessarily limited to an H⁺-donating species.
- The most strikingly different concept of the Stewart model is that the serum bicarbonate is not used as the measure of

buffering capacity. This model uses the **strong ion difference** as a fundamental **measure of** the presence of **buffers.**

The Strong Ion Difference

- Strong ions (SIDs) are the ions in the blood that can be considered as **completely dissociated** in solution **The SID is analogous to the buffer base of a solution.** The SID is calculated as follows:

$$[SID] = \{[Na^+] + [K^+]\} - \{[Cl^-] - [lactate]\}$$

- The remaining anions in solution are the buffers, which can be thought of as the bicarbonate plus the nonbicarbonate buffers, denoted $[A^-]$. $[A^-]$ is the sum of negative charge (buffering capacity) of albumin and phosphate.

$$[SID] = [HCO_3^-] + [A^-]$$

- The SID is considered more reflective of the concentrations of buffers and not only the serum bicarbonate.
- The Stewart equation describes the pH in terms of three independent variables: The SID, $[A_{tot}]$, and PCO_2, where A_{tot} is the concentration of weak acids (see later). This is in contrast to the Henderson–Hasselbalch equation, which relates pH to $[HCO_3^-]$ and PCO_2.
- The SID under normal conditions can be thought of as the sum of the buffer anions (bicarbonate and nonbicarbonate buffer anions) and should be about 40 mEq/L.
- A high SID denotes metabolic alkalosis, and a low SID denotes metabolic acidosis.
- The expected SID (SIDe) is the SID that would be predicted based on the pH, PCO_2, and A_{tot} (in this case, A_{tot} is approximated based on the albumin and phosphate). This relationship is given below.

$$[SIDe] = (1{,}000 \times 2.46 \times 10^{-11} \times PCO_2/10^{-pH}) + [albumin] \times (0.123 \times pH - 0.631) + [phosphate] \times (0.309 \times pH - 0.469)$$

- The **apparent SID (SIDa)** is the strong ion difference that is normally present in the serum: Na⁺, K⁺, and Cl⁻.

$$[SIDa] = \{[Na^+] + [K^+]\} - [Cl^-]$$

- When the SIDa and SID differ, there is a strong anion gap, which is described next.

Strong Ion Gap

- The strong ion gap (SIG) is as an evaluation of **unmeasured anions,** analogous to the traditional anion gap. The strong anion gap is **normally zero** and is defined as follows:

$$SIG = anion\ gap - [A^-]$$

where A^- is the composite of nonbicarbonate buffers in the blood. *[A⁻] = 2.8 (albumin in g/dL) + 0.6 (phosphate in mg/dL) at a pH of 7.4*

$$SIG = [SID_e] - [SID_a]$$

- **SIG** exceeding zero (**high SIG**) signifies presence of **unmeasured anions.** This is analogous to the traditional anion gap, with a correction factor for the presence of hypoalbuminemia. The traditional anion gap is rarely corrected for disturbances in phosphate although the contribution of deviations in phosphate is much smaller than that of albumin (see previous equation).

- A **low SID** is consistent with **metabolic acidosis.** The metabolic acidosis are **further subdivided** based on a **high SIG** (analogous in many ways to a high anion gap) and a **low SIG** (analogous to a low or normal anion gap). In this regard, the two approaches approximate each other. The use of the SIG may be advantageous over the use of the standard anion gap, given that the anion gap can have a wide range of values and is thus somewhat imprecise. This is especially true in settings where nonbicarbonate buffers deviate from normal—for example, the patient with acidosis, sepsis, and acute renal failure with serum albumin of 1.9, phosphorus of 7.0, and hemoglobin of 7.2 mg/dL. Clearly, in this extreme, the assumption that only changes in serum bicarbonate species reflect the metabolic component of the acidosis may not hold true.

Stewart versus Traditional Approach

- The advantage of the Stewart approach is that nonbicarbonate buffers are considered in quantifying acid-base disturbances.
- However, accurate quantification of acid-base status is only part of managing acid-base disturbances. Correctly diagnosing acid-base disorders and **treating** them appropriately is the **ultimate goal;** in this regard, we do not find considerable advantage of the Stewart approach over more traditional methodologies. It is important that the clinician understand the limitation of any of the acid-base models.

Volatile Acidity

- Volatile acidity plays a very important role in determining the systemic pH both in **primary respiratory disturbances** and in **compensation** to metabolic disturbances, as will be discussed
- Carbon dioxide is soluble in water and, in solution, reacts with water molecules to form carbonic acid, which can then further react as follows:

$$CO_2 + H_2O \Leftrightarrow H_2CO_3 \Leftrightarrow H^+ + HCO_3^-$$

- H_2CO_3 **is the acid portion** of the bicarbonate buffer; however, its concentration is **proportional to the partial pressure of** CO_2, and, therefore, its direct measurement of H_2CO_3 is not necessary. By the previous equilibrium expressions, a high PCO_2 will increase the concentration of H_2CO_3, and a low PCO_2 will decrease the concentration of H_2CO_3.
- The PCO_2 in the circulation is the sum of its production and excretion. The production of CO_2 is not frequently altered; however, the excretion of CO_2—occurring only through respiration—is variable based upon the minute ventilation.

Mechanisms of Compensation

- The buffering systems and respiratory compensation are very rapid, whereas renal compensation may take days.

- In response to systemic changes in pH, compensatory mechanisms act to counteract the primary disturbance (Fig. 18.2A and B) gives an overview of the compensatory responses to the primary acid-base disturbances.
- In response to **metabolic acidosis,** there is increased ventilation to decrease PCO_2; the kidney responds by increasing the excretion of H^+, thereby generating more HCO_3^- (see Fig. 18.2A). The opposite response occurs during **metabolic alkalosis,** except that the kidneys are usually not able to respond to the increase in HCO_3^- appropriately, as failure of the kidney to respond to elevated HCO_3^- is necessary for the development of metabolic alkalosis (this is described later).
- The response to **elevated PCO_2 (respiratory acidosis)** is to increase the renal excretion of H^+, which leads to increased HCO_3^- production (see Fig. 18.2B)
- In response to **decreased PCO_2 (respiratory alkalosis),** the excretion of H^+ decreases, and less bicarbonate is produced, thereby decreasing serum bicarbonate. Only the chronic phase is depicted in Figure 18.2B.
- An important point is that a **compensatory response will never normalize the pH** or lead to a recovery of the pH past neutrality. If this has occurred, there must be another acid-base disturbance present.

Determining which Acid-base Disturbances Are Present

- The approach to acid-base disorders is summarized in Figures 18.3 and 18.4. A key is to identify **the primary disturbance.**
- Once the primary disturbance is identified, the next step is to **assess the adequacy of compensation.** Table 18.2 gives the expected values of PCO_2 and HCO_3^- after compensations for primary disturbances.
- In the setting of **respiratory disorders, acute compensation occurs over hours,** whereas the **chronic compensation occurs over days.**
- If there is only **one disturbance, the compensation is adequate.**
- If the compensation is inappropriate (patient has a derangement that is not all explained by compensation), a **second disorder is present.**
- Recall that a compensation will never normalize the pH or "compensate" past the point of neutrality. In these cases, a mixed acid-base disorder is present.
- An additional clue that a mixed acid-base disorder is present is an elevated anion gap when a metabolic acidosis is not suspected. For this reason, it is good practice to **calculate the anion gap** in all critically ill patients.

METABOLIC ACIDOSIS

Causes of Anion Gap Acidosis

- The common etiologies of elevated anion gap metabolic acidosis are listed in Table 18.3.

Diabetic Ketoacidosis

- Diabetic ketoacidosis occurs when a deficit of insulin activity leads to altered cellular metabolism and glucose utilization

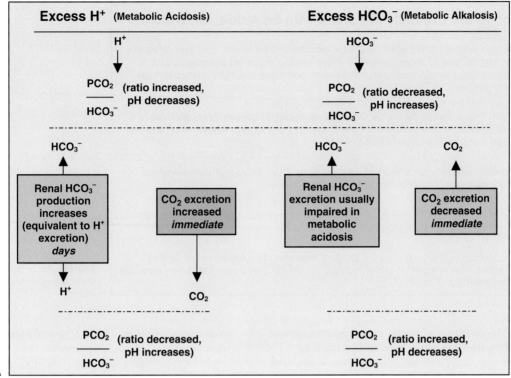

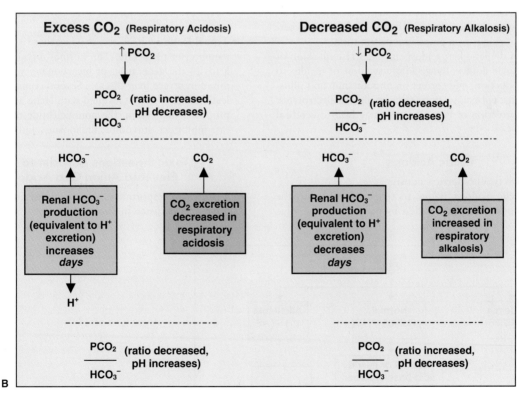

FIGURE 18.2. **A:** Primary metabolic acid-base disturbances and compensatory mechanisms. **B:** Primary respiratory acid-base disturbances and compensatory mechanisms.

Approach to the Critically Ill Patient with an Acid-base Disorder

The first step is to determine which acid-base disorder(s) are present, the cause of each disorder, and the degree of compensation. There are four important variables to look at when determining the acid-base status of a patient and these should be evaluated in all critically ill patients:

- Arterial pH: This is always the starting point. Avoid making judgments in the absence of a measured arterial pH. The pH is the negative logarithm of the concentration of H^+ and the physiologic range for this value is 7.38 to 7.44

- Arterial PCO_2: Indicates the amount of volatile acidity. The PCO_2 generally reflects the respiratory response or contribution to the acid-base disorder.

- Serum bicarbonate: Indicative of the degree of fixed acids present (lower means more fixed acids present). Normal value is 24 mEq/L.

- Serum anion gap ($= [Na^+] - \{[Cl^-] + [HCO_3^-]\}$): A measure of conjugate bases (anions) present above what is expected under "normal" conditions. Has a wide variability, normal is usually between 8 and 12 mEq/L.

FIGURE 18.3. Approach to the critically ill patient with an acid-base disorder.

is impaired. The deficiency of insulin causes the **liberation of fatty acids** and pathophysiologic **keto acid** production.
- A decrease in circulatory volume, deficits in free water, with concurrent hypokalemia and hypophosphatemia may occur. Even though total body **potassium stores are decreased,** the **serum potassium** concentration is frequently **elevated** on presentation owing to the effects of insulin deficiency, hyperglycemia, and acidosis on potassium distribution.
- Treatment of diabetic ketoacidosis includes re-expansion of the extracellular **fluid volume,** administration of insulin to halt acid production, and correction of **potassium** and **phosphorus** deficits, with close monitoring of plasma electrolytes.
- Too-rapid correction of blood glucose may lead to cerebral edema.

Lactic Acidosis
- There are two types of lactic acidosis:
  - **Type A lactic acidosis** is due to **tissue hypoxia** and the formation of excess lactic acid, a by-product of anaerobic

cellular metabolism. This is frequently seen in sepsis, profound anemia, shock, hypotension, and bowel and limb ischemia. Carbon monoxide poisoning can present with nonspecific symptoms and lead to lactic acidosis by inhibiting oxygen utilization in the tissues.
  - Type A lactic acidosis is often associated with **poor outcomes** if the cause is not quickly reversed.
- **Type B lactic acidosis** occurs when there is insufficient liver metabolism of lactate. The normal metabolism of lactate leads to the generation of bicarbonate, which is compromised in severe liver disease. Several commonly used **medications** have been associated with lactic acidosis including propofol, metformin, the nonnucleotide reverse transcriptase inhibitors, stavudine, didanosine, and zidovudine.

Toxic Ingestions Associated with Elevated Anion Gap Acidosis

- Ingestions are important causes of acidosis in the critical care setting and are listed in Table 18.3

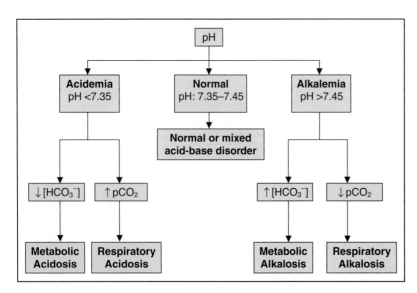

FIGURE 18.4. General approach to acid-base disorders. (From Ayus JC. MKSAP 14, 2006, Nephrology Section. Medical Knowledge Self Assessment Program. American College of Physicians; 2006. Copyrighted by the American College of Physicians.)

TABLE 18.2

COMPENSATIONS FOR ACID-BASE DISORDERS

Metabolic acidosis	• For every 1 mmol/L decrease in HCO_3^- → 1 mm Hg decrease in PCO_2 • Expected $PCO_2 = 1.5\ (HCO_3^-) + 8 \pm 2$ • PCO_2 should approach last two digits of pH
Metabolic alkalosis	• For every 1 mmol/L increase in HCO_3^- → 0.7 mm Hg increase in PCO_2
Respiratory acidosis	• **Acute:** For 10 mm Hg increase in PCO_2 → 1 mmol/L increase in HCO_3^- • **Chronic:** For 10 mm Hg increase in PCO_2 → 4 mmol/L increase in HCO_3^-
Respiratory alkalosis	• **Acute:** For every 10 mm Hg decrease in PCO_2 → 2 mmol/L decrease in HCO_3^- • **Chronic:** For every 10 mm Hg decrease in PCO_2 → 4 mmol/L decrease in HCO_3^-

- The presence of ingested alcohols or other solvents can be inferred by measurement of the **osmolal gap** calculated as follows:

(Measured serum osmolality) − (Claculated serum osmolality)

where the calculated serum osmolality is obtained as follows:

$$2 \times [Na^+](mEq/L) + \text{Urea nitrogen (mg/dL)}/2.8 + \text{Glucose (mg/dL)}/18$$

- The osmolal gap is normally approximately **10 mOsm/kg H_2O.** The normal osmolal gap is a reflection of substances normally present in the serum that exert oncotic forces. These are plasma proteins and ions found in smaller quantities, such as calcium and magnesium.
- An **elevated osmolal gap** is an indication that an **unmeasured osmole** is present and can be used to quantify the level of ethylene glycol or methanol, although direct measurement of these toxins is indicated if their presence is suspected. Therapy should not be delayed while waiting for results.

Renal Failure

- Renal failure can run the spectrum of causing either anion gap or non–anion gap acidosis.
- Usually associated with mixed type of metabolic acidosis, and glomerular filtration rate of <20 mL/minute, anion gap is caused by elevation in organic acids.

TABLE 18.3

COMMON CAUSES OF ELEVATED ANION GAP METABOLIC ACIDOSIS

Lactic acidosis
Diabetic ketoacidosis
Renal failure
Ingestions
- Methanol
- Ethylene glycol
- Paraldehydes
- Salicylates

Causes of Non-anion Gap Acidosis

- There is a primary **decrease in the serum bicarbonate** and an associated **increase in the serum chloride** (Table 18.4).

Gastrointestinal Loss below the Stomach

- **Diarrhea:** There is **loss of bicarbonate** via the intestinal tract, and is typically associated with volume depletion and hypokalemia. In very severe cases, circulatory collapse can occur, and an anion gap (lactic) acidosis may supervene upon the non–anion gap acidosis.
- **Pancreatic or biliary fistula:** These disorders can lead to the loss of bicarbonate-rich solutions and, if correction of the underlying fistula is not possible, treatment with alkali salts may be needed.

Ureterointestinal Diversions

- In a ureterointestinal diversion, urine in the intestine leads to reabsorption of chloride and water. Consequently, the absorption of chloride can induce secretion of bicarbonate into the intestine. Additionally, urease-positive bacteria in the intestine metabolizes the urea in the urine to form ammonium that, when absorbed, liberates excess acid after it is metabolized in the liver. Also, chronic pyelonephritis is common in the diverted kidney, and a superimposed distal renal tubular acidosis (RTA) may occur.

Renal Causes

- One of the key etiologic questions is whether the kidney is appropriately responding to the acidosis by excreting the acid load or whether the cause of the acidosis is improper acid excretion by the kidney. This allows one to differentiate **renal from nonrenal** causes of the acidosis. The **urine anion gap** is a convenient method to assess urinary acid excretion.
- $[Na^+] + [K^+] - [Cl^+]$ = urinary anion gap.
- If the **urine anion gap is positive or close to zero,** this suggests that (a) there is very little ammonium in the urine and the **kidney is not appropriately excreting acids.** If the urine **anion gap is highly negative,** this suggests that (b) there is a large amount of ammonium in the urine and the **kidney is excreting acids** appropriately.

Renal Tubular Acidosis

- Renal tubular acidosis (RTA) is a heterogeneous mix of disorders that is characterized by defects in urinary acid excretion in the setting of intact renal function. **Proximal (type 2) RTA** is caused by a decrease in proximal bicarbonate

TABLE 18.4

ETIOLOGIES OF NON–ANION GAP METABOLIC ACIDOSIS

Extrarenal source	**Renal source**
Gastrointestinal disorders	
• Diarrhea	• Renal tubular acidosis
• Pancreatic and biliary fistulas	• Renal failure
• Laxatives, cholestyramine	• Hypoaldosteronism
• Ureterointestinal diversions (ileal conduit)	

reabsorption. **Distal (type 1) RTA** is caused by impairment of distal acidification.

- RTA often presents with profound acidosis and **hypokalemia.** It is important to treat the hypokalemia first with potassium chloride before correcting the acidosis, as administration of bicarbonate in the setting of severe potassium depletion can lead to fatal hypokalemia as potassium is taken up by cells when H^+ exits the cells.

- **Type 4 RTA** is a clinical syndrome of hyperkalemia and hyperchloremic metabolic acidosis caused by a **lack of aldosterone effect** on the kidney and is seen most commonly in the following settings: diabetes, advanced age, acquired immunodeficiency syndrome, interstitial nephritis, obstructive uropathy, postrenal transplant status, use of angiotensin-converting enzyme inhibitors and heparin (both of which impair aldosterone production), and use of cyclosporine.

- RTA should be suspected if the renal response to systemic acidemia is impaired as evidenced by a **positive urine anion gap.**

- The next step is to **determine the type.** The most practical starting point is to differentiate a **proximal from a distal RTA.** Proximal RTA demonstrates lack of bicarbonate reabsorption with wasting of bicarbonate in the urine until a steady state is reached in which the serum bicarbonate drops to a level at which the reabsorptive capacity of the proximal tubule is no longer overwhelmed. At this point, there is **no longer any bicarbonate in the urine.** For this reason, in a patient with proximal RTA, the **serum bicarbonate will be low;** however, the **urine pH will be low**—this is because the distal acidification mechanisms are functional. If such a patient is given an alkali load, serum bicarbonate is temporarily increased, and bicarbonate "spills" into the urine because the filtered load of bicarbonate exceeds the reabsorptive threshold, which leads to an **increase in the urine pH.** Once the alkali load is stopped, serum bicarbonate drops, bicarbonate no longer appears in the urine, and the urine pH can now drop to its maximally acidic level of approximately 5.5. This is the basis for the **provocative testing** to demonstrate a **proximal RTA,** and also explains why these patients often require a tremendous amount of alkali to achieve normal serum pH.

- **Hypoaldosteronism:** Similar to type 4 RTA acidosis, hypoaldosteronism can lead to excretion of sodium and absorption of K^+ and H^+, leading to metabolic acidosis.

- **Renal failure:** The kidneys have the capacity to excrete acids until kidney function deteriorates to below a glomerular filtration rate of approximately 20 mL/minute. The resulting acidosis is of a mixed type, and it is generally associated with an elevated anion gap. Chronic metabolic acidosis should be treated to prevent bone demineralization, which may occur with time. The goal of treatment is to maintain normal acid-base status.

Treatment of Metabolic Acidosis

Treatment of Anion Gap Metabolic Acidosis

- The treatment is focused on reversing the pathogenesis of the endogenous acid production and eliminating excess acid.

- Treatment with **bicarbonate** replacement therapy remains **controversial,** especially in lactic acidosis. The approach of using alkali therapy assumes that there is a detriment to a low pH (or serum bicarbonate) above and beyond the harm

caused by the underlying condition. Bicarbonate may lead to the generation of CO_2 during buffering and, as CO_2 readily diffuses across cell membranes, intracellular acidosis has been shown to worsen.

Treatment of Non–anion Gap Metabolic Acidosis

- Bicarbonate therapy is generally indicated in non–anion gap acidosis as the primary disturbance is a decrease in bicarbonate. This is contrasted to anion gap acidosis where correction of the underlying cause is the primary concern. Oral bicarbonate or oral citrate solutions are agents for chronic therapy for non–anion gap acidosis. For acute presentations, especially in patients who may not be able to tolerate prolonged hyperventilation, intravenous bicarbonate therapy may be used.

Medications and Metabolic Acidosis

- **Lactic acidosis** has been reported with all **nonnucleoside reverse transcriptase inhibitors** used to treat human immunodeficiency virus; this effect is related to the drug's inhibition of mitochondrial function, with resultant anaerobic metabolism. The newer-generation anticonvulsant **topiramate** and antiglycemic agent **metformin** may cause a metabolic acidosis. The propofol infusion syndrome is a dangerous complication sometimes seen with the use of this drug and associated with head injury, use of propofol for more than 48 hours, use in children, and concomitant use of catecholamines and steroids.

METABOLIC ALKALOSIS

- **Metabolic alkalosis occurs when there is an excess of buffers present, raising the systemic pH** and serum bicarbonate. Without an impairment of the renal capacity to excrete bicarbonate, the kidneys would simply excrete the bicarbonate load. The most common reason for **impairment of renal excretion of bicarbonate** is **chloride deficiency and renal failure.**

- In general, metabolic alkaloses are generated by either **bicarbonate intake** in excess of loss or by the primary **loss of H^+.**

"Chloride-sensitive or Responsive" Metabolic Alkalosis

- **The hallmark is spot** urine Cl^- <20 mEq/L.

- The key factors are **hypovolemia** (also called **contraction alkalosis**) and/or Cl^- **deficiency** resulting in **active sodium-bicarbonate absorption and excretion of H^+** by the kidneys from the effects of secondary hyperaldosteronism.

- **Nasogastric suction, vomiting, and diuretics** are very frequent causes of metabolic alkalosis. Volume depletion stimulates **aldosterone** secretion enhancing sodium reabsorption in the distal tubule, which is coupled with secretion of potassium and H^+. Therefore, a urine that is paradoxically acidic is generated despite alkalemia.

- Hypokalemia develops in the setting of vomiting or nasogastric suction not due to gastrointestinal losses (as the stomach contents are not rich in potassium) but through **renal losses** due to potassium bicarbonate excretion and secondary hyperaldosteronism. In these settings, renal losses of sodium and potassium are obligatory to excrete bicarbonate. In this situation, the **urinary chloride** (not the urinary sodium) better reflects the **effective blood volume** of the patient.

"Chloride-insensitive or Unresponsive" Metabolic Alkalosis

- **The hallmark is** spot urine chloride >40 mEq/L.
- A common etiology is the use of **loop diuretics** (furosemide) that inhibits the sodium-potassium-chloride cotransporter in the thick ascending limb. This increases distal tubular sodium concentration and stimulates the aldosterone-sensitive sodium pump to increase sodium resorption in exchange for K^+ and H^+. Loss of H^+ and K^+ will result in metabolic alkalosis. Excessive use of diuretics may result in hypovolemia and contraction alkalosis (i.e., chloride-sensitive metabolic alkalosis).
- Other causes of chloride-insensitive metabolic alkalosis are **hyperaldosteronism**—both primary and secondary—such as might be seen with renovascular disease and **mineralocorticoid (steroid)** use. Rare causes of chloride-insensitive metabolic alkalosis are Bartter and Gitelman syndromes.

Renal and Extrarenal Compensation

- Respiratory compensation for a metabolic alkalosis involves respiratory suppression and an increase in the PCO_2 (see Fig. 18.2A and Table 18.2).
- Respiratory compensation for severe metabolic alkalosis has practical limits, as respirations can be suppressed only to a certain degree.

Treatment of Metabolic Alkalosis (Table 18.5)

- In patients with chloride-sensitive metabolic alkalosis, treatment usually consists of **replacing volume and chloride**—usually with **normal saline.**
- **Potassium chloride** is almost always indicated when hypokalemia is also present, although potassium concentrations may increase as the alkalosis is corrected.
- **Carbonic anhydrase inhibitors** may be used if one is confident that patient is not hypovolemic, K^+ has been replaced, has adequate renal function, and does not have a sulfa allergy.
- In severe, symptomatic metabolic alkalosis—a pH >7.6 **hemodialysis**—may be indicated and can be used to correct alkalemia, especially when associated with renal failure. The use of **acidic solutions** is rarely indicated.

TABLE 18.5

TREATMENT OF METABOLIC ALKALOSIS

Chloride sensitive	• IV normal saline volume expansion • Discontinue diuretics if possible • H_2 blockers or proton pump inhibitors in cases of nasogastric suction and vomiting
Chloride resistant	• Remove offending agent • Replace potassium if deficient
Extreme alkalosis	• Hemodialysis • NH_4Cl or HCl can also be used

RESPIRATORY ACID-BASE DISORDERS

- Approximately **15,000 mmol/day** of CO_2 is produced.
- Carbon dioxide enters the plasma and forms carbonic acid, which subsequently dissociates to **bicarbonate and H^+**. The bulk of this CO_2 generated is transported to the lungs in the **form of bicarbonate.** The H^+ produced in the process is exchanged across the erythrocyte cell membrane and is buffered intracellularly.
- In the alveoli, this process is reversed, and the **bicarbonate combines with H^+**, liberating CO_2, which is then excreted through respiration.
- Carbon dioxide is the **main stimulus for respiration,** which is activated by small elevations in the PCO_2.
- Hypoxia is a minor stimulus for respiration and is typically effective when the PO_2 is in the range of 50 to 55 mm Hg.
- Derangements in respiratory CO_2 excretion lead to alterations in the ratio of PCO_2 to bicarbonate in the serum and, therefore, alter systemic pH (Henderson–Hasselbalch relationship).

Respiratory Acidosis

- Respiratory acidosis results from the primary retention of carbon dioxide (in relationship to CO_2 production).
- The common etiologies of respiratory acidosis are listed in Table 18.6.

TABLE 18.6

CAUSES OF RESPIRATORY ACIDOSIS

Airway obstruction	• Foreign body, aspiration • Obstructive sleep apnea • Laryngospasm or bronchospasm
Neuromuscular disorders of respiration Acute	• Myasthenia gravis • Guillain-Barré syndrome • Botulism, tetanus, drugs • Hypokalemia, hypophosphatemia (respiratory muscle impairment) • Cervical spinal injury
Chronic	• Morbid obesity (aka Pickwickian syndrome) • Central sleep apnea
Central respiratory depression	• Drugs (opiates, sedatives), anesthetics • Oxygen administration in acute hypercapnia • Brain trauma or stroke
Respirator disorders Acute	• Severe pulmonary edema • Asthma or pneumonia • Acute respiratory distress syndrome
Chronic	• Chronic obstructive pulmonary disorder • Pulmonary fibrosis • Chronic pneumonitis

- In respiratory acidosis, the extracellular buffering capacity is severely limited because bicarbonate cannot buffer carbonic acid. Intracellular buffers—**hemoglobin and other intracellular proteins**—serve as the protection against acute rises in PCO_2, and buffering occurs within 10 to 15 minutes.
- **Renal compensation** occurs and stimulates secretion of protons in the distal nephron-enhanced reabsorption of bicarbonate. Full compensation may take 3 to 4 days (see Table 18.2).
- An increase in **alveolar ventilation** is ultimately required to eliminate excess CO_2 and therefore to re-establish equilibrium
- After sustained hypercapnia that has elicited an appropriate renal response (i.e., a compensatory increase in serum bicarbonate), bicarbonaturia accompanies the return of the PCO_2 to normal. **Chloride intake** must be sufficient to replenish the deficit that developed during the renal compensation to the chronic respiratory acidosis, which induces a negative chloride balance. If chloride is deficient, the serum bicarbonate will remain persistently elevated, a phenomenon termed **posthypercapnic metabolic alkalosis.**
- **Clinical presentation:** Acute respiratory acidosis can produce headaches, confusion, irritability, anxiety, and insomnia, although the symptoms are difficult to separate from concomitant hypoxemia. Symptoms may progress to asterixis, delirium, and somnolence. The severity of the clinical presentation correlates more closely with the **rapidity** of the development of the disturbance rather than the absolute PCO_2 level.

Treatment

- An increase in **effective alveolar ventilation** is necessary through either reversal of the underlying cause or, if necessary, mechanical ventilation.
- The administration of bicarbonate in respiratory acidosis when a coexisting metabolic acidosis is not present is potentially harmful.
- During chronic respiratory acidosis, renal compensation leads to a near-normalization of the arterial pH. The objective is to ensure adequate oxygenation and, if possible, to increase alveolar ventilation. The administration of excessive oxygen and use of sedatives should be avoided because these treatments can depress the respiratory drive.
- Mechanical ventilation may be indicated when there is an acute exacerbation of chronic hypercapnia. If mechanical ventilation is used, the PCO_2 should be **decreased gradually,** avoiding precipitous drops, as rapid correction may cause severe alkalemia. Also, this may increase the cerebrospinal fluid pH, because carbon dioxide rapidly equilibrates across the blood–cerebrospinal fluid barrier. This complication can lead to serious neurologic problems, including seizures and death.
- **Permissive hypercapnia:** It has been shown that ventilator strategies to reduce tidal volume and decrease stretch trauma will reduce ventilator-associated lung injury and improve outcomes Further studies will be needed to delineate the specific role of respiratory acidosis with or without buffering in the management of acute lung injury, cardiac function, and outcomes.

Respiratory Alkalosis

- Respiratory alkalosis is due to a primary increase in ventilation or decrease in CO_2 production.

- The lowered PCO_2 in turn reduces carbonic acid levels, which decreases systemic pH. Proteins, phosphates, and hemoglobin liberate H^+. These liberated protons subsequently react with bicarbonate to form carbonic acid. At the level of the erythrocyte, a shift of chloride to the extracellular compartment ensues, as bicarbonate and cations enter in exchange for protons.
- The net effect results in a **2-mEq/L decrease** in the serum bicarbonate for every **10 mm Hg decrease** in the PCO_2 that occurs in the **acute** setting (see Table 18.2).
- Persistent respiratory alkalemia elicits a renal response, which leads to a net decrease in the secretion of H^+. The kidneys decrease proximal reabsorption of bicarbonate and a decrease in the excretion of titratable acids and of ammonium. This compensatory response reaches peak in 3 to 4 days.
- **Clinical presentation:** Respiratory alkalosis may lead to a wide range of clinical manifestations ranging from alteration in consciousness, perioral paresthesias, muscle spasms, coronary and cerebral vasoconstriction, cardiac arrhythmias, and bronchoconstriction.
- In addition, alkalemia also can affect metabolism of divalent ions. By stimulating **glycolysis**, alkalemia causes phosphate to shift from the extracellular space into the intracellular compartment as glucose-6-phosphate is formed. **Ionized calcium** may decrease due to increased binding of calcium to albumin.
- Shifting of the O_2 dissociation curve to the left may impair unloading of O_2 to the tissues.

Treatment

- The underlying cause for respiratory alkalosis should be sought in order to tailor the treatment (Table 18.7).
- **Cirrhosis** can lead to respiratory alkalosis through impaired clearance from the circulation of progesterones and estrogens, similar to pregnancy.
- In **psychogenic hyperventilation,** rebreathing air using a bag increases the systemic PCO_2 and can treat alkalemia. Specific therapy, other than treatment of the underlying cause, is typically not necessary.

TABLE 18.7

CAUSES OF RESPIRATORY ALKALOSIS

Hypoxia	• High altitude • Congestive heart failure • Severe V/Q mismatch
Lung diseases	• Pulmonary fibrosis • Pulmonary edema • Pneumonia • Pulmonary embolism
Drugs	• Salicylates • Progesterone • Nicotine
Direct stimulation of respiratory drive	• Psychogenic hyperventilation • Cirrhosis • Gram-negative sepsis • Pregnancy (progesterone) • Excessive mechanical ventilation • Neurologic disorders (e.g., pontine tumors)

APPROACH TO ACID-BASE DISORDERS

- There is no simple algorithm to use in the approach to an acid-base disorder. Complex acid-base problems should be suspected when the values cannot be explained by a **single disorder and its compensation.** An example of this might be a patient with lactic acidosis and an alkaline pH.
- Start with the pH value to determine the primary disturbance.
- Assess the compensatory response using clinical judgment whether this is "acute" or "chronic."
- A mixed acid-base disorder should always be suspected if the pH is normal or the "compensation" has surpassed the normal pH.

- Mixed metabolic and respiratory acidosis occurs when the respiratory compensation is insufficient for the degree of decrease in bicarbonate.
- The presence of an increased anion gap despite normal serum bicarbonate levels should raise suspicion for mixed metabolic acidosis and metabolic alkalosis.
- Non–anion gap metabolic acidosis and anion gap metabolic acidosis can coexist.
- After the differential diagnosis of each disturbance, ask whether the disturbance needs to be treated.
- Administer treatment with close observation of electrolytes, fluid status, and acid-base status.

CHAPTER 19 ■ THE HOST RESPONSE TO INJURY AND CRITICAL ILLNESS

INITIAL THOUGHTS

- The stress response
  - Biphasic physiologic response
  - When uninterrupted by complications, has predictable characteristics
    - Lasts 7 to 10 days (Fig. 19.1)
    - Initiated by a global depression of energy expenditure and metabolism.
      - A 24-hour phase immediately following injury
    - Followed by a period of hypermetabolism that persists 5 to 7 days
      - Driving force lies with the need to mount an immune or inflammatory response to combat infection and facilitate repair
      - Most markers for ongoing inflammation/metabolism peak post injury day 2 and return to baseline around day 7.
    - These events must take place or the organism will not survive.
- Normal stress response may be altered by coexisting disease or interrupted by adverse events.
  - Recurrent bleeding
  - Systemic inflammatory response syndrome (SIRS)
  - Progression of SIRS to sepsis
- Organism may then enter a state of persistent hypermetabolism.
  - Continued inflammation postulated to lead to organ dysfunction and immune incompetence (Fig. 19.2)
  - Onset of immune incompetence marks transition from hyperfunctional to hypofunctional state: most ICU deaths result from this.
    - Patients at higher risk for nosocomial infections.
    - Demonstrates pervasive endocrinopathy (Fig. 19.3)

THE NORMAL STRESS RESPONSE

- Prolonged immobilization post injury
  - Urinary excretion of sulfur, nitrogen, phosphorus, and calcium elevated
- Body temperature follows characteristic pattern (Fig. 19.1).
  - First 24 hours following injury, temperature decreases
  - The temperature then rises, peaking post injury day 3 and returning to baseline by post injury day 7
  - Temperature change correlates with alterations in O_2 consumption and CO_2 production.
- Paradigm by which the body responds to injury
  - Not immediate fatal damage
    - Compensatory reaction—vasoconstriction shunts blood away from periphery and to central organs, notably heart and brain.
    - Promotes short-term survival
    - Hypothermia and oliguria associated with global decrease in oxygen consumption and energy expenditure
    - Termed the "ebb" phase of traumatic shock
  - When clear death not imminent, a second aspect of response emerges
    - Attempt to repair tissue damage
      - Accomplished by the activity of WBCs
      - Neutrophils react first, followed by macrophages
      - Characterized by phagocytosis and lysis of bacterial, viral, or fungal invaders and removal of cellular debris

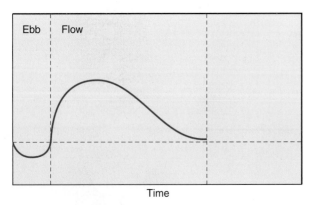

FIGURE 19.1. The stress response. (Reprinted with permission from Kohl BA, Deutschman CS. The inflammatory response to surgery and trauma. *Curr Opin Crit Care.* 2006;12(4):325–332.)

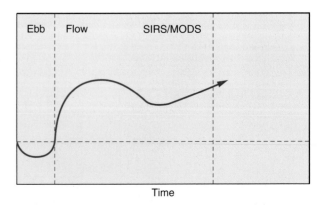

FIGURE 19.2. Continued inflammation, which has been postulated to lead to organ dysfunction and immune incompetence. SIRS, systemic inflammatory response syndrome; MODS, multiple organ dysfunction syndrome.

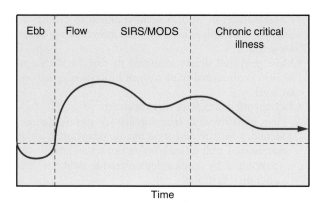

FIGURE 19.3. The onset of immune incompetence marks a transition from a hyperfunctional to a hypofunctional state in which patients are at higher risks for nosocomial infections and demonstrate a pervasive endocrinopathy. SIRS, systemic inflammatory response syndrome; MODS, multiple organ dysfunction syndrome.

- Cytokines—secreted by macrophages, lymphocytes, and antigen-presenting cells (APCs)
  - Growth factors that facilitate repair of damaged tissue
  - Process requires enormous amounts of energy, with a 2- to 20-fold increase in O_2 consumption and resting energy expenditure (REE)
  - Body temperature rises, O_2 consumption and CO_2 production increase
  - Associated increase in glucose requirements
  - After first 24 hours, hepatic glycogen stores get depleted
    - Glucose is further generated by hepatic gluconeogenesis—breaking down protein
  - Due to thrombosis in damaged tissue, most injured areas are avascular.
    - Substrate delivery to these regions
      - Requires capillary tight junctions to separate
      - This allows fluid and substrate to "leak" from the vasculature
    - Increased vascular permeability
      - Results in redistribution of extracellular fluid and plasma proteins to form edema and exudate
      - Causes glucose/other nutrients to
        - Move down concentration gradients across the extracellular matrix to areas of damage
    - This part of the response is the "flow" phase
- Initiation of the flow phase is partly hormonally modulated
- Results in initial dramatic release of endogenous catecholamines
- Supplemented by alterations in growth hormone and insulin-like growth factor
- Causes suppression of thyroid and gonadal axes
- ACTH secretion heightened
  - Increased corticotropin-releasing hormone
  - Arginine vasopressin (AVP)
  - Catecholamines
  - Angiotensin II
  - Serotonin
  - Some inflammatory cytokines (interleukin [IL]-1, IL-2, IL-6, and tumor necrosis factor [TNF])

- ACTH stimulates adrenal production of glucocorticoids and mineralocorticoids
  - Glucocorticoids/glucagon promote glucogenesis, glycogenolysis, and induce peripheral insulin resistance
  - Leads to increased glucose production
  - In turn, increases insulin secretion, producing an "insulin-resistant" state
- Tissue repair initiated by these activities
  - Fibroblasts at edge of wound divide, migrate toward center, and produce collagen,
  - Surviving capillaries bud, and new capillaries also migrate toward center.
    - Wound edges fuse and consist of vascularized granulation tissue.
    - Mediated by increased fibroblast growth factors, epidermal growth factor, platelet-derived growth factor, and vascular endothelial growth factor

DEVIATION FROM THE NORMAL STRESS RESPONSE

- Aspects of the process may become excessive or unbalanced.
- Converts adaptive response to pathologic one
- Risk factors that predispose to the development of an abnormal response include:
  - Inadequate or delayed resuscitation
  - Persistent inflammatory or infectious sources
  - Baseline organ dysfunction
  - Age more than 65 years
  - Immunosuppression
  - Alcohol abuse
  - Malnutrition
  - Invasive instrumentation
- Two common occurrences in surgical/trauma population
  - Hemorrhage, uncorrected fluid loss, or under-resuscitation
    - Results in recurrence of shock, vasoconstriction, decreased perfusion and cardiac output, and impaired tissue substrate delivery
    - Treatment
      - Identification and treatment of underlying cause and correction of fluid imbalance
  - Prolonged hypermetabolism
    - Persistence of a hyperdynamic circulation and secretion of immunologic markers
    - Elevation of serum potassium, magnesium, phosphate, and marginal urine output
      - Indicate prolonged/renewed stress response and warn of a new or recurrent abnormality
    - Commonly referred to as SIRS
      - If SIRS suspected to be from infectious cause
        - Condition referred to as *sepsis* or *sepsis syndrome*
      - Initially, normal stress response, SIRS, and sepsis may mimic each other
      - Differentiation lies in time course and etiology of metabolic perturbations (Table 19.1)
- Sepsis
- Most common cause of death in noncardiac intensive care units
  - Increasing use of broad-spectrum antibiotics, immunosuppression, and invasive technology may be responsible

TABLE 19.1

DIAGNOSTIC CRITERIA FOR SEPSIS IN ADULTS

Suspected or documented infection

General variables
Fever (T >38.3°C)
Hypothermia (T <36°C)
Heart rate (>90 bpm or >2 SDs above normal for age)
Tachypnea
Altered mental status
Edema or positive fluid balance (>20 mL/kg over 24 h)
Hyperglycemia (plasma glucose >120 mg/dL or 7.7 mmol/L) without DM

Inflammatory variables
Leukocytosis (WBC >12,000 cells/μL)
Leukopenia (WBC <4,000 cells/μL)
Normal WBC count with >10% immature forms
Plasma C-reactive protein >2 SDs above the normal value
Plasma procalcitonin >2 SDs above the normal value

Hemodynamic variables
Arterial hypotension (SBP <90 mm Hg, MAP <70 or SBP ↓ >40 mm Hg or <2 SDs below normal)
SvO_2 >70%
Cardiac index >3.5 L/min/m^2

Organ dysfunction variables
Arterial hypoxemia (PaO_2/FiO_2 <300)
Acute oliguria (urine output <0.5 mL/kg/h for at least 2 h)
Creatinine increase >0.5 mg/dL
Coagulation abnormalities (INR >1.5 or aPTT >60 s)
Ileus
Thrombocytopenia (platelets <100,000 cells/μL)
Hyperbilirubinemia (plasma total bilirubin >4 mg/dL or 70 mmol/L)

Tissue perfusion variables
Hyperlactatemia (>1 mmol/L)
Decreased capillary refill or mottling

T, temperature; SDs, standard deviations; DM, diabetes mellitus; WBC, white blood cell; SBP, systolic blood pressure; MAP, mean arterial pressure; SvO_2, mixed venous saturation; PaO_2, arterial partial pressure of oxygen; FiO_2, fraction of inspired oxygen; INR, international normalized ratio; aPTT, activated partial thromboplastin time.
From Levy MM, Fink MP, Marshall JC, et al. 2001 SCCM/ESICM/ACCP/ATS/SIS international sepsis definitions conference. *Crit Care Med.* 2003;31(4):1250–1256.

- Incidence of sepsis in United States estimated as 240 to 300 cases of severe sepsis per 100,000 people
  - Increased from 74 cases per 100,000 people in 1979
- Mortality rate:
  - Is 17.9% for sepsis
  - Is 28.6% for severe sepsis
  - Up to 50% in those with septic shock and comorbid conditions
- Etiology of sepsis has changed over time
  - In 1970s and 1980s, gram-negative bacteria were predominant.
  - Gram-positive organisms are now the leading pathogens
  - Fungal organisms are also on the rise.
- Likely predisposes to organ dysfunction
  - When overt, process is referred to as *multiple organ dysfunction syndrome (MODS).*

- Abnormalities in MODS seem confined to cellular and organ dysfunction as histology and infrastructure are preserved.
- Most proximal defect identified to date in SIRS/sepsis/MODS is abnormality of oxygen utilization at subcellular level.
- Two theories to explain this advanced
  - First, impairment of microcirculatory autoregulation
  - Second, adequate perfusion but an alteration in cellular metabolism with an inability to extract and use oxygen
    - Supported by studies demonstrating defect in mitochondrial function
  - In either case, the result is a block in cellular metabolism with inability of cells and organs to respond to external stimuli.
    - Progressive loss of hormonal responsiveness
    - Liver becomes unresponsive to insulin and glucagons.
    - Cardiovascular system becomes less responsive to catecholamines
  - Thus, the hyperfunctional state cannot be maintained.
    - Acute lung injury progresses to acute respiratory distress syndrome.
    - Hypotension from vasoplegia is compounded by cardiac dysfunction that requires vasopressors and inotropic and chronotropic support.
    - Renal function decreases to a point that renal replacement therapy must be considered.
    - Hepatic dysfunction results in severe ascites and coagulopathy, and potentially profound encephalopathy.
    - Immune incompetence coupled with a pervasive endocrinopathy places patient at higher risk for nosocomial infections.
      - In this state, most deaths from sepsis occur.
- Major contributor to development of complications is the presence of comorbidities
  - Chronic comorbid conditions present in over 50% of septic patients.
    - Associated with increased mortality
  - Comorbid conditions reported to increase risk of normal stress response
    - Diabetes mellitus (DM)
    - Human immunodeficiency virus (HIV)
    - Chronic liver disease
    - Cancer
  - Other factors increasing likelihood of sepsis include:
    - Men more likely than women
    - African–Americans more likely than Caucasians
    - Septic non-Caucasians are more likely to have concomitant DM, HIV, chronic renal failure, and alcohol abuse.
    - Septic Caucasians had higher incidences of cancer and chronic obstructive pulmonary disease (COPD)
      - Presence of one comorbidity increased the risk of developing at least one organ system failure by 30%.
      - The risk of developing organ failure increased by 39% for two comorbidities.
      - Three or more comorbidities presented a 45% chance of developing acute organ failure.

TREATMENT OR PREVENTION

- Treatment of pre-existing disorders/comorbidities will alter the stress response.

- Perhaps the reason why perioperative β-blockade, in appropriate patients, improves outcome
- Attempts to alter the course of prolonged state constituting SIRS, sepsis, MODS, and chronic critical illness are more problematic.
- Most approaches have failed in patients.
- Some successes
  - In the pediatric burn population, REE decreased and net muscle protein balance increased with administration of propranolol.
    - Several murine experiments in septic or hemorrhagic shock increased mortality from immunosuppression after β-blockade.
  - Adequate analgesia
    - Epidural and intravenous

  - Opiates, α-blockers, NSAIDs, and local anesthetics
  - Shown to both decrease inflammation and improve immune function
  - Early goal-directed resuscitation was shown to improve outcome in a single-center trial.
  - Protocol using insulin infusion to maintain serum glucose levels between 80 and 110 mg/dL was shown to reduce mortality and complications in a surgical ICU in a single institution.
    - Similar results not observed in medical ICU
      - Benefit of insulin confined to patients in the MICU for more than 3 to 5 days
  - Likely "optimal" goal for glucose control has moved to a range of 100 to 140 mg/dL.
    - Data need to be confirmed.

CHAPTER 20 ■ MULTIPLE ORGAN DYSFUNCTION SYNDROME

IMMEDIATE CONCERNS

- Multiple organ dysfunction syndrome (MODS)
- A leading cause of death in critically ill and injured patients
- MODS is a disease of medical progress.
  - Broader use of intensive care unit (ICU) resources
  - Improvements in single organ–directed therapy
    - Mechanical ventilation and renal replacement therapy
  - Has reduced early mortality after major physiologic insults
  - The result is longer ICU stay after severe sepsis and trauma.
    - Inflammation and tissue injury may result in MODS.
- MODS represents a systemic disorder.
  - Immunoregulation
  - Endothelial dysfunction
  - Hypermetabolism
  - Varying manifestations in individual organs
- Mortality of MODS
  - Increases as the number of failing organs increases
    - Suggests that changes in function of all organs of equal significance in outcome
- Organs differ in host defense functions and sensitivity to host-derived inflammatory mediators or reductions in oxygen delivery ($\dot{D}O_2$).
  - Thus, diagnosis and therapy focus on prevention.
  - Changes in cellular oxygen (O_2) supply and metabolism may cause and complicate MODS
    - Consequences can include the following:
      - Direct hypoxic organ damage
      - Secondary ischemia/reperfusion (I/R) injury mediated by neutrophils and reactive O_2 species

  - Enhanced injury by activation of cytokines, including tumor necrosis factor-α
- Initial and subsequent therapy follows a two-tiered approach.
  - Targeting systemic factors contributing to ongoing inflammation and single organ-related problems
    - Stabilizing $\dot{D}O_2$
    - Addressing life-threatening derangements in acid-base balance and gas exchange
    - Prompt correction of hemodynamic instability to defined end points that correlate with resolution of tissue O_2 debt minimizes ischemia-related organ damage.
    - Element of time is a critical factor.
      - Delays in completing initial resuscitation, eliminating foci of infection or devitalized tissue, or treating *de novo* organ-specific problems, (i.e., oliguria) worsen outcome.
      - Late-phase (e.g., >72 h) problems involve acquired immunosuppression, predisposition to secondary infection, and hypermetabolism, which impairs wound healing and host defense.

INITIAL ESSENTIAL DIAGNOSTIC TESTS AND PROCEDURES

Hemodynamic and Metabolic Monitoring

- Assess adequacy of initial resuscitation efforts by noninvasive measures including the following:
- Skin color and temperature

- Arterial blood pressure and pulse rate
- Respiratory rate
- Mental status
- Urine output
- Determine whether metabolic acidosis is present from arterial blood gas and plasma bicarbonate determinations.
  - If acidosis present, establish whether the anion gap and plasma lactate concentrations increased.
- Consider invasive hemodynamic monitoring by arterial and central vascular catheterization.
  - Central venous pressure estimates right heart filling.
    - May not accurately gauge left ventricular preload with tricuspid insufficiency, pre-existing heart disease, pulmonary hypertension, or adult respiratory distress syndrome (ARDS)
  - Exclude myocardial infarction as cause of hemodynamic instability.
    - Electrocardiography, creatine kinase isoenzyme, and troponin I levels
- Targeted hemodynamic management:
  - Accomplished by invasive or noninvasive means
    - Pulmonary artery catheterization
    - Arterial pulse contour analysis
    - Esophageal Doppler
  - Mixed/central venous O_2 saturation and lactate concentrations—if the latter are initially elevated
    - Monitored to determine the adequacy of resuscitation and assist in titration of therapy
- Hemodynamic instability despite adequate fluid resuscitation in severe sepsis
  - Treated with inotropes as indicated
  - Hemoglobin level should be raised to 10 mg/dL in early stages of resuscitation.

Evaluation for Infection

- Suspected sepsis upon ICU admission before antibiotic initiation
  - Immediate blood cultures—including fungal where appropriate
  - Gram stains and cultures of urine
  - Adequate sputum specimen
    - "Adequate is defined by 25 or more leukocytes per low-power field" or tracheobronchial washings.
    - Wound discharges
    - Suspicious skin lesions–culture by aspiration and biopsy
    - Fluid collections should be studied
      - Perform thoracentesis and paracentesis within 12 hours or less.
      - Determine pH.
      - Perform Gram stain, culture, cell count, cytologic studies, glucose level, and other chemistries as needed.
  - Evaluate patient for all infectious/potential noninfectious etiologies of MODS.
- Suspected nosocomial sepsis
  - Reculture blood, urine, and sputum.
  - Evaluate all sites of vascular cannulation and remove catheters, if possible.
  - Consider fiberoptic bronchoscopy to obtain protected brush specimen or bronchoalveolar lavage samples in patients with pneumonia.

- Exclude infective endocarditis or endovascular infection by echocardiography and scintigraphic scanning for high-grade or recurrent bacteremia.
- Serially monitor renal, pancreatic, and hepatic function:
  - Exclude acalculous cholecystitis or pancreatitis by abdominal ultrasound.
  - Perform computed tomography of the sinuses, chest, abdomen, and pelvis when appropriate to define fluid collections.
- Maintain high index of suspicion for opportunistic fungal infection.
  - For example, *Candida* spp. despite negative blood culture results

Initial Therapy

- Resuscitation of hemodynamic instability should be rapidly initiated.
  - Crystalloid or colloid infusions
  - Followed by replenishment of the red cell mass
- Vasopressors
  - Dopamine, norepinephrine, vasopressin
  - Titrated to systolic blood pressure of 90 to 100 mm Hg or mean pressure of 70 mm Hg or higher
- With septic shock and hypotension despite "adequate" fluid resuscitation
  - Is patient resuscitated?
  - Evaluate for evidence of adrenal insufficiency.
    - Random cortisol level <12 μg/dL
    - Artificial adrenocorticotropic hormone (ACTH) stimulation study
  - Initiate therapy with low-dose corticosteroids if indicated.
    - 50 mg every 6 hours or 10 mg/hour continuous infusion
      - Our preference is the latter.
    - Begin wean about 48 hours after hemodynamic stability obtained.
- If response to catecholamine therapy is inadequate
  - Evaluate and treat ionized hypocalcemia and severe metabolic acidosis.
- If shock persists despite rapid and aggressive fluid resuscitation
  - Consider endotracheal intubation and mechanical ventilation, irrespective of arterial blood gas values.
  - Achieve proper titration of ventilatory therapy, which averts respiratory muscle fatigue and arrest by reducing shock-related increases in the O_2 cost of breathing.
- Evaluate and treat oliguria.
  - Differentiate prerenal causes by obtaining serum and urine Na^+, creatinine, and urea nitrogen to calculate fractional excretion of sodium (FeNa) or urea nitrogen.
- Stabilize long-bone fractures early.
- Initiate broad-spectrum antimicrobial therapy.
  - Coverage against methicillin-resistant *Staphylococcus aureus, Staphylococcus epidermidis,* and *Pseudomonas aeruginosa*
  - Add coverage for suspected anaerobic intra-abdominal sepsis.
- Begin antifungal therapy when high risk for fungal sepsis present.
  - Despite negative results on blood culture

TABLE 20.1

COMPARISON OF THE PHYSIOLOGIC AND BIOCHEMICAL PARAMETERS USED BY FOUR SCORING SYSTEMS FOR ORGAN DYSFUNCTION AND FAILURE

Organ system	Sequential organ failure assessment (SOFA)	Multiple organ dysfunction score (MOD)	Logistic organ dysfunction (LOD)	Brussels
Cardiovascular	Blood pressure and vasopressor use	Blood pressure and adjusted heart rate	Blood pressure and heart rate	Blood pressure, fluid responsiveness, and acidosis
Pulmonary	PaO_2/FiO_2 and mechanical ventilation	PaO_2/FiO_2	PaO_2/FiO_2 and mechanical ventilation	PaO_2/FiO_2
Hepatic	Bilirubin	Bilirubin	Bilirubin and prothrombin time	Bilirubin
Hematologic	Platelets	Platelets	Platelets and white blood cell count	Platelets
Renal	Creatinine and urine output	Creatinine	Creatinine, blood urea nitrogen, or urine output	Creatinine
Central nervous system	Glasgow coma score (GCS)	GCS	GCS	GCS

Reprinted from Bernard GR. Quantification of organ dysfunction: seeking standardization. *Crit Care Med.* 1998;26:1767–1768, with permission.

- When clinical findings suggestive
  - Extensive colonization by *Candida*
  - Nonintertriginous skin rash
  - Myositis
  - Retinitis
- Prompt re-exploration for suspected intra-abdominal sepsis and abscess formation

EPIDEMIOLOGY OF MULTIPLE ORGAN DYSFUNCTION SYNDROME

- MODS is leading cause of death for patients in the ICU.
- Death rate remains high for patients who survive ICU admission.
- Financial costs are significant.
  - More than 60% of ICU resources consumed by these patients.
- Individual organ dysfunction may result from a direct insult, pulmonary aspiration of gastric contents (primary MODS), or associated with a systemic process, shock, or pancreatitis (secondary MODS).
- Alterations in organ function a continuum rather than a discrete, dichotomous event indicating the failure of an organ
  - Several organ dysfunction scores have been developed to predict the clinical outcome of these patients (Table 20.1).

- Changes in the **sequential organ failure assessment (SOFA)** score are a good indicator of prognosis.
  - In a study of 352 consecutive patients, increased SOFA score during first 48 hours of intensive care predicted a mortality rate of at least 50%.
- The overall rate of MODS, defined as severe acquired dysfunction in two or more organ systems
  - 43% for patients without a diagnosis of sepsis
  - 73% of those with a diagnosis of severe sepsis
- There is a direct relationship between number of organs failing and ICU mortality (Fig. 20.1).
  - Single-organ failure has ICU mortality rate of 6%.
  - Four or more failing organs has mortality rate of 65%.
  - Organ failure in patients with severe sepsis generally carried a higher mortality than in those patients without a diagnosis of severe sepsis.
    - For individual organ systems in the group of patients with severe sepsis
      - Failure of the coagulation system has highest mortality–52.9%
      - Hepatic system–45.1%
      - Central nervous system–43.9%
      - Cardiovascular system–42.3%
      - Renal system–41.2%
      - Respiratory failure–34.5%

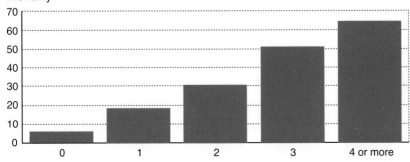

FIGURE 20.1. Relationship between the number of failed organs on admission and intensive care unit mortality. (Reproduced from Vincent J-L, Sakr Y, Sprung CL, et al. Sepsis in European intensive care units: results of the SOAP study. *Crit Care Med.* 2006;34:344–353, with permission.)

- Certain subsets of ICU patients at greater risk of MODS:
  - Patients older than 65 years (older than 55 years in trauma patients)
  - Increased severity of illness as assessed by APACHE II scores (20 or more)
  - Those carrying the diagnosis of sepsis or acute lung injury (ALI) on admission

Pathophysiology

- MODS usually occurs in patients with signs of a generalized inflammatory response (systemic inflammatory response syndrome).

Derangements in Oxygen Delivery and Consumption

- Usually, oxygen consumption (VO_2) is determined by metabolic demand and is independent of DO_2.
  - When DO_2 is reduced, VO_2 is maintained by increased oxygen extraction by the tissues.
  - If DO_2 is reduced to the point where the metabolic need cannot be met, VO_2 becomes "supply dependent."
    - Point at which VO_2 decreases is called the critical DO_2.
- More recent recognition that supply dependency may be occurring locally in patients.
  - Increasing appreciation that the regional circulation and microcirculation—arterioles, capillary bed, and postcapillary venules—play a crucial role in the pathogenesis of organ dysfunction in shock
  - Heterogeneous microcirculatory abnormalities occur due to changes in the activation state and shape of endothelial cells, alterations in vascular smooth muscle tone, activation of the clotting system, and changes in red and white blood cell deformability.
  - The surface receptors and mediators associated with these changes are now being identified, and include oxidants, lectins, proteases, vasoactive products of inducible nitric oxide synthase, and altered adrenergic receptor sensitivity.
  - Alterations in microvascular circulation have been demonstrated in congestive heart failure, cardiogenic shock, hemorrhage, and sepsis.
    - Tissue (skeletal muscle) oxygen saturation in septic patients is no different than that observed in healthy controls or postsurgical patients.
      - Microvascular compliance and skeletal muscle oxygen consumption is reduced, and postischemic reperfusion time is increased compared to controls.
    - Orthogonal polarization spectral imaging—a technique by which perfusion of small and large vessels in the microcirculation of mucosal surfaces can be seen and quantified–has been utilized to show the fraction of perfused small vessels in patients with severe heart failure, cardiogenic shock, or sepsis is significantly lower than in those critically ill patients without those conditions.
  - Functional cellular hypoxia—"cytopathic hypoxia"—or metabolic failure is a condition where the cell is incapable of utilizing oxygen to produce despite adequate oxygen delivery.
    - In patients with sepsis and in animal models of sepsis, oxygen tension in the intestine, bladder, and skeletal mus-

cle is elevated, suggesting that the problem is not one of inadequate DO_2 but one of oxygen utilization.
- The defect in oxygen utilization likely resides in the mitochondrion.
  - Mechanism by which cytopathic hypoxia or metabolic failure occurs has not been fully elucidated.
  - However, nitric oxide and its metabolite, peroxynitrite, are mediators that are released during sepsis and are inhibitors of the mitochondrial electron transport chain.

Role of Inflammatory and Vasoactive Mediators

- Early clinical series emphasized the implication of uncontrolled infection in the development of MODS.
  - Clear now that MODS can occur either with extensive tissue injury such as that seen with trauma, pancreatitis, or sepsis
  - Large amount of evidence available that implicates the release of inflammatory mediators in the pathogenesis of MODS (Table 20.2)
- The coagulation system
  - Lipopolysacchiarride (LPS) and many proinflammatory mediators will activate the coagulation system.

TABLE 20.2

INFLAMMATORY MEDIATORS IMPORTANT IN THE PATHOGENESIS OF SEPSIS AND THE MULTIPLE ORGAN DYSFUNCTION SYNDROME

Complement (C3a, C5a)
Neutrophil products
Proteases
Neutral proteases
Elastase
Cathepsin G
Collagenase
Acid hydrolase
Cathepsins B and D
β-glucuronidase
Glucosaminase
Oxygen radicals
Superoxide anion
Hydroxyl radical
Hydrogen peroxide
Peroxynitrite
Bradykinin
Lipid mediators
Prostaglandins
Thromboxane A_2
Prostaglandin I_2
Prostaglandin E_2
Leukotrienes (LTB$_4$, LTC$_4$, LTD$_4$, LTE$_4$)
Platelet-activating factor (PAF)
Cytokines
Tumor necrosis factor-α (TNF-α)
Interleukins (IL-1, IL-6, IL-8)
High-mobility group 1 (HMG-1)
Macrophage migration inhibition factor (MIF)
Nitric oxide

Reprinted from Heard SO, Fink MP. Multiple-organ dysfunction syndrome. In: Murray MJ, Coursin DB, Pearl RG, et al., eds. *Critical Care Medicine. Perioperative Management*. Philadelphia: Lippincott Williams & Wilkins; 2002, with permission.

- Coagulation in sepsis or inflammatory states is initiated primarily by the extrinsic tissue factor–dependent pathway.
- Same mediators activate the fibrinolytic system, but subsequent increases in plasminogen activator inhibitor-1 and thrombin-activatable fibrinolysis inhibitor effectively suppress fibrinolysis.
- Important inhibitors of coagulation such as antithrombin, tissue factor pathway inhibitor, protein C, protein S, and endothelial-bound modulators—heparan sulfate and thrombomodulin—may be down-regulated.
- Consequently, there is a net *procoagulant tendency* with the potential for the development of disseminated intravascular coagulation.
- Recombinant human activated protein C has been shown to reduce the relative risk of death in patients with severe sepsis by more than 19%, at least in part by its inhibition of the coagulation cascade.

Prevention and Treatment of Multiple Organ Dysfunction Syndrome

- (Table 20.3) lists suggested strategies for the prevention of multiple organ dysfunction syndrome.

Resuscitation

- An episode of circulatory shock is probably the most common event that occurs before the development of MODS.
- Timely restoration of intravascular volume and oxygen delivery is important in preventing or abrogating MODS in high-risk patients.
- Controversy continues regarding the correct fluid for resuscitation and the optimal circulating hemoglobin concentration.
  - Crystalloid solutions are efficacious and cheaper than colloid solutions—there is no overall difference in outcome—death, length of stay, or organ dysfunction—when the two groups were compared.
  - Subgroup analysis demonstrated an increased relative risk of death for trauma patients who received albumin, whereas the relative risk of death for severe sepsis patients was higher if saline was used.
- Assessing the adequacy of tissue oxygenation can often be difficult.
  - Clinical parameters used most often, including arterial blood pressure, skin color, temperature, urine flow, mixed venous oxygen saturation, and blood-lactate concentrations, may be unreliable.
  - Use of the pulmonary artery catheter to guide therapy has not been shown to be of benefit in a large number of studies.
    - Pulmonary capillary wedge pressure does not accurately reflect ventricular volume, even in normal volunteers.
    - Less invasive and probably safer monitors have been developed for monitoring cardiac output that compare favorably with the accuracy of the thermodilution method—systolic blood pressure variation, pulse pressure variation, stroke volume variation, or left ventricular end-diastolic area (as assessed by transesophageal echocardiography).

TABLE 20.3

SUGGESTED STRATEGIES FOR THE PREVENTION OF MULTIPLE ORGAN DYSFUNCTION SYNDROME

1. **Prevention of hospital-acquired infection**
   a. Prevention of catheter-related bloodstream infections
      - Implementation of educational initiatives
      - Use of chlorhexidine solution for skin preparation
      - Use of maximum barrier precautions
      - Avoidance of the femoral insertion site
      - Removal of catheter as soon as possible when no longer needed
   b. Strict infection control measures and hand hygiene
2. **Metabolic control and support**
   a. Strict glucose control
   b. Early enteral nutrition
3. **Early and appropriate treatment of infection and trauma**
   a. Early goal-directed therapy for severe sepsis
   b. Early and aggressive resuscitation of trauma victims
   c. Prompt eradication of documented sources/foci of infection
   d. Early fracture stabilization in multiple trauma
   e. Appropriate empiric antibiotic therapy according to consensus guidelines where available, with earliest possible de-escalation of therapy according to culture results
4. **Prevention of acute lung injury (ALI), acute respiratory distress syndrome (ARDS), and ventilator-associated and aspiration pneumonia**
   a. Elevation of the head of bed to 30 degrees in all patients without spine precautions
   b. Stress gastritis prophylaxis according to consensus guidelines
   c. Lung protective ventilation strategies in patients with ALI/ARDS
   d. Implementation of weaning protocols
   e. Daily sedation holidays
   f. Chlorhexidine oral rinse
   g. Selective decontamination of the digestive tract
5. **Prevention of acute renal failure**
   a. Normal saline administration to prevent contrast-induced nephropathy, with the addition of sodium bicarbonate or N-acetylcysteine as indicated
   b. Discontinuation of nephrotoxic drugs whenever possible; consider once-daily dosing regimens for aminoglycoside antibiotics

- Aggressive resuscitation in the ICU may be too late. Early (i.e., in the emergency department before hospital admission), goal-directed therapy can reduce mortality and organ dysfunction in patients with severe sepsis and septic shock.

Mechanical Ventilation

- The method by which patients are mechanically ventilated can contribute to organ dysfunction.
- Overdistension of the lung through the use of large tidal volumes will cause lung injury, stimulate the release of inflammatory mediators, and effect derangements in organs other than the lung.
- Small tidal volumes (6 mL/kg) in ALI and ARDS patients will decrease mortality and increase ventilator-free and organ failure–free days.

- Cyclic "opening" and "closing" of collapsed airways during tidal ventilation is also thought to cause lung injury.
  - Use of positive end-expiratory pressure above the lower inflection point of the respiratory system compliance curve may reduce mortality and the number of failed organs compared to controls.
- Fluid management is also an important component in the care of the patient with ARDS or ALI.
  - Restrictive fluid strategy where cumulative fluid balance is kept close to zero in these patients improves the oxygenation index and increases the number of ventilator-free days without increasing the number of other organ failures.

Acute Renal Failure

- Acute tubular necrosis accounts for more than 75% of the cases of acute renal failure in the ICU.
- Mortality rate ranging from 40% to 80%
- Most common insult that predisposes ICU patients to acute tubular necrosis is persistent prerenal azotemia.
- In the critically ill patient, there is often more than one insult to the kidney: sepsis; exposure to aminoglycosides, amphotericin B, or radiocontrast agents; and the administration of nonsteroidal anti-inflammatory agents.
  - Efforts to minimize these insults to the kidneys should be maximized.
    - Timely resuscitation as mentioned previously is very important to prevent renal ischemia.
    - If aminoglycosides must be used to treat infection, once-daily dosing.
    - Liposomal preparations of amphotericin B reduces the risk of renal damage.
    - If patients are to receive contrast agents, hydration with sodium bicarbonate solutions have been shown to reduce the risk of subsequent renal dysfunction.
      - Although N-acetylcysteine has been purported to reduce the risk of contrast-induced acute renal failure, the observed results may be a reflection of the activation of creatinine kinase or an increase in the tubular secretion of creatinine.

Debridement of Necrotic Tissue and Fracture Stabilization

- Presence of dead or devitalized tissue appears to predispose patients to the development of MODS.
- Timely debridement of dead tissue is important in the prevention of the syndrome.
- Early surgical fixation of major lower-extremity fractures results in a lower incidence of ARDS and pneumonia.
  - "Damage control" orthopedics has gained popularity and is a concept whereby fractures are initially treated with external fixation. Definitive therapy occurs later when the patient is more stable.
    - Inflammatory response appears to be attenuated in these patients, and the incidence of organ dysfunction is no higher compared to patients undergoing definitive therapy.

Infection

- Sepsis is an important cause (or correlate) of MODS.
  - The presence of infection must be excluded in critically ill patients with signs of deteriorating organ function.

- Empiric administration of broad-spectrum antibiotics is often necessary in the patient with suspected infection.
  - Failure to administer correct antibiotic(s) in a timely fashion can increase the risk of death.
- Intra-abdominal sepsis: Early and adequate drainage of intra-abdominal sepsis is important to prevent the development of MODS.
  - Without clinical or radiologic evidence of intra-abdominal infection, "blind" laparotomy in the patient with worsening MODS is unlikely to be fruitful.
- Pulmonary sepsis: Ventilator-associated pneumonia can play a role in the development and course of MODS.
  - Preventive measures include noninvasive positive pressure ventilation, elevation of the head of the bed, continuous subglottic suctioning, weaning protocols, optimization of sedation with daily "wake-ups" for the patient, and chlorhexidine oral rinse.
  - Selective digestive decontamination is a technique by which topical nonabsorbable antibacterial and antifungal agents are applied to the oropharynx and proximal bowel in mechanically ventilated patients to reduce the incidence of nosocomial infections, organ dysfunction, and mortality.
  - A meta-analytic review of 57 randomized controlled trials demonstrated a favorable effect on bloodstream infections and mortality.
  - Fears concerning the emergence of resistance organisms do not appear to be well founded.
- Catheter-related sepsis: Catheter-related bloodstream infections may contribute to the development and propagation of MODS. Proven strategies to reduce the risk of catheter-related bloodstream infections include hand washing prior to catheter insertion, use of maximum barrier precautions (cap, mask, sterile gloves and gown, and a large sterile drape that covers the patient), use of an aqueous chlorhexidine skin preparation solution, avoiding the femoral site for catheter insertion, and removing catheters when no longer needed.
  - If these measures are ineffective in reducing the risk of infection, catheters with antiseptic surfaces or impregnated with antibiotics or the use of chlorhexidine dressing sponges can reduce the risk of infection.
- Other sources of sepsis: Many other sources of infection in critically ill patients may contribute to the development of MODS.
  - Purulent sinusitis, suppurative thrombophlebitis, otitis media, perirectal abscess, epididymitis, prostatitis, calculous or acalculous cholecystitis, meningitis or brain abscess (particularly after instrumentation of the central nervous system), prosthetic intravascular graft infection, lower- or upper-urinary tract infection, and endocarditis.
  - Physical examination and appropriate laboratory and radiographic studies should exclude these conditions.

Nutritional Support

- Malnutrition can contribute to the morbidity and mortality of sepsis and MODS.
- Early nutritional support may be beneficial in patients at risk for developing MODS.
  - Consensus is that enteral feeding is preferable to the parenteral route.

- Overfeeding should be avoided.
- Current guidelines for support of hypermetabolic patients with sepsis or MODS include a total caloric intake (exclusive of protein) of 20 to 25 kcal/kg/day—2 to 5 g/kg/day of glucose, plus 0.5 to 1.0 g/kg/day of fat, and 1.2 to 1.5 g/kg/day of protein.
- Specialty formulas: A number of enteral nutritional formulas are available that provide specific nutrients: glutamine, peptides, arginine, omega-3 fatty acids, nucleic acids, and antioxidants (e.g., vitamins E and C, β-carotene). Arginine is the substrate for NO synthase and is important in lymphocyte proliferation and wound healing.
- The Canadian Critical Care Clinical Practice Guideline Committee recommends that arginine and other "select" nutrients not be used for enteral nutrition.
  - In patients with ARDS, a formula supplemented with fish oil, borage oil, and antioxidants should be used.
  - Although routine use of glutamine is discouraged, in patients with trauma and burns, enteral glutamine should be considered.

CHAPTER 21 ■ SHOCK: GENERAL

• *Shock* is defined as an acute clinical syndrome resulting when cellular dysoxia occurs, ultimately leading to organ dysfunction and failure. Cellular dysoxia or inadequate tissue perfusion is critical in diagnosing shock, as there are many other causes of organ dysfunction and failure that are not resultant from shock.

• Note the emphasis on shock as a syndrome, as this constellation of signs and symptoms predictably follows a well-described series of pathophysiologic events. Its clinical presentation is complex (Table 21.1) and varies widely based on the underlying etiology, the degree of organ perfusion, and prior organ dysfunction.

CLASSIFICATION OF SHOCK

• Current classification of shock is based on cardiovascular parameters. The categories include hypovolemic, cardiogenic, extracardiac obstructive, and distributive. Table 21.2 represents an adaptation of this system. It is important to appreciate that most shock states incorporate different components of each of the aforementioned shock categories.

TABLE 21.1

CLINICAL RECOGNITION OF SHOCK

Organ system	Symptoms or signs	Causes
CNS	Mental status changes	↓ Cerebral perfusion
Circulatory		
Cardiac	Tachycardia	Adrenergic stimulation, depressed contractility
	Other dysrhythmias	Coronary ischemia
	Hypotension	Depressed contractility secondary to ischemia or MDFs, right ventricular failure
	New murmurs	Valvular dysfunction, VSD
Systemic	Hypotension	↓ SVR, ↓ venous return
	↓ JVPs	Hypovolemia, ↓ venous return
	↑ JVPs	Right heart failure
	Disparate peripheral pulses	Aortic dissection
Respiratory	Tachypnea	Pulmonary edema, respiratory muscle fatigue, sepsis, acidosis
	Cyanosis	Hypoxemia
Renal	Oliguria	↓ Perfusion, afferent arteriolar vasoconstriction
Skin	Cool, clammy	Vasoconstriction, sympathetic stimulation
Other	Lactic acidosis	Anaerobic metabolism, hepatic dysfunction
	Fever	Infection

CNS, central nervous system; MDFs, myocardial depressant factors; VSD, ventricular septal defect; SVR, systemic vascular resistance; JVPs, jugular venous pulsations.
From Jimenez EJ. Shock. In: Civetta JM, Taylor RW, Kirby RR, eds. *Critical Care.* 3rd ed. Philadelphia: Lippincott–Raven Publishers; 1997:359.

TABLE 21.2

SHOCK CLASSIFICATIONS

Hypovolemic
Hemorrhagic
–Trauma, gastrointestinal, retroperitoneal
Nonhemorrhagic
–Dehydration, emesis, diarrhea, fistulae, burns, polyuria, "third spacing," malnutrition, large open wounds

Cardiogenic
Myocardial
–Infarction, contusion, myocarditis, cardiomyopathies, pharmacologic
Mechanical
–Valvular failure, ventricular septal defect, ventricular wall defects
Arrhythmias

Obstructive
Impairment of diastolic filling
–Intrathoracic obstructive tumors, tension pneumothorax, positive-pressure mechanical ventilation, constrictive pericarditis, pericardial tamponade
Impairment of systolic contraction
–Pulmonary embolism, acute pulmonary hypertension, air embolism, tumors, aortic dissection, aortic coarctation

Distributive
–Septic, anaphylactic, neurogenic, pharmacologic, endocrinologic

From Jimenez EJ. Shock. In: Civetta JM, Taylor RW, Kirby RR, eds. *Critical Care.* 3rd ed. Philadelphia: Lippincott–Raven Publishers; 1997:359; and Kumar A, Parrillo JE. Shock: classification, pathophysiology, and approach to management. In: Parrillo JE, Dellinger RP, eds. *Critical Care Medicine.* 2nd ed. St. Louis: Mosby, Inc.; 2002:371.

CHAPTER 22 ■ CARDIOGENIC SHOCK

- Cardiogenic shock is defined as inadequate tissue perfusion due to primary ventricular failure. Its incidence has remained fairly stable, and ranges from 6% to 8%. In the United States, it is the most common cause of mortality from coronary artery disease. Despite medical advances, it remains the number one cause of in-hospital mortality in patients experiencing a transmural myocardial infarction, with rates ranging between 70% and 90%. Other causes include myocarditis, cardiomyopathy, valvular diseases, and arrhythmias (Table 22.1).
- The most common inciting event in cardiogenic shock is an acute myocardial infarction. Historically, once 40% of the myocardium has been irreversibly damaged, cardiogenic shock may result. From a mechanical perspective, decreased cardiac contractility diminishes both stroke volume and cardiac output (Table 22.2). These lead to increased ventricular filling pressures, cardiac chamber dilatation, and ultimately univentricular or biventricular failure with resultant systemic hypotension. This further reduces myocardial perfusion and exacerbates ongoing ischemia. The end result is a vicious cycle with severe cardiovascular decompensation. Similar to hypovolemic shock, a significant systemic inflammatory response has been implicated in the pathophysiology of cardiogenic shock (Fig. 22.1).

ESSENTIAL DIAGNOSTIC TESTS AND PROCEDURES

- Bedside clinical criteria that provide evidence of reduced organ perfusion include oliguria, confusion, peripheral cyanosis, and evidence of peripheral vasoconstriction.
- An accurate definition of cardiogenic shock also requires persistence of the shock state after correction of extra-cardiac conditions, such as hypovolemia or a variety of metabolic abnormalities including significant disturbances in acid–base metabolism, electrolyte abnormalities, or arrhythmias.
- The pulmonary artery occlusion pressure (PAOP) is frequently in excess of 18 mm Hg, and the cardiac index (CI) is usually less than 2.2 L/minute/m^2.

LEFT VENTRICULAR ACUTE MYOCARDIAL INFARCTION

- The Killip classification uses pure clinical bedside evaluation of the patient to establish prognostic indicators to predict the mortality associated with an acute myocardial infarction using the physical findings of congestive heart failure.
- *Class I* patients developed no overt signs of congestive heart failure, and these individuals had a low in-hospital mortality rate. This subgroup represented approximately 40% to 50% of all patients who presented with an acute MI. The in-hospital fatality rate was approximately 6%.
- *Class II* patients demonstrated evidence of impaired ventricular function as manifest by persistent bibasilar rales and an audible third heart sound. This subset of patients accounted for approximately 30% to 40% of patients with acute MI. The in-hospital mortality rate of 17% was triple relative to class I patients.
- *Class III* patients were characterized by the development of acute pulmonary edema, which was seen in approximately 10% to 15% of patients admitted to the hospital. A significant mortality rate of 38% was seen in this group treated conservatively before the thrombolytic era.
- *Class IV* patients had established cardiogenic shock with hypotension and signs of organ hypoperfusion. Cardiogenic shock occurred in 5% to 10% of infarct patients in this series but was associated with a high in-hospital mortality rate of 80%, which was a function of both severity of the underlying illness plus the limited availability of definitive treatment at the time this classification was proposed.

TABLE 22.1

SHOCK CLASSIFICATIONS

Hypovolemic
Hemorrhagic
–Trauma, gastrointestinal, retroperitoneal
Nonhemorrhagic
–Dehydration, emesis, diarrhea, fistulae, burns, polyuria, "third spacing," malnutrition, large open wounds

Cardiogenic
Myocardial
–Infarction, contusion, myocarditis, cardiomyopathies, pharmacologic
Mechanical
–Valvular failure, ventricular septal defect, ventricular wall defects
Arrhythmias

Obstructive
Impairment of diastolic filling
–Intrathoracic obstructive tumors, tension pneumothorax, positive-pressure mechanical ventilation, constrictive pericarditis, pericardial tamponade
Impairment of systolic contraction
–Pulmonary embolism, acute pulmonary hypertension, air embolism, tumors, aortic dissection, aortic coarctation

Distributive
–Septic, anaphylactic, neurogenic, pharmacologic, endocrinologic

From Jimenez EJ. Shock. In: Civetta JM, Taylor RW, Kirby RR, eds. *Critical Care*. 3rd ed. Philadelphia: Lippincott–Raven Publishers; 1997:359; and Kumar A, Parrillo JE. Shock: classification, pathophysiology, and approach to management. In: Parrillo JE, Dellinger RP, eds. *Critical Care Medicine*. 2nd ed. St. Louis: Mosby, Inc.; 2002:371.

TABLE 22.2

SHOCK HEMODYNAMIC PARAMETERS

	CVP	PCWP	CO	SVR	S$\overline{V}O_2$
Hypovolemic	↓↓	↓↓	↓↓	↑	↓
Cardiogenic					
Left ventricular myocardial infarction	Nl or ↑	↑	↓↓	↑	↓
Right ventricular myocardial infarction	↑↑	Nl or ↑	↓↓	↑	↓
Obstructive					
Pericardial tamponade	↑↑	↑↑	↓ or ↓↓	↑	↓
Massive pulmonary embolism	↑↑	Nl or ↓	↓↓	↑	↓
Distributive					
Early	Nl or ↑	Nl	↓ or Nl or ↑	↑ or Nl or ↓	Nl or ↓
Early after fluid administration	Nl or ↑	Nl or ↑	↑	↓	↑ or Nl or ↓
Late	Nl	Nl	↓	↑	↑ or ↓

CVP, central venous pressure; PCWP, pulmonary capillary wedge pressure; CO, cardiac output; SVR, systemic vascular resistance; S$\overline{V}O_2$, mixed venous oxygen saturation; Nl, normal.
From Jimenez EJ. Shock. In: Civetta JM, Taylor RW, Kirby RR, eds. *Critical Care.* 3rd ed. Philadelphia: Lippincott–Raven Publishers; 1997:359; and Kumar A, Parrillo JE. Shock: classification, pathophysiology, and approach to management. In: Parrillo JE, Dellinger RP, eds. *Critical Care Medicine.* 2nd ed. St. Louis: Mosby, Inc.; 2002:371.

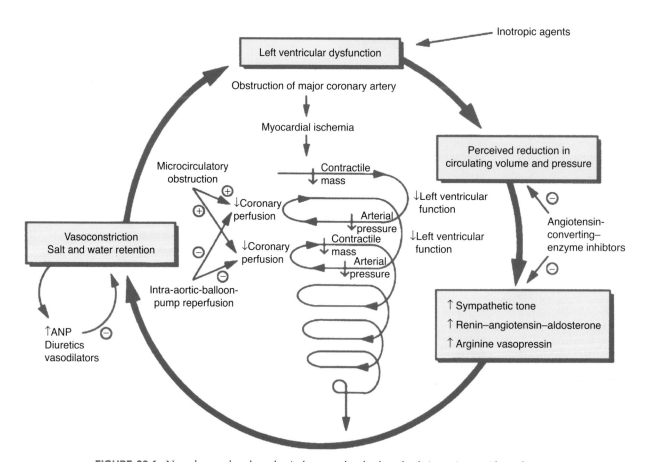

FIGURE 22.1. Neurohumoral and mechanical events that lead to death in patients with cardiogenic shock. ANP, atrial natriuretic peptide. (Reproduced with permission from Pasternak RC, Braunwald E. Acute myocardial infarction. In: Wilson JD, Braunwald E, Isselbacher KJ, eds. *Harrison's Principles of Internal Medicine.* 12th ed. Vol. 1. New York: McGraw-Hill; 1991:953–964; and Francis GS. Neuroendocrine manifestations of congestive heart failure. *Am J Cardiol.* 1988;62(Suppl):9A–13A).

RIGHT VENTRICULAR INFARCTION

- Although isolated right ventricular (RV) infarction is rare, evidence of RV infarction and RV dysfunction is found in up to half of all infarcts and is clinically significant in nearly half of all inferior infarcts.
- The clinical diagnosis of RV infarction should be considered when elevated jugular venous pressure is accompanied by hypotension, while the lung fields are clear. But the diagnosis may be difficult to establish clinically unless hemodynamic measurements, special electrocardiographic leads, echocardiography, or nuclear imaging are performed.
- Right-sided precordial leads obtained by electrocardiography that demonstrate at least 1-mm ST elevation is approximately 70% sensitive in the diagnosis of RV infarction and confers a particularly poor prognosis. Echocardiography is an easily obtainable noninvasive study that demonstrates RV dilation and impairment of wall motion of the right ventricle.
- Radionuclide angiography currently is considered to be the most sensitive means to diagnose RV infarction, although more recent data suggest that magnetic resonance imaging is comparable.
- A decrease in RV ejection fraction that is associated with wall motion abnormalities is more than 90% sensitive in the diagnosis of an RV infarction. Hemodynamic studies that are supportive of significant ischemic involvement of the right ventricle are manifest by increases in right atrial pressures plus demonstration of resistance to diastolic filling, as shown by blunting of the y-descent that follows tricuspid valve opening. A "square root" sign or "dip and plateau" pattern in the diastolic pressure curve is commonly demonstrated in RV infarctions but is not specific and may be associated with pericardial tamponade or restrictive cardiomyopathy.
- Cardiogenic shock in patients with RV infarction frequently represents a substantial loss of functioning myocardium and carries a poor prognosis. RV infarction accompanied by cardiogenic shock is frequently associated with a variety of conduction abnormalities, including a high-grade atrioventricular block or significant rhythm disturbances.
- The treatment of RV infarction complicated by cardiogenic shock centers around maintaining RV filling pressures and assurance of adequate volume. Hemodynamic measure-ments may facilitate the estimate of volume loading required. Nitrates, diuretics, and other predominantly vasodilating compounds should be avoided. Atrial fibrillation is frequently poorly tolerated by these patients and may require immediate electrical cardioversion. The use of digitalis in acute RV infarction, even in the presence of atrial fibrillation, is controversial. Adequate inotropic support with vasodilating inotropic agents such as dobutamine is used if cardiac output fails to optimize after adequate volume loading. Percutaneous revascularization should be considered as it has been shown to improve outcomes.

MECHANICAL DEFECTS

- A variety of mechanical defects that may be associated with cardiogenic shock in the peri-infarction stage are summarized in Table 22.3.

Free Wall Rupture and Tamponade

- Free wall rupture is a major complication of myocardial infarction and is difficult to diagnose premortem. The prevalence of this complication is unknown but may occur in up to 8% of all myocardial infarctions with approximately one-third occurring in the first 24 hours after the onset of the ischemic event and the peak incidence between days 5 and 7.
- Cardiac rupture is a catastrophic event resulting in sudden cardiac death unless a pseudoaneurysm forms. Hemopericardium with cardiac tamponade is difficult to diagnose early enough to institute definitive therapy. Cardiac tamponade after acute myocardial infarction also may be secondary to hemorrhagic pericarditis, but massive hemopericardium is usually due to cardiac rupture with rapid development of electromechanical dissociation and death.
- The diagnosis of free wall rupture is difficult but should be suspected with sudden hypotension, elevated jugular venous pressures, muffled heart sounds, and a pulsus paradoxus. Echocardiography can document the presence of pericardial fluid and occasionally demonstrates the perforated free wall.
- The classic signs of tamponade are present on echocardiography and are caused by the rising intrapericardial pressure compressing the right atrium and right ventricle, resulting

TABLE 22.3

COMPLICATIONS OF MYOCARDIAL INFARCTION

Characteristic	Ventricular septal rupture	Papillary muscle rupture	Papillary muscle dysfunction
Incidence	Unusual	Rare	Common
Murmur			
Type	Pansystolic	Early to pansystolic	Variable
Location	Left sternal border (95%)	Apex → axilla (50%)	Apex
Thrill	>50%	Rare	No
Clinical presentation	Left and right ventricular failure	Profound pulmonary edema	None to moderate left ventricular failure
Catheterization	O_2 step-up in right ventricle	Large left atrial V wave	Mild to moderate elevation of left atrial pressure

With permission from Crawford MH, O'Rourke RA. The bedside diagnosis of the complications of myocardial infarction. In: Eliot RS, ed. *Cardiac Emergencies*. Mount Kisco, NY: Futura; 1962.

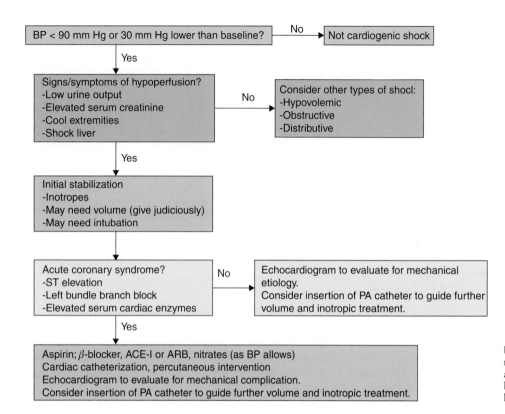

FIGURE 22.2. Management algorithm for cardiogenic shock. ACE-I, angiotensin-converting enzyme inhibitor; ARB, angiotensin II receptor blocker; PA, pulmonary artery.

in equalization of pressures and right ventricular diastolic collapse. Definitive therapy involves pericardiocentesis in addition to volume and pressure support with early surgical intervention being necessary for salvage. Untreated free wall rupture is universally fatal, although isolated instances of successful aggressive intervention with surgical therapy have been reported.

Left Ventricular Aneurysm

- Left ventricular aneurysm is a relatively common complication of MI and may occur in up to 15% of survivors.
- A true aneurysm has a wide base with the ventricular walls composed entirely of myocardium, compared with a pseudoaneurysm, which generally has a narrow base with the walls consisting of pericardium and thrombotic debris. True aneurysms have a relatively low risk of free wall rupture but are associated with increased mortality due to sudden death from ventricular arrhythmias, emboli from mural thrombus, and progressive loss of left ventricular function.
- Aneurysms may develop early in the postinfarction period and can be asymptomatic or present with significant deterioration of left ventricular function. The presence of left ventricular aneurysm may be inferred by persistent ST elevation in the absence of chest pain or enzyme leakage.

THERAPY

- The clinical manifestations of cardiogenic shock are a function of the underlying cause, and mechanical defects must be aggressively sought because of the need for definitive therapy. Clinical recognition of the shock syndrome frequently

requires prompt and aggressive stabilization procedures to be instituted before the definitive diagnosis of the underlying etiology (Fig. 22.2). A history and physical examination should be obtained with special attention to mental status, jugular venous pulsations, quality and intensity of heart sounds, presence and localization of a murmur, and presence of oliguria.
- Diagnostic tests such as electrocardiogram, portable chest radiograph, arterial blood gases, and echocardiography frequently provide adequate clinical information to make a diagnosis and initiate stabilization therapy. A quarter of patients presenting with cardiogenic shock secondary to predominant left ventricular dysfunction do not have evidence of pulmonary congestion.

Surgical Intervention

- Surgical intervention in myocardial infarction has been used to limit infarct size by direct revascularization or to correct the mechanical defects of an acute ischemic event such as ventricular septal defect (VSD), acute mitral insufficiency, free wall rupture, or left ventricular aneurysm. Evidence is accumulating that early revascularization (<6 h) by direct percutaneous transluminal coronary angioplasty (PTCA), intravenous or intracoronary thrombolytic agents, or bypass surgery in selected patients represents the treatment of choice.

OBSTRUCTIVE SHOCK

- In obstructive shock, external forces compress the thin-walled chambers of the heart, the great vessels, or any combination thereof. These forces impair either the diastolic filling or the systolic contraction of the heart. Large obstructive intrathoracic tumors, tension pneumothoraces, pericardial tamponade, and constrictive pericarditis limit ventricular filling, while pulmonary emboli and aortic dissection impede cardiac contractility.

- The hemodynamic parameters witnessed in obstructive shock include increases in central venous pressure and systemic vascular resistance and decreases in cardiac output and mixed venous oxygen saturation (see Table 22.2). The pulmonary capillary wedge pressure and other hemodynamic indices are dependent on the obstructive cause. In pericardial tamponade, there is equalization of the right and left ventricular diastolic pressures, the central venous pressure, and the pulmonary capillary wedge pressure (increased). However, following a massive pulmonary embolus, right ventricular failure leads to increased right heart pressures and a normal or decreased pulmonary capillary wedge pressure.

DISTRIBUTIVE SHOCK

- Distributive shock is characterized by a decrease in peripheral vascular tone. Septic shock is the most common form. Additionally, distributive shock includes the other oft-quoted classes of shock including anaphylactic, neurogenic, and adrenal shock (see Table 22.1).
- Physiologically, all forms of distributive shock exhibit a decreased systemic vascular resistance (see Table 22.2). Subsequently, these patients experience a relative hypovolemia as evidenced by a decreased (or normal) central venous pressure and pulmonary capillary wedge pressure. The cardiac output is initially diminished; however, following appropriate volume.

CHAPTER 23 ■ SEPSIS AND SEPTIC SHOCK

- Current and previous definitions follow:
- *Infection:* A microbial phenomenon characterized by an inflammatory response to the presence of microorganisms or the invasion of normally sterile host tissue by these organisms.
- *Bacteremia:* The presence of viable bacteria in the blood. The presence of other organisms in the blood should be described in like manner—viremia, fungemia, and so on. Bacteremia can either be transient, sustained, or intermittent.
- *Systemic inflammatory response syndrome (SIRS):* The systemic inflammatory response to various severe clinical insults, including but not limited to infection. Various other clinical insults include pancreatitis, ischemia, multiple trauma and tissue injury, hemorrhagic shock, immune-mediated organ injury, and exogenous administration of inflammatory mediators such as tumor necrosis factor or other cytokines. Previous criteria for SIRS are enumerated in Table 23.1. The more recent revision to sepsis definitions removed these SIRS criteria while retaining the concept. However, some understanding of these criteria remains crucial for the intensivist/clinical researcher, as most trials in the last 15 years have been predicated on patients having three or more of these criteria.
- *Sepsis:* The systemic response to infection. This response is similar to SIRS, except that it is considered to result from an infection. The previously accepted definition required at least two of the four SIRS criteria in the presence of documented or suspected infection. The recent revision of the criteria enumerates multiple potential diagnostic criteria for sepsis (Table 23.2) and no longer specifically requires the discarded elements of the SIRS criteria.

- *Severe sepsis:* Sepsis associated with organ dysfunction, perfusion abnormalities, or hypotension. Organ system dysfunction can be described by organ failure scoring systems.
- *Septic shock:* Sepsis with hypotension despite adequate fluid resuscitation, in conjunction with perfusion abnormalities. Standard abnormalities in an adult include mean arterial pressure <60 mm Hg, systolic blood pressure <90 mm Hg, or a drop in systolic blood pressure >40 mm Hg from baseline.
- *Multiorgan dysfunction syndrome* (MODS): The presence of altered organ function in an acutely ill patient, such that homeostasis cannot be maintained without intervention. Primary MODS is the direct result of a well-defined

TABLE 23.1

DEFINITION OF SYSTEMIC INFLAMMATORY RESPONSE SYNDROME

Systemic inflammatory response syndrome (SIRS): The systemic inflammatory response to a wide variety of severe clinical insults manifests as two or more of the following conditions:
- Temperature >38°C or <36°C
- Heart rate >90 beats per minute (bpm)
- Respiratory rate >20 breaths per minute or $PaCO_2$ <32 mm Hg
- White blood cell count >12,000/μL, <4,000/μL, or 10% immature (band) forms

From Bone R. American College of Chest Physicians/Society of Critical Care Medicine Consensus Conference: definitions for sepsis and organ failure and guidelines for the use of innovative therapies in sepsis. *Crit Care Med.* 1992;20:864–874.

TABLE 23.2

REVISED DIAGNOSTIC CRITERIA FOR SEPSIS

Infection,[a] documented or suspected, and some of the
following:

General variables
  Fever (core temerpature >38.3°C)
  Hypothermia (core temperature <36°C)
  Heart rate >90 min or >2 SD above the normal value for
    age
  Tachypnea
  Altered mental status
  Significant edema or positive fluid balance (>20 mL/kg over
    24 h)
  Hyperglycemia (plasma glucose >120 mg/dL or
    7.7 mmol/L) in the absence of diabetes

Inflammatory variables
  Leukocytosis (WBC count >12,000 μL)
  Leukopenia (WBC count <4,000 μL)
  Normal WBC count with >10% immature forms
  Plasma C-reactive protein >2 SD above the normal value
  Plasma procalcitonin >2 SD above the normal value

Hemodynamic variables
  Arterial hypotension[b] (SBP <90 mm Hg, MAP <70, or an
    SBP decrease >40 mm Hg in adults or <2 SD below
    normal for age)
  SvO_2 >70%[b]
  Cardiac index >3.5 L/min/m^{2b}

Organ dysfunction variables
  Arterial hypoxemia (PaO_2/FiO_2 <300)
  Acute oliguria (urine output <0.5 mL/kg/h or 45 mmol/L
    for ≥2 h)
  Creatinine increase >0.5 mg/dL
  Coagulation abnormalities (INR >1.5 or aPTT >60 s)

Ileus (absent bowel sounds)
  Thrombocytopenia (platelet count <100,000 μL)
  Hyperbilirubinemia (plasma total bilirubin >4 mg/dL or
    70 mmol/L)

Tissue perfusion variables
  Hyperlactatemia (>1 mmol/L)
  Decreased capillary refill or mottling

WBC, white blood cell; SBP, systolic blood pressure; MAP, mean
arterial blood pressure; $S\overline{v}O_2$ mixed venous oxygen saturation;
INR, international normalized ratio; aPTT, activated partial
thromboplastin time.
[a]Infection defined as a pathologic process induced by a microorganism.
[b]$S\overline{v}O_2$ sat >70% is normal in children (normally, 75%–80%), and CI
3.5–5.5 is normal in children; therefore, *neither* should be used as
signs of sepsis in newborns or children.
From Levy MM, Fink MP, Marshall JC, et al. 2001 SCCM/ESICM/
ACCP/ATS/SIS International Sepsis Definitions Conference. *Crit Care
Med.* 2003;31(4):1250–1256.

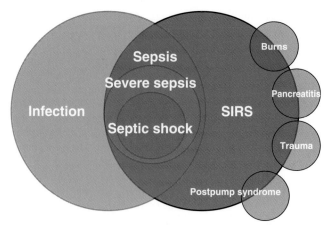

FIGURE 23.1. Venn diagram showing the relationship between infection and other sepsis-associated terms. The intersection of systemic
inflammatory response syndrome (SIRS) and infection defines sepsis.
Severe sepsis is a subset of sepsis defined by the presence of organ failure. Septic shock is a subset of severe sepsis in which the organ failure is
cardiovascular (i.e., shock). Patients with certain inflammatory conditions (e.g., extensive burn injury, pancreatitis, major trauma, postpump
syndrome) may demonstrate a "septic" appearance (i.e. SIRS) without
the presence of infection required for a diagnosis of sepsis. (Adapted
from Bone R. American College of Chest Physicians/Society of Critical
Care Medicine Consensus Conference: definitions for sepsis and organ
failure and guidelines for the use of innovative therapies in sepsis. *Crit
Care Med.* 1992;20:864–874.)

rather than two SIRS criteria) in their entry criteria. The concept of a compensatory anti-inflammatory response has also
been introduced after the demonstration that traditional anti-
inflammatory mediators were also elevated during sepsis.

- The complex interaction between the infecting organism, host
cellular and humoral response, cellular alteration. and clinical
manifestation of organ dysfunction are illustrated in Figure
23.2 and Table 23.3.

DIAGNOSIS OF SEPSIS

- To ensure maximally rapid implementation of effective therapy, an initial presumptive diagnosis of severe sepsis and
septic shock is mandated. The criteria for this presumptive
diagnosis should be highly inclusive and based primarily on
clinical criteria.
- The initial presumptive diagnosis of sepsis with organ dysfunction (severe sepsis) may be made in the presence of the
following elements:
  - Suspected infection based on a minimal clinical constellation
  of localizing (e.g., dyspnea, cough, purulent sputum production, dysuria, pyuria, focal pain, local erythema) and systemic signs and/or symptoms of infection and sepsis (Tables
  23.4 and 23.5). Supportive/confirmatory findings should
  follow (Table 23.6).
  - Clinical evidence of organ dysfunction (e.g., hypotension
  with peripheral hypoperfusion, oliguria, hypoxemia, obtundation)
  - Similarly, an initial diagnosis of septic shock is established in
  the presence of suspected infection with sustained hypotension without a definitive alternate explanation. Key laboratory values to differentiate infection from septic shock are
  listed in Table 23.7.

insult in which organ dysfunction occurs early and can be
directly attributable to the insult itself. Secondary MODS
develops as a consequence of a host response and is identified within the context of SIRS.

- The relationship of many of these conditions to each other
is demonstrated in Figure 23.1. An understanding of sepsis
definitions has become increasingly important, as most clinical trials in the last two decades have used the modified version of the 1991 sepsis definitions (usually requiring three

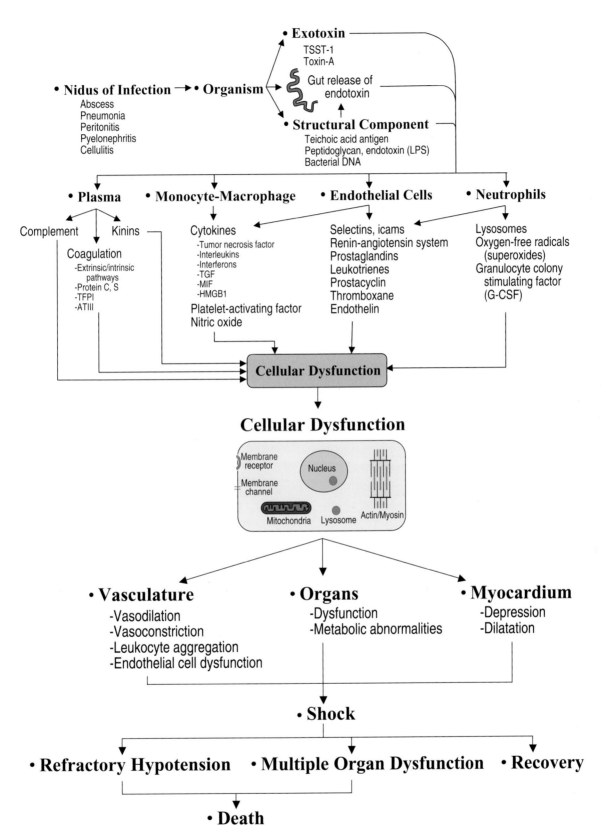

FIGURE 23.2. Pathogenesis of sepsis and septic shock. ATIII, antithrombin III; DNA, deoxyribonucleic acid; HMGB1, high-mobility group box 1 protein; LPS, lipopolysaccharide; MIF, macrophage migration inhibitory factor; TFPI, tissue factor pathway inhibitor; TGF, transforming growth factor; Toxin A, *Pseudomonas* toxin A; TSST-1, toxic shock syndrome toxin 1. (Adapted from Parrillo JE. Pathogenic mechanisms of septic shock. *N Engl J Med.* 1993;328:1471–1477.)

TABLE 23.3

ORGAN SYSTEM DYSFUNCTION IN SEPSIS AND
SEPTIC SHOCK

Central nervous system	Septic encephalopathy Critical illness polyneuropathy/myopathy
Heart	Tachycardia Supraventricular tachycardia Ventricular ectopy Myocardial depression
Pulmonary	Acute respiratory failure Adult respiratory distress syndrome
Kidney	Prerenal failure Acute tubular necrosis
Gastrointestinal	Ileus Erosive gastritis Pancreatitis Acalculous cholecystitis Colonic submucosal hemorrhage Transluminal translocation of bacteria/ antigens
Liver	Intrahepatic cholestasis
Hematologic	Disseminated intravascular coagulation Thrombocytopenia
Metabolic	Hyperglycemia Glycogenolysis Gluconeogenesis Hypertriglyceridemia
Immune system	Neutrophil dysfunction Cellular immune (T-cell/macrophage) depression Humoral immune depression

TABLE 23.4

CLINICAL SYMPTOMS AND SIGNS FOR PRESUMPTIVE
DIAGNOSIS OF SEVERE SEPSIS AND SEPTIC SHOCK

Fever or hypothermia
Chills, rigors
Tachycardia
Widened pulse pressure
Tachypnea or hyperpnea
Confusion, decreased level of consciousness or delirium
Decreased urine output
Hypotension

MANAGEMENT OF SEVERE SEPSIS AND SEPTIC SHOCK (THE SEPSIS SIX-PACK)

- Six major areas in the evaluation and treatment of severe sepsis can be identified (Table 23.8). These include the following:
- Fluid resuscitation
  - Initial resuscitation of septic patients should be aimed at rapid intravascular volume expansion.
  - Initial fluid resuscitation should be titrated to specific clinical end points. Suggested initial targets are heart rate ≤100 beats/minute, systolic blood pressure (≥90 mm Hg), mean arterial pressure (≥60–65 mm Hg), urine output (≥0.5 mL/kg/hour).
  - Initial fluid resuscitation should be achieved using isotonic crystalloid solutions.
- Antimicrobial therapy
    Empiric antibiotic regimens should approach 100% coverage of pathogens for the suspected source of infection (Table 23.9).

TABLE 23.5

LOCALIZING CLINICAL SYMPTOMS AND SIGNS IN SEVERE INFECTIONS

	History	Physical exam
Central nervous system	Headache, neck stiffness, photophobia	Meningismus (neck stiffness), focal neurologic signs (weakness, paralysis, paresthesia)
Head and neck	Earache, sore throat, sinus pain, or swollen lymph glands	Inflamed or swollen tympanic membranes or ear canal, sinus tenderness, pharyngeal erythema and exudates, inspiratory stridor, and cervical lymphadenopathy
Pulmonary	Cough (especially if productive), pleuritic chest pain, and dyspnea	Dullness on percussion, bronchial breath sounds, and localized crackles
Cardiovascular	Palpitations, syncope	New regurgitant valvular murmur
Intra-abdominal	Abdominal pain, nausea, vomiting, diarrhea, purulent discharge	Abdominal distention, localized tenderness, guarding or rebound tenderness, and rectal tenderness or swelling
Pelvic/genitourinary	Pelvic or flank pain, vaginal or urethral discharge, and urinary frequency and urgency	Costovertebral angle tenderness, pelvic tenderness, pain on cervical motion, and adnexal tenderness
Skin/soft tissue/joint	Localized limb pain or tenderness, focal erythema, edema, and swollen joint	Focal erythema or purple discoloration (subcutaneous necrosis), edema, tenderness, crepitus in necrotizing infections (*Clostridia* and Gram-negative infections), petechiae, purpura, erythema, ulceration, and bullous formation and joint effusion

Adapted from Sharma S, Mink S. Septic shock. http://www.emedicine.com/MED/topic2101.htm. 2007. Accessed Dec. 1, 2007.

TABLE 23.6

SUPPORTIVE/CONFIRMATORY FINDINGS FOR SEVERE SEPSIS AND SEPTIC SHOCK

Leukocytosis, leukopenia, increased immature white blood cell (WBC) forms, toxic granulation, Dohle bodies

Thrombocytopenia ± increased INR or PT

Increased D-dimer or fibrin split products

Increased serum bilirubin, AST/ALT, C-reactive protein

Serum procalcitonin elevation

Metabolic acidosis with anion gap

Serum lactate elevation

Respiratory alkalosis or acidosis

Mixed venous saturation >70%

Diagnostic imaging findings

Positive microbiologic or pathologic samples for abnormal presence of microorganisms, leukocytes, or tissue necrosis

---

INR, international normalized ratio; PT, prothrombin time; AST/ALT, aspartate aminotransferase/alanine aminotransferase.

Intravenous administration of broad-spectrum antimicrobials should be initiated immediately (preferably <30 minutes) after the clinical diagnosis of septic shock.

Antimicrobial therapy should be initiated with dosing at the high end of the therapeutic range in all patients with life-threatening infection.

Multidrug antimicrobial therapy is preferred for the initial empiric therapy of septic shock.

Empiric antimicrobial therapy should be adjusted to a narrower regimen within 48 to 72 hours if a plausible pathogen is identified or if the patient stabilizes clinically (i.e., resolution of shock).

Where possible, early source control should be implemented in patients with severe sepsis, septic shock, and other life-threatening infections (Table 23.10).

- Vasopressors and inotropes
  - Rapid volume expansion (500 mL isotonic crystalloid every 10–30 minutes) should be continued until clinical and physiologic treatment targets are met.
  - Vasopressor/inotropic support is required if fluid infusion alone fails to achieve physiologic response targets. Norepinephrine and dopamine are both effective as initial therapy. Dobutamine is indicated for patients with low cardiac index or other evidence of hypoperfusion after achievement of adequate blood pressure. Milrinone can be used as an alternate agent if the response to dobutamine is suboptimal. Continuous infusion of vasopressin (0.01–0.04 U/minute) exerts a strong pressor effect and may be beneficial in catecholamine-resistant septic shock after adequate volume resuscitation. Administration of low- or renal-dose dopamine (1–4 µg/kg/minute) to maintain renal or mesenteric blood flow in sepsis and septic shock is not recommended.
- Invasive and noninvasive monitoring
  - Patients with established septic shock should have continuous monitoring of blood pressure, oxygen saturation, electrocardiogram, and urine output in a closed intensive care unit (ICU) staffed with full-time dedicated intensivists and critical care–trained nurses.
  - Patients requiring vasopressor agents for a prolonged period or at high dose should be strongly considered for

TABLE 23.7

KEY LABORATORY VALUES IN INFECTION/SEPSIS VERSUS SEPTIC SHOCK

	Sepsis	Septic shock
Hb	N or ↓ (chronic disease)	↑ (hemoconcentration)
WBC	↑ + left shift	↑, N or ↓ –marked left shift with metamyelocytes, toxic granulation, and/or Dohle bodies
Platelets	N or ↑	N or ↓
PT/INR	N or ↑ (malnutrition)	↑↑
Fibrinogen	N or ↑	N or ↓
Fibrin split products/ D-dimer activity	↑	↑↑
Glucose	N or ↑	↑↑
Cr/BUN	N or ↑	↑↑
Bilirubin	N, late ↑	↑, late ↑↑
AST/ALT	N	↑-↑↑
Albumin	N or ↓ (malnutrition)	↓↓ (endothelial leakage/interstitial redistribution)
ABG	respiratory alkalosis	metabolic acidosis
HCO₃⁻	N	↓
Lactate	N	↑-↑↑
C-reactive protein	↑	↑↑
Procalcitonin	↑	↑↑
Blood culture positivity	5%–10%	30%–40%

↑ increase; ↑↑ marked increase; ↓ decrease; ↓↓ marked decrease; N, normal;. Hb, hemoglobin; WBC, white blood cell count; PT, prothrombin time; INR, international normalized ratio; Cr/BUN, serum creatine and blood urea nitrogen; AST/ALT, serum aspartate transaminase and alanine transaminase; ABG, arterial blood gas; HCO₃⁻, serum bicarbonate concentration.

TABLE 23.8

TIME LINE OF IMPLEMENTATION OF RECOMMENDED DIAGNOSTIC AND THERAPEUTIC INTERVENTIONS

	Resuscitation	Antimicrobials	Vasopressors/inotropes	Monitoring	Specific therapy	Supportive therapy
First hour	• Initiate crystalloid fluid resuscitation (500 mL every 10–15 min), titrating to HR <100, MAP ≥65 mm Hg, and urine output ≥0.5 mL/h	• Initiate empiric, broad-spectrum, high-dose antimicrobial therapy with two or more cidal drugs where possible		• Implement continuous monitoring of ECG, arterial saturation, blood pressure and UO		• Supplemental oxygen • Consider intubation and mechanical ventilation prior to overt respiratory distress
1–8 h	• Titrate fluid resuscitation to elimination of base deficit and normalization of serum lactate	• Initiate radiographic investigation for localization and delineation of infection • Implement source control if necessary	• Initiate vasopressor therapy if circulatory shock persists following adequate fluid resuscitation • Initiate inotropes if CI or are persistently decreased	• ICU transfer with full monitoring support • Arterial catheter assessment • If shock persists with >2 L crystalloid resuscitation, venous catheter assessment ± placement (goal CVP ≥8 mm Hg)		• Consider low-dose steroid therapy ± ACTH stimulation test
8–24 h	• Dynamic evaluation of resuscitative goals (based on clinical and invasive monitoring end points)		• Consider vasopressin if shock refractory to first-line vasopressors persists	• If persistently pressor dependent after 3–5 L crystalloid infusion, CVP ≥8 achieved, suspicion of intravascular volume depletion or limited cardiovascular reserve, PAC placement (initial goal PWP 12–15 mm Hg) • May be inserted earlier if clinically indicated	• Consider initiation of drotrecogin-alfa (activated) if single organ failure with APACHE II ≥25, two or more organ failures in absence of APACHE score	• Initiate enteral feeding • Consider intensive insulin therapy
>24 h		• Narrow antimicrobial regimen depending on isolation of pathogenic organisms and/or clinical improvement • Reassess necessity for or efficacy of source control		• Consider PAC in vasopressor-dependent patients with progressive respiratory, renal, or multiple organ dysfunction		• Intensive hemodialysis therapy for renal failure • Low-pressure, volume-limited ventilation for ARDS

HR, heart rate; MAP, mean arterial blood pressure; ECG, electrocardiography; UO, urine output; ICU, intensive care unit; ACTH, adrenocorticotropin hormone; Cl, chloride; S̄vO₂, mixed venous oxygen saturation; CVP, central venous pressure; APACHE, Acute Physiology and Chronic Health Evaluation; PAP, pulmonary artery pressure; PWP, pulmonary wedge pressure; PAC, pulmonary artery catheter; ARDS, acute respiratory distress syndrome; CI, cardiac index.

TABLE 23.9

INDICATION FOR EXTENDED EMPIRIC ANTIBIOTIC THERAPY OF SEVERE SEPSIS AND SEPTIC SHOCK

↑ Gram-negative coverage	• Nosocomial infection • Neutropenic or immunosuppressed • Immunocompromised due to chronic organ failure (liver, renal, lung, heart, etc.)
↑ Gram-positive coverage (vancomycin)	• High-level endemic MRSA (community or nosocomial) • Neutropenic patient • Intravascular catheter infection • Nosocomial pneumonia
Fungal/yeast coverage (triazole, echinocandin, amphotericin B)	• Neutropenic fever or other immunosuppressed patient unresponsive to standard antibiotic therapy • Prolonged broad-spectrum antibiotic therapy • Positive relevant fungal cultures • Consider empiric therapy if high-risk patient with severe shock

MRSA, methicillin-resistant *Staphylococcus aureus*.

TABLE 23.10

COMMON SOURCES OF SEVERE SEPSIS AND SEPTIC SHOCK REQUIRING URGENT SOURCE CONTROL

Toxic megacolon or *C. difficile* colitis with shock
Ischemic bowel
Perforated viscus
Intra-abdominal abscess
Ascending cholangitis
Gangrenous cholecystitis
Necrotizing pancreatitis with infection
Bacterial empyema
Mediastinitis
Purulent tunnel infections
Purulent foreign-body infections
Obstructive uropathy
Complicated pyelonephritis/perinephric abscess
Necrotizing soft tissue infections (necrotizing fasciitis)
Clostridial myonecrosis

insertion of an arterial pressure catheter for continuous blood pressure monitoring and to facilitate frequent measurements of arterial blood gases and chemistry.

• If volume resuscitation requirements exceed 2 L, placement of a central venous catheter for monitoring of central venous pressure (CVP) and for vasopressor/inotrope infusion should be considered. An initial target CVP of ≥8 mm Hg is recommended.

• Initiation of invasive cardiac monitoring using a pulmonary artery catheter should be considered if there has been an inadequate response to fluid resuscitation (3–5 L or CVP 8–12 mm Hg), if there is clinical suspicion of intravascular fluid volume overload, or if the patient has impaired cardiac function. An initial target of pulmonary capillary wedge pressure (PWP) of 12 to 15 mm Hg will ensure that hypovolemia is absent in most patients, but higher pressures may be required in certain subgroups.

• In patients with vasopressor-requiring shock who develop progressive organ failure or hypoxemic respiratory failure, pulmonary artery catheterization may be a useful clinical management tool. However, invasive monitoring using a pulmonary artery catheter is not recommended for routine use in all patients with severe sepsis.

• Specific therapy
  • Recombinant human-activated protein C should be administered in patients with suspected sepsis with organ dysfunction. Acceptable criteria include, but are not nec-

essarily limited to, a minimum of one organ dysfunction with an acute physiology and chronic health evaluation (APACHE) II score ≥25; or if an accurate APACHE II score is unavailable, the presence of two or more organ dysfunctions.

  • Intravenous immune globulin should be considered for patients suffering from streptococcal toxic shock syndrome.
  • Immunosuppressive doses of corticosteroids are contraindicated in the management of sepsis and septic shock.

• Miscellaneous supportive therapy
  • Intensive renal replacement therapy (daily intermittent dialysis or continuous renal replacement therapy) is indicated for severe sepsis or septic shock with renal failure.
  • Intensive insulin therapy maintaining a blood glucose of 4.4 to 6.1 mmol/L (80–110 mg/dL) may be beneficial in critically ill ICU patients with severe sepsis.
  • Stress dose steroids may be administered at presentation to selected patients with septic shock
  • Low-volume (6–8 mL/kg ideal body weight), pressure-limited ventilation is indicated in patients with sepsis-associated acute lung injury or acute respiratory distress syndrome pending the result of an adrenocorticotropic hormone stimulation test.
  • Endotracheal intubation and mechanical ventilation should be considered early in the management of all patients with sepsis and organ failure.
  • Enteral feeding should be considered within 24 hours of admission to the ICU for most patients with sepsis and septic shock. Parenteral feeding should be used only if enteral feeding is not possible despite best efforts.
  • Intravenous administration of sodium bicarbonate is not indicated for sepsis-associated metabolic acidosis with a pH ≥ 7.15.

CHAPTER 24 ■ HYPOVOLEMIC AND HEMORRHAGIC SHOCK

- Hypovolemic shock represents a state of decreased intravascular volume. Inciting events include internal or external hemorrhage, significant fluid losses from the gastrointestinal tract (emesis, high-output fistulae, or diarrhea) or urinary tract (hyperosmolar states), and "third spacing" ("capillary leakage" into the interstitial tissues or the corporeal cavities). Additional etiologies include malnutrition and large open wounds (burns and the open abdomen).
- The pathophysiology of shock is dependent upon its classification. Hypovolemic shock is characterized by a decrease in intravascular volume with resultant decreases in pulmonary capillary wedge pressure and cardiac output. There is a subsequent increased sympathetic drive in an attempt to increase peripheral vasculature tone, cardiac contractility, and the heart rate. These initially beneficial measures ultimately turn detrimental, as their resultant hypermetabolic state predisposes tissues to localized hypoxia. Furthermore, the aforementioned increased peripheral vascular tone may result in tissue ischemia through an inconsistent microcirculatory flow. In cases of severe hypovolemic shock, a significant inflammatory component coexists.
- Hypovolemic shock can be due to hemorrhagic and nonhemorrhagic sources. Hemorrhage is the most frequent cause of hypovolemic shock and is most commonly due to blood loss after trauma or major surgery (Table 24.1).
- Nonhemorrhagic sources of hypovolemic shock can also occur. Although not the focus of this chapter, these are due to external fluid losses such as dehydration, vomiting, diarrhea, polyuria, uncontrolled diabetes mellitus leading to osmotic diuresis, and acute adrenocortical insufficiency. Disorders that lead to interstitial fluid redistribution such as thermal injury, trauma, and anaphylaxis can also lead to hypovolemic shock. Finally, disorders that cause increased vascular capacitance (venodilation) can lead to a relative hypovolemia and include sepsis, anaphylaxis, and the release of toxins/drugs leading to vasodilation.
- There is a progressive hemodynamic deterioration with ongoing blood loss. This classic progression is delineated in Table 24.2. Total blood volume is estimated at approximately 70 mL/kg in the average adult, or nearly 5 L for a person weighing 70 kg.

TABLE 24.1

MAJOR ETIOLOGIES OF HEMORRHAGIC SHOCK

- I. **Trauma (blunt or penetrating)**
  - Intrathoracic
  - Intraperitoneal
  - Retroperitoneal
  - Soft tissue or fractures
- II. **Gastrointestinal**
  - Upper gastrointestinal tract
    - Peptic ulcer disease, reflux esophagitis, variceal bleeding, erosive gastritis, aortoduodenal fistula
  - Lower gastrointestinal tract
    - Hemorrhoids, tumor, arteriovenous malformation, diverticulitis, ulcerative colitis, Crohn's disease, ischemia
  - Hemobilia
    - Biliary tumor, iatrogenic injury or manipulation, penetrating trauma
  - Pancreatic
    - Pancreatitis, iatrogenic injury, or manipulation
- III. **Retroperitoneal (non-trauma)**
  - Abdominal aortic aneurysm

POTENTIAL PITFALLS

- Despite these guidelines, several potential pitfalls exist that can make the diagnosis more difficult. Concurrent medication, such as β-blockers, may attenuate the physiologic response to hemorrhage. In the presence of β-blockade, tachycardia may be blunted or may not occur at all. Prior hydration status and use of diuretics can also alter the rate at which these signs present. Pregnant patients have a significantly increased total blood volume, and thus can lose up to 1,000 mL of blood before presenting with any clinical signs of hemorrhage. Blood is diverted from the placenta by vasoconstriction; the mother's total blood circulation is maintained at the expense of the fetus. Elderly patients may have atrial arrhythmias leading to a high ventricular response, making tachycardia less sensitive in this patient population. Concurrent use of antiplatelet or anticoagulant medication can cause relatively small injuries to bleed excessively, and identification and intervention may be delayed. Although unloading of the baroreceptors and activation of the sympathetic nervous system usually lead to tachycardia, some patients may respond to traumatic hemorrhage with bradycardia as a result of a vagal nerve–mediated transient sympathoinhibition due to acute and sudden blood loss. Finally, a significant reduction in skin blood flow (i.e., cool, clammy skin) is an early ominous sign of shock in view of selective cutaneous vasoconstriction. Intervention and resuscitation must be imminent upon presentation of these signs and symptoms.

CIRCULATORY CHANGES

- Hemorrhage results in a predictable pattern of events that begins with acute changes in circulating blood volume and

TABLE 24.2

CLINICAL CLASSES OF HEMORRHAGIC SHOCK

	Class I	Class II	Class III	Class IV
Blood loss (mL)	<750	750–1,500	>1,500–2,000	>2,000
Estimated blood loss	<15%	15%–30%	>30%–40%	>40%
Heart rate (beats per minute)	<100	>100	>120	>140
Systolic blood pressure	Normal	Normal	Decreased	Decreased
Pulse pressure	Normal	Decreased	Decreased	Decreased
Capillary refill	Delayed	Delayed	Delayed	Delayed
Respiratory rate (breaths per minute)	14–20	20–30	30–40	>35
Urine output (mL/h)	>30	20–30	5–15	Minimal
Mental status	Slightly anxious	Anxious	Confused	Confused and lethargic

culminates in a final common pathway shared by all classifications of shock (Fig. 24.1).

OXYGEN BALANCE

- Critical oxygen delivery is a function of cellular needs for oxygen and the ability of cells to extract oxygen from the arterial blood. Many factors contribute to this equation. During hemorrhage, tissue oxygen needs may increase due to increased respiratory muscle activity and increased catecholamine circulation. However, some evidence suggests that catecholamines down-regulate the metabolic needs of cells during hypovolemic shock.

- Regional blood flow is modified during hypovolemic shock in an attempt to maintain oxygen delivery to critical tissues. In

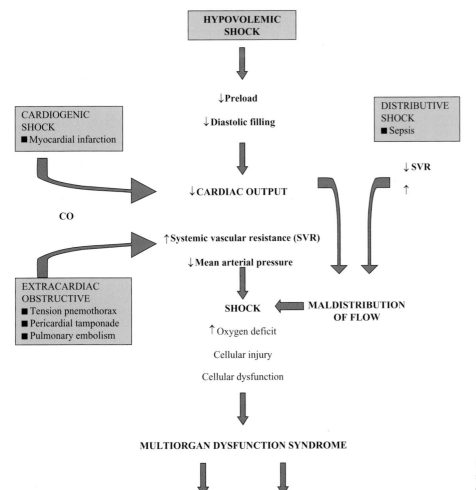

FIGURE 24.1. Final common pathway of shock. Hemorrhagic shock results in acute changes in circulating blood volume that culminates in a final common pathway shared by all classifications of shock.

ANAEROBIC GLYCOLYSIS   AEROBIC GLYCOLYSIS

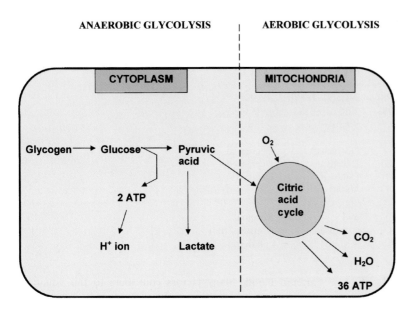

FIGURE 24.2. Cellular mechanisms during anaerobic and aerobic glycolysis. In anaerobic conditions, pyruvic acid cannot enter the citric acid cycle within the mitochondria and is instead shunted to the production of lactate. This process produces only two molecules of adenosine triphosphate (ATP), as opposed to the 36 molecules of ATP produced from glucose in the mitochondria during aerobic glycolysis. Hydrolysis of ATP molecules in anaerobic conditions results in the production of hydrogen ions that cannot be cleared, leading to intracellular acidosis. (Adapted from Mizock BA, Falk JL. Lactic acidosis in critical illness. *Crit Care Med.* 1992; 20[1]:80.)

addition, the individual needs of various tissues may vary during hemorrhagic shock. For instance, the oxygen needs of the kidney may decline during hemorrhage because a fall in renal perfusion leads to a fall in glomerular filtration and a decrease in energy-consuming tubular absorption. In contrast, the gut may experience an increased oxygen debt early due to the high oxygen need of the mucosa, along with redistribution of blood away from the gut to more critical tissues. The severity of oxygen debt during hypovolemic shock has been shown to be a major determinant of survival in animals and in patients following trauma, hemorrhage, and major surgery.

CELLULAR RESPONSE

- During hypovolemic shock, the oxygen deficit in the tissues causes a fall in the mitochondrial production and concentration of high-energy phosphates because of greater breakdown than production, failure of the Na and K pump with rapid decrease of transmembrane potential and heat shock protein production. The process is exacerbated by Ca++ influx that further inhibits cellular respiration (Fig. 24.2).

NEUROHUMORAL RESPONSE

- In response to hemorrhage and hypovolemia, a complex neurohumoral response is initiated in an attempt to maintain blood pressure and retain fluid (Fig. 24.3).

MACRO CIRCULATION

- Regional autoregulation takes place by a delicate balance of endogenous vasodilators and vasoconstrictors. Endothelial cells produce potent vasodilators such as endothelium-derived relaxing factor (nitric oxide [NO]), heme oxygenation–derived carbon monoxide (CO), and metabolic byproducts in tissues, including carbon dioxide (CO_2), potassium, and adenosine. The complex interplay of these mechanisms for vasodilation and vasoconstriction ultimately

determines the regional redistribution of blood flow to organs following hemorrhagic shock.

MICROCIRCULATION

- Alterations in microvascular function and flow (vessels < 100–150 μm) are affected through precapillary and postcapillary sphincters, which are sensitive to both extrinsic and intrinsic control mechanisms.

METABOLIC AND HORMONAL RESPONSE

- The early hyperglycemic response to trauma/hemorrhage is the combined result of enhanced glycogenolysis, caused by the hormonal response to stress including elevated epinephrine, cortisol, and glucagon levels; increased gluconeogenesis in the liver, partly mediated by glucagon; and peripheral resistance to the action of insulin. Without energy for glycolysis, the cell depends on lipolysis and the autodigestion of intracellular protein for energy. Eventually these sources become inefficient, leading to hypertriglyceridemia, increased β-hydroxybutyric acid and acetoacetate levels, and changes in the amino acid concentration pattern.

INFLAMMATORY RESPONSE AND TISSUE INJURY

- Following hemorrhage and resuscitation, macrophages, including lung macrophages and Kupffer cells in the liver, may release proinflammatory cytokines including tumor necrosis factor (TNF)-α and interleukin (IL)-1, -6, and -8. During reperfusion, cytokines may induce and amplify the inflammatory response to ischemia and may further induce local and remote organ damage. Thromboxane, prostaglandins, leukotrienes, platelets activating factor (PAF), complement

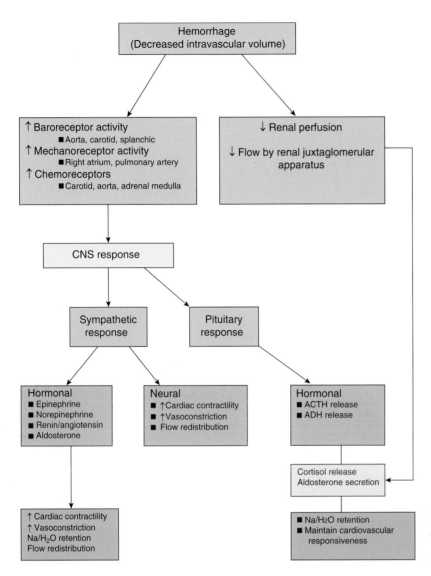

FIGURE 24.3. Neurohormonal response to hemorrhage. Hemorrhage results in a decrease in the circulating intravascular volume, which initiates a complex cascade of compensatory events. CNS, central nervous system; ACTH, adrenocorticotropic hormone; ADH, antidiuretic hormone.

fragments and oxygen radicals contribute to the inflammatory cascade and neutrophil and endothelial cell activation.

IMMUNE FUNCTION

- Despite the initiation of the inflammatory cascade, hypovolemic shock and resuscitation depress the immune system by suppressing the function of lymphocytes, macrophages, and neutrophils, depressing both humoral and cellular immune responses, decreasing antigen presentation and delayed hypersensitivity to skin-test antigens, and increasing susceptibility to sepsis. The immune consequences of hemorrhage and resuscitation differ among cell populations.

Immediate Management

Airway and Breathing

- Most patients with fully developed shock require tracheal intubation and mechanical ventilation, even if acute respiratory failure has not yet developed. If the initial response to

resuscitation is sustained (Table 24.3), then close observation of the airway may be appropriate while additional workup and treatment are pursued. However, in a patient who is not responsive or has a transient response (see below) to fluid resuscitation, control of the airway early is necessary prior to respiratory collapse.
- In addition, if diagnostic and therapeutic interventions, such as angiography and embolization, are required during resuscitation to control hemorrhage, early airway control should be obtained. Once the airway is secured, it is important to closely monitor techniques of ventilation. Studies have shown that there is a tendency of rescue and medical personnel to hyperventilate patients during resuscitation. Hyperventilated patients have been shown to have an increased mortality when compared to non-hyperventilated patients in the setting of severe traumatic brain injury.

Circulation

- The management steps to restore adequate circulation are threefold:
  - Secure access to the bloodstream to initiate infusion of fluids and blood products.

TABLE 24.3

RESPONSE TO INITIAL FLUID RESUSCITATION AND PATIENT MANAGEMENT

	Rapid response	Transient response	No response
Vital signs	Return to normal	Transient response, recurrent hypotension, and/or tachycardia	Remains abnormal
Estimated blood loss	Minimal (10%–20%)	Moderate (20%–40%)	Severe (>40%)
Additional crystalloid	Unlikely	Yes	Yes
Need for blood transfusion	Unlikely	Moderate to high	Immediate
Blood preparation	Type and cross-match (30–60 min)	Type-specific (10–20 min)	Emergency blood release (immediate type O Rh-negative blood)
Operative intervention	Possible	Likely	Highly likely
Early presence of surgeon	Yes	Yes	Yes

Adapted from American College of Surgeons Committee on Trauma. Shock. In: *Advanced Trauma Life Support.* 7th ed. American College of Surgeons Chicago, IL; 2004:79.

- Control obvious sources of hemorrhage and prevent ongoing hemorrhage.
- Assess extent of shock and hemorrhage.
- Resuscitative thoracotomy is occasionally indicated for exsanguinating hemorrhage (Table 24.4).

LETHAL TRIAD OF RESUSCITATION: HYPOTHERMIA, ACIDOSIS, AND COAGULOPATHY

- Patients with severe hemorrhagic shock requiring massive resuscitation are at risk for exhaustion of their physiologic

TABLE 24.4

INDICATIONS AND CONTRAINDICATIONS FOR EMERGENCY DEPARTMENT RESUSCITATIVE THORACOTOMY

Indications

Salvageable post-injury cardiac arrest
- Patients sustaining witnessed penetrating trauma with <15 min of prehospital cardiopulmonary resuscitation (CPR)
- Patients sustaining witnessed blunt trauma with <5 min of prehospital CPR

Persistent severe post-injury hypotension (systolic blood pressure ≤60 mm Hg) due to:
- Cardiac tamponade
- Hemorrhage—intrathoracic, intra-abdominal, extremity, cervical
- Air embolism

Contraindications
- Penetrating trauma: CPR >15 min, and no signs of life[a]
- Blunt trauma: CPR >5 min, and no signs of life[a] or asystole

[a]No signs of life = no pupillary response, respiratory effort, or motor activity.
Adapted from Cothren CC, Moore EE. Emergency department thoracotomy for the critically injured patient: objectives, indications, and outcomes. *World J Emerg Surg.* 2006;1:4.

reserves, leading to irreversible shock and the inability to recover despite ongoing resuscitation. The common denominator in these patients is the development of the "lethal triad," "bloody vicious cycle," or "spiral of death"—terms used to describe the combination of profound acidosis, hypothermia, and coagulopathy (Fig. 24.4). Each of these factors has been independently associated with increased risk of death. There also seems to be a cumulative synergistic effect for each of these risk factors in patients with hemorrhagic shock.
- In particular, *acute traumatic coagulopathy* is present in 25% to 30% of critically injured patients on arrival to the emergency department. The presence of coagulopathy may be even higher in patients with severe closed head injury, with an incidence of 21% to 79% when stratified by injury severity score (ISS). It has also been shown that the presence of early coagulopathy is an independent predictor of mortality following trauma. Early acute traumatic coagulopathy appears to be due to alterations in the thrombomodulin–protein C pathway rather than consumption of coagulation factors; however, additional work needs to be done to clarify these mechanisms.
- *Hemostatic resuscitation* employs blood components *early* in the resuscitation process to restore both perfusion and normal coagulation function while minimizing crystalloid use. Lactated Ringer solution and normal saline resuscitation have been shown to increase reperfusion injury and leukocyte adhesion. As such, standard crystalloid resuscitation

Metabolic Components of Shock

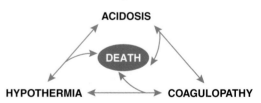

FIGURE 24.4. Lethal triad of hemorrhagic shock. The development of acidosis, hypothermia, and coagulopathy during resuscitation from hemorrhagic shock is described as the "lethal triad," "bloody vicious cycle," or "spiral of death." Each of these factors has been independently associated with mortality. There is a cumulative synergistic effect for each of these variables, such that irreversible shock may develop if all factors are present.

may worsen, presenting acidosis and coagulopathy in severely injured patients. Several retrospective studies in trauma have shown that survival is associated with an increased use of clotting factors. Many other studies have recommended more aggressive use of clotting factors to treat and correct underlying coagulopathy.

- Although additional prospective studies need to be completed, there seems to be increased literature supporting early aggressive resuscitation with clotting factors while minimizing crystalloid use during massive resuscitation. Current military experience has moved to using thawed plasma as the primary resuscitation fluid in at least 1:1 or 1:2 ratios with packed red blood cells. Continued resuscitation occurs with a massive transfusion protocol at a ratio of 6 units of plasma, 6 units of packed red blood cells, 6 units of platelets, and 10 units of cryoprecipitate. Recombinant factor VIIa is occasionally used along with early red cell transfusion to promote early hemostasis.

CHAPTER 25 ■ NEUROGENIC SHOCK

- Once other systemic reasons for shock have been ruled out, neurogenic shock should be considered. Three mechanisms can lead to neurogenic shock (Fig. 25.1):
- *Vasodilatory (distributive) shock* from autonomic disturbance with interruption of sympathetic pathways, with associated parasympathetic excitation, which causes profound vasodilatation and bradycardia, as seen in spinal cord injury or diseases of the peripheral nervous system (Guillain-Barré syndrome).
- *Cardiogenic shock,* as frequently seen in subarachnoid hemorrhage (SAH) with stunned myocardium after a catecholamine surge or ischemic stroke, especially those involving the right insula. Peripheral and pulmonary vasoconstriction, platelet aggregation and myocardial dysfunction all participate to the genesis of hemodynamic instability (Fig. 25.2).
- Hypopituitarism/adrenal insufficiency.
- Although some subtypes of neurogenic shock occur more frequently with certain disease entities—for example, cardiogenic neurogenic shock after SAH, vasodilatory neurogenic shock with spinal cord injury—significant overlap exists between different disease entities (intracerebral hemorrhage, SAH, traumatic brain injury, ischemic stroke), and one cannot establish a firm rule by which neurogenic shock occurs. Interestingly, only some patients with neurologic injuries experience true neurogenic shock, and it remains difficult to predict in whom this will be seen.

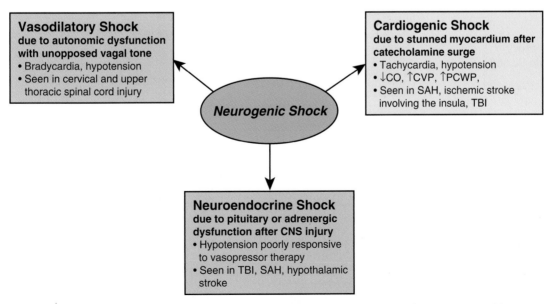

FIGURE 25.1. Neurogenic shock consists of three pathomechanisms. CNS, central nervous system; CO, cardiac output; CVP, central venous pressure; PCWP, pulmonary capillary wedge pressure; SAH, subarachnoid hemorrhage; TBI, traumatic brain injury.

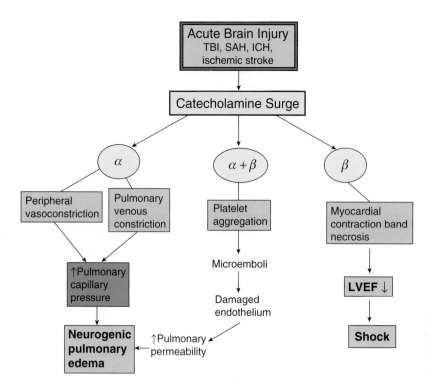

FIGURE 25.2. Summary of the pathophysiology of the cardiogenic type of neurogenic shock. ICH, intracerebral hemorrhage; LVEF, left ventricular ejection fraction; SAH, subarachnoid hemorrhage; TBI, traumatic brain injury.

- Clinical manifestations are illustrated in Figure 25.3 and are based on the relative weight of the three components described previously.

MANAGEMENT

- Two important reasons for early and proactive treatment of patients in neurogenic shock are as follows:

- Prevention of secondary brain injury from hypoxia and hypotension
- The fact that neurogenic shock, especially cardiogenic and neuroendocrine forms, is easily treatable and transient, with potentially good outcomes despite the moribund appearance of the patient in the acute phase.
- Once the diagnosis of neurogenic shock has been established and the pathophysiology (subtype) has been understood, treatment tailored to the specific subtype is initiated.

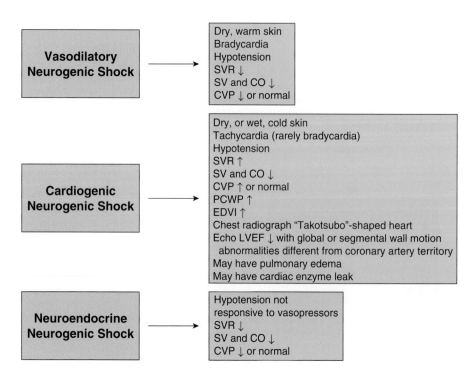

FIGURE 25.3. Clinical manifestations of the different types of neurogenic shock. CO, carbon monoxide; CVP, central venous pressure; EDVI, end-diastolic volume index; PCWP, pulmonary capillary wedge pressure; SV, stroke volume; SVR, systemic vascular resistance.

In all cases, euvolemia is of utmost importance and must be achieved before any other treatment can be successful.

- In general, vasopressor treatment as a continuous infusion is initiated and titrated to a goal mean arterial pressure and cerebral perfusion pressure (CPP). As an important management tool, an intracranial pressure measurement device is very helpful, allowing the indirect measurement of CPP. We recommend a goal CPP of ≥65 to 70 mm Hg.

- Vasodilatory neurogenic shock can be difficult to treat. In general, vagal tone predominates; however, in this state, patients frequently have peripheral α-adrenoceptor hyperresponsiveness, limiting the use of norepinephrine, epinephrine, ephedrine, and phenylephrine. In fact, sympathomimetics should be avoided as they can lead to severe blood pressure fluctuations.

- As arginine vasopressin (AVP) does not affect α- or β-adrenergic receptors, but acts on V_1 receptors, AVP may have an advantage over catecholamines or phenylephrine in this form of neurogenic shock. It has not been studied in neurogenic shock, however, and it remains unclear whether AVP may have adverse effects on neurologically ill patients. This

concern is based on animal studies indicating that vasopressin may promote the development of vasospasm in SAH, and indirect experimental studies showing a reduction in brain edema with vasopressin antagonists. No prospective human study has been undertaken to confirm or dismiss this concern, and the only retrospective study on the use of vasopressin in SAH did not show any of these potentially adverse effects. In addition to vasopressors, a temporary demand pacemaker and/or atropine may be required in cases of refractory bradycardia and hypotension.

- In cardiogenic neurogenic shock, some form of inotropic support may be necessary, either in the form of a dobutamine, milrinone, or norepinephrine infusion. Once diagnosed, neuroendocrine neurogenic shock from primary, or more often secondary, adrenal insufficiency is treated with steroid replacement therapy. We use the same dosing as in adrenal insufficiency in septic shock: hydrocortisone, 50 mg intravenously every 6 hours. As previously discussed, a cortisol stimulation test is usually not helpful, and empiric treatment after a random cortisol level should be initiated.

CHAPTER 26 ■ ANAPHYLACTIC SHOCK

- Anaphylaxis is severe, has a rapid onset, and is potentially fatal—a systemic allergic reaction that occurs after contact with an allergy-causing substance. Activation of mast cell and basophil populations by either IgE-dependent (i.e., anaphylactic reactions) or IgE-independent (i.e., anaphylactoid reactions) mechanisms results in the release of multiple mediators capable of altering vascular permeability and vascular and bronchial smooth-muscle tone and recruiting and activating inflammatory cell cascades.

- Anaphylaxis is a severe, systemic allergic reaction characterized by multisystem involvement, including the skin, airway, vascular system, and gastrointestinal tract. Severe cases may result in complete obstruction of the airway and cardiovascular collapse by vasogenic shock. Anaphylaxis accounts for about 500 to 1,000 deaths per year in the United States. The most common causes of anaphylaxis include insect stings, foods, drugs, and physical factors/exercise. Idiopathic anaphylaxis (where no causative agent is identified) accounts for up to two-thirds of patients referred to allergy/immunology specialty clinics.

- Foods such as shellfish, eggs, nuts, and milk account for one-third of food-induced anaphylactic episodes. Cardiovascular collapse is the most common hemodynamic manifestation. Vasodilation and increased capillary permeability, causing decreased preload and relative hypovolemia up to 37% of circulating blood volume, can rapidly lead to cardiac arrest if not promptly corrected. Hypoxemia from upper-airway obstruction or bronchoconstriction and myocardial ischemia can contribute to the rapid deterioration.

THERAPEUTIC MANAGEMENT

- *Rapidly assess and maintain the airway, breathing, and circulation.* If airway obstruction is imminent, perform endotracheal intubation; if unsuccessful, consider needle-catheter cricothyroid ventilation, cricothyrotomy, or tracheostomy. Patients in anaphylactic shock should be placed in a recumbent position with the lower extremities elevated, unless precluded by shortness of breath or vomiting.

- *Remove the inciting agent* (i.e., remove Hymenoptera stinger). Epinephrine by intramuscular (IM) injection should be administered early to all patients with signs of a systemic reaction, especially hypotension, airway swelling, or definite difficulty breathing at a dose is 0.2 to 0.5 mg (1:1000) IM to be repeated every 5 to 15 minutes in the absence of clinical improvement. Consider gastric lavage and administration of activated charcoal if the inciting agent was ingested.

- For aggressive crystalloid resuscitation, guidelines similar to those for septic shock can be used.

- A continuous use of epinephrine intravenously should be started immediately if hypotension persists despite IV fluids and IM epinephrine.

- There are no prospective randomized clinical studies evaluating the use of other therapeutic agents in anaphylactic shock or cardiac arrest. Adjuvant use of antihistamines (H_1 and H_2 antagonist), inhaled β-adrenergic agents, and intravenous corticosteroids has been successful in the management of a patient with anaphylaxis, and may be considered for the cases refractory to the foregoing measures.

CHAPTER 27 ■ SEDATION AND NEUROMUSCULAR BLOCKADE

PERSPECTIVE

- Anxiety is the human emotion that helps anticipate and prepare for real or perceived threats.
  - Results in release of endogenous catecholamines with an accompanying increase in heart rate, blood pressure, tremulousness, and so on
  - Can lead to agitation (i.e., anxiety coupled with confusion and movement and, if the confusion is severe enough, delirium).
    - Increasingly, there is recognition that the spectrum of anxiety, agitation, and delirium may be a manifestation of systemic inflammatory response syndrome and multiorgan dysfunction syndrome.
      - Brain is the end organ affected.
  - Thus, anxiety warrants increasing attention to monitoring its severity and treatment and to assessing the effects of therapy.

FEATURES

Anxiety

- Often described as heightened sense of awareness, apprehension, dread, or anticipation
  - Latter is important characteristic, for anxiety is an emotional state; the individual "anticipates" a threat, and anxiety prepares the individual for "fight or flight"
- Has its anatomic construct in the limbic system
  - Associated with the release of catecholamines
    - Leads to the tremulousness, sweating, tachycardia, and tachypnea—all the hallmarks of anxiety
    - At extreme, an individual may have a "panic attack"
- Anxiety and pain are often a continuum, with the perception of one increasing the perception of the other.
  - Anxiety may lead to insomnia
  - Insomnia (and sleep deprivation) can increase the perception of anxiety
  - Sleep interruption occurs for several reasons
    - Excessive noise levels in many intensive care units (ICUs) at night
    - Patient care activities
    - Measurement of vital signs
    - Laboratory tests, radiographs, and so on
  - Intubated/mechanically ventilated patients
    - Even more likely to have interrupted sleep
    - Experience discomfort from the mode of mechanical ventilation and/or tracheal suctioning and hypercarbia and hypoxia

Agitation

- Defined in the 2001 Agitation Consensus Conference
  - "Continual movement characterized by constant fidgeting, moving from side to side, pulling at dressings and bed sheets, and attempting to remove catheters or other tubes"
  - Associated with some degree of cognitive impairment—disorientation, confusion, confabulation, and so on
  - Different from anxiety as agitated patient displays purposeless movement and has some degree of cognitive dysfunction
  - At risk of injuring themselves and, in some circumstances, injuring health care providers
- Factors associated with agitation include:
  - Advanced age
  - Neuropsychiatric comorbidities
  - Seriousness of illness
  - Pain
  - Drugs that have unrecognized interactions/side effects
- Agitation is associated with
  - Increased length of stay
  - Iatrogenic infections
  - Self-extubation
- Prolonged anxiety, depending on the cause, if left untreated may lead to agitation
  - Tools to monitor agitation and the effects of interventions are listed in Table 27.1
  - Some use a variant of the Ramsay Sedation Scale and the Motor Activity Assessment Scale to monitor for agitation (Table 27.2)

Delirium

- Delirium's hallmark is cognitive dysfunction, commonly manifested as disorientation
  - This used to be termed "ICU syndrome," a diagnosis of exclusion.
  - Prevalence of delirium
    - Coronary care unit: as low as 7%
    - Medical ICU: as high as 70% to 80%

TABLE 27.1

SEDATION SCALES

ATICE	Adaptation to the Intensive Care Environment
MSAT	Minnesota Sedation Assessment Tool
RSS	Ramsay Sedation Scale
RASS	Richmond Agitation-Sedation Scale
SAS	Sedation Agitation Scale
VICS	Vancouver Interaction and Calmness Scale

TABLE 27.2

MOTOR ACTIVITY ASSESSMENT SCALE

Score	Description	Definition
0	Unresponsive	Does not move with noxious stimulus
1	Responsive only to noxious stimuli	Opens eyes *or* raises eyebrows *or* turns head toward stimulus *or* moves limbs with noxious stimulus
2	Responsive to touch or name	Opens eyes *or* raises eyebrows *or* turns head toward stimulus *or* moves limbs when touched or name is loudly spoken
3	Calm and cooperative	No external stimulus is required to elicit movement, *and* the patient is adjusting sheets or clothes purposefully and follows commands
4	Restless and cooperative	No external stimulus is required to elicit movement, *and* patient is picking at sheets or clothes or uncovering self and follows commands
5	Agitated	No external stimulus is required to elicit movement, *and* patient is attempting to sit up *or* moves limbs out of bed *and* does not consistently follow commands
6	Dangerously agitated, uncooperative	No external stimulus is required to elicit movement, *and* patient is pulling at tubes or catheters *or* thrashing side to side *or* striking at staff *or* trying to climb out of bed *and* does not calm down when asked

Reprinted from Devlin JW, Boleski G, Mlynarek M, et al. Motor Activity Assessment Scale: a valid and reliable sedation scale for use with mechanically ventilated patients in an adult surgical intensive care unit. *Crit Care Med.* 1999;27:1271–1275, with permission.

- Manifestations include a variety of psychomotor symptoms/ signs
  - Hypoactive (listlessness) to hyperactive (combative behavior) is seen
  - A mixed picture may be noted, with patients cycling between overly sedated states to hyperactive, agitated states
  - Delirious patient at risk for developing
    - Long-term cognitive impairment
    - Greater length of ICU and hospital stay
    - Increased mortality

TABLE 27.3

ANXIETY ASSOCIATED WITH AN INCREASED INCIDENCE OF SEVERAL DISEASE STATES/PROCESSES

Myocardial ischemia
Asthma
Pain
Agitation
Delirium

TABLE 27.4

PHYSICAL EXAMINATION

Tachypnea
Tachycardia
Confusion
Abdominal distention (ileus, full bladder)
Movement

EVALUATION

- Anxiety is a valid emotional response to hospitalization in an ICU.
  - Overexuberant response to the stressors in the ICU environment can be detrimental.
  - Anxious patients have an increase in the incidence of several disease states/processes (Table 27.3).
  - Patients are examined daily to look for signs that increase anxiety likelihood (Table 27.4).
  - Laboratory evaluation (Table 27.5) is helpful in looking for causes.
- When a patient admits to excessive anxiety, first attempt is to decrease the anxiety through nonpharmacologic means (Table 27.6).
  - Recognize that the ICU environment must be calm and nurturing.
  - Attention to such details must be paid
    - Room temperature
    - Noise levels
    - Sleep disturbance—the bane of most modern ICUs
- 60% to 70% of patients in the ICU for longer than 48 hours require pharmacologic therapy (Table 27.7).
  - Opioids, benzodiazepines, haloperidol, propofol, and dexmedetomidine are treatment mainstays.

TREATMENT

Nonsteroidal Anti-inflammatory Drugs

- Nonsteroidal anti-inflammatory drugs are not sedative but, by decreasing pain, they decrease pain-associated anxiety.
  - When cyclo-oxygenase-2 inhibitors coupled with gabapentin or its precursor, pregabalin, they have analgesic and sedative properties if given preoperatively *per os* to patients who are anticipated to be admitted postoperatively to the ICU.

TABLE 27.5

LABORATORY EVALUATION

Complete blood count (anemia, leukocytosis/leukopenia)
Arterial blood gases (hypoxia, hypocarbia/hypercapnia)
Electrolytes[a]
Glucose
Creatinine/blood urea nitrogen

[a]To include calcium and magnesium.

TABLE 27.6

NONPHARMACOLOGIC THERAPY FOR ANXIETY-PRODUCING EVENTS

Thorough explanation of situation/findings
Reassurance
Increased presence of family members
Decreased noise
Decreased nocturnal interruptions
Assisted ventilation for hypercarbia
Cardioversion for hemodynamically significant
    tachyarrhythmias
Decrease/stop tube feedings if (partial) ileus
Foley catheter for bladder distention
Re-establishment of sleep cycle

- A combination of 400 mg of celecoxib and 150 mg of pregabalin improved patients' sedation levels by approximately 33% for up to 24 hours postoperatively.

Opioids

- Opioids have not only analgesic but also anxiolytic properties.
  - Morphine is anxiolytic.
    - Not nearly as effective as newer opioids
    - Because of the buildup of active metabolites in patients with renal insufficiency, it is not recommended for patients in the ICU.
    - Fentanyl and remifentanil are more than 90% effective in providing adequate sedation for intubated and mechanically ventilated patients in the ICU.
      - With equal efficacy and differences in cost, fentanyl is recommended in most patients, except those with significant renal/hepatic impairment (Table 27.8).

Benzodiazepines

- Benzodiazepines potentiate gamma-amino butyric acid (GABA) effects via the benzodiazepine receptor and suppress central nervous system (CNS) activity.
  - They have hypnotic, muscle-relaxant, anticonvulsive, and antegrade and variable retrograde amnestic properties.
  - No analgesic properties

TABLE 27.7

THERAPY FOR ANXIETY-PRODUCING EVENTS

Supplemental oxygen for hypoxia
Minimize dose of supplemental catecholamines
Continue any of patients' psychotropic medications, if
    appropriate
Opioids
Benzodiazepines
Haloperidol
Propofol
Dexmedetomidine
Ketamine

TABLE 27.8

OPIOIDS AS SEDATIVE DRUGS IN THE INTENSIVE CARE UNIT

Drug[a]	Bolus dose	Infusion
Fentanyl	1 μg/kg	1–2 μg/kg/h
Remifentanil	—	9 μg/kg/h

[a]Side effects: Hypotension, nausea and vomiting, respiratory depression.

- Similar to the opioids, they produce respiratory depression in a dose-dependent fashion.
- Benzodiazepines are metabolized in the liver with the metabolites excreted by the kidneys.
  - Half-lives ($t\frac{1}{2}$) are prolonged, and active metabolites may accumulate.
  - Commonly, benzodiazepines are administered by continuous infusion.
    - Context-sensitive $t\frac{1}{2}$ is more germane but independent of the method of administration because of the potential prolonged effect.
    - Daily "off" period should be established to avoid overdosage.
    - Commonly used ICU benzodiazepines are diazepam, midazolam, and lorazepam (Table 27.9).

Additional Cautions and Recommendations Regarding Benzodiazepine Use

- The US Food and Drug Administration has administered black box warnings for benzodiazepines.
  - Anyone administering these respiratory depressants must be skilled in airway management and resuscitation.
  - Must have the benzodiazepine antagonist flumazenil available in the ICU
    - Flumazenil has maximum effect within 5 to 10 minutes after IV administration and has a mean $t\frac{1}{2}$ of approximately 1 hour.
    - Usually given in 0.1 to 0.2 mg increments, repeated every 5 to 10 minutes, to a total dose of 1 mg
    - Recommended that infusions of benzodiazepines be stopped for a daily drug "holiday"
      - Infusion stopped typically every morning around 7:00 or 8:00 AM.
      - Infusion remains off until the patient exhibits symptoms or signs that warrant restarting the infusion.
  - Ramsey Sedation Scale can be used to monitor sedation (Table 27.10).
  - Several others exist that may be used are more comprehensive (see Table 27.1).
  - Once these medications are completely discontinued, up to one-third of the patients will exhibit signs of withdrawal.
    - Thus, discontinue the benzodiazepines slowly over several days.
    - Treat side effects of withdrawal—tachycardia and hypertension—with a beta-blocker or an alternative drug, including chronic low doses of benzodiazepines if beta-blockers are contraindicated.

TABLE 27.9

BENZODIAZEPINES USED FOR ANXIOLYSIS IN THE ICU

Drug (classification)	$t_{1/2}$ (h)	Active metabolite(s) ($t^{1/2}$)	Intermittent IV bolus	Continuous IV infusion
Diazepam (long-acting)	20–50	Desmethyldiazepam (30–200)	1–2 mg (max 0.1–0.2 mg/kg)	—
Lorazepam (intermittent-acting)	10–20	None[a]	0.5–2 mg (max 4 mg)	Up to 0.025 mg/kg/h
Midazolam (short-acting)	1–2.5	1-hydroxy midazolam	0.5–2 mg (max 0.1 mg/kg)	Up to 0.05 mg/kg/h

[a] 3–0-phenolic glucuronide is the inactive metabolite.

Propofol

- Propofol (di-isopropylphenol)
- Highly lipophilic compound formulated in an isotonic oil in water emulsion (Intralipid) unrelated to other sedative/anesthetic agents.
  - Side effects include hypertriglyceridemia and bacterial contamination of infusions.
  - Addition of ethylenediaminetetraacetic acid or bisulfite as preservatives decreases the incidence of bacterial overgrowth.
  - Rare side effect is propofol infusion syndrome
    - Metabolic acidosis and ventricular fibrillation in children and in young adults with neurologic injury receiving >100 μg/kg/minute for more than 12 to 24 hours.
  - Propofol probably most commonly used IV anesthesia induction agent.
    - Advocated for use in moderate sedation (endoscopy suite) protocols
    - Rapid onset and offset, few residual aftereffects, and low side-effect profile makes it often used for short-term sedation in the ICU.
  - Propofol has no analgesic properties.
    - For patients with pain, an analgesic drug should be co-administered.
- Propofol has also been used to treat status epilepticus and to induce sleep in the ICU.

Dexmedetomidine

- Alpha-2 (α_2) agonists, such as methyldopa and clonidine, long known to have sedative properties.

TABLE 27.10

RAMSEY SEDATION SCALE

Patient:		
Awake	1.	Anxious or agitated
	2.	Cooperative/tranquil
	3.	Responds to commands only, response to glabellar tap
Asleep	4.	Brisk
	5.	Sluggish
	6.	None

From Ramsay MAE, Savege TM, Simpson BRJ, et al. Controlled sedation with alphaxalone-alphadolone. *Br Med J.* 1974;2:656–659, with permission.

- Clonidine is administered epidurally for its antinociceptive effects in the spinal cord.
- Dexmedetomidine is an α_2 agonist that binds to α_2 receptors in the locus ceruleus.
  - α_2/α_1 ratio of approximately 1,620:1
    - Approximately seven times more avidly than clonidine
    - Binding to the α_2 receptor releases norepinephrine and decreases sympathetic activity
    - Net effect is sedation, analgesia, and amnesia
- Dexmedetomidine is unique compared to the other anxiolytic drugs because patients are not only calm but appear to be sleeping.
  - Commonly used to sedate patients after cardiac surgery and after neurosurgical procedures
  - Patients who abuse alcohol, cocaine, and marijuana may benefit the most because dexmedetomidine treats many of the symptoms and signs of withdrawal.
- Dexmedetomidine not associated with respiratory depression, unlike opioids or benzodiazepines.
  - Because of its central alpha agonist, hypotension can and does occur.
  - Low-dose dexmedetomidine (6 μg/kg/hour for 10 minutes followed by an infusion of 0.2 μg/kg/hour) is as effective as higher doses (0.6 μg/kg/hour), with fewer side effects.
    - Concern of a hyperdynamic state if dexmedetomidine used for more than 24 hours and discontinued abruptly
      - Similar to the one that develops when clonidine is stopped abruptly after long-term use
- Dexmedetomidine is FDA approved for 24-hour use.
  - Many clinicians are using it for longer than 24 hours.
  - Dexmedetomidine the most expensive of common sedatives.

Butyrophenones

- Neuroleptic drugs also known as antipsychotic drugs or major tranquilizers
- Induce apathy, a state of mental detachment in patients with psychoses or delirium
- Inhibit dopamine-mediated neurotransmissions in CNS and decrease the frequency of hallucinations, delusions, and other abnormal thoughts
- Patients may develop a characteristic flat affect.
- Active in the chemoreceptor trigger zone in the brainstem and thus are effective antiemetics
- Also used to treat hiccups

- A synergistic anxiolytic drugs when used with benzodiazepines
- Haloperidol used most often to treat delirium in the ICU
  - Has a wide therapeutic margin
    - Rare but important side effects including hypotension, extrapyramidal symptoms, anticholinergic effects (tachycardia, urinary retention, ileus), neuroleptic malignant syndrome, and seizures
      - Hypotension after a dose of haloperidol almost always seen in patients who are hypovolemic
      - Extrapyramidal symptoms are more often seen in younger patients and in patients with depleted dopamine stores (e.g., patients with Parkinson disease).
  - Initial dose of haloperidol
    - Usually 0.5 to 2 mg administered parenterally
    - Depending on the patient's size, age, and degree of agitation/delirium, 5 mg can be given.
    - Has a slow onset, so peak effects may not be seen for 15 to 30 minutes
      - Repeat doses then administered at 30- to 60-minute intervals
      - Recurrence of agitation or an increase in delirium is an indication for repeat doses, which may be increased if the initial dose was inadequate
      - Tardive dyskinesia or neuroleptic malignant syndrome can occur even during the short duration of therapy used in the ICU.
    - Because of its anticholinergic effects, may prolong the QT in a dose-dependent fashion
      - Resulting in arrhythmias and torsades de pointes
      - Those receiving haloperidol should have electrocardiogram monitored
- Retrospectively in mechanically ventilated ICU patients, those receiving haloperidol had significantly lower mortality than those who did not

Other Agents

- *Barbiturates:* Have pronounced effects on the CNS, lowering intracranial pressure and raising the seizure threshold
- Used to induce a "barbiturate coma" in patients with increased intracranial pressure and terminate seizures
- Administered by IV bolus to produce hypotension
- Because of lipid solubility, if given by continuous infusion, accumulate in fat stores
  - Thus have a duration of action that can be significantly long (i.e., days to weeks)
  - Infrequently administered by continuous infusion for long-term use except as salvage for elevated
- *Ketamine:* A phencyclidine derivative nonbarbiturate, rapid-acting, general anesthetic
- Administered parenterally
- Induces "dissociative anesthesia" because it interrupts association pathways of the brain before blocking sensory pathways
  - Patients may perceive pain, but it does not bother them.
  - Because it is a phencyclidine derivative, 10% to 20% of adult patients may have psychological sequelae including hallucinations.
- Used as a general anesthetic because it raises cardiac output, pulse rate, and arterial and venous pressures

- Maintains pharyngeal and laryngeal reflexes without suppressing respiration
- A bronchodilator and advocated as the anesthetic agent of choice in patients with reactive airways disease
- Dose
  - 1-mg/kg bolus of ketamine can be administered, followed by an infusion of 1.0 mg/kg/hour, titrated up to 4.5 mg/kg/hour
  - Administer a benzodiazepine to reduce the frequency of psychologic sequelae
  - Ketamine is contraindicated in patients with cardiac ischemia or raised intracranial pressure.

Neuromuscular Blockade

- Even with effective doses of anxiolytic drugs, some patients remain delirious and agitated, and a further increase in the dose of anxiolytic drugs is proscribed because of side effects.
- Such patients, along with those with closed-head injuries, tetanus, and ALI, may require other therapeutic modalities.
- If patient is tracheally intubated, mechanically ventilated, and receiving adequate sedation, chemical paralysis with a neuromuscular blocking agent (NMBA) is an option (Table 27.11).

Monitoring

- Before administering NMBAs, patients must be mechanically ventilated, sedated, and monitored.
- Most practitioners will first implement sedation therapy to the point that the patient is unconscious before initiating NMBA therapy.
- Monitoring the depth of blockade and the necessity of blockade is essential in minimizing these side effects.
  - Assessing the degree of blockade by measuring the amount of block of the neuromuscular receptor with a twitch monitor is the preferred technique.
    - An electrical stimulus is applied to a peripheral motor nerve, and the effects of the stimulus on the motor group supplied by that nerve are observed (Figs. 27.1 and 27.2).
    - Most often performed using a twitch stimulator that generates a stimulus of up to 160 mA intensity that lasts 10 ms and is repeated every 500 ms so that four stimuli (train-of-four [TOF]) are delivered
      - Effects can be visualized, but the preferred technique is for the observer to palpate the response.

TABLE 27.11

INDICATIONS FOR THE MANAGEMENT OF PATIENTS WITH NEUROMUSCULAR BLOCKING AGENTS

Closed-head injury with raised intracranial pressure
Tetanus
Decreased $S\bar{v}O_2$ in hypermetabolic, agitated states

Purpose:

To describe the process of utilizing a nerve stimulator to stimulate the ulnar nerve, usually with tactile assessment of a neuromuscular twitch, usually tactile assessment of an abducted thumb, to assess the degree of neuromuscular block.

Definitions:

Neuromuscular block: the process by which the postsynaptic acetylcholine receptor is depressed and variably response to release of acetylcholine in the neuromuscular junction cleft

Peripheral nerve stimulation: electrical stimulation, usually from 40 to 120 mA at a peripheral nerve, usually the ulnar, either at the elbow or at the wrist

Train-of-four: a specific type of nerve stimulation in which the nerve stimulator delivers an electrical stimulus to the nerve lasting 10 ms and repeated every 500 ms for a total of 4 stimuli

Equipment:

1.   Peripheral nerve stimulator
2.   Two electrode pads (electrocardiogram pads may be used)

Procedure:

1.   Clean the area where the electrode pads will be placed with alcohol to remove any skin oils. This will reduce the resistance at the skin and decrease the amount of current needed to stimulate the nerve. If the resistance of the skin is still high, then an abrasive compound can be used to remove dead skin.
2.   Place two electrodes over the ulnar nerve, usually 3 to 5 cm apart.
3.   Attach electrodes to the leads, usually the positive electrode proximally.
4.   Cover the fingers and abduct the thumb. Increase the amperage of the stimulator until 4 twitches of the thumb are palpated by tactile assessment. Stimuli should not be delivered more frequently than every 20 seconds. Once 4 twitches are palpated, a supramaximal stimulus can be delivered by increasing the amperage 10% to 30% over the amperage required to palpate 4 twitches.

Goals:

1.   To achieve a level of train-of-four of 2 to 4. If with 3 or 4 twitches the patient either spontaneously triggers the ventilator or exhibits muscular activity that adversely affects oxygenation or airway or intracranial pressure, then increased neuromuscular block is required.
2.   A train-of-four of 1 to 0 indicates that the degree of neuromuscular block is too great, and the dosage of neuromuscular blocking agent should be decreased.

FIGURE 27.1. Protocol for monitoring degree of neuromuscular block using a nerve stimulator and assessment of the train-of-four twitch. (Reproduced from Murray MJ, Oyen L, Bazzell CM. Use of sedatives, analgesics, and neuromuscular blockers. In: Parillo JE, Dellinger RP, eds. *Critical Care Medicine: Principles of Diagnosis and Management.* 2nd ed. St. Louis, MO: Mosby; 2001:296–311, with permission.)

○ Probably easiest to measure the TOF response by stimulating the ulnar nerve at the wrist

○ Goal of therapy is to provide a sufficient amount of drug so that the patient has only one to two twitches,

as opposed to none (overblocked) or three to four (possibly underblocked) twitches.

Complications of Neuromuscular Blocking Agents

● One of the most feared complications of neuromuscular block is accidental extubation.

  ● Should a paralyzed patient become accidentally extubated, time is of the essence, especially in patients with adult respiratory distress syndrome

  ● Ventilation must begin immediately with a mask and anesthesia bag using 100% oxygen while steps are taken to reintubate the patient.

● Another complication is profound weakness once the drug is discontinued.

  ● Approximately 10% of patients who receive NMBAs will develop a myopathy from which it takes days or weeks to recover.

  ● Known as critical illness myopathy (CIM)

  ● Cause of CIM in ICU multifactorial

    ○ Prolonged use of NMBAs in the ICU is one of the causative factors

    ○ Corticosteroids are also known to produce myopathy

    ○ Daily assessments must be made to determine whether NMBA use is justified, and the TOF should be maintained at one to two twitches

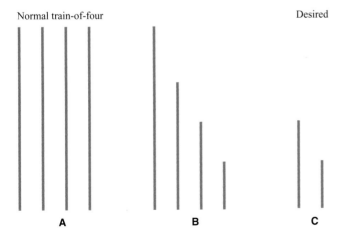

FIGURE 27.2. Train-of-four monitoring. **A:** With the twitch stimulator at 40 to 10 mA, four twitches are measured. **B:** As the neuromuscular blocking agent (NMBA) takes effect, the second, third, and fourth twitches are weaker/fade. **C:** The goal with additional time or drug is to have one to two twitches.

Agents: Aminosteroids

- *Pancuronium:* A long-acting, nondepolarizing, aminosteroidal compound
  - Produces effective block for up to 90 minutes after a bolus dose of 0.06 to 0.08 mg/kg
  - Intermittent boluses often administered but can be used as a continuous infusion, titrating the dose to one or two twitches by TOF monitor
  - Induces vagolysis, limiting its use in patients who cannot tolerate an increase in heart rate
  - With renal or liver failure, pancuronium's effects are prolonged because of the increased elimination $t^1/_2$ of pancuronium and its 3-hydroxypancuronium metabolite, which has one-third to one-half the activity of pancuronium.
- *Vecuronium:* Related to pancuronium, but an intermediate-acting NMBA without the vagolytic properties of pancuronium
  - IV bolus dose of 0.08 to 0.10 mg/kg produces block within $2^1/_2$ to 3 minutes that typically lasts 35 to 45 minutes.
  - After a bolus, may be administered as a continuous infusion of 0.8 to 1.4 μg/kg/minute, titrating the rate to the degree of block desired
    - The 3-desacetylvecuronium metabolite has 50% of the pharmacologic activity of the parent compound
      - Patients with hepatic dysfunction may have increased plasma concentrations of both the parent compound and the active metabolite, causing prolonged block.
      - Renal dysfunction also prolongs the duration of block.
      - Associated with CIM, especially in patients receiving corticosteroids
- *Rocuronium:* A newer aminosteroidal NMBA, with an intermediate duration of action and a rapid onset
  - A bolus of 0.6 to 0.1 mg/kg results in a block almost always achieved within 2 minutes, with maximum block occurring within 3 minutes.
- Continuous infusions are administered at 8 to 10 μg/kg/minute.
  - Rocuronium's metabolite, 17-desacetylrocuronium, has approximately only 5% to 10% activity compared to the parent compound.
    - Renal failure should not have an effect on duration of action, but hepatic failure may prolong rocuronium's duration of action.

Agents: Benzylisoquinolinium Compounds

- *Atracurium:* An intermediate-acting NMBA with minimal cardiovascular side effects
  - Associated with histamine release at higher doses
  - Unique metabolism (ester hydrolysis and Hofmann elimination) so that renal or hepatic dysfunction does not affect its duration of block

- Has been associated with persistent neuromuscular weakness as has been reported with other NMBAs
- *Cisatracurium:* One of atracurium's 16 isomers
  - An intermediate-acting benzylisoquinolinium NMBA
  - Produces few cardiovascular effects
  - Has fewer tendencies to produce mast cell degranulation than does atracurium
  - Bolus doses with a 0.10 to 0.2 mg/kg result in paralysis in an average of 2.5 minutes, and recovery begins at approximately 25 minutes.
  - Maintenance infusion rates should be started at 2.5 to 3.0 μg/kg/minute.
  - Metabolized by ester hydrolysis and Hofmann elimination, so duration of block should not be affected by multiorgan dysfunction syndrome.
  - Not yet been reports of significantly prolonged recovery associated with cisatracurium
    - Mean peak plasma laudanosine concentrations are lower in patients receiving cisatracurium as compared to patients receiving clinically equivalent doses of atracurium.
    - Laudanosine at high doses produces seizures in animals.
      - A case of seizures in a human receiving atracurium or cisatracurium has not been reported.

Recovery

- Patients receiving an NMBA should have daily drug holidays.
- When NMBA is no longer required, it is discontinued.
- With all the NMBAs, the TOF should normalize (four twitches) within 3 to 4 hours
- If not, the patient may have a CIM associated with the NMBA (with an increased incidence in patients receiving corticosteroids and patients with sepsis, etc.).
- If, after 24 hours, the patient has inadequate strength, additional studies should be done to include an assessment of the antibiotics the patient is receiving, electrolytes (calcium, magnesium, phosphorus), and temperature (hypothermia prolongs neuromuscular block).
- If no comorbid condition accounts for the degree of neuromuscular block, a neurology consult should be considered.
  - Electromyography is typically performed (to rule out critical illness polyneuropathy).
  - In some circumstances, a muscle biopsy is obtained.
  - Patients with CIM secondary to the neuromuscular blockade will have loss of myosin.
  - Treatment is supportive with maintenance of sedation, mechanical ventilation, physical therapy, skin care, eye care, and so on.

CHAPTER 28 ■ NUTRITIONAL ISSUES

IMMEDIATE CONCERNS

- There is no medical evidence that starvation is therapeutic.
  - More than 25 years ago, it was noted that the catabolic response to multiple injuries resulted in loss of up to 20% of normal body weight within 3 weeks despite some oral intake started during the first week.
  - Catabolic rapid wasting of large weight-bearing muscle groups of critically injured patients in a hospital setting has been noted (Table 28.1).
  - Critical illness most frequently compromises a patient's ability to normally take in adequate nutrition; critical care technology offers several alternative routes of providing nutritional support (Table 28.2).
    - Intravenous routes—total parenteral nutrition (TPN) and peripheral parenteral nutrition
    - Enteral routes with various formulae tailored to the patient's unique requirements

NUTRITIONAL ASSESSMENT

- Critically ill patients are at risk for nutritional deficiencies.
  - Diagnostic criteria for various protein and calorie-deficient states are noted in Table 28.3.
  - Because of the risk that a critically ill patient with underlying nutritional deficiency will develop marasmic kwashiorkor, they are screened for chronic undernutrition on admission to the hospital/intensive care unit.
    - One such screening tool, the Malnutrition Universal Screening Tool (MUST), provides a numerical index.
      - 0: minimal risk
      - 1: medium risk
      - 2: high risk of malnutrition
      - Urgency of instituting nutritional support increases for patients with a score of 1 and especially 2.
      - MUST evaluates

- Patients' body mass index (weight in kilograms [kg] divided by height in meters squared [m^2])
- Prehospital involuntary weight loss as a percent of body weight
- Potential for critical illness-induced starvation for the next 5 days.
  - Many biochemical markers are available to track a patient's nutritional state.
    - Albumin concentration—a good prognostic marker of a patient's *chronic* nutritional state
      - Perioperative mortality has been shown to increase when albumin concentration is <30 g/L.
      - Serum albumin has a long serum half-life and, hence, does not reflect acute responses to nutritional therapy.
    - Estimates of whole-body potassium
      - Total body potassium represents lean cellular mass and can be a useful measurement of changes in lean tissue mass that occur rather slowly.

TABLE 28.1

EBB–FLOW PHASE OF RESPONSE TO INJURY

	Ebb	Catabolic flow	Anabolic flow
O_2 consumption	↓	↑↑	↑
Nitrogen balance	↓	↓↓	↑
Cortisol	↑	↑	
Epinephrine	↑↑↑		
Insulin	↑	↑	↑↑
Glucagon	↑↑	↑↑	↑
Glucose	↑	↑	

TABLE 28.2

COMMONLY USED ROUTES OF NUTRITION

		Parenteral	
Enteral	Central	Peripheral	
Advantages			
Uses gut barrier to control water and electrolyte absorption; natural relationship for hepatic "first pass" metabolism; cost-effective	Uninterrupted nutrient administration; can be continued in operating room; rapid change in formula possible; does not interfere with oral drug administration; does not depend on gut motility	Avoids central venous catheter	
Disadvantages			
Frequent interruptions for NPO status; interference with drug absorption (e.g., phenytoin); frequent feeding tube complications	Hyperosmolar, hyperglycemic coma; expensive; central venous line complications/infections	Partial nutritional support to supplement low levels of enteral intake	

NPO, nothing by mouth.

TABLE 28.3

INDICES OF MALNUTRITION: PROTEIN–ENERGY MALNUTRITION

% IBW	Undernutrition 80%	Marasmus less than 60%	Kwashiorkor 60%–80% with edema	Obesity
BMI	18.5–20	<18.5	<18.5	30
Unplanned weight loss past 3–6 mo	5%–10%			<5%
Acute disease effect	Iatrogenic starvation	Prolonged underfeeding with catabolic illness	Severe protein-energy deprivation, usually prolonged fasting with catabolic diseases	Eating
Arm circ. (cm)	23.5	<23.5	<23.5	32.0
MUST score	1	2	2	0
Edema	–	–	+	–
Cause	Low nutrition intake, chronic illness	Low protein calorie intake	Low protein intake	Excess energy intake
T-lymphocyte count (cells/μL)	<1,800	<800	<800	2,000

IBW, ideal body weight; BMI, body mass index; circ., circumference; MUST, Malnutrition Universal Screening Tool.

– Similarly, 24-hour creatinine production is a marker of total skeletal muscle mass.
– Both of these markers change relatively slowly and may not be useful to monitor the patient's response to nutritional therapy for critical illness.
○ Water balance
○ Visceral proteins such as prealbumin, transferrin, and retinol-binding protein
– Short half-lives make these useful to monitor protein synthetic response to nutritional support therapy.
• Nitrogen (N) balance via a 24-hour urine urea nitrogen excretion is a useful technique to monitor response to nutritional support (Table 28.4).
○ If the patient's blood urea nitrogen is not stable, corrections for retained N must be performed.

• Energy expenditure may be calculated by the Harris–Benedict equation or measured directly with an indirect calorimeter (Table 28.5).
• Overall monitoring of a patient's response to nutrition support performed by a battery of the tests described earlier
• Daily weights are tracked to monitor a patient's response to nutritional support.
○ Initially, weight gain will represent an increase in total body water, which will start decreasing (diuresing) as the patient becomes anabolic.
○ During the anabolic phase, the patient will initially lose weight via diuresis of water, then gain weight as lean body mass.
○ Obese patients may continue to lose weight from fat stores if they are fed a high-protein, restricted calorie diet.

TABLE 28.4

ASSESSMENT OF DAILY NITROGEN BALANCE

Nitrogen intake = protein administered in g/day divided by 6.25 = g N/day
[0.1 g protein = 0.16 g N (6.25 g protein contains 1 g N)]
Urine urea nitrogen = 80% of total urine nitrogen
1 g (16.6 mMol) urea = 28/60 g nitrogen[a]
1) 24-h urine urea N in g/day = (A) in g
2) Measure of proteinuria, if any = Y

$$Y \times 0.16 = (B) \text{ in g}$$

3) Correction for any rise of BUN assuming no change in body weight in kg
Rise in blood urea (in 24 h) = Z in g $\cdot$ L^{-1}
Z in g $\times$ 60% body weight $\times$ 28/60 = Z $\times$ body weight $\times$ 0.28 = (C) in g
(A) + (B) + (C) = nitrogen loss
N balance = (nitrogen intake – nitrogen loss)

BUN, blood urea nitrogen.
[a]28 is molecular weight of N in urea and 60 is total molecular weight of urea (i.e., 1 g urea = 0.47 g N).

TABLE 28.5

INDIRECT CALORIMETRY—DAILY ENERGY EXPENDITURE

Kcal/day = 3.94 $\times$ VO_2 (L/24 h) + 1.11 $\times$ VCO_2 (L/24 h) $\times$ 2.17 UN (g/24 h)
VO_2 = [($FiO_2 \times V_I$) – ($F_EO_2 \times V_E$)] $\times$ 1,440 min/24 h
VCO_2 = ($F_ECO_2 \cdot V_E - F_ICO_2 \cdot V_I$) $\times$ 1,440 min/24 h
$$V_1 = \frac{V_E[(1 - F_EO_2) - F_ECO_2]}{(1 - F_1O_2)} \text{ Haldane correction}$$
VO_2 = oxygen consumption (L/24 h)
VCO_2 = carbon dioxide production (L/24 h)
V_I = inspired ventilation (L/min)
V_E = expired ventilation (L/min)
FiO_2 = mole fraction inspired oxygen
FeO_2 = mole fraction expired oxygen
F_ICO_2 = mole fraction inspired carbon dioxide (assumed to be 0)
F_ECO_2 = mole fraction expired carbon dioxide
UN = 24-hour urinary nitrogen loss (g/24 h)

- Functional measurements that indirectly depend on the nutrition response, such as immunologic function, can be followed.
  - Severely malnourished patient exhibits immunocompromise by skin test anergy, low absolute lymphocyte count, low T-cell lymphocyte count, difficulty mounting a fever, and increased susceptibility to infections.
  - These functions should improve with aggressive nutritional support.

Timing of Nutritional Support

- Once the decision is made to provide nutritional support for the critically ill, one has to decide on the best route of administration—parenteral or enteral.
- One to two decades ago, parenteral nutrition (TPN) was thought to be associated with a higher mortality rate than enteral nutrition in patients who had abdominal trauma.
  - More recently, the major difference between total enteral nutrition (TEN) and TPN was the fact that enteral-fed patients had more frequent interruptions of nutrition).
- There has been grave concern that TPN puts a patient at risk for serious infection complications.
  - Bloodstream infections are relatively rare during TPN.
  - TEN patients have a significantly higher incidence of feeding tube complications than TPN patients have from central venous catheter complications.
  - Inadequate nutritional intake (<7 kcal/kg/day) was associated with sepsis.
  - Those who received TEN were equally likely to have infectious complications as those who received TPN.
    - Starting early and adequate nutrition support to prevent infectious morbidity is important.
  - An alleged benefit of early enteral feeding is to maintain the integrity of the gut mucosal lining and thus limit translocation of microorganisms from intestinal lumen to bloodstream.
    - This may not be correct, as bacterial translocation from the gut to the bloodstream is not the source of bloodstream infections in patients who are fed parenterally.
  - TEN does have some demonstrated advantages over TPN.
    - Lower cost
    - Using gut absorption to regulate total body water balance
    - Ability to utilize larger molecules as a food source
  - TPN has advantages over TEN that include fewer interruptions for NPO status prior to procedures and no interference with drug absorption.

Nutritional Support for Specific Organ Dysfunction

Hepatic Failure

- One of the most vexing morbidities requiring prescriptions for nutritional support
  - Nitrogen from amino acid metabolism remains as ammonia because it is not metabolized to urea in severe disease.
  - Hyperammonemia leads to secondary neurologic dysfunction including hepatic coma.

- Protein needs to be administered in amounts to replace catabolic losses but not high enough to lead to high levels of ammonia.
- Sorbitol may be administered enterally to try to lower ammonia by increasing gut motility and decreasing intestinal transit time to decrease the absorption of proteins and ammonia from bacterial metabolism of intraluminal amino acids.
- Hepatic glycogen stores are also depleted in end-stage hepatic failure.
  - Maintenance of normoglycemia is extremely difficult.
  - High glucose feedings may be required to compensate for lack of hepatic glucose production.

Renal Failure

- Rising blood levels of the nitrogenous waste product urea and creatinine are the hallmarks
- Acute renal failure is rather common in critically ill patients in response to intrarenal insults from circulating inflammatory mediators and changes in renal perfusion.
  - Modern critical care uses renal replacement therapy.
    - Either hemodialysis or continuous venovenous hemoperfusion to maintain acceptable levels of urea, creatinine, and electrolytes until the kidney regains its function.
    - One of the few evidence-based therapies that enhances the repair of acute renal failure is nutritional support with adequate protein for renal healing.

Glycemic Control

- Hyperglycemia is a common occurrence in critically ill patients.
- Not all hyperglycemic critically ill patients have diabetes.
- The hormonal milieu of the stress response tends to cause hyperglycemia.
  - Among the hormones that increase plasma glucose are growth hormone, cortisol, glucagon, and epinephrine.
  - A diagnostic hallmark of sepsis is glucose intolerance/ insulin resistance.
    - Normoglycemia has a significant improvement in outcome effects that persists for several months after recovery.
    - These effects included decreased intensive care unit length of stay, reduced infectious complications, and survival.
      - It is recommended that critically ill patients be managed with normal glucose levels.
      - Insulin infusion is the best method to manage glucose concentrations.

Brain Injury

- The injured brain is characterized by an impairment of the blood–brain barrier.
- Causes increased susceptibility to changes in plasma concentrations of glucose and electrolytes.
- Important goal is the prevention of edema in the injured brain.
- Nutritional goals for the head-injured patient include avoidance of hyperglycemia, hyperosmolar state, and maintenance of normal sodium and potassium.
  - Hyperglycemia, even with normal osmolality, is detrimental to the injured brain by causing cerebral edema in ischemic areas of the brain.

- Occurs when one glucose molecule diffuses into the brain and is anaerobically metabolized to two lactic acid molecules that are highly polar and do not diffuse out into the bloodstream.
  - The interior of the cell increases in osmolality (more nondiffusible particles) relative to plasma and attracts increased cell water.
- Sodium replacement is important in brain-injured patients.
  - Many patients with brain injuries develop hyponatremia.
    - Tends to increase the risk of cerebral edema from excess plasma water and decreased serum osmolality
      - Cerebral salt-wasting syndrome or inability to conserve sodium in the kidney needs to be differentiated from syndrome of inappropriate antidiuretic hormone secretion.

- Cerebral salt-wasting patients tend to be hypovolemic and need extra sodium replacement in their nutrition support.
- Syndrome of inappropriate antidiuretic hormone patients tend to be hypervolemic and generally need fluid restriction to correct their serum sodium levels.
- Brain-injured patients require adequate protein to compensate for their increased demands to provide brain healing.
- Metabolic rate should be measured directly
- Caloric needs met by appropriate amounts of nutritional support
  - Some concern about excitatory amino acids having deleterious effects on the injured brain but unclear that nutritional support affects the central nervous system concentration of these amino acids.

CHAPTER 29 ■ PRACTICAL ASPECTS OF NUTRITIONAL SUPPORT

WRITING A TOTAL PARENTERAL NUTRITION ORDER

- Life-threatening errors continue to occur in the preparation and delivery of total parenteral nutrition (TPN).
- Many errors are related to the ordering process.
- One solution—albeit imperfect—is to use an institution-specific standardized TPN form.
- The ultimate goal of nutritional support is to minimize loss of lean body mass, especially in patients with burns, sepsis, acute respiratory distress syndrome, and trauma.
  - Energy expenditure of the critically ill patient depends on the underlying disease state and on the nutritional status of the patient before the injury or illness.
  - The Harris–Benedict equation, widely used to estimate the basal energy expenditure, may be excessive and can lead to overfeeding.
    - The American Society of Parenteral and Enteral Nutriiton (ASPEN) guidelines and American College of Chest Physicians (ACCP) suggest using a total energy requirement of 25 kcal/kg/day.
    - An adjusted body weight should be used in the calculation for the obese.
  - Protein requirements for critically ill patients with normal renal function range from 1.3 to 2 g/kg/day (moderate to severe stress), using the premorbid body weight or the adjusted body weight if obese.
    - In acute renal failure patients, ASPEN recommended protein amounts are as follows:
      - 0.8 to 1.2 g/kg/day if patients are not dialyzed

      - 1 to 1.4 g/kg/day in patients receiving dialysis
      - 1.5 to 2.5 g/kg/day in patients undergoing continuous renal replacement therapy (CRRT)
    - For chronic kidney disease, the ASPEN recommends 0.5 to 0.6 g of protein per kilogram per day.
    - ACCP recommends no change in the amount of protein given to patients with acute renal failure versus patients with normal kidney function (i.e., 1.2 to 2 g/kg/day).
    - In chronic renal failure, the ACCP recommends 0.5 to 0.8 g of protein per kilogram per day.
- There are three different ways parenteral nutrition (PN) can be ordered.
  - If the patient has only peripheral venous access, peripheral parenteral nutrition (PPN) is used.
    - Compared to TPN, PPN is lower in osmolarity (<900 mOsm/L) to minimize thrombophlebitis.
  - For formulas to be given via central line, TPN can be administered in two ways.
    - A two-in-one TPN formula, which is protein and dextrose in one bag, with the intravenous fat emulsions hung separately.
    - A three-in-one TPN formula, in which all three fuel substrates (amino acids [AAs], dextrose, and fats) are mixed in one bag.
    - Each has advantages and disadvantages. ASPEN guidelines do not favor one formulation over another.
      - For two-in-one formulas, fat is administered separately, usually three times a week.
      - To calculate the total caloric contributions, the amount of calories per week from fat is totaled and then divided

TABLE 29.1

RESPIRATORY QUOTIENT AND CALORIES PER GRAM OF DIFFERENT FUEL SUBSTRATES

Fuel substrates	RQ	Kilocalories per gram
Fats	0.7	9 kcal/g; Intralipid 10% contains 1.1 kcal/mL and 20% contains 2 kcal/mL due to the presence of phospholipids
Proteins	0.8	4 kcal/g (these are not factored into the total calories administered per day)
Carbohydrates	1	3.4 kcal/g

by 7 days per week to obtain the calories per day. For example, Intralipid 20% 500 mL containing 1,000 kcal is given three times a week. The caloric contribution per day would be 3,000 kcal/week ÷ 7 days/week, which equals 429 kcal/day from fat.

– This amount is then added to the known calories provided by the dextrose and AAs in the two-in-one formula (Table 29.1).

• Most institutions have default amounts of additives (electrolytes) to facilitate the ordering process.

• Ordering electrolytes and other additives is as much an art as it is a science.

• With practice, one can develop a "feel" for how patients will respond to the additives depending on their condition.

○ The most difficult part of the ordering process is how much electrolyte to add initially; subsequent adjustments are easier with adjustments to increase, decrease, or keep the additives the same, depending on the laboratory values (Table 29.2).

Initiating Parenteral Nutrition

• ASPEN guidelines suggest ≤150 to 200 g/day of glucose initially to ensure tolerance.

• Prudent to infuse only 1 L of the TPN on the first day at 42 mL/hour.

• Achieve goal rate on day 2 or 3, depending on the patient's tolerance.

• Central line placement must be verified by radiography before initiating TPN.

• TPN should be administered through a dedicated infusion port via an infusion pump that is equipped with protection from "free flow" and has reliable alarms.

• To reduce the chance for infusing particulates, microorganisms, and pyrogens, a 1.2-μ filter may be used in a three-in-one formula.

• A 0.22-μ filter may be used for a two-in-one formula.

• PPN formula is not as calorie dense and contains less protein; therefore, it may be initiated at goal rate.

TABLE 29.2

PARENTERAL NUTRITION (PN) ADDITIVES AND SUGGESTED AMOUNTS

Electrolytes/additives	Suggested amounts	Comments
Sodium	1–2 mEq/kg/d	Assess the current IV fluid the patient is receiving and how the sodium level is responding (i.e., if the patient is receiving lactated Ringer solution [130 mEq/L], and Na^+ is within desired range, then add 130 mEq/L in the PN). Patients no longer requiring fluid resuscitation will need 1/2 normal saline or 80 mEq/L of Na^+ in PN.
Potassium	1–2 mEq/kg/d	Major intracellular cation. There is obligatory daily loss. Assess current repletion and patient's response as this will guide the clinician on how much to add to the PN.
Chloride	Default salt	This is the "acidifying" salt; acidemia is preferable in most situations to alkalemia (improved unloading of O_2 to the tissues). It can be given as either NaCl or KCl.
Acetate (Ac)	Add if patient has metabolic acidosis	May be useful in patients with metabolic acidosis secondary to renal failure; acetate is metabolized into bicarbonate in the body. Bicarbonate is not compatible in the PN solution. It can be given as NaAc or KAc.
Calcium gluconate	10–15 mEq/d	Use ionized calcium as a guide rather than total calcium.
Magnesium sulfate	8–20 mEq/d	Intracellular cation. It can accumulate in renal failure; 1 g = 8 mEq.
Phosphorus	20–40 mMol/d	Major intracellular anion. May be given as KPO_4 (4.4 mEq K^+/3 mMol PO_4^-) or $NaPO_4$ (4 mEq Na^+/3 mMol PO_4^-) depending on cation deficiency. Amount of calcium or phosphorus in total PN is limited by the calcium-phosphate solubility curve.
Trace elements	Standard amount daily	Adjust to twice a week in patients with severe renal failure and severe hepatic failure.
Insulin	Add 50%–70% of insulin sliding scale needs	Use amounts of insulin used by the sliding scale used in the last 24 h to guide how much to add to the PN bag. Start conservatively with 50%–70% of total insulin used during last 24 h.
H_2 blocker	Add total daily dose	Continuous infusion of H_2 blocker is superior in keeping pH elevated compared to intermittent dosing.[a] Protein pump inhibitors are not compatible in total PN.

[a]Ballesteros MA, Hogan DL, Koss MA, et al. Bolus or IV infusion of ranitidine: effects on gastric pH and acid secretions. A comparison of efficacy and cost. *Ann Intern Med.* 1990;112:334–339.
From Merritt R, ed. The ASPEN Nutrition Support Practice Manual. 2nd ed. Silver Spring, MD: ASPEN; 2005.

- PN administration set must be changed every 24 hours using aseptic techniques and universal precautions.
  - If the PN does not contain fat emulsions, the administration set may be changed every 72 hours.
    - The administration set used in infusing the IV fat separately must be discarded after use or at least every 12 hours.

Transitional Feeding and Weaning Parenteral Nutrition

- The transitional period is when enteral feeding is started and PN is discontinued.
  - Young patients with no history of malignancy, and were well nourished before PN was started can have it discontinued as soon as they are able to tolerate solid food.
  - Generally, PN can be discontinued once 60% of energy needs is met enterally.
  - In older debilitated patients who have a history of malnutrition and malignancy, transitioning to enteral feeds may be more challenging.
  - Calorie counts help to guide the reduction or discontinuation of PN.
  - Factors such as aspiration risk, appetite, strength, and ileus play a role in whether patients successfully transition to enteral feeds.
- Terminating TPN is just the opposite of initiating.
  - Major concern is rebound hypoglycemia from rapid cessation of PN.
    - Recommended that the TPN be decreased by half for 1 to 2 hours before discontinuation if the current infusion rate is >42 mL/hour.
    - This allows body to adjust its insulin secretion to decreasing amounts of circulating dextrose and avoid hypoglycemia.
    - Weaning of PN is not necessary in patients receiving oral nutrition.
- If problems occur with the TPN bag that render it not usable (e.g., a leak in the bag) and the patient is on a rate >42 mL/hour, dextrose 10% or dextrose 10% with 0.9% sodium chloride should be infused at the same rate as the TPN to avoid rebound hypoglycemia.
  - In the same scenario, dextrose 5% may be substituted in place of PPN, not because of rebound hypoglycemia but more for maintaining caloric intake.

Cyclic Parenteral Nutrition

- PN that is infusing 24 hours a day means.
  - Patient is tethered to the IV pole, limiting mobility.
  - Getting the patient to eat more may be problematic because the satiety center is constantly being stimulated.
    - Reduced oral intake can be expected if more than 25% of caloric needs is provided by PN.
  - Cyclic PN may be a good option.
    - Cyclic or nocturnal PN has the same volume infused over a shorter period (12 or 14 hours) starting in the evening and finishing in the morning.

- Allows patients to be more mobile during the day and have more of an appetite.
- May see less deterioration of liver function.
- Nutritional goal needs to be defined.
  - Full support means that the total amount of protein and calories will be provided. In this case, it is important to make sure that the TPN is already concentrated, as the patient will be receiving the same volume that was previously given over 24 hours over a shorter period of time.
  - If the goal is to have the patient eat more but not get behind in nutrition, one can provide 50% of assessed needs as cyclic PN while the patient is fed orally or enterally.
  - An important aspect of cyclic TPN is calculating the tapered flow rate to minimize harmful fluctuations of blood sugar.
  - One simplified method of calculating the tedious cyclic PN rate comes from Stanford University:
    - $v = r + 2r + 4r (t - 4) + 2r + r$, where t = cyclic PN time, v = volume infused, and r = rate of PN
    - $v = 6r + 4rt = 16r$
    - $v = 4rt - 10r$
    - $v = r(4t - 10)$
    - $r = v/(4t - 10)$
    - $r = 1,500$ mL$/(4[12$ hours$] - 10)$
    - $r = 39.47$ or $\sim$40 mL/hour
  - For example, the patient will be receiving a total of 1,500 mL ("v") of PN formula X over 12 hours ("t"). To calculate the cyclic TPN rate ("r"), the formula uses the model (r mL/hour × 1 hour) + (2r mL/hour × 1 hour) + [4r mL/hour × (cyclic PN time − 4)] + (2r mL/hour × 1 hour) + (r mL/hour × 1 hour). Therefore, the cyclic TPN will be ordered as follows: 40 mL/hour × 1 hour, then 80 mL/hour × 1 hour, then 160 mL/hour × 8 hour, then 80 mL/hour × 1 hour, then 40 mL/hour × 1 hour, then stop.
  - It is important that there be a "ramp up" and "ramp down" during cyclic TPN infusion to avoid significant glucose fluctuations. Glucose may be drawn 60 minutes after the maximal infusion rate or 60 minutes after discontinuation of cyclic PN to make sure the patient is tolerating.

Hidden Sources of Kilocalories

- Inadvertent hypercaloric feeding can result in increased carbon dioxide production, hyperglycemia, and hepatomegaly.
- Propofol, which is suspended in 10% Intralipid, contributes 1.1 kcal/mL.
  - Patient receiving 50 μg/kg/minute (assuming a 70-kg patient) can easily receive an extra 554 kcal/day.
- Dextrose concentration in the dialysate fluid of patients receiving CRRT.
  - Diffusion greatly influences dextrose absorption across the hemofilter.
    - Daily caloric contribution ranges from 123 to 2,388 kcal depending on the dextrose concentration of 0.5% to 4.25% in the dialysate solution.

○ Approximately 43% to 45% of dextrose can be absorbed by the body across the hemofilter.

Electrolyte Abnormalities

- Refeeding syndrome is an imbalance of electrolytes and vitamins, micronutrients, and fluids that occurs within the first few days of refeeding malnourished patients as nutrients replete the intracellular space.
  - The hallmark biochemical findings include the following:
    - Hypophosphatemia (intracellular shift plus depletion of phosphorus substrate to synthesize adenosine triphosphate)
    - Hypomagnesemia (intracellular shift plus magnesium is a cofactor in many enzymatic functions)
    - Hypokalemia (intracellular shift of potassium with insulin secretion as a response to dextrose infusion)
  - Patients may exhibit respiratory distress, cardiac arrhythmias, congestive heart failure, hemolytic anemia, or paresthesias, or they may die.
  - The three most important steps in preventing refeeding are as follows:
    - Identify high-risk patients (chronic alcoholism, kwashiorkor, marasmus, rapid refeeding) and those receiving high TPN rates.
    - Baseline electrolytes must be checked before the initiation of PN and low magnesium, phosphorus, or potassium levels must be corrected immediately.
    - The TPN rate should be advanced slowly (<150 g/day of carbohydrates) as tolerated over several days before going to the goal rate.
  - Patients receiving enteral nutrition could be advanced more aggressively if needed, provided that electrolytes are monitored closely and repleted in a timely manner.
- Replacing electrolytes is both a science and an art, because patients respond differently.
  - Table 29.3 will help guide the clinician in managing electrolyte imbalances that occur. There are two things to remember when adjusting the electrolytes in PN: First, the degree of metabolic derangements must be determined before any adjustments are made. Second, PN should not be used to replace electrolytes rapidly, but should be used for maintenance.

Monitoring

- Potential for serious complications is high in patients receiving PN unless careful monitoring is conducted.
  - Appropriate monitoring can be cost-effective by avoiding complications.
  - Suggested protocols for monitoring PN in adults are shown in Table 29.4.

WRITING ENTERAL ORDERS

- Ordering enteral feedings is less complex than ordering PN but just as confusing with many different formulas.

- Enteral feeding should be started as early as possible, as it is a "pharmacotherapy" for the gut (improves mesenteric blood flow and maintains gut integrity).
  - Feeding early, defined as 48 hours within mechanical ventilation onset, is associated with a 20% decrease in intensive care unit (ICU) mortality and a 25% decrease in hospital mortality.
  - When choosing enteral formulas, consideration depends on the patient's digestive capability, fluid restriction status, electrolyte balance, nutrient requirements, disease state, and possible routes available for administration.
- Enteral formulas may be categorized.
  - The monomeric (which contain free amino acids with or without peptides, with modified fat)
  - The polymeric
    - Most enteral formulas fall in the semisynthetic polymeric formulas, which are more cost-effective but require patients to have digestive capability.
    - Monomeric formulas are for patients with malabsorption, such as short-gut syndrome.
      ○ Because of the cost, polymeric formulas should be tried first.
      ○ For instance, in patients with pancreatitis, instead of using monomeric formulas, adding pancreatic enzyme tablets may help with polymeric tube feed tolerance. If the patient continues to have absorption issues, monomeric formulas could be substituted.
- Enteral formulas also vary by caloric density.
  - In patients with chronic renal failure with fluid restriction, a high caloric-density polymeric (high caloric-to-fluid ratio) may be helpful.
  - Enteral formulas also differ in the amount of protein, the carbohydrate-to-fat ratio, and the fiber content.
  - Each enteral feed formula has known amounts of kilocalories per milliliter and grams per liter of protein.
    - Once caloric and protein needs are assessed, the volume needed can be calculated.
    - Enteral feeding formulas are fixed, but there are protein powders available if supplemental protein is necessary.
- Before starting any enteral feeds, feeding tube placement must be confirmed by abdominal radiography and documented in the orders.
  - Once the enteral feeding formula has been selected, indicate initial strength (e.g., full or half-strength), initial rate in milliliters per hour, and desired progression regimen, followed by the goal rate.
    - Rate can be started at 10 to 20 mL/hour and be advanced by 10 to 20 mL/hour every 8 hours as tolerated until goal reached
      ○ As long as residual is <200 mL via nasogastric tube, or <100 mL via gastrostomy tube, in 4 hours.
      ○ Many institutions have converted to a "closed system" to reduce the risk of microbial contaminations by minimizing the number of times the formula is manipulated
        – These enteral feedings thus start at full strength as a "closed system" will make it difficult to order partial-strength formulas.
  - When the patient is ready to transition over to a regular diet, similar strategies employed with the cyclic PN can be used.

TABLE 29.3

AN EXAMPLE OF MANAGEMENT GUIDELINES FOR METABOLIC COMPLICATIONS IN ADULTS INDUCED BY
PARENTERAL NUTRITION

Hyperglycemia	>200 mg/dL	Once daily requirements of insulin are known from the insulin sliding scale, add 50%–75% into TPN. Consider insulin drip if blood sugar is uncontrolled, or if patient is edematous with unreliable absorption of subcutaneous insulin. Goal blood sugar is 80–140 mg/dL in critically ill surgical patients
Hypoglycemia	<80 mg/dL	If related to sudden discontinuance of TPN, administer D10W or D10NS at the same rate as the TPN. If related to insulin in TPN, initiate continuous glucose supplement (e.g., D10W). If glucose is still below desirable level, discontinue TPN and hang D10W or D10NS at the same rate as the TPN
Hypernatremia	>150 mEq/L	If hypovolemic, give isotonic or hypotonic fluid depending on degree of hypovolemia. If euvolemic or hypervolemic, reduce sodium from TPN and/or other source. If patient is symptomatic, consider discontinuing TPN and starting D10W at the same rate as the TPN
Hyponatremia	<130 mEq/L	If hypervolemic, restrict fluid intake ± diuretics; if euvolemic/hypovolemic, increase sodium content in TPN; if hypovolemic, give additional isotonic fluid
Hyperkalemia	>5 mEq/L	If TPN related and patient symptomatic, discontinue TPN and initiate D10W or D10NS at the same rate as the TPN. If patient is asymptomatic, decrease K^+ in TPN and other sources.
Hypokalemia	<3.5 mEq/L	Give KCl bolus either IV or enterally (4 mEq for each 0.1 <4.5 of K^+; maximum IV KCl concentration is 20 mEq/50 mL via central venous access and 10 mEq/50 mL via peripheral vein). Add K^+ in TPN
Hypermagnesemia	>2.6 mEq/L	If TPN related and patient is symptomatic, discontinue TPN and start D10W or D10NS at the same rate as the TPN. If patient is asymptomatic, decrease Mg^{2+} in TPN
Hypomagnesemia	<1.8 mEq/L	Give magnesium bolus either IV or enterally (1 g $MgSO_4$ = 8 mEq; 1 tablet magnesium oxide = 6 mEq). Maximum rate of IV infusion is 1 g in 7 min. (If level is <1, give 4 – 6 g IV or enteral equivalent; if level is >1 but <1.8, give 2 – 4 g IV or enteral equivalent). Increase Mg^{2+} in TPN
Hypercalcemia	>10.2 mg/dL	If TPN related and patient is symptomatic, discontinue TPN and initiate D10W or D10NS at the same rate as the TPN. If patient is asymptomatic, decrease Ca^{2+} in TPN. Check ionized calcium in critically ill patients
Hypocalcemia	<8.5 mg/dL	Correct for hypoalbuminemia [True Ca^{2+} = Ca^{2+} observed + 0.8 (4 – albumin observed)]. Increase Ca^{2+} in TPN if corrected Ca^{2+} is trending low. If hemodynamically unstable and/or critically ill, obtain an ionized calcium level (normal range 1.05 – 1.35 mg / dL). Give calcium chloride bolus via slow IV push if ionized calcium is low (<1.05) and patient is symptomatic (e.g., hypotensive). 1 g $CaCl_2$ = 13.6 mEq; 1 g calcium gluconate = 4.7 mEq
Hyperphosphatemia	>4.8 mg/dL	If TPN related and patient is symptomatic, discontinue TPN and run D10W or D10NS at the same rate as the TPN. If patient is asymptomatic, decrease phosphate (PO_4^-) in TPN
Hypophosphatemia	<2.4 mg/dL	Phosphorus replacement should be given over 6 h to avoid hypotension. If level is <1, give 30 mMol PO_4^- × 2 doses IV plus check phosphorus level 1 h after end of infusion; if level is ≥1 but <1.8, give 30 mMol PO_4^- × 1 dose or enteral equivalent and check phosphorus level 1 h after end of infusion; if level is ≥1.8 but <2.4, give 15 mMol PO_4^- or enteral equivalent. One packet of Neutra-Phos enterally = 8 mMol of PO_4^-. Increase phosphorus in TPN
Metabolic acidosis	pH <7.4 HCO_3^- <23	Consider increasing acetate-to-chloride ratio
Metabolic alkalosis	pH >7.4 HCO_3^- >29	Consider increasing chloride-to-acetate ratio

TPN, total parenteral nutrition; D10W, dextrose 10%; D10NS, dextrose 10% with 0.9% sodium chloride.

- Patient may be converted to bolus feeding of full-strength enteral formula with increases of 60 to 120 mL every 8 to 12 hours as tolerated up to goal volume.
  - Bolus feedings are more physiologic, allowing the brain to stimulate sensations of hunger and satiety.
  - When patient is able to consume 60% of nutritional needs by mouth discontinue the tube feeds.

"Designer" Enteral Feedings: Facts and Myths

- Specialized formulas contain modified protein and other ingredients to assist patients in stressed states.
- Sometimes the ratio of carbohydrate to fat, and the sources of fat, may also be altered to achieve desired effects.

TABLE 29.4

MONITORING PARAMETERS FOR CRITICALLY ILL ADULT PATIENTS ON
PARENTERAL NUTRITION

Parameter	Frequency
Na^+, K^+, Cl^-, HCO_3^-, BUN, serum creatinine	Daily
Ca^{2+}, Mg^{2+}, phosphorus, liver function tests	Two to three times per week
Serum triglycerides	Weekly
CBC with differential	Weekly
Input/output	Daily
Prealbumin	Weekly
Indirect calorimetry	As needed. Highly recommended in the following patients: Difficult to estimate accurately caloric requirements, inadequate response to nutrition support, and clinical signs of over- or underfeeding
24-h urine urea nitrogen	As needed. Highly recommended in the following patients: Difficult to estimate accurately protein requirements, inadequate response to nutrition support, and clinical signs of over- or underfeeding
Weight	Daily
Serum glucose	As needed to keep blood sugar control of 80–140 mg/dL

BUN, blood urea nitrogen; CBC, complete blood count.
From Merritt R, ed. *The ASPEN Nutrition Support Practice Manual.* 2nd ed. Silver Spring, MD: ASPEN; 2005.

Hepatic Formula

- Specialized hepatic formulas (e.g., NutriHep) differ from the standard formulas in two ways
  - Actual protein content is usually lower (around 40–46 g/L).
  - Ratio of branched-chain amino acids (BCAAs) to aromatic and ammonia-forming amino acids is higher in the hepatic formula.
    - Theory is that in liver dysfunction, depletion of BCAAs might enhance passage of ammonia-forming amino acids across the blood–brain barrier, resulting in the synthesis of false neurotransmitters.
    - By giving a higher BCAA formula, the altered ratio is returned to a more normal state.
  - Although there are conflicting data, there is evidence of the beneficial effects of "special hepatic formulas" to support their use in the treatment of malnourished patients with advanced cirrhosis.
    - Based on the available studies and cost consideration of up to 20 times more, the "hepatic formula" should be restricted to patients who present with grade II or higher encephalopathy or whose grade of encephalopathy worsens with the advancement standard enteral formulation.

Renal Formula

- Formulas in this class (e.g., Nepro) are more calorie-dense and low in electrolytes and mineral contents (especially potassium and phosphorus)
  - These modifications are to provide adequate nutrients but minimize complications such as uremia, fluid overload, and electrolyte accumulation.
  - Older renal formulas differ from standard amino acids in that they were designed for patients who could not tolerate dialysis or for whom dialysis was being avoided.

- Thus, the formulas tend to be enriched with essential amino acids. The rationale with this admixture is that the urea from essential amino acids would be recycled to produce nonessential amino acids.
- Evidence supporting the use of the older renal formulas is scant and of poor quality.
  - Cost of the older renal formulas is 10 to 15 times that of standard polymeric formulas.
- These formulas have now been replaced with standard polymeric proteins, as most patients with acute renal failure are now being dialyzed or are receiving CRRT.
  - The new renal formulas are more calorie dense (usually 2 kcal/mL) with minimal electrolytes or additives (K^+, Mg^{2+}, PO_4^-) that could accumulate in renal failure.
  - They are appropriate for patients whose serum electrolyte and mineral levels are difficult to control.

Pulmonary Formula

- Respiratory quotient (RQ) is defined as the molecules of carbon dioxide produced per molecule of oxygen consumed (VCO_2/VO_2).
- Pulmonary formulas (e.g., PulmoCare) are designed to decrease CO_2 by providing the fuel substrate with the lower respiratory quotient (see Table 29.1).
  - To achieve this, the manufacturer decreases the carbohydrate-to-fat ratio to achieve fat calories of about 38% to 55%.
  - By decreasing the carbohydrates (RQ = 1)–to–fat (RQ = 0.7) ratio, the assumption is that CO_2 production is reduced.
    - Studies looking at the benefit of high-fat enteral feeds are poor.
    - More recent evidence suggests that reducing total calories is more important than the source of calories, in terms of reducing CO_2 production (as the RQ of lipogenesis or overfeeding is 1–1.2).

- The source of fat has also changed over the years. Whether the data from the earlier studies can be extrapolated to reflect the effect of the modern formulas on CO_2 remains to be answered.

Metabolic Stress (Critical Care) Formula

- The critical care formulas (e.g., Perative) are somewhat similar to the hepatic formulas in that both have a high percentage of BCAAs, which are the preferred substrate of muscles during critical illness.
  - Differences include higher protein content and fewer aromatic amino acids in the critical care formulas compared to the hepatic formulas.
  - The data on use are equivocal from the standpoint of nutritional markers.
    - Overall, BCAA-enriched enteral formulas are not the current standard of practice.
    - This class of enteral formula, like the immunomodulating formulas, may contain immune-enhancing agents (i.e., arginine) and must be used cautiously in critically ill septic patients.

Immunomodulating Formula

- A subset of the metabolic stress formulas
- Designed to reduce inflammatory response (e.g., acute respiratory distress syndrome [ARDS])
- These so-called immunomodulating formulas are standard enteral formulas fortified with omega-3 fatty acids, nucleotides, arginine, and/or glutamine.
  - Oxepa contains no glutamine and arginine but does contain 55% of calories as fat, of which the omega-6–to–omega-3 ratio is optimized to 2:1.
  - Impact has 25% of calories as fat, has arginine and glutamine, and contains 17.1% BCAAs in protein, and the omega-3–to–omega-6 ratio is 1.4:1.
  - Immun-Aid has 36% protein as BCAAs, contains arginine and glutamine, has 20% fat calories, and has an omega-6–to–omega-3 ratio of 2.1:1 (ratio similar to Oxepa).
- Theory behind this class of enteral feeds is that by minimizing omega-6 fatty acids and optimizing the ratio of omega-6 to omega-3 fatty acids, the inflammatory response is reduced, resulting in less lung injury.
  - Based on the early clinical trials and meta-analyses, which have mainly looked at Immun-Aid and Impact, it appears that surgical patients benefited most from this class of enteral formula.
    - One prospective, double-blind, placebo-controlled, randomized trial in 165 critically ill patients with severe sepsis found that this formula decreased mortality (19.4% absolute risk reduction) and ventilator days.
    - Another prospective, randomized, controlled trial looking at enteral diet enriched with EPA + GLA in 100 patients with acute lung injury concluded that the formula reduced ventilator days.
    - Despite the many pieces of evidence pointing toward the benefit of immunomodulating formulas, it does have to be used with caution and at the right time.

Glycemic Control Formula

- Glycemic control enteral formulas are similar to the pulmonary formulas in design.

- Carbohydrate (35%–40%)-to-fat (40%–50%) ratio is reduced compared to standard formulas.
  - With varying ratios of omega-6 to omega-3 fatty acids (e.g., Glucerna)
  - Results in a greater proportion of fat calories than recommended (American Heart Association recommends ≤30% of calories from fat)
  - Various soluble fibers and/or soy polysaccharides are also added to the glycemic enteral formulas
- Clinical trials limited
  - High fat content in the glycemic formulas can decrease stomach emptying.
    - Tolerance to these formulas may be decreased even more in patients with diabetic gastroparesis.
    - If glycemic control is needed, consider insulin infusion.

Timing of Specialized Enteral Feeding (Immunonutrition) and Manipulation of Immune and Inflammatory System

- Immunonutrition enteral feedings (e.g., Impact and Immun-Aid) are formulas containing nutrients that have been shown to influence immunologic and inflammatory responses in humans.
  - Immune-enhancing agents usually include the following:
    - Glutamine
    - Arginine
    - Omega-3 fatty acids
    - Nucleotides
    - Antioxidants
- An extensive meta-analysis to determine whether immunonutrition is safe and effective in critically ill patients found a trend toward higher mortality in the critically ill patients.
  - Recommendation that immunonutrition not be used in critically ill patients until more clinical trials are conducted.
- A randomized multicenter trial comparing parenteral and early enteral nutrition containing immune-enhancing formula (Perative) in patients with and without severe sepsis noted in an interim analysis that mortality in severely septic patients receiving immune-enhancing enteral formulas was significantly higher than in those receiving parenteral nutrition (44.4% vs. 14.3%), and the study was aborted.
  - In patients without sepsis, there was no 28-day mortality difference between the patients receiving parenteral nutrition versus immune-enhancing enteral formulas.
  - However, those receiving immunonutrition had fewer episodes of septic shock, and the ICU length of stay was 4 days shorter.
- Thus, immunonutrition formulas should be used with caution in critically ill septic patients.
  - Based on expert opinions, the immune-modulating nutrient likely to be responsible for the excess harm is arginine (see later), which has not been well studied in a randomized, clinical fashion in critically ill patients.
  - In the critically ill nonseptic patients, immune-enhancing formulas appear to be beneficial if started within 48 hours.

Immunomodulators

- *Glutamine:* Normally nonessential, glutamine becomes conditionally essential during times of high stress as evidenced by a decrease in glutamine concentration in the body during this period.

- Comes in the free form (unstable in solution, so only found in dried form) and protein-bound form as seen in all protein sources used in enteral formulas.
- Important amino acid because of its involvement in many vital functions, such as the following:
  - Gluconeogenesis
  - Synthesis of glycogen, nucleotides, nucleic acid, and urea
  - Ammoniagenesis
  - Ammonia reduction
  - Also the preferred fuel substrate for rapidly dividing cells in both the small intestine mucosa and the immune system
  - Plays a big part in the antioxidation process, as it is the precursor of glutathione, a strong antioxidant
- Critically ill patients need about 30 g/day (0.5 g/kg/day) of glutamine to meet both basal and increased enterocyte requirements.
- Meta-analysis of 14 randomized trials concluded that glutamine supplementation in critically ill patients may be associated with a reduction in complication and mortality rates.
  - Supplementation in surgical patients may be associated with a reduction in infectious complication rates and shorter hospital stay without any adverse effect on mortality.
  - Parenteral glutamine is more effective than enteral glutamine.
- The effectiveness and benefits of glutamine supplementation are still not conclusive.
- *Arginine:* Like glutamine, considered to be a conditionally essential amino acid
  - About 5% to 6% comes from intake of proteins, and the rest is synthesized by the body via the urea cycle.
  - Arginine is important in the following:
    - Ammonia detoxification
    - Production of nitric oxide
    - Purported to enhance wound healing in humans, mainly via improvements in *in vitro* markers of immune function (e.g., CD4 count), rather than outcome measures like infection rates.
  - Optimal dose of arginine in the critically ill patient is unknown.
    - However, up to 30 g/day is generally well tolerated by relatively healthy people.
    - Arginine supplementation may increase nitric oxide production, which can lead to vascular smooth-muscle dilation.
      - Should use arginine-containing formulas with caution in critically ill septic patients
- *Nucleotides:* The structural units for nucleic acids and various enzymes involved in energy transfer and essential for the formation of new cells (e.g., intestinal epithelium) and in the synthesis of protein, lipids, and carbohydrates.
  - Of interest because supplementation of infant formulas with nucleotides was noted to enhance bifidobacteria growth in the gastrointestinal tract, which decreases the colonic lumen pH and inhibit growth of enteric bacteria.
  - Studies involving nucleotide use in humans are limited.
    - Studies available often involve immune-enhancing diets fortified with nucleotides, making it difficult to determine the effects of the nucleotides *per se.*
  - A prospective, controlled trial studied the effects of nucleotide-supplemented formula in 26 severely malnourished children (younger than 4 years old) found that insulin-like growth factor, growth factor–binding protein-3 were notably affected, which could stimulate the catch-up growth of severely malnourished infants and toddlers.
- *Structured lipids:* Triglycerides are three fatty acid chains attached to a glycerol backbone. Structured lipids are triglycerides with combinations of long-, medium-, and short-chain fatty acids on a single glycerol backbone not found in nature.
  - Intent is to make a product that has improved absorption (compared to long-chain triglycerides), minimizes immune dysfunction, and provides essential fatty acids.
  - Not yet commercially available in IV forms, although it has been a component of immunomodulating enteral formulas.
- *Antioxidant therapy:* Antioxidants such as vitamin C, vitamin E, selenium, and β-carotene are often found in immunomodulating formulas.
  - Role of antioxidant supplementation during critical illness is unclear.
  - Critically ill patients often have low serum concentrations of some antioxidants, the significance of which is unclear.
  - Good evidence now to suggest that reactive oxygen species induce direct oxidative tissue injury by means of peroxidation of cellular membranes, oxidation of critical enzymatic and structural proteins, and induction of apoptosis.
    - Thus, importance of antioxidants seems obvious.
    - A prospective, observational clinical trial looking at 595 critically ill surgical patients (91% trauma patients) were administered vitamin E 1,000 international units every 8 hours via nasogastric tube and vitamin C 1 g IV every 8 hours.
      - Found that early administration of vitamin E and vitamin C reduced the incidence of organ failure by 57% and shortened the ICU stay by 1 day
    - Another randomized study looking at 37 burned patients (>30% of body surface area) concluded that high-dose vitamin C (66 mg/kg/hour) for 24 hours reduced resuscitation fluid volume requirements, body weight gain, wound edema, and the severity of respiratory dysfunction.

CHAPTER 30 ■ TOXICOLOGY

HISTORY

- The American Association of Poison Control Centers (AAPCC) maintains the National Poisoning and Exposure Database (NPED).
  - Database suffers from many obvious limitations.
    - Many exposures go unreported.
    - In one study, only 12% of poisoning deaths identified by the medical examiner were reported to poison centers.
    - Those reported are usually unconfirmed.
  - The NPED categorizes exposures based on outcome, designating effects as minor, moderate, or major.
    - *Major effects* are those where the patient exhibits signs or symptoms as a result of exposure that is life-threatening or results in significant disability or disfigurement; this category constitutes a large portion of ICU toxicology cases.
    - In 2005, the AAPCC received nearly 2.5 million reports of exposures.
      - 16,545 major effects
      - 1,261 deaths (0.005% of total exposures)
- Herein, any substance introduced to the body will be referred to as a *xenobiotic.*
  - Terms *drug* and *pharmaceutical* identify the subgroup of xenobiotics that are commercially produced.
  - A *toxin* is a xenobiotic produced by a biologic system, such as plant, animal, or fungi.
  - An *exposure* occurs whenever a human comes into contact with a xenobiotic.
    - Exposures may be dermal, oral, ophthalmic, or inhalational.
  - *Poisoning, intoxication,* and *toxicity* characterize the harmful consequences of a xenobiotic exposure.

DIAGNOSIS AND GENERAL APPROACH TO THE POISONED PATIENT

- By the time the patient reaches the ICU, initial stabilization will have already occurred.
  - Nevertheless, the initial approach to the poisoned patient deserves mention.
  - "Treat the patient, not the poison."
  - The management of the poisoned patients begins with the following:
    - Addressing airway compromise, breathing difficulty, and circulatory problems

- Vital signs should be obtained, and cardiac and respiratory monitoring should be applied and supplemental oxygen used as needed.
  - Significant abnormalities or oxygen desaturation should be addressed immediately.
- Bedside serum glucose concentration should be rapidly obtained in any patient with altered sensorium or an abnormal neurologic examination.
  - Hypoglycemia may present with almost any altered mental status, including agitation, delirium, coma, seizure, or focal neurologic deficit.
  - Though common and easy to correct, this may be life threatening.
- A thorough physical examination will identify the presence of a toxic syndrome, or "toxidrome" (Table 30.1).
- Electrocardiogram (ECG) should be obtained.
  - Several well-defined exposures (such as tricyclic antidepressants) will be identified based on a characteristic ECG
  - Xenobiotics such as cocaine or lidocaine can produce life-threatening dysrhythmias via direct myocardial effect.
    - Xenobiotics can also produce dysrhythmias by causing an electrolyte abnormality.
    - Exposure to hydrofluoric acid, even dermally, can result in hypocalcemia, resulting in QTc prolongation and torsades de pointes
- History should attempt to identify the specific xenobiotic exposure, the amount, the time and reason for exposure, and general medical history.
  - A specific antidote may be warranted based on the history (Table 30.2).
- Thoughtful use of laboratory studies is important.
  - Electrolyte abnormalities complicate many severe poisonings.
  - Serum chemistries are warranted for all critically ill patients.
  - Blood gas analysis and aminotransferases are judiciously used.
  - Routine urine toxicologic screen rarely aids in management and is not recommended.
    - Urine toxicologic screen generally focuses on select drugs of abuse and omits the vast majority of potential toxins.
    - Assays included in the commonly used qualitative urine screen have either too many false-positive or false-negative results.
      - Fentanyl, a synthetic opioid, will not produce a positive result on an opiate screen.
      - Dextromethorphan may yield a positive result for phencyclidine.

TABLE 30.1

TOXIDROMES

Group	BP	P	R	T	Mental status	Pupil size	Peristalsis	Diaphoresis	Primary treatment
Anticholinergic	−/↑	↑	+/−	↑	Delirium	↑	↓	↓	Benzodiazepines
Cholinergic	+/−	+/−	−/↑	−	Normal/depressed	+/−	↑	↑	Atropine, oximes
Ethanol, sedative-hypnotic	↓	↓	↓	−/↓	Depressed	+/−	↓	−	Airway support
Opioid	↓	↓	↓	↓	Depressed	↓	↓	−	Naloxone
Sympathomimetic	↑	↑	↑	↑	Agitated	↑	−/↑	↑	Benzodiazepines
Withdrawal from ethanol or sedative-hypnotic	↑	↑	↑	↑	Agitated, disoriented	↑	↑	↑	Benzodiazepines
Withdrawal from opioids	↑	↑	−	−	Normal, anxious	↑	↑	↑	Opioids

BP, blood pressure; P, pulse; R, respirations; T, temperature.
Adapted with permission from Flomenbaum NE, Goldfrank LR, Hoffman RS, et al. Initial evaluations of the patient: vital signs and toxic syndromes. In: Flomenbaum NE, Goldfrank LR, Hoffman RS, et al., eds. *Goldfrank's Toxicologic Emergencies.* 8th ed. New York: McGraw-Hill; 2006:37–41.

- Acetaminophen concentration should be obtained after all overdoses where self-harm was intended, even **if the history is negative for acetaminophen ingestion.**

Determining the Need for Intensive Care Unit Admission

- Criteria that are traditionally used to determine whether patients need critical care may not apply to poisoned patients.
- Dangerous xenobiotic poisonings may appear well but require precautionary ICU admission and monitoring.
- Factors that influence the need for critical care can be divided into three general categories:
  - Patient characteristics
  - Xenobiotic characteristics
  - Hospital unit capabilities
- Unstable poisoned patients require ICU care.
- Patients with significant laboratory abnormalities, unresponsiveness, inability to protect the airway, hypotension, dysrhythmias, or conduction abnormalities are admitted to the ICU.
  - Pre-existing medical conditions—severe liver or renal insufficiency, congestive heart failure, or pregnancy—may also influence disposition.
- Disposition for minimally symptomatic patients is determined by the xenobiotic involved.
  - Most important considerations are the potential for deterioration or the requirement for a therapeutic agent with potentially adverse effects.
  - Sustained-release products, potentially lethal doses, or xenobiotics that may cause dysrhythmias have the potential to cause rapid clinical deterioration.
  - Thus, asymptomatic patients with exposure to calcium channel blockers or sulfonylureas often are admitted to the ICU for observation.
  - When xenobiotics require therapy with potentially adverse effects—such as high-dose atropine for organic phosphorus insecticides—ICU admission is appropriate.

- Hospital capabilities influence patient disposition.
  - Time-consuming nursing activities—hourly bedside glucose checks or the administration of drug infusions—may not be possible on general inpatient units and are indications for ICU admission.
  - If admitting team or nursing staff is not familiar with the complications associated with a particular xenobiotic exposure, ICU admission may also be indicated.

NONOPIOID ANALGESICS: ACETAMINOPHEN, NONSTEROIDAL ANTI-INFLAMMATORY DRUGS, AND SALICYLATES

Acetaminophen

- More than 100,000 reports of acetaminophen exposure were received by the NPED in 2005.
- Vast majority of exposures do not result in significant morbidity.
- Only 333 were fatal and another 3,310 considered major.
- Although the data set is controversial, acetaminophen is estimated to be responsible for 51% of all cases of acute liver failure in the United States.
- Acetaminophen ingestions require ICU admission when hepatotoxicity is established.
- **Mechanism of action and metabolism:** Acetaminophen is an analgesic and antipyretic with less anti-inflammatory activity than the nonsteroidal anti-inflammatory drugs (NSAIDs).
- Analgesic effects are mediated by central cyclo-oxygenase-2 and prostaglandin synthase inhibition.
- Less than 5% is eliminated unchanged in urine.
- Metabolism of acetaminophen occurs principally in the liver.
  - Ninety percent of absorbed acetaminophen undergoes hepatic conjugation with either glucuronide or sulfate to produce inactive metabolites.

TABLE 30.2

SELECTED ANTIDOTES WITH COMMON DOSES

Xenobiotic	Antidote and dose
Acetaminophen	**N-acetylcysteine- IV:** 150 mg/kg infused over 60 min, followed by 50 mg/kg over 4 h, then 100 mg/kg over 16 h **Oral:** 140 mg/kg, followed by 70 mg/kg every 4 h for 17 doses
β-Adrenergic antagonists	**Atropine (for bradycardia):** 0.5–1 mg IV **Glucagon:** 3–5 mg IV (50 μg/kg in children) up to 10 mg/h **Calcium:** 13–25 mEq of Ca^{2+} IV bolus (10–20 mL of 10% calcium chloride or 30–60 mL of 10% calcium gluconate) **Hyperinsulinemia/euglycemia:** Insulin 0.5–1 U/kg/h accompanied by 0.5 g/kg/h dextrose, titrated to maintain euglycemia
Calcium channel blockers	**Atropine (for bradycardia):** 0.5–1 mg IV **Calcium:** 13–25 mEq of Ca^{2+} IV bolus (10–20 mL of 10% calcium chloride or 30–60 mL of 10% calcium gluconate) **Glucagon:** 3–5 mg IV (50 μg/kg in children) up to 10 mg/h **Hyperinsulinemia/euglycemia:** Insulin 0.5–1 U/kg/h accompanied by 0.5 g/kg/h dextrose, titrated to maintain euglycemia
Cholinergic compounds	**Atropine:** 1 mg IV (0.05 mg/kg in children) doubled every 2 min until muscarinic symptoms are controlled **Pralidoxime:** Adults: 1–2 g IV over 30 min followed by 500 mg/g infusion for sickest patients. Children: 20–50 mg/kg (max 1–2 g) infused IV over 30–60 min and then 10–20 mg/kg/h (max 500 mg/h)
Cyanide	**Adults:** 1. Sodium nitrite: 300 mg (10 mL of a 3% conc.) infused IV over 2–5 min 2. Sodium thiosulfate: 12.5 g (50 mL of a 25% conc.) infused IV over 10–20 min or as a bolus 3. Hydroxocobalamin IV 70 mg/kg (up to 5 g) **Children:** 1. Sodium nitrite: 6–8 mL/m^2 (0.2 mL/kg of a 3% conc., up to adult dose) infused IV over 2–5 min 2. Sodium thiosulfate: 7 g/m^2 (0.5 g/kg, up to adult dose) infused over 10–30 min or as a bolus
Cyclic antidepressants	**Sodium bicarbonate:** 1 mEq/kg IV bolus, followed by infusion of 150 mEq in 1 L of D5W, infused at twice maintenance rate
Digoxin	**Digoxin-specific Fab:** Known level: # of vials = [wt (kg) × level (ng/mL)/100] rounded up to nearest vial. Empiric dosing: Acute: 10–20 vials. Chronic: Adults, 3–6 vials; children, 1–2 vials. Usually given as IV infusion over 30 min (administer as IV bolus for asystole)
Ethylene glycol, methanol	**Fomepizole:** 15 mg/kg infused IV over 30 min; next 4 doses at 10 mg/kg every 12 h; additional doses at 15 mg/kg every 12 h if needed **Ethanol (when fomepizole not available):** 0.8 g/kg infused IV over 20–60 min, followed by initial infusion of 100 mg/kg/h
Methemoglobin	**Methylene blue:** 1–2 mg/kg IV over 5 min followed by a 30 mL fluid flush
Salicylates	**Sodium bicarbonate:** 150 mEq in 1 L of D5W, infused at twice maintenance rate. Activated charcoal, 1g/kg every 4 h
Sulfonylurea-related hypoglycemia	**Octreotide:** 50 μg SQ every 6 h. Children: 1.25 μg/kg (up to adult dose) SQ every 6 h

Adapted with permission from Flomenbaum NE, Goldfrank LR, Hoffman RS, et al., eds. *Goldfrank's Toxicologic Emergencies.* 8th ed. New York: McGraw-Hill; 2006.

- Remainder (5%–15%) is oxidized by the cytochrome P450, forming N-acetyl-p-benzoquinoneimine (NAPQI), a toxic oxidant.
  - Thiol-containing compounds, such as reduced glutathione, are used as electron donors to detoxify NAPQI.
- **Toxicity:** Single dose generally thought to be required to produce toxicity is ≥150 mg/kg.
- In overdose, absorption may be delayed.
- Peak absorption generally occurs at 2 hours and rarely after 4 hours.

- Absorption is further delayed in the presence of peristalsis-decreasing opioid or anticholinergic coingestants or if the acetaminophen is formulated for extended release.
- In overdose, metabolism by sulfation becomes saturated, and the formation of NAPQI exceeds that which can be detoxified by available glutathione.
  - As toxic metabolite is formed in the liver, hepatic toxicity is the key clinical feature.
  - N-acetylcysteine (NAC), the key to management of acetaminophen poisoning, acts as a precursor to glutathione synthesis, a substrate for sulfation; it directly

binds to NAPQI itself; and enhances the reduction of NAPQI to acetaminophen.

- **Clinical manifestations:** Acute acetaminophen toxicity has been divided into four clinical stages. Not every untreated patient will advance through each, and spontaneous improvement is possible at any point.
  - *Stage I:* Patient is either asymptomatic or has nonspecific clinical findings (nausea, vomiting, malaise), and no laboratory abnormalities are recognized.
  - *Stage II:* This begins with onset of liver injury, 24 to 36 hours after ingestion.
    - Symptoms are similar to other causes of hepatitis.
    - Initial laboratory findings include elevated aminotransferases (aspartate aminotransferase [AST]/alanine aminotransferase [ALT]), but progress to signs of hepatic dysfunction, including prolonged prothrombin time (PT), metabolic acidosis, and hypoglycemia.
  - *Stage III:* Time of peak hepatotoxicity is usually 72 to 96 hours from ingestion. AST and ALT may ultimately exceed 10,000 IU/L, but creatinine, lactate, phosphate, and PT are better prognostic indicators.
    - Fatalities usually occur within 3 to 5 days of ingestion.
  - *Stage IV:* Hepatic regeneration will be histologically and functionally complete in survivors
- **Management:** NAC is the key to managing acetaminophen poisoning. Decontamination with activated charcoal should be considered only if significant coingestants are expected.
  - Oral protocol for acute ingestions is a 140 mg/kg loading dose, followed by 17 doses of 70 mg/kg every 4 hours for a total of 72 hours.
  - IV regimen is 150 mg/kg over 45 minutes, followed by 50 mg/kg over 4 hours, and then 100 mg/kg over 16 hours.
  - Both regimens have equal efficacy for simple acute ingestion.
    - IV regimen has shorter course and is the only route that has been studied adequately in patients with hepatic failure.
    - Parenteral NAC carries the risk of anaphylactoid reactions.
  - Simple, acute ingestion occurs when a single dose of acetaminophen is ingested over a short period of time, within 24 hours of presentation.
    - Little controversy in managing this type of ingestion
      - Serum acetaminophen concentration should be plotted against the number of hours after ingestion on the Rumack–Matthew nomogram to determine whether treatment with NAC is necessary.
        - Currently recommended line intersects 150 μg/mL at 4 hours, incorporating a 25% safety margin over the original nomogram line, which was itself nearly 100% sensitive for predicting hepatoxicity.
        - Treatment initiated within 8 hours of ingestion has complete efficacy in preventing hepatotoxicity.
        - NAC should be started immediately in any patient with suspected acetaminophen poisoning when the laboratory result for the acetaminophen concentration is not expected to be available within 8 hours of the initial ingestion.
        - Once the serum acetaminophen concentration is available, the decision whether to continue the NAC can be made based on the nomogram (Fig. 30.1).
          - If any uncertainty with regard to the exact time of ingestion, the physician should use the most conser-

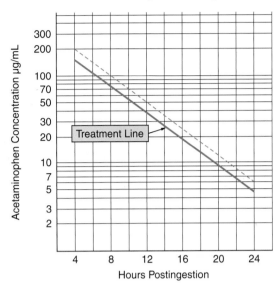

Acetaminophen Nomogram

FIGURE 30.1. Acetaminophen nomogram. (Adapted with permission from Hendrickson RG, Bizovi KE. Acetaminophen. In: Flomenbaum NE, Goldfrank LR, Hoffman RS, et al., eds. *Goldfrank's Toxicologic Emergencies.* 8th ed. New York: McGraw-Hill; 2006: 523–543.)

vative estimate (i.e., the earliest possible time) when using the nomogram.
- Indications less clear for the use of NAC for hepatoxicity after suspected chronic acetaminophen use
- The vast majority of people who take acetaminophen have no adverse clinical manifestations. Clinical trials involving daily dosing of 4 g of acetaminophen in both alcoholics and nonalcoholics showed that patients have either normal aminotransferase concentrations or very minor increases.
  - Nonetheless, NAC should be administered to all patients with suspected acetaminophen hepatotoxicity until the diagnosis has been excluded.
  - Nomogram cannot be used for patients who present more than 24 hours after ingestion.
    - In such cases, NAC should be started immediately upon presentation.
      - If the patient has both undetectable acetaminophen concentration and normal aminotransferases, acetaminophen overdose is highly unlikely, and NAC need not be continued
      - If either acetaminophen or aminotransferase concentrations are elevated (even minimally so), the patient should be administered 20 hours of IV NAC.
- When acetaminophen-induced hepatoxicity is encountered, IV NAC should be administered as described previously.
  - Maintenance dose should be continued until clinical improvement, liver transplantation, or death.
  - Even in the presence of fulminant hepatic failure, IV NAC has been shown to decrease mortality, cerebral edema, and the need for vasopressors.
- **Hepatic transplantation:** Generally, patients with significant acetaminophen poisoning will have AST and ALT concentrations >1,000 IU/L by 24 to 48 hours after ingestion.
- Several prognostic criteria are available.

- The King's College Hospital Criteria suggest that pH <7.3 after resuscitation or the combination of PT >100, creatinine >3.3 mg/dL, and grade III or IV encephalopathy are predictive of death in the absence of a transplantation.
- Serum phosphate is a good predictor.
  - A 48-hour serum phosphate concentration >1.2 mMol/L has been shown to be sensitive and specific for predicting the need for transplant and the probability of death from acetaminophen hepatotoxicity.
  - Presumably, a low or normal phosphate concentration is evidence that the phosphate is being utilized by hepatocytes for adenosine triphosphate (ATP) generation.

Salicylates and Other Nonsteroidal Anti-inflammatory Drugs

- ICU admission is required when patients present with metabolic acidosis and hemodynamic instability or if they require bicarbonate infusion or frequent measurements of salicylate concentration.
- **Mechanism:** Therapeutic effects result from the inhibition of cyclo-oxygenase, a mediator of prostaglandin synthesis.
  - Salicylates uncouple oxidative phosphorylation, meaning that some of the proton gradient across the mitochondrial matrix is dissipated in the formation of heat, rather than ATP, forcing the production of lactate.
- **Clinical manifestations of salicylate poisoning:** Acute salicylate poisoning may cause epigastric pain, nausea, and vomiting. Salicylates induce hyperventilation (both tachypnea and hyperpnea) by direct stimulation of the brainstem respiratory center.
  - Neurologic signs and symptoms of salicylate poisoning range from mild to severe and include tinnitus, delirium, coma, and seizure.
  - Initial feature of toxicity is primary respiratory alkalosis.
  - A primary metabolic acidosis is characterized by the presence of lactic acid, ketoacids, and salicylic acids.
  - Net result is an increased anion gap metabolic acidosis.
    - In adults, the presence of an acidemia or even normal pH indicates advanced poisoning.
  - Chronic salicylate poisoning presents with the same signs and symptoms as acute poisoning but typically occurs in elderly patients taking supratherapeutic amounts of salicylate to treat a chronic condition.
    - It often is not suspected.
    - Elderly salicylate-poisoned patients presenting with metabolic acidosis and an altered sensorium may initially be misdiagnosed with sepsis, dehydration, or cerebrovascular accident if a salicylate concentration is not obtained.
- Serum salicylate concentrations correlate loosely with toxicity because the principal site of poisoning is the central nervous system (CNS).
  - Threshold for toxicity is usually considered to be 30 mg/dL when tinnitus develops.
  - Chronically poisoned patients have a lower salicylate concentration for the same degree of illness because much of their total body burden has redistributed into the CNS.
  - Degree of poisoning is determined by evaluating the serum concentration in context of the patient's clinical appearance, laboratory results, and acuity of ingestion.

- **Management of salicylate poisoning:** The key principles for management of salicylate poisoning are to minimize absorption, speed elimination, and minimize redistribution to tissues.
- Gastric emptying is attempted if a significant amount of drug is expected to be in stomach.
  - Activated charcoal, 1 g/kg, should be administered every 4 hours if it can be given safely.
  - Salicylates cause pylorospasm and may form concretions in overdose, leading to delayed absorption.
    - Multiple-dose activated charcoal prevents delayed absorption and may speed elimination of salicylates by disrupting the drug's enteroenteric circulation.
    - Serum chemistry, venous or arterial blood gas, and salicylate concentration should be obtained every 2 hours until the salicylate concentration demonstrates an interval decrease.
- Moderately poisoned patients (increased anion gap or a salicylate concentration greater than 40 mg/dL) should also have blood and urine alkalinized with sodium bicarbonate.
  - As a weak acid (pKa 3.5), salicylates will be ionized in an alkaline environment and "trapped" (i.e., unable to passively move through lipid membranes).
  - Alkalinization is achieved with infusion of sodium bicarbonate of 150 mEq in 1 L of D5W at twice the maintenance rate (ideal body weight in kg + 40 = maintenance rate in milliliters per hour).
    - Urine pH should be maintained from 7.5 to 8.0 and systemic arterial pH between 7.45 and 7.55.
    - Replete potassium, as low serum potassium will cause preferential reabsorption of potassium over hydrogen ions in the proximal tubule and compromise attempts to alkalinize the urine.
    - Endotracheal intubation and sedation should be avoided whenever possible.
      - Tachypnea and hyperpnea of salicylate poisoning does not necessarily represent "tiring" and produces a helpful alkalosis.
      - If intubation is unavoidable, patients should be administered 1 to 2 mEq/kg of bicarbonate prior to the procedure, intubated quickly and hyperventilated afterward.
- Early consultation with a nephrologist is recommended for seriously ill patients.
- Extracorporeal elimination is reserved for patients who are very ill, those who cannot tolerate alkalinization, or those with serum concentrations so elevated that their clinical status is expected to deteriorate.
  - Hemodialysis is used for severe acid-base disturbances, mental status changes, inability to tolerate alkalinization (renal failure or congestive heart failure), and serum concentrations of 100 mg/dL after acute poisoning and 60 mg/dL in chronic poisoning (Table 30.3).
- **Clinical manifestations of NSAID poisoning:** NSAIDs are considered safer than salicylates in therapeutic dosing.
- Acute overdose of NSAIDs can cause gastric injury.
  - Chronic NSAID use is associated with interstitial nephritis, nephritic syndrome, or analgesic nephropathy; acute overdose sometimes accompanied by a reversible azotemia caused by vasoconstriction from decreased prostaglandin production.

TABLE 30.3

INDICATIONS FOR HEMODIALYSIS IN SALICYLATE POISONING

Renal failure
Congestive heart failure (relative)
Acute lung injury
Persistent CNS disturbances
Progressive deterioration in vital signs
Severe acid-base or electrolyte imbalance, despite appropriate treatment
Hepatic compromise with coagulopathy
Salicylate concentration (acute) >100 mg/dL or (chronic) >60 mg/dL

CNS, central nervous system.
Adapted with permission from Flomenbaum NE. Salicylates. In: Flomenbaum NE, Goldfrank LR, Hoffman RS, et al., eds. *Goldfrank's Toxicologic Emergencies.* 8th ed. New York: McGraw-Hill; 2006:550–564.

- In severe overdose, the most consequential effects are elevated anion gap metabolic acidosis, coma, and hypotension.
- **Management of NSAID poisoning:** Activated charcoal should be administered if the patient presents within several hours of overdose.
  - Good supportive care is the mainstay of therapy after overdose.
  - Elimination is not increased with alkalinization.
  - High degree of protein binding precludes removal with hemodialysis.
    - Hemodialysis has been used to correct acidemia and electrolyte abnormalities in patients with multiorgan system failure.

Psychiatric Medications

- Represent a disproportionate number of poisonings in the United States
- Antidepressants, antipsychotics, and sedative-hypnotics accounted for more than half of all deaths reported to poison control centers in 2005.
  - High mortality figure is a function of the prevalence of these ingestions, as these drugs do not have a high case-fatality rate.
  - With sound supportive care, most patients can be managed successfully.

Antipsychotic Medications

- Antipsychotics are categorized as either typical or atypical.
- Typical antipsychotics, which include haloperidol, chlorpromazine, and thioridazine, antagonize dopamine primarily at the D_2 receptor.
- Newer medications, atypical drugs, are exemplified by clozapine, olanzapine, quetiapine, risperidone, and ziprasidone.
  - Have less dopaminergic antagonism
  - More serotonergic effects than the typicals

- When antipsychotic medications produce coma, conduction abnormalities, or hyperthermia, patients require ICU admission.
- **Clinical manifestations of overdose:** All antipsychotics produce sedation in overdose, though respiratory depression is usually not consequential.
  - Varying degrees of muscarinic and α-adrenergic antagonism occur, often resulting in tachycardia and moderate hypotension.
    - Many of the typical antipsychotics have type IA antidysrhythmic properties.
    - Most typicals and a few of the atypical drugs (notably ziprasidone) can cause QTc prolongation and torsades de pointes.
  - Management of overdose generally requires only supportive care.
- **Clinical manifestations of the neuroleptic malignant syndrome:** The dopamine antagonism required for control of psychosis can cause a group of distinct movement disorders that range in severity from mild to life threatening.
  - Conditions—dystonia, akathisia, parkinsonism, tardive dyskinesia, and neuroleptic malignant syndrome (NMS)—are more likely to occur in the presence of the typicals, although the atypicals can cause them as well.
- NMS is the most consequential of the movement disorders associated with the antipsychotics.
  - Characterized by altered mental status, muscular rigidity, hyperthermia, and autonomic dysfunction
    ○ Symptoms usually begin within weeks of starting treatment but occur in individuals taking the drug chronically.
    ○ Risk factors include the following:
      – Young age
      – Male gender
      – Extracellular fluid volume contraction
      – Use of high-potency antipsychotics
      – Depot drug preparations
      – Concomitant lithium use
      – Rapid increase in dose, or simultaneous use of multiple drugs
    ○ Diagnosis is not always clear because there is no reference standard.
      – Differential diagnosis of hyperthermia and altered mental status is very broad, including:
        - Infection
        - Environmental hyperthermia
        - Hyperthyroidism
        - Serotonin syndrome
        - Ethanol and sedative-hypnotic withdrawal
        - Sympathomimetic intoxication
        - Anticholinergic intoxication
  - Management of NMS
    ○ Immediate treatment of life-threatening hyperthermia: Ice-water immersion and paralysis by neuromuscular blockade should not be delayed if temperature is >106°F (41.1°C).
      – In instances of environmental hyperthermia, a delay of cooling longer than 30 minutes has been associated with significant morbidity and mortality.
        - Benzodiazepines should be titrated to sedation and muscle relaxation.

- Rhabdomyolysis, electrolyte disorders, and hypotension should be aggressively treated.
- Bromocriptine, a centrally acting dopamine agonist given at 2.5 to 10 mg three to four times a day is of theoretical benefit but has not been well studied.
  - NMS may not be controlled for days after the introduction of bromocriptine.
  - After signs and symptoms begin to improve, bromocriptine should be decreased by no more than 10% a day as decreasing the dose too rapidly may precipitate a relapse of NMS.
- No evidence for the antidotal use of dantrolene in the management of NMS
  - Dantrolene drug of choice in malignant hyperthermia, a disorder affecting the sarcoplasmic reticulum seen in susceptible individuals receiving inhalational anesthetics or succinylcholine
    - May be confused with neuroleptic malignant syndrome because of their similar names and clinical manifestations

Benzodiazepines

- In 2005, the AAPCC received reports of 3,018 major effects and 243 fatalities from benzodiazepines.
- These are widely used for their sedative, anxiolytic, and anticonvulsant properties.
- All effects result from increasing the frequency of opening of γ-aminobutyric acid (GABA)-mediated chloride channels in the CNS.
- In overdose, these drugs produce somnolence, coma, and minimal decreases in blood pressure, heart rate, and respiratory rate.
- **Management of benzodiazepine overdose:** Supportive
- Care focuses on supporting airway and blood pressure while waiting for the drug elimination.
  - Flumazenil, a competitive benzodiazepine antagonist, plays a limited role.
    - It can precipitate withdrawal in individuals who are tolerant to benzodiazepines and induce seizures in those with seizure disorders.
    - Flumazenil may be indicated in patients without tolerance to benzodiazepines who suffer from a pure benzodiazepine overdose; overdoses in children may meet these criteria.
    - When indicated, flumazenil should be given IV, 0.1 mg/min, up to 1 mg.
    - Dosing may be repeated if the clinical response is inadequate.
      - Duration of the effect of flumazenil is shorter than the effect of the benzodiazepine, so recurrence of symptoms should be expected.
      - Alternatively, redosing or a continuous IV infusion at 0.1 to 1.0 mg / hour may be administered.
- If any doubt as to whether the patient has tolerance to benzodiazepines, flumazenil should not be administered

Cyclic Antidepressants

- Until introduction of the selective serotonin reuptake inhibitors, the cyclic antidepressants were the principal pharmacologic treatment available for depression.

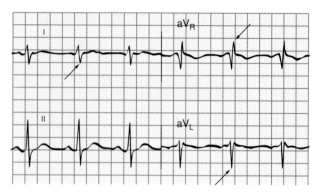

FIGURE 30.2. Terminal elevation of aVR and QRS prolongation. (Adapted with permission from Clancy C. Electrocardiographic principles. In: Flomenbaum NE, Goldfrank LR, Hoffman RS, et al., eds. *Goldfrank's Toxicologic Emergencies.* 8th ed. New York: McGraw-Hill; 2006:51–62.)

- Roughly 12% of the 11,198 reported cyclic antidepressant exposures in 2005 had either a major outcome or fatality.
- The cyclic antidepressants (CAs) differ slightly from one another in their receptor affinities but can be treated as a group.
  - CAs are usually absorbed within hours of ingestion.
  - Antimuscarinic effects may delay absorption in overdose.
    - Drugs also exhibit α-adrenergic antagonism, inhibition of reuptake of norepinephrine, and anticholinergic properties.
    - CAs act as type IA antidysrhythmics, blocking sodium entry into myocytes during phase 0 of depolarization.
- **Clinical manifestations:** Important CNS effects include lethargy, delirium, coma, and seizures. Tachycardia and hypotension develop early in toxicity.
  - IA antidysrhythmic properties cause prolongation of the QRS interval.
  - CAs also produce a characteristic rightward shift of the axis in the terminal portion of the QRS, best seen as an R wave in the terminal 40 msec of lead aVR (Fig. 30.2).
- **Management:** Gastrointestinal decontamination should be considered in every patient. If the history suggests a recent large ingestion, gastric lavage may be attempted.
  - Acute ingestions of 10 to 20 mg/kg of most CAs can cause significant poisoning.
  - Activated charcoal should be administered.
  - Serum drug concentrations do not correlate well with toxicity.
  - The ECG is the most important diagnostic test when managing CA overdose.
    - QRS duration is an indicator of severity of poisoning.
    - No patients with QRS <160 msec had ventricular dysrhythmias, and no patients with a QRS duration <100 msec had seizures.
  - Sodium bicarbonate should be administered if the QRS duration is ≥100 msec.
    - High sodium concentration and alkaline pH of sodium bicarbonate solution are responsible for salutary effects.
      - Sodium load increases the sodium gradient across the poisoned myocardial sodium channel, resulting in a narrowing of the QRS complex.
      - Bicarbonate raises the pH, reducing CA binding to the sodium channel.

○ Sodium bicarbonate should be administered as a 1 to 2 mEq/kg bolus during continuous ECG monitoring.

○ If the complex narrows, sodium bicarbonate can be administered as an infusion.

○ If the complex remains unchanged, the diagnosis of CA poisoning should be reconsidered.

• Sodium bicarbonate infusion may be performed by adding 150 mEq of bicarbonate to 1 L of D5W and infusing at twice the maintenance rate.

○ Arterial pH should be targeted to 7.50 to 7.55.

○ Occasional repeat boluses of 1 to 2 mEq/kg may be necessary.

○ Hypertonic sodium chloride (3% NaCl) may be indicated when the QRS complex widens and the serum pH precludes further alkalinization.

○ Hyperventilation may be used to induce alkalemia in intubated CA-poisoned patients.

○ If hypotension persists despite fluid resuscitation and vasopressors become necessary, norepinephrine may be superior to dopamine.

• Seizures should be rapidly controlled.

• Convulsions result in a metabolic acidosis, causing even more avid binding of the CA to the cardiac sodium channels, potentially resulting in more cardiotoxicity.

○ Benzodiazepines, propofol, or barbiturates are appropriate.

○ Phenytoin, a type IA antidysrhythmic, may worsen cardiac toxicity and is not indicated.

• Therapy should continue until vital signs and ECG improve.

• Unless there is significant secondary injury (such as from shock), those who survive to 24 hours are expected to make a complete recovery.

• Because of protein binding, hemodialysis is ineffective.

Lithium

• Used in the treatment of bipolar affective disorders

• Patients will require ICU admission when they have signs of CNS toxicity, do not tolerate fluid therapy, or have serum concentrations >2 mMol/L.

• Of 5,559 exposures reported to the AAPCC, 5.7% were classified as major or fatal.

• **Pharmacology:** Thought to increase serotonin release and increase receptor sensitivity to serotonin and modulate the effects of norepinephrine on its second-messenger system

• Kidney handles lithium (Li) and sodium similarly.

• Li is freely filtered by the glomerulus, and 80% is reabsorbed, with 60% occurring in the proximal tubule.

• Immediate-release Li preparations produce peak serum concentrations within hours; sustained-release Li may not peak for 6 to 12 hours.

• Li generally accepted therapeutic range is 0.6 to 1.2 mMol/L.

○ In overdose and therapeutic dosing, clinical signs and symptoms are a better guide than the serum concentration.

• **Clinical manifestations of overdose:** Acute and chronic Li toxicity have similar neurologic features; acute toxicity usually associated with significant gastrointestinal (GI) manifestations

• Acute toxicity occurs when an individual without a body burden of Li takes a supratherapeutic dose of drug.

• Chronic toxicity is usually the result of decreased elimination of drug in a patient who is receiving a fixed dose (e.g., after developing renal insufficiency).

• Acute-on-chronic toxicity occurs when a patient with a pre-existent total body drug takes a supratherapeutic dose.

• In acute toxicity, a large ingestion of Li—a GI irritant—will initially cause GI symptoms, such as vomiting and diarrhea.

• Neurotoxicity (which is clinically more significant) will be delayed until the drug has been absorbed and is redistributed into the CNS.

• In chronic toxicity, GI symptoms may be absent.

• Neurotoxicity manifests as movement disorders and alterations in mental status.

• Mild toxicity: Only a fine tremor is present.

• More advanced poisoning: Fasciculations, hyperreflexia, dysarthria, and nystagmus may be seen.

• Mental status changes range from confusion to coma and seizures.

• Nephrogenic diabetes insipidus and hypothyroidism occur after chronic therapeutic Li use but are not features of overdose.

• The syndrome of irreversible Li-effectuated neurotoxicity (SILENT) is a chronic neurologic disorder with many of the same features of Li neurotoxicity.

• SILENT persists even when body burden of Li eliminated.

• Mechanism is not completely elucidated but may involve demyelination.

• SILENT has been reported both as a result of chronic therapeutic use and as a sequela of Li intoxication.

• **Management:** GI decontamination should be considered after acute Li toxicity.

• Li does not bind to activated charcoal, so its use is only considered when a mixed overdose is suspected.

• For sustained-release preparation ingestion, whole-bowel irrigation has been shown to decrease serum Li concentration.

• Whole-bowel irrigation is performed by administering 2 L of polyethylene glycol orally every hour (25 mL/kg/hr in children) until rectal effluent clear.

• In both acute and chronic toxicity, IV fluids are given to optimize volume.

○ Volume-depleted patient will have decreased GFR and increased Li reabsorption.

○ When fluid deficits are restored, 0.9% saline can be administered at twice the maintenance rate or approximately 200 mL/hour in adults to aid in Li elimination.

• Extracorporeal elimination may be necessary to treat Li toxicity.

• Li can be removed by hemodialysis due to its low volume of distribution and limited protein binding.

• Li concentrations may rebound after dialysis—movement from intracellular to extracellular compartments—but tissue burden has actually decreased.

• Hemodialysis is performed when signs of significant end-organ damage, when lithium cannot be eliminated without dialysis, or when the serum concentration is elevated such that severe toxicity is highly likely.

○ Recommend dialysis in the following:

– Significant CNS toxicity such as clonus, obtundation, coma, or seizures

- Patient with milder toxicity cannot eliminate lithium efficiently (renal insufficiency) or tolerate saline resuscitation (congestive heart failure)
- Serum Li concentration >4.0 mMol/L after acute poisoning or >2.5 mMol/L after chronic poisoning
- Repeat dialysis may be necessary, so reapply the preceding criteria 4 hours after dialysis is completed to determine whether dialysis should be repeated.
  ○ Common clinical pitfall is to deny dialysis to patients with an elevated Li concentration and signs of toxicity because consecutive concentrations have shown small decrease.
    - Unfortunately, duration of exposure to the toxic Li levels may predispose the patient to SILENT.
    - Though not adequately studied, it seems prudent to hemodialyze.

TOXICOLOGIC BRADYCARDIA: DIGOXIN, β-ADRENERGIC ANTAGONISTS, AND CALCIUM CHANNEL BLOCKERS

- In 2005, the AAPCC NPED reported more than 30,000 exposures to cardioactive steroids (including digoxin), β-adrenergic antagonists, and calcium channel blockers.
  - Among these were 1,085 major outcomes and 167 fatalities.
  - These xenobiotics have narrow therapeutic index, drawing a fine line between therapeutic dosing and poisoning.

Digoxin

- Digoxin is a cardioactive steroid derived from the foxglove plant.
  - Digoxin and digitoxin are the only pharmaceuticals in the class.
  - Plants such as oleander, yellow oleander, dogbane, and red squill contain cardioactive steroids with similar toxicity.
    - Some of these plants cause a great deal of morbidity worldwide.
  - Of 2,828 reported exposures to cardiac steroid medications in 2005, 7.4% classified as major or fatal.
- **Mechanism:** Multiple therapeutic and toxic cardiovascular effects, all of which result from inhibition of the Na^+-K^+-ATPase
  - Na^+-K^+-ATPase extrudes sodium from the myocardial cell, creating a sodium gradient that drives an Na^+-Ca^{2+}-antiporter moving calcium extracellularly.
  - Inhibition of Na^+-K^+-ATPase by digoxin increases intracellular Ca^{2+}, which therapeutically triggers Ca^{2+}-mediated Ca^{2+} release from the sarcoplasmic reticulum; commonly called Ca-mediated Ca release.
- Slows conduction through the sinoatrial (SA) and atrioventricular (AV) nodes
  - Probably through direct and vagally mediated mechanisms
  - In therapeutic use, decreases heart rate and increases inotropy
  - In overdose, the increased intracellular Ca^{2+} brings the cell closer to threshold, resulting in increased automaticity.

- Does not exert its therapeutic and toxic effects until it redistributes from the serum into the myocardium
  - Has large volume of distribution, precluding elimination by hemodialysis
  - Mostly eliminated renally, although some hepatic metabolism
  - Maximal effect from therapeutic dose:
    ○ Seen at 4 to 6 hours when administered orally
    ○ Seen at 1.5 to 3 hours when given IV
- **Clinical manifestations:** Poisoning can be either acute or chronic.
  - Acute toxicity occurs when an individual without a tissue burden of digoxin ingests a supratherapeutic dosage of the drug.
  - Chronic toxicity usually occurs when an individual on a fixed dose of the drug loses the ability to excrete it effectively.
  - Both syndromes have similar cardiovascular manifestations.
    - Acute toxicity may feature more prominent GI symptoms.
  - Acute poisoning may result in nausea, vomiting, and abdominal pain, whereas chronic poisoning develops more insidiously.
    - In addition to GI symptoms, chronic poisoning may present with weakness, confusion, or delirium.
  - Bradycardia with a preserved blood pressure typically occurs in digoxin toxicity.
    - ECG is the most important test in establishing the diagnosis.
      ○ No single ECG manifestation is consistently seen in patients with digoxin toxicity.
      ○ Almost any rhythm is possible, with the exception of a rapidly conducted supraventricular rhythm.
      ○ Most common rhythm disturbance on initial ECG is the presence of ventricular ectopy.
        - ECG could potentially exhibit increased automaticity from elevated resting potential, conduction disturbance from AV and SA nodal block, both, or neither.
        - Ectopy may degrade into ventricular tachycardia or ventricular fibrillation.
        - If conduction disturbance predominates, the ECG may demonstrate sinus bradycardia or varying degrees of AV block.
- Therapeutic range for digoxin is usually reported as 0.5 to 2.0 ng/mL.
  - Serum digoxin concentration is interpreted in the context of the history and ECG.
  - Digoxin cardiotoxin and serum concentrations do not necessarily reflect the degree of poisoning.
  - Digoxin requires several hours to redistribute from the serum to the tissues.
    ○ Shortly after an acute ingestion, the serum concentration may overestimate toxicity.
    ○ A mild increase in serum concentration in a patient chronically on digoxin may underestimate the high extent of the increased tissue burden.
  - Serum potassium concentration a better predictor of illness after acute ingestions.
    ○ In the pre–digoxin-specific antibody fragment era, no mortality when the potassium concentration was less than 5.0 mEq/L
    ○ 50% mortality when the potassium concentration was 5.0 to 5.5 mEq/L

- **Management of toxicity:** Acute toxicity can cause vomiting, so activated charcoal and gastric lavage may be of limited value.
  - Atropine can be given IV in 0.5-mg doses for bradycardia.
    - Probably not important to "correct" the heart rate if the blood pressure is preserved
  - If necessary, potassium should be supplemented.
    - Hypokalemia inhibits the function of the Na^+-K^+-ATPase, and thereby exacerbates digoxin poisoning.
    - A pitfall in managing digoxin-poisoned patients is the administration of calcium in response to the recognition of hyperkalemia.
      - When hyperkalemia is the result of an increase in total body burden of potassium, such as in renal failure, calcium is the treatment of choice.
      - However, calcium administration is not recommended in the setting of digoxin poisoning where extracellular distribution of potassium is the result of a poisoned Na^+-K^+-ATPase, not an increase in total body potassium.
      - Here, increasing extracellular calcium may accentuate toxicity.
- Digoxin-specific immune fragments
  - Digoxin-specific antibody fragments (Fab) is the most important intervention in digoxin-poisoned patients.
    - Prepared by cleaving the Fc fragment from IgG
    - Resulting Fab fragments less immunoreactive than the whole IgG antibodies
      - Causes allergic reaction in 0.8% of patients
  - Should be administered to anyone with the following:
    - Digoxin-induced cardiotoxicity
    - Serum potassium concentration ≥ 5.0 mEq/L after an acute overdose
    - Serum digoxin concentration ≥ 15 ng/mL at any time or ≥ 10 ng/mL at 6 hours after ingestion
  - Given by IV infusion and dosed according to serum concentration (Table 30.4)
    - In presence of suspected severe toxicity, treatment should not be dependent on nor await serum digoxin concentration results.
    - First clinical effect of Fab should be seen within 20 minutes and a maximal response within several hours.
    - After immune-specific antibody fragment administration, the serum digoxin concentration determined by most laboratories will be a total digoxin concentration.

  - This will include the antibody-bound digoxin, a result without clinical utility.
  - Free digoxin concentration would be useful.

β-Adrenergic Antagonists and Calcium Channel Blockers

- In 2005, 18,207 reports to NPED of exposures to β-adrenergic antagonists
  - Including 60 fatalities and 525 major outcomes
- 10,500 reports of exposures to calcium channel blockers
  - Including 75 fatalities and 384 major outcomes

β-Adrenergic Antagonists

- Receptors are coupled to G proteins, which activate adenyl cyclase, resulting in increased production of ATP from cyclic adenosine monophosphate.
  - Cyclic adenosine monophosphate activates protein kinase A, which initiates a series of phosphorylations.
  - Phosphorylation of L-type calcium channels on cell membranes increases intracellular calcium, which allows more activation of the SR and further calcium release from the SR, causing muscle contraction.
  - Calcium influx brings pacemaker cells closer to threshold.
  - Net result is increased inotropy and chronotropy.
- Most β-adrenergic antagonists are exclusively metabolized or biotransformed in the liver and then renally eliminated.
  - Exception to the rule is atenolol, which is exclusively renally eliminated.
- **Clinical manifestations of overdose:** All β-adrenergic antagonists have the potential to produce dose-dependent bradycardia and hypotension.
  - β-Adrenergic antagonists differ from one another in their selectivity for α-, β_1-, and β_2-adrenergic receptors.
    - Drugs with α- and β-adrenergic antagonist effects, such as labetalol and carvedilol, produce more hypotension and afterload reduction.
    - The more β_1-selective drugs, including metoprolol and atenolol, have less potential for β_2-related adverse effects such as bronchospasm.
    - The more lipid-soluble β-adrenergic antagonists, such as propranolol, penetrate the CNS more readily, causing obtundation or seizures prior to hemodynamic collapse.
    - Membrane-stabilizing activity, similar to type I antidysrhythmic activity, produces lengthening of the QRS interval, tachydysrhythmias, and hypotension.
      - Membrane-stabilizing effect usually is associated with propranolol and other lipid-soluble drugs but is observed after overdose with others.
  - Sotalol and acebutolol can produce QTc prolongation due to potassium channel blockade, which may result in torsades de pointes.

Calcium Channel Blockers

- The calcium channel blockers (CCBs) are formulated as both immediate and sustained release, but in overdose, the effects of either type may be prolonged.
- CCBs undergo hepatic metabolism.
- Three major classes of CCBs
  - Dihydropyridines (including amlodipine, nifedipine, and others ending with the suffix "-pine")

TABLE 30.4

DIGOXIN-SPECIFIC FAB DOSE CALCULATION

When serum digoxin concentration (SDC) known:
No. of vials = [SDC (ng/mL) × patient weight (kg)]/100

When SDC unknown, dose known:
No. of vials = Amount ingested (mg)/0.5 mg/vial

When both SDC and dose unknown (acute poisoning):
Empiric therapy
10–20 vials (adult or pediatric)

When both SDC and dose unknown (chronic poisoning):
Empiric therapy
Adult: 3–6 vials
Pediatric: 1–2 vials

- Phenylalkylamines (verapamil)
- Benzothiazepine (diltiazem)
- More clinically useful to divide them into two classes: the dihydropyridines and the nondihydropyridines
  - All the drugs inhibit function of L-type calcium channels.
  - Dihydropyridines have greater affinity for calcium channels in vascular smooth muscle than the myocardium.
- **Clinical manifestations of overdose:** The most consequential clinical features of CCB overdose are cardiovascular. All of the CCBs produce hypotension with reflex tachycardia.
  - Effects on heart rate and contractility vary based on the class of the particular drug.
    - Diltiazem produces little peripheral blockade but suppresses contractility and conduction through the SA and AV nodes, resulting in bradycardia and decreased inotropy.
    - These effects can be much more difficult to treat than the peripheral vasodilation of the dihydropyridines.
      - In severe poisoning, heart block or complete cardiovascular collapse results.
    - Verapamil, active in the peripheral vasculature and in the myocardium, produces a combination of the effects of the dihydropyridines and diltiazem.
      - This is considered to be the most dangerous of the CCBs, although any of them can cause death in overdose.
  - CCBs have effects outside the cardiovascular system.
    - Blockade of L-type calcium channels in pancreatic β-islet cells trigger blockade of insulin release and may result in hyperglycemia.
- **Management of overdose of β-adrenergic antagonists and CCBs:** Patients who initially present without symptoms may rapidly become very ill.
  - These overdoses should be taken very seriously and treated aggressively.
  - Many antidotes have been investigated, with varying degrees of clinical success.
    - Patients with β-adrenergic antagonist and CCB overdose do not benefit from hemodialysis.
    - No single antidote exists for either β-adrenergic antagonists or CCBs.
  - Optimal treatment
    - GI decontamination should be considered in all patients.
      - Gastric lavage may be indicated if there are pills still expected to be in the stomach (usually in the first hour or two after ingestion).
      - Activated charcoal should be administered.
      - Whole-bowel irrigation with polyethylene glycol is indicated for patients with a history of ingesting sustained-release drugs.
    - Initial management for hypotension
      - IV crystalloid fluid
      - IV atropine, 0.5 mg to 1 mg, may be given for bradycardia, though studies of atropine efficacy in CCB toxicity not definitive.
    - Calcium has a role in calcium channel blocker toxicity and β-adrenergic antagonist poisoning.
      - Increasing extracellular calcium helps to overcome calcium channel blockade and increase intracellular calcium, typically with greater improvement in blood pressure than heart rate.
      - The ideal dosing of calcium is not yet established.
        - IV bolus of 13 to 25 mEq of Ca^{2+} (10–20 mL of 10% calcium chloride or 30–60 mL of 10% calcium glu-

conate) can be followed by repeat boluses or an infusion of 0.5 mEq/kg/hour of Ca^{2+}.
        - Calcium concentration should be closely monitored.
    - Glucagon, an endogenous polypeptide hormone released by pancreatic α cells
      - Glucagon has significant inotropic effects mediated by its ability to activate myocyte adenylate cyclase without the β-adrenergic receptor.
      - Calcium channel opening occurs "downstream" from adenylate cyclase; glucagon may not be as effective for overcoming calcium channel blockade.
      - Glucagon should be given IV, at an initial dose of 3 to 5 mg (50 μg/kg in children), up to 10 mg.
      - The total initial dose that produces a response should be given hourly as an infusion.
        - Glucagon may cause hyperglycemia or vomiting, but neither complication should limit the therapy if effective.
    - Hyperinsulinemia/euglycemia therapy should be instituted early in patients with moderate to severe poisoning.
      - Insulin is a positive inotrope and may independently increase Ca^{2+} entry into cells.
      - Insulin may allow the myocardium, which usually relies on fatty acids, to use more carbohydrate for metabolism.
      - Ideal dose is not known.
        - Recommend IV bolus of 1 unit/kg, followed by an infusion of 0.5 to 1 unit/kg/hour.
        - Initial bolus should be preceded by a 1 g/kg bolus of dextrose, followed by an infusion to maintain euglycemia.
          - Initial infusion of 0.5 g/kg/hour of dextrose can be instituted and adjusted based on the subsequent glucose concentration.
  - In severe poisoning, all of the preceding measures should be performed.
    - In addition, institute inotropes and vasoactive drugs.
    - Intra-aortic balloon counterpulsation should also be considered if cardiac output is severely compromised.
      - Technique may be ideal for these patients because cardiac output can recover in a relatively short period of time.

TOXIC ALCOHOLS

Mechanism of Toxicity

- *Toxic alcohols* refers in particular to methanol and ethylene glycol, which are the most important chemicals in the class because they are both of high potential toxicity and wide availability.
- In 2005, NPED received the following:
- 6,220 reports of exposure to ethylene glycol, including 5.4% classified as major or fatal
- 2,276 exposures to methanol, with 3.2% major or fatal
- Toxic alcohols have numerous industrial and consumer uses.
- Methanol is commonly found in windshield wiper fluid.
- Ethylene glycol is in automobile antifreeze.
- Isopropanol is a ubiquitous topical disinfectant.
- Specific laboratory testing is usually not available for these chemicals; establishment of the diagnosis of toxic alcohol

poisoning will necessitate skilled use of the serum osmolarity and anion gap.

- Toxic alcohols are readily absorbed and have a volume of distribution similar to total body water.
- Parent compounds and the toxic metabolites are dialyzable.
- It is the metabolites that produce significant toxicity.
  - Methanol and ethylene glycol are metabolized in a stepwise fashion by alcohol dehydrogenase (ADH) and aldehyde dehydrogenase (ALDH) to the clinically important metabolites formic acid (methanol) and glycolic, glycoxylic, and oxalic acid (ethylene glycol).
  - Isopropanol is less clinically consequential, as it is converted by ADH to acetone, which is an end product rather than a substrate of ALDH.
- ADH preferentially metabolizes ethanol over all other alcohols.
  - No significant metabolism of toxic alcohols will occur while high concentrations of ethanol are present.
  - When ADH is inhibited, the parent compounds are eliminated very slowly without metabolism.
    - Absent ADH, ethylene glycol is renally eliminated with a half-life of 8.5 hours, whereas methanol, which is eliminated as a vapor, has a half-life of 30 to 54 hours.
- When suspected, toxic alcohol poisoning requires ICU admission.
  - Patients may be obtunded and require therapeutic medication infusions and hemodialysis.

Clinical Manifestations

- The physical examination may be unremarkable.
  - All toxic alcohols can produce significant CNS depression.
  - Compensatory tachypnea may be present if there is a metabolic acidosis.
- Acetone, generated from ADH metabolism of isopropanol, produces nausea, hypotension, hemorrhagic gastritis, and tachycardia, but these are not usually life threatening.
- Formate, a methanol metabolite, can produce blindness from toxicity to the retina and optic nerve.
- Laboratory studies can suggest—not establish or exclude—the diagnosis of toxic alcohol poisoning.
  - Metabolites of methanol or ethylene glycol may cause an elevated anion gap metabolic acidosis.
  - The hallmark laboratory finding of isopropanol poisoning is ketonemia without acidosis.
  - Ethylene glycol may cause nephrotoxicity when the primary metabolite oxalic acid precipitates as calcium oxalate crystals in the renal tubules.
  - Osmolar gap, the difference between the measured and unmeasured osmoles, may be increased when the serum contains toxic alcohol osmoles.
    - Very high osmolar gap does suggest the presence of toxic alcohol.
    - Low or normal gap does not exclude the presence of ethylene glycol or methanol.
    - The "normal" osmolar gap varies widely in population, from—0 to 10, such that very high concentrations of toxic alcohols might not be apparent when the gap is calculated.

- Fluorescence of the urine or presence of calcium oxalate crystals in the presence of ethylene glycol poisoning is neither sensitive nor specific.
- Fluorescein is added to some brands of ethylene glycol–based antifreeze to facilitate detection of radiator leaks.
  - Woods lamp may be used to detect urine for fluorescence as a screen for ethylene glycol.
    - However, a large group of children not exposed to ethylene glycol had urinary fluorescence.
  - Because of limitations of laboratory studies, treatment should be started empirically as soon as the diagnosis is considered.

Management

- Several clinical presentations suggest poisoning with a toxic alcohol, and each requires different management considerations.
- First type presents without acidosis and either a history of ingesting ethylene glycol or methanol or a very elevated osmolar gap.
  - Immediately begin an ADH inhibitor.
  - Obtain toxic alcohol concentrations (when available).
    - Decision to continue treatment or begin hemodialysis can be made based on the presence of a toxic alcohol in a high concentration.
    - If result is not expected in a timely manner, dialysis should be presumptively performed.
- Second scenario presents with an unexplained elevated anion gap metabolic acidosis that is not explained by the presence of lactate, ketoacids, or uremia.
  - Diagnosis should be considered.
  - ADH inhibition and hemodialysis should be instituted.
  - A helpful test in this scenario is a serum ethanol concentration.
    - As long as there is elevated ethanol concentration present in the serum, toxic alcohols cannot be converted into their metabolites.
    - Thus, if a patient has a very elevated ethanol concentration, the elevated anion gap metabolic acidosis cannot be explained by toxic alcohol poisoning, unless the ethanol was consumed only hours after the ingestion of the toxic alcohol.
- In the third scenario, if a serum toxic alcohol concentration is available, the diagnosis can be established rapidly, and management is straightforward.
  - If the serum concentration of methanol is <25 mg/dL—or ethylene glycol <50 mg/dL—and there is no metabolic acidosis, treatment is not necessary.
- If treatment is required, the clinician must determine whether to use an ADH inhibitor alone or in conjunction with hemodialysis.
  - Two important considerations when determining whether hemodialysis is necessary
    - First concern is the presence of toxic metabolites such as formate. Although these metabolites cannot easily be measured directly, the presence of a metabolic acidosis suggests that some of the parent compound has already been metabolized to a toxic metabolite, and dialysis should be employed.

○ Second consideration is the duration of time needed to eliminate the toxic alcohol without dialysis.
  – Half-life of methanol is approximately 2 days when ADH is inhibited.
  – If the initial serum concentration is 200 mg/dL, about 6 days in an ICU may be necessary to reach a concentration of 25 mg/dL.
  – In contrast, if dialysis were performed, the patient may require only a day of hospitalization, depending on the reason for ingestion of the alcohol.
• Two ADH inhibitors available are fomepizole and ethanol.
  ○ Though more expensive, fomepizole is the treatment of choice.
  – Fomepizole is administered by empiric weight-based dosing, whereas ethanol infusion requires serum concentrations to be obtained frequently.
  – Fomepizole does not cause CNS or respiratory depression.
  – Fomepizole is given as a 15 mg/kg IV loading dose, followed in 12 hours by 10 mg/kg every 12 hours for 48 hours.
  – If continued dosing is required, the infusion rate should be increased to 15 mg/kg.
  ○ When fomepizole is unavailable, ethanol should be given IV, or orally if necessary.
  ○ Loading dose of ethanol is 0.8 g/kg over 20 to 60 minutes, followed by an initial infusion of 100 mg/kg/hour.
  ○ The goal of ethanol therapy is to maintain an ADH inhibitory concentration of 100 mg/dL.
  ○ Serum ethanol concentration should be obtained frequently and the rate adjusted accordingly.
• Hemodialysis is performed for patients with concentrations of methanol >25 mg/dL or ethylene glycol >50 mg/dL when toxic metabolites are shown to be present (indicated by metabolic acidosis), or when ADH inhibition alone would require an unreasonable amount of time.
  ○ ADH blockade should continue during hemodialysis; fomepizole should be dosed every 4 hours; and ethanol should be administered at a rate of 250 to 350 mg/kg/hour.
  ○ Several hemodialysis sessions may be needed to remove the toxic alcohol, depending on the initial concentration.
  ○ Symptoms of isopropanol can usually be managed with fluids and supportive care alone, although rarely, hemodialysis may be indicated.
• Folate is a cofactor in the conversion of formic acid to a nontoxic metabolite, and thiamine and pyridoxine assist in transforming toxic metabolites after ethylene glycol poisoning.
  ○ Therefore, 1 to 2 mg/kg of folic acid given every 4 to 6 hours in the first 24 hours of methanol poisoning
  ○ Thiamine hydrochloride (100 mg IM or IV) and pyridoxine (100 mg/day IV) administered for ethylene glycol poisoning
• Reasonable to administer sodium bicarbonate to a target pH of 7.2 to shift the equilibrium from formic acid to the less toxic formate

CHOLINERGIC COMPOUNDS

Mechanism of Toxicity

• Acetylcholine is the neurotransmitter found throughout the parasympathetic nervous system, in the sympathetic nervous system at the level of the ganglia and sweat glands, and at the neuromuscular junction (Fig. 30.3).

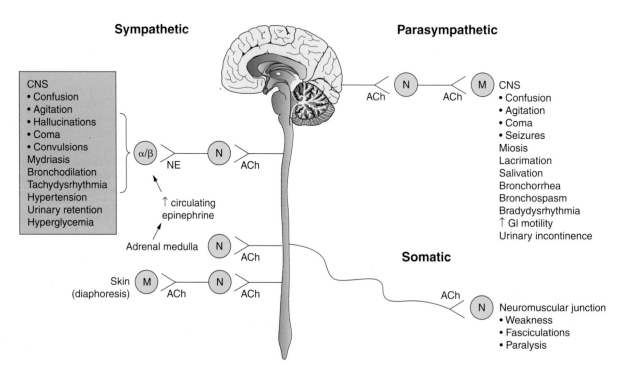

FIGURE 30.3. Sympathetic and parasympathetic nervous system. (Adapted with permission from Clark RF. Insecticides: organic phosphorous compounds and carbamates. In: Flomenbaum NE, Goldfrank LR, Hoffman RS, et al., eds. *Goldfrank's Toxicologic Emergencies.* 8th ed. New York: McGraw-Hill; 2006:1447–1459.)

- *Cholinergic syndrome* describes the condition of excess acetylcholine characterized by the sum of the parasympathetic, somatic, and sympathetic effects.
- Cholinergic compounds are used as medications, pesticides, and weapons.
- In 2005, the AAPCC received reports of 10 fatalities and 62 major effects related to organophosphate and carbamate insecticides.
  - World Health Organization estimates at least 1 million unintentional poisonings and 2 million suicide attempts annually worldwide from these insecticides.
- Acetylcholine is inactivated in the synapse by acetylcholinesterase (AChE).
  - Inhibition of AChE causes an excess of the neurotransmitter in the synapse.
  - Two most important classes of AChE inhibitors
    - The carbamates—inactivate AChE by carbamylation
    - The organic phosphorous compounds—inactivate AChE by phosphorylation
    - Carbamates and organic phosphorous compounds both are absorbed by ingestion, by inhalation, and through skin.
  - Some generalizations can be made about the two classes.
    - Organic phosphorous compounds have a greater delay to onset of action.
      ○ After ingestion, peak concentrations reported at 6 hours
      ○ Many organic phosphorous agents activated in the liver
        – Resulting in a further delay to peak action
    - Many of the carbamates have peak concentrations within 40 minutes of ingestion.
    - Organic phosphorous compounds are generally very lipophilic.
      ○ Redistribution from fat allows measurable serum concentrations for up to 48 days.
      ○ Carbamates may be almost completely eliminated within days.
    - Organic phosphorous compounds exhibit peripheral and CNS effects, whereas the carbamates do not readily cross into the CNS.
    - Most important
      ○ Organic phosphorous compounds exhibit "aging" whereby the reversible inhibition of AChE becomes permanent.
        – Aging can take minutes to days, depending on the particular compound.
      ○ Carbamates, in contrast, spontaneously hydrolyze from the active site of AChE and do not age.
- ICU admission is required for those with respiratory compromise, hemodynamic instability, or the need for administration of large amounts of atropine.

Clinical Manifestations

- Diagnosis is often established by recognition of the muscarinic signs.
  - Includes salivation, lacrimation, urination, defecation, bradycardia, bronchorrhea, and bronchospasm
  - Acetylcholine initially acts as an agonist.
    - In excess, acetylcholine becomes an antagonist at the neuromuscular junction, producing weakness, fasciculations, and paralysis.
    - Simulation of nicotinic receptors at the sympathetic ganglia produces tachycardia and mydriasis.

Management

- The first management priorities involve the following:
  - Securing the airway when necessary
  - Decontaminating the patient's skin to protect caregivers and prevent further absorption
  - After initial stabilization, administering atropine
    - Tachycardia is not a contraindication to atropine.
    - The goal is reversal of the muscarinic symptoms.
    - Titrate to effect the resolution of bronchospasm and bronchorrhea.
    - The initial dose of 1 mg IV atropine (0.05 mg/kg in children) can be doubled every 2 minutes until muscarinic signs are controlled.
    - There is variation in amount of atropine required, ranging from one to hundreds of milligrams.
- If CNS anticholinergic toxicity develops prior to resolution of peripheral muscarinic signs
  - The peripherally acting antimuscarinic agent, glycopyrrolate, may be given.
  - Initial dose is 1 mg IV and then titrate to symptomatic relief.
  - A common clinical pitfall is to interpret froth from the patient's mouth as a sign of cardiogenic pulmonary edema and respond with fluid restriction.
    - On the contrary, cholinergic-poisoned patients have large volume losses from diaphoresis and bronchorrhea.
- Oximes are used to supplement antimuscarinic therapy.
  - Improve both muscarinic and nicotinic signs, primarily by restoring activity to phosphorylated AChE
  - Will not restore activity once aging has occurred, so must be administered early
  - Recommended for both organic phosphorous compounds and carbamates because oximes may have salutary effects after carbamate poisoning and because the toxic agent in question is not always known with certainty
  - Even in carbaryl poisoning, adequate atropinization overcomes any deleterious effect of pralidoxime.
    - Pralidoxime (2-PAM) is the oxime most frequently available in the United States.
    - Administer 1 to 2 g IV over 30 minutes (20–40 mg/kg in children, to a maximum of 2 g).
    - Significant poisoning may require a continuous infusion of 500 mg/hour (10–20 mg/kg/hour in children, up to adult dose).
- Diazepam should be administered to patients severely poisoned by organic phosphorous compounds.
  - Although human data are not available, animal studies show a survival benefit possibly unrelated to the GABAergic effects of diazepam.
  - Severely poisoned patients will require endotracheal intubation.

Diagnostic Studies

- AChE inhibitor poisoning is a clinical diagnosis.
  - RBC cholinesterase and butyrylcholinesterase are inhibited by carbamates and organic phosphorous compounds.
    - Activity may remain depressed after clinical signs and symptoms have resolved.
    - These tests may have a clinical role in mild cases when the diagnosis is unclear.

- Electromyography may be a sensitive indicator of toxicity before clinically apparent symptoms have occurred.

Delayed Manifestations

- In the acute setting, the physician should be vigilant for recurrence of cholinergic signs after apparent resolution and for a distinct form of toxicity called the *intermediate syndrome*.
- *Intermediate syndrome*
  - Syndrome is so named because it occurs after acute, but before delayed, toxicity that may occur 24 to 96 hours after organic phosphorous poisoning.
  - The syndrome consists of upper-body weakness, cranial nerve palsies, and areflexia.
  - Syndrome appears to be self-limited but can last up to 30 days and be severe enough to require intubation.
  - Continue pralidoxime infusion at 500 mg/hour when this diagnosis is considered.
  - Organic phosphorous compounds are very lipophilic; redistribution from fat stores may result, causing delayed toxicity days after apparent resolution.
  - Considered discharge when the patient has been asymptomatic without additional treatment for 1 to 2 days.

CYANIDE

Mechanism

- Cyanide salts are widely available and may be used in suicidal or homicidal poisoning.
  - Jewelers, laboratory workers, and industrial workers have ready access to cyanide.
    - Relationship to these industries may be an important historical clue.
    - Cyanide poisoning should also be considered in all fire victims.
      - Cyanide is released when certain synthetic and natural fibers undergo combustion.
- Cyanide poisoning most frequently occurs after the ingestion of a cyanide salt or inhalation of the gas hydrogen cyanide.
  - In both forms, cyanide is rapidly absorbed.
  - Most important toxic effect of cyanide is inhibition of cytochrome oxidase of the electron transport chain.
    - Despite the presence of oxygen, cells cannot offload electrons from nicotinamide adenine dinucleotide (NADH) to oxygen, and generate ATP, resulting in anaerobic metabolism and producing lactic acid.
  - Small quantities of cyanide are detoxified by the enzyme, rhodanese.
    - Rhodanese catalyzes the transfer of sulfur from thiosulfate, yielding thiocyanate.
    - Poisoning results when this system is overwhelmed by large concentrations of cyanide.

Clinical Manifestations

- History may be very helpful in establishing diagnosis.
- Cyanide poisoning should be considered in anyone who rapidly loses consciousness after ingestion or inhalational exposure.

- Signs and symptoms resemble those of hypoxia, with no cyanosis.
  - Headache
  - Lethargy
  - Seizures
  - Coma

Management of Cyanide Poisoning

- Requires treatment before laboratory confirmation is available
- As soon as considered
  - 100% oxygen should be administered.
  - IV access should be established.
  - Fluids should be given.
  - Remainder of treatment depends on the route of exposure.
    - Symptoms of cyanide poisoning are similar to those associated with hypovolemia or carbon monoxide poisoning.
    - Diagnosis is difficult to establish with certainty.
    - Laboratory studies will show a lactic acidosis.
      - Plasma lactate concentration >8 mMol/L in patients with clinical suspicion of poisoning was 94% sensitive and 70% specific for cyanide toxicity.
    - The cyanide antidote kit consists of amyl nitrite, sodium nitrite, and sodium thiosulfate.
      - Nitrites derive their efficacy by generating methemoglobin, which has a greater affinity for cyanide than cytochrome oxidase.
        - If reduced oxygen-carrying capacity suspected (due to anemia or carboxyhemoglobinemia), omit nitrites.
        - Avoid nitrites in patients after smoke inhalation.
          - Such individuals may not tolerate further compromise in their oxygen distribution associated with an increase in methemoglobin.
        - Amyl nitrite is a volatile liquid.
          - Ampule encasing is broken and held in front of the patient's mouth for 15-second intervals with 15-second breaks.
        - Once IV access is established, sodium nitrite can replace the amyl nitrite.
          - Sodium nitrite is administered 10 mL IV in adults (0.2 mL/kg in children).
          - In 2 hours, the dose can be repeated at half the initial dose.
          - A methemoglobin concentration should be obtained 30 minutes after nitrite administration: target concentration of 20% to 30%.
        - Sodium thiosulfate, the final component of the kit, functions by providing substrate to rhodanese, facilitating conversion of cyanide to thiocyanate.
        - Dose is 50 mL in adults and 1.65 mL/kg in children.
        - Drug may be repeated in 2 hours at half the initial dose if symptoms persist.
        - Hydroxocobalamin
          - Available in the United States shortly
          - Combines with cyanide to form cyanocobalamin (vitamin B_{12})
          - Synergistic with thiosulfate
          - Hydroxocobalamin should be given IV at 70 mg/kg (to a maximum of 5 g) in a separate infusion site from thiosulfate.

CYANIDE, THIOCYANATE, AND NITROPRUSSIDE

- Nitroprusside contains an iron molecule coordinated to five cyanide molecules and one molecule of nitric oxide.
  - Cyanide molecules slowly liberated after nitroprusside is infused
    - Usually at a rate that can be detoxified by endogenous pathways
  - Risk factors for accumulation of cyanide are:
    - Prolonged infusion
    - High infusion rate
    - Poor nourishment
  - If diagnosis suspected
    - Discontinue infusion.
    - Administer hydroxocobalamin and thiosulfate.
- More likely complication of nitroprusside use is thiocyanate toxicity.
  - Thiocyanate causes no symptoms at low concentrations.
  - Cleared renally
    - Bioaccumulation occurs in patients with impaired renal function.
  - Symptoms are as follows:
    - Delirium
    - Hallucinations
    - Seizures
    - Rash
  - Serum thiocyanate concentrations checked after 48 to 72 hours of infusion in the following:
    - Patients receiving >2 μg/kg/minute nitroprusside
    - Those with renal insufficiency
    - Discontinue infusion if thiocyanate concentration is >10 mg/dL.
    - Dialysis effective for thiocyanate accumulation.
      - Reserve for the most severely compromised patients.

METHEMOGLOBIN

Mechanism

- Results from the formation of "dyshemoglobin"
  - Caused by inappropriate oxidation of heme iron
  - Normally, iron in deoxyhemoglobin remains in the reduced ferrous state: Fe^{2+}.
    - Heme is available to bind oxygen.
    - After oxygen binds, iron assumes the oxidized ferric state: Fe^{3+}.
  - Methemoglobin is formed normally in small quantities when hemoglobin iron moiety is exposed to oxidative stress.
    - Methemoglobin is converted to the ferric state in the absence of binding oxygen.
    - It is unable to bind oxygen and increases the affinity of normal hemoglobin for oxygen.
    - Result of methemoglobin formation is as follows:
      - Decreased oxygen delivery
      - Leftward shift in the oxygen dissociation curve
      - Low-level methemoglobin production may be a protective mechanism against oxidant damage to erythrocytes.
      - Major mechanism of methemoglobin reduction is catalyzed by enzyme, methemoglobin reductase

(cytochrome b_5 reductase), using NADH generated from the Embden-Meyerhof glycolytic pathway.
- Congenital methemoglobinemia
  - Rare condition caused by methemoglobin reductase deficiency
  - Enzyme also relatively deficient until approximately 4 months, making infants prone to methemoglobin formation
- Most individuals with methemoglobinemia treated and discharged from ED
  - May require ICU admission when it recurs after initial treatment
    - Either from continued absorption of an inducer or
    - Continued metabolism of a drug to a methemoglobin inducer

Clinical Manifestations

- Diagnosis commonly confirmed by co-oximetry
  - May be established presumptively based on symptoms and signs and via pulse oximetry
  - Symptoms of methemoglobinemia those associated with hypoxia
    - Severity of symptoms determined by concentration of methemoglobin and the patient's underlying comorbidities
      - At low concentrations (0%–15%), patients may be asymptomatic.
      - At moderate concentrations (20%–50%), patients may manifest decreased exercise tolerance and dyspnea.
      - At high concentrations (50%–70%), metabolic acidosis, seizures, and coma result.
      - Concentrations greater than 60% or 70% can cause death in previously healthy individuals.
  - Cyanosis, an important physical examination finding, occurs when methemoglobin concentration is 1.5 g/dL.
    - This corresponds to a concentration of 10% in an individual with a total hemoglobin concentration of 15 g/dL.
    - In contrast, 5 g/dL of deoxyhemoglobin is required to produce cyanosis, corresponding to an oxygen saturation of 66% in the same patient.
      - Thus, patients who are cyanotic from methemoglobinemia will not appear as ill as those who are cyanotic from impaired oxygenation.
  - Pulse oximetry aids in diagnosis before co-oximetry has been obtained.
    - Methemoglobin interferes with pulse oximetry somewhat predictably.
    - Pulse oximetry reads absorbance of light at 660 nm and 940 nm, so chosen because they are the best to distinguish the absorption spectra of oxyhemoglobin and deoxyhemoglobin.
    - Based on the ratio of absorption between the two wavelengths, the pulse oximeter uses an algorithm to estimate the percentage of total hemoglobin as oxyhemoglobin.
    - Methemoglobin has greater absorption than either oxyhemoglobin or deoxyhemoglobin at those wavelengths.
    - When present in modest concentrations, the pulse oximeter will no longer be able to meaningfully calculate oxygen saturation.
    - In the clinical setting, methemoglobin does consistently generate readings between 70% and 90%.

- SaO_2 derived from arterial blood gas analysis is not measured in the same fashion as SpO_2, and will not reflect the methemoglobin concentration.
  - SaO_2 is a calculated saturation based on the pO_2 and should be normal in the setting of methemoglobinemia.
    - Difference between the SpO_2 and SaO_2 may suggest methemoglobinemia.

Methemoglobin Inducers

- Acquired methemoglobinemia is most frequently seen after drug exposure.
  - It can also be found in infants without drug exposure who are ill with a metabolic acidosis or diarrhea.
  - Drugs associated with methemoglobin formation are extensive.
  - Dapsone, nitrites, nitrates, benzocaine, and sulfonamides are consistently implicated in producing methemoglobinemia (Table 30.5).

TABLE 30.5

COMMON ETIOLOGIES OF METHEMOGLOBINEMIA

Hereditary
Hemoglobin M
Cytochrome b_5 reductase deficiency

Acquired: medications
Amyl nitrate
Benzocaine
Dapsone
Lidocaine
Nitric oxide
Nitroglycerin
Phenacetin
Phenazopyridine
Prilocaine
Quinones
Sulfonamides

Acquired: other xenobiotics
Aniline dye derivatives
Butyl nitrite
Chlorobenzene
Fire
Food adulterated with nitrites
Food high in nitrates
Isobutyl nitrite
Naphthalene
Nitrate
Nitrite
Nitrophenol
Nitrous gases
Silver nitrate
Trinitrotoluene
Well water (nitrates)

Pediatric
Reduced nicotinamide adenine dinucleotide (NADH)
 methemoglobin reductase activity in infants (<4 mo)
In association with low birth weight, prematurity,
 dehydration, acidosis, diarrhea, and hyperchloremia

Adapted with permission from Price D. Methemoglobin inducers. In: Flomenbaum NE, Goldfrank LR, Hoffman RS, et al., eds. *Goldfrank's Toxicologic Emergencies.* 8th ed. New York: McGraw-Hill; 2006:1734–1745.

- It is not entirely clear why some individuals develop methemoglobinemia after exposure to these drugs and others do not.
  - There is clearly a dose-response effect, and host factors such as coexisting medical illness and metabolic variables play a role in methemoglobin development.

Management of Methemoglobinemia

- When cyanosis is recognized and methemoglobinemia is considered
- Administer 100% oxygen by nonrebreather mask.
- Unless patient is asymptomatic, methylene blue should be administered IV, 1 to 2 mg/kg over 5 minutes.
  - Methylene is reduced by nicotinamide adenine dinucleotide phosphate to leukomethylene blue.
  - Leukomethylene blue, in turn, reduces methemoglobin to hemoglobin.
  - Clinical improvement is seen within minutes of administration.
  - Because the medication itself has a blue color, SpO_2 may transiently worsen.
  - Repeat dose of methylene blue may be required if the methemoglobin concentration is high or if there is ongoing oxidative stress.
- Some recommend against giving methylene blue, an oxidizing agent, to individuals with glucose-6-phosphate dehydrogenase (G6PD) deficiency.
  - Patients with this condition suffer from hemolytic anemia when exposed to drugs that create oxidative stress.
  - Because G6PD is required to activate methylene blue, a deficiency in the enzyme may lead to a lack of efficacy of the antidote.
  - Administration of methylene blue is appropriate when clinically indicated unless there is a strong history of G6PD deficiency.
    - In these cases, hyperbaric oxygen or exchange transfusion should be considered.
    - If the G6PD-deficient patient presents with severe methemoglobinemia, methylene blue should be administered and the patient monitored closely for hemolysis.

Dapsone-induced Methemoglobinemia

- Both dapsone and its hydroxylamine metabolites are responsible for methemoglobin formation.
  - Cytochrome P450 conversion of dapsone to these metabolites inhibited by cimetidine
  - Cimetidine administered IV, 300 mg every 6 hours, to these patients

CARBON MONOXIDE

Mechanism

- The AAPCC received more than 16,000 reports of carbon monoxide (CO) exposure, including 176 major effects and 66 fatalities.
- These figures underestimate morbidity and mortality from carbon monoxide, considered the leading cause of poisoning death in the United States.

- CO is as follows:
  - Hemotoxin
  - Neurotoxin
  - Cardiac toxin
  - Inhibitor of cytochrome oxidase
- CO binds to hemoglobin with greater affinity than does oxygen and causes a leftward shift of the oxyhemoglobin dissociation curve.
  - This causes a decrease in the delivery of oxygen to cells.
  - Although the formation of carboxyhemoglobin can impair oxygen delivery sufficiently to cause mortality, inhibition of oxygen delivery does not fully explain why carboxyhemoglobin concentrations of 50% are often fatal whereas a similar degree of anemia might be well tolerated.
  - Formation of carboxyhemoglobin is inadequate to explain the chronic cardiac and neurologic sequelae of CO.
    - CO inhibition of cytochrome oxidase persists for days after carboxyhemoglobin concentration has normalized
    - CO is associated with damage to the brain endothelium, resulting in lipid peroxidation.
    - CO also binds to myoglobin with high affinity, making it a direct skeletal and cardiac muscle toxin.
- CO results from the incomplete combustion of carbonaceous fuels.
  - It is tasteless, odorless, and colorless.
  - Initial clue to the presence of CO in the home may be the alarm from a CO detector.
  - Methylene chloride, an important source of CO that is not a product of combustion, is hepatically metabolized to CO by the liver.
    - Methylene chloride is used as a paint stripper and can be absorbed dermally, inhalationally, or by ingestion.
    - Unlike other sources of CO poisoning, where carboxyhemoglobin begins to decline as soon as the patient is removed from the exposure, peak carboxyhemoglobin concentration will occur hours after exposure to methylene chloride as the parent compound is metabolized to CO.
- CO poisoning does not usually require ICU admission.
  - ICU admission necessary only for the following:
    - patients who are comatose or obtunded
    - patients with signs of cardiotoxicity
    - patients with significant burns or other comorbidities

Clinical Manifestations

- Initially complaints are of headache, nausea, and dizziness.
  - CO poisoning may be misdiagnosed as a viral illness.
  - Diagnosis should be considered when more than one person in a home presents with the same symptoms.
- Alteration in mental status, coma, seizures, and syncope are signs of severe poisoning.
  - Indicators of tissue hypoxia, such as tachypnea, tachycardia, and ECG changes, may be seen.
  - CO can cause dysrhythmias or an acute myocardial infarction (MI).
- Intensity of signs and symptoms is related to duration and severity of exposure and comorbid conditions.

- Pulse oximetry will interpret carboxyhemoglobin as hemoglobin: SpO_2 will be falsely normal.
- Diagnosis of CO poisoning
  - Aided by obtaining the carboxyhemoglobin concentration, which can be taken from either a venous or arterial sample
  - Normal carboxyhemoglobin concentration less than 5%
    - In smokers, may be up to 10%
  - Carboxyhemoglobin concentrations are an indicator of exposure but do not correlate with degree of toxicity.
    - With delay from exposure to measurement of carboxyhemoglobin, the concentration loses further value as a clinical tool.
    - More likely if the patient has been receiving supplemental oxygen, which decreases the half-life of carboxyhemoglobin the level will have decreased.

Chronic Sequelae

- For survivors of an acute CO exposure, there may be significant chronic neurologic and cardiovascular effects.
  - Delayed neurologic sequelae follow the resolution of initial symptoms.
    - Sometimes days to weeks later
    - Include dementia, movement disorders, and memory impairment

Diagnostic Studies

- In patients with chest pain, shortness of breath, palpitations, or neurologic deficits indicating severe exposure
- ECG should be performed.
- Serum cardiac markers should be obtained.
- Pregnancy status should be determined in women of childbearing age.
- Elevated serum cardiac markers during moderate and severe acute toxicity predict long-term mortality.
  - Pathophysiology of chronic cardiovascular effects of carbon monoxide poisoning probably involves CO poisoning of cardiac myoglobin but needs further study.
- Within 12 hours of exposure, loss of consciousness occurs, and changes on a computed tomography (CT) scan of the brain may be seen.
  - Findings include the following:
    - Symmetric, low-density changes in the globus pallidus, putamen, and caudate nuclei
    - Normal CT scan a good prognostic indicator
      - A negative CT within 1 week of admission associated with good outcome

Management

- When diagnosis is considered, administer 100% oxygen.
- Obtain carboxyhemoglobin concentration.
- Without supplemental oxygen, the half-life of carboxyhemoglobin in blood is 4 to 6 hours.
- With oxygen, it ranges from 1 to 2 hours.
- Most important decision is whether to administer hyperbaric oxygen (HBO).
  - HBO decreases the half-life of carbon monoxide even more rapidly than 100% normobaric oxygen, but this is not clinically important.

- Value of HBO is its potential to decrease morbidity, not mortality.
  - Specifically, HBO may reduce delayed neurologic sequelae by preventing brain lipid peroxidation and regenerating CNS cytochrome oxidase after CO exposure.
- The use of HBO for CO poisoning is controversial.
  - Large randomized clinical trials report mixed results.
  - All of the trials conducted to date have limitations, and the ideal trial may never be performed because of the ethical concerns of randomizing patients to nonhyperbaric therapy.
  - In light of the demonstrable benefit of HBO and the relative safety of the therapy, we recommend HBO in patients with moderate to severe poisoning as early as safely possible.
    - Delay greater than 6 hours may associated with worse outcome.
  - Indications for HBO are as follows:
    - Ayncope, coma, seizure, or any other hard neurologic findings
    - Signs of cardiac ischemia or dysrhythmias
    - Carboxyhemoglobin >20%

Pregnancy and Carbon Monoxide

- Because fetal circulation relies on maternal oxyhemoglobin for oxygenation, any disturbance in maternal oxygen delivery will be magnified in the fetus.
  - Fetal hemoglobin has less affinity for CO than adult hemoglobin, but there is a high incidence of fetal CNS damage and spontaneous abortion after severe maternal poisoning.
  - Pregnant women with lesser exposures have normal pregnancies and deliver healthy children.
  - All prospective trials of HBO have excluded pregnant women, but we recommend treating these patients similarly to those who are not pregnant.

CAUSTICS

Mechanism

- Chemicals that produce damage during contact with tissues
- Generally acid or alkali
- Commercially available as toilet bowl cleaners, drain cleaners, and other products
  - Commonly encountered alkalis include the following:
    - Ammonium hydroxide (ammonia)
    - Sodium hydroxide (lye, found in drain cleaners)
    - Hydrochloric acid and sulfuric acid, which are both used as drain cleaners, with the latter used in automobile batteries as well
- Alkali drain cleaners accounted for more than 3,677 reported exposures in 2005, more than any other caustic chemical. Of these, 46 were major and 5 fatal.
- Damage caused by caustics is determined by pH, quantity, duration of contact, and the titratable alkaline (or acid) reserve.
  - Ingested caustics can potentially produce damage to the oropharynx, esophagus, stomach, and respiratory tract.

- Acid and alkali produce different injuries.
  - Alkaline exposure produces dissociated OH^- ion, resulting in fat saponification, membrane dissolution, and cell death—a process known as liquefactive necrosis.
  - Acid exposure releases H^+ ions, producing an eschar and desiccation, a process referred to as *coagulation necrosis*.
  - Both acid and alkali produce stomach and esophageal injury.
- Esophageal burns can be described by a commonly used classification system.
  - Grade I burns demonstrate hyperemia without ulceration.
  - Grade II burns demonstrate ulcers but do not damage periesophageal tissues.
    - Grade II lesions are subdivided into IIa (noncircumferential) and IIb (circumferential) lesions.
  - Grade III describes burns with deep ulceration and damage to surrounding tissues.
  - Classification of the burn predicts chronic sequelae.
    - Grade IIb and III injuries may heal with strictures and dysphagia and may perforate.
    - When esophageal perforation is suspected, or when there is airway injury, patients are admitted to the ICU.

Clinical Manifestations

- Lack of oral burns does not exclude significant esophageal injury.
  - Presence of oral lesions does not guarantee visceral burns.
- Physical examination after caustic ingestion can be deceiving.
  - Visceral burns present in 37.5% of patients without oral burns and 50% of patients with oral burns.
  - Drooling, odynophagia, and abdominal pain are common findings after significant caustic exposure.
  - Abdominal pain or tenderness occur in fewer than half of patients with gastric injury.
  - Pulmonary aspiration may lead to coughing and respiratory distress.
  - Absorption of acid from the stomach may cause acidemia after ingestion.
  - Alkalis are not systemically absorbed in consequential amounts.
  - Metabolic acidosis may be present if significant injury has occurred.

Management

- Endoscopy should be performed in all adult patients presumed to have significant exposures to establish the severity of the burn.
  - If endoscopy is normal, the patient can be safely discharged.
  - Patients with severe injury are rapidly stabilized and referred for surgical care before their condition worsens.
  - Endoscopy should be performed as early as possible, ideally within 12 hours.
    - Wound strength is weakest between 5 days and 2 weeks after ingestion, when the perforation risk is greatest.
- Exception to universal endoscopy may be a subset of pediatric exposures.

- No serious esophageal injuries are found in patients who lacked stridor or the combination of vomiting and drooling.
- Presence of endoscopic evidence of perforation mandates immediate surgery.
  - Other indications for operative repair include the following:
    - Pleural effusions
    - Ascites
    - Serum pH <7.2
- With grade I injury, the patient can be started on a soft diet and the diet advanced as tolerated.
- Presence of grade II esophageal burns with gastric sparing warrants placement of a nasogastric tube under direct visualization.
- More severe injury may require parenteral nutrition or a jejeunostomy.
- Silicone rubber esophageal stents have been used to prevent stricture.
- Administer antibiotics that cover anaerobic bacteria and gram-positive and gram-negative aerobic organisms when perforation considered.
  - Piperacillin/tazobactam are appropriate choices as are levofloxacin and clindamycin.
  - Corticosteroids are recommended to help prevent scarring and stricture formation in grade II lesions.
    - Most recent meta-analysis could not find a benefit for the administration of corticosteroids following exposure to caustics.

HYDROFLUORIC ACID

Mechanism

- Hydrofluoric acid (HF), a weak acid, has no important tissue-corrosive properties.
  - HF dissolves metal oxides and glass, making it useful in rust removal and glass etching.
  - HF is stored in plastic, not glass.
- HF is an important dermal, ophthalmic, pulmonary, and systemic toxin.
  - HF penetrates deeply into tissues before dissociating into protons and fluoride ions.
  - Protons cause some damage.
  - Most important toxic effects result from fluoride ions binding the divalent cations calcium and magnesium.
    - This leads to neuropathic pain and cell death.
- HF ingestions and exposures resulting in electrolyte abnormalities require ICU admission.

Clinical Manifestations

- Clinical syndrome distinct from the caustic agents and requires specific therapy.
  - In small dermal exposures, HF produces severe pain with limited dermal findings.
  - Large exposures by any route, including dermal, can produce severe hypocalcemia and death.
- Most unintentional HF exposures are dermal.

- Severity of HF exposure is determined by the duration of exposure, concentration, and extent of surface area exposed.
  - Low fluoride concentration solutions may cause severe pain beginning hours after the exposure.
    - Physical examination is unremarkable.
    - Area that appears normal or merely mildly erythematous may be extremely painful.
  - High-concentration industrial preparations may cause immediate pain, with hyperemia and ulceration.
  - Ophthalmic exposures result in pain, chemosis, and damage to conjunctiva and corneal epithelium.
- Most consequential effects of HF poisoning are systemic.
  - Dermal exposures to concentrated HF covering only 2.5% body surface area have resulted in systemic toxicity.
  - Typical fatal dermal exposures are larger.
  - Lengthening of the QRS and QT intervals or presence of peaked T-waves may be early indicators of toxicity.
    - Proximal cause of death is usually dysrhythmias; ventricular fibrillation and sudden cardiac arrest are described.

Management

- Most important concern in small dermal injuries is pain control.
- Mainstay of therapy is calcium gluconate.
  - Derives its efficacy from binding fluoride ions.
  - Calcium chloride should be used only topically, as extravasation causes tissue damage.
  - Analgesics and regional anesthesia are not contraindicated.
    - Calcium has the advantage of halting tissue damage in addition to providing pain relief.
  - After decontamination with water, calcium gluconate gel should be applied to the injured area.
    - If hands involved, gel can be held in contact by placing it in a sterile glove and putting the glove on the hand.
    - Gel is prepared by mixing 25 mL of 10% calcium gluconate in 75 mL of water-based lubricant.
    - If wound is located where compartment syndrome is not a concern, 0.5% calcium gluconate can be injected intradermally, 0.5 mL/cm^2.
  - If these techniques fail to give relief
    - There is a role for careful use of intra-arterial calcium gluconate.
    - Obvious advantage of this route is that calcium can be administered directly and by continuous infusion to affected area.
      - Add 10 mL of 10% calcium chloride to 40 mL of 0.9% sodium chloride and infuse over 4 hours.
- Nasogastric tube should be carefully placed, and any material in the stomach should be aspirated and followed by instillation of a calcium solution.
  - Benefits of this practice are not established, but it seems reasonable.
- IV calcium and magnesium should be given liberally, and electrolytes should be obtained hourly.
  - One gram calcium gluconate contains 4.5 mEq of elemental calcium.
  - One gram calcium chloride contains 13.6 mEq.
    - Both calcium salts can produce vasodilation and dysrhythmias when administered too quickly.

- ○ IV calcium should be administered no faster than 0.7 to 1.8 mEq/minute.
- ○ Dysrhythmias should be expected in severely poisoned patients.
- ○ Place defibrillator pads on the patient and perform continuous cardiac monitoring.
- ○ In animal models, quinidine was protective after lethal doses of IV fluoride.
- ○ When systemic toxicity occurs, electrolyte abnormalities are most severe in the first several hours of toxicity.
  - – If no signs or symptoms of systemic toxicity for 24 hours, transfer to lower level of care.

ANTIDIABETIC AGENTS

Mechanism

- Diabetes is characterized by an inability to maintain normal blood glucose concentration due to deficiency of insulin, resistance to insulin, or a combination of both.
- Medications used to treat diabetes are collectively known as *antidiabetic agents*.
- Subset of these drugs is properly called *hypoglycemic agents*.
  - Hypoglycemics include insulin and those drugs that promote the release of endogenous insulin.
  - Hypoglycemic agents and antidiabetic agents are not synonymous, because many diabetic medications (metformin, thiazolidinediones) cannot produce hypoglycemia.
- In 2005, the AAPCC received reports of 8,695 exposures to sulfonylureas and biguanides, including 244 major exposures and 28 deaths.
- The antidiabetics are diverse, but there are some important generalizations.
  - Sulfonylureas, meglitinides, and thiazolidinediones are very highly protein-bound and thus not amenable to extracorporeal removal.
  - Insulin and metformin are completely renally eliminated.
    - Most of the sulfonylureas have active hepatic metabolites with urinary excretion of both active metabolites and the parent drug.
- Most important pharmacokinetic parameter of the hypoglycemics is duration of action.
  - Duration of action of insulin and the sulfonylureas is greatly increased in overdose.
  - In overdose, the formation of depots of the drug in tissues can slow release and greatly prolong the duration of action.
    - ○ Vascularity of the site of injection will also influence the duration of hypoglycemia.
    - ○ Sulfonylureas generally have a duration of action of 12 to 24 hours in therapeutic doses.
      - – Chlorpropamide, a first-generation sulfonylurea, may promote insulin release for up to 72 hours.
      - – Duration of action is prolonged in overdose, resulting in delayed hypoglycemia.
      - – Meglitinides, intended to prevent postprandial hyperglycemia, induce insulin release for only 1 to 4 hours.
        - Appears likely that duration of action would be increased in overdose.

Clinical Manifestations

- Most important signs and symptoms of the aptly classified hypoglycemics are manifestations of decreased serum glucose.
- Diagnosis of hypoglycemia is established by interpreting a serum glucose concentration in the context of a patient's clinical status.
  - Threshold for symptoms of hypoglycemia ranges between 78 mg/dL in poorly controlled diabetics and 53 mg/dL in nondiabetics.
- Manifestations of hypoglycemia can be classified as either autonomic or neuroglycopenic.
  - Autonomic symptoms include tremor, diaphoresis, hunger, and nausea.
  - Neuroglycopenic features of hypoglycemia can manifest as almost any conceivable neurologic deficit, including the following:
    - ○ Coma
    - ○ Agitation
    - ○ Seizure
    - ○ Hemiplegia
    - ○ Mild confusion
    - ○ Autonomic symptoms, which precede neuroglycopenic symptoms, serving as a warning of hypoglycemia
      - – Autonomic symptoms may be blunted or absent in diabetics or patients taking β-adrenergic antagonists.
- Less clinically important—electrolyte abnormalities
  - Hypokalemia
  - Hypomagnesemia
  - Hypophosphatemia
  - Reported more frequently in very large insulin overdoses
- Metformin does not produce hypoglycemia itself but is often formulated with drugs that do, such as glipizide or glyburide.
  - Metformin and its biguanide predecessor, phenformin, are associated with lactic acidosis by promoting anaerobic metabolism and inhibit lactate metabolism.
  - Lactic acidosis is rare but is more likely in the setting of liver disease, renal insufficiency, heart failure, other acute illness, or acute overdose.
  - Hepatotoxicity is reported from therapeutic use of thiazolidinediones and acarbose.

Management

- Rapid bedside serum glucose concentration is obtained when hypoglycemia considered.
  - If diagnosis is established, 1 g/kg IV dextrose should be given.
  - Children should receive 25% dextrose solution and infants 10% dextrose solution.
  - When normal mental status is restored, patient should be fed.
    - Each 50-mL vial of 50% dextrose supplies 100 kcal of short-lived simple carbohydrate.
    - A meal will supply hundreds of "sustained-release" kilocalories.
    - Glucagon should not be administered unless IV access is delayed and the patient cannot be fed.
      - ○ Glucagon will not be effective in patients with depleted glycogen stores.

- Recurrent insulin-induced hypoglycemia should be treated with a dextrose infusion.
  - 10% to 20% solution and titrate to maintain glucose in a normal range
  - 5% dextrose solution inappropriate for glucose maintenance
- Octreotide, a somatostatin analog, is indicated for hypoglycemia following sulfonylurea use.
  - It is given subcutaneously, 50 μg every 6 hours (4–5 μg/kg/day in divided doses in children).
  - Dextrose alone might not be sufficient to manage sulfonylurea-induced hypoglycemia.
    - This drug class potentiates endogenous β-islet cell insulin release, supplemental dextrose will induce more insulin release, with transient corrections and subsequent recurrence of hypoglycemia.
    - Octreotide inhibits the β-islet cell calcium channel, inhibiting sulfonylurea-induced insulin release.
      - No significant adverse effects result from short-term octreotide use.
      - Octreotide should be continued for 24 hours.
      - After octreotide is discontinued, the patient should be observed for 24 hours.
  - Limited data in the literature regarding meglitinide toxicity
    - Mechanism of action similar to the sulfonylureas, the meglitinides are shorter acting
    - Less likely to produce recurrent hypoglycemia but no data to support this assumption
- Metformin-associated lactic acidosis should be considered in the following:
  - Patients taking an overdose
  - Children exposed to more than one or two tablets
  - Patients who take metformin therapeutically and also have renal insufficiency, hepatic insufficiency, heart failure, or another acute illness
- Diagnosis is established by obtaining a serum chemistry, lactate concentration, and serum pH.
  - Primary therapy is supportive.
  - Role of bicarbonate in metformin-associated lactic acidosis is unclear; supplemental bicarbonate should be used to maintain the pH above 7.1.
  - Metformin is highly protein bound, but hemodialysis can be used to correct refractory acidosis.
- Adults and children should be observed for 24 hours, even in the absence of hypoglycemia.
- Patients who present with hypoglycemia from long-acting forms of insulin should be observed for 24 hours.

NATURAL TOXINS

Plants

- In 2005, 76 major outcomes resulting from plant exposure were reported to the AAPCC.

Belladonna Alkaloids

- Plants such as jimsonweed (*Datura stramonium*) contain numerous anticholinergic compounds.
  - These are used recreationally, often in the form of teas, for their hallucinatory effects.

- Toxicity is identified by the presence of anticholinergic symptoms: tachycardia; hyperthermia; dry, flushed skin; urinary retention; and agitation.
- One hundred jimsonweed seeds contain nearly 6 mg of atropine and similar alkaloids.
- In addition to supportive care, physostigmine can be given when the diagnosis is relatively certain, administered 1 to 2 mg IV slowly over 5 minutes.
  - Physostigmine should be discontinued and the diagnosis reconsidered if cholinergic symptoms develop.
  - If there is improvement or no change in the patient's condition, physostigmine can be readministered after a 10- or 15-minute delay.

Nicotine and Nicotinelike Alkaloids

- Nicotine poisoning occurs from inhaled, transdermal, and ingested nicotine.
- Dose of 1 mg/kg can be lethal in an adult.
- A cigarette contains 13 to 30 mg of nicotine, most not delivered to the smoker.
  - Largest portion of the nicotine is pyrolysed but not inhaled.
  - 5 to 7 mg of nicotine remains in the cigarette butt, a potentially lethal dose for a child.
- Workers handling tobacco can be poisoned from nicotine as well.
- Signs and symptoms of nicotine toxicity result from activation and then inhibition (from overstimulation) of nicotinic receptors:.
  - GI signs include nausea, vomiting, and diarrhea.
  - Early cardiovascular toxicity involves hypertension from nicotinic stimulation of the sympathetic ganglia, but hypotension eventually occurs.
  - Most important signs and symptoms result from nicotinic agonist effects at the neuromuscular junction. Early toxicity causes fasciculation, which gives way to paralysis.
- Management is supportive.
  - Vasoactive agents may be necessary to maintain blood pressure.
  - Intubation may be indicated to support respiration during paralysis.

Cicutoxin

- Cicutoxin is found in *Cicuta* spp. such as water hemlock.
  - Toxin is found throughout the plant, which is often eaten by adults who misidentify it as wild parsley, turnip, or parsnip.
  - Mechanism of cicutoxin poisoning is unclear.
  - Early symptoms are primarily GI and begin soon after ingestion.
  - Later, cicutoxin can cause status epilepticus, renal failure, and rhabdomyolysis.

Sodium Channel–altering Plants

- Aconitine, from *Aconitum* spp., opens sodium channels, increasing cellular excitability.
  - Increased sodium influx delays repolarization, which in turn delays conduction.
    - Slow conduction of peripheral nerves can lead to decreased sensation, weakness, paralysis; in the CNS, seizures.
    - Vagal and cardiac myocyte sodium channel effects lead to bradycardia, atrioventricular blockade, increased automaticity, or asystole.

- Aconitine is found in *Aconitum napellus* (monkshood) and Chinese herbal remedies.
- Management is supportive.
  - GI decontamination should be performed.
  - Cardiac complications have been successfully managed with ventricular assist device.

Mushrooms

- Forty-six major outcomes and six deaths from mushroom ingestions were reported to poison control centers in 2005.
  - Vast majority of mushroom exposures do not result in significant morbidity, and most of the fatalities that occur are caused by only a few of the many mushroom species in North America.
  - Identification of mushrooms is challenging and best left to the mycologist.
  - Each of the clinically important toxic mushrooms causes a distinct clinical syndrome that should be identified.
- **GI toxin–containing mushrooms:** Most reported exposures are to mushrooms containing gastrointestinal toxins.
  - Most notable clinical feature of ingestion of these mushrooms is the development of vomiting and diarrhea within several hours of ingestion.
  - Mushrooms that cause GI symptoms within 6 hours belong to this category and usually do not cause life-threatening symptoms.
    - Early onset of vomiting after exposure to GI toxin–containing mushrooms clinically differentiates them from the cyclopeptide-containing mushrooms.
  - Treatment of exposure to these mushrooms is supportive, and symptoms are generally self-limited.
  - These mushrooms rarely lead to toxicity requiring ICU admission.
- **Cyclopeptide-containing mushrooms:** Three of five fatalities from mushrooms in 2004 were related to cyclopeptide-containing mushrooms.
  - Mortality from these mushrooms is high.
  - Most prominent member of this group is *Amanita phalloides* and other *Amanita* spp.
    - *Amanita phalloides* contains numerous cyclopeptides.
    - Most important are a group called the amatoxins, which are heat-stable and present in lethal concentrations in mushrooms as small as 20 g.
  - *Clinical manifestations and management:* Amatoxins cause endocrine, renal, and CNS injury, but the hepatic effects are the most consequential.
    - Patients are asymptomatic for the first few hours after ingestion.
    - Within 5 to 24 hours, patients develop watery diarrhea.
    - Hepatic toxicity is evident on day 2 with elevations in bilirubin, AST, and ALT.
      - Signs of fulminant hepatic failure such as encephalopathy and coagulopathy follow.
      - Hypoglycemia results not just from hepatic failure but from direct pancreatic toxicity.
    - Cyclopeptides may also cause decreased levels of thyroid hormone and increased calcitonin.
    - Patients do not seek help until symptoms develop; it is common for patients to present to a health care facility with volume depletion and early hepatic injury.
  - Good supportive care and prevention of secondary complications are the keys.
  - Activated charcoal should be administered 1 g/kg every 2 to 4 hours to adsorb any toxin remaining.
  - No data support its use in *Amanita* poisoning, but NAC effectively treats hepatic failure from other hepatotoxins, such as acetaminophen.
    - Administer NAC IV, according to the acetaminophen protocol: 150 mg/kg over 45 minutes, 50 mg/kg over 4 hours, and 100 mg/kg over 16 hours. Continue the final infusion until the patient expires, definitively recovers, or receives liver transplant.
  - Silibinin, extracted from milk thistle, improved hepatic markers and mortality in a dog model of *Amanita* poisoning but was not beneficial in a meta-analysis of human studies.
    - In light of its experimental benefits, recommend orally administered silibinin, 20 to 50 mg/kg/day.
    - Silibinin is not a Food and Drug Administration–approved drug but is available at health food stores.
  - High-dose penicillin had some effectiveness in a dog model of *Amanita* poisoning, possibly by blocking hepatocyte uptake of amatoxin.
    - Therapy includes IV penicillin G, 1 million units/kg/day in divided doses.
  - The criteria for liver transplantation have not been clearly established.
  - Some consider transplantation for those with encephalopathy and prolonged PT, persistent hypoglycemia, metabolic acidosis, increased serum ammonia, aminotransferases, and hypofibrinogenemia.
- **Gyromitrin-containing mushrooms:** These are found throughout the United States and contain gyromitrin (N-methyl-N-formyl hydrazone), which is hydrolyzed to monomethylhydrazine (MMH).
  - MMH inhibits the formation of pyridoxal-5′-phosphate (PLP), an enzyme cofactor synthesized from pyridoxine (vitamin B_6).
  - PLP is a cofactor for glutamic acid decarboxylase, the enzyme in the CNS that converts glutamate to GABA.
  - Inhibition of PLP by monomethylhydrazine results in excessive excitation relative to inhibition.
  - *Clinical manifestations and management:* The initial phase of toxicity, occurring 5 to 10 hours after ingestion, is manifest by nonspecific clinical features including nausea, vomiting, diarrhea, and headache, and ultimately leads to intractable seizures.
    - Ingestions of *Gyromitra* spp. should receive activated charcoal, 1 g/kg.
    - Seizures may not respond to benzodiazepines alone.
      - If *Gyromitra* spp. ingestion is considered or if a patient presents with seizures after mushroom ingestion, pyridoxine 70 mg/kg IV should be given.
      - This serves as substrate for pyridoxine phosphokinase, allowing some PLP to be generated despite inhibition by MMH.
- **Allenic norleucine–containing mushrooms:** The nephrotoxic *Amanita smithiana* contains the amino acid toxins allenic norleucine (amino-hexadienoic acid) and possibly 1–2-amino-4-pentynoic acid.
  - All known exposures to these mushrooms have occurred in the Pacific Northwestern United States.

- These mushrooms are important exceptions to the "rule" that mushrooms that cause early GI toxicity do not cause significant end-organ damage later.
- *Clinical manifestations and management:* Initial symptoms, which include nausea, vomiting, diarrhea, and abdominal cramping, may begin within an hour of ingestion.
  - Most important clinical features of toxicity develop later.
    - Acute renal failure, indicated by elevations in blood urea nitrogen and creatinine, manifest 4 to 6 days after ingestion.
  - Activated charcoal should be administered when patients present after ingesting mushrooms from the Pacific Northwest.
  - Management of nephrotoxicity is supportive.
  - Patients who required hemodialysis underwent the procedure two to three times per week for approximately 1 month.
- **Orellanine- and orellinine-containing mushrooms:** *Cortinarius orellanus,* found in North America, contains the toxin orellanine, which is converted by photochemical degradation to another toxin, orellinine.
- Orellanine and orellinine are important causes of mushroom-induced nephrotoxicity.
- Orellanine is activated by the P450 system.
  - Molecules generate oxidative damage by sustained redox cycling.
- *Clinical manifestations and management:* Symptoms begin 24 to 36 hours after ingestion.
  - Headache, chills, polydipsia, nausea, and vomiting have been reported.
  - Early laboratory findings of hematuria, leukocyturia, and proteinuria indicate interstitial nephritis.
    - Later, renal failure develops, characterized histologically by tubular damage and fibrosis of tubules with relative glomerular sparing.

- Hepatotoxicity is uncommon.
- Management is supportive.
  - Administer activated charcoal if patients present early.
  - Some patients will rapidly improve, whereas others require chronic hemodialysis.

TREATMENT REFUSAL

- Patents with toxicologic emergencies are often suicidal and self-destructive and may have an altered level of consciousness.
- We have an ethical obligation to our patients to allow them to guide their own treatment.
- This may mean the patient will decide against the physician's recommendation.
  - To refuse care, the patient must demonstrate the capacity to understand his or her condition and the implications of treatment refusal.
  - Refusal must be voluntary in the absence of a medical or psychiatric condition precluding the ability to make such a decision.
  - The hospital has the right to physically restrain a person who has an altered level of consciousness for the purpose of evaluation and intervention.
- There is potential for legal liability whenever the medical staff physically restrain a patient, retain a patient against his or her will, or allow a patient to refuse a life-saving therapy.
  - Staff can reduce liability by thoroughly documenting the patient's decision-making process and by involving psychiatric consultation in determining the patient's capacity.
- When in doubt, the physician should consult the hospital's legal department.

CHAPTER 31 ■ SUBSTANCE ABUSE AND WITHDRAWAL: ALCOHOL, COCAINE, OPIOIDS, AND OTHER DRUGS

INTRODUCTION

- Ethanol, illicit drugs, and prescription drugs used for nonmedical purposes are significant medical and social problems.
- The 2005 National Survey on Drug Use and Health found that 22.7% of Americans, or 55 million individuals, were binge drinkers.
  - Includes 16 million heavy drinkers (five or more drinks on the same occasion at least 5 different days in the prior 30 days).

- Pain relievers were used nonmedically by 4.7 million Americans, and 3.5 million used stimulants or cocaine.
- Casual or habitual use of these drugs contributes to acute and chronic illness.
- Also underlies many forms of injury, including vehicular accidents, falls, near-drowning, thermal injuries, homicide, and suicide.
- Other critical illnesses may be impacted by either substance use or substance withdrawal.

ETHANOL

Mechanism

- Alcohol abuse and alcoholism (a dependence on alcohol) are major social, economic, and public health problems throughout the world.
  - Alcoholism is the third leading cause of death in the United States.
    - Reduces life expectancy by 10 to 12 years
    - Men who imbibe more than 14 drinks per week or 4 drinks at one time or women who have more than 7 drinks per week or 3 drinks at one time are at risk for alcohol abuse and dependence.
- Ethanol is rapidly absorbed unaltered from stomach and small intestine.
  - Presence of food (especially milk and fatty foods) in the stomach delays absorption.
  - Presence of water enhances absorption.
  - Primarily metabolized in the liver
    - Less than 10% is excreted by the lungs or kidneys or through the skin.
    - Several hepatic enzyme systems independently metabolize ethanol to acetaldehyde.
      - Primary degradation pathway is in the hepatic cytosol by alcohol dehydrogenase, with nicotinamide adenine dinucleotide as a cofactor.
      - Acetaldehyde generated by this process is in turn metabolized through the Krebs cycle to carbon dioxide and water with 7 kcal/g liberated.
      - Most people can metabolize about 150 mg ethanol/kg body weight/hour.

Acute Toxicity

- Common features of acute ethanol intoxication are shown in Table 31.1.
- Intoxication with ethanol depends on the rate of rise of the blood alcohol level and the length of time the level is maintained.
  - Blood alcohol levels of 20 to 30 mg/dL are often associated with a mild euphoria, delayed reaction time, decreased inhibition, and alteration in judgment.
  - Most exhibit gross intoxication at levels above 150 mg/dL.
  - Obtundation often develops at levels above 300 mg/dL.
  - Death may result from respiratory depression, aspiration, or cardiovascular collapse when levels exceed 400 to 500 mg/dL.
- Ethanol is a sedative-hypnotic drug and exerts its primary effects on the central nervous system (CNS).

Assessment and Treatment of Acute Intoxication

- Treatment of acute ethanol intoxication is primarily supportive.
  - Careful examination is needed to detect complications.
    - First priority is assessment and stabilization of the airway and ventilation.

TABLE 31.1

CLINICAL MANIFESTATIONS OF ALCOHOL INTOXICATION

Central nervous system
Decreased inhibition
Slowed reaction time
Visual disturbance
Incoordination
Slurred speech
Diplopia
Nystagmus
Lethargy, stupor, coma

Cardiovascular
Vasodilation
Cardiac dysrhythmias
Myocardial depression

Respiratory
Hypoventilation
Aspiration

Metabolic
Hypoglycemia
Electrolyte abnormalities
Hypophosphatemia
Hypomagnesemia
Acid-base disturbance
Respiratory acidosis
Metabolic alkalosis (vomiting)
Metabolic acidosis (alcoholic ketoacidosis)

Gastrointestinal
Gastritis
Increased incidence of peptic ulcer
Pancreatitis
Alcoholic hepatitis

Hematologic
Suppression of all bone marrow cell lines

Other
Suppression of antidiuretic hormone (diuresis)
Increased sweating
Altered temperature regulation

- Respiratory rate, depth of respirations, SpO$_2$, mental status, gag reflex, and presence of vomitus should be rapidly evaluated.
- Arterial blood gas analysis should be obtained if hypoventilation is a concern but is not obvious on clinical examination.
- Intubation is indicated in the obtunded or comatose patient who is unable to protect his or her airway and when aspiration has occurred or is likely.
- Positive pressure ventilation should be instituted to correct alveolar hypoventilation and hypoxemia.
- With altered mental status, 50 to 100 mg of thiamine and 25 g of glucose should be administered intravenously.
  - If the patient responds to the administration of glucose or if blood glucose levels are low, a continuous infusion of glucose should be given.
  - Intravenous (IV) naloxone may be administered if concomitant opioid use is suspected.
- Hypotension should be treated initially with volume resuscitation.

- Gastrointestinal (GI) bleeding should be considered in the hypotensive patient, and further assessment may include a rectal examination and insertion of a nasogastric tube.
- GI decontamination is of limited utility because the majority of alcohol is already absorbed.
  ○ Ethanol is not adsorbed by activated charcoal, but charcoal may be administered if ingestion of other toxic drugs is suspected.
- Hypothermia, fluid, electrolyte, and acid-base disturbances are corrected, depending on the clinical presentation.
- Creatine phosphokinase level is warranted in the patient with trauma or prolonged muscle compression to evaluate for rhabdomyolysis.
- Ethanol blood level may be helpful in documenting the severity of intoxication and estimating the duration of impairment.
  ○ A low ethanol level in the setting of a patient with a depressed level of consciousness should prompt an evaluation for other etiologies.
- Chest x-ray is often necessary to assess for evidence of aspiration or other complications such as pneumonia.
- Consider obtaining computed tomography of the head if there is any suspicion of subdural hematoma or other intracranial injury.
- Hemodialysis has been used in cases of massive ethanol ingestion.
- Chronic alcoholic may also develop alcoholic ketoacidosis.
  - Typically preceded by binge drinking followed by a period of abstinence for 1 to 3 days with nausea, vomiting, and insufficient nutrient intake.
  - Liver produces excessive ketones in response to starvation, results in an anion gap acidosis.
  - Pancreatitis is frequently present in these patients.
  - Blood glucose may be low or high in this setting but is rarely above 300 mg/dL unless chronic glucose intolerance is present.
  - Condition responds to volume replacement and administration of glucose.
    - Insulin is not needed.
  - Thiamine administered before glucose to avoid precipitation of acute beriberi and Wernicke–Korsakoff syndrome.

Alcohol Withdrawal

- Chronic excessive alcohol ingestion depresses central α and β receptors and potentiates the inhibitory neurotransmitter γ-aminobutyric acid (GABA).
- Brain adapts with a functional increase in N-methyl D-aspartate (NMDA) receptors part of an excitatory system.
- When alcohol consumption stops, excess excitatory receptors and removal of GABA-mediated inhibitory effects contribute to the hyperadrenergic state seen in alcohol withdrawal.
- Alcohol withdrawal syndromes occur during the initial period of abstinence.
  - In hospitalized patients, symptoms of alcohol withdrawal may occur in up to 40% of those who drink excessive amounts of alcohol.

- Prevention of alcohol withdrawal syndromes has been shown to improve morbidity and mortality and shorten hospital and intensive care unit length of stay.
- Four stages of alcohol withdrawal have been described, but symptoms are a continuum of neuropsychiatric and hemodynamic manifestations (Table 31.2).
- A key distinction is to determine whether the patient has an intact or altered sensorium.
- Benzodiazepines act as an alcohol substitute to dampen the excitatory neuronal activity, and additional benefits include prevention of seizures and delirium tremens.
  - Choice of benzodiazepine in hospitalized patients may depend on severity of hepatic dysfunction, desired duration of action, and available routes of administration.
  - All benzodiazepines are effective when appropriate doses are used.
  - Fixed dosing and symptom-triggered regimens have been used effectively.
    ○ Fixed dosing may be more appropriate in critically ill patients until other conditions have stabilized.
    ○ Treatment duration beyond 7 days is seldom required.
- All patients with alcohol withdrawal should receive supportive measures in addition to pharmacologic intervention.
  - Thiamine (vitamin B_1) should be given IV or orally to prevent Wernicke encephalopathy.
  - Magnesium sulfate may be needed to correct hypomagnesemia.

Seizures

- Approximately 5% to 10% of patients with untreated mild alcohol withdrawal symptoms progress to seizures.
- Those with several detoxification admissions are at higher risk of seizures than patients with fewer detoxification admissions.
  - This association has been termed the "kindling effect"—accumulation of multiple episodes lowers the seizure threshold.
- Most alcohol withdrawal seizures are brief and self-limited in duration.
  - Usually generalized tonic-clonic but focal seizures may also occur.
  - Multiple seizures (two to six episodes) occur in approximately 60% of patients and within a 12-hour period.
  - May be difficult to distinguish withdrawal seizures from a pre-existing seizure disorder or new onset of a nonalcohol-related seizure.
- Other causes such as hypoglycemia, metabolic abnormalities, trauma, infection, and other drug intoxication must be considered.
- CT scan of the head should be obtained for new-onset seizure, persistent neurologic deficits, or evidence or suspicion of trauma
- Alcohol withdrawal seizures can be terminated with benzodiazepines.
  - The risk of a recurrent seizure is 13% to 24%.
  - Lorazepam (2 mg) significantly reduces the risk of recurrent seizure.
  - Phenytoin has no effect.
  - Fewer than 3% of patients develop status epilepticus, and they should be treated with benzodiazepines or propofol. Phenytoin is not as effective.

TABLE 31.2

STAGES OF ALCOHOL WITHDRAWAL AND TREATMENT

Symptoms	Time frame[a]	Treatment
Tremulousness		
Hyperactivity, tremor	Onset within hours	Benzodiazepines (oral or IV)
Diaphoresis, nausea	Peak 10–30 h	Supportive measures
Mild tachycardia, hypertension	Subside in ~40 h	Fluid and electrolytes PRN
Clear sensorium		Quiet environment
		Thiamin, folate, vitamins
Seizures		
	Onset 6–48 h	Lorazepam 2–4 mg IV; repeat as needed
	Peak 13–24 h	Diazepam 10–20 mg IV
		Supportive measures as above
Hallucinations		
Auditory	Onset 8–48 h	Benzodiazepines (oral or IV)
Visual	May last 1–6 d	Supportive measures as above
Tactile		
Delirium tremens		
Coarse tremors, agitation	Onset 60–96 h	Benzodiazepines IV as needed
Altered sensorium (delusions, hallucinations, confusion)		Diazepam
Fever, tachycardia		Lorazepam
Hypertension		Midazolam
Circulatory collapse		Alternative treatments
		Propofol
		Barbiturates
		β-blockers

[a]Time after last drink.

Delirium Tremens

- DTs are most severe manifestation of alcohol withdrawal and should be cared for in intensive care unit setting.
  - Untreated DT carries a mortality of 15% but declines to 1% if treated.
  - Accumulation of multiple prior withdrawal episodes leads to more severe DT with each episode.
  - DT patients have more severe autonomic hyperactivity than milder stages of withdrawal and manifest delirium that may fluctuate.
  - Fluid requirements may be increased due to increased insensible losses (fever, diaphoresis) and lack of oral intake.
  - High-dose IV benzodiazepines (diazepam, lorazepam, midazolam) administered at frequent intervals or as a continuous infusion are needed to control the hyperadrenergic symptoms.
    - Individualize dose to achieve light somnolence.
    - Benzodiazepines bind at the GABA—benzodiazepine receptor, and once these receptors are saturated, additional drug cannot bind.
      - Propylene glycol diluent in benzodiazepines may result in a lactic acidosis with prolonged administration
      - Daily dose reductions of 25% can be initiated after the second or third day of treatment.
      - Propofol infusions may be useful for patients who are refractory to benzodiazepines.

- Dual activity similar to alcohol (GABA agonist and NMDA antagonist properties) that may explain its efficacy.
- Other sedative-hypnotic drugs such as paraldehyde and barbiturates are effective in treating DT but are not commonly used.
- Neuroleptic agents are inferior to benzodiazepines and should not be used as single agents for treatment of DT.
- Neuromuscular blockers may be considered to control agitation when high-dose sedatives ineffective.
- Cardiac monitoring is necessary to detect arrhythmias early and institute therapy.
  - Torsade de pointes may develop owing to hypomagnesemia or prolongation of the QTc interval and should be treated aggressively with IV magnesium sulfate.
  - Beta blockers may be needed to treat hypertension or tachycardia.
    - Propranolol may worsen delirium.
- Thiamine supplementation (100 mg/day) is recommended for 3 days
- DTs usually last 2 to 5 days.
  - In 5% to 10% of cases, DT lasts longer than a week.
  - Elderly alcoholics have a longer withdrawal period with more symptoms than younger alcoholics.
  - Small percentage of patients remain delirious for several weeks and require continuing treatment.

- After head trauma, a subdural hematoma can evolve subacutely in the alcoholic patient.
  - Repeat imaging of the brain may be warranted 7 to 10 days into a course of protracted delirium to rule out a slowly accumulating subdural hematoma.

COCAINE

Mechanism

- Cocaine (benzoylmethylecgonine) is an alkaloid derived from leaves of *Erythroxylon coca.*
  - Second most commonly used illicit drug and the most frequent cause of drug-related deaths.
  - Eighteen- to twenty-five-year-olds are the most common users.
- Cocaine is available in two forms.
  - Cocaine hydrochloride—prepared by dissolving alkaloidal cocaine in hydrochloric acid resulting in a white water-soluble powder, crystals, or granules.
    - This form of cocaine is used intranasally (snorting), orally, or intravenously.
  - Free-base or crack cocaine—heating cocaine hydrochloride in sodium bicarbonate or ammonia makes the hard crystallized cocaine base called crack because of the popping sound it makes when heated.
    - Smoking crack cocaine has become a widespread practice due to the rapid absorption across the alveolar surface.
- Peak effects range from 1 to 90 minutes depending on administration route.
  - Inhalational and IV uses result in the most rapid peak effects and shortest duration of action.
  - Rapidly metabolized by hepatic and plasma cholinesterases and nonenzymatic hydrolysis to ecgonine methyl ester and benzoylecgonine, which are excreted in urine.
  - Urinary excretion of unchanged cocaine ranges from 1% to 15%.
    - ○ Half-lives of most metabolites range from 45 to 90 minutes.
  - Subjective rating of euphoria declines within minutes after constant concentrations are achieved, demonstrating rapid desensitization and acute tolerance.
  - Duration of positive urinary metabolites is somewhat dependent on the assay technique, the activity of plasma cholinesterases, and the duration and dosing of cocaine use.
- Cocaine's lipophilic nature, rapid distribution into and out of the CNS, suggests a highly abusive profile (rush and crash) and increased incidence of kindling.
- Major neurochemical actions of cocaine are as follows:
  - CNS stimulation with release of dopamine
  - Inhibition of neuronal norepinephrine and dopamine uptake, resulting in generalized sympathetic nervous system stimulation
  - Release of serotonin or blockade of serotonin reuptake
  - Inhibition of sodium current in neuronal tissue, resulting in a local anesthetic effect

Toxicity

- Numerous morbidities have been associated with acute and chronic cocaine use (Table 31.3).

TABLE 31.3

CLINICAL MANIFESTATIONS OF COCAINE USE

Anesthetic effects
Localized numbness
Central neuronal depression
Coma

Central nervous system
Euphoria
Alertness
Tremor
Sleeplessness
Paranoia
Psychosis
Headache
Seizures
Stroke
Transient ischemic events
Intracerebral hemorrhage
Cerebral vasculitis
Cognitive dysfunction

Cardiovascular
Tachycardia
Arrhythmias
Hypertension
Myocardial ischemia and infarction
Myocarditis
Aortic dissection or rupture
Sudden death
Cardiomyopathy
Atherosclerosis
Vasculitis

Renal
Induction of renal atherogenesis
Renal failure
Renal infarction
Scleroderma renal crisis

Respiratory
Pulmonary edema
Pulmonary hypertension
Respiratory arrest
Pulmonary vascular occlusion, pulmonary infarction
Pneumothorax
Pneumomediastinum
Hemoptysis

Gastrointestinal
Mesenteric ischemia, infarction
Gastrointestinal perforations

Metabolic
Weight loss
Hyperthermia
Rhabdomyolysis

Other complications
Nasal mucosal injury
Nasal septal perforation
Chronic rhinitis
Deep venous thrombosis
Dystonic reaction
Skin ischemia

Obstetric
Spontaneous abortions
Abruptio placentae
Intrauterine growth retardation
Prematurity

Diagnosis of Acute Intoxication

- Patients with cocaine intoxication may present with a variety of primary complaints such as altered mental status, chest pain, syncope, palpitations, seizures, or attempted suicide.
- Characteristic findings of CNS stimulation such as agitation, mydriasis, sweating, hypertension, and tachycardia often present.
- Effects of other drugs, the presence of complications, and delays in presentation may obscure typical sympathomimetic manifestations.
- Other conditions such as meningitis, encephalopathy, epilepsy with status, and thyrotoxicosis may mimic cocaine intoxication.
- Confirmation of acute or recent cocaine exposure is made by urine toxicology testing.

Treatment for Acute Intoxication

- Benzodiazepines the pharmacologic agents of choice for control of cocaine-induced agitation.
  - Agitation and psychosis of cocaine overdose usually can be managed with titrated doses of IV diazepam, 5 to 20 mg; lorazepam, 2 to 4 mg; or midazolam, 5 to 10 mg slowly.
  - Haloperidol not recommended as a first-line agent because of the lack of experimental support and potential to lower the seizure threshold.
  - Adequate hydration and correction of electrolyte abnormalities important.
- **Cardiovascular:** No large clinical trials have evaluated treatment strategies for cocaine-associated ischemia
  - Treatment of cardiac toxicity is directed at reversing physiologic effects that cause ischemia or arrhythmias.
    - Aspirin should be administered as an antiplatelet agent for suspected myocardial ischemia unless there is evidence of cerebral hemorrhage.
    - Oxygen may help to limit myocardial ischemia.
    - Benzodiazepines and nitroglycerin are considered first-line agents for relief of chest pain, but small clinical studies have yielded conflicting results on the benefit of combining the agents.
    - Alpha blockers such as phentolamine are recommended as a second-line treatment for unrelieved pain, but rarely.
    - β-blockers in the management of myocardial ischemia are debated.
      - Concern of worsening vasospasm or hypertension due to unopposed stimulation of α receptors
  - Most patients with cocaine-associated chest pain will not have infarction.
    - Managed in chest pain or observation units similar to other chest pain patients.
    - Low-risk patients with normal cardiac markers can be risk-stratified safely with stress testing.
  - Therapy for cocaine-induced myocardial infarction should consist of oxygen, aspirin, and nitroglycerin as required for pain relief.
    - If pain persists, patients are candidates for reperfusion therapy.
      - Primary percutaneous angiography is preferred in patients with evidence of ST-elevation myocardial infarction.
      - Thrombolytic therapy has been safely used in cocaine-associated myocardial infarction and may be considered if invasive reperfusion not available.
- Arrhythmias associated with cocaine use are usually transient. Standard therapy should be considered for sustained arrhythmias unresponsive to control of pain and agitation.
- Sustained hypertension in acute cocaine intoxication is not common due to the short physiologic effects of the drug.
  - IV labetalol is a reasonable option if the blood pressure needs to be lowered due to its α- and β-blocking effects.
  - Cocaine-intoxicated patients should be considered to have acute elevations in blood pressure, and there should be little concern about cerebral hypoperfusion with immediate lowering of blood pressure to normal levels.
- **Central nervous system:** Seizures induced by cocaine are best controlled with IV benzodiazepines.
  - Other standard antiepileptics can be added for refractory cases.
  - Neuromuscular blocker use warrants continuous EEG monitoring.
  - Interventions for ischemic strokes associated with cocaine use should be carefully considered.
    - Etiology may involve vasoconstriction as well as thrombosis; the decision to use thrombolytic agents in patients presenting within 3 hours of symptom onset may be more difficult.
    - Vascular imaging may be helpful.
    - Blood pressure is not usually severely elevated, but if sustained hypertension is present, current guidelines should be followed for lowering blood pressure.
    - Neurosurgical consultation should be sought for intracranial hemorrhages to evaluate for possible interventions.
    - Patients with subarachnoid hemorrhage should be evaluated for vascular malformations that may be treatable.
- **Pulmonary:** Most pulmonary toxicities associated with cocaine are managed with usual care or supportive care.
  - Bronchospasm and asthma should be treated with inhaled β-agonists and corticosteroids if indicated.
  - Pneumomediastinum can be followed without hospital admission for most patients.
  - Small pneumothoraces may also resolve without intervention.
  - Noncardiogenic pulmonary edema may require supplemental oxygen and mechanical ventilation but resolves within a few days.
- **Hyperthermia/rhabdomyolysis:** Hyperthermia associated with cocaine use should be treated aggressively by rapid cooling.
  - Control of coexisting agitation, psychosis, or seizures is essential.
  - No evidence that pharmacologic agents such as dantrolene are of benefit in cooling patients with life-threatening hyperthermia.
  - Patients with hyperthermia, severe agitation or motor activity, seizures, and obtundation require evaluation for rhabdomyolysis.
    - Aggressive fluid resuscitation to replete the intravascular volume and enhance urine output initiated prior to definitive diagnosis.
    - Serial tests of electrolytes, renal function, and creatine kinases are needed to monitor the severity and response.

- **Body packers/stuffers:** Individuals may ingest packets of cocaine or any illicit drug for the purpose of transport or concealment.
  - Body stuffers swallow small amounts of drug (wrapped or unwrapped) in order to avoid arrest.
    - Drugs are not prepared for passage through the GI tract and drug is frequently absorbed.
    - Toxicity is usually mild.
  - Body packers swallow larger quantities of drug in multiple packets that are specially prepared for smuggling to withstand transit through the GI tract.
    - Abdominal radiographs often show the location of the packets and allow tracking.
    - Negative result on plain abdominal radiograph does not rule out body packing.
      - Abdominal CT scan may be needed to visualize the packets.
  - Most body packers are asymptomatic and can be managed conservatively until the packets have been completely evacuated.
    - Activated charcoal given every 4 to 6 hours can reduce the lethality of oral cocaine.
    - Whole-bowel irrigation may assist with passage of the packets.
    - Body packers with signs and symptoms of drug toxicity, *in vivo* degradation, or gastrointestinal obstruction require emergent surgical intervention.

Cocaine Withdrawal

- Psychological and biochemical dependency on cocaine may be intense.
- Brain becomes dopamine deficient.
- Short period of cocaine abstinence can result in a withdrawal state.
- Clinical effects of cocaine withdrawal include the following:
  - Depression
  - Fatigue
  - Irritability
  - Sleep and appetite dysfunction
  - Psychomotor agitation or retardation
  - Craving for more cocaine
- A period of prolonged somnolence and decreased arousal can occur after binge use of cocaine
  - Often necessitates evaluations to rule out complications associated with cocaine use
  - Supportive environment and professional drug counseling are warranted.

OPIOIDS

Mechanism

- Opioids include all drugs with morphine-like properties and/or that bind to opioid receptors.
  - At least five opioid receptors with various physiologic roles, including analgesia, ventilatory depression, drug dependence, bradycardia, dysphoria, hallucinations, sedation, and miosis

TABLE 31.4

CLASSIFICATION OF OPIOID AGENTS

Opioid agonists
Natural opium derivatives
Codeine
Morphine
Semisynthetic opioids
Heroin
Hydrocodone
Hydromorphone
Oxymorphone
Oxycodone
Synthetic opioids
Diphenoxylate
Fentanyl
Levorphanol
Loperamide
Meperidine
Methadone
Propoxyphene
Tramadol

Pure opioid antagonists
Nalmefene
Naloxone
Naltrexone

Agonists–Antagonists
Butorphanol
Nalbuphine
Pentazocine

- Classified as receptor agonists or antagonists, or combined because they stimulate one type of receptor and antagonize another (Table 31.4)
- Opioid dependence characterized by repeated self-administration of the drug and encompasses physiologic dependence and addictive behavior.
- Exposure to opioids causes neural changes that produce tolerance, dependence, and withdrawal.

Toxicity

- All opioids are associated with toxicity.
- Most fatal overdoses occur with IV administration.
- Diagnosis of opioid toxicity made by characteristic clinical findings, exposure history, qualitative toxicology assay, and response to naloxone.
- Qualitative urine assays may not detect all opioid derivatives (e.g., fentanyl).
- Opioid intoxication is characterized by a clinical syndrome of depressed level of consciousness, respiratory depression, and miosis.
  - Manifestations are variable depending on the drug used and presence of other drugs or alcohol.
  - Miosis is not seen with meperidine and propoxyphene toxicity.
  - The primary toxic manifestations of opioids are mediated by the μ and κ receptors in the brain, which cause CNS depression.
  - Common clinical effects of these drugs are shown in Table 31.5.

TABLE 31.5

CLINICAL MANIFESTATIONS OF OPIOID INTOXICATION

Central nervous system
Analgesia
Apathy
Lethargy
Seizures
Coma
Ventilatory depression
Nausea
Emesis
Miosis

Respiratory
Histamine release—bronchospasm
Pulmonary edema

Cardiovascular
Arteriolar and venous dilation
Preload reduction
Hypotension

Gastrointestinal
Decreased peristalsis
Decreased hydrochloric acid secretion
Constipation

Other
Histamine release—urticaria, pruritus
Muscle rigidity (fentanyl)
Urinary retention

- The most worrisome feature of CNS depression is hypoventilation.
  - Tidal volume decreases first, then respiratory rate falls.
- Seizures may be associated with meperidine, propoxyphene, and tramadol toxicity or result from hypoventilation and hypoxemia due to other opioids.
- Arteriolar and venous dilatation with opioid use can precipitate preload reduction, a fall in cardiac output, and hypotension.
- Opioid-induced release of histamine from mast cells can precipitate bronchospasm, urticaria, and pruritus.
- Other respiratory complications include the following:
  - Aspiration of gastric contents
  - Noncardiogenic pulmonary edema
  - Asthma exacerbation (heroin)
  - Pulmonary hypertension
  - Acute respiratory distress syndrome
  - Septic pulmonary emboli
- IV-injected illicit opioids may be mixed with microcrystalline cellulose, talc, or cellulose.
  - These are capable of producing angiothrombosis and a foreign-body granulomatous reaction in the lung.
- Decreased GI peristalsis and increased ileocecal and anal sphincter tone are responsible for the constipation frequently seen with opioid use.
- Urinary retention may be caused by increased detrusor muscle tone.
- Local infections, endocarditis, and other systemic infections are especially common in the IV user.

Treatment for Acute Intoxication

- The most common cause of death in opioid overdose is ventilatory failure.
  - Immediate priority in acute opioid intoxication is airway management and ventilation.
  - If reversal of respiratory depression cannot be accomplished quickly with naloxone, intubation may be necessary.
  - Naloxone, a pure opioid antagonist, reverses all of the opioid-induced CNS and ventilatory depressant effects.
    - Dose required to reverse opioid effects depends on the amount and type of opioid administered.
      - Initial dose of naloxone is 0.4 to 2 mg; the lower dose should be administered initially in patients suspected of chronic addiction to avoid precipitating acute withdrawal symptoms.
      - We dilute 0.4 mg in a total of 10 mL, resulting in a concentration of 40 mcg/mL and administer 1 to 2 mL at a time, initially.
      - Additional doses of naloxone can be given based on the patient's response.
        - Can be administered intramuscularly, by sublingual injection, or through an endotracheal tube
        - Goal of therapy is to restore adequate spontaneous respirations rather than complete arousal.
      - CNS depression not reversed by 20 mg of naloxone, alternate causes should be aggressively addressed.
        - Hypoglycemia
        - Hypothermia
        - Head trauma
        - Close observation of the patient after naloxone administration is warranted because its effects last approximately 60 to 90 minutes.
          - May require repeated bolus injections of naloxone or a continuous infusion to maintain adequate respirations, particularly with long-acting opioids.
          - Infusion dose is one-half to two-thirds of the initial naloxone dose that reversed respiratory depression given hourly.
- Isotonic fluids should be administered for hypotension due to opioids.
- Noncardiogenic pulmonary edema is usually self-limited (24–36 hours) and managed with supportive care that may include intubation and mechanical ventilation.
- Seizures unresponsive to naloxone should be treated with IV benzodiazepines.
  - Refractory seizures may suggest either body packing or another complication.
- Potential for acetaminophen toxicity should be considered in patients ingesting opioids formulated with acetaminophen.

Acute Opioid Withdrawal

- Chronic administration of exogenous opiates is thought to lead to diminished endogenous opioid peptides.
  - When exogenous opiates discontinued, opioid withdrawal may occur.
  - The clinical manifestations of opioid withdrawal are outlined in Table 31.6.

TABLE 31.6

CLINICAL MANIFESTATIONS OF OPIOID
WITHDRAWAL

Early
Yawning
Lacrimation
Rhinorrhea
Sneezing
Sweating

Intermediate
Restless sleep
Piloerection
Restlessness
Irritability
Anorexia
Flushing
Tachycardia
Tremor
Hyperthermia

Late
Fever
Nausea
Vomiting
Abdominal pain
Diarrhea
Difficulty sleeping
Muscle spasm
Joint pain
Involuntary ejaculation
Suicidal ideation

- Onset of symptoms varies with the drug abused.
  - Within 6 to 12 hours of the last dose with short-acting opioids such as heroin
  - Within 36 to 48 hours with long-acting opioids such as methadone
  - Withdrawal is rarely life threatening and usually does not require intensive care.
- If necessary to control withdrawal symptoms
  - Most opioids in sufficient dosage will alleviate symptoms.
  - Methadone, buprenorphine, and clonidine have been used to treat acute opioid withdrawal.
  - Methadone and buprenorphine have been used to treat opioid addiction chronically.
    - Methadone can cause constipation, respiratory depression, dizziness, sedation, nausea, and diaphoresis.
    - Oral buprenorphine is restricted in the United States to qualified physicians who treat opioid dependence.
      - Has low toxicity in high doses, partly because its μ-antagonist effects limit the opioid effects of sedation, respiratory depression, and hypotension
      - Is more effective than clonidine and similar to methadone for management of opioid withdrawal
    - Clonidine is used to suppress the autonomic effects of opioid withdrawal.
      - Doses of 0.1 to 0.3 mg orally can suppress the signs and symptoms of opiate withdrawal within 24 hours and shorten acute withdrawal reactions by 3 to 4 days.
      - Side effects are hypotension, drowsiness, dry mouth, and bradycardia.

Heroin Body Packers

- Heroin body packers should be managed similar to cocaine body packers (preceding section).
- If evidence of systemic absorption from leaking packets, treat opioid toxicity with a continuous infusion of naloxone.

AMPHETAMINES AND DERIVATIVES

Mechanism

- Amphetamines, methamphetamines, and similar derivatives are the most commonly abused CNS stimulants along with cocaine.
- Usually abused for the euphoric effects or to enhance performance.
  - Amphetamines by increasing release and inhibiting reuptake of dopamine and serotonin in the brain.
  - Minor chemical substitutions enhance drug's hallucinogenic properties.
  - Production of these drugs from readily available ingredients in clandestine laboratories has resulted in increased supply throughout the United States.
    - Methamphetamine can be made from common ingredients such as rock salt, paint thinner, lantern fuel, battery acid, lye, ammonia, lithium, ether, rubbing alcohol, iodine, and cold medicines containing pseudoephedrine.
  - Methamphetamine in a crystalline form (commonly called ice, crank, glass, or crystal) one of the most popular drugs in this class.
    - Can be orally ingested, smoked, snorted, or injected IV
    - An amphetamine-like drug, 3–4-methylenedioxymethamphet-amine (MDMA), is a designer drug (commonly known as Ecstasy, XTC, or MDMA) that acts simultaneously as a stimulant and hallucinogen.
      - Results in greater serotonin release in the brain with inhibition of serotonin reuptake
      - Most amphetamines are detected on qualitative urine toxicology assays but a negative result does not rule out amphetamine intoxication or abuse.

Toxicity

- Drugs cause release of catecholamines, which result in a sympathomimetic/adrenergic syndrome.
  - Compared to cocaine, the "high" and physiologic effects last longer (hours to several days depending on the agent used).
- Clinical presentation is characterized by tachycardia, hyperthermia, agitation, hypertension, and mydriasis.
  - Hallucinations (visual and tactile), hypervigilance, and acute psychoses (often paranoia) are frequently observed.
  - MDMA leads to increased verbosity and sociability.
  - MDMA use is associated with bruxism that is often countered by sucking on a pacifier or lollipop.
  - Often associated with behaviors resulting in trauma and risky sexual encounters.

- Acute adverse medical consequences are similar to those seen with cocaine abuse (preceding discussion).
- Long-term use of these drugs may result in dilated cardiomyopathy and "meth mouth."
  - Meth mouth refers to a pattern of oral signs and symptoms of methamphetamine abuse, thought to include rampant caries and tooth fracture, leading to multiple tooth loss and edentulism.
  - Burn injuries from methamphetamine laboratory explosions are associated with a higher incidence of inhalational injury and greater use of critical care resources.
- Complications of MDMA use are usually a result of the drug effects and nonstop physical activity.
  - Effects of MDMA last 4 to 6 hours.
  - Medical complications include the following:
    - Hyperthermia
    - Hyponatremia
    - Rhabdomyolysis
    - Seizures
    - Renal failure
    - Arrhythmias
    - Syncope
    - Cerebral infarction/hemorrhage
    - Hepatotoxicity
    - Serotonin syndrome
    - Death

Management

- Primarily supportive
  - Gastric lavage is not recommended because absorption after oral ingestion is usually complete when patients present.
  - Activated charcoal may be considered if a recent oral ingestion is known to have occurred.
  - Careful assessment for complications should be made, including measurement of core temperature, obtaining electrocardiogram, searching for evidence of trauma, and evaluating laboratory data for evidence of renal or hepatic dysfunction and rhabdomyolysis.
  - IV hydration for possible rhabdomyolysis is warranted in individuals with known exertional activities pending creatine phosphokinase results.
  - Patients should be placed in a quiet, calm environment, and benzodiazepines, often in high doses, are used for controlling agitation.
    - Haloperidol is reserved for patients with inadequate response to benzodiazepines.

Withdrawal

- Acute withdrawal from amphetamines is similar to cocaine.
- Symptoms include fatigue, depression, anxiety, motor retardation, hypersomnia (followed by insomnia), increased eating, and drug craving.
  - Although uncomfortable, the manifestations are not dangerous.
  - Patients may become suicidal during withdrawal and should be evaluated for this possibility.
  - Symptoms may persist for months.

γ-HYDROXYBUTYRATE

Mechanism

- γ-Hydroxybutyrate (GHB) is a naturally occurring metabolite of GABA found in the brain.
  - Commonly a drug of recreational abuse
  - One of several agents characterized "date rape" drug.
  - Promoted to build muscle, improve performance, produce euphoria, and enhance sleep.
  - Available as a colorless, odorless liquid with a mild salty taste easy to mask in drinks.
    - GHB absorbed from stomach within 10 to 15 minutes.
    - Readily crosses the blood–brain barrier where it interacts with GHB and γ-aminobutyric acid type B (GABA$_B$) receptors
    - Stimulatory effects occur from resulting increased dopamine levels in the brain and sedative effects by potentiation of endogenous opioids
- γ-Butyrolactone (GBL), also known as 2(3H)-furanone-dihydro, and 1,4 butanediol (BD), also called tetramethylene glycol, are abused with the same adverse effects as GHB.
  - Both agents are metabolized systemically to GHB.

Acute Toxicity

- Manifestations of GHB toxicity are dose-related and include the following:
  - Agitation
  - Coma
  - Seizures
  - Respiratory depression
  - Vomiting
- Other effects include amnesia, tremors, myoclonus, hypotonia, hypothermia, decreased cardiac output, and bradycardia.
- Dose of 20 to 30 mg/kg can produce euphoria and sleepiness and coma may result from doses of $\geq$40 to 60 mg/kg.
  - Concomitant use of ethanol results in synergistic CNS and respiratory depressant effects.
  - Deaths attributed to GHB and related agents usually result from respiratory depression, hypoxemia, or aspiration.
- GHB is not routinely detected by urine toxicology assays but can be detected in plasma or urine by gas chromatographic-mass spectrophotometric techniques.
  - Rapid clearance precludes detection beyond 12 hours after a dose.
  - Diagnosis is usually determined by the clinical course and history of exposure elicited after the patient recovers.
  - Hallmark of GHB intoxication is rapid onset of toxicity and sudden, rapid recovery rather than gradual recovery seen with ethanol or benzodiazepine intoxication.

Assessment and Treatment of Acute Intoxication

- No antidote for GHB, GBL, or BD toxicity.
- Primary management for ingestion of these drugs is supportive care with particular attention to airway protection.

- In some cases, intubation and mechanical ventilation are required.
- Gastric lavage and activated charcoal are not warranted because of the small amounts involved and the rapid absorption.
- Naloxone and flumazenil are of no benefit.
- Atropine may be needed for symptomatic bradycardia.
- Mild intoxication may be observed in the emergency department and released after symptoms resolve.
  - Rapid recovery of consciousness from an obtunded condition in a few hours is frequently observed.
  - Patients requiring intubation and mechanical ventilation can be expected to resolve within 2 to 96 hours unless complications such as aspiration or anoxic injury have occurred.
  - Concomitant use of alcohol may prolong the CNS depression.
  - Physostigmine reported to awaken patients with GHB intoxication, its use is not recommended.

γ-Hydroxybutyrate Withdrawal

- Sedative withdrawal syndrome after high-dose frequent use (every 1–3 hours) of GHB, GBL, and BD has been described.
- Mild symptoms such as anxiety, insomnia, nausea, vomiting, and tremors begin within 6 hours of the last dose.
- May progress to severe delirium with autonomic instability (usually mild) requiring hospitalization and sedation.
- Patients may experience auditory, visual, and tactile hallucinations.
- Symptoms requiring treatment may be as long as 2 weeks.
- Benzodiazepines are the initial choice for management and high doses may be required.
  - Propofol and barbiturates have also been used successfully.

PHENCYCLIDINE

Mechanism

- Phencyclidine (PCP) is a psychoactive drug used as a hallucinogen that can be administered by oral ingestion, nasal insufflation, smoking, or IV injection.

- A dissociative agent that blocks the NMDA receptors leading to an inhibition of sensory perception.
- Sympathomimetic effects result from inhibition of norepinephrine and dopamine reuptake.

Clinical Manifestations

- Signs and symptoms reported with PCP use are variable depending on the route of abuse, susceptibility of the user, and concomitant drug use
- Behavioral effects of PCP include coma, catatonia, psychosis, and confusion.
  - Agitation may be intermittent and unexpected.
  - Misperception of reality can lead to violent behavior, risk-taking behavior, and accidents resulting in trauma.
  - Nystagmus (horizontal, vertical, and/or rotatory) and miosis are characteristic findings with PCP intoxication along with ataxia.
  - Medical complications can include hyperthermia, rhabdomyolysis, and seizures.
  - Dystonic reactions occur rarely.
  - PCP is usually detected on urine qualitative toxicology tests.

Management

- Includes control of agitation using a quiet, nonstimulatory environment and benzodiazepines as needed
  - Haloperidol may be beneficial for frank psychosis.
  - Physical restraints are often needed until adequate sedation is achieved.
  - Tachycardia and hypertension, if present, usually respond to control of agitation.
- Activated charcoal does adsorb PCP, but most patients present after GI absorption is complete.
- Urinary acidification enhances PCP excretion but is not recommended.
- Possibility of rhabdomyolysis should be evaluated, and early fluid therapy should be considered while awaiting test results.

CHAPTER 32 ■ ENVENOMATION

SNAKES NATIVE TO THE UNITED STATES

General

- The United States has two broad categories of venomous snakes.
  - First, and less common, is the coral snake, members of the family Elapidae, with two general and several species.
    - The only venomous snake in North America that is not a pit viper, does not have "cat eye"–shaped pupils, and a rather small head.
    - Only 1% to 2% of all U.S. snakebite envenomations involve coral snakes, yet this small number accounts for a somewhat disproportionate amount of human morbidity and mortality.
  - Secondly, the pit vipers account for about 95% of U.S. snakebites.
    - Members of the family Crotalidae and comprise rattlesnakes, water moccasins, and copperheads.
    - Pit vipers are composed of three genera and numerous species.
      ○ They have two heat-sensing pits approximately halfway between their nostrils and eyes.
      ○ Because of their considerable venom apparatus, they appear to have heads significantly larger than one might expect, given the size of their bodies.
  - Remaining 2% to 3% of all U.S. snakebites are inflicted by exotic venomous snakes.
  - Identification of offending animals should be done if possible but without undue risk of further bites to the victim or others.
    - U.S. pit viper and coral snake antivenoms are polyvalent, so it is only necessary to identify a snake to the family level.
    - Identification charts are available, and experts such as local herpetologists may be consulted in certain cases.

Coral Snake Envenomation

General

- Rather small and brilliantly colored secretive reptiles
- Often found around newer housing projects and may be encountered in one's garden or yard
  - Not aggressive, supporting stories that children may play with them for hours to days without being bitten
  - Cannot open their mouths as widely as the pit vipers, so they typically bite only at the tips of fingers or the webbed space between the thumb and first finger

- Envenomation requires hanging on to this small anatomic part for 10 to 30 seconds to work venom into the skin, an activity most victims will not tolerate.
- Several nonpoisonous distant look-alikes with which it is sometimes confused
  - Coral snake (in the United States) has a black nose, with alternating rings of red, yellow (sometimes white), and black encircling the entire body of the snake.
  - Coral snake envenomation is complicated by the fact that, in direct contradistinction to pit viper envenomation, there is little or no local tissue damage.
    - Characteristic triad of immediate local pain, swelling, and discoloration characteristic of pit viper envenomation does not develop.
    - However, it is possible to misconstrue a serious bite from a coral snake as one from either a "dry bite" by a venomous snake or a bite by a nonvenomous snake.
    - Can lead to an unfortunate outcome

Symptoms and Manifestations

- Symptoms may be delayed up to 12 hours.
  - Dangerous and can progress rapidly should they occur
  - Observe patients for 24 hours to determine whether an envenomation has occurred.
- Venom chiefly neurotoxic so signs and symptoms are declared in approximately the following ascending order and frequency:
  - Mild numbness in the bitten extremity
  - Euphoria, often precipitously followed by cranial nerve symptoms
    - Diplopia being the one that the patient most often first notices.
    - Distinct flat dysarthria (similar to patients with myasthenia gravis) is the one that health care professionals usually first notice.
  - Stridor
  - Inability to swallow
- Finally, respiratory arrest may rapidly ensue.
  - During progression from dysarthria to respiratory arrest, aspiration pneumonia is extremely common and constitutes one of the major morbidities and mortalities of coral snake envenomation.
  - Should cranial nerve involvement be noted to develop, prophylactically and preemptively intubate to protect airway.
- Lacking the large fangs characteristic of pit vipers, this snake's puncture wounds are notoriously not prominent.
- Squeeze the bite site: One may see minute, pinpoint accumulations of blood welling up from the tissue, indicating that the teeth of the coral snake have successfully entered the subcutaneous tissue, allowing venom deposition.
- Triad of risk factors, if any two are present, warrant strong consideration for the infusion of three to five vials of antivenom:

- Snake is positively identified as a coral snake.
- History of the snake "hanging on" the bitten site for at least 15 to 30 seconds
- One can observe pinpoints of blood after applied pressure to the bitten area.
- Typically do not administer antivenom for the presence of only one feature of this triad, but typically observe the patient for about a day.
- Natural history of duration of respiratory arrest is approximately 7 to 10 days before the effects of the venom naturally abate.
  - Mentation is not affected.
  - Patient is totally flaccid.
  - Long-term sequelae after either successful treatment or the natural history of the envenomation syndrome may include several months of dysesthesias and paresthesias in bitten extremity but generally fade after several months to a year.

Antivenom Administration

- Antivenom Wyeth (Antivenin [Micrurus fulvius] [equine origin]) is no longer being manufactured.
  - Present statements and future predictions on how to treat envenomation by coral snake difficult
  - If antivenom can be procured, if symptoms deemed either imminent or present, three to five vials of the antivenom given IV about every 8 to 12 hours until symptoms stop progressing.
  - Single treatment is usually sufficient.
  - If symptoms develop ≥1 hour before antivenom administration
    - Notoriously difficult to reverse the neurologic blockade
    - Repeated administration of antivenom futile and probably unwise
  - Antivenom, prepared in Mexico (Coralmyn, Bioclon) available in emergencies
    - Call regional poison center (1.800.222.1222) to assist in acquisition, as most products in the United States are held by zoos.

Pit Viper Envenomation

General

- *Crotalus:* The family Crotalidae consists of three genera found within the United States. The largest genus, composed of some 15 to 20 species and subspecies, is *Crotalus,* the rattlesnakes.
  - Most serious bites those of the eastern diamondback rattlesnake (*Crotalus adamanteus*) and the western diamondback rattlesnake (*Crotalus atrox*)
- *Sistrurus:* Two other species of rattlesnakes in the genus *Sistrurus. Sistrurus catenatus* (also known as the massasauga) is mostly encountered in the upper Midwest from western Pennsylvania and New York across to Michigan and Iowa.
  - *Sistrurus miliarius* (also known as the pygmy rattlesnake) is seen chiefly in Florida and up into the Atlantic coast states.
  - Bites are characterized by a very low morbidity and virtually zero mortality.
    - Antivenom used only occasionally (approximately 10% of the time).

- *Agkistrodon:* The third genus of the family Crotalidae is *Agkistrodon.*
  - The copperhead (*Agkistrodon contortrix*) is the most common pit viper from Georgia up through the Atlantic Coast states. Antivenom administered to only 0% to 11% of victims.
  - *Agkistrodon piscivorus* (water moccasin) is also in the Atlantic Coast states, in Florida, and westward through Alabama and Mississippi and into eastern Texas. Neither species of *Agkistrodon* is extremely venomous. Bites characteristically cause significant edema but virtually no mortality. Antivenom used in only about 25% of victims of water moccasin envenomations.
    - Chiefly for patients either at the extremes of age or with significant comorbidities

Range of Venom Effects

- Bites from these species of pit vipers vary enormously.
  - Variability of the virulence is due to the variability of the venom.
  - Individual members of a species, kept over time, display variability in their venom pattern.
    - Important when one considers the antivenom that is currently available. CroFab (Crotalidae polyvalent immune Fab [ovine] [FabAV], Therapeutic Antibodies, Inc., Nashville, TN) is a mixture of Fab fragments prepared from purified immunoglobulins produced by sheep repeatedly injected with venom from one of the following four snakes: *Crotalus atrox, Crotalus adamanteus, Crotalus scutulatus,* or *Agkistrodon piscivorus.*
      - Fab fragments from all four preparations are then mixed together to produce a polyvalent mixture.
      - Variable degrees of immunogenicity and responses from the sheep.
      - Not all venom components will be neutralized to exactly the same degree.

Symptoms and Manifestations

- A near-immediate onset of a symptom triad occurs in victims of pit viper envenomation.
  - Pain
  - Swelling
  - Discoloration
- Digestive enzymes such as phosphatases, hyaluronidases, proteinases, phospholipases, and other substances dissolve connective tissue and proteins, and attack nerve endings.
- Edema is largely brought about by disruption of the endothelium of capillaries and lymphatics due to a variety of proteins that directly attack the endothelial integrity of the microcirculation.
- Lack of pain, swelling, and discoloration usually indicate that the victim is one of the 15% to 30% of pit viper victims in which the reptile did not inject venom.
  - So-called "dry bites" do not require antivenom.
    - Some patients may be envenomated by a pit viper, fail to have any local signs, yet may be clearly ill as attested by their profuse weakness, fasciculations, diaphoresis, hypotension, nausea, vomiting, diarrhea, mental status alterations (which include confusion and stupor), and the oft-mentioned "metallic taste" experienced by several victims.

- This occurs in approximately 5% to 10% of envenomations.
  - Attributed to injection of the venom more or less directly into a vessel or a muscular bed rich in capillaries such that venom goes more directly into the circulatory system.

Clinical and Laboratory Findings

- Coagulopathic findings—clinical and laboratory—are of great interest to those who treat pit viper envenomations.
  - Laboratory coagulation defects are far most pronounced within the *Crotalus* genus and rarely encountered in the *Agkistrodon* and rarely, if ever, in the *Sistrurus* genera.
- Laboratory coagulation abnormalities due to a thrombin-like enzyme that has been referred to as crotalase.
  - Enzyme rapidly, efficiently, and partially cleaves fibrinogen by cleaving the B-peptide off the β-subunit, as does thrombin.
  - Neither cleaves the A-peptide from the α-subunit nor activates factors V, VIII, or XIII
  - This partially clotted fibrinogen forms a loose gel that is exquisitely sensitive to any proteolytic activity, so visible thromboses or organ manifestations of systemic thromboses are not encountered.
  - Crotalase neither activates platelets nor consumes antithrombin III.
  - Crotalase does not activate plasminogen directly (i.e., *in vitro* or *in vivo*) but does so indirectly, most likely by release of endothelial-secreted tissue plasminogen activator.
    - Plasma levels of tissue plasminogen activator spike in a reflex response to the deposition of the partially formed fibrin on the endothelial surface, and a brisk fibrinolysis occurs.
      - Essentially, the total body fibrinogen complement (some 15 g) is nearly totally converted into fibrin degradation products (FDPs) within an hour.
      - Crotalase is necessary in only extremely small amounts to totally defibrinogenate an adult human, resulting in plasma fibrinogen levels <50 mg/dL.
      - Coagulation end point (visible fibrin clot) of routine coagulation tests, such as prothrombin time (PT) and partial thromboplastin time (PTT) so impaired that many interpret this as the blood being "incoagulable."
      - Thrombin generation via the intact coagulation cascade is **totally retained** save for the lack of the visible clot.
      - Intact thrombin generation serves to afford intact hemostasis, despite incoagulable *in vitro* PTs and PTTs.
    - Defibrinogenation syndrome is reversed by the administration of fibrinogen in the form of approximately 8 to 10 units of cryoprecipitate.

Postmortem Findings

- Death from American pit viper envenomation is rare, and full autopsies are even rarer.
- In 16 deaths of about 1,000 cases of North American envenomations reported up to 1989
  - Central nervous system edema and hemorrhage were reported in a few cases.
  - Cerebral hemorrhage was deemed the cause of death in only one.

- Mortality rate from severe, complicated rattlesnake envenomation was approximately 1.4%.
- Most common cause of death was progressive shock leading to multiorgan failure and death hours to a few days later.

Prehospital Treatment

- The key to good and effective therapy with minimal chance of loss of life, limb, or function is prompt transportation to a medical care facility.
- Initial scene management
- Prevent further bites
- Calm the patient
- If successful transport is anticipated within an hour, it is probably best to forgo any local therapy other than to gently splint the bitten extremity, keeping it at or slightly below heart level, and transport the patient.
- Topical cold packs may provide some relief of severe pain.
- Incising or excising the wound, the application of electrical currents, or other traumatic manipulations are contraindicated.
  - Suction devices remove at best 2% of the venom load, are likely to be clinically insignificant, and, if used, should not delay transport.
  - The use of a tourniquet with pressure sufficient to impede either arterial or venous flow is contraindicated.
  - A lymphatic constriction band (ideally a blood pressure cuff inflated to 15 to 25 mm Hg, a band that allows a finger to pass easily beneath) or a properly applied pressure immobilization bandage may be considered if there are immediate life-threatening effects or a prolonged (>1 hour) transport time.

Hospital Treatment

- Approximately 5,000 to 10,000 bites occur in the United States each year.
  - Death from envenomation by North American pit vipers occurs only about five to 10 times (0.1%) per year, representing approximately a 99.9% survival rate.
  - Table 32.1 outlines the essentials of appropriate management of such patients.

Immediate Management

- *Confirm the bite:* Confirm that the patient was bitten by a snake and, particularly, a venomous snake.
  - With the exception of coral snake envenomation, this usually includes the presence of puncture wounds.

TABLE 32.1

INITIAL EVALUATION AND DIAGNOSTIC POINTS

- Confirm patient was bitten by a venomous snake; determine snake species if possible.
- Evaluate for local signs of envenomation:
  - Pain
  - Swelling
  - Discoloration
- Evaluate for systemic signs of envenomation:
  - Alterations in vital signs, nausea, vomiting, diarrhea
  - Fasciculations
  - Coagulation abnormalities
  - Altered mental status

TABLE 32.2

CLINICAL CHARACTERISTICS OF ENVENOMATION THAT POTENTIALLY AID IN IDENTIFICATION OF OFFENDING *CROTALUS* SPECIES

Common name	Scientific name	Distribution	Neurologic symptoms	Coagulopathic findings	Rhabdomyolysis
Eastern diamondback	*Crotalus adamanteus*	Southeastern United States	+	Prolonged PT/PTT; minimal thrombocytopenia	+
Canebrake	*Crotalus horridus atricaudatus*	Eastern United States	Nil	Nil	++++
Mojave	*Crotalus scutulatus*	Desert southwest United States	+++	Nil	++++
Timber	*Crotalus horridus horridus*	Eastern United States	Nil	Prolonged PT/PTT; moderate to severe thrombocytopenia	Nil

PT, prothrombin time; PTT, partial thromboplastin time.
+ = usually minimally present; ++ = usually moderately present; +++ = usually extensively present; ++++ = always present.

- Not uncommon to see snakes with one fang or even three or four, as their fangs maturate and move forward, replacing one another with time.
- Vast majority of patients will have the prompt triad of pain, swelling, and discoloration confined to the bite site almost within minutes of the event but up to 2 hours later in unusual cases.
- *Determine the genus and species:* Next, one should try to determine the family and/or genus and species of snake if at all possible.
  - Majority of victims know precisely that they were in the same area as a venomous snake and the snake's common name.
  - Another 25% to 30% will bring the snake to the health care facility in conditions ranging from badly mutilated to quite alive.
  - Several online links, such as http://www.pitt.edu/~mcs2/herp/SoNA.html, are available to assist identification.
  - One can occasionally augment identification of an offending snake by the symptom complex its bite produces (Table 32.2).
  - Prognosis generally species dependent but also related to the time to presentation, time to antivenom administration, the health of the host, and other factors.
- *Determine systemic signs and manifestations:* Assuming the patient does have signs of local envenomation, next in order is to determine whether there are any systemic signs of envenomation.
  - No one dies of local envenomation but only from systemic manifestations.
  - Systemic symptoms such as nausea, vomiting, diarrhea, and diaphoresis and fasciculations—particularly in *Crotalus* envenomations—portend the possibility of a more serious outcome.
  - Many coagulation abnormalities seen in *Crotalus* envenomations are often spectacular in their laboratory manifestations.
  - Altered mental status to include a noticeable stupor and a metallic taste is often reported in serious envenomations.
- *Assign degree of severity:* In attempting to assign a degree of severity from mild to moderate to severe, one must recognize

- That the envenomation syndrome is progressive
- Evaluation is ongoing and time-dependent
- The *rate of change* in signs, symptoms, and other manifestations is important
  - Not only in grading the severity of the bite but in grading the effect—or lack of effect—of the administration of antivenom

Antivenom Administration

- Indications for the use of antivenom vary.
  - Severe envenomations are often apparent by the time they arrive at emergency care, primarily because of the rapidity with which the venom initially gains entry into the circulatory system.
    - In our experience, it is quite rare to see one progress from moderate envenomation to severe envenomation.
    - Severely envenomated patients may be considerably hypotensive with lethargy, nausea, and vomiting, and require immediate and aggressive therapy (Table 32.3).
    - Suggested therapy is outlined in Table 32.4.
      ○ At least one large-bore intravenous access site must be obtained and blood drawn for a variety of tests.
    - It is useful to outline the leading edge of proximal progression of the swelling with some type of ink pen.
      ○ In this manner, one can observe whether the swelling is progressive. Whereas some relatively slow progression is tolerated—particularly if one elects not to treat the patient or if antivenom is not immediately available—more rapid swelling, particularly with concomitant systemic symptoms, usually justifies prompt and aggressive therapy.
- In a situation involving our native reptiles, antivenom is not administered to patients who have no envenomation.
  - About 10% to 15% of people with minimal envenomation, half of those patients with moderate envenomation, and all patients with severe envenomation are administered antivenom.
  - There are several reasons for not administering antivenom to all, or nearly all, victims:
    - The extremely low mortality rate of envenomation by snakes native to the United States

TABLE 32.3

SEVERITY OF ENVENOMATION BY PIT VIPERS

Grade	Frequency	Initial findings	FabAV vials in first 24 h
No envenomation	15%–30%	No local, systemic, or laboratory abnormalities 2 h after bite	0
Minimal envenomation	20%–40%	Local and slowly progressive swelling without systemic or severe laboratory abnormalities	0–6
Moderate envenomation	20%–40%	Rapidly progressive local swelling; systemic symptoms of nausea, vomiting, diarrhea, diaphoresis, fasciculations, moderate hypotension, and moderate hemostatic abnormalities, but without bleeding	6–18
Severe envenomation	5%–10%	Severe systemic symptoms as above plus severe hypotension and lethargy; severe hemostatic abnormalities and possible bleeding	12–24 or more

- The—admittedly very low—rate (<0.01%) of serious and mild (14%) allergic reactions
- The modest rate (15%) of serum sickness–like late reactions (occurring typically 8–12 days after administration) to FabAV
- The cost of antivenom treatment can easily exceed $50,000.
- Antivenom is more efficacious the earlier it is administered.
  - If the decision made to employ the drug, do it promptly.
  - Control of the envenomation syndrome is adjudged by the slowing, or preferably the cessation, of progressive local swelling.
- Hemorrhagic bleb formation at the site of the bite is *not* an important sign in and of itself, although it generates much attention.
  - These should be left alone or, if one thinks that bursting is imminent, the blebs should be topically sterilized and lanced.
- Compartment syndromes seen very rarely.
  - Indications for surgical intervention are justified by pressure measurements in only about 1% to 2%.
  - Reliable signs of compartment syndrome are total lack of function and exquisite pain of the muscles contained

within a compromised compartment and often an intense hardness of the site.
- The mainstay for treatment for North American pit viper envenomation is ovine FabAV for bites in both adults and children.
  - The Fab portions of sheep immunoglobulins are made by enzyme cleavage and elimination of the Fc fragment and by further enzymatic cleavage of the resulting $F(ab')_2$.
  - Pretreatment skin or conjunctival testing is neither required nor recommended prior to the administration of FabAV.
- Some species of snakes, particularly the timber rattlesnake (*Crotalus horridus horridus*), have a principle in their venom that causes significant thrombocytopenia, which is resistant to reversal by antivenom therapy.
  - If platelet counts are significantly falling and/or are <10,000 to 20,000 cells/μL
    - Administration of (additional) antivenom and infusion of platelets may be indicated.
    - With most Crotalid envenomation, there is a mild thrombocytopenia in the range of 50,000 to 150,000 cells/μL that is thought to be due to passive entrapment of platelets within the previously described soft fibrin network and does not support diagnosis of disseminated intravascular coagulation (DIC).
    - Platelet count often will rebound within the day as the soft fibrin network is quickly cleaved by endogenously generated plasmin.

TABLE 32.4

SUMMARY OF THERAPEUTIC MEASURES FOR PIT VIPER ENVENOMATION

- Obtain IV access and administer crystalloid as indicated.
- Obtain CBC, PT, PTT, and platelet count every 6–12 h.
- Estimate severity of envenomation:
  - Species of snake
  - Age, health status of victim
  - Rate of progression of signs/symptoms
- Administer FabAV per Table 32.3.
- Follow rate of progression of signs/symptoms after FabAV administration.
- Determine tetanus vaccination status.
- Seek consultation from experts or a poison center (1.800.222.1222), especially if less experienced in treating snake envenomation.

CBC, complete blood count; PT, prothrombin time; PTT, partial thromboplastin time.

Surgical Procedures

- Surgical procedure for the wound is rarely indicated.
- Antibiotics are generally not employed, as they are of questionable assistance, and their routine use is not recommended.
- Tetanus vaccination status should be ascertained as being up to date.

Observation

- Best to have the extremity clearly visible so as not to compromise the evaluation
  - No covering dressings or wraps are recommended.
  - Once the patient is at the hospital and receiving antivenom, the extremity should be elevated above the level of the heart.
  - Monitoring is usually best performed in the ED.

- Subsequent admission to the intensive care unit (ICU) may be needed, although ICU therapy should not be considered a standard of care.
- Usual length of hospitalization required is 4 to 6 days.
- For up to 24 hours, we often observe patients—either in the emergency department or in the hospital—who are deemed to have no envenomation or mild envenomations and who do not receive antivenom because of the very high incidence of concurrent inebriation, which would allow for the possibility of inadequate history or incomplete evaluation and follow-up.

Prognosis

- Nearly all North American pit viper bites result in some near-instantaneous local tissue destruction.
  - Should not be expected to be totally absent or to resolve, even with the very best and most rapid care
- Most edema and swelling that does occur after antivenom treatment lasts only for a month or two, with longer recovery times seen in older or debilitated patients.
- In general, there is a total return of function to the bitten extremity.
  - Some patients can experience mild stiffness, atrophy, and weakness for up to a year or more.
- Patients who are bitten by snakes tend to continue their risky behavior, resulting in the finding that re-envenomation is not rare.

SNAKES NONNATIVE TO THE UNITED STATES

Major Problems

- The severity and spectrum of effects in envenomation varies widely.
  - Life-threatening effects may be seen, and fatalities do occur.

Epidemiology

- About 3,000 snake species in the world
  - Fewer than 300 are dangerous to humans.
  - Venomous reptiles include the families Atractaspididae Colubridae, Crotalidae, Elapidae, Helodermatidae, and Hydrophiidae.
  - Between 40 and 50 nonnative snake envenomations occur yearly in the United States.
  - Certain families, genera, and species are more commonly encountered.
    - Cobras (family Elapidae) account for one-third of all nonnative venomous snake exposures, and 86% of Elapids
      - *Naja naja, Naja nigricollis,* and *Ophiophagus hannah* are the most commonly involved Elapid species.
    - Viperids account for 46% of all nonnative venomous snake exposures.
      - *Bothrops, Bitis,* and *Lachesis* genera accounting for 33%, 19%, and 11% of these, respectively.
      - *Bothrops goodmanni, Bothrops schlegeli, Bitis gabonica,* and *Lachesis mutus* the most commonly encountered viperid species.

- Almost one-third of nonnative envenomations develop major to moderate symptoms and signs of disease, and are admitted to an ICU.
- Case fatality rate of approximately 1% is significantly greater than in native snakebites
- Males are involved in 84% of bites, a percentage similar to that in native bites.
  - Almost 15% are ages 17 years or less, and approximately 7% are ages 5 years or younger, most likely as a result of private collections in home settings.
- Potential penalties for possession of venomous animals in some jurisdictions may result in the withholding of critical information.
- A qualified herpetologist should be consulted for the identification of nonnative snakes that are otherwise unidentified.
  - Presence of a puncture and typical appearance of the site, progression of findings, and consistent laboratory abnormalities of a snakebite, indicate the possibility even with no history.

Pathophysiology

- The venom glands of poisonous snakes are modifications of salivary glands.
- The venom of a single snake is a complex mixture of enzymes, nonenzymatic proteins and peptides, and other substances.
- Some of these components may be found in all venomous snakes, with mixed clinical effects. The most important deleterious components of snake venom are shown in Table 32.5.
- Elapid venoms vary widely among species but contain more neurotoxins and cardiotoxins, resulting in various expressions of nerve and cardiac toxicity.
- Sea snakes have venom similar to elapids.

Diagnosis and Monitoring

- **Size and species:** In general, larger snakes contain and deliver more venom.
  - Fatal envenomations may result from juvenile snakes.
- **Quantity injected:** As many as 30% of Crotalid bites and 50% of Elapid bites may result in no envenomation.
  - When venom is injected, the amount may be reduced by poor penetration of the fang or high tissue pressures, as in fingertips.
  - Volume of available venom may also be reduced by recent previous feedings.
- **Bite location:** Tissues and anatomic areas with a low capacity for swelling or which are functionally important, such the fingers or hand, are particularly at risk of both short- and long-term impairment.
- Destructive effects of proteolytic enzymes may directly damage tissues.
- Tissue pressures may be significantly elevated, and vascular compromise may occur.
- Lower-extremity bites may damage venous valves and produce long-term dependent edema.
  - Decreased mobility and mobilization after a bite may predispose to deep venous thrombosis or other morbidities.

TABLE 32.5

SOME COMPONENTS OF SNAKE VENOM

Component	Viperid	Elapid	Effect
Proteinases	+++	+	Tissue destruction; hematologic effects
Hyaluronidase	++	++	Hydrolyzes connective tissue stroma; promotes spread
Cholinesterase	+	++	Catalyzes hydrolysis of acetylcholine
Phospholipase A_2	+++	+	Hemolysis; may potentiate neurotoxins; myonecrosis
Phosphodiesterase	+	+++	Unknown
Neurotoxins	+	+++	Flaccid paralysis; muscle fasciculation
Cardiotoxins	+	+++	Depolarizing; depression; rhythm disturbances

+ = usually minimally present; ++ = usually moderately present; +++ = usually extensively present.

- **Age and health of the victim:** Those at greatest risk of morbidity and mortality include patients with long delays to treatment, those with significant comorbid conditions, and those at the extremes of age.
  - Because of smaller body mass, children receive a relatively greater dose of venom.
- **Symptoms and manifestations:** As snakes can, to some extent, control whether and how much venom to deliver and as other factors may affect the quantity and specific components available and delivered, it is difficult to make an *a priori* determination of the clinical potential of the envenomation.
- *Local effects:* Snake venom that produces local effects causes pain and edema at the bite site, erythema, ecchymosis, and occasional bleb formation. Later, the increased membrane permeability and cellular destruction produced by proteases result in spreading edema both distally and proximally and may cause tissue necrosis.
  - If there is concern for elevated tissue or compartmental pressures, they should be measured directly (Stryker Intra-Compartmental Pressure Monitor System, Stryker United Kingdom; COACH Transducer, MIPM GmbH, Mammendorf, Germany).
  - Local venom effects will respond to adequate amounts of antivenom with cessation of progression of proximal edema and reduced tissue pressures.
  - Locally acting venom components are usually exhausted by 24 to 36 hours.
    - Resulting tissue injury may continue to develop over days to weeks.
  - Starting on the second day after envenomation, the clinical appearance of the bitten extremity, with increased heat and inflammation of the lymphatics, may be difficult to distinguish from an infective process.
- *Hematologic effects:* Coagulation alterations result from proteases acting on various parts of the coagulation cascade and may occur singly or in any combination.
  - Fibrinogenolysis may occur, resulting in decreased levels of fibrinogen and increased levels of fibrin degradation products.
  - Platelet inhibition, aggregation, or consumption may occur with abnormal function and/or decreased platelet counts.
  - Intravascular hemolysis has also been reported with some snake venoms.
  - The coagulation defects may result in local or systemic bleeding, including life-threatening hemorrhage.

- Laboratory tests, including a complete blood count (CBC) with platelet count, PT/INR, PTT, fibrinogen, and fibrin degradation products (or d-dimers)
- Most patients who will develop hematologic abnormalities will demonstrate them within 1 to 2 hours, although early use of antivenom may mask this finding.
  - Normal hematologic values at 6 hours suggests an absence of such effects.
- *Neurologic effects:* These may result from Atractaspid, Elapid, Helodermid, Hydrophiid, or Viperid envenomations.
  - Clinical effects can include sweating, numbness, paresthesias, convulsions, coma, muscle fasciculation, muscle weakness, and respiratory arrest.
    - Respiratory muscle paralysis is the primary cause of death with most Elapid and Hydrophiid venoms.
    - Coma may be secondary to hypovolemia or to a direct effect of the toxin.
    - Neurologic effects may develop rapidly, with respiratory arrest occurring within 15 to 30 minutes, but also may be delayed by many hours.
    - Measures such as the application of a pressure immobilization bandage (PIB) may also delay the onset of neurotoxicity.
    - Once neurologic effects occur, they may progress very rapidly.
    - Patients should be observed for a sufficient period of time, and preparations to manage the airway should be readily available.
      - Both antivenom and cholinergic agonists will generally stop the progression of effects and have been reported to result in either dramatic or more rapid improvement than would otherwise be expected.
      - Extubation criteria are based on standard tests of respiratory sufficiency.
- *Nonhematologic systemic effects:* Type I hypersensitivity reactions to venom (IgE or non–IgE mediated) with or without hypotension may occur; incidence is approximately 1%.
  - Characterized by wheezing, urticaria, laryngeal edema, and/or hypotension
  - Airway compromise from laryngeal edema may also occur
  - Incidence of type I hypersensitivity to antivenoms varies from <5% to 25%.
  - Other systemic findings common in snakebites are nausea, vomiting, diaphoresis, and pulmonary edema, especially in more severe cases.

○ Usually resolve in response to antivenom and rarely persist beyond the immediate postbite period.
- Type III hypersensitivity reactions—"serum sickness"—may occur in any patient who has received antivenom and are the result of circulating immune complexes.
  ○ Usually occur between 5 and 21 days after receiving antivenom and vary widely in incidence by antivenom utilized, from less than 5% to 100%

Diagnosis

- The diagnosis of snakebite may be a clinical one and should be suspected in any unknown presentation with any of the foregoing clinical manifestations.
- Immunoassays and bioassays have been used to identify various snake venoms in tissue within endemic areas; these are not available in the United States.
- A local zoo or aquarium may be of assistance in identifying the snake.

Management

- The management of clinically significant snake envenomation can be divided into first aid, specific antivenin therapy, and supportive therapy (Table 32.6)

TABLE 32.6

DIAGNOSTIC PEARLS

- Up to 30% of Viperid and 50% of Elapid bites do not result in envenomation.
- Signs and symptoms of envenomation may be delayed by many hours.
- Identification of the snake to the species level is required for antivenom selection.
- Viperid venoms usually produce (a) local tissue injury and (b) hematologic abnormalities and may also include (c) cardiovascular effects and (d) neurologic effects.
- Elapid venoms usually produce (a) neurologic toxicity, progressing to respiratory muscle paralysis, and may also include (b) local tissue injury and (c) hematologic abnormalities.
- Type I hypersensitivity reactions (anaphylaxis) may occur to venom or antivenom.
- Anaphylaxis, cardiotoxins, or fluid loss may produce hypotension.
- Local tissue injury may result in severe swelling, pain, and elevated tissue and/or compartmental pressures. Functional impairment, necrosis, and tissue loss may occur.
- Hematologic effects include impairment or consumption of platelets, fibrinogenolysis, hypofibrinogenemia, prolongation of PT/PTT, procoagulant effects, and other abnormalities, either singly or in combination; also, significant bleeding may occur.
- Neurologic effects include diplopia, ptosis, fasciculations, respiratory muscle paralysis, and arrest. Viperids may cause weakness but usually not respiratory compromise.
- Other venom effects include tachycardia, nausea, vomiting, diaphoresis, and anxiety.
- Wound infection is uncommon, documented in fewer than 5% of cases.
- Local effects may continue or recur for the first 24–36 h, and hematologic effects may continue or recur for up to 3 wk.

PT, prothrombin time; PTT, partial thromboplastin time.

TABLE 32.7

PREHOSPITAL MANAGEMENT

- A pressure immobilization bandage (PIB, a crepe bandage wrapped at lymphatic pressure tension from the distal to proximal aspects of an extremity) or lymphatic constriction band (a blood pressure cuff inflated to 15 to 25 mm Hg) will retard progression of venom into the general circulation.
- Prehospital management is indicated with Elapids; in Viperids with early, severe, systemic effects; and possibly when there are long transport times
- The bitten body part should otherwise be kept gently splinted, slightly below heart level. It may be lowered further if systemic effects are seen, and elevated for excessive swelling.
- At least one large-bore IV should be initiated.
- The offending snake should be identified to the species level, if possible.
- If available, antivenom should accompany the patient.
- The victim should be rapidly transported by emergency medical services to a health care facility.
- Contraindicated management approaches
  - Arterial or venous tourniquets
  - Incision, excision, heat, cold, electricity, or other local wound manipulations
  - Suction devices, which are not effective and should not delay transport to definitive care

---

- **Online antivenom index:** Initiation of efforts to obtain the appropriate antivenom should not wait until symptoms or signs develop; should be done immediately
  - The online antivenom index is a resource for determining the appropriate antivenom(s) for any given snake and maintains a continuously updated listing of zoo antivenom stocks and contact information; accessible by regional poison centers (1-800-222-1222).
- **First aid:** In general, the patient should get away from the snake, and the snake should be secured by a qualified individual (Table 32.7).
  - Pre-existing medical information, information regarding the biting species, and any available antivenom should be transported with the patient.
  - Bitten body part should be splinted to slow the passage of venom into circulation.
  - With envenomations from known neurotoxic snakes, generally the Elapids and sea snakes, the application of a PIB (a wide crepe bandage wrapping the entire extremity from distal to proximal at lymphatic compression pressures) or a lymphatic constriction band (i.e., a blood pressure cuff inflated to 15–25 mm Hg) has been shown to slow central compartment spread of venom and reduce the risk of out-of-hospital respiratory arrest, and thus should be routinely employed.
  - Hypotension, airway compromise, or other signs of a severe type I hypersensitivity reaction are examples of appropriate indications for the use of a PIB or lymphatic constriction band in a Viperid bite.
  - Prior to arrival at a hospital and administration of antivenom, the bitten area should be kept at or slightly below the level of the heart.
    ○ Dependent position may be used if rapid, severe systemic effects are occurring.

TABLE 32.8

HOSPITAL BITE SITE AND WOUND MANAGEMENT

- If previously applied, a pressure immobilization bandage (PIB) or lymphatic constriction band (LCB) should not be removed until antivenom is being administered or a decision has been made to observe without antivenom.
- Wash the bite site, apply antibiotic ointment, leave it otherwise uncovered, and provide tetanus immunization updating as needed.
- Once antivenom has been initiated, or a decision has been made not to administer it, keep a bitten extremity elevated with periodic assessment of edema (and tissue pressures if indicated), and monitor for development or progression of systemic symptoms.
- Management of progressive tissue edema and elevated tissue or compartmental pressures is by adequate amounts of antivenom and elevation, if tolerated.
- Frankly necrotic tissue should be debrided.
- There is little to no role for dermotomy or fasciotomy.

- Transport to a health care facility should be by paramedic ambulance.
- Initiation of two, large-bore intravenous lines is a sensible precaution.
- **Hospital care:** Basic wound care should be provided, including updating the tetanus status. After period of observation—8 to 24 hours—depending on the species of the snake, if the victim demonstrates no signs or symptoms of envenomation, release from the hospital (Tables 32.8 through 32.10).
- **Surgical management:** Frankly devitalized tissue, usually becoming evident several days following an envenomation, should be debrided.
  - Because high concentrations of venom have been found in blisters overlying the bite area, unroofing these should be considered.
  - Fasciotomy or dermotomy have been advocated for compartment syndrome or tense tissue edema potentially affecting blood flow.

TABLE 32.9

HOSPITAL ANTIVENOM MANAGEMENT

- Antivenom is the definitive management of snake envenomation, when it is available.
- Antivenom for an exotic species can be located via the Online Antivenom Index. Poison centers (1-800-222-1222) can assist.
- When available, species-specific antivenom should be used.
- Skin testing is indicated if recommended by the manufacturer.
  - Skin tests are neither sensitive nor specific to predict hypersensitivity reactions.
  - A positive reaction does not preclude antivenom administration.
  - Skin testing should not delay administration of antivenom in a life- or limb-threatening envenomation.
- Exotic antivenoms are imported under Investigational New Drugs licenses and, if used, appropriate reports need to be made to the hospital's institutional review board (IRB) and the Food and Drug Administration (FDA).

TABLE 32.10

HOSPITAL SYMPTOMATIC MANAGEMENT

- Hypotension
  - May be due to a type I hypersensitivity reaction to venom or to antivenom, cardiotoxins, or fluid loss.
  - Management is with Trendelenburg positioning, crystalloid fluid expansion, pressors, anaphylaxis treatments (epinephrine, H_1 and H_2 blockers), and antivenom (if believed to be secondary to venom).
- Neurologic effects
  - Should be managed with antivenom and mechanical airway support as needed.
  - Cholinergic agonists, such as neostigmine, may be used as adjunctive or substitute managements of muscle weakness in some Elapid envenomations.
- Hematologic effects
  - Severe or multicomponent abnormalities are managed primarily with antivenom.
  - Blood products are reserved for clinically significant hemorrhage and are given with additional antivenom if needed.
  - Some effects (e.g., platelet aggregation) may be readily reversed, while other processes (e.g., fibrinogenolysis) may be stopped, with components returning to normal levels by their natural replenishment.
- Other systemic effects are managed with symptomatic and supportive care.
  - Parenteral opioids may be required for pain.
- Recurrence of local and/or hematologic venom effects may occur.
  - Patients at high risk should be closely monitored, especially after discharge.
  - Additional antivenom should be considered for recurrent local effects in the first 24 h or recurrent severe or multicomponent hematologic abnormalities.

- **Other supportive therapies:** These include basic wound care and updating tetanus status.
  - Ventilatory support and hemodialysis may be necessary for pulmonary and renal complications of severe envenomation.
  - Corticosteroids may be used for hypersensitivity reactions to venom or antivenom.
  - Antibiotics are indicated for documented infection or in the presence of frank necrosis.
- **Hypersensitivity reactions:** If a type-I hypersensitivity reaction develops, the antivenom infusion should be stopped.
  - Anaphylactoid reactions are primarily related to rate of infusion, and stopping the infusion often results in rapid improvement.
  - Anaphylactic reactions (i.e., those IgE-mediated) are often dramatic and continue to progress after the infusion has been stopped.
  - Standard managements should be used. If symptoms persist, the patient should be treated with H_1 (e.g., diphenhydramine, 50 mg IV) and H_2 (e.g., ranitidine, 50 mg IV) blockers. Wheezing may respond to β-adrenergics by nebulizer (e.g., albuterol). If there is hypotension or laryngeal edema, epinephrine, either subcutaneously or intravenously, should be considered.
  - Antivenom should be withheld until the reaction has subsided and then a determination made whether to restart it.

TABLE 32.11

POSTDISCHARGE MANAGEMENT

- Physical therapy may be helpful in minimizing the extent and duration of functional impairment.
  - Type III hypersensitivity reactions ("serum sickness"):
  - They usually develop between 5 and 14 d following antivenom administration.
  - The incidence varies from fewer than 5% to greater than 80% of cases depending on the antivenom, host, and other factors.
  - Nonsteroidal anti-inflammatory drug analgesics and antihistamines are usually sufficient for symptomatic care.
  - Severe reactions may have renal involvement and require steroids and, in rare cases, rehospitalization.
- Patients with significant hematologic abnormalities, especially those treated with Fab antivenoms, may be at risk of recurrent effects after discharge.
  - Close follow-up is necessary for at least 2 to 4 d to detect recurrence.
  - Consider readministration of antivenom for clinical bleeding or multicomponent or severe hematologic abnormalities, especially with comorbid conditions.

○ If restarted, the patient should receive pretreatment with H_1 and H_2 blockers and the infusion begun more slowly.
- **Postdischarge considerations:** Desirable to see patients at least once post discharge to monitor for persistent or recurrent hematologic effects if indicated or tissue injury and its sequelae.
  - To refer for physical or occupational therapy in order to maximize functional recovery
  - Patients should also be cautioned about the possible risk of sensitization to snake venoms or antivenoms regarding possible future envenomations (Table 32.11).

SPIDERS AND SCORPIONS

Spiders

- In the United States, only two groups of spiders are typically considered medically significant.
- These are the widow or *Latrodectus* spiders and the brown spiders belonging to the *Loxosceles* genus.

Widow Spiders (Latrodectus Genus)

- Widow spiders, including the well-known black widow, belong to the *Latrodectus* genus
- Widow spiders are found throughout most of the country but are most common in the southeast, with the black widow (*Lactrodectus mactans*) believed to cause most envenomations.
- The female black widow, more harmful to humans than the male, as her fangs are longer and better able to penetrate human skin, has a shiny black round abdomen and a characteristic bright red hourglass marking on her underside.
- Considered shy spiders and can be found in dark, secluded areas such as under leaf litter
- All widow spiders worldwide are believed to have similar venom characteristics and similar clinical symptoms.

- **Pathophysiology:** The primary component of widow spider venom that causes human clinical effects is α-latrotoxin.
  - Binds to neuronal tissue and causes neurotransmitter release in at least two ways:
    - Binds to and helps form ion channels, which allow calcium and other ions to leak, causing a calcium-dependent release of neurotransmitter
    - Binds to the latrophilin receptor on neuronal tissue, and causes a calcium-independent release of synaptic vesicles
- **Diagnosis:** Diagnosis is primarily clinical and historical, as there are no laboratory tests to confirm envenomation.
  - Bite victims will recall a painful pin pricklike bite, but the bite can be painless.
    - Historically are associated with outhouse use
    - Can also occur when dressing or putting on shoes, especially if they are left outside, or even while in bed
- **Clinical effects–local:** Can produce mild local irritation
  - Bite is classically described as two small punctures with a small area of erythema surrounding a minimally blanched area centrally, producing a "halo" or "target" effect.
  - Local injection of venom is not believed to cause necrotic wounds.
  - Superinfection is uncommon.
- **Clinical effects–systemic:** The more medically significant effects after widow envenomation are the constellation of systemic symptoms known as *latrodectism*
  - Symptoms begin within an hour after the bite.
    - Local muscle cramps can progress to involve larger muscle groups, spreading continuously from the site of the bite.
    - Abdominal muscles can be involved, leading to abdominal rigidity that can imitate the peritoneal signs of a perforated viscus and which may result in an incorrect diagnosis in the young child or uncommunicative adult.
    - Priapism
    - Compartment syndrome
    - Elevations in creatine kinase
    - Myocarditis
    - Hypertension has been reported and could be life threatening in susceptible populations.
- **Management:** Though the *Latrodectus* venom is very potent, the volume of venom is minuscule.
  - No role for tourniquets, incision, or excision at the venom injection site
  - Initial control of pain and muscle contraction should be accomplished through administration of opiates and benzodiazepines.
  - IV calcium has not been shown to provide significant benefit and is no longer considered a first-line agent.
  - An antivenom specific to *L. mactans* is available ([*L. mactans*] Black Widow Spider Antivenin, Equine Origin, Merck & Co., Inc).
    - Risk of hypersensitivity reactions, including anaphylaxis and serum sickness
    - Use of antivenom is controversial.
      ○ Most would agree that when dealing with patients in the extremes of age, pregnant patients, or those with intractable muscle cramping and pain, the use of antivenom should be strongly considered.
      ○ The dose for adults or children is the contents of one restored vial (2.5 mL) of antivenom.
        – Can be given as an intramuscular injection but is typically administered as a slow IV infusion

– Can be redosed if needed, but one vial of antivenom is usually sufficient
- Evidence for cross-reactivity of antivenoms produced to various *Latrodectus* species, including a purified F(ab′)₂ antivenom produced in Australia to the red-backed spider (*Latrodectus hasselti*) by CSL Limited and which possesses an improved safety profile compared with the U.S. product
  - This antivenom is not currently approved for use in the United States; consultation with a regional poison center (1-800-222-1222) can be beneficial.
- **Follow-up:** Unless antivenom is administered, in which case monitoring for serum sickness should be arranged, there are no long-term sequelae expected from a widow spider envenomation.

Brown Spiders (Loxosceles Genus)

- *Loxosceles* spiders are found primarily in the southern half of the United States.
- *Loxosceles reclusa* species ("brown recluse") is the most common and medically important in the United States.
  - Considered shy spiders, hiding in woodpiles and dark corners, only biting when threatened
    - More common in warmer months and are often presumed to occur when a spider is caught next to skin by clothing or linens
- **Pathophysiology:** Venom from *Loxosceles* spiders is a complex mixture of cytotoxic components that indirectly cause impressive, delayed local symptoms and have the potential for causing human systemic toxicity.
  - Hyaluronidase in the venom causes significant tissue destruction, allowing spread.
  - Sphingomyelinase D in *Loxosceles* venom is believed responsible for the dermal inflammation seen after bites.
- **Diagnosis:** Because the bite is usually painless and thus unnoticed at the time, unless a *Loxosceles* bite is witnessed and positive identification of the spider occurs, the diagnosis is typically a historical and clinical one.
  - The necrotic wounds found with *Loxosceles* spider bites can mimic numerous other common cutaneous conditions, such as bites by other spiders or other insects, soft-tissue bacterial infections, or a vasculitis.
    - Broad differential, including these, as well as conditions such as erythema nodosum, pyoderma gangrenosum, pyogenic granuloma, and herpes infections, should be reviewed before a necrotic wound is attributed to a *Loxosceles* spider in the absence of a known bite.
  - Positive laboratory identification by ELISA or hemagglutination is possible to confirm *Loxosceles* envenomation in research settings but is not at this time clinically useful.
- **Clinical effects–local:** Unlike the widow spiders, the majority of clinical effects seen from *Loxosceles* spiders are a result of local tissue injury.
  - Characteristic necrotic wounds are described as having a "red, white, and blue" appearance.
  - Local tissue inflammation occurs over the first day after envenomation, causing skin erythema.
    - In the center of this reddened skin, a small necrotic or "blue" area develops that is surrounded by a halo of blanched tissue appearing gray or "white."
    - Often the wound is not noted until it begins to cause significant pain or the necrotic area becomes prominent.
- **Clinical effects–systemic:** Rarely, a *Loxosceles* spider bite can lead to a clinical syndrome known as *systemic loxoscelism*.

- Cases, many of them in children, begin as low-grade febrile illness with arthralgias and other nonspecific symptoms.
  - Within 24 to 48 hours after the bite, these symptoms can progress to a potentially life-threatening illness characterized by hemolysis and shock.
  - Systemic loxoscelism should be in the differential of unexplained hemolysis associated with shock.
- **Management:** Many pharmacologic and surgical treatments have been proposed in the management of the necrotic dermal wounds associated with *Loxosceles* spiders, but none has been proven to have significant effects in preventing or reversing damage.
  - Early attempts to "core" out affected areas to prevent venom spread result in poor wound healing and worsened scarring.
  - Systemic loxoscelism should be treated with symptomatic and supportive care.
    - Aggressive fluid resuscitation
    - Blood product transfusion
    - Vasopressor use

Nonnative Spiders

- The funnel web spiders (*Hadronyche* and *Atrax* spp.), native to Australia, and the banana spider (*Phoneutria* spp.), native to South America, are considered far more dangerous than the native *Latrodectus* and *Loxosceles* spiders.
- These can be found through collectors or as accidental stowaways in goods transported internationally.
  - The funnel web spider venom contains a potent neurotoxin that can cause fasciculations, weakness, and autonomic instability, with coma and pulmonary edema complicating the clinical course.
    - An antivenom available in Australia has been successfully used in severe envenomations.
  - The South American spiders belonging to the genus *Phoneutria* have a neurotoxic venom that can cause pain and neurologic and gastrointestinal symptoms and shock and pulmonary edema in severe cases.
    - An equine antivenom is available in South America.
  - Antivenoms may be located in the United States through the Online Antivenom Index, with the assistance of a regional poison center (1.800.222.1222).

Scorpions

- In United States, only one medically significant species of scorpion, *Centruroides exilicauda* (formerly *Centruroides sculpturatus*)
  - Found in the southwestern United States, primarily in southern Arizona, it is commonly known as the bark scorpion.
  - Stings occur by the tail, with the venom containing neurotoxins and other components.
    - Pediatric patients are at greatest risk of having clinically significant symptoms associated with such a scorpion sting.
    - Symptoms can be minor with only some local paresthesias but, for some, symptoms can be severe, including cardiac manifestations such as tachycardia and hypertension, neurologic manifestations such as roving eye movements and agitation, and respiratory manifestations, including tachypnea and stridor.
    - Cholinergic symptoms such as hypersalivation have also been reported.

- Treatment options in the past have included a goat-derived antivenom, limited to use within the state of Arizona.
  - No longer produced, however, and existing supplies are rapidly dwindling.
  - A F(ab')$_2$ antivenom is currently in clinical trials.
  - Continuous midazolam infusion, ventilatory support, and otherwise supportive and symptomatic care are current mainstays of treatment.
  - Atropine for excessive cholinergic signs has been recommended.

MARINE ANIMALS

Stingray

- Eleven different species of stingray are found in U.S. waters, seven of which are found in the Atlantic Ocean.
- Have long, sharp, serrated barbs along the dorsal surface of their tails, which can cause significant tissue damage and death, even without envenomation
- The tail barbs are covered in an integumentary sheath that covers two ventrolateral venom glands.
  - Their venom is a complex mixture that includes phosphodiesterase, nucleosidases, and serotonin.

Clinical Effects

- Burning pain at the wound site typically intensifies with time, and local symptoms may last up to 48 hours.
  - Venom can cause initial vasodilation and edema at the bite site, then vasoconstriction with hemorrhagic necrosis of tissue, and inflammatory infiltrate.
    - Cardiac conduction abnormalities ranging from bradycardia to atrioventricular nodal blocks with dysrhythmias and cardiac arrest from asystole have been reported.
    - Venom effects also include nausea/vomiting/diarrhea and abdominal pain and ataxia, seizure, coma, hypotension, and respiratory distress.

Treatment

- Treatment is symptomatic and supportive.
- Radiographic imaging and local wound exploration are necessary to evaluate for retained foreign body in the wound.
- Tetanus prophylaxis should be administered if needed.
- Prophylactic antibiotics to cover marine microorganisms should be considered, as secondary bacterial infections are common.
- Pain control with narcotic analgesia is often required.
- Immersion of the limb in hot water (110°F, 43°C) may aid in pain relief.
- Care should be taken to not produce thermal injury.
- Consider an observation period of at least 4 hours to ensure that symptoms do not progress to systemic effects.

Scorpaenoidea

- Group is composed of a number of venomous fish, and is the most common marine source of human envenomation, both in the wild and in home aquaria.
  - Found in the warm waters of the Gulf of Mexico and Florida Keys, as well as the Pacific, including around Hawaii, and the Indian Ocean

- Includes
  - Lionfish (*Pterois*)
  - Zebrafish (*Danio*)
  - Scorpionfish (*Scorpaena*)
  - Stonefish (*Synanceja*)
- Venom apparatus is a collection of spines along the body of the fish, each composed of paired venom glands covered by an integumentary sheath.
  - Dorsal spines are typically the most numerous and can inject the most venom.
  - Venom of the fish in this phylum is a complex mixture, and most contain significant amounts of inflammatory mediators such as thromboxane and prostaglandins.
    - The chemical makeup and potency of venom vary by species within this group, and clinical effects range from very severe (stonefish) to mild (lionfish).
    - Stonefish is by far the deadliest of this group; however, outside of zoos, educational institutions, and private aquaria, it is not likely to be encountered in the United States. It lives in the temperate and warm waters of the Australian and Indo-Pacific and east African coast.
    - Lionfish, zebrafish, and scorpionfish although not found wild in U.S. coastal waters, are a favorite of exotic fish collectors, and stings can result from pets kept in home aquaria.

Clinical Effects

- Majority of reported stings occur on hands and fingers, followed by local, excruciating pain.
  - Local swelling common, with few reported vesicular lesions at the bite site
  - Systemic symptoms are much less commonly reported but include nausea, sweats, chest and abdominal pain, and rarely hypotension.
  - Local effects, especially numbness, may persist long after the sting, and often wounds are very slow to heal, usually resulting in granulomatous and fibrous scarring.

Treatment

- Treatment is primarily by symptomatic and supportive care.
  - Exception is the stonefish, for which there is an antivenom.
    - Can be located by contacting a regional poison center (1.800.222.1222)
  - Good wound care is also essential.
    - Spines may break off during envenomation, and the wound should be closely inspected for any retained foreign body.
    - Immersion of the limb in nonscalding hot water (110°F, 43°C) may aid in pain relief.
    - Unroofing of any blisters that form at the envenomation site is indicated as the vesicle may contain venom and contribute to persistent effects.
    - Tetanus immunization or booster should be administered as needed.
    - Antibiotics should be given if secondary infection develops.

Sea Snakes

- Approximately 50 species of sea snakes in several subfamilies
- Found primarily in the warm tropical waters of the Indo-West Pacific

- None are found in the Atlantic Ocean or Caribbean Sea.
- Envenomations are likely the result of such snakes being kept in zoos or academic institutions or kept by private collectors.
- Venom is similar to Elapid venom, with neurotoxicity—and potentially respiratory arrest—as the primary clinical effect. See the earlier section, **Snakes Not Native to the United States,** for management considerations.

Invertebrates

- Five phyla—Cnidaria, Porifera (sponges), Echinodermata (sea urchins, starfish), Mollusca (octopi and cone snails), and Annelida (bristle worms)—constitute the venomous invertebrates.
- More than 10,000 species in the phylum Cnidaria (formerly Coelenterata), and several hundred are dangerous to humans.
  - Includes jellyfish (class Scyphozoa), the Portuguese man-of-war and other sea hydroids (class Hydrozoa), and the sea anemones and fire corals (class Anthozoa)
  - All possess envenoming apparatus in the form of nematocysts.
- In jellyfish and hydroids, nematocysts are primarily on the tentacles, and each tentacle can contain thousands.
  - Each nematocyst is a spiral-coiled dart-like structure within venom sacs. Venom is injected when the barb penetrates the flesh of its prey.
  - Nematocysts that have become detached from the tentacle, tentacles of dead jellyfish, or detached tentacles can all still cause envenomation upon contact.
- The Portuguese man-of-war (*Physalia physalis*) is found in the Atlantic waters off the southern coast of the United States, especially from July through September.
  - Actually a complex colony of multiple hydroids
    - Body is pale blue and bell or bottle shaped and the tentacles may grow to more than 100 feet in length.
    - Venom is especially complex and also contains neurotoxins.
- The severity of the sting depends on the organism, the number of successful discharges, and the composition of the venom.
  - Like the majority of venoms, Cnidaria venoms are complex mixtures of many substances.
    - Commonly found chemicals include histamine, serotonin, alkaline and acid phosphatases, proteases, hyaluronidase, nucleosidases, hemolysins, and inflammatory mediators, among others.

Clinical Effects

- Most organisms in this grouping, with the exception of the Portuguese man-of-war, cause only mild local effects in humans.
  - Local effects consist of burning pain at the site of the sting, which may be severe, with swelling, erythema, and possible vesicle formation and ulceration of the area.
  - Regional lymphadenopathy may be seen.
  - Secondary infection and scarring are common.
- Anaphylactoid reactions can occur as well.
- Systemic effects, if any, are mild, but immune reactions such as erythema nodosum and reactive arthritis have been reported.
- Irukandji syndrome is a constellation of both local and systemic symptoms that occur in a delayed fashion after envenomation by an Australian jellyfish (*Carukia barnsi*).
  - Reports of a similar syndrome occurring in swimmers and divers off the coast of southern Florida, likely after exposure to another organism in the same genus, although the responsible organism has not yet been identified
- With envenomation by the Portuguese man-of-war
  - Immediate intense local pain at the sting site, with development of large, linear, erythematous welts where tentacles have contacted the skin
    - Often leave significant scarring
    - Systemic effects include nausea and vomiting, headache, and myalgias and may progress to muscle weakness, respiratory distress, and cardiovascular collapse in severe envenomations.
    - Intense pain and occasional paralysis caused by many stings from this jellyfish can result in drowning.
    - Multiple stings can be fatal.
- Fire coral (*Millepora*) is not a true coral, rather a relative of fresh water hydra, but has nematocysts to envenomate its prey.
  - Stings cause local burning pain, urticaria, and intense pruritus.
  - Wheals may take weeks to heal completely and may leave hyperpigmented scars.
- Scyphozoa contain the "true" jellyfish, including the deadly box jellyfish (*Chironex fleckeri* or sea wasp), which is not found in U.S. waters, and is present here in zoo, institutional, and possibly private collections only.
- Usually found in tropical climates of the Indian and Pacific Oceans, including the coastal waters of Australia
- Box jellyfish is so named because of its four translucent panels that roughly form a box.
  - Sting of the box jellyfish is painful and can cause death within minutes.
    - Mortality rate in native settings is 15% to 20%.
    - An antivenom is available and should be stocked by the institutions that house these creatures; antivenom can be located by contacting the regional poison center (1.800.222.1222).
- Scyphozoa also include sea nettles (*Dactylometra quinquecirrha*), which pose a greater chance of exposure to swimmers of this country.
  - Sting in most cases is a minor annoyance.
  - Systemic symptoms similar to those seen with Physalia envenomations have been reported.

Treatment

- Swimmers and divers in waters endemic for venomous animals and health care providers caring for victims of envenomations should wear gloves and clothing for personal protection.
  - If stung, any nematocysts still on the skin should be inactivated with 5% acetic acid (vinegar) and then removed by "shaving" the area with a dull-edged knife or the edge of a credit card.
    - Shaving cream may aid in the shaving process.
    - Adhesive tape may also be effective at removing unseen nematocysts.
    - Papain meat tenderizer has been reported to improve symptoms and may be used with caution.
    - Alcohol or fresh water may cause the remaining nematocysts to fire and should not be used.
    - A few species' nematocysts will fire in the setting of acetic acid, including the American sea nettle, the little mauve stinger jellyfish, and the hairy or lion's mane jellyfish.

○ For these few, a slurry of baking soda should be applied for at least 10 minutes over the affected area.

○ If tentacles remain attached to the skin, a vinegar or baking soda slurry should be applied, then shaving cream and scraping as for nematocysts to remove the tentacles.

• Many components of the venoms of these organisms are heat-labile, and immersion of the affected area in non-scalding hot water (110°F, 43°C) may aid in pain relief.

• Tetanus prophylaxis should be given as needed.

• Third-generation cephalosporin used for secondary infection

• Pain should be treated with both nonsteroidal anti-inflammatory drugs and opioids as needed.

• Persistent pruritus and swelling should be treated with antihistamines.

• Systemic steroids have not been shown to be of any benefit.

Sea Lice (Seabather's Eruption)

• The prolific time period for the appearance of sea lice is March through June on the southeast coast of Florida.

• Contact dermatitis can develop with exposure to the larvae of sea lice (*Linuche unguiculata*).

• The larvae attach to the fibers in bathing suits and cause a rash in the distribution of the swimwear, thus "seabather's eruption."

• The rash is pruritic, erythematous, and maculopapular and typically resolves spontaneously in hours to days without sequelae.

• Topical treatment with antihistamines and calamine lotion may give relief.

Sponges

• Some sponges contain spicules composed of calcium carbonate and silica, which can cause local irritation and itching of skin upon contact.

• Also known as "skin diver's" or "sponge fisherman's" disease

• The fire, red, and bun sponges also have toxins in their coatings that can cause local irritation, which may be painful and pruritic and produce erythema.

• Pain and paresthesias after contact may persist for weeks.

Treatment

• Remove spicules with adhesive tape or the edge of a dull knife or credit card.

• Washing the area with 5% acetic acid may aid in symptom control.

• Antihistamines and nonsteroidal antiinflammatory drugs may be used for symptom control.

Mollusca

Conus Snails

• Cone shell snails have an ejectable tooth at the end of a long flexible proboscis and envenomate their prey by sinking this tooth deep into the flesh.

• Venom contains primarily neurotoxins that act by ion channel effects.

• **Clinical effects:** Clinical effects include local burning pain, numbness, and paresthesias.

• Systemic effects of perioral paresthesias, cranial nerve palsies, coma, respiratory muscle paralysis, and cardiovascular collapse are reported.

• Majority of human envenomations are mild and limited to local effects.

• About 15 deaths have been reported.

• **Treatment:** Treatment is primarily symptomatic and supportive.

Toxic Octopi

• Other marine animals may cause serious, and at times fatal, envenomations.

• Bite of the blue-ringed octopus introduces tetrodotoxin, a potent neurotoxin also found in the puffer fish, and several other neurotoxins, including maculotoxin.

• This organism is of importance, as it may be found in zoo aquaria and the home aquaria of private collectors in the United States.

• The giant monster octopus should not be of concern in the United States.

Clinical Effects

• Clinical effects include local pain, numbness, and paresthesias, which may also involve distant sites such as the lips and tongue.

• Cranial nerve palsies can be seen.

• In severe envenomations, muscle weakness progressing to respiratory paralysis and cardiovascular collapse occurs.

Treatment

• Treatment is primarily symptomatic and supportive care.

• Respiratory and cardiovascular support may be required.

• No antivenom is available.

Echinodermata

• Crown of thorns (*Acanthaster planci*) is found primarily in the Indo-Pacific Oceans.

• Of little concern in the United States except when encountered in zoo, academic institution, and private collector aquaria

• Sharp, rigid spines over the dorsum of the organism can cause deep puncture wounds, even through gloves.

• Venom delivered is a complex mixture of inflammatory mediators, histamine, and others including toxic saponins, with hemolytic and anticoagulant effects.

Clinical Effects

• Local effects predominate, such as burning pain and local hemorrhagic injury.

• Secondary infection and retained foreign body from broken spines are not uncommon.

• Systemic symptoms are rarely reported but may include nausea and vomiting.

• Immersion of the limb in nonscalding hot water (110°F, 43°C) may aid in pain relief, as the venom components are heat-labile.

Sea Urchins

- Many sea urchins have long, sharp spines composed of calcium carbonate that cause local injury, but most are not venomous.
- Deep tissue injury and extension of spines into organs and joint spaces may cause tissue destruction and morbidity from secondary infection.
  - If it is a venom-containing species, the gland is located at the end of the spines and in their pedicellaria (the mouthlike apparatus at the end of a stalk used to gather food).
  - Venom is composed of a mixture of steroid glycosides, serotonin, proteases, and others.

Clinical Effects

- Local pain, erythema, and edema are typically self-limited.
- Partial paralysis of the envenomated limb has been reported with exposure to some species.
- Rare systemic symptoms are noted in the literature.

Treatment

- Affected area should be immersed in nonscalding hot water (110°F, 43°C).
- Oral analgesics
- Local wound care and removal of any embedded spines as needed
- Care is otherwise symptomatic and supportive.

Annelid Worms

- The common bristle worm, found in Floridian and Caribbean waters, causes intense local inflammation with edema, erythema, and urticaria.
- No systemic reactions have been reported, and the toxin is unknown.
- Removal of any bristles adherent to the skin and otherwise simple symptomatic and supportive care are the mainstays of treatment.

CHAPTER 33 ■ PERIOPERATIVE PULMONARY FUNCTION TESTING AND CONSULTATION

- The **quantification** of pulmonary function has specific applications to clinical medicine in the intensive care unit setting, such as the following:
  - Confirming a clinical **diagnosis** of obstructive versus restrictive ventilatory defects in a patient with respiratory insufficiency or failure.
  - Following the course of the patient's **disease and the response** to treatment.
  - Enhancing **decision making** for patients about to undergo thoracoabdominal surgery.
  - Developing an **anesthetic and postoperative plan** for a patient with pulmonary disease

ROUTINE PULMONARY FUNCTION TESTING

- Although no test is "routine," there are three types of measurement and assessment of lung function that define the pulmonary status of a patient: (a) **spirometry**, (b) measurement of **lung volumes**, and (c) measurement of lung **diffusing capacity.**

Spirometry

- Spirometry is the most basic technique to assess lung function, and the most valuable.
- The patient is asked **to inhale to total lung capacity (TLC)** and then to **forcefully exhale** into a device that measures volume versus time. The ability to perform a forceful exhalation is key to obtaining an adequate study.
- To ensure that patient effort and cooperation are maximal, the procedure is repeated **three times,** and the spirometric curves are superimposed and compared.
- A patient with pulmonary impairment may have difficulty with this procedure, and an understanding technician is necessary.
- The patient is asked to use a **metered dose inhaler (beta$_2$ agonist)** and then repeat the forced vital capacity maneuver three more times to assess response to bronchodilators (Fig. 33.1).
- The results are compared to data provided by examining a normal population of men and women and seek to answer two additional questions: whether the patient has an **obstructive** or a **restrictive** physiologic defect.
- **Restrictive defects** are associated with a decrease in the **forced vital capacity** (FVC) of at least **20%** of the predicted value.
- **Obstructive defects** are revealed when the ratio of the forced expiratory volume in 1 second (FEV_1) divided by the FVC (the **FEV_1/FVC ratio**) is <85%. Other indications of obstructive lung disease include (a) the peak expiratory flow rate, a useful assessment in asthmatics, and (b) **maximal midexpiratory flow rate** measured at the midpoint of the FVC. The slope of the line between 25% and 75% of the FVC (**FEF 25%–75%**) is a better indication of obstructive lung disease due to chronic bronchitis (Fig. 33.2).

- Another method of representing a **maximal forced expiratory maneuver** depicts the FVC versus flow rather than versus time (Fig. 33.3). The forced exhaled volume between TLC and residual volume (RV) is the **maximal expiratory flow curve.** If the patient is asked to fully **inhale** back to TLC once the expiratory maneuver is completed, the flow–volume relationship is referred to as a **flow–volume loop.** This study is especially useful for diagnosing intrathoracic and extrathoracic upper airway obstruction.
- **Maximum voluntary ventilation** (MVV) is a test that involves repeated breaths and vigorous breathing for 10 to 12 seconds. The MVV is reported in liters per minute. Although it is only a rough index, the MMV assesses both **airway** status and respiratory muscle **endurance.**

Lung Volumes

- The lung volume study is completed by once again using the spirometer and coaching the patient to a full respiratory maneuver. Then, after quiet tidal breathing, the patient is asked to exhale to **RV**, then inspire fully to **TLC** and, after a second interval of quiet tidal breathing, fully inspire to TLC and expire to RV. Knowing the functional residual capacity **(FRC)** from the dilution studies (see below), all of the lung volume compartments can be calculated (see Fig. 33.2).

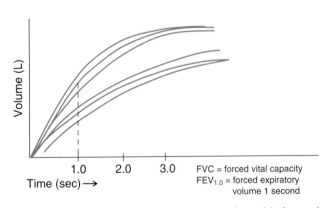

FIGURE 33.1. Three forced exhalations are performed before and after bronchodilator inhalation to assess immediate response. The maximum measured exhaled volume is FVC. The exhaled volume at 1 second is $FEV_{1.0}$. The $FEV_{1.0}$/FVC ratio is reduced with an obstructive ventilatory deficit.

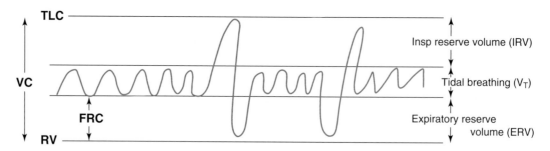

FIGURE 33.2. Compartmentalization of lung volume is achieved by noting the volume excursion during tidal breathing and repeated inhalation and exhalation. The functional residual capacity is measured using gas wash-in or wash-out techniques. TLC, total lung capacity; VC, vital capacity; FRC, functional residual capacity; RV, residual volume.

- There are two methods to measure residual volume: the **nitrogen washout** technique and the **inert gas helium** technique.
- RV, FRC, and TLC can be viewed as a system of concentric circles (Fig. 33.4).
- An **obstructive** ventilatory defect is characterized by **hyperinflation,** with a greater effect on **RV and FRC** than on TLC.
- A restrictive ventilatory defect can be either intrinsic or extrinsic. An **intrinsic restrictive** defect is characterized by a concentric reduction (each volume decreases by the same percentage). An **extrinsic restrictive** defect shows a disproportionate loss of volume "off the top" with the major change in TLC. The postoperative patient who has had a surgical procedure in the thorax or upper abdomen shows the latter change in physiology. Though transient, the extrinsic restrictive ventilatory change, especially when superimposed on a patient with obstructive physiology, can be significant.

Diffusing Capacity

- Diffusing capacity studies assess gas transfer at the **alveolo-capillary membrane.**

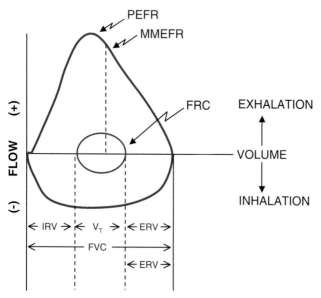

FIGURE 33.3. The relationship between a recording of flow and volume during a forced vital capacity (FVC) maneuver. ERV, expiratory reserve; FRC, functional residual capacity; IRV, inspiratory reserve; MMEFR, maximal midexpiratory flow rate; PEFR, peak expiratory flow rate; V_T, tidal volume.

- Oxygen is the gas transfer of interest, but making this measurement is difficult because there is always a back pressure or gas tension in the blood that must be compared to alveolar gas.
- This problem can be overcome by introducing a gas that is not normally in the bloodstream, specifically small amounts of **carbon monoxide** (CO). As CO is not a physiologic gas, this measurement is referred to as the *diffusing* capacity, not *diffusion* capacity.
- The measurement can be made in two ways, and there is controversy over which test gives superior information. The two methods include introducing CO into a breathing circuit and measuring the change in tidal breathing to a steady state and similarly inhaling CO with a single breath.
- If the tissue of an adult lung were microdissected and spread out, it would cover the space of a football field. Thus, one of the reasons for a decrease in diffusing capacity (as opposed to a **thickened alveolar-capillary membrane**) is **loss of effective surface area** for gas transfer. This is a pathognomonic change seen in patients with emphysema.
- When (a) **spirometry,** (b) **lung volumes,** and (c) **diffusing capacity** are all evaluated, there is a characteristic pattern of physiologic changes that identifies patient status and diagnosis, which is important in the care of the perioperative patient (Table 33.1).
- There is value in identifying the patients with obstructive lung disease who have emphysema, as opposed to chronic bronchitis, in assessing and designing postoperative therapy. Table 33.1 summarizes the findings for the various physiologic states.

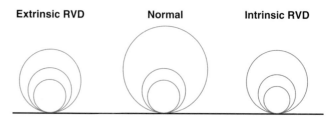

FIGURE 33.4. Changes in lung volumes with extrinsic and intrinsic restriction ventilatory defects (RVD) are compared to normal. An extrinsic RVD mainly alters the total lung capacity (TLC) with minimal alteration of the functional residual capacity (FRC) and the residual volume (RV). An intrinsic RVD results in concentric reduction of the TLC, FRC, and RV.

TABLE 33.1

PATTERNS OF PULMONARY PATHOLOGY MEASURED BY PULMONARY FUNCTION TESTS

		OVD_E	OVD_{CBR}	OVD_A	RVD_I	RVD_E
Spirometer	FVC	NL or ↓	NL or ↓	NL or ↓	↓	↓
	$FEV_{1.0}$/FVC	↓	↓	↓	NL or ↑	NL
	BD responder	0	10%	25%	0	0
	TLC	↑	NL or ↑	NL or ↑	↓	↓
	RV/TLC	↑	↑	NL or ↑	N	↓
	DLCO	↑	NL	NL or ↑	↓	NL
	PaO_2	NL or ↓	↓	NL or ↓	↓	NL or ↓
	$PaCO_2$	NL	↑	NL or ↑	NL	NL

OVD, obstructive ventilatory defect; OVD_E, emphysema; OVD_{CBR}, chronic bronchitis; OVD_A, asthma; RVD_I, intrinsic restrictive ventilatory defect; RVD_E, extrinsic restrictive ventilatory defect; FVC, forced vital capacity; $FEV_{1.0}$, forced expiratory volume at 1 second; BD, bronchodilator; TLC, total lung capacity; RV, residual volume; DLCO, diffusion capacity of the lung for carbon monoxide; PaO_2, arterial partial pressure of oxygen; $PaCO_2$, arterial partial pressure of carbon dioxide.

Arterial Blood Gas Analysis

- **Arterial blood gas** analysis is often ordered, but the usefulness is limited to an analysis of trends and diagnosis of underlying chronic disease.
- Prognostic value is limited, and for resectional lung surgery, postoperative arterial blood gases are often improved.

PREOPERATIVE PULMONARY FUNCTION TESTING

Resectional Lung Surgery

- The main indication for lung resection remains the removal of a lung cancer. These patients usually have a history of smoking. Presence of **obstructive lung disease** is not uncommon in these patients.
- Imaging studies have advanced such that the extent of the disease is well documented before surgery. However, until the surgeon explores the chest, the extent of the necessary resection for cure is not known.
- Preoperative evaluation should determine whether the patient can tolerate a pneumonectomy with guidance from pulmonary function testing as outlined in Table 33.2.

TABLE 33.2

PULMONARY FUNCTION INDICATING PHYSIOLOGICAL TOLERANCE FOR SURGERY UP TO AND INCLUDING PNEUMONECTOMY

Pulmonary function	Physiologic tolerance
FVC	50% predicted, or >3.0 L
$FEV_{1.0}$	2.0 L
$FEV_{1.0}$/FVC	50%
RV/TLC	<59%
DLCO	50% predicted
MVV	50% predicted

FVC, forced vital capacity; $FEV_{1.0}$, forced respiratory volume at 1 second; RV, residual volume; TLC, total lung capacity; DLCO, diffusion capacity of the lung for carbon monoxide; MVV, maximum voluntary ventilation.

- If the foregoing criteria are not met and surgical resection, including pneumonectomy, is being considered, the next step is to perform **split-lung function testing** and ascertain the contribution of the right versus the left lung to overall pulmonary function.
- Since the 1970s, the radionuclide **ventilation perfusion lung scans** have been used to determine split-lung function. For example, if the preoperative $FEV_{1.0} = 1.6$ L, and the scan reveals 60%/40% left lung versus right lung, and the right lung is being considered for resection, then:

$$1.6 \text{ L} \times .60 = .96 \text{ L, the calculated postoperative } FEV_{1.0}$$

- It was observed that the diseased lung often made little or no contribution to overall lung function, and the postoperative lung function was *better* than predicted. Therefore it was suggested that the requirement for the predicted postoperative $FEV_{1.0}$ be lowered from **1.0 L to 800 mL**, the level below which they noted respiratory failure and cor pulmonale occurring in the chronic obstructive pulmonary disease patients.

Non-cardiothoracic Surgery

- Whereas quantitative assessment of pulmonary function is useful for **thoracic surgery** patients, there is little evidence to suggest that measurement of pulmonary function should be obtained solely for the purpose of perioperative management of patients undergoing other types of surgery.
- Although certain types of surgery, such as upper-abdominal, non-resectional thoracic, and cardiac surgery, often cause severe alterations in pulmonary function (the FVC may be reduced as much as 50% the first postoperative day), little is added by the pulmonary function tests to the history and physical examination in terms of considering risk.

PREDICTING POSTOPERATIVE PULMONARY COMPLICATIONS

- **Postoperative pulmonary complications** are usually defined as newly developed **atelectasis, pneumonia, pulmonary thromboembolism,** and **acute respiratory failure** requiring mechanical ventilation *after* surgery.
- **Predicting** pulmonary complications cannot be done based solely on the measurement of pulmonary function but needs to include **patient risk factors**.

- The National Veterans Surgical Quality Improvement Program developed a multifactorial risk index for predicting postoperative pneumonia and respiratory failure after major non-cardiac surgery:
  - **Smoking status:** The duration of smoking cessation to achieve benefit appears to be at least 4 weeks, possibly as long as 8 weeks.
  - **Chronic obstructive lung disease,** as defined by history and physical examination (spirometry has not been shown to be useful in prognosis).
  - Measures of **general health status** include the presence/measures of comorbid conditions, functional status, and recent weight loss.
  - **Cognitive impairment** of any etiology
  - **Previous stroke**
  - Type and location of the **anticipated surgical procedure**
  - **Age:** a risk factor when controlled for comorbid conditions
  - Long-term **steroid therapy**
  - Recent moderate-to-heavy **alcohol** intake.
  - Impaired **renal function.**
  - **Large transfusion requirement:** generally >6 units of packed red blood cells, plus other blood products
- The use of **general anesthesia** for surgical procedures and the **duration** (more than 4 hours) have been associated with increased risk of **Postoperative pulmonary complications.** Advances in **anesthesia** technology and skills have allowed investigators to reframe the question. Does the presence of adequate **neuroaxial blockade** during a surgical procedure reduce risk? The anesthetic plan can include spinal anesthesia, epidural anesthesia, combined spinal/epidural anesthesia, and combined light levels of general anesthesia (the "epigeneral"). It does appear that the presence of neuroaxial blockade, either alone or in combination with general anesthesia, is associated with fewer deaths and complications.
- **Postoperative pain management** is an important goal that also enables a patient to complete deep breathing maneuvers.

STRATEGIES TO REDUCE POSTOPERATIVE PULMONARY COMPLICATIONS AFTER NONCARDIOTHORACIC SURGERY

- The general approach has included **cessation of smoking** and an attempt to maximize pulmonary function with the use of **bronchodilators** (both beta-2-agonists and parasympatholytic agents), treatment of underlying **infections** or purulent sputum, and coaching to learn **deep-breathing exercises.** Bronchodilators are continued throughout the anesthetic and surgical procedure.
- *Studies with good evidence:* **lung expansion** interventions including incentive spirometry, deep breathing exercises, and continuous positive airway pressure are useful in preventing PPCs.
- *Studies with fair evidence:* **selective** rather than routine use of **nasogastric tubes,** the use of **short-acting** intraoperative **neuromuscular blocking agents** (e.g., rocuronium vs. pancuronium) is associated with improved outcomes.
- *Studies with conflicting evidence:* Cessation of smoking, use of epidural anesthesia and analgesia, and laparoscopic ver-

sus open abdominal surgery demonstrate conflicting results. As noted above, the presence or absence of neuroaxial blockade—not the anesthetic choice—may be the determining factor. Laparoscopic procedures result in less pain and a lesser reduction in the FVC. Finally, although **malnutrition** is associated with increased risk, routine total enteral or parenteral nutrition may not reduce the risk.
- The value of **preoperative pulmonary function testing** has been repeatedly called into question. Preoperative pulmonary function testing is safe and noninvasive but should not be routinely performed; rather, it should be limited to a specific indication supported by changes in the anesthetic or surgical procedure.

Breathing Patterns

- Normal **tidal breathing** begins at FRC, a point where the tendency for the chest wall to spring outward is balanced by the tendency of the lung to collapse. The balance of these two forces occurs when there is complete apposition of the pleural surfaces. A tidal breath is an energy-transferring mechanism, the reason why exhalation is usually a passive phenomenon returning the lung volume to the normal FRC.
- Patients in respiratory distress alter their tidal **breathing patterns** according to the added load placed on the respiratory system. Patients with a **resistive load** will slow inspiratory or expiratory flows and **diminish the respiratory rate,** in an effort to obtain the best combination of rate and tidal volume/flow, to work against the imposed load. Patients with alterations in **compliance** reach the best combination of rate and tidal volume, which results in a **rapid respiratory rate** and smaller tidal volumes. In the latter patients, tracheal intubation, mechanical ventilation, and the addition of positive end expiratory pressure are used to support the patient.
- The reoccurrence of **rapid, shallow breathing** is used to assess the ability to wean a patient from positive pressure ventilation. The so-called *spontaneous breathing trial* involves watching the patient breathe with very low levels of positive pressure support, presumably enough to overcome the endotracheal tube resistance prior to extubation. Thus, rapid shallow breathing patterns, which can be measured by the rapid shallow breathing index, are used to assess the feasibility of weaning from ventilatory support (see Chapter 95).

SUMMARY

- Pulmonary evaluation is a critical step in managing patients with lung disease who are undergoing elective surgeries or are admitted to the ICU for respiratory insufficiency or failure. It allows confirmation of pathophysiology (restrictive vs. obstructive), follow response to treatment, assist with decision making regarding surgery and anesthesia, and plan for patient education and postoperative course.
- It is still not clear whether risk stratification can be assessed with the use of sophisticated or simple exercise tests and measurements.
- Efforts should be directed to anticipate and correct patient's physiologic response to surgery and improve outcome.

CHAPTER 34 ■ PREOPERATIVE EVALUATION OF THE HIGH-RISK SURGICAL PATIENT

- The perioperative mortality rate for **elective** surgical procedures is low, ranging from 0.001% to 1.9%.
- Age and the **American Society of Anesthesiologist (ASA) physical status classification** systems are good predictors of perioperative complications (Table 34.1).
- **Age >70 years and ASA** physical status ≥II are strong predictors of postoperative pulmonary complications.
- The **strength** of the ASA classification is its simplicity and its application to all age groups, medical conditions, and degrees of health. The **weakness** is its inability to distinguish among disorders of different systems and to cumulate risk based on multiple disorders.
- A **multidimensional model** of perioperative risk may be useful, including ASA physical status, surgical risk/invasiveness, physical factors affecting mask ventilation, intubation predictors, and a list of optional risk indicators. The acronym **ASPIRIN** is applied to this model.
- Initial assessment begins with **history and physical examination.** The data obtained from the history and physical examination allow for **preoperative testing based on clinical risk categorization.**
- Following the implementation of the **American College of Cardiology/American Heart Association (ACC/AHA) guidelines** for preoperative cardiac risk assessment allows cardiac testing to be done in a cost-effective manner.

CARDIOVASCULAR SYSTEM

Noncardiac Surgery

Of the approximately 44 million patients undergoing noncardiac surgery in the United States yearly, 30% either have, or are at risk for, **coronary artery disease** (CAD) with a 2.8-fold increase in adverse postoperative cardiac events.

- ACC/AHA Task Force on Practice Guidelines has recommendations on the perioperative cardiovascular evaluation for noncardiac surgery; the update is available at the following Web site: **www.acc.org/qualityandscience/clinical/statements.htm**
- The ACC/AHA guideline is an eight-step algorithm that incorporates **clinical predictors** based on the patient's history and physical examination, **surgery-specific risk,** and the functional capacity or **exercise tolerance** (Fig. 34.1).
- In the event of an **emergency procedure,** patients should be taken to surgery with no preoperative testing.
- If an elective or urgent procedure is planned, the decision making proceeds down steps 2 and 3 of the algorithm (see Fig. 34.1). If the patient has had a coronary revascularization procedure within the last 5 years with no recurrent symptoms or signs, no further workup is necessary. A cardiac evaluation performed within the last 2 years with no deterioration in cardiac status also negates the need for further workup.
- Steps 5 through 8 of the algorithm (see Fig. 34.1) integrate the **clinical predictor, surgery-specific risk,** and the **functional capacity** to determine whether the patient warrants further cardiac workup.
- The presence of major clinical predictors demands intense further workup and may result in delay or cancellation of elective surgery. Intermediate clinical predictors increase the risk of perioperative cardiovascular complications, whereas minor clinical predictors have not been proven to independently increase cardiac risk (Table 34.2).
- The nature and duration of the surgical procedure are strong predictors of cardiovascular morbidity and mortality (Table 34.3).
- Finally, the **functional capacity** of the patient must be evaluated, as it is a strong predictor of perioperative outcome. Functional capacity is expressed in **metabolic equivalents (METs),** where one MET is 3.5 mL/kg/min of oxygen consumption in a 70 kg, 40-year-old man at rest. Increasing levels of activity correlate with increasing METs, with strenuous sports requiring >10 METs (Table 34.4).
- Inability to perform **at least 4 METs** is associated with increased perioperative cardiac risk.
- Based on the aforementioned **triad of clinical predictors, functional capacity, and surgery-specific risk,** a decision is made regarding whether the patient can proceed to surgery or whether additional investigations to delineate the ischemic burden are required (Table 34.5).
- Delineation of the **ischemic burden** can be broadly achieved by two methods. The first method involves coronary vasodilatation and induction of a "steal" phenomenon by pharmacologic agents, followed by a nuclear imaging technique

TABLE 34.1

AMERICAN SOCIETY OF ANESTHESIOLOGISTS'
PHYSICAL STATUS CLASSIFICATION

Physical status	Definition
I	Healthy patient
II	Mild systemic disease; no functional limitation
III	Severe systemic disease; definite functional limitation
IV	Severe systemic disease that is constant threat to life
V	Moribund patient; unlikely to survive 24 h with or without surgery
VI	Brain-dead patient; organ donor
E	Emergency procedure

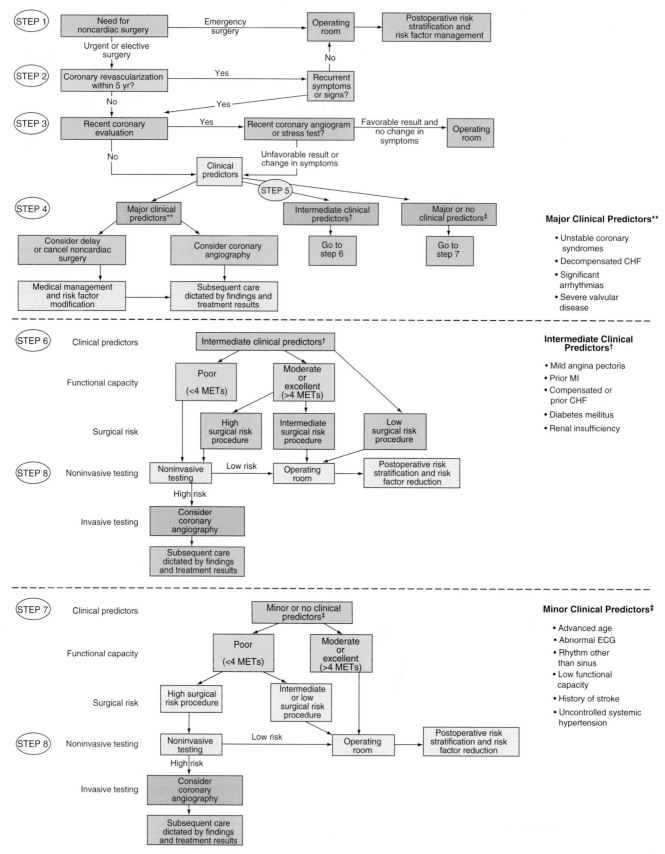

FIGURE 34.1. Stepwise approach to preoperative cardiac assessment. (Reproduced with permission from Eagle KA, Berger PB, Calkins H, et al. ACC/AHA Guideline Update for Perioperative Cardiovascular Evaluation for Noncardiac Surgery: a report of the American Heart Association/American College of Cardiology Task Force on Practice Guidelines [Committee to Update the 1996 Guidelines on Perioperative Cardiovascular Evaluation for Noncardiac Surgery]. *Circulation.* 2002;105:1257–1267.)

TABLE 34.2

CLINICAL PREDICTORS OF INCREASED PERIOPERATIVE CARDIOVASCULAR RISK (MYOCARDIAL INFARCTION, CONGESTIVE HEART FAILURE, DEATH)

Major
Unstable coronary syndromes
Acute or recent MI[a] with evidence of important ischemic risk by clinical symptoms or noninvasive study
Unstable or severe[b] angina (Canadian class III or IV)[c]
Decompensated heart failure
Significant arrhythmias
High-grade atrioventricular block
Symptomatic ventricular arrhythmias in the presence of underlying heart disease
Supraventricular arrhythmias with uncontrolled ventricular rate
Severe valvular disease

Intermediate
Mild angina pectoris (Canadian class I or II)
Previous MI by history or pathologic Q waves
Compensated or prior heart failure
Diabetes mellitus (particularly insulin-dependent)
Renal insufficiency

Minor
Advanced age
Abnormal ECG (left ventricular hypertrophy, left bundle-branch block, ST-T abnormalities)
Rhythm other than sinus (e.g., atrial fibrillation)
Low functional capacity (e.g., inability to climb one flight of stairs with a bag of groceries)
History of stroke
Uncontrolled systemic hypertension

MI, myocardial infarction; ECG, electrocardiogram.
[a]The American College of Cardiology National Database Library defines recent myocardial infarction as >7 days but ≤1 month (30 days).
[b]May include "stable" angina in patients who are unusually sedentary.
[c]Campeau L. Grading of angina pectoris. *Circulation.* 1976;54:522–523.
From Eagle KA, Berger PB, Calkins H, et al. ACC/AHA Guideline Update for Perioperative Cardiovascular Evaluation for Noncardiac Surgery: a report of the American Heart Association/American College of Cardiology Task Force on Practice Guidelines (Committee to Update the 1996 Guidelines on Perioperative Cardiovascular Evaluation for Noncardiac Surgery). *Circulation.* 2002;105: 1257–1267, with permission.

TABLE 34.3

CARDIAC RISK[a] STRATIFICATION FOR NONCARDIAC SURGICAL PROCEDURES

High (reported cardiac risk often >5%)
* Emergent major operations, particularly in the elderly
* Aortic and other major vascular surgery
* Peripheral vascular surgery
* Anticipated prolonged surgical procedure associated with large fluid shifts and/or blood loss

Intermediate (reported cardiac risk generally <5%)
* Carotid endarterectomy
* Head and neck surgery
* Intraperitoneal and intrathoracic surgery
* Orthopedic surgery
* Prostate surgery

Low[b] (reported cardiac risk generally <1%)
* Endoscopic procedures
* Superficial procedures
* Cataract surgery
* Breast surgery

---

[a]Combined incidence of cardiac death and nonfatal myocardial infarction.
[b]Do not generally require further preoperative cardiac testing.
From Eagle KA, Berger PB, Calkins H, et al. ACC/AHA Guideline Update for Perioperative Cardiovascular Evaluation for Noncardiac Surgery: a report of the American Heart Association/American College of Cardiology Task Force on Practice Guidelines (Committee to Update the 1996 Guidelines on Perioperative Cardiovascular Evaluation for Noncardiac Surgery). *Circulation.* 2002;105: 1257–1267, with permission.

* Currently, angioplasty is followed by placement of either a bare-metal or a drug-eluting stent; stents reduce both the acute risk of major complications and long-term restenosis rate. After placement of a stent, patients require **antiplatelet therapy** for 1 to 12 months, depending on the type of stent. The presence of antiplatelet therapy adds a new dimension of complexity to the patient presenting for noncardiac surgery after **percutaneous coronary intervention.**
* Elective surgery should be **delayed** for more than **6 weeks** to allow for endothelialization of the stent and discontinuation of antiplatelet therapy. In the event of **urgent surgery** and severe CAD, **angioplasty alone** with no stent placement can be performed. This obviates the need for prolonged antiplatelet therapy and the risk of perioperative bleeding.

Perioperative β-Blockade Therapy

* β-Blockers help to correct the imbalance between **myocardial oxygen demand and supply.** They have additional plaque-stabilizing, antiarrhythmic, anti-inflammatory, and altered gene expression effects.
* There may be a subgroup where there is potential harm with β-blocker use. Insufficient data are available regarding the use of β-blockade therapy in low–cardiac risk patients undergoing intermediate or high-risk surgery.
* Patients on β-blockers at home should be continued on β-blockers. Patients with a positive stress test undergoing vascular surgery should be started on β-blockers (ideally a week before surgery and titrated to heart rate-decreasing effect).

(dipyridamole-thallium scan). The second method involves increasing myocardial oxygen demand (by exercise stress or pharmacologically with dobutamine) and evaluating electrocardiographic or echocardiographic data for evidence of ischemia.

* The negative-predictive value of both tests is high. However, the positive-predictive value of dobutamine stress echocardiography is higher.
* Once the degree of myocardial ischemia is quantified, patients can either undergo **perioperative medical optimization or revascularization** by either percutaneous coronary intervention or surgery. It is important to note that to obtain benefit from a preoperative coronary intervention, the risk of noncardiac surgery must supersede the **combined risk** of both coronary catheterization and subsequent revascularization procedure.

TABLE 34.4

ESTIMATED ENERGY REQUIREMENTS FOR VARIOUS ACTIVITIES

1 MET	Can you take care of yourself? Eat, dress, or use the toilet? Walk indoors around the house? Walk a block or two on level ground at 2 to 3 mph (3.2–4.8 km/h)?
4 METs	Do light work around the house like dusting and washing dishes? Climb a flight of stairs or walk up a hill? Walk on level ground at 4 mph (6.4 km/h)? Run a short distance? Do heavy work around the house like scrubbing floors or lifting or moving heavy furniture? Participate in moderate recreational activities like golf, bowling, dancing, doubles tennis, or throwing a baseball or football?
>10 METs	Participate in strenuous sports like swimming, singles tennis, football, basketball, or skiing?

MET, metabolic equivalent.
Adapted from the Duke Activity Status Index and AHA Exercise Standards.
From Eagle KA, Berger PB, Calkins H, et al. ACC/AHA Guideline Update for Perioperative Cardiovascular Evaluation for Noncardiac Surgery: a report of the American Heart Association/American College of Cardiology Task Force on Practice Guidelines (Committee to Update the 1996 Guidelines on Perioperative Cardiovascular Evaluation for Noncardiac Surgery). *Circulation.* 2002;105:1257–1267, with permission.

TABLE 34.5

SUMMARY OF ACC AND AHA GUIDELINES FOR CARDIAC EVALUATION BEFORE NONEMERGENT, NONCARDIAC SURGERY

Risk of surgery	Major clinical predictors	Clinical predictors			
		Intermediate clinical predictors		Minor clinical predictors	
		Poor functional capacity	Good functional capacity	Poor functional capacity	Good functional capacity
High Emergent major operations, particularly in the elderly Aortic and other major vascular surgery Peripheral vascular surgery Anticipated prolonged surgical procedures associated with large fluid shift and/or anticipated blood loss	Postpone or delay surgery	Testing indicated	Testing indicated	Testing indicated	Testing not indicated
Intermediate Carotid endarterectomy Head and neck surgery Intraperitoneal and intrathoracic surgery Orthopedic surgery Prostate surgery	Postpone or delay surgery	Testing indicated	Testing not indicated	Testing not indicated	Testing not indicated
Low Endoscopic procedure Superficial procedures Cataract surgery Breast surgery	Postpone or delay surgery	Possible testing	Testing not indicated	Testing not indicated	Testing not indicated

ACC, American College of Cardiology; AHA, American Heart Association.
From Akhtar S, Silverman DG. Assessment and management of patients with ischemic heart disease. *Crit Care Med.* 2004;32(Suppl):S126, with permission.

- Although there is debate on the use of perioperative β-blockade use, ACC/AHA 2006 Guideline Update on Perioperative Cardiovascular Evaluation for Noncardiac Surgery: Focused Update on Perioperative Beta-Blocker Therapy has some recommendations until future results from multicenter trials are available (1).

Cardiac Surgery

- There are no standardized definitions for risk thresholds; many of the assessments of statistical risk are based on **odds ratios**. In addition, multiple risk factors frequently coexist, making risk profiling for the individual patient difficult. Steady improvement in cardiac surgical outcomes has been attributed to improving surgical technique, perioperative care, and patient selection.
- Cardiac risk evaluation can be performed by risk assessment tools based on large databases, such as the **EuroSCORE** and the **Society for Thoracic Surgeons** database.
- The **Society for Thoracic Surgeons** database working group has published their analysis of independent risk factors in valvular surgery (Table 34.6).
- **Scoring systems** have a role in predicting both perioperative and long-term mortality and intensive care unit resource use. They provide a framework for identifying and modifying preoperative risk.
- **EuroSCORE** is a compilation of risk factors as weighted by the Parsonnet, EuroSCORE, and Society of Cardiothoracic Surgeons databases. The percentages quoted in Table 34.7 are for *individual* risk factors in each section. Risk factors may be additive and/or synergistic.

Preoperative Risk Modification for Cardiac Surgery

- Preoperative risk modification involves **optimization of comorbidity** and limiting cardiopulmonary bypass–related myocardial injury.

Comorbidity

- **Renal dysfunction and failure** are significant risk factors in both valvular and coronary artery bypass graft (CABG) surgery. Increase in plasma creatinine of one-and-a-half times from baseline with short periods of oliguria may carry a 90-day mortality of 8%. Patients with **cardiogenic shock or an emergent indication** for surgery often have acute renal failure; these patients have a high risk of death perioperatively with a mortality above 40%.
- Survival rates at 8 years in dialysis-dependent patients were 45.9% for CABG, 32.7% for **percutaneous coronary intervention,** and 29.7% for no surgical intervention.
- **Diabetics** undergoing cardiac surgery are at increased risk of prolonged ventilation, postoperative sepsis, renal failure, and cognitive dysfunction. The perioperative management of diabetes and hyperglycemia in cardiac surgery is controversial. Insulin has been used in two strategies: tight glycemic control and as part of glucose-insulin-potassium regimens (GIK). Meta-analysis of GIK therapy indicates that trials using tight glycemic control gave the best results. This observation needs validation by other randomized trials.
- **Congestive cardiac failure** represents a complex neurohumoral syndrome that develops in response to altered cardiac

TABLE 34.6

PERIOPERATIVE RISK FACTORS FOR VALVULAR CARDIAC SURGERY

Surgical factors	Odds ratio	Patient factors	Odds ratio
High risk			
Aortic root replacement	2.78		
Isolated tricuspid replacement	2.26	4 Comorbidities	2
Emergent operation	2.11		
Multiple valve replacement	2.06		
Moderate risk			
Concurrent operation	1.58		
Reoperation	1.61	Age ≥70 years	1.88
Valve replacement vs. repair	1.52	3 Comorbidities	1.68
		Endocarditis	1.59
Low risk		Coronary artery disease	1.58
Isolated mitral replacement	1.47		
Year <1999	1.34	2 Comorbidities	1.41
Isolated pulmonic replacement	1.29	CHF	1.39
Isolated aortic replacement	1	Female gender	1.37
		Ejection fraction <0.35	1.34
		Average per comorbidity	1.19

Procedural risk is compared to the lowest-risk procedure—isolated aortic valve replacement.
The odds ratio for perioperative mortality during valvular surgery is compared to the lowest-risk valvular procedure (aortic valve replacement; odds ratio 1, mortality 5.6%).
CHF, congestive heart failure.
From Rankin JS. Determinants of operative mortality in valvular heart surgery. *J Thorac Cardiovasc Surg.* 2006;131:547, with permission.

TABLE 34.7

PERIOPERATIVE RISK FACTORS FOR CABG ACCORDING TO SCORING SYSTEM

Parsonnet score	EuroSCORE	UKSCTS complex Bayes
High risk (17%–40% mortality)		
Cardiogenic shock	Postinfarct septal rupture	Emergency surgery
Acute renal failure	Thoracic aortic surgery	LV EF <30%
Acute structural defect (e.g., VSD)	LV EF <30%	Dialysis
>80 y old	ARF	Creatinine >200 μmol/L (2.3 mg/dL)
	Preop IABP or inotropes	
	Preop ventilation	
	Active endocarditis	
	Reoperation	
	Age ≥75 y	
Significantly elevated risk (9%–17% mortality)		
75–79 y old	CABG plus major symptoms	Age >75 y
Third reoperation	Emergency	One or more previous operations
Dialysis dependency	Systolic PAP >60 mm Hg	BSA <1.70 m^2
Rare circumstances	Recent MI <90 days	
Recently failed intervention <24 h	IVI nitrates on arrival in theater	
PA pressure ≥60 mm Hg	Serum creatinine >200 μmol/L (2.3 mg/dL)	
AV pressure gradient ≥120 mm Hg	Neurology affecting ADL	
	Peripheral vascular disease	
	Age 70–74 y	
Elevated risk (3%–9% mortality)		
MV surgery PAP <60 mm Hg	LV EF 30%–50%	Age 71–75 y
AV surgery gradient <120 mm Hg	Chronic pulmonary disease	Left main stem disease
Recently failed intervention >24 h	Female	Diabetes
Aneurysmectomy	Age 65–69 y	Urgent surgery
Second reoperation		LV EF 30%–49%
Age 70–74 y		Hypertension
LV EF <30%		
Hypertension		
BMI >35		
IABP preoperative		
Female		

CABG, coronary artery bypass grafting; UKSCTS, United Kingdom Society of Cardiothoracic Surgeons; VSD, ventricular septal defect; LV EF, left ventricular ejection fraction; ARF, acute renal failure; IABP, intra-aortic balloon counter pulsation; PAP, pulmonary artery pressure; BSA, body surface area; MI, myocardial infarction; IVI, intravenous infusion; PA, pulmonary artery; AV, atrioventricular; ADL, activities of daily living; MV, mitral valve; BMI, body mass index.

function. The stages of this condition have been classified by the ACC/AHA (Table 34.8). In the perioperative period, decompensated stage C or D heart failure represents an independent risk factor for cardiac complications.

Myocardial Preservation Interventions

- Several nonpharmacologic and pharmacologic interventions can be initiated preoperatively to improve intraoperative and postoperative outcomes.
- **Intra-aortic balloon counterpulsation (IABP)** is a nonpharmacologic intervention that can be commenced preoperatively in the appropriate group of patients (Table 34.9).
  - Good evidence exists for the benefits of IABP in **CABG patients** with ischemia or with an ejection fraction <25% undergoing nonelective operation or reoperation or who have New York Heart Association class III to IV symptoms.
  - The efficacy of IABP for **valvular surgery** is poor and is associated with a twofold increase in mortality regardless of timing of use. This probably reflects the fact that the ven-

tricular dysfunction is either nonreversible or only partially reversible.
- IABP improves **cardiac output by approximately 20%** if set to maximal efficiency.
- **Pharmacologic therapies** include preoperative statins, β-type natriuretic peptide, calcium channel sensitizers, and antioxidant therapy.
  - **HMG CoA reductase inhibitors**, known as **statins**, have several beneficial effects. Their mechanism of action is via a lipid-dependent and a lipid-independent pathway. Statins inhibit atherogenesis, thrombosis, and inflammation and maintain endothelial integrity. Preoperative statin therapy was associated with a 1.1% absolute reduction in mortality after CABG (OR 0.25; CI 0.07–0.87), and cessation of statin therapy after surgery was associated with an increased in-hospital and late cardiac mortality.
  - **Brain natriuretic peptide.** Nesiritide is a recombinant form of brain natriuretic peptide that decreases pulmonary artery pressures and myocardial oxygen consumption and

TABLE 34.8

ACC/AHA CLASSIFICATION OF HEART FAILURE

Stage A	Patients at high risk of developing heart failure (HF) because of the presence of conditions that are strongly associated with the development of HF. Such patients have no identified structural or functional abnormalities of the pericardium, myocardium, or cardiac valves and have never shown signs or symptoms of HF.
Stage B	Patients who have developed structural heart disease that is strongly associated with the development of HF but who have never shown signs or symptoms of HF.
Stage C	Patients who have current or prior symptoms of HF associated with underlying structural heart disease.
Stage D	Patients with advanced structural heart disease and marked symptoms of HF at rest despite maximal medical therapy and who require specialized interventions.

ACC, American College of Cardiology; AHA, American Heart Association.

increases coronary blood flow and urine output. Nesiritide is used in two clinical settings: inotrope-resistant cardiac failure and postcardiac surgery patients with high pulmonary pressures and low cardiac output syndrome.

- **Calcium sensitizers.** Levosimendan is a calcium-sensitizing inodilator that improves myocardial contractility without increasing oxygen demand. It also decreases pulmonary vascular resistance in patients with heart failure and may be more effective than dobutamine in the management of severe congestive heart failure insofar as hemodynamic and mortality benefit. This drug offers enormous promise in the preoperative period in patients with severe congestive cardiac failure and poor cardiac output.
- **Antioxidants. Reactive oxygen species,** both within myocardial cells and those derived from the systemic circulation, are thought to overwhelm local endogenous antioxidant systems during bypass. They initiate **cellular damage, necrosis,** and **apoptosis** during cardiopulmonary **bypass and reperfusion. Allopurinol,** which inhibits xanthine oxidase,

TABLE 34.9

INDICATIONS FOR INTRA-AORTIC BALLOON COUNTERPULSATION

- Ongoing unstable angina refractory to medical therapy
- Acute myocardial ischemia/infarction associated with percutaneous transluminal angioplasty (PTCA)
- Perioperative low cardiac output syndrome
- Cardiogenic shock after myocardial infarction
- Congestive heart failure
- Bridge to transplant
- Ischemic ventricular septal defect
- Acute mitral valve insufficiency
- Poorly controlled perioperative ventricular arrhythmias

a significant source of reactive oxygen species outside the myocardium, has been studied in 10 human CABG trials, with 8 trials showing benefit. Despite these encouraging data, allopurinol has not received widespread support. Other antioxidants used are **superoxide dismutase, desferrioxamine, mannitol, vitamins C and E, and N-acetylcysteine.**

There has been an improvement in the ability to identify and **categorize the high-risk cardiac patient** presenting for cardiac surgery. As more data are accrued, **risk profiling** is becoming more accurate. This will allow for cost-effective implementation of promising preoperative interventions in the appropriate patient.

PULMONARY SYSTEM

The **definition** of postoperative pulmonary complications include respiratory failure, atelectasis, pneumonia, pulmonary edema, and pulmonary thromboembolic disease.
- Predicting the likelihood of postoperative pulmonary complications requires preoperative **pulmonary-risk stratification.**

Preoperative Evaluation

- After the history and clinical examination, patients can be classified into two groups: those with **known pulmonary disease** and those with **suspected pulmonary disease.** Both groups require an assessment of their functional classification and the degree of pulmonary reversibility.
- Laboratory investigations with a good predictive value for postoperative pulmonary complications include **blood urea nitrogen >21 mg/dL, creatinine >1.5 mg/dL,** and **albumin <3.0 g/dL.**
- The utility and cost-effectiveness of routine **preoperative chest x-ray** has been extensively debated. Only patients with **known cardiopulmonary disease,** and patients **older than 50 years** undergoing procedures with **high pulmonary risk** should have a preoperative chest radiograph.
- **Spirometry** has been evaluated as a predictive tool for pulmonary disorders in noncardiothoracic surgery. There are no studies to guide spirometry evaluation in the perioperative period for **restrictive** pulmonary disorders. In **obstructive** pulmonary disorders, there are conflicting data on the utility of spirometry; however, it may identify patients at higher risk for postoperative pulmonary complications.
- In **lung resection surgery,** spirometry forms the cornerstone of the evaluation process in both Europe and North America. Other parameters evaluated are the cardiopulmonary reserve and the lung parenchymal function (Fig. 34.2). A simplified algorithm integrating these parameters assists in the preoperative workup for lung resection surgery (Fig. 34.3).
- When the information gathered from history, physical examination, and special investigations is examined, a *risk profile* can be constructed from the guidelines published by the American College of Physicians (Table 34.10).
- The relationships between individual risk factors in each risk category have not been fully elucidated; they may be either additive or synergistic. Once a risk profile is formulated, risk modification strategies should be implemented.

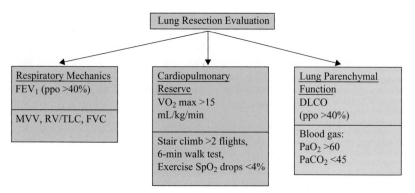

FIGURE 34.2. The best validated test is shown in the first box. Alternative tests are shown below. DLCO, total diffusion capacity for carbon monoxide; FEV_1, forced expiratory volume at 1 second; FVC, forced vital capacity; MVV, maximal voluntary ventilation; PaO_2, arterial partial pressure of oxygen; $PaCO_2$, arterial partial pressure of carbon dioxide; ppo, predicted postoperative value based on the number of lung segments remaining after resection; RV/TLC, residual volume divided by total lung capacity; SpO_2, pulse oximetric oxygen saturation; VO_2, oxygen uptake/consumption.

Preoperative Management of Pulmonary System

Restrictive Pulmonary Disorders

- Characteristics of restrictive disorders include the presence of mechanical volume limitations.
- Restrictive pulmonary disorders are substantially less common than obstructive disorders. These disorders are static in nature unless bronchial hyperreactivity coexists (e.g., hypersensitivity pneumonitis). The restriction can be either pulmonary or extrapulmonary.
  - Pulmonary/parenchymal causes of pulmonary restriction include pulmonary edema, adult respiratory distress syndrome, atelectasis, sarcoidosis, hypersensitivity pneumonitis, silicosis, tuberculosis, and lung resection.
  - Extrapulmonary causes include pleural effusion, pneumothorax, kyphoscoliosis, and increased abdominal pressure (ascites, pregnancy, obesity).
- In the extrapulmonary group, management of the mechanical volume effects (such as drainage of pleural effusion) can improve the perioperative pulmonary status of the patient.
- Lung protective ventilation using positive end-expiratory pressures and low tidal volumes of 6 to 8 mL/kg has become the standard of care for acute respiratory distress syndrome

and other disorders of static compliance found in this group of conditions.

Obstructive Airway Disease

- Obstructive pulmonary disorders are recognized by **fixed airway obstruction,** the presence of bronchial hyperreactivity, and a predisposition to infection.
- In nonoptimized patients with chronic obstructive pulmonary disease, a component of reversible airway obstruction or **bronchial hyperreactivity** (similar to asthma) makes them prone to **acute exacerbations** of airway obstruction triggered by upper- and lower-airway infections.
- Obstructive pulmonary disorders are associated with **increased risk** of postoperative pulmonary complications, and this risk is amplified when reversible airway obstruction is present.
- The key element in the management is appropriate treatment of the reversible component of the airway disease. β_2-Agonists have a salutary effect on airway hyperreactivity in obstructive airway disease. **Preoperative steroid** therapy, even of short duration, has been shown to decrease the incidence of wheezing after intubation. The concern for negative effects on wound healing and increased infection rates have not been borne out in the literature. Cochrane review in 2001 showed that **methylxanthines** (theophylline nor aminophylline) did

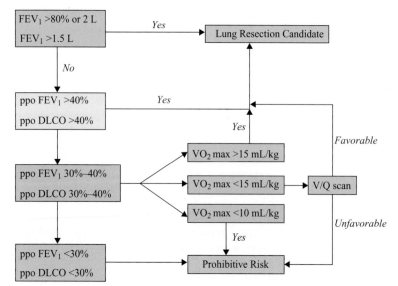

FIGURE 34.3. Simplified algorithm for the preoperative evaluation for lung resection surgery. DLCO, total diffusion capacity for carbon monoxide; FEV_1, forced expiratory volume at 1 second; ppo, predicted postoperative value based on the number of lung segments remaining after resection; VO_2, oxygen uptake/consumption; V/Q, ventilation/perfusion ratio.

TABLE 34.10

RISK FACTORS FOR RESPIRATORY COMPLICATIONS

High risk	OR	Strength of evidence	Indeterminate risk	OR	Strength of evidence
Patient-related risk factors					
Age 60–69 y	2.09				
Age 70–79 y	3.04	A	Diabetes		C
ASA class ≥2	2.55–4.87	A	Obesity		D
CHF	2.93	A	Asthma		D
Functionally dependent	1.65–2.51	A	Obstructive sleep apnea		I
			Corticosteroid use		I
Moderate risk			HIV infection		I
COPD	1.79	A	Arrhythmia		I
Weight loss	1.62	B	Poor exercise capacity		I
Low risk					
Impaired sensorium	1.39	B			
Cigarette use	1.26	B			
Alcohol use	1.21	B			
Abnormal findings on chest exam	NA	B			
Procedure-related risk factors					
High risk			**Indeterminate risk**		
Aortic aneurysm repair	6.9	A			
Thoracic surgery	4.24	A	Hip surgery		D
Abdominal surgery	3.01	A	Gynecologic or urologic surgery		D
Upper abdominal surgery	2.91	A	Esophageal surgery		I
Neurosurgery	2.53	A			
Prolonged surgery	2.26	A			
Moderate risk					
Head and neck surgery	2.21	A			
Emergency surgery	2.21	A			
Vascular surgery	2.1	A			
General anesthesia	1.83	A			
Low risk					
Perioperative transfusion >4 units	1.47	B			
Special investigations					
High risk			**Indeterminate risk**		
Albumin level <3.5 g/dL	2.53	A	BUN level >7.5 mmol/L (21 mg/dL)	NA	B
Chest radiography	4.81	B	Spirometry		I

A, good evidence that the factor is an independent predictor; B, at least fair evidence that the factor is an independent predictor; C, at least fair evidence that the factor is *not* a predictor; D, good evidence that the factor is *not* a predictor; I, evidence is lacking, conflicting, or indeterminate.
OR, odds ratio; ASA, American Society of Anesthesiologists; CHF, congestive heart failure; HIV, human immunodeficiency virus; COPD, chronic obstructive pulmonary disease; BUN, blood urea nitrogen; NA, not available.
Adapted from Smetana G. Preoperative pulmonary risk stratification for noncardiothoracic surgery: systematic review for the American College of Physicians. *Ann Int Med.* 2006;144:581, with permission.

not offer any advantage over β_2-agonists in the setting of acute bronchospasm.

- **Infection** increases **airway reactivity** and results in demonstrable spirometry abnormalities for **6 to 8 weeks after infection.** Elective surgery should ideally be delayed in patients with underlying bronchial hyperreactivity.
- The American Thoracic Society and the Global Initiative for Chronic Obstructive Lung Disease have issued guidelines for the assessment and management of obstructive lung disorders and their acute exacerbations. Modification for preoperative patient is presented in Figure 34.4.
- The most important intervention on a global scale is **smoking cessation** and prevention of exposure to second-hand smoke. Another intervention that can be started in the preoperative period is **nutritional support** with preferably enteral nutri-

tion with an immune-repleting formula for the malnourished undergoing elective gastroenterology and oncologic surgery. Benefits may include a decrease in the incidence of nosocomial sepsis and hospital length of stay.

RENAL SYSTEM

- The incidence of intensive care unit–associated **acute renal failure (ARF)** varies between 15% and 35%. In the United States, the incidence of **end-stage kidney disease (ESKD)** varies between 331 and 343 cases per million population. The preoperative evaluation and management of the patient with renal disease is complicated by the coexistence of multiple medical and surgical problems.

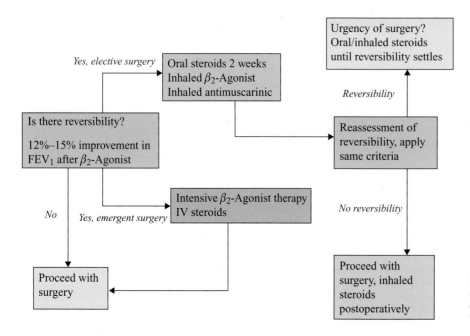

FIGURE 34.4. Preoperative optimization of obstructive airways disease. FEV$_1$, forced expiratory volume at 1 second; IV, intravenous.

Chronic Renal Failure

Risk Evaluation and Stratification

- Preoperative renal risk evaluation and stratification are based on (a) **comorbid** medical condition of the patient, (b) pre-existing **renal function,** and (c) the **procedure-specific** renal risk.

Comorbid Status

- Comorbid conditions that increase the risk of chronic renal insufficiency include a spectrum of **cardiovascular, endocrine, hepatic, autoimmune,** and **congenital disorders. Diabetes mellitus** is the leading cause of ESKD, with **hypertension, glomerulonephritis,** and **polycystic kidney disease** being the other major diagnoses.
- **CAD** is common in patients with diabetes mellitus and may be **asymptomatic** due to an associated autonomic neuropathy. A high index of suspicion for untreated CAD should be maintained for patients with diabetic nephropathy. Therefore, the preoperative workup of the diabetic patient with renal dysfunction should be done within the framework of the ACC/AHA algorithm discussed previously.
- **Hypertension** is the second leading cause of ESKD in the United States. Aggressive control of the blood pressure to approximately 125/75 mm Hg in patients with diabetic renal disease is recommended by the National Kidney Foundation
- **Polycystic kidney disease** is an inherited disorder that is characterized by multiple cysts in the kidney and the liver. It is responsible for 4% to 5% of ESKD in the United States. Important extrarenal manifestations of polycystic kidney disease include intracranial aneurysm in approximately 10% of patients, whereas 26% of patients have evidence of mitral valve prolapse.
- Once comorbid conditions and their related complications are identified, an attempt must be made to **quantify the degree of renal dysfunction.**

Pre-Existing Renal Dysfunction

- The National Kidney Foundation-Kidney Disease Outcomes Quality Initiative recently proposed a standardized classification system to assess the severity of pre-existing chronic renal disease. It is based on an estimation of the glomerular filtration rate (GFR) and the documentation of renal injury (Table 34.11).
- The GFR can be estimated using either **mathematical models** or by determining the **clearance of insulin or other filtration markers.** To estimate the GFR, either the Cockroft–Gault equation or the formula derived from the Modification of Diet in Renal Disease Study can be used. The latter formula, although mathematically more complex, uses readily available data to provide a more accurate estimate of the GFR than the Cockroft–Gault equation:

$$\text{GFR (mL/min/1.73 m}^2) = 170 \times [P_{cr}]^{-0.999} \times [age]^{-0.176} \times [0.762 \text{ if patients is female}] \times [1.18 \text{ if patient is black}]$$

where SUN is serum urea nitrogen and Alb is albumin.

The presence of pre-existing renal dysfunction increases the incidence of **perioperative morbidity and mortality** in high-risk surgery. On multivariate analysis, preoperative creatinine (P_{Cr}) ≥ 2.8 mg/dL was strongly associated with postoperative ARF

TABLE 34.11

STAGES OF CHRONIC KIDNEY DISEASE

Stage	Definition
1	GFR ≥ 90 mL min/1.73 m^2 with evidence of kidney damage
2	GFR 60–89 mL/min/1.73 m^2 with evidence of kidney damage
3	GFR 30–59 mL/min/1.73 m^2
4	GFR 15–29 mL/min/1.73 m^2
5	GFR ≤ 15 mL/min/1.73 m^2 or dialysis dependent

GFR, glomerular filtration rate.

(OR 10.3; 95% CI 12–411, p <0.0001). Of the patients who developed ARF, the mortality rate was 49%.

Procedure-related Risk

- Procedure-related renal risk is an important determinant of perioperative renal failure. **Cardiac** and **major vascular procedures** are associated with a high incidence of ARF. The development of renal failure is associated with increased mortality, hospital length of stay, and cost. A 7.9% incidence of ARF and 0.7% incidence of ARF requiring renal replacement therapy have been reported with CABG patients. The mortality for patients who developed ARF was 14% compared with 1% among those who did not develop ARF. Off-pump CABG, by avoiding cardiopulmonary bypass, has less damaging effects.
- Renal insufficiency or failure exists in many patients presenting for major vascular surgery. In vascular surgery, the location of the arterial reconstruction, the duration of the aortic cross-clamp, and the emergent nature of the procedure are all strong predictors of postoperative renal complications. Reported incidence of acute postoperative renal dysfunction for thoracoabdominal reconstruction varies between 13% and 25%, whereas renal failure rates for abdominal aortic reconstruction are much lower at approximately 1.5% to 2%.

Acute Renal Failure

- ARF is a common complication of critical illness and is associated with significant morbidity and mortality. To standardize the definition of ARF, the **RIFLE classification,** which includes criteria for serum creatinine, GFR, and urine output, has been validated (Table 34.12). Multivariate logistic regression analysis demonstrates that the RIFLE classification is an independent risk factor assessment for 90-day mortality.

Classification

- ARF is divided into three categories based on its pathophysiology. They are prerenal, postrenal, and intrarenal ARF.

Prerenal Acute Renal Failure

- Prerenal ARF is reversible renal insufficiency due to renal hypoperfusion, usually associated with hypovolemia. If the renal hypoperfusion is left untreated, acute tubular necrosis (ATN) secondary to ischemia will develop. Laboratory data include **low urine Na^+, fractional excretion of Na^+ <1%,** and bland urine sediment.

Postrenal Acute Renal Failure

- Postrenal ARF is due to **obstruction of urine** flow at any level of the urine collecting system. Postrenal ARF can be diagnosed promptly by either ultrasound or computed tomography scan, and relief of the obstruction usually results in prompt reversal of the renal insufficiency.

Intrarenal Acute Renal Failure

- Intrarenal ARF is divided into five groups based on the underlying pathology. **Acute tubular necrosis (ATN)** is injury and subsequent death of the tubular epithelium. ATN is caused by either ischemia or nephrotoxic agents. **Acute interstitial nephritis** is an inflammation of the renal interstitium and the tubules. It may occur secondary to infections or drugs, such as the penicillins or cephalosporins. **Acute glomerulonephritis, acute vascular syndromes,** and **intratubular obstruction** are other causes. The differential diagnosis of intrarenal ARF should be guided by history and physical exam and examination of the urine sediment. The presence of tubular epithelial cells and granular **cast** is suggestive of ATN, whereas the presence of red cell cast indicates glomerulonephritis. Eosinophiluria suggests the presence of interstitial nephritis; however, it is not diagnostic.
- ARF is characterized by retention of nitrogenous waste products, fluid and electrolyte abnormalities, acid-base disorders, and impairment of the hematologic and coagulation systems. The preoperative evaluation of these patients must, therefore, take into account these specific changes and the increased risk they pose during the perioperative period.

Preoperative Evaluation of Renal Failure

- The **history and physical examination** should be directed toward evaluating the severity of the **comorbid conditions** and the complications related to the acute renal dysfunction. Signs and symptoms of uncompensated **cardiac failure and pericarditis** should be elicited.
- Uremia is associated with nausea, vomiting, and recurrent episodes of hiccoughing. Severe nausea and vomiting may result in **dehydration,** and a thorough evaluation of the patient's volume status must be performed.
- **Anemia** in renal failure is multifactorial in nature. Bleeding from platelet dysfunction, malnutrition, and decreased

---

TABLE 34.12

THE RIFLE CLASSIFICATION SCHEME FOR ACUTE RENAL FAILURE

	GFR criteria	Urine output criteria	Mortality
Risk	Increased plasma creatinine × 1.5 or GFR decrease >25%	<0.5 mL/kg/h × 6 h	8%
Injury	Increased plasma creatinine × 2 or GFR decrease >50%	<0.5 mL/kg/h × 12 h	21.40%
Failure	Increased plasma creatinine × 3 or acute plasma creatinine ≥350 μmol/L (4 mg/dL) or acute rise ≥44 μmol/L (0.5 mg/dL)	<0.3 mL/kg/h × 24 h or anuria × 12 h	32.50%
Loss	Persistent acute renal failure with complete loss of kidney function × 4 weeks		
ESKD	End-stage kidney disease (× 3 mo)		

GFR, glomerular filtration rate; ESKD, end-stage kidney disease.

erythropoietin production all contribute toward the low red cell mass.

- **Electrolyte abnormalities** are common in renal failure. Hyperkalemia, hyperphosphatemia, and hypocalcemia is the typical electrolyte profile seen in renal failure. Hypocalcemia may manifest as cramps, paraesthesia and, in severe cases, with mental status changes.

Diagnostic Testing

- **Complete blood count** helps to assess the severity of the **anemia, morphology of the red blood cells,** and the platelet count. There is an acquired platelet dysfunction that results in an increased risk of bleeding. To assess the degree of **platelet function,** either a bleeding time or, more accurately, a platelet function assay can be performed.
- The **basic metabolic panel** helps to determine the electrolyte profile.
- An **electrocardiogram** must be performed to determine whether ischemia, ventricular hypertrophy, or strain pattern is present. **Hyperkalemia** is characterized by tall peaked T-waves, widened QRS complex, and shortened QT interval. The electrocardiogram of patients with **pericardial effusion** may demonstrate small QRS complexes and the presence of electrical alternans (change in QRS amplitude with each heartbeat).
- A **chest radiograph** may reveal signs of pulmonary edema, cardiomegaly, or a large pericardial effusion.
- Examination of the urine and determination of the **urine indices** provides invaluable data in helping to differentiate prerenal from intrarenal ARF (Table 34.13).
- The **fractional excretion of urea** is a useful index to differentiate prerenal from intrarenal failure if diuretic therapy has been initiated:

$$FE_{UN} = [(\text{urine nitrogen/blood urea nitrogen})/ \\ (\text{urine creatinine/plasma creatinine})] \times 100$$

- Fractional excretion of urea nitrogen is primarily dependent on passive forces and is, therefore, less influenced by diuretic therapy. In contrast, diuretic therapy will falsely raise the FE_{Na+} under prerenal conditions.

Primary and Secondary Prevention

- **Primary prevention** of ARF refers to clinical strategies that reduce the occurrence of ARF in patients with or without chronic renal disease.
- **Secondary injury** is additional renal injury developing in the face of a primary insult to the renal system.

TABLE 34.13

CRITERIA TO DIFFERENTIATE PRERENAL FROM INTRARENAL FAILURE

	Prerenal	Intrarenal
Urine Na$^+$	<20 mEq/L	>40 mEq/L
FE_{Na+}	<1%	>2%
FE_{UN}	<35%	>50%
Urine/plasma creatinine	>40	<20
Urine/plasma osmolarity	>1.3	<1.1
Urine/plasma urea	>8	<3

- The principles of management of patients with ARF are to maintain an adequate **mean arterial pressure,** maintain an appropriate **cardiac output,** ensure **euvolemia,** and **avoid nephrotoxic agents.**
- The **mean arterial pressure** required to maintain adequate renal perfusion pressure **may vary.** Patients with a long history of hypertension may require a higher mean arterial pressure to maintain perfusion.
- **Low cardiac output states** induce renal ischemia and reduce the glomerular filtration rate. It is important to restore cardiac output. This may require placement of monitors such as a **pulmonary artery catheter** or a transesophageal echocardiography probe to determine cardiac output.
- **Volume expansion** has been shown to prevent contrast-induced nephropathy and attenuate the tubular injury associated with rhabdomyolysis. High-risk patients should receive an intravenous bolus of 3 mL/kg of the study solution over an hour, before radiocontrast injection, followed by a continuous infusion of 1 mL/kg/hour during the procedure and for 6 hours after the procedure.
- In conclusion, the best evidence to date suggests that nonpharmacologic therapy strategies are more effective than drugs in reducing the risk of ARF. High-risk patients should be identified early and secondary renal injury aggressively prevented.

NEUROLOGIC SYSTEM

Ischemic Cerebrovascular Disease

- The incidence of perioperative stroke in patients undergoing nonvascular surgery under general anesthesia is <0.5%. However, the mortality associated with a perioperative stroke may be as high as 26%.

Carotid Stenosis

- The risk of a perioperative stroke increases in the presence of carotid stenosis or a history of transient ischemic attack. The presence of carotid stenosis of at least 50% is associated with a perioperative stroke rate of approximately 3.6%. Although higher than the general population stroke rate, this risk does not appear sufficient to mandate prophylactic carotid endarterectomy (CEA).
- Patients with carotid disease who present with transient ischemic attacks have a 10% risk of stroke during the subsequent year.
- The benefit of antiplatelet therapy in reducing perioperative stroke during CEA is unresolved. However, a dose range of aspirin 50 to 1,300 mg/day is commonly used.

Surgery-Specific Risk

- Noncarotid procedure associated with the highest risk of perioperative neurologic injury is **cardiac surgery.** Studies report a 3% incidence of stroke in CABG procedures, 8% in isolated valve surgery, and 11% in combined CABG-valve surgery. Advanced age and female gender are additional risk factors. The single most important factor for cerebral injury during cardiac surgery is macroembolization of atheromatous debris during aortic manipulation. Every attempt should be made to identify the high-risk patient with a large atheromatous burden by using epiaortic echocardiography and **minimizing manipulation** of the aorta.

Preoperative Evaluation

- The history and physical examination of the patient with cerebrovascular disease require a thorough assessment of the cardiovascular and neurologic system.
- Patients with carotid artery stenosis are at an increased risk of **CAD**. Severe correctable CAD is evident in approximately 26% of patients with cerebrovascular disease, whereas only 9% of patients have normal coronary anatomy.
- Studies, though, have demonstrated the rate of medical complications in patients undergoing **CEA** to be low, with perioperative medical complications occurring in fewer than 10%, and only 0.4% had severe complications. Perioperative nonfatal and fatal myocardial infarction occurred in only 1% of the patients and was associated with a mortality rate of approximately 0.2%. Therefore, recommending a CABG procedure to a patient with symptomatic carotid disease and asymptomatic CAD is not justified
- The ACC/AHA guidelines for noncardiac surgery list **CEA as an intermediate-risk procedure** where the perioperative cardiac risk is <5%.

- **Hypertension** is a prevalent and treatable risk factor for stroke. Treatment of systolic and diastolic hypertension results in a 36% and 42% stroke reduction, respectively. Knowledge of preoperative blood pressure is important in management strategy, as patients with long-standing hypertension may need a higher mean arterial pressure to ensure adequate cerebral perfusion. Poor control of blood pressure after CEA increases the risk of **cerebral hyperperfusion syndrome.** This complication occurs due to impairment of cerebral autoregulation and can result in intracerebral hemorrhage and white-matter edema. Patients with severe preoperative carotid stenosis and chronic hypertension are at greatest risk for this complication. Blood pressure should be carefully monitored and aggressively treated if symptoms of hyperperfusion syndrome develop.

Reference

1. Fleisher LA, Beckman JA, Brown KA, et al. ACC/AHA 2006 Guideline Update on Perioperative Cardiovascular Evaluation for Noncardiac Surgery: Focused Update on Perioperative Beta-blocker Therapy. A Report of the American College of Cardiology/American Heart Association Task Force on Practice Guidelines (Writing Committee to Update the 2002 Guidelines on Perioperative Cardiovascular Evaluation for Noncardiac Surgery). *J Am Coll Cardiol.* 2006;47:2343.

CHAPTER 35 ■ ANESTHESIA: PHYSIOLOGY AND POSTANESTHESIA PROBLEMS

INTRODUCTION

- The overall **risk of death** from anesthesia is between 1 in 112,000 and 1 in 450,000.
- The characteristics of anesthetic injuries have changed over the past years, with an increase in problems related to **cardiovascular issues** and a decrease in those related to the respiratory system.

INHALATIONAL AGENTS

- The goal of inhalational anesthesia is to develop a critical partial pressure of the agent within the brain. **Brain levels** are determined by several factors presented: delivery of inhaled agents, uptake from lungs, and distribution to tissues.
- The **brain tissue partial pressure** is responsible for the depth, and some of the side effects of anesthesia, and correlates closely with the end-tidal partial pressure of the inhaled agents.

Delivery of Inhaled Agents

- The inspired concentration is important to the rate of rise of anesthetic agent concentration in the lungs; this relationship is termed the **concentration effect.**
- **The second gas effect.** When large amounts of an anesthetic agent such as nitrous oxide are rapidly taken up, the lungs do not collapse. Instead, a subatmospheric alveolar pressure is generated as a result of the rapid removal of this gas by the pulmonary blood flow. A passive inflow of additional gas (another anesthetic agent) from the anesthesia circuit replaces that which is taken up. This second gas may have a partial pressure increase which is more rapid than when it is administered alone.
- **Alveolar ventilation** ($\dot{V}_A$) is another important factor in delivery of inhaled agents.

Uptake of Inhaled Agents from the Lungs

- **Solubility** is the extent to which the anesthetic dissolves in blood and tissues; the more soluble the agent, the more it is dissolved in the pulmonary blood and the longer it takes to reach the necessary partial pressure in the lungs and brain.

- A high **cardiac output** increases uptake and decreases the alveolar partial pressure of the agent. This effect is greater with more soluble inhalational anesthetics. A longer induction time is required for a patient with a high cardiac output.

- **Alveolar–to–central mixed venous anesthetic partial pressure gradient.** This factor relates the size of the anesthetic "sink" to the increase or decrease in uptake from the lungs. At the beginning of induction when the tissue anesthetic level is zero, most of the anesthetic agent in the arterial blood is removed. Thus, the venous anesthetic partial pressure is much lower than that in the arterial blood, and a large uptake of anesthetic occurs as the venous blood passes through the lungs. The alveolar partial pressure of the anesthetic agent is accordingly reduced. However, as the tissue sinks become filled, the alveolar to venous anesthetic partial pressure difference decreases.

Distribution

Tissue Solubility and Blood Flow

- The greater the solubility of an anesthetic in a tissue, the larger the capacity of that tissue for the agent. If the tissue has a large capacity but low blood flow, equilibration takes a long time; if the tissue has a small capacity and large blood flow, equilibration is rapid. The vessel-rich group is composed of the **brain, liver, heart, and kidneys.** An intermediate group includes **muscle and skin.** The vessel-poor group incorporates **skeletal elements, ligaments, and cartilage. Fat** has a poor blood supply but a great capacity. At the end of surgery, the factors that affect elimination of the agent from the body are the same as those that govern the uptake and distribution at the beginning. Factors that **lengthen the period of emergence** are hypoventilation, increased cardiac output, use of a highly soluble anesthetic agent, and an increased alveolar-to-venous anesthetic concentration gradient.

Diffusion Hypoxia

- Diffusion hypoxia may occur at the conclusion of an anesthetic if the patient is allowed to breathe room air while large quantities of nitrous oxide diffuse into the alveoli and dilute the oxygen that is present. This problem is significant only for approximately 10 minutes and can be alleviated by having the patient breathe 100% oxygen after discontinuation of the nitrous oxide.

Effects of Illness

Changes in Ventilation

- Organ system dysfunction can affect the uptake and distribution of inhaled anesthetic agents. In a hyperventilated patient, each 1 mm Hg decrease in the $PaCO_2$ caused by an increase in $\dot{V}_A$, leads to a 3% to 4% decrease in cerebral blood flow (CBF). A change in the length of time of anesthetic induction results from three factors: increased $\dot{V}_A$, decreased CBF, and solubility of the inhaled agents used for induction. The induction time for a moderately soluble agent such as halothane is decreased because the increased $\dot{V}_A$ produces a more rapid rise in end-tidal halothane partial pressure that offsets the

decrease in CBF. For a relatively nonsoluble agent such as nitrous oxide, induction time is increased because the modest increase in end-tidal nitrous oxide partial pressure obtained by hyperventilation is more than offset by the decrease in CBF.

Changes in Cardiac Output

- A decrease in cardiac output yields an increase in the agent's end-tidal partial pressure, whereas a decrease in CBF decreases transfer of the agent from the lungs to the brain.

Inhalational Agents and Organ System Function

- The differential effects of various inhalation agents on organ system function must be compared at equipotent doses. The **minimum alveolar concentration (MAC)** is the amount of an inhalational agent that prevents movement in 50% of patients in response to surgical incision. In neonates, the MAC is less than in children, adolescents, and young adults. After approximately 31 years of age, the MAC value begins to decrease; theoretically, the value for a patient 100 years of age is only 25% to 50% that of a young adult.

Circulatory Effects

- **Blood pressure** is decreased with the use of all inhalational agents. This may be due to decreased **contractility,** as with halothane, or due to decreased **systemic vascular resistance,** as with isoflurane or desflurane.

Cardiac Rhythm

- Of the several methods for evaluation of the effects of inhalational agents on cardiac rhythm, a common procedure is to determine the dose of epinephrine required to produce three or more premature ventricular contractions in 50% of normal patients breathing oxygen and anesthetized at 1.25 MAC (Table 35.1).

Respiratory Effects

- All inhalational agents are respiratory depressants. Decreases in minute ventilation at 1 MAC of various agents are presented in Table 35.1.

Hepatic Effects

- Up to 20% of patients may demonstrate mild disturbances in liver function after anesthesia with halothane presenting as **abnormalities of liver function** tests. They may be due to other physiologic disturbances such as hemodynamic abnormalities during surgery or blood transfusion. This has been one of the reasons for the marked reduction in the use of halothane as a common anesthetic agent.

Renal Effects

- All potent inhalation agents result in a dose-dependent decrease in renal blood flow from 25% to 50%, glomerular filtration rate from 23% to 40%, and urine flow from 35% to 67%.

Immune Function

- Anesthesia and surgery may impair immune system function, at least *in vitro*. Relevance to clinical outcome is debated.

TABLE 35.1

RESPIRATORY AND CIRCULATORY EFFECTS OF THE INHALATIONAL AGENTS

	N_2O	Halothane	Enflurane	Isoflurane
Respiratory				
$\dot{V}_A$	↓	↓	↓↓↓	↓↓
% awake response to CO_2	↓↓	↓↓	↓↓	↓↓
% awake response to hypoxia	—	↓	↓↓	↓↓
Circulatory				
% awake ballistocardiogram	—	↓	↓↓	θ
% awake cardiac output	θ	↓	↓	θ
% awake stroke volume	θ	↓	↓↓	↓
μg/kg epinephrine for three or more PVCs	—	2.1–3.7	10.9	6.7

—, no data; θ, no change; ↓, decrease of ≤33%; ↓↓, decrease of ≤66%; ↓↓↓, decrease of ≥66%; PVCs, premature ventricular contractions; N_2O, nitrous oxide; $\dot{V}_A$, expired volume per minute; CO_2, carbon dioxide.

INTRAVENOUS AGENTS

Narcotics

General Considerations

- Opiates have been used for pain for thousands of years. There are specific binding sites for opiates in the central nervous system The opiate receptor complex with three major receptor groups have been described: μ, δ, and κ. The main drugs available for pain relief are relatively selective for the μ-receptor.
- A wide variety of narcotic drugs are available including morphine, meperidine, methadone, fentanyl, alfentanil, sufentanil and, more recently, remifentanil.
- Problems with morphine include recall, **histamine release,** prolonged postoperative respiratory depression, hypertension, and increased blood and fluid requirements because of vasodilation.
- Synthetic drugs related to the phenylpiperidines, such as fentanyl, sufentanil, alfentanil, and remifentanil, do **not induce histamine release,** nor do they increase blood and fluid requirements.
- **Remifentanil** has a time to effect that is very rapid (**half-life 8–20 minutes**), and because it is metabolized by plasma esterase, is independent of liver or renal function. This makes the drug ideal for situations in which rapid discontinuation of a drug is required to enable assessment of consciousness, such as in neurosurgical procedures.
- Narcotics cannot be depended upon to provide complete anesthesia, which requires **amnesia, hypnosis, and muscle relaxation** to enable safe surgery. The addition of intravenous hypnotics and muscle relaxants, or inhaled agents, is required.

Pharmacokinetics/Pharmacodynamics

- Pharmacokinetic data for four commonly used opioids are summarized in Table 35.2.
- Similarities between the redistribution and elimination half-lives and the clearance and steady-state volume of distribution are noteworthy. The major difference is in **lipid solubility,** which correlates with **potency.**

- **Peak respiratory depressant effect** of morphine occurs at 15 to 30 minutes after injection, and 5 to 10 minutes after fentanyl. The respiratory depressant effect from morphine usually lasts longer, although that of fentanyl can be seen **after the analgesic effect has dissipated.** Remifentanil is unique in that it has a rapid onset and offset of effect, even when delivered for a prolonged infusion.

Hemodynamic Effects

- **Hypotension** can be a significant problem with morphine in a dose of 1 to 4 mg/kg. During induction of anesthesia with morphine, systolic blood pressure may decrease to less than 70 mm Hg in 10% of patients. Possible mechanisms include vagal-induced bradycardia, vasodilation, and splanchnic blood sequestration. Some of the effects of morphine seem to result from **histamine release.**
- **Fentanyl** 30 to 100 μg/kg rarely causes hypotension even in patients with poor left ventricular function, perhaps because it does not cause histamine release. When blood pressure decreases with fentanyl, it is often secondary to a decrease in heart rate and is attenuated with a vagolytic agent.
- **Remifentanil** has a beneficial hemodynamic profile, similar to fentanyl.

Respiratory Effects

- Significant dose-dependent respiratory depression can occur with opioids.
- Opioids block (a) **hypoxic ventilatory drive** and (b) the drive seen with increased airways resistance. The pontine and medullary centers for respiratory rhythmicity are impaired, resulting in increased respiratory pauses and delayed exhalation, producing irregular and periodic breathing.
- Morphine can trigger **bronchospasm** due to histamine release.

Neurologic Effects

- Morphine, at a dose of 1 to 3 mg/kg with 70% nitrous oxide, has no effect on **CBF, cerebral metabolic rate for oxygen** ($CMRO_2$), or **cerebral metabolic rate for glucose** (CMR_G).
- Fentanyl, in a model of traumatic brain injury, did not lead to a reduction in CBF despite a decrease in arterial blood pressure.

TABLE 35.2

SELECTED PHARMACOKINETIC DATA FOR FOUR OPIOIDS

	Morphine	Fentanyl	Sufentanil	Remifentanil
Lipid solubility[a]	1	580	1778	50
$t^{1}/_{2}\ \pi$ (min)	0.9–2.4	1–3	0.5–2	1
$t^{1}/_{2}\ \alpha$ (min)	10–20	5–20	5–15	6
$t^{1}/_{2}\ \beta$ (h)	2–4	2–4	2–3	0.06
Clearance (mL/kg/min)	10–20	10–20	10–12	40–70
Vd_{ss} (L/kg)	3–5	3–5	2.5	0.2–0.3

$t^{1}/_{2}\ \pi$, rapid redistribution half-life; $t^{1}/_{2}\ \alpha$, slow redistribution half-life; $t^{1}/_{2}\ \beta$, elimination half-life; Vd_{ss}, steady-state volume of distribution.
[a]Proportional to ease with which agent crosses blood–brain barrier and, hence, potency.

Gastrointestinal Effects

• Nausea and vomiting may occur secondary to stimulation of the chemoreceptor trigger zone in the area postrema of the medulla.
• There may be increased gastrointestinal secretions, decreased motility, and increased smooth muscle tone of the gastrointestinal tract and the sphincter of Oddi.

Barbiturates

General Considerations

• **Thiobarbiturates** (e.g., **sodium thiopental and methohexital**): The chemical structure of these barbiturates confer ultrashort onset and offset action compared with other barbiturates.
• Sodium thiopental usually comes in a 2.5% solution with a pH greater than 10, causing the drug to be irritating if accidental extravasation occurs.
• Methohexital is two to three times more potent than thiopental.

Pharmacokinetics/Pharmacodynamics

• The pharmacokinetics of thiopental, and other commonly used nonnarcotic, intravenous anesthetic agents, are summarized in Table 35.3.
• Thiopental is a highly lipophilic agent and, with a standard clinical dose of 3 to 5 mg/kg, loss of consciousness occurs within one arm–brain circulation time (i.e., 10–15 seconds). The short duration of action of this drug—**5 to 10 minutes**—

is secondary to its **redistribution** from the brain to muscle, skin and, to a lesser extent, fat. The elimination half-life of the drug is long, making thiopental into a long-acting drug when a large enough dose has been given to saturate the redistribution compartment. **Hepatic metabolism** is important for its inactivation.

• **Methohexital** is only slightly less lipid soluble than sodium thiopental. The onset and duration of loss of consciousness are approximately the same as with thiopental because of its rapid redistribution, with an elimination half-life of 3 to 5 minutes. Because it is more dependent on **hepatic blood flow** for clearance, any changes in blood flow are more significant for its final elimination.

Neurologic Effects

• The mechanisms of action of the barbiturates are multiple and dose related. It facilitates the action of inhibitory—GABA—neural transmitters and inhibition of excitatory neural transmitter action. It may be used to reduce intracranial pressure and improve cerebral hemodynamics while providing a degree of brain protection.

Cardiorespiratory Effects

• Thiopental increases coronary blood flow, heart rate, and myocardial oxygen consumption with a **decrease in the inotropic state** of the myocardium. The result is a 10% to 25% decrease in cardiac output, blood pressure, and stroke volume at clinically relevant doses.

TABLE 35.3

SELECTED PHARMACOKINETIC DATA FOR NONOPIOID INTRAVENOUS ANESTHETICS

	Thiopental	Propofol	Diazepam	Lorazepam	Midazolam	Ketamine
$t^{1}/_{2}\ \alpha$ (min)	2–4	2–4	10–15	3–10	7–15	7–17
$t^{1}/_{2}\ \beta$ (h)	10	1–3	20–40	10–20	2–4	2–3
Clearance (mL/kg/min)	2.6–2.8	20–40	0.2–0.5	0.7–1	4–8	18–20
Vd_{ss} (L/kg)[a]	1.4–2.8	2.8–7.1	0.85–1.4	0.7–1.3	1–1.8	2.8–3.6

$t^{1}/_{2}\ \alpha$, slow redistribution half-life; $t^{1}/_{2}\ \beta$, elimination half-life; Vd_{ss}, steady-state volume of distribution.
[a]Assume a 70-kg person.
Modified from White PF. Propofol: pharmacokinetics and pharmacodynamics. *Semin Anesth*. 1988;7(Suppl):4.

- **Venous tone** may also decrease, resulting in decreased preload.
- At doses of 3 to 5 mg/kg, the responses to carbon dioxide elevation and hypoxia are impaired.

Immune Effects

- In patients who are given continuous barbiturate infusion, there may be an effect on immune function and they may be more prone to develop infections.

Propofol

General Considerations

- Propofol is a sedative–hypnotic agent that may be used for induction and maintenance of anesthesia. The agent is **not an analgesic** but is reported to have minimal amnestic effects.
- An alkylphenol, propofol is virtually insoluble in aqueous media and thus is provided in a 1% weight/volume (**Intralipid**) emulsion. The emulsion is composed of 1% di-isopropylphenol (propofol), 10% soybean oil, 2.25% glycerol, and 1.2% purified egg phosphatide.

Pharmacokinetics/Pharmacodynamics

- The basic pharmacokinetic data of propofol are shown in Table 35.3. Propofol is extensively distributed into vessel-rich tissues and ultimately redistributed to lean muscle and fat. Accumulation occurs with repeated bolus injections or continuous infusion.
- In comparing propofol with the other agents in Table 35.3, one observes the high clearance and the short elimination half-life. This is one of the reasons that the agent is so appealing.
- A propofol dose of **2 to 2.5 mg/kg** results in loss of consciousness in less than 60 seconds. Intravenous injection of 1 to 1.5 mg/kg in the elderly or a patient who has been given narcotic or benzodiazepine premedication is often sufficient for induction.

Neurologic Effects

- The mechanisms of action of propofol are unclear. It can cause desynchronization of the awake electroencephalographic (EEG) pattern when a loading dose of 2.5 mg/kg followed by an infusion of 100 to 200 μg/kg/minute are used.
- More than 150 μg/kg/minute results in EEG burst suppression lasting 15 seconds or longer; the EEG returns to the awake state within 11 minutes after the drug infusion is discontinued.
- There a dose-related **decrease in CBF and CMRO$_2$** and progressive EEG suppression with increasing dose of propofol, which may be useful in patients with **intracranial disease.**

Cardiovascular Effects

- A dose-dependent decrease in systolic, diastolic, and mean arterial blood pressure is observed; this effect is enhanced by narcotic premedication. Profound **cardiovascular depression** may be seen in elderly, hypovolemic patients and those with impaired ventricular function.

Respiratory Effects

- **Apnea** is seen on induction with propofol in 30% to 60% of unpremedicated patients and in virtually 100% of those premedicated with narcotics. The respiratory response to hypoxia is significantly blunted.

Other Effects

- Up to 58% of patients with an intravenous catheter in the dorsum of the hand report **pain on injection.**
- A syndrome of severe hemodynamic compromise with bradycardia (even asystole) combined with severe metabolic acidosis called the **propofol infusion syndrome** has been described, initially in children and now in adults.
- The pathophysiology of the propofol infusion system is unclear, and various theories have been suggested: (a) **mitochondrial function** leading to extreme metabolic acidosis and rhabdomyolysis, (b2) **genetic predisposition** of mitochondria to dysfunction, or (c) problems with **lipid metabolism,** particularly in patients who have a low carbohydrate input. Risk factors include a **high dose** of the drug and its **prolonged** administration.
- **Acute lung injury** has also been reported possibly due to the effects of the lipids inciting an inflammatory response.

Benzodiazepines

General Considerations

- Commonly used benzodiazepines **diazepam, lorazepam, and midazolam** are presented in Table 35.3. Diazepam and lorazepam are insoluble in water. Midazolam, because of its imidazole ring, is water-soluble at a pH <4. Lorazepam is less lipid-soluble than diazepam, and its **slow entry into the central nervous system** may be a reason for its slower onset of action.

Pharmacokinetics/Pharmacodynamics

- **Diazepam's** sedative properties make it useful as a premedicant; peak plasma levels are seen 30 to 60 minutes after an oral dose. Intramuscular injection is painful, and absorption is erratic. With **hepatic disease,** the volume of distribution increases and metabolism decreases, resulting in an **increase in the half-life from 40 to 80 hours.** With significant renal disease, an increase in the unbound fraction of diazepam results in a twofold to threefold increase in hepatic clearance and a resultant decrease in the half-life.
- **Lorazepam** is useful in oral, intramuscular, and intravenous forms. This agent is directly metabolized in the liver to inactive, glucuronide-conjugated metabolites. The kinetics of this drug are unaltered by age or renal disease, but hepatic disease increases the half-life.
- **Midazolam** can be administered by intramuscular, intravenous, or oral routes. The drug undergoes extensive metabolism to active and inactive metabolites.

Neurologic Effects

- Benzodiazepines have multiple, dose-dependent effects on the central nervous system and potentiate **inhibitory GABA neurotransmission.** Loss of consciousness occurs 2 to 3 minutes after an intravenous induction. Antegrade amnesia is seen with all of the benzodiazepines but more so with lorazepam.

Cardiorespiratory Effects

- When used alone, negative cardiovascular effects are rare; however, cardiovascular depression has been observed when used in conjunction with other anesthetic agents.
- Decrease in the ventilatory response to carbon dioxide may occur.

Ketamine

Pharmacokinetics/Pharmacodynamics

- Ketamine is the only arylcyclohexylamine used in anesthesia. It is structurally related to phencyclidine, known in street vernacular as "angel dust." Its pharmacokinetics are summarized in Table 35.3.
- After an intravenous dose of 2 mg/kg, consciousness is lost in little more than one arm–brain circulation time and returns 10 to 15 minutes later.
- Recovery of consciousness results from rapid drug redistribution into muscle and other tissues. However, 95% of the injected drug is metabolized by the **liver,** and less than 5% is recovered unchanged in the urine.

Neurologic Effects

- The exact mechanism of action of ketamine is not well understood. Specific arylcyclohexylamine receptors in the brain may be related to the μ subclass of opioid receptors.
- Ketamine increases CBF and so must be used with caution in individuals with **elevated intraccranial pressure (ICP).**

Cardiovascular Effects

- There is an increase in systemic blood pressure and cerebrovasodilation resulting in increased intracranial pressure.
- Ketamine is often thought not to be a myocardial depressant. Nonetheless, with sympathetic blockade or in patients in prolonged shock with a significantly stressed autonomic nervous system, cardiac depression can be seen with ketamine.
- **Pulmonary vascular resistance** and right ventricular stroke work are frequently increased.

Respiratory Effects

- Although **not** commonly thought of as a respiratory depressant when used in anesthetic doses of 1 to 2 mg/kg, a moderate decrease in the PaO_2 may occur. The ventilatory response to carbon dioxide is maintained, and ketamine potentiates the bronchodilatory effects of catecholamines.
- It also increases **oral secretions** so that an anticholinergic agent may be necessary.

Other Effects

- **Postanesthetic emergence reactions**—nightmares and hallucinations—may occur in 5% to 30% of patients. A benzodiazepine and 2 mg/kg (or less) maximal doses of ketamine seem to decrease the incidence of this problem.

Etomidate

- Due to maintenance of **hemodynamic stability,** etomidate is commonly used in the induction of anesthesia or for intubation of critically ill patients.

- Etomidate causes a **dose-dependent reduction in contractility** in both normal and failing heats, but this decrease is **minimal** and not of clinical significance.
- The major problem is adrenal suppression when used in a prolonged infusion, but adrenal failure has also been demonstrated after a single dose.

Dexmedetomidine

- Dexmedetomidine is a highly selective, short-acting **central α_2-agonist.** It provides a dose-dependent degree of sedation, analgesia, anxiolysis, and sympatholysis. When used in postoperative patients in the intensive care unit, dexmedetomidine can provide better sedation with fewer narcotics than propofol. It may also facilitate extubation in patients who may otherwise require large amounts of benzodiazepines. The place of this agent in intensive care medicine practice is increasing.

POSTANESTHESIA PROBLEMS

- Postanesthetic complications have been found to occur in 5% to 30% of patients; the wide range results from lack of uniform criteria defining complications, different practices in individual institutions, and strictness of monitoring, and varies with the populations studied.

Hypoxemia

- Postoperative hypoxemia may result from diverse etiologies:
  - **Hypoventilation** may be caused by residual anesthetic or muscle relaxant.
  - **Upper-airway obstruction** due to a decreased level of consciousness is a common reason for hypoxemia and hypercarbia.
  - **Pulmonary edema** may result from heart failure, noncardiogenic pulmonary edema, aspiration, acute respiratory distress syndrome, infection, trauma, transfusion reaction, or neurogenic pulmonary edema from head injury.
- Postoperative hypoxemia can lead to acute complications such as **cardiac ischemia.**

Negative-pressure Pulmonary Edema

- Pulmonary edema may develop after a **strenuous inspiratory effort** against an **obstructed airway.** This type of pulmonary edema may appear immediately or up to 10 hours after the episode of airway obstruction. It is most commonly associated with **laryngospasm** during anesthetic induction or during emergence from anesthesia.
- A common explanation is that the **massive negative intrapleural pressure** generated during airway obstruction shifts the balance in the Starling forces toward a large fluid transudation from the intravascular to the interstitial space.
- Typically, the patient is a **young, vigorous adult** who sustains an episode of laryngospasm either before intubation or after tracheal decannulation.

- The radiologic picture is bilateral alveolar and interstitial **edema** (rarely unilaterally), with normal heart size but enlarged vascular pedicle.
- **Treatment** is **supportive.** Patients should be given oxygen to maintain an arterial saturation of at least 90%. Some patients require reintubation and mechanical ventilation with positive pressure to ensure oxygenation and to reduce work of breathing;
- Despite pulmonary edema, intravascular volume may be depleted. Diuretics should be used only if volume overload is suspected. In most cases, the edema resolves within 24 hours.

Pain and Perioperative Stress

- Early postoperative pain remains a serious concern. Up to 75% of patients receiving parenteral narcotics may have significant residual pain after the drug is administered.
- Uncontrolled pain can lead to serious physiologic consequences. **Sympathetic nervous system stimulation** leads to elevated plasma catecholamine levels, tachycardia, hypertension, increased systemic vascular resistance, and an increase in **myocardial oxygen consumption.** In the patient with underlying coronary artery disease, this may result in ischemia or infarction.
- Surgical procedures on the upper abdomen and thorax may have profound effects on the respiratory system. The ability to deep–breathe (sigh) and cough is impaired due to pain, resulting in **atelectasis** and retained secretions. Decreased oxygenation and the potential for pulmonary parenchymal **infection** may follow.

Stress Response

- **General anesthesia** should be viewed as a potential for **stress response** as there is an increase in corticotropin, corticosteroids, β-endorphins, and catecholamine levels in response to intubation, skin incision, intra-abdominal manipulation, and on emergence from anesthesia. **High-dose narcotic techniques,** commonly used in cardiac anesthesia or for patients with ischemic heart disease, have been shown to blunt the endocrine response to stress.
- **Regional anesthesia** attenuates the stress response to surgery by avoiding the direct neural activation and transmission of noxious stimuli from the traumatized area (which general anesthesia does not do).
- **Combined anesthesia:** A common approach is to use regional anesthesia, with control of the airway by intubation, inhalational agents, and positive-pressure ventilation. The possible advantages of combined anesthesia over a purely general technique are controversial.
- **Maintenance of cardiac output and oxygen delivery** to meet the increased demands of the tissues and avoid cellular hypoxia is an important concept. Literature needs to stress the importance of **time factor** when resuscitative goals are studied. This topic is discussed in other chapters (see Chapters 7 and 8).

Delirium

- Delirium and **acute confusional states** can be very disturbing for patients and family members and impose a significant risk to patients. Incidence ranges from 0% to 73%.
- **Risk factors** include age, preoperative cognitive impairment, use of anticholinergic agents, benzodiazepines and general anesthesia.
- The reasons for postoperative delirium are many (Table 35.4).

Treatment

- Treatment depends on the etiology and removing the offending agent (see Table 35.4). **Haloperidol,** an antipsychotic with no anticholinergic properties, may be given. Haloperidol has minimum hypotensive property and is not an antidepressant. Side effects include extrapyramidal symptoms and, rarely, torsades de pointes.

Residual Neuromuscular Blockade

- Residual neuromuscular blockade usually presents in one of three ways: (a) delayed return to consciousness, which should

---

TABLE 35.4

ETIOLOGY OF POSTOPERATIVE MENTAL STATUS ALTERATION

Drugs	In the patient emergently anesthetized from the emergency department, street drugs such as alcohol, narcotics, and cocaine may have been present on induction; residual neuromuscular blockade must also be considered.
Postseizure	A seizure under anesthesia may be easily missed. One must consider the delayed emergence as a possible postictal event.
Glucose	Hyperglycemia or hypoglycemia can result in altered mental status.
Metabolic causes	Hypoxia, hypercarbia, hypernatremia or hyponatremia, hypercalcemia, and hypothermia (usually at or below 31°C) are several examples.
Trauma	Again, in the patient emergently anesthetized from the emergency department, head trauma must be considered.
Infection	Agitation in an infected patient is sometimes seen; this is no less so in the postoperative period.
Psychogenic causes	Rarely, a patient will feign unconsciousness for some secondary gain. This may be diagnosed only after other life-threatening and treatable causes have been ruled out.
Hemodynamic instability	Hypotension, and sometimes severe hypertension, may cause mental status changes. The former may result from hypovolemia, anaphylaxis, sepsis, or ischemia.
Pain	Pain at the operative site, a full bladder, or gastric distention can result in agitation.

ETIOLOGY OF POSTOPERATIVE HYPERCAPNIA

I. **Central respiratory depression**
   Intravenous (narcotic) anesthetics
   Inhaled anesthetic agents

II. **Respiratory muscle dysfunction**
   Site of incision (upper abdominal, thoracic)
   Residual neuromuscular blockade
   Use of drugs that enhance neuromuscular blockade
      (gentamicin, clindamycin, neomycin, furosemide)
   Physiologic factors that prevent reversal of neuromuscular
      blockade (hypokalemia, respiratory acidosis) or
      enhance the blockade (hypothermia, hypermagnesemia)

III. **Physical factors**
   Obesity
   Gastric dilation
   Tight dressings
   Body cast

IV. **Increased production of carbon dioxide**
   Sepsis
   Shivering
   Malignant hyperthermia

V. **Underlying hyperthermia**
   Chronic obstructive pulmonary disease with CO_2
      retention
   Neuromuscular—chest cage dysfunction (kyphoscoliosis)
   Acute or chronic respiratory failure of any etiology

Modified from Feeley TW. The recovery room. In: Miller RD, ed. *Anesthesia.* 2nd ed. New York: Churchill Livingstone; 1986:1921; and Wyngaarden JB, Smith LH Jr, eds. *Cecil Textbook of Medicine.* 18th ed. Philadelphia: WB Saunders; 1988:417, 472, 474.

ETIOLOGY OF PROLONGED NEUROMUSCULAR BLOCKADE

I. **Nondepolarizing neuromuscular blocking agents**
   Intensity of neuromuscular blockade
   Renal failure (decreased metocurine and pancuronium
      excretion)
   Hepatic failure (decreased pancuronium and vecuronium
      excretion)
   Residual potent inhaled anesthetic agent
   Inadequate dose of reversal agents
   Hypothermia
   Acid–base state
   Hypokalemia, hypermagnesemia
   Drugs
   Antibiotics (gentamicin, clindamycin, and multiple other
      drugs with several mechanisms)
   Local anesthetics
   Antiarrhythmics (quinidine)
   Furosemide
   Dantrolene
   Trimethaphan (possibly)
   Underlying diseases (myasthenia gravis, myasthenic
      syndrome, familial periodic paralysis)

II. **Depolarizing neuromuscular blocking agents
   (succinylcholine)**
   Decreased effective pseudocholinesterase
   Phase II block
   Hypermagnesemia
   Local anesthetics

Modified from Miller RD, Savarese JJ. Pharmacology of muscle relaxants and their antagonists. In: Miller RD, ed. *Anesthesia.* 2nd ed. New York: Churchill Livingstone; 1986:889.

have been noted prior to leaving the operating room; (b) respiratory difficulty with hypercapnia (Table 35.5); and (c) muscle weakness (Table 35.6).

- Several **risk factors** for the development of **prolonged paralysis** are renal failure, concomitant drug use, length of administration, monitoring technique used, and the use of steroids in patients receiving steroid-based drugs such as pancuronium or vecuronium.

Diagnosis

- Most anesthesiologists monitor the depth of neuromuscular blockade with a **twitch-stimulating device** or a group of clinical signs. Nevertheless, some patients remain with residual neuromuscular blockade. This condition may take the form of an apparent alteration in mental status (see Table 35.4)
- The key point is to **recognize the problem,** with early intubation if necessary.

Treatment

- If residual neuromuscular blockade is present, reversal may be necessary. If prolonged blockade results from succinylcholine, which can occur in patients with pseudocholinesterase deficiency, reversal agents will not be of any benefit. The diagnosis is made by measuring pseudocholinesterase activity in plasma,
- If a **nondepolarizing blocking agent** was used, reversal may be attempted with anticholinesterases and anticholinergics (Table 35.7).

Malignant Hyperthermia

- Manifestations of malignant hyperthermia (MH) may be divided into **early, late, and postcrisis** phases (Table 35.8). The differential diagnosis of MH includes sepsis, light anesthesia, thyrotoxicosis, myotonias, neuroleptic malignant syndrome, and pheochromocytoma.

REVERSAL AGENTS USED WITH NEUROMUSCULAR BLOCKING AGENTS

Anticholinesterase	Anticholinergic
Neostigmine 35–70 μg/kg (maximum, 5 mg)	Atropine 20 μg/kg or
Edrophonium 500–1,000 μg/kg	Glycopyrrolate 10 μg/kg
Pyridostigmine 175–350 μg/kg (maximum, 20 mg)	

Modified from Miller RD, Savarese JJ. Pharmacology of muscle relaxants and their antagonists. In: Miller RD, ed. *Anesthesia.* 2nd ed. New York: Churchill Livingstone; 1986:889.

TABLE 35.8

SIGNS OF MALIGNANT HYPERTHERMIA

Early signs	Late signs	Postcrisis signs
Skeletal muscle rigidity	Hyperpyrexia—may exceed 43°C (109.4°F)	Muscle pain, edema
Tachycardia and hypertension	Cyanosis	Central nervous system damage
Elevated PetCO$_2$	Serum electrolyte abnormalities	Renal failure
Acidosis	Elevated serum creatinine phosphokinase	Continued electrolyte imbalance
Dysrhythmias	Myoglobinuria	
	Coagulopathy	
	Cardiac failure and pulmonary edema	

PetCO$_2$, end tidal partial pressure of carbon dioxide.

Background

- MH is a pharmacogenetic clinical syndrome that usually occurs during general anesthesia. The incidence varies; fulminant cases are seen from 1 in 250,000 to 1 in 62,000 anesthetics.
- Its onset may be **delayed** for several hours

TABLE 35.9

ACUTE THERAPY FOR MALIGNANT HYPERTHERMIA

I. **Discontinue all anesthetic agents.**
   Hyperventilate with an FiO$_2$ of 1.0.
   CO$_2$ is increased so hyperventilate to achieve a normal PaCO$_2$.

II. **Dantrolene**
   Intravenously 2 mg/kg every 5 min to a total of 10 mg/kg
   Effective dosage should be repeated every 10–15 h for at least 48 h.

III. **Sodium bicarbonate**
   Initial dose (mEq) = (base excess × [body weight in kg])/4
   Give half the calculated dose; repeat as determined by arterial blood gas studies.

IV. **Control fever**
   Iced fluids
   Surface cooling
   Cooling of body cavities with sterile iced saline
   Heat exchanger with a pump oxygenator
   Dantrolene

V. **Monitor urinary output**
   At least 0.5 mL/kg/h
   If myoglobinuria is present, at least 1 mL/kg/h

VI. **Further therapy**
   Guided by blood studies, temperature, and urine output
   (Blood studies include blood gases, electrolytes, liver profile, coagulation studies [including DIC studies], serum hemoglobin and myoglobin, and urine hemoglobin and myoglobin.)

DIC, disseminated intravascular coagulation; FiO$_2$, fraction of inspired oxygen.
Modified from Askanazi J. Principles of nutritional support. In: Barash PG, Deutsch S, Tinker J, eds. *Refresher Courses in Anesthesiology.* Vol. 14. Philadelphia: JB Lippincott; 1986:1.

- The hallmark is rapidly **increasing temperature** caused by uncontrolled skeletal muscle metabolism that can result in rhabdomyolysis and death. Oxygen consumption can increase threefold, whereas blood lactate may increase 15- to 20-fold.
- The mechanism involves myoplasmic calcium accumulation and a failure of calcium uptake by the sarcoplasmic reticulum.
- A 24-hour per day **emergency phone number** for consultations has been set up by the Malignant Hyperthermia Association of the United States (**1-209-634-4917**).
- Evaluation of **susceptibility** includes a family history and measurement of baseline creatine kinase level, which is elevated in 70% of those affected.
- The definitive test is a **muscle biopsy** for contracture studies after exposure to halothane, caffeine, halothane plus caffeine, or potassium. A new approach is **genetic testing.**

Diagnosis

- Diagnosis must be considered in the presence of unexplained tachycardia, tachypnea, arrhythmias, mottling, cyanosis, hyperthermia, muscle rigidity, diaphoresis, or hemodynamic instability.
- The presence of more than one sign must initiate arterial and central venous blood gas analysis for metabolic and respiratory **acidosis** and **hyperkalemia.**
- Central **venous oxygen** and **carbon dioxide partial pressures** change more dramatically than do those of arterial blood.

Treatment

- The mortality rate of MH has decreased from 70% to less than 5% when recognized and treated appropriately because of improved therapy (Table 35.9).
- With fulminant MH, PaCO$_2$ above 60 mm Hg, base excess more than –5 mEq/L, and a body temperature that is increasing by approximately 1°C every 15 minutes, specific therapy with **dantrolene** is required.
- The mechanism of action of dantrolene is not completely clear, but it is known to affect the ryanodine receptor, which is a major calcium release channel of the skeletal muscle sarcoplasmic reticulum, thus **decreasing the intracellular calcium.** Because of dantrolens's poor water solubility, the **preparation** for intravenous use requires the full attention of at least one person. Help must be requested.

CHAPTER 36 ■ INITIAL MANAGEMENT OF THE TRAUMA PATIENT

- How does initial trauma care differ from other critical care treatment? **Time is the key,** as common traumatic injuries are rapidly lethal. Initial management of the trauma patient requires a different focus.
- **Prioritization,** aided by careful planning and a team approach, contributes to patient survival.

THE TEAM

- Treatment plan starts **before** the next trauma patient arrives.
- A multiply injured patient may require **several simultaneous interventions.**
- Having a team of **physicians, nurses, technicians, therapists, and aides** allows for parallel rather than sequential treatment.
- Adding personnel (e.g., x-ray technicians, respiratory therapists, surgical specialists) to your team can reduce treatment delays.
- Critically reviewing trauma resuscitations in your facility will reveal any needed additions or deletions of members to your team.
- Take a lesson from the National Association for Stock Car Auto Racing (NASCAR). A NASCAR team can change four tires and fill the gas tank in about a minute. To **function as a team,** you need to **practice as a team.**
- **Mock trauma drills** allow you to do it **over and over again** until you do it right. Do you have more than one chest tube set? How long does it take to get the drugs for a rapid sequence induction and intubation? Do you even have a pediatric endotracheal tube? Your team will need to establish intravenous (IV) access and administer fluid, gather baseline vital signs, and complete the primary survey in this time frame of minutes.
- Do team members understand the big picture (what needs to be done for the patient) beyond their specific assignments? Are they prepared to **shift roles** when necessary?

TRIAGE

- Called to the **scene of an accident,** paramedics initially triage the victims. They determine whom to transport and when and where to take them (following established community protocols). The number of patients and severity of their injuries are weighed against available resources.
- In a **mass casualty event,** you may need to evacuate the emergency department (ED) to make room for incoming patients. The seriously injured will be brought in slowly as patients with minor injuries flood into your waiting room. It is important that the vital role of making these initial triage decisions

be done by someone who is **experienced in trauma management.**
- Triage is **most effective at "ground zero,"** a site in the field where patients are gathered prior to transport. If roads and communications are disrupted, much of the initial trauma care may need to be provided at that site.
- Paramedics play a **critical role** even when triage is not an issue. Their observations may be the only **medical history** that is ever available.

PRIORITIZATION

- **"Airway, breathing, and circulation"** is worth repeating over and over as you struggle to revive a trauma victim. **An obstructed airway is lethal** within minutes. Securing an airway can buy enough time to address many other injuries.
- In a deteriorating patient **not responding to resuscitation,** it is more important to look for airway obstruction repeatedly (even in intubated patients).
- After ensuring **airway, breathing, and circulation,** "D" is a reminder to consider **disability** (i.e., to perform a **rapid neurologic assessment**). At the bare minimum, this should include an assessment of the **patient's pupils** (size and reaction to light), **extremity motion (looking for lateralizing signs),** and **Glasgow coma scale.**
- "E" reminds you to **expose** the patient. Cutting off clothes may seem wasteful until you miss an unsuspected wound. Slight tracheal deviation may be the only sign of a tension pneumothorax. The odds of identifying this are vastly improved if the patient is exposed.
- Placing a **warmed blanket** allows you to quickly cover and uncover a patient. This mitigates hypothermia caused by cold IV fluid, field exposure, and ED exposure.
- In trauma, **coagulopathy is multifactorial.** Ongoing bleeding, attempted clotting, and crystalloid resuscitation lead to the direct loss, consumption, and dilution of platelets and clotting factors. With mild **hypothermia, platelets adhere poorly.** Below 33°C, **coagulation enzymes fail.** Once the core body temperature drops below 32°C, trauma patients have a 100% mortality. Hypothermia is a preventable cause of death mitigated by simple measures such as active warming blankets and warming the fluids and temperature of the ED trauma bay/operating room.

THE PRIMARY SURVEY

- The primary survey focuses on high-priority injuries, those that are **rapidly lethal and rapidly correctable** (Table 36.1).

TABLE 36.1

THE FOCUS OF THE PRIMARY SURVEY

Rapidly lethal and rapidly correctable injuries	Initial treatment
Airway obstruction	Obtain a secure airway
Tension pneumothorax	Needle thoracostomy
Open pneumothorax	Support ventilation
Cardiac tamponade	Decompression
Peripheral arterial injuries	Direct pressure

Airway Obstruction and Airway Management

- Failure in airway maintenance rapidly leads to death. Apart from the rare patient with severe facial trauma who requires an immediate cricothyroidotomy, trauma patients' airway should be approached in the standard fashion.
- Assume that all patients are at risk for a respiratory arrest and for a **cervical spine** injury and are likely to have a **full stomach.**
- If you have any doubt, err on the side of intubating the patient.

Airway Management and the Cervical Spine

- Any patient who rapidly decelerates (e.g., motor vehicle accident, fall) requires spinal stabilization.
- Protecting the spine is occasionally at odds with needed intervention. This conflict is best overcome by assigning one team member to maintain in-line **stabilization** (not traction) while other team members perform necessary interventions.
- **Cervical spine clearance** criteria are controversial and may require a C-spine series or computed tomography of the neck, to rule out fractures, followed by flexion/extension views or magnetic resonance imaging of the neck, to rule out ligamentous injuries. In an alert, cooperative patient who has no neck tenderness, no distracting injury, and a normal neurologic examination, the collar may be safely removed based on clinical exam.
- Clearing the C-spine is **not an immediate priority** and should be delayed until patients are stable.

Pneumothorax and Tension Pneumothorax

- **Pneumothorax** is one of the most common thoracic injuries. Air usually enters the pleural space from a lung injury. During normal inspiration, the diaphragm contracts, intrapleural pressure falls, and the lung expands via the bellows effect. If the pleural space contains trapped air, the lung cannot fully expand. Blood then circulates through nonaerated alveoli, leading to hypoxia.
- In **tension pneumothorax,** inspiration pulls air into the pleural space, but expiration compresses the lung and obstructs air egress. As pleural pressure builds, the mediastinum is **pushed to the contralateral side** (**shifting the trachea**), eventually kinking the superior vena cava and inferior vena cava.

- Venous pressure then rises (distending the neck veins), and **venous return falls.** As preload drops, **cardiac output drops,** and then blood pressure drops.
- Patients **die from cardiogenic shock, not hypoxia,** although hypoxia may also be present.
- **Do not wait for chest radiograph** confirmation. In rapidly deteriorating patients, chest tube insertion may take too long. Use the largest IV catheter immediately available (ideally 14- or 16-gauge). Place the catheter in the **second or third intercostal space, in the midclavicular line,** aiming toward the back.
- Regardless of whether the patient had a tension pneumothorax, the outcome will be a simple pneumothorax. A **chest tube** should then be placed in the fifth intercostal space in the midaxillary line.
- **Volume loading** should be done simultaneously for treating a tension pneumothorax. Increasing the venous volume (and pressure) will overcome the venous obstruction (until the mediastinum shifts further).

Open Pneumothorax and Flail Chest

- There is a large hole into the chest. As the patient tries to breathe, air moves in and out through the hole, therefore the name "sucking chest wound."
- Intrapleural pressure never falls, so the ipsilateral lung never expands.
- There are two treatment options: (a) **Cover the hole** and create a simple pneumothorax, which can then be treated with tube thoracostomy, or (b) intubate the patient so **positive pressure ventilation** will expand both lungs regardless of the presence of an open pneumothorax.
- **Flail chest has similar pathophysiology.** If three or more ribs are broken in two places, the "flail" segment moves in and out as the patient tries to breathe. There are three choices: (a) Place a chest tube, (b) intubate, or (c) do both.

Cardiac Tamponade

- **Beck's triad (hypotension, jugular venous distention, and muffled heart sounds)** and **pulsus paradoxus** (an exaggerated drop in systolic blood pressure of >10 mm Hg with inspiration) are the hallmarks of cardiac tamponade. These clinical signs are **less reliable in trauma.** Hypotension is nearly universal, hypovolemia may prevent jugular venous distention, and ED noise obscures heart sounds.
- The widespread adoption of focused abdominal **sonography** for trauma has made it easier to identify cardiac tamponade.
- As blood enters the rigid pericardial sack, it **prevents the heart from filling** during diastole. **Venous return** is **obstructed,** venous pressure rises, and cardiac output falls. The rapid infusion of IV fluid will transiently raise the blood pressure. Decompression is key, followed by definitive correction of the underlying injury.
- **Pericardiocentesis** has been used effectively for trauma. The technique is outlined in Chapter 16. However, the preferred treatment is subxiphoid pericardial window or emergency room thoracotomy. Decompression buys time but rarely addresses the underlying injury. Patients should, therefore,

ESTIMATED FLUID AND BLOOD LOSSES BASED ON PATIENT'S INITIAL PRESENTATION

	Class I	Class II	Class III	Class IV
Blood loss (mL)	Up to 750	750–1,500	1,500–2,000	>2,000
Blood loss (% blood volume)	Up to 15%	15%–30%	30%–40%	>40%
Pulse rate	<100	>100	>120	>140
Blood pressure	Normal	Normal	Decreased	Decreased

From American College of Surgeons Committee on Trauma. *ATLS Advance Trauma Life Support for Doctors.* Chicago: American College of Surgeons; 2004:74 (Table 1).

be expeditiously taken to the operating room for median sternotomy or anterolateral thoracotomy.

Peripheral Arterial Injuries

- Significant arterial bleeding from extremity laceration is sometimes **"audible."** **Direct pressure** is the treatment of choice with peripheral arterial injuries. Tourniquets cut off collateral circulation and are best reserved for those situations where you need to stop bleeding while carrying the victim to safety. Direct clamping is instantaneously effective but may be difficult in the emergency room. A clamp may crush the artery, reducing the length available for a primary anastomosis and may damage adjacent nerves and veins.

Resuscitation

- Resuscitation starts in the field and continues after arrival to ED.
- It is rare for patients to develop congestive heart failure from resuscitation in the emergency room even if they have underlying cardiac disease.
- Under-resuscitation is common. Young, athletic patients may be able to **compensate** for significant blood loss without tachycardia or hypotension. Essential **hypertension and heart block** also make it difficult to interpret vital signs in the elderly.
- As a sign of shock, tachycardia is more sensitive than hypotension; however, tachycardia may reflect pain rather than blood loss. With the foregoing caveats, **continuously monitoring the vital signs** is the best way to gauge the efficacy of ongoing resuscitation (Table 36.2).
- As a general guide, a **palpable carotid pulse** implies that the blood pressure is at least **60 mm Hg;** a **femoral pulse** implies that the blood pressure is over **70 mm Hg;** and a **radial pulse** implies **80 mm Hg.**

Intravenous Access

- **"Two large-bore IVs,** placed at different sites," is a tenet of trauma resuscitation. "Large bore" implies that the line can be used to rapidly transfuse blood.

- Commercial **warming equipment** (e.g., Level 1 or Rapid Infusion System) and simple pressure bags can greatly increase the transfusion pressure. Large IV catheters (No. 6 or No. 8 French) are readily available and can be placed easily using the Seldinger technique.
- A shorter length and larger diameter IV access are advantageous.
- If you place femoral lines in patients with pelvic trauma, you may find one of your lines infusing into the peritoneal cavity through a lacerated iliac vein. Whenever possible, **place IV lines away from the site of trauma.**

Colloid, Crystalloid, and Blood Substitutes

- Restoring volume can be achieved with colloid or crystalloid. Restoring oxygen-carrying capacity requires red cells.
- **Crystalloid** should be used first in trauma resuscitation. It must be isotonic either normal saline (0.9% NaCl) or Ringer lactate. Crystalloid equilibrates throughout the interstitial and intracellular spaces. As a consequence, 3 L of crystalloid is needed to replace 1 L of blood.
- If patient remains hypotensive after 2 L of crystalloid, O-negative or type-specific blood should be started.

Permissive Hypotension

- In models of uncontrolled hemorrhagic shock, aggressive resuscitation may increase mortality by increasing the bleeding from unsecured injured vessels. Improved outcome in younger patients with penetrating torso trauma has been reported with permissive hypotension, but this treatment should not be extrapolated to other types of patients until further studies are done.

THE SECONDARY SURVEY

This chapter has explored the initial management of the trauma patient. After ruling out injuries that are *rapidly lethal and rapidly correctable,* many **other injuries remain.** Some may be severe, contributing to death and disability. To avoid missing these injuries, the **secondary and tertiary survey** should be thorough, detailed, and compulsive.

CHAPTER 37 ■ SECONDARY AND TERTIARY TRIAGE OF THE TRAUMA PATIENT

The previous chapter covers the initial assessment and care of the injured trauma patient. The patient will make the transition to the more comprehensive capabilities of the inpatient setting. This chapter is focused on **transport, transfer of care to the intensive care unit (ICU) team, the gathering of additional information, continued resuscitation, and a more complete and thorough assessment of the patient's injuries, including commonly missed injuries.**

TRANSPORT

- Appropriate equipment, monitoring, and adequate personnel are necessary for **safe transport** (Table 37.1).

COMMUNICATION

- Communication between areas of transfer, between and among nursing staff, physicians, and even hospital administrators, is essential.
- Early **communication with the family** allows the family members to transition to an emotional state where they are capable of dealing with the issues at hand. From the family, a thorough **history** may be obtained with attention to **chronic diseases, anticoagulant use** (aspirin, warfarin, clopidogrel, etc.), and patient **allergies.** Finally, **informed consent** should be obtained for any planned invasive procedures.
- The **social worker** has the ability to obtain insight into **family dynamics** and resources. They may interact with **law enforcement** officials and get a thorough description of the circumstances surrounding the issue, even as the acute resuscitation and management phase is taking place.

INITIAL INTENSIVE CARE UNIT CARE

Reassessing the ABCs while Maintaining Vital Function

- Arrival in the ICU represents a time for **reassessment** of patient status, particularly the **ABCs (airway, breathing, circulation).**
- The **airway** may be assessed in standard fashion: in the non-intubated patient, by patient's ability to **speak;** in intubated patients, by confirmation of endotracheal tube placement using of end-tidal carbon dioxide and chest radiograph.
- Assessment of **breathing** should consist of both auscultation of the lungs and confirmation of adequate oxygen saturation via pulse oximetry.

- Evaluation of **circulatory status** should include auscultation of the heart, confirmation of pulses, measurement of blood pressure, and verification of adequate intravenous access.
- Two large-bore **intravenous lines** should be present, although a large-bore central venous line (e.g., a No. 9 French introducer) may be preferred in the critically injured patient as it is less likely to become dislodged, allows central venous pressure measurements, and can provide a port of entry for a right heart catheter should this be desired. The authors recommend a subclavian approach due to the lesser incidence of catheter-related bloodstream. The femoral vein may also be utilized for rapid access; however, femoral venous catheters should be removed within 24 hours due to the risk of deep vein thrombosis.

PERSISTENT SHOCK

- In the trauma patient, persistent shock is **hemorrhage** until proven otherwise, and a meticulous search for hidden sources of bleeding is indicated, such as **scalp lacerations** (bleeding edges can be quickly sutured with a large monofilament suture) and **fractures,** which should be aligned and temporarily splinted to avoid further bleeding.

Management of the Patient in Persistent Hemorrhagic Shock

- Resuscitation of the bleeding patient in shock is best performed with **blood and fresh frozen plasma in a 1:1 ratio.** In patients requiring more than 10 units of blood replacement, it is helpful to have a **massive transfusion protocol** in place to guide management (Fig. 37.1).
- Patients requiring massive transfusions may benefit from **recombinant factor VIIA,** although studies demonstrating a survival benefit are lacking.

Goal-directed Therapy

- Goal-directed therapy refers to the use of resuscitation end points (**cardiac index, oxygen delivery (DO_2I), mixed venous O_2 saturation**) to guide management of the patient in shock.
- Though controversial, there is a general consensus that maintenance of tissue oxygenation is beneficial in preventing the sequelae of shock. Debate has centered on the specific end points that should be utilized, whether a pulmonary artery catheter should be used, and whether normal or supranormal oxygen delivery values should be pursued. This topic is discussed in other chapters (see Chapters 7 and 23).

TABLE 37.1

AMERICAN COLLEGE OF CRITICAL CARE MEDICINE/SOCIETY OF CRITICAL CARE MEDICINE GUIDELINES FOR INTRAHOSPITAL TRANSFER OF THE CRITICALLY ILL PATIENT

Pretransport coordination	Continuity of care ensured by physician-to-physician and/or nurse-to-nurse communication to review patient condition and the treatment plan
	Confirmation by the receiving location that it is ready to receive the patient
	Coordination of appropriate hospital personnel (e.g., respiratory therapy) to be available on patient arrival
Accompanying personnel	Minimum of two people
	In unstable patients, a physician with training in airway management, advanced cardiac life support (ACLS), and critical care training or equivalent
Accompanying equipment	A blood pressure monitor (or standard blood pressure cuff), pulse oximeter, and cardiac monitor/defibrillator to accompany every patient without exception
	When available, a memory-capable monitor with capacity for storing and reproducing patient bedside data
	Airway management equipment and oxygen source to supply for projected needs and 30-minute reserve
	Basic resuscitation medications (epinephrine, antiarrhythmic agents)
	If employing a transport ventilator, must have alarms to indicate disconnection and excessively high airway pressures and must have a backup battery power supply
Monitoring during transport	At a minimum, continuous electrocardiographic monitoring, continuous pulse oximetry, and periodic measurement of blood pressure, pulse rate, and respiratory rate

Adapted from Warren J, Fromm RE Jr, Orr RA, et al. 2004. Guidelines for the inter- and intrahospital transport of critically ill patients. *Crit Care Med.* 2004;32:256.

Schedule for Massive Transfusion Protocol Shands at the University of Florida					
Shipment	Red Blood Cells	Plasma	Platelet Dose	**Cryo	***rFVIIa
*1	10 (O-Neg)	4(AB)			
2	10	4	1	10	rFVIIa
3	10	4	1		
4	10	4	1	10	rFVIIa
5	10	4	1		
6	10	4	1	10	

The shipment number refers to the allotment of blood components (Red Blood Cells, Plasma, Platelets, Cryoprecipitate, and rFVIIa) provided at each step of massive transfusion. At the conclusion of each step, the decision must be made by the team providing care whether or not to order the next shipment of blood products.

Definition of massive transfusion

Massive transfusion at Shands at the University of Florida is defined as a presumed need for the transfusion of at least 10 units of packed red blood cells (PRBC) in an adult patient or at least five (5) units of PRBC in a child within a short time frame (i.e. two (2)-hour time period).

Adult	Greater than 10 units
6-12 year old child	Greater than or equal to 5 units
4-5 year old child	Greater than or equal to 3 units
2-3 year old child	Greater than or equal to 2 units
0-1 year old child	Greater than or equal to 1 unit

*Shipment 1 is located in the Satellite Blood Bank Refrigerator, located in the Emergency Department and Operating Room.
**Cryo=Cryoprecipitate
***Recombinant Factor VIIa (rFVIIa) is not routinely shipped and must be ordered from Pharmacy. These are recommended intervals if rFVIIa is clinically warranted.

FIGURE 37.1. The massive transfusion protocol of the Acute Care Surgery Service of Shands Hospital at the University of Florida (Appendix A).

- Values obtained **through right heart catheterization** are considered the "gold standard" physiologic measurements to which noninvasive cardiovascular measurements are compared. The primary therapeutic end-point value obtained through right heart catheteriza$_t$ion is DO_2I, which is a **function of cardiac index, hemoglobin, and oxygen saturation.**

BLUNT CARDIAC INJURY

- **Cardiac function** is **essential** in delivering oxygen to the tissues, and delayed recognition of myocardial dysfunction will lead to tissue ischemia and poor outcome.
- Blunt cardiac injury (BCI) may be classified according to descriptors of the specific abnormalities and can range from minor clinical manifestations to fulminant cardiac failure and death:
  - BCI **with minor electrocardiogram (ECG) or enzyme abnormality**
  - BCI **with complex arrhythmia**
  - BCI **with coronary artery thrombosis**
  - BCI **with free wall rupture**
  - BCI **with septal rupture**
  - BCI **with cardiac failure**
- BCI must be suspected in any case involving thoracic trauma and may coexist with rib/sternal fractures, hemopneumothorax, and pulmonary contusion.
- **Clinical exam** may show hypotension, visual sequelae of chest trauma (abrasions, bruising, seatbelt sign, or steering wheel imprint), flail chest, rib fractures, sternal fractures, findings consistent with cardiac tamponade such as abnormal heart sounds (muffling, distance, S_3, S_4, murmurs, bruits, or rubs), and jugular venous distention.
- **Bedside sonography** in trauma focused abdominal sonography in trauma (FAST) exam should be performed to look for fluid in the pericardium. There are no **ECG findings** that are pathognomonic for BCI; however, the finding of an abnormal ECG should prompt further workup. With regard to the **chest radiograph,** there are no findings that will definitively demonstrate cardiac injury, but they often prove useful by demonstrating some of the associated injuries that may accompany BCI.
- **Troponin I** testing may have a sensitivity ranging from 23% to 100% and a specificity of 85% to 97%.
- The value of **formal echocardiography** has been studied in BCI. In patients with hemodynamic instability, it is felt that transthoracic echocardiography may provide diagnostic information; however, transesophageal echocardiography also allows evaluation of the aorta.
- The patient with BCI accompanied by hypotension may benefit from use of **right heart catheterization** to maintain cardiac index and tissue perfusion.

Management

- Management consists of treating hypotension, arrhythmias, and pump failure.
- **Complex arrhythmia** occurring from 2% to 30% may consist of atrial dysrhythmia, ventricular dysrhythmia, or commotio cordis (myocardial concussion). Commotio cordis is a rare entity where a blow to the chest results in an immedi-

ate rhythm disruption without myocardial structural damage and may be the cause of **sudden death** in young people.
- **Cardiac failure** with BCI is less commonly seen. Supportive care with volume and inotropic agents is the mainstay of management in these patients. In extreme cases, use of intra-aortic balloon counterpulsation pump has been used, but the benefits and risks of heparinization in a trauma patient must be considered.
- **Myocardial wall rupture** is rare. Should this injury be suspected or the diagnosis confirmed with echocardiography, immediate operation via open thoracotomy is the sole management option.
- **Coronary artery thrombosis** with BCI is uncommon. The diagnosis is made via findings of ST-segment changes consistent with myocardial ischemia after blunt chest trauma. Management is similar to that employed when a patient presents with a myocardial infarction of another etiology. Percutaneous angioplasty, stenting, and bypass are available options. Some patients may have had a myocardial infarct first that precipitated the accident.

EXTREMITY COMPARTMENT SYNDROME

- Secondary and tertiary survey should identify fractures that may not be life-threatening but may lead to severe disability if not recognized. The extremities are divided into several fascial compartments that contain the musculature, blood vessels, and nerves that supply the respective limbs. During trauma and/or due to resuscitation, increased pressure causes impairs lymphatic, venous, and arterial flow and may lead to muscle necrosis and permanent nerve damage.

Clinical Suspicion

- Extremity compartment syndrome most commonly occurs in fractures of the **tibial shaft or distal radius,** followed by soft-tissue injuries **without fracture.** Though compartment syndrome is most commonly associated with fracture within a closed space, an open fracture does not preclude the presence of a compartment syndrome. Patients taking anticoagulant medications are at increased risk.

Diagnosis and Monitoring

- The presence of the **"six P's"** (pain, pulselessness, pallor, pressure, paresthesias, and paralysis) are the keys to diagnosis, although originally described for acute arterial occlusion rather than compartment syndrome.
- **Pain during passive range-of-motion** exercises is often the first sign of a developing problem. **Pulselessness** is a late finding once compartmental pressures have become great enough to overcome arterial pressure. **Paresthesias** are potentially ominous signs, as they may represent muscle or nerve ischemia;
- As the clinical diagnosis can sometimes be difficult and/or unclear, **monitoring devices** have been developed to evaluate intracompartmental pressures. Patients demonstrating a ΔP **value of 20 mm Hg** between measured compartment pressure and diastolic blood pressure should undergo fasciotomy.

Management

- **Fasciotomy** in the extremity is accomplished through either a single incision on the anterolateral calf or incisions on the medial and lateral calf, with subsequent division of the fascial compartments.
- After fasciotomy, a popular method of dressing the patient is with **vacuum-assisted closure** although wet-to-dry dressings with saline will provide adequate coverage. In cases where the patient has developed muscle necrosis, debridement will be necessary at an interval operation between fasciotomy and closure. Closure may be accomplished primarily, if tension allows, or by secondary intention. Skin grafting is the final option and should be considered any time that tension precludes closure by the first two techniques.

ABDOMINAL COMPARTMENT SYNDROME

- Abdominal compartment syndrome (ACS) occurs from increased intra-abdominal pressure either from a primary cause (bleeding) or from resuscitation. There is hypoperfusion secondary to a **low cardiac output** (from impaired venous return) and **high peak inspiratory pressure** with **hypercarbia,** and there is **oliguria.** The surgical technique performed for damage control is a continuum that includes primary resuscitation, damage control celiotomy, secondary resuscitation, and delayed reconstruction. If ACS is recognized late or goes unrecognized, it can lead to multiple organ failure and death.

Clinical Suspicion, Diagnosis, and Monitoring

- A normal intra-abdominal pressure is approximately 5 mm Hg but may be higher with obesity. **Bladder pressure** may be measured by injecting 50 to 100 mL of sterile saline into the aspiration port of the Foley drainage tube. The catheter is then clamped distal to the aspiration port, and a 16-gauge needle is used to connect a pressure transducer to the aspiration port of the catheter. The pressure transducer should be zero-referenced to the level of the **midaxillary line** or the symphysis pubis.
- For continuous, indirect intra-abdominal pressure measurement, a balloon-tipped catheter in the stomach or a continuous bladder irrigation method is recommended (Fig. 37.2). A pressure of 25 mm Hg or higher is associated with organ dysfunction and considered clinical intra-abdominal hypertension.
- The inaugural World Conference on Abdominal Compartment Syndrome held in Australia in December 2004 produced consensus definitions as follows:
  - **Intra-abdominal hypertension** is defined by either one or both of the following: (a) an intra-abdominal pressure ≥12 mm Hg, recorded by a minimum of three standardized measurements conducted 4 to 6 hours apart; (b) an **abdominal perfusion pressure** (abdominal perfusion pressure = mean arterial pressure–intra-abdominal pressure) ≤60 mm Hg, recorded by a minimum of two standardized measurements conducted 1 to 6 hours apart.

TABLE 37.2

GRADING OF INTRA-ABDOMINAL HYPERTENSION

Grade	Intra-abdominal pressure (mm Hg)
I	12–15
II	16–20
III	21–25
IV	>25

Adapted from World Society of Abdominal Compartment Syndrome. http://www.wsacs.org/.

- Intra-abdominal hypertension is graded as described in Table 37.2.
- ACS was defined as the presence of an intra-abdominal **pressure ≥20 mm Hg,** with or without an **abdominal perfusion pressure <50 mm Hg,** recorded by a minimum of three standardized measurements conducted 1 to 6 hours apart and single or multiple **organ system failure** that was not previously present.

Management

- Aggressive, nonsurgical, critical care support is of utmost importance and should include continuous cardiorespiratory monitoring and aggressive intravascular fluid replacement. *Excessive* fluid resuscitation, however, is **detrimental. Hypertonic** lactated or saline resuscitation may reduce the risk of secondary ACS due to lower fluid volume requirements during the acute resuscitation phase.
- Nonsurgical management of ACS is listed in Table 37.3.
- **Decompressive laparotomy** is the gold standard for treatment of ACS. Mesh can be used for temporary abdominal closure. Skin closure itself may be associated with increased intra-abdominal pressure, so care must be taken when selecting this option.

TABLE 37.3

COMPONENTS OF NONSURGICAL MANAGEMENT OF THE ABDOMINAL COMPARTMENT SYNDROME

Gastric decompression
Rectal enemas
Colonic prokinetic agents (neostigmine)
Continuous venovenous hemofiltration with aggressive ultrafiltration
Paralysis
Botulinum toxin into the internal anal sphincter
Paracentesis
Gastrointestinal prokinetic agents (cisapride, metoclopramide, domperidone, erythromycin)
Furosemide with or without use of human albumin 20%
Sedation
Body positioning

Adapted from Sugrue M. Abdominal compartment syndrome. *Curr Opin Crit Care.* 2005;11:333.

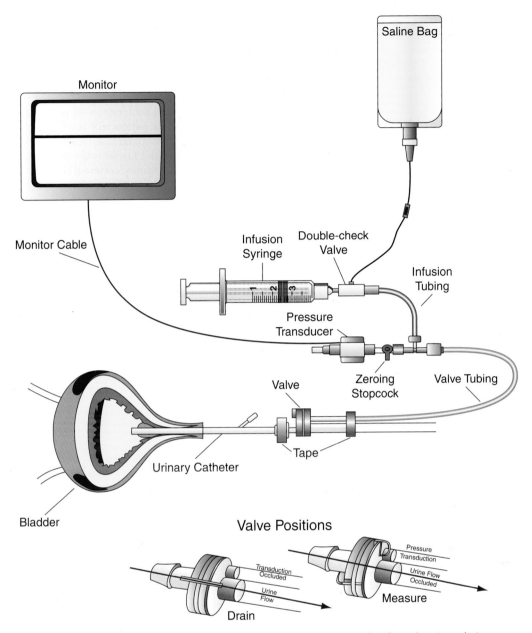

FIGURE 37.2. Intra-abdominal pressure monitoring device. The device is placed into the urinary drainage circuit. By changing the valve from "drain" to "measure," intermittent measurements may be taken. This device allows measurement of intra-abdominal pressure without breaking or interrupting the urinary drainage circuit.

- Permanent abdominal closure is usually planned for a time after the acute phase of resuscitation when edema has subsided.

Potential Complications if Abdominal Compartment Syndrome is not Diagnosed in a Timely Manner

- Multiple organ dysfunction results from inadequate oxygen delivery to the tissues with low cardiac output and ventilatory failure. Prolonged bowel ischemia is associated with intestinal necrosis. The mortality rate is high is not promptly recognized and treated.

PELVIC FRACTURES

- Pelvic fractures often are indicative of a **high-energy** impact as the pelvic ring is an extremely stable bony structure; thus, pelvic fractures rarely occur in isolation.
- Mortality rate is about 10% in all patients and up to 80% with hemodynamic instability.
- Patients involved in motorcycle crashes, pedestrian injuries, falling from heights >15 feet, and in automobile accidents are high risk.
- Pelvic pain, pain on hip rotation, pain on pelvic compression, the presence of blood at the urethral meatus, and finding a perineal and/or scrotal hematoma have all been associated with pelvic fractures and warrant further investigation.

- Pelvic fractures represent another **"hidden" source** of hemorrhage, as patients may bleed >20 units into the retroperitoneal space; thus, a patient with an appropriate mechanism of injury and unexplained hypotension should have the diagnosis of pelvic fracture considered.

Diagnosis

- Plain film radiographs done in the ED usually identifies pelvic fractures but computerized tomography is superior to plain films and offers the advantage of identifying active hemorrhage at the site of pelvic fracture, in the form of a contrast **"blush"** on arterial phase imaging. The presence of a blush should prompt mobilization of the interventional radiology team.

Management

- Beyond the usual components of the trauma resuscitation, management of the patient with severe pelvic fracture is aimed at **control of hemorrhage** and fixation of fractures.
- One of the first and fastest ways to decrease bleeding after pelvic fracture is through **external compression** of the pelvis. Circumferential wrapping of the pelvis with a bed sheet and clamping the sheet anteriorly is one technique. **"Pelvic binders"** are also commercially available.

SHANDS
at the University of Florida

Trauma and Emergency Surgery
Tertiary Survey Form *(page 1 of 2)*

Patient Name: MR#:

Physical Examination	Lacerations / Abrasions / Burns *(Document Location / Size)*

Date:

Admission Date: Admission Time:

HPI Recap (MOI, Interventions, Hospital Course):

Past Med / Surg Hist:

Social Hist:

Physical Examination | Lacerations / Abrasions / Burns (Document Location / Size)

VS:

T: P: BP: R:

GCS:

Eyes: Verbal: Motor:

HEENT:

Neck:

CV:

Resp / Chest:

Abd / Rectal:

GU:

Extremities:

Neuro (CN, Extremities):

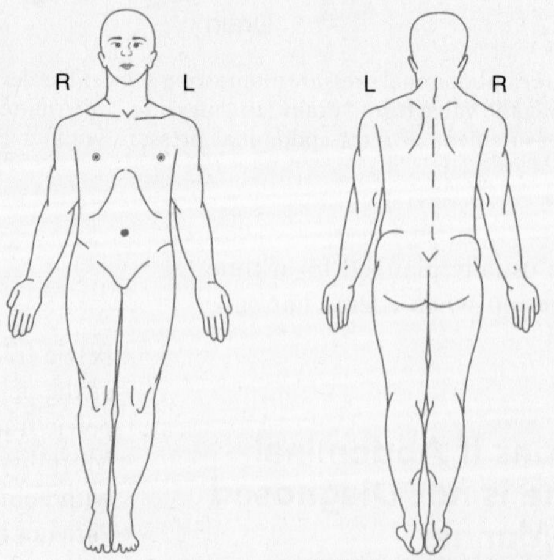

FIGURE 37.3. The tertiary survey instrument of the Acute Care Surgery Service of Shands Hospital at the University of Florida (page 1).

- An **external fixator** may be applied reasonably rapidly, particularly in the case of a posterior ring disruption where a C-clamp may be used; fixations involving anterior disruptions may require the operating room.
- **Preperitoneal and retroperitoneal packing** have recently been receiving attention. This procedure can be performed rapidly and decreases the need for emergent angioembolization. Decreased transfusion requirements and a reduction in mortality have been observed. This method is helpful when angioembolization is not immediately available for hemodynamically unstable patients.
- In cases where computed tomography (CT) demonstrates a potential arterial source of bleeding (a blush), **angioembolization** should be performed. These techniques involves obtaining arterial access, selective cannulation of the iliac vessels, and instillation of contrast dye to localize the bleeding source under fluoroscopic visualization. Upon identification of an actively bleeding site (noted by extravasation of contrast), embolization is performed through the injection of Gelfoam or coils. Angioembolization is extremely successful in the control of hemorrhage.

Delayed Diagnosis

- The evaluation of the critically injured patient does not always allow for immediate identification of all the injuries. Limitations in the examination of the patient due to mental status changes, and injuries that do not manifest on initial studies, lead to delays in diagnosis and possibly mortality.

SHANDS
at the University of Florida

Trauma and Emergency Surgery
Tertiary Survey Form *(page 2 of 2)*   Patient Name: _____ MR#: _____

Consults / Interventions (include dates):
Neurosurgery:
Orthopaedics:
Plastics / ENT / OMFS:
Urology:
Others:

Radiologic Findings (Please provide *FINAL READS*):
Plain Films
CXR:
Pelvis:
T/L/S Spine:
Extremities:
CT / MR
Chest:
Abdomen / Pelvis:
Other:
Laboratory Trends:

Plan:

MD Signature _____ MD# _____ Date / Time _____
TRE Attending:
I have seen this patient with _____ *and agree with plan and assessment.*

FIGURE 37.4. The tertiary survey instrument of the Acute Care Surgery Service of Shands Hospital at the University of Florida (page 2).

COMMONLY MISSED INJURIES

- 4% to 6% of **musculoskeletal injuries** are missed in multisystem trauma patients and rank number one in the missed-injury list. Risk factors include significant multisystem trauma, physiologic instability, altered sensorium, quickly applied splints for a less serious injury, poor-quality initial radiographs; and inadequate significance being applied to minor signs and symptoms.

- Injuries involving **retroperitoneal structures** have a strong potential for presenting in delayed fashion. Although CT scan has allowed for early detection of retroperitoneal hematomas, **pancreatic and duodenal** injuries can remain undetected in the initial survey.

- **Pancreatic injuries** occur in <5% of blunt abdominal traumas; however, they carry with them a substantial morbidity and mortality. In the alert patient, exam findings are typically nonspecific, with vague abdominal pain, epigastric discomfort, nausea, vomiting, and fever. Laboratory testing provides equally imprecise findings as an **elevated amylase** may hint at the diagnosis, but is not specific. CT findings are often subtle and may be delayed after injury.

- **Duodenal injuries** occur in <5% of blunt abdominal trauma and are equally challenging to diagnose, with similar features as pancreatic injury. Physical exam demonstrates ambiguous abdominal pain. Patients have nausea and vomiting, with development of progressively increasing tachycardia and fever. Laboratory findings are nonspecific, with elevated amylase levels suggestive of, but not diagnostic for, duodenal injury. Repeat CT scan may detect retroperitoneal air and extravasated oral contrast.

- Jejunal and ileal injuries may go undetected because the findings may be subtle. Small-bowel injuries affect 0.9% of blunt trauma victims but have a high morbidity (29%) and mortality (19%).

- Physical examination is nonspecific with abdominal pain, nausea, vomiting, and later, signs and symptoms of peritonitis if perforation occurs. CT scan may show **unexplained free abdominal fluid with no solid-organ injury, bowel wall thickening** or, in the case of a perforation, free air or extravasated gastrointestinal contrast material. **Diagnostic peritoneal lavage (DPL)** may be helpful in this group of patients. It is recommended that patients with positive microscopic, white cell count, or biochemical criteria on DPL undergo exploratory laparotomy. The technique of DPL is described in Chapter 16.

THE ROLE OF THE TERTIARY SURVEY INSTRUMENT

- A **formal trauma tertiary survey** allows for the detection of missed injuries, should be done **in the first 24 hours after injury, and may detect 56% of all missed injuries** and 90% of all clinically significant missed injuries.

- Examples of our Acute Care Surgery **Service's tertiary survey form** are seen in Figures 37.3 and 37.4.

- We take advantage of the tertiary survey instrument to review and record the patient's mechanism of injury, medical history, physical examination findings, laboratory trends, final radiologist reads on imaging findings, the interventions that have been performed up to that point in time, and the patient's immediate plan of care.

- When many issues are being handled in the ICU, this **systematic approach to secondary and tertiary survey** assists in detecting missed injuries.

CHAPTER 38 ■ SURGICAL AND POSTSURGICAL BLEEDING

GENERAL OVERVIEW AND IMMEDIATE CONCERNS

- In patients experiencing life-threatening hemorrhage, a defined approach for prompt recognition of the underlying cause is used.

- First, attention is directed toward **stabilizing the patient.** This includes securing an adequate airway, ventilation, vascular access, and restoring intravascular volume.

- There should be immediate dialogue with individuals involved in the intraoperative management of the patient.

Bleeding related to **technical factors** that can be associated with the conduct of any surgical procedure ("**surgical bleeding**") must be considered.

- A generalized slow oozing of blood from raw surfaces (often termed "**nonsurgical bleeding**") is often a manifestation of a systemic disorder of hemostasis.

- The evolving coagulopathy may proceed swiftly in critically ill patients. Qualitative abnormalities of **platelet** function, depletion of both platelets and plasmatic **coagulation factors,** and **hypothermia** contribute to the coagulopathic state.

- Early recognition of the clinical symptoms and signs attributable to **hypovolemia,** (restlessness, anxiety, shortness of breath, pallor, tachycardia, and oliguria) is compulsory. **Hypotension is a *late* sign** of significant hypovolemia.

- It is important to differentiate the **inherited (primary)** coagulation disorders, which are associated with a history of bleeding diatheses, from the more commonly **acquired (secondary)** coagulation disorders, which are the consequence of pathologic conditions and numerous medications.

- In parallel with the ongoing resuscitation of the bleeding patient, attention must be directed toward expeditiously **determining the need for surgical re-exploration.**

CAUSES OF POSTOPERATIVE BLEEDING

- Postoperative bleeding, often termed **local hemostatic failure** or **surgical bleeding,** is a known potential complication of any surgical procedure.

- The vast majority of patients affected typically present within the **immediate perioperative period.** Subtle signs may be evident in the postanesthesia care unit and generally become apparent within the first 8 hours after surgery.

- A high index of suspicion is necessary given that the **signs are nonspecific** in the postoperative period, Tachycardia may be from pain and anxiety, mental status changes from narcotic administration, or oliguria could be from anticipated third-space fluid sequestration after major surgery. **Hypotension is a late sign!**

- On occasion, **localized symptoms** may be elicited. Kehr sign is referred pain to the right shoulder due to blood under the right hemidiaphragm.

- **Serial hemoglobin** levels may assist in determining the degree of bleeding, but isolated, single values can be difficult to interpret due to either hemoconcentration or hemodilution.

- Certain surgical procedures are not associated with exsanguinating hemorrhage but can be life threatening. An expanding neck hematoma results in airway obstruction from both mechanical compression and from mural edema caused by lymphatic obstruction. The cause is frequently venous bleeding compounded by hypertension and liberal preoperative use of antiplatelet medications. Acutely reopening the incision and evacuating the hematoma is often lifesaving, although endotracheal intubation or rarely cricothyroidotomy may be required as a temporizing measure until the airway edema resolves.

- Caution must be exercised in interpreting **drain output** as drains can malfunction or tubings can obstruct with clot.

- There is no single criterion available to direct re-exploration for control of postoperative bleeding, and this decision is based on considering a number of variables. **The timing of the active bleed relative to the operative procedure,** its **duration,** its **rate,** the potential for additional **complications,** the patient's age as a surrogate for **physiologic reserve,** and **other comorbid diseases** must be considered.

- The most **conservative treatment** is to **return to the operating room** with **early control** of surgical bleeding. It is desirable to **correct any coagulopathy** prior to returning to the operating room. However, situations characterized by exsanguinating hemorrhage from failure of local surgical hemostasis may not allow for correction of the coagulopathy because of rapid ongoing consumption of coagulation factors and platelets.

- There are certain circumstances where operative re-exploration is obligatory, despite the fact that the bleeding may be self-limiting. A vascular anastomosis with a contained leak must be repaired to avert the consequences of false aneurysm formation and later rupture.

- There are some instances where bleeding is optimally addressed **without surgical intervention.** Some bleeding is amenable to arteriography with embolization or endoscopic control.

EVALUATION OF BLEEDING: CLINICAL HISTORY AND THE UTILITY OF DIAGNOSTIC TESTING

History

- A detailed **history and physical examination** are the most important preliminary steps in elucidating the cause of surgical bleeding and should be done simultaneously with resuscitative efforts. Collateral history from family members and previous medical records is helpful.

- A **history** of easy bruisability, excessive gingival bleeding after brushing of teeth, bleeding diathesis with dental extractions, hypermenorrhagia, frequent spontaneous epistaxis, melenic stools or spontaneous hematuria, petechiae or purpura, hemarthroses, and a family history of bleeding disorders may indicate a congenital or familial coagulation disorder, such as hemophilia A or B or von Willebrand disease.

- The **family pedigree** may provide important clues as to the presumptive disease process based on the pattern of inheritance, whether autosomal or sex-linked, dominant or recessive. Suspicion for a congenital disorder of coagulation is further raised by a **history of blood transfusions** required for common ambulatory procedures such as dental extractions, circumcisions, tonsillectomies, or biopsies. Due to differences in gene penetrance, not all individuals afflicted with inherited coagulation disorders are diagnosed at an early age, and coagulopathy may become unmasked when confronted by a major surgical procedure or trauma.

- A history of **liver disease or heavy ethanol consumption** should alert the clinician to the possibility of acquired plasmatic factor deficiencies, in addition to thrombocytopenia resulting from secondary hypersplenism with platelet sequestration.

- A thorough **medication history** is essential for many medications that interfere with hemostasis (aspirin, nonsteroidal anti-inflammatory agents, warfarin, ticlopidine, clopidogrel, or semisynthetic penicillins). Popular **supplements** that may aggravate bleeding are ginkgo, garlic, ginger, ginseng, feverfew, and vitamin E.

- **Nutritional assessment** is paramount, and careful evaluation for the presence of a **vitamin K deficiency** is obligatory, as this may occur in patients on parenteral nutrition or with cancer cachexia

- Other variables that may affect the integrity of the coagulation system include previous irradiation, renal failure, and sepsis, which affect the coagulation cascade at multiple points.

Physical Exam

- Physical findings may assist in distinguishing localized surgical bleeding from systemic bleeding resulting from a coagulopathy.
- Presence of petechiae, purpura, and mucosal bleeding is often indicative of thrombocytopenia, a qualitative functional disorder of platelets or increased vascular fragility. Ecchymoses or spontaneous, nontraumatic hemarthrosis is consistent with plasmatic coagulation factor abnormalities or deficiencies such as hemophilia. Both platelet and plasmatic coagulation disorders are associated with hematomas.
- **Hepatic** insufficiency or failure can be presumptively identified by recognizing jaundice, ascites, angiomas, palmar erythema, asterixis, congestive splenomegaly, and testicular atrophy.
- **Splenomegaly** itself may also be associated with hematologic dyscrasias and malignancies associated with hemostatic abnormalities (lymphomas and leukemias).
- **Connective-tissue or collagen vascular disorders** that result in increased vascular fragility may manifest with petechiae, joint abnormalities, and a history of delayed wound healing. These conditions focus attention on the increased risk for a perioperative bleeding complication, which underscores the need for vigilance both intraoperatively and postoperatively.
- The **possibility of sepsis** as an underlying cause for the development of a coagulopathy must always be entertained in the postoperative, critically ill patient.

Coagulation Tests

- The establishment of a definitive diagnosis of a coagulation disorder rests on a **limited battery of laboratory tests,** usually **quantitative platelet count, prothrombin time (PT), activated partial thromboplastin time (PTT), fibrinogen level, thrombin time (TT),** and **template bleeding time.**
- The **PTT** provides a global measure of the activity of factors XII, XI, IX, and VIII in addition to the common pathway factors shared by the extrinsic system (factors X, V, II, and I) and, therefore, identifies many of the inherited disorders of bleeding, typically a deficiency of factor VIII (hemophilia A), IX (hemophilia B), or von Willebrand factor, vWF (von Willebrand disease). It is worth noting that factor XII deficiency is not associated with any significant bleeding tendency despite abnormal prolongation of the PTT. Enzymatically active vWF is a necessary cofactor for optimum functioning of the factor VIII procoagulant protein.
- The **PT** exclusively evaluates factor VII, which is one of the vitamin K-dependent factors (in addition to factors II, IX, and X). Therefore, the PT is prolonged in individuals on warfarin therapy.
- Factor levels reflect a dynamic equilibrium, and **fibrinogen** is an acute-phase protein that increases in response to stress. The TT is a **qualitative measure of fibrinogen levels** and will be prolonged if the fibrinogen level is <100 mg/dL, by the presence of dysfibrinogenemia associated with liver disease, and also by circulating inhibitors. Its most useful role clinically is in the **detection of circulating heparin** not detectable by changes in the PT.

DISORDERS OF PLASMATIC COAGULATION FACTORS: OVERVIEW

- Hemostasis involves a **complex interplay** between elements of the **vascular endothelium, plasmatic coagulation factors, platelets, and the fibrinolytic system.**
- Primary isolated disorders of the fibrinolytic system as a cause of major bleeding are rare in the critically ill patient and are covered elsewhere.
- Disorders of the clotting system can be broadly classified as **congenital or acquired.**
- **Acquired coagulopathies are relatively common** in the postoperative intensive care unit patient, and these disorders can be operationally separated into those involving **platelets,** the **plasmatic coagulation factors,** or both.

Platelet

- Surgical and postsurgical bleeding may therefore result from either **quantitative (thrombocytopenia)** or **qualitative (abnormal function) platelet disorders.**

Quantitative Platelet Disorders

- Defined as a platelet count $<140 <10^9/L$ may be attributed to (a) a **decrease in production** of platelets (aplastic anemia, hypoplastic bone marrow, chemotherapy, space-occupying lesions of the bone marrow as seen with malignancy), (b) **ineffective production** (vitamin B_{12} or folic acid deficiency states), (3) **platelet sequestration** (primary or secondary hypersplenism), or (d) **increased destruction or consumption** (hemorrhage, microangiopathic processes such as thrombotic thrombocytopenic purpura, disseminated intravascular coagulation [DIC], hemolytic-uremic syndrome, immune destruction due to antiplatelet antibodies such as in posttransfusion purpura or idiopathic thrombocytopenic purpura), or dilution of circulating platelet volume (massive blood transfusion).
- Platelet counts of $50 <10^9/L$ or higher are generally considered adequate for surgical hemostasis in the absence of an associated qualitative functional defect. Counts **below 20 $<10^9/L$** are associated with increased risk for **spontaneous hemorrhages.**

Qualitative Platelet Disorders

- Qualitative bleeding disorders are not measured by the standard battery of coagulation tests. The template bleeding time is. not commonly used. This test has been attended by poor reproducibility.
- Defects may be **inherited** (Bernard–Soulier syndrome, abnormal release mechanism, Glanzmann thrombasthenia, storage pool disease, or von Willebrand disease) or **acquired** (uremia, drugs, myeloproliferative disorders).
- Numerous drugs are associated with inhibition of platelet function. It is generally recommended that antiplatelet medications, such as aspirin, ticlopidine, and clopidogrel, are discontinued approximately **7 to 10 days** prior to surgery. For **nonsteroidal anti-inflammatory agents,** some investigators advocate 2 days of abstinence.

- Discontinuing the antiplatelet drug combined with use of **desmopressin** and **platelet transfusions** has been beneficial in treating bleeding encountered in these situations.
- **Hypothermia** is another common cause of acquired qualitative platelet defect.
- There is a qualitative platelet function defect related to the **degree of uremia.** Use of desmopressin and cryoprecipitate may be helpful temporizing measures until dialysis is initiated. Conjugated estrogens have also been used with some success, but the effects are not immediate.
- Petechiae, purpura, and mucosal oozing, characteristic of thrombocytopenic states, may also be observed in qualitative platelet disorders and in conditions associated with increased vascular fragility.

Coagulation Factors

- Disorders involving plasmatic coagulation factors are generally caused by either (a) a **decrease in production** of clotting factors or (b) **an increase in consumption** of circulating coagulation factors.

Decreased Production

- Decreased production of circulating plasmatic coagulation factors occurs secondary **to liver failure** (with the exception of factor VIII); **vitamin K deficiency** (seen with oral antibiotic usage, which depresses gut flora in the setting of nutritional deficiency); **malabsorption** syndromes (seen in celiac sprue, chronic diarrheal conditions, or **obstructive jaundice**); and use of **warfarin.**
- In these situations, therapy is acutely centered on replacement of coagulation factors, most commonly with use of **fresh frozen plasma (FFP).** Vitamin K is administered parenterally in patients with deficient states or to reverse the effects of warfarin, although the effects are not generally seen for 24 to 36 hours after administration.

Impaired Function

- The effect of **hypothermia** on antagonizing normal functioning of the hemostatic mechanism globally has been described under qualitative platelet abnormalities, but all enzymatic processes function optimally in a narrow temperature range. Reliance solely on the values of the PT, PTT, or TT is misleading since these assays are performed by both manual and automated **laboratory methods at 37°C.**
- **External warming measures** include blankets generating heated air, warming of all fluid infusions, heated humidifier in ventilated patients, and warming the environment.
- Normal physiologic processes (fibrinolytic system) exist to control for unremitting clot formation. Impaired function of the coagulation cascade may be the result of various disorders that are characterized by **circulating anticoagulants,** abnormal protein products, or accumulation of proteinaceous breakdown products that affect the normal function of coagulation proteins.
- Collagen vascular diseases, such as systemic lupus erythematosus, is an example. In these patients an antibody is produced (**lupus anticoagulant**) that affects the coagulation cascade at the juncture of the intrinsic and extrinsic systems,

resulting in **prolongation of both the PT and PTT** *in vitro.* Paradoxically, these patients tend to be **hypercoagulable,** and if clinically significant bleeding is noted, it is attributable to associated thrombocytopenia and increased vascular fragility.
- When there are elevated titers of either the **lupus anticoagulant or anticardiolipin antibodies,** or both, these patients may present with manifestation of the antiphospholipid antibody syndrome with generalized microvascular thrombosis, thrombocytopenia, gangrene of the extremities, multiorgan failure, and death. Plasmapheresis, anticoagulation, and immunosuppressive therapy serve as the foundation of treatment.
- Other commonly acquired inhibitors or circulating anticoagulants include **factor VIII inhibitors and factor IX inhibitors,** related primarily to prior frequency of transfusion with plasma-derived blood concentrates and alloimmunization. Exogenously administered **heparin,** the prototype for anticoagulation therapy, binds to circulating **antithrombin III** and catalyzes its ability to neutralize the action of a number of coagulation factors. The end result is interference with the normal coagulation cascade.
- Disorders characterized by the production of abnormal globulins, often referred to collectively as the **paraproteinemias** (associated with multiple myeloma and Waldenstrom macroglobulinemia), also result in interference with coagulation proteins and inhibition of fibrin polymerization. In these conditions the PT, PTT, and TT are prolonged. **Fibrinogen/fibrin degradation products** also inhibit fibrin polymerization, as does uremia, with prolongation of the PT, PTT, and TT. Treatment of the coagulopathy associated with all of these conditions consists of replacement of deficient coagulation factors when bleeding is dominant and definitive treatment directed at the underlying disease process.

Increased Destruction or Consumption

- The most common cause of increased destruction of plasmatic coagulation factors has been variously termed **DIC, defibrination syndrome, or consumptive coagulopathy.** This syndrome is characterized by a hemorrhagic diathesis with unrestrained clotting and fibrinolysis in the vascular microcirculation, initiated by activation of the intrinsic or the extrinsic system, or both.
- The end point is normalization of the PT, PTT, TT, and platelet count.
- The underlying pathophysiology has been best elucidated with Gram-negative infections, with **endotoxin** (cell wall lipopolysaccharide) triggering the intrinsic system by activation of factor XII directly and by factor XII exposure to subendothelial collagen. **Traumatic injuries** (particularly involving brain, bone, or liver), thermal injuries, and severe crush injuries, as well as surgical procedures may produce a consumptive coagulopathy. Secondary infection and hemorrhagic shock further serve to aggravate the coagulopathy, especially if acidosis, hypothermia, or tissue ischemia and necrosis develops.
- **Obstetric complications** can result in some of the most profound and challenging instances of DIC from amniotic fluid embolism, abruptio placentae, retained dead fetus, and eclampsia. There is massive systemic release of tissue thromboplastin that generates a fulminant course characterized by bilateral renal cortical necrosis to frank cardiopulmonary collapse, shock, multiorgan failure, and death.

- The **laboratory diagnosis of DIC** is readily established with routinely available tests. **The PT, PTT, and TT are all prolonged,** and the **platelet count is decreased.** Depending on the severity of the disease process, **fibrinogen** may not be detectable. Fibrinogen/fibrin **degradation products** are elevated, and the peripheral blood smear often reveals the presence of schistocytes. Factors I (fibrinogen), V, VIII, and XIII tend to be markedly depressed. In milder forms, fibrinogen levels may not be significantly decreased.

- Optimum management of DIC requires aggressive treatment of the **underlying disease process** and supportive therapy with coagulation factor and platelet replacement. FFP and platelet concentrates are the two most common blood products used as a temporizing measure.

- Stored or banked whole blood is a reasonable source of most clotting factors if the units are <24 hours old. The biologic half-life of factors V, VII, VIII, and IX are on the order of 24 hours or less; hence whole blood stored for longer than 24 hours may not provide adequate amounts of these coagulation factors.

TREATMENT

- An important concept is **not to fall behind** in factor replacement. Due to the lag time in receiving laboratory values, in clinical conditions where the patient is actively bleeding, initiation of FFP and platelets should be started early with red cell transfusion.

- In patients with known warfarin use and a small bleed in an uncompromising area (skull), FFP should be used *before* patients develop increasing intracranial hemorrhage.

- **FFP** is the most commonly used blood component for plasmatic coagulation abnormalities since it provides **all necessary coagulation factors** in concentrations that approach those found in normal plasma.

- **Cryoprecipitate,** a component made from thawing FFP in the cold under specialized conditions, is rich in **factors XIII, VIII, I, vWF, and fibronectin.** It has been used in factor VIII–deficient states (**hemophilia A**) if virally inactivated plasma-derived or recombinant factor VIII concentrates are not readily available; in **von Willebrand** disease recalcitrant to desmo-pressin and if virally inactivated plasma derived factor VIII concentrate rich in vWF is not readily available; in **hypofibrinogenemic or dysfibrinogenemic conditions;** in hemorrhage associated with massive blood transfusions; in **DIC;** in **factor XIII deficiency** (FFP is also used); in bleeding **uremic** patients with qualitative platelet function defects unresponsive to desmopressin therapy; or as a **topically** applied surgical sealant ("fibrin glue").

- For specific coagulation disorders, such as hemophilia A, hemophilia B (deficiencies of factor VIII and IX, respectively), and von Willebrand disease, virally inactivated plasma-derived factor concentrates are commercially available, as are recombinant products, and these are the blood components of choice if available for use.

- For deficiencies of the **vitamin K-dependent factors (II, VII, IX, X), prothrombin complex** concentrates are also commercially available, as is recombinant factor VII for isolated factor VII deficiency states.

- Platelet concentrates are used for both **quantitative (thrombocytopenias) and qualitative platelet disorders** associated with significant bleeding.

- Patients transfused with any blood component, whether FFP, cryoprecipitate, plasma-derived factor concentrates, or platelet concentrates, incur similar risks of complications attributed to all types of blood component therapy such as febrile and allergic reactions, transmission of blood-borne pathogens (human immunodeficiency virus, hepatitis B and C), immunosuppression, transfusion-related pulmonary injury, and hemolytic transfusion reactions if a substantial volume of ABO-incompatible units is transfused. Therefore, judicious use of blood component therapy must always be adhered to.

SUMMARY

Postoperative bleeding requires immediate recognition of early shock, resuscitation, and differentiation between surgical and nonsurgical bleed. Knowledge of coagulation and appropriate replacement of blood and blood products is essential. Careful history and evaluation of the patient helps to identify primary or secondary coagulation disorders.

CHAPTER 39 ■ ABDOMINAL TRAUMA: NONOPERATIVE MANAGEMENT AND POSTOPERATIVE CONSIDERATIONS

INTRODUCTION

- The intensivist should be familiar with the implications of specific injuries including guidelines for nonoperative management, postoperative care, and expected postinjury complications and their sequelae.
- It should not be assumed that the emergency department evaluation was comprehensive and accurate. A repeated history and physical examination performed in light of imaging studies and pertinent intraoperative findings, called the tertiary survey (see Chapter 37), should be performed.
- Further information is obtained from family members, and the physician has time for a more meticulous physical examination. Key elements include the patient's medical history, specifically issues such as cardiopulmonary disease and medications.
- Some patients will require imaging upon arrival to the intensive care unit (ICU); patients with intracranial or thoracic injury may go emergently to the operating room (OR) prior to computed tomography (CT) scanning of the abdomen. These patients, once hemodynamically stable in the ICU, should undergo CT scanning to delineate any associated intra-abdominal injuries. Even in patients who undergo exploratory laparotomy, CT of the abdomen may be necessary to diagnose spine fractures and to evaluate the retroperitoneum.
- Routine postadmission studies include repeat chest film and laboratory studies. A chest film is important to determine central line catheter, tube thoracostomy, and endotracheal tube positions, as any of these could become dislodged with transport. The chest radiograph may also show interval change in a patient's hemothorax, pneumothorax, or pulmonary contusion. Based upon physical exam findings in the tertiary survey, further imaging of extremities may also be required.
- Once the patient has been fully evaluated by the treating ICU physicians and associated imaging and laboratory results obtained, there is concurrent cardiopulmonary resuscitation, and there is treatment of known injuries, ongoing evaluation for missed injuries, and monitoring for the sequelae of recognized injuries.

POSTINJURY RESUSCITATION

- ICU management undergoes distinct phases because there are differing goals and priorities.
- The period of acute resuscitation, typically lasting for the first 12 to 24 hours, combines several principles: optimizing tissue perfusion, ensuring normothermia, and restoring coagulation.
- There are a multitude of management algorithms aimed at accomplishing these goals—the majority involves goal-directed resuscitation (1) with initial volume loading to attain adequate preload, followed by judicious use of inotropic agents or vasopressors.
- Although the optimal hemoglobin (Hb) level remains debated, during shock resuscitation a Hb >10 g/dL optimizes oxygen delivery. A more judicious transfusion trigger of Hb <7 g/dL in the euvolemic patient after the first 24 hours of resuscitation limits adverse inflammatory effects and improves mortality, but the optimum hemoglobin level may vary depending on the patient's cardiac function.
- A challenging aspect of early care is balancing cardiac preload vs. promoting an abdominal compartment syndrome or tissue edema with fluids. During this initial treatment period, a low urine output is usually suggestive of a low preload and not an indication for diuretics.
- Invasive monitoring with pulmonary artery catheters (PACs) may be a critical adjunct in the multiply injured patient. PACs allow minute-to-minute monitoring and additional information on volume status, cardiac function, peripheral vascular tone, and response to intervention. Cardiac indices (CIs) and oxygen delivery (DO$_2$) become important variables in the ongoing ICU management. Resuscitation to values of DO$_2$I >500 mL/minute/m^2 and CI >3.8 L/minute/m^2 are the goals (1).
- PACs allow rapid titration of vasoactive agents. Although norepinephrine is the agent of choice for patients with low systemic vascular resistance unable to maintain a mean arterial pressure >60 mm Hg (1), patients may have an element of myocardial dysfunction requiring inotropic support. In patients with ongoing need for pressors, one should evaluate for adrenal insufficiency.
- Adequate resuscitation is mandatory, especially when future return to the OR is necessary. Specific goals of resuscitation whether patient needs further surgery or not include core temperature >35°C, base deficit less negative than 6, and normal coagulation indices.
- Although correction of base deficit and lactate values is desirable, how quickly this should be accomplished requires careful consideration. Adverse sequelae of aggressive crystalloid resuscitation include increased intracranial pressure, worsening pulmonary edema, and intra-abdominal visceral and retroperitoneal edema resulting in secondary abdominal compartment syndrome.
- Exogenous bicarbonate, occasionally given to improve cardiovascular function and response to vasoactive agents if the

TABLE 39.1

GENERAL GUIDELINES FOR OPERATIVE OR
RADIOLOGIC INTERVENTION DURING
NONOPERATIVE MANAGEMENT OF SOLID ORGAN
INJURIES

LIVER: Hemodynamically unstable with 4 units of packed red
blood cells (PRBCs) in 6 h or 6 units PRBCs in 24 h
SPLEEN: Hemodynamically unstable with need for initial
transfusion related to splenic injury rather than associated
trauma

serum pH is <7.2, obfuscates the acid-base balance, and **lactate** may be a more reliable indicator of adequate perfusion.

NONOPERATIVE MANAGEMENT OF TRAUMA

Blunt Liver and Spleen Injuries

- The liver and spleen are the most commonly injured solid organs after trauma, occurring in approximately 10% to 15% of all trauma admissions. Although the liver is more often injured, splenic injuries tend to be more precarious clinically.
- Nonoperative management of solid organ injuries is pursued in **hemodynamically stable** patients who do not have overt peritonitis or other indications for laparotomy. CT findings of high-grade injuries, a large amount of hemoperitoneum, contrast extravasation, and pseudoaneurysms are not absolute contraindications for nonoperative management; however, these patients are at **high risk for failure** and are more likely to need **angioembolization.** There is no age cutoff for nonoperative management.
- A multidisciplinary approach including angiography with selective **angioembolization** and **endoscopic retrograde cholangiopancreatography (ERCP)** with stenting has resulted in decreased nonoperative failure rates and improved survival in liver and splenic injuries.
- If a patient is going to fail nonoperative management, the **time to failure** is different for liver versus spleen injuries. Typically liver injuries rebleed within the first hours of admission, whereas splenic laceration may have delayed rupture or bleeding weeks after the original injury.
- **General guidelines for operative intervention or angioembolization** are noted in Table 39.1.
- Repeat imaging in patients with complex hepatic injuries can be performed with bedside ultrasound. Patients with evidence of right upper quadrant fluid collections or clinical deterioration (increasing abdominal pain, worsening liver function tests, unexplained fever) should undergo CT scanning.

Pancreatic Injuries

- With the recent evolution of nonoperative management for solid organ injuries, a nonresectional management schema has been developed for select pancreatic injuries. Observation of **pancreatic contusions,** particularly those in the head of the

pancreas that may involve ductal disruption, includes **serial exams** and monitoring of serum amylase.
- Patients with pancreatic injuries involving the major ducts, **originally a strict indication for operative intervention,** may now be managed with **ERCP and stenting** in select patients; durability of this approach is currently under investigation.

Duodenal Hematomas

- After blunt trauma, duodenal wall hematomas may **obstruct** the lumen. Clinical exam findings include epigastric pain associated with either emesis or high nasogastric tube (NGT) output; CT scan imaging with oral contrast failing to pass into the proximal jejunum is diagnostic.
- Nonoperative management includes continuous NGT decompression and nutritional support with total parenteral nutrition. A marked drop in NGT output heralds resolution of the hematoma, which typically occurs within **2 weeks;** repeat imaging to document these clinical findings is optional.
- If the patient does not improve clinically or radiographically within **4 weeks,** operative evaluation is warranted.
- If **perforation** is suspected by clinical deterioration or imaging with retroperitoneal free air or contrast extravasation, immediate surgery is needed.

Penetrating Wounds

- Patients with abdominal gunshot wounds violating the peritoneum undergo **emergent laparotomy** due to an approximate 90% visceral injury rate.
- Select patients with isolated low-energy gunshot wounds to the **right upper quadrant** are observed; CT scan imaging must delineate the **track of the bullet,** which should be confined to the parenchyma of the liver, and the patient must be hemodynamically **stable** with a benign clinical examination. In some cases, **laparoscopy** will be done to assess the penetrating liver injury and ensure the viscera are not violated.
- Patients with abdominal stab wounds to the back or flank with negative CT imaging or an isolated kidney injury are also managed nonoperatively.
- Regardless of the trauma surgeon's decision for operative versus nonoperative management, it is essential that these patients undergo **repeated abdominal examination.**
- Observation for a **missed small- or large-bowel injury** is critical; clinical findings in such patients include a rising white blood cell count, fever, tachycardia, and increasing abdominal pain or frank peritonitis.
- In patients with isolated liver injuries, complications are similar to those for patients with blunt injuries, namely bleeding and bile leaks or biliary sepsis.

COMPLICATIONS OF NONOPERATIVE INJURY MANAGEMENT

Liver

- **Bile leak or biloma** occurs in up to 20% of patients. Clinical presentation includes abdominal distention, intolerance of enteral feeds, and elevated liver functions tests. CT scanning effectively diagnoses the underlying problem, and the vast majority are treated with **percutaneous drainage and ERCP with sphincterotomy.**

- Occasionally, laparoscopy or laparotomy with drainage of biliary ascites is indicated if ileus and fever persist.
- **Hemobilia** (connection between a blood vessel and the biliary tree) manifests with **right upper quadrant pain, jaundice, and upper gastrointestinal bleeding.** Angiography and embolization may be needed to control the brisk gastrointestinal bleeding.
- **Delayed rupture** of a subcapsular hematoma with hemorrhage is infrequent.
- Patients undergoing angioembolization for liver trauma must be carefully monitored for **hepatic necrosis** and may occasionally require delayed formal hepatic resection.

Spleen

- The most common problem is **delayed bleeding.** Patients undergoing splenic embolization can fail with rebleeding and 13% of patients requiring splenectomy. Successful angioembolization patients typically have **significant pain** associated with their "splenic infarct," and up to **20% develop splenic abscesses.**

ONGOING EVALUATION FOR INJURIES (HOW TO AVOID A MISSED INJURY)

- With the paradigm shift from operative to nonoperative management of trauma, the clinician must have a heightened sense of awareness to avoid missing an occult injury. CT scan imaging is not 100% accurate; repeat CT scan imaging, diagnostic peritoneal lavage (DPL), ultrasound, and even laparotomy may be necessary for definitive evaluation.
- **Missed bowel injuries** are the most commonly pursued injury, not due to their frequency (<5% of blunt trauma) but rather their associated **morbidity** caused by even short delays in diagnoses.
- DPL should be considered if a patient's initial CT scan of the abdomen shows **free fluid without evidence of a solid organ injury** to explain such fluid; if there is increasing intra-abdominal fluid on bedside ultrasound even with a solid-organ injury but a stable hematocrit; and/or in patients with unexplained clinical deterioration.
- DPL at the bedside is done, with specific laboratory values indicating need for laparotomy (Table 39.2). Attention should be paid to elevations in white blood cells (WBCs), bilirubin, alkaline phosphatase, and amylase when pursuing a diagnosis of bowel injury. Red blood cell count is not the issue, as DPL is not being done to rule out bleeding.
- Missing a **rectal injury** may be life threatening in patients with pelvic fractures. If a **rectal exam** has been omitted in the trauma bay, the intensivist should ensure that this exam is done. Flexible sigmoidoscopy is easy to perform at the bedside; endoscopic evaluation should rule out **blood within the canal, clear intestinal perforation, or ischemic mucosa.**
- **Pancreatic contusions,** with or without associated ductal disruption, are difficult to diagnose in patients with blunt

TABLE 39.2

A POSITIVE DIAGNOSTIC PERITONEAL LAVAGE AFTER BLUNT TRAUMA DEFINED BY SPECIFIC LABORATORY VALUES

Laboratory study	Positive value
White blood cell	>500 cells/μL
Red blood cell	>100,000 cells/μL
Amylase	>19 IU/L
Alkaline phosphatase	>2 IU/L
Bilirubin	>0.1 mg/dL

abdominal trauma. The initial CT scan may show nonspecific stranding of the pancreas. Associated fluid around the pancreas should prompt further invasive studies such as **ERCP** or magnetic resonance cholangiopancreatography to rule out a biliary or pancreatic duct injury. Serial determinations of amylase/lipase may be considered and prompt a repeat CT scan, a duodenal C-loop study, a DPL, or an ERCP depending upon the suspected lesion.

POSTOPERATIVE MANAGEMENT OF SPECIFIC INJURIES

- Communication between the operating surgeon and the intensivist is critical and should include **intraoperative findings and procedures, any tenuous operative repairs, anticipated problems or complications, the need for repeat operative exploration, and location of drains.** The **intraoperative estimated blood loss** and associated blood product transfusion requirements are essential data to anticipate events in the postoperative period.
- Remember that injuries **can be missed** even with prior operative intervention.

Liver and Spleen Injuries

- Life-threatening bleeding from the liver is most often controlled with perihepatic liver packing or sometimes with additional Foley catheter tamponade of deep lacerations. Immediate concerns in the postoperative period are **rebleeding** and **parenchymal ischemia.**
- Signs of **rebleeding** are a falling hematocrit, blood clots accumulating under a temporary abdominal closure device, and bloody output from the Jackson–Pratt drains. Patients with recurrent hemorrhage may be treated with angioembolization or may necessitate repeat operative packing depending on the rate of bleeding.
- **Hepatic ischemia** is usually due to either a prolonged intraoperative Pringle maneuver (with anticipated resolution of ischemia) or hepatic artery ligation (which may result in liver necrosis). Patients are typically returned to the OR for pack removal 24 to 48 hours after initial injury.
- Other complications are intra-abdominal **abscess, biloma, and hemobilia,** and "liver fever" for the first 5 postinjury days.
- Operative intervention for splenic injuries includes splenectomy and splenorrhaphy. **Postoperative hemorrhage** may be

due to the splenic hilar vessel tie loosening, a missed short gastric artery, or recurrent bleeding from the spleen if splenic repair was used.

- An immediate postsplenectomy increase in platelets and WBCs is normal; however, beyond postoperative day 5, a **WBC count >15,000** should prompt a thorough search for underlying infection.
- Other complications are unrecognized iatrogenic injury to the **pancreatic tail** during rapid splenectomy resulting in pancreatic ascites or fistula.
- Left upper quadrant abscess after splenectomy may occur, but presumptive drainage does not prevent this complication.
- Routine care also includes **immunizations** for encapsulated organisms (*Streptococcus pneumoniae, Haemophilus influenzae,* and *Meningococcus*) usually just prior to discharge, optimally at 2 to 3 weeks postsplenectomy.

Gastrointestinal Injuries

- Operative intervention for either penetrating or blunt gastrointestinal injuries entails primary repair, resection with primary anastomosis, or resection with a stoma diversion. If an **ileostomy or colostomy** was required, one should inspect it daily to ensure it is pink without evidence of necrosis. Postoperative complications include anastomotic leak, prolonged ileus, and bowel obstruction.
- A devastating complication is an **anastomotic leak** with intra-abdominal contamination or sepsis and presents with increasing abdominal pain, fevers, and respiratory. CT scan is diagnostic, and repeat operation is often required.
- Important questions for the intensivist after operative intervention for pancreatic injuries include how much of the pancreas was resected (potential for diabetes), is there a pancreaticoenteric anastomosis (potential for leak), was the pancreatic stump closed with either staples and/or fibrin glue, was the spleen preserved, and where were drains placed?
- Postoperative complications include **pancreatic fistula, pseudocyst, abscess, pancreaticoenteric leak, and pancreatitis.** The most common of these is a pancreatic fistula seen in 7% to 20% of patients with isolated pancreatic trauma and up to 35% of patients with combined pancreatic and duodenal injuries. CT scan imaging should be performed to evaluate for an intra-abdominal fluid collection. Drainage by interventional radiology is performed for fistula diagnosis and control. Pancreatic fistulae after trauma are managed in a fashion identical to those occurring after elective pancreatic resection.

Abdominal Vascular Injuries

- Vascular injuries can produce rapid exsanguination and threaten extremities or may be a clinically silent time bomb due to temporary retroperitoneal tamponade. Few result in a delayed diagnosis, particularly with CT scanning, and hence the focus of the intensivist is in postoperative management.
- Main causes of patient morbidity and mortality are associated **soft-tissue and nerve injuries** once the vascular repair has been accomplished. Therefore, optimizing the patient's hemodynamic status, maintaining euthermia, and correcting coagulopathy are critical points of resuscitation.

- Prosthetic graft infections are rare complications, but preventing bacteremia is imperative.
- There are specific injuries that require additional care: (a) **Abdominal aortic injuries** are repaired using either a polytetrafluoroethylene patch or interposition grafting; the patient's **systolic blood pressure should not exceed 120 mm Hg for at least the first 72 hours postoperatively;** (b) patients requiring **ligation of an inferior vena cava injury** often develop marked bilateral lower extremity edema; to limit the associated morbidity, the patient's legs should be wrapped with ACE bandages from the toes to the hips and elevated at a 45- to 60-degree angle; (c) **superior mesenteric vein injuries, either ligation or thrombosis** after venorrhaphy results in marked **bowel edema;** fluid resuscitation should be aggressive and abdominal pressure monitoring routine in these patients; and (d) in complex hepatic trauma, the **right or left hepatic artery or the portal vein may be selectively ligated;** persistent elevation in liver transaminases indicates secondary liver **necrosis** and may necessitate delayed resection. Of note, if the right hepatic artery is ligated intraoperatively, **cholecystectomy** must be performed to prevent gangrenous gallbladder.

Abdominal Wounds

- Wounds sustained from trauma or from surgery should be **examined daily** for progression of healing and signs of infection. Complex soft-tissue wound care includes wet-to-dry dressing changes twice daily, or application of the wound vacuum-assisted closure.
- One should carefully watch for **infection,** development of necrotizing fasciitis, subcutaneous abscess, or associated undrained hematoma.

Damage Control Surgery

- Damage control surgery (DCS) is an abbreviated operation the goals of which are to control hemorrhage, limit contamination from enteric sources, and enable rapid transport to the ICU for correction of adverse physiology. There are standard indications for performing the DCS abbreviated laparotomy in patients with unresolved metabolic failure (Table 39.3).
- Intraoperative techniques of DCS include perihepatic packing, balloon tamponade of deep liver lacerations, segmental

TABLE 39.3

INTRAOPERATIVE INDICATIONS TO PERFORM DAMAGE CONTROL SURGERY

Factor	Level
Body temperature Acid-base status	Temperature <35°C
Arterial pH	pH <7.2
Base deficit (BD)	BD < −15 mmol/L in patient <55 y
	BD < −8 mmol/L in patient >55 y
Serum lactate	Lactate >5 mmol/L
Coagulopathy	PT or PTT >50% of normal

PT, prothrombin time; PTT, partial thromboplastin time.

stapled bowel resection left in discontinuity, ligation of abdominal venous injuries, shunting of abdominal arterial injuries, and pancreatic drainage.

- After DCS, the surgeon will "close" the abdomen with a **temporary closure** device using either a plastic intravenous bag or wound vacuum-assisted closure dressing. The temporary abdominal closure allows egress of abdominal contents and contains the edematous bowel while providing excellent decompression.
- Upon transfer to the ICU, aggressive resuscitation of the patient is performed to reverse metabolic failure. This includes vigorous **rewarming** through heating the room, infusion of fluids and blood products through a warming device, and use of a active warming blankets. Continuous **arteriovenous rewarming** may be warranted for refractive temperatures <34°C. **Restoration of a normal cardiovascular state** is attained by infusion of fluids and blood products and judicious use of vasopressor agents. Finally, the patient's **coagulopathy** must be reversed with appropriate blood products including fresh-frozen plasma, cryoprecipitate, and platelets. Occasionally, recombinant activated factor VII (rFVIIa; NovoSeven, NovoNordisk, Denmark) is needed.
- Ideally, **physiologic correction** should occur within **12 to 24 hours** of admission to the ICU, with planned return to the OR for definitive repair.
- There are several specific management points of the patient with an open abdomen that deserve mention. Despite a widely open abdomen, patients can develop **abdominal compartment syndrome;** Patients with an open abdomen lose between **500 and 2,500 mL/day** of abdominal effluent.

Abdominal Compartment Syndrome

- Diagnosis and management are also presented in Chapter 37.
- Organ failure can occur over a wide range of recorded bladder pressures; there is **not a single measurement** of bladder pressure that prompts therapeutic intervention, except >35 cm H_2O. Rather, emergent decompression is warranted in the patient with intra-abdominal hypertension with **end-organ dysfunction**.
- **Mortality** is directly affected by abdominal decompression, with 64% mortality in patients undergoing presumptive decompression, 70% mortality in patients with a delay in decompression, and 89% mortality in those without decompression.

Reference

1. Moore FA, McKinley BA, Moore EE, et al. Inflammation and the Host Response to Injury, a large-scale collaborative project: patient-oriented research core—standard operating procedures for clinical care. III. Guidelines for shock resuscitation. *J Trauma.* 2006;61:82–89.

CHAPTER 40 ■ NEUROLOGIC INJURY: PREVENTION AND INITIAL CARE

HEAD INJURY

Nearly 1.4 million people sustain a **traumatic brain injury** (TBI) per year in the United States, 235,000 are hospitalized, and approximately 50,000 die. In children younger than 14 years, TBI results in 2,685 deaths per year, with 37,000 hospitalizations and 435,000 emergency department visits. TBI death rate for males is 3.3 times higher than for females and highest in persons at age 75 years or older.

Subdural Hematoma

- Subdural hematomas (SDHs) are more common than epidural hematomas and were seen in 25% of patients with severe head injury. SDH typically results from tearing of the bridging veins between the brain and the draining venous sinuses. The mechanism usually involves high-velocity acceleration and deceleration forces.
- Imaging shows a **crescent-shaped hyperdensity** that follows the contours of the brain.
- Acute SDH carries a **poor prognosis** and is one of the most lethal of all head injuries. Fifty to 60% of patients with SDH die, and only 19% to 38% will achieve functional recovery despite surgical treatment.
- Early evacuation within the first 4 hours of injury decreased mortality from 90% to 30% in a single study of 82 consecutive comatose patients. This suggested that preventable secondary injury was the cause of the high mortality, despite multiple studies, these findings have not been replicated.

Epidural Hematomas

- An epidural hematoma requires a great impact force and is often associated with a skull fracture that disrupts the **middle meningeal artery** in the supratentorial space or causes injury to the venous sinuses in the posterior fossa.

- Classically, patients present awake and alert, known as the lucid interval, and quickly lapse into unconsciousness.
- Imaging shows a **lenticular-shaped hyperdensity.**
- With rapid evacuation, epidural hematoma has a relatively **good prognosis,** and the mortality rate is 5% to 10%. Factors determining mortality and functional outcome include age, best motor response on the Glasgow coma score (GCS), hematoma volume, and degree of midline shift.

Cerebral Contusions

- Cerebral contusions result from direct impact of the brain on the skull. These are known as **coup injuries.** Alternatively, acceleration/deceleration injury of the brain against the contralateral side of the direct impact causes **contrecoup injuries.** The most common areas of contusion are the frontal, temporal lobes, and occipital regions. These lesions are **hyperintense areas** within the parenchyma on computed tomography (CT) scan.
- Clinical deterioration or elevation in intracranial pressure (ICP) requires urgent repeat cerebral imaging.

Intraparenchymal Hemorrhage

- Intraparenchymal hemorrhage (IPH) is **hyperintense** on CT scan. It is a focal process and less diffuse than a contusion, as it is caused by direct vascular injury or by stretching of the vessels with brain shift and distortion.
- Hemorrhage in the **upper brainstem (midbrain and pons),** known as Duret hemorrhages, can occur with rapidly evolving **transtentorial herniation** and may be due to stretching of the perforating arterioles or from venous thrombosis and infarction. Spontaneous causes of IPH are hypertensive hemorrhagic stroke or hemorrhaging due to arteriovenous malformation, aneurysm, amyloid angiopathy, or tumor. In the setting of hemorrhage in the basal ganglia, cerebellum, or thalamus, the clinician should consider the differential of spontaneous IPH as a possible **cause** of the traumatic event, **rather than the result.**

Subarachnoid Hemorrhage

- Subarachnoid hemorrhage (SAH) occurs in 21% to 53% of patients with severe TBI and worsens outcome. In contrast to aneurysmal SAH, traumatic SAH (**tSAH**) is less likely concentrated in the basal cisterns and is usually found over the hemispheric convexities. The presence of tSAH in the basal cisterns is predictive value of unfavorable outcome of up to 70%.

Intraventricular Hemorrhage

- Intraventricular hemorrhage in isolation is not commonly seen in closed-head injury. However, like traumatic SAH, it has been associated with **worsened outcome. Obstructive hydrocephalus** may result and may require cerebrospinal fluid (CSF) diversion by external ventricular drainage.

Diffuse Axonal Injury

- Diffuse axonal injury occurs in approximately half of patients with severe closed-head injury. Sudden acceleration-deceleration impact causes rotational forces and **shear injury to axons.** The axon may not be entirely transected, but axoplasmic transport is disrupted, causing swelling and disconnection and Wallerian degeneration. Outcome is worsened with severe diffuse axonal injury.

PHYSIOLOGIC PRINCIPLES

- The **Monro–Kellie hypothesis** describes the skull as a semiclosed compartment containing brain and interstitial fluid (80%), CSF (10%), and blood (10%). Compensatory mechanisms to decrease cerebral blood or CSF volume (decreased synthesis) become active where ICP and volume increase.
- **Cerebral perfusion pressure (CPP)** is determined by the difference of the mean arterial pressure (MAP) and ICP. CPP supplants MAP goals. Normal ICP is <10 mm Hg.
- Brain Trauma Foundation guidelines recommend **CPP >60 mm Hg and ICP between 20 and 26 mm Hg.** Prior to placement of an intracranial monitor, recommendations are to maintain a **MAP of 90 mm Hg** or greater.

Evaluation

- On arrival at the intensive care unit (ICU), the initial focus is on **respiratory** and **hemodynamic** stability. In addition examination of the head for scalp lacerations, which can be a major source of bleeding and orbital, facial, and depressed skull fractures, basilar skull fractures with raccoon eyes, and middle fossa or temporal bone fractures with postauricular ecchymosis known as the Battle sign seen. **Cervical spine precautions** are maintained.
- Repeated neurologic monitoring includes the vital signs with special attention to extremes in blood pressure. **Hypotension** may result in secondary injury, whereas **hypertension,** not always associated with bradycardia, can be a sign of impending cerebral herniation. If ICP rises, cerebral autoregulation elevates MAP to maintain an adequate CPP.
- A rapid neurologic assessment includes **level of consciousness** and ability to speak or understand language by assessing the ability to follow simple commands. Vision is assessed by asking the patient to count fingers placed in the right or left visual field with one eye covered or to mimic finger movements.
- In patients with a lower level of consciousness, **vision** is assessed by blinking to a visual threat. Pupillary response to light (cranial nerves [CN] II, III), corneal reflex (CN V, VII), and gag and cough (CN IX, X) responses assess **cranial nerve** and brainstem function.
- **Oculocephalic maneuvers** (CN III, VI, VIII) should not be performed in patients who have a risk of **cervical spine fracture. Ice water caloric** response (CN III, VI, VIII) can be performed if the tympanic membranes are intact. The head of the bed should be up at 30 degrees, and 60 to 90 mL of ice water instilled into the otic canal. A normal response is a slow lateral deviation to the side stimulated with ice water and nystagmus with the fast phase to the opposite ear. Absence may be caused by medications or **brainstem injury.**

TABLE 40.1

GLASGOW COMA SCALE

Score	Eye opening	Best verbal	Best motor
1	No response	No response	No response
2	To pain	Incomprehensible	Extensor
3	To speech	Inappropriate	Flexor
4	Spontaneous	Disoriented	Withdraws to pain
5	—	Oriented	Localizes pain
6	—	—	Obeys command

From Teasdale G, Jennett B. Assessment of coma and impaired consciousness: a practical scale. *Lancet.* 1974;2:81–84.

- **Motor response** is assessed by verbal commands to move the limbs. In patients with lower levels of consciousness, motor responses are elicited by painful stimuli delivered to the sternum or fingernail bed. During **painful stimulation,** the examiner should also reassess facial movement for asymmetry. If flexion is noted, pain is applied to the supraorbital ridge or by trapezius squeeze to test for localization.
- In the lower extremities, it is important to recognize a **triple flexion response,** which is described by the flexion of the ankle, knee, and hip. Triple flexion is a **spinal reflex to painful stimulation** of the legs or feet. It is stereotyped in appearance independent of the location of pain delivery on the lower extremity. It does not reflect brainstem or upper–spinal cord function. Patients who are brain dead or with higher cord complete lesions can triple-flex lower extremities.
- The GCS has been divided into three categories: (a) a **GCS of 8 or less** is defined as severe head injury, (b) a **GCS of 9 to 12** represents moderate head injury, and (c) a **GCS of 13 to 15** is mild or minor (Table 40.1).
- The **best GCS** after adequate fluid resuscitation and stabilization has previously been shown to be predictive of outcome. A **change between the field and arrival GCS** can be predictive of outcome.
- **Laboratory evaluation** of patients with head injury include complete blood count with platelet counts, partial thromboplastin time, prothrombin time, electrolytes with blood urea nitrogen, creatinine, glucose, and liver function tests, toxicology screen. Arterial blood gas and lactic acid levels help assess volume status and whether ventilation is adequate.

Imaging

- **Noncontrast head CT** is the fastest, most widely available noninvasive imaging technique to determine this. All patients with altered mental status and/or focal neurologic findings should have an initial CT scan performed.
- Progressive intracranial hemorrhage consistent with an evolving contusion is seen in 14% to 38%. Although worsening CT findings do not necessarily require treatment, 54% of patients may require neurosurgical intervention, including ICP monitoring or craniotomy subsequent to the findings on a repeat scan.
- In stable patients without clinical neurologic deterioration, the utility of repeat imaging is debated. Risk factors for progression include associated tSAH, SDH, older age, and prolonged partial thromboplastin. A large initial contusional or intraparenchymal hemorrhage size and effacement of cisterns are strongly predictive of failure of nonoperative management.

SECONDARY BRAIN INJURY PREVENTION: TREATMENT AND MANAGEMENT

- After immediate impact and anatomic damage, **secondary damage** at the cellular level from inflammation, edema, free radicals, and excitatory neurotransmitters can worsen outcome.
- Contributing factors include **hypoxemia, hypotension, seizures, fever, and intracranial hypertension.** Immediate postinjury care focuses on the prevention of these problems.

Hypoxemia and Respiratory Management

- Hypoxia, defined as **a PaO_2 <60 mm Hg or O_2 saturation less than 90%,** can independently **increase mortality from 27% to 50%** and increase poor outcome from 28% to 71%. Early intubation can prevent aspiration, and minimizing hypoxic and hypercapnic events is recommended. A **GCS of 8 or less** is the usual threshold for endotracheal intubation.
- Hyperventilation with resultant **hypocapnia causes cerebral vasoconstriction** and a reduction in cerebral blood flow (CBF). Prolonged hypocapnia appears to slow neurologic recovery, and hyperventilation of $PaCO_2$ less than 35 mm Hg should be avoided.
- $PaCO_2$ as low as 30 mm Hg may be necessary for brief periods for immediate treatment of intracranial hypertension.
- **Pulmonary infections** were seen in 41% of patients registered in the Traumatic Coma Data Bank. Bedside management includes adequate pulmonary toilet and strategies such as elevation of the head of the bed to decrease the risk for ventilator-associated pneumonia.

Neurogenic Pulmonary Edema

- Neurogenic pulmonary edema (NPE) results from central sympathetic stimulation. TBI causes a **sympathetic discharge,** which **increases systemic and pulmonary vascular pressures.** The resultant increase in pulmonary capillary pressure increases the hydrostatic pressure and causes pulmonary capillary injury; this in turn causes leakage of fluid and protein and pulmonary hemorrhages.
- Clinical signs include dyspnea, tachypnea, tachycardia, and chest pain if the patient is awake. Chest radiography shows a bilateral alveolar filling process.
- There are two distinct forms of NPE. The classic form appears **early,** within minutes to a few hours after acute brain injury. A **delayed form** of NPE slowly progresses over 12 to 72 hours after injury. Treatment is supportive and often requires supplemental oxygen and positive pressure ventilation.

Hypotension

- Hypotension, defined as systolic blood pressure <**90 mm Hg,** independently worsens mortality. Adequate fluid resuscitation with euvolemia is essential. Once an ICP monitor is placed, the optimal blood pressure is determined by a CPP ≥60 mm Hg.

Contraction Band Necrosis

- After head trauma, subarachnoid hemorrhage, seizures, or stroke, patients may have **cardiogenic shock** with global hypokinesis associated with transient cardiac arrhythmias and repolarization changes.
- **Arrhythmias** may include supraventricular tachycardias, sinus bradycardia, atrioventricular block, atrioventricular dissociation, nodal rhythms, and paroxysmal ventricular tachycardia.
- **Myofibrillar degeneration** (also known as **contraction band necrosis** or coagulative myocytolysis) is seen. It is postulated that centrally mediated sympathetic or exogenous catecholamine stimulation of the myocardium results in cellular calcium overload and results in the formation of the contraction bands predominantly located in the subendocardium affecting the conducting system, which results in the associated arrhythmias.

Posttraumatic Vasospasm

- After TBI, **focal cerebral ischemia** as a result of **posttraumatic vasospasm** can occur in 24% to 36% of patients and may manifest as lateralizing neurologic deficits such as hemiparesis and aphasia between 2 to 37 days after injury.
- If vasospasm is suspected, cerebral angiography can confirm the diagnosis. The effectiveness of treatment of posttraumatic vasospasm with modalities used after aneurysmal SAH (e.g., hypervolemic, hypertensive therapy, or nimodipine) has not been assessed.

Fever

- **Hyperthermia accelerates neuronal injury** by increasing basal energy requirements (neuronal discharges), excitatory neurotransmitters, free radial production, calcium-dependent protein phosphorylation, ICAM-1 and inflammatory responses, DNA fragmentation, and apoptosis, causing blood–brain barrier changes as seen by extravasation of protein tracers.
- Therapeutic hypothermia lowers ICP by **reducing the cerebral metabolic rate 7% for each degree Celsius decrease.** This treatment can be lifesaving and result in reasonable neurologic recovery.
- **Pentobarbital coma** and/or **neuromuscular blockade** may be necessary to achieve cooling without shivering. New techniques for intravascular and topical cooling are available.
- Complications of hypothermia include **arrhythmias, hypotension, bradycardia, thrombocytopenia, and pneumonia.**

Hyperglycemia

- Hyperglycemia causes **brain-tissue acidosis,** and early hyperglycemia has been associated with worsened neurologic outcome after TBI. Although tighter glucose control with TBI is theoretically reasonable, based on current evidence, it is not clear that aggressive treatment of hyperglycemia in the neurologic and neurosurgical population improves outcome.

Coagulopathy

- Brain is rich in tissue thromboplastin and may cause a **disseminated intravascular coagulopathy.** Associated coagulopathy and thrombocytopenia increases mortality in TBI.
- Although there are no guidelines for correction of coagulopathy or thrombocytopenia, usual practice is to transfuse **platelets** for values <100,000/mL and fresh-frozen plasma for an **elevated** thromboplastin time **or a** prothrombin time **international ratio of 1.5 or more.** Other alternatives such as activated factor VII or prothrombin complex concentrate may be effective emergently.

INTRACRANIAL PRESSURE MONITORING AND MANAGEMENT

- Normal ICP is <10 mm Hg. ICPs **>20 mm Hg to 25 mm Hg** should be treated.
- Maneuvers for management of ICP begin with those with fewer potential side effects and progress to more invasive treatments with higher complication risk (Fig. 40.1).
- **Elevation of the head of bed to >30 to 45 degrees** not only decreases the risk of ventilator-associated pneumonia but can also facilitate cerebral venous drainage and lower ICP. In orthostatic, hypovolemic patients, however, head of bed elevation can lower MAP. Adequate fluid resuscitation is necessary.
- Adequate **pain therapy** with opioids and adequate **sedation** with sedative-hypnotics decrease ICP. Constant infusion may be hemodynamically better tolerated than bolus administration.
- $PaCO_2$ <35 mm Hg should be avoided except in the situation of impending herniation or refractory intracranial hypertension.
- **Osmotic therapy** is a mainstay in ICP management. Mannitol or hypertonic saline are both effective. However, repetitive dosing by the preceding agents may worsen the volume of injured brain. Doses of **0.25 g/kg to 1 g/kg of mannitol** are effective. An osmolar gap of >10 from baseline may be a better indicator for maximizing mannitol administration. **Hypertonic saline** may be more effective and have a longer duration of action on lowering ICP than mannitol. Doses include **250 mL of 3% or 7.5% saline or 30 mL of 23.42% saline.**
- **Neuromuscular blockade** lowers ICP by decreasing muscle tone, especially during shivering. Shivering increases the metabolic rate and generates carbon dioxide. After administering neuromuscular blockade, an arterial blood gas should be obtained to ensure that the $PaCO_2$ has not dropped below 35 mm Hg. Neuromuscular blockade also cools the patient. The patient is unable to effectively clear secretions, and empiric pulmonary toilet with frequent suctioning is often necessary.
- **Barbiturate-induced coma** lowers the cerebral metabolic rate. This results in lowered cerebral blood volume and ICP. Thiopental or pentobarbital infusions can be used. Thiopental in long-term infusion, because of its lipophilicity, may take over a week to clear after the infusion is stopped. For

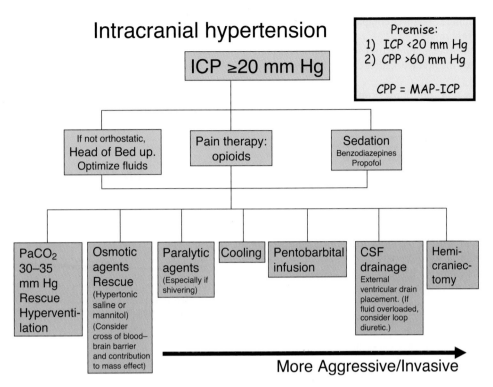

Intracranial hypertension

ICP ≥20 mm Hg

Premise:
1) ICP <20 mm Hg
2) CPP >60 mm Hg

CPP = MAP-ICP

If not orthostatic, **Head of Bed up.** Optimize fluids

Pain therapy: opioids

Sedation
Benzodiazepines
Propofol

$PaCO_2$ 30–35 mm Hg Rescue Hyperventilation

Osmotic agents Rescue (Hypertonic saline or mannitol) (Consider cross of blood–brain barrier and contribution to mass effect)

Paralytic agents (Especially if shivering)

Cooling

Pentobarbital infusion

CSF drainage External ventricular drain placement. (If fluid overloaded, consider loop diuretic.)

Hemi-craniec-tomy

More Aggressive/Invasive

FIGURE 40.1. Algorithm for management of intracranial hypertension. CCP, cerebral perfusion pressure; CSF, cerebrospinal fluid; ICP, intracranial pressure.

pentobarbital, **20 mg/kg is given as a slow loading dose** followed by a maintenance infusion of **1 mg/kg per hour.** The loading dose may significantly lower mean arterial pressure. Often fluids and vasopressor administration may be necessary. **Electroencephalography** is critical to **titrating the dose** during barbiturate coma.

- Side effects include **hypotension** from peripheral vasodilation, **decreased cardiac inotropy,** and ileus. Cough reflex is diminished, and decreased bronchociliary activity and slowed leukocyte chemotaxis increase the risk for pneumonia. A quiescent hypothalamus that no longer modulates body temperature and hypothermia occurs.
- **Loop diuretics** have been used to help manage ICP by decreasing CSF production in the choroids plexus. Loop diuretics will decrease volume status and should not be used in hypovolemic patients.
- For **refractory intracranial hypertension,** placement of an **external ventricular drainage** allows for CSF drainage. Hemicraniectomy may be lifesaving and a viable option depending on the patient.

Brain Tissue Oxygenation

- Hypoxic brain injury causes secondary damage. **Jugular bulb oximetry ($SjvO_2$)** is a global measure of the balance between oxygen delivery to the brain and oxygen consumption. Local **brain tissue partial pressure oxygen ($PBtO_2$)** is measured by a polarographic Clark-type microcatheter.
- An increase in cerebral oxygen delivery is reflected by increases in $SjvO_2$ and $PBtO_2$. Oxygen delivery to the brain is manipulated by increases in blood pressure, cardiac output,

and red blood cell transfusion. Optimal $SjvO_2$ is generally accepted as **50% oxygen saturation.** The optimal $PBtO_2$ has not been established but should be maintained **>15 mm Hg to 25 mm Hg.**

OTHER INTENSIVE CARE UNIT CONSIDERATIONS

Antibiotic Prophylaxis

- **Fractures of the skull base and severe facial trauma** can result in a CSF leak. Studies conflict as to whether prophylactic antibiotics decrease the risk of infection, and there are no guidelines or recommendations. Constant surveillance for meningitis is essential.
- After penetrating head trauma, a **CSF leak** is the primary predictor of intracranial infection. Current recommendations are to treat with empiric broad-spectrum antibiotics after penetrating brain injury.
- For clean neurosurgical procedures, such as external ventricular drain placement or craniotomy, guidelines have been established by the Surgical Infection Prevention and Surgical Care Improvement Projects that recommend cefazolin within 1 hour prior to surgical incision.

Posttraumatic Seizures

- Early posttraumatic seizures occur **within 7 days of injury.** Three percent to 6 percent of patients with closed-head injury

suffer early posttraumatic seizures compared to 8% to 10% with penetrating brain injury.
- **Antiseizure medications** (e.g., phenytoin and carbamazepine) are recommended for the **first week** after closed and penetrating brain injury.
- There is no evidence that continuing prophylactic antiseizure medications beyond a week prevents late seizures.

Thromboprophylaxis

- After major head injury, the **risk for deep vein thrombosis (DVT) is as high as 54%.**
- Patients undergoing major neurosurgical procedures receive thromboprophylaxis in the form of **intermittent pneumatic compression** devices with or without **graduated compression stockings** (grade 1A). Acceptable alternatives include subcutaneous unfractionated **heparin** (grade 2B) or postoperative low-molecular-weight heparin (LMWH, grade 2A). In high-risk neurosurgery patients, the combination of mechanical and pharmacologic prophylaxis is recommended (grade 2B).
- In patients who are not neurosurgical candidates, a grade 1A recommendation is that trauma patients receive LMWH as soon as it is considered safe to do so. Inferior vena cava filters are not considered acceptable primary prophylaxis in trauma patients (grade 1C).

Nutrition

- After severe TBI, patients have a hypermetabolic, catabolic state, with rapid weight loss associated with a negative nitrogen balance and protein wasting.
- **Early parenteral or enteral nutrition** can speed neurologic recovery and decrease disability and mortality. Early enteral nutrition with glutamine and probiotics may decrease the infection rate and length of ICU stay. Arginine and glutamine modulate gut permeability. There is some debate whether glutamine should be used in brain injury patients due to the potential increase in cerebral glutamate with neuroexcitatory properties and cell damage.
- Current guidelines in severe TBI are to replace 140% of resting metabolism in nonparalyzed patients and 100% of resting metabolism expenditure in paralyzed patients within 7 days.

Stress Gastritis

- Stress gastritis was seen in 91% of 44 comatose mechanically ventilated patients within 24 hours of head injury. **Sucralfate, H$_2$-antagonists, proton pump inhibitors, or antacids** in patients with mechanical ventilation may be effective; none are recommended over another with regard to risk of ventilator-associated pneumonia.

Prognosis

- Survivors of TBI variably suffer from long-term cognitive, motor, sensory, and emotional deficits. These manifest as weakness, incoordination, emotional lability, impulsivity, and difficulty with vision, concentration, memory, judgment, and mood.
- **Independent predictors of outcome** include older age at time of injury, the postresuscitation GCS, injury severity score, pupillary response on admission, and CT scan findings of diffuse edema, subarachnoid hemorrhage, subdural hematoma, partial obliteration of the basal cisterns, or midline shift.

Spinal Cord Injury

- The annual incidence of acute spinal cord injury (SCI) in North America is between 27 and 47 cases per million, cases per million; in the United States about 11,000 cases per year.

Management

- Primary SCI results from cord compression. Secondary injury results from systemic and local vascular insults, which may be a result of hypotension, electrolytes changes, edema, and excitotoxicity.

Immobilization

- Spine immobilization can be uncomfortable, carries potential morbidity of pressure sores and risk of aspiration, and may limit respiratory function; however, it is the usual treatment for all patients with a mechanism of injury that may cause spinal injury.
- Various methods for complete spine immobilization can be used, but a rigid cervical collar with supportive blocks on a rigid backboard is effective.

Radiologic Evaluation

- No cervical radiologic evaluation is recommended in **awake, alert, nonintoxicated** trauma patients who have **no neck pain or tenderness** and no distracting injury. The CT scan is better than magnetic resonance imaging (MRI) for evaluating bones; however, flexion/extension radiographs in an awake patient or MRI **within 48 hours** of injury can best detect ligamentous injury.
- Newer-generation CT scanners are sensitive, and some centers no longer perform plain radiographs. However, current American Association of Neurological Surgeons standards are for an anteroposterior, lateral, and odontoid cervical spine series supplemented with CT scan in the initial evaluation. In an awake patient with neck pain, options to clear the cervical spine include normal flexion/extension films or a normal MRI within 48 hours of injury. In obtunded patients with normal cervical spine films, options to clear the spine include (a) dynamic flexion/extension studies under fluoroscopy, (b) normal MRI obtained within 48 hours of injury, or (c) the discretion of the treating physician.

Hemodynamic Support

- Systemic hypotension, which contributes to secondary SCI, can result from trauma-related hypovolemia and from neurogenic shock. **Neurogenic shock** is defined as the loss of sympathetic innervation that causes loss of peripheral vasoconstriction and cardiac compensatory mechanisms of tachycardia and increased stroke volume and cardiac output. Augmentation of **mean arterial pressures to 85 to 90 mm Hg for 5 to 7 days** after injury improves outcome.

- Treatment typically includes **volume** resuscitation with crystalloid or red blood cell transfusion if the patient is anemic. **Vasoactive medications** such as norepinephrine, dopamine, and phenylephrine are used as needed. Volume-resistant hypotension is fivefold more common among patients with complete SCI above the thoracic sympathetic innervation.
- In the subset of patients requiring vasopressors and inotropes, central venous catheters and invasive monitoring with arterial catheters should be used.

Surgical Intervention

- The timing of surgical decompression, reduction of bony structures, and fusion in the treatment of acute SCI remains in debate. There is little agreement on optimal timing. Early surgery may be associated with shorter hospitalizations and reduced pulmonary complications.

Pharmacologic Intervention

- After acute SCI, a cascade of biochemical processes is activated that produces excitatory amino acids, calcium fluxes, free radicals, acidosis, protein phosphorylation, phospholipases, and apoptosis, which can further injure surrounding tissue. Pharmacologic agents targeted to interrupt this cascade may provide neuroprotection by preventing secondary injury.
- **Methylprednisolone at 30 mg/kg bolus followed by 5.4 mg/kg/hour infusion for 23 hours** given within 8 hours of injury reported significant improvement in motor function and pin and light touch at 6 months compared to those treated after 8 hours and those treated with naloxone or placebo. There are criticisms of this study, and other trials have not shown benefit of early steroid usage.
- Increased complications from steroid usage such as a higher rate of respiratory complications including pneumonia, gastrointestinal hemorrhage, sepsis, and longer hospital stays have been reported.

Pulmonary Support

- The most common cause of death in patients with SCI is due to **pneumonia, pulmonary emboli, and septicemia.** Patients with high-level cervical injuries (C3–5) may fatigue over the first few hours to days. Early measurements indicating the need for elective endotracheal intubation include the use of **vital capacity** (<20 mL/kg) and **negative inspiratory force (less negative than –20 cm H_2O).** Hypoxia and hypercapnia are late signs of respiratory failure, and intubation should not await these findings.

Associated Vascular Injury

- Blunt cervical spinal trauma can result in **vertebral artery injury** and cause posterior circulation ischemia. Incidence varies from 0.05% to 1% and may depend on screening methods. Mortality ranges from 23% to 28%.
- Patients at risk include those with **cervical fractures with subluxation** or with a **fracture through the transverse foramen,** especially those with displaced or complex midface or

mandibular fracture, a basilar skull fracture involving the carotid canal or sphenoid sinus, near-hanging resulting in cerebral hypoxia, and cervical vertebral body fraction or distraction injury.

- Suspicion should be high if the patient develops a **lateralizing neurologic deficit with normal initial CT scan,** or evidence of a recent ischemic stroke on cerebral imaging. Although CT angio with a 16-channel detector shows high sensitivity for screening, the gold standard is four-vessel cerebral angiography. Aspirin or heparin therapy should be initiated if no contraindications are present.

Thromboprophylaxis

- **Prophylactic anticoagulation** for all patients with acute SCI is a grade 1A recommendation from the American College of Chest Physicians. The recommended anticoagulation is LMWH once primary hemostasis is achieved or a combination of intermittent pneumatic compression and either low-dose unfractionated heparin or LMWH. If anticoagulation is contraindicated, it is recommended that intermittent pneumatic compression with or without graduated compression stockings be used (grade 1C).
- The period of highest risk for deep vein thrombosis is in the first few months after injury. For this reason, duration of treatment is recommended for **at least 6 to 12 weeks.** Warfarin is recommended for the rehabilitative phase of SCI. Vena caval filters are not recommended as primary prophylaxis. There are no prospective randomized studies of the safety of anticoagulation after spinal surgery.

Nutritional Support and Metabolic Changes

- As described earlier, traumatic injury is associated with a hypermetabolic, catabolic state with nitrogen loss.
- In SCI victims, indirect calorimetry will be more accurate than the Harris–Benedict equation to determine metabolic needs.

Autonomic Dysreflexia

- Autonomic dysreflexia is a life-threatening hypertensive emergency that typically occurs in patients with motor-complete SCI **above the T6 neurologic level,** typically seen in the **rehabilitative phase** of SCI described as early as 4 days after injury.
- **Noxious stimuli** including fecal impaction, bladder distention, or pain to the lower extremities increases **sympathetic outflow below the injury level.** Resultant vasoconstriction of the splanchnic bed forces blood into the system circulation and increases blood pressure. Reflex parasympathetic outflow rostral to the injury allows flushing of the skin above the level of the lesion and bradycardia.
- Recognition of this entity and detection and removal of the inciting noxious stimulus is primary. Blood pressure treatment traditionally included ganglionic blockers, although intravenous antihypertensives such as nicardipine or nitroprusside can be effective.

Prognosis

- Incomplete injury has a better prognosis than those that are complete. MRI shows that complete SCI was associated with more substantial maximum canal compromise, spinal cord compression, length of lesion, hemorrhage, and cord edema and poorer prognosis.

- Two clinical entities described in SCI are pertinent to prognosis: (a) **Spinal shock** is a transient loss of spinal cord sensorimotor function, patients present with **flaccid paralysis** and loss of all spinal cord reflexes including the bulbocavernosus, cremasteric, and deep-tendon reflexes, and **priapism** can be seen due to local **unopposed parasympathetic outflow;** if there is no anatomic injury, function returns within hours to days; (b) **central cord syndrome,** in which the motor deficit in the **upper extremities** is disproportionately **worse** than that in the lower extremities, occurs with bowel and bladder dysfunction and variable sensory loss below the level of injury. The natural history of central cord syndrome is good neurologic recovery.

CHAPTER 41 ■ ORTHOPEDIC TRAUMA

- Bony and soft-tissue injuries often complicate trauma. Patients treated suboptimally are at risk for myriad complications such as fat embolism syndrome, pulmonary embolus, soft-tissue infection, and multiple organ failure. There is little prospective randomized data to guide treatment decisions in patients with bony injuries.
- **Fracture stabilization** is an operative procedure of significance. Some patients may be too critically ill or injured at the time of initial presentation to tolerate definitive fracture fixation. The critical care staff must be well versed in the management principles that govern musculoskeletal injuries, as they will often have important roles to play in decision making.
- Orthopedic surgeons and/or anesthesiologists may not have sufficient information on total patient physiology to make these decisions without input from the critical care staff.
- **Fractures missed** at the time of initial presentation can cause significant morbidity or mortality (see Chapter 37). Careful ongoing assessment of an intubated obtunded patient is critical. A delayed diagnosis can produce substantial disability that is lifelong. Even worse, unrecognized ischemia and/or compartment syndrome can place a limb at jeopardy, requiring amputation later. Unrecognized ischemia can also produce life-threatening electrolyte abnormalities such as hyperkalemia and/or be the source of multiple organ failure.

TREATMENT OPTIONS FOR FRACTURES

- Fractures that are not associated with life-threatening bleeding are *not* the highest priority. However, all long-bone fractures should be **splinted** as part of the initial management. Every time the patient is moved, unsplinted fractures are displaced, producing **blood loss and pain and risking secondary nerve or vascular injury.**
- Rigid fracture fixation is generally obtained via **open reduction/internal fixation (ORIF)** or closed **intramedullary (IM)** nail fixation.
- **ORIF** involves directly exposing the fracture fragments. Overlying muscles must often be divided for exposure, fracture manually reduced, and rigid fixation is achieved with plates and screws or rods. This also allows for debridement of nonviable and/or contused muscle and irrigation of the fracture hematoma.
- **Closed IM nailing** involves making a small incision proximally or distally in the extremity, then the fracture fragments are reduced under fluoroscopic visualization. A nail is then driven up the medullary canal over the guide wire.
- Either of these can produce **systemic inflammatory response syndrome (SIRS)** and/or **acute lung injury.**
- **External fixation** involves placing an external frame that spans the fracture, limiting fracture movement. It can be rapid and noninvasive and result in substantially less blood loss than ORIF or IM nailing and is reserved for unstable patients.
- **Open fractures** require an initial debridement and irrigation of the fracture fragments as a minimum. This is done to reduce the rate of early soft tissue infection and late osteomyelitis.

OPTIMAL TIMING OF FRACTURE FIXATION

- The definition of **early fracture fixation** usually implies within **24 hours of injury.** Paradoxically, the advantages are most pronounced in patients with multiple system injury who are at risk for any operative procedure. Judgment is needed to weigh **risks and benefits** to early fracture fixation.
- Nonoperative management requires that the patient remain supine in bed. In some patients, inability to elevate head of bed may aggravate intracranial pressure. There is higher risk of atelectasis, pneumonia, aspiration, pain, bleeding, SIRS, and thromboembolic complications.
- **Fracture hematoma** may be a **metabolically active organ,** capable of producing **SIRS and multiple organ failure.** Early fracture fixation allowed for irrigation of the fracture hematoma.
- Caution should be exercised in patients with **traumatic brain injury,** and conflicting results have been reported, with some studies demonstrating worse neurologic outcome whereas others have not.

- Several factors should be considered: (a) the risk of anesthesia and the magnitude of the operative procedure; (b) does the patient have a reasonable nonoperative option—could a lesser procedure be adequate? (c) finally, is the patient in optimal condition? Can cardiac performance be improved with volume and/or inotropes? Will 1 to 2 days allow ventilatory requirements to be reduced? Would a delay improve renal function? Only when all of these questions are answered can an intelligent decision about the **optimal time and fracture fixation** be made.

Damage Control Orthopedics

- Traditional teaching was to repair all injuries at the time of initial surgical procedure. Unfortunately, this often required prolonged operative care, and patients would develop a **lethal triad of acidosis, coagulopathy, and hypothermia** and die in the intensive care unit of acute organ failure within 24 hours.
- Many trauma centers began using a staged approach where **only lifesaving procedures are performed at the time of the initial procedure.** The patient was then admitted to the intensive care unit and resuscitated. Between 1 and 3 days later, the patient was taken back to the operating room to care for all the other injuries. This resulted in improved outcome.
- The same principles can be applied to bony injuries and is called **damage control orthopedics (DCO).** There are clear advantages to early fracture fixation. Yet, some patients may not be best served by such technique. A technique that would achieve many of the advantages of fracture fixation without the disadvantages of definitive surgery would be advantageous for some patients.
- For that subset of patients whose physiologic condition precludes primary definitive operative stabilization of fractures (early total care), **external fixation** can be a useful technique for temporary stabilization of long-bone fractures.
- Such external fixation is advantageous because it can be applied rapidly, with minimal blood loss and with sufficient restoration of stability to prevent ongoing soft-tissue injury and to prevent ongoing release of inflammatory mediators. Effective limitation of secondary effects of shock has been demonstrated with this type of initial DCO approach.
- DCO may be effective in patients with **polytrauma and lung or brain injury.** For the majority of patients with femoral shaft fractures, including most polytrauma patients, primary reamed femoral nailing **within 24 hours of injury** remains the gold standard of treatment.
- Defining the "at-risk" patients who are unable to tolerate early reamed nailing is difficult, but if adequate resuscitation and normalization of serum lactate are achieved, damage control should rarely be necessary.
- In borderline patients who are physiologically unstable because of severe chest or head injury or inadequate resuscitation, temporizing external fixation and damage control orthopedics may be advantageous.

COMPARTMENT SYNDROME

- Compartment syndrome occurs when there is increased tissue pressure within a confined osseofascial space. This increased pressure compromises blood flow and subsequently results in tissue damage if left untreated.
- The clinical diagnosis of compartment syndrome can be elusive. In the alert patient, pain is typically the first symptom. **Sensory deficits** may occur late and are typically in the distribution of the sensory nerve traversing the affected compartment. **Motor weakness** is a late and ominous sign. **Loss of palpable pulses** is very late and rare.
- In the patient who is not awake and alert, the diagnosis of compartment syndrome requires extreme vigilance and a high degree of clinical suspicion. The diagnosis in these patients requires frequent physical examination and tissue pressure measurements.
- Many techniques have been described, but the simplest and most widely used is the **STIC Device** (Stryker Corporation, Kalamazoo, MI). The handheld STIC catheter utilizes a disposable syringe and needle and, after zeroing the monitor, insertion of the needle through the fascia of the compartments.
- There is some debate concerning the measured pressure at which the diagnosis of compartment syndrome should be made and fasciotomy performed. Many advocate the use of absolute values of >30 to 35 mm Hg. Others have stressed the importance of the difference between **diastolic pressure and measured compartment pressure** with a Δp <30 mm Hg.
- In the patient who is **at risk** of compartment syndrome, tight casts, splints, and dressings should be avoided. The optimal position is to place the affected extremity at the level of the heart to optimize both arterial and venous flow.
- **Surgical decompression** is the treatment.
- In the patient at high risk for the development of compartment syndrome, **prophylactic fasciotomy** may be appropriate. If the patient will be unexaminable, unable to complain of symptoms, and unavailable for serial measurements of compartment pressures, prolonged hypotension, arterial vascular repairs, or concomitant venous injury, fasciotomy should not be delayed because venous insufficiency may exaggerate edema and increase the risk of the development of compartment syndrome.
- Once fasciotomies are performed, **sterile dressings or a closed vacuum suction** device should be applied and the wounds re-examined in about 48 hours. Muscle with borderline or questionable viability should be left and re-examined in 24 to 48 hours.
- **Complications** of untreated compartment syndrome include **muscle necrosis, irreparable nerve damage, and limb loss.** When treatment is delayed more than 12 hours, amputation rates may be more than 20%.
- **Myonecrosis** can result in the release of large amounts of myoglobin particularly during the reperfusion phase after fasciotomy. **Myoglobin** can precipitate **renal failure** via three mechanisms: decreased renal perfusion, renal tubular obstruction due to cast formation, and direct toxic effects of myoglobin on the kidney. Treatment is aggressive hydration and maintenance of high-volume urine output. Some have advocated the use of mannitol and urine alkalinization.

FAT EMBOLISM SYNDROME

- Fat embolism syndrome (FES) is most commonly associated with long bone fractures. Although fat embolism may occur in up to 90% of trauma patients, **FES occurs in only 2% to 5%** of patients with long-bone fractures characterized by both pulmonary and systemic fat embolism and includes a spectrum from subclinical to mild to fulminant presentations.

- Clinical FES typically involves multiple organ systems; however, involvement of the **pulmonary, neurologic, hematologic, and dermatologic systems** is the most common.
- Fat embolization can occur at the time of fracture and long-bone fixation. Elevated pressures during reaming of the intramedullary canal appear to be temporally associated with embolization to the pulmonary circulation when studied with echocardiography. Once fat is liberated into the circulation and embolizes, the pulmonary microvasculature becomes occluded. Smaller globules may traverse the pulmonary microvasculature and reach the systemic circulation, leading to the common neurologic manifestation of FES. Although the **pulmonary, cerebral, retinal, and skin microcirculations** are typical clinical manifestations of FES, fat embolization can affect **any microcirculatory bed.**
- **Acute lung injury and adult respiratory distress syndrome** may result from fat emboli occluding pulmonary capillaries, and biochemical alterations directly damage the pulmonary capillary endothelium.
- Biochemical fat embolization is associated with the **release of free fatty acids. free fatty acids** in the lung are locally hydrolyzed in pulmonary circulation by lipoprotein lipase, which releases toxic substances that injure the capillary endothelium and may initiate disseminated intravascular coagulation and platelet aggregation, further compounding **systemic inflammation.**
- Fat emboli that pass through the pulmonary vasculature result in systemic embolization, most commonly in the **brain and kidneys. Cerebral FES** is rare, yet potentially lethal. Neurologic symptoms vary from confusion to encephalopathy with coma and seizures. In severe cases, **intracranial pressure (ICP) monitoring** may be helpful. A clinical diagnosis may be difficult as cerebral FES may be masked by other clinical scenarios. **Diffuse encephalopathy, petechial hemorrhages, localized cerebral edema, and white-matter changes** may be seen with magnetic resonance imaging, whereas computed tomography scan may be normal.
- **Treatment is supportive.**
- The outcome in patients with FES who receive supportive care is generally favorable, with mortality rates of <10%. Pulmonary, neurologic, and retinal abnormalities generally resolve completely.

PELVIC FRACTURES

- Pelvic fractures occur from high-impact trauma and are associated with mortality rates ranging from 10% to 50%. The principles of pelvic fracture management after the initial assessment of "airway, breathing, and circulation" include **detection of associated injuries** (especially intraperitoneal bleeding source), **stabilization of pelvic fracture** in patients who demonstrate signs of hemorrhage (external compression devices), **early embolization** of pelvic arterial bleed, and **avoiding coagulopathy** and hypothermia by vigilant monitoring and treatment.
- **Older patients** (≥60 years) have a higher likelihood of **arterial bleeding** with more transfusion requirement. After control of life-threatening issues such as bleeding, careful assessment of other injuries that may cause significant morbidity such as rectal and vaginal tears and bladder and urethral injuries need to be assessed.
- **Missed open pelvic fractures** will lead to sepsis. Pelvic exam in females and rectal exam should be done in all patients.
- Adequate hydration, monitoring for abdominal compartment syndrome, and vigilant secondary and tertiary survey are necessary. Some patients require **more than one embolization** to control hemorrhage.

CHAPTER 42 ■ FACIAL TRAUMA

GENERAL ISSUES

- Comprehensive management and treatment of facial trauma involves airway control, control of bleeding, reduction of swelling, prevention of infection, repair of soft-tissue lacerations, and repair of fractures to restore function and esthetic form to the face.
- Essential component of initial care begins with the ABCs (airway, breathing, circulation) and cervical spine assessment.
- As with any other trauma patient, the facial trauma patient should be evaluated in a systematic and comprehensive fashion in cooperation with the trauma team.

- Abdominal, thoracic, cervical spine, and neurosurgical emergencies take priority over maxillofacial injury.

AIRWAY

- Early airway control and neurologic assessment of a potential head injury are critical because the eyes and oropharynx are the "shock organs" of the face, and development of facial edema will obscure the pupils and obstruct the upper airway. Immediate treatment of maxillofacial trauma patients is indicated in the following situations: (a) airway compromise, (b) severe hemorrhage, (c) large open wounds, (d) superior orbital fissure and orbital apex syndrome, (e) mandibular condylar impaction into the cranial fossa, and (f) if urgent surgical procedures need to be performed by other services.

- Definitive treatment of facial fractures can be delayed as much as 2 weeks after injury as long as the fractures do not violate the cranial space.
- Spinal injuries are increased fourfold if there is a clinically significant head injury (Glasgow coma scale score <9).
- The following subsets of patients require immediate securing of airway to prevent respiratory failure: patients with (a) Glasgow coma score <9, (b) sustained seizure activity, (c) unstable midface trauma, (d) direct injuries to the airway, (e) aspiration risk or unable to maintain an airway, and (f) oxygenation problems.
- The airway should be cleared of debris, foreign bodies (teeth), blood, and secretions. The classic "chin lift" or "jaw thrust" maneuvers are commonly employed for assessment of airway patency and to remove obstruction of the tongue base. However, jaw thrust and chin lift may cause distraction of at least 5 mm in a cadaver with C5–6 instability.
- Manual in-line axial stabilization must, therefore, be maintained throughout. Bag-and-mask ventilation also produces significant degrees of cervical spine movement at zones of instability. The "sniffing the morning air" position for standard endotracheal intubation should similarly be avoided as it flexes the lower cervical spine and extends the occiput on the atlas. Atlanto-occipital extension is necessary to visualize the vocal cords. Patients with unstable C1 or C2 injuries are at risk.
- The hard C-collar may interfere with intubation efforts. The front part of the collar can be removed to facilitate intubation as long as manual stabilization remains in effect.
- The safest method of securing an endotracheal tube remains debatable. Orotracheal intubation is the fastest and surest method although the Advanced Trauma Life Support recommends a nasotracheal tube in the spontaneously breathing patient and orotracheal intubation in the apneic patient. With caution, patients may be safely intubated orally with a modified rapid sequence induction technique with preoxygenation and cricoid pressure.
- Nasotracheal intubation is (relatively) contraindicated in patients with potential skull base fractures or unstable midface injuries that typically involve the naso-orbito-ethmoid complex. Any paranasal manipulation (including insertion of a nasogastric tube) may produce or recreate local hemorrhage, making airway manipulations difficult or impossible. Inadvertent placement and contamination/violation of the cranial space are also possible.
- The need for a surgical airway should be recognized and obtained without delay. A percutaneous needle cricothyroidotomy with high-flow oxygen is indicated in emergency situations when standard tracheotomy is not feasible or advisable. The potential for carbon dioxide retention with this technique must be remembered and the levels in arterial samples monitored.
- Cricothyroidotomy is contraindicated in laryngeal or tracheal trauma, cervical infection, and young children but is necessary if unable to intubate. A standard tracheotomy is essential in unstable patients who require prolonged maxillomandibular fixation for fracture stabilization and management.

HEMORRHAGE

- Because the face and neck have a rich vascular supply, injuries in these areas can lead to substantial blood loss. Major hemorrhage can result from large scalp wounds, nasal or midface fractures, and penetrating wounds.
- Hence, external hemorrhage can usually be controlled by direct pressure to the wound and/or bleeding areas. Pressure can also be applied proximal to major arteries if direct pressure to the wound is not effective.
- Scalp wounds can be rapidly approximated with 2.0 nonabsorbable sutures (nylon, Prolene) or staples if available. Sutures should be placed away from the wound edge to ensure hemostasis as the galea tends to retract.
- Nasal fractures and midface fractures can result in tearing of the ethmoidal arteries. Most of these can be controlled with direct pressure or packing. Nonintubated patients with nasal packing in place should have the head of the bed elevated 30 degrees and be observed and monitored for respiratory distress. Continued bleeding may not be apparent on the nasal side of the packing. Nasal packing easily slips posteriorly with swallowing or out with movement or sneezing. The posterior oropharynx should be checked regularly.
- Fractures of the posterior maxillary wall, as in LeFort I and II fractures, may be associated with profuse bleeding from the internal maxillary artery. Bleeding from this artery can be very difficult to control by gauze packing.
- Hypoxemia and hypercarbia can cause respiratory and cardiac complications. Airway obstruction and asphyxiation can occur if the nasal packing slips back into the airway, particularly during sleep. Complications may occur if a pack compresses the eustachian tube. Rarely, infections can develop in the nose, sinus, or middle ear after nasal packing and lead to toxic shock syndrome.
- When tight nasal/oral packing fails in unstable patients, supraselective arteriography and embolization are the treatment of choice in institutions where this modality is available. Ligation of the external carotid artery is a last resort in the unstable multitrauma patient who cannot be transported. However, due to collateral circulation of the face, ligation is seldom truly effective. Best control of hemorrhage is obtained by exploratory surgery and fixation of fractures. In patients with isolated LeFort fractures, open reduction/internal fixation is the first line of treatment.

WOUND MANAGEMENT

- There are some basic rules that apply in treating soft-tissue injuries. Soft-tissue injuries are only properly evaluated after the wound is cleaned of dirt, foreign bodies, debris, and dry blood.
- Facial nerve function should be assessed in all patients with facial lacerations, and nerve function should be documented *prior* to anesthetic use. Ideally, repair of the facial nerve should occur as soon as possible but no later than 72 hours unless the wound is heavily contaminated.
- In patients with deep lacerations of the cheek, the wound should also be explored for injury to the parotid duct (Stensen duct). One may see saliva in the wound if the duct is lacerated. The parotid duct is repaired over a stent to prevent stenosis.

- Optimum timing of facial laceration repair is a topic of debate. After tetanus prophylaxis, soft-tissue repair can be performed within 12 to 24 hours provided the wounds are irrigated, cleaned, and kept moist.

Cranial Nerve Exam

- Olfaction (cranial nerve one [CN I]) is typically not examined in the acute trauma bay setting but reserved for later trauma surveys (tertiary survey). Damage to CN I should be considered with the naso-orbito-ethmoid complex and frontal sinus fractures if disruption of the cribriform plate is present.
- Pupillary responses (CN II, III) may be difficult to examine in patients with extensive orbital trauma, as the eyelid swells rapidly. Next, examine with a flashlight. Note the direct constriction of the illuminated pupil and the consensual constriction of the opposite pupil. In an afferent pupillary defect, there is decreased direct response in the affected eye. This can be demonstrated by moving the flashlight back and forth between the eyes, with a lag of 2 to 3 seconds. The afferent defect becomes evident when the flashlight is moved from the normal to the affected eye because the affected eye will dilate in response to light. Brief pupillary oscillations of the stimulated pupil (hippus) are normal and should be distinguished from pathologic response. Finally, test the pupillary response to accommodation, by moving an object (e.g., finger) from far to near. The pupils should constrict. The direct response of the ipsilateral pupil is absent in lesions to the ipsilateral optic nerve, the pretectal area, the ipsilateral sympathetic nerves traveling with CN III, or the pupillary constrictor muscle of the iris. The consensual response is impaired (contralateral pupil illuminated) in lesions of the contralateral optic nerve, the pretectal area, the sympathetic nerves, or the pupillary constrictor of the iris. Accommodation is affected for the same reasons and in pathways from optic nerve to the visual cortex. Accommodation is spared in injury to the pretectal area
- Extraocular movements (CN III, IV, VI) are readily checked by asking patients to look in all directions without moving their head and asking them if they experience any diplopia in any direction. Test "smooth pursuit" by slowly moving an object or finger up and down and sideways. Test convergence by asking the patient to fixate on an object that is moved toward a point between the eyes. During these tests, look closely for nystagmus and dysconjugate gaze.
- Facial sensation and muscles of mastication (CN V) are tested using a soft object or finger in the forehead, cheek, and lower jaw line to capture all three branches of the nerve. Test the masseter muscles during jaw clench. In facial fractures, the most commonly affected nerve is the Vb branch, which may indicate maxillary, orbital, or zygomaticomaxillary complex fractures.
- Muscles of facial expression and taste (CN VII) are tested by looking for asymmetries in spontaneous facial expressions such as blinking, smiling, and squinting. Taste testing is usually not performed. Facial weakness can be caused by lesions of upper motor neuron in the contralateral cortex or in descending nerve pathways (ipsilateral). Upper motor neurons to the upper face cross over to both facial nuclei so in intracranial injury or stroke, motor functions of the upper face remain intact. Lower motor neuron lesions typically cause weakness to the entire ipsilateral face.

- Hearing and vestibular sense (CN VIII) are seldom checked in the acute setting. Vestibular sense is typically not tested except in patients with vertigo.
- Palate elevation and gag reflex (CN IX, X) are tested by an intraoral exam and observing palatal motion when the patient says "aaah." Observe the gagging motion when the posterior pharynx is touched. The gag reflex is usually checked in patients with suspected brainstem pathology.
- Sternocleidomastoid and trapezius muscles (CN XI) are examined by asking the patient to shrug the shoulders and turn the head from side to side. Of note is that bilateral upper motor neuron projections control the sternocleidomastoid, analog to the bilateral CN VII projections controlling the upper face.
- Tongue (CN XII) will deviate toward the weak side. Lesions of the motor cortex cause contralateral tongue weakness as opposed to lower motor lesions or lesions of the tongue muscles.

Fractures

Nasal Fracture

- Due to its prominence, the nose is the most commonly fractured bone in the facial skeleton. Nasal fracture diagnosis is often a clinical, and not a radiologic, diagnosis as evidenced by mobility, swelling, flattened or deviated nose, epistaxis, septal deviation/hematoma, and mouth breathing. Septal hematoma must be ruled out in every patient. A septal hematoma forms between the septal cartilage and perichondrium from which it gets its blood supply. It appears as edema and ecchymosis of the septum with narrowing of the nasal airway on speculum exam. Septal hematoma is treated with incision and drainage. Failure to treat can lead to a septal abscess, intracranial complications, or delayed saddle nose deformity due to cartilage loss.
- Leakage of cerebrospinal fluid (CSF) indicates a fracture through the cribriform plate of the ethmoid bone. This potentially carries a risk of meningitis. There is controversy on the use of prophylactic antibiotics. Epistaxis is treated by packing the nose as discussed earlier. If this is not successful, an epistaxis catheter can be inserted to control bleeding from branches of the anterior ethmoidal artery. Treatment of most noncomminuted nasal fractures is closed reduction. Manipulation is required to restore an obstructed nasal airway and for restoration of facial cosmesis. The ideal timing for manipulative treatment varies. If reduction is not performed within the first few hours after injury, treatment is delayed 3 to 5 days for swelling to resolve. After a prolonged period (7–14 days), manipulation becomes increasingly difficult as the nasal bones will be difficult to move into place without osteotomies and a formal rhinoplasty may be required.

Naso-ethmoid-orbital Fracture

- Naso-ethmoid-orbital fractures are evidenced by (a) flat nasal bridge with splaying of nasal complex and crepitus, (b) saddle-shaped deformity of nose ("punched-in" look), (c) telecanthus (increased distance between the medial canthi), (d) circumorbital edema and ecchymosis ("raccoon eyes"), (e) subconjunctival hemorrhage, (f) epistaxis, (g) CSF rhinorrhea, or (h) supraorbital/supratrochlear nerve paresthesia.

- With true nasoethmoidal fractures, a CSF leak should be assumed even if not clinically evident.
- Closed manipulation of naso-orbito-ethmoid injuries notoriously gives a poor result, with a high incidence of persistent or recurrent deformity postoperatively.

Orbital Blowout Fracture

- The term *orbital blowout fracture* is reserved for a fracture of the bones of the orbit. This may involve the orbital floor, walls, or roof. The majority of cases involve the orbital floor and medial wall, as these areas comprise the thinnest bone of the orbit.
- Often, the thin bone of the floor displaces downward into the maxillary antrum, remaining attached to the orbital periosteum as one fragment ("trap door"). The periorbital fat herniates through the defect, thereby interfering with the inferior rectus and inferior oblique muscles, which are contained within the same fascia sheath. This prevents upward movement and outward rotation of the eye, and the patient experiences diplopia on upward gaze. This clinical finding should be distinguished from true "entrapment," which indicates impingement of the ocular muscles. Those patients will present with pain, tenderness around the eye, swelling, and subjective diplopia in all outer fields of gaze.
- Ophthalmologic evaluation is advised if significant eye trauma is detected. If the patient is unresponsive, an afferent pupillary defect may uncover occult visual loss. If indicated clinically, tonometry may be used to assess intraocular pressure.
- Complications of unrecognized orbital floor fracture are as follows:
  - Posttraumatic persistent enophthalmos
  - Hypoglobus (inferior displacement of the orbit)
  - Persistent diplopia
  - Lower eyelid retraction (ectropion) and scleral show
  - Persistent edema of the lower eyelid

Zygoma Fractures

- Prominent zygoma is the second most commonly fractured facial bone.
- Clinical features of zygomaticomaxillary complex fractures are as follows:
  - Swelling and bruising over the cheek or flattening
  - Step-off deformity at the orbital rim
  - Periorbital ecchymosis
  - Subconjunctival hemorrhage
  - Para-/anesthesia of the infraorbital nerve
  - Trismus and restricted lateral excursion
  - Para-/anesthesia of Z-facial/temporal nerves
- Because the zygoma articulates superficially with the maxilla, frontal, and temporal bones, zygomatic fractures in the past have been referred to as tripod or trimalar fractures. However, the fourth articulation with the sphenoid really makes it a quadripod fracture.
- Owing to traction on the infraorbital nerve, patients often complain of upper lip/tooth numbness. Trismus may be present as the masseter muscle pulls the malar fragment down, which impinges on the mandible.
- For the zygoma, timing of repair is 5 to 7 days after injury to allow tissue edema and swelling to subside. After 10 days, masseter contracture may complicate closed reduction of the zygoma.

Midfacial Skeleton: LeFort Fractures

- LeFort fractures tend to result from anterior forces. The fracture possibilities and combinations thereof are numerous; hence, classification schemes fail to describe them all.
- The LeFort I fracture essentially separates the lower maxilla, including the alveolar ridge and teeth, from the rest of the midface.
- The LeFort II fracture is a pyramidal fracture that includes the entire piriform aperture in the distracted midface. The fracture line includes the frontonasal suture, passes through the inferomedial orbit, and runs between the zygoma and maxilla for a larger area of dissociation.
- The LeFort III fracture is a suprazygomatic fracture through the lateral orbit. The fracture line extends from the dorsum of the nose and the cribriform plate along the medial and lateral wall of the orbit to the ZF suture line. This is also known as craniofacial dissociation, as the bones of the midface are essentially completely disarticulated from the cranium.
  - All complete LeFort fractures will create mobility of the maxilla, especially the upper alveolus (tooth-bearing portion of the maxilla). Hence, all will lead to subjective (and objective) malocclusion in varying degrees of severity.
- Comminuted fractures and fractures with malocclusion are treated with maxillomandibular fixation and/or by open reduction/internal fixation. Truly rigid fixation of the midface, unlike the mandible, is unattainable owing to the thin bones and correspondingly thin plates.

Unfortunately, many trauma patients are obtunded or intoxicated and unable to provide any subjective information. Physical examination alone is inconclusive in the majority of cases. On physical examination, the examiner should note presence and location of lacerations, ecchymoses, and gross asymmetry. Palpation is done to assess instability, crepitus, tenderness, bony stepoffs, and canthal tendon disruption. The trigeminal nerve should be tested. Ophthalmologic examination deserves special mention. Many authors believe that it is impractical to expect ophthalmologic consultation on every patient with facial injury. Most physicians are able to test visual acuity (subjective and objective), pupillary function, ocular motility, anterior chamber exam (to look for hyphema), and funduscopic exam. Ophthalmologic consultation should then be obtained as indicated. Last, but not least: Although cosmesis is not an immediate concern, it is of great concern to patients, especially once the acute trauma experience has worn off. Long-term goals and appearance outcomes should, therefore, be discussed with every patient on an individual basis to avoid misunderstandings and misconceptions.

CHAPTER 43 ■ BURN INJURY: THERMAL AND ELECTRICAL

BURN PHYSIOLOGY AND THE EFFECTS ON ORGAN SYSTEMS

- Burn injury has a systemic effect on the patient, and each organ system responds to this injury in a predictable manner proportional to the extent of burn.

Cardiovascular System

- Resultant fluid losses and increased capillary permeability lead to hypovolemia.
- The loss of fluid leads to decreased cardiac preload and decreased cardiac output.
- Early and late inflammatory mediators influence myocardial contraction and relaxation in the first 24 to 48 hours after burn injury.
- Multiple formulas exist for fluid management (see later). Myocardial depression can be supported pharmacologically with the use of inotropic agents.

Pulmonary System

- The pulmonary response is characterized by transient pulmonary hypertension, decreased lung compliance, and hypoxia, mediated by multiple factors including inflammation, acid-base imbalance, airway injury, and chest wall restriction.
- Chest burns with edema formation result in decreased chest wall compliance, restricted ventilation, and increased airway pressures; burn wound escharotomy of the chest wall may be indicated.
- Burn wound infection may lead to lung dysfunction secondary to inflammatory mediator release.
- Complications associated with intubation after burn injuries include ventilator-associated pneumonia and tracheal stenosis. Extubation at the earliest opportunity afforded by the patient's physiology—and his or her operative schedule—is important in reducing this complication.
- Smoke inhalation injury affects between 10% and 30% of burn patients and is associated with increased mortality over that predicted by age and extent of burn alone. High-frequency percussive ventilation has been used to treat patients with severe inhalation injury with promising results.

Renal System

- Renal failure has been reported in up to 20% of burn injury patients, with a clinical picture related to the size and severity of burn injury. The time course of renal failure falls into early or late categories.
- Early acute renal failure appears to be directly associated with clinical events such as delayed resuscitation, underresuscitation, hypotension, and rhabdomyolysis. Rhabdomyolysis is often associated with electrical injury.
- Late episodes of acute renal failure are more commonly associated with sepsis, toxic drugs, and pre-existing medical conditions.
- Treatment includes adequate fluid resuscitation initiated as early as possible, monitoring urine output as a measure of renal perfusion. Sepsis from lines, wound, pneumonia, or urinary tract should be controlled by replacing the lines, excising the burn wound, and providing adequate antibiotic therapy for pneumonia and urinary tract infection.
- When needed, renal replacement therapy should be instituted.

Gastrointestinal Tract and Liver

- Ileus presents in patients with burns exceeding 20% total body surface area (TBSA).
- Using the gastrointestinal tract with some—even minimal—level of feeding is advocated early after injury and is usually well tolerated. Tube feeding should be instituted for patients with large burns where the patient is unable to tolerate sufficient intake.
- Gastroduodenal stress ulceration has markedly decreased with the use of antacids, H_2-antagonists, and proton pump inhibiting medications.
- Poor perfusion of the gut during resuscitation may lead to segmental ischemia in the watershed areas of the intestine leading to perforation. The use of vasoactive medications during burn resuscitation or during prolonged septic events may increase this risk.
- Normal gut flora have been identified as an infection source, and maintaining gut integrity with nutritional support in the form of glutamine supplementation has been studied. Selective gut decontamination has been shown to reduce bacterial translocation from the gut. Clinical success with this approach is not well documented.
- Intra-abdominal hypertension, as defined by a bladder pressure of 30 mm Hg or greater is the precursor to the abdominal compartment syndrome. Respiratory compromise with increasing peak airway pressures, renal compromise with decreased renal perfusion and urine output, and increased mortality have been observed. Burn patients with >30% burn injury are at risk for this complication. We recommend monitoring bladder pressures. Reduced fluid administration, sedation, and chemical paralysis of the patient are the initial treatments. Escharotomies and peritoneal drainage

make up the next most invasive line of management and, ultimately, abdominal decompression through a laparotomy may be needed to relieve the symptoms.

Central Nervous System

- Autoregulation of cerebral blood flow is effective to a point and then begins to fail as resuscitation proceeds, suggesting that the cerebrovascular system has a limited reserve to tolerate the effects of burn injury.

Endocrine System

- The elevations in stress-related hormones are noted in a time- and burn size-dependent manner after injury.
- The hypothalamus responds by secreting antidiuretic hormone that acts on the collecting ducts of the kidney to facilitate the reabsorption of water into the blood.
- The anterior pituitary releases adrenal corticotropic hormone, which stimulates the release of the mineralocorticoid aldosterone and glucocorticoid cortisol.
- The adrenal medulla releases the tyrosine-derived neurotransmitters adrenaline and noradrenaline.
- Several medications are available that can modify the endocrine response to burn injury and include use of oxandrolone and beta-blockade to modify the metabolic response.

Hematopoietic System

- The red blood cell (RBC) mass in the burn patient declines in a burn size- and severity-dependent fashion.
- Initial heat injuries to the RBCs and sequestration of blood in the burn eschar are early factors in the loss of RBCs. Damage to RBCs secondary to the inflammatory response to the burn wound is a later development.

Immune System

- The risk of infection and its complications are directly related to the size of the burn injury and additional factors such as inhalation injury and pre-existing medical conditions. Burned skin loses its barrier function against the environment, and normal skin flora and environmental pathogens are able to gain access to the system.
- Damaged skin is the most obvious portal for bacterial entry. Burn-related hypotension and peripheral vasoconstriction may permit intestinal hypoperfusion and translocation of normal gastrointestinal flora into the systemic circulation. Other portals of entry are intubations of the respiratory, vascular, and genitourinary systems.

Musculoskeletal System

- Bone loss is due to (a) an increase in glucocorticoids that inhibit bone formation and osteoblast differentiation;(b) hypercalciuria secondary to hypoparathyroidism; and (c) vitamin-D deficiency.
- Muscle loss is secondary to an intense catabolic state initiated by the inflammatory response. Intravenous pamidronate

administration may help preserve bone mass in children with >40%surface area burns.

FLUID RESUSCITATION

- Aided by the use of the rule of nines and Lund–Browder charts, a patient's TBSA of burn and weight measurements are used to determine his or her initial fluid requirement. One half of the fluid requirements calculated are given in the first 8 hours after the burn injury, with the remaining amount administered over the subsequent 16 hours (Table 43.1).
- Adequate resuscitation is measured by end organ perfusion. A surrogate measure of the success of fluid administration is the measurement of urine output to a rate of 0.5 to 1.0 mL/kg using the ideal weight. The combination of blood pressure, heart rate, oxygenation, and central venous pressure are used in tandem to determine the adequacy of treatment.
- Postburn tissue edema will decrease the accuracy of cuff blood pressure measurements, and the vasoconstriction caused by catecholamine release will adversely affect the accuracy of indwelling arterial lines.
- Urinary rates of one-third the predicted value or less of the patient's body weight over 2 consecutive hours should prompt an increase in intravenous fluid administration.
- Patients running one-third or more over their expected urine output may benefit from decreased fluid administration.
- A graded increase or decrease of the intravenous fluid rate of 20% per hour is a measured and conservative response to these situations.
- Those patients who do not respond as expected to calculated fluid administration or who require more than 6 mL/kg per percent of TBSA burn should be considered for more invasive monitoring. A decision can be made to either support the cardiac output or reduce the peripheral vascular resistance, or both.
- Insensible water losses become more significant with larger TBSA burns and peak on the third day after burn. An estimation of insensible water losses may be calculated as follows:

$$\text{Insensible water loss (in mL/h)} = (125 + \%\text{TBSA burned}) \times \text{TBSA (in m}^2)$$

The total body surface area involved may be estimated using the formula of DuBois and DuBois as follows:

$$\text{BSA} = (W^{0.425} \times H^{0.725}) \times 0.007184$$

where W is the weight in kilograms and H is the height in centimeters. Initially, the replacement fluid should free water and then be altered based on electrolyte measurements.

TABLE 43.1

COMMON RESUSCITATION FORMULAS

	Common burn formulas		
	Evans formula	Brooke formula	Parkland formula
Colloid	1.0 mL/kg/%	0.5 mL/kg/%	None
Crystalloid	1.0 mL/kg/%	1.5 mL/kg/%	4.0 mL/kg/%
Free water	2,000 mL	2,000 mL	None

ELECTRICAL INJURY

- Electrical injuries can be divided into those due to low voltage (<1,000 volts), and those due to high voltage (≥1,000 volts).
- Electrical energy interacts with human anatomy following the basic principles of physics. Current flowing through tissue is related to the voltage drop across the resistance of that tissue. Heat produced by this current can be represented mathematically as follows:

$$J(\text{heat in Joules}) = I^2 \times R \times T$$

where I is current, R, resistance, and T, time in seconds. Differing tissues would create varying degrees of heat and subsequent damage; interestingly, clinical findings do not wholly support this concept. The highest resistance is found in the bone, fat, and tendons, whereas the lowest resistance has been identified in the muscles, blood, and nerves; skin has an intermediate resistance.
- Contact wounds on the hands and feet are common. Each of the contact areas might have a low cross-section, releasing more heat in that area; as the current crosses the "bottleneck" areas of the ankles and wrists with more tissue damage generated at these sites. At its most extreme, heat released by high-voltage injuries produces coagulation necrosis of the tissues and varying other effects on the organs as the electricity passes through.
- Arc injuries are less common but just as destructive. Electricity can travel 2 to 3 cm/10,000 volts and may travel 10 feet or more to its target. Temperatures at the contact points range from 2,000°C to 4,000°C, with spikes of up to 20,000°C; this intense temperature leads to severe and deep tissue damage.
- With high-voltage injuries, cardiac standstill and ventricular fibrillation are the most lethal cardiac injuries. Other electrocardiography includes atrial fibrillation, focal ectopic arrhythmias, supraventricular tachycardia, right bundle branch block, and nonspecific ST-T segment changes. These clinical findings are thought to be associated with direct myocardial muscle damage, coronary vasospasm, and coronary endarteritis.
- Renal injury is usually due to rhabdomyolysis. Large quantities of muscle protein, hemoglobin, and other tissue proteins released from the tissues coagulated by high voltage and current are filtered into the renal tubules, causing acute renal failure with oliguria or polyuria. Up to 15% of patients injured in high-voltage accidents will suffer from this type of renal injury.
- Central nervous system injury ranges from instant death to more subtle findings. Altered levels of consciousness with varying degrees of recovery have been reported, whereas progressive neurologic deterioration has been noted in both the central and the peripheral nervous systems. With high-voltage injuries, progressive deterioration of the microvascular nutrient vessels to the nerves has been identified and is thought to lead to ischemia, necrosis, and fibrosis of the injured nerve; progressive loss of function can be seen as a late developing problem.

INHALATION INJURY

- The pathophysiology associated with smoke inhalation injury falls into three categories: (a) upper-airway injury, (b) asphyxiant gases and hypoxic environments, and (c) carbonaceous particle deposition.
- The diagnosis of inhalation injury is based on several site-specific and clinical findings surrounding each burn patient. Closed-space injuries or explosions, noxious fumes noted at the scene, and facial burns are some findings associated with inhalation injury, with the elderly being more susceptible.
- Signs and symptoms of a true airway burn injury include hoarseness; stridor and/or wheezing; carbonaceous sputum; singed nasal hair, eyebrows, or facial hair; and edema or inflammatory changes in the upper airway. The resultant upper-airway edema formation can threaten the airway and the patient's breathing.
- Asphyxiant gases and hypoxic environments lead to the second area of pathology associated with inhalation injury. In fires involving structures, the ambient oxygen level markedly decreases leading to carbon monoxide–generation-a byproduct of incomplete combustion. Carbon monoxide binds tightly to hemoglobin, reducing the amount of oxygen delivered to end organs, causing hypoxic injury. Cyanide generation is associated with burning plastics; this molecule is highly lethal. Treatment of carbon monoxide intoxication includes a high concentration of oxygen and, sometimes, hyperbaric oxygen. Cyanide poisoning treatment includes delivery of oxygen and a three-part regimen to bind the cyanide compound in the blood.
- The flame-generated toxins that are bound to the carbon particles will induce a chemical tracheal bronchitis. The clinical sequelae include bronchorrhea, bronchospasm, distal airway obstruction, and atelectasis and pneumonia. Epithelial injury leads to sloughing of the mucosa and blockage of the airways with this cellular debris. Air trapping in this situation leads to atelectasis and the development of barotrauma and pneumonia.
- Endotracheal intubation to protect the airway should be performed early Patients suffering from carbon monoxide exposure and showing clinical signs of intoxication should be treated with 100% oxygen to displace the molecule from hemoglobin. In severe neurologic symptoms, hyperbaric oxygen therapy should be administered if readily available.
- Cyanide toxicity presents clinically with lethargy, nausea, headache, weakness, and coma. Cyanide combines with cytochrome oxidase, thereby blocking oxygen use and inhibiting high-energy phosphate compound production. Cyanide toxicity begins at 0.1 μg/mL of serum and quickly leads to death at concentrations of 1 μg/mL. Laboratory studies show a decreased arterial-venous oxygen difference with severe metabolic acidosis; this acidosis is unresponsive to fluids and oxygen administration. S-T segment elevations may be seen mimicking a myocardial infarction.
- Treatment of cyanide toxicity includes the administration of 100% oxygen and a three-part medication regimen: (a) administration of amyl nitrate pearls, by inhalation for 15 to 30 seconds every minute, (b) 10 mL 3% sodium nitrate solution (300 mg) intravenously over 3 minutes, repeated at one-half the dosage in 2 hours if symptoms persist or recurrent signs of toxicity are present, (c) sodium thiosulfate 50 mL of a 25% solution (12.5 gm) intravenously over 10 minutes, repeated at one-half the dosage in 2-hour intervals if persistent or recurrent signs of toxicity are present.

INFECTION CONTROL

- The new challenge in burn injury is the concurrent development of infection in a compromised host.
- The advent of topical antibiotic/anti-infective agents addressed this new area of pathology. Subsequent movement toward early wound excision and skin grafting led to improvements in the rates of wound sepsis and its complications. Although the burn wound has become less of a risk for infection, other portals of entry have persisted in plaguing the burn patient. With our current methods of intubating the respiratory, vascular, and genitourinary systems, we expose the burn patient to other portals of entry for pathogens.

NUTRITION

- Basic principles are (a) an assessment of the patient's initial nutritional status, (b) monitoring of his or her nutritional status throughout the hospital course, and (c) adjustments based on the monitoring measures.
- Nutritional assessment should begin with measurement of the patient's weight, estimation of the patient's calorie and protein needs, measurement of the patient's serum albumin, prealbumin, and C-reactive protein levels. Pre-existing illnesses should prompt the practitioner to make adjustments in the rate of feeding, use of additional medications, and the need for additional nutrient support.
- Glutamine supplementation has been shown to improve morbidity and mortality when administered to critically ill patients. Glutamine affects the immune system, the antioxidant status, glucose metabolism, and heat shock protein response.

WOUND MANAGEMENT

- The patient should be covered with a clean sheet and blanket to conserve body heat and minimize burn wound contamination during transport to the hospital.
- The application of ice or cold water soaks, when initiated within 10 minutes after burning, may reduce tissue heat content and lessen the depth of thermal injury. Care must be taken to avoid causing hypothermia and limiting this form of therapy to 10% or less burn of the body surface area.
- Daily wound care involves cleansing, debridement, and dressing of the burn wound. On the day of injury, the burn wound is best cleansed by means of hydrotherapy. Hydrotherapy is accomplished by means of showering, immersion, or use of a spray table.
- Immersion hydrotherapy often is used for patients in a less acute stage who have a moderate or smaller injury. Soaking promotes removal of therapeutic creams and exudate, debridement of loose eschar, and active participation by the patient in range-of-motion exercises. Immersion hydrotherapy should be avoided in patients with an extensive thermal injury as this process may spread contamination. The consensus is that a hydrotherapy session of 30 minutes or less is optimal for patients with acute burns.

- Mechanical debridement is accomplished through application and removal of gauze dressings, hydrotherapy, irrigation, and use of scissors and tweezers. Wet-to-dry or wet-to-moist dressings are sometimes used to debride exudative wounds.
- Mafenide acetate (Sulfamylon), silver sulfadiazine (Silvadene), and silver nitrate are the three most commonly used topical antimicrobial agents for burn wound care.
- Mafenide acetate burn cream is an 11.1% suspension in a water-soluble base. This compound diffuses freely into the eschar and is the preferred agent in heavily contaminated burn wounds or in situations where burn wound care has been delayed by several days. This agent is highly effective against Gram-negative organisms, including most *Pseudomonas* species. Hypersensitivity reactions occur in 7% of patients and pain or discomfort lasting 20 to 30 minutes.
- Mafenide inhibits carbonic anhydrase, resulting in a diuresis of bicarbonate with development of metabolic acidosis. Inhibition of this enzyme rarely persists for >7 to 10 days, and the severity of the acidosis may be minimized by alternating applications of mafenide with silver sulfadiazine cream every 12 hours.
- Silver sulfadiazine burn cream is a 1% suspension in a water-miscible base. Unlike mafenide, silver sulfadiazine has limited solubility in water and limited ability to penetrate into the eschar. This agent is painless on application, and serum electrolytes and acid-base balance are not.
- Silver sulfadiazine occasionally induces neutropenia by a mechanism thought to involve direct bone marrow suppression; white blood cell counts usually return to normal after discontinuation. With continual use, resistance to the sulfonamide component of silver sulfadiazine is common, particularly in certain strains of *Pseudomonas* and many *Enterobacter* species.
- A 0.5% silver nitrate solution has a broad spectrum of antibacterial activity imparted by the silver ion. This agent does not penetrate the eschar, as the silver ions rapidly precipitate on contact with any protein or cationic material. The dressings are changed twice daily and moistened every 2 hours with the silver nitrate solution to prevent evaporation from increasing the silver nitrate concentration to cytotoxic levels within the dressings. Transeschar leaching of sodium, potassium, chloride, and calcium should be anticipated and replaced. Hypersensitivity to silver nitrate has not been described.
- Mafenide acetate, silver sulfadiazine, and 0.5% silver nitrate are effective in the prevention of invasive burn wound infection. Because of their lack of eschar penetration, silver nitrate soaks and silver sulfadiazine burn cream are most effective when applied soon after burn injury.
- Acticoat is a new burn wound dressing. It consists of a urethane film onto which nanocrystalline elemental silver is deposited. When moistened, application of this dressing to the wound results in a sustained release of elemental silver, which is bactericidal and fungicidal. The mechanism of action is probably much like that of silver nitrate dressings; however, Acticoat does not cause transeschar leaching of electrolytes. The silver does not penetrate the eschar, limiting its use on heavily contaminated wounds. The use of Acticoat is currently limited to partial-thickness burns.
- Aquacel Ag hydrofiber is another dressing containing elemental silver, though at a much lower concentration. When compared to silver sulfadiazine on partial-thickness burns,

this dressing was associated with an increased rate of re-epithelization and was slightly more cost-effective.

PAIN MANAGEMENT AND ANXIOLYSIS

- An appropriate rationale is to titrate the drug dose to the desired effect rather than to rely on a particular textbook dose for all patients. Owing to the development of drug tolerance, opioid analgesic dose may exceed those recommended in standard dosing guidelines.
- Anxiety, in itself, can exacerbate acute pain. This has led to the common practice in many burn centers of using anxiolytic drugs in combination with opioid analgesics.

TEAM APPROACH

- This multidisciplinary care spans the early resuscitative phases of care through the long-term rehabilitation and reconstructive phases. Team members include burn surgeons, plastic and reconstructive surgeons, critical care specialists, anesthesiologists, critical care burn nurses, physical therapists, occupational therapists, clinical nutritional specialists, psychologists, social workers, and pastoral care support personnel.
- This concept of team care, originating in the 1950s when the first burn centers opened, has persisted to this day and is a model of coordinated, interdisciplinary, outcome-driven patient care.

CHAPTER 44 ■ TEMPERATURE-RELATED INJURIES

- The balance between heat generation and dissipation is the key to maintaining optimal body temperature. Under normal circumstances, body temperature is 37°C under the tongue, 38°C in the rectum, 32°C at the skin, and 38.5°C in the central liver. Significant deviation from normal body temperature is a critical condition that requires prompt diagnosis, treatment, and normalization of the temperature alteration.

HYPOTHERMIA

- Hypothermia is defined as a core temperature below 35°C (95°F): Mild hypothermia is that between 35°C and 32°C, moderate hypothermia between 32°C and 28°C, and severe hypothermia below 28°C.
  - Table 44.1 outlines the classification of severity and clinical manifestations.
  - Hypothermia is considered to be an underrecognized condition, especially in the aged with inadequate home heating and inappropriate clothing for actual ambient temperatures.
  - Several confounding factors can further impair temperature control (Table 44.2).
- Accidental hypothermia is defined as a spontaneous decrease in core temperature, often caused by a cold environment.
  - Mortality rates for accidental hypothermia have been reported to range between 10% and 80%.

Clinical Syndromes

Cardiovascular

- A sympathetic response increases myocardial oxygen consumption and causes tachycardia and peripheral vasoconstriction—that is, diminished pulses, pallor, acro-

cyanosis, and cold extremities—in patients with mild hypothermia (core temperature of 32°C–35°C).
- Blood pressure and heart rate are initially increased and followed by bradycardia, which further deteriorates at 32°C, and consequently, cardiac output, myocardial contractility, and arterial pressure fall.
- Electrocardiographic (ECG) findings include the Osborne J-wave after the QRS complex as hypothermia becomes more severe (Fig. 44.1) The Osborne J-wave is an important diagnostic feature, (also seen in central nervous system lesions and sepsis), but it is frequently absent.
- Atrial and ventricular fibrillation are common, and electrical defibrillation during hypothermia is often ineffective.
- Hypothermic myocardium is irritable, making placement of pulmonary artery or other central catheters dangerous.

Respiratory System

- Respiratory rate falls. The patient becomes apneic or has an agonal respiratory pattern when the body temperature is <28°C.

Central Nervous System

- The electroencephalogram becomes flat at 19°C to 29°C (12). Cerebrovascular autoregulation remains intact until the core temperature falls to below 25°C, but mentation starts to drop at 30°C. Dysarthria and hyperreflexia occur below 35°C, and hyporeflexia occurs below 32°C.

Coagulation

- Hypothermia produces coagulopathy via three major mechanisms: (a) the enzymatic coagulation cascade is impaired, (b) platelet dysfunction occurs, and (c) enhanced plasma fibrinolytic activity is seen.

TABLE 44.1

CLASSIFICATION OF HYPOTHERMIA

Core temperature	Consciousness	Shivering	Heart rate	ECG	Respiration
Mild (35°C–33°C)	Normal	+	Normal	Normal	Normal
Moderate (33°C–30°C)	Depressed (stupor)	–	Slight decrease	Prolongation	Depressed
Severe (30°C–25°C)	Confusion	–	Decreased	Osborne J-wave	Apneic/agonal
25°C–20°C	Coma	Muscle rigidity	Decreased	Atrial fibrillation	Apneic
Below 20°C	Coma	Muscle rigidity	Asystole	Ventricular fibrillation	Apneic

ECG, electrocardiogram.

- Because coagulation tests, such as prothrombin time or partial thrombin time, are performed at 37°C in the laboratory, a major disparity between clinical coagulopathy and the reported values is frequently observed.
- A disseminated intravascular coagulation (DIC) type of syndrome is also reported.

Renal System

- Exposure to cold induces a diuresis irrespective of the state of hydration. Centralization of the blood volume—due to the initial peripheral vasoconstriction—stimulates the diuresis.
- Hypothermia depresses renal blood flow by 50% at 27°C to 30°C, and the renal cellular basal metabolic rate decreases. As a result, renal tubular cell reabsorptive function decreases, and the kidney excretes a large amount of dilute urine. This

is termed *cold diuresis*, resulting in a decreased blood volume and progressive hemoconcentration.

Glucose Metabolism

- Blood glucose concentration commonly increases because pancreatic function, insulin activity, and/or response to insulin decrease, along with activated function of the autonomic nervous system in hypothermia. At the same time, hemoconcentration results in elevated serum glucose concentration.

Therapeutic Approach

Pre-Hospital Treatment

- Even if a patient is found down, cold, stiff, and cyanotic, the patient is not necessarily dead, and rescue efforts should not be given up while the patient is cold.
- As ventricular fibrillation or asystole may be induced by any stimuli, such as tracheal intubation, comatose patients should be treated with extreme care.
- The initial primary focus of prehospital treatment is to avoid further loss of heat. Removal of wet clothing and applying dry insulating covers and an aluminized space blanket may be used.
- The patient should be kept horizontal to minimize the circulatory and sympathetic change. Vigorous rubbing should be avoided because it induces vasodilation, which may be followed by hypotension or "rewarming shock." Hot water bottles or hot packs may be used if available but should be used cautiously to avoid burn injury.
- Resuscitation using the ABCs—airway, breathing, circulation—of basic life support are implemented if needed.
- Warmed (42°C–46°C), humidified oxygen during bag-mask ventilation (20) and warmed intravenous fluids should be given if possible.
- Death should not be declared below 32°C.

In-Hospital Treatment

- Indicated monitoring includes an ECG, Doppler evaluation of pulses, and temperature.
- General laboratory studies include electrolytes, complete blood count, coagulation studies (prothrombin time and partial thromboplastin time), blood urea nitrogen, creatinine, amylase, calcium, magnesium, and glucose concentrations.
- Radiologic examinations are indicated.

TABLE 44.2

CAUSES OF HYPOTHERMIA

Clinical cause	Associated disorders
Central nervous system	Head trauma, tumor, stroke, Wernicke encephalopathy, Shapiro syndrome, Parkinson disease, multiple sclerosis, sarcoidosis, acute spinal cord transection, paraplegia
Metabolic	Hypoglycemia, hypothyroidism, hypoadrenalism, panhypopituitarism, diabetic ketoacidosis, anorexia nervosa
Integument	Burns, erythroderma, ichthyosis, psoriasis, exfoliative dermatitis
Infection	Sepsis
Chronic diseases	Chronic heart failure, chronic renal failure, chronic hepatic insufficiency, advanced age
Environmental exposure	Outdoor activities and physical or metabolic exhaustion, cold water immersion, inadequate indoor heating (particularly in the elderly and infirm), operating room
Pharmaceuticals/drugs	Ethanol, muscle relaxants, phenothiazines, barbiturates, tricyclic antidepressants, lithium (toxic dose), α-adrenergic agonist (clonidine), anticholinergic drugs, β-adrenergic blocker

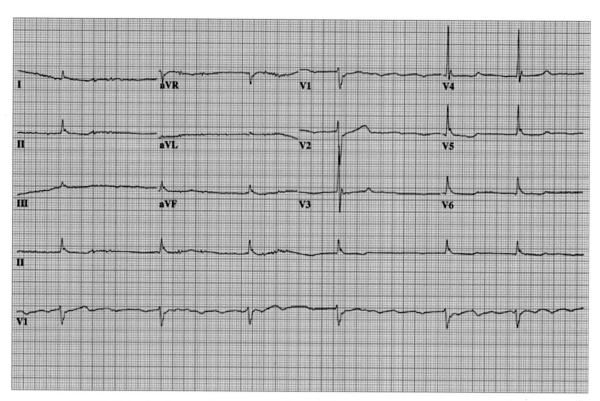

FIGURE 44.1. The electrocardiogram (ECG) shows atrial fibrillation with a very slow ventricular response, prominent (Osborne) J-waves (late, terminal upright deflection of QRS complex; best seen in leads V3–V6), and nonspecific QRS widening. (Adapted from O'Keefe J, Hammill S, Freed M, et al. *The Complete Guide to ECGs.* 2nd ed. Royal Oak, MI: Physicians' Press; 2002.)

- Patients with hypothermia are usually dehydrated, which should be corrected with IV fluids warmed to 43°C.
- The glucose-containing solutions should be used with caution as hypothermic patients are usually hyperglycemic owing to hypoactivity of insulin.
- Techniques of rewarming are presented in Table 44.3.
- Percutaneous or open-chest cardiopulmonary bypass is recommended for pulseless hypothermic patients.
- Bronchopneumonia secondary to aspiration is a common complication. Oral intake of warm or hot drink should be avoided because obtunded, hypothermic patients may have suppressed airway protective mechanisms, including cough or gag reflexes.
- Prophylactic tracheal intubation may be considered if suppression of these reflexes is present. When the trachea is intubated, warmed (42°C–46°C), humidified oxygen should be administered.

HYPERTHERMIA

- Table 44.4 outlines the major causes, which may be classified as hyperthermia or fever.

Environmental Hyperthermia: Heat Stroke

- Heat stroke is a medical emergency, characterized by a high body temperature, altered mental status, and hot dry flushed skin.

- It may lead to multisystem organ dysfunction with hemorrhage and necrosis in the lungs, heart, liver, kidneys, brain, and intestines.
- Mortality in the last 50 years has remained between 10% and 50%.
- There are several heat-related illnesses (see Table 44.5).
  - *Heat syncope* is fainting due to peripheral vasodilation secondary to high ambient temperature.
  - *Heat cramp* refers to muscular cramping occurring during exercise in heat, which is related to electrolyte deficiency; it is usually benign.
  - *Heat exhaustion* or prostration refers to patient's collapsing from dehydration, salt depletion, and hypovolemia. Anorexia, nausea, and vomiting frequently occur. Salt-depletion heat exhaustion usually occurs when an unacclimatized person exercises and replaces only water. Water-depletion heat exhaustion is usually observed in an acclimatized person who has inadequate water intake during exposure to extreme heat. Serum sodium concentration may be normal or mildly elevated. The core temperature may or may not be raised (usually mild to moderate, <38°C) and tissue damage does not occur.
  - *Heat stroke* occurs when the core body temperature rises against a failing thermoregulatory system and rectal temperature exceeds 40.6°C. Exertional heat stroke occurs in previously healthy young people exercising in hot and humid climates without being acclimatized. Nonexertional heat stroke occurs during extreme heat waves, the elderly being particularly vulnerable (Table 44.6).

TABLE 44.3

REWARMING METHODS

Classification		Methods	Effects
Passive	External	Adding an insulating layer (e.g., blanket, sleeping bag)	0.1°C–0.7°C increase/h
		Increasing ambient temperature	Effective when body temperature is above 32°C
Active	External	Hot water bottles	1°C–4°C increase/h
		Heating blanket	Internal rewarming recommended to avoid rewarming shock
		Infrared lamp	
		Submersion in a warm water tank	5°C–7°C increase/h
	Internal (core)	Warmed crystalloid fluids or blood transfusion	1.5°C–2°C increase/h
		Gastric lavage	Warmed fluids administration required due to loss of circulatory blood volume caused by cold diuresis
		Rectal lavage	
		Cystic lavage	
		Airway rewarming	
	(invasive)	Peritoneal dialysis	3°C–15°C increase/h
		Thoracic cavity lavage	
		Hemodialysis	
		Cardiopulmonary bypass	
		Percutaneous cardiopulmonary support	

Temperature Regulation

- Normal heat production is primarily due to metabolic activity in the liver and skeletal muscle, with the liver generating most body heat at rest and muscle being the major source with exercise or shivering.

TABLE 44.4

HYPERTHERMIA AND FEVER

Hyperthermia
Environmental exposure
Malignant hyperthermia
Neuroleptic malignant syndrome
Thyroid storm
Pheochromocytoma
Serotonin syndrome
Iatrogenic hyperthermia
Brainstem/hypothalamic injury
Drugs
Diuretics
Anticholinergics
Phenothiazines
Antidepressants
Lithium
Antihistamines
Ethanol
Salicylates
β-adrenergic blockers

Fever
Inflammatory disorders
Infection
Allergic reactions
Collagen diseases
Neoplasm
Inherited and metabolic diseases
Factitious fever

- Heat elimination occurs by four major mechanisms, as we have discussed in hypothermia.
- Heat stroke is mostly defined as a core temperature above 40.6°C, but neurologic impairment may occur at lower temperatures. Neurologic manifestations include slurred speech, delirium, stupor, lethargy, coma, seizures, ataxia, dysmetria, and dysarthria. Cerebral edema, and localized brain hemorrhages may occur with irreversible brain damage at above 42°C. Cerebellar impairment may persist after recovery.
- Cardiovascular manifestations include tachydysrhythmia and hypotension. Cardiac complications include myocardial pump failure, tachydysrhythmia, high cardiac output, and myocardial infarction. ECG abnormalities are also observed. Sinus tachycardia and QT prolongation are followed by non-specific ST-T wave changes, suggesting cardiac ischemia.
- Lactic acidosis may occur, and restoration of the circulating volume may lead to worsening lactic acidosis as skeletal muscle is reperfused. Patients typically hyperventilate to compensate for the acute acidosis with an acute respiratory alkalosis. This may lead to heat-induced tetany.
- Significant dehydration is noted in most patients with exertional heat stroke with elevated blood urea nitrogen and creatinine levels or hemoconcentration. Sodium, potassium, phosphate, calcium, and magnesium serum concentrations are frequently low in the early period. Sodium, potassium,

TABLE 44.5

HEAT SYNDROMES

Syndrome	Temperature	Manifestation
Heat syncope	Normal	Faintness
Heat cramps	Normal	Muscle cramps
Heat exhaustion	Normal to 39°C	Faintness, weakness
Heat stroke	>40.6°C	Gross neurologic impairment

TABLE 44.6

EXERTIONAL AND NON-EXERTIONAL HEAT STROKE
SYNDROMES

	Exertional	Nonexertional
Age	Young	Elderly
Precipitating event	Heat, strenuous activity	Heat
Underlying process	None	Medical illness, drug therapy
Onset	Rapid	Slow
Sweating	Present	Absent

and magnesium are lost through increased sweating. Hypokalemia may be as a result of catecholamine release or may occur secondary to hyperventilation. Cellular death begins to occur throughout the body at temperatures above 42°C. Hyperkalemia may occur if significant skeletal muscle damage or cellular lysis develops. If significant rhabdomyolysis develops, injured cells release phosphate, which reacts with serum calcium and may lead to hypocalcemia.

- Renal dysfunction is well documented in exertional heat stroke, with the incidence of acute renal failure approximately 25%. Acute renal failure may be caused by direct heat damage, renal hypoperfusion, or rhabdomyolysis. The incidence of renal failure is about 35% with exertional heat stroke and about 5% in classic nonexertional heat stroke, with which rhabdomyolysis is less likely to coexist.
- Liver damage is very frequently seen and is probably related to splanchnic redistribution.
- Hematologic complications include hemolysis, thrombocytopenia, and DIC Hemorrhagic complications may be petechial hemorrhages and ecchymoses, which may represent direct thermal injury or may be related to the development of DIC.
- Pulmonary edema may be caused by a limited cardiac function or may develop secondary to the acute respiratory distress syndrome. Pulmonary aspiration may be observed in obtunded patients.

Therapeutic Approach

- Heat stroke requires prompt oxygen therapy, rapid cooling, and cautious hydration.
- Tracheal intubation should be considered if the patient is obtunded or in respiratory distress.
- Oxygen delivery is often less than normal, and pulmonary shunt fraction is increased.
- Rapid cooling is accomplished by external techniques: immersion in ice water or application of cooling blankets, wetting the skin with water or alcohol, followed by the use of fans to facilitate evaporation and heat dissipation.
- Both techniques usually reduce core temperature below 40°C in 1 hour.
- Significant disadvantages of immersion are impairment of access to the patient and limited monitoring, intense vasoconstriction, and increased cardiac afterload.
- More aggressive cooling techniques include gastric lavage with iced saline, cold hemodialysis, and cardiopulmonary bypass.

- The efficacy of rapid infusion of large-volume ice-cold fluid (LVICF) intravenously with 30 mL/kg of LVICF (lactated Ringer solution at 4°C) over 30 minutes may decrease core temperature by 1.7°C immediately after infusion.
- Core body temperature should be monitored closely at the rectum, bladder, or tympanic membrane.
- Vital signs, neurologic functions, urine output, and laboratory measurements should also be monitored closely. Laboratory measurements include arterial blood gas and serum electrolyte concentrations, especially potassium, which may increase significantly and result in life-threatening hyperkalemia. Glucose–insulin therapy should be instituted emergently in patients with ECG changes.
- Volume deficit is not a prominent feature in classic nonexertional heat stroke. Central venous catheter and pulmonary artery catheter placement may be invaluable to assess volume depletion, peripheral vascular vasodilation, or primary myocardial dysfunction, especially in patients with limited cardiac reserve.
- Hypotension usually responds to intravenous fluids but, if an inotropic drug is needed, dobutamine is the drug of choice for heat stroke.
- Seizures occur commonly in heat stroke patients and should be treated with intravenous diazepam or other benzodiazepines.
- DIC may be treated with continuous infusion heparin therapy although its utility seems uncertain.

Malignant Hyperthermia and the Neuroleptic Malignant Syndrome

- Malignant hyperthermia (MH) and the neuroleptic malignant syndrome (NMS) are disorders of rising body temperature related to an imbalance between heat production and heat dissipation.
- Main features include hyperthermia, muscle rigidity, metabolic acidosis, and autonomic disturbances.
- Both MH and NMS are uniquely characterized by their association with various drugs, although they are distinctive from each other; associated drugs are listed in Table 44.7. An additive in commercial succinylcholine, chlorocresol, has been reported as an additional trigger in MH.
- The in vitro halothane–caffeine contracture test on skeletal muscle helps to identify susceptible individuals.
- For MH, the mortality rate was initially 70%; earlier diagnosis and use of dantrolene have reduced it to <5%.
- A decrease in mortality has been reported; NMS has had a 76% mortality and a 15% mortality since 1980.
- Free inbound ionized calcium can be released from the storage sites, which normally maintain skeletal muscle relaxation by sequestering calcium from the muscle contractile apparatus. The administration of anesthetics may unpredictably trigger rapid calcium release into the myoplasm, followed by the development of muscle contracture, rigidity, and increased muscle metabolic activity. This process can cause core body temperature to rise vigorously at a rate of 1°C every 5 minutes.
- A common pathophysiology of NMS and MH has been suggested based mainly on three points: (a) NMS and MH have clinical features in common, such as hyperthermia, rigidity, an elevated creatine kinase concentration, and a mortality rate

TABLE 44.7

DRUGS ASSOCIATED WITH MALIGNANT
HYPERTHERMIA AND THE NEUROLEPTIC
MALIGNANT SYNDROME

Classification	Associated drugs
MALIGNANT HYPERTHERMIA	
Volatile anesthetics	Halothane, cyclopropane, enflurane, methoxyflurane, isoflurane, sevoflurane, desflurane, diethyl ether
Depolarizing muscle relaxants	Succinylcholine, decamethonium
Antidysrhythmics	Lidocaine
NEUROLEPTIC MALIGNANT SYNDROME	
Phenothiazines	Fluphenazine, chlorpromazine, levomepromazine, thioridazine, trimeprazine, methotrimeprazine, trifluoperazine, prochlorperazine, promethazine, alimemazine
Butyrophenones	Haloperidol, bromperidol, droperidol
Thioxanthenes	Thiothixene, zuclopenthixol
Dibenzazepines	Loxapine
Dopamine-depleting drugs	Alpha-methyltyrosine, tetrabenazine, amoxapine
Dopamine agonist withdrawal	Levodopa, levodopa/carbidopa, amantadine
Serotonin dopamine antagonists	Risperidone
Serotonin-depleting drugs	Paroxetine

of 10% to 30%; (b) sodium dantrolene has been successfully in both syndromes; and (c) abnormal findings have been observed in *in vitro* contractility tests in patients with either of the syndromes.

- MH may occur shortly after induction of anesthesia, at any time during the administration of anesthetics, or postoperatively.
- Trismus is the initial event in 50% of patients, and other early signs are tachycardia and hypercapnia due to increased metabolism. These are followed by whole-body rigidity and a marked increase in core body temperature.
- Sympathetic system overactivity produces tachycardia, hypertension, and mottled cyanosis. These symptoms precede hyperthermia, hyperkalemia, hypercalcemia, and lactic acidosis.
- Capnography may provide an early warning, as carbon dioxide production is remarkably increased while MH is in progress.
- Core body temperature can rise at a rate of 1°C every 5 minutes.
- Anesthesia should be aborted if these signs appear or if MH is suspected.
- Laboratory evaluation reveals increased serum myoglobin, creatine kinase (>20,000 U/L), lactate dehydrogenase, and aldolase levels. Dark urine reflects myoglobinemia and myoglobinuria.
- A clinical grading scale for the prediction of MH is summarized in Tables 44.8A and 44.8B.
- NMS should be suspected in patients given any neuroleptic drugs who subsequently develop signs of muscular rigidity, dystonia, or unexplained catatonic behavior, followed by

TABLE 44.8A

SCORING RULES FOR THE MALIGNANT HYPERTHERMIA (MH) CLINICAL GRADING SCALE

MH INDICATORS
Review the list of clinical indicators. If any indicator is present, add the points applicable for each indicator while observing the double-counting rule below, which applies to multiple indicators representing a single process.
If no indicator is present, the patient's MH score is zero.

DOUBLE-COUNTING
If more than one indicator represents a single process, *count only the indicator with the highest score.* Application of this rule prevents double-counting when one clinical process has more than one clinical manifestation.
Exception: The score for any relevant indicators in the final category of Table 44.8B ("other indicators")*should* be added to the total score without regard to double-counting.

MH SUSCEPTIBILITY INDICATORS
The italicized indicators listed below apply only to MH susceptibility. Do not use these indicators to score an MH event. To calculate the score for MH susceptibility, add the score of the italicized indicators below to the score for the highest-ranking MH event.
Positive family history of MH in relative of first degree
Positive family history of MH in relative not of first degree
Resting elevated serum creatinine kinase
Positive family history of MH together with another indicator from the patient's own anesthetic experience other than elevated serum creatine kinase

INTERPRETING THE RAW SCORE: MH RANK AND QUALITATIVE LIKELIHOOD

Raw score range	MH rank	Description of likelihood
0	1	Almost never
3—9	2	Unlikely
10—19	3	Somewhat less than likely
20—34	4	Somewhat greater than likely
35—49	5	Very likely
50+	6	Almost certain

TABLE 44.8B

CLINICAL INDICATORS FOR USE IN DETERMINING THE MALIGNANT HYPERTHERMIA (MH) RAW SCORE

Process	Indicator	Points
Process I: Rigidity	Generalized muscular rigidity (in absence of shivering due to hypothermia, or during or immediately following emergence from inhalational general anesthesia)	15
	Masseter spasm shortly following succinylcholine administration	15
Process II: Muscle breakdown	Elevated creatine kinase >20,000 IU after anesthetic that included succinylcholine	15
	Elevated creatine kinase >10,000 IU after anesthetic without succinylcholine	15
	Cola-colored urine in perioperative period	10
	Myoglobin in urine >60 μg/L	5
	Myoglobin in serum >170 μg/L	5
	Blood/plasma/serum K >6 mEq/L (in absence of renal failure)	3
Process III: Respiratory acidosis	PETCO$_2$ >55 mm Hg with appropriately controlled ventilation	15
	Arterial PaCO$_2$ >60 mm Hg with appropriately controlled ventilation	15
	PETCO$_2$ >60 mm Hg 15 with spontaneous ventilation	
	Arterial PaCO$_2$ >65 mm Hg with spontaneous ventilation	15
	Inappropriate hypercarbia (in anesthesiologist's judgment)	15
	Inappropriate tachypnea	10
Process IV: Temperature increase	Inappropriately rapid increase in temperature (in anesthesiologist's judgment)	15
	Inappropriately increased temperature >38.8°C (101.8°F) in the preoperative period (in anesthesiologist's judgment)	10
Process V: Cardiac involvement	Inappropriate sinus tachycardia	3
	Ventricular tachycardia or ventricular fibrillation	3
Process VI: Family history (used to determine MH susceptibility only)	*Positive MH family history in relative of first degree[a]*	15
	Positive MH family history in relative not of first degree[a]	5
Other indicators that are not part of a single process[b]	Arterial base excess more negative than −8 mEq/L	10
	Arterial pH <7.25	10
	Rapid reversal of MH signs of metabolic and/or respiratory acidosis with IV dantrolene	5
	Positive MH family history together with another indicator from the patient's own anesthetic experience other than elevated resting serum creatine kinase[a]	10
	Resting elevated serum creatine kinase[a] (in patient with a family history of MH)	10

[a]These indicators should be used only for determining MH susceptibilty.
[b]These should be added without regard to double-counting.

hyperpyrexia. Other symptoms include unstable blood pressure, confusion, coma, and delirium (Table 44.9).

Complications

- Complications arising from MH and NMS are rhabdomyolysis (with renal failure), hepatic necrosis, and ventricular fibrillation. Cerebral edema with seizures is uncommon but may be seen. Patients with NMS are at risk for aspiration

pneumonia because of dystonia and the inability to handle secretions.

Therapeutic Approach

- Successful treatment of MH and NMS depend on prompt withdrawal of the suspected drugs. It may take 5 to 7 days to return to the patient's baseline because neuroleptics cannot be removed by dialysis, and blood concentrations decline slowly.
- General symptomatic treatment, such as hydration, nutrition, and reduction of fever, is essential.
- Dantrolene should be administered emergently to prevent further release of calcium from the sarcoplasmic reticulum. The dose is 2 mg/kg intravenously every 5 minutes to a total dose of 10 mg/kg until the episode terminates. Dantrolene also decreases temperature in NMS and thyroid storm.
- Acidosis should be treated aggressively with intravenous administration of bicarbonate, 2 to 4 mEq/kg.
- Hyperkalemia should be treated with insulin and glucose infusion and with diuresis.

TABLE 44.9

CRITERIA FOR GUIDANCE IN THE DIAGNOSIS OF NEUROLEPTIC MALIGNANT SYNDROME

Category	Manifestations
Major	Fever, rigidity, elevated creatine kinase concentration
Minor	Tachycardia, abnormal arterial pressure, tachypnea, altered consciousness, diaphoresis, leukocytosis

- Fever should be controlled by iced fluids, surface cooling, and cooling of body cavities with sterile iced fluids. Cold dialysis and cardiopulmonary bypass may also be applicable if other measures fail.
- Mannitol infusion—0.5 g/kg—with or without furosemide should be used to establish a diuresis and prevent the onset of acute renal failure from myoglobinuria.

- Further therapy is guided by blood gases, electrolytes, temperature, arrhythmia, muscle tone, and urinary output.
- Lab analyses include electrolytes, creatine kinase concentrations, liver enzymes, blood urea nitrogen, lactate, glucose, serum hemoglobin and myoglobin, coagulation profile, and urine hemoglobin and myoglobin.

CHAPTER 45 ■ EVALUATING THE ACUTE ABDOMEN

An acute abdomen is any problem in which the patient's pain or other physical findings originate from an abdominal lesion resulting in serious morbidity or mortality without appropriate therapy. Early recognition of the acute abdomen and initiation of definitive surgical or medical therapy often determine the outcome. A high index of suspicion is required in the critically ill patient who may not be able to give a lucid history, and physical findings may be masked by narcotics, steroids, and other therapy administered.

ANATOMY

Knowledge of the sensory nerve supply of the abdomen is particularly important in evaluating the abdomen in critically ill patients.

Visceral Pain

- Visceral pain is transmitted via both sympathetic and parasympathetic nerves.
- The pain is poorly localized, typically unpleasant, and associated with autonomic symptoms such as tachycardia, bradycardia, and diaphoresis.
- The primary stimulus is stretching of hollow viscera or solid organ capsules.
- Visceral pain shares common pathways and areas of the sensory cortex with somatic pain, which explains referred pain to remote dermatomes (e.g., shoulder pain caused by diaphragmatic irritation).
- Abdominal pain becomes more localized when the parietal peritoneum, with its rich somatic sensory supply, is affected by the underlying inflammatory process.
- Knowledge of the **blood supply** of the abdomen is also important given the extensive diagnostic and therapeutic applications of angiography in acute abdominal pathology.
- The foregut (esophagus to duodenum) is supplied by branches of the celiac trunk.
- The midgut (jejunum to distal transverse colon) is supplied by branches of the superior mesenteric artery (SMA).

- The hindgut (descending colon and rectum) is supplied by branches of the inferior mesenteric artery.
- **Collateral circulation** exists between branches of the mesenteric vessels.
- The **marginal artery of Drummond** connects the SMA and inferior mesenteric artery along the mesenteric border of the colon.
- The **arc of Riolan** connects the middle colic artery with the ascending branch of the left colic artery.
- The internal iliac artery contributes to colonic circulation through a connection between the middle and superior rectal arteries.
- An embolus tends to lodge distal to the origins of the most proximal branches of the SMA, namely the inferior pancreaticoduodenal, the middle colic, and the proximal jejunal branches. The proximal jejunum and the transverse colon are typically spared in acute ischemia due to SMA embolism compared to thrombosis.

HISTORY

- **A careful evaluation of the characteristics of abdominal pain is essential.** Its nature, onset, associated symptoms, radiation, and other characteristics are useful in localizing and delineating the cause. The history should include a complete surgical history, family history, and a list of medications. It should also include allergies, ethanol use, immunosuppressive drugs, and a history of human immunodeficiency virus (HIV), hepatitis, or chemotherapy.
- Diabetic and immune-suppressed patients, particularly those on steroids, can present with advanced intra-abdominal sepsis before peritoneal signs become obvious.
- Gastrointestinal bleeding or perforation may occur as a consequence of taking steroids or nonsteroidal anti-inflammatory agents.
- As we become more globalized, awareness of infectious disease from emerging countries is necessary for evaluation of disparate symptoms. The presence of a percutaneous endoscopic gastrostomy or other tubes should alert the physician

to the possibility of a problem related to tube misplacement or obstruction.
- **Abdominal symptoms can be masked by other disease processes.**
  - Diabetic ketoacidosis or syncope may have an underlying abdominal catastrophe as a precipitating factor.
  - Inferior myocardial infarction, pericarditis, and lower lobe pneumonia may present with upper abdominal pain.
  - Porphyria and sickle cell crises can mimic abdominal catastrophes, although they rarely cause admission to the intensive care unit.

PHYSICAL EXAMINATION

- Abdominal examination in the critically ill patient can be challenging, as many patients will be unconscious, intubated, combative, comatose, narcotized, or paralyzed. The standard routine of inspection—palpation, percussion, and auscultation—should be followed. Vital signs, including blood pressure (with the patient sitting if possible), pulse, respiratory rate, and rectal or core temperature, should be taken.
- Inspection of the abdomen can give many clues:
  - The Gray–Turner sign, flank ecchymosis, was initially described with hemorrhagic pancreatitis but can occur with other causes of retroperitoneal bleeding.
  - The Sister Mary Joseph nodule indicates abdominal or breast malignancy that spread along the round ligament to the umbilicus.
  - Dilated abdominal wall veins indicate advanced portal hypertension.
  - A large abdominal aortic aneurysm may be discerned as a pulsating upper abdominal mass in a thin patient.
  - Absent or hypoactive bowel sounds is a nonspecific sign as many patients will have ileus associated with their critical illness. Bowel sounds are frequently absent in paralyzed patients, despite the fact that muscular paralysis should not eliminate autonomic bowel function. Hyperactive sounds or "rushes" are most common with small-bowel obstruction. The presence of bowel sounds, however, does not always correlate with normal bowel function.
- The presence of guarding or rigidity indicates peritoneal irritation.
  - Rebound may not be present in a postoperative patient with significant abdominal pathology.
  - Patients' response to the presence of blood in the peritoneal cavity can vary from guarding and rigidity to a soft abdomen.
  - In obese patients, assessment for abdominal wall rigidity is unreliable, and they may have groin or incisional hernias that are not easily discerned.
  - Patients with mesenteric ischemia have pain that is out of proportion to the findings of the physical exam.
  - Rectal and pelvic examinations are frequently avoided in the ICU; however, they are mandatory to discover low pelvic abscesses and masses, prostatic infection, and bloody stools.
- The physical examination of the acute abdomen should be performed by an experienced physician on a regular basis.
  - An isolated examination is not nearly as useful as **sequential examinations by the same observer** to carefully document

any progression of tenderness, muscular rigidity, and the overall trend toward improvement or deterioration.
- The physician who will ultimately make the decision whether surgical intervention is required should be involved as early as possible.
- The presence of abdominal distention in the setting of decreased urine output and increased ventilator pressures should lead to a possible diagnosis of **abdominal compartment syndrome** and immediately to a measurement of intra-abdominal pressures using bladder pressure manometry.

LABORATORY EVALUATION

- **Laboratory tests should be viewed as adjuncts in the evaluation of patients,** often providing useful information but rarely being diagnostic.
  - A hemogram, including hematocrit, hemoglobin, and white blood cell (WBC) count with differential
  - Urinalysis, including specific gravity and analysis for bacteria, bile, and reducing substances
  - Serum amylase, especially fractionated into isoenzymes, is helpful in diagnosing intra-abdominal catastrophe when it is elevated but is not specific.
  - Serum lipase is a more specific marker of acute pancreatitis than amylase and is less influenced by other intra-abdominal problems; calcium and phosphorus values are also helpful in determining the severity of pancreatitis.
  - Serum bilirubin elevation is associated with sepsis, resolving hematoma, hemolysis, and hepatobiliary disease.
  - Liver enzymes, such as serum glutamate oxaloacetic transaminase, serum glutamic pyruvic transaminase, and alkaline phosphatase, may be helpful but are rarely diagnostic by themselves.
- **Depending excessively on laboratory findings is costly and occasionally misleading.**
  - Severe sepsis can cause a leukopenia with a shift to the left that will be missed without a differential count.
  - Patients with indwelling Foley catheters often have asymptomatic bacteriuria and mild hematuria; a full workup of "benign bacteriuria" may delay the diagnosis of the true cause of sepsis.
- **Laboratory data are most useful in the management and correction of fluids, electrolytes, and acid-base derangements.** Persistent acidosis and arterial hypoxemia suggest severe metabolic problems that may be a reflection of unresolved third-space losses from untreated abdominal sepsis or ischemia. These causes are frequently overlooked in the early workup of these problems.

RADIOGRAPHIC STUDIES

- Although **plain portable radiographs** of the abdomen are obtained on most patients with suspicious abdominal findings, their yield is relatively low and their quality is frequently suboptimal.
  - Most useful is determining the position of intra-abdominal tubes such as nasogastric tubes and drains.
  - Examine abnormal intraluminal and extraluminal gas patterns.

- The absence of gas may be found with ischemic bowel.
- Small-bowel obstruction and colonic volvulus present with massive gaseous distention.
  - An upright or left lateral decubitus film to discover air-fluid levels and free air above the liver should be obtained.
- A retrospective study of 1,000 patients presenting to the emergency room with acute abdominal pain compared the use of plain films to computed tomography (CT) scans.
  - 588 of 871 (68%) of abdominal radiographs were interpreted as nonspecific, no free air was found, and films were most sensitive for foreign bodies (90%) and bowel obstruction (49%).
  - CT was predictive of bowel obstruction in 75% and pancreatitis in 60%.
  - 120 patients had both exams: Abdominal films were negative in 20%, nonspecific in 76%, and abnormal in 4%.
- **Ultrasonography** has emerged as a dependable adjunctive diagnostic tool.
  - Can be brought to the bedside
  - Useful in demonstrating intra-abdominal blood or fluid and performing percutaneous drainage, such as percutaneous cholecystostomy
  - Less invasive and less expensive than CT scan
  - Limitations are as follows:
    - Acalculous cholecystitis
      ○ The gallbladder can be distended with poor contractility in patients in admitted to an ICU for extended periods.
      ○ Ultrasound is not specific unless a radionuclide study using a hepatobiliary iminodiacetic acid (HIDA) scan confirms abnormal gallbladder filling.
  - Ultrasound can be difficult to interpret in patients with distended bowel gas
- **CT scan** has become the most widely used tool to examine the abdomen for abnormalities.
  - CT scanning is more accurate than any other modality for diagnosing intra-abdominal fluid collections.
  - It is especially useful in liver, splenic, renal, and retroperitoneal abscesses but may not be as useful as ultrasound in the diagnosis of right upper quadrant and pelvic masses.
  - Plain films have a low yield as compared to CT scan in the diagnoses of processes such as pneumatosis intestinalis, a finding very suggestive of bowel necrosis.
  - Increasingly useful as a therapeutic modality
    - CT drainage of abscesses, ascites, and pancreatic collections
    - CT-guided nephrostomy tube insertions
  - Optimal use of CT scan requires oral contrast, which may be difficult for the critically ill patient to ingest and retain and may be an aspiration risk.
  - CT scanning requires transporting the patient to the scanner accompanied by the nurse, therapist, and sometimes physician; the possibility exists of an untoward event during transport.
- A **Gastrografin swallow** is still an excellent tool to differentiate a gastric leak after gastric bypass surgery or persistent leak from a perforated ulcer.
- **Diagnostic peritoneal lavage** is still useful to drain tense ascites and determine the source and infectious nature of abdominal fluid. The presence of bacteria, bile, and >500 WBCs/mm^3 can be inferred to indicate an acute abdominal process requiring immediate laparotomy.

THERAPY

- **Surgical consultation** should be obtained early in the evaluation of intra-abdominal problems as treatment in the acutely ill frequently requires surgical intervention. Acute abdominal catastrophe may be the first event in the precipitous cascade of multiple organ system failure. Unrecognized abdominal sepsis is associated with multiple organ system failure in 44% of cases. Early aggressive surgical therapy, vigorous fluid replacement, and appropriate antibiotic regimens are necessary.
  - Adequate volume resuscitation and electrolyte correction are vital to prepare the patient.
  - Patients who are volume-contracted may be hyponatremic, hypochloremic, hypokalemic, and alkalotic because of vomiting, nasogastric suctioning, and third-space losses.
  - Resuscitation with isotonic fluid, such as normal saline, is required to prevent anesthetic disaster.
  - Only after volume and salt repletion will their chloride-dependent alkalosis resolve.
  - Hypokalemia should be corrected cautiously until oliguria is resolved.
- **The specific management of disease entities should be based on well-established surgical principles.** However, the explosion of minimally invasive surgery has led to a new era in surgical intervention.
  - Acute cholecystitis
    - Can be treated conservatively for 24 to 48 hours
    - If the signs and symptoms do not improve within 48 hours or if cholangitis appears, an endoscopic retrograde cholangiopancreatography can be performed to drain the common duct.
      - A percutaneous cholecystostomy or a laparoscopic cholecystectomy can be performed in most cases.
  - Perforated ulcers can now be treated laparoscopically in some surgeons' hands.
  - Ruptured abdominal aneurysm can be addressed with endovascular aortic repair.
    - This repair can be performed under local anesthesia with bilateral groin cutdown, avoiding the significant morbidity of open procedures.
    - Initial studies imply that the overall morbidity, mortality, and ICU stay may be lower than that of open procedures.
- The use of **CT scan and ultrasonic-guided drainage** and catheter decompression of intra-abdominal abscesses had revolutionized care in some postoperative patients.
  - Results in excellent control of the septic source with a low morbidity
  - Often preferable to secondary exploratory laparotomy
  - If a patient persists in a downward clinical course, exploration with wide drainage of abscesses may be necessary.
- **Stress ulceration without perforation** may be prophylactically treated with antacids, H2 blockers, and sucralfate, although aggressive pH control may lead to an increase in nosocomial pneumonia. Bleeding, though rare, requires operative intervention if it cannot be contained with conservative measures. This carries a high mortality rate of 50% but approaches 100% if multiple transfusions have created dilutional or hypothermic coagulopathies; the best treatment is prevention.
- **Antibiotics** are not a panacea for intra-abdominal sepsis, and abscesses will form despite adequate coverage. Usually

adjunctive to prevent systemic sepsis, the prolonged use of antibiotics for localized abscesses instead of surgical or radiologic drainage can lead to morbidity and increased mortality. Guidelines for the use of antimicrobial agents are published by several medical societies.

SPECIFIC DISEASE STATES

Any stable patient in an ICU developing sudden shock or sepsis must be examined closely for an intra-abdominal cause.

- **Appendicitis,** the most common abdominal condition in surgery, is rarely seen in the ICU.
- **Pancreatitis** and **acalculous cholecystitis** are seen, especially after open-heart surgery.
- **Ileus** and **colonic pseudo-obstruction** are frequent in elderly patients after orthopedic procedures.
- **Mechanical ventilation** carries a high risk for **gastrointestinal bleeding,** ileus, and unrecognized **perforation.**
- **Stress ulcer perforation** and ileus are insidious causes of respiratory failure and sepsis in any patient with a **spinal injury.**

Acquired Immunodeficiency Syndrome

Immunocompromised hosts require special attention when presenting either with abdominal pain or sepsis of unknown origin. Fever and nonspecific abdominal pain are frequently noted, although peritoneal signs may be lacking in severely immunocompromised patients.

- Acute abdominal pain is a complaint in 12% to 45% of patients with HIV infection presenting to the emergency room.
- Cytomegalovirus (CMV), gastroenteritis, lymphoma, Kaposi sarcoma, and mycobacterial disease were frequent causes of abdominal pain in HIV patients in early studies.
- There has been a significant reduction in these opportunistic infections, especially peritonitis secondary to atypical mycobacterium and fungi.
- The frequency of pulmonary, cardiac, gastrointestinal, and renal disease that is not directly related to the underlying HIV has increased.
- The HIV patient continues to present with non–HIV-related problems, such as appendicitis, diverticulitis, and pancreatitis.

  Patients presenting with overt AIDS have a constellation of problems that are unique to this population. **Prognosis is somewhat dependent on the CD4 count and viral loads.** CD4 counts <200 cells/mm^3, total lymphocyte count <1,000 cells/mm^3, and viral loads >75,000 RNA copies/mL are associated with higher morbidity and mortality.

- Earlier studies reported increased morbidity and mortality in patients with AIDS, whereas recent data yield 10% to 19% operative mortality for emergency surgery.
- Acute appendicitis in AIDS patients may be routine or secondary to opportunistic organisms.
- WBC count may be low or normal.

Perforation

- Bowel perforation secondary to CMV or Kaposi sarcoma has decreased since the advent of retroviral therapy.

- Diligence is required to ensure perforation has not occurred.
- CMV perforations are more common in the ileum and colon secondary to ischemic lesion.
- Acute bowel obstruction suggests disseminated disease and has a poor prognosis if the cause is age–related.
- Recent data point to lymphoma and disseminated mycobacterial disease as causes.
- Colonic disease, especially **toxic megacolon,** has been seen with *Clostridium difficile* colitis, especially in patients with CMV infection. Megacolon can be a significant prognostic indicator in advanced age and may best be treated with colonoscopy for short-term management of the severely ill.
- **Acute hepatobiliary disease** secondary to opportunistic disease can present difficult diagnostic problems in patients with CD4 counts <100 cells/mm^3. Acalculous cholecystitis is more common in HIV/AIDS patients than in the normal population.
- **Neutropenic patients with cancer** also present a diagnosis and therapeutic challenge. In patients who underwent emergency celiotomy for suspected intra-abdominal disease, the most common disease reported was neutropenic enteropathy (61%), with postoperative mortality up to 32%.

Biliary Disease

- Primary biliary tract disease in critically ill patients appears as calculous or acalculous cholecystitis. Calculous disease may present as acute cholecystitis, cholangitis, or pancreatitis. The typical presentation of right upper quadrant pain, a positive Murphy sign, and fever may be absent in critically ill patients. Leukocytosis is common, although nonspecific. The presence of stones in the gallbladder in patients with nonspecific symptoms is not pathognomonic of acute biliary disease.

Acute Acalculous Biliary Disease

- A concomitant of critical illness, it has been reported in 1% of surgical patients and 0.2% of postoperative cardiac patients.
- Risk factors include use of narcotics for more than 6 days, gastric suction, prolonged ileus with nothing by mouth, ventilatory support longer than 24 hours, multiple recent operations, more than 10 blood transfusions, open wound or abscesses, and intravenous hyperalimentation for more than 3 days.
- Presence of five of these risk factors in a patient with acute abdominal findings should lead to a search for acalculous biliary disease.
- Right upper quadrant pain may be present in 30%, peritonitis in only 24%; persistent fever is the most consistent finding.
- Up to 65% of patients with acalculous cholecystitis have elevated bilirubin; however, a control group of patients receiving multiple transfusions had similar hyperbilirubinemia.
- Liver enzymes are elevated in fewer than 50%.
- The presence of fever, mild elevation of bilirubin, sludge on ultrasound, and nonvisualization on HIDA are accurate indications of acute acalculous cholecystitis in critically ill patients.
- Treatment of choice is cholecystectomy if the patient is able to tolerate a major procedure.
- Use of percutaneous cholecystostomy has been reported in severely ill patients.
- The mortality rate is as high as 40% secondary to the multiplicity of the patient's problems.

Hepatobiliary Iminodiacetic Acid Scan

- 95% accurate in the diagnosis of acute cholecystitis
- Derivatives of iminodiacetic acid rapidly taken up by the hepatocytes and excreted into the bile even with elevations of bilirubin up to 6 g/dL
- Requires moving the critically ill patient to the radiology suite for up to 4 hours
- Caution urged in patients receiving hyperalimentation, which severely limits usefulness of the test.

Abscess

Intra-abdominal abscesses develop as a complication of secondary peritonitis that is the result of a perforation of a hollow viscus. Examples include colonic resection complicated by anastomotic leak, diverticular disease, appendicitis, inflammatory bowel disease, and malignancy.

- Abscess should be suspected in any patient deteriorating after abdominal surgery.
- The clinical picture can be vague, peritonitis is rare, and bowel function may be normal.
- Nonspecific manifestations such as fever, chills, malaise, and leukocytosis should raise the suspicion.
- Abscesses that incorporate the anterior abdominal wall are associated with a palpable tender mass.
- Retroperitoneal abscesses can develop from cecal perforation, lymphatic and hematogenous spread of bacteria, or infected pancreatic necrosis.
- Hiccup, unexplained pleural effusion, and a raised hemidiaphragm on chest radiograph may indicate subphrenic abscess.
- Diarrhea and urinary retention may indicate a pelvic abscess.
- CT scan, preferably with oral and intravenous contrast, is the standard diagnostic modality.
- Bedside ultrasonography may be useful in unstable patients.

The **bacterial flora** are related to the organ involved, the host defenses, and the duration of the critical illness. The flora of the normal stomach and duodenum are very sparse.

- Mainly swallowed oral organisms such as microaerophilic streptococci and *Streptococcus viridans,* lactobacillus, fusiform bacteria, and *Candida* species.
- Flora grow and change remarkably if there is gastric outlet obstruction, achlorhydria, or acid-suppressive therapy.
- Small-bowel flora consist mainly of Enterobacteriaceae, *Enterococcus* species, and anaerobic species.
- Colonic flora are extremely dense.
  - Account for one-sixth of the dry weight of stools
  - Contains both aerobic and anaerobic bacteria
    - Aerobic bacteria are much more abundant; primarily gram-negative (e.g., *Escherichia coli, Klebsiella* species, *Enterococcus* species, and *Proteus* species)
    - Anaerobic bacteria include *Bacteroides fragilis, Eubacterium* species, and *Bifidobacterium* species.
- Intra-abdominal abscesses are typically polymicrobial, but anaerobes are difficult to grow on cultures.
- Surgical consultation should be obtained, and **the decision to operate is based on individual patient conditions.** The efficacy of CT-guided percutaneous drainage of intra-abdominal abscesses has long been established. Antibiotic therapy is based on empiric coverage of gram-positive, gram-negative,

and anaerobic bacteria normally present within the gut rather than culture results. Antifungal agents are not given even if fungi are seen on cultures unless the patient is immunosuppressed or has recurrent intra-abdominal infection.

- **Mortality** from intra-abdominal sepsis is 24%, ranging from 7.5% for single abscess to 43% for patients with multiple abscesses and peritonitis. Mortality correlates directly with acute physiology score, malnutrition, age, and shock. Only early recognition, appropriate use of antibiotics, and prompt drainage can improve on these data.

Pneumoperitoneum

The most common cause of pneumoperitoneum is abdominal surgery. Free air may persist for weeks after laparotomy, although air from laparoscopy is frequently absent at 48 hours. Pneumoperitoneum in a patient who does not have a recent history of laparotomy or laparoscopy should be presumed to be due to a perforated viscus until proven otherwise.

- Perforation of the stomach or duodenum due to peptic ulcer disease is more likely to cause an obvious pneumoperitoneum than perforation of the colon due to diverticular disease.
- Other conditions that may cause pneumoperitoneum are a recent percutaneous endoscopic gastrostomy and barotrauma to the lung.
- Pneumoperitoneum has been observed in up to 10% of patients who suffer severe chest trauma with extra-alveolar air, such as pneumothorax and pneumomediastinum.

Pneumoperitoneum should be evaluated in the context of the patient's overall condition. In unconscious or paralyzed septic patients with no obvious source of sepsis, pneumoperitoneum should prompt an exploratory laparotomy. Diagnostic peritoneal lavage may be considered if the risk of operative exploration is too high or the index of suspicion is low.

Pseudo-Obstruction of the Colon

Isolated colonic ileus without mechanical obstruction was first described by **Ogilvie.**

- The abdomen is distended and tympanitic without signs of peritonitis, fever, or leukocytosis.
- Most common risk factors are old age, bed rest, prolonged narcotic use, mechanical ventilation, multiple trauma, abdominal and pelvic operations, orthopedic operations, and spinal cord injuries.
- The cause is unknown, but hyponatremia and hypokalemia may play a role in the development of this condition.
- On radiograph, the colon appears diffusely distended, including the rectum, and the small bowel is usually not seen.
- The cecum, being the widest segment of the colon, is at risk for necrosis and perforation if the diameter reaches 12 cm.
- **Mechanical obstruction should be ruled out** with a Hypaque enema; this hyperosmolar water-soluble enema helps to cleanse the colon and, unlike barium, does not interfere with a subsequent colonoscopy.

Initial management consists of decompressing the stomach and colon with nasogastric and rectal tubes. Electrolyte abnormalities, especially hypokalemia, should be promptly corrected. If there is no response to these measures, neostigmine, a parasympathomimetic, may be given to stimulate colonic motility.

- 1 to 2 mg intravenously and can be repeated in 3 hours
- Should be done under cardiac monitoring as it may result in severe bradycardia
- Should not be given if the patient's baseline heart rate is <60 beats/minute, the systolic blood pressure is <90 mm Hg, or if there is a significant heart block or bronchospasm

The next step in management, if the previous measures fail, is colonoscopic decompression. This is **associated with a higher-than-normal risk of perforation.**

- Should be used gently and with the goal of decompression only
- Not necessary to advance the colonoscope all the way to the cecum
- Recurrence is seen in up to 40% of patients, and colonoscopy can be repeated.
- **Surgery is reserved for patients who fail all other measures and those with complications or impending cecal rupture** (i.e., diameter >**12 cm**). The operation of choice is right hemicolectomy with primary ileocolic anastomosis if there is no evidence of necrosis or perforation, in which case an ileostomy with mucus fistula should be performed.

Abdominal Compartment Syndrome

The abdominal compartment syndrome (ACS) is a condition in which the **intra-abdominal pressure rises to a point that impairs respiratory, renal, and cardiovascular function.** The diagnosis of ACS is made when there is abdominal distention associated with high ventilator pressures, oliguria, and elevated urinary bladder pressures (>25–30 cm H_2O). It is believed that severe edema of the abdominal wall, bowel wall, and the retroperitoneum occurs as a result of massive fluid shifts associated with the severe systemic inflammation that accompanies reperfusion of tissues after shock states.

- Described mainly in the trauma population but can occur in any patient who receives a massive resuscitation for a profound shock state
- The abdomen not necessarily the site where the original pathology occurs (e.g., severe burns, sometimes described as secondary ACS).

Treatment

Treatment consists of abdominal decompression using a midline celiotomy and keeping the abdomen open using various dressing mechanisms over the bowel. For a detailed discussion of the ACS, see Chapter 39. More abdomens are now kept open if fascial closure is expected to increase abdominal pressure.

- Renal and pulmonary functions are not compromised, and the integrity of fascial edges is preserved.
- Gives the opportunity for frequent bedside washouts and debridements such as with infected pancreatic necrosis.

Once the swelling has resolved, the abdomen should be closed as soon as possible either by primary fascial closure or using one of the commercially available biologic or synthetic grafts. Prolongation of the open abdomen management is associated with increased risk of fistula formation.

Bariatric Surgery

- It is estimated that more than 130,000 bariatric procedures will be performed in the United States each year. Many of these patients have sleep apnea, hypoventilation, or other physiologic abnormalities that require ICU care in the immediate postoperative period. Anastomotic leak after gastric bypass and duodenal switch are potentially fatal, rapid recognition, diagnosis, and treatment are necessary to minimize patient risk.
- Abdominal pain is frequently not a major symptom, although shoulder (referred) pain may be present.
- The **hallmarks of dilatation and leak** are persistent tachycardia, tachypnea, fever, anxiety, and hiccups, usually accompanied by a mild leukocytosis with or without fever.
- Because this is also found in patients with **pulmonary emboli,** it is vital that the diagnosis of leak be made early.
- Immediate **Gastrografin swallow** with adequate volume of contrast should be performed
- The presence of a large gastric bubble without leak requires immediate decompression to prevent gastric perforation or an anastomotic disruption.
- A leak must be addressed immediately with drainage either percutaneously for small and contained leaks or operative intervention to attempt to repair and drain the area of concern.

Acute Mesenteric Ischemia

- The presence of physical signs indicating peritoneal irritation is extremely important because they portend impending or progressive gangrene and are associated with significant mortality. Leukocytosis out of proportion to the physical findings, elevated hematocrit, unexplained acidosis, and blood-tinged fluid on peritoneal lavage are all signs of advancing intestinal necrosis. **Numerous causes** exist for acute intestinal ischemia:
- Embolus (50%–60%) or thrombus (25%–35%) of the SMA must be differentiated from nonmesenteric thrombosis (10%–20%) and acute mesenteric venous occlusions (5%).
- Colonic and rectal ischemias have been reported after abdominal aortic aneurysmectomy in which the inferior mesenteric artery was ligated.
- **A characteristic of gut ischemia is the disparity between the patient's pain and abdominal findings.**
- Common signs and symptoms include pain (75%–90%), nausea and vomiting (50%–60%), abdominal distention (56%–80%), peritoneal signs (60%), ileus (50%), and shock and fever (30%).
- Upper gastrointestinal bleeding is less common.
- Leukocytosis (WBC count of 20,000/mm^3) is seen in fewer than 50% of patients.
- A mild elevation in amylase is common.
- Plain radiographs are useful to exclude the other processes; signs of intestinal ischemia on plain radiograph are a grave prognosticator with 90% mortality.
- **Patients at highest risk** are those older than 50 years with either valvular or atherosclerotic heart disease, congestive heart failure (especially if there is poor control with digitalis and diuretics), hypovolemia, hypotension of any cause,

recent myocardial infarction or cardiogenic shock, or cardiac arrhythmias. Dialysis patients seem to be at added risk for right colon ischemia.

- Once the diagnosis is suspected, **vigorous fluid resuscitation is necessary** to maintain adequate blood flow and pressure head in the mesenteric vessels. Occasionally, dextran has been used to expand plasma and to decrease sludging. Digitalis should be used cautiously. Gastrointestinal decompression with a nasogastric tube and proper hemodynamic monitoring are necessary to adequately resuscitate these precarious patients. Early heparinization should be used if immediate surgery is not undertaken.

- **CT scans** have improved in both availability and reliability and may demonstrate clot or ischemia. **Emergency selective arteriography** is still the keystone of the diagnostic and therapeutic approach to acute mesenteric ischemia.

  - Arteriography can differentiate occlusive from nonocclusive disease.
  - There are reports of successful thrombolysis of clot in the SMA; however, acute occlusion is best treated by immediate surgical restoration of circulation by embolectomy or aortosuperior mesenteric artery bypass.
  - Examination of the bowel for ischemia, which will require resection, is essential to avoid unnecessary morbidity and mortality.

- **Nonocclusive mesenteric ischemia** is diagnosed when mesenteric vasoconstriction on angiogram is seen in the patient with a clinical picture suggestive of intestinal ischemia.

  - Shock and vasopressors make interpretation of the arteriogram difficult.
  - Treatment is begun in the radiology suite by the administration of papaverine (30–60 mg/hour) through a catheter placed selectively in the SMA; it is continued for 24 hours, and an arteriogram is repeated.
  - Heparin may be used concomitantly.
  - If peritoneal signs are present and abdominal exploration is necessary to examine the viability of the bowel, vasodilators and local anesthetics can be injected directly into the base of the mesentery.

- **Systemic antibiotics are indicated** because of the high incidence of positive blood cultures resulting from compromised bowel, but may mask peritoneal signs.

- **Second-look operations** are frequently used at 24 to 48 hours to determine viability of remaining bowel, though survival is not necessarily improved by this technique.

- **Mortality** rate for acute mesenteric ischemia remains at 70% to 80%.

  - Embolus in the SMA is still associated with a 44% to 90% mortality rate.
  - Nonocclusive ischemia without peritoneal signs has a more favorable outcome
  - Peritonitis is associated with mortality rates of 60% to 90%.
  - Logistic regression yields an odds ratio of 22 for peritonitis and 14.9 for hypotension as independent predictors of mortality.
  - Death occurs from MSOF secondary to ischemia (65%), sepsis (25%), pulmonary failure (8%), and stroke (2%).

- High index of suspicion for ischemia followed by an early, aggressive, and rapid diagnostic workup seems to be the only method for improving this abysmal mortality rate.

SUMMARY

Acute abdominal problems are frequent among ICU patients. The physician must maintain a high level of suspicion that an abdominal problem is present when faced with a deteriorating critically ill patient. History and physical examination must guide the use of more invasive and expensive tests. Laboratory tests are usually adjunctive and rarely diagnostic. Radiographic procedures, especially ultrasound and CT scans, when appropriately used, can be helpful. Surgical consultation should be obtained early in a patient's course, because treatment frequently requires surgical intervention. Only by maintaining constant vigilance can critical care practitioners guide their patients through the multiple perturbations created by acute abdominal problems.

CHAPTER 46 ■ THE DIFFICULT POSTOPERATIVE ABDOMEN

The practice of surgery inevitably carries the risk of postoperative complications and difficult therapeutic choices. In this chapter, we address some of the most vexing operative dilemmas involved in the management of the postoperative abdomen. The core principles of careful surgical technique and meticulous patient management, including wound care, nutritional management, and timing of recurrent interventions, are key in treating these obstacles.

ADHESIONS

- Adhesive connections may occur between loops of bowel, intra-abdominal structures and the abdominal wall, and the pelvis and nearby structures (bowel, gynecologic organs, etc.).
  - Most (94%–98%) of abdominal adhesions are acquired, either from operative therapy or via inflammatory processes (e.g., Crohn's disease, cancer).

- The remaining 2% to 6% of adhesions are congenital and largely consist of Ladd bands.
- In the reoperative abdomen, adhesions are present in 30% to 40% of patients.
- Adhesions result from trauma to tissues, relative ischemia, infection within the abdominal cavity, inflammatory processes, or the presence of foreign bodies such as suture, talc from gloves, and lint from sponges.
- **Adhesion formation** tends to follow predictable patterns, and the degree of adhesion formation is profoundly affected by the type of surgery performed.
  - Laparoscopic surgeries have been shown to have a 15% adhesion rate.
  - In open laparotomies, 50% result in adhesion formation.
  - Adhesions form more commonly after surgery to the small and large bowel than with other intra-abdominal organs, especially in surgeries involving bowel distal to the transverse colon or gynecologic organs.
  - Areas most frequently affected are the undersurface of the midline incision and at the operative site.
  - Owing to its tendency to migrate to regions of inflammation, the omentum is the most frequently involved organ (57%) and may be used to wrap anastomoses or to protect abdominal contents from a healing midline incision.
  - Small- and large-bowel adhesions continue to result in the highest morbidity and account for approximately 75% of postoperative bowel obstruction cases and 12% to 17% of hospital admissions after previous abdominal surgery.
  - One-fourth of these admissions occur within the first year after surgery, and 2% to 5% of small-bowel obstructions due to adhesions will require operative adhesiolysis.
- **To minimize adhesions,** principles of good surgical technique are the best defense.
  - Gentle tissue handling with strict hemostasis
  - Minimization of intraperitoneal trauma
  - Frequent irrigation to dilute or to remove contaminants
  - Use of small, nonreactive suture material
  - Raw surfaces or anastomoses should be protected by autologous tissue, either with a tongue of omentum or via mobilized local tissue flaps.

Barriers to Adhesiogenesis

- Despite meticulous technique and conscientious efforts to prevent adhesions, they will continue to form with attendant postoperative morbidity and mortality. Research efforts have focused on developing materials to minimize the occurrence and severity of adhesions. The most common method of decreasing the number and strength of adhesions is with one of a variety of barrier materials. Regardless of which product is ultimately chosen, the ideal barrier would be nonreactive in vivo, would be active during the key healing stages, and would then be reabsorbed by the body when no longer needed. Research interest in this area remains high as adhesion-related morbidity continues to plague surgical patients.

FISTULAS

- A fistula is an abnormal communication between two spaces. In the abdomen, varieties of fistulas differ tremendously and include such types as pancreatic fistulas, biliary fistulas, fistulas between two intra-abdominal organs (i.e., colovesical fistulas), and enterocutaneous fistulas. The natural history of a fistula begins as a leak from bowel or other intra-abdominal organ.
- The ultimate **type of fistula** depends on whether the leak is uncontrolled, partially controlled, or well controlled.
  - Uncontrolled leak will result in peritonitis, which requires surgical exploration and correction.
  - Partially controlled leak may result in an intra-abdominal abscess, which will require definitive therapy.
  - Controlled leaks result in fistulas, the management of which can be a long-term challenge for both surgeon and patient.

Enterocutaneous Fistulas

- An enterocutaneous fistula is an abnormal communication between lumen of bowel and the skin.
  - Spontaneous fistulas are uncommon, but causes may include malignancy, inflammatory processes such as Crohn's disease, or vascular insufficiency, as seen in radiation enteritis.
  - The iatrogenic fistula is the most common (accounts for 71%–90% of fistula's) resulting from inadvertent enterotomies, intra-abdominal infections, direct injury or bowel desiccation in the open abdomen, misplaced stitches, or anastomotic breakdown.
  - Impaired tissue perfusion from hypotension or vascular disease may predispose to this complication, as will infections, steroids, and malnutrition.
  - A seeming wound infection opened at bedside will result in copious drainage of discolored, watery material or frank succus.
  - Passage of gas from the midline wound is diagnostic of an enterocutaneous fistula.
  - Patients will usually demonstrate signs of advancing infection including increasing temperature and white blood cell count and persistent ileus.
- Less commonly, patients may develop profound shock due to electrolyte imbalances and sepsis, necessitating emergent re-exploration. If the patient presents with drainage or an obvious fistula but is hemodynamically stable, conservative management is warranted, at least in the short term.

Conservative Management of the Enterocutaneous Fistula

- Management is predicated on controlling output, managing electrolyte fluxes and nutritional deficiencies, and maximizing the potential for spontaneous closure (Fig. 46.1).
  - Aggressive fluid resuscitation and close monitoring of electrolyte balance are mandatory to maintain stability.
  - Nutritional replacement should begin immediately; this patient population is exceptionally prone to malnutrition from protein losses, increased metabolic demands, and limited or no oral intake.
  - Parenteral nutrition is nearly mandatory to provide early and aggressive nutritional repletion, to allow close management of electrolyte and protein balances, and to decrease volume transit past the fistula in the gastrointestinal tract.
- Perhaps a greater challenge in this patient population is control of fistula output.

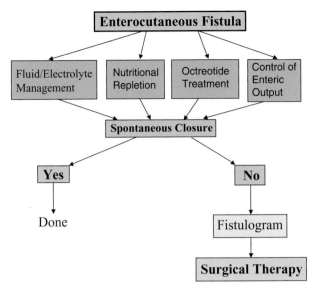

FIGURE 46.1. Management strategy for enterocutaneous fistulas.

- Enteric contents are extremely caustic to the skin and surrounding tissues.
- An immediate goal is to isolate enteric contents from the skin.
- For a simple enterocutaneous fistula, a stoma appliance may be all that is needed.
- Fistulas present in open wound beds, including on granulating abdomens, are not amenable to the placement of a simple stoma appliance.
- In these situations, a close association between the surgeon, patient, and wound care nurse/enterostomal therapist is mandatory to control fistula output.
- Once initial control is achieved, it may be possible to close fistulas surgically or to skin-graft the region.

Spontaneous Closure

- The goal of conservative therapy is to achieve spontaneous closure of the fistula, which is **dependent largely on inherent characteristics of the fistula.**
  - Most fistulas that close without intervention will do so in the first 3 to 6 weeks.
  - Fistulas with **long tracts and narrow mouths** are most likely to resolve.
  - **Low-output fistulas,** defined as having an output <500 mL/day, have a higher likelihood of closure.
  - A fistula that is not closed by 3 months is unlikely to close without surgical therapy.
- Additionally, many **patient factors** have been associated with failure of the fistula to close spontaneously. Factors that will virtually ensure patency of the fistula include the following:
  - Presence of a **foreign body** in the fistula tract
  - Close association between the fistula and an abscess
  - Association with a **malignancy**
  - **Distal bowel obstruction** leading to increased pressure and transit through the fistulous tract
  - **Epithelialization** of the tract
  - Short neck with wide fistula mouth
  - Long-standing fistulas with high outputs, which are unlikely to close spontaneously

- The patient and surgeon are not completely at the mercy of physiology and chance while awaiting spontaneous closure.
- A positive nitrogen balance and a transferrin level >200 mg/dL are associated with successful closure.
- Use of octreotide or other somatostatin analogue (100 μg intravenously every 8 hours) may decrease secretion in the gastrointestinal tract.
  - Somatostatin inhibits the secretion of most gastrointestinal hormones.
  - Enhances fluid and electrolyte absorption, thereby decreasing intraluminal volume and potentially decreasing fistula output.
  - Despite the theoretical benefits of somatostatin use, clinical studies have revealed mixed results on effectiveness.
  - As side effects are relatively mild, including gastrointestinal discomfort and increased biliary sludge, we recommend trying a somatostatin analogue in conjunction with other conservative therapies while waiting for a fistula to close spontaneously.
  - However, somatostatin analogues should not be relied on as a primary therapy to close fistulas.

Surgical Therapy

If after approximately 3 months a fistula has failed to resolve, the likelihood of closure without operative intervention is poor.

Criteria for Closure

- Defining the fistula tract via fistulogram to detect the length of the tract, tortuosity, tract diameter, and which segment of the gastrointestinal tract is involved.
- A computed tomography scan may also be helpful in defining intra-abdominal abscesses, malignancy, and hernias.
- It is imperative that the patient's nutrition be maximized at the time of repair.
- Fistula output should be controlled, as healthy skin at the time of operation will improve the success of abdominal wall reconstruction.
  By delaying operative repair until all criteria are met, successful closure rates improve from 50% to 94%, and mortality decreases from 50% to 4%.

Operative Intervention

- Extensive, dense adhesions may make access to the fistula very difficult.
- Risk of multiple enterotomies in approaching the segment involved in fistulization
- Attempts to oversew the fistula primarily may be appealing due to simplicity and avoidance of an anastomosis but has a dismal failure rate and often results in a larger fistula.
- **Definitive surgical therapy** remains complete lysis of intra-abdominal adhesions and resection of the involved segment with an anastomosis performed between two healthy segments of intestine.
- The complete lysis of adhesions allows careful inspection of small bowel to rule out downstream obstruction or other pathology.

The Open Granulating Abdomen

- A superior option for the patient is the **split-thickness skin graft.**
  - Skin graft rarely results in fistula closure.

- Decreases the metabolic demands in an already stressed body
- Provides a good base for appliances to control fistula output
- In general, the split-thickness skin graft, with or without fistula closure, is more successful in low-output fistulas.
- High-output fistulas will stress a fistula repair, leading to recurrent fistulization, or will interfere with adherence of the grafted skin and ultimately digest the skin graft.

The Pancreatic Fistula

- The pancreatic fistula is of an entirely different nature.
  - Most often result from trauma or iatrogenic injury, though a small percentage will be the result of pancreatitis.
  - The **cardinal principles** of management are diagnosis of the fistula and wide drainage.
  - A pancreatic fistula may drain **100 to 1,000 mL of fluid per day;** the resulting **pancreatic ascites** may cause abdominal pain, fevers, and a plethora of vague symptoms including abdominal bloating, hiccups, intolerance to oral intake, and abscess.
  - Pancreatic fluid contains a large amount of **bicarbonate** compared to plasma (70–90 mEq/L) and may lead to **nonanion gap metabolic acidosis.**
  - All patients respond differently to a pancreatic leak, and whereas some may present in profound shock, other patients may tolerate large-output pancreatic fistulas with few signs or symptoms.
  - Variability in clinical presentation is poorly understood but is likely due to the degree of enzymatic activation of the leaking fluid.
  - The most common method of diagnosis is by computed tomography scan.
  - If the patient is of reasonable body habitus and transport is hazardous, an ultrasound may provide equivalent information.
- For most patients, the **initial treatment is simply drainage.**
  - In the modern era, interventional radiology is invaluable in placing these drains.
  - If at initial operation, there is concern for postoperative leak; wide drainage with a closed-system drain should be established before closing the patient's abdomen.
  - Wide drainage of pancreatic secretions should allow time for the patient to stabilize and prevent damage to other abdominal organs.
  - Frequently, patience to allow long-term drainage to resolve will permit spontaneous closure of the pancreatic fistula.
- Adjuncts such as **total parenteral nutrition and octreotide** may be helpful in decreasing secretory stimulation to the pancreas.
  - Octreotide, administered 100 μg subcutaneously every 8 hours begun immediately after procedures deemed at high risk for pancreatic fistulas may help reduce fistula output, lower serum amylase and lipase levels, and help earlier return of positive nitrogen balance.
  - It is reasonable to pursue this therapy for a time-limited course (approximately 1 week) to improve chances of nonoperative resolution.

Management

- Conservative management with drains is generally pursued for up to 6 months and has a success rate of up to 97%.

- Depending on the cause of the fistula, intervention may be indicated on an earlier basis.
- If drainage fails to resolve the fistula, an imaging study should be pursued to define the duct and to determine whether an obstructive process is mandating fistula patency.
  - Magnetic resonance cholangiopancreatography and endoscopic retrograde cholangiopancreatography may provide equivalent information.
  - Endoscopic retrograde cholangiopancreatography is preferred; it allows the opportunity to identify pathology of the pancreatic duct and intervene.
- Stenting of a proximal obstruction may be adequate to allow prograde drainage of pancreatic secretions and closure of the fistula.
- When all less-invasive therapies fail, exploratory laparotomy remains the gold standard for definitive therapy.
  - Options at laparotomy depend on the level of the injury.
  - Primary duct repair is unlikely in most circumstances.
  - A distal duct fistula (perhaps secondary to a splenectomy) is well treated by distal pancreatectomy.
  - If the leaking duct is sufficiently large, as is seen in relation to a ductal obstruction, a pancreaticojejunostomy may be performed to allow for a low-resistance drainage pathway.
  - Pancreatic fistulas involving the proximal duct are most often iatrogenic or related to trauma and are troublesome to deal with, in light of other major structures in the region.
    - A pancreaticoduodenectomy (Whipple procedure) will resect the leaking portion of pancreas and allow reconstruction.
    - The Whipple procedure should be entertained only in patients with good physiologic reserve.
    - As noted, an attempt at conservative therapy and complete preoperative imaging and optimization are mandatory as these procedures are a major commitment for surgeon and patient.
- Despite the wealth of surgical options, most pancreatic fistulas will resolve with appropriate drainage, and thus, surgical correction is an end-stage option for correction of the fistula.

ABDOMINAL COMPARTMENT SYNDROME

Since its first description in the 1980s, abdominal compartment syndrome has become an increasingly recognized clinical entity. Although classically described as a primary entity, in current surgical therapy it is usually seen after a **massive fluid resuscitation** from trauma, burns, intraoperative resuscitation, pancreatitis, or sepsis. As the abdomen is a limited potential space, increasing interstitial edema and free fluid in the abdomen result in increased intra-abdominal pressure, which is transmitted to organs in both the thorax and abdomen.

- Capillary leak occurs secondary to sepsis or reperfusion injury in the splanchnic circulation and results in massive interstitial edema.
- In operative cases requiring large-volume resuscitations, the abdomen is frequently left open postoperatively until edema decreases enough to allow tension-free primary closure.
- In this way, compartment syndrome and its sequelae are avoided.

- The first clue to abdominal compartment syndrome is a distended and tense abdomen, but the key to diagnosis is a high index of suspicion.

The Physiologic Effects

- Compression of the inferior vena cava by abdominal contents and fluid results in decreased preload and a subsequent **decrease in cardiac output.**
- This ultimately leads to increased systemic vascular resistance and decreased stroke volume.
- Clinically, patients will become increasingly tachycardic and hypotensive.
- Increased abdominal volume also places pressure on the diaphragm, resulting in **high peak ventilatory pressures** (>30–35 mm Hg) and decreased ventilation with hypercapnia and hypoxemia.
- If ventilated with a pressure-control ventilatory method, the patient will demonstrate low tidal volumes.
- Compression of the ureters and bladder and renal vein compression leads to **diminished urine output** and renal injury and **elevated bladder pressures** (>25–30 mm Hg).
- **Bladder pressure** may be transduced for definitive diagnosis.
  - An arterial pressure line is attached to the patient's Foley catheter.
  - Approximately 60 mL of sterile saline is introduced.
  - Abdominal pressures >15 mm Hg are indicative of abdominal compartment syndrome.
  - When the transduced pressure reaches 25 to 30 mm Hg, a decompressive laparotomy is indicated as therapy for abdominal compartment syndrome.
  - Decompressive laparotomy may be indicated at lower intra-abdominal pressures depending on the patient's clinical condition.
- After decompressing the abdominal contents, the abdomen is left open with a **temporary abdominal closure** until swelling diminishes enough to allow closure.
  - Decompressive laparotomy for abdominal compartment syndrome is lifesaving.
  - Associated with a 42% to 68% mortality rate although this is dependent on the severity score.

The Open Abdomen

- Two increasingly recognized trends in surgery have led to a change in perspective over the last 20 years, where the open abdomen is no longer a catastrophe but rather a tool in the surgeon's armamentarium.
  - Primary and secondary abdominal compartment syndrome
  - "Damage control laparotomies" have become increasingly common in treating major abdominal trauma.
- **Damage control laparotomy** is aimed at limiting intraoperative times for deteriorating patients.
  - Allows transfer to the intensive care unit for vigorous resuscitation
  - Major vascular hemorrhage is controlled, either by ligation or packing.
  - Gross bowel contamination is controlled through ligation, often leaving the gastrointestinal tract in discontinuity.

"THE BLOODY VICIOUS CYCLE"

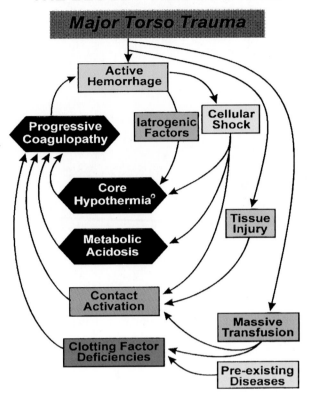

FIGURE 46.2. The "bloody vicious cycle" of coagulopathy, hypothermia, and metabolic acidosis.

- The abdomen is then closed in a rapid and temporary manner, with a plan to return when the patient is more stable to effect definitive repair.
- An aggressive strategy for treatment of patients who develop the deadly triad of coagulopathy, hypothermia, and metabolic acidosis (Fig. 46.2)

Management

Management of the open abdomen involves three primary decision-making stages—initial operative management, decision to close primarily versus a planned ventral hernia, and definitive closure of the planned ventral hernia.

- The original temporary abdominal dressing is known as the Bogota bag initially described from its use in Colombia during the 1980s and consists of covering the abdominal contents with a sterile saline bag to protect the bowel until re-exploration.
- A derivation of the Bogota bag is a widely used method of temporary abdominal closure in current practice.
  - A plastic drape, such as a sterile cassette cover, is placed over the bowels to prevent them from injury and under the fascia to contain the abdominal contents.
  - A sponge or blue towel, with two large Jackson-Pratt drains (Cardinal Health, McGaw Park, IL), is then placed over the plastic drape to allow egress of blood and edema fluid.
  - An adhesive drape is placed over the abdomen to maintain sterility, contain contents, and prevent free drainage of fluid (Fig. 46.3)
- After an appropriate resuscitation period, typically 24 to 48 hours, the patient is returned to the operating room.

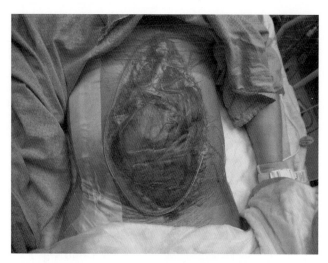

FIGURE 46.3. A temporary abdominal closure, using a sterile cassette cover and drains, as used in our practice.

- If definitive therapy is complete, the decision to close primarily depends on the quantity of intra-abdominal edema and the quality of the fascia.
- **Whenever possible, primary tension-free closure of fascia is ideal.**
- High-tension closures not only result in elevated intra-abdominal pressures but lead to ischemia of the involved fascia with subsequent breakdown and the risk of dehiscence.
- If it is not possible to close the fascia, or if further trips to the operating room are indicated, the surgeon should choose a temporary closure that prevents lateral retraction of the fascia and facilitates later primary closure.
- **Vacuum-assisted fascial closure,** most commonly by KCI (KCI Wound VAC System, Kinetic Concepts, Inc., San Antonio, TX) involves a pie-crusted plastic drape with incorporated sponge, a separate wound sponge, and adhesive dressing with suction tubing.
  - The sponge suction provides constant medial tension, without disrupting the fascia, to prevent lateral retraction.
- Management of the patient's volume status may be as important as the method of temporary closure in allowing later reapproximation of the fascia. Regardless of which method is chosen, most studies have indicated a high rate of primary closure if the patient has a net negative fluid balance at the time of operation.
  - Net negative volume balance is extremely difficult to achieve in critically ill trauma patients requiring large-volume resuscitations.
- A large percentage of these patients will go on to planned giant ventral hernias.

Short Bowel Syndrome

- Short bowel is an outcome of intra-abdominal catastrophe resulting in extensive surgical resection. Short bowel is defined as a **gastrointestinal length of 2 m or less. The cause may vary greatly between children and adults.** Regardless of the cause, a patient's ultimate outcome is largely determined by the length of remaining small bowel and the presence or absence of the colon.
  - Children most commonly end with short gut syndrome after a congenital or neonatal process such as necrotizing enterocolitis, intestinal atresia, volvulus, or gastroschisis.
  - Adults acquire short gut syndrome after extensive surgical resection necessitated by malignancy, trauma, obstruction, or vascular insufficiency.
  - Presence of the colon can extend the functional capacity of the remaining bowel.
  - To have the **potential for enteral autonomy,** a patient requires at least 150 cm of small bowel or 60 to 90 cm if the colon is present.
  - Presence of the **ileocecal valve** is also important in maintaining hydration and modulating gastrointestinal transit time.
  - There may be difficulty meeting nutritional requirements and dependence on parenteral nutrition.
  - Patients will complain of weight loss, diarrhea, and steatorrhea.
  - Gastric emptying abnormalities and rapid transit times are due to short intestinal length.
  - Dehydration is a constant threat if the colon is absent due to an inability to reabsorb the approximately 4 L of gastrointestinal secretions per day.
  - Loss of absorption results in deficiencies in B_{12}, fat-soluble vitamins, and bile salts.
  - Patients are also prone to cholelithiasis and nephrolithiasis due to altered absorption of bile salts and oxalate, peptic ulcers due to increased gastric secretions, liver dysfunction and line sepsis from parenteral nutrition.

Management

- A surgeon's role in managing short gut starts in the operating room with the very first incision.
  - At the initial operation, make every effort to preserve bowel length and the ileocecal valve.
  - In some cases, it may be safest to limit resection and return at a later date to inspect marginally viable bowel.
  - Initial postoperative therapy is often supportive, as this patient population is critically ill after emerging from the operating room.
  - Early central venous access with immediate institution of parenteral nutrition aids in healing and prevents malnutrition.
  - The long-term management of short gut patients then requires a multidisciplinary team involving physicians and nurses, nutritionists, patients, and their families.
- Patients with short gut generally fall into two groups: those with insufficient length (usually <45–60 cm) who require lifelong parenteral nutrition and those with adequate length to potentially adapt and become partially or totally enterally independent.
  - Adaptation is a process whereby the absorptive surface of the gut alters to increase digestive capacity and improve nutritional potential.
  - In most cases, the ability is dependent on time and the nature of the remaining bowel.
  - The ileum is capable of adapting to many jejunal functions, but the reverse is less successful.
  - Recombinant growth hormone has been used to improve adaptation by promoting mucosal hyperplasia and increasing villous surface area.

- The process is further enhanced by high-carbohydrate, low-fat diets.
- Glutamine has also been proven beneficial and works synergistically with growth hormone.
- Glutamine, and trophic feeds, stimulate enterocytes and enhance cell proliferation.
- Even in patients who are completely parenterally dependent, low-rate trophic feeds maintain mucosal health.
- Preservation of colonic length improves fluid reabsorption, leading to a more normal bowel regimen and improving the success of adaptation and weaning from parenteral nutrition.
- Conservative therapies such as medication and diet modification are the first line of therapy.
- If inadequate, segmental interposition (surgery) may be attempted:
  - Approximately 10 cm of small bowel is reversed and interposed in the gastrointestinal tract. The antiperistaltic flow slows transit time.
  - When small bowel length is inadequate, a colonic limb may be interposed; this option is much less favored and rarely performed.
- Creation of an artificial valve is also a possibility for those lacking a native ileocecal valve.
- Surgical therapy for short bowel syndrome is pursued infrequently and is generally referred to tertiary centers with extensive experience managing these challenging patients.
- In some cases, patients may have adequate remaining length for enteral independence but suffer from poor function secondary to obstruction, pseudo-obstruction, or dilation.
- A final option in pursuit of enteral independence is **small bowel transplantation.**

Radiation Enteritis

Of patients undergoing abdominal and pelvic radiation, 50% to 75% will have some symptoms related to the therapy in the months to years after treatment. The most common symptoms are vague abdominal pain, diarrhea, rectal bleeding, and tenesmus. In 1% to 15%, bothersome symptoms will progress into actual radiation enteritis.

- The incidence of injury is dependent on such factors as volume of irradiated small bowel, total dose delivered, and dose per fraction, and type of radiation being delivered.
- Symptoms most commonly occur during therapy and may be abrogated by decreasing the radiation dose by 10%.
- In the case of late radiation enteritis, workup should include dismissing recurrence of the initial neoplasm.
- Affected bowels may develop strictures, perforate, or develop fistulas.

- Sitz baths and stool softeners are effective initial treatments for rectal and anal symptoms.
- Opiates, antispasmodics, and anticholinergics will decrease diarrhea.
- Steroid enemas and sucralfate (by mouth or by rectum) can diminish irritation of the mucosa, which results in rectal pain and bleeding.
- If malnourished from chronic enteritis, total parenteral nutrition may be necessary, especially if operative intervention is entertained.

Techniques to Diminish or Prevent Radiation Injury

- Simple nonsurgical methods include patient positioning, multiple field techniques, and bladder distention.
- Intra-operative efforts are designed to decrease the volume of small bowel included in the radiation field postoperatively.

Treatment of Radiation Enteritis Complications

- The most common indication for surgery remains obstruction, but other indications include excessive bleeding, intractable diarrhea, pain, fistulas, and persistent abscess.
- Any surgical intervention should use the least invasive procedure required to address the issue.
- Excessive handling and adhesiolysis of radiated tissues commonly results in unplanned enterotomies and may interrupt an already tenuous blood supply.
- If dense adhesions prevent access to the involved segment, a gastrointestinal bypass may be necessary; this will predispose a patient to blind loop syndrome and bleeding but may be a better option than attempting to mobilize frozen bowel.
- Chronic proctopathy may include rectal pain and bleeding and affects 2% to 5% of patients.
  - First-line therapies of sucralfate and steroid enemas are of limited benefit.
  - Endoscopic coagulation of bleeding with electrocautery or laser has been successful but requires multiple treatment sessions.
  - The most effective nonoperative therapy remains the topical application of 4% formalin, with 85% of patients responding after two instillations or less.
  - Strictures should undergo serial dilation; if unsuccessful or the indication is intractable pain, severe incontinence, or profound bleeding, a diverting colostomy may be necessary.
  - In worst case situations, abdominoperineal resection may be pursued.
  - In the event of fistulas, the fistula tract and involved tissue at either end must be resected and the sites closed.
  - An interposition flap of omentum or muscle should then be placed to protect the repair sites.

CHAPTER 47 ■ CRITICAL CARE OF HEPATOPANCREATOBILIARY SURGERY PATIENTS

- Hepatopancreatobiliary (HPB) surgery is composed of surgery of the liver, bile duct, and pancreas, and may include portal decompressive procedures for complications of portal hypertension. Patients are admitted to the intensive care unit (ICU) for a variety of reasons following HPB surgery, including maintenance or restoration of normal physiology immediately after extensive surgery and the subsequent management of complications that develop. Recurring issues that are relatively specific to HPB surgery patients will be discussed.

LIVER ANATOMY AND PHYSIOLOGY

Liver anatomy has been described by various methods, surgical anatomy is based on the segmental nature of vascular and bile duct distribution.

- The liver is approximately 4% to 5% of total body weight but responsible for **20% to 25% of body oxygen consumption** and 20% of total energy expenditure.
- Liver has a dual blood supply, 75% from the portal vein and 25% from the hepatic artery.
  - Total blood flow to the liver is approximately 1.5 L/minute/1.73 m^2.
  - There is autoregulation of hepatic arterial flow but not of the portal venous system.
  - Decreasing portal venous flow increases hepatic arterial flow; with complete portal occlusion or diversion, hepatic arterial flow does not completely compensate, and total liver blood flow is diminished.
  - Portal flow is increased by food intake, bile salts, secretin, pentagastrin, vasoactive intestinal peptide (VIP), glucagon, isoproterenol, prostaglandin E$_1$, E$_2$, and papaverine.
  - Serotonin, angiotensin, vasopressin, nitrates, and somatostatin decrease portal flow.
- The portal pedicle divides into right and left branches and supplies the liver in a segmental fashion.
- Venous drainage is through the hepatic veins, which drain directly into the inferior vena cava.
- **Hepatic segmentation** is based on the distribution of the portal pedicles and their relation to the hepatic veins. The three hepatic veins run in the portal scissurae and divide the liver into four sectors, which are, in turn, divided by the portal pedicles running in the hepatic scissurae. Segmental anatomy becomes important in considering surgical resection when essentially any segment or combination of segments can be resected if attention is paid to maintaining vascular and biliary continuity to the remaining segments.
- Common liver resections are performed that may require ICU admission after surgery.

- Right or left hepatectomy, about 50% of liver volume is removed.
- Right or left trisectionectomy, up to 80% of the liver is removed.
- If <40% of the liver is resected in patients with normal underlying liver function, then relatively little derangement of liver physiology is noted.
- The **liver performs many functions,** including uptake, storage, and eventual distribution of nutrients from the blood or gastrointestinal tract, as well as synthesis, metabolism, and elimination of a variety of endogenous and exogenous substrates and toxins (including narcotics and other drugs).
- **Bile,** composed of inorganic ions and organic solutes, is formed at the canalicular membrane of the hepatocyte, as well as in the bile ductules, and is secreted by an active process that is relatively independent of blood flow.
  - The major organic components of bile are the conjugated bile acids, cholesterol, phospholipid, bile pigments, and protein.
  - Approximately 600 to 1,000 mL of bile is produced per day.
  - Bile secretory pressure is 10 to 20 cm saline, with maximal secretory pressures of 30 to 35 cm in the presence of complete biliary obstruction.
  - Bilirubin, a degradation product of heme, is eliminated almost entirely in the bile.
  - Complete obstruction of one of the right or left hepatic ducts alone will cause marked liver enzyme abnormalities, but rarely causes jaundice.
- The **liver synthesizes many of the major human plasma proteins** including albumin, γ-globulin, and many of the coagulation proteins.
  - Liver dysfunction can have a profound effect on coagulation.
  - In obstructive jaundice, there is decreased activity of factors II, V, VII, IX, and X, secondary to a lack of **vitamin K-dependent** posttranslational modification.
  - Reversal of coagulation abnormalities by exogenous administration of vitamin K allows differentiation between synthetic dysfunction and lack of vitamin K absorption secondary to obstructive jaundice.
- After resection, there is a reduction in functional liver mass and potential ischemia/reperfusion injury to the liver remnant.
  - Reduction below 25% functional liver volume has been associated with an increased risk of both liver failure and mortality in patients with normal presurgical liver function.
  - Preoperative portal vein embolization (PVE) of the liver to be resected is done percutaneously.
  - Diversion of portal flow and its hepatotrophic factors to the future liver remnant (FLR) causes growth and hypertrophy

of about 30% over a 6-week period and has been shown to reduce the complications associated with subsequent extended liver resections.

SURGICAL PROCEDURES

Liver Resection

- The liver is a tremendously vascular organ, intra- or postoperative complications are often related to excessive blood loss. While liver resection may be performed, in many cases without the need for interruption of blood flow to the liver, it is sometimes necessary to reduce blood flow to prevent excessive blood loss.
- Selective inflow control can be established by division or occlusion of the vascular structures supplying the segment(s) of liver to be removed.
  - This maintains blood flow to the segment of the liver being preserved, but is generally only useful in smaller resections.
- **Total inflow occlusion** (Pringle maneuver) clamps the entire inflow of the liver at the hepatoduodenal ligament, and has been shown to reduce blood loss during the parenchymal transection phase of the resection.
  - **Warm ischemic injury** is a concern, but abundant data show that the normal liver can tolerate inflow occlusion up to 1 hour; this may also hold true for some cirrhotic livers.
  - Clamp times are expected to be <30 minutes for formal hepatectomies, but may be higher for more complex parenchymal transections.
  - In such cases, total occlusion is carried out in 15-minute increments with 5-minute reperfusion intervals.
  - **Ischemic preconditioning** involves inflow occlusion for 10 minutes, 15 minutes reperfusion, and then sustained clamping for up to 1 hour.
  - Intermittent clamping is associated with more blood loss than ischemic preconditioning; however, the protective results of ischemic preconditioning in ischemia reperfusion injury have not been uniform across age groups, and may not be as effective in livers that have been exposed to preoperative chemotherapy.
- **Total vascular isolation** of the liver with both inflow occlusion and occlusion of the supra- and infrahepatic vena cava can be useful for technically demanding cases where the vena cava or proximal hepatic veins are involved with tumor.
  - Safe for up to 60 minutes in normal liver, but can be accompanied by varying degrees of hemodynamic instability.
  - When required, we carry out as much of the operation as possible prior to isolation of the liver to reduce the ischemic time and the period of hemodynamic instability.
- The most troublesome bleeding sources during liver resection are usually from hepatic vein branches, which may be minimized by maintaining the central venous pressure (CVP) below 5 mm Hg during the period of hepatic transection.
  - Cooperation of the anesthetist in minimizing volume loading, and occasionally using pharmacologic agents to reduce CVP, is essential.

- If total vascular isolation is to be used, volume loading prior to caval clamping is required to avoid an acute decrease in cardiac output at the time the clamps are applied.
- Knowledge of the **details of intraoperative conduct** of the operation is therefore important to the physicians who are to manage the postoperative care of the liver resection patient in the ICU setting.
- Was inflow occlusion or vascular isolation required, and for how long? Prolonged clamp times are associated with greater liver dysfunction.
- Was the patient maintained with a low CVP throughout the course of the surgery? The patient may need volume expansion on arrival to the ICU.
- How much liver remains, and is it normal? If the percentage of remaining liver is <25% in normal livers or <40% in cirrhotic livers or livers with bile duct obstruction, then the chance of liver failure and the need for its management are higher.
- Was there significant blood or fluid requirements? Patients may need a period of ventilation while fluid shifts and equilibrates.

Pancreatic and Bile Duct Surgery

In general, procedures on the pancreas or biliary tree should not be associated with major intraoperative hemodynamic changes or alterations in physiology. The more common indications for admission to the ICU after pancreatic or biliary surgery are either an underlying medical condition or the development of a postoperative complication.

- With **portal vein resection or repair,** it is more likely that the patient will require ICU care.
  - Technical difficulties can arise in which damage occurs to, or resection is required of, the portal vein.
  - Requires variable durations of portal venous outflow obstruction from the gut, which are usually short and well tolerated, but can increase the amount of fluid third-spaced into the bowel wall.
  - Can lead to massive transfusion requirements and hypotension.
- Pancreatic or bile leaks, which can lead to sepsis, will be discussed later in the chapter.

Portal Decompressive Procedures

- Surgical portal decompressive procedures, although a rarity since the introduction of the **transjugular intrahepatic portosystemic shunt (TIPS),** remain indicated in select patients with variceal bleeding and preserved liver function who have failed medical management and are not transplant candidates.
  - The high-pressure portal system is surgically connected to the low-pressure caval circulation.
  - Reduction of portal flow in patients with borderline liver function can precipitate liver dysfunction or failure.
  - The fraction of portal flow diverted into the systemic circulation is not cleared by the liver until it returns by the arterial circulation.
  - Shunts that divert most or all of the portal flow are more likely to induce encephalopathy than those shunts that are selective or partial.

- One special case scenario is **Budd-Chiari syndrome,** in which the hepatic venous outflow is obstructed, usually due to thrombosis secondary to a hypercoagulable state.
- Blood inflow cannot exit through the blocked hepatic veins.
- A functional side-to-side shunt is performed (portacaval, mesocaval) that allows hepatic arterial blood to flow into the sinusoids, exit through the portal vein, and then through the shunt into the systemic circulation.
- It is not uncommon for liver function to deteriorate initially after the shunt is performed, with subsequent gradual improvement and liver regeneration.
- In some cases, the shunt may **precipitate acute liver failure,** making urgent liver transplantation the only option.

IMMEDIATE POSTOPERATIVE MANAGEMENT

- Postoperative fluid management is important in the care of patients after major hepatobiliary surgery. Most liver resections are performed with low central venous pressure and low intravascular volume to minimize bleeding; postoperatively, these patients may have signs of hypovolemia with low urine output and low blood pressure. Volume re-expansion should be gentle, as partial liver resection leads to hypoalbuminemia, and pulmonary edema and ascites can develop with aggressive resuscitation.
  - Physiology is similar to patients with cirrhosis.
  - **Albumin,** if the serum albumin is <2.9 mg/dL, may be useful in the resuscitation of patients after liver resection.
  - Fresh frozen plasma can be used for volume expansion; however, it is generally reserved for abnormalities in coagulation.
  - Serial **lactate levels** are helpful in the postoperative management of patients after liver resection.
  - Elevated lactic acid levels may be a sign of hypovolemia, but the lack of response to volume can indicate liver dysfunction.
- After liver resection, **glucose metabolism** is altered due to both a reduction in functional liver mass and the relative dysfunction of the remaining liver secondary to ischemia reperfusion injury if vascular control has been used during the procedure.
  - Normally, as glycogen stores are depleted, the liver uses gluconeogenesis to provide glucose.
  - Resulting from altered hepatic physiology, hypoglycemia may occur, although lethal hypoglycemia is rare.
  - Tight glucose control to reduce risk of sepsis requires closer monitoring and may necessitate reduced insulin dosing to prevent hypoglycemia after major liver resection.
- Patients who have undergone shunt surgery require a different approach than patients undergoing other types of hepatobiliary surgery.
  - More aggressive fluid management is required immediately postoperatively to maintain **circulating intravascular volume** and reduce the risk of shunt thrombosis.
  - Maintenance fluid should be 0.45% saline solution with 5% dextrose to provide the liver with carbohydrate.
  - After the immediate postoperative period, patients are also at risk for ascites formation, so excessive sodium should be minimized and additional volume expansion—if needed—should be albumin or fresh frozen plasma.

- Diuretics, a combination of 100 mg of spironolactone for every 40 mg of Lasix, can be reinstituted after the immediate postoperative period.
- Antibiotics are administered for 48 hours postoperatively to minimize infection from bacterial translocation.
- **Encephalopathy** is rare in patients after liver resection, unless they are in liver failure or have preexisting liver disease.
  - The presence of asterixis can be an early sign.
  - Treat with lactulose and dietary protein restriction.
  - Infection, dehydration, and bleeding, as well as narcotic use can trigger decompensation that leads to encephalopathy.

Hypophosphatemia

- The exact mechanism of the hypophosphatemia seen after hepatic resection remains unclear.
- Utilization during liver regeneration and a renal wasting mechanism has been proposed.
- Clinical consequences include respiratory depression, diaphragmatic insufficiency, seizures, and cardiac irritability.
- Hepatocellular regeneration is dependent on adenosine triphosphate (**ATP**) and may be impaired if phosphate is not repleted.
- Significant postoperative hypophosphatemia (<2.5 mg/dL) increases complications after liver resection.
- Phosphate should be replaced with potassium or sodium phosphate preparations, or added to parenteral nutrition solutions.

Liver Function: Assessment and Support

Liver function should be carefully monitored after major liver resections and shunt surgery, as liver failure is a risk in any major hepatobiliary surgery.

- Risk increases with the extent of hepatectomy and with preoperative liver disease or cirrhosis.
- **Liver function tests** may not show elevation until the patient has significant liver failure.
- Mechanical injury and partial devascularization elevates transaminases in the 200 to 300 units/dL range post resection.
- Prothrombin time and lactate are helpful in evaluating early postoperative liver dysfunction.

Elevated total and indirect bilirubin are also useful indicators of postoperative liver dysfunction. However, isolated elevation of total bilirubin in the presence of normal liver function can have other etiologies.

- Perioperative blood transfusions can lead to hemolysis and direct **hyperbilirubinemia.**
- Bile leaks or obstruction can also lead to an elevated serum bilirubin.
- Many popular anesthetics, antibiotics, and other drugs can cause hepatotoxicity and elevation of the serum bilirubin and need to be reduced or stopped if liver failure occurs.

When postoperative liver dysfunction develops, it is important to exclude sepsis, drug toxicity, biliary obstruction or leak, and anatomic causes of liver failure.

- Ultrasound can evaluate for portal vein, hepatic arterial, or hepatic vein thrombosis or obstruction, which may be amenable to surgical intervention.

- In the absence of these conditions, liver failure is likely related to a preexisting liver disease and/or the extent of resection.
- Treatment is then supportive, with correction of coagulopathy, encephalopathy, and ascites.
- Systemic antibiotics or gut decontamination may be beneficial, since the liver Kupffer cells play a role in decreasing bacterial translocation from the portal blood flow, and patients with liver failure or biliary leak or obstruction may have an increased risk of bacteremia and sepsis.

Although definitive clinical data are lacking, both **N-acetylcysteine and prostaglandin (PG) E₁** have been used to ameliorate postoperative liver damage in both liver resection and transplant patients.

- N-acetylcysteine is given as a continuous IV infusion, 40 mL of 10% solution mixed in 250 mL D5W, over 16 hours.
  - Decrease liver injury after acetaminophen overdose.
  - Lessen ischemia reperfusion injury of the liver.
- Prostaglandin is given as a continuous IV infusion, starting at 0.15 μg/kg/hour, titrated up to 1 μg/kg/hour based on systemic hypotension.
  - Linked to improvement of ischemia reperfusion injury and liver damage.

Coagulopathy

Coagulopathy is common after liver resection.
- Increase in prothrombin time directly proportional to the extent of liver resection.
- Attributed to impaired synthesis and clearance of clotting factors, inhibitors, and regulatory proteins.
- Underlying liver disease and cirrhosis often have **thrombocytopenia and qualitative platelet defects.**
- Intraoperative hypothermia and perioperative transfusions, while not routine, are not uncommon during major hepatobiliary surgery, and can contribute to postoperative coagulopathy.

Because of the vascular nature of hepatobiliary surgery combined with postoperative coagulopathy from decreased liver function, serial hemoglobin and prothrombin levels should be followed for postoperative bleeding.
- In general, we would obtain a hematocrit and international normalized ratio (INR) on ICU arrival and then repeat them, every 6 hours, for the next 24 hours.
- The surgeon should be notified of excessive bloody output from the drains, increasing abdominal distention, or hemodynamic instability.
- If INR goes above 2.0 it should be corrected both with vitamin K and fresh frozen plasma.
- Any patient who is bleeding should have his or her coagulopathy completely corrected.
- For severe bleeding, both aprotinin (currently not available until further safety studies are done) and activated factor VII are safe in patients during and after liver resection.
- Patients who fail to stop bleeding after correction of their coagulopathy require return to the operating room for exploration.
- The surgical team should be made aware of any patient who requires transfusion immediately after surgery.
- Once the postoperative coagulopathy has resolved or stabilized, all patients should be given subcutaneous heparin or low-molecular-weight heparin with sequential compression devices to prevent the formation of deep venous thrombosis.

Pain Management and Sedation

Major hepatobiliary surgery can result in significant pain after surgery.
- Resultant from the large subcostal incision
- Altered pharmacokinetics, metabolism of many common medications, and coagulopathy, in particular after partial liver resection or shunt surgery, can make postoperative pain management a challenging proposition.
- With narcotics and sedatives that require hepatic clearance, oversedation is a common problem that arises in the ICU after liver resection.
- A standard dose of narcotics given to a patient who has had 80% of the liver resected may well cause prolonged respiratory depression and signs and symptoms of encephalopathy.
- **Narcotics should be used at the minimum dose required to achieve pain control.**
- After liver resection, basal rates on patient-controlled anesthesia pumps should be avoided, as metabolism of narcotics is difficult to forecast.
- **Benzodiazepines** also have altered clearance after liver resection, and should be administered **at a lower dose** or, if possible, avoided altogether.
- In patients requiring ongoing endotracheal intubation and mechanical ventilation, the level of sedation can be more easily titrated and reversed with sedative agents such as propofol rather than narcotics.
- **Epidural** pain management may be the optimal analgesic technique after liver resection.
  - Contraindicated in many patients because of postoperative coagulopathy
  - Good pain control with small risk of oversedation requiring naloxone in living donor partial hepatic resection
  - Useful in select patients who do not have underlying liver disease and who are not undergoing extensive resections.

Nutrition

- The role of the liver in protein and carbohydrate metabolism makes proper postoperative nutrition imperative after major hepatobiliary surgery, in particular after partial liver resection when liver function is temporarily reduced.
- Preoperative biliary obstruction, malignancy, and cirrhosis are higher risk for nutrition-related complications after major liver or bile duct surgery.
- Preoperative nutritional risk factors associated with postoperative complications include weight loss >14% lean body mass over 6 months, serum albumin <3 g/dL, hematocrit <30%, total body potassium <85% of normal, <25th percentile for midarm circumference, and skin test anergy.
- Preoperative bilirubin, albumin, prealbumin, prothrombin time, and transferrin, as well as replacement of vitamin and trace mineral deficits, may also be important preoperatively.
- As with most critically ill patients, **early enteral nutrition has been associated with improved outcomes.**

- In hepatobiliary surgery, both enteral and parenteral nutrition have been associated with improved outcomes, especially in high-risk patients.
- Parenteral nutrition has an increased risk of wound infection and catheter sepsis.
- Enteral nutrition improves gut flora, prevents gastrointestinal atrophy and loss of immunocompetence.
- In patients who have undergone routine liver resection or shunt surgery, low-volume enteral feeds can be started almost immediately after surgery.
- Unless the feeding tube is placed distal to the anastomosis, hepaticojejunostomies or pancreatic surgery must await the return of bowel function prior to starting feeds.
- Consult with the operating surgeon before starting enteral feeds in any patient, particularly those with enteric reconstruction.
- Patients with major pancreatic surgery (pancreaticoduodenectomy, subtotal or total pancreatectomy) may require pancreatic enzyme supplementation with enteral feeds or when resuming oral intake.
- Patients with **chronic liver disease or cirrhosis** often have severe metabolic derangements that make nutritional management difficult.
  - Depletion of fat-soluble vitamins, in particular vitamin K, leads to coagulopathy and diminished antioxidant response.
  - Chronic liver disease stimulates a catabolic state with proteolysis and cachexia.
  - Protein loss can be exacerbated by dietary restriction for encephalopathy.
  - Branched-chain amino acids do not reduce encephalopathy.
  - Cirrhosis patients have abnormal glucose tolerance and insulin levels, along with elevated ammonia levels, hypophosphatemia, and hypoalbuminemia.
  - All Child's B or C cirrhotic patients should be fed enterally when hospitalized.
  - The caloric needs of these patients are increased, and goal kcal is 25 to 25 kcal/kg/day, with administration of protein at 1 to 1.5 g/kg dry weight in nonencephalopathic patients and 0.5 g/kg dry weight in encephalopathic patients.
  - Patients with ascites need sodium restriction of 2 g/day and a fluid restriction of 1 to 1.5 L/day, in combination with diuretics if tolerated.
- **Patients with preoperative obstructive jaundice**
  - Such patients often have decreased hepatic protein synthesis and catabolism as well as chronic, low-grade endotoxemia and sepsis.
  - Malabsorption of fat and fat-soluble vitamins from obstruction of bile flow, leads to weight loss, anorexia, coagulopathy, and a diminished antioxidant response.
  - Mandatory biliary decompression prior to surgery is controversial but allows malnutrition and sepsis to resolve.
  - Two weeks of alimentation (both parenteral and enteral) **prior to operation** is associated with a lower risk of infection, morbidity, and mortality.
  - Standard nutrition is acceptable as hepatic dysfunction is usually not present.
  - A low-fat diet and replacement of fat-soluble vitamins is appropriate in patients where bile flow is not restored.
  - Medium-chain triglyceride absorption is not bile salt–dependent.
- Partial liver resections also cause metabolic abnormalities secondary to the regenerating liver.

- Postoperative parenteral nutrition should be supplemented with protein and fat, but low on glucose to improve hepatic regeneration.
- Hepatic mitochondria switch to **fat from glucose** as their preferred energy source in hepatic regeneration.
- Hypertonic glucose and insulin infusions should be avoided immediately after resection, as hyperglycemia and insulinemia suppress fatty acid release and decrease ketone body production by the liver.
- The evidence for administration of fat/ketone bodies or infusions of glucose and insulin directly into the portal vein after liver resection to accelerate regeneration is lacking.
- General goals are 30 kcal/kg/day, with 1.0 to 1.5 g/kg protein; glucose approximating 5 mg/kg/minute, and fat should not exceed 30% of the calories.
- Patients with cancer may need an increase of up to 35 kcal/kg/day and 2 g/kg protein.

Renal Failure

- Acute renal failure occurs in 10% of major hepatobiliary surgery patients and significantly increases postoperative mortality.
- Risk factors include postoperative sepsis, preoperative uremia, preoperative anemia, malignant disease, and preoperative jaundice.
- About 10% of patients with preoperative obstructive jaundice develop postoperative renal failure.
  - Both dehydration and endotoxin production from bile duct obstruction have been postulated to cause renal failure in these patients.
  - Mannitol, bile salts, hydration, and lactulose may decrease endotoxin absorption, and may be beneficial in the prevention of renal failure.
  - Preoperative biliary drainage helps lessen the perioperative inflammatory response.
- Adequate hydration, treatment of sepsis, and avoidance of nephrotoxic drugs are mandatory.
- Supportive care and dialysis are needed until renal function returns.
- Patients with advanced cirrhosis or postoperative liver failure can develop **hepatorenal syndrome** (HRS).
  - This outcome is more significant in the acute care of patients with liver failure or after liver transplantation.
  - Hepatorenal syndrome is a diagnosis of exclusion, with decreased renal function associated with urine sodium <10 mg/dL combined with urine osmolality greater than plasma osmolality that does not respond to volume administration.
  - The cause is likely multifactorial, but is primarily related to circulatory disturbances in patients with advanced liver disease, reduced liver function, and portal hypertension.
  - Systemic vasodilatation and low mean arterial pressure result in renal vasoconstriction and a reduction in the glomerular filtration rate.
  - Although liver transplantation remains the only cure for HRS, vasoconstrictors, albumin infusions, and transhepatic portosystemic shunts are able to reduce HRS and may prevent its development in patients with spontaneous bacterial peritonitis.

POSTOPERATIVE COMPLICATIONS FOLLOWING LIVER RESECTION

- The morbidity associated with liver resection is reported to range between 30.7% and 47.7%.
- In addition to the standard complications associated with all major operations, liver resection is associated with specific problems including bleeding, bile leaks, liver insufficiency, ascites, pleural effusions, and infections. Risk factors of complications following liver resection include increased blood loss, increased number of segments resected, increased preoperative bilirubin, increased prothrombin time, prolonged operative time, resection of segment VIII, diabetes, and concomitant surgical procedures.

Mortality

- The in-hospital mortality due to liver resection has decreased over the last two decades, and high-volume centers have reported rates of 0% to 5% despite increased mean age and comorbidities.
  - This decrease is attributed to improved surgical technique, intraoperative anesthesia management, and perioperative care.
  - Risk factors include hypoalbuminemia, thrombocytopenia, preoperative total bilirubin >6 mg/dL, serum creatinine >1.5 mg/dL, cholangitis, major hepatic resection, increased number of segments resected, synchronous abdominal procedure, major comorbid illness, diabetes mellitus, and blood transfusion requirements.
  - Specific surgical strategies to decrease mortality include minimizing blood loss and transfusions, and avoiding ischemic injury to the remnant liver.
  - Specific posthepatectomy strategies include minimizing ongoing liver injury by maintaining tissue oxygenation, early nutritional support to facilitate liver regeneration, and replenishing phosphate levels.

Bleeding

- Bleeding was once the "Achilles heel" of liver resection surgery but has decreased dramatically over the last two decades due to a better appreciation of liver anatomy, surgical technique, and improved anesthesia management.
  - Estimated blood loss has decreased from 750 mL to 300 mL and perioperative transfusion rates from 28.3% to 17.3%.
  - Risk factors for increased bleeding from liver resection include cirrhosis, portal hypertension, increased segments resected, coagulopathy, thrombocytopenia, and elevated central venous pressure during resection.
  - Strategies include appropriate patient selection—especially avoiding resection in patients with portal hypertension—and maintenance of central venous pressure under 6 mm Hg, Pringle maneuver, preoperative correction of coagulopathy and thrombocytopenia, use of fibrin sealant on raw liver surfaces, use of intraoperative ultrasound to locate the hepatic venous branches, and utilization of selective hepatic vascular exclusion.

Bile Leak

- Biliary leaks occur in 3.6% to 17% of liver resection cases and are associated with increased mortality and concomitant complications.
  - Risk factors include older age, preoperative leukocytosis, left-sided hepatectomy, prolonged operative time, resection for peripheral cholangiocarcinoma, and resection of segment IV.
  - For hepatocellular carcinoma (HCC) resection, risk factors for bile leaks included central tumor location and preoperative transarterial chemoembolization (TACE).
  - The efficacy of fibrin glue to decrease bile leak is debatable.
- Most bile leaks following liver resections without biliary reconstructions are small and can be managed nonoperatively.
  - If a drain was not placed during the procedure, a percutaneous drain prevents abdominal sepsis and controls the leak.
  - Broad-spectrum antibiotics are started for fevers, leukocytosis, or positive bile cultures.
  - Persistent drainage for 2 to 3 days of more than 100 mL of bilious fluid confirms an active leak, and is managed with endoscopic retrograde cholangiopancreatography (ERCP), sphincterotomy, and stent placement.
    - These measures may define the location of the leak and facilitate enteric biliary drainage and leak closure.
    - When leaks are at the resected hepatic duct stump, a stent traversing the leak may further facilitate leak closure, although the main principle of treatment is to reduce the pressure in the biliary tree and allow spontaneous closure.
    - Early endoscopic management of biliary leaks can minimize hospital length of stay and are not associated with late biliary complications.
  - Endoscopically placed nasobiliary tubes to decompress the biliary system allows easy repeat cholangiograms and later removal.
  - Although most leaks will close with time with these measures, they may persist for months.
- Around 0% to 32% of patients ultimately require reoperation because the leak cannot be controlled, and these procedures are associated with a high mortality rate.
  - Biliary enteric drainage is performed on patients in whom ERCP cannot be performed for technical reasons, or with persistent leaking despite ERCP.
  - Important factors contributing to a good outcome are early reoperation, control of the biliary fistula before surgery, and utilization of healthy bile duct edges for enteric anastomosis.
- Hemobilia may complicate bile leaks or liver resections or may occur secondary to trauma.
  - Hemobilia is an open communication from a branch of the hepatic artery to the biliary tree and leads to intermittent, and sometimes exsanguinating, gastrointestinal (GI) bleeding.
  - Identification is made when blood is seen exiting the ampulla when endoscopy is performed for upper GI bleeding.
  - Computed tomography (CT) scanning with arterial phase contrast can localize the bleeding within the liver; however, management is by angiographic embolization.

Liver Failure and Dysfunction

- **Liver failure** complicates liver resection in up to 12% of cases, and occurs when inadequate functional liver volume is left after resection. This complication occurs primarily in patients undergoing resection for hepatocellular carcinoma with underlying liver disease, and is often a consequence of patient selection and choice of operation.
  - Risk factors for hepatic insufficiency in cirrhotics include major resections, especially right lobectomy, portal hypertension, long-standing jaundice, Childs-Pugh Turcotte (CPT) score greater than A, and hepatic steatosis.
  - Preoperative chemotherapy, routine in colorectal cancer metastases, with newer agents such as irinotecan, oxaliplatin, and Avastin cause an increase in both hepatic steatosis as well as steatohepatitis, which can contribute to postoperative liver dysfunction.
- By assessing the patient's **functional liver status,** the surgeon can estimate the maximum amount of liver mass that can be resected while preserving adequate functional liver volume.
  - In a normal liver, up to 75% of total liver volume can be resected safely.
  - In general, Child-Pugh class C is a contraindication to any sort of resection.
  - Early Child's class B patients without portal hypertension may undergo minor resections—from wedge resection to a single segmentectomy—but may be better served by nonsurgical local ablation techniques.
  - Child-Pugh class A patients who are considered for major hepatectomy—resection of four or more segments—should undergo assessment of both liver and physiologic status.
  - Model for End-Stage Liver Disease (MELD) score ≥11 predicts liver failure following HCC resection.
  - Portal hypertension, defined as a hepatic vein pressure gradient (HVPG) >10 mm Hg, and as suggested by signs such as esophageal varices, anatomic portosystemic shunts, and ascites, has been associated with increased morbidity and mortality following major resection.
  - Thrombocytopenia with platelet counts <100,000 cells/μL has been associated with in-hospital mortality following liver resection.
  - The indocyanine green (ICG) clearance test, commonly used in Asia, is one method of quantifying liver function.
    - ICG retention at 15 minutes (ICGR15) of <20% allows safe, limited liver resection.
    - A value <14% is associated with near-zero operative mortality.
  - In Child-Pugh class A patients with right-sided lesions curable by major resection but whose liver reserve may be inadequate, preoperative ipsilateral portal vein embolization increases the remnant contralateral liver volume.
    - This is generally performed in patients with a predicted function liver remnant of <25% in noncirrhotics or <40% in patients with significant fibrosis and/or cirrhosis.
- Liver failure following liver resection presents clinically with encephalopathy and asterixis.
  - Severe cases appear similar to fulminant liver failure, presenting with marked acidosis, jaundice, and hemodynamic instability; the patient ultimately succumbs to multiorgan failure and sepsis.
- In mild cases, treatment is supportive, with judicious fluid management, optimization of tissue oxygenation, infection prophylaxis, and nutritional support if recovery is prolonged.
- The goal in the mild and salvageable cases is to promote immediate liver functional recovery from the insults inherent to liver resection; to promote liver regeneration with nutritional and electrolyte repletion, particularly phosphate; and to minimize the chance of infectious complications.
- N-acetylcysteine may improve hepatic oxygen delivery and extraction in patients for non–acetaminophen-induced liver failure.

Ascites and Pleural Effusion

- Ascites occurs in up to 9% of liver resections and is associated with decreased survival, as it is a surrogate marker of liver insufficiency and because of its potential contribution to prerenal insufficiency.
  - Risk factors for both ascites and pleural effusion include right lobectomy, diabetes mellitus, poor nutritional status and hypoalbuminemia, left-sided cardiac insufficiency, and liver and renal insufficiency.
- Pleural effusion, usually occurring on the right side and frequently accompanying ascites, is found following liver resection in 3.8% to 21% of cases and is usually asymptomatic, requiring no treatment.
  - Effusion may develop from underlying ascites that crosses the diaphragm.
  - The same pathophysiologic processes of fluid overload and hypoproteinemia that cause ascites may also contribute to the development of pleural effusion.
  - Risk factors specifically associated with pleural effusion include resection for HCC with underlying liver disease, subphrenic collections, postoperative liver insufficiency with ascites, and duration of inflow occlusion.
  - Strategies to prevent postresection ascites and pleural effusion include avoiding overhydration, including gentle diuresis; preventing renal insufficiency by avoiding nephrotoxic drugs and hypotension; early detection and treatment of infection; maintaining adequate nutrition; and the use of perioperative drains. The appropriate selection of patients and resection to maintain adequate liver function, especially in patients with hepatomas and underlying liver disease, will minimize the risk of liver failure and subsequent ascites.

COMPLICATIONS FOLLOWING BILE DUCT RESECTION/RECONSTRUCTION

- Perhaps the most extensive hepatobiliary operations are performed for proximal extrahepatic cholangiocarcinomas, with mounting evidence demonstrating significantly improved survival following extended liver and bile duct resections and reconstructions.
- Perioperative mortality following extended liver and biliary resections ranges from 1.3% to 16%. Complications following these procedures occur in 51% to 81%, and many patients have multiple complications.

- Complications include **bile duct leaks, bleeding, liver failure, pleural effusions, wound infection, and sepsis.**
- Each of these complications can also be found in liver resections alone, share the same risk factors, and can be approached with the same preventative strategy and treatment.
- Liver failure following extended resections for obstructive cholangiocarcinoma may have a unique pathophysiology and, hence, preventative strategy.
  - Prolonged biliary obstruction causes significant hepatocellular dysfunction, with up to 27.6% liver failure in patients who undergo extended liver and biliary resections and reconstructions, this is frequently fatal.
  - Resection of up to 75% of the liver and vascular reconstruction that requires an increased duration of ischemia is often necessary to resect hilar cholangiocarcinoma.
- Strategies to optimize functional liver volume prior to extended liver resections are essential.
  - Preoperatively biliary decompression, using percutaneous transhepatic cholangiocatheterization, is somewhat controversial.
    - May introduce infectious agents into an otherwise sterile biliary tree
    - May be avoided in patients who can undergo surgery within 2 to 3 weeks after the onset of jaundice
  - Contralateral portal vein embolization may be performed to increase the remnant liver volume prior to resection.
  - Decreased liver failure rates are observed when these are employed.

COMPLICATIONS FOLLOWING PANCREATIC SURGERY

- The mortality rate following pancreaticoduodenectomy (PD) ranges between 2.7% and 6.9%.
  - Risk factors for perioperative mortality include elevated serum bilirubin, the diameter of the pancreatic duct, increased intraoperative blood loss, pancreatic fistulae, and older age.
- Complications are seen to occur in 22.1% to 30.2% of PDs, and include **pancreatic fistulae, delayed gastric emptying, bleeding, abdominal abscesses, and wound infections.**
- **Pancreatic fistulae** are a dreaded complication of PD, occurring in 12% to 18% of patients.

- Risk factors for pancreatic fistulae include small duct size, soft pancreas texture, duration of surgery >8 hours, diabetes mellitus, lower creatinine clearance, preoperative jaundice, and increased intraoperative blood loss.
- Pancreatic fistulae are associated with a mortality rate ranging to 19%.
- Patients often die secondary to massive erosive *bleeding* from sepsis and pancreatic enzyme accumulation.
- **Bleeding** occurs in 1% to 8.8% of PD patients and carry a mortality rate of 47% to 50%.
- Strategies to prevent pancreatic fistulae following PD, including the use of octreotide, fibrin sealants, pancreatic stents, and different methods and sites of pancreatic anastomosis, have not proven effective.
- Pancreatic fistulae are initially detected on postoperative day 6 as abdominal pain, fever, nausea/vomiting, and leukocytosis.
- Fistulae are then confirmed by CT scan demonstrating fluid collection behind the pancreatic anastomosis, elevated serum amylase, drain output >50 mL/day, and drain amylase 10-fold greater than serum amylase.
- Management is initially conservative, with bowel rest, total parenteral nutrition, antibiotics, and monitoring of clinical signs and symptoms and drain output.
  - If repeat imaging demonstrates increased accumulation of fluid and the patient does not respond to conservative measures, another drain may be placed percutaneously to prevent progression to abdominal sepsis.
  - About 80% to 90% of patients seal pancreatic fistulae with these measures.
  - Uncontrolled leaks and abdominal sepsis may require surgery, usually for completion pancreatectomy.
  - Life-threatening erosive intra-abdominal **bleeding can occur,** usually from the stump of the gastroduodenal artery, small arterial branches to the pancreas or, rarely, the portal vein occurs in a small group of patients.
    - This presents with signs and symptoms of sepsis and hypovolemia, such as fever, abdominal pain, hypotension, anemia, and bloody drain output.
    - Patients are treated by rapid resuscitation and angiography for potential **embolization** of the bleeding arterial branch.
    - If arterial bleeding cannot be controlled in this manner, or if the bleeding is venous, the patient is explored for hemostasis and completion pancreatectomy.
    - Surgery in this setting is associated with a high mortality of up to 36%.

CHAPTER 48 ■ CRITICAL CARE OF THE THORACIC SURGICAL PATIENT

Thoracic surgical patients are among the most complicated admissions to intensive care due to their preoperative status, variety of operations, airway and pleural appliances, and requirements for postoperative interventions. Information transfer is key, including operative procedure, the expected medical course, and the predictable potential complications.

PREOPERATIVE CONSIDERATIONS: IDENTIFYING THE HIGH-RISK PATIENT

- The patient undergoing thoracic surgery is frequently older, with concurrent medical problems and often debilitated owing to cancer and associated malnutrition.
  - Pulmonary abnormalities commonly arise from prior occupational exposure, tobacco use, or a primary disease process. History of asthma, wheezing, or allergic airway responses identify patients in whom bronchodilator management may be needed in the postoperative period.
  - With severe chronic obstruction, the best predictors of postoperative ventilation requirements are arterial pO_2 <70% of that predicted for age and the presence of dyspnea at rest.
  - Factors associated with postoperative pneumonia after elective surgery include low preoperative serum albumin values, high American Society of Anesthesiologists physical status classification, smoking history, prolonged preoperative stay, longer operative procedure, and thoracic or upper abdominal site for surgery.
- **Preoperative pulmonary function tests**
  - By themselves are not reliable predictors of postoperative pulmonary function. The forced expiratory volume in 1 second (FEV_1) is an indicator of effective cough and ability to clear secretions. A postoperative FEV_1 is affected by inspiratory muscle strength, elastic recoil, and degree of obstructive air trapping, as well as any surgical removal of lung tissue.
  - FEV_1 decrease may not be proportional to the extent of resection with an obstructed lobar or mainstem bronchus.
  - An FEV_1 of 800 mL is commonly used as a cutoff value for a postpneumonectomy.
  - Forced vital capacity and functional residual capacity (FRC) can fall to <60% of preoperative values on the first postoperative day; return to baseline can take up to 14 days.
  - Any decline in FRC contributes to physiologic shunting and hypoxemia.
- **Advanced age** is frequently cited as a surgical risk factor.
  - Elderly patients have a number of age-related changes in pulmonary function, including decreased elastic recoil and progressive stiffening of the chest wall, increase in the ratio of FRC to total lung capacity, and diminished vital capacity and FEV_1.

- The activity of upper-airway reflexes is blunted, which may result in impaired clearance of secretions and the ability to protect the airway.
- **Obesity** results in decreases in FRC and expiratory reserve volume.
  - The expiratory reserve volume drops below closing volume, resulting in perfused, unventilated segments of lung and a widened alveolar-arterial (A-a) pO_2 gradient.
  - Patients are more likely to cough poorly, retain secretions, and develop basilar atelectasis.
- **Cigarette smoking** contributes to perioperative morbidity via its effects on the cardiovascular system, mucus secretion and clearance, and small-airway narrowing.
  - Cessation should occur at least 8 weeks prior to elective surgery.
  - Smoking cessation *just prior* to surgery may actually increase the risk of postoperative pulmonary complications, probably due to transient increases in sputum volume.
  - Expectations of postoperative respiratory failure allow increased awareness of unanticipated cardiovascular or respiratory deterioration.
- A very large patient population from the Veterans Affairs Medical Centers provided a database to learn what factors play a role in predicting postoperative respiratory failure.
  - These factors are all assigned a point status (Table 48.1); more points increase the probability of postoperative respiratory failure (Table 48.2).
  - Women were excluded from data collection in this study, but the factors noted do not have gender specificity.

OPERATING ROOM EVENTS THAT AFFECT INTENSIVE CARE UNIT CARE

- The pace of postoperative recovery depends on the amount and types of anesthetic agents given as premedication and during the operative procedure. Anesthetic delivery is constrained by patient factors.
  - The need for high inspired oxygen concentrations, particularly during one-lung anesthesia, limits the ability to use nitrous oxide and an early extubation goal limits the use of opioids.
  - Regional techniques (spinal, epidural) can supplement general anesthesia but are generally not applicable because of the difficulty in providing a high enough spinal level.
  - Controlled ventilation is necessary to sustain respiration during open thorax procedures.
  - An awake, comfortable, and extubated patient at the end of the procedure avoids stress on fresh suture lines from positive pressure ventilation and coughing or bucking.

TABLE 48.1

RESPIRATORY FAILURE RISK INDEX

Preoperative predictor	Point value
Type of surgery	
Abdominal aortic aneurysm	27
Thoracic procedure	21
Neurosurgery, upper abdominal or peripheral vascular	14
Neck procedure	11
Emergency surgery	11
Albumin (<30 g/L)	9
Blood urea nitrogen (>30 mg/dL)	8
Partially or fully dependent functional status	7
History of chronic obstructive pulmonary disease	6
Age (y)	
≥70	6
60–69	4

Adapted from Arozullah AM, Daley J, Henderson WG, et al. Multifactorial risk index for predicting postoperative respiratory failure in men after major noncardiac surgery. *Ann Surg.* 2000;332:242–253.

- **Selective endobronchial intubation** isolates the right and left airways to permit operation on a quiet, collapsed lung. One-lung ventilation alters the ventilation/perfusion relationship, as blood to the unventilated lung causes a right-to-left shunt, thus reducing arterial saturation.
  - The nonoperative side is used for selective intubation in lobectomies and pneumonectomies.
  - In pediatric patients, very small adults, and laryngectomy patients, a bronchial blocker can be placed under fiberoptic guidance in place of selective intubation.
  - Collapse and hypoxic pulmonary vasoconstriction limit perfusion of the unventilated lung.
  - The double-lumen endotracheal tube (DLETT) is large and has the potential to cause airway trauma and edema. It may shift its position and suctioning through it is difficult; it is usually replaced by a single-lumen tube when continued mechanical ventilation is required post-operatively.
  - Selective intubation may be continued to protect against soilage (pus or blood) and provide alternate positive end-expiratory pressure (PEEP) to a lung of different compliance in emphysematous patients undergoing single-lung transplantation.
- A flexible tube changer and a pediatric fiberoptic bronchoscope are essential tools that should be available in the ICU for placement and adjustment of double-lumen tubes.

IMMEDIATE POSTOPERATIVE ISSUES

- Usual postoperative monitoring includes intermittent blood pressure determinations, continuous electrocardiography, and pulse oximetry. In selected patients, assessing intravascular volume status and cardiopulmonary function may be facilitated with central venous pressure or pulmonary artery catheters. A checklist of immediate considerations in the postoperative thoracic patient is helpful (Table 48.3).
- **Chest tubes** are inserted to drain the surgical site, except in pneumonectomy patients where the standard practice is to avoid a chest tube. The patient will arrive with at least one chest tube; daily chest radiographs are usually obtained while chest tubes are in place.
  - Air leak from the thorax is demonstrated by bubbles in the water seal bottle.
  - Tube(s) should drain blood and some clots; large quantities suggest continued bleeding.
  - Should never be clamped owing to risk of unrecognized bleeding or tension pneumothorax.
  - Except for those in pneumonectomy spaces, are set to −20 cm H_2O of suction.
  - A chest radiograph will confirm endotracheal, nasogastric, and chest tube placement and identify any pneumothorax, mediastinal shift, or significant atelectasis.
  - Routine chest radiographs are not necessary after an uncomplicated removal of chest tubes.
- Hourly output from chest tubes should be recorded and the operative team notified if drainage is >100 mL/hour for more than 4 hours, or if >200 mL in any 1-hour observation period.
- Expected drainage from major procedures in the first 24 hours is roughly 300 to 600 mL, tapering to <200 mL by the second day.
- The level of fluid in the water seal chamber should fluctuate with each respiration (assuming no air leak) and serves as confirmation of chest tube patency.

TABLE 48.2

RESPIRATORY FAILURE RISK INDEX SCORES AND OUTCOMES

Class	Point total	N (%)	Predicted probability of PRF (%)	Observed phase I (% RF)	PRF phase II (% RF)
1	≤10	39,567 (48%)	0.5	0.5	0.5
2	11–19	18,809 (23%)	2.2	2.1	1.8
3	20–27	13,865 (17%)	5.0	5.3	4.2
4	28–40	7,976 (10%)	11.6	11.9	10.1
5	>40	1,502 (2%)	30.5	30.9	26.6

PRF, postoperative respiratory failure; RF, respiratory failure.
Phase I indicates patients enrolled between October 1, 1991, and December 31, 1993, and phase II indicates patients enrolled between January 1, 1994, and August 31, 1995.
Adapted from Arozullah AM, Daley J, Henderson WG, et al. Multifactorial risk index for predicting postoperative respiratory failure in men after major noncardiac surgery. *Ann Surg.* 2000;332:242–253.

IMMEDIATE ICU CONSIDERATIONS IN THE THORACIC SURGICAL PATIENT

Preparation
- Supplemental oxygen or mechanical ventilator ready.
- Bedside monitoring: ECG, pulse oximetry; possible arterial, central, or PA line.
- Infusion pumps if inotropes, vasopressors, or vasodilators in use.
- Wall suction to connect to pleural drainage system.

On arrival in ICU
- Connect patient to bedside monitors and ventilator (if needed).
- Check and secure all connections to chest tubes and assess function.
- Auscultate breath sounds and observe chest excursion; suction if necessary.
- Assess adequacy of circulation (BP, HR, pulse oximetry).
- Assess adequacy of oxygenation and ventilation (via ABG or noninvasive devices).
- Consider need for lung-protective ventilation if trauma/sepsis/operative issues.
- Fluid management: confirm need for continued maintenance fluid; generally keep "dry."
- Monitor inputs and outputs; label all chest tubes and chart outputs.
- Control pain with intravenous analgesics and/or regional anesthetics/analgesics.
- Order any necessary laboratory studies and chest radiograph.

Information to be obtained from operating room team
- Patient name, age, gender, and brief history.
- Operation performed and any major problems encountered.
- Circulatory and ventilatory requirements as determined in OR.
- Current drug infusions and titration plans; timing and dose antibiotics.
- Anesthetic agents given and plans for awakening/extubation (if relevant).
- Fluids and blood products given; urine output during case.
- Estimated blood loss, assessment of hemostasis at closing, and blood products available including surgical salvage if any.
- Laboratory results (e.g., ABGs, Hct) obtained during operating room.

ICU, intensive care unit; ECG, electrocardiogram; PA, pulmonary artery; BP, blood pressure; HR, heart rate; ABG, arterial blood gas; OR, operating room; Hct, hematocrit.

- Most pulmonary resections have mild to moderate air leaks, which are problems only if the lung does not completely expand or a significant amount of tidal volume is lost.
- Additional pleural drainage or changes in mechanical ventilation may be required to minimize the air leak and optimize ventilation. Ventilation techniques such as smaller volumes at higher rates, pressure-controlled inverse ratio ventilation, or high-frequency oscillation may sometimes minimize leaks.
- Once all air leaks resolve and drainage is <100 mL/24 hours, chest tubes may be removed during the expiratory phase of ventilation or while the patient performs a Valsalva maneuver.

INDICATIONS FOR CONTINUED POSTOPERATIVE VENTILATION

Airway compromise due to edema or bleeding
Inadequate pulmonary reserve after surgery
Compromised myocardial function, especially with perioperative infarction
Expected large fluid shifts with thoracoabdominal procedures
Severe neurologic impairment
Continued bleeding with likelihood of return to operating room
Esophageal surgery patients (risk for reflux and aspiration—delay extubation until airway reflexes have fully recovered as for full stomach intubation)

- PEEP is sometimes used in an effort to decrease postoperative drain output, especially from mediastinal drains in cardiac patients.

Extubation and Airway Concerns

- Extubation can often be accomplished in the operating room, but continued ventilation may be necessary in the presence of concurrent cardiac illness, inability to protect the airway, malnutrition, or coexisting lung disease.
- Endotracheal intubation for 24 hours postoperatively decreases pneumonia from silent aspiration and decreases the operative mortality rate in high-risk patients.
- Measurement of maximal inspiratory pressure (often called negative inspiratory force, is helpful in determining respiratory muscle strength, particularly after thymectomy for myasthenia gravis and after long-acting neuromuscular blocking agents intraoperatively.
- Ideally, the patient should be awake and following instructions and have an adequate gag reflex (signifying airway protection) and cough (for secretion clearance).
- Measured extubation parameters include a respiratory rate to tidal volume (f/Vt) ratio of <100, a maximal inspiratory pressure >25 cm H_2O, and oxygen saturation >92% on FiO_2 <50% at PEEP <5 cm H_2O. Although many patients will not meet these criteria, it is usually best to attempt weaning and extubation rather than risk the complications of continued mechanical ventilation.
- Indications for continued ventilator support are presented in Table 48.4.
- **High-frequency jet ventilation** has a role in the operating room during "shared airway" procedures (i.e., laryngoscopy, bronchoscopy, microlaryngeal procedures, and airway surgery). In the intensive care unit, particularly for hypoxemic respiratory failure, its role is poorly defined except for the case of a bronchopleural fistula. High-frequency jet ventilation allows ventilation at lower airway pressures, minimizing air passing through the fistula and promoting healing. With decreased pulmonary compliance, the benefit of lowering airway pressure may be lost.

Postoperative Fluid Management

- Thoracic surgery patients present unique issues in fluid management due to the potential for pulmonary edema that

affects 4% to 27% of patients. Procedures involving the mediastinum experience even more profound fluid shifts. Operative, insensible (600–1,200 mL/day in a 70-kg adult), and interstitial and intracavitary (6 to 8 mL/kg/h) losses provide valuable information when anticipating needs.
- Intraoperative handling of the lung, fresh frozen plasma, prolonged one-lung ventilation, collapse and re-expansion of the lung, and increases in postresection pulmonary artery pressures prime the lung for a more profound inflammatory response and potential fluid accumulation.
- Traditional markers include urine output (usually >0.5 mL/kg/hour), mental status, blood pressure, heart rate, blood lactate level, capillary refill time, venous oxygen saturation, filling pressures, and cardiac performance. If a state of poor perfusion persists, invasive devices allowing for precise hemodynamic monitoring and oxygen consumption need consideration to establish goals of therapy.
- Resection patients, especially right-sided pneumonectomy with high ventilatory pressures during surgery, are at increased risk for postpneumonectomy pulmonary edema and crystalloid infusion is ideally limited to 20 mL/kg for the first 24 hours.

Pain Management

- The pain after thoracotomy is one of the most intense of any surgical procedure. Adequate pain control is important not only to ensure patient comfort but also to avoid potential complications and reduce the risk of long-term postthoracotomy pain.
  - Without satisfactory pain relief, the patient is unable to breathe deeply, which decreases vital capacity and functional residual capacity. Splinting also occurs, making it more difficult to clear secretions and increases the likelihood of developing respiratory failure.
  - Pain elevates catecholamine levels and increases myocardial oxygen consumption.
- **Pain management options**
  - The mainstay of postoperative pain control is systemic analgesics in the form of **opioids;** intravenous route provides the most predictable responses but side effects like respiratory depression, nausea/vomiting, and ileus are an issue.
  - **Nonopiate medications** such as nonsteroidal anti-inflammatory drugs—including the parenteral prostaglandin inhibitor, ketorolac—are reasonable adjuncts. Nonsteroidal anti-inflammatory drugs may exacerbate renal dysfunction and pose a risk with postoperative healing.
  - **Neuraxial opioids and local anesthetics** via the epidural or intrathecal route provide excellent regional pain control. Epidural catheters are the preferred route when local anesthetics, either with or without opioids, are infused in this manner. Pulmonary complications decrease relative to that with systemic opioids, and initiation prior to the operation allows for better postoperative pain management. Hypotension due to sympathetic blockade is a potential side effect when local anesthetics such as bupivacaine are administered, and it may be necessary to decrease the dose or eliminate the local anesthetic from the infusion completely.
  - **Intercostal and paravertebral nerve blocks** may be performed intraoperatively or postoperatively, lasting up to 12 hours; repetitive dosing may be needed and can be accomplished with cryoablation of the intercostal nerves during the surgery. Intercostal nerve blocks are relatively contraindicated in postpneumonectomy patients due to the risks of entering and contaminating the empty chest cavity; splinting on the pneumonectomy side may actually reduce atelectasis in the remaining lung.
  - **Intrapleural catheters** inserted in the posterior pleural cavity can deliver local anesthetic such as bupivacaine or lidocaine via intermittent bolus or continuous infusion. Not a viable option in the setting of pleural effusion or pleural fibrosis. Complications include technical difficulties during placement, pneumothorax, toxicity to the anesthetic, and tachyphylaxis to the local anesthetic with time.
  - Transcutaneous electrical nerve stimulation, heat and cold application, music therapy, and relaxation are additional techniques.
  - Prolonged mechanical ventilation may benefit from dexmedetomidine.

Specific Patient Populations

- **Thoracic trauma:** Patients are typically evaluated and treated for acute, life-threatening injuries prior to their arrival in the ICU. Typical blunt injuries to the chest include rib fractures, flail chest, hemothorax, pneumothorax, tension pneumothorax, pulmonary contusion, cardiac contusion, and aortic disruption. Penetrating trauma such as gunshots and stabbings are less predictable in terms of the injuries generated and therefore require a case-by-case assessment in terms of management issues. Uncontrolled hemoptysis or cavitary lesions after penetrating injury require emergent surgical intervention. Mortality increases in thoracic trauma with increasing age, lower Glasgow coma scale scores, liver injury, splenic injury, more than five rib fractures, and long-bone fractures. Mortality rates typically are between 9% and 20% in the United States; with out-of-hospital traumatic arrest, <10% survive to hospital discharge. Maintaining a high degree of vigilance is paramount for diagnosing potential missed injuries.
- **Rib fractures**
  - The most common type of chest trauma, by themselves are rarely life-threatening but may serve as indicators for more severe intrathoracic or intra-abdominal injuries.
  - Pain may be significant and impairs usual respiratory mechanics, leading to splinting, hypoventilation, atelectasis, and potentially pneumonia as pulmonary toilet is compromised.
  - First and/or second rib fractures indicate a large transfer of energy to the thoracic cage and should raise further suspicion for other intrathoracic problems such as aortic rupture or tear.
  - The implications of age begin at 45 years; those with four or more rib fractures have more in-hospital complications such as increased ventilator and ICU days.
  - For the elderly, defined as 65 years of age and older, mortality increases by 19% with each rib fracture and the risk of pneumonia by 27%.
  - Epidural analgesia is associated with a decreased incidence of nosocomial pneumonia and shorter duration of mechanical ventilation in patients with three or more rib fractures.

- **Flail chest** occurs when two or more adjacent ribs are fractured at two or more sites leading to a paradoxical movement during inspiration, manifested as an inward collapse. Pain control is important to avoid splinting and to facilitate pulmonary toilet. Positive pressure ventilation, whether invasive or noninvasive, may be required to stent open the affected lung region and thereby avoid atelectasis.
- **Hemothorax** is a collection of blood in the pleural cavity. Large collections, >200 mL, of blood are needed to be seen on chest radiograph. The mainstays of therapy are ensuring adequate circulating blood volume and tube thoracostomy to drain blood from the pleural space. Inadequate hemothorax drainage may progress to empyema or fibrothorax.
  - Thoracotomy is required if bleeding continues at a significant rate, defined as initial 1,500 mL out or 250 mL/hour for 4 hours or if the patient's vital signs suddenly decompensate.
  - Retained hemothorax can be addressed with further large-diameter tube thoracostomy, open thoracotomy, or video-assisted thoracoscopy. Less invasive than thoracotomy and just as effective, video-assisted thoracoscopy is the intervention of choice unless there are extensive adhesions. Early surgical drainage decreases the duration of tube drainage, hospital stay and cost.
  - Fibrinolytic therapy offers a possible alternative, especially if the time from injury to therapy is delayed, with a response rate of up to 92% in terms of resolution.
- **Pneumothorax** is the accumulation of air, originating from the lung, between the visceral and parietal pleura and is the most common complication of trauma.
  - Treatment with tube thoracostomy is indicated when the size is >20% on chest x-ray, the patient is on positive pressure ventilation, or there are signs and symptoms of hypoxia and dyspnea.
  - If after tube placement the lung does not completely re-expand and there is a persistent air leak, it is important to search for a more severe tracheal or bronchial injury, as this situation would require surgical intervention.
- **Tension pneumothorax,** a life-threatening condition requiring immediate therapy, occurs when air accumulates under pressure, causing impaired venous return and cardiac output. Ipsilateral absence of breath sounds and tracheal and mediastinal deviation away from that side are the hallmarks, especially in the presence of severe hypotension. Initial therapy includes needle decompression, followed by tube thoracostomy.
- **Pulmonary contusion** is a result of blunt force transmitted across the thorax. The mechanism is related to compression and re-expansion of the lung tissue, leading to capillary disruption with interstitial and intra-alveolar edema, decreased compliance, and hypoxemia due to a shunt physiology. Care is largely supportive in this population, with close attention to pain management and pulmonary toilet.
- **Cardiac contusion** is a potential complication of blunt chest trauma; its exact incidence is unclear, as different studies used varying criteria to make the diagnosis. It is typically well tolerated in mildly injured patients but may lead to fatal arrhythmias or cardiogenic shock if severe.
  - Motor vehicle accidents are the most common cause; with rapid deceleration, the heart moves freely and can strike the internal sternum with a substantial amount of force.

TABLE 48.5

ELECTROCARDIOGRAPHIC FINDINGS IN CARDIAC CONTUSION

Nonspecific abnormalities
  Pericarditis-like ST-segment elevation or PTa depression
  Prolonged QT interval

Myocardial injury
  New Q wave
  ST-T segment elevation or depression

Conduction disorders
  Right bundle branch block
  Fascicular block
  Atrioventricular (AV) nodal conduction disorders (1st-, 2nd-, and 3rd-degree AV block)

Arrhythmias
  Sinus tachycardia
  Atrial and ventricular extrasystoles
  Atrial fibrillation
  Ventricular tachycardia
  Ventricular fibrillation
  Sinus bradycardia
  Atrial tachycardia

Adapted from Sybrandy KC, Cramer MJM, Burgersdijk C. Diagnosing cardiac contusion: old wisdom and new insights. *Heart.* 2003;89:485–489.

- Biomarkers Troponin I and T are specific to the myocardium and may avoid false-positives by relying solely on creatine kinase as patients often have diffuse muscular damage.
- Treatment involves cardiac monitoring and stabilization of the traumatically induced injuries, supporting blood pressure and cardiac output as indicated. Electrocardiographic findings in cardiac contusion are presented in Table 48.5. Echocardiographic findings in this same setting are presented in Table 48.6. A therapeutic algorithm for blunt chest trauma is presented in Figure 48.1.
- **Aortic disruption:** Only 13% to 15% of these patients reach the hospital alive; those who do have a 30% chance of subsequent rupture and death. Diagnostic modalities include chest radiograph, aortography (the gold standard), computed tomography scan, and transesophageal echocardiography. Treatment is immediate repair of the injury.

TABLE 48.6

ECHOCARDIOGRAPHIC FINDINGS IN ACUTE CARDIAC CONTUSION

Transthoracic echocardiography
- Regional wall motion abnormalities
- Pericardial effusion
- Valvular lesions
- Right and left ventricular enlargement
- Ventricular septal rupture
- Intracardiac thrombus

Transesophageal echocardiography
- Aortic endothelial laceration or aortic dissection
- Aortic rupture

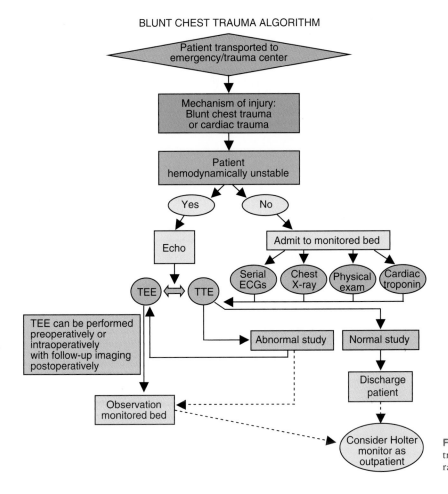

BLUNT CHEST TRAUMA ALGORITHM

FIGURE 48.1. Therapeutic algorithm. ECGs, electrocardiograms; TEE, transesophageal echocardiography; TTE, transthoracic echocardiography.

- **Lung volume reduction surgery** is used to improve the pulmonary dynamics of patients with severe emphysema by palliating dyspnea and improving functional status. This population is prone to more postsurgical complications than most other thoracic surgery patients due to their underlying fragile nature. Anticipated complications include arrhythmias, prolonged respiratory failure, air leaks, pneumonia, and ICU readmission.
- **Esophageal surgery** patients undergo procedures that traumatize the lung, the interposed stomach, and the diaphragm. Patients who undergo esophageal resection for carcinoma tend to be malnourished. Increasing patient age and decreasing performance on spirometry predict increased risk of pulmonary complications including atelectasis, pneumonia, aspiration, and retained secretions.
  - Aspiration risk is minimized by having patients undergo a thorough swallowing evaluation, including radiographic testing, prior to initiating oral intake.
  - The most dangerous complication, occurring in as many as 11% of patients, is leakage from the surgical site. Risk factors include high estimated intraoperative blood loss, cervical location of the anastomosis, and the development of postoperative adult respiratory distress syndrome. Use of thoracic epidural analgesia is associated with a decreased occurrence rate. Mortality is historically high, but improved with modern surgical techniques. Early identification is important, and endoscopy provides a safe method for determining the integrity of the graft and whether surgery is necessary to avoid loss of the graft.

Respiratory Therapy

- Thoracic patients often have significant underlying chronic obstructive pulmonary disease, impaired mucociliary clearance, excessive secretions, and/or increased closing volumes, all of which predispose to atelectasis.
- The respiratory therapist plays an important role in providing secretion management and chest physiotherapy (percussion and vibration) and should begin as soon as the patient has recovered sufficiently from anesthesia to cooperate.
- Other modalities include adequate hydration, aerosolized bronchodilators, humidified oxygen, and early treatment of tracheobronchial tree infection. Mucolytic agents (such as N-acetylcysteine) help with thick secretions but may cause bronchospasm.
- Oral or nasotracheal suctioning is used in selected extubated patients, but discomfort and the possibility of complications (hypoxemia, vagal-mediated bradycardia, or cardiac arrest) limit routine use. Inadequate clearance of secretions often requires flexible bronchoscopy, which is of greatest benefit in the extubated patient who cannot adequately be suctioned.
- A mini-tracheostomy (bedside percutaneous cricothyroidotomy for suctioning) can provide access to the lower airway in patients with thick secretions.
- If pulmonary parenchymal involvement is confined to one lung, altering body position and use of specialized beds can improve gas exchange by changing the relationships between ventilation and perfusion.

TABLE 48.7

POSTOPERATIVE COMPLICATIONS AFTER ANY THORACIC PROCEDURE

Airway edema/stridor
Arrhythmias (especially atrial fibrillation, multifocal atrial tachycardia)
Arytenoid dislocation
Aspiration of gastric contents
Atelectasis
Bronchospasm
Bronchopleural fistula
Chylothorax
Congestive heart failure
Deep venous thrombosis
Empyema
Hemorrhage
Hemothorax
Infection (superficial, deep)
Lobar collapse
Lobar torsion
Myocardial infarction
Pain and splinting
Pleural effusion
Pneumothorax
Pulmonary embolus
Re-expansion pulmonary edema
Respiratory failure
Retaining secretions
Subcutaneous emphysema
Tension pneumothorax

From Higgins TL. Selected issues in postoperative management. In: American College of Chest Physicians: *The ACCP Critical Care Board Review*. Northbrook IL; 1998:323–334, with permission.

Complications

- **Laryngeal and glottic edema** frequently occur after airway manipulation or intubation with a double-lumen endotracheal tube (Table 48.7). A critical airway may be converted to an adequate airway by the administration of Heliox, a helium and oxygen mixture. Upright or sitting position, racemic epinephrine and corticosteroids are traditional treatments used. Serious laryngeal edema can be detected by an absent cuff leak. If there are any doubts, the endotracheal tube should be removed only under direct laryngoscopic or fiberoptic observation, with a percutaneous tracheostomy set immediately at hand.
- The **recurrent laryngeal nerves** branch from the vagus nerves as they enter the chest. Injury can result from excessive traction, aggressive dissection, or the operative sacrifice of these nerves. Mediastinoscopy, anterior mediastinotomy, left pulmonary resection with subaortic exenteration, and resections of mediastinal tumors are common operations in which the recurrent laryngeal nerve may be damaged.
  - Early airway and laryngeal edema may allow adequate coaptation of the vocal cords, preventing identification of injury until after ICU discharge, when ineffective cough or aspiration of secretions becomes apparent.
  - If there is permanent damage, injection with Teflon may be considered.

- Aggressive chest physiotherapy, careful airway management, and temporary avoidance of oral feeding may eliminate the need for intervention until nerve function has recovered.
- Intermittent noisy inspiration and painful swallowing suggest **arytenoid dislocation,** an uncommon cause of postextubation respiratory failure. Treatment consists of surgical reduction, before the cricoarytenoid joint becomes fibrosed in poor position.
- Postoperative **air leaks** most often result from distal fistulae between tiny bronchioles or respiratory units and the pleural cavity. Repositioning or insertion of chest tubes into undrained spaces ensure complete expansion of the lung help them close.
  - A substantial persistent air leak or incomplete expansion of the lung suggests a significant bronchopleural fistula. Major proximal airway problems such as failure of the anastomosis, disruption of a bronchial closure, or retained secretions or foreign bodies can be identified by bronchoscopy.
  - Any fistula within the first 7 postoperative days is likely to be due to a technical problem.
  - Fistulae at 1 to 6 weeks are more often due to an empyema or local peribronchial abscess.
  - Late fistulae, >6 months after the operation, are frequently due to recurrent carcinoma.
- **Early postoperative bronchopleural fistula in a pneumonectomy patient** is a surgical emergency. A chest radiograph will show loss of fluid from the pneumonectomy space. Typical presentation is sudden expectoration of copious amounts of pink, frothy sputum, which may be misdiagnosed as pulmonary edema.
  - The patient should be positioned with the operated or pneumonectomy side down to trap remaining fluid in the pneumonectomy space and prevent drowning.
  - Management will likely include bronchoscopy and immediate reoperation.
- **Empyema** is initially treated with closed tube drainage and antibiotic therapy.
  - Any bronchopleural fistula is identified and treated.
  - A chest radiograph helps to determine whether the mediastinum is fixed or whether it has shifted and compressed the contralateral remaining lung. If the mediastinum is stable, open drainage in the form of rib resection and marsupialization of the pneumonectomy cavity (Clagett window or Eloesser flap) may be performed.
  - With time, the cavity shrinks in size, and the window or flap may be closed.
- **Postoperative hypoxemia** is common and may be due to sepsis, adult respiratory distress syndrome, pneumonia, or pulmonary embolization.
  - If pulmonary embolization is suspected, ventilation/perfusion scanning, spiral computed tomography, or pulmonary angiography should be done and treatment initiated. If anticoagulation or lytic therapy is contraindicated, an inferior vena caval filter should be placed.
  - Systemic tumor emboli, though uncommon, may be seen after pulmonary resections for primary bronchogenic carcinomas or metastatic sarcomas.
- **Massive postoperative hemorrhage** from the pulmonary vein or artery and requiring emergent reoperation can present

TABLE 48.8

COMPLICATIONS OF SPECIFIC THORACIC PROCEDURES

Procedure	Complications
Anterior mediastinotomy (Chamberlain)	Damage to recurrent laryngeal nerve (particularly left)
Bronchoscopy/mediastinoscopy	Bleeding from major vessels if torn, air leak with biopsy of bronchus
Bronchopleural fistula repair	Persistent leak, dehiscence
Bronchopulmonary lavage	Respiratory distress/contralateral spillage
Bullectomy	Tension pneumothorax, air leak
Chest wall reconstruction	Blood loss, altered chest wall compliance, unstable chest, infection of prosthetic material
Clagett window	Air leak
Collis-Belsey	Gastric leak, splenic injury
Decortication	Blood loss, air leak(s)
Esophageal dilatation	Esophageal perforation, pleural effusion, airway obstruction
Esophagoscopy	Esophageal perforation
Esophagogastrectomy	Third-spacing of fluids, anastomotic leak, gastric devascularization, splenic injury, gastric torsion
Heller myotomy	Esophageal tear
Lobectomy	Bronchial leak, lobar collapse, lobar torsion
Mediastinal tumor excision	Airway obstruction with sedation/anesthesia, damage to recurrent laryngeal nerve
Nissen fundoplication	Esophageal obstruction (with tight wrap), splenic injury
Pectus repair	Costochondritis, unstable sternum
Pleuroscopy	Pharyngeal laceration, air leak
Pneumonectomy	Atrial arrhythmias (atrial fibrillation, MAT), mediastinal shift, cardiac torsion, air embolism, disrupted bronchus
Thoracic aortic aneurysm	Paraplegia, bleeding, aortobronchial fistula, esophageal injury
Thymectomy	In myasthenics, possible weakness and respiratory failure
Lung transplant	Rejection (day 5), reperfusion injury, infection, overdistention of native lung, dehiscence
Tracheal resection	Fixed neck flexion postoperatively, dehiscence, air leak

MAT, multifocal atrial tachycardia.
From Higgins TL. Selected issues in postoperative management. In: American College of Chest Physicians: *The ACCP Critical Care Board Review*. Northbrook, IL; 1998:323–334, with permission.

as significant shock. Slower hemorrhage results from small bleeding vessels in the mediastinum or chest wall.

PULMONARY PARENCHYMAL COMPLICATIONS

- **Tracheoesophageal fistula:** A communication occurs between the anterior esophageal wall and membranous (posterior) wall of the trachea after prolonged intubation due to pressure exerted from the cuff of the endotracheal or tracheostomy tube leading to tissue necrosis.
  - Tracheoesophageal fistula should be suspected when feedings are aspirated from the airway.
  - Surgical revision is definitive therapy but may not be practical in patients still requiring positive pressure ventilation.
  - Stenting of the esophagus allows for temporary sealing of the fistula until the patient is a suitable candidate for final surgical repair.
- **Tracheoinnominate fistula:** A rare life-threatening complication with massive bleeding, it is seen 48 hours or more after tracheostomy requires urgent action.
  - Initial steps include hyperinflation of the tracheostomy cuff or direct arterial compression with a finger to tamponade the bleeding.

- Bronchoscopy is the diagnostic procedure of choice, followed by surgery to divide the innominate artery, with subsequent separation of the trachea from the divided artery by viable tissue.
- **Atelectasis** is the most common complication after thoracic surgery.
- Potential contributors include hypoventilation, splinting, bronchospasm, poor cough, retained secretions, pneumothorax, and trauma to the lung during the surgical procedure.
- Symptoms include fever, tachypnea, arrhythmias, hypoxia, or respiratory failure.
- Efforts to avoid atelectasis include frequent suctioning of the tracheobronchial tree, chest percussion and postural drainage, humidification of inspired gases, frequent patient rotation, bronchodilators, pain control, coughing, deep breathing, bronchoscopy for removal of mucus plugs or secretions, invasive or noninvasive positive pressure ventilation, and early ambulation.
- Chest physiotherapy uses clapping and vibration to stimulate coughing and move secretions, potentially decreasing hospital costs due to shorter lengths of stay; incentive spirometry does not provide the same benefit.
- **Lobar collapse and torsion**
  - Lobar collapse most commonly occurs in either the right upper lobe after double-lumen endotracheal intubation or in the right middle lobe after right upper lobectomy.

- Lobar torsion occurs as the result of a lung segment twisting about its hilar structures with infarction occurring if the process is not recognized and treated. The right middle lobe and lingula are at greatest risk after thoracotomy.

PLEURAL COMPLICATIONS

- Pneumothorax occurs as described earlier.
- **Pleural effusions** should be evaluated via thoracentesis if persistent. If the fluid is transudative, the underlying cause needs to be addressed. Exudative fluid induces a high suspicion for empyema. If pleural effusions and pneumothoraces do not resolve, more definitive therapy such as pleurodesis needs to be entertained.
- **Thoracic duct injury** is a known complication after dissection in the posterior mediastinum and may result in chylothorax, high in triglycerides and chylomicrons. The leakage site is localized with lymphangiography or computed tomography scanning, and the clinical situation will dictate the type of management. Management initially includes chest tube drainage and parenteral nutrition to decrease thoracic duct output, with surgery reserved for failure of conservative management.
- Complications of specific thoracic procedures are presented in Table 48.8.

CHAPTER 49 ■ POSTOPERATIVE MANAGEMENT OF THE ADULT CARDIOVASCULAR PATIENT

CARDIOPULMONARY BYPASS (CPB)

- Development of the heart–lung machine over the last 50 years has made complex repairs of intracardiac structures and the great vessels feasible. The most basic components are a venous cannula, a venous reservoir, a pump, an oxygenator, a heat exchanger, a filter, and an arterial cannula (Fig. 49.1). A cardioplegia delivery system, ultrafiltration unit, cardiotomy suction system, left ventricular vent, and cell saver system are some of the other components.
- Interaction between the patient's blood and the large plastic surface area of the CPB circuit triggers the inflammatory cascade; this activates plasma enzyme systems and blood cells, dilutes plasma proteins, causes coagulopathy, produces emboli, and leads to release of an array of vasoactive mediators that affect vascular motor tone and endothelial permeability (Table 49.1).
- The post-CPB inflammation is typically self-limited; vasomotor mediators reach peak levels within 24 hours of surgery and subside over ensuing days.

Immediate Concerns

- Almost all patients are in a state of controlled shock because of fluid shifts and changes in vascular tone. A checklist is useful to ensure that essential tasks are accomplished within the first 30 minutes of a patient's arrival in the ICU (Table 49.2).
- The first step should be a quick assessment of the ABCs (airway, breathing, circulation), electrocardiogram, and pressure measurement catheters to verify that they are connected and calibrated.

- Sign-out of patient information from the perioperative team to the ICU team ensures the safe transition of care. Important details may include ease of intubation, perioperative ventricular function, inotropic and vasopressor requirement, optimal

TABLE 49.1
VASOACTIVE SUBSTANCES RELEASED FOLLOWING CARDIOPULMONARY BYPASS
Aldosterone
Angiotensin II
Atrial natriuretic peptide
Complement: C3a, C4a, C5a, C5b-9
Electrolytes: Ca^{2+}, Mg^{2+}, K^+
Endothelin-1
Epinephrine
Glucagon
Histamine
Interleukins: IL-1, IL-6, IL-8, IL-10
Leukotrienes: LTB_4, LTC_4, LTD_4
Lysosomal enzymes
Nitric oxide
Norepinephrine
Oxygen free radicals
Platelet-activating factor
Prostacyclins
Prostaglandin E_2
Proteases
Renin
Serotonin
Thromboxane A_2
Thyroid hormones: T_3, T_4
Vasopressin

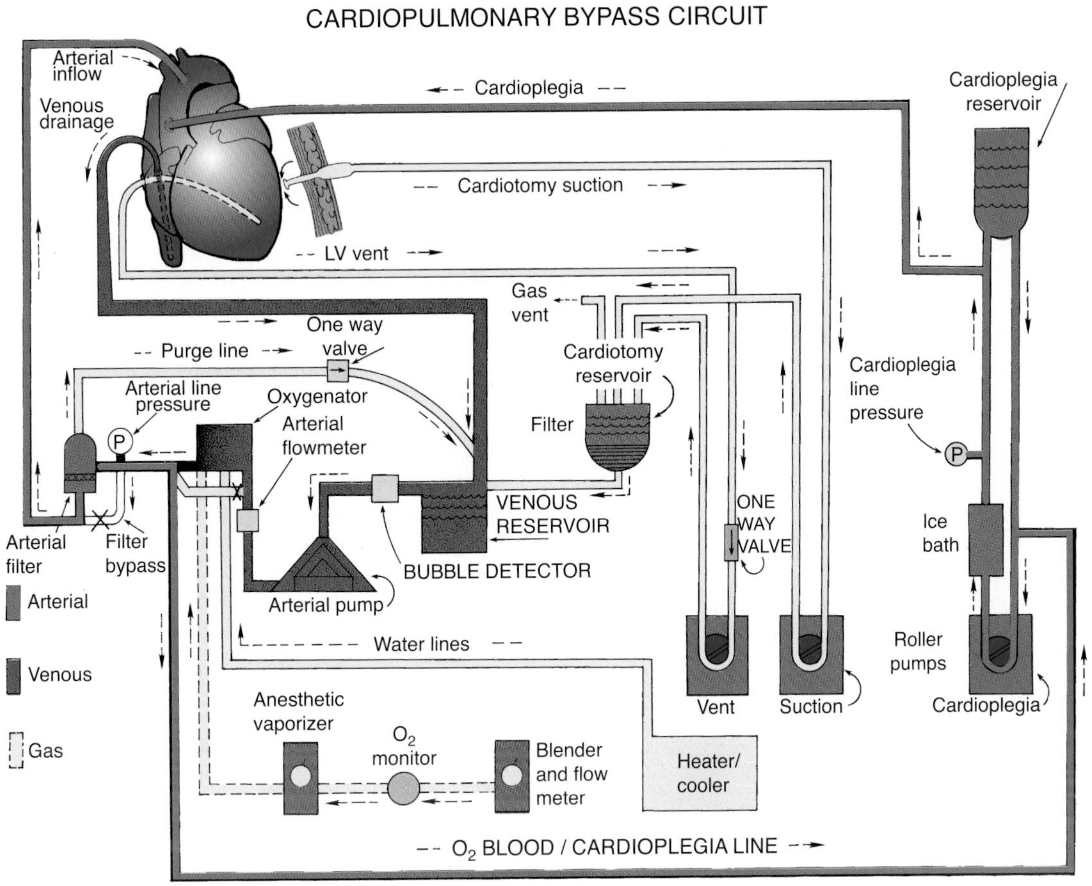

CARDIOPULMONARY BYPASS CIRCUIT

FIGURE 49.1. Schematic of a typical cardiopulmonary bypass circuit. (Reproduced from Wellons HA Jr, Zacour RK. Cardiopulmonary bypass. In: Kaiser LR, Kron IL, Spray TL, eds. *Mastery of Cardiothoracic Surgery.* 2nd ed. Philadelphia, PA: Lippincott Williams & Wilkins; 2007:312, with permission.)

volume status, completeness of revascularization, and suspected coagulopathy.

- Mechanical ventilation is continued and significant arterial-alveolar (A-a) gradients are common; hence high concentrations of oxygen (70%–80%) are routine until adequate oxygenation is confirmed. Tidal volume in the absence of acute lung injury is set at 8 mL/kg of predicted body weight.
- Although affected by severe atherosclerosis, skin temperature, pulse amplitude, and capillary refill time provide essential information about the adequacy of cardiac output. Palpable peripheral pulses are an excellent indicator of systemic perfusion. Mental status and central nervous system assessment is also part of the initial exam.
- A portable chest radiograph is obtained to determine the proper placement of the endotracheal tube, monitoring catheters, and nasogastric tube. Look closely for evidence of a pneumothorax, hemopneumothorax, and areas of lung collapse or atelectasis.

Initial Therapy

- The first hour is a critical and unstable time. The goals are to maintain adequate systemic perfusion, adequate oxygenation and ventilation, and control cardiac rate and rhythm.
- Hypothermia, especially below 35.5°C, reduces the threshold for ventricular tachycardia or fibrillation; serum potassium

levels should be maintained in the 4.5- to 5.0-mmol/L range to prevent ventricular irritability. Avoid correcting acidosis with rapid IV sodium bicarbonate that can acutely lower serum potassium.

- Monitor closely for inappropriate dieresis, which occurs commonly after CPB and may require rapid replacement of crystalloid and electrolyte losses. Mediastinal drain output is also closely observed. If rapid hemorrhage is suspected, transfusion therapy is initiated and the operating team should be made aware of any massive hemorrhage.

The First 8 Hours after Cardiopulmonary Bypass

- The *golden period* frequently follows when the patient's hemodynamics are adequate and the patient is relatively stable. Cardiorespiratory performance should be optimized so that the decreasing cardiac function that characterizes the following 16 hours does not jeopardize end organ perfusion. Inotropes should be cautiously weaned despite adequate hemodynamics in anticipation of this deterioration.
- Nonemergent cardiovascular surgery patients can usually be extubated safely during this period. The major criteria for extubation are adequate central nervous system function, stable hemodynamics without malignant arrhythmias, normothermia, low A-a gradient, adequate pulmonary mechanics, and

TABLE 49.2

TASKS TO BE COMPLETED WITHIN THE FIRST 30 MINUTES OF A PATIENT'S ARRIVAL TO THE ICU FOLLOWING CARDIOVASCULAR SURGERY

Establish monitoring
    Arterial waveform
    Central venous and pulmonary artery waveforms
    ECG
    Mixed venous oxygen saturation
    Pulse oximetry

Mark and record urometer and mediastinal drains

Re-establish mechanical ventilation

Assess airway control and bilateral air entry
    70%–100% FiO_2
    Tidal volume 8 mL/kg of predicted body weight
    Respiratory rate 14 breaths/min

Directed physical exam
    Airway
    Ventilation
    Adequacy of blood pressure and cardiac output
    Abdomen
    Peripheral pulse exam

Studies
    Arterial blood gas, electrolytes, ionized calcium,
        hematocrit, platelet count, and coagulation studies
    Chest radiograph

Transfer responsibility of patient care from perioperative team to ICU team

Verbal sign-out of patient's clinical history and perioperative course

ICU, intensive care unit; ECG, electrocardiogram; FiO_2, fraction of inspired oxygen.

no ongoing mediastinal hemorrhage. Early extubation is not suitable for patients with deep hypothermic circulatory arrest, long CPB periods, poor ventricular function, unstable hemodynamics, or a large anticipated transfusion requirement.

The Next 16 Hours after Cardiopulmonary Bypass

- Changes in heart compliance
  - Clinically, the heart seems to become noncompliant or "stiff" leading to reduced cardiac output at any given filling pressure. One usually observes a rise in pulmonary artery pressure and pulmonary artery occlusion pressure (PAOP), and a reduction in the systemic arterial pressure, cardiac output, and mixed venous oxygen saturation.
  - Patients with a low cardiac output syndrome before the onset of changes in compliance often develop hemodynamic instability.
- Time course
  - The usual time course is a steady deterioration in cardiac performance between the 8th to 12th hours following CPB. The condition stabilizes and generally persists over the next 12 to 24 hours, followed by a gradual improvement over the next 48 hours.
  - Once unstable, far more interventions are required to return to a steady state than if problems are anticipated and

stability maintained. Even if cardiac output remains low during this time, it is better tolerated than marked swings in hemodynamics.
- Optimizing the determinants of cardiac output
  - Heart rate and rhythm. The ventricles are stiff and noncompliant, so slower heart rates do not necessarily lead to increased filling and improved stroke volume. Optimal heart rates of 90 to 110 beats/minute are typically necessary. Atrial fibrillation may be poorly tolerated as the noncompliant ventricles depend on atrial contraction for filling; sinus rhythm should be restored.
  - Volume loading to a PAOP beyond 12 to 14 mm Hg is unlikely to lead to significant increases in stroke volume due to noncompliance (unless the patient has an underlying stiff myocardium). Once in this range, attention should be turned to other determinants of cardiac output to improve cardiac performance.
  - Afterload reduction improves cardiac performance without increasing myocardial oxygen consumption ($M\dot{V}O_2$), but institute cautiously to avoid hypotension. Renal function in older patients may be particularly sensitive to decreases in perfusion pressure. Patients with recent right ventricular infarcts and right ventricular stunning are also sensitive to hypotension.
- Patients with a relatively normal cardiac output before surgery often poorly tolerate a cardiac index <2.0 L/minute/m^2, venous PO_2 <30 mm Hg, or $S\bar{V}O_2$ <50%. Although costly in terms of $M\dot{V}O_2$, enhancement of cardiac contractility is an effective method to augment cardiac output until reversible cardiac dysfunction related to CPB and reperfusion effects have resolved. Moderate doses of inotropes are generally well tolerated by completely revascularized patients and those with valvular disease, but can cause myocardial ischemia in incompletely revascularized patients. Myocardial ischemia
  - Increases in heart rate, filling pressures, and contractility to support patients during this period may cause myocardial ischemia from increased $M\dot{V}O_2$.
  - An electrocardiogram should be obtained immediately after surgery and as clinically indicated thereafter. Continuous telemetry should be monitored closely for ischemic changes in the ST segment.
  - Cardiac enzymes are usually not helpful in this early period because they typically rise in all cardiovascular surgery patients. Although, an unusually high enzyme level or a sudden change in the usual pattern of enzyme leak may be useful.
  - If acute graft closure is suspected after a coronary artery bypass, echocardiography should show a new segmental wall motion abnormality. Comparison with intraoperative transesophageal studies is particularly useful. If bypass graft failure of a large myocardial territory is suspected, coronary angiography with either percutaneous or open surgical reintervention may be indicated.

The Second 24 Hours after Cardiopulmonary Bypass

- Cardiovascular function typically improves; small increases in the mixed venous oxygen saturation ($S\bar{V}O_2$) and cardiac output, together with a noticeable decrease in fluid requirements, herald this recovery phase. Invasive monitoring with arterial and pulmonary artery catheters should be maintained until patients demonstrate recovery.

- Patients with normal preoperative systolic ventricular function usually tolerate weaning of inotropes, the amount of active intervention is largely determined by the function of other organ systems such as the lungs and kidneys. Patients with preoperative decompensated left ventricular function should have slow wean inotropes, active diuresis, and substitution of oral afterload-reducing drugs, particularly angiotensin-converting enzyme (ACE) inhibitors.
- If not extubated in the early postoperative period, the patient should be continuously re-evaluated for extubation to limit their risk for ventilator-associated complications.
- For patients who have undergone routine elective procedures, transfer to a step-down telemetry ward may be considered. Important criteria include adequate central nervous system (CNS) function, no or trivial requirement for inotropes, no dependence on temporary pacemaker leads, and good pulmonary toilet.

The Third 24 Hours after Cardiopulmonary Bypass

- Patient care is focused on the transition from ICU to ward care. Compliance in the left ventricle should improve rapidly accompanied by a decrease in interstitial pulmonary water. Improved cardiac performance at lower filling pressure can be anticipated. Mobilization of third-spaced fluid occurs, and active diuresis should be instituted as is physical rehabilitation with emphasis on pulmonary toilet and early ambulation.
- Oral medications oriented more toward long-term cardiovascular risk reduction, such as β-blockers, aspirin, and statins, are started. ACE inhibitors are favored in patients with valvular heart disease, particularly those with adverse left ventricular remodeling preoperatively. IV insulin is transitioned to long-acting subcutaneous regimens.

Catheters and Tubes

- Mediastinal drains, pacing wires, arterial lines, Foley catheters, and pulmonary artery catheters often can be removed. If continuous invasive cardiac monitoring is still necessary, a central venous pressure (CVP) catheter will measure right ventricular filling pressure. The association of CVP and PAOP will be known by this point (although this may change), and left heart filling pressures can be estimated. Venous saturation from the superior caval–atrial junction correlate closely with the $S\overline{V}O_2$ in the absence of a left-to-right shunt.

Arrhythmias

- Despite rapid improvements in this period, atrial arrhythmias including flutter and fibrillation are prominent. The atrial contribution to cardiac output remains high and a rapid heart rate may not be well tolerated.
- Patients undergoing elective cardiovascular procedures are frequently on β-blockers preoperatively. Amiodarone and atorvastatin have also shown promise for prophylaxis against atrial fibrillation. Postoperatively, all patients are begun on low-dose metoprolol as soon as inotropes are discontinued and up-titrated as the blood pressure and heart rate permit. For patients with depressed left ventricular function who require prolonged inotropic support, amiodarone may be used for arrhythmia prophylaxis.
- The mainstays of atrial fibrillation treatment in the hemodynamically stable patient include diuresis, aggressive repletion of serum potassium and magnesium, IV amiodarone loading, and IV β-blockers.
- IV calcium channel blockers and procainamide are used occasionally in certain circumstances. Procainamide is useful in heart transplant recipients who are still on inotropic support to avoid long-acting agents such as amiodarone, which may have a prolonged slowing effect on sinus and atrioventricular node function.
- Hemodynamic instability with the onset of atrial fibrillation should be treated with synchronized direct-current cardioversion. Whenever feasible, rapid atrial pacing should be attempted to suppress by overdrive pacing atrial flutter with a 2:1 block.

Monitoring and Managing Cardiovascular Performance

Arterial Blood Pressure

- Most adults require a mean arterial pressure (MAP) of at least 50 to 55 mm Hg for overall systemic perfusion, especially cerebral and renal perfusion. Older patients, particularly with severe atherosclerotic disease, may require a MAP of 65 mm Hg or higher depending on their baseline.
- Pulse pressure is a useful indicator of systemic perfusion and left ventricular ejection volume. Poorer ventricular ejection is observed when the dicrotic notch is at the base of the arterial pressure trace compared to when it is located midway up the down slope of the tracing, resulting in a larger area under the arterial pressure curve.
- Harmonic augmentation characterized by a sharp, spiked arterial pressure tracing with virtually no dicrotic notch suggests an increase in peripheral vascular tone.
- A central arterial pressure reading provides a better and more reliable assessment of overall hemodynamic function and cardiac output.

Heart Rate and Rhythm

- Normally, the atrial contraction or "kick" contributes approximately 5% of the cardiac output. However, in the postoperative patient, this may be as high as 30%. Minimizing the incidence of atrial fibrillation and maintaining sinus rhythm are as important after cardiovascular surgery.

Pacemakers

- Temporary epicardial atrial and ventricular pacing wires are commonly placed at the completion of cardiovascular procedures and can be invaluable both diagnostically and therapeutically. Heart rates of 90 to 110 beats/minute are important to optimize cardiac output of poorly compliant ventricles immediately following cardiovascular surgery and can also suppress premature ventricular beats. Patients with temporary heart block following surgery can have A-V synchrony restored with dual-mode pacing/sensing (DDD) pacemakers.
- An atrial pacing wire may be needed to determine the cardiac rhythm and differentiate supraventricular tachycardia. Simply connect the atrial pacing wire to the right arm ECG

limb lead and observe the rhythm of leads I, II, or III. The contour of the left and right atrial waveforms is another way of determining sinus rhythm.

Ventricular Preload

- The load that determines resting muscle length is primarily manipulated by fluid administration. Maintain cardiac preload at an adequate but not excessive level with the left ventricular end-diastolic pressure (PAOP) between 12 and 14 mm Hg.

Fluid Administration

- Increasing right and left ventricular filling pressures to their upper limits (16–20 mm Hg) exacerbates several problems that are difficult to manage later, especially pulmonary dysfunction. Immediately after CPB, colloid oncotic pressure is reduced by as much as 50% and returns to normal over a 2-week period of time. In addition, neutrophil and endothelial activation following CPB increase pulmonary vascular permeability, promoting increased pulmonary interstitial water accumulation and pulmonary edema.

Crystalloids and Colloids

- The focus of this debate concerns the administration of crystalloid versus colloid (blood products, albumin, or hydroxyethyl starch) solutions. Sole reliance on crystalloid solutions such as Ringer lactate may result in an inordinate amount of fluid administration to maintain adequate preload. In patients without hemorrhage we use up to 2 L of crystalloid, before 5% albumin is given.
- When the hematocrit is low (<22%) and the patient is bleeding or is hemodynamically unstable, blood products are indicated. If coagulation factors are abnormal and bleeding continues, fresh frozen plasma and platelets should be considered. The threshold to give blood is lowered in patients with incomplete revascularization, low cardiac output, and signs of inadequate oxygen delivery such as low mixed venous oxygen saturation, that is, $S\overline{V}O_2$.

Ventricular Afterload

- Afterload reduction offers the most efficient means to improve cardiac output at little or no expense to myocardial oxygen demand; judicious volume loading should be performed to avoid hypotension and hemodynamic collapse. Especially in patients with severely depressed systolic ventricular function, the ejection fraction can be dramatically improved by a reduction in systemic vascular resistance (SVR) and peripheral vascular resistance (PVR). The extent of afterload reduction that is necessary greatly depends on ventricular performance.

Vasodilators

- Nicardipine hydrochloride (1–15 mg/h), a peripheral acting calcium channel blocker, acts as a direct systemic arterial vasodilator. It is our primary afterload-reducing agent because it is reasonably evanescent, avoids cyanide toxicity, and is less associated with pulmonary artery shunting and ventilation–perfusion (V-Q) mismatch than sodium nitroprusside.
- Sodium nitroprusside increases venous capacitance and directly vasodilates the systemic and pulmonary arterioles. Its advantage is its fast onset of action (15–20 s), allowing rapid titration (0.3–10 μg/kg/min). It can be associated with cyanide toxicity as well as pulmonary artery shunting and V-Q mismatch.
- Nitroglycerin (0.5–2 μg/kg/min) is a venous and arterial vasodilator but primarily a preload-reducing agent with mild afterload-reducing effects including on the coronary arterial tree. An additional advantage with right ventricular failure is its effects on the pulmonary vasculature. It decreases myocardial oxygen consumption and may be especially useful with incomplete revascularization.

Pulmonary Artery Vasodilators

- Right ventricular failure may be the primary cause of low cardiac output in patients who have after right ventricular myocardial infarction, heart transplantation, pulmonary endarterectomy, or CPB in patients with a long-standing history of congestive heart failure.
- The inhaled prostacyclin analogue iloprost is our preferred specific pulmonary artery vasodilator. An important advantage is its ease of administration, it can be delivered intermittently by a nebulizer to either intubated or extubated patients.
- Inhaled nitric oxide has vasodilatory activity restricted to the pulmonary artery tree because of its short half-life but requires continuous delivery by a specialized system and can be used only in intubated patients.
- Hypercapnia and hypoxia should be strictly avoided with marginal or severe right ventricular dysfunction due to their pulmonary vasoconstrictive effects. High FiO_2 can be considered a form of pulmonary vasodilator in this subset of patients.

Vasoconstrictors

- Vasodilation is especially common after prolonged CPB, a period of circulatory arrest, or preoperative treatment with ACE inhibitors. Vasoconstrictors are first-line treatment for low SVR with adequate volume and contractility.
- Phenylephrine hydrochloride (20–180 μg/min), an α-specific catecholamine, acts as a pure peripheral vasoconstrictor. It has a relatively short half-life and can be easily titrated for goal parameters, such as mean arterial blood pressure.
- Vasopressin (1–10 units/h) also acts as a pure peripheral vasoconstrictor. Because of its longer half-life, it is less suited for minute-to-minute changes in blood pressure but may be particularly useful in patients treated preoperatively with ACE inhibitors. Its mechanism of action is synergistic with norepinephrine.

Contractility

- The specific conditions under which the operation was conducted, including repairs performed, completeness of revascularization, length of cardiopulmonary bypass, and myocardial preservation can profoundly influence myocardial contractility.

Inotropes

- Few pharmacologic agents affect only one determinant of cardiac performance; this is especially true of inotropes. A major goal after CPB is to gain cardiac output with as little increase in myocardial oxygen consumption as possible.
- Epinephrine (0.01–0.10 μg/kg/min), can be particularly useful to support right ventricular function. Above these levels it also has vasoconstrictor and chronotropic effects.

- Norepinephrine (0.01–0.10 μg/kg/min), has stronger vaso-constrictor effects in this range and is associated with improved coronary and splanchnic blood flow.
- Isoproterenol (0.005 and 0.02 μg/kg) is a relatively weak inotrope with primarily chronotropic properties. Used primarily in heart transplant to achieve tachycardia of 100 to 120 beats/minute because of the normal coronary arteries, diastolic dysfunction, and right ventricular distention common in this population.
- Milrinone (optional 50 μg/kg loading dose, then 0.1–0.75 μg/kg/min) is a phosphodiesterase inhibitor with potent inotropic and vasodilatory effects commonly used in patients with pre-existing ventricular systolic dysfunction. It is frequently given in combination with a vasoconstrictor agent.
- Dopamine hydrochloride (3–5 μg/kg/min) can be used to decrease SVR and augment cardiac contractility when a more potent catecholamine is not required. In this dosage range, it also stimulates dopaminergic receptors in the kidney enhancing renal perfusion, although prevention of renal failure has not been documented.
- Dobutamine (3–5 μg/kg/min) has inotropic and vasodilatory effects similar to milrinone. At higher doses, it has α stimulatory effects and acts as a vasoconstrictor.

Cardiac Output and Cardiac Index

- A pulmonary artery catheter measures cardiac output by thermodilution, facilitates calculation of SVR, PVR, pulmonary and intracardiac shunts, and estimates left ventricular end-diastolic pressure (LVEDP) by PAOP. Cardiac output should always be normalized by conversion to cardiac index.
- An index of 2.0 L/minute/m^2 or more is usually sufficient to maintain end organ performance. Chronic low cardiac output pathology may tolerate a lower index in the immediate postoperative period.
- Higher body temperature, agitation, or other concomitant conditions such as sepsis, may lead to cardiac index requirements >2.0 L/minute/m^2. Postoperative stress normally produces cardiac indices approaching 3.5 to 4.0 L/minute/m^2.

Mixed Venous Saturation

- Continuous display of $S\overline{V}O_2$ affords one the opportunity to observe acute and gradual changes in cardiac performance, increasing oxygen consumption ($\dot{V}O_2$), or both.
- Acute changes in $\dot{V}O_2$ and cardiac performance are especially demonstrable during episodes of agitation, tracheal suctioning, and rapid extracellular volume shifts.
- $S\overline{V}O_2$ varies with cardiac output, hemoglobin, SaO_2, and oxygen consumption and is a balance between oxygen delivery and oxygen consumption.
- Equipment used to measure physiologic parameters such as the arterial pressure and $S\overline{V}O_2$ must be calibrated regularly.

Serum Lactate

- As an indicator of anaerobic metabolism, serum lactate can provide information about the adequacy of cardiac performance in meeting the body's oxygen requirement. Several problems, however, limit its ability to assess cardiac performance.
- On arrival to the ICU, lactate values may range between normal (<2.0 mmol/L) to as high as 8 to 9 mmol/L. As body temperature normalizes, serum lactate may actually rise despite improving hemodynamics because underperfused

vascular beds open and release lactate into the systemic circulation.
- The difficulty is whether to attribute a rise in serum lactate to a washout phenomenon or to a diminution of cardiac performance. Evaluation of the cardiac index, $S\overline{V}O_2$, and SVR in conjunction with serial serum lactate determinations helps to resolve this dilemma. Lactate levels should decrease after 8 hours if perfusion is adequate.

Serum Ionized Calcium and Potassium

- Serial measurement of Ca^{2+} is especially helpful when solutions containing protein such as blood, fresh frozen plasma, albumin, or plasma protein solutions are administered. Protein binds calcium and may diminish that which is available for myocardial function.
- Maintenance of adequate serum potassium is crucial, especially after the usually brisk diuresis following CPB and in conjunction with diuretic therapy. Potassium chloride should be considered a first-line agent for prevention and treatment of arrhythmias.

Urine Output

- Initially brisk, urine output alone should not be relied on to judge cardiac performance as it is influenced by numerous variables including high serum glucose, denatured plasma protein fractions, and diuretics during CPB.
- Later, urine output may be influenced by stress hormones such as antidiuretic hormone, aldosterone, and cortisol, which conserve intravascular volume.
- Almost all patients have excess total body water but intravascular volume is variable because of third-spacing related to increased capillary permeability and post-CPB inflammation.
- Diuretic therapy is directed to low normal filling pressures, as long as hemodynamics are not compromised, to minimize interstitial lung water and improve pulmonary function. Diuresis should be performed cautiously when ventricular compliance is poor, especially with concentric ventricular hypertrophy, and cardiac function may be especially preload dependent.

Special Concerns

- Bleeding
  - Severe postoperative bleeding occurs in 3% to 5% of patients who undergo CPB.
  - **Causes**
    - Inadequate surgical hemostasis should always be suspected.
    - At least half have acquired hemostatic defects including activation of fibrinolysis, decreased clotting factors, and transient platelet dysfunction.
    - Preoperative use of antiplatelet agents such as clopidogrel and aspirin are associated with increased postoperative transfusion requirements.
  - **Treatment**
    - Antifibrinolytic agents, such as epsilon aminocaproic acid, are begun intraoperatively to decrease transfusions in high-risk subpopulations. No evidence supports use in the postoperative period. Aprotinin is not available.
    - Recombinant activated factor VII and XIII replacement is an emerging strategy.

- Isolated activated partial thromboplastin time elevation may indicate heparin rebound reversible with protamine sulfate administration.
  - Point-of-care platelet function assays may be useful for directing platelet transfusion, even in patients without thrombocytopenia.
- Blood loss of >3 mL/kg/hour for several consecutive hours prompts a return to the operating room. Evacuation of the mediastinal hematoma frequently improves coagulopathy even when no surgical bleeding is identified. Brisk hemorrhage should be re-explored even before coagulopathy is corrected to prevent cardiac tamponade and hemodynamic collapse.
- **Cardiac tamponade.** Two fairly reliable signs of cardiac tamponade are increased or exaggerated cycling of the systolic blood pressure during positive pressure ventilation, and equalization of right and left atrial and pulmonary artery diastolic pressures. Blood clots on the acute margin of the right ventricle may substantially affect cardiac performance without atrial pressure equalization. A reduction in $S\overline{V}O_2$ and decreased urine output will also be observed. The diagnosis may be suspected with abrupt cessation of drain output and confirmed by echocardiography. In severe low-output states, tamponade must be ruled out by exploration in the operating room or a limited opening of the chest at bedside. Percutaneous drainage is not useful in the immediate postoperative period.
- Thrombocytopenia
  - Platelet counts <100,000/μL are common and managed by removal of offending agents. Causes include platelet activation and consumption during CPB, mechanical destruction by intravascular devices, and inadequate production.
  - If counts fall more than 50% or a thrombotic event occurs between 4 and 14 days of heparin exposure, heparin-induced thrombocytopenia (HIT) should be excluded. If diagnosed or strongly suspected, a nonheparin anticoagulant such as lepirudin or bivalirudin should be considered to prevent thrombotic complications.
  - For patients who require long-term anticoagulation for DVT, warfarin can be started once platelet levels are in the normal range.
- Ventilator management
  - Ventilator management after cardiac surgery is directed toward optimizing pulmonary function without compromising hemodynamics. Acute hemodynamic changes may indicate patient distress. Patient dyssynchrony with the ventilator should prompt assessment of sedation and analgesia.
  - Positive end-expiratory pressure (PEEP) above 8 to 10 cm H_2O, may affect chamber filling and decrease cardiac performance. With high PEEP, intravascular volume may be necessary to raise the effective LVEDP, though the amount of pressure transmitted through diseased lungs may vary.
  - Nitroprusside and to a lesser extent nicardipine in heavy smokers or patients with severe chronic lung disease may increase pulmonary shunting and cause hypoxia. Bronchodilators and PEEP rarely correct this and alternative agents such as nitroglycerin (3–5 μg/kg/min) or hydralazine should be used.
  - Acute respiratory distress syndrome (ARDS) is much less frequent due, in part, to shorter CPB times and the use of membrane oxygenators. When ARDS does occur, it may be accompanied by multiple organ dysfunction syndrome or sepsis.
- Diuretics
  - Diuresis is desirable during the recovery period to reverse hemodilution and improve pulmonary function, but should always be closely monitored. A 24-hour diuresis goal is set with reassessments to avoid hypovolemia.
  - Excessive diuresis of 500 to 1,500 mL over several hours may rapidly deplete intravascular volume, reduce cardiac performance and promote increased SVR.
  - Relatively small doses of furosemide (10–20 mg) every 4 to 8 hours as needed spares the patient rapid volume shifts and produces a gradual negative fluid balance. In patients with marginal ventricular or renal function, a continuous infusion at doses up to 20 mg/hour may be necessary.
  - Intermittent doses of thiazide diuretics are a useful adjunct to therapy.
- Renal failure
  - Acute tubular necrosis may develop with an extremely low cardiac output or hypotension during the first 24 hours after CPB. Most respond to adequate volume maintenance and diuretic therapy and can be kept in a nonoliguric renal failure. Some, especially those with a preoperative creatinine clearance <50 mL/minute, may develop oliguric or anuric renal failure.
  - **Diuretics.** Patients with oliguria should be given a test bolus of furosemide (60–120 mg) and be evaluated for a urine response >50 mL/hour. A continuous infusion up to 20 mg/hour with intermittent doses of thiazide diuretics usually maintains urine output and avoids gross volume overload. Avoiding hypovolemia is also essential.
  - **Ultrafiltration.** Patients with renal failure and volume overload who fail initial diuretic therapy may be candidates for ultrafiltration to remove excess salt and water without clinically significant effects on hemodynamics or electrolyte balance. Standard central or peripheral venous catheters can be used for access.
  - **Dialysis.** Intravascular volume overload and inadequate clearance of potassium are the principal indications for dialysis. The overall goal is to remove excess water and solutes while maintaining cardiovascular stability, this is best achieved with continuous venovenous hemodialysis (CVVHD). CVVHD offers good clearance and accurate control of ultrafiltration that is adaptable to the patient's hemodynamic requirements. Average filter life is 16 to 24 hours, heparin should be administered to prolong filter life if postoperative bleeding is not a concern.
  - Patients should be transitioned to conventional hemodialysis only after a significant period of myocardial recovery. Blood flow rates of at least 200 mL/hour are required and result in large volume shifts over a several-hour period.
- Central nervous system complications
  - The incidence of cerebrovascular accidents (CVAs) with focal neurologic sequelae is 2% to 5% but may be lower with advancements in intraoperative technique including routine use of epiaortic ultrasound. Advanced age, history of CVA, peripheral vascular disease, valvular surgery, and procedures requiring a period of circulatory arrest are associated with a higher incidence of central nervous system events.
  - Patients should be continuously assessed for focal motor deficits and the ability to comprehend and follow simple

commands. Focal deficits should prompt noncontrast computed tomography (CT) of the brain to rule out hemorrhagic mass lesions. Magnetic resonance imaging (MRI) may be useful to identify smaller embolic foci. Fresh post-CPB patients are usually poor candidates for thrombolysis because of their risk for bleeding. The treatment for major embolic CNS events is usually supportive. Higher blood pressures may lead to greater perfusion through collaterals in patients with severe occlusive cerebrovascular disease.

- Untoward psychological and cognitive sequelae are more prevalent than focal CVAs. The precise cause of neuropsychological complications remains unclear, however microemboli, especially air, are related to both severe and subtle postoperative neuropsychological deficits.
- **Delirium.** Postcardiotomy delirium is typically preceded by a lucid interval, usually 36 to 48 hours from the time patients awaken from anesthesia. This syndrome is characterized by confusion, disorientation, and disordered thinking and perception. Severe manifestations may include visual and auditory illusions, hallucinations, and paranoid ideation. Treatment consists of undisturbed rest, frequent reorientation, ensuring patient safety, reassurance to both the patient and family, and haloperidol. Avoid benzodiazepines because of the paradoxical excitatory response seen occasionally in the elderly. Subtle changes in mentation and thinking processes occur frequently during the first few weeks after surgery and usually resolve by the sixth postoperative month.
- Sedation and paralysis
  - Shivering, agitation, or both can cause a marked increase in $\dot{V}O_2$ and reduction in $S\bar{V}O_2$, especially in low cardiac output states. Once gross neurologic function is assessed in the immediate postoperative period, these are best treated with narcotic agents. Meperidine is particularly efficacious, although its mechanism is unknown.
  - If early extubation is expected, propofol has a short half-life and is useful for temporary sedation. A combination of narcotic and benzodiazepine infusions are used for prolonged periods of mechanical ventilation. Fentanyl has limited effects on myocardial contractility and the peripheral vasculature.
  - In rare instances, such as severe pulmonary artery hypertension and right heart failure, a paralytic agent may be indicated to prevent any respiratory effort, which can trigger increased pulmonary artery pressures and precipitate hemodynamic collapse. Because of their association with critical illness neuropathy, we prefer to avoid paralytic agents and treat these patients with deep sedation. When required, vecuronium has a lesser chronotropic effect than pancuronium.
- Mechanical cardiac assistance
  - **Intra-aortic balloon pumps (IABP).** When patients fail to respond to moderately high-dose inotropic drug combinations such as epinephrine and milrinone, IABP therapy should be considered early and can be instituted at the bedside by a percutaneous technique. The IABP improves cardiac performance primarily by afterload reduction and augmentation of systemic diastolic pressure, thereby increasing coronary artery perfusion pressure. Its main contraindications are aortic insufficiency and aortoiliac occlusive disease. Complications and adverse effects include platelet consumption, catheter sepsis, and lower extremity ischemic complications.

- **Ventricular assist devices (VAD) and total artificial hearts.** VADs replace the function of either or both ventricles until myocardial recovery occurs or cardiac transplantation can be performed. End-stage congestive heart failure patients who are not transplant candidates may have a VAD placed as destination therapy. Currently, total artificial heart therapy remains experimental and is limited to research protocols.
  - In some cases, extracorporeal membrane oxygenation (ECMO) is indicated for profound cardiorespiratory failure.
- Blood glucose control
  - For cardiac surgery patients, tight blood glucose control (blood glucose 80–110 mg/dL) reduces the incidence of mediastinitis, atrial fibrillation, ischemia, length of stay, hospital costs, and mortality in both diabetic and nondiabetic patients. Nearly all adult patients require an intravenous insulin infusion through the immediate postoperative period if normoglycemia is to be maintained.
  - Once taking an oral diet, the patient is transitioned to a long-acting insulin formulation to cover basal needs and fast-acting insulin based on the percentage of meals consumed.
- Catheter sepsis
  - Bloodstream infections have particularly significant implications in cardiovascular surgery patients as prosthetic intravascular devices are frequently implanted during surgery and multiple invasive monitoring catheters are used.
  - The incidence of sepsis increases when invasive monitoring catheters are left in place longer than 72 hours, for straightforward cases they should be removed by this time. All peripheral lines are changed with transfer to the intermediate care floor.
  - The critically ill, who require prolonged invasive monitoring, are observed closely for signs of sepsis such as fever and leukocytosis, with a low threshold to remove old lines. Rewiring catheters is avoided, new catheter insertion at a different site is preferred.
- Clinical pathways
  - Coronary artery bypass grafting (CABG) procedures were among the first to benefit from clinical pathways to improve the continuity and coordination of care. CABG procedures are common, usually elective, have typical recovery milestones, and require coordination of multidisciplinary provider teams, which make pathways extremely useful to support both clinical and administrative management. Pathways for other cardiovascular procedures including heart valve surgery and transplantation have been developed as well.
  - When successfully implemented, they encourage the use of clinical guidelines, follow a timeline, improve multidisciplinary teamwork, reduce variations in patient care, and improve clinical outcomes.
  - It is important that clinical pathways not discourage personalized care and that they function well even in the face of unexpected changes in a patient's condition.
- Cardiac surgery databases
  - Institutional and multi-institutional databases are useful tools to track outcomes following cardiovascular operations, conduct clinical research, and guide continuous quality improvement. The data collected is clinical, administrative, or both.

- Data is also used by various regulatory bodies and third-party payers to monitor health care quality and costs; in the future it will also be used for pay-for-performance initiatives.
- The Society of Thoracic Surgeons Cardiac Database is the largest clinical cardiothoracic surgery database in the world and currently has more than 500 participating sites. This allows risk modeling for common procedures and provides individual institutions with comparative outcomes data and national benchmarks.
- All databases are limited by the variable quality of collected data, which in many instances is self-reported. Comparison of outcomes is also subject to selection bias not corrected by imprecise risk models.

Special Clinical Scenarios

- Off-pump coronary artery bypass (OPCAB) surgery
  - OPCAB avoids diffuse inflammatory response, multiorgan dysfunction, and neurocognitive complications that may follow after CPB (Table 49.3).
  - There are several important differences for expedited care after OPCAB surgery.
    - Decreased need for inotropic support, most likely from avoidance of global ischemia and reduced myocardial stunning.
    - Euvolemia is more likely in the immediate postoperative period as systemic inflammatory response and capillary leak related to CPB are avoided.
    - A relatively hypercoagulable state as opposed to the coagulopathy typical after CPB. This reduces postoperative hem-

---

TABLE 49.3

BENEFITS OF OFF-PUMP CORONARY ARTERY BYPASS GRAFTING DEMONSTRATED IN PROSPECTIVE, RANDOMIZED STUDIES

Myocardial protection
   Reduced release of cardiac enzymes
   Decreased need for inotropic support
   Fewer postoperative arrhythmias
Pulmonary function
   Decreased requirement for mechanical ventilation
Renal protection
   Improved preservation of glomerular filtration and renal
     tubular function
Coagulation
   Decreased coagulopathy
   Decreased transfusion requirement
Inflammation
   Reduced release of cytokines
   Reduced complement activation
   Decreased incidence of postoperative infections
Neurocognitive function
   Improved early postoperative neurocognitive function
Resource utilization
   Decreased total resource utilization

Reproduced from Song HK, Puskas JD. Off-pump coronary artery bypass surgery. In: Kaiser LR, Kron IL, Spray TL, eds. *Mastery of Cardiothoracic Surgery.* 2nd ed. Philadelphia, PA: Lippincott Williams & Wilkins; 2007:455, with permission.

---

orrhage and transfusion requirements but has the potential to adversely affect graft patency. In addition to daily aspirin as with conventional CABG, clopidogrel (75 mg/d) is started once chest tube drainage has been low for 3 consecutive hours.
- Persistent or massive hemorrhage is more likely surgical and not related to factor or platelet deficiency.
- One of the major benefits to the healthcare system benefits is the potential for reduced resource use, especially length of mechanical ventilation and ICU stay.
- Thoracic aortic surgery
  - Patients undergoing surgery for disorders of the thoracic aorta present critical care providers with several unique challenges, including neurologic complications, hemodynamic disturbances, and malperfusion syndromes. Several of these conditions are caused by the period of circulatory arrest that the patient undergoes during the conduct of the surgical repair whereas others are caused by the specific anatomy of the underlying thoracic aortic pathology.
  - **Circulatory arrest sequelae.** Aortic arch procedures usually have a period of circulatory arrest during the operation, which increases the risk for neurologic complications. Elderly patients with prolonged (>30 min) hypothermic circulatory arrest typically have neurologic dysfunction resulting in agitation and delirium. Although transient, it may necessitate a several-day period of supportive care including mechanical ventilation.
    - Circulatory arrest is also associated with profound coagulopathy. This is especially problematic with long suture lines and friable aortic tissue, hypertension should be avoided. Surgical bleeding should always be suspected with brisk hemorrhage.
    - Complex vascular repairs with long bypass times and circulatory arrest may develop profound vasodilatory shock recalcitrant to vasopressors. The cause is unclear but may be related to bacterial translocation of intestinal flora. Patients should be volume resuscitated and supported with vasopressors and inotropes as needed. With profound vasodilation, intravenous steroids and methylene blue allows reduction of high dose vasopressors.
  - **Spinal cord ischemia.** This occurs during thoracoabdominal aneurysm repair and is exacerbated by postoperative hypoperfusion, particularly when the artery of Adamkiewicz is not reconstituted. Anterior spinal artery syndrome results with impaired lower extremity motor function and, to a lesser degree, impaired sensation. When suspected, a lumbar drain should be placed if not already done intraoperatively. Cerebrospinal fluid (CSF) drainage for pressures 10 mm Hg or higher, and maintaining the mean arterial blood pressure 85 to 100 mm Hg has led to reversal of acute lower extremity neurologic findings. MRI is useful for confirming the diagnosis but should not be delay initiation of treatment.
  - **Malperfusion syndromes.** In patients with aortic dissection, branch orifices become obstructed by the dissected intimal flap or inadequate perfusion by the false lumen causing malperfusion of virtually any limb or end organ, depending on the anatomic extent of the dissection. Patients with ascending aorta involvement (Stanford type A) typically undergo emergency surgery whereas patients with only descending aorta involvement (Stanford type B) are treated initially with medical therapy. After repair of an ascending aortic dissection, patients are frequently left with residual

dissection involving the descending aorta; therefore malperfusion syndromes may develop in both groups. Patients should undergo serial peripheral pulse, neurologic, and abdominal exams; serial arterial blood gases, liver enzymes, and lactate levels are useful when visceral malperfusion is suspected. Angiography and interventional techniques such as fenestration or stenting can frequently be used to diagnose and treat malperfusion during the same procedure. Laparotomy may be occasionally required for visceral malperfusion that progresses to bowel infarction.

CHAPTER 50 ■ MANAGEMENT OF THE PEDIATRIC CARDIAC SURGICAL PATIENT

The successful collaboration of numerous disciplines including pediatric cardiac surgery, anesthesia, cardiology, and intensive care over the past several decades have led to an increase in the complexity of cardiac lesions repaired, with a simultaneous reduction in surgical mortality. This chapter focuses on the key principles for successful management of the pediatric cardiac surgical patient, including assessment of the preoperative status and operative course, postoperative stabilization, subsequent evaluation of the repair, and support of myocardial function.

CARDIAC INTENSIVE CARE: A SPECIALIZED ENVIRONMENT

- The pediatric cardiac intensive care unit (CICU) must be equipped with bedside monitors able to display vital signs and transduce several pressures simultaneously as many patients have several intracardiac catheters for postoperative hemodynamic monitoring. Storing at least 24 hours of hemodynamic data and alarms is often important for reconstructing critical events and trending a patient's recovery or deterioration over time.
- Ventilators capable of supporting patients of all sizes (from premature neonates through adults) should be readily available. Specialized ventilators such as the oscillator should be also available for patients with coexisting lung disease. There should be several ventilators capable of delivering inhaled nitric oxide, essential in treatment of pulmonary hypertension (PH), as multiple patients commonly receive this therapy simultaneously.
- Bedside blood gas analysis testing devices are the norm at many institutions. If unavailable, a laboratory turnaround time of <15 to 30 minutes is necessary.
- A portable electrocardiogram (ECG) machine and defibrillator are essential devices for bedside diagnosis, cardioversion, and emergency defibrillations. Most contemporary battery-operated temporary pacemakers can deliver rapid atrial pacing to terminate tachyarrhythmia including re-entrant supraventricular tachycardia and atrial flutter.
- Echocardiography allows for rapid assessment of residual lesions or tamponade. A mediastinal cart or tray for emergent bedside sternotomy is required and also facilitates emergency cannulation for extracorporeal membrane oxygenation (ECMO).

POSTOPERATIVE ASSESSMENT AND STABILIZATION

Transition from the Operating Room

- Patients are the most vulnerable to decompensation during the first several hours after cardiopulmonary bypass (CPB). The medical decision making and patient management should be provided by the anesthesia and surgical team until a complete exchange of information occurs.
- Key operative events are details of the repair, length of CPB including any special techniques used such as deep hypothermic circulatory arrest or low-flow regional perfusion; abnormal rhythms; or significant bleeding after CPB.
- Key anesthesia events are airway issues such as difficulty with bag-mask ventilation or tracheal intubation; type of anesthesia given, including cumulative dose of narcotics and benzodiazepines; current vasoactive and inotropic support;, and blood and colloid products administered.
- If the sternum is left open, it is important to know whether this is for excessive bleeding, poor myocardial function, or difficulty with ventilation, as each has different implication for management strategies in the first postoperative hours.
- The initial assessment of the repair typically includes transesophageal or epicardial echocardiography, intracardiac saturation to assess for residual shunts, and hemodynamic pressure measurements. If a second CPB run is required to correct residual lesions, this can have important effects on myocardial function. The physical exam should focus on clinical cardiac output and evidence for residual lesions.
- Murmurs are expected after some procedures (e.g., aortopulmonary shunt) but abnormal in others (e.g., ventricular septal defect [VSD] repair).
- Cavopulmonary connections such as the bidirectional Glenn or Fontan procedure should have a quiet precordial exam;

murmurs may indicate outflow tract obstruction or atrioventricular valve regurgitation.

- Arterial blood gas interpretation requires understanding of the patient's physiology. With two-ventricle physiology in the absence of significant pulmonary pathology, a high arterial partial pressure of O_2 (PaO_2) is expected on 100% oxygen (O_2). Mild hyperventilation ($PaCO_2$ 30–35 mm Hg) may be indicated in PH to reduce pulmonary vascular resistance (PVR).
  - Patients with large left-to-right shunts preoperatively may have significant alveolar–arterial gradients from pulmonary edema.
  - After right ventriculotomy, right ventricular (RV) dysfunction and elevated central venous pressures may cause right-to-left shunt through a patent foramen ovale with PaO_2 <100 mm Hg regardless of the fraction of inspired oxygen (FiO_2).
  - PaO_2 35 to 45 mm Hg is targeted in single-ventricle patients to prevent pulmonary overcirculation and systemic undercirculation. Pulmonary overcirculation may be treated with hypoventilation ($PaCO_2$ 45–50 mm Hg) to increase PVR.
  - Metabolic acidosis should raise concern for low cardiac output syndrome requiring judicious intravascular volume supplementation, increased inotropic support, and maximization of oxygen-carrying capacity. If the cause is unclear or initial measures fail to improve cardiac output, urgent bedside echocardiography should be performed to evaluate the repair and myocardial function and look for possible tamponade.
- Higher initial ICU lactate (9.4 vs. 5.6 mmol/L) and levels that continue to rise >0.75 mmol/L/hour are associated with poorer outcome (death or use of ECMO).
- Prothrombin time (PT), partial thromboplastin time (PTT), fibrinogen, and platelet count should be normal and aggressively corrected for bleeding. Protamine can be given for a prolonged PTT, but if all coagulation parameters are corrected excessive bleeding persists, an antifibrinolytic such as tranexamic acid or ε-aminocaproic acid may be considered. Aprotinin is currently not available until further studies are done. Activated factor VIIa has been used for refractory bleeding in post-CPB ECMO. Pronounced bleeding despite aggressive pharmacologic and blood product transfusion may be surgical, and brisk bleeding that stops abruptly with a concurrent rise in intracardiac pressures is likely tamponade; both require chest exploration.
- A chest radiograph performed minutes after arrival will verify tracheal tube, nasogastric tube, pacing wire, and intracardiac catheter placement; assess cardiac size and rule out a significant pneumothorax or hemothorax. A right or common atrial catheter enters the right atrial (RA) appendage and is directed inferiorly. A left atrial (LA) catheter usually enters a right pulmonary vein taking a horizontal course, alternatively it enters the LA appendage and courses inferiorly. A pulmonary artery (PA) catheter enters the right ventricular outflow tract and is directed superiorly into the main PA. An RV catheter tip sits in the body of the RV.
- A 12- or 15-lead ECG should be performed to assess rhythm and atrioventricular (AV) conduction. Lack of AV synchrony can contribute to a low cardiac output state; temporary pacing for AV nodal block or an ectopic junctional rhythm may be needed. The QRS complex should be assessed for new

abnormalities including bundle branch block. Complete right bundle branch block is common after VSD closure but not usually of hemodynamic significance. Assess the ST segment for signs of ischemia, especially after procedures that include coronary artery reimplantation.

- After the initial assessment and stabilization, a plan is made for weaning inotropes, ventilatory support, analgesia, and sedation over the subsequent hours to days.
  - Older children with short CPB support times, stable hemodynamics, and minimal chest bleeding (e.g., conduit revisions, subaortic membrane resections, septal defect closures) can be extubated when they awaken from anesthesia.
  - Neonates and younger infants often undergo more complex repairs and will need more gradual weaning of support over 24 to 48 hours. Those undergoing complex neonatal single-ventricle palliation often require several days of stabilization and diuresis before their sternums can be closed.

Hemodynamic Monitoring

- Intracardiac catheters are invaluable and have a low risk of complications.
  - Transthoracic RA catheters are also known as common atrial catheters in single-ventricle patients, as common atrium is either created or congenitally present.
  - Transthoracic LA catheters are typically used in young infants with complex two-ventricle or a mitral valve repair to assess LV and mitral valve function and intravascular volume.
  - Transthoracic PA catheters are placed for selected repairs including truncus arteriosus and tetralogy of Fallot (TOF). With intraoperative transesophageal echocardiography, these catheters are less common and reserved for procedures where the incidence of postoperative PH is high, such as repair of obstructed total anomalous pulmonary venous return.
  - Transthoracic RV catheters are more common; entering through the RA appendage the tip crosses the tricuspid valve to assess RV and PA pressures after complex PA reconstructions.
  - In contrast to adults, children rarely have flow-directed PA (Swan-Ganz) catheters placed due to both small patient size and the need for unobstructed access for intracardiac repairs.
- Mean RA pressure ranges from 0 to 8 mm Hg; mean LA pressure is typically 1 to 2 mm Hg higher; abnormal pressures have multiple causes (Tables 50.1 and 50.2). Postoperative pressures are higher owing to CPB effects on the myocardium and the volume of fluid received but should not exceed 15 mm Hg.
  - The onset is important as gradually increasing pressures often indicate a clinical problem such as low cardiac output or tamponade physiology is evolving. A sudden change without changes in rhythm or other vital signs may indicate a technical problem with the catheter or transducer.
  - The morphology of the atrial tracing is also helpful. Large A waves, referred to as *cannon A waves*, result from loss of AV synchrony when the atrium contracts against a closed AV valve as in AV block or junctional rhythm. Large V waves occur during ventricular contraction with an incompetent AV valve.

TABLE 50.1

CAUSES OF ELEVATED OR REDUCED RIGHT ATRIAL PRESSURE

Elevated
Volume overload
Right ventricular dysfunction
   Systolic dysfunction
   Diastolic dysfunction or noncompliance
Tricuspid stenosis
Tricuspid regurgitation
Tamponade
Loss of atrioventricular synchrony from heart block, junctional rhythm
Tachyarrhythmia
Catheter or transducer malposition or malfunction

Reduced
Volume depletion
   Inadequate preload
   Bleeding
Catheter or transducer malposition or malfunction

- Low atrial filling pressures in the setting of low arterial blood pressure or cardiac output should be treated with volume expansion. Typically, 5 to 10 mL/kg of colloid or crystalloid is the initial dose to restore preload.
- Causes of abnormal PA or RV pressures are listed in Table 50.3. Normal mean PA pressures are 10 to 20 mm Hg; considerable postoperative variation is possible but should not exceed 25 to 30 mm Hg. Elevated pulmonary pressures are not well tolerated for long periods of time; quickly correct hypocarbia and acidosis, which increase PVR. Inhaled nitric oxide is useful for PH and low cardiac output. The RV systolic pressure, often expressed as a percentage, should be <30% to 50% of the systemic systolic pressure.
- Causes of abnormal RA, LA, and PA saturations are listed in Table 50.4. Accurate interpretation relies on precise knowl-

TABLE 50.2

CAUSES OF ELEVATED OR REDUCED LEFT ATRIAL PRESSURE

Elevated
Volume overload
Left ventricular dysfunction
   Systolic dysfunction
   Diastolic dysfunction or noncompliance
Mitral stenosis
Mitral regurgitation
Left-to-right shunt
Tamponade
Loss of AV synchrony from heart block, junctional rhythm
Tachyarrhythmia
Catheter or transducer malposition or malfunction

Reduced
Volume depletion
Catheter or transducer malposition or malfunction

AV, atrioventricular.

TABLE 50.3

CAUSES OF ELEVATED OR REDUCED PULMONARY ARTERY PRESSURE

Elevated
Primary pulmonary hypertension
Anatomical obstruction
   Pulmonary artery stenosis
   Pulmonary vein stenosis
   Mitral stenosis
Left atrial hypertension
   Ventricular dysfunction
   Mitral valve disease
Hypoxia
   Lung disease (edema, atelectasis)
   Pleural effusion
   Pneumothorax
Acidosis
   Hypoventilation
   Metabolic
Left-to-right shunt
Hyperviscosity (polycythemia)
Catheter or transducer malposition or malfunction

Reduced
Intravascular volume depletion
Obstruction to pulmonary blood flow
Catheter or transducer malposition or malfunction

edge of the catheter tip location and the patient's physiology. RA and PA saturation data are a useful assessment of the patient's cardiac output and oxygen extraction.

- Normal superior vena cava (SVC), RA, and PA saturations with two-ventricle physiology and no intracardiac shunt are approximately 70% to 80%; true mixed venous saturation is in the PA. Elevation after atrial or ventricular septal defect repair indicates a residual left-to-right shunt. An absolute PA saturation of >80% while receiving an FiO_2 <0.4 is predictive of a residual intracardiac shunt of >1.5:1.
- With normal cardiac output and fully saturated systemic arterial blood, the arteriovenous O_2 saturation difference will be 25% to 30%. RA saturation is commonly around 60% after CPB with adequate oxygen delivery and perfusion.
- Lower RA saturations are expected in single-ventricle physiology from intracardiac right-to-left shunting and systemic O_2 desaturation. As long as the arteriovenous saturation difference is ≤30%, the cardiac output should be normal.
- Typically, LA and PA catheters are removed within the first 48 hours while still intubated and with chest tubes in place to monitor for bleeding. Although significant bleeding is rare, catheters are removed with blood available at the bedside. RA catheters may remain in place up to 2 weeks but as soon as clinically indicated.

Postoperative Rhythm and Pacing

- Sinus **bradycardia**, normal in children during sleep and with high vagal tone, is generally well tolerated in the absence of long sinus pauses. Hypothermic patients with core temperatures of 32°C to 34°C will remain bradycardic until their temperature rises. At risk are those undergoing atrial baffles such

TABLE 50.4

CAUSES OF ABNORMAL RIGHT ATRIAL, LEFT ATRIAL, AND PULMONARY ARTERY SATURATION

Location	Elevated	Reduced
Right atrium	Left-to-right atrial shunt Anomalous pulmonary venous return Increased venous oxygen content Decreased oxygen extraction Catheter tip position (near inferior vena cava)	Low cardiac output (increased O_2 extraction) Increased oxygen consumption (fever, high catecholamines) Decreased arterial saturation with normal O_2 extraction Catheter tip position (near coronary sinus) Anemia
Left atrium	Normal is fully saturated	Right-to-left atrial shunt Decreased pulmonary vein saturation (lung disease, arteriovenous malformation)
Pulmonary artery	Left-to-right cardiac shunt Catheter tip wedged (left atrial sample)	Low cardiac output (increased O_2 extraction) Increased oxygen consumption (fever, high catecholamines) Decreased arterial saturation with normal O_2 extraction Anemia

as a lateral tunnel-type Fontan for a single-ventricle defect or atrial switch procedures for transposition of the great arteries. Sinus venosus and primum atrial septal defect repairs also commonly have slower sinus rates. Extremely bradycardic patients can be treated with pacing with temporary epicardial wires.

- Conduction system injury occurs with surgery near the AV node such as VSD repair, AV canal repair, resection of subaortic muscle, and TOF repair. Usually this manifests as bundle branch block, and more significant block, such as complete heart block, is rare. The majority resolve without need for permanent pacemaker placement.
- Common **tachycardias** include supraventricular, junctional, and ectopic tachycardias. High catecholamine states, intracardiac catheters and suture lines, and electrolyte abnormalities all contribute to the appearance of postoperative tachyarrhythmias in previously asymptomatic patients. Most tachyarrhythmias will improve with time.
  - The onset of tachycardia may provide useful information regarding its etiology. A sudden onset with sustained heart rate and minimal variability is likely to be re-entrant, whereas a gradual increase in heart rate with some beat-to-beat variability is likely to be automatic.
  - Temporary epicardial atrial wires can be used to obtain intracardiac atrial electrograms to examine the relationship of the P waves to the QRS complex (Fig. 50.1). Atrial wires can also terminate re-entrant rhythms by overdrive pacing. The indication for treatment is a hemodynamic change causing low cardiac output or blood pressure. A summary of common antiarrhythmics used after congenital heart surgery is provided in Table 50.5.
  - For re-entrant and ectopic supraventricular tachycardias, β-blockers are first-line therapy and well tolerated. Digoxin is considered with apparent accessory pathways that are not pre-excited or for rate control in rapid atrial rhythms. Second-line agents include procainamide and amiodarone. Amiodarone is used with caution, given the high incidence of serious side effects including circulatory collapse and proarrhythmia. Refractory cases may be treated with the class III agent sotalol or class IC agents flecainide or propafenone. The length of treatment, at least 1 to 3 months, will vary with the nature of the tachycardia.

- Junctional ectopic tachycardia is a narrow complex rhythm occurring in the first 24 to 48 hours and is almost always self-limited. Most common after VSD closure in TOF and AV canal repairs, the typical ECG finding is AV dissociation (Fig. 50.2) with a more rapid ventricular rate (typically >180 bpm), but there can be retrograde P waves with a 1:1 relationship. Lack of AV synchrony can cause elevated atrial pressures and low cardiac output with hypotension. Atrial overpacing (if <180 bpm) can restore AV synchrony and improve hemodynamics. Reduce catecholamine states by weaning vasoactive infusions; providing sedation, analgesia, and possibly paralysis; and avoiding hyperthermia with active cooling. The best pharmacologic therapy is procainamide in combination with cooling. Amiodarone should be used with caution. Once normal sinus rhythm is restored, a gradual rewarming and removal of deep sedation and/or paralysis can occur. Pharmacologic support should then be weaned over 24 to 48 hours.

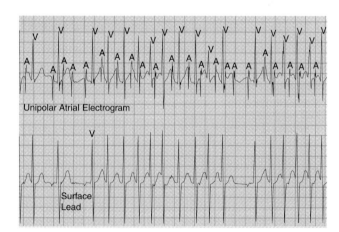

FIGURE 50.1. The use of an atrial electrocardiogram to diagnose ectopic atrial tachycardia. The surface electrocardiogram (*lower tracing*) reveals an irregular, narrow complex rhythm. Atrial depolarizations (P waves) are not easily discernible. The unipolar atrial electrocardiogram (*upper tracing*) reveals a rapid ectopic atrial tachycardia with many blocked atrial premature beats. Atrial depolarization is denoted by "A" and ventricular depolarization is denoted by "V."

TABLE 50.5

COMMON ANTIARRHYTHMIC AGENTS USED AFTER CONGENITAL HEART SURGERY

Drug name	Class/mechanism/indications	Dosing	Considerations/side effects
Adenosine	Blocks AV node; termination of re-entrant SVT	0.1–0.2 mg/kg rapid IV push (max 6 mg)	Sinus arrest (have pacing available); hypotension; bronchospasm
Procainamide	IA, prolongs atrial refractory period; atrial tachycardia (re-entrant SVT, atrial fib/flutter)	5–15 mg/kg IV load (30 min) 20–80 μg/kg/min IV infusion	Myocardial depressant; vasodilator; monitor levels; lupus syndrome with long-term use
Esmolol	II, β-blocker; re-entrant SVT, ectopic atrial tachycardia, ventricular tachycardia	0.1–0.5 mg/kg IV load 50–250 μg/kg/min IV infusion	Myocardial depressant; bradycardia; hypotension; bronchospasm
Amiodarone	III, prolongs atrial and ventricular refractory periods; atrial, junctional, ventricular tachycardia	5 mg/kg IV load (60 min) 5–15 μg/kg/min IV infusion 5–10 mg/kg/day PO	Potent vasodilator and myocardial depressant; proarrhythmic (torsades); hepatic, thyroid, and pulmonary toxicity
Lidocaine	IB, prolongs ventricular refractory period; prevents ventricular ectopy, tachycardia, and fibrillation	1 mg/kg slow IV push 20–50 μg/kg/min IV infusion	Monitor levels; seizures at toxic levels
Verapamil	IV, Ca channel blocker, prolongs AV node refractory period; re-entrant SVT	0.1 mg/kg/dose slow IV push 3–4 mg/kg/day PO divided q8h	Myocardial depressant; avoid in infants; do not use concurrently with β-blockers
Digoxin	Prolongs AV node refractory period; atrial tachycardia except WPW syndrome	20–60 μg/kg IV/PO digitalizing 4–10 μg/kg IV/PO divided q12h	Multiple medication interactions; AV block and proarrhythmic at toxic levels
Propranolol	II, β-blocker; oral treatment atrial tachycardia	2–4 mg/kg/day PO divided q6–8h	Hypotension; hypoglycemia; bronchospasm
Sotalol	III, β-blocker, prolongs atrial and ventricular refractory period; oral treatment, atrial and ventricular tachycardia	80–200 mg/m^2/day PO divided q8–12h	Myocardial depressant
Flecainide, Propafenone	IC, prolongs atrial and ventricular refractory period; oral treatment of atrial tachycardia	Flec: 2–6 mg/kg/day divided q8h Prop: 150–300 mg/m^2/day	Myocardial depressant; proarrhythmic; monitor QRS prolongation

AV, atrioventricular; SVT, supraventricular tachycardia; WPW, Wolf-Parkinson-White; Flec, flecainide; Prop, propafenone.

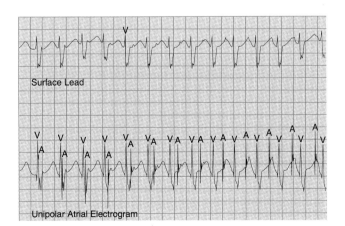

FIGURE 50.2. The use of an atrial electrocardiogram to diagnose junctional ectopic tachycardia. The surface electrocardiogram (*upper tracing*) reveals a regular, narrow complex rhythm with possible atrioventricular (AV) disassociation. The unipolar atrial electrocardiogram (*lower tracing*) demonstrates AV dissociation with a ventricular rate that is more rapid than the atrial rate. This is junctional ectopic tachycardia. Atrial depolarization is denoted by "A" and ventricular (or junctional) depolarization is denoted by "V."

- Ventricular ectopy can occur, especially with electrolyte abnormalities. Monomorphic premature ventricular beats or ventricular bigeminy or trigeminy is usually benign and self-limited. Sustained ventricular tachycardia that is rapid and polymorphic is dangerous and concerning for myocardial ischemia. Treatment with lidocaine and cardioversion should be attempted, but an urgent evaluation of myocardial function and perfusion must be pursued or a cardiac arrest may be imminent.

Respiratory and Ventilatory Management

- Ventilatory support and weaning should be individualized to the physiology and hemodynamic status of each patient using a set of guiding principles. Frequent reassessment and ventilatory adjustments should be expected.
- **Positive pressure ventilation** has effects on preload. Increasing tidal volumes and positive end-expiratory pressure increase intrathoracic pressure, limiting systemic venous return and increasing afterload to the RV.

- With limited RV function, elevated mean airway pressures may result in high right-sided filling pressure, poor RV function, hepatomegaly, ascites, and pleural effusions. With fluid overload and impaired gas exchange, increasing ventilatory support is tempting but may worsen the clinical status. Cavopulmonary connections and passive pulmonary blood flow are also compromised with positive pressure ventilation.
  - A strategy of a larger tidal volume (15 mL/kg) with a lower ventilatory rate may minimize afterload and give the RV an opportunity to eject or the PA additional filling time during a longer expiratory phase. Encourage spontaneous breathing with less mandatory ventilator breaths or extubation if possible.
- Positive pressure has the opposite effect on the LV: The increased intrathoracic pressure decreases transmural pressure across the myocardium to reduce LV afterload. Patients with LV dysfunction have increased pulmonary edema and decreased lung compliance; positive pressure ventilation helps decrease work of breathing and oxygen consumption. A judicious amount of positive end-expiratory pressure at 3 to 5 cm H_2O maintains lung volumes at functional residual capacity to minimize PVR from atelectasis.
- The **mode of ventilation** used depends on the experience of the CICU team, pressure and volume ventilation are equally acceptable. Novel techniques such as high-frequency oscillatory ventilation and airway pressure release ventilation are used successfully with primary lung disease but have limited use after congenital heart surgery due to higher mean airway pressures.
- Prior to extubation, the patient should be awake, not tachypneic for age, hemostatic, and evaluated for significant residual cardiac lesions and the adequacy of myocardial function. Support is weaned to no or few mandatory breaths (4–6 per minute) and an FiO$_2$ of ≤0.4; spontaneous tidal volumes should be 6 to 8 mL/kg.
- Problems encountered after extubation include atelectasis, stridor, and diaphragm paresis or paralysis. Chest physiotherapy and occasionally bronchoscopy may be employed to re-expand atelectatic segments of lung. Stridor, usually self-limited, can be treated with nebulized racemic epinephrine and steroids.
  - Persistent stridor or a weak cry can be a manifestation of recurrent laryngeal nerve injury with vocal cord paresis or paralysis; formal assessment of swallowing function to prevent recurrent aspiration may be required.
  - In phrenic nerve injury, an elevated hemidiaphragm with ipsilateral lung collapse is seen on the postextubation chest radiograph. Decreased (paretic) or paradoxical (paralyzed) movement of the diaphragm on fluoroscopy confirms the diagnosis; the injury usually recovers with time. Ultrasound is less reliable in distinguishing a paretic from a paralyzed diaphragm. Older children often tolerate the injury; neonates and infants may require a hemidiaphragm plication.
- **Noninvasive forms of respiratory support** are being used more commonly. Continuous positive airway pressure and bilevel positive airway pressure delivered with nasal or full-face masks provide positive pressure without a tracheal tube. Utilities include avoiding reintubation for increased work of breathing and providing postextubation systemic afterload reduction.

Sedation, Analgesia, and Neurologic Monitoring

- The strategy should be tailored to the age and anatomy of the patient, type of repair and operative course, and anticipated postoperative course.
- High-dose **narcotics** alleviate the stress response associated with cardiac surgery and CPB; fentanyl (up to 25 μg/kg) can be administered to neonates with minimal hemodynamic effect. Patients with marginal hemodynamics and complex repairs or palliations are initially deeply sedated with continuous fentanyl infusions and usually paralyzed to minimize the stress response and oxygen consumption.
- Of the common **muscle relaxants,** rocuronium has the shortest onset, making it useful for intubation, whereas vecuronium is employed for continuous paralysis. Pancuronium is the longest-acting agent and is cleared by the kidneys. Cisatracurium undergoes Hofmann degradation (i.e., independent of renal and hepatic function); it may be the best choice in multisystem organ failure. The significant side effects of succinylcholine, including severe bradycardia, have limited its routine use.
- Hemodynamically stable patients who require a longer ventilatory course for diuresis or pulmonary recovery benefit from continuous infusions of a narcotic and benzodiazepine though tolerance may develop after 5 to 7 days and require transition to methadone and lorazepam, longer-acting oral agents, for a weaning taper after extubation.
  - Morphine is the most common narcotic used, but fentanyl (shorter-acting) and hydromorphone are alternatives. Bolus dosing of fentanyl may result in an idiosyncratic chest wall rigidity reaction requiring rapid muscle relaxation.
  - Midazolam is the most common benzodiazepine, having sedative and amnestic properties. Lorazepam and diazepam are administered in bolus doses rather than infusions.
- After extubation, transition to oral agents, including acetaminophen, ibuprofen, and oxycodone. Older patients can benefit from narcotic-based patient-controlled analgesia. Short courses of the nonsteroidal anti-inflammatory drug ketorolac (eight doses or less) can be used with normal coagulation and renal function.
- Propofol, a popular sedating agent in adult ICUs, has a rapid onset of action and clearance. It has no analgesic properties, however, and is a potent vasodilator and negative inotrope, limiting use with decreased myocardial function. There are reports of myocardial failure and acidosis in children, so propofol is restricted to short-term use in older patients with two-ventricle physiology and normal myocardial function who are anticipated to extubate within 6 to 12 hours.
- Dexmedetomidine, an α_2 agonist, is given as a continuous infusion to decrease narcotic and benzodiazepine requirements. It does not depress respiration, and patients do not develop tolerance. Some patients develop bradycardia, which resolves when the infusion is discontinued. A relative contraindication may be high-grade AV nodal block or concurrent medications that slow conduction at the AV node such as digoxin.
- For procedural anesthesia in the CICU, ketamine is an excellent agent. It is a dissociative anesthetic with rapid onset, excellent analgesia, and minimal effects on respiratory drive at lower doses, although airway secretions can be increased.

Heart rate and blood pressure are preserved through central stimulation and diminished postganglionic reuptake. A benzodiazepine is given concurrently for hallucinations in older children. Etomidate causes minimal cardiovascular depression and is ideal intubation in a hemodynamically compromised patient. Chloral hydrate is a hypnotic agent that can be safely given by mouth or per rectum for nonpainful procedures such as echocardiography.

- Neurologic monitoring is evolving as the incidence of abnormalities after CPB is likely to be higher than reported. Postoperative electroencephalographic seizures occur in up to 11% to 20% of neonates and may be related to the duration of deep hypothermic circulatory arrest. Periventricular leukomalacia (as a marker of brain injury) is found on brain magnetic resonance imaging in >50% of neonates after congenital heart surgery. Most appear to resolve over time, but the long-term implications on cognition and development are still being determined.

- Near-infrared spectroscopy to monitor transcutaneous cerebral oxygen saturation may help identify periods of vulnerability to central nervous system injury. The measured saturation is a combination of mixed venous (85%) and arterial (15%), normally 70% in acyanotic lesions. A decrease of 20% from baseline is associated with increased seizures and coma, and prolonged cerebral desaturation <45% is associated with an increased incidence of periventricular leukomalacia.

Fluids and Nutrition

- Post-CPB inflammation significantly increases total body water and edema with diffuse capillary leak; ultrafiltration and steroids are given during the operation to minimize this. Fluid management and diuretic therapy in the first 24 to 48 hours after cardiac surgery have a significant impact on the patient's hemodynamic status and recovery.

- During the first 24 hours, many patients are oliguric despite adequate atrial filling pressures. Longer CPB, increased complexity of the repair, and preoperative renal dysfunction contribute to the duration of oliguria. Restrict fluids to one-half calculated maintenance for at least 24 hours if oliguria does not improve. Preload should be maintained using intermittent boluses, 5 to 10 mL/kg, of crystalloid or colloid solutions. Anecdotally, neonates benefit from volume expansion with 5% albumin over crystalloid.

- Electrolytes should be normalized; replace potassium cautiously with oliguria to avoid hyperkalemia. Maintain high normal ionized calcium levels (1.2–1.3 mmol/L) with bolus dosing (10 mg/kg CaCl or 100 mg/kg Ca gluconate) or a continuous infusion especially in myocardial dysfunction, neonates, and patients with 22q11.2 deletions (DiGeorge syndrome) with hypoparathyroidism. Magnesium should be repleted to avoid developing ventricular dysrhythmias.

- **Diuretics** are introduced after 12 to 24 hours as bolus doses or a continuous infusion. Use earlier with large left-to-right shunts and pulmonary edema to clear excess lung water and wean from the ventilator, but delay after 24 hours in hemodynamically unstable patients with frequent preload repletion. Furosemide is administered as 1 to 2 mg/kg IV doses every 6 to 12 hours; a continuous infusion (1 mg/kg load, 0.1 to 0.3 mg/kg/h) is useful in hemodynamically fragile or significant fluid overload patients. If output remains inadequate, chlorothiazide (5 to 10 mg/kg dose IV every 6 to 12 hours) or metolazone (0.1 to 0.4 mg/kg enterally once daily) are common second agents added. Newer agents include fenoldopam (Table 50.6), a selective dopamine receptor agonist, and nesiritide (Table 50.7), a natriuretic peptide.

- Hypochloremic metabolic alkalosis and hypokalemia and hyponatremia are common when receiving furosemide and/or chlorothiazide.

- Chloride can be repleted with arginine chloride, potassium chloride, or sodium chloride (only if hyponatremic from sodium loss and not congestive heart failure).

- Neonates with shunted single-ventricle physiology can develop a compensatory respiratory acidosis; metabolic alkalosis, and hypochloremia should be normalized prior to extubation.

- Significant **renal dysfunction** beyond 72 hours is uncommon. Consider renal replacement therapy when function continues to worsen despite maximizing cardiac output. Often a peritoneal dialysis catheter placed to gravity drainage can improve fluid balance without dialysis. Indications for dialysis include life-threatening electrolyte abnormalities including hyperkalemia, persistent metabolic acidosis, severe fluid overload impairing ventilation or sternal closure (if open), and rising blood urea nitrogen levels >100 mg/dL. If required, dialysis can be accomplished with peritoneal exchanges or continuous venovenous hemofiltration. Conventional hemodialysis is usually not well tolerated with myocardial dysfunction. Significant ongoing renal dysfunction can have a poor prognosis with >50% mortality.

- Adequate **nutrition** is required for adequate wound healing and recovery but is often compromised for several days due to hemodynamic instability and fluid restrictions. Use of promotility agents, metoclopramide, and postpyloric feeding tubes can enable enteral feeding. Enteral feedings should be restarted as soon as feasible; however, an absolute contraindication is necrotizing enterocolitis. Relative contraindications are the presence of an umbilical artery catheter, high-dose vasoconstrictive agents, and paralysis.

- Neonates with left-sided obstructive lesions, aortopulmonary shunts, and cyanotic lesions are at increased risk for necrotizing enterocolitis. Enteral feedings in these patients should advance slowly with close observation for feeding intolerance such as emesis and abdominal distention.

- If enteral feedings are not feasible, use total parenteral nutrition to avoid a catabolic state. A histamine-2 antagonist should be routinely prescribed for protection against gastric mucosal bleeding from stress and nasogastric tubes until full-volume enteral feeds are re-established.

Infection Issues

- In the first 24 hours, fever is common, does not represent infection, and should be treated to minimize oxygen consumption. All patients receive at least three doses of a second-generation cephalosporin IV as prophylaxis. Treatment is extended in high-risk patients such as those with an open sternum, with immune deficiency, or receiving mechanical circulatory support.

- Fevers that persist or arise after the first 24 hours should be evaluated with a physical exam focused on the sternal

TABLE 50.6

SUMMARY OF CATECHOLAMINES AND DOPAMINERGIC AGENTS

Name	IV dose range	Peripheral vascular effect			Cardiac effect		Comment
		Alpha	Beta$_2$	Dopa	Beta$_1$	Beta$_2$	
Dopamine	2–4 µg/kg/min	0	0	2+	0	0	Increasing doses produce increasing alpha effect; splanchnic vasodilator
	4–10 µg/kg/min	0	2+	2+	1–2+	1+	
	10–20 µg/kg/min	2–4+	0	0	1–2+	2+	
Epinephrine	0.01–0.05 µg/kg/min	1+	1–2+	0	2–3+	2+	Increasing doses produce increasing alpha effect
	0.1–0.5 µg/kg/min	4+	0	0	4+	3+	
Dobutamine	2–10 µg/kg/min	1+	2+	0	3–4+	1–2+	Dose-dependent effect similar to dopamine; increasing doses associated with tachycardia and dysrhythmias
Isoproterenol	0.1–0.5 µg/kg/min	0	4+	0	4+	4+	Potent inotrope and chronotrope; vasodilator; increasing doses produce tachycardia and increased oxygen consumption
Norepinephrine	0.01–0.1 µg/kg/min	4+	1+	0	2+	1+	Moderate inotrope; increases systemic vascular resistance
Phenylephrine	0.01–0.5 µg/kg/min	4+	0	0	0	0	Increases systemic vascular resistance; no inotropy
Fenoldopam	0.05–1 µg/kg/min	0	0	yes	0	0	Dopaminergic receptor agonist; little chronotropic or inotropic effect; may increase renal blood flow

IV, intravenous.
From Castanada AR. *Cardiac Surgery of the Neonate and Infant.* Philadelphia: W. B. Saunders, 1994.

TABLE 50.7

SUMMARY OF NONCATECHOLAMINE VASOACTIVE AGENTS

Name	IV dose range	Peripheral vascular effect	Cardiac effect	Comment
Calcium		Vasoconstrictor	Inotropic effect; depends on iCa level	Slows sinus node and AV node conduction
Chloride	10–20 mg/kg			
Gluconate	50–100 mg/kg			
Milrinone	50 µg/kg load 0.25–1 µg/kg/min	Systemic and pulmonary vasodilator	Diastolic relaxation, decreases afterload	Minimal tachycardia
Amrinone	1–3 mg/kg load 5–20 µg/kg/min	Systemic and pulmonary vasodilator	Diastolic relaxation, decreases afterload	Minimal tachycardia, lowers platelet count, longer half-life than milrinone
Nitroprusside	0.5–5 µg/kg/min	NO donor, relaxes smooth muscle, dilates pulmonary and systemic vessels	Decreases afterload	Reflex tachycardia
Nitroglycerin	0.5–10 µg/kg/min	NO donor, venodilator, more preload effect than nitroprusside	Decreases preload and afterload, may decrease myocardial wall stress	Minimal tachycardia, sometimes used as a coronary vasodilator
Vasopressin	0.0003–0.003 U/kg/min	Potent vasoconstrictor	Weak inotrope	Used to increase systemic blood pressure
Tri-iodothyronine	0.05–0.1 µg/kg/hour	Vasodilation	Inotrope	Tachycardia
Nesiritide	0.01–0.03 µg/kg/min	Natriuresis	Diastolic relaxation	Hyponatremia
Digoxin	6–10 µg/kg/day	Increases systemic vascular resistance	Inotrope	Slows sinus node and AV node conduction

IV, intravenous; iCa, ionized calcium; NO, nitric oxide; AV, atrioventricular.

incision, blood cultures obtained from indwelling intravascular catheters, and a urine culture. If tracheal secretions are copious and/or discolored, suggesting a respiratory source, an aspirate is obtained for Gram stain and culture. Chronically ventilated patients are often colonized; a qualitative change in secretions or increase in white blood cells on Gram stain may indicate infection.

- If the clinical suspicion for infection is high, IV antibacterial coverage should be broadened while awaiting culture results. Nosocomial infections are a significant cause of morbidity in the ICU; maintain sterile technique while inserting or manipulating catheters and remove them as soon as feasible.

- Mediastinitis is a serious postoperative infection, commonly Staphylococcus *aureus* affecting 2% of patients. Risk factors include prolonged open sternum and need for multiple chest re-explorations. Prompt antibiotic treatment with debridement and use of muscle flaps has decreased morbidity and mortality.

Low Cardiac Output Syndrome

- Low cardiac output syndrome (LCOS) is common after congenital heart surgery with CPB, especially in neonates and young infants. Many factors are thought to contribute to decreased cardiac output, including myocardial ischemia from aortic cross-clamping and associated reperfusion injury, inflammation from CPB, ventriculotomies, and the existence of hemodynamically significant residual lesions. There is an expected decrease in cardiac output that occurs over the first 6 to 12 hours after CPB with a nadir of <2 L/minute/m^2 in the youngest patients. With appropriate recognition, the significant morbidities and occasional mortality related to LCOS can be prevented. Milrinone combined with dopamine is currently the combination therapy most commonly used to prevent and treat LCOS.

Recognition of Low Cardiac Output

- There are several clinical symptoms and signs of LCOS that should be immediately recognized (Table 50.8). Hypotension and metabolic acidosis are late findings; they require immediate attention, or a cardiac arrest may be imminent. Auscultation for pathologic murmurs caused by residual obstructions, shunts, or valvar regurgitation is important. Hepatomegaly and ascites may indicate right heart failure, especially with right ventriculotomies.

- Echocardiogram can assess ventricular systolic function and rule out tamponade. Large residual shunts, severe valvular regurgitation, outflow tract obstructions, and venous baffle obstructions are generally poorly tolerated. If the patient has an open sternum or if chest dressings obstruct transthoracic echocardiographic windows, a transesophageal echocardiogram should be performed.

- Occasionally, the etiology of LCOS is not obvious by echocardiography or needs additional clarification before considering reoperation. Cardiac catheterization is safe, even with ECMO, and diagnoses important lesions addressed with interventional catheter procedures or reoperation in a majority of patients.

TABLE 50.8

SIGNS OF LOW CARDIAC OUTPUT SYNDROME

Physical exam/signs
Tachycardia
Hypotension
Narrowed pulse pressure/diminished pulses
Cool extremities
Central hyperthermia
Diminished heart sounds
Hepatomegaly
Pleural effusion and ascites
Oliguria
Elevated central venous pressure/left atrial pressure

Laboratory
Anion gap acidosis
Elevated lactate
Low mixed venous saturation
Indices of abnormal end organ function
Cardiomegaly on chest radiograph

Treatment

- Concurrent with ruling out correctible residual lesions, immediate therapy should be initiated. The goals of therapy are to maximize oxygen delivery and minimize oxygen consumption. Transfuse red blood cells in anemia to increase oxygen-carrying capacity. Optimize cardiac output by repleting intravascular volume and utilizing pharmacologic agents to increase inotropy and decrease afterload (see Tables 50.6 and 50.7). Neuromuscular blockade, deep sedation or anesthesia, and active cooling are used to minimize oxygen consumption.

- Continual reassessment of the response to therapy by physical exam focused on perfusion, and monitored parameters such as urine output and acidosis are required.

Pharmacologic Therapy

- Catecholamines (see Table 50.6) have been the first-choice pharmacologic agents for increasing cardiac output. Almost all patients receive dopamine immediately after CPB to stimulate coronary β receptors and increase contractility (initial dose 3 to 7 μg/kg/min); higher doses (>10 μg/kg/min) stimulate α receptors causing peripheral vasoconstriction. Low to moderate doses of epinephrine (0.02–0.1 μg/kg/min) increase contractility and cause mild peripheral vasoconstriction. Dobutamine acts primarily on coronary β receptors and is most often used in chronic congestive heart failure (e.g., dilated cardiomyopathy); high doses are associated with arrhythmias and tachycardia. Isoproterenol stimulates β receptors and is both an inotrope and chronotrope. it increases oxygen consumption and peripheral vasodilation and is not commonly used in LCOS. Norepinephrine and phenylephrine (pure α agonist) are predominantly α-receptor agonists; their use is limited to patients with profound hypotension.

- Arginine vasopressin, a noncatecholamine vasoconstrictor, promotes vascular smooth-muscle constriction without causing tachycardia. Its role in cardiogenic shock is unclear.

- Patients requiring continued high doses of these potent vasoconstricting agents to support systemic blood pressure should be considered for mechanical circulatory support.

- Relatively noncompliant neonatal myocardium may be more susceptible to catecholamine-driven increases in tachycardia, afterload, and oxygen consumption.
- Afterload reduction is increasingly recognized as the principal form of pharmacologic support for the myocardium after CPB. The type III phosphodiesterase inhibitors enhance myocyte contractility, peripheral vasodilation, and diastolic relaxation. Milrinone is tolerated well by postoperative neonates, and it promotes increased cardiac output, lower atrial pressures, and decreased pulmonary and systemic vascular resistance; it also has a shorter half-life and fewer antiplatelet effects than amrinone. A large, multicenter trial of milrinone after congenital heart surgery found prophylactic milrinone at 0.75 μg/kg/minute had a relative risk reduction of 55% for LCOS compared to placebo. The vasodilators nitroprusside and nitroglycerine, nitric oxide donors, can decrease afterload and improve cardiac output, but they have no direct inotropic effects on the heart.
- Other agents include thyroid hormone, B-type natriuretic peptide, and glucocorticoids. All patients develop low thyroid hormone levels approximately 24 hours after CPB; this typically recovers by 5 to 7 days. Replacing tri-iodothyronine may increase cardiac output, blood pressure, and time to negative fluid balance and extubation. Infusions of nesiritide, a synthetic form of BNP, in adults with heart failure decreases atrial pressures and systemic vascular resistance and improves cardiac output, but pediatric findings are less convincing. Hydrocortisone decreases the inotrope requirements in neonates and infants receiving high-dose catecholamines (>0.15 μg/kg/min epinephrine) after congenital heart surgery, possibly due to a relative adrenal insufficiency after CPB.

Extracorporeal Membrane Oxygenation

- The principal mode of mechanical circulatory support in the postoperative pediatric cardiac patient is venoarterial (cardiac) ECMO, ideally before the development of severe end organ dysfunction or cardiac arrest. The overall goal is to provide myocardial rest; indications are listed in Table 50.9. Cannulation can be initiated via an open sternum with direct

TABLE 50.9

INDICATIONS FOR VENOARTERIAL
EXTRACORPOREAL MEMBRANE OXYGENATION

Low cardiac output
Cardiomyopathy with progressive dysfunction
Myocarditis
Failure to wean from cardiopulmonary bypass
Sudden cardiac arrest

Cyanosis
Marked intracardiac shunting with inadequate oxygenation
Acute obstruction to pulmonary flow (shunt thrombosis)
Pulmonary hemorrhage from pulmonary venous hypertension
Respiratory failure

Arrhythmia
Refractory primary arrhythmias
Postoperative arrhythmia

Support during interventional procedures
Intervention that creates life-threatening physiology

atrial and aortic cannulation when the patient fails to wean from CPB or suffers a postoperative cardiac arrest. Alternatively, the neck or groin vessels can be accessed if there is more time for cannulation.
- The expected course of myocardial recovery after CPB is 3 to 5 days. If unable to wean from ECMO after this time and there are no residual cardiac lesions to be corrected, the possibility of cardiac transplantation should be explored. Most patients cannot be supported with ECMO for longer than 2 to 4 weeks owing to complications. Smaller ventricular assist devices are becoming available to bridge infants and young children to transplantation. Poor outcomes are seen in those who fail to wean from CPB, those with cavopulmonary connections, and adult congenital patients. The results of cardiac ECMO for all indications through July 2006 as reported to the international registry of the Extracorporeal Life Support Organization were 60% survival through decannulation and 42% survival to discharge.

SUPPORT OF THE MYOCARDIUM AFTER CARDIAC TRANSPLANTATION

- Myocardial function of the donated heart will depend on the circumstances leading to donor status, the level of vasoactive support preharvest, and the ischemic time. Recipient factors include preoperative PVR, end organ function, and the overall condition of the patient.
- The transplanted heart is denervated and tends to be bradycardic in the immediate postoperative period; pacing wires should be placed. Alternatively, isoproterenol can be used as a chronotrope, but it increases oxygen consumption and can cause arrhythmias and systemic hypotension at higher doses.
- All cardiac transplant patients should have both right and left atrial pressures monitored to differentiate right heart failure (RHF) caused by elevated PVR from biventricular failure due to graft ischemia or acute rejection. RHF is an important cause of morbidity and mortality after cardiac transplantation and should be treated aggressively.

Pulmonary Hypertension and Right Heart Failure

- Primary RHF and PH leading to secondary RHF are significant causes of postoperative morbidity. Primary RHF should be anticipated after right ventriculotomies for RV outflow tract reconstruction or conduit placement where the hypertrophied noncompliant RV may develop both systolic and diastolic dysfunction. Those at risk for PH and secondary RHF include patients with pulmonary arterial or venous obstruction, heart transplant recipients with elevated PVR from preoperative LA hypertension, and patients with preoperative PH from large left-to-right shunts.
- Patients expected to have a reactive pulmonary vascular bed should have a transthoracic PA or RV catheter placed intraoperatively. In the absence of direct PA pressure measurement, signs of PH include elevated right-sided filling pressures with normal or low left-sided filling pressures and tachycardia. Right-to-left shunts can become more cyanotic. As the right heart fails, physical exam will reveal poor perfusion, hepatomegaly, and possibly a loud tricuspid regurgitation murmur.

- In a pulmonary hypertensive crisis, signs of poor left heart filling including systemic hypotension and bradycardia occur. In the immediate postoperative period, evaluate for residual anatomic problems; residual pulmonary venous obstruction, PA stenosis, or significant left-to-right shunts can cause PH unresponsive to medical therapies.
- If PH is anticipated, patients may benefit from leaving the foramen ovale patent or even creating a new atrial level communication to allow the RV decompression. With the right-to-left shunt, systemic cardiac output will be preserved at the expense of mild cyanosis, which is usually well tolerated and transient.
- The post-CPB inflammatory response, PA endothelial dysfunction, and alveolar hypoxia from edema and atelectasis all contribute to PH but should be time-limited processes. The strategies for medical treatments are outlined in Table 50.10.
- Inhaled nitric oxide (iNO) is a selective pulmonary vasodilator without significant systemic hemodynamic effects usually delivered via a tracheal tube but can also be delivered via a face mask or nasal cannula. A reduction in PA pressure is usually seen at doses of up to 40 parts per million; higher doses may increase toxicity (from methemoglobinemia) without any additional benefit. With PH caused by severe LV dysfunction, pulmonary vasodilation can increase pulmonary blood flow and LA pressures, which may volume-overload the LV, causing further dysfunction.
  - The most responsive patients appear to be those who have relief of pulmonary venous obstruction such as with repair of obstructed total anomalous pulmonary venous return or congenital mitral stenosis.
  - It is an ideal agent to prevent RV failure in a transplanted heart due to elevated PVR.
- Once PA pressures have normalized and diuresis is achieved, iNO can be slowly weaned off. Rapid iNO weaning (e.g., dose lowered at intervals <4 to 6 hours), especially below doses of 5 parts per million, can result in "rebound" PH. If unable to wean off iNO, transition to sildenafil.
- Intravenous vasodilators are not selective for the pulmonary vasculature, but some agents still have a role in treating PH and RV dysfunction. Milrinone is used to afterload reduce

TABLE 50.10

TREATMENT OF POSTOPERATIVE PULMONARY HYPERTENSION

Encourage/administer
Investigate for residual shunts, obstructions to pulmonary blood flow
Supplemental oxygen
Mild alkalosis (pH 7.45–7.5)
Mild hyperventilation (pH 7.45–7.5)
Sedation and analgesia, consider paralysis
Inotropic support of right ventricle
Intravenous vasodilators
Inhaled nitric oxide

Avoid
Metabolic acidosis (pH <7.30)
Hypoventilation or respiratory acidosis
Agitation and pain
Alveolar hypoxia
Atelectasis or alveolar overdistention
Polycythemia

the RV and provide inotropic support and diastolic relaxation. Prostaglandin derivatives such as prostacyclin, delivered either nebulized or as an IV infusion, can be beneficial but are limited by systemic vasodilatory effects.
- Nonspecific vasodilators such as nitroprusside, tolazoline, and isoproterenol should be used infrequently for treatment of PH. Oral therapies for adults with chronic primary PH, including calcium channel blockers and endothelin receptor blockers, have not been adequately studied in children in the postoperative setting, but may have a future role.

SINGLE-VENTRICLE PHYSIOLOGY

- There are many variations of single-ventricle anatomy, but the defects can be broadly divided into those with obstruction to pulmonary blood flow (tricuspid or pulmonary atresia) or obstruction to systemic blood flow. Most will need a palliative operation; either an aortopulmonary shunt when pulmonary flow is obstructed or a stage I (Norwood) operation with aortic arch reconstruction and an aortopulmonary shunt or RV–PA conduit when systemic flow is obstructed. Occasionally, a patient will have two well-developed unobstructed outflow tracts and require a PA band shortly after birth as first-stage palliation.
- Most neonates with single-ventricle anatomy require prostaglandin E_1 to maintain adequate pulmonary or systemic blood flow via the ductus arteriosus. The single ventricle's output occurs in parallel rather than in series; output to the systemic and pulmonary circulations is dependent on the vascular resistance of each. The single ventricle's workload is the sum of the outputs to these two circulations so that the single ventricle does the work of two ventricles. During the postnatal transition, PVR falls rapidly, so these patients often develop excessive pulmonary blood flow and compromised systemic flow within a few days of birth. This is commonly referred to as pulmonary overcirculation.

Shunted Single-ventricle Physiology

- Irrespective of the operation, the principles of balancing the parallel circulations are the same. An acceptable balance of pulmonary-to-systemic blood flow can be defined as sufficient pulmonary blood flow to provide adequate systemic oxygenation without pulmonary overcirculation. An RV-PA conduit is less likely to create overcirculation compared to an aortopulmonary shunt, as pulmonary blood flow occurs only in systole but can still occur.
- Assuming normal pulmonary venous saturations of 100% and normal oxygen extraction with a mixed venous saturation of 60%, a systemic and PA saturation of 80% would result in a pulmonary blood flow (Qp)–to–systemic blood flow (Qs) ratio of 1:1 and correlate with a PaO₂ of 40 mm Hg. Typically, the Qp:Qs ratio is higher than this, and as it progresses toward 2:1, the single ventricle becomes volume-overloaded; ratio >2:1 may be associated with low systemic output, hypotension, and acidosis.
- The ability to monitor Qp:Qs accurately at the bedside is limited. Arterial saturations and mixed venous saturations can be measured, but pulmonary venous saturations are assumed. The degree of postoperative lung disease is highly variable, assuming that pulmonary venous saturations are normal can

erroneously underestimate pulmonary blood flow and the degree of overcirculation in patients with low systemic oxygen saturations. Patients with complete cardiac mixing, high systemic saturations (>90%) and high arterial PaO_2 (>50 mm Hg) with low blood pressure and metabolic acidosis should be treated for pulmonary overcirculation.

- Strategies to treat pulmonary overcirculation focus on increasing PVR and decreasing pulmonary blood flow. Transfusing the patient to a hematocrit of 45% to 50% will increase blood viscosity and PVR. Minimizing inspired oxygen to a room air level and/or lower (e.g., FiO_2 of 17%–19%) with the addition of nitrogen also increases PVR. Allowing the $PaCO_2$ to rise (e.g., to 45–50 mm Hg with a pH <7.34) with hypoventilation or by the addition of carbon dioxide to the ventilator circuit has a similar effect but may increase oxygen delivery to the brain as measured by increased mixed venous saturations in the SVC and decreased arteriovenous saturation difference.

- High SVR should be avoided, as it increases pulmonary blood flow and the afterload on the single ventricle. High upper-extremity blood pressures and oxygen saturations should raise the suspicion of residual coarctation of the aorta in single-ventricle patients and aortic arch obstruction. Large-dose catecholamines should be avoided, and afterload reduction with milrinone should be optimized.

- If a patient remains in a low cardiac output state despite ventilatory and pharmacologic strategies to limit pulmonary blood flow, surgical options such as narrowing the pulmonary conduit or aortopulmonary shunt with clips should be considered.

- Excessive cyanosis is less common after patients are palliated with an aortopulmonary shunt, but it does occur. Possible etiologies include lung disease, elevated PVR, obstruction to pulmonary blood flow, and low mixed-venous saturation from increased oxygen consumption or low cardiac output.

- When a shunt-dependent postoperative patient suddenly develops oxygen desaturation and bradycardia, it should raise the suspicion of acute shunt thrombosis. These patients need emergent cannulation for ECMO and shunt revision. Many patients with shunted single-ventricle physiology have labile hemodynamics for the first several postoperative hours to days. Delayed sternal closure is an accepted strategy that provides rapid access for additional procedures such as clipping of the shunt and emergent ECMO cannulation.

Cavopulmonary Connections

- The transition to a SVC-PA connection, which is called a bidirectional Glenn (BDG) shunt, is typically performed when the patient is 3 to 6 months old. The BDG is the first of a two-stage conversion to a total cavopulmonary circulation with separation of pulmonary and systemic blood flow (Fontan circulation) to reduce volume load and work for the single ventricle. Systemic hypertension and irritability are common after the BDG; this may be secondary to intracranial hypertension from elevated SVC pressures. Mild hypertension preserves cerebral blood flow during the transition to passive pulmonary blood flow through the BDG. Systemic hyperten-

sion associated with bleeding or marked hypertension (>120 mm Hg systolic blood pressure) should be treated.

- Cyanosis associated with elevated SVC pressure occasionally occurs after BDG. If there is a low transpulmonary gradient with elevated atrial pressures, ventricular function should be optimized with inotropes. If the atrial pressures are low and the transpulmonary gradient is >10 mm Hg, this suggests either anatomic obstruction to pulmonary blood flow or elevated PVR.

- The role of carbon dioxide and its effects on PVR and pulmonary blood flow are complex in BDG patients. Modest hypoventilation with elevated carbon dioxide increases arterial PaO_2, presumably by increasing pulmonary blood flow via greater cerebral blood flow from cerebral autoregulation. The vasodilatory role of carbon dioxide in the brain predominates over any increase in PVR from hypoventilation and lower blood pH. The data for use of nitric oxide in these patients are mixed.

- Positive pressure ventilation and increased intrathoracic pressures may play a role in limiting passive pulmonary blood flow, so early extubation is advocated. An SVC pressure >20 mm Hg that is unresponsive to medical therapies is concerning for the successful transition to BDG physiology. Postoperative cardiac catheterization to assess for reversible causes and consideration of possible takedown of the BDG should be pursued.

- The final stage is the completion of the cavopulmonary connection with a Fontan operation performed with either a lateral tunnel baffle through the common atrium or an extracardiac conduit, usually when the patient is 2 to 3 years old and weighs 10 to 15 kg. Postoperative concerns are usually focused on PVR and cardiac output, with an ideal Fontan baffle pressure at 10 to 15 mm Hg and a transpulmonary gradient of <10 mm Hg.

- A Fontan baffle pressure >20 mm Hg is worrisome. Elevated Fontan baffle and atrial pressures indicate low cardiac output or tamponade physiology. An elevated Fontan baffle pressure with a low atrial pressure indicates either high PVR or obstruction in the Fontan pathway; these patients should be promptly investigated and treated.

- Low Fontan baffle and atrial pressures indicate inadequate intravascular volume status. The passive pulmonary blood flow of the Fontan circulation is preload dependent, so hypovolemia will quickly lead to low cardiac output and hypotension.

- Patients undergoing Fontan operations often have sinus node dysfunction with junctional rhythm. AV synchrony is preserved with mechanical pacing to maximize cardiac output.

- Surgical fenestration allows right-to-left shunt to decompress the Fontan baffle and causes mild oxygen desaturation but preserves cardiac output by increasing preload to the ventricle. The Fontan circulation is highly sensitive to elevations in PVR, so acidosis, alveolar hypoxia, and atelectasis should be avoided. As the patient diureses and is extubated from positive pressure ventilation, PVR decreases, and the arterial oxygen saturation improves as less blood is shunted right to left. The fenestration may be electively closed with an occluder device during cardiac catheterization at a later time with good intermediate functional outcomes.

CHAPTER 51 ■ VASCULAR SURGERY IN THE INTENSIVE CARE UNIT

- Patients requiring open vascular or endovascular procedures are elderly and have comorbidities that complicate their overall care. The perioperative care of the vascular surgery patient requires meticulous attention to detail and knowledge about the possible pitfalls these patients can encounter to achieve acceptable perioperative outcomes. A key element is the recognition of vascular pathology as a systemic disease and not just a focal anatomic problem regardless of the procedure.
- **Atherosclerosis** affects the blood vessels of all circulatory beds: cardiac, peripheral, and cerebral. Patients with leg ischemia are at significantly higher risk over the general population for having myocardial infarctions and/or cerebrovascular accidents. The average patient with claudication has an estimated mortality rate of 50% over 5 years, predominantly from cardiovascular causes. Evidence suggests increased inflammation in vascular patients. These patients have elevated levels of C-reactive protein, interleukin-6 (IL-6), and soluble intercellular adhesion molecule-1. Elevated C-reactive protein is a predictor of cardiovascular events among patients with peripheral artery disease.
- **Tobacco use** exceeds 50% and often approaches 90% in patients with peripheral artery disease. Patients with vascular occlusive disease have a high incidence of **chronic obstructive pulmonary disease, occult cardiac disease, diabetes,** and **renal insufficiency.** The adverse pulmonary sequelae of vascular procedures are frequently related to the ravages of smoking. Endovascular therapy, despite decreased durability, may be appropriate for patients based on their condition and ability to tolerate general anesthesia. Similarly, spinal or epidural anesthesia, rather than general anesthesia, may be more appropriate.
- **Coronary artery disease** is present in up to 93% of patients undergoing the most common vascular procedures (abdominal aortic aneurysm [AAA] repair, carotid endarterectomy, peripheral bypass). Additionally, most vascular surgery procedures for occlusive or aneurysmal disease are considered "high-risk." Much attention has been given to preoperative risk stratification and how to minimize the risk of perioperative cardiac events in the vascular surgery patient.
  - The American Heart Association/American College of Cardiology goals should be targeted, including a blood pressure <140/90 mm Hg, serum low-density lipoprotein <100 mg/dL, and hemoglobin A_{1C} <7%.
  - To achieve these goals, patients should be on an aspirin, a β-blocker dosed judiciously to a target heart rate of 70 to 75, an angiotensin-converting enzyme inhibitor, or other antihypertensive therapy.
  - The electrocardiogram should be monitored continuously for any changes suggestive of ischemia.

- Coronary revascularization (percutaneous or open) before elective major vascular surgery has not been shown to decrease the overall mortality.
- A preoperative cardiology consultation may be useful to help determine existing cardiac function.
- There is increasing evidence that all patients with vascular disease, regardless of cholesterol levels, benefit from **statin therapy** due to its anti-inflammatory, immunomodulatory, and anticoagulant effects.
- Perioperative continuation of statin therapy is recommended due to a rebound effect and a possible increase in cardiovascular complications with abrupt discontinuation.
- Cardiac dysrhythmias are often caused by ischemia, electrolyte disturbances, or fluid shifts in the postoperative period. Patients should be monitored closely for such events.
- **Renal insufficiency,** as determined by creatinine clearance, may be present in vascular patients without prior known elevated serum creatinine. Perioperative mortality after most vascular procedures is increased in patients with renal failure. Nephrotoxic effects of the IV contrast commonly used in revascularization procedures make postoperative renal dysfunction a constant threat. Strict monitoring of fluid balance, maintenance of serum electrolytes, appropriate dosing of nephrotoxic medications, adequate hydration, and resumption of chronic diuretics may minimize the chance of postoperative renal dysfunction.
- **Diabetes mellitus** is present in the majority of vascular patients. This group is at higher risk for postoperative vascular and nonvascular complication. Patients with diabetes have a higher rate of postoperative amputations after peripheral bypass surgery for tissue loss and a higher rate of wound infections. Additionally, patients with diabetes can manifest angina as nausea, diaphoresis, or "indigestion." Euglycemia should be maintained, utilizing a constant IV infusion of insulin if necessary.
- **Hypercoagulability** is present in a subset of patients with vascular disease. Suspicion for a hypercoagulable state should be raised with patients with seemingly advanced atherosclerotic disease at a younger age. A careful history can assist with determining these patients, but when identified, they should be started on appropriate anticoagulation. A hematology consultation should be obtained but may be of somewhat limited value in the setting of the acute thrombotic event.

VASCULAR CARE IN THE INTENSIVE CARE UNIT

- The routine assessment of the vascular intensive care unit (ICU) patient includes not only all the usual cardiovascular, pulmonary, and metabolic parameters but frequent and detailed physical exams. Objective assessment of distal perfusion should be performed regularly, even hourly, in the immediate postoperative period. This assessment includes looking at the extremity for cutaneous signs of malperfusion, assessing motor function, and palpating the major muscle groups for tenseness, which may signify compartment syndrome in patients who are too sedated to relate the classic "pain with passive motion." All incisions should be inspected for signs of early wound complications such as infection, separation, or hematoma.

- **Extremity perfusion** should be assessed by checking for palpable pulses; if none is found, Doppler signals must be auscultated to assess the perfusion.
  - Normal Doppler signals are described as *triphasic.*
  - Doppler signals distal to an obstruction may be characterized as *biphasic* or *monophasic* with the latter suggesting significantly diminished blood flow.
  - Extremity perfusion is assessed prior to leaving the operating room (OR). The quality and location of each Doppler signal or palpable pulse should be communicated and recorded as a reference.
  - A worsening exam or inability to detect the signal may potentially constitute an emergent trip back to the operating room to restore perfusion.
  - Bedside ankle-brachial index measurements is an objective marker of extremity perfusion. Any change of more than 0.15 is significant and should be reported, independent of any other clinical event.
- **Compartment pressure** monitoring devices are advocated by some centers. We perform fasciotomies emergently if compartment syndrome is even suspected. Fasciotomies can be performed in the ICU setting using Bovie electrocautery and sterile scissors.
  - The two-incision technique—a medial infrageniculate incision releasing the deep and posterior compartments—and a lateral incision release the anterior and lateral compartments.
  - The underlying muscle should bulge when released, thereby confirming the diagnosis.
  - The wound should be left open and treated with routine dressing changes with subsequent closure in several days to weeks when the swelling abates.
  - Metabolic sequelae of compartment syndrome may consist of cellular lysis with release of potassium and myoglobin that may cause systemic hyperkalemia and acute renal failure.
  - We routinely check urine myoglobin and administer aggressive IV fluids to ensure brisk urine output of at least 100 mL/hour. Electrolytes are checked frequently, and continuous telemetric cardiac monitoring is employed.
- All **vascular surgery wounds** should be examined daily for signs of infection. Groin wounds can be problematic, with wound complications in up to 44%. Most wound breakdowns can be treated with local wound therapy at the bedside. However, wound breakdown with exposure of the underlying vascular graft or anastomosis is a serious vascular wound complication due to the devastating potential for anastomotic disruption. In this situation, patients should be scheduled for the OR for exploration and attempted reclosure of the wound, preferably with autogenous tissue such as a sartorius or rectus flap. Additionally, it is imperative that all health care personnel treating the patient be aware of exposed vasculature. A "blowout precaution" protocol may be instituted wherein patients are kept at bedrest and blood is typed and crossed. Any bleeding from the wound is a potential emergency. Immediate pressure should be placed on the wound, the patient stabilized, and the operating team notified. Direct pressure on the wound should be maintained until the patient is intubated and anesthetized, the surgeon scrubbed in, and the operative field prepped (even if this includes the team member's gloved hand being prepped into the field).

- **Meticulous skin care** is mandatory for the vascular patient. Even modest duration of pressure on the heel by the bed mattress can lead to skin breakdown and turn a successful revascularization into an amputation. As the vast majority of vascular patients have compromised distal perfusion, heels may be elevated off the bed by placing pillows under the leg to distribute leg weight over a larger surface area. There is no substitute for frequent inspection of all pressure-sensitive areas ,and this should be part of the physician's and nurse's practice.
- **Pharmacologic prophylaxis** against thromboembolic events is the routine. All vascular patients in an ICU have a propensity for developing venous thromboembolic events as dictated by Virchow's triad. Venous stasis is inevitable in the postsurgical patient due to relative immobility. Endothelial injury occurs during the course of the surgical procedure. Many patients require systemic anticoagulation after vascular surgical procedures such as with distal bypasses when there is compromised outflow or less than ideal conduit. The need for systemic anticoagulation must be balanced with the risk of bleeding complications, and usually we hold off full anticoagulation until postoperative day 2 or 3. Patients are monitored for any decline in platelet counts, and if seen, a heparin antibody panel is sent. If the clinical suspicion is high, we stop all heparin and switch to anticoagulation with other agents.
- **Stress gastritis** is a constant threat in the vascular ICU patient. Consideration of either histamine-receptor blockers or proton pump inhibitors, irrespective of any clinically detected gastrointestinal hemorrhage, is suggested.
- **Ventilator-associated pneumonia** has been well documented to increase in-hospital mortality, length of stay, and overall cost of hospitalization. We employ routine suctioning, aggressive bronchoscopy to control secretions, and head elevation for all our intubated patients. Once extubated, activity is encouraged, and adequate pain control is important for patients with an abdominal or a thoracic incision.
- **Acute limb ischemia** in the ICU setting can have disastrous consequences. The pathologic differential includes embolic events (usually from cardiac or aortic sources) or *in situ* thrombosis of preexisting atherosclerotic lesions.
  - If identified acutely, there may be a role for intra-arterial thrombolysis, although this modality is limited due to excessive bleeding risk in the postsurgical patient.
  - When an ischemic extremity is identified, patients should immediately be fully anticoagulated.
  - More aggressive intervention, either catheter-based therapy or open surgical thrombectomy, should be entertained.
  - If the acute arterial occlusion is associated with motor or sensory deficits, an emergent exploration is indicated.
  - On rare occasions, patients present with acute lower-extremity paralysis secondary to acute infrarenal aortic occlusion. Absence of femoral pulses is a clue to the

vascular nature of the paralysis. These patients typically require emergent procedures, and despite operative success, the perioperative mortality rate exceeds 50%.
- **Common ICU causes of arterial occlusion** include sequelae of invasive monitoring, usually intra-arterial lines.
  - Brachial artery cannulations for cardiac catheterizations have an overall complication rate as high as 36%.
  - Arterial lines can impair distal perfusion. In this situation, the first step is to remove the catheter and to observe for restoration of perfusion.
  - The collateral blood supply and distal perfusion should also be assessed, and a motor and sensory assessment of the affected limb should be performed.
  - Choices of therapy include observation, systemic anticoagulation, local thrombolysis, and operative thrombectomy with the potential for bypass.
- **Invasive arterial and venous monitoring** is a challenge in the vascular ICU patient.
  - Lower-extremity IV and arterial lines are contraindicated in patients with peripheral arterial occlusive disease.
  - Patients with dialysis-access fistulae should have that extremity kept free of IVs, central venous catheters, invasive arterial lines, and noninvasive blood pressure cuffs.
  - If a patient is likely to require future permanent vascular access, duplex ultrasonography should be used to identify a potential arm. Invasive lines in this arm should be avoided.
- **Various bleeding complications** can occur in the postoperative vascular wound. These can range from simple "skin edge" bleeding to frank exsanguination.
  - Skin edge bleeding may be a nuisance and may be treated with manual compression, application of silver nitrate, or a simple suture.
  - Hematomas are monitored closely. Recurrent blood transfusion requirements, overlying skin or wound compromise, deleterious mass effects, and hemodynamic instability are all indications for operative evacuation of the hematoma.
  - Patients who have had percutaneous interventions (usually through the groin at the common femoral artery) should also be monitored for hematomas.
  - Attempted femoral artery punctures that are aimed more cephalad may in fact be external iliac artery punctures. Compression may be ineffective due to the retroperitoneal location of the arteriotomy. A progressive hematoma in such a location more often requires surgical repair (open or endovascular).

SPECIFIC CONDITIONS

Aneurysmal Disease

The natural history of aneurysms of the aorta is to expand and rupture. An unstable condition develops as expansion of the aortic diameter leads to further aortic wall thinning and, by the Law of Laplace, increased wall tension. Increased wall tension promotes further aortic dilatation, and the vicious cycle continues until the aortic wall ruptures.

Infrarenal Abdominal Aortic Aneurysm

- Approximately 90% of the extracranial aneurysms involve the infrarenal aorta.

- Most aneurysms are asymptomatic and are discovered during radiographic workup of other problems.
- Symptomatic aneurysms frequently present with back or abdominal pain. These symptoms may herald impending rupture and thus require urgent repair.
- Operative repair is recommended when the aortic aneurysm diameter reaches 5.5 cm in asymptomatic males.
- Preoperative preparation includes a single dose of preoperative antibiotics for all patients and arterial lines, central lines, and Foley catheters for most patients.

Endovascular Repair
- Depending on patient anatomy and institutional expertise, abdominal aortic aneurysm repair can be performed via an endovascular approach. This approach is appealing in terms of reduced physiologic insult to the patient. These patients rarely require admission to the ICU but are monitored for hematomas and lower-extremity pulses. The devices used to deploy endovascular stents can be as large as No. 26 French, and these are introduced through femoral or external iliac arteries. There is a possibility of local arterial damage or dislodging of plaque that may embolize distally.

Open Repair
- Open aneurysm repair, conversely, requires surgical ICU monitoring postoperatively. The overall perioperative mortality is approximately 5%. Bleeding is the main concern due to the aorta-to-graft anastomosis. Perfusion of the lower extremities is an additional concern due to arterial occlusion during the procedure. Lower-extremity ischemic events after open abdominal aortic aneurysm repairs occur in 2% to 5% of patients. Any inability to detect a Doppler signal or palpate a pulse when there previously was one is a potential surgical emergency.
- *Postoperative complications*
  - **Prolonged postoperative ileus** may occur in up to 11% of patients. A retroperitoneal approach may be shorten the duration of postoperative ileus.
  - Nonischemic diarrhea may occur in 7.1% of patients.
  - **Colonic ischemia** has an estimated prevalence of 0.6%. It typically presents as bloody stools 3 to 5 days postoperatively but may occur as early as the first 24 hours after surgery. Additional signs of colonic ischemia are fever, abdominal pain, thrombocytopenia, unexplained leukocytosis, or lactic acidosis.
  - Any suspicion of colonic ischemia should prompt endoscopic evaluation, with the caveat that endoscopy cannot evaluate for transmural ischemia.
  - In the appropriate clinical setting, mucosal ischemia may justify operative exploration with possibly colon resection and end colostomy.
  - Broad-spectrum antibiotics to include gram-negative and anaerobic coverage are used.
  - Patients with colonic ischemia require intensive invasive ICU monitoring, as they often progress to multisystem organ failure.
  - **Pancreatitis** and **cholecystitis** may also complicate aneurysm surgical repair.
  - Pancreatitis is self-limited and likely related to direct surgical trauma during aortic exposure.
  - Cholecystitis may be ischemia-related or may be a variant of acalculous cholecystitis seen in ICU patients. Treatment

options range from percutaneous cholecystostomy to surgical cholecystectomy.

- **Postoperative renal dysfunction** can be as high as 5.4% after open infrarenal aortic surgery, but dialysis requirement is much less at 0.6%. The exact etiology of the renal dysfunction after infrarenal clamping is largely speculative but may involve migration of atheroemboli leading to acute tubular necrosis.
- Renal dysfunction is lower in patients with infrarenal versus suprarenal aortic cross-clamping.
- In the early postoperative period, oliguria is most frequently due to intravascular depletion and not intrinsic renal dysfunction.
- Patients with baseline renal insufficiency or those who do not respond appropriately to IV fluid challenges should be investigated for acute tubular necrosis or other intrinsic cause of oliguria.
- **Thrombocytopenia** may occur in the absence of other causes (e.g., colon ischemia). Although an inciting event or agent is not always identifiable, there are several likely etiologies. Unless there is evidence of ongoing bleeding, mild thrombocytopenia is usually well tolerated.
- Perioperative cardiac events occur in 15% for any perioperative cardiac event is observed in patients with AAAs. Patients with AAAs may have coronary artery disease and are at risk for postoperative myocardial infarctions (5.2%), heart failure (8.9%), and dysrhythmia requiring treatment (10.5%). Unless contraindicated, patients undergoing open aneurysm repair should be on a medical regimen consisting of a β-blocker with a target heart rate of 70 to 75, a statin (independent of serum cholesterol levels), and some form of antiplatelet therapy, usually aspirin.

Ruptured Aortic Aneurysms

- Operative mortality rate of ruptured AAA is near 50% versus <5% in elective cases. With ruptured AAA, there are impressive fluid shifts that transpire during such an emergent operation, independent of overt blood loss. These fluid shifts, associated with the hypotension and the physiologic strain of an emergent procedure, contribute to a tenuous postoperative course. The incidence of colonic ischemia is significantly higher after ruptured aneurysm repair compared to elective open aneurysmorrhaphy, and some authors recommend empiric and routine endoscopic evaluation of the colonic mucosa.

Juxtarenal or Suprarenal Aortic Aneurysms

- Aneurysms that extend to the level of the renal arteries or involve the paravisceral aorta are technically more challenging.
- Postoperative complications escalate dramatically due to renal and possibly mesenteric ischemia-reperfusion.
- Depending on the length of intraoperative ischemia, there is a resultant release of pro- and anti-inflammatory cytokines that drives a systemic inflammatory reaction resulting in multisystem organ failure.
- There is considerable third spacing of fluid in the first 24 hours. Attempts to improve mortality and morbidity by a hybrid approach involving multiple visceral bypasses and endovascular repair of the aneurysm have met with mixed results.
- Adequate pain control is key in these patients.

Infected Aortic Graft

- One of the more dreaded complications of aortic surgery is infection of the prosthesis. Graft infection is a serious problem and should be investigated and treated aggressively.
- Early postoperative graft infection is rare. The majority occur months to years later, with unexplained fevers.
- Infection may also present as gastrointestinal bleeding (a manifestation of an aortoenteric fistula) or a draining sinus in the groin.
- The causative organism is usually *Staphylococcus*.
- Computed tomography (CT) scan shows fluid around an aortic graft.
- Broad-spectrum antibiotics, IV resuscitation, and close hemodynamic monitoring should be undertaken. Patients should be medically optimized and prepared for a staged procedure. The initial step is usually an extra-anatomic bypass with subsequent laparotomy and excision of the aortic graft. In good operative candidates, a single-stage aortic replacement using autogenous tissue (syndactylized bilateral femoral veins) or cadaveric vessels can be performed. Patients are routinely sent to the ICU as some may become floridly septic after manipulation of the infected retroperitoneum.

Arterial Occlusive Disease

Aortoiliac Occlusive Disease

- The most durable surgical solution for aortoiliac occlusive disease is an aortobifemoral bypass.
- Peripheral pulses are regularly monitored. Any deviation from the immediate postoperative pulses is a potential emergency as it may represent a graft thrombosis.
- Distal embolization involves ischemia of the toes (trash foot). Management is expectant, and most often this resolves with minimal or no permanent tissue loss.
- Patients < 55 years of age are believed to have better long-term vascular durability for infrarenal aortic reconstruction with autogenous tissue rather than Dacron grafts.
- Redo aortic surgery is fraught with intraoperative and postoperative complications. Extra-anatomic bypasses may be performed, usually axillobifemoral.
- As endovascular technology evolves, many iliac lesions are treated with angioplasty and possible stent placement.

Infrainguinal Bypasses

- The incisions that are made are significant, and may not only be located on the extremity being reperfused but may be on either leg or either arm as a site of vein harvest.
- The patency of infrainguinal bypass grafts using autogenous tissue is superior to that using prosthetic tissue.
- The main sources of morbidity from these procedures are arterial occlusion, bleeding, and wound complications.
- The mortality from peripheral bypasses is estimated to be between 2% and 8%.
- Mortality is primarily cardiac. Aggressive cardiac medical management, judicious use of antiplatelet therapy, and careful fluid status monitoring are essential.
- Bypass is associated with a reperfusion syndrome. The reperfused extremity should be monitored for compartment

syndrome, and electrolytes and urine myoglobin should be monitored.

Carotid Endarterectomy

- Carotid endarterectomy decreases the chance of a future cerebrovascular accident in certain patients with carotid stenosis. The key outcome variable is perioperative stroke related to disruption of cerebral blood flow or embolic event from clamping an atherosclerotic vessel.
- Aspirin should be continued in the recovery phase. Full anticoagulation is seldom indicated unless carotid occlusion has occurred.
- A new neurologic deficit may manifest itself upon awakening or occur in the early postoperative period. This should be investigated with imaging or a return to the OR.
- Large postoperative fluctuations in blood pressures occur due to carotid bulb baroreceptor "stretch." Blood pressure should be targeted to the "normal range" of 120 to 140 mm Hg.
- Wound hematoma is of concern as a moderate hematoma can cause carotid compression and resultant bradycardia or airway compression. The operating team should be alerted if hematoma is suspected.
- Several cranial nerves are intimately associated within the field of dissection. Thus, a detailed head and neck exam is mandatory at regular intervals.
- Particular attention should be paid to assessing the function of the marginal mandibular nerve and the hypoglossal nerve.
- Headache and seizure activity may be manifestations of cerebral reperfusion syndrome. This is rarely seen in the immediate postoperative period but may cause readmission for blood pressure control in the weeks after carotid endarterectomy.
- Patients with these symptoms should receive a CT scan due to the incidence of intracranial bleeding that accompanies these symptoms.

Mesenteric Revascularization

- Mesenteric ischemia, whether acute or chronic, can have lethal consequences. The restoration of intestinal perfusion sets in motion a cascade of inflammatory cytokines that frequently progress to the systemic inflammatory response syndrome, multisystem organ failure, and even death.
- After restoration of blood flow, patients typically have a period of hemodynamic stability for 24 to 48 hours after the procedure.
- After 48 hours, some patients show signs of unrelenting systemic inflammation with a continuation of fluid third spacing and progressive thrombocytopenia.
- Efforts to predict which patient will progress to clinical deterioration have been unsuccessful.
- Like any other revascularization bypass, the patency of the mesenteric graft should be assessed objectively. Duplex ultrasound is noninvasive and is highly sensitive.
- Despite all the usual supportive measures, the average postoperative length of stay is more than 3 weeks.

Aortic Dissections

- Dissections start as an intimal flap, and blood escapes the true lumen and channels down the aorta, shearing apart the layers of the wall.
- Dissections of the ascending aorta (Stanford type A) are cardiac surgical emergencies, as potential retrograde dissection can cause coronary malperfusion or cardiac tamponade.
- Dissections of the descending aorta (Stanford type B) are usually treated medically with aggressive blood pressure control.
- Four indications for operative intervention are branch vessel malperfusion (usually celiac, superior mesenteric, renal, or iliac), inability to control hypertension, persistent pain related to the dissection, or aneurysmal degeneration.
- Dissections can be repaired via open techniques or endovascularly.
- Postoperative blood pressure control is paramount.

Hemodialysis

- Although the annual mortality of patients on hemodialysis approaches 25%, many patients in the ICU are on chronic hemodialysis with functional fistulae.
- The extremity with the fistula should be preserved from invasive and noninvasive monitoring devices, and all IVs and central lines should be placed away from that extremity if possible.
- If a fistula is present, the extremity distal to it is at risk of ischemic events and should be monitored closely.
- Tunneled catheters should not be used as an IV line except in dire circumstances. Limiting their use to their intended purpose will decrease the chance of infection.
- It is routine practice to "lock" the catheter with concentrated heparin to decrease mechanical catheter complications. Flushing this heparin "lock" will systemically anticoagulate the patient.

Vascular Trauma

The care of the trauma patient with vascular injuries shares many of the same principles as care of other vascular surgery patients with the exception that this cohort frequently, but not always, lacks the systemic comorbidities of the typical atherosclerotic vascular patient.

- Most extremity vascular injuries are associated with orthopedic fractures and dislocations (e.g. posterior knee dislocation and popliteal artery injury).
- Extremity pulses should be assessed in the secondary survey as part of the Advanced Trauma Life Support evaluation and clearly documented.
- The same assessment is merited in any patient recovering from an orthopedic procedure.
- Any change in pulse exam or hard sign of vascular injury mandates radiographic evaluation, usually with an arteriogram or, alternatively, with a CT angiogram.

Penetrating extremity trauma associated with hard signs of vascular injury (decreased distal perfusion, active arterial hemorrhage, or a rapidly expanding hematoma) should be evaluated immediately after lifesaving measures are undertaken.

- Operative exploration with visual inspection of the vessel should be performed.
- If injured, it is either repaired or blood flow is rerouted around the "blast field."
- Venous injuries are ligated unless easily repaired.
- Revascularization of an extremity malperfused for >6 hours increases the likelihood of a reperfusion syndrome and/or compartment syndrome.

- Fasciotomy is prudent if there is any question of reperfusion injury.
- Severe musculoskeletal damage beyond that which is salvageable can be treated with simple ligation and amputation.
- Trauma to an artery and adjacent vein can cause an arteriovenous fistula. This can present months after the inciting trauma with unexplained extremity swelling, distal ischemic symptoms, heart failure, or an audible bruit over an extremity.

Aortic trauma is increasing, possibly due to the increased use of CT scans in trauma management. With the resolution of the current scanners, we are seeing a number of intimal injuries and short segments of dissection that previously were not detected.

- In the absence of hemodynamic compromise, most intimal injuries or short dissections of the in the infrarenal aorta and iliac vessels can be observed.
- In the abdomen, any central periaortic hematoma should be operatively evaluated.
- Initial care thoracic aortic injuries of is directed toward treating the urgent life-threatening injuries and controlling blood pressure with β-blockers.
- Thoracic aortic injuries are increasingly treated with endovascular devices. Though open surgical repair is still a viable option, in most series the morbidity is clearly greater.

Penetrating neck trauma can involve the carotid artery, which can be exposed readily in certain locations (zone 2).

- In the stable patient with a zone 2 injury, perform the global assessment of the patient ,including abdominal sonography and IV resuscitation, and then take the patient to the OR for exploration.
- For more proximal or distal injuries (zones 3 and 1), angiography (standard contrast angiography or CT angiography) plays a vital role in both diagnosing and planning either open or endovascular treatment.

Blunt cerebrovascular injury injuries are relatively rare (<1% of blunt trauma patients), and controversy remains about the best way to diagnose and treat these patients. The Eastern Association for the Surgery of Trauma guidelines recommend screening, preferably with angiography, for blunt trauma patients who present with the following:

- Cervical spine fractures
- LeFort II or III fractures
- Petrous bone fracture
- Fracture through the foramen transversum
- Glasgow coma scale <8 or diffuse axonal injury

Additionally, any patient with an unexplained neurologic deficit should prompt further investigation.

The general consensus is that these lesions should be treated with either full anticoagulation or an antiplatelet agent that should continue for 3 to 6 months. Occasionally, pseudoaneurysms are seen, and endovascular repair seems to be the evolving treatment modality for this lesion. Morbidity from this lesion remains high as many patients present with a deficit.

CHAPTER 52 ■ CNS VASCULAR DISEASE

IMMEDIATE CONCERNS

Stress Points

- Strokes may be ischemic, resulting from the occlusion of small or large arteries, or hemorrhagic, resulting from the rupture of a conducting artery or an intraparenchymal arteriole.
- An abrupt focal lateralizing neurologic deficit attributable to a cerebrovascular distribution is the hallmark of ischemic stroke.
- A depressed level of consciousness is rarely the presenting symptom of ischemic stroke and much more commonly occurs in the setting of a hemorrhagic event.
- Patients with acute ischemic stroke may be candidates for thrombolytic therapy, but the therapeutic window is extremely narrow, so timely diagnosis and evaluation are of the utmost importance.

Essential Diagnostic Tests and Procedures

- A computed tomography (CT) scan of the brain is critical for the initial evaluation and management of the stroke patient.

Additionally, when available, CT angiography and perfusion studies may aid in diagnosis and management.

- Magnetic resonance imaging (MRI) is more sensitive than CT, but it is usually less available urgently, and patients must remain still for a much longer period of time.
- Vascular ultrasound allows rapid bedside assessment of abnormal flow within the major intracranial and extracranial arteries and can provide valuable immediate information about the vascular physiology to supplement the anatomic information provided by the CT scan.
- A transthoracic or transesophageal echocardiogram may identify potential cardiac sources of cerebral emboli.
- An electrocardiogram followed by continuous cardiac telemetry monitoring is often necessary to identify arrhythmias associated with stroke.
- A lumbar puncture may be necessary to rule out subarachnoid hemorrhage (SAH) in patients in whom the diagnosis is strongly suspected, but CT is unrevealing.

Initial Therapy

- Thrombolytics are the mainstay of treatment of acute ischemic stroke in eligible patients.

- Careful attention to blood pressure may reduce complications such as hemorrhage.
- Supportive care, with special attention paid to prevention of aspiration pneumonia and deep-vein thromboses, is essential to reduce mortality associated with stroke.
- Rapid initiations of secondary preventive therapies are effective in reducing risk for recurrent stroke.
- Certain patients, such as those with large ischemic or hemorrhagic strokes, will require monitoring of intracranial pressure and, potentially, decompressive surgery.

DIFFERENTIAL DIAGNOSIS

Stroke Symptoms

- Most patients who suddenly develop a lateralized focal neurologic problem have, in fact, had a stroke (Table 52.1).
- When the presentation differs from this definition, further investigation and supportive evidence should be sought before establishing the diagnosis.
- Many stroke symptoms may occur alone, unaccompanied by other evidence of neurologic damage, that are not an expression of vascular disease.
- Most of the errors in the diagnosis of stroke occur in patients with altered mental status. Beware of attributing such nonfocal symptoms to strokes without corroborating historic or diagnostic evidence.

Diseases Most Commonly Mistaken for Stroke

- Epilepsy mimics stroke more often than any other condition (Table 52.2).
- Intracranial hemorrhage, encephalitis, or other structural brain lesions, such as tumors, may produce focal deficits identical to ischemic stroke.
- Drug intoxication, alcohol, or metabolic abnormalities constitute the next largest group of mistaken diagnoses in patients suffering confusion and neurologic deficits.
- Extreme electrolyte or serum glucose derangements can produce temporary focal deficits.
- Migraine may produce several transient neurologic symptoms that may be misinterpreted as stroke.
- Occasionally, peripheral nerve lesions, such as Bell palsy, may appear suddenly and mimic an ischemic stroke.

TABLE 52.1

SYMPTOMS SELDOM RESULTING FROM CEREBROVASCULAR DISEASE

Vertigo alone	Confusion
Dysarthria alone	Memory loss
Dysphagia alone	Delirium
Diplopia alone	Coma
Headache	Syncope
Tremor	Incontinence
Tonic-clonic motor activity	Tinnitus

TABLE 52.2

CONDITIONS MOST FREQUENTLY MISTAKEN FOR STROKE

Seizures	Peripheral neuropathy and Bell palsy
Metabolic encephalopathy	Multiple sclerosis
Cerebral tumor	Hypoglycemia
Subdural hematoma	Encephalitis
Cerebral abscess	Migraine
Vertigo, Ménière disease	Psychogenic illness

Ischemic Stroke

Pathogenesis

- Ischemic stroke occurs when the supply of blood to brain tissue is acutely interrupted.
- Autoregulation of the cerebral vasculature adjusts vascular resistance to maintain normal blood flow in the setting of blood pressure changes.
- Once these vessels are maximally dilated, further drops in systemic pressure will reduce cerebral blood flow.
- Normal cerebral blood flow in the cortical mantle is about 50 mL/100 g tissue per minute. When cerebral blood flow drops below 20 mL/100 g tissue per minute, synaptic failure occurs, and patients become symptomatic.
- When cerebral blood flow drops below 10 mL/100 g tissue per minute, metabolic failure and irreversible cell death occur.
- A potentially salvageable area of brain tissue is referred to as the *penumbra*. This occurs in regions with diminished flow that will survive longer but not indefinitely. The purpose of acute stroke therapies is to salvage the penumbra.
- The causes of disruptions of arterial flow can be separated into three major categories based on cause: (a) large-vessel atherothrombotic disease, (b) small-vessel (lacunar) infarction, and (c) cardiogenic embolism.

Large-vessel Atherothrombosis

- Large-vessel atherothrombosis encompasses approximately 15% of all strokes; of these, two-thirds are of extracranial internal carotid artery (ICA) origin, and one-third are due to intracranial atheromatous disease.
- Atheromatous vascular plaques may fragment, exposing an ulcerated surface that is highly thrombogenic and leading to local occlusion or creation of emboli material.
- Atherosclerotic lesions tend to occur at bifurcations or sharp turns in the vessel where flow turbulence is increased. The prototypic example of this is carotid stenosis at the origin of the ICA.
- Intracranially, common sites include the distal vertebral artery, the midbasilar artery, the siphon of the ICA, and the proximal middle cerebral artery (MCA).

Lacunar Strokes

- Lacunar strokes represent approximately one-fourth of all such events. The primary risk factor for lacunar infarction is hypertension.
- These strokes are caused by occlusion of a single perforating arteriole, typically to those that supply deep brain structures like the thalamus, pons, or basal ganglia.

- The result is a small infarction (<1 cm^3) that undergoes liquefaction necrosis.

Cardiogenic Embolism

- Embolism causes ~60% of all ischemic strokes, of which only one-third have a definitively known clinical source.
- Cerebral emboli may be composed of atherosclerotic plaque material, clotted blood or, in rare cases, air or fat.
- Emboli tend to follow the straightest path formed by the most blood. Therefore, most emboli will affect distal branches of the MCA.
- Cerebral emboli may originate from atheromatous disease of the carotid arteries or the aortic arch or from material in the heart.
- Atrial fibrillation is the most common cardiac cause, but others include valvular heart disease, intracardiac thrombus, atrial myxoma, dilated cardiomyopathy, patent foramen ovale, especially when accompanied by an atrial septal defect, and endocarditis.
- Air emboli are usually iatrogenic and result when a large amount of air enters the venous circulation and bypasses the lungs through a patent foramen ovale, thereby entering the arterial circulation.
- Fat emboli are generally the result of long-bone fractures in severe trauma.
- The definitive source should be identified as it can alter the management of secondary stroke prevention.

Arterial Dissections

- Arterial dissections are the most common cause of stroke in young patients (<50 years old) who are unlikely to have typical risk factors.
- Arterial dissections may arise spontaneously or follow a traumatic head or neck injury.
- These lesions typically arise at the petrous portion of the ICA or at cervical level 1 to 2 in the vertebral artery.
- Dissection may also lead to subarachnoid hemorrhage when a pseudoaneurysm forms after the artery passes intradurally.

CLINICAL EVALUATION

History

- The history, when available, is the key instrument in diagnosing neurologic disease. If the patient is unable to provide a reliable history, historic details should be sought from witnesses, family, emergency medical services (EMS) records, or any available sources.
- The key historic element in ischemic cerebrovascular disease is *sudden* onset of symptoms, which are typically maximal at onset.
- Additional history should be focused on obtaining the exact time of symptom onset, as current acute stroke treatment protocols depend on this for inclusion.
- If the onset was not witnessed, the time when last known to be normal is used.
- Aside from time of onset, factors that may place the patient at increased risk for bleeding must be sought. Tables 52.3, 52.4, and 52.5 list common inclusion and exclusion criteria for intravenous (IV)-tPA (tissue plasminogen activator).

TABLE 52.3

INCLUSION CRITERIA FOR tPA USE

1. Symptoms consistent with acute ischemic stroke, with a clearly defined onset of <3 hours before rt-PA will be given. (If the onset was not witnessed, the ictus is measured from the time the patient was last seen to be at baseline.)
2. A significant neurologic deficit is expected to result in long-term disability.
3. A noncontrast CT with no evidence of hemorrhage or well-established infarction.

tPA, tissue plasminogen factor; CT, computed tomography.
From Adams HP Jr, Del Zoppo G, Albert MJ, et al. Guidelines for the early management of adults with ischemic stroke: a guideline from the American Heart Association/American Stroke Association Stroke Council, Clinical Cardiology Council, Cardiovascular Radiology and Intervention Council, and the Atherosclerotic Peripheral Vascular Disease and Quality of Care Outcomes in Research Interdisciplinary Working Groups: the American Academy of Neurology affirms the value of this guideline as an educational tool for neurologists. *Stroke.* 2007;38(5):1655–1711, with permission.

- Once a decision regarding acute treatment has been made, attention can be directed to identifying conditions that may have caused the patient's stroke.

Neurologic Examination

- The neurologic examination will allow the clinician to quickly determine which brain areas are dysfunctional and further narrow the differential diagnosis.
- The first step in localization of vascular lesions is determining whether the signs and symptoms arise from the anterior circulation or the posterior circulation.
- The two symptoms that most accurately reflect carotid (anterior) circulation disease are aphasia and monocular blindness.
- The areas responsible for language reside in the dominant (nearly always left) hemispheric cortex, within the territory of the MCA; a stroke causing aphasia must, therefore, involve this circulation.
- Similarly, the blood supply of the eye arises largely from the ophthalmic artery, a direct branch from the carotid artery.

TABLE 52.4

ABSOLUTE CONTRAINDICATIONS TO tPA USE

1. Mild or rapidly improving deficits
2. Hemorrhage on CT, well-established acute infarct on CT, or any other CT diagnosis that contraindicates treatment, including abscess or tumor (excluding small meningiomas)
3. A known CNS vascular malformation or tumor
4. Bacterial endocarditis

tPA, tissue plasminogen factor; CT, computed tomography; CNS, central nervous system.
From Adams HP Jr, Del Zoppo G, Albert MJ, et al. Guidelines for the early management of adults with ischemic stroke: a guideline from the American Heart Association/American Stroke Association Stroke Council, Clinical Cardiology Council, Cardiovascular Radiology and Intervention Council, and the Atherosclerotic Peripheral Vascular Disease and Quality of Care Outcomes in Research Interdisciplinary Working Groups: the American Academy of Neurology affirms the value of this guideline as an educational tool for neurologists. *Stroke.* 2007;38(5):1655–1711, with permission.

TABLE 52.5

RELATIVE CONTRAINDICATIONS TO tPA USE

1. Significant trauma within the past 3 months (including CPR with chest compressions within the past 10 days)
2. Ischemic stroke within 3 months
3. History of intracranial hemorrhage, or symptoms suggestive of subarachnoid hemorrhage
4. Major surgery within the past 14 days
5. Minor surgery within past 19 days, including liver and kidney biopsy, thoracentesis, and lumbar puncture
6. Arterial puncture at a noncompressible site within past 14 days
7. Pregnancy (and ≤10 days postpartum)
8. Gastrointestinal, urologic, or respiratory hemorrhage within past 21 days
9. Known bleeding diathesis (includes renal and hepatic insufficiency)
10. Peritoneal dialysis or hemodialysis
11. PTT >40s, PT >15 (INR >1.7), platelet count <100,000
12. Seizure at onset of stroke (This relative contraindication is intended to prevent treatment of patients with a deficit due to postictal Todd paralysis or with seizure due to some other CNS lesion that precludes thrombolytic therapy. If rapid diagnosis of vascular occlusion can be made, treatment may be given.)
13. Glucose <50 or >400 mg/dL (This relative contraindication is intended to prevent treatment of patients with focal deficits due to hypoglycemia or hyperglycemia. If the deficit persists after correction of the serum glucose, or if rapid diagnosis of vascular occlusion can be made, treatment may be given.)
14. Systolic BP >180 mm Hg *or* diastolic BP >110 mm Hg, despite basic measures to lower it acutely
15. Consideration should be given to the increased risk of hemorrhage in patients with severe deficits (NIHSS >20), age >75, or early edema with mass effect on CT.

tPA, tissue plasminogen factor; CPR, cardiopulmonary resuscitation; PTT, partial thromboplastin time; PT, prothrombin time; INR, international normalized ratio; CNS, central nervous system; BP, blood pressure; NIHSS, National Institutes of Health Stroke Scale; CT, computed tomography.

- Posterior circulation syndromes that result from strokes are usually more complex than those in the cerebral hemispheres.
- Strokes involving the brainstem often manifest with cranial nerve dysfunction (dysarthria, dysphagia, diplopia).
- Crossed signs, with motor or sensory deficits affecting one side of the face and the opposite side of the body, may occur as major decussations in these pathways and occur in the pons and medulla.
- The unique vascular anatomy of the basilar artery may lead to bilateral neurologic deficits.
- Classic lacunar syndromes include pure motor hemiparesis, pure hemisensory symptoms, dysarthria–clumsy hand syndrome, and ataxia-hemiparesis (pontine infarct).

Vascular System Examination

- The neurologic examination complements the history, but physical examination of the vascular system itself is usually surprisingly unrewarding.

- The presence of carotid bruits is of low sensitivity and specificity for predicting vascular disease. Many bruits reflect benign conditions.
- Clinical decisions should be based on definitive assessment of blood vessels using ultrasound or angiography.
- Examination of the heart should focus on detecting thrombogenic diseases, including myocardial infarction, congestive heart failure, arrhythmias, prosthetic valves, and bacterial endocarditis.

Laboratory Studies: General

- Laboratory studies may narrow the differential diagnosis and reveal relevant comorbid conditions.
- Studies that need to be obtained immediately to determine a patient's candidacy for thrombolytic therapy include an electrolyte battery, glucose, platelet count, cardiac enzymes, human chorionic gonadotropin, and coagulation parameters.
- Severe hyponatremia, hypernatremia, or glucose disturbances can cause neurologic dysfunction that may mimic stroke.
- Coagulation parameters and a platelet count will identify patients who may be at greater risk for bleeding.
- A fasting lipid profile should be obtained for potential vascular risk factor modification.
- In patients older than 50 years, an erythrocyte sedimentation rate and C-reactive protein are essential if giant-cell arteritis is suspected.
- In patients for whom an unusual cause of stroke is suspected (young patients or minimal vascular risk factors), investigation of prothrombotic states may be performed.
- Toxicology screening should be performed on hospital admission, with attention directed to amphetamines, phencyclidine, ephedrine, and cocaine.

Imaging Studies

- **Computed tomography**
  - A noncontrasted CT scan of the brain is the standard initial evaluation for stroke.
  - CT is very sensitive to the presence of hemorrhage and is the only radiologic test necessary to determine eligibility for IV-tPA.
  - CT is not sensitive for detection of an acute cerebral infarction, and the lack of abnormality within the first 24 hours should be expected.
  - The view of the posterior fossa is also quite limited, and any changes (with the exception of hemorrhage) seen within the brainstem or cerebellum should be confirmed with MRI.
  - When available, CT angiography (CTA) and perfusion studies can be obtained with very little additional time and provide valuable additional information regarding the patency of blood vessels and blood flow to individual large-vessel territories.
  - The angiographic results from CTA are closest to the traditional gold standard exam: digital subtraction catheter angiography.
  - When examining the carotid arteries, the results from CTA are often sufficient to differentiate a high-grade stenosis (60%–99%) that is treatable from complete occlusion that is not.

- **Magnetic resonance imaging**
  - MRI is far more sensitive for acute infarction than CT. Diffusion MRI sequences can detect ischemia within minutes of onset.
  - MRI is of special value in brainstem and posterior circulation strokes, as the images are not obscured by bony artifacts as with CT.
  - Multiple MRI sequences allow for much more specific differentiation between ischemic brain and other structural abnormalities. In addition, MRI can display flow-related enhancement of the vasculature, resulting in a magnetic resonance angiogram (MRA).
  - MRA tends to slightly overestimate the degree of stenosis, and thus is not usually sufficient to differentiate high-grade stenosis from occlusion.
  - Disadvantages of MRI and MRA include reduced availability and substantially longer scanning times, which place some limitations on their use.
- **Digital subtraction catheter angiography**
  - Digital subtraction catheter angiography is no longer used as a routine screening test as the quality of noninvasive imaging techniques has improved.
  - Indications now include precisely delimiting critical vascular stenoses and examination of arterial dissections, arteriovenous malformations, and aneurysms.
- **Carotid ultrasound**
  - Carotid ultrasound provides a rapid noninvasive assessment of carotid artery disease, based on abnormalities of either flow (Doppler) or morphology (B-mode).
  - Ultrasound, however, suffers from the same limitation as MRA in differentiating high-grade stenosis and occlusion.
  - Lesions of the more distal internal carotid artery may also be difficult to visualize in some patients.
- **Transcranial Doppler**
  - Transcranial Doppler allows rapid bedside assessment of abnormal flow within the distal ICA and major intracranial arteries.
  - The 2-MHz ultrasonic signal can penetrate various bony "windows" in most patients, and its gated character allows identification of arteries by "depth" of the reflected signal.
  - Transcranial Doppler can examine proximal portions of all major branches of the circle of Willis but is insensitive for pathology beyond the A1, M1, or P1 segments.
  - Newer applications include detection of microemboli and online monitoring of arterial flow during invasive procedures, such as carotid endarterectomy.
  - Disadvantages include major dependency on operator skill and the prevalence of acoustically inadequate bony windows.
- **Transthoracic echocardiography (TTE) and transesophageal echocardiography**
  - TTE is essential to evaluate cardiac function.
  - Physicians must attend not only to a visualized thrombus but to other pathologic states associated with systemic embolization, including left ventricular wall motion abnormalities, chamber dilatation, valvular disease, ejection fraction, and septal defects.
  - TTE can be routinely performed and is a superior study for the detection of ventricular apex pathology, left ventricle thrombus, and views of prosthetic valves.
  - TEE provides much greater resolution and is more sensitive for pathology of the left atrial appendage, intra-atrial

septum, atrial aspect of mitral-tricuspid valves, and the ascending aorta.
  - TEE is an invasive procedure that requires sedation but can be performed safely on most patients.

MANAGEMENT

Acute Therapy

- The immediate goal is to determine whether the patient is a candidate for thrombolytic therapy; thus attention should be focused on obtaining the relevant history and performing a neurologic examination.
- Patients with acute stroke are often markedly hypertensive, and one should be cautious in aggressively treating elevated blood pressure before a more complete assessment of the patient has been completed.
- Blood pressure goals are determined by type of stroke, cause, and the presence of comorbid conditions, such as coronary artery disease (CAD).
- All patients should be evaluated with the National Institutes of Health Stroke Scale, which can help to exclude a patient from potentially harmful therapy on the basis of the stroke being too small or too severe.
- **Thrombolytic therapy**
  - Currently, thrombolytic treatment with tPA in eligible stroke patients is the standard of care.
  - Multiple trials indicate that patients treated with tPA within 3 hours of onset were ≥30% more likely to have minimal or no disability at 3 months compared with placebo.
  - To optimize the risk-benefit ratio, strict inclusion criteria (see Table 52.3) for the administration of thrombolytic therapy in acute stroke patients are followed.
  - Absolute exclusion criteria have been established as well (see Table 52.4).
  - Additionally, there is a long list of *relative* contraindications to thrombolytic therapy (see Table 52.5).
  - Most patients who experience intercerebral hemorrhage (ICH) after tPA therapy have severe baseline insults and were already destined for a poor outcome; thus, the hemorrhage does little to alter the final outcome.
  - The dose of tPA is 0.9 mg/kg, with a maximum dose of 90 mg; 10% is given as a bolus over 1 minute, and the remaining 90% is infused over 60 minutes.
  - All invasive procedures, including placement of nasogastric tubes, urinary bladder catheters, central venous lines, arterial lines, intramuscular injections, and rectal temperature probes, must be avoided for 24 hours.
  - After treatment, patients should be monitored in an intensive care unit for more than 24 hours. Vital signs and neurologic exams should be checked frequently.
  - Blood pressure should be strictly controlled for 24 hours, keeping the systolic blood pressure <180 mm Hg and the diastolic blood pressure <105 mm Hg.
  - The benefit of therapeutic hypothermia is yet to be confirmed, but euthermia is clearly associated with better outcome.
- **STAT head CT**
  - A STAT head CT should be performed for any worsening neurologic status.
  - Should an intracerebral hemorrhage develop after thrombolysis, several steps must be taken emergently.

- Neurosurgery should be contacted for possible hematoma evacuation, and anticoagulation should be reversed.
- **Intra-arterial approach for thrombolytic therapy**
  - The use of thrombolytic interventions outside of the 3-hour time window is controversial.
  - Trials that have extended the therapeutic window beyond 3 hours for IV therapy have failed to show convincing benefit as the risk of hemorrhage rapidly increases with time.
  - According to the American Stroke Association guidelines, intra-arterial thrombolysis is an option for treatment of selected patients who have major stroke of <6 hours' duration due to occlusion of the MCA and who are not otherwise candidates for IV-tPA.
  - The availability of intra-arterial thrombolysis should not preclude the administration of IV-tPA in otherwise eligible patients.
  - Treatment requires immediate access to cerebral angiography and qualified interventionalists.
  - Recommendations for blood pressure control after tPA use are presented in Table 52.6.
  - Management of post-tPA hemorrhage is presented in Table 52.7.

Supportive Care

- Early initiation of physical, occupational, and speech therapy services hastens functional recovery from stroke.

TABLE 52.6

BLOOD PRESSURE CONTROL AFTER tPA

1. Management of blood pressure during and after treatment with tPA or other acute reperfusion intervention:
   a. Monitor blood pressure every 15 min during treatment and then for another 2 h, then every 30 min for 6 h, and then every hour for 16 h;
   b. For systolic 180–230 mm Hg or diastolic 105–120 mm Hg:
      i. Labetalol 10 mg IV over 1 to 2 min, may repeat every 10 to 20 min, maximum dose of 300 mg; or
      ii. Labetalol 10 mg IV followed by an infusion at 2 to 8 mg/min
   c. For systolic >230 mm Hg or diastolic 121 to 140 mm Hg:
      i. Labetalol 10 mg IV over 1 to 2 min, may repeat every 10 to 20 min, maximum dose of 300 mg; or
      ii. Labetalol 10 mg IV followed by an infusion at 2 to 8 mg/min; or
      iii. Nicardipine infusion, 5 mg/h, titrate up to desired effect by increasing by 2.5 mg/h every 5 min to maximum of 15 mg/h
      iv. If blood pressure not controlled, consider sodium nitroprusside.

tPA, tissue plasminogen factor.
From Adams HP Jr, Del Zoppo G, Albert MJ, et al. Guidelines for the early management of adults with ischemic stroke: a guideline from the American Heart Association/American Stroke Association Stroke Council, Clinical Cardiology Council, Cardiovascular Radiology and Intervention Council, and the Atherosclerotic Peripheral Vascular Disease and Quality of Care Outcomes in Research Interdisciplinary Working Groups: the American Academy of Neurology affirms the value of this guideline as an educational tool for neurologists. *Stroke.* 2007;38(5):1655–1711, with permission.

TABLE 52.7

MANAGEMENT OF POST-tPA HEMORRHAGE

1. Blood should be sent STAT for CBC, PT, PTT, platelets, fibrinogen and D-dimer (this should be repeated every 2 h until bleeding is controlled).
2. Give 2 U of fresh frozen plasma every 6 h for 24 h after the thrombolytic agent was given.
3. Give cryoprecipitate (20 U); if the fibrinogen level is <200 mg/dL at 1 h, repeat the cryoprecipitate dose.
4. Give 4 U of platelets.
5. Give protamine sulfate (1 mg/100 U heparin given in the last 3 h);
   a. A test dose of 10 mg slow IV push over 10 min should be given while observing for anaphylaxis;
   b. Then the remaining dose by slow IV push, up to a maximum dose of 50 mg.
6. Institute frequent neurologic checks, as well as management of increased ICP, as needed.
7. Aminocaproic acid (Amicar) can be given as a last resort, in a dose of 5 g in 250 mL normal saline IV over 1 h.

CBC, complete blood count; PT, prothrombin time; PTT, partial thromboplastin time; IV, intravenous; ICP, intracranial pressure.
From Adams HP Jr, Del Zoppo G, Albert MJ, et al. Guidelines for the early management of adults with ischemic stroke: a guideline from the American Heart Association/American Stroke Association Stroke Council, Clinical Cardiology Council, Cardiovascular Radiology and Intervention Council, and the Atherosclerotic Peripheral Vascular Disease and Quality of Care Outcomes in Research Interdisciplinary Working Groups: the American Academy of Neurology affirms the value of this guideline as an educational tool for neurologists. *Stroke.* 2007;38(5):1655–1711, with permission.

- Dysphagia is common after stroke. All patients should be screened for dysphagia before being allowed to take anything by mouth, as aspiration pneumonia is a substantial contributor to mortality after stroke.
- Early mobilization not only prevents deep vein thromboses but speeds rehabilitation.
- Deep vein thrombosis prophylaxis with low-molecular-weight heparin is safe and more effective than unfractionated heparin in stroke patients.
- For most stroke patients with acute hypertension, aggressively lowering the blood pressure may cause more harm than benefit.
- The general practice is to refrain from intervening until the pressure exceeds an arbitrary limit of 220 mm Hg systolic or 120 mm Hg diastolic. In patients having received thrombolytics, the tolerable limit is lower (<180 mm Hg systolic or <105 mm Hg diastolic).
- Control of hyperglycemia is recommended as persistent hyperglycemia (blood glucose level >200 mg/dL) during the first 24 hours after stroke is associated with poor neurologic outcomes.
- Although most patients eventually improve after a stroke, early clinical deterioration is not uncommon. Neurologic causes of clinical deterioration include progressive or recurrent stroke, hemorrhagic transformation of the infarct, and local cerebral edema.
- Cerebral edema is the most common cause of deterioration and may cause fatal herniation in large MCA infarctions, especially in the young, women, and in patients with involvement of additional vascular territories.

- Corticosteroids do not appear helpful and hyperglycemia associated with their use may worsen clinical outcome.
- Decompressive surgery, including hemicraniectomy and durotomy with temporal lobe resection, for treatment of brain edema after stroke is controversial.

INTRACEREBRAL HEMORRHAGE

Pathogenesis

- Primary ICH involves bleeding, usually of arterial origin, into normally perfused brain and thus must be distinguished from hemorrhagic transformation of an initially ischemic stroke.
- The expanding hematoma causes direct injury to local brain tissue and dysfunction in surrounding regions.
- In younger patients, hypertension is by far the more common cause and, as such, ICH tends to occur in the same brain areas where other hypertensive pathologies occur.
- In contrast, lobar ICHs occur more commonly in the elderly population and are often associated with cerebral amyloid angiopathy in the absence of hypertension.
- ICH may also occur in the setting of trauma, use of illicit drugs or over-the-counter medications, excessive alcohol consumption, an underlying vascular abnormality, brain tumor, or a bleeding diathesis.

Clinical Evaluation

- Rapid diagnosis of ICH is essential, as progression during the first several hours is the norm.
- The hallmark is sudden-onset focal neurologic deficit, which progresses over minutes to hours. Headache, increased blood pressure, and impaired level of consciousness are common features that complete the presentation.
- History gathering should be directed at elucidating the presence of risk factors as outlined earlier. Other considerations include the use of antithrombotic medications (e.g., aspirin or warfarin) or hematologic disorders that predispose to bleeding.
- The patient's coagulation parameters should be checked immediately and corrected if abnormal.
- Once stabilized, the patient should undergo a noncontrast head CT immediately to verify brain hemorrhage. CT angiography may also be helpful in detecting aneurysms, arteriovenous malformations, underlying tumors, or abscesses.
- MRI will also provide information about the hemorrhage but is time-consuming and potentially dangerous for an unstable patient.
- Catheter angiography should be considered in a young patient with an ICH with no history of hypertension, as an occult arteriovenous malformation or aneurysm may be responsible.
- Cardiac arrhythmias represent another potentially catastrophic secondary complication of ICH, especially those that occur in the right hemisphere insular region. Dysfunction of this area has a propensity for causing abnormal cardiac electrical activity and "cerebrogenic sudden death."
- Patients with such lesions must have close cardiac monitoring in the intensive care unit during their first several days after hemorrhage.

Management

- The mainstays of medical treatment of acute ICH are correction of any coagulopathy and avoidance of hypertension.
- Beyond the first few hours after onset, aggressive lowering of blood pressure may be potentially harmful (Table 52.8). When necessary, certain pharmacologic agents may be used (Table 52.9). Attention must be focused on maintaining the cerebral perfusion pressure >70 mm Hg to avoid secondary ischemia.
- Seizures—occasionally nonconvulsive—occur commonly after ICH. Prophylactic anticonvulsant medications may be considered for patients. If seizures are confirmed, they should be treated aggressively.
- Treatment of increased ICP should initially focus on more conservative noninvasive measures.
- An implanted ICP monitor should be considered for those patients with large hematomas to guide whether to place an intraventricular drain or perform a surgical evacuation.
- In general, patients with a Glasgow Coma Score of 4 or more have a uniformly poor outcome, regardless of whether surgery is performed, and thus these patients should be treated medically.
- Patients with cerebellar hemorrhages >3 cm in diameter should be considered for emergency decompression, especially if there are signs of brainstem compression, hydrocephalus, or neurologic deterioration.
- Patients who deteriorate despite maximal medical therapy may benefit from surgical decompression, but results from clinical trials have been mixed.

TABLE 52.8

SUGGESTED RECOMMENDED GUIDELINES FOR TREATING ELEVATED BLOOD PRESSURE IN SPONTANEOUS ICH

1. If SBP is >200 mm Hg or MAP is >150 mm Hg, then consider aggressive reduction of blood pressure with continuous intravenous infusion, with frequent blood pressure monitoring every 5 min.
2. If SBP is >180 mm Hg or MAP is >130 mm Hg and there is evidence of or suspicion of elevated ICP, then consider monitoring ICP and reducing blood pressure using intermittent or continuous intravenous medications to keep cerebral perfusion pressure >60 to 80 mm Hg.
3. If SBP is >180 mm Hg or MAP is >130 mm Hg and there is not evidence of or suspicion of elevated ICP, then consider a modest reduction of blood pressure (e.g., MAP of 110 mm Hg or target blood pressure of 160/90 mm Hg) using intermittent or continuous intravenous medications to control blood pressure, and clinically re-examine the patient every 15 min.

ICH, intercerebral hemorrhage; SBP, systolic blood pressure; MAP, mean arterial pressure; ICP, intracranial pressure.
From Broderick J, Connolly S, Feldmann E, et al. Guidelines for the management of spontaneous intracerebral hemorrhage in adults: 2007 update: a guideline from the American Heart Association/American Stroke Association Stroke Council, High Blood Pressure Research Council, and the Quality of Care and Outcomes in Research Interdisciplinary Working Group. *Circulation.* 2007;116(16): e391–413, with permission.

TABLE 52.9

INTRAVENOUS MEDICATIONS THAT MAY BE CONSIDERED FOR CONTROL OF ELEVATED BLOOD PRESSURE IN PATIENTS WITH ICH

Drug	Intravenous bolus dose	Continuous infusion rate
Labetalol	5–20 mg every 15 min	2 mg/min (maximum 300 mg/d)
Nicardipine	NA	5–15 mg/h
Esmolol	250 μg/kg IVP loading dose	25–300 μg $\cdot$ kg^{-1} $\cdot$ min^{-1}
Enalapril	1.25–5 mg IVP every 6 h[a]	NA
Hydralazine	5–20 mg IVP every 30 min	1.5–5 μg $\cdot$ kg^{-1} $\cdot$ min^{-1}
Nipride	NA	0.1–10 μg $\cdot$ kg^{-1} $\cdot$ min^{-1}
Nitroglycerin	NA	20–400 μg/min

ICH, intercerebral hemorrhage; NA, not applicable; IVP, intravenous push.
[a]Because of the risk of precipitous blood pressure decrease, the first test dose of enalapril should be 0.625 mg.
From Broderick J, Connolly S, Feldmann E, et al. Guidelines for the management of spontaneous intracerebral hemorrhage in adults: 2007 update: a guideline from the American Heart Association/American Stroke Association Stroke Council, High Blood Pressure Research Council, and the Quality of Care and Outcomes in Research Interdisciplinary Working Group. *Circulation.* 2007;116(16): e391–413, with permission.

- Patients with lobar hemorrhages secondary to amyloid angiopathy have exceptionally friable cortical blood vessels and are poor surgical candidates.
- ICH causes approximately 10% of first-time strokes. The 30-day mortality rate is high at 35% to 50%, with half of the deaths occurring within the first 2 days.
- Outcome in ICH is dependent on several factors, including the location and size of the hemorrhage, the presence of intraventricular blood or hydrocephalus, the age of the patient, the Glasgow Coma Scale on presentation, and the cause of the hemorrhage.

SUBARACHNOID HEMORRHAGE

- SAH is a relatively uncommon but often devastating type of stroke.
- Incidence is estimated at 30,000 patients per year in the United States, with a mortality that exceeds 50%.
- Whereas head trauma is the most frequent cause of subarachnoid hemorrhage, aneurysmal rupture results in the greatest morbidity and mortality.
- Most commonly, patients perceive a sudden severe headache with rapid impairment of consciousness.
- Focal neurologic symptoms such as hemiparesis, sensory loss, or diplopia may occur if loculation of subarachnoid blood or intraparenchymal extension of the hemorrhage develops.
- The most important features of the neurologic examination are the assessment of level of consciousness, cranial nerve function, and motor function.

Diagnosis

- Diagnosis of SAH is based on neuroimaging or cerebrospinal fluid (CSF) analysis.
- Brain CT scan is a very sensitive indicator of the presence of subarachnoid blood.
- Brain parenchyma itself most commonly displays no acute abnormalities.

- Erythrocyte concentration in CSF below approximately 30,000 cells/μL may not result in the diagnostic increased density within CSF on CT scans.
- In approximately 10% of patients, diagnosis requires CSF analysis through lumbar puncture.
- In addition to elevated erythrocyte count, CSF xanthochromia and elevation of CSF D-dimer can often be detected in true subarachnoid hemorrhage.
- The latter two findings may help distinguish bloody CSF from a "traumatic tap," as these serve as markers of the breakdown of thrombosis or blood products.
- Serial cell counts should always be obtained, however, whenever SAH is suspected.
- Cell counts in SAH should be roughly equivalent in all tubes, whereas a declining count is usual in traumatic punctures.
- Lumbar puncture should be avoided in any patient with a depressed level of consciousness until CT scan excludes a focal mass (such as intraparenchymal or subdural hemorrhage).
- If bacterial meningitis is a concern, blood cultures should be obtained and antibiotics started while awaiting results of the CT scan.

Management

- Patients with acute SAH are at high risk for a multitude of complications (Table 52.10) that usually mandate admission to an intensive care facility.
- All patients should be placed on strict bed rest, with appropriate precautions for deep venous thrombosis and aspiration.
- Patients with progressive lethargy may require intubation for airway protection and mechanical ventilation.
- Until the aneurysm has been ablated, blood pressure should be kept in the normotensive range, and isotonic intravenous fluids should be used to maintain normovolemia.
- All patients should be started on nimodipine at 60 mg every 4 hours (duration 21 days), either orally or through a nasogastric tube, for prevention of vasospasm.
- The practice of prophylactic anticonvulsants has recently come into question, as recent data suggest that patients who

TABLE 52.10

COMPLICATIONS OF SUBARACHNOID HEMORRHAGE

Complication	Clinical features	Diagnostic tests	Therapy
Increased ICP	Decreased alertness, worsened headache, herniation syndrome	ICP monitor	Mannitol, steroids, hyperventilation
Hydrocephalus	Decreased alertness, worsened headache, herniation syndrome	CT scan	Ventriculostomy drainage or shunt
Vasospasm	Delayed focal neurologic deficit	TCD, angiography	Nimodipine, hypervolemia, hypertension, angioplasty
Rebleed	Worsened neurologic condition, especially level of consciousness	CT scan, lumbar puncture	Ablation of aneurysm
Seizure	Sudden behavioral change or uncontrolled motor activity	EEG	Anticonvulsants
Hyponatremia	Confusion, seizure	Serum electrolytes	Isotonic fluids to achieve euvolemia or hypervolemia
Infection	Confusion, lethargy	Panculture, chest radiograph, urinalysis	Appropriate antibiotic

ICP, intracranial pressure; CT, computed tomography; TCD, transcranial Doppler; EEG, electroencephalogram.

were on prophylactic anticonvulsants had significantly more in-hospital complications and worse clinical outcomes.
- Electrocardiogram changes and elevations in cardiac enzymes, troponin, and CK-MB are commonly seen in SAH patients and may represent the phenomenon of stunned myocardium, in which case management should be aimed at optimizing left ventricular function to support cardiovascular and cerebrovascular perfusion.
- Serum electrolytes are closely monitored, as hyponatremia may be seen in more than 30% of patients after SAH; however, hypernatremia can occur as well and is significantly associated with clinical outcome.
- Serum glucose levels should also be closely monitored, as hyperglycemia has been significantly associated with mortality and poor functional outcome in SAH patients.
- Because fever in SAH patients has been associated with mortality and poor clinical outcome and has even been linked to vasospasm, patients should be kept normothermic.
- Platelet levels should be monitored, as a relatively significant incidence of heparin-induced thrombocytopenia has been reported in SAH patients.

Complications

- In those patients surviving the initial hemorrhage, *the leading factor associated with mortality is rebleeding from the aneurysm.* A second bleed from an aneurysm is associated with a 74% mortality rate.
- Untreated aneurysms rebleed at a rate of 4% on day 1, then 1% to 2% a day for the next 4 weeks. Thus, early treatment to secure a ruptured aneurysm is critical.
- Aneurysmal clipping is best performed either early (0 to 3 days) or late (11 to 14 days). Outcome is worse when performed at 7 to 10 days after the onset of SAH.
- Early treatment of the ruptured aneurysm also allows aggressive management of vasospasm, manipulations that would increase the risk of rebleeding from an unsecured aneurysm.
- After rebleeding, vasospasm is the next leading cause of mortality and morbidity from an SAH.

- The exact cause of arterial vasospasm after SAH is unknown, but its incidence does appear to be correlated with the density of blood products seen on CT scan.
- Severe vasospasm may result in cerebral infarction within the vascular distribution of the involved artery.
- The risk for vasospasm begins about 3 days after the bleed and may persist for 3 weeks.
- Transcranial Doppler is a sensitive indicator of the presence and degree of vasospasm within proximal arteries, although it may not detect vasospasm restricted to smaller peripheral vessels.
- The calcium channel blockers nimodipine and nicardipine can reduce the incidence of vasospasm and associated cerebral infarction.
- Studies with statin therapy (HMG Co-A inhibitors) have demonstrated promising results with reduced rates of vasospasm and better clinical outcomes.

Management after Aneurysm Ablation

- Triple-H therapy—hypertension, hypervolemia, hemodilution—is the first-line therapy against vasospasm.
- Once vasospasm occurs, IV fluids should be pushed to the tolerance of the patient (<400 mL/h).
- As congestive heart failure is a potential complication, central pressure monitoring—at a minimum—should be used in patients at risk; optimal central venous pressure is 8 to 12 mm Hg.
- Other modalities of monitoring, from pulse-waveform variability to placement of a pulmonary artery catheter may be necessary to properly care for these patients.
- If hypervolemic therapy is not adequate to control vasospasm, hypertension can be initiated by cessation of antihypertensives or use of vasopressors (e.g., phenylephrine, 0.1–5 μg/kg/min, or vasopressin, 0.01–0.04 U/min), targeting mean arterial pressures of 120 to 140 mm Hg (systolic blood pressure 180–200 mm Hg).
- Triple-H therapy does not increase the risk of rupture of other, incidentally found, aneurysms in patients with multiple aneurysms.

- Acute hydrocephalus occurs in approximately 20% of survivors of SAH.
- The likelihood of hydrocephalus increases with worsening grade of hemorrhage.

- Ventriculostomy drainage is recommended for patients with acute hydrocephalus and decreased level of consciousness; improvement can be expected in >50% of patients.

CHAPTER 53 ■ UROLOGIC SURGERY AND TRAUMA

IMMEDIATE CONCERNS

- Primary emergency considerations in urology from the critical care perspective include hemorrhagic, obstructive, infectious, and ischemic processes, in addition to a wide variety of general postoperative difficulties that may warrant emergent intervention. Oncologic emergencies also arise in urology and may require urgent critical care management.
- **Gross hematuria** may require immediate critical care intervention depending on the magnitude of the hematuria and details of the individual case.
  - Gross hematuria may have a defined cause (e.g., known radiation cystitis, recurrent benign prostatic hypertrophy [BPH]-related bleeding) or may be a new sign.
  - Immediate urologic intervention is necessary if the patient has clot retention, is bleeding severely, has significant pain, is infected, has coagulopathy, or has underlying medical factors that increase risk of further complications.
  - Vital signs, physical examination, and basic laboratory studies including complete blood count (CBC), coagulation functions, electrolyte and renal function testing, urinalysis, and culture will often lead to a diagnosis and determine the need for immediate intervention.
  - In the setting of gross hematuria and a distended bladder, a catheter must be inserted. The catheter should be irrigated using 60 to 120 mL of normal saline.
  - A three-way catheter for continuous bladder irrigation (CBI) in the setting of continuing bleeding may be used to keep the catheter patent in this situation, but this decision is best made along with urologic consultation.
  - Risks of CBI include bladder rupture if the outflow lumen becomes occluded without recognition and the inflow of irrigant continues.
  - Early cystoscopy can provide diagnosis and definitive intervention.
  - Other hemorrhagic urologic problems requiring immediate critical care intervention include renal or perirenal bleeding (e.g., spontaneous hematoma or renal tumor) or scrotal hematoma.

Urosepsis

- Sepsis of the urinary tract or urogenital origin may present in a most precipitous and potentially life-threatening manner, or may be indolent.

- The combination of infection and obstruction of the urinary tract is a surgical emergency requiring immediate action.
- Septic shock may unfold rapidly in such situations with a significant mortality rate, even in the otherwise healthy host.
- Other infectious states requiring urgent critical care intervention include renal or perirenal abscess, scrotal abscess, acute epididymo-orchitis, and Fournier gangrene.

Obstruction of the Urinary Tract and Urinary Retention

- May require critical care intervention independent of the presence or absence of hematuria or infection.
- Upper or lower tract obstruction can result in acute or chronic renal failure, mandating prompt drainage to control metabolic instability.
- Acute urinary retention with bladder distention must be promptly relieved by introduction of a catheter into the bladder, preferably by a transurethral route, or alternatively by a suprapubic route if the urethra is impassable.

Ischemic States

- The quintessential example is that of testicular torsion. The other condition of critical care relevance is the ischemic kidney.
- Delayed diagnosis of torsion is a common cause of unnecessary testicular loss. After 8 hours, the likelihood of testicular salvage decreases significantly.
- A high index of suspicion is necessary when addressing "the acute scrotum," with accurate history and physical examination forming the core of this assessment.
- When clinical suspicion of acute testicular torsion is high, surgical exploration should not be delayed to obtain confirmatory imaging that is not readily and rapidly available.
- The differential diagnosis of the acute scrotum includes incarcerated or strangulated inguinal hernia for which urgent surgical management is also critical.
- The kidney begins to undergo irreversible loss of function following approximately 30 minutes of warm ischemia time; thus, rapid action is necessary.

Oncologic Emergencies

- Often involve hemorrhagic, obstructive, and infectious problems. Other emergencies include neurologic compromise and pain management issues.
- Prostate cancer may metastasize preferentially to the skeletal system and may cause sudden neurologic compromise from spinal cord compression.
- Manifestations include sensory loss, paralysis, and loss of urinary, bowel, and sexual function; when observed, immediate neurosurgical consultation should be obtained.
- Antiandrogen therapy may be of great value when prostate cancer patients present with complications such as neurologic or urinary obstructive compromise. Intramuscular luteinizing hormone–releasing hormone agonists may be started immediately.
- An antiandrogen drug such as bicalutamide should be commenced simultaneously or prior to the luteinizing hormone–releasing hormone analog to prevent transient worsening from the androgen flare.

POSTOPERATIVE MANAGEMENT

- Both major and minor urologic surgery may present critical care issues that require rapid and accurate assessment and intervention. Currently, many urologic procedures that have traditionally been performed through open surgical approaches are now commonly being approached by laparoscopic, robotic, and other minimally invasive techniques, which bring with them their own set of postoperative challenges.

Upper Abdominal Surgery

- **Patient position and selection of incision** are relevant to the postoperative management to anticipate the types of problems that may arise postoperatively.
  - In flank surgery, it is not uncommon to encounter a "down-lung" syndrome, with postoperative atelectasis involving the lung positioned downward against the operating table.
  - Occasionally lobar or complete lung atelectasis may be noted and may require bronchoscopic intervention.
  - Excellent pulmonary toilet is critical following upper abdominal and flank urologic surgery and ideally should be initiated preoperatively.
  - Postoperative pain from flank surgery can be a major problem and can require expert pain management intervention, continuous epidural analgesic strategies, subcutaneous pain pumps, and patient-controlled intravenous analgesics.
  - Appropriate pain control is also key to minimizing pulmonary complications by aiding respiratory and coughing efforts.
- **Early postoperative hypoadrenal state** should be considered after surgery involving removal or manipulation of the adrenal gland.
  - The critical care specialist should know if the adrenal was removed along with a nephrectomy procedure and whether there is any reason to suspect hypofunction or absence of the contralateral gland.

- **Acute renal insufficiency** may occur following any major surgery, and is of particular concern following renal surgery.
  - Partial nephrectomies may be performed using warm or cold ischemia techniques.
  - When the latter approach is used, vascular control of the kidney is obtained and the patient's kidney is packed in saline slush. The excisional procedure is completed in a setting of local hypothermia.
  - Some degree of postoperative acute tubular necrosis may still occur despite the cold ischemia technique.
  - The clinical relevance of the acute tubular necrosis depends largely on the state of the contralateral kidney, and standard management principles for acute renal insufficiency are applicable.
- **Postoperative bleeding** may be manifested by hemodynamic changes, acute anemia, physical findings such as palpable flank hematoma or ecchymosis, or radiologic findings of blood in the renal fossa, chest (after a transthoracic procedure) or peritoneal cavity (after a transperitoneal procedure).
  - Following a partial nephrectomy, significant postoperative bleeding most commonly arises from arterial branch vessels within the renal parenchyma at the resection site.
  - If significant bleeding occurs following renal surgery, expectant management with transfusion, correction of any coagulopathy, angiographic embolization, CT scanning to assess the specific anatomic site of bleeding and judge the size of the hematoma, and/or a return to the operating room for re-exploration are options to be considered.
  - The choice between these measures is individualized based on the severity of the bleeding, patient condition and physiologic reserve, and access to imaging, interventional radiologic and surgical resources.
  - If there is evidence that major early postoperative bleeding occurs that may be due to an uncontrolled renal pedicle, rapid surgical re-exploration is the best approach.
  - If bleeding occurs subacutely and renal parenchymal bleeding is suspected, interventional radiology is usually favored.
  - The patient should be maintained in a fluid-resuscitated state when a renal bleeding issue is evolving, with the hemoglobin at a level that would allow the patient to tolerate continued blood loss without catastrophic decompensation.
- **Urinary extravasation** following upper urinary tract surgery may be manifested by increased drainage from suction drains for which creatinine determination confirms the fluid's identity as urine.
  - Urologic input should be sought as to whether the region is well drained, whether the leak is expected, and whether intervention versus observation is indicated.

Pelvic Surgery

- Critical care issues typically relate to standard postoperative abdominal surgical concerns such as pain, bleeding, and ileus.
- Procedures requiring postoperative critical care include exenterative procedures for malignancies (radical prostatectomy or cystectomy), simple open prostatectomy for benign prostatic hyperplasia, and reconstructive pelvic surgeries for incontinence.

- Management of tubes and drains and recognizing when urinary extravasation arises in the postoperative period is important.
- Bleeding following major urologic pelvic surgery may result in Foley catheter occlusion with clot. The acceptable degree of hematuria and management of catheter drainage failure should be established with the urologist.
- The possibility of anastomotic leakage or a missed injury to the ureter exists in the radical prostatectomy patient. If suspected, the fluid should be sent for creatinine level to determine if a urine leak is present.
- Radical cystectomy is the procedure carrying the greatest deep vein thrombosis risk of the urologic operations, as an extensive pelvic lymphadenectomy is also typically included.
- Many urologic oncologists will start low-molecular-weight heparin regimens 24 hours after surgery if there are no bleeding issues.

Endoscopic Upper and Lower Urinary Tract Surgery

- The above category includes diagnostic cystoscopy (rigid, flexible), cystoscopic surgery (bladder biopsy, transurethral resection of prostate or bladder tumor [TURP, TURBT]), ureteroscopy, and percutaneous renal access surgery (percutaneous nephrostolithotripsy).
- Postprocedure infection can occur after lower tract endoscopy, but the risk is small if the urine is sterile preprocedure. Prophylactic oral antibiotics are often administered for all endourologic procedures to minimize the infection risk.
- Cystoscopic surgery using glycine or sterile water can result in significant hyponatremia if major absorption occurs.
- As hyponatremia develops, the patient may develop altered mental status, bradycardia, hypertension, and respiratory compromise. If under general endotracheal anesthesia, foamy material may be noted in the breathing circuit.
- Severe hyponatremia may cause cerebral edema and grand mal seizures, and may be life threatening.
- Diuretics with normal saline or hypertonic saline administered intravenously may be indicated. The more abrupt the development of the hyponatremia and the lower the serum sodium, the more dramatic the clinical manifestations are.
- Minimal intraperitoneal resectoscopic injuries may be manageable with catheter drainage alone. If problems arise (abdominal distention, persistent extravasation) with this nonoperative approach, laparoscopic or open surgical repair should be performed.
- Bleeding may be a problem following either TURP or TURBT. Often three-way catheter CBI is employed following these procedures.
- For TURP procedures, catheter traction may help control bleeding from within the prostatic fossa, whereas for TURBT procedures, catheter traction is of no value. Only the urologist should implement or adjust the traction system.
- If a catheter needs to be changed in the early postoperative period following a TURP or TURBT, this should be done by the operating urologist's team or on their specific order.
- Laser energy to ablate, vaporize, or coagulate tissue endoscopically for TURP and TURBT usually result in less bleeding than the traditional approaches. Complications usually relate to obstruction following catheter removal or to iatrogenic injury from misdirected laser energy.
- **Upper tract endoscopy** (ureteroscopy, percutaneous nephroscopy) has progressed greatly in the last two decades, with the current instrumentation allowing complex upper tract procedures to be performed with low morbidity.
  - Problems that the critical care provider may encounter usually relate to ureteral perforation, gross hematuria with stent occlusion, or obstructive problems from stone fragments.
  - Percutaneous nephrostolithotomy or nephrolithotomy may be accompanied by problems related to having surgery in the prone position, a high access traversing or affecting the chest, and postoperative bleeding.
  - If entry into the upper pole calyx is needed for stone access, a supracostal puncture may be required (above the 12th rib). The risk exists to traverse the chest cavity resulting in pneumothorax or hydrothorax, which may require tube thoracostomy postoperatively.
  - Significant bleeding can occur intraoperatively, perioperatively, or days or weeks postoperatively at the time of nephrostomy removal. Occasionally angiographic embolization may be necessary for major renal bleeding.
  - When removing a nephrostomy tube following percutaneous nephrostolithotomy or nephrolithotomy, a tamponade catheter should be immediately available to place into the tract and inflate if dangerous bleeding ensues following tube removal.
  - Extracorporeal shock wave lithotripsy involves the noninvasive fragmentation of renal or ureteral calculi with a shock wave generator system under fluoroscopic or ultrasound guidance. Following extracorporeal shock wave lithotripsy, colic can occur due to passage of fragments. Whether manageable expectantly or requiring stent insertion depends on the stone burden, the amount of debris created, the size of residual fragments, the degree of symptoms, and whether there are signs of infection and septic shock.
- **Laparoscopy** in urologic surgery has come into its own in recent years and has become a major element of our approach to a wide range of surgical tasks that previously were performed solely through major open approaches.
  - In many centers, the open radical retropubic prostatectomy has been nearly replaced by the robotic-assisted laparoscopic prostatectomy.
  - Potential issues include postoperative ileus, CO_2 retention, venous CO_2 embolism, postoperative bleeding, unrecognized intraoperative iatrogenic injury, and trochar and port-site complications.
  - Two potential major sites of postoperative bleeding in laparoscopic renal surgery are the renal pedicle and the renal parenchyma.
  - Bleeding can occur immediately postoperatively or in a more delayed fashion. When precipitous and life threatening, a quick return to the operating room with either laparoscopic or open re-exploration may be the most appropriate course.
  - If the patient's condition and rate of bleeding allows for further evaluation, postoperative CT scanning to determine if there is a renal or perirenal hematoma may be relevant prior to a surgical effort.
  - If bleeding occurs from the cut surface of the kidney following either open or laparoscopic partial nephrectomy, angiography with subselective embolization is often the preferred approach.

- **Drains** left within the abdomen following laparoscopic procedures are often placed intraperitoneally, as opposed to the case in extraperitoneal flank surgery, where the drain is often not within the peritoneal cavity. As such, intraperitoneal drains may drain retained irrigant or peritoneal fluid in copious amounts following surgery.
  - If there is uncertainty as to the significance of increased drain output, fluid may be sent for chemical analysis (creatinine to determine if fluid is urine, amylase to rule out pancreatic fluid leak).
  - Leakage of urine following laparoscopic urologic surgery may not require immediate intervention if the leak is well drained. If action is needed, postoperative ureteral stent insertion (along with a urethral Foley catheter or in some cases nephrostomy insertion) will often allow the collecting system to heal without sequelae.
- **Unrecognized bowel injury** must be appreciated during and after laparoscopic urologic surgery, especially if electrocautery is extensively utilized.
  - The presentation of such complications may be subtle, with low-grade fever; minimal diffuse tenderness, which may be consistent with the expected postsurgical state, or delayed return of bowel function or persistent anorexia.
  - A high degree of suspicion is important when patients fail to thrive following laparoscopic surgery. Postoperative CT scanning may demonstrate a fluid collection in an unexpected location or inflammatory changes in or near the intestine that is unanticipated.
- **Genital surgery** issues that may arise in the critical care setting may relate to penile, sphincter, and testicular prosthetic implants, neurologic stimulater implants, or complications of the wide range of other genital procedures urologists perform.
  - Dressings on the genitalia should be inspected for bleeding or excessive tightness, which can cause vascular compromise, especially if applied circumferentially around the penis.
  - Any major local complaint by a patient following genital surgery should be referred to the urologic surgeon for input.
  - Other genital surgery procedures can be complicated by bleeding or infection. If marked swelling occurs following genital surgery, the urologist should be immediately made aware.

UROLOGIC TRAUMA

- The urologist's experience in elective urologic surgery; endoscopic, radiologic, and open surgical intervention; reconstructive approaches; and management of complications may be very helpful to the trauma and critical care teams when faced with the multiply injured patient or with solitary urologic organ trauma. When no urologist is available, the critical care provider must have a working knowledge of the approach to the most common and important types of urologic trauma.

Iatrogenic Injury Management

- For bladder injuries, simple closure is feasible as long as the injury involves the upper bladder segment, the trigone is uninvolved, and there is not significant tissue loss.
- A generously sized Foley catheter should be used (No. 20 French or larger) to allow drainage of bloody efflux and allow efficient irrigation when needed.
- If the bladder wall surrounding the injury is markedly abnormal (fibrotic, friable, irradiated), a two-layer closure may not be feasible and a one-layer, interrupted closure with heavy suture may be performed.
- If there is involvement of the trigone, ureteral orifices, or intramural ureters, the situation is more complex, and ureteral stent insertion or ureteral reimplantation may be needed.
- Prophylactic insertion of externalized ureteral catheters prior to complex pelvic or retroperitoneal surgery may be helpful in avoiding surgical injury to the ureter.
- For iatrogenic ureteral injuries, the repair approach depends on the level of injury, whether there is loss of ureteral length, the condition of the ureter and surrounding tissue, and the comfort of the surgeon.
- Traditionally, if the ureter is transected caudal to the crossing of the internal iliac artery, a reimplant rather than a primary anastomosis should be performed.
- Reimplantation can be performed with or without a psoas hitch depending on ureteral length and bladder status.
- For injuries in the mid- or upper ureter, primary, spatulated anastomosis performed over an indwelling stent is the preferred solution.
- If primary repair is not possible, the options include ligation followed by nephrostomy insertion and planned delayed reconstruction, transureteroureterostomy, renal autotransplantation, or ileal ureteral replacement.

Penetrating and Blunt Trauma to the Genitourinary System

General Evaluation

- Diagnosis of urinary tract injury is typically based on history and mechanism of injury, physical examination, laboratory assessment, and the findings on imaging studies. Any patient with a history of gross hematuria following trauma should be imaged, unless of course he or she is unstable and/or must be taken directly to surgery.
  - Current literature supports obtaining imaging studies for patients with microscopic hematuria and hypotension at any time following trauma, as well as those patients with significant deceleration mechanisms of injury and other injury factors that portend a high risk of urinary tract injury such as lower posterior rib fracture, transverse spinal process fracture, or pelvic or femur fracture.
  - The contrast-enhanced CT scan of the abdomen and pelvis has become the standard study of choice for assessment of hematuria, for staging of injuries in the trauma setting, and for the evaluation of renal or ureteral injuries.
  - The "shock room intravenous pyelogram" has fallen out of favor and provides much less information than the CT scan.
  - Bladder injuries may be suspected based on the presence of gross hematuria following pelvic trauma with confirmation by either standard radiographic or CT cystography. Adequate bladder filling must be accomplished to demonstrate extravasation and minimize false-negative studies.
  - When urethral injury is suspected (following pelvic fracture or perineal or genital trauma), especially when blood is

exiting from the urethra or present at the urethral meatus, retrograde urethrography should be performed prior to any attempt at urethral catheterization.

- For genital trauma, scrotal ultrasonography may be of great value in diagnosing testicular rupture from blunt forces; in penetrating genital trauma, surgical exploration is usually necessary and one can usually forego imaging studies.
- **Urethral injuries** should be suspected in cases of pelvic fracture, particularly with severe pubic diastasis and vertical shear injuries. A urethrogram that demonstrates contrast extravasation is diagnostic.
  - The standard approach remains suprapubic tube insertion. Suprapubic cystostomy insertion may be accomplished using trochar-based percutaneous systems if the bladder is adequately distended. If not, an open surgical approach in the operating room is preferable.
  - Blunt trauma to the perineum with complete urethral rupture is also best handled with suprapubic diversion.
  - Penetrating injuries to the urethra can also be managed in a delayed fashion with suprapubic diversion, or, if the injury is readily apparent, direct suture repair with fine absorbable suture may be attempted in the stable patient.
  - All such injuries can be managed in a delayed fashion as long as proximal urinary diversion is achieved acutely.
- **Extraperitoneal bladder injuries** from blunt trauma are diagnosed on cystography, and can usually be managed with catheter drainage alone.
  - Adequate-bore catheters (No. 20 French or larger) are preferable to evacuate grossly bloody efflux. If there is failure of catheter management, surgical repair may be necessary.
  - Surgical repair to such an injury is approached through a high midline cystotomy to avoid entering into a fresh retropubic hematoma, which may produce problematic bleeding.
  - Other cases of extraperitoneal bladder injury that benefit from surgical repair include those that involve communication with a vaginal or rectal injury.
  - A suprapubic tube, in addition to the urethral Foley catheter, may be left indwelling in cases in which the repair is tenuous or prolonged tube drainage is anticipated.
  - In the uncomplicated case, a contrast cystogram at approximately 10 to 14 days after injury and prior to catheter removal ensures complete healing before stressing the bladder.
- For **intraperitoneal bladder injuries**, direct suture repair is required. These injuries invariably occur in the bladder dome, and result from sudden compression of the full bladder.
- **Ureteral injury** is usually noted upon abdominal exploration in the penetrating trauma setting, or may be noted on preoperative CT scanning.
  - It is necessary to obtain a delayed excretory phase on the CT such that the excreted contrast column has transited the entire ureter, or the risk of missing a ureteral injury is significant.
  - For gunshot wounds to the middle and upper ureter, limited debridement to viable ureter, careful extra-adventitial mobilization, and spatulated suture anastomosis is appropriate.
  - For distal ureteral injuries, reimplantation into the bladder ("ureteroneocystostomy") is a more dependable approach.
  - Ureteral injuries from blunt trauma are rare. Exceptions would include the pediatric population, where ureteropelvic

avulsion injuries or renal pelvic lacerations may occur following blunt injuries.

- When major injury occurs to the urinary tract following seemingly trivial trauma, one should be suspicious of the presence of previously existent underlying pathology of the urinary tract such as neoplasm or ureteropelvic junction obstruction.
- **Renal injuries** are typically staged by contrast-enhanced CT using the American Association for the Surgery of Trauma Organ Injury Scaling system.
  - Renal injuries are managed according to a multifactorial decision process that considers grade and whether they are due to blunt or penetrating forces, and is based on patient clinical status and hemodynamic stability.
  - For **blunt renal injury**, grade I, II, and III injuries are routinely managed nonoperatively.
  - Grade IV injuries require a selective approach, largely influenced by hemodynamic parameters and degree of progressive blood loss, and often warrant monitoring to address whether continued bleeding or urinoma formation occurs.
  - The majority of such injuries in most series do not require early exploration. Observation of extravasation from the collecting system is not, in itself, a strong indication for surgical exploration. If there is extensive medial extravasation on CT, retrograde pyelography may be indicated to exclude a major injury to the renal pelvis or proximal ureter.
  - Grade V injuries from blunt trauma routinely require surgical exploration and often nephrectomy, and most reported results of attempts to manage true grade V injuries nonoperatively have not resulted in good outcomes.
  - Renal pedicle injuries, which are considered in both the grade IV and V groups, require careful consideration to select appropriate management. When the kidney suffers a pedicle stretch injury from deceleration trauma, resulting in arterial intimal disruption, the artery can thrombose, resulting in renal devascularization.
  - If the vessels are thrombosed but not avulsed or lacerated, the decision of whether to operate to revascularize the kidney depends on how much time has elapsed, which predicts renal salvage, as well as the patient's other injuries and ability to tolerate a laparotomy. After 30 minutes of warm ischemia, irreversible renal damage begins; by 3 hours, the kidney is not retrievable.
  - If there is a pedicle avulsion injury, surgery is mandatory to prevent delayed catastrophic bleeding.
- For **penetrating renal trauma**, the standard approach is operative exploration and repair; departure from this approach is appropriate when complete staging information is available that predicts a favorable outcome for a specific injury with a nonoperative approach, the patient is hemodynamically stable, and careful monitoring for failure of nonoperative management can be carried out. Criteria and a plan for changing to an operative strategy should exist.
- When comparing the approach to blunt versus penetrating trauma, one must consider the high likelihood of there being associated injuries in penetrating trauma.
- Proactive angiography may be considered when weighing the safety of a nonoperative approach to the penetrating renal injury in selected cases, and admission to the ICU is essential to monitor for renewed bleeding.
- **Genital injuries** require specialized care and should be handled by practitioners experienced in genital surgery. As a

general principle, a very conservative approach to genital debridement should be maintained, with tissues of questionable viability reassessed in a delayed fashion.

- Nearly all penetrating genital injuries should be surgically explored acutely, assuming the patient is sufficiently stable to undergo a reconstructive effort.
- Penetrating penile injuries are repaired surgically by closing lacerations in the corpus cavernosum, urethral repair, and skin and soft tissue reconstruction. Penetrating testicular injuries can usually be repaired by closing the tunica albuginea of the testis after debriding nonviable testicular parenchyma.
- Blunt fracture of the penis, which results from forcible flexing of the penile shaft during erection (often due to trauma during intercourse), should be explored and repaired acutely, upon presentation, to achieve the most favorable cosmetic and functional outcome.
- For blunt scrotal injury, it is often useful to assess the patient with scrotal ultrasonography to determine if testicular rupture is present. Ultrasound is quite accurate for detecting testicular rupture: loss of capsular continuity or marked heterogeneity of testicular parenchyma is predictive of rupture. Testicular salvage is enhanced by early exploration and repair.

Damage Control Strategies for the Management of Urologic Injury in the Unstable Patient

- Many urologic injuries are quite amenable to initial management by applying damage control strategies. With the exception of severe renal or bladder bleeding cases, urinary tract injuries do not directly result in early mortality. When, in the surgeon's judgment, the patient would not tolerate the magnitude of reconstructive effort needed to deal definitively with a urologic injury at initial laparotomy (due to pattern of injury, hypothermia, acidosis, coagulopathy, or other parameters that mandate a damage control approach), certain temporary solutions may be very desirable.
  - Renal injuries that are incompletely staged or unstaged may be approached with delayed assessment and exploration, as long as a determination is made that early, exsanguinating bleeding from the injury is unlikely.
  - In the absence of significant bleeding from the renal fossa into the peritoneal cavity, a large midline hematoma, or an expanding or pulsatile renal hematoma, one can elect to leave the perinephric hematoma undisturbed and either obtain postoperative imaging during the resuscitation phase following initial laparotomy or explore during a second-look procedure.
  - If the kidney is already surgically exposed, hemostasis for major bleeding from parenchyma or branch renal vessels can be rapidly obtained.
  - If a major reconstructive effort is still needed in the unstable patient, packing the kidney and returning for reconstructive interventions later is also an option.
  - Ureteral injuries may be initially managed with externalized stenting, ligation, or simple local drainage.
  - A similar approach can be utilized for extensive bladder injuries: the ureteral orifices can be catheterized, the

catheters externalized, and the pelvis packed, leaving bladder reconstruction to be performed at a more suitable time, following appropriate resuscitation.

- Urethral and genital injuries are also amenable to damage control approaches, generally involving tube urinary diversion, placement of moistened dressings, and tissue preservation until definitive reconstruction following appropriate resuscitation.

URINARY DIVERSION MANAGEMENT FROM THE CRITICAL CARE PERSPECTIVE

- Beyond the considerations regarding tube diversion or drainage, some patients under the critical care team's care may have undergone, either acutely or remotely, a surgical urinary diversion procedure. Problems include urinary outflow obstruction, intra-abdominal urinary extravasation, infectious complications, and problems with the intestinal anastomosis.
- One can divide urinary diversion procedures into conduits and reservoirs. Conduits are simple surgical reconstructions that allow urine to exit to the outside and do not involve an internal urinary reservoir.
  - An **ileal conduit** is one of the most commonly encountered urinary diversions. In this procedure, a segment of distal ileum is isolated from the fecal stream, followed by a small bowel anastomosis to re-establish intestinal continuity. One end of the isolated segment is closed, and the other end is brought to the skin of the abdominal wall as a stoma. The ureters are sutured into the conduit intra-abdominally to route the urinary stream externally.
  - **Other conduits** employed in urologic surgery may utilize other bowel segments, including jejunum and descending or transverse colon, especially when there has been extensive pelvic irradiation that has damaged the ileum and lower small intestine.
- **Reservoirs (neobladders)** involve the use of larger segments of intestine to fashion a neobladder internally, along with some form of urinary efflux mechanism, often designed to create a continent diversion that the patient can catheterize (and not wear a urinary collection appliance) or that is sutured to the native urethra (in the male or female) to allow restoration of voiding (an "orthotopic neobladder").
- Reservoir urinary diversions can develop certain other potentially serious problems including "pouchitis," pouch rupture, and formation of pouch calculi.
- The issue of pouch rupture deserves specific mention as this must be promptly recognized. Any patient with signs of abdominal infection or sepsis who has a neobladder should raise the suspicion of pouch rupture. This entity can also be seen in patients who have had an augmentation cystoplasty, in which a segment of bowel is added to the native bladder to increase capacity or deal with severe and intransigent overactive bladder symptoms.
- Such patients should have urgent urologic assessment, which may involve contrast imaging studies (CT or "pouchography") to rule out urinary leakage intra-abdominally. Broad-spectrum antibiotics should be instituted early in

such cases, as the urine is often colonized and intra-abdominal infection may be developing.

- Many such cases can be managed with tube drainage of the neobladder alone, though in some cases surgical exploration and repair, and/or evacuation of infectious fluid from the abdominal cavity are necessary.
- Depending on the type of urinary diversion and the specific segment of the gastrointestinal tract used for the reconstruction, these patients may be at risk for dehydration, and specific electrolyte and metabolic disturbances.
- Jejunal conduits may result in hyponatremic, hypochloremic metabolic acidosis; this process may be clinically manifested by nausea, vomiting, anorexia, and muscular weakness.
- When ileum and colon are utilized for the urinary diversion, hyperchloremic metabolic acidosis may be seen. Clinically this may produce weakness, anorexia, vomiting, or Kussmaul breathing, and may progress to coma.
- When gastric segments are utilized for urinary diversion, dehydration and hyponatremic metabolic alkalosis may occur, requiring replacement of sodium and chloride through intravenous salt administration.
- Abnormal bile salt metabolism following ileal resection, can affect fat digestion and uptake of vitamins A and D.
- Malabsorption and steatorrhea and a propensity to develop cholelithiasis may also be associated with ileal resection.
- Gastric or ileal resection may cause vitamin B_{12} deficiency, which can lead to megaloblastic anemia and peripheral nerve dysfunction; B_{12} nutritional supplementation may be indicated.

UROSEPSIS AND COMPLEX UROGENITAL INFECTION IN THE CRITICAL CARE SETTING

Specific Infectious Processes of the Upper and Lower Urinary Tract

- The combination of obstruction and infection of the upper and lower urinary tract requires urgent drainage, antibiotic therapy, and supportive care.
- Initial empiric antibiotic therapy for presumed urosepsis must address the likely offending organisms and must consider the "worst-case scenario" from the bacteriologic standpoint.
- While awaiting culture data, Gram's stain findings can also be very helpful in selecting initial therapy. Broad-spectrum antibiotics that cover aerobic gram-negative rods and the typical gram-positive cocci that appear as uropathogens are critical.
- If the patient has been recently instrumented, has been recently hospitalized, or has other risk factors for having sepsis due to atypical or resistant pathogens, coverage should be expanded accordingly.
- It may be necessary in certain situations to consider the presence of anaerobic infections of the genitourinary system. Sepsis following transrectal prostate biopsy may introduce the risk of anaerobic infection. Additionally, anaerobic infection of the urinary tract has also been described outside the setting of iatrogenic rectal violation, so this uncommon scenario is worth bearing in mind.

- Staphylococcal infections of the urinary system do also occur, particularly in the elderly or immunocompromised population, or in patients who have iatrogenic manipulation.
- When a gram-positive coccus is noted on stained urine or infectious fluid, vancomycin is an appropriate empiric choice for sepsis of urinary tract origin, as both *Enterococcus* and *Staphylococcus* species are usually covered.
- Fungal organisms should be considered especially in the diabetic patient and in the patient who has had extensive antibiotic therapy. Empiric fluconazole is appropriate.
- In addition to supportive care and antibiotic management, prompt drainage of the urinary tract is critical in certain conditions of urinary infection and urosepsis. Rapid decline in clinical status may ensue if there is a delay in instituting prompt drainage of an infected, obstructed system.
- When either upper or lower tract obstruction is present with urosepsis, prompt imaging of the urinary tract should be obtained (noncontrast CT of the abdomen and pelvis or renal ultrasound, bladder ultrasound to exclude retention).
- One major potential diagnostic pitfall occurs when a patient has complete unilateral upper tract obstruction with a negative urinalysis, as no urine from the obstructed system enters the bladder, and the urinary tract origin of sepsis is therefore not suspected.
- Emphysematous pyelonephritis and cystitis are infections of the kidney and bladder, respectively, which result in gas formation within the tissues.
- The presence of gas in the urinary tract may be due to gas-forming infection, previous instrumentation, or fistula. The clinical situation will usually lead to the correct etiology.
- The most commonly seen organism in such infections is *Escherichia coli*, which may enter into a state of facultative anaerobic metabolism, especially in a diabetic when severe hyperglycemia is present.
- These patients may become severely ill and require aggressive resuscitation and sometimes drainage procedures or occasionally urgent nephrectomy; urologic consultation is essential.
- Emphysematous cystitis reflects the same bacteriologic basis and propensity for the diabetic patient as for the renal counterpart. Bladder catheter drainage and aggressive antibiotic management will usually correct the process.
- Renal and perinephric abscesses are the important causes of urosepsis, and one must have a high index of suspicion in the setting of incomplete resolution of upper tract urinary infection with standard antibiotic regimens, prompting imaging to detect an undrained source of relapsing or persistent infection.
- CT scanning is significantly superior to ultrasound for imaging the perinephric space, and is preferable when an abscess is suspected.
- Small renal parenchymal abscesses not causing a septic picture may resolve with antibiotic treatment alone.
- When multiloculated or when inadequately drained by the percutaneous route, an open surgical drainage procedure may be necessary.
- Acute bacterial prostatitis can present with a septic picture. Common symptoms include dysuria, frequency, urgency, chills and fever, elevated white blood count on CBC, and infected urine.
- If the patient is emptying adequately, antibiotic administration is usually adequate without catheter drainage. If the patient is in acute urinary retention, bladder drainage is

needed; one can proceed either with a gentle attempt at Foley catheter passage per urethra or with percutaneous suprapubic cystostomy placement.

- For patients presenting with acute prostatitis or other complex lower tract infection who do not respond appropriately to antibiotic therapy, or for those with suspicious findings on a digital rectal examination, prostatic abscess should be suspected.
- Transrectal ultrasound or CT scanning of the pelvis will usually confirm the presence of a prostatic abscess when present, and can also guide therapy by revealing whether the abscess cavity may be best drained through a transurethral, transperineal, or transrectal route.

Urologic Involvement in Complex Soft-Tissue Infectious Processes

- Urologic involvement with such entities as perirectal abscess or Fournier gangrene is common. Fournier gangrene may be idiopathic with no identifiable point of origin, or may be due to extension from primary rectal, urinary, intra-abdominal, or retroperitoneal processes. These patients require a combination of aggressive antibiotic therapy, metabolic and fluid resuscitation, and prompt and aggressive surgical debridement and drainage. These infectious processes can progress very rapidly, and delays in bringing the patient to surgery may result in loss of otherwise salvageable tissues and increased mortality.
  - Diabetics are at increased risk for this disease. When there is genital, perineal, or groin involvement in such processes, several applicable management principles may be of value.
  - Broad-spectrum ("triple antibiotic") regimens that cover aerobes, anaerobes, and gram-positive and gram-negative organisms should be started, as polymicrobial infection is the norm.
  - Aggressive surgical debridement and drainage by close collaboration between the urology and general surgery teams may aid functional and organ preservation, and subsequent reconstructive efforts.
  - When an abscess or necrotizing process extends into the region of the perineum or genital soft tissues, incision or debridement of scrotal or penile skin and underlying dartos may be necessary.
  - In the scrotum, we try to establish a dissection plan just superficial to the parietal tunica vaginalis and keep this membrane, which surrounds the testes, intact.
  - The testes are rarely involved in these soft tissue infections, and preserving the parietal tunica vaginalis directly will aid in subsequent wound management and avoid the pain and desiccation that occurs when the testis is exposed externally.
  - If the surgeon must enter the scrotal wall for drainage of a local abscess, it is best to avoid deep incision into the tunica vaginalis compartment to avoid preventable injury to the scrotal contents.
  - On the penis, necrotic skin and dartos may be debrided up to the coronal sulcus when necessary, taking care to stay superficial to the Buck fascia (deep fascial layer) of the penis, to avoid injury to the corpora and the dorsal neurovascular bundle.
  - Fournier gangrene may occasionally arise from a urethral source (such as a periurethral abscess or perforated stricture or diverticulum). Debridement of urethral tissue should be avoided unless it is grossly necrotic, as a superficial exudate may create the appearance of marginally perfused tissue; such changes can be reassessed on take-back to the operating room.

CHAPTER 54 ■ CRITICAL CARE AND TRANSPLANTATION: OVERVIEW

- Critical care and clinical organ transplantation have developed in parallel over the past several decades. While organ transplantation has emerged as the treatment of choice for an ever-growing number of patients with end-stage organ failure, the intensive care unit (ICU) has become the venue where much of this care is rendered. The modern intensivist plays an important role in the care of the critically ill patient awaiting transplant, the postoperative management of the transplant recipient, and the identification and management of the potential deceased organ donor.

- The success of organ transplantation can be attributed to a number of factors. These include better patient selection and preoperative preparation, standardization of surgical techniques, advances in immunosuppression and graft surveillance, and improved postoperative care. This success, in part reflective of advances in critical care medicine, poses a great challenge to the skills of the intensivist and the resources of the ICU. The continuing shortage of organs available for transplantation translates into longer waiting times for recipients, during which their condition may further deteriorate. Additionally, organ allocation algorithms—especially heart, lung, liver, and intestine—in the United States emphasize the "sickest first" philosophy, which states that the highest priority for organs should go to those most in danger of imminent death. Finally, the shortage of organs has forced the transplant community to consider the use of organs from less-than-ideal donors. The organs from these marginal or "expanded criteria" donors, though used with caution, must be considered to minimize deaths on the waiting list. The impact on the ICU is clear: More transplants are being performed on critically ill patients with an organ pool that now includes compromised organs.

- A prerequisite to the success of organ transplantation is the availability of suitable organs. Deceased organ donors are, and will continue to be in the foreseeable future, our most important organ source. A crucial consideration of the ICU staff should be the timely recognition of the potential organ donor, both those who are brain-dead and those for whom death is imminent, and the early involvement of organ procurement organization (OPO) personnel to facilitate the process. The assessment of the potential organ donor, a clear understanding of donation after brain death and cardiac death protocols, and donor management are skills of the intensivist that are fundamental to the organ procurement process and the subsequent transplants performed.

INTESTINAL TRANSPLANTATION

- Intestinal transplantation has emerged as an accepted therapy for complicated intestinal failure. Standardization of surgical techniques, better management of the intestinal failure patient, improvements in immunosuppression, and advances in graft surveillance have led to better patient and graft survival. Survivors are almost always able to be completely tapered from parenteral nutrition.

- The intestine can be transplanted as an isolated organ or as part of a composite graft depending on the needs of the patient. The multivisceral graft includes, en bloc, the stomach, liver, duodenum, pancreas, and small intestine. This graft can be modified to include or exclude the liver, spleen, colon, or a kidney. Each modification has critical care implications, especially when the recipient requires a liver as part of the transplantation.

- The number of intestinal transplants has been increasing, as illustrated in Figure 54.1. Many variables affect outcome and, in recent years, patient and graft survival have been improving. Patient survival from data over the past 15 years are shown in Figure 54.2.

DONOR RECOGNITION AND ASSESSMENT

- Transplantation depends on organ donation. OPOs are charged with the responsibility of deceased organ donor recognition and assessment. Medical professionals are required to cooperate with OPO personnel to ensure that all potential organ and tissue donors are identified and afforded the opportunity to donate. It is recommended that OPO and hospital staff collaborate by establishing criteria as to when it is the earliest appropriate time to consult the OPO.

- The critical care physician's first priority is to provide excellent patient care. Additionally, he or she should recognize, when brain death is imminent or when withdrawal of support measures are considered, that there is an opportunity through organ donation to help other patients. Timing is critical: Approaching a family too early is inappropriate and too late threatens the potential for organ donation.

- To assist in defining the appropriate time to consider OPO involvement, the United Network for Organ Sharing (UNOS) has devised the term *imminent neurologic death*. This term describes the patient with an irreversible brain injury who may fit the general criteria of a potential organ donor but has not been legally declared brain-dead. It is appropriate to notify the OPO when a patient meets this definition and displays an absence of at least three of the following neurologic functions as a result of the brain injury (not pharmacologic sedation or other confounding variables):
  - Pupillary reaction
  - Response to cold calorics

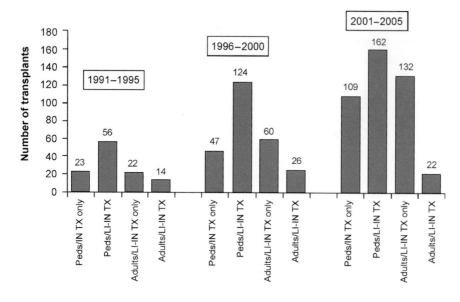

FIGURE 54.1. Number of intestinal transplants by age group and era. TX, transplant; LI, liver; IN, intestine; Peds, pediatric patients. (Source: 2006 Annual Report of the U.S. Organ Procurement and Transplantation Network and the Scientific Registry of Transplant Recipients: Transplant Data 1996–2005. Rockville, MD: Health Resources and Services Administration, Healthcare Systems Bureau, Division of Transplantation. The data and analyses reported in the 2006 Annual Report of the U.S. Organ Procurement and Transplantation Network and the Scientific Registry of Transplant Recipients have been supplied by the United Network for Organ Sharing and Arbor Research under contract with the Department of Health and Human Services. The authors alone are responsible for reporting and interpreting these data; the views expressed herein are those of the authors and not necessarily those of the U.S. government).

- Gag reflex
- Cough reflex
- Corneal reflex
- Doll's eyes reflex
- Response to painful stimuli
- Spontaneous breathing
- In short, when the diagnosis of brain death is being considered and the clinical assessment has begun to confirm that diagnosis, the OPO should be notified.
- There are two important implications of the preceding statement that warrant clarification. First, OPO personnel are permitted access to patients' medical records per an exemption in the Health Insurance Portability and Accountability Act. Second, the critical care provider is not required to notify the patient's family that the OPO has been consulted. If they wish, critical care providers can inform the family and/or introduce the idea of organ donation. It is not recommended that they discuss the process and options in detail. That task should be left to OPO personnel who are specially trained to approach grieving families and are qualified to obtain informed consent for organ and tissue donation.

ORGAN DONATION PROCESS

- There are fundamentally two types of potential donors who can be considered from the critical care population: ventilator-dependent patients who will be withdrawn from life-sustaining measures and patients who are declared clinically brain dead. In the former circumstance, it is possible to offer the option of organ donation after cardiac death, provided certain criteria are met. In the latter, donation may occur in the presence of circulation after the patient has been declared clinically brain dead. This is termed *organ donation after brain death*. As guidelines, the UNOS has published the Critical Pathway for the Organ Donor and the Critical Pathway for Donation after Cardiac Death.

DONOR MANAGEMENT

- In many ways, management of the organ donor resembles that of the critically ill patient, with an important distinction. The goal for the critically ill patient is recovery, prolonging

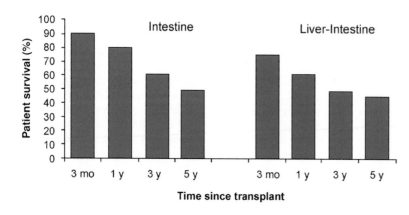

FIGURE 54.2. Patient survival after intestinal transplant, 1991–2005. (Source: 2006 Annual Report of the U.S. Organ Procurement and Transplantation Network and the Scientific Registry of Transplant Recipients: Transplant Data 1996–2005. Rockville, MD: Health Resources and Services Administration, Healthcare Systems Bureau, Division of Transplantation. The data and analyses reported in the 2006 Annual Report of the U.S. Organ Procurement and Transplantation Network and the Scientific Registry of Transplant Recipients have been supplied by the United Network for Organ Sharing and Arbor Research under contract with the Department of Health and Human Services. The authors alone are responsible for reporting and interpreting these data; the views expressed herein are those of the authors and not necessarily those of the U.S. government).

life, and improving its quality. The goal of donor management is maximization of the number and quality of transplantable organs. Once brain death has been determined, OPO personnel play an instrumental role in donor management. Brain death is associated with grossly impaired body temperature regulation, profound hypernatremia due to diabetes insipidus, impaired blood pressure regulation, coagulopathy, endocrine dysfunction, and electrolyte and acid-base disturbances. Physiologic derangement may have been the manifestation of the inciting injury or insult; this is often worse at the time of cerebral edema, herniation, and brain death.

- Donor maintenance has become more sophisticated in recent years. Each OPO has detailed protocols and care pathways for organ donor optimization. Each has a medical director and/or critical care physician as a consultant or as an active participant in the process. The OPO community under the direction of the Health Resources and Services Administration has developed its "best practices" for donor monitoring and maintenance. Fluids administered and urine output and any other fluid losses are measured. Monitoring routinely includes the use of arterial catheters for blood pressure monitoring, central venous pressure monitoring, and sometimes pulmonary artery catheter placement. Arterial oxygenation is monitored via continuous pulse oximetry.

- Fluid warmers and other warming devices are utilized as needed to maintain normothermia. Mechanical ventilation modalities geared toward maintaining oxygenation and ventilation while minimizing pulmonary injury are utilized. Hemodynamic derangement is addressed with fluids (crystalloid, colloid, and blood products) and the administration of vasopressors, inotropes, or antihypertensives as indicated. A standardized battery of laboratory tests is obtained, and detected abnormalities are corrected, if possible. Acid-base abnormalities are corrected, and hypernatremia and hyperglycemia are treated. Antibiotics, corticosteroids, endocrine replacement, and other medications are given to the donor in accordance with detailed management protocols. Cultures, viral serologies, blood type, and human leukocyte antigen studies are performed to assess donor and recipient compatibility.

ASSESSMENT OF DONOR'S ORGAN FUNCTION

- Coincident with monitoring and correction of physiologic derangement, the donor organs are evaluated for transplantation. A thorough history is obtained and the medical record reviewed. Emphasis is placed on detection of infection, presence or a history of malignancy, and comorbid conditions that can affect organ viability.

- Each organ is considered individually, and specific tests are available to measure function or detect impairment. The heart is evaluated by an assessment of the donor's hemodynamic status, sometimes with the aid of a pulmonary artery catheter, need for vasopressors or inotropic drugs, transthoracic echocardiography and, in selected cases, coronary angiography. Lung assessment includes serial arterial blood gas measurement, chest radiography, and flexible bronchoscopy. The kidneys are evaluated by urine output, serum creatinine measurement and, for some OPOs, a calculation of the glomerular filtration rate. After procurement, a renal cortical biopsy can yield important information regarding organ quality. Some OPOs and TCs preserve kidneys with a pulsatile perfusion machine.

- Some transplant surgeons use the performance parameters of the kidney(s) on the pump as an adjunct measure of quality. There are few specific indicators of pancreas viability and quality. Euglycemia without the need for significant amounts of exogenous insulin is preferable. Elevated serum amylase may raise concern that the gland is not suitable because of pancreatitis.

- The liver is assessed by transaminase and bilirubin measurements. Serum albumin and coagulation studies are measures of liver function. A liver biopsy obtained percutaneously before procurement or in the operating room at the time of organ recovery can be useful for detecting inflammation, necrosis, fibrosis, or steatosis. There are no specific standardized methods for the evaluation of the donor intestine.

CHAPTER 55 ■ HEART TRANSPLANTATION

- The number of patients on the waiting list for a heart and the number of transplantations performed has decreased significantly over the past decade Over the same time, deaths on the waiting list have declined, and survival results after heart transplantation remain high (Fig. 55.1). These data reflect the improvements in transplantation, better medical management of interventional techniques for patients with heart disease, and the development of more effective mechanical support devices.

PERIOPERATIVE CARE OF HEART TRANSPLANTATION

Hemodynamic Markers of Heart Failure

- Knowing the risk of dying and the prognosis of patients receiving optimal medical therapy is critical to the determination of transplant candidacy and timing. Cardiopulmonary

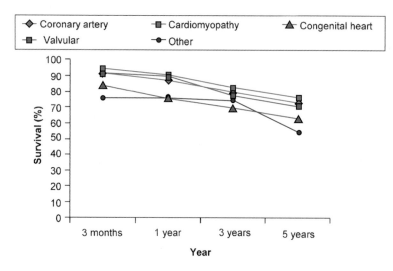

FIGURE 55.1. Patient survival after heart transplant by diagnosis. (Source: 2006 Annual Report of the U.S. Organ Procurement and Transplantation Network and the Scientific Registry of Transplant Recipients: Transplant Data 1996–2005. Rockville, MD: Health Resources and Services Administration, Healthcare Systems Bureau, Division of Transplantation. The data and analyses reported in the 2006 Annual Report of the U.S. Organ Procurement and Transplantation Network and the Scientific Registry of Transplant Recipients have been supplied by the United Network for Organ Sharing and Arbor Research under contract with the Department of Health and Human Services. The authors alone are responsible for reporting and interpreting these data; the views expressed herein are those of the authors and not necessarily those of the U.S. government).

testing as a measure of oxygen consumption is routinely used to determine candidacy for transplantation. The currently accepted indication for transplantation is a peak VO_2 <10 mL/kg per minute in patients with adequate β-blockade who achieved anaerobic threshold. Patients with a VO_2 between 10 and 14 mL/kg per minute are more problematic, and decisions to list for transplantation should be individualized. The use of VO_2 as a discriminatory variable requires experience and attention to detail in testing performance. It is important to note that patients tolerating β-blockade demonstrate improved survival with equivalent VO_2. It is also notable that appropriate patient selection assumes maximal effort to achieve a plateau of performance. In populations with limited functional status a respiratory exchange ratio >1.05 is generally considered a maximal exercise test. Peak VO_2 also varies with age and gender and is normalized for body weight, with heavier patients having a lower VO_2 at comparable levels of performance. In the era prior to widespread use of β-blockers and angiotensin-converting enzyme inhibitors, a VO_2 maximum of <50% was shown to be a significant predictor of cardiac death. Nonetheless, isolated peak VO_2 should not be used as the sole criterion for transplant eligibility.

- Right heart catheterization provides information on cardiac output, ventricular filling pressures, and pulmonary vascular resistance (PVR) and is an absolute prerequisite to consideration for transplantation. A pulmonary vascular resistance greater than 5 Wood units, an indexed PVR greater than 6 Wood units, or a transpulmonary gradient greater than 16 to 20 mm Hg have been considered relative contraindications to transplant (1 Wood Unit = 80 dynes · s/cm^5). Candidacy for transplantation is less dependent on the absolute measures of PVR than on the responsiveness of the pulmonary vascular bed to therapy. Heart failure patients with pulmonary artery systolic pressures greater than 50 mm Hg and either a PVR >3 Wood units or a transpulmonary gradient >15 mm Hg are routinely challenged with multiple vasodilators to ascertain whether the elevated pulmonary pressures are reactive. Most patients with acute decompensated heart failure have elevated left-sided filling pressures with secondary pulmonary venous hypertension. Pharmacologically unloading the left ventricle with sodium nitroprusside while maintaining a systolic blood pressure of >85 mm Hg is generally considered evidence of a reactive vascular bed and does not preclude transplantation.

- A significant minority of patients have evidence of fixed pulmonary hypertension.
- Patients without evidence of an anatomic substrate are treated with aggressive diuresis and short-term inotropy with the phosphodiesterase inhibitor milrinone. If subsequent provocative testing demonstrates continued non-reactivity, dobutamine is added to the inotropic support for synergy. Such vasodilatory conditioning generally improves pulmonary vascular resistance, but these patients remain at higher risk for acute cardiac death prior to transplant and, in our experience, remain at significant risk for elevated pulmonary artery pressures after transplantation. It is important to recognize that the reversibility of PVR in patients with low left ventricular ejection fraction cannot be assessed without unloading the left ventricle. Fixed pulmonary hypertension has been effectively treated with mechanical circulatory support, allowing isolated cardiac transplantation in patients initially thought to require a combined heart–lung procedure.
- Renal dysfunction is among the most significant clinical variables complicating the decision to transplant and one of the most significant morbidities after transplant.
- Currently, renal dysfunction is rarely a contraindication to transplant and have actively pursued combined heart and kidney transplant in patients at high risk for end-stage renal disease in the early postoperative interval. Outcomes for combined transplant are comparable to those of isolated cardiac allografts. Regardless of approach, the decision to exclude patient candidacy secondary to significant renal dysfunction or to simultaneously transplant a renal allograft requires careful consideration of the cause of preoperative renal insufficiency, the degree to which renal insufficiency is irreversible, and the probability of progressive renal failure after transplant.

Neurohormonal Markers of Heart Failure

- The natural history of heart failure is characterized by systemic neurohormonal activation in response to the structural and functional remodeling of decreased ejection fraction and progressive volume overload. Optimal medical therapy of heart failure is designed to ameliorate these neurohormonal changes: β-blockade of adrenergic pathways, diuresis to reduce volume overload and natriuretic hormone production, and various inhibitors of the renin–angiotensin system including angiotensin-converting enzyme inhibitors and angiotensin receptor blockade.

- Analysis of the Randomized Evaluation of Strategies for Left Ventricular Dysfunction trial data demonstrated that temporal increases in brain natriuretic and N-terminal atrial natriuretic peptide during medical therapy were associated with concurrent reductions in ejection fraction and increases in end-diastolic and systolic volume.

- Brain natriuretic is often used as a marker to evaluate the adequacy and response to acute heart failure therapy and consider it a physiologic marker of volume overload. C-reactive protein (CRP), a nonspecific marker of inflammation, is considered a sensitive marker of the neurohormonal milieu in acute heart failure and a more sensitive marker of prognosis. In patients with decompensated heart failure, CRP is most elevated (CRP >15%–18 mg%) and associated with poor outcomes regardless of ejection fraction.

Heart Failure Survival Score

- The Heart Failure Survival Score is a clinical descriptor derived from a Cox proportional hazards regression model of noninvasively derived measurements describing ambulatory patients with advanced heart failure. The prognostic variables include resting heart rate, mean systemic blood pressure, left ventricular ejection fraction, serum sodium, peak oxygen consumption, intraventricular conduction delay defined as a QRS complex >120 ms, and the presence or absence of ischemic cardiomyopathy (see Table 55.1). Based on the absolute value of the sum of weighted variables, three risk-stratified groups were identified: high risk (score <7.19, 35% 1-year survival with medical therapy), medium risk (score 7.20–8.09, 60% 1-year survival), and low risk (score >8.10, 88% 1-year survival with medical therapy).

Organ Allocation

The current allocation system for donor hearts is designed to prioritize patients with the most urgent medical need of transplantation—potential recipients with mechanical circulatory assist devices and patients requiring multiple inotropes or a single high-dose inotrope (dobutamine >7.5 μg/kg/min or milrinone >0.5 μg/kg/min) are listed as status 1A. Patients requiring a single continuous low-dose inotrope to maintain hemodynamics and end organ perfusion are listed as 1B. Patients with end-stage heart disease who fail to meet either of these criteria are listed as status 2. Because of the increasing efficacy of medical therapy, the survival benefit of transplantation to United Network for Organ Sharing status 2 patients has been questioned.

POSTOPERATIVE COMPLICATIONS

Acute Allograft Loss

- Within 30 days of transplantation, causes of death include graft failure (primary and/or nonspecific) accounting for 40%, multiorgan system failure (14%), and noncytomegalovirus (non-CMV) infection (13%)

Right Ventricular Dysfunction and Allograft Failure

- Whereas acute right ventricular (RV) failure at the time of allograft implantation is an uncommon but highly morbid condition with historical mortalities approaching 30% to 50%, RV dysfunction after allograft implantation is common. Nearly 20% of orthotopic heart transplants demonstrate some degree of RV dysfunction as manifested by tricuspid regurgitation. Tricuspid regurgitation has recently been shown to be a predictor of late survival after cardiac transplantation, suggesting that early RV dysfunction is a marker of poor outcome. The etiology of transplant RV dysfunction is poorly understood but is clearly multifactorial and includes primary aspects of donor organ biology (e.g., primary RV graft dysfunction), inherent injury secondary to the procurement process (e.g., ischemia–reperfusion injury), and specific characteristics of recipient pathophysiology (e.g., elevated pulmonary vascular resistance).

- Heart donors with cerebrovascular accident as the cause of death have consistently demonstrated a significant

---

TABLE 55.1

HEART FAILURE SURVIVAL SCORE (HFSS)

Coronary artery disease (yes = 1, no = 0)	(...... × 0.6931) =	+
Intraventricular conduction delay (yes = 1, no = 0)	(...... × 0.6083) =	+
Left ventricular ejection fraction (%)	(...... × 0.0464) =	+
Heart rate (bpm)	(...... × 0.0216) =	+
Na$^+$ concentration (mmol/L)	(...... × 0.0470) =	+
Mean arterial pressure (mm Hg)	(...... × 0.0255) =	+
Peak VO$_2$ (mL/kg/min)	(...... × 0.0546) =	+
	HFSS = ...	

High risk <7.19 (35% 1-y survival), medium risk 7.20–8.09 (60% 1-y survival), and low risk >8.10 (88% 1-y survival).
From Aaronson KD, Schawartz JS, Chen TM, et al. Development and prospective validation of a clinical index to predict survival in ambulatory patients referred for cardiac transplant evaluation. *Circulation.* 1997;95:2660.

negative impact on 1-year post-transplantation mortality, and experimental data have supported the concept that donor brain death contributes to RV dysfunction after cardiac transplantation. Animal studies have demonstrated a significant decrease in RV function after transplantation in hearts retrieved from a brain-dead donor whereas RV function is maintained or increased after implantation of normal hearts even in recipients with chronic pulmonary hypertension. Furthermore, large animal models assessing the intrinsic myocardial mechanics of transplanted hearts independent of the severe changes in peripheral loading conditions that accompany the catecholamine storm of brain death (elevated peripheral and pulmonary vascular resistance) demonstrate a nearly 40% reduction in RV contractility without a similar decrease in left ventricular contractility. This suggests that RV dysfunction is primarily related to the status of the donor heart, and although elevated pulmonary vascular resistance will increase the severity of postoperative RV dysfunction, it is unlikely that elevated PVR independently creates RV dysfunction.

- The early biology of transplanted hearts is defined by denervation and diastolic dysfunction. Loss of afferent parasympathetic vagal tone and corresponding lowering of myocardial catecholamine levels in response to sympathetic denervation results in higher resting heart rates and a blunted response to hypovolemia and decreased preload. A poorly understood but useful consequence of denervation is increased presynaptic sensitivity to β-adrenergic stimulation. The transplanted heart is also "stiff," and restrictive physiology is expected in the immediate postoperative period. Elevated diastolic ventricular filling pressures generally diminish within weeks of transplantation, but persistent diastolic dysfunction may represent donor–recipient size mismatch, myocardial injury from harvest ischemia, intrinsic characteristics of the donor heart (e.g., hypertension), or evidence of rejection.

- Because of limited therapies, prophylaxis for acute allograft dysfunction is a preferable clinical strategy. It is our practice to start inhaled nitric oxide (NO) (20 ppm) prior to weaning from cardiopulmonary bypass to lower pulmonary vascular resistance in patients with preoperative PVR >3 Wood units. All patients exit the operative theater on low- to moderate-dose epinephrine (0.02–0.06 µg/kg/min), and patients receiving chronic afterload reduction preoperatively (e.g., intravenous milrinone) are simultaneously started on low-dose norepinephrine (0.02–0.04 µg/kg/min). Patients are atrially paced (92 beats per minute [bpm]), or atrio-ventricular (AV) sequentially paced, in the immediate postoperative period. In the absence of significant tricuspid regurgitation and RV dysfunction, NO is weaned in the immediate postoperative period, and patients are generally extubated within 6 hours of exiting the operating room. Caution should be used in weaning NO, as rebound pulmonary hypertension has been observed. We have not found this to be a significant clinical problem outside the pediatric population. Inotropic support is maintained for the initial 24 hours and weaned off between 24 and 36 hours as determined by clinical exam.

- Clinical exam and echocardiogram effective for evaluating ventricular function, filling pressures, and RV strain and right heart catheters are generally placed for specific diagnostic questions and rarely guide clinical management. Right heart catheterization and biopsy is performed in general within 7 to 14 days of transplant.

Ischemia–reperfusion Injury

- Traditional views hold that the obligatory ischemia of organ procurement induces endothelial dysfunction, lipid peroxidation with loss of membrane integrity, free radical superoxide production, dysregulation of intracellular and mitochondrial calcium flux, and neutrophil activation with allograft infiltration. Reperfusion at the time of allograft implantation is thought to extend the inflammatory injury with subsequent apoptosis and delayed cell death contributing to graft dysfunction

Rejection and Immunosuppression

- With the exception of homozygous twins, all allografts are incompatible. This incompatibility is defined by the predominant mechanism of allorecognition—humoral or cellular—and the temporal pattern of allograft rejection. *Hyperacute rejection* occurs within minutes to hours of allograft reperfusion and is a rare form of perioperative graft loss caused by preformed antibodies directed against donor human leukocyte antigen or endothelial antigen. Complement activation results in intravascular thrombosis and ischemic graft dysfunction. There is no medical therapy, as graft loss is nearly immediate, and salvage requires mechanical circulatory support (extracorporeal life support [ECLS] or ventricular assist device [VAD]) and consideration for retransplantation.

- *Acute rejection* is historically considered a T cell–mediated process with perivascular infiltration of lymphocytes and macrophages and variable degrees of myonecrosis. It can occur anytime after transplantation but is most commonly diagnosed within the first 6 months—nearly 60% of heart recipients—and is the most common form of rejection within days to weeks after allograft implantation.

- *Chronic rejection* is characterized by circumferential myointimal proliferation and progressive coronary artery vasculopathy. Nearly half of all heart transplants demonstrate angiographically recognizable cardiac allograft vasculopathy (CAV) by year five.

BALANCED RISK: IMMUNOSUPPRESSION AND INFECTION

- Coronary artery vasculopathy is a probable complication of under-immunosuppression, whereas early infection and late malignancy are probable complications of over-immunosuppression. These opposing problems represent the major failure of contemporary thoracic transplantation.

- In spite of institutional preferences, all protocols shared immunosuppressive strategies for the *induction* of immune tolerance at the time of allograft implantation and for the *maintenance* of chronic immune suppression over time. *Rescue* (antirejection) therapy in response to histologic rejection remains very problematic, as there is no direct relationship between microscopic evidence of allograft rejection, allograft dysfunction, and patient survival.

- A list of most common solid transplantation immunosuppression drugs is available elsewhere in this book.

Infection Prophylaxis and Perioperative Risk

- Pneumonia is the most common presentation with a historical incidence of approximately 14% to 28% and an overall mortality of 23% to 31%. Hospitalization at the time of transplantation, postoperative endotracheal intubation for more than 1 day after transplantation, reintubation after transplantation, evidence of pretransplant pulmonary infection, use of antilymphocyte induction therapy, and prolonged and excessive use of steroids (>80 mg/day during the first month) are considered significant risk factors. It is important to note that nearly 20% of heart transplantations occur in patients on mechanical assist devices and that nearly half of all VAD recipients experience infectious complications.
- However, the recent deaths of organ recipients receiving allografts from patients with undiagnosed trypanosomal infection (*www.CDC.org*) underscores the increasing globalization of the donor population and the need for increasingly sophisticated screening technologies. A common prophylaxis treatment of bacterial, viral, and fungal pathogens are listed below:
  - Vancomycin (10–15 mg/kg every 12 h) and piperacillin/tazobactam (3.375 gm IV every 6 h) are empiric bacterial prophylaxis. Therapy is stopped at 72 hours after review of donor cultures.
  - Cytomegalovirus seropositivity is not a contraindication for either donor or recipient. Leukocytes are the source of CMV infection, and seronegative blood products should be used in seronegative patients and patients with seronegative allografts. Primary infection, a seropositive (CMV+) organ into a seronegative (CMV–) recipient, is associated with the greatest risk of CMV disease. These patients receive prophylaxis with CMV immune globulin (CytoGam, CMV-IVIG) at 150 mg/kg IV for 7 days followed by valganciclovir (Valcyte) for 1 year (450 mg twice daily [BID] dosed for renal function). Seropositive patients who receive either CMV-positive or CMV-negative allografts are at moderate to low risk of reactivation disease as are seronegative recipients of CMV-negative transplants. These patients receive prophylactic coverage for 6 months with Valcyte (450 mg orally BID. Any patient receiving treatment for histologic rejection receives 6 months of prophylactic Valcyte in the context of increased immunosuppression. Active CMV disease is treated with CytoGam (50–150 mg/kg IV daily) and

a relative withdrawal of immunosuppression to facilitate immunocompetence.

- Hepatitis B surface antigen seropositivity in potential recipients has been associated with hepatic inflammation or cirrhosis in 37% of heart recipients and is a relative contraindication to transplantation. Currently, all patients receive hepatitis B vaccine prior to transplantation (HBsAg-positive, HBsAb IgM–positive, HBcAb-negative). We routinely use HBcAb-positive donor hearts in the context of HBsAg seronegativity as we consider this a sign of prior exposure and not active disease.
- Positive hepatitis C serologies (Hep C Ab+), if confirmed by nucleic acid testing, is considered evidence of active donor infection. It is our practice not to use organs from donors with presumed active hepatitis C because of high conversion rates (>50%) in recipients and poor outcomes. Active hepatitis C in patients with end-stage heart disease is not an absolute contraindication to transplant. Favorable hepatitis C viral genotype and low to undetectable viral titre by quantitative polymerase chain reaction (PCR) identifies a group of patients with outcomes comparable to those of thoracic transplant recipients without viral infection. We have also challenged hepatitis C seropositive patients before transplant with low-dose calcineurin inhibitors (target level of 5–8 ng%) and mycophenolate (1,000 mg BID). Patients without a significant rise in viral titer by quantitative PCR over 3 months have not demonstrated evidence of active viral disease after transplantation.
- All patients receive trimethoprim/sulfamethoxazole (*Septra*) for *Pneumocystis carinii* prophylaxis. Fluconazole (100 mg orally every week) is given for mucocutaneous candidiasis prophylaxis as long as patients are receiving steroids, and patients with evidence of fungal colonization (e.g., *Aspergillus* spp.) are maintained on voriconazole.
- In the absence of allograft dysfunction, the decision to treat moderate histologic (2R) rejection with pulse steroids deserves discussion. There are no compelling data that treatment of mild to moderate rejection significantly influences allograft survival, and there is significant evidence that increased steroids and antilymphocyte therapy increase the incidence of infection. Given the variability of histologic interpretation and the inherent possibility of non-representative biopsy tissue, the decision to treat histological rejection should be approached with caution as this represents the most significant variable in transplant infections.

CHAPTER 56 ■ LUNG TRANSPLANTATION

- The past decade has seen a steady increase in the percentage of older patients on the waiting list. Over the past several years, the average waiting time to transplant has decreased, the number of deaths on the list has decreased, and the number of transplants has increased (Fig. 56.1). These data are the product of changes in lung allocation policy, better patient management while on the list, and the efforts of organ procurement organizations (OPOs) and hospitals to recognize and optimize potential lung donors.

PERIOPERATIVE CARE OF LUNG TRANSPLANTATION

- The typical recipient is an adult 50 to 64 years of age. Recipient diagnosis and criteria for "ideal" lung donors are listed in Figure 56.2 and Tables 56.1 and 56.2, respectively. Median waiting time to transplant is nearly 7 months. Survival rates after lung transplant have gradually improved the main determinants of outcome including recipient age, diagnosis, history of prior transplant, and severity of illness at the time of transplant. Adjusted survival rates at 1, 3, and 5 years are currently 85%, 66%, and 51%, respectively.
- Once the recipients have been declared eligible for lung transplantation (Table 56.3), there are four lung transplant surgical procedures being considered: (i) single-lung transplantation (SLT), (ii) bilateral sequential lung transplantation (BLT), (iii) combined heart–lung transplantation (HLT), and (iv) bilateral lobar transplantation from living related donors. Although recipient history of previous talc pleurodesis still gives many transplant centers pause, a history of other chest surgeries is not a contraindication to lung transplantation.
- Historically, SLT used to be the most applied technique, but lately, more centers are adopting BLT as the transplant procedure of choice.

- Table 56.4 details the numerous side effects, interactions, and dosing of the immunosuppressive medications.

PULMONARY FUNCTION AND GAS EXCHANGE

- Both SLT and BLT patients have significant improvement in pulmonary function tests (PFTs) and in gas exchange post transplantation. The peak improvement in PFTs is achieved at 1 to 3 months after SLT, but after BLT, improvement may not be achieved until 4 to 6 months post transplant. The factors associated with the delay in achieving peak values are reperfusion injury, postoperative pain, altered chest wall mechanics, and respiratory muscle dysfunction after transplant surgery.
- After SLT in patients with chronic obstructive pulmonary disease (COPD), the forced expiratory volume in 1 s (FEV_1) significantly improves to about 45% to 60% of the predicted value, and lung volumes approach the normal predicted values. The chest radiograph in COPD recipients of SLT shows hyperinflated native lung with a flat diaphragm and mild herniation across the midline. The transplanted allograft is a normal-sized lung—although it appears small compared to the native lung—with a physiologically domed diaphragm.
- After SLT in patients with idiopathic pulmonary fibrosis (IPF), the vital capacity improves to about 70% to 80% of the predicted value. Compared to a fibrotic native lung on the contralateral side, the chest radiograph shows a normal-sized lung allograft. After BLT, the chest radiograph and spirometry values approximate predicted values for the recipient size (Fig. 56.3). After lung transplantation, arterial oxygenation rapidly returns to normal, but hypercapnia may take a

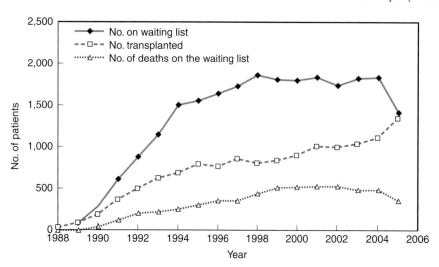

FIGURE 56.1. In the United States: number of lung transplants, number of patients waiting, and deaths on the waiting list, 1988 to 2005 (ages 18–64 years). (Adapted from 2005 Annual Report of the U.S. Organ Procurement and Transplantation Network and the Scientific Registry of Transplant Recipients: transplant data 1994–2006).

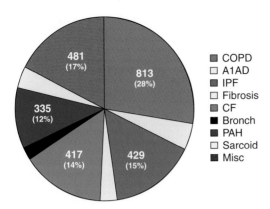

FIGURE 56.2. Adult patients on the waiting list in the United States in 2005, by indication. COPD, chronic obstructive pulmonary disease; A1AD, alpha 1-antitrypsin deficiency; IPF, idiopathic pulmonary fibrosis; CF, cystic fibrosis; PAH, pulmonary arterial hypertension. (Adapted from 2005 Annual Report of the U.S. Organ Procurement and Transplantation Network and the Scientific Registry of Transplant Recipients: transplant data 1994–2006).

few days before returning to normal. Supplemental oxygen is unnecessary for most patients at the time of hospital discharge.

HEMODYNAMICS

- Both SLT and BLT result in immediate and sustained normalization—or near normal in SLT—of pulmonary artery

TABLE 56.1

DISEASE-SPECIFIC GUIDELINES FOR REFERRAL

Chronic obstructive pulmonary disease
FEV_1 (forced expiratory volume in 1 s) <25% of predicted postbronchodilator, especially when associated with mild or moderate pulmonary artery hypertension
Frequent severe exacerbations
BODE index (body mass index [B], airflow obstruction [O], dyspnea [D], and exercise capacity [E]) of ≥7)

Cystic fibrosis
FEV_1 <30% of predicted
$PaCO_2$ >50 mm Hg
Frequent severe exacerbations
Rapid decline in lung function (especially in females)

Idiopathic pulmonary fibrosis
Vital capacity (VC) <65% predicted
10% decline in VC or in diffusion capacity in the last 12 mo
Initiation of oxygen therapy

Pulmonary arterial hypertension
NYHA (New York Heart Association) functional class III or IV
Cardiac index <2 $L/min/m^2$
Mean right atrial pressure >12 mm Hg
Failure of medical therapy to improve hemodynamic indexes or functional class

Eisenmenger syndrome
NYHA III or IV despite optimal medical therapy (especially if patients are discontented with their current quality of life)

TABLE 56.2

CRITERIA FOR "IDEAL" LUNG DONORS

PaO_2 >300 mm Hg on FiO_2 = 1.0 and 5 cm H_2O continuous positive airway pressure
Less than 20 pack-years smoking history
Clear chest radiograph
Minimal secretions on bronchoscopy
Negative viral serology (HIV, hepatitis B and C infections)
Age younger than 55–60 years

pressures in PPH recipients, barring significant reperfusion injury. This is associated with near total or total resolution of the associated tricuspid valve insufficiency and is accompanied by an immediate increase of the cardiac output with a gradual remodeling of the right ventricle. The right ventricle decreases in size and regains normal function over the next few days to weeks. This hemodynamic improvement is sustained after successful transplantation. The advantage of BLT over SLT for patients with pulmonary vascular disease is that airway injury is better tolerated in BLT. Due to the resultant severe ventilation/perfusion mismatch, airway injury (caused by pneumonia, or acute or chronic rejection) results in profound hypoxemia in patients with severe pulmonary hypertension who undergo SLT.

EXERCISE CAPACITY

- Peak exercise performance, as measured by cycle ergometry, is characteristically reduced in both SLT and BLT

TABLE 56.3

GENERAL GUIDELINES FOR SELECTION OF RECIPIENTS

Indications
End-stage lung disease with average life expectancy <2 y
Failed medical and surgical therapy
Severe functional limitation, but ambulatory
Upper age limit has recently been liberalized to include ≤69 years

Absolute contraindications
Significant extrapulmonary end organ damage
Acute critical illness
History of cancer in the last 5 y
Active psychosis or history of noncompliance with therapy
Cigarette smoking in the last 6 mo
History of substance abuse with risk factors for recidivism
Nonambulatory, with poor rehabilitation potential
Inadequate social support
Systemically active collagen vascular diseases
Extrapulmonary infections (human immunodeficiency virus, hepatitis B, C active infections)

Relative contraindications
Mechanical ventilation
Extensive pleural adhesions from previous surgical procedures (especially talc)
Airway colonization with bacteria panresistant to all antibacterials
Body mass index >30

TABLE 56.4

COMMONLY USED IMMUNOSUPPRESSIVE MEDICATIONS

Drug	Dosing and adjustments	Side effects	Drug interactions
Cyclosporine and tacrolimus	Every 12 h	Commonly occur with both: nephrotoxicity, hypertension, neurotoxicity (tremors, headaches, rarely seizures), hyperkalemia, hyperlipidemia, hypomagnesemia Occur only with tacrolimus: myalgias, hyperglycemia Occur only with CyA: hemolytic-uremic syndrome, hirsutism, gingival hyperplasia	Blood levels are increased with all macrolide antibiotics (except azithromycin), azole antifungals, and calcium channel blockers (except nifedipine). Blood levels are decreased by anticonvulsants and rifampin.
Sirolimus	Every 24 h	Cytopenias, hyperlipidemia (mainly hypertriglyceridemia)	Same drug interactions as tacrolimus and cyclosporine: Blood levels are increased with all macrolide antibiotics (except azithromycin), azole antifungals (voriconazole contraindicated with sirolimus), and calcium channel blockers (except nifedipine). Blood levels are decreased by anticonvulsants and rifampin.
Azathioprine	Every 24 h Decrease dosage in the event of renal or hepatic insufficiency.	Cytopenias, hepatotoxicity, pancreatitis, nausea	Increased bone marrow suppression with allopurinol, ganciclovir, and antithymocyte globulin.
Mycophenolate mofetil	Every 12 h Decrease dosage in the event of renal or hepatic insufficiency.	Abdominal cramps, diarrhea, vomiting, cytopenias	No significant interactions.
Prednisone	0.3–0.5 mg/kg/d in the first 3 mo, then tapered afterward.	Hypertension, hyperglycemia, weight gain, myopathy, osteoporosis, cataracts, mood swings, and hyperlipidemia	No significant interactions.

recipients as late as 1 or 2 years after the surgery. These patients have subnormal peak work rate, peak oxygen consumption, and early lactate threshold on incremental exercise testing. Maximal oxygen consumption is significantly

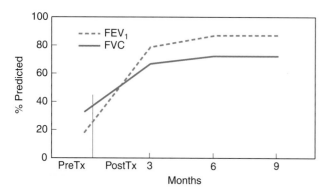

FIGURE 56.3. Spirometry values in cystic fibrosis patients undergoing bilateral lung transplantation (BLT) ($n = 5$). FEV_1, forced expiratory volume in 1 second; FVC, forced vital capacity. (Courtesy of Division of Pulmonary Medicine, University of Florida, Gainesville, FL).

increased after lung transplantation, but it typically is 40% to 60% of the maximal predicted value. Interestingly, the limitation to exercise is not cardiac or ventilatory in nature, and, surprisingly, the maximal oxygen consumption attained during exercise testing is similar whether the recipients are of SLT or BLT. Reduced mitochondrial oxidative capacity and peripheral oxygen use in the skeletal muscles of lung transplant recipients may be secondary to the deconditioning associated with chronic lung diseases or cyclosporine-associated impairment in skeletal muscle mitochondrial respiration.

COMPLICATIONS AFTER LUNG TRANSPLANTATION

- Most allografts have reperfusion lung injury manifesting as pulmonary edema within the first 24 hours after transplantation. The injury is mild to moderate, and the edema is transient in most cases. However, in 5% to 10% of cases, the lung injury is severe enough to cause acute respiratory distress syndrome or severe primary graft failure.

- It is presumed to reflect ischemia–reperfusion injury, but hyperacute rejection (caused by preformed antibodies in the recipient) is the cause for the severe injury in a small subset of patients with this complication. The chest radiograph and clinical scenario are almost identical in all these etiologic factors, that is, all have widespread interstitial and alveolar infiltrates in the allograft(s) and severe hypoxemia. The diagnosis of reperfusion injury is established by excluding other causes of graft dysfunction: hyperacute or acute rejection, pneumonia, volume overload, and thrombosis of the pulmonary venous anastomosis.
- Inhaled nitric oxide, independent lung ventilation, and extracorporeal membrane oxygenation have been attempted with variable success. The mortality rate reportedly ranges between 40% and 60% in cases of severe hypoxemia. The clinical course in survivors is protracted, but some of the survivors are able to ultimately attain normal allograft function. Variables associated with increased mortality in patients with reperfusion lung injury are age, severity of gas exchange impairment, and severity of hemodynamic failure.

Airway Complications

- Airway complications requiring intervention occur in 7% to 15% of bronchial anastomosis.
- Most airway complications manifest in the first 100 days after transplantation. They may present as wheezing, exertional dyspnea, or decline in FEV_1. As the bronchial arteries are not reconnected at the time of transplantation, the bronchial mucosa distal to the anastomosis could be affected by bronchial artery reperfusion injury. This manifests as bronchial mucosal injury with ischemic mucosal surface. The mucosal injury may heal with minimal sequelae, thereby resulting in airway stricture, or, if the bronchial artery ischemia injures the underlying cartilaginous support of the bronchus, it may cause bronchomalacia. Alternatively, bronchial stenosis may be caused by overgrowth of the scar tissue at the site of the bronchial anastomosis. Thus, airway complications may be at the anastomotic site or a few centimeters distally.
- Bronchial mucosal injury has the bronchoscopic appearance of a pseudomembrane, which is sometimes superinfected with fungal organisms. Most airway complications are amenable to correction with stent placement, balloon dilation, or cautery.

Infections

- Infection, the most common cause of death in the first 12 months after lung transplantation, is also a common cause of death in patients afflicted with obliterative bronchiolitis (OB).
- Most recipients will have at least one infection requiring therapy with an antimicrobial agent during the first 12 months after transplantation.
- Respiratory tract pathogens are the most common source of bacterial infections after transplantation. Microbes from donor lungs cause a significant number of early episodes of bacterial pneumonia, but the incidence has decreased because antibacterial prophylaxis is used at the time of trans-

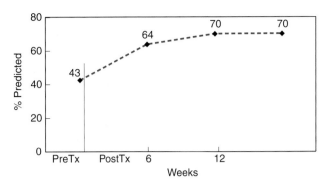

FIGURE 56.4. Vital capacity in idiopathic pulmonary fibrosis patients after single lung transplant (n = 7). (Courtesy of Division of Pulmonary Medicine, University of Florida, Gainesville, FL).

plantation. *Pseudomonas* and the *Enterobacteriaceae* cause most bacterial infections after discharge from the transplant hospitalization; infections caused by *Staphylococcus* and Haemophilus are also common. Viral infections are the second most common cause of infections; cytomegalovirus (CMV) infection is the most common among the viral causes. The incidence of CMV infection or reactivation has been reported to be 40% to 75%, which is much higher than that for other solid organs. The patients at highest risk of infection and morbidity are CMV-seronegative recipients from a seropositive lung donor. The case fatality rate of CMV infection is reported to be about 5%. Herpes simplex (HSV) and varicella-zoster (VZ) infections are also quite common. HSV and VZ are mostly caused by reactivation of a latent viral infection. Acquired respiratory viral infections are mostly secondary to respiratory syncytial virus (RSV), influenza, and parainfluenza viruses. These viral infections may cause cough, wheezing, or, in extreme cases, acute respiratory distress syndrome. Parvovirus has been reported to cause refractory anemia in recipients of solid organ transplants.
- The most common cause of fungal infection is *Candida albicans,* with *Aspergillus* a close second. The lung allograft is a common site of infection; the spectrum of disease ranges from necrotic bronchitis (Fig. 56.4) to invasive fungal pneumonia. The incidence of *Pneumocystis carinii* pneumonia (PCP), approximately 80% prior to prophylaxis, has decreased to between 5% and 10% since the institution of long-term prophylaxis.

Acute Rejection

- Acute rejection denotes the infiltration of the allograft by lymphocytes; severity of the rejection is classified by pathologic criteria.
- Acute rejection may present as decline in airflows, cough, oxygen desaturation with exercise, or, rarely, as low-grade temperature elevation. The chest radiograph may be clear and unchanged or may represent a pulmonary edema pattern. While the classic triple maintenance immunosuppressive regimen remains cyclosporine (CyA), prednisone, and AZA, acute rejection episodes are treated with a course of pulse steroids consisting of three daily doses of methylprednisolone, dosed at 15 mg/kg/day, followed by oral prednisone taper and optimization of the CyA and AZA doses. Patients

TABLE 56.5

STAGING OF BRONCHIOLITIS OBLITERANS
SYNDROME (BOS)

BOS-p (potential BOS): 10%–19% decline in forced
expiratory volume in 1 s (FEV_1) compared with the peak
FEV_1

Stage 1: 20%–33% decline in FEV_1 compared with the peak
FEV_1

Stage 2: 33%–50% decline in FEV_1 compared with the peak
FEV_1

Stage 3: >50% decline in FEV_1 compared with the peak FEV_1

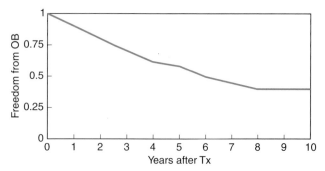

FIGURE 56.5. Freedom from obliterative bronchiolitis (OB). (From Taylor DO, Edwards LB, Boucek MM, et al. Registry of the International Society for Heart and Lung Transplantation: twenty-third official adult heart transplantation report—2006. *J Heart Lung Transplant.* 2006;25(8):869–879).

resistant to pulse steroid therapy are treated with antilymphocyte antibodies—polyclonal antithymocyte globulin or monoclonal OKT3—and are often switched from CyA to tacrolimus.

Chronic Rejection (Bronchiolitis Obliterans)

- *Chronic lung rejection* is used synonymously with *bronchiolitis obliterans syndrome* (BOS). BOS is a progressive and irreversible decline in airflow, ultimately resulting in respiratory failure. The disease has a variable course: some patients experience a rapid decline in airflow, whereas others experience either slow progressive decline or intermittent decline in airflow punctuated by long periods of stable lung function. BOS is staged by the magnitude of the loss of lung function. BO is the histologic equivalent of chronic lung rejection, and the histologic diagnosis is difficult because transbronchial biopsy specimens are not sufficiently sensitive for diagnosis.
- After the exclusion of other factors confounding bronchoscopy and transbronchial biopsy, the diagnosis is made by pulmonary function tests. Bronchoscopy is performed to exclude anastomotic complications, infections, acute rejection, or disease recurrence in the allograft. If the decline in FEV_1 is >20% compared to the peak FEV_1 attained after transplantation, and the bronchoscopy—with transbronchial biopsy—excludes confounding factors, the clinical scenario is then diagnostic of BOS. Moreover, if the decline in FEV_1 is associated with acute rejection on transbronchial biopsy but does not reverse with augmentation of immunosuppression, it is also consistent with BOS (Table 56.5).
- BOS occurs in approximately 50% of recipients 5 years after transplantation (Fig. 56.5). It is the most common cause of death in patients surviving >1 year. The median survival after

the diagnosis of BOS approximates 2 years. In most patients, BOS is characterized by a relentless decline in airflows, albeit at variable rates in different patients, and ultimately results in respiratory failure. In SLT recipients, BOS is associated with a significantly lower survival when it occurs in IPF patients rather than COPD patients. Recurrent episodes of acute lung rejection are a definite risk factor for BOS; CMV pneumonitis is a probable risk factor. In a retrospective study, mismatching at the HLA-A locus was found to be a risk factor for BOS.

- BOS presents as cough that later becomes productive, followed by progressive exertional dyspnea. The chest radiograph is clear, but in the advanced stages will show bronchiectasis and interstitial infiltrates. Studies have shown that augmentation of immunosuppression will not reverse the decline in most cases; furthermore, it probably places patients at increased risk of infection, with very little impact on the natural history of the disease. Retransplantation has been attempted for this complication but with variable success.

Posttransplant Lymphoproliferative Disease (PTLD)

- The reported incidence of PTLD after lung transplantation varies between 2% and 6%. The presentation and pattern of organ involvement is related to the time of onset. In the first year, intrathoracic involvement is the most common presentation; gastrointestinal tract involvement predominates later. The incidence of PTLD increases in proportion to the intensity of immunosuppression, especially when antilymphocyte antibodies are used.

CHAPTER 57 ■ LIVER TRANSPLANTATION

- Liver transplantation remains the only therapy for end-stage, chronic liver disease and irreversible, fulminant liver failure. It is increasingly being performed for patients with localized, unresectable hepatocellular carcinoma with promising results. Since 2002, the number of patients waiting for liver transplantation has slowly increased to near 13,000. The age distribution of those waiting has changed more dramatically, with ages between 50 and 64 years making up the majority (Fig. 57.1).
- The total number of liver transplants being performed has steadily increased over the past decade, with 6,441 transplants in 2005. This increase is primarily due to the increase in deceased donor livers available for transplant. Living donor liver transplantation (LDLT) accounted for 5% of liver transplants performed in 2005, down from a peak of 10% in 2001 (Fig. 57.2). This decrease may be due in part to the increased utilization of extended criteria donor (ECD) livers and concerns about the morbidity and mortality risks associated with living donor liver transplantation.
- Liver allocation for adults depends primarily on disease severity as determined by the Model for End-Stage Liver Disease (MELD) (Table 57.1). The MELD formula uses easily obtained laboratory data—total bilirubin, serum creatinine, and international normalized ratio—and is highly predictive of death on the waiting list. Important exceptions are made for selected patients with hepatocellular carcinoma and other groups of patients for whom the MELD score does not reflect disease severity. Despite performing transplants in much older patients, utilizing more ECD livers, and employing an allocation system that gives priority to the sickest patients, the results of liver transplantation continue to be encouraging.

PERIOPERATIVE CARE OF LIVER TRANSPLANTATION

Cardiovascular Issues

- The cardiac physiology of liver failure is characterized as a hyperdynamic profile with a high cardiac output. If there is any degree of dysfunction, it has been assumed in the past that the patient suffered from alcohol chronic toxicity, which is responsible for 30% of dilated cardiomyopathies. However, it is becoming evident that a significant amount of systolic dysfunction and even more diastolic dysfunction is present in patients with ESLD of all causes, including nonalcoholic. In addition, the potential for coronary artery disease has been underappreciated previously in the potential liver transplant patient. Current studies suggest that the prevalence of coronary artery disease in patients with ESLD is at least as common and probably more so than in the general population. Patients may also be less symptomatic despite moderate to severe coronary heart disease. At least 50% of patients with coronary artery disease will suffer significant morbidity and mortality while undergoing a liver transplantation.
- Patients with liver failure demonstrate blunted cardiac response to stimuli such as hemorrhage, hypovolemia, and administration of inotropic drugs.
- Adrenergic receptor desensitization occurs so the normal inotropic and chronotropic responses to isoproterenol and dobutamine are attenuated.

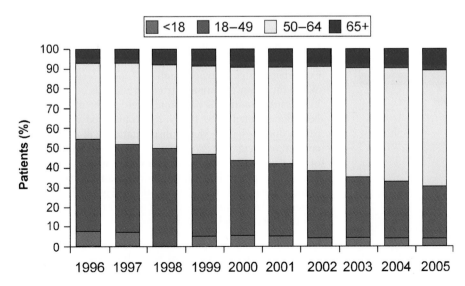

FIGURE 57.1. Age distribution of patients listed for liver transplant per year. (Source: 2006 Annual Report of the U.S. Organ Procurement and Transplantation Network and the Scientific Registry of Transplant Recipients: Transplant Data 1996–2005. Rockville, MD: Health Resources and Services Administration, Healthcare Systems Bureau, Division of Transplantation. The data and analyses reported in the 2006 Annual Report of the U.S. Organ Procurement and Transplantation Network and the Scientific Registry of Transplant Recipients have been supplied by the United Network for Organ Sharing and Arbor Research under contract with the Department of Health and Human Services. The authors alone are responsible for reporting and interpreting these data; the views expressed herein are those of the authors and not necessarily those of the U.S. government.)

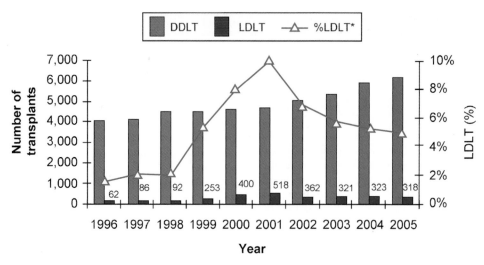

FIGURE 57.2. Number of liver transplants performed by donor type per year. DDLT, deceased donor liver transplant; LDLT, living donor liver transplant. (Source: 2006 Annual Report of the U.S. Organ Procurement and Transplantation Network and the Scientific Registry of Transplant Recipients: Transplant Data 1996–2005. Rockville, MD: Health Resources and Services Administration, Healthcare Systems Bureau, Division of Transplantation. The data and analyses reported in the 2006 Annual Report of the U.S. Organ Procurement and Transplantation Network and the Scientific Registry of Transplant Recipients have been supplied by the United Network for Organ Sharing and Arbor Research under contract with the Department of Health and Human Services. The authors alone are responsible for reporting and interpreting these data; the views expressed herein are those of the authors and not necessarily those of the U.S. government.)

Pulmonary Disorders in Liver Failure

- Approximately 40% of cirrhotic patients have hepatopulmonary syndrome, with approximately 8% to 15% developing impaired oxygenation. Essentially, the patient develops pulmonary arteriovenous dilations due to the increased presence of vasodilators. The gold standard in diagnosis is a contrast echocardiogram demonstrating intrapulmonary shunting. There is no effective treatment for this disease, but transplantation results in an 85% resolution or significant improvement. The duration of time until that improvement occurs can be quite variable, anywhere between a few days to 14 months postoperatively. Unfortunately, there are no good indicators to predict reversibility. Baseline room air arterial oxygenation of ≤50 mm Hg has been shown to worsen survival despite liver transplantation.

MODEL FOR END-STAGE LIVER DISEASE

$0.378 \times 00D7$; $\log_e$ (bilirubin) [mg/dL]
+
$1.120 \times \log_e$ (INR)
+
$0.957 \times \log_e$ (creatinine) [mg/dL]
+
0.643
Add the above 4 numbers and multiply by 10.
Round to the nearest integer.

INR, international normalized ratio.
From United Network for Organ Sharing. MELD/PELD calculator documentation. www.unos.org/resources, with permission. Accessed October 12, 2007.

- Conversely, portopulmonary hypertension is essentially pulmonary hypertension, which occurs in 2% to 5% of cirrhotic patients. It does not correlate with the degree of portal hypertension or liver failure. Using a cutoff of 40 mm Hg for right ventricular systolic pressure, the sensitivity of echocardiogram is 80% and the specificity is 96%.
- The treatment of portopulmonary hypertension is not at all the same as for other types of pulmonary artery hypertension. At the present time, diuretics and epoprostenol have been the best studied and the most likely to provide benefit. Recommended therapies for pulmonary artery hypertension, such as anticoagulation, calcium channel blockers, β-blockers, and endothelin receptor antagonists, can have adverse effects either on the prognosis of portopulmonary hypertension or on liver failure in general. A transjugular intrahepatic portosystemic shunt is contraindicated in this setting. Sildenafil may have some benefit, but it does increase the production of endogenous nitric oxide and can further exacerbate systemic hypotension.
- When the mean pulmonary artery pressure is >50 mm Hg, liver transplantation is contraindicated, as the mortality has been documented to be 100%. It is considered a contraindication due to the fact that transplantation will decrease the amount of circulating prostaglandins and result in worsening of the disease. Below a mean pulmonary artery pressure of 35 mm Hg, proceeding with liver transplantation can occur without delay. Between 35 and 50 mm Hg, optimizing the patient's status with diuretics and epoprostenol is indicated prior to liver transplantation.

Hepatorenal Syndrome

- Hepatorenal syndrome (HRS) is a functional type of renal impairment that occurs in 11.4% of patients with liver failure within 5 years of the first episode of significant ascites. There are two types, which are both potentially reversible with liver transplantation. HRS 1 is rapidly progressive, with a doubling of initial creatinine to above 2.5 mg/dL or 50% reduction of creatinine clearance to less than 20 mL/minute, which occurs in less than 2 weeks. The mortality rate is nearly 100% within 10 weeks of development. HRS 2 is associated with a more moderate, steady decline in renal function. The 1-year probability of survival is 38.5% with HRS 2, but the mean survival of HRS 1 is only 7 $\pm$ 2 days. A more complete discussion of this topic is found in the chapter on liver failure. Therefore, the focus here will be regarding the goals of therapy during liver transplantation in patients with HRS.

- The most successful management to prevent further injury during surgery is to alter the physiology that led to the development of HRS. The effect of peripheral and splanchnic vasodilation from cytokines and nitric oxide, as well as the intrarenal vasoconstriction that occurs in response to intravascular depletion are both aspects of liver failure that combine to produce this syndrome. Obviously, euvolemia is a primary goal, and in most studies looking at prevention and improvement of HRS, albumin is used as an adjuvant therapy.
- Vasopressin analogues administered with albumin to patients with both types of HRS have been shown to improve glomerular filtration rate and creatinine levels.
- The major risk associated with vasopressin analogues is the potential for ischemia, which has been shown to be clinically significant with only ornipressin. Terlipressin is not currently available in the United States, however.
- The combination of octreotide and midodrine has been shown to have some beneficial effects on renal function and mortality in HRS; however, patients treated with vasopressin had improved survival rates and were more likely to receive a liver transplant. There is no literature that has investigated the combined effects of all three agents. In a very small study, norepinephrine had comparable efficacy to vasopressin without any adverse side effects. In patients with liver failure who develop hypotension, norepinephrine and vasopressin are agents that should be considered first line with less concern regarding renal side effects. Patients who do not respond to the above therapies will likely require some form of renal replacement therapy. Continuous venovenous hemodialysis (CVVHD) is the treatment of choice since it causes less hypotension, with a decreased potential to create ongoing injury compared to hemodialysis performed three times a week. However, once a patient has received any type of dialysis for HRS lasting longer than 12 weeks, there is a risk that renal dysfunction will either continue after transplantation or will recur within a few years.

Fulminant Hepatic Failure

- The abrupt onset of liver failure within 8 weeks in a previously healthy patient has been the traditional definition of fulminant failure, but modern discussion centers on potentially decreasing the time period to 2 weeks to correlate with the prognosis. There are several potential causes, but acetaminophen is by far the most common. The mortality rate is 80% without liver transplantation.
- Table 57.2 summarizes the King's College criteria for liver transplantation. The MELD score has a higher sensitivity and negative predictive value, but a very high false-positive rate

---

TABLE 57.2

KING'S COLLEGE CRITERIA FOR LIVER TRANSPLANTATION IN FULMINANT HEPATIC FAILURE

Acetaminophen
- pH <7.3 (irrespective of encephalopathy)

Or all three of the following:
- Grade III or IV encephalopathy
- PT >100 sec or INR >6.5
- Serum creatinine >3.4 mg/dL

All other causes
- PT >100 s or INR >6.5 (irrespective of encephalopathy)

Or any three of the following:
- Age <10 or >40 years
- Cause: non–A, non–B hepatitis; halothane; idiosyncratic drug reaction; Wilson disease
- Length of time from jaundice to encephalopathy >7 days
- PT >50 seconds or INR >3.5
- Serum bilirubin >17.5 mg/dL

PT, prothrombin time; INR, international normalized ratio.
From O'Grady JG, Alexander GJ, Hayllar KM, et al. Early indications of prognosis in fulminant hepatic failure. *Gastroenterology.* 1989;97: 439–445, with permission.

---

so it may be better to use it in conjunction with King's College criteria to avoid transplantation in patients who may recover spontaneously.

- Infection occurs in 80% of patients with fulminant hepatic failure (FHF), and thus a high index of suspicion and regular surveillance are important. Some centers use prophylactic antibiotics, but this increases the risk of fungal infections, which occur in 30% of patients with FHF. Hemodynamically, FHF is associated with a high cardiac output and vasodilation similar to sepsis, making infection difficult to discern. Optimizing intravascular volume is the main goal in management, but vasopressors may be necessary. Fluid management may be complicated by renal failure since this occurs in 40% to 50% of patients.
- Encephalopathy inversely correlates with prognosis. Table 57.3 summarizes the four stages of encephalopathy that are seen in FHF. Cerebral edema occurs in most cases that progress to stage 4. Typical symptoms of cerebral edema

---

TABLE 57.3

HEPATIC ENCEPHALOPATHY IN FULMINANT HEPATIC FAILURE

Stage	Mental status	EEG
I	Confusion, slow mentation and affect, slurred speech, disordered sleep	Normal
II	Accentuation of stage I, drowsy, inappropriate, loss of sphincter control	Slowing
III	Marked confusion, sleeps mostly but arousable, incoherent	Abnormal
IV	Not arousable; may or may not respond to painful stimuli	Abnormal

EEG, electroencephalograph.
From Sass DA, Shakil AO. Fulminant hepatic failure. *Liver Transplant.* 2005;11(6):594–605, with permission.

are the Cushing reflex, decerebrate rigidity, dysconjugate eye movements, and a loss of pupillary reflexes. Intracranial pressure (ICP) monitoring should be considered if the patient develops stage 3 or 4 encephalopathy due to the development of increased ICP in the setting of systemic hypotension. Cerebral perfusion pressure (CPP) of >60 mm Hg is necessary to maintain intact neurologic function. Liver transplantation in the setting of CPP <40 mm Hg for 2 hours or more is contraindicated. Concern for intracranial bleeding associated with the placement of an ICP monitor has precluded use in most liver transplant centers. Recently, factor VIIa has been shown to be effective in transiently correcting coagulopathy to allow for safer placement of this monitor. Patients with elevated ICP are candidates for mannitol, mild hyperventilation, and barbiturate or propofol infusions while maintaining systemic blood pressure in an attempt to optimize CPP.

BLOOD PRODUCT USE

- Patients with liver failure have a decrease in all factors except von Willebrand. Platelets are also reduced secondary to hypersplenism, bone marrow suppression, and decreased thrombopoietin production in ESLD. Attempts to correct coagulation defects in patients undergoing liver transplantation result in a hypervolemic state, which can lead to an increase in blood transfusion.
- Thromboelastography is used because most serum component markers of coagulation do not reflect the intricate dynamics of whole blood clotting to guide transfusion.
- Aprotinin use in liver transplantation has been shown to decrease red blood cell transfusion in several randomized trials. During the anhepatic phase of surgery, the suprahepatic and infrahepatic vena cava may be cross-clamped. This is a stage during which there is rapid increase in tissue-type plasminogen activator in the absence of α-2-antiplasmin and plasminogen activator inhibitor. Therefore, plasmin activity increases, and fibrinolysis can ensue. Aprotinin acts to inhibit plasmin. The concern regarding the use of aprotinin on a prophylactic basis is due to scattered case reports of thrombotic episodes such as clots on pulmonary artery catheters and an increased rate of vein graft occlusions in cardiac surgery.
- Given the crude understanding of coagulation in the presence of liver disease, potential aprotinin administration should be reserved for documented fibrinolysis during the reperfusion stage. The lowest effective dose documented in the literature is 500,000 kallikrein inactivation units (KIU) as a bolus, with 150,000 KIU/hour, with equal efficacy to higher doses in limiting the number of blood products transfused. If pulmonary embolism occurs, supportive care and thrombolysis may lead to better outcomes compared to embolectomy.
- Factor VIIa is a novel way to increase the thrombin burst and acutely improve coagulation on a short-term basis secondary to rapid factor consumption. Theoretically, it requires an activated platelet so coagulation occurs at the site of bleeding and not systemically. It has been studied in cirrhotic patients in trials for gastrointestinal bleeding and liver transplantation. Neither showed any difference in the degree of bleeding or required transfusions. However, cirrhotic patients are likely to be factor VII deficient. There has been no dose-ranging study to look at efficacy related to the degree of serum levels achieved.

FLUIDS AND ELECTROLYTES

- Along the lines of avoiding hypervolemia, minimizing fluid use is the goal during liver transplantation. There is no particular type of fluid that conclusively shows benefit. ESLD patients have a decreased ability to metabolize lactate and are prone to lactic acidosis, especially during the required interruption of blood flow for performing the vascular anastomosis of the liver transplant. The exclusive use of lactate-containing solution is likely unwise.
- Hyponatremia at $\leq$127 mEq/L occurs in 3.5% of liver transplant candidates. A change in serum sodium approaching 20 mEq/L is much more likely to produce central pontine myelinolysis than a change closer to 7 mEq/L. Central pontine myelinolysis is a source of mortality after liver transplantation. Normal saline solutions are actually somewhat hypernatremic and hyperchloremic to serum, and excessive use will lead to hyperchloremic acidosis. Albumin administration has shown benefit during paracentesis and in the long-term management of patients with ESLD. Patients with significant renal dysfunction and/or those undergoing dialysis at the time of transplantation will most likely require CVVHD during liver transplantation. Although this is helpful to manage electrolyte abnormalities, it is not quick. This is particularly the case with metabolic acidosis in which patients often require the addition of a dilute bicarbonate infusion, which may be faster and safer. However, CVVHD can be used to both remove and administer fluid expeditiously. A heating system should be used during CVVHD since serum is exchanged at about the rate of 22 to 30 L in 24 hours, and patients can become hypothermic, which can exacerbate baseline coagulopathy. To prevent the system from developing clots, citrate is often used, as opposed to heparin, in patients with significant coagulopathy. Between this condition and the amount of citrate that may be administered from blood products, calcium supplementation is often required.

POSTTRANSPLANT COMPLICATIONS

Primary Nonfunction

- There is no clear definition or uniform diagnostic criteria for this diagnosis, but generally it includes patients who die or require retransplantation within 1 week without a definite technical or immunologic cause. Patients appear to rapidly go back into hepatic failure with high levels of aminotransferases, prolonged prothrombin time, hepatic encephalopathy, hypoglycemia, and lactic acidosis.
- There are currently no definitive preventative strategies or treatments. Donor age older than 50 years and macrovesicular steatosis of >60% are possible risk factors, but these have not been shown to be consistently so.

Vascular Occlusion

- Studies concerning the incidence of portal vein thrombosis (PVT) at the time of liver transplant show that it occurs in about 12% of patients. The presence of a pre-existing thrombosis makes surgery more challenging and increases the risk of

TABLE 57.4

IMMUNOSUPPRESSIVE MEDICATION IN LIVER TRANSPLANTATION

Medication	Side effects
Steroids	Acne, obesity, hypertension, bone loss, hyperglycemia, bone disease, cataracts, adrenal suppression, muscle wasting
Calcineurin inhibitor (cyclosporine, tacrolimus)	Neurotoxicity, nephrotoxicity, hypertension, hyperglycemia, lipid abnormalities
Mycophenolate	Nausea, diarrhea, leukopenia, thrombocytopenia, anemia
Azathioprine	Gastrointestinal ulceration, myelosuppression
MTOR inhibitor (sirolimus, everolimus)	Increased cholesterol and triglycerides, proteinuria, potentially nephrotoxic[a]
Murine monoclonal antibody (OKT3)	Fever, rigor, headache, dyspnea, nausea, diarrhea, flash pulmonary edema
Rabbit polyclonal antibody (thymoglobulin)	Similar to OKT3, leukopenia, thrombocytopenia, serum sickness
Anti-interleukin-2 receptor (basiliximab)	Minimal to none

[a]Patients on sirolimus and a calcineurin inhibitor in combination may exhibit more nephrotoxicity than is seen with the latter drug alone.
From Hirose R, Vincenti F. Immunosuppression: today, tomorrow and withdrawal. *Semin Liver Dis*, 2006;26(3):201–210, with permission.

rethrombosis after transplantation, but it has not been shown to alter mortality. The incidence of PVT presenting after transplantation is less than 1%. In addition to a prior history of PVT, the risk factors include a hypercoagulable state, perioperative hypotension, and allograft cirrhosis. Acutely, it can lead to hepatic failure, but chronically there is a more insidious presentation involving portal hypertension with ascites and varices. Hepatic vein thrombosis is very unusual except in patients who have undergone transplantation for Budd-Chiari syndrome with subtherapeutic anticoagulation, and it typically takes months to years to develop.

- The most common vascular complication is hepatic artery thrombosis (HAT), which occurs somewhere between 3% and 9%. In addition, mortality is common without retransplantation, with an incidence of about 30%. If HAT is tolerated by the liver surviving solely on portal flow, then complications occur usually after 1 month with the development of bile duct strictures since virtually all biliary perfusion comes from the hepatic artery. For patients who cannot be supported solely on portal flow, their presentation is much more acute with severe graft dysfunction or primary nonfunction.

- Risk factors for HAT include small caliber or complex arterial structure of both the donor and recipient. Increased donor age and a recipient/donor ratio greater than 1.25 can put the recipient at risk for HAT. Medical issues that may predispose to HAT include cytomegalovirus infection, rejection, tobacco use, and hypercoagulable states. Urgent revascularization can be attempted for early presentation of HAT-associated graft dysfunction. This can be accomplished angiographically or surgically. However, about 50% of patients in this scenario will require retransplantation. Patients who do receive some type of intravascular therapy have difficulty maintaining long-term hepatic artery patency.

Rejection

- Not only is rejection less common in liver transplantation than in other solid organ transplants, but less rejection occurs in the latter group when performed in the setting of a con-

current or previous liver transplant. Nonetheless, transplantation tolerance is not attainable consistently. It has been shown that patients can be weaned off corticosteroid immune suppression 3 to 4 months after transplantation, but complete cessation of immune suppression is associated with about a 30% incidence of rejection. The commonly used immunosuppressive agents in liver transplantation, with their side effects, are listed in Table 57.4.

- Acute rejection occurs within the first 5 to 15 days after transplantation. It is manifested by fever, graft enlargement, tenderness, leukocytosis with increased eosinophils, and reduced bile production. Biopsies are done only when symptoms are present because the morphologic features consistent with acute rejection can be present in a significant percentage of patients in the early posttransplant period. Treatment for acute rejection is 3 to 5 days of 500 to 1,000 mg of methylprednisolone daily, with about 75% resolution. A second course is sufficient for treatment in an additional 10%. The rest require some type of antilymphocyte therapy, with a rare case requiring retransplantation. Patients who develop rejection in the setting of complete immunosuppressive cessation have been shown to have an increased risk of steroid-resistant rejection.

- Early complications of the biliary tract are leaks and strictures. Anastomotic leaks and strictures are the most serious and are usually related to ischemic necrosis of the donor distal bile duct. These can be managed with endoscopic or percutaneous stenting and require surgery only if a major leak is present. The vast majority of these problems present within the first 2 months after transplantation.

Live Donor or Living-Related Liver Transplantation

- Unique to this type of transplantation is small-for-size syndrome. Essentially, the patient has poor bile production, delayed synthetic function, prolonged cholestasis, and intractable ascites. These patients are at risk for sepsis and have an increased mortality. A similar situation may affect patients who receive a split liver.

CHAPTER 58 ■ PANCREATIC TRANSPLANTATION

- Pancreas transplantation offers selected diabetic patients the prospect of glucose control, avoiding—and, in some cases, reversing—the devastating complications of the disease. Most pancreata are transplanted simultaneously with a kidney (SPK), although a significant fraction are transplanted alone (PTA) or at some time after a kidney (PAK) transplant. Deceased donor pancreas remains a relatively underutilized organ resource; only 19% of available deceased donor pancreata are recovered and transplanted. A few percent are procured, processed, and transplanted as islet cell transplants. The reasons for this underutilization are multifactorial, and include regional variation in the number of potential recipients, donor and organ quality, and competition for kidneys with other patients.

- In 2005, 903 SPK transplants, 344 PAK transplants, and 195 PTA transplants were performed. These totals have changed little over the last several years. Figure 58.1 depicts the trend for SPK transplants over the past decade. Similarly, patient and graft survival has improved, with 5-year patient survival approaching 90%.

- There are three broad categories of recipients: SPK, PAK, and PTA.

  - *SPK transplants:* Most SPK transplants have been done with both organs coming from the same cadaveric donor. Because a large number of patients are waiting for a kidney, unless priority is given to SPK candidates, waiting times tend to be long (years). Thus, to avoid two operations and a long wait, a simultaneous kidney and segmental pancreas transplant from a living donor can be done. Only a few centers offer this option. There has been a report from Japan of successful islet transplantation from a live donor. Therefore, a simultaneous living-donor islet kidney transplant may become a viable option in the future. If a living donor is suitable for or only willing to give a kidney, another option is a simultaneous living-donor kidney and cadaveric pancreas transplant. For these options, the living kidney donor usually must be available on a moment's notice (the same as for the recipient), as the cadaveric pancreas must be transplanted soon after procurement. Alternatively, a recipient of a scheduled living-donor kidney transplant could also receive a cadaveric pancreas simultaneously if one became available fortuitously. If not, and only a kidney is transplanted, the recipient becomes a PAK candidate.

  - *PAK transplants:* For nephropathic diabetic patients who have already undergone a kidney transplant from a living or a cadaveric donor, a PAK transplant can be performed. Most PAK transplants today are done in patients who previously received a living-donor kidney because suitable uremic diabetic patients without a living donor will undergo a cadaveric pancreas transplant. Although a PAK means a uremic diabetic patient requires two operations to achieve both a dialysis-free and insulin-independent state, the two

transplants done separately are smaller procedures than a combined transplant. The interval between the living-donor kidney and cadaveric pancreas transplant depends on several factors, including recipient recovery from the kidney transplant and donor availability, but the outcome is similar for all intervals more than 1 month. PAK is the largest pancreas transplant category at the University of Minnesota.

  - *PTA:* For recipients with adequate kidney function, a solitary pancreas transplant can be performed from either a living or a cadaveric donor. Because the waiting time for a cadaveric pancreas is relatively short at the present time, living-donor pancreas transplants are done infrequently, but are particularly indicated if a candidate has a high panel-reactive antibody and a negative cross-match to a living donor. Most PTA candidates have problems with glycemic control, hypoglycemic unawareness, and frequent insulin reactions. A successful PTA not only obviates these problems, but also improves the quality of life, and may ameliorate secondary complications, thus increasing the applicability of PTA.

PERIOPERATIVE CARE OF PANCREAS TRANSPLANTATION

- After an uncomplicated pancreas transplant, the recipient is transferred to the postanesthesia care unit or the surgical intensive care unit. Centers that have a specialized monitored transplant unit (with central venous and arterial monitoring capabilities) transition the postoperative recipients through the postanesthesia care unit to the transplant unit. Others transfer directly to the surgical intensive care unit for the first 24 to 48 hours. Care during the first few hours after transplant is similar to care after any major operative procedure. Careful monitoring of vital signs, central venous pressure, oxygen saturation, and hematologic and laboratory parameters is crucial. The following factors are unique to pancreas recipients and should be attended to:

- *Blood glucose levels:* Any sudden, unexplained increase in glucose levels should raise the suspicion of graft thrombosis. An immediate ultrasound examination must be done to assess blood flow to the graft. Maintenance of tight glucose control (<150 mg/dL) using an IV insulin drip is important to "rest" the pancreas in the early postoperative period.

- *Intravascular volume:* Because the pancreas is a "low-flow" organ, intravascular volume must be maintained to provide adequate perfusion to the graft. Central venous pressure monitoring is used to monitor intravascular volume status. In some cases, such as patients with depressed cardiac function, pulmonary artery catheter monitoring may be required during the first 24 to 48 hours. If the hypovolemia is

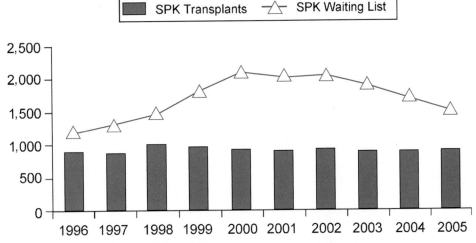

FIGURE 58.1. Number of simultaneous pancreas–kidney transplants (SPK) and size of active waiting list per year. (Source: 2006 Annual Report of the U.S. Organ Procurement and Transplantation Network and the Scientific Registry of Transplant Recipients: Transplant Data 1996–2005. Rockville, MD: Health Resources and Services Administration, Healthcare Systems Bureau, Division of Transplantation, Tables 1.7 and 8.1a. The data and analyses reported in the 2006 Annual Report of the U.S. Organ Procurement and Transplantation Network and the Scientific Registry of Transplant Recipients have been supplied by the United Network for Organ Sharing and Arbor Research under contract with the Department of Health and Human Services. The authors alone are responsible for reporting and interpreting these data; the views expressed herein are those of the authors and not necessarily those of the U.S. government.)

associated with low hemoglobin levels, then washed packed red blood cell transfusions should be given. Otherwise, colloid or crystalloid replacement can be used.

- *Maintenance IV fluid therapy:* The choice of IV fluid is usually 5% dextrose in half normal saline. The use of dextrose is not contraindicated and may be of benefit, as long as IV insulin is used to maintain good blood glucose control. In SPK recipients, whose IV rate is based on urine output, dextrose should be eliminated if the urine output is high (more than 500 mL/h). Maintenance solution for bladder drainage (BD) recipients should include 10 mEq of HCO_3 added to each liter to account for the excess HCO_3 loss. Sodium lactate can be used as an alternative.
- *Antibiotic therapy:* Broad-spectrum antibiotic therapy (with strong gram-negative coverage) and antifungal therapy are instituted before the incision is made in the operating room, and then continued for 3 days (for antibiotics) and 7 days (for antifungal), respectively. At the University of Minnesota, since the introduction of this protocol, we have noted a decrease in postoperative abdominal infections. Cytomegalovirus (CMV) and antiviral prophylaxis is similar to that for other solid organs.
- *Octreotide:* The use of octreotide in pancreas recipients helps reduce the incidence of technical complications. This benefit should be weighed against evidence, in rat studies, that shows decreased pancreatic islet blood flow with octreotide use, although clinically no detrimental effects of octreotide use have been documented. A dose of 100 to 150 μg IV or subcutaneously three times a day is administered for 5 days after transplant. Dose adjustments may be made for nausea, which is the predominant side effect.
- *Anticoagulation:* The use of low-dose heparin in the early postoperative period (days 0–5) decreases the risk of graft thrombosis. An intraoperative dose of 70 units/kg is given, followed by an IV infusion of 3 units/kg started at 4 hours

postoperatively and gradually increased up to 7 units/kg (depending on hemodynamic stability and hemoglobin levels). Enteric-coated aspirin (8 mg) is started on day 1 and continued for 6 months. At the University of Minnesota, this protocol decreased the thrombosis rate from about 12% to 6%, but increased the relaparotomy rate due to bleeding from 4% to 6%. Segmental pancreas transplants (as in living-donor transplants) have a higher thrombosis risk and therefore therapeutic heparinization (with a target partial thromboplastin time of 50) for 5 days and Coumadin therapy (with a target international normalized ratio of 2–2.5) are recommended for 6 months. The higher risk of thrombosis is due to the smaller vessels in a segmental graft.

IMMUNOSUPPRESSION

- One common immunosuppression regimen is shown in Table 58.1.

SURGICAL COMPLICATIONS

- *Bleeding:* Postoperative bleeding is a frequent reason for early relaparotomy in pancreas recipients. The incidence ranges from 6% to 8%. This risk is increased by the use of anticoagulation in the immediate postoperative period. Frequent physical examinations and monitoring of hemoglobin help detect bleeding early. Heparin may be temporarily suspended to stabilize the patient. If bleeding continues, early operative intervention is indicated. If bleeding stops or slows down, heparin should be restarted at a lower rate and judiciously increased as tolerated.
- *Thrombosis:* The incidence of thrombosis after transplant ranges from 5% to 13%. The risk is increased after segmental

TABLE 58.1

UNIVERSITY OF MINNESOTA STANDARD IMMUNOSUPPRESSION PROGRAM FOR PANCREAS TRANSPLANTATION

SPK Transplantation	PAK & SPLK Transplantation	PTA	Rejection
Antithymocyte globulin (1.25 mg/kg)[a] 5 doses First dose intraoperative Give methylprednisolone 500 mg, 250 mg, and 100 mg before first, second, and third doses, respectively.	Antithymocyte globulin (1.25 mg/kg)[a] 7 doses First dose intraoperative Give methylprednisolone 500 mg, 250 mg, and 100 mg before first, second, and third doses, respectively.	Antithymocyte globulin (1.25 mg/kg)[a] 7–10 doses First dose intraoperative Give methylprednisolone 500 mg, 250 mg, and 100 mg before first, second, and third doses, respectively.	Methylprednisolone Day 0: 500 mg IV Day 1: 250 mg IV Day 2: 125 mg IV **Antithymocyte globulin** 1.25 mg/kg IV[a] × 5–7 d Give premedication. Monitor ALC.[b] *Resistant rejection*
Tacrolimus 2 mg PO BID Start when creatinine <3 mg/dL or postoperative day 5, whichever is later. If tacrolimus is delayed. continue TMG until tacrolimus levels are therapeutic: levels 8–10 ng/mL for 3 mo, then 5–8 ng/mL.	Tacrolimus 2 mg PO BID Start postoperatively. If tacrolimus is delayed, continue TMG until tacrolimus levels are therapeutic: levels 8–10 ng/mL for 3 mo, then 5–8 ng/mL.	Tacrolimus 2 mg PO BID Start postoperatively. If tacrolimus is delayed, continue TMG until tacrolimus levels are therapeutic: levels 8–10 ng/mL for 3 mo, then 5–8 ng/mL.	OKT3 qd × 5–7 doses First dose = 5 mg IV Subsequent doses = 2.5 mg IV Give premedication. Monitor CD3.[c]
Mycophenolate Start postoperatively, 1 g PO BID.	Mycophenolate Start postoperatively, 1 g PO BID.	Mycophenolate Start postoperatively, 1 g PO BID.	**Note:** Renal rejection on the steroid avoidance protocol should be treated with thymoglobulin (mild) or OKT3 (moderate/severe or vascular).

SPK, simultaneous pancreas–kidney; PAK, pancreas after kidney; SPLK, simultaneous cadaver pancreas–live-donor kidney; PTA, pancreas transplantation alone; TMG, antithymocyte globulin; ALC, absolute lymphocyte count.
[a]Round up antithymocyte globulin dose to the nearest 25.
[b]**ALC levels:** If zero, hold antithymocyte globulin; if 0.1, give half-dose antithymocyte globulin; if 0.2 or above, give full dose.
[c]**CD3 levels** (if using OKT3): Monitor effectiveness of antibody therapy. Absolute CD3 level should drop to <100 mm^3. Antithymocyte globulin and OKT3 require "premedication."

pancreas transplants because of the small caliber of vessels. Most thromboses are due to technical reasons. A short portal vein (requiring an extension graft) or atherosclerotic arteries in the pancreas graft increases the risk for thrombosis. In the recipient, a narrow pelvic inlet with a deeply placed iliac vein, atherosclerotic disease of the iliac artery, a technically difficult vascular anastomosis, kinking of the vein by the pancreas graft, significant hematoma formation around the vascular anastomosis, and a hypercoagulable state are some of the factors that increase the risk for thrombosis. The most common form of hypercoagulable state is factor V Leiden mutation in the Western population. The incidence ranges from 2% to 5% but may be as high as 50% to 60% in patients with a history (self or family) of thrombosis. Other causes of hypercoagulable state include antithrombin deficiency, protein C or S deficiency, activated protein C resistance, and anticardiolipin antibodies.

- *Duodenal leaks:* The incidence of duodenal leaks ranges from 4% to 6%. A leak from the anastomosis of the duodenum to the bowel almost always leads to a relaparotomy. Gross peritoneal contamination due to an enteric leak necessitates a graft pancreatectomy. The diagnosis is made by elevated pancreatic enzymes associated with acute abdomen. The differ-

ential diagnosis is pancreatitis, abdominal infection, or acute severe rejection. A Roux-en-Y anastomosis to the pancreatic duodenum may be preferred if the risk of leak is thought to be increased during intraoperative inspection of the pancreas. Other novel techniques such as a venting jejunostomy (Roux-en-Y) have been used in selected recipients.

- Duodenal leaks in BD recipients are usually managed nonoperatively with prolonged catheter decompression of the urinary bladder. The diagnosis is made using plain or computed tomography cystography. The size and extent of the leak cannot always be assessed by the imaging studies. Large leaks may require operative intervention, such as a repair or enteric conversion.

- *Major intra-abdominal infections:* The incidence of intra-abdominal infections requiring reoperation ranges from 4% to 10%. Opening the duodenal segment intraoperatively, with associated contamination, predisposes to this high rate. Fungal and gram-negative infections predominate. With the advent of advanced interventional radiologic procedures to drain intra-abdominal abscesses, the incidence of reoperations is fast decreasing. If the infection is uncontrolled or widespread, then graft pancreatectomy followed by frequent washouts may be necessary.

- *Renal pedicle torsion:* Torsion of the kidney has been reported after the SPK transplants. The intraperitoneal location of the kidney (allowing for more mobility) predisposes to this complication. Additional risk factors are a long renal pedicle (more than 5 cm) and a marked discrepancy between the length of artery and vein. Prophylactic nephropexy to the anterior or lateral abdominal wall is recommended in intraperitoneal transplants to avoid this problem.
- *Others:* Other surgical complications that may require laparotomy also decreased from 9% to 1%. Improved anti-infective prophylaxis, surgical techniques, immunosuppression, and advances in interventional radiology have all contributed to this disease.

NONSURGICAL COMPLICATIONS

- *Pancreatitis:* The incidence of posttransplant pancreatitis varies based on the type of exocrine drainage. BD recipients with abnormal bladder function are at increased risk secondary to incomplete bladder emptying or urine retention causing resistance to the flow of pancreatic exocrine secretions. Other causes of pancreatitis include drugs (corticosteroids, azathioprine, cyclosporine), hypercalcemia, viral infections (CMV or hepatitis C), and reperfusion injury after prolonged ischemia. Pancreatitis is usually manifested by an increase in serum amylase and lipase with or without local signs of inflammation. The treatment usually consists of catheter decompression of the bladder for a period of

2 to 6 weeks, depending on the severity. In addition, octreotide therapy may be used to decrease pancreatic secretions. The underlying urologic problem, if any, should be treated. If repeated episodes of pancreatitis occur, an enteric conversion of exocrine drainage may be indicated.
- *Rejection:* The incidence of rejection is discussed in the Results section earlier in this chapter. The diagnosis is usually based on an increase in serum amylase and lipase and a decrease in urine amylase in BD recipients. A sustained significant drop in urinary amylase from baseline should prompt a pancreas biopsy to rule out rejection. In ED recipients, one has to rely on serum amylase and lipase only. A rise in serum lipase has recently shown to correlate well with acute pancreas rejection. Other signs and symptoms include tenderness over the graft, unexplained fever, and hyperglycemia (usually a late finding). Diagnosis can be confirmed by a percutaneous pancreas biopsy. In cases in which percutaneous biopsy is not possible due to technical reasons, empiric therapy may be started. Rarely, open biopsy is indicated. Transcystoscopic biopsy, which was used in the past, has been largely abandoned.
- *Others:* Other findings include infectious complications such as CMV, hepatitis C, extra-abdominal bacterial or fungal infections, posttransplant malignancy such as posttransplant lymphoproliferative disorder, and other rare complications such as graft–versus–host disease that occur in pancreas transplantation. The diagnosis and management of these complications is similar to those of other solid-organ transplants.

CHAPTER 59 ■ RENAL TRANSPLANTATION

- More than 46,000 patients were on the active waiting list for a kidney transplant in 2005. In that year, approximately 16,000 kidney transplantations were performed. The total number of kidney transplantations has gradually increased, as has the fraction of those kidneys transplanted with other organs. Live-donor kidneys accounted for approximately 41% of those transplants, and the remainder of transplanted kidneys originated from deceased donors. Policy changes continue to refine deceased donor kidney allocation to better utilize this scarce resource. Additionally, novel live donor–recipient matching strategies have been developed that offer the prospect of some relief to this shortage. As shown in Figure 59.1, the disparity between the number of those waiting for a kidney and those transplanted continues to increase despite increases in both living and deceased organ donation over the last decade.
- Kidney transplantation confers a clear survival advantage for patients with end-stage renal failure compared to long-term hemodialysis. For live-donor kidney recipients, 5-year patient and graft survival are 90% and 80%, respectively

PERIOPERATIVE CARE IN KIDNEY TRANSPLANTATION

- Renal transplantation is carried out in the standard fashion through an incision that exposes the iliac fossa. The donor renal vessels are sutured in an end-to-side fashion to the external iliac artery and vein, and a ureteroneocystostomy is created. Patients are monitored with continuous electrocardiography and central venous pressure in the immediate postoperative period. Blood pressures are carefully monitored, as most patients have underlying hypertension, and administration of immunosuppressive medications such as corticosteroids can affect blood pressure control. In addition, pain, catecholamine release, and fluid status may contribute to difficulties with blood pressure control. Though adequate blood pressure control is important for the integrity of the renal arterial anastomosis, it is equally important to avoid hypotension and therefore prevent renal hypoperfusion and graft thrombosis.

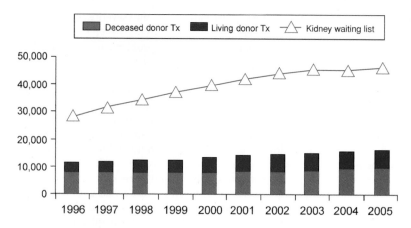

FIGURE 59.1. Number of kidney transplantations and size of active waiting list per year. TX, transplant. (Source: 2006 Annual Report of the U.S. Organ Procurement and Transplantation Network and the Scientific Registry of Transplant Recipients: Transplant Data 1996–2005. Rockville, MD: Health Resources and Services Administration, Healthcare Systems Bureau, Division of Transplantation, Tables 1.7 and 5.1a. The data and analyses reported in the 2006 Annual Report of the U.S. Organ Procurement and Transplantation Network and the Scientific Registry of Transplant Recipients have been supplied by the United Network for Organ Sharing and Arbor Research under contract with the Department of Health and Human Services. The authors alone are responsible for reporting and interpreting these data; the views expressed herein are those of the authors and not necessarily those of the U.S. government.)

- Urine output is carefully monitored on an hourly basis via an indwelling urinary catheter. This urinary catheter also serves to protect the ureteroneocystostomy during the early postoperative period. Any increase in intravesical pressure due to incomplete emptying of the bladder could compromise the newly created anastomosis between the ureter and bladder. Hematuria occurring early after transplantation may be due to bleeding at the ureteral anastomosis, in the bladder, or along the urethra. This can be managed with gentle flushing of the urinary catheter with 20 to 30 mL of sterile saline. Changing the urinary catheter to one of a larger caliber may also help remove clots. Three-way urinary catheters are also used to facilitate continuous bladder irrigation should other measures fail to treat the hematuria.

- Blood glucose monitoring is also done on a regular basis. Many transplant recipients have underlying diabetes mellitus, and all patients may have hyperglycemia exacerbation related to administration of steroids and other immunosuppressive agents. Use of continuous insulin infusion and frequent blood glucose monitoring may be necessary to maintain good glycemic control. Optimal control of hyperglycemia in the postoperative period and in critically ill patients has been shown to decrease morbidity and mortality.

- Particular attention should be paid to the volume and electrolyte status, as the urine output in the immediate posttransplantation period can vary from oliguria (frequently due to delayed graft function) to several liters as a result of generous fluid replacement during the surgery and also due to solute-induced osmotic diuresis. Live-donor allografts typically have excellent immediate function and may have prompt and marked diuresis. Most transplantation centers utilize a center-specific protocol with a fixed-rate maintenance of intravenous fluids usually with 0.9% normal saline at 50 mL/hour or 100 mL/hour together with replacement fluid at two-thirds or one-half of previous hour urine output. Some recipients may need hourly fluid replacement on a milliliter-for-milliliter basis to keep up with fluid losses. Kidneys from expanded donors or donation after cardiac death or with longer cold ischemia times may not have immediate function due to acute tubular necrosis (ATN). These recipients should be kept on a maintenance volume of intravenous fluids, and the central venous pressure can be used to guide fluid status (Fig. 59.2). Other factors to consider would include the timing of the last dialysis and the amount of urine produced by the patient before transplantation. Hemodialysis treatment shortly before the transplantation surgery may render a recipient relatively hypovolemic during the perioperative period. Patients who have not yet been started on renal replacement therapy or who make a normal amount of urine may not have issues with hypovolemia.

- Postoperative evaluation of electrolytes should include monitoring of serum sodium, potassium, bicarbonate, calcium, magnesium, and phosphorous. Though some patients require bicarbonate supplements, potassium supplements are usually not necessary. However, supplementation may be required in patients with large-volume posttransplantation diuresis.

- Prophylaxis with subcutaneous heparin to prevent deep venous thrombosis and H_2 receptor blockers or proton pump inhibitors to prevent gastric and/or duodenal ulcers are often administered. Patients should be evaluated for the need for dialysis based on their electrolyte, metabolic, and volume status.

Early Complications

- The most common complication early after transplantation is an inappropriately low urine output. The differential diagnosis includes (a) obstruction of urine flow anywhere between the renal pelvis and the collection bag; (b) graft hypoperfusion; (c) urinary leak; (d) renal parenchymal disease, usually ATN; and (e) acute rejection in immunologically sensitized patients. If a brisk diuresis was observed in the operating room or has been recorded in previous hours, a sudden reduction in urine flow should immediately raise suspicion of a mechanical problem. Graft thrombosis is rare, but any hope of graft salvage requires immediate return to the operating room.

Delayed Graft Function and Acute Tubular Necrosis

- Delayed graft function (DGF) or acute renal dysfunction in the immediate posttransplantation period has been a serious and frequent problem in cadaver renal transplantation and occurs in up to 30% of the recipients and up to 35% to 40% in expanded-criteria-donor and donation-after-cardiac-death kidney recipients, respectively. However, this diagnosis should be considered only after all other causes are eliminated. ATN is the most common histologic feature in patients with DGF. The risk factors associated with an increased incidence of DGF include donor hypovolemia or hypotension, particularly in the presence of nephrotoxic drugs or

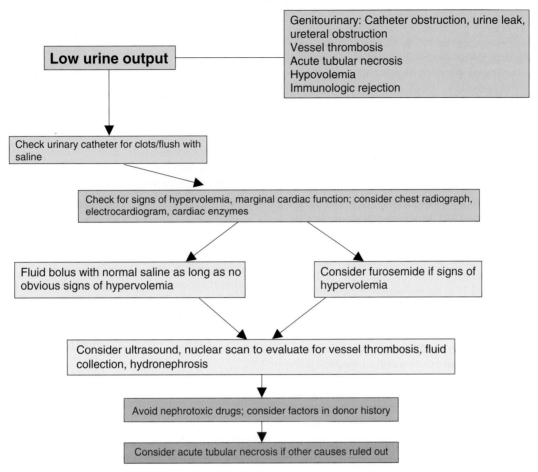

FIGURE 59.2. Algorithm for management of low urine output after renal transplantation.

vasopressors; prolonged cold or warm ischemia times; kidneys procured from older donors and from donors with hypertension or vascular occlusive disease; injury incurred during procurement, preservation, or implantation; and a high (>50%) panel reactive antibody level in the recipient. Live-donor kidneys are much less likely to have DGF than deceased donor kidneys. The pathophysiology leading to DGF is complex and incompletely understood and appears to be due to ischemia–reperfusion injury. The short-term and long-term deleterious effects on graft survival that have been demonstrated in patients developing this disorder relate to its association with acute and chronic rejection. Therefore, protocols were developed to administer antilymphocyte antibodies for the preemptive treatment of acute rejection, during this period of graft dysfunction, when a diagnosis of rejection could be difficult. This led to the development of protocols termed *sequential quadruple immunosuppressive therapy,* where patients receive antibody induction followed by maintenance immunosuppression, usually with three agents.

IMMUNOLOGIC CAUSES OF EARLY GRAFT DYSFUNCTION

- Hyperacute rejection is a rare and largely preventable cause of immediate graft failure. It is caused by preformed antibodies present in the recipients' serum at the time of transplantation against donor antigens. These antibodies are the consequence of previous exposure to donor antigens due to blood transfusions, prior transplantation, or pregnancy. It also occurs when transplantation is attempted across ABO-incompatible barriers. The events that lead to hyperacute rejection may occur with such rapidity that the kidney becomes visibly ischemic while the patient is still on the operating table. It always occurs within 24 hours of transplantation. Renal histology shows fibrin thrombi occluding the glomerular capillaries and small vessels with extensive tissue necrosis. Although plasmapheresis and anticoagulation have been advocated, there is no established effective treatment and interventions are seldom successful. A kidney with hyperacute rejection should always be removed promptly. The current cross-match techniques, because of their increased sensitivity, have greatly diminished the incidence of hyperacute rejection. *Antibody-mediated (CD4-positive) acute rejection* is another form of early rejection that can occur in previously sensitized patients but with an initial negative cross-match. This form of acute rejection is potentially reversible if diagnosed early and treated aggressively with plasmapheresis and intravenous immunoglobulin.

Immunosuppression

- The different phases of immunosuppressive therapy after transplantation are (a) induction immunosuppression in the immediate posttransplantation period when potent therapy is required to prevent rejection; (b) maintenance immunosuppression for long-term therapy to prevent allograft rejection but at the same time preserving host defense mechanisms against infections; and (c) intensification of the immunosuppressive therapy for the treatment of an acute rejection episode.

- Antilymphocyte antibodies are ideally suited for use as induction immunosuppressive agents and some for the treatment of acute rejection. They have been available for use as immunosuppressive agents since the late 1960s. All early forms of antilymphocyte antibodies were polyclonal, which are made by injecting human lymphocytes into horses, goats, rabbits, or sheep. In contrast to polyclonal antibodies, a monoclonal antibody is highly specific and recognizes a single antigen epitope. They have a greater potency at lower doses and have a more predictable and consistent effect. Monoclonal antibodies that are currently approved for use in transplantation are directed either at cell surface receptors such as the CD3/T-cell receptor complex (OKT3), or the interleukin-2 (IL-2) receptor (IL-2R; daclizumab and basiliximab). Current maintenance immunosuppression protocols often use the combination of a calcineurin inhibitor, an antimetabolite, and corticosteroids. However, the principles of the different regimens are similar: more intense immunosuppression in the induction phase with gradual reduction in immunosuppression in the maintenance phase. The immunosuppression protocol and institution implements should provide a balance between preventing rejection and avoiding the consequences of overimmunosuppression such as infection and malignancy.

MINIMIZING OPPORTUNISTIC INFECTIONS IN THE TRANSPLANT RECIPIENT

Viral Infections

- Cytomegalovirus is the most important viral infection affecting transplant recipients. Treatment options are available in Table 59.1. Other viral infections that may occur in the immunosuppressed renal allograft recipient include Epstein-Barr virus, which may lead to the development of Epstein-Barr virus–positive lymphomas; herpes simplex virus (types I and II); hepatitis B virus; hepatitis C virus; varicella-zoster virus; and the influenza virus. Treatment of viral infections depends on the type of virus and the extent of the disease. All transplant recipients should receive an annual influenza immunization.

Fungal Infections

- Fungal infections are a major concern in the immunosuppressed renal allograft recipient. As with the general population, *Candida albicans* infections resulting from endogenous flora are common. However, with immunosuppression, these infections can rapidly develop into more serious infections. Other fungal pathogens seen in transplant recipients include nocardiosis, aspergillosis, *Cryptococcus,* histoplasmosis, coccidiomycosis, blastomycosis, and mucormycosis. Treatment of fungal infections include the use of antifungals specific to the organism, surgical excision (especially in the case of mucormycosis), and reduction in the overall immunosuppression. Careful consideration should be given to the choice of the antimicrobial agent because of drug interactions (azole antifungals) or additive nephrotoxicity (amphotericin B). Invasive fungal infections in transplant recipients are associated with a high risk of graft loss and mortality. Early diagnosis and aggressive treatment can preserve organ function and can be lifesaving.

Other Opportunistic Infections

- Urinary tract infections are a frequent complication of renal transplantation. Although urinary tract infections are frequently asymptomatic, they constitute the major source of bacteremia in this patient population. Therefore, all urinary tract infections, even asymptomatic ones, should be treated appropriately. Fortunately, renal dysfunction is an uncommon complication of urinary tract infections in the transplant recipient. It usually occurs with severe pyelonephritis involving the allograft, usually in the setting of ureteric obstruction or vesicoureteral reflux. Chronic urinary tract infections may require daily prophylactic antibiotic administration.
- Renal allograft recipients, especially patients with poor allograft function with a background of intensive acute and chronic immunosuppressive therapy for recurrent rejection episodes, are susceptible to a large range of infections. Empiric treatment should be initiated at the first sign of infection, as infections can be aggressive and worsen rapidly.

GASTROINTESTINAL COMPLICATIONS

- A wide variety of gastrointestinal complications may occur after transplantation due to infections with organisms such as cytomegalovirus (CMV), *Candida* spp., and

TABLE 59.1

CYTOMEGALOVIRUS (CMV) RISK STRATIFICATION AND TREATMENT OPTIONS

Risk status	Donor CMV IgG serostatus	Recipient CMV IgG serostatus	Usual drug of choice	Dose	Duration
High	Positive	Negative	Valganciclovir	450 mg QD	90–180 d
Moderate	Positive	Positive	Valganciclovir	450 mg QD	90 d
	Negative	Positive	Valganciclovir	450 mg QD	90 d
Low	Negative	Negative	Valacyclovir	500 mg BID or TID	30 d

Clostridium difficile; adverse effects associated with immuno-suppressive agents; posttransplantation complications of pre-existing conditions such as diverticulitis; and other complications such as acute appendicitis, gastrointestinal bleeding, colonic or small-bowel perforations, pancreatitis, and ischemic colitis.

Peptic Ulcer Disease

- Gastroduodenal ulcers presenting after transplantation can be attributed to a variety of causes including pre-existing ulcer history, viral pathogens (CMV in 15%, herpes simplex in 2%), and immunosuppressive agents, mainly corticosteroids.

Bowel Perforations

- Colonic perforation should be suspected in the presence of one or more of the following: abdominal pain, fever, increased white blood cell count, tenderness, and pneumoperitoneum. These clinical criteria may be blunted in the presence of poor renal function, use of high-dose corticosteroids, or the overall state of immunosuppression

Acute Pancreatitis

- Acute pancreatitis is an infrequent but severe complication after renal transplantation. A review of the literature has documented an incidence of 2.3% with a mortality rate of 61.3% in 3,253 renal transplant recipients. Several etiologic factors have been considered. Azathioprine has been reported to cause pancreatitis with rapid improvement after cessation and with recurrence of symptoms with reinstitution. Corticosteroids and cyclosporine have also been reported to cause pancreatitis; however, this association is not as convincing. Other causes of pancreatitis include hyperparathyroidism, CMV infection, biliary tract disease, alcoholism, and hyperlipidemia.

HEMATOLOGIC COMPLICATIONS

- Neutropenia is a frequent complication after transplantation, often as a result of the adverse effects of immunosuppressive medications. Antithymocyte globulin can cause transient decreases in neutrophils that often rebound after cessation of therapy. Maintenance immunosuppression with mycophenolic acid, sirolimus, and prophylaxis with ganciclovir and cotrimoxazole contribute to the development of neutropenia due to their myelosuppressive effects. Careful dose reduction of these agents and/or use of granulocyte-stimulating factors are often required for persistent neutropenia. Of particular importance is that neutropenia can be a sign of CMV infection; therefore, this should always be excluded in transplant recipients with persistent neutropenia.
- Anemia is a frequent occurrence in the early posttransplantation period as a result of pre-existing anemia of end-stage renal disease, surgical blood loss, and immunosuppressive medications. Thrombocytopenia is also a frequent occurrence in renal allograft recipients and often is caused by the immunosuppressive medications. Antithymocyte globulin, valganciclovir, and dapsone can cause transient decreases in platelets. Withholding doses or dose adjustments of the responsible agent may be required for thrombocytopenia. Platelet recovery is rapid, often returning to baseline within days

CARDIAC AND VASCULAR DISEASES

- The management of transplantation patients with coronary artery disease is similar to that of other patients and should include noninvasive exercise or resting diagnostic testing, coronary arteriography, or both. Of particular note: If cardiac catheterization is necessary, femoral arterial puncture on the ipsilateral side to the renal transplant should be avoided whenever feasible to reduce the risks of mechanical injury and atheroembolization to the renal allograft.

Cerebrovascular and Peripheral Vascular Disease

- Cerebrovascular disease occurs in 1% to 3% of all renal allograft recipients. There is also an increased risk of peripheral vascular disease. A thorough history to elicit symptoms associated with cerebrovascular and peripheral vascular disease and examination of the carotid arteries and peripheral circulation should be performed annually, and the presence of a carotid bruit should be further investigated with duplex ultrasonography and magnetic resonance angiography. In the presence of more than 60% stenosis of the carotid artery, the patient should be referred to the neurovascular surgeon for further evaluation.
- Successful transplantation does not reduce the rate of atherosclerosis initiated in renal failure. Factors contributing to the high incidence of vascular disease include hypertension, hyperlipidemia, obesity, cigarette smoking, and the presence of pre-existing diabetes mellitus or the development of posttransplantation diabetes mellitus.

Hypertension

- Hypertension is a common complication of renal transplantation and remains an important risk factor for mortality from cardiovascular disease. Posttransplantation hypertension is a major risk factor for graft survival. It is unclear, however, whether this is because of the deleterious effects of hypertension on the structure and function of the renal allograft or whether hypertension is a marker of underlying renal disease. The causes of hypertension in renal transplant recipients include acute and/or chronic allograft rejection; recurrent or *de novo* transplant glomerulonephritis; transplant renal artery stenosis; high renin output state from diseased native kidneys; immunosuppressive agents such as steroids, cyclosporine, and tacrolimus; obesity; hypercalcemia; and new-onset essential hypertension.

Hyperlipidemia

- Elevations in triglycerides, low-density lipoproteins, apolipoprotein B, and total cholesterol levels are common. The pathogenesis of hyperlipidemia in renal transplant recipients is poorly understood and appears to be multifactorial. The numerous factors that have been shown to be associated with hyperlipidemia after renal transplantation are age, body weight, gender, pretransplantation lipid levels, renal dysfunction, proteinuria, concomitant use of diuretics or β-blockers, diabetes, steroid use, and cyclosporine and sirolimus use.

New-onset Diabetes after Transplantation

- New-onset diabetes after transplantation (NODAT) has been reported in 3% to 40% of transplant recipients with an even higher incidence occurring in African Americans, Hispanics, and patients with a family history of diabetes mellitus, increasing with recipient age and weight. NODAT has been attributed to the use of immunosuppressive agents, especially with tacrolimus and corticosteroids; however, cyclosporine has also been implicated. Patients with NODAT have a poor outcome in terms of patient and graft survival, with increased mortality resulting from cardiovascular and possibly infectious complications.

GRAFT DYSFUNCTION AND GRAFT FAILURE

- The differential diagnosis of acute allograft dysfunction can be divided into (a) early, occurring <90 days after transplantation, and (b) late, occurring >90 days after transplantation. It can be further differentiated into medical and surgical problems as outlined in Table 59.2. Some of the more common medical and surgical problems are discussed below.

TABLE 59.2

CAUSES OF GRAFT DYSFUNCTION AND FAILURE

	Early (0–90 days after transplantation)	Late (>90 days after transplantation)
Medical	Hyperacute rejection	Acute rejection
	Delayed graft function	Calcineurin inhibitor toxicity
	Acute rejection	Chronic rejection
	Acute calcineurin inhibitor nephrotoxicity	Dehydration
	Dehydration	Other drug toxicities
	Other drug toxicities	Infection
	Infection	BK virus nephropathy
	De novo/recurrent disease	*De novo*/recurrent disease
Mechanical	Lymphocele	Renal artery stenosis
	Ureteric obstruction	Ureteric obstruction
	Urine leak	Urine leak
	Vascular thrombosis	Vascular thrombosis

Acute Rejection

- Factors significantly associated with the development of acute rejection are human leukocyte antigen (HLA) mismatch, anti-HLA antibodies reactive to >50% of a lymphocyte panel, retransplantation, African American race, and recipient age younger than 16 years. The classic clinical features associated with acute rejection are fever, oliguria, weight gain, edema, hypertension, and the presence of an enlarged, tender graft. However, these features are frequently absent, and the most common presentation may be an asymptomatic rise in serum creatinine. An increase in serum creatinine >20% is often the cardinal feature of rejection. Percutaneous needle biopsy of the allograft is the most reliable method of diagnosis of acute rejection. The principles and the management of acute rejection include rapid diagnosis, accurate classification, and prompt administration of antirejection therapy.

Chronic Rejection

- Chronic rejection is characterized clinically by a progressive decline in renal function, persistent proteinuria, and hypertension. The course of chronic rejection is slow and insidious. Chronic rejection often occurs in conjunction with other histologic causes of allograft dysfunction: acute rejection, calcineurin inhibitor nephrotoxicity, and recurrent or *de novo* glomerular diseases. There is no treatment for chronic rejection at the present time.

Urologic Complications

- Urologic problems have been reported in between 2% and 20% of all renal transplantations. These complications can include urinary retention, urine leak, and ureteral stenosis.

Vascular Complications

- Vascular complications including vessel thrombosis or stenosis have been reported in 2% to 12% of all renal transplants. Vascular complications in general are significantly associated with ATN and graft loss. Early graft dysfunction should be evaluated for vascular complications with ultrasound with Doppler.

Lymphocele

- A lymphocele is a collection of lymphatic fluid around the allografted kidney that can occur due to leakage of small lymphatic channels around the iliac vessels at the time of the transplantation. The incidence of lymphoceles has been reported from 0.02% up to 26% after renal transplant. Consequences of lymphoceles can include distention due to the fluid collection and venous or ureteral obstruction and graft compromise. Treatment of lymphoceles can include percutaneous techniques with drainage and sclerosis of the cavity or may include operative marsupialization via the laparoscopic or open technique. Laparoscopic techniques are less invasive, have less morbidity, and are generally the first line of therapy.

Stones

- Calculi may have been present in the donor kidney or may develop after transplantation. Predisposing factors include obstruction, recurrent urinary tract infection,

hypercalciuria, hyperoxaluria, internal stents, and non-absorbable suture material. Open removal of a calculus from the transplanted kidney is rarely necessary. Complete stone removal is usually possible by standard urologic techniques.

CHAPTER 60 ■ CRITICAL CARE ASPECTS OF STEM CELL TRANSPLANTATION

- Bone marrow and blood cell transplants are widely used to treat aplastic anemia, leukemias, lymphomas, myeloma, and immunodeficiency disorders. Transplants are also increasingly used to treat other bone marrow disorders such as sickle cell disease and thalassemia. Morbidity and mortality associated with transplants usually result from regimen-related toxicity, such as adverse effects of drugs and radiation given pretransplant, complications of graft-versus-host disease (GVHD), and infections resulting from bone marrow failure.
- Pretransplant evaluation of recipients typically includes the following:
  - Measurement of the left ventricular ejection fraction, which should be at least 40%
  - Pulmonary function tests, including diffusing capacity (DLCO), and forced vital capacity, which should be more than 50% of predicted
  - Hepatic transaminases, which should be less than twice normal
  - Creatinine clearance, which should be more than 50 mL/minute
  - A pretransplant performance score consistent with an independent life

PERIOPERATIVE CARE OF STEM CELL TRANSPLANTATION

- In the setting of allotransplants, the pretransplant conditioning regimen needs to moderate or eliminate recipient immunity to prevent graft rejection. When the allotransplant recipient has cancer, the pretransplant conditioning regimen must also eradicate it. Most allotransplant conditioning regimens contain cyclophosphamide and busulfan, or total-body radiation. Antilymphocyte antibodies, such as antilymphocyte globulin, antithymocyte globulin, or alemtuzumab (anti-CD52), are often used in reduced-intensity conditioning regimens or in alternative donor transplants. In immunodeficiency disorders—for example, severe combined immunodeficiency, pretransplant conditioning is not necessary, as the host is already immune deficient.
- For autotransplants, the choice of pretransplant conditioning regimen is based on anticancer effect, a steep dose-response curve, lack of cross-resistance with other drugs, and low non-bone marrow dose-limiting toxicities. In general, these regimens contain alkylating drugs, such as melphalan or cyclophosphamide, combined with two or three other drugs. Immunosuppression is unnecessary and an unwanted side effect of therapy. Radiation is not used in autotransplants, as the effective anticancer doses exceed non-bone marrow dose-limiting toxicity.
- Pretransplant conditioning regimens are typically empirically determined (Table 60.1).

BONE MARROW AND BLOOD CELL INFUSION

- Bone marrow and blood cells may be frozen in dimethyl sulfoxide for later use. The intracellular contents of cells destroyed in the freezing and thawing processes—and dimethyl sulfoxide itself—may cause hypotension, anaphylaxis, or dysrhythmias, including transient heart block. To avoid complications, subjects are premedicated with diphenhydramine hydrochloride (Benadryl) and methylprednisolone sodium succinate (Solu-Medrol). Intubation equipment and epinephrine should be available at the bedside when cells are infused. If hypotension occurs, the infusion is slowed or temporarily interrupted until the blood pressure stabilizes. If the bone marrow or blood cells have not been frozen, the risk of anaphylaxis is similar to a standard blood transfusion, and premedication is unnecessary.
- Approximately 1.2% of cultures obtained during these processes are found to contain bacteria. Most cultures show coagulase-negative *Staphylococcus spp.*, which colonize the skin; pathogenic gram-negative bacteria are occasionally present. Thus, despite positive culture results, most centers reinfuse the stem cells after appropriate antibiotic coverage.

FLUIDS AND HYPOTENSION

- High-dose chemotherapy and radiation damage vascular endothelial cells, resulting in extravascular leakage of fluids. Furthermore, GVHD and cytokines such as tumor necrosis

TABLE 60.1

TOXICITY OF CONDITIONING REGIMEN DRUGS

Drug/dose	Extramedullary dose-limiting toxicity	Other toxicities
BCNU	Interstitial pneumonitis	Renal insufficiency, encephalopathy, nausea, vomiting, VOD
Busulfan	Mucositis, VOD	Seizures, rash, hyperpigmentation, nausea, vomiting, pneumonitis
CCNU (lomustine)	Interstitial pneumonitis	Renal insufficiency, encephalopathy, nausea, vomiting, VOD
Cyclophosphamide	Heart failure	Hemorrhagic cystitis, SIADH, nausea, vomiting, pulmonary edema, interstitial pneumonitis
Cytarabine	Mucositis, cerebellar ataxia	Pulmonary edema, conjunctivitis, rash, fever, hepatitis, toxic epidermal necrolysis
Cisplatin	Renal insufficiency, peripheral neuropathy	Nausea, vomiting, renal tubular acidosis, hypomagnesemia
Carboplatin	Ototoxicity, hepatitis	Renal insufficiency, hypomagnesemia, peripheral neuropathy
Etoposide	Mucositis	Nausea, vomiting, hemorrhagic cystitis, pneumonia, hepatitis
Ifosfamide	Encephalopathy, renal insufficiency	Hemorrhagic cystitis, renal tubular acidosis
Melphalan	Mucositis	Nausea, vomiting, hepatitis, SIADH, pneumonitis, renal insufficiency
Mitoxantrone	Cardiotoxicity	Mucositis
Paclitaxel	Mucositis	Peripheral neuropathy, bradycardia, anaphylaxis
Thiotepa	Mucositis	Intertriginous rash, hyperpigmentation, nausea, vomiting

VOD, veno-occlusive disease; SIADH, syndrome of inappropriate antidiuretic hormone.

factor, interleukin 2, and interferon-gamma contribute to a posttransplant capillary leak syndrome.

- If hypotension develops, emphasis should be placed on early invasive cardiovascular monitoring, inotropic support, and irradiated packed red blood cell transfusion to maintain intravascular oncotic pressure. Aggressive hydration may precipitate pulmonary and peripheral edema, even with normal pulmonary artery wedge pressure and right atrial pressure.

ELECTROLYTE BALANCE

- Electrolyte abnormalities are common in transplant recipients, resulting from the underlying disease, prophylactic hydration for hemorrhagic cystitis, diarrhea, parenteral nutrition, renal insufficiency, diuretics, and other medications.

BLOOD PRODUCT TRANSFUSIONS

- Subjects receiving transplants are immunocompromised and at risk for transfusion-associated GVHD. All cellular blood products contain white blood cells, including immune-competent T cells, and should be irradiated (25 Gy).
- Furthermore, all allotransplant recipients should receive cytomegalovirus-negative (CMV-negative) blood product transfusions, especially when the recipient is CMV-seronegative
- In the allotransplant setting, special consideration is needed regarding ABO compatibility between recipient and donor. This complexity of blood product transfusion support should be viewed in terms of whether there is a major or minor ABO incompatibility between the recipient and donor (Tables 60.2 and (60.3). Despite using ABO-compatible platelets, many subjects fail to respond to platelet transfusions early after transplant. Causes include fever, hepatic veno-occlusive disease (VOD), drugs, infection, disseminated intravascular

coagulation, and microangiopathic hemolytic anemia related to cyclosporine and/or GVHD.

INFECTION PREVENTION

- Standards for prevention of infection vary from strict isolation in laminar airflow (LAF) rooms to none. In LAF rooms, the subject is in a sterile environment; anyone who enters must be gloved and gowned, and the patient's food is sterilized or has a low microbial content secondary to autoclave or microwave treatment. Prophylactic oral antibiotics are given to destroy enteric pathogens, which not only are reservoirs for infection, but also may function as superantigens that increase the severity of GVHD.
- The minimal standards to prevent bacterial infections include the following:
  - A transplant unit set aside from general hospital, patients, and visitor traffic
  - High-efficiency particulate air filtration to prevent iatrogenic *Aspergillus* species infection
  - Careful handwashing before entering a patient's room
  - A diet without fresh salads, vegetables, or fruits, as these may be contaminated with gram-negative bacteria, or without pepper, as this may be contaminated with an *Aspergillus* species. Bacterial prophylactic measures are generally discontinued when the neutrophil count is $>0.5 \times 10^9$ cells/L.
- Tactics to prevent fungal infections include the use of oral triazoles such as itraconazole or fluconazole, given orally or intravenously for the first month after transplant.
- Subjects with prior aspergillus infection are at high risk of recurrence, especially in the presence of the following:
  - Prolonged neutropenia after transplant
  - A more advanced cancer state
  - A 6-week or shorter interval from beginning systemic anti-*Aspergillus* therapy to the transplant
  - Severe acute GVHD

TABLE 60.2

DONOR-RECIPIENT ABO INCOMPATIBILITY

Major ABO incompatibility	Minor ABO incompatibility	Major and minor ABO incompatibility
Recipient has antibody to donor	Donor has antibody to recipient	Recipient has antibody to donor and donor has antibody to recipient
Immediate hemolysis Prevent by RBC depletion of marrow	Prevent by plasma depletion of marrow	Prevent by RBC and plasma depletion of marrow
Delayed hemolysis Occurs 2–4 weeks after SCT + Direct antiglobulin test Risk increased with high recipient isohemagglutinin titer	Occurs day 9–day 16 after SCT + Direct antiglobulin test Risk increased with T cell–depleted marrow	+ Direct antiglobulin test
Delayed erythropoiesis Plasma exchange, erythropoietin, steroids		Plasma exchange, erythropoietin, steroids

RBC, red blood cell; SCT, stem cell transplantation; +, positive.

- Persons with prior aspergillosis should receive amphotericin, voriconazole, or caspofungin early after transplant.
- Herpes simplex reactivation is usually prevented by using intravenous or oral acyclovir for the first month after transplant. Treatment thereafter results in frequent acyclovir resistance and delays the development of natural immunity.

FEVER AND NEUTROPENIA

- In transplant recipients with fever—temperature $\geq 38^\circ$C—and a neutrophil count $<0.5 \times 10^9$ cells/L—one should

TABLE 60.3

ABO TYPE OF BLOOD COMPONENTS USED IN PATIENTS WHO HAVE RECEIVED AN ABO-INCOMPATIBLE TRANSPLANT

Donor	Recipient	Red cells	Platelets[a]	FFP
Major ABO incompatibility				
A	O	O	A	A
B	O	O	B	B
AB	O	O	A	AB
AB	A	A	A	AB
AB	B	B	B	AB
Minor ABO incompatibility				
O	A	O	A	A
O	B	O	B	B
O	AB	O	A	AB
A	AB	A	A	AB
B	AB	B	B	AB
Major and minor ABO incompatibility				
A	B	O	B	AB
B	A	O	A	AB

FFP, fresh frozen plasma.
[a] Occasionally, owing to nonavailability of platelets of the requested group, group O platelets (labeled as "low titer," (i.e., low titer of anti-A and anti-B) may be used for patients of any group).
When full ABO conversion has taken place, all patients receive products of their new ABO group.

try to identify an infection source using a chest radiograph, blood and urine cultures, and physical examination with emphasis on line sites and perineal, oropharyngeal, and sinus regions. Usually, no focal source is found, and broad-spectrum antibiotics are begun. The choice of antibiotics may include an antipseudomonal penicillin, aminoglycoside, and vancomycin or a third-generation antipseudomonal cephalosporin. Recurrent or persistent fever for 3 to 5 days without source in a person with granulocytes $<0.5 \times 10^9$ cells/L is an indication for empiric antifungal therapy with amphotericin.

MUCOSITIS

- The severity of mucositis depends on the components of the preconditioning regimen. The non–bone marrow dose-limiting toxicity of etoposide, busulfan, cytarabine, thiotepa, and paclitaxel is mucositis. Radiation also contributes to mucositis.
- Management of mucositis includes good oral hygiene using, for example, saline, chlorhexidine, and nystatin rinses, and topical analgesics. Opioids are often needed and should be given intravenously by schedule or using patient-controlled analgesia. Severe mucositis may require prophylactic intubation for airway protection. Ultimately, the resolution of mucositis generally correlates with recovery of the neutrophil count bone marrow.

DIARRHEA

- Diarrhea in transplant recipients may be caused by high-dose chemoradiotherapy, other drugs such as antibiotics, and bacterial or viral infections, and GVHD. The pretransplant conditioning regimen is the most common cause of diarrhea within 2 to 3 weeks after transplantation. Nevertheless, an infectious cause should always be considered. including *Clostridium difficile* and *Escherichia coli* (0157:H7), CMV, herpes simplex, adenoviruses, rotaviruses, echoviruses, astroviruses, Norwalk virus, Coxsackie virus, *Strongyloides* spp., *Giardia* spp., and *Cryptosporidium* spp.. GVHD also causes diarrhea; the diagnosis can be confirmed by intestinal biopsy showing loss of crypts, vacuolization of crypt epithelium, karyorrhectic apoptotic debris, microabscesses and, in severe cases, ulceration and denudation of the epithelium.

- Therapy is directed toward appropriate antibiotics for infections and immunosuppression for GVHD. Conditioning regimen- and GVHD-associated diarrhea may respond to octreotide, a somatostatin analogue whose mechanism of action is partly through the inhibition of secretory hormones. Some viral infections—for example, CMV—respond to ganciclovir, foscarnet, or cidofovir.

HEMORRHAGIC CYSTITIS

- Hemorrhagic cystitis, occurring 2 to 3 weeks after transplant, usually results from drugs in the pretransplant conditioning regimen, such as cyclophosphamide, ifosfamide, or etoposide. Prophylaxis for hemorrhagic cystitis includes hydration and diuretics to maintain urine output at 0.2 mL/kg/hour.
- Complications of hemorrhagic cystitis are uncontrolled bleeding and clotting of the ureters or urethra, resulting in acute kidney failure. Obstruction of the ureters by clots may be asymptomatic or cause kidney colic from ureteral spasm. Severe pain may occur in the back or flank and radiate into the groin or genitals.
- Therapy of hemorrhagic cystitis consists of using a Foley catheter to irrigate the bladder with normal saline at 250 mL/hour to prevent intravesicular clotting. Platelets should be maintained at more than 50×10^9 cells/L with platelet transfusions, and red blood cell transfusion should be given to replace blood loss.
- Hemorrhagic cystitis seen more than 2 weeks after transplant can result from pre-transplantation conditioning or viral infection due to, for example, adenovirus, CMV, JC or BK viruses of the bladder epithelium. Except for CMV, there are no effective antiviral drugs.

VENO-OCCLUSIVE DISEASE OF THE LIVER

- VOD of the liver is caused by drugs and/or radiation in the pretransplant conditioning regimen within 1 to 3 months after transplant.

TABLE 60.4

CLINICAL CRITERIA FOR VENO-OCCLUSIVE DISEASE OF THE LIVER

McDonald criteria— Seattle	Jones criteria—Johns Hopkins
Before day 30: Any two of the following	*Before day 21: Any two of the following*
Bilirubin >27 μmol/L = 1.7 mg/dL	Bilirubin >34 μmol/L = 2.0 mg/dL
Hepatomegaly	Hepatomegaly
Ascites or weight gain	Ascites
	Weight gain

- VOD, with a reported incidence of 1% to 56%, is a clinical diagnosis suggested by elevated bilirubin, weight gain, ascites, and tender hepatomegaly (Table 60.4). Therapy for VOD is predominantly supportive, but its prognosis is poor when bilirubin is more than 15 to 20 mg/dL.

RESPIRATORY FAILURE

- Transplant recipients who develop respiratory failure and require mechanical ventilation have a poor prognosis. Respiratory failure within the first 30 days is usually caused by pretransplant conditioning, regimen-related epithelial cell damage, and/or infection.
- Early in the course of respiratory distress, efforts should be directed to preventing intubation. Although not evaluated in prospective studies and therefore of unproven benefit, management may include early invasive hemodynamic monitoring, red blood cell transfusions to maintain hemoglobin more than 12 g/dL, ultrafiltration to decrease intravascular volume, and anticytokine monoclonal antibodies or cytokine receptor antagonists. Use of high-dose corticosteroids is controversial. Transplant recipients are especially susceptible to pulmonary infections because of bone marrow failure, immunosuppressive drugs, mucositis, aspiration, and bronchial epithelial cell damage with impaired ciliary motility. Gram-negative and -positive pneumonias are common in the first 30 days after transplantation. Fungal infections of the lung also occur early after transplant, and isolation of *Aspergillus* species in a nasal or sputum culture should prompt initial therapy with amphotericin, voriconazole, or caspofungin.

TABLE 60.5

GRAFT-VERSUS-HOST DISEASE, GRAFT FAILURE, AND DISEASE-FREE SURVIVAL FOR TRANSPLANTS WITH SIBLING-MATCHED OR UNRELATED DONORS

Degree of HLA match	GVHD grade III or IV (%)	Acute Chronic GVHD (%)	Graft failure (%)	DFS-AML or all in remission (%)	DFS-CML in chronic phase (%)	DFS-AML or all in relapse (%)	DFS-CML in transformation (%)	DFS-AA (%)
Sibling 6/6	7–15	30–35	<2	50–60	60–80	20	10–35	78–90
Related 5/6	25–30	50	7–9	40–60	60–80	20	10–35	25–40
Related 4/6	45–50	50	21	10–40	—	10	10–30	—
Haplo-identical	50–100	>50	20	10–40	—	10	10–30	—
Unrelated 6/6	45–50	55	6	45	40	20	20	30–40

GVHD, graft-versus-host disease; DFS, disease-free survival; AML, acute myelogenous leukemia; CML, chronic myelogenous leukemia; ALL, acute lymphoblastic leukemia; AA, aplastic anemia.

- Viral pneumonia is rare early after transplant; the most common etiologic agent when this does occur is herpes simplex.

HEART FAILURE

- Heart failure may result from volume overload or impairment of left ventricular function from sepsis or toxicity from pretransplant conditioning regimen drugs such as cyclophosphamide, ifosfamide, and/or anthracyclines. The end result is loss of voltage, heart failure, and/or pericardial effusion. Therapy is usually supportive or aimed to reverse ventricular decompensation as described elsewhere without a reason to alter therapy.

KIDNEY FAILURE

- Renal insufficiency is usually a multifactorial process whose cause includes the underlying disease—for example, cast nephropathy in myeloma, a prerenal decrease in glomerular filtration, intrinsic renal dysfunction, or postrenal obstruction. The most common reason for renal insufficiency early in the posttransplant period is drug-related, especially with use of aminoglycosides, cyclosporine, and amphotericin. Postkidney transplant renal failure may result from hemorrhagic cystitis with ureteral or urethral obstruction due to blood clots, retroperitoneal hemorrhage, urate nephropathy, or drugs that undergo intratubular crystallization and obstruction such as acyclovir, ciprofloxacin, and triamterene.

GRAFT FAILURE (ENGRAFTMENT)

- Generally, graft failure is defined as a neutrophil count $\leq 0.5 \times 10^9$ cells/L by day 28. Causes of graft failure include too few normal hematopoietic cells, damage to the bone marrow microenvironment, immune-mediated graft rejection, or drug- or virus-related immunosuppression.

TABLE 60.6

INCIDENCE OF GRADES III–IV ACUTE GRAFT-VERSUS-HOST DISEASE IN CHRONIC MYELOGENOUS LEUKEMIA ACCORDING TO THE NUMBER OF MISMATCHED CLASS I AND CLASS II ALLELES

	0 Class I (%)	1 Class I (%)	≥2 Class I (%)	Total (%)
0 Class II	32	29	36	32
1 Class II	45	31	55	45
≥2 Class II	67	67	86	74
Total	34	30	44	35

Note: There were 467 chronic myelogenous leukemia unrelated donor–recipient pairs.

- The minimal number of bone marrow or blood cells needed for sustained engraftment is unknown. There are several reasons for this:
  - It is not known what hematopoietic cells are responsible for sustained engraftment.
  - Different hematopoietic cells may operate under different circumstances and in different persons.
  - After autotransplants, there is no need for sustained engraftment in the context of autologous bone marrow recovery.
  - There is no validated method to identify the hematopoietic cell or cells responsible for sustained engraftment.
- Because of these limitations, surrogate markers are used to assess the hematopoiesis-restoring functionality of grafts. Most commonly used are CD34 and mononuclear cells.

ACUTE GRAFT-VERSUS-HOST DISEASE

- The principle manifestations of acute GVHD are rash, diarrhea, and jaundice, present individually or in combination. Acute GVHD is an allogeneic response mediated by donor

TABLE 60.7

GRADING OF ACUTE GRAFT-VERSUS-HOST DISEASE

Organ	Grade	Severity of individual organ involvement description
Skin	+1	A maculopapular eruption involving <25% of the body surface
	+2	A maculopapular eruption involving 25%–50% of the body surface
	+3	Generalized erythroderma
	+4	Generalized erythroderma with bullous formation and often with desquamation
Liver	+1	Moderate increase of AST (150–750 IU) and bilirubin (2.0–3.0 mg/dL)
	+2	Bilirubin rise (3.1–6.0 mg/dL) with or without an increase in AST
	+3	Bilirubin rise (6.1–15 mg/dL) with or without an increase in AST
	+4	Bilirubin rise (>15 mg/dL) with or without an increase in AST
Gut		Diarrhea, nausea, and vomiting graded +1 to +4 in severity. The severity of gut involvement is assigned to the most severe involvement noted.
	+1	Diarrhea >500 mL/d
	+2	Diarrhea >1,000 mL/d
	+3	Diarrhea >1,500 mL/d
	+4	Diarrhea >2,000 mL/d or severe abdominal pain with or without ileus

AST, aspartate transaminase.

TABLE 60.8

OVERALL GRADE OF GRAFT-VERSUS-HOST DISEASE[a]

Grade	Skin	Gut		Liver	ECOG performance
I	+1 to +2	0		0	0
II	+1 to +3	+1 to +2	and/or	+1 to +2	0 to 1
III	+2 to +4	+2 to +4	and/or	+2 to +4	2 to 3
IV	+2 to +4	+2 to +4	and/or	+2 to +4	3 to 4

ECOG, Eastern Cooperative Oncology Group.
[a]If no skin disease, the overall grade is the higher single organ grade.
Adapted from Glucksberg H, Storb R, Fefer A, et al. Clinical manifestations of graft versus host disease in human recipients of marrow from HL-A-matched sibling donors. *Transplantation.* 1974;18:295–304.

T cells, which recognizes recipient tissues as foreign. The incidence and severity of acute GVHD increase with increasing recipient age and human leukocyte antigen (HLA) and non-HLA disparity between the recipient and donor (Tables 60.5 and 60.6).

• Skin involvement in acute GVHD results in a maculopapular, erythematous rash, often beginning on the palms and soles and which may become systemic. In severe cases, acute GVHD with skin involvement may be pruritic with bullae. The skin involvement in acute GVHD may be precipitated by exposure to sunlight and/or drugs. Histologically, one can see the dermal-epidermal border disrupted by vacuolar degeneration of epithelial cells, dyskaryotic bodies, acantholysis (i.e., separation of cell–cell contact), epidermolysis (separation of the epidermal and dermal layers), and lymphocytic infiltration. These clinical and histologic findings are not unique to acute GVHD and may occur from drug allergy or the effects of the high-dose chemotherapy and radiation used in the pretransplant conditioning regimen.

• Gastrointestinal involvement with acute GVHD results in diarrhea, often accompanied by cramping abdominal pain. In severe cases, the diarrhea may be bloody or associated with a paralytic ileus. Histologically, lymphocytes and apoptotic cells are present, and intestinal crypts are lost, which leads to epithelial denudation. Evaluation of gastrointestinal tract signs and symptoms should include stool cultures for bacteria, fungi, and viruses, especially CMV. Sigmoidoscopy with biopsy may be helpful if the diagnosis is in doubt and platelet levels are sufficient. Acute GVHD with hepatic involvement presents as jaundice and an elevated alkaline phosphatase with or without elevated transaminases. The differential diagnosis includes VOD or infections with CMV or *Candida* spp. and may require a transjugular liver biopsy for accurate diagnosis. In acute GVHD, the liver biopsy may show T-cell infiltration of the portal triad, with apoptosis of epithelial cells lining the biliary tree.

• Acute GVHD and infections from immunosuppression are major causes of early death after allotransplant. Consequently, acute GVHD prophylaxis is needed for all allotransplant recipients.

• Clinical staging of acute GVHD considers individual tissue/organ involvement scores, which are combined for an overall grade (Tables 60.7 and 60.8). Grade 1 acute GVHD is not clinically important and requires no specific therapy. Grades 2 through 4 acute GVHD are typically treated with corticosteroids such as methylprednisolone, 1 to 2 mg/kg/day, with or without cyclosporine. Acute GVHD unresponsive to this approach has a poor prognosis.

CHAPTER 61 ■ THE OBSTETRIC PATIENT: GENERAL

- Review is focused mainly on the most life-threatening pathophysiologic processes (Tables 61.1 and 61.2):
  - Thrombosis and thromboembolism
  - Hypertensive disease of pregnancy
  - Hemorrhage
  - Amniotic fluid embolism
  - Peripartum cardiomyopathy
  - Pulmonary edema

PHYSIOLOGIC CHANGES ASSOCIATED WITH PREGNANCY

Body Constitution

- Optimal weight gain in pregnancy is currently a matter of debate
  - Generally, weight gain of 6 kg attributed to fetus, placenta, and uterus
  - Remainder attributed to increase in maternal blood, interstitial fluid volume, and fat
  - Gestational weight gain of more than 12 kg in women of normal prepregnant weight is related to the lowest risk for complications during delivery

- Women who exceed 18 kg of weight gain during pregnancy are considered at greater risk for maternal (preeclampsia, gestational diabetes) and fetal (increased incidence of operative delivery) complications

Metabolism and Respiration

- Key physiologic changes of respiration in pregnancy are:
  - Increased minute ventilation—caused by increased respiratory center sensitivity and drive
  - Compensated respiratory alkalosis
  - Low expiratory reserve volume
    - Vital capacity and measures of forced expiration are well preserved
  - Women with severe lung diseases tolerate pregnancy well
    - Except for those with pulmonary hypertension or chronic respiratory insufficiency from parenchymal or neuromuscular disease
  - Lung volumes measured in pregnant women and compared to nonpregnant women or those in the postpartum state
    - Well preserved in the majority of cases
    - Residual volume tends to decrease slightly, which leads to a small increase or stability of the vital capacity

TABLE 61.1

DIRECT MATERNAL DEATHS, 2000–2002[a]

Cause of death	1985–87	1988–90	1991–93	1994–96	1997–99	2000–02
Thrombosis and thromboembolism	32	33	35	48	35	30
Hypertensive disease of pregnancy	27	27	20	20	15	14
Hemorrhage	10	22	15	12	7	17
Amniotic fluid embolism	9	11	10	17	8	5
Deaths in early pregnancy: Total	22	24	18	15	17	15
Ectopic	16	15	8	12	13	11
Spontaneous miscarriage	5	6	3	2	2	1
Legal termination	1	3	5	1	2	3
Other	0	0	2	0	0	0
Genital tract sepsis	6[b]	7[b]	9[b]	14[c]	14[c]	11[c]
Other direct total	27	17	14	7	7	8
Genital tract trauma	6	3	4	5	2	1
Fatty liver	6	5	2	2	4	3
Other	15	9	8	0	1	4
Anaesthetic	6	4	8	1	3	6
Total number of deaths	139	145	128	134	106	106

[a]Deaths reported to the Enquiry only and excluding other deaths identified by ONS.
[b]Excluding early pregnancy deaths due to sepsis.
[c]Including early pregnancy deaths due to sepsis.
From Confidential Enquiry into Maternal and Child Health (CEMACH), Chiltern Court (Lower ground floor), 188 Baker Street, London. Publication 2004: Why Mothers Die 2000–2002.

TABLE 61.2

INDIRECT MATERNAL DEATHS, 2000–2002[a]

Causes of indirect deaths	1985–87	1988–90	1991–93	1994–96	1997–99	2000–02
Cardiac	22	18	37	39	35	44
Psychiatric	N/A	N/A	N/A	9	15	16
Other indirect	62	75	63	86	75	90
Indirect malignancies	N/A	N/A	N/A	N/A	11	5
Total number of indirect deaths	84	93	100	134	136	155

N/A, not available.
[a]Deaths reported to the Enquiry only and excluding other deaths identified by ONS. From Confidential Enquiry into Maternal and Child Health (CEMACH), Chiltern Court (Lower ground floor), 188 Baker Street, London. Publication 2004: Why Mothers Die 2000–2002.

- Most consistent change in static lung volumes with pregnancy is the reduction in the functional residual capacity (FRC) and expiratory reserve volume
  - As uterus enlarges, FRC decreases by 10% to 25% of the previous value, starting about the 12th week of pregnancy
  - Normal reduction in FRC is accentuated further in the supine position
  - Reduction in FRC is due to a decrease in chest wall compliance, up to 35% to 40%
- Lung compliance remains normal
- Expiratory muscle strength is in the low-normal range
- Decreased chest wall compliance is the result of the enlarging uterus increasing the abdominal pressure, leading to reduced FRC
- Diaphragm elevates about 4 cm, and the circumference of the lower rib cage increases about 5 cm
- Decreased FRC leads to an increased area of apposition of the diaphragm to the chest wall, which improves the coupling of the diaphragm and chest wall
  - Thus, increased tidal volume of pregnancy achieved without an increase in the respiratory excursions of the diaphragm
- Rib cage undergoes structural changes
  - Progressive relaxation of the ligamentous attachments of the ribs causes the subcostal angle of the rib cage to increase early in pregnancy
    - Persists for months into the postpartum period
    - Increased elasticity mediated by the polypeptide hormone, relaxin, increased during pregnancy and responsible for the softening of the cervix and relaxation of the pelvic ligaments

Changes in Arterial Blood Gases

- Hormonal changes of pregnancy lead to remarkable respiratory changes throughout its course (Table 61.3)
- Mean arterial PO_2 during pregnancy consistently >100 mm Hg
  - No alterations of dead space-to-tidal volume ratio (V_D/V_T) and shunt.

Cardiovascular System

- Most important hemodynamic change in the maternal circulation during pregnancy is an increase in the cardiac index of more than 30% (Tables 61.4 and 61.5)

Red Blood Cell, Plasma, and Blood Volume

- Increased plasma volume evident by sixth week of gestation
  - By the end of the first trimester of 15% above nonpregnant women
  - Subsequently a steep increase of this parameter until 28 to 30 weeks of gestation to a final volume at term of 55% above the nonpregnant level
- Red blood cell mass decreases during first 8 weeks of gestation
  - Increases to nearly 30% above the nonpregnant level at term
- Result in 45% increase of total blood volume and a reduction of the hemoglobin concentration and hematocrit to values of approximately 11.6 g/100 mL and 35.5%, respectively
- Estrogens, progesterone, and placental lactogen elevate aldosterone production either directly or indirectly, and are responsible for the increase of plasma volume during pregnancy
  - Hyperaldosteronism of pregnancy can result in retention up to 500 to 900 mEq of sodium and an increase of 6,000 to 8,000 mL of total body water, 70% of which is extracellular
  - Elevated red blood cell volume after 8 to 12 weeks can be attributed to increased serum erythropoietin
  - Erythropoiesis may also be stimulated by prolactin, progesterone, and placental lactogen

TABLE 61.3

BLOOD GAS ANALYSIS IN LATE PREGNANCY[a]

pH	7.44	HCO_3^- (mMol / L)	20
PaO_2 (mm Hg)	103	BE (mMol / L)	2.5
$PaCO_2$ (mm Hg)	30		

[a]Averages.
Data from Templeton A, Kelman GR. Maternal blood-gases, PAO_2–PaO_2, physiological shunt and V_D/V_T in normal pregnancy. *Br J Anaesth.* 1976;48:1001.

TABLE 61.4

HEMODYNAMIC CHANGES IN PREGNANCY

	% Change[a]		
	Pregnancy	Labor and delivery	Postpartum
Cardiac output	+30–50	+50–65[b]	+60–80
Heart rate	+10–15	+10–30[b]	−10–15
Stroke volume	+20–30	+40–70	+60–80
Blood volume	+20–80	—	+0–10
Plasma volume	+44–55	—	+0–30
Red cell volume	+20–30	—	−10
Oxygen consumption	+20	+40–100[b]	−10–15
Systemic vascular resistance	−10–25	—	—
Systemic blood pressure:			
Systolic	−5	+10–30[b]	+10
Diastolic	−10	+10–30[b]	+10
Pulmonary vascular resistance	−30	—	—
Pulmonary artery occlusion pressure (PAOP)	0	—	—
Colloid oncotic pressure (COP)	−10	—	—
COP—PAOP	−25	—	—

[a]Percentage change from nonpregnant state.
[b]Percentage change without regional anesthesia (local anesthetic).

Plasma Proteins and Colloid Osmotic Pressure

- Total serum protein concentration decreases from a nonpregnant value of 7.3 to 6.5 g/100 mL at term gestation
  - Change due primarily to a decline of the albumin concentration
    - Decreases from a nonpregnant level of 4.4 to 3.4 g/100 mL at term
    - Maternal colloid osmotic pressure decreases in parallel with the decline in serum albumin concentration from nonpregnant values of 25 to 26 to approximately 22 mm Hg at term

Aortocaval Compression

- Angiographic studies show that the aorta and inferior vena cava can be significantly compressed by the gravid uterus in the supine position
  - Complete obstruction of the inferior vena cava at the level of the bifurcation in 80% of patients in late pregnancy
  - Partial obstruction of the aorta at the level of the lumbar lordosis (L3–L5) demonstrated in patients between the 27th week of pregnancy and term gestation
  - Term pregnant woman, when placed in the lateral decubitus position, exhibits a right ventricular filling pressure (central venous pressure) similar to that of a nonpregnant woman
    - Suggests that venous return in this position is maintained by the collateral circulation despite partial caval obstruction
    - In plain supine position right atrial pressure falls substantially, demonstrating that collateral circulation cannot compensate for complete or nearly complete caval obstruction
    - Evident by 20 to 28 weeks of gestation
    - Results in a decrease of stroke volume and cardiac output of approximately 25%

- 20% reduction of uterine blood flow
- Reliably improved by a tilt to the left of at least 25 degrees
- Despite the reduction of cardiac output and stroke volume, a position change from lateral to supine can be associated with elevation of blood pressure
  - Results from an increase of systemic vascular resistance
    - Due to compression of the aorta by the gravid uterus
    - Enhanced sympathetic nervous system outflow

TABLE 61.5

NORMAL CARDIAC SYMPTOMS AND SIGNS IN PREGNANCY

Symptoms
Fatigue
Dyspnea
Decreased exercise tolerance
Light-headedness
Syncope

Signs
General:
  Distended neck veins
  Peripheral edema
  Hyperventilation
Heart:
  Loud S_1; increased split S_1
  Loud S_3
  Systolic ejection murmur
  Continuous murmurs (venous hum, mammary souffle)
Chest radiograph:
  Increased pulmonary vasculature
  Horizontal position of heart
Electrocardiogram:
  Left axis deviation
  Nonspecific ST-T–wave changes
  Mild sinus tachycardia

- In approximately 5% of women a substantial drop in blood pressure occurs ("supine hypotensive syndrome")
  - Associated with bradycardia (usually following a transient tachycardia) and maternal symptoms, low systemic perfusion such as of pallor and sweating, possibly followed by cardiocirculatory collapse
  - May be exacerbated by neuraxial block, the preferred method of providing anesthesia in pregnant women
- Based on the observations above, the intensivist should always consider in his or her emergency treatment plan the proper positioning of the pregnant patient and its influence on hemodynamics.

THROMBOSIS AND THROMBOEMBOLISM IN PREGNANCY

- Venous thromboembolism (VTE)
- Includes deep venous thrombosis (DVT) and pulmonary embolism, occurs in approximately 1 in 1,000 pregnancies
- Women five times more likely to develop VTE during pregnancy than during a nonpregnant state
  - Fatal pulmonary embolism (PE) remains a leading cause of maternal mortality in the Western world
  - Rate of PE in pregnancy is five time greater than that for nonpregnant women of the same age
    - Seen in about 1 in 100 deliveries
    - Risks even higher in the puerperium

Risk Factors and Predisposition to Venous Thrombosis

- Compared to nonpregnant females, pregnant women have a 10-fold risk of a thrombotic episode (Table 61.6)
- Pregnancy associated with increased clotting potential, decreased anticoagulant properties, and decreased fibrinolysis
  - Accompanied by two to three times increased concentration of fibrinogen
  - 20% to 1,000% increase in factors VII, VIII, IX, X, and XII, all of which peak at term
  - Levels of von Willebrand factor (vWf) increase up to 400% by term
  - Free protein S levels decline significantly (up to 55%) during pregnancy due to increased circulating levels of carrier molecular, complement four binding proteins

TABLE 61.6

RISK FACTORS FOR VENOUS THROMBOEMBOLISM (VTE) DURING PREGNANCY

Cesarean delivery
History of prior VTE
Family history of VTE
Inherited or acquired thrombophilia
Obesity
Older maternal age
Higher parity
Prolonged immobilization

- Thus pregnancy associated with increase in resistance to activated protein C
- Levels of plasminogen activation inhibitor-1 increase three to four times during pregnancy
  - Plasma plasminogen activation inhibitor-2 values-- negligible before pregnancy--reach concentrations of 160 mg/L at delivery
- Pregnancy also associated with venous stasis in the lower extremities due to compression of the inferior vena cava and pelvic veins by the enlarging uterus and hormone-mediated increases in deep vein capacitance secondary to increased circulating levels of estrogen and local production of prostacyclin and nitric oxide
- Important hereditary risk factors that can increase DVT risk are:
  - Antithrombin III deficiency
  - Protein S and C deficiency
  - G1691A mutation of the factor V gene
  - G20210A mutation of the factor II gene

Diagnosis of VTE During Pregnancy

- In pregnant women presenting with:
  - Lower extremity edema
  - Back pain
  - And/or chest pain
- Prevalence of VTE is less than in the general population because of the high frequency of these complaints in the pregnant woman
  - D-dimer assays--used to exclude VTE in healthy nonpregnant individuals--usually positive late in pregnancy
  - Radiologic studies not been validated in pregnancy
    - Potential risks to the fetus, particularly in terms of ionizing radiation exposure, need to be considered
  - Compression ultrasonography (CUS) of the proximal veins has been recommended as the initial test for suspected DVT during pregnancy
    - When results equivocal or an iliac vein thrombosis is suspected, magnetic resonance venography (MRV) can be used
- Approach to the diagnosis of PE is similar in the pregnant and nonpregnant
  - Ventilation/perfusion (V/Q) scanning confers relatively low radiation exposure to the fetus, a risk less than that of missing a diagnosis of PE in the mother
  - When V/Q study is indeterminate in a pregnant woman without demonstrated lower extremity thrombosis, it is usually followed by angiography.
    - Brachial approach carries less radiation exposure to the fetus than spiral CT

Prevention of Thrombosis During Pregnancy

- Optimal anticoagulation regimen not established
  - Low-molecular-weight heparins (LMWHs) the anticoagulant of choice
    - They do not cross the placenta (like unfractionated heparin [UFH])
    - Have better bioavailability

- Carry less risk of osteoporosis and heparin-induced thrombocytopenia than UFH
  - LMWHs safe alternatives to UFH as anticoagulants during pregnancy
- Recent practice trend to switch patients to the longer-acting, subcutaneous UFH a few weeks before delivery to allow use activated partial thromboplastin time as a diagnostic test to assess anticoagulation pre- and postlabor
- VTE prophylaxis with elastic compression stockings may be used for entire pregnancy
  - Appropriate for in-hospital patients at increased risk of VTE, and may be combined with the use of LMWH
- Vena cava filter placement a potentially important but poorly evaluated therapeutic modality in the prevention of pulmonary emboli
  - Randomized trials to establish the appropriate role of vena cava filters in the treatment of venous thromboembolic disease are lacking

Thrombolytic Therapy for Pulmonary Embolism

- Indications for thrombolytic therapy for PE controversial
- Incidence of intracranial hemorrhage as high as 2% to 3% with systemic thrombolytic therapy
  - Fatality rates in patients with PE presenting in cardiogenic shock as high as 30%
    - Thrombolytic therapy should be considered in this circumstance, although evidence is limited
  - Approximately 10% of symptomatic pulmonary emboli are rapidly fatal
    - 2% of patients were first diagnosed with PE at autopsy
    - Of patients diagnosed with PE before death, 5% to 10% have shock at presentation
      - Associated with a mortality of 25% to 50%
    - Echocardiographic evidence of right ventricular dysfunction at presentation
      - Suggested as indication for thrombolytic therapy
      - Recent randomized trial failed to demonstrate a survival benefit with thrombolysis in patients with this finding.
      - Mortality rates with conventional therapy are conflicting.
        - Routine thrombolysis cannot be justified in all patients.

HEMORRHAGE

- Peripartum hemorrhage remains a significant cause of maternal and fetal morbidity and mortality.
  - In industrialized nations, massive obstetric hemorrhage ranks among the top three causes of maternal death despite modern improvements in obstetric practice and transfusion services.
- Peripartum hemorrhage includes a wide range of pathophysiologic events.
  - Antepartum bleeding occurs in nearly 4% of pregnant women.
    - Causes of serious antepartum bleeding are:
      - Abnormal implantation (placenta previa, accreta)

TABLE 61.7

MANAGEMENT OF SEVERE POSTPARTUM HEMORRHAGE

Conservative Management
General Measures
  Administration of supplemental oxygen
  Placement of adequate intravenous access lines
  Intravenous hydration
  Blood typing and cross-matching
  Placement of arterial line for repeated blood sampling
Pharmacologic Measures
  Oxytocin
  Methylergonovine
  15-Methyl prostaglandin F_2-α

Surgical Management
Vascular Ligation
  Uterine artery
  Hypogastric artery
  Ovarian artery
Hysterectomy
  Supracervical
  Total

- Placental abruption
- Uterine rupture
- Main reason for postpartum bleeding:
  - Uterine atony when myometrial contraction is inadequate
    - Blood flow perfusing the uterus at term is up to 600 mL/minute
- Patients with hemodynamic instability or massive hemorrhage require prompt resuscitative measures (Table 61.7):
  - Administration of supplemental oxygen
  - Placement of two large-bore intravenous (IV) lines
  - IV hydration
  - Blood typing and cross-matching for the replacement of packed red blood cells (PRBCs)
  - Delay in the correction of hypovolemia, diagnosis and treatment of impaired coagulation, and surgical control of bleeding are avoidable factors in most maternal mortality cases caused by hemorrhage.
  - If transfusion must be given before full cross-matching, type-specific uncross-matched blood can be used.
  - If placenta not delivered when hemorrhage begins, it must be removed
    - Placenta accreta diagnosed if placental cleavage plane indistinct
    - In this situation, the patient should be prepared by the intensivist or the anesthesiologist for probable urgent hysterectomy
    - Firm bimanual compression of uterus (with one hand in the posterior vaginal fornix and the other on the abdomen) can limit hemorrhage until help obtained
  - Hemorrhage after placental delivery:
    - Should prompt vigorous fundal massage while the patient is rapidly given 10 to 30 units of oxytocin in 1 L of intravenous crystalloids
      - Uterotonic agents such as oxytocin routinely used in management of uterine atony
      - If fundus does not become firm, uterine atony is the presumed (and most common) diagnosis

- While fundal massage continues
- Patient may be then given 0.2 mg of methylergonovine (Methergine) intramuscularly (IM), with dose repeated at 2- to 4-hour intervals if necessary
  - May cause undesirable adverse effects such as cramping, headache, and dizziness
  - Coexisting severe hypertension is an absolute contraindication to its use
- Injectable prostaglandins may also be used when oxytocin fails
- Prostaglandin E and prostaglandin F_2 stimulate myometrial contractions
  - Have been used IM or IV for refractory hemorrhage due to uterine atony
  - Carboprost (Hemabate), 15-methyl prostaglandin F_2-α, may be administered IM or intramyometrially in dose of 250 μg every 15 to 90 minutes, to a maximum dose of 2 mg
    - 68% of patients respond to a single carboprost injection; 86% respond to a second dose
    - Oxygen desaturation has been reported with the use of carboprost, so patients should be monitored by pulse oximetry
- Use of a hydrostatic balloon has been advocated as an alternative to uterine packing for controlling hemorrhage due to uterine atony
  - Inflated Rusch balloon can conform to the contour of the uterine cavity and provides an effective tamponade
  - Life-threatening hemorrhage can also be treated by arterial embolization by interventional radiology
  - Finally, in cases of continuing hemorrhage, surgical techniques can be used to avoid a hysterectomy, such as bilateral uterine artery ligation or internal iliac artery ligation

AMNIOTIC FLUID EMBOLISM (AFE)

- Entry of amniotic fluid into the maternal circulation recognized in 1926
- True incidence of AFE not known, estimated to be between 1 in 8,000 and 1 in 80,000 pregnancies

Clinical Presentation

- Classic presentation of amniotic fluid embolism is described as a sudden, profound, and unexpected cardiovascular collapse followed, in many cases, by irreversible shock and death
  - Only known predisposing factor to this life-threatening complication is multiparity, which accounts for 88% of the cases
  - A smaller percentage of cases (51%) had respiratory-related presenting symptom
  - Hypotension is present in 27% of surviving cases
  - Coagulopathy comprising 12%
  - Seizures 10%
  - Fetal bradycardia (17%) and hypotension (13%) the next most common presenting features (Table 61.8)

TABLE 61.8

CLINICAL PRESENTATION OF AMNIOTIC FLUID EMBOLISM

Acute cardiorespiratory collapse
Acute respiratory distress
Hypotension
Hemorrhage/coagulopathy
Seizures
Fetal distress

Etiology and Pathophysiology

- Squamous cells can appear in the pulmonary blood of heterogenous populations of both pregnant and nonpregnant patients who have undergone pulmonary artery (PA) catheterization
  - Presence of these cells probably the result of contamination by epithelial cells derived from the cutaneous entry site of the PA catheter
  - Isolated finding of squamous cells in the pulmonary circulation of pregnant patients, with or without coexisting thrombotic pulmonary embolism, seen as a contaminant and not indicative of maternal exposure to amniotic fluid
- Amniotic fluid could act as a direct myocardial depressant
  - *In vitro* observation document that amniotic fluid decreases myometrial contractility
  - Humoral factors, including proteolytic enzymes, histamine, serotonin, prostaglandins, and leukotrienes, may contribute to the hemodynamic changes and consumptive coagulopathy associated with AFE
  - Pathophysiologic mechanism similar to distributive or anaphylactic shock

Diagnosis and Management

- AFE syndrome a diagnosis of exclusion (Table 61.9)
- Treatment is essentially supportive
  - Hemodynamic instability treated with optimization of preload by rapid volume infusion

TABLE 61.9

DIFFERENTIAL DIAGNOSIS OF AMNIOTIC FLUID EMBOLUS: EXCLUSION CRITERIA

Thrombosis
Air embolus
Septic shock
Acute myocardial infarction
Peripartum cardiomyopathy
Anaphylaxis
Aspiration
Placental abruption
Transfusion reaction
Local anesthetic toxicity

- α-receptor agonist such as phenylephrine useful to maintain adequate aortic perfusion pressure (90 mm Hg systolic) while volume is infused
- Coagulopathy treated with aggressive administration of blood component therapy
- If maternal cardiopulmonary resuscitation (CPR) must be initiated, and the fetus is sufficiently mature and is undelivered at the time of the cardiac arrest, a perimortem cesarean section should be immediately instituted.

PERIPARTUM CARDIOMYOPATHY (PPCM)

- A rare disease of unknown cause that strikes women in the childbearing years and is associated with a high mortality rate

Definition

- PPCM defined by the development of left ventricular or biventricular failure in the last month of pregnancy or within 5 months of delivery in the absence of other identifiable cause
- In the United States can affect women of various ethnic backgrounds at any age
  - More common in women 30 years of age
- Strong association of PPCM with gestational hypertension and twin pregnancy
  - Raise level of suspicion for this condition in pregnant women who develop symptoms of congestive heart failure

Etiology and Diagnosis

- Possible causes proposed for PPCM
  - Myocarditis
  - Abnormal immune response to pregnancy
  - Maladaptive response to the hemodynamic stresses of pregnancy
  - Stress-activated cytokines
  - Prolonged tocolysis
- Diagnosis of PPCM requires the exclusion of more common causes of cardiomyopathy
  - Confirmed by standard echocardiographic assessment of left ventricle systolic dysfunction
  - Including depressed fractional shortening and ejection fraction documentation

Treatment and Prognosis

- Initiated using standard clinical protocols for heart failure
  - Angiotensin-converting enzyme inhibitors should be avoided prenatally
- Long-term clinical prognosis is usually defined within 6 months after delivery
  - Approximately half of 27 women studied had persistent left ventricular dysfunction beyond 6 months, with a cardiac mortality rate of 85% over 5 years
- As compared with the group in whom cardiac size returned to normal by the same time interval, with no mortality
  - Identification of the underlying cause of heart failure in the pregnant patient is important factor influencing long-term survival

CHAPTER 62 ■ CARDIAC DISEASE AND HYPERTENSIVE DISORDERS IN PREGNANCY

HYPERTENSIVE DISEASE OF PREGNANCY

Diagnosis

- Hypertensive disorders of pregnancy include:
  - Chronic hypertension
  - Preeclampsia/eclampsia
  - Preeclampsia superimposed on chronic hypertension
  - Gestational hypertension
- Preeclampsia is a pregnancy-specific, multisystem disorder that is characterized by the development of hypertension and proteinuria after 20 weeks of gestation (Table 62.1)
  - Complicates approximately 5% to 7% of pregnancies

- Incidence of 23.6 cases per 1,000 deliveries in the United States
- Diagnostic criteria for preeclampsia include:
  - New onset of elevated blood pressure and proteinuria after 20 weeks of gestation
  - Severe preeclampsia indicated by more substantial blood pressure elevations and a greater degree of proteinuria
    - Other features of severe preeclampsia include oliguria, cerebral or visual disturbances, and pulmonary edema or cyanosis (Tables 62.2 through 62.4)
- Chronic hypertension defined by elevated blood pressure that predates the pregnancy
  - Is documented before 20 weeks of gestation or is present 12 weeks after delivery

TABLE 62.1

RISK FACTORS FOR PREECLAMPSIA

Maternal	Fetal
• First pregnancy • New partners • Age younger than 18 y or older than 35 y • Chronic hypertension • Prior history of preeclampsia • Family history of preeclampsia • Pregestational diabetes • Obesity • Thrombophilias • Systemic erythematosus • Renal disease	• Multiple gestations • Molar pregnancies (can cause preeclampsia at <20 wk gestation) • Fetal hydrops • Triploidy

• Eclampsia, a severe complication of preeclampsia, is a new onset of seizures in a woman with preeclampsia

Therapy

• Initial therapeutic goals during labor are focused on preventing seizures and controlling hypertension.
  • Magnesium sulfate is the medication of choice to prevent eclamptic seizures for either preeclampsia or eclamptic seizures.
    • Shown to be superior to phenytoin (Dilantin) and diazepam (Valium) for the treatment of eclamptic seizures.

TABLE 62.2

PHYSICAL EXAMINATION OF SEVERELY PREECLAMPTIC PATIENT

- **Funduscopic**
  - Arteriolar spasm (focal or diffuse)
  - Retinal edema
  - Retinal hemorrhages (superficial and flame shaped, or deep and punctate)
  - Retinal exudates (hard or "cotton wool")
  - Papilledema
- **Cardiovascular**
  - Heart failure (rales, elevated jugular venous pressure, S_3) or aortic dissection
  - New or increased murmur of mitral regurgitation
  - Bruits
- **Neurologic**
  - Hypertensive encephalopathy: Disorientation
  - Depressed consciousness (Glasgow coma scale <13)
  - Focal deficits, generalized or focal seizures
- **Abdominal**
  - Palpation for liver tenderness or increase in size
- **Fetal**
  - Assessment of fetal well-being (fetal heart rate strip, biophysical profile)

• With systolic blood pressures of 160 to 180 mm Hg or higher, or diastolic blood pressures of 105 to 110 mm Hg should receive immediate antihypertensive therapy
  • Treatment goal is to lower systolic pressure to 140 to 150 mm Hg and diastolic pressure to 90 to 100 mm Hg
  • Hydralazine (Apresoline) and labetalol (Normodyne, Trandate) are the antihypertensive drugs most commonly used.
  • Nifedipine (Procardia) and sodium nitroprusside (Nitropress) are potential alternatives.
    ○ Use is associated with significant adverse effects and risk of overdose.
    ○ Similarly, labetalol should not be used in women with asthma or congestive heart failure.
    ○ Angiotensin-converting enzyme inhibitors are also contraindicated.
    ○ In women with preeclampsia, blood pressure usually normalizes within a few hours after delivery but may remain elevated for 2 to 4 weeks.

Care and Management of the Hypertensive Parturient

• Some with severe preeclampsia will require admission in the intensive care setting for invasive monitoring and close supervision.
  • Typical indications include:
    • Severe increase in blood pressure, with diastolic blood pressures >115 to 120 mm Hg or a systolic blood pressure >200 mm Hg refractory to initial antihypertensive therapy
    • Oliguria refractory to repeated fluid challenges
    • Eclamptic seizures
    • Respiratory insufficiency with pulmonary edema
• Initial physical examination should include a neurologic assessment, funduscopic examination, auscultation of the heart and lungs, and palpation of the abdomen (Tables 62.2 and 62.3)
• If magnesium sulphate is given, it should be continued for 24 hours following delivery or at least 24 hours after the last seizure.
  • Regular assessment of urine output, maternal reflexes, respiratory rate, and oxygen saturation is paramount while magnesium is infused.
  • Loading dose of 4 g should be given by infusion pump over 5 to 10 minutes, followed by a further infusion of 1 g/hour maintained for 24 hours after the last seizure.
  • Gradual antihypertensive therapy can be accomplished with a 25% reduction of mean arterial pressure within minutes to 2 hours, to 160/100 mm Hg (Table 62.5).

The Role of Arterial Lines, Central Venous Pressure Monitors, and Pulmonary Artery Catheters in Preeclamptic Patients

• Most severe preeclamptic patients have normal or hyperdynamic left ventricular (LV) function with normal pulmonary artery pressure.
  • Central venous pressure (CVP) monitoring is usually adequate to assess volume status and LV function.

TABLE 62.3

CLINICAL FEATURES OF PREECLAMPSIA

Symptoms	Headache	The headache that characterizes preeclampsia is typically frontal in location, throbbing in character, persistent, and not responsive to mild analgesia.
	Visual phenomena	The visual disturbances that characterize preeclampsia are presumed to be caused by cerebral vasospasm and are typically scintillations or scotomas. Longer-lasting visual field deficits and rarely transient blindness can result from edema, posterior reversible encephalopathic syndrome, and even infarction in the occipital region of the brain. Serous retinal detachments can also occur in preeclampsia and are related to retinal edema. Magnesium, which is commonly used to prevent seizures in preeclamptic women, can cause mild visual blurring or double vision but should not cause scotomas, scintillations, or visual loss.
	Epigastric pain	The epigastric or right upper quadrant discomfort that occurs in preeclampsia can be marked and may be out of proportion to the degree of liver enzyme abnormalities. It is believed to be caused by edema in the liver that stretches the hepatic capsule. In rare cases, it may be caused by hepatic infarction or rupture.
	Edema	Edema is present in more than 30% of normal pregnancies and is thus not a reliable sign of preeclampsia. Rapid weight gain (more than 1 pound per week in the third trimester) or edema in the hands or facial area (nondependent edema) is best viewed as a sign that should lead the clinician to evaluate the patient for other, more specific, evidence of preeclampsia.
Signs	Hypertension >140/90 mm Hg	Hypertension in preeclampsia is due to vasospasm and can be very labile. Ideally, blood pressure should be measured in the sitting position with a manual cuff, with the brachial artery at the level of the heart. There is a literature suggesting that some automated blood pressure cuffs may be less reliable in preeclampsia and that either a manual cuff or arterial line should be used to verify blood pressure in preeclamptic patients with severe hypertension. Although a rise in systolic/diastolic blood pressure of 30/15 mm Hg was once considered a criterion for diagnosing preeclampsia, it is now recognized that this definition lacks both sensitivity and specificity.
	Epigastric or right upper quadrant tenderness	Abdominal pain in preeclampsia is attributed to hepatic capsular stretching from edema. The degree of tenderness is often out of proportion to the degree of elevation of liver function tests. Epigastric tenderness is suggestive of severe preeclampsia and is associated with an increased risk of both maternal and fetal adverse outcomes.
	Hyperreflexia	Clonus is an important sign of preeclampsia but should be distinguished from the very brisk reflexes commonly seen in normal pregnancies.
	Retinal artery vasospasm on funduscopy	Retinal vasospasm, retinal edema (in the form of soft exudates), hemorrhage, and exudative retinal detachment are uncommon findings in preeclampsia. Papilledema is rare.

- Severely preeclamptic patients may develop cardiac failure, progressive and marked oliguria, or pulmonary edema.
  - In such cases, a pulmonary artery (PA) catheter may be helpful for proper diagnosis and treatment, because right and left ventricular pressures may not correlate.
    - The rather limited literature about their use in obstetric populations is questioned.
    - No clear consensus exists as to their role in the management of preeclampsia.
    - Risks—especially on labor and delivery units where the personnel have less experience in their placement and interpretation—seem to outweigh the evidence justifying their use.
    - An urgent bedside echocardiogram may guide care.
- An arterial catheter monitor may be indicated for protracted severe hypertension during therapy with potent antihypertensive agents.
- Most patients satisfying the criteria for intensive care unit admission should be monitored with central venous access and an arterial catheter.

FETAL MONITORING IN THE INTENSIVE CARE SETTING

- Electronic fetal monitoring (EFM) is used in the management of labor and delivery in nearly three of four pregnancies in the United States.
- Apparent contradiction between the widespread use of EFM and expert recommendations to limit its routine use indicates that a reassessment of this practice is warranted.
- Question of whether fetal monitoring is of any substantial use in the critically ill mother or the mother undergoing surgery.
- Continuous cardiotocography (CTG) during labor is associated with a reduction in neonatal seizures, but no significant differences in cerebral palsy, infant mortality, or other standard measures of neonatal well-being.
  - This monitoring technique was associated with an increase in cesarean sections and instrumental vaginal births.

TABLE 62.4

LABORATORY FEATURES OF PREECLAMPSIA

Complete blood count with elevated hemoglobin and/or thrombocytopenia	The "elevation of hemoglobin" seen with preeclampsia (which may manifest as a hemoglobin of 12 g/dL at 37 wk when it would be expected to be closer to 10 g/dL because of the physiologic dilutional anemia that is seen in pregnancy) is due to hemoconcentration. Much less commonly, hemoglobin may fall with preeclampsia due to a microangiopathic hemolytic anemia.
	Platelet consumption in preeclampsia can cause an increased mean platelet volume and thrombocytopenia and is an important manifestation of severe disease.
	In severe cases of preeclampsia or HELLP (a subset of preeclampsia), schistocytes (fragmented red cells) may be seen on peripheral smear and can lead to a mild drop in hemoglobin. Brisk hemolysis is rare, however, and should lead to the consideration of HUS or TTP.
Elevated serum creatinine	Typically serum creatinine is <0.8 mg/dL (70 μmol/L) in pregnancy and values greater than this are considered abnormal.
	Renal function impairment is caused by decreased renal blood flow and glomerular filtration rate secondary to swelling of intracapillary glomerular cells, fibrin deposition along the basement membranes, and afferent arteriolar spasm.
Elevated serum uric acid	Typically, serum uric acid is <5.0 mg/dL (280 μmol/L) in pregnancy. Uric acid is the most sensitive test for identifying preeclampsia, but it is still only elevated in approximately 80% of preeclampsia cases. Uric acid rises in this setting due to impaired excretion of uric acid in the renal tubules that is caused by preeclampsia-related changes in the renal microcirculation. Although an important sign of preeclampsia, the elevated uric acid level is distinct from an elevated creatinine, AST, or decreased platelet count in that the uric acid level is not generally believed to have any direct clinical consequences and should not be used as a marker of disease severity.
Elevated liver enzymes	Mild elevations of AST, typically <100 U/L, suggest hepatic involvement. Greater levels may be due to severe preeclampsia, HELLP syndrome, hepatic infarction, hepatic rupture, or superimposed acute fatty liver of pregnancy.
Proteinuria	Proteinuria is an essential diagnostic feature of preeclampsia. Urine dipsticks are routinely used to screen for proteinuria in asymptomatic patients. However, dipsticks lack the needed sensitivity and specificity to make them a reliable test for proteinuria in patients in whom the diagnosis of preeclampsia is suspected because of the presence of other features of this disease. When preeclampsia is suspected, a 24-hour urine test for proteinuria with creatinine and creatinine clearance should be obtained. Proteinuria is present if there is more than 300 mg of protein excreted over 24 hours. Total urinary creatinine should be measured to assess the adequacy of urine collection. The creatinine clearance can be used in conjunction with the serum creatinine as a measure of renal function.
	The use of a random spot urinary protein-to-creatinine ratio to diagnose proteinuria in pregnancy has had many advocates, but it remains unclear at this time whether this test can replace the 24-hour urine in pregnant patients with suspected preeclampsia.
DIC screen	Severe preeclampsia can rarely cause DIC, but it is almost always seen in association with thrombocytopenia. Checking INR, PTT, and fibrinogen degradation products is usually only done if the patient with preeclampsia has thrombocytopenia or is undergoing an invasive procedure.

AST, aspartate aminotransferase; DIC, dissemination intravascular coagulation; HUS, hemolytic uremic syndrome; INR, international normalized ratio; PTT, partial thromboplastin time; TTP, thrombotic thrombocytopenic purpura.

TABLE 62.5

ANTIHYPERTENSIVE THERAPY IN PREECLAMPSIA

- **Labetalol (Normodyne, Trandate)**
IV bolus, 20–40 mg IV. May repeat in 10 min. Usual effective dose is 50–200 mg, or continuous infusion of 2 mg/min (this regimen avoids reflex tachycardia).
- **Nitroglycerin**
Start at 10 μg/min (6 mL/h). Titrate by 10–20 μg/min to 400 μg/min until desired effect.
- **Hydralazine (Apresoline)**
Initial dose: 5 mg IV. Maintenance: 5–10 mg IV every 20–30 min.
- **Other Antihypertensive Options**
Nicardipine, nitroprusside, phentolamine, fenoldopam, diazoxide

- When considering the use of EFM, the intensivist should consider the effects of many sedative, hypnotic, or analgesic drugs routinely used in the critical care setting on fetal heart rate variability.
- No systematic studies have been performed concerning the value of CTG during general anesthesia for nonobstetric surgery.
- It is assumed that uneventful sedation and analgesia provide adequate oxygenation and circulatory stability without having any influence on the fetus.

PULMONARY EDEMA IN PREGNANCY

- Pulmonary edema is a rare but well-documented complication of tocolytic therapy in pregnant women.
- Incidence of pulmonary edema related to β-mimetic tocolysis is estimated to be 0.15%.

- Etiology of the pulmonary edema is unclear, but is likely multifactorial.
  - Both cardiogenic and noncardiogenic mechanisms have been proposed.
  - Possible cardiogenic causes include:
    - Fluid overload
    - Catecholamine-related myocardial necrosis
    - Cardiac failure secondary to reduced diastolic compliance
    - Down-regulation of β-receptors

Treatment

- Immediate recognition and appropriate therapy can ameliorate the course of respiratory insufficiency in patients who develop pulmonary edema during tocolytic treatment.
- Therapy involves discontinuing the medication, ensuring adequate ventilation and oxygenation, correcting fluid imbalance and hypotension, and maintaining adequate cardiac output.
  - Continuous assessment of the fetus' well-being is necessary.

Tocolytic Therapy

- The development of pulmonary edema during the course of β-adrenergic agonist treatment for preterm labor is an indication for discontinuing the treatment.
  - Either switching to a different type of labor-inhibiting drug or terminating all efforts to prevent preterm delivery
  - Magnesium sulfate, calcium channel blockers, or oxytocin antagonists are the most frequently used alternatives.

Ventilatory Support

- Mechanical ventilation principles are not different for the pregnant patient and are being standardized by evidence-based medicine and consensus conferences.

Fetal Considerations

- Fetal well-being must be interpreted within the context of maternal respiratory failure.
- Minimally, intermitted fetal monitoring is indicated.
- If refractory maternal hypoxemia and acidosis presents, and results in fetal distress, cesarean delivery to salvage the fetus should be considered.

CARDIAC DISEASE

Who is Most at Risk, and When is That Risk Greatest?

- Table 62.6 classifies the risk of various cardiac lesions in pregnancy.
- "Risk" for these patients refers to congestive heart failure, arrhythmias, stroke, and death.
  - About 13% of cardiac patients will suffer one of these outcomes in pregnancy.
  - The presence of pulmonary hypertension (PHTN) is always associated with increased risk.
    - Risk is commensurate to degree of severity of PHTN.
  - Other factors associated with an increased risk of cardiac complications in pregnancy include the following:

- **New York Heart Association (NYHA) functional class:** Perhaps most important predictor of pregnancy outcome
  - NYHA class I and II cardiac disease generally have a good prognosis during pregnancy.
  - NYHA class III and IV more likely to experience complications and may require special management at time of delivery.
- **Left-sided obstructive cardiac lesions:** Lesions such as aortic stenosis may result in difficulty accommodating the increased blood volume and cardiac output seen in pregnancy, and become increasingly symptomatic.
  - Regurgitant valvular lesions result in less difficulty in pregnancy.
    - Cardiac output (CO) in these cases may benefit from the decrease in systemic vascular resistance seen in pregnancy
- **Cyanosis**
- **LV systolic dysfunction**
- **Prior cardiac events or previous arrhythmia**
- Although pregnant women with cardiac disease may experience complications at any point during pregnancy, there are three periods of particular risk:
  - At the end of the second trimester when CO is increased to its peak
  - At time of labor and delivery when cardiac work may be increased dramatically by both pain and the autotransfusion of blood from the placenta and uterus with each contraction
  - During the first 72 hours following delivery when the uterine involution and resolution of pregnancy-related edema leads to mobilization of large amounts of fluid

General Management of Cardiac Patients during Pregnancy

- Management includes good preconception counseling to assess and inform the patient of the risks associated with a pregnancy.
  - No woman should be told that she "should never get pregnant."
  - But a clear discussion of the risk is essential
    - With severe PHTN or Eisenmenger syndrome, patient should be strongly cautioned against pursuing a pregnancy.
    - Women with congenital heart disease (CHD) need to be informed that they are at increased risk of giving birth to a child with CHD.
  - If she decides to pursue pregnancy after a clear discussion of risk:
    - Cardiac status must be clearly delineated and optimized.
    - Necessary investigations or interventions should be carried out prior to conception.
    - Regular visits with a medical specialist and an obstetrician trained in the care of high-risk pregnancies to watch for evidence of heart failure and arrhythmias are essential.
    - Consultation with an obstetric anesthesiologist prior to delivery is also prudent.
- Most cardiac medications can be used in pregnancy when indicated (Table 62.7).
  - Angiotensin-converting enzyme inhibitors, angiotensin receptor blockers, and warfarin are known or strongly suspected to be human teratogens.

TABLE 62.6

PERIPARTUM RISK OF VARIOUS CARDIAC LESIONS

Risk category	Lesion
Lower-risk lesion	Mitral valve prolapse
	Mitral valve prolapse with regurgitation
	Atrial septal defect
	Ventricular septal defect with normal pulmonary pressures
	Trace to mild valvular regurgitation
	NYHA class I
	History of SVT with recent good control
	Pacer
Intermediate-risk lesion	Stable ischemic heart disease
	Mild to moderate pulmonary hypertension
	Moderate to severe valvular insufficiency
	NYHA class II
	Cardiomyopathy with ejection fraction 30%–50%
	Poorly controlled SVT
High-risk lesion	Unstable ischemic heart disease
	Moderate to severe left ventricular obstruction (e.g., aortic <1.5 cm^2 or mitral valvular stenosis <2 cm^2, peak gradient lV outflow tract of >30 mm Hg)
	NYHA class III
	Cardiomyopathy with ejection fraction $<30\%$
	Dilated aortic root/Marfan/Ehlers-Danlos
	Moderate pulmonary hypertension
	History of ventricular tachycardia with or without AICD
	Mechanical prosthetic heart valve
	History of TIA or CVA
Highest-risk lesion	Pulmonary hypertension >80 mm Hg
	Eisenmenger syndrome
	NYHA class IV
	Cyanosis

AICD, automated implantable cardioverter-defibrillator; CVA, cerebrovascular accident; NYHA, New York Heart Association; SVT, supraventricular tachycardia; TIA, transient ischemic attack.
Items above can be used to calculate a risk index with 1 point being assigned for each and 0, 1, and >1 points being associated with a risk of some cardiac event during the entire pregnancy of 5%, 27%, and 75%, respectively. (Risk calculation adapted from Siu S, Sermer M, Colman JM, et al. Prospective multicenter study of pregnancy outcomes in women with heart disease. *Circulation.* 2001;104:515).

- Angiotensin-converting enzyme inhibitors/angiotensin receptor blockers: fetal anomalies, fetal loss, oligohydramnios, cranial ossification abnormalities, and neonatal renal failure
- Should not be used at any time in gestation
- Warfarin associated with a high risk of miscarriage and anomalies of the eyes, hands, neck, and central nervous system
- Amiodarone has had mixed data with respect to its safety in pregnancy, with some reports of congenital hypothyroidism, goiter, prematurity, hypotonia, and bradycardia.
- Studies
  - Ultrasound has a long history of safe use in pregnancy.
  - Radiation exposure associated with plain film radiographs, nuclear medicine scans, angiography, and computed tomography scans are all well below what is deemed acceptable during pregnancy.
  - Contrast agents appear to be well tolerated by the fetus.
  - Magnetic resonance imaging has not been associated with any ill effects in human pregnancies.
    - Fetal well-being is dependent on maternal well-being; more harm will generally be caused to a mother and

her fetus by withholding necessary investigations than by obtaining them.
- Mode of delivery should not generally be determined by medical concerns.
  - Need for cesarean deliveries is generally dictated by obstetric concerns.
  - Vaginal deliveries are generally viewed as the safest and best option for cardiac patients.
  - Keep neutral fluid balance over the course of their delivery period.
  - Monitors
    - Intra-arterial lines are advisable for cardiac lesions for which moment-to-moment monitoring of blood pressure might be desirable, such as severe aortic stenosis.
    - Pulmonary artery catheter in the laboring patient remains unclear.
- Bacterial endocarditis prophylaxis is no longer recommended by the American Heart Association for vaginal or cesarean deliveries.
  - Organisms associated with delivery unlikely to cause endocarditis.

TABLE 62.7

COMMONLY USED CARDIAC MEDICATIONS AND THEIR SAFETY IN PREGNANCY

	Use generally justifiable for this indication in pregnancy	Use justifiable in special circumstances for this indication in pregnancy	Use almost never justifiable for this indication in pregnancy
Arrhythmia	Digoxin β-Blockers (all probably safe but most avoid propranolol and atenolol, which may cause intrauterine growth restriction) Calcium channel blockers, especially verapamil and diltiazem (less known about amlodipine) Adenosine Quinidine Procainamide Lidocaine	Amiodarone Disopyramide, mexiletine, and flecainide (less is known about these agents in pregnancy but there is no evidence at this point of human teratogenesis; they should generally be considered second-line agents in pregnancy)	
Ischemia	Nitrates Low-dose (<100 mg) ASA β-Blockers Heparin (unfractionated or low molecular weight) Tissue plasminogen activator Streptokinase	HMG-coA reductase inhibitors ("statins") have concerning animal pregnancy data, but very limited reported human experiences thus far have been encouraging; should only be used in pregnancy when short-term benefits are clear Abciximab (and other glycoprotein IIb/IIIa inhibitors) dipyridamole, ticlopidine, and clopidogrel lack published human data; they are probably safe but should only be used in pregnancy when short-term benefits are clear	Warfarin
Heart failure	Furosemide Digoxin Hydralazine β-Blockers Dopamine Dobutamine	Nitroprusside (fetal cyanide toxicity possible at high doses)	ACE inhibitors Angiotensin II receptor blockers
Hypertension	Labetalol β-Blockers Nifedipine Hydralazine Methyldopa	Thiazide diuretics (in this category for the treatment of hypertension because of effects of blood volume in pregnancy) Clonidine, prazosin, verapamil, diltiazem, and amlodipine (in this category for the treatment of hypertension because of limited data on safety and the availability of many good alternatives with more data) Nitroprusside (fetal cyanide toxicity possible at high doses)	ACE inhibitors Angiotensin II receptor blockers

ASA, acetylsalicylic acid; ACE, angiotensin-converting enzyme.

Specific Lesions

Mitral Stenosis

- Rheumatic heart disease a common form of heart disease in pregnancy despite its declining incidence in the developed world.
- Mitral stenosis accounts for approximately 90% of the rheumatic valvular lesions in pregnancy.
- Often presents for the first time in pregnancy
- Risk factors include atrial fibrillation, pulmonary edema, and thromboembolic stroke.

- Most patients will experience some worsening of symptoms during pregnancy.
- Avoidance of tachycardia, increased PA pressure, decreased systemic vascular resistance, and increased central blood volume are essential to patient management.
- Many patients will benefit from β-blockade to improve filling time during pregnancy.
- Echocardiograms in these patients should be done once every trimester and with any change in status in these patients.

- Pulmonary edema should be treated with diuretics and β-blockade.
- Atrial fibrillation should be treated promptly to decrease tachycardia and the associated risk of a low cardiac output state or degeneration into more malignant dysrhythmias.
  - Rate control, full anticoagulation with heparin, and consideration of either medical or electrical cardioversion remain the core management principles.
- For labor, vaginal delivery or cesarean, excellent pain control is important and is best achieved with early establishment of regional anesthesia.

Aortic Stenosis

- Aortic stenosis (AS) is a valvular lesion rarely seen during pregnancy
  - Can be of rheumatic or congenital origin
  - Mild to moderate AS generally well tolerated in pregnancy.
  - Severe AS (defined as <1.0 cm^2) carries a significant fetal and maternal risk.
    - Rate of complication varies from 10% to 31%.
    - Symptomatic aortic stenosis should be repaired prior to pregnancy
  - Monitoring
    - Arterial lines are strongly advised.
    - PAC, while not proven, may be of benefit.
    - With severe AS, regional anesthesia has been avoided because of the resulting local anesthetic–induced sympathectomy, which can lead to bradycardia and decreased venous return.
      - Good results have been obtained in patients with severe AS managed during labor with a carefully titrated epidural anesthetic.

Mitral and Aortic Insufficiency

- Mitral insufficiency is the second most common valvular lesion seen in pregnancy.
  - Typically due to rheumatic heart disease
- Aortic insufficiency is less common.
  - May be due to rheumatic, infectious, or rheumatologic conditions
- When found in isolation, these lesions do well in pregnancy unless there is associated ventricular decompensation.
  - Treatments when symptomatic include diuretics, digoxin, or calcium channel blockers.
  - Angiotensin receptor blockers should not be used despite the benefits of afterload reduction.
  - Increases in systemic vascular resistance, decreased heart rate, atrial arrhythmias, and myocardial depressants may be poorly tolerated.
  - Most important peripartum issue for these patients is early regional anesthesia to prevent pain-associated increases in systemic vascular resistance.

Congenital Heart Disease

- Approximately 25% of heart disease in pregnancy is congenital.
- Categorized as left-to-right shunt, right-to-left shunt, and aortic lesions.
  - **Left-to-right Shunt**

- Most common CHD lesions are atrial septal defects (ASDs) and ventricular septal defects (VSDs), usually well tolerated in pregnancy.
- Risk of cardiac complications greatest in large defects.
  - CHF (due to increased blood volume in pregnancy leading to cardiac decompensation), atrial arrhythmias, shunt reversal (occurring due to sudden systemic hypotension), and thromboembolic disease are all possible complications seen with ASD and VSD in pregnancy.
- When symptomatic septal defects present in pregnancy principles of management include:
  - Acetylsalicylic acid (ASA) 81 mg daily to prevent thromboembolism
  - Diuretics and digoxin to treat heart failure
  - Avoidance of hypotension with epidural administration or postpartum blood loss
  - Rapid rate control with any arrhythmia
- **Right-to-left Shunt and Pulmonary Hypertension**
  - High-risk congenital disorders in pregnancy include right-to-left shunts.
    - Eisenmenger syndrome (any congenital heart lesion with a bidirectional or right-to-left shunt at the atrial, ventricular, or aortic level)
    - Any other lesions associated with significant PHTN
    - Women with uncorrected cyanotic heart disease have increased spontaneous abortion rates, pulmonary embolization, congestive heart failure, and CHDs in the fetus
    - High hematocrit (≥65%) not only an indication of the severity of the cardiac disease
      - Has a poorer prognosis secondary to complications from hyperviscosity (decreased cardiac output, organ hypoperfusion, and thrombosis)
  - With Eisenmenger syndrome, reveals maternal mortality rates of 25% to 52%
    - Fetal loss as high as 44%
    - If they continue with the pregnancy, they may warrant hospitalization from 20 weeks onward.
    - Oxygen should be administered for dyspnea, and prophylactic heparin should be considered throughout pregnancy and for 6 weeks postpartum.
    - Mode of delivery should be determined on the basis of obstetric indications.
    - PAC can carry additional risks in patients with significant PHTN.
      - Should probably be avoided in these patients
    - Active efforts should be made to avoid sudden decreases in systemic vascular resistance, blood volume, and venous return. Increased pulmonary vascular resistance promotes right-to-left shunting.
      - Hypercapnia and hypoxia are to be avoided.
    - Best peripartum anesthesia not clear.
      - If regional anesthesia is used, care must be taken to prevent precipitous drops in venous return.
      - With PHTN and/or Eisenmenger syndrome, observe patients for 72 hours postpartum in a cardiac setting.
        - Many maternal deaths associated with these conditions occur during this period.

Aortic Disease

- Coarctation of the aorta and aortic manifestations of Marfan syndrome pose significant problems in pregnancy.

- Physiologic changes during pregnancy may promote aortic dissection in either of these conditions.
- Patients with coarctation of the aorta may also suffer from worsening hypertension or congestive heart failure in pregnancy.
- Marfan syndrome is often associated with aortic dilation, aortic valve regurgitation, and mitral valve disease.
  - Aortic dissection occurs in about 10% of patients with Marfan syndrome who become pregnant.
    - Most likely to occur if the aortic root measures beyond 4.5 cm in diameter
    - Ideally, the aorta is repaired prior to pregnancy.
    - Otherwise, serial echocardiography during pregnancy to watch for worsening dilation
    - Activity of patients with significant aortic dilation in pregnancy should be limited.
    - Patients should be prescribed β-blockers to decrease shear stresses on the vessel wall.
    - It is common practice for women with aortic roots dilated beyond 4.0 cm to deliver by cesarean to avoid additional stressors on the aorta associated with the pain and pushing of a vaginal delivery
    - The majority of dissections in these patients occur prior to labor's onset.
- Aortic coarctation in pregnancy associated with
  - Increased risk of worsening hypertension
  - Less commonly, congestive heart failure or preeclampsia
  - Much less likely to be associated with aortic dissection than Marfan syndrome
    - However, dissection can and does occur.
  - Keep blood pressure <160/100 mm Hg but not below 120/70 mm Hg
    - There may be a significant gradient between blood pressure measurement in the arm and the estimated blood pressure of the placenta circulation that is distal to the aortic narrowing.
    - β-blockers are the preferred antihypertensives.
  - Can undergo a vaginal delivery but should have a limited second stage (i.e., prolonged pushing should be avoided by the use of vacuum extractor or forceps)

Tetralogy of Fallot

- The most common cyanotic congenital heart disease
  - Consists of
    - Ventricular septal defect
    - Overriding aorta
    - Infundibular pulmonary stenosis
    - Secondary right ventricular hypertrophy
  - Uncorrected patients have significant complications in pregnancy.
    - Biventricular failure
    - Arrhythmias
    - Stroke
    - Risk of shunt reversal with worsening cyanosis
  - Preconception surgical repair should be undertaken if at all possible.
    - Those who proceed with a pregnancy unrepaired should be managed like patients with Eisenmenger syndrome.
    - Patients who have had surgical repair and have a good functional status generally tolerate pregnancy well.

- Main risks are right-sided heart failure and arrhythmias.
  - Volume status should be watched throughout pregnancy.
  - Complaints of palpitations or syncope are investigated with an event monitor.
  - Delivery should include cardiac monitoring.

Other Repaired Congenital Heart Conditions

- An increasing number of women with congenital heart problems that were repaired in childhood are reaching adulthood and undergoing pregnancy.
- Generally, course in pregnancy is predictable by the parameters outlined earlier.
- The majority have a good pregnancy outcome for both themselves and their infants if they enter the pregnancy with a good functional status.

Peripartum Cardiomyopathy (PPCM)

- Defined by National Heart, Lung, and Blood Institute as the new onset of systolic dysfunction occurring in the absence of other plausible causes anytime between the final month of pregnancy up to 5 months postpartum
- Incidence between 1 in 3,000 and 1 in 15,000 pregnancies
- May be increasing
- Most commonly found in
  - Women who have twins
  - Women who have preeclampsia/eclampsia
  - Older multiparous women
  - Not clear if race is an independent risk factor for PPCM
    - Clear that African American women are more likely to die of PPCM than Caucasian women when it does occur
    - Generally, one-third of these patients have complete resolution in the year following delivery.
      - One-third are left with residual cardiac dysfunction.
      - One-third have progressive cardiac decompensation.
- Mortality rate is between 9% and 56%.
  - Highest in patient subset with persistent cardiomegaly beyond 6 months
  - May be due to end-stage heart failure, arrhythmia, or thromboembolism
- Pathologic findings include
  - Four-chamber enlargement with normal coronary arteries and valves
  - Light microscopic findings include myocardial hypertrophy and fibrosis with scattered mononuclear infiltrates.
- Clinical signs include symptoms of ventricular failure with possible associated arrhythmias and/or pulmonary emboli.
- Treatment
  - Bed rest
  - Sodium restriction
  - Diuresis
  - Preload/afterload reduction with a calcium channel blocker and hydralazine while pregnant and an angiotensin-converting enzyme inhibitor postpartum.
  - With ejection fraction <35%, consider anticoagulation with low-molecular-weight heparin while pregnant, and warfarin postpartum.
  - Antidysrhythmics should be utilized in a manner similar to what would be done for any patient with an idiopathic cardiomyopathy.
- Evidence that peripartum cardiomyopathy may recur or worsen with subsequent pregnancies.

Hypertrophic Cardiomyopathy

- During pregnancy, course of hypertrophic cardiomyopathy (HCM) variable:
  - While the normal increase of blood volume is beneficial, the decrease in systemic vascular resistance and the increase in heart rate may be detrimental.
  - Complications are not common but include
    - Congestive heart failure
    - Chest pain
    - Supraventricular tachycardias, ventricular tachycardia, and sudden death
    - Can occur at any point in pregnancy or labor as a result of stress, pain, and increased circulating catecholamines
      - Immediate postpartum period can increase risk due to blood loss and decrease in systemic vascular resistance
  - Atrial fibrillation and supraventricular tachycardias are a common feature of this cardiac anomaly.
    - Cardioselective β-blockers and verapamil are usually administered.
    - Tocolytics, sympathomimetic agents, and digoxin should be avoided in these patients, as they may increase the risk of arrhythmia.
  - Peripartum period should include cardiac monitoring and use of forceps or vacuum extractor to minimize pushing.
  - Regional anesthesia should be done incrementally.
    - With agents that minimize the risk of a sudden drop in preload

Ischemic Heart Disease in Pregnancy

- Myocardial infarction (MI) in pregnancy is uncommon.
  - Incidence estimated to be between 1 in 10,000 and 1 in 35,700
  - Does appear to be increasing
- Risk factors include
  - Advancing age
  - Preeclampsia
  - Multiparity
  - Chronic hypertension
  - Diabetes
- MI associated with pregnancy occurs at any time during gestation.
  - 38% occurred antepartum
  - 21% intrapartum
  - 41% in the first 6 weeks postpartum
  - Maternal mortality rate ranges from 7% to 35%.
    - Disproportionate number of deaths occurring among the antenatal cases
    - A large portion of pregnancy-associated MI not due to atherosclerotic heart disease but to coronary artery *in situ* thrombus formation, dissection, or spasm.
- Diagnosis of ischemic heart disease in pregnancy
  - Requires considering it as part of the differential diagnosis
  - Even in absence of traditional risk factors
  - Creatine phosphokinase (CPK) and creatine kinase-MB (CK-MB) can be mildly elevated following a cesarean delivery.
  - Troponin is a more specific marker of cardiac disease in the peripartum period.

- Stress testing can be safely carried out in pregnancy, including nuclear imaging.
  - Diagnostic coronary angiography is performed on pregnant women for the same indications as for nonpregnant patients.
- Treatment of coronary artery disease is largely unchanged in pregnancy.
  - None of the medications commonly used to treat ischemic heart disease have been shown to cause adverse effects in the fetus.
    - Broad experience with low-dose aspirin, nitrates, β-blockers, and heparins in pregnancy
    - Paucity of data regarding use of clopidogrel and glycoprotein IIb/IIIa inhibitors limit their use in pregnancy.
  - Coronary angiography, angioplasty and stenting, and thrombolysis have been and can be carried out safely throughout pregnancy.
  - Management of laboring patients with ischemic heart disease is the same as for other cardiac patients and has strong parallels with the management of the cardiac patient undergoing general surgery.

Cardiac Arrhythmias in Pregnancy

- Arrhythmias appear to be more common than in the nonpregnant population.
  - Hormonal changes, stress, and anxiety are contributing factors.
  - Most arrhythmias are not serious unless associated with organic heart disease.
- **Atrial fibrillation** occurring in pregnancy is usually associated with an underlying disease such as mitral stenosis, peripartum cardiomyopathy, hypertensive heart disease, thyroid disease, or atrial septal defects.
  - With acute atrial fibrillation and hemodynamic changes
    - Direct current cardioversion
    - Cardioversion appears to have no adverse effects on fetus
    - Most require medical management with rate-controlling or rhythm-restoring antidysrhythmics.
      - β-Adrenergic blockers—metoprolol
      - Calcium channel blockers—diltiazem or verapamil
      - Agents such as procainamide or digoxin
      - All safe during pregnancy
      - Amiodarone is not a first-line agent for hemodynamically stable atrial fibrillation.
        - Possible effects on the fetal thyroid
        - Use in pregnancy not absolutely contraindicated.
        - Anticoagulation for atrial fibrillation has same indications as in nonpregnant patients.
          - Must use heparin (usually in the form of subcutaneous low-molecular-weight heparin).
          - Warfarin is associated with adverse fetal effects throughout gestation.
- **Supraventricular tachycardia (SVT):** SVTs during pregnancy can occur with or without organic heart disease.
  - Four percent of women with SVT report that the condition was first identified during pregnancy.
  - Up to 22% state pregnancy exacerbated the condition.
  - Absent underlying cardiac disease, not usually associated with increased morbidity

- With underlying structural cardiac disease or cardiomyopathy, SVT can lead to heart failure and death.
- Treatment protocols for supraventricular tachycardia remain unchanged in pregnancy and include carotid sinus massage, adenosine, calcium channel blockers, β-blockers, and direct current cardioversion.
- **Ventricular arrhythmias:** During pregnancy, these may be associated with cocaine use, peripartum or any other form of cardiomyopathy, ischemic heart disease, and digitalis toxicity,
  - Antiarrhythmic agents for which we have the most pregnancy data are lidocaine, β-blockers, and procainamide,
    - Amiodarone is associated with increased risk of fetal thyroid disease.
      - Should not be considered a first-line agent
    - Implantable defibrillators can and should be used when indicated in pregnancy.
- **Bradycardia:** Bradyarrhythmias during pregnancy are rare.
  - May result from
    - Lyme disease
    - Hypothyroidism
    - Myocarditis
    - Drug-induced congenital or acquired heart blocks
  - Permanent pacemakers are indicated for hemodynamically significant bradycardia.
    - With pre-existing pacemakers
      - May need to increase baseline rate to mimic normal physiologic changes of pregnancy
- **Antiarrhythmic Drugs:**
  - Table 7 classifies the commonly used antiarrhythmic agents on the basis of what is known about their safety in pregnancy.
  - Treatment should never be withheld from a pregnant woman based on theoretic fears of fetal harm.

Cardiac Surgery during Pregnancy

- Nonurgent cardiac surgery should take place during second trimester.
  - Deferring until after first trimester avoids period of organogenesis and risk of miscarriage.
  - Third-trimester surgery carries risk of precipitating preterm labor.
    - Surgery that is important to a patient's short-term well-being and survival should be done at any point.
  - Coronary artery bypass grafts, valvuloplasties, valvular replacements, and aortic root replacements have all been done in pregnancy with good outcomes for both mother and baby.
  - When medical management can ameliorate the disease process, surgery may be postponed.
    - Until at least 4 to 6 weeks postpartum
    - Decisions should be based on the best plan of action for the mother's safety rather than a cultural discomfort related to performing surgery in pregnancy.
- Special intraoperative considerations in pregnant patients include:
  - Fetal monitoring during and after surgery
  - Maintenance of high flow and systemic mean arterial pressure (during cardiopulmonary bypass)
  - Uterine displacement devices if patient in supine position for median sternotomy
    - Pregnant women fare well with open-heart procedures; fetal mortality rate can be high.
      - Better results seen in closed-heart procedures.
      - Postoperatively, fetal monitoring should be continued and maternal analgesia maintained to avoid precipitating labor from accelerated postoperative pain.

Pregnancy after Prosthetic Valve Surgery

- Mechanical heart valve prostheses pose significant risk during pregnancy.
- Secondary to coagulation status
- Fewer maternal and fetal complications occur with bioprosthetic valves.
  - Need for reoperation on these valves for degenerative changes means not commonly used in reproductive women
- Typically low-molecular-weight heparin (LMWH)
  - Anticoagulant agent of choice during pregnancy
  - Molecular weight prevents placental crossover.
  - Not teratogenic
  - Anticoagulant of choice in pregnancy except for mechanical heart valves
    - Unclear whether LMWH provides same level of protection against mechanical valve thrombosis as warfarin.
    - Warfarin and its derivatives are associated with increased risk of CNS anomalies and warfarin embryopathy.
      - Risk may be worth taking to prevent the catastrophic consequences of valve thrombosis.
      - Can use LMWH during the period of organogenesis; switch to warfarin for the majority of the pregnancy and then switch back to LMWH close to term to avoid both fetal and maternal bleeding associated with delivery.
      - Conversely, can use LMWH with frequent anti-Xa levels.

Cardiac Transplant Patients

- Increasing number and survival of heart transplant recipients
- Increasing numbers of women recipients have become pregnant.
- Pregnancy experience with solid tissue transplants has a 25% risk of maternal complications.
  - 44% to 50% of these complications are hypertension.
  - 29% risk of miscarriage
  - 41% risk of prematurity
  - 22% risk of rejection
  - 13% risk of worsening renal function
- Women who have undergone cardiac transplantation are encouraged to wait 2 years after transplantation before becoming pregnant.
- Drugs used to prevent rejection should be continued during pregnancy.
  - Evidence of their safety is accumulating.
- Peripartum management should be dictated by the quality of LV function

Cardiopulmonary Resuscitation in Pregnancy

- Cardiopulmonary resuscitation (CPR) in pregnancy poses unique problems.
  - Third trimester and particularly near term, the gravid uterus impairs venous return.
    - During CPR, the uterus should be displaced (i.e., left uterine tilt).
    - If defibrillation is required, the left breast needs to be displaced because of marked enlargement during pregnancy.
    - Unlikely but theoretical possibility of electrical arcing between a defibrillator and fetal monitoring devices.
      ○ Devices should be removed prior to defibrillation.
- Otherwise, ACLS protocols, including medications and the use of the defibrillator, should be followed as done in nonpregnant woman.
- Data about the risk and benefits of an emergency cesarean delivery in the context of maternal resuscitation are very limited.
  - If fetus has reached more than about 24 weeks gestation
    - Emergency cesarean should be considered a part of the resuscitative efforts.
    - Evacuation of the gravid uterus may improve efficacy of chest compressions and improve the outcome for both mother and baby.
    - Present recommendations are
      ○ Consideration of cesarean delivery in pregnant women more than 24 weeks gestation
      ○ In cardiac arrest and failed to respond to 5 minutes of aggressive and appropriate resuscitative efforts
- Major causes of maternal cardiac arrest are:
  - Trauma
  - Cardiac arrest
  - Embolism
  - Other causes are:
    - Sepsis
    - Magnesium overdose
    - Complications of eclampsia
    - Result of an unanticipated difficult intubation
- General treatment of the pregnant patient in cardiac arrest is no different than any other patient, including drug dosages and defibrillation settings.
  - Chest compressions and ventilations should be performed with the recommended sequence.
  - Slight left tilt of the pregnant patient during CPR enhances venous return after 24 weeks of gestation.
  - Because of the reduced pulmonary reserve, pregnant women do not tolerate hypoxia well.
  - IV fluid should be running wide open on pressure bags, and blood products should be considered if hemorrhage is suspected.
  - Once the age of the fetus is determined, a decision can be made whether to proceed with a perimortem cesarean section.
    - Fetus can tolerate hypoxia longer than normal, but the decision to proceed with a cesarean delivery should be made within 4 minutes.
  - Management of the airway in the obstetric patient may be especially challenging.
    - Main mechanisms for airway problems are inadequate ventilation, esophageal intubation, and difficult intubation.
    - Unanticipated difficult airway may require alternative airway management attempts including the laryngeal mask airway or the Combitube.
    - If cricothyrotomy becomes necessary, this maneuver should be initiated in a timely fashion to minimize the chance of maternal hypoxic brain damage.

CHAPTER 63 ■ HEMORRHAGIC AND LIVER DISORDERS OF PREGNANCY

MAJOR PROBLEMS

- Maternal mortality
  - Defined as deaths occurring during pregnancy or within 6 weeks postpartum
  - Cause of death identified as complications related to pregnancy, delivery, or the puerperium (ICD-9 codes 630–676)
  - Decreased significantly over the past century
    - From 850 deaths in 1900 to 7.5 deaths per 100,000 in 1982
    - Rate has remained stable between 1982 and 1996
- Hemorrhage and hypertensive disorders the major contributors to maternal death rates
  - Hemorrhagic disorders can become life threatening quickly

HEMORRHAGIC CONCERNS

- Significant bleeding in pregnancy can be quantified by total amount
  - Postpartum hemorrhage is established when:

- Greater than 500 mL for vaginal deliveries
- More than 1 L for cesarean deliveries
- Clinical symptoms and signs with respect to the blood loss are considered in the management

PLACENTAL COMPLICATIONS

Placental Abruption

- Placental abruption (abruptio placentae):
  - Condition in which placenta separates from implantation site of uterus prior to delivery of fetus
  - Area of hemorrhage along the decidua basalis expands as the bleeding progresses
  - Hematoma may be concealed or present clinically with vaginal bleeding
  - Underlying mechanism may be related to:
    - Vascular damage caused by pre-eclampsia
    - Trauma
    - Cocaine/alcohol use
    - Chorioamnionitis
  - Risk factors for abruption include:
    - Maternal or paternal (second-hand) smoking
    - Multiparity
    - Prior caesarean delivery
    - African American ethnicity
  - Incidence ranges between 0.4% and 0.8%
    - A 15% recurrence rate for a subsequent pregnancy
    - A 20% recurrence rate for two previous episodes
- Classic clinical manifestations include:
  - Vaginal bleeding
  - Abdominal pain/uterine irritability
  - Fetal heart rate abnormalities or fetal distress
  - None or all of these symptoms may be present
  - Ultrasound has limited usefulness as it reveals a retroplacental blood clot in only 15% of cases, thus giving a high false-negative rate
- Treatment:
  - Fluid resuscitation
  - Adequate oxygenation
  - Close fetal monitoring
  - Critical to anticipate additional postpartum complications, such as uterine atony, to limit further hemorrhage

Placenta Previa

- Occurs with improper implantation of the placenta such that it overlies the internal os of the cervix during the third trimester
- Incidence of placenta previa approximately 0.5%
- Risk factors include:
  - Prior placenta previa
  - History of cesarean delivery
  - History of suction curettage
  - Maternal age older than 35 years
  - African American or nonwhite ethnicity
  - Cigarette smoking
- Clinical symptoms include:
  - Painless vaginal bleeding beginning in the second or third trimester

- Ultrasound then performed to confirm or rule out the diagnosis
- Management expectant unless maternal bleeding or fetal heart rate abnormalities/fetal distress necessitates imminent delivery via cesarean section
- If the patient is stable—meaning no bleeding—and the fetal surveillance is reassuring, the patient is closely monitored on pelvic rest
- Nothing per vagina, no vaginal examination, no intercourse
- Until fetal lung maturity or 37 weeks' gestation, then cesarean delivery is performed
- Risks of placenta previa include other placental implantation abnormalities:
  - Placenta accreta
  - Placenta increta
  - Placenta percreta
- Physician must be aware of these risks at the time of delivery and be prepared for a possible cesarean hysterectomy (hysterectomy performed at the time of the cesarean delivery) if necessary

HEMOLYSIS, ELEVATED LIVER ENZYMES, AND LOW PLATELETS (HELLP) SYNDROME AND DISSEMINATED INTRAVASCULAR COAGULATION (DIC)

- HELLP thought to be a distinct variant, rather than a progression, of the pre-eclampsia/eclampsia continuum
  - Incidence is rare: 310 per 100,000 pre-eclamptic patients
  - Associations with genetic mutations of the Fas gene and regulation of the immune system
  - Risk factors have been shown to include:
    - African Americans
    - History of prior pregnancy with HELLP
  - Recurrence rate has been reported as 14%
- A disease with significant morbidity and mortality, both maternal and perinatal
- Maternal death 1.1%
- Significant maternal morbidity included:
  - DIC (21%)
  - Placental abruption (16%)
  - Acute renal failure (7.7%)
  - Pulmonary edema (6%)
  - Rare occurrences of subcapsular liver hematoma and retinal detachment
    - Case reports of hepatic rupture have been documented
- Fetal outcome typically related to the necessity to proceed with preterm delivery
- Neonatal outcomes include risk of intensive care requirements, mechanical ventilation, sepsis, and intraventricular hemorrhage
- Clinical features and laboratory evaluation of HELLP not firmly defined
  - Generally, findings reflect disease process on the vascular supply of the maternal liver
  - Hemolysis can be noted by an abnormal peripheral smear, elevated serum bilirubin, low serum haptoglobin levels, elevated lactate dehydrogenase (LDH) of subtypes LDH1/LDH2, or a fall in the hemoglobin

- Elevated liver enzymes, generally aspartate transaminases (AST), alanine transferase (ALT) and/or bilirubin present
- However, no strict definition of the degree of elevation
- Also great variability in establishing the criteria for low platelets
  - Varying from 150,000 to <50,000 cells/μL
  - Patients with HELLP have altered vascular reactivity
  - Methods of prediction of HELLP by Doppler ultrasound have been examined, revealing a decrease in dual hepatic blood supply preceding the onset of HELLP
  - Objective parameters for DIC include:
    o Prolonged prothrombin time (PT) and activated partial thromboplastin time (aPTT)
    o Elevated fibrinogen degradation products
    o Elevated D-dimers
    o As fibrinogen is increased in a normal pregnancy, the value in DIC may decrease to "normal" (nonpregnant) values, so it is not used as an objective parameter
- Treatment of HELLP includes:
  - Supportive care in a facility suited for such high-level care
  - Prompt delivery of the fetus is indicated if the patient is beyond 34 gestational weeks or sooner if disease has progressed to multiorgan dysfunction, DIC, liver infarction or hemorrhage, renal failure, suspected placental abruption, or a nonreassuring fetal status
  - More controversy regarding the recommendations if the pregnancy is <34 weeks gestation and there are only mild to moderate laboratory abnormalities
    - Expectant management and corticosteroids for fetal lung maturity are given with delivery after completion of the course of steroids
    - Significant debate over use of steroids for *treatment* of the laboratory abnormalities of HELLP
    - Benefit of plasma exchange therapy has been shown to improve treatment outcome
    - Heparin therapy is associated with further bleeding complications
    - Transfusion of both packed red cells and component therapy as indicated
    - Fluid replacement and oxygenation are critical

LIVER CONCERNS

Physiologic Changes Associated with Pregnancy

- Pregnancy-related hormones and fetal enzymes significantly affect the maternal liver
- Changes in liver profile reveal:
  - Decreased serum albumin secondary to the dilutional effect of a 50% increase in maternal plasma volume
  - Increased serum alkaline phosphatase due to placental/fetal production
  - Markers of liver injury—aspartate aminotransferase, alanine aminotransferase, and lactate dehydrogenase—will not change in normal pregnancy
  - Bilirubin and γ-glutamyl transpeptidase are both significantly lowered
- One main hormone causing alterations in hepatic physiology is estrogen

- Produces increase in hepatic rough endoplasmic reticulum
  - Increases the production of proteins
- Approximate 12 times increase in estradiol through pregnancy related to multiple factors:
  - Changes in the binding hormones
  - Changes in metabolism and production
- Stimulates approximate six times increase in production of sex hormone–binding globulin
- Estrogen also has an inverse relationship with bile salt production and bile flow
  - Change in both composition of the bile and in the rate of cholesterol and phospholipid production
  - Produce an increased lithogenicity
- Progesterone mainly affects an increase of smooth endoplasmic reticulum and an increase in cytochrome P-450
  - Also notable smooth muscle relaxation of the gallbladder and biliary ductal system
  - Can produce slow wave dysrhythmia in the gastrointestinal tract

Hyperemesis Gravidarum (HG)

- HG a condition characterized by serious and persistent vomiting that limits fluid intake and adequate nutrition
- Clinical manifestations include:
  - Weight loss >5% of prepregnancy weight
  - Weakness
  - Dehydration
  - Ketosis
  - Muscle wasting
- HG occurs in approximately 0.3% to 2.0% of pregnancies
  - Seems to affect a diverse population with multiple risk factors
    - Associated with various hormone levels including:
      o Human chorionic gonadotropin
      o Estrogen
      o Prolactin
      o Thyroxine
      o Androgens
      o Cortisol
      o Maternal prostaglandins
    - Other factors identified include:
      o Prior history of HG with previous pregnancies
      o Female fetal gender
      o Maternal age
      o Maternal weight
      o Smoking
      o *Helicobacter pylori* may or may not have a role
  - Chronic medical conditions contribute to risk:
    o History of gastritis
    o Allergies
    o Gallbladder disease
- Complete differential diagnosis includes multiple systems:
  - Obstetric and gynecologic conditions: molar pregnancy, degenerating uterine leiomyoma, or ovarian torsion
  - Gastrointestinal causes: gastroenteritis, gastroparesis, achalasia, biliary tract disease, hepatitis, intestinal obstruction, peptic ulcer disease, pancreatitis, and appendicitis
  - Urinary tract conditions: pyelonephritis, uremia, and kidney stones

- Metabolic diseases: hyperthyroidism, diabetic ketoacidosis, porphyria, and Addison disease
- Neurologic disorders, drug reactions, and psychiatric conditions are other considerations
- HG may or may not be protective against adverse outcomes
  - Relationship between HG and low birth weight that is mostly attributed to poor maternal weight gain
  - Additionally worsened maternal morbidity and mortality are also noted
    - Wernicke encephalopathy
    - Central pontine myelinolysis
    - Severe liver injury
    - Splenic avulsion
    - Pneumomediastinum following esophageal rupture
    - Acute kidney injury
- Treatment for HG is primarily supportive:
  - Antiemetics
  - Fluid therapy
  - Electrolyte replacement
  - Natural remedies: pyridoxine (vitamin B$_6$) and ginger shown to be effective
  - Behavior modification with avoidance of strong odors/scents and adjustment of diet may be tried
    - If these measures are inadequate, hospitalization and treatment with steroids and parenteral nutrition may be necessary

Intrahepatic Cholestasis of Pregnancy (ICP)

- ICP the most frequent of the pregnancy-related liver diseases
- Occurs in approximately 1% of pregnancies
- Characterized by:
  - Progressive pruritus of cholestasis
  - Elevated fasting bile salts >10 μmol/L:
    - Chenodeoxycholic acid
    - Deoxycholic acid
    - Cholic acid
  - Elevated amino transferases
- Clinical manifestations:
  - Begin in the late second or third trimester
  - Most often will resolve spontaneously within 2 to 3 weeks postpartum
  - Direct cause is unknown, a strong familial component recognized
  - ICP affects specific populations at different rates:
    - Occurs in <0.2% of pregnancies in women of North American and Central/Western European descent
    - Scandinavian and Baltic populations show a rate of 1% to 2%
    - Chilean and Bolivian populations have shown rates of 5% to 15%
  - Severe form of ICP with bile acid levels >40 μmol/L
    - In the Swedish population is associated with a frame shift mutation in the gene coding for the adenosine triphosphate (ATP) binding cassette transporter
      - Specifically the ABCB4_5 gene variant (formerly known as multidrug resistance gene 3 [MDR3])
    - Mutations in the bile salt export pump (BSEP) can also predispose to ICP
    - Other possible causes relate to "leaky gut" theories

- Based on the increased absorption of bacterial endotoxins and the enterohepatic circulation of cholestatic metabolites of sex hormones and bile salts
    - Also an association with low maternal serum estrogen
- Fetal complication rates:
  - Directly related to maternal serum bile acids
  - Levels >40 μmol/L associated with:
    - Preterm delivery
    - Fetal asphyxial events
    - Meconium staining
    - Case reports of neonatal respiratory distress syndrome and fetal death are noted
    - Maternal morbidity and mortality are low
- Treatment:
  - Supportive measures for pruritus with antihistamine is inadequate
    - Has limited effectiveness and fails to address the bile acid elevation and fetal concerns
  - Cholestyramine, S-adenosylmethionine, and dexamethasone were the treatments of choice
  - Newer work advocates use of ursodeoxycholic acid (UDCA), a tertiary bile acid
    - Initial use of UDCA was with bear bile in traditional Chinese medicine for the treatment of liver disease
    - UDCA effective in reducing bile acids and bilirubin
    - Fetal risks are decreased, but not eliminated
    - Careful fetal monitoring and delivery at fetal lung maturity should be considered
    - Ondansetron being evaluated as a treatment for pruritus
      - No data are noted on fetal benefits of that antiemetic

Acute Fatty Liver Disease of Pregnancy (AFLP)

- AFLP a rare but potentially fatal disease that occurs in the third trimester
- Mean gestational ages vary between 34.5 and 37 weeks
- Incidence documented as between 1 in 6,659 births to 1 in 15,900 births
- Characterized by:
  - Significant malaise
  - Nausea/vomiting
  - Anorexia
  - Abdominal pain
  - Jaundice
- Clinical signs include:
  - Hypertension
  - Jaundice
  - Elevated serum transaminases
  - Coagulopathies
  - Thrombocytopenia
  - Hypoglycemia
- High index of suspicion should be maintained if signs and symptoms are noted
- Imaging studies are often performed but have limited usefulness:
  - Ultrasound may show nonspecific changes
  - Computed tomography has a high false-negative rate
  - Liver biopsy is the gold standard in confirming the diagnosis

○ Rarely necessary and carries significant maternal risk in setting of DIC
- Disease has significant risks with respect to morbidity and mortality
  - Older work reported maternal and perinatal mortality rates as high as 75% and 85%, respectively
    ○ While maternal mortality rate has fallen significantly, fetal mortality remains as high as 66%.
  - Maternal morbidity includes:
    ○ Coagulopathies (specifically DIC)
    ○ Hepatic encephalopathy
    ○ Respiratory compromise (pulmonary edema or respiratory arrest)
    ○ Renal insufficiency

- There is an associated genetic component with mitochondrial trifunctional protein mutations
- Treatment is supportive:
  - Management in an intensive care unit
  - Delivery is recommended as efficiently as possible
  - Hypoglycemia should be treated with dextrose-containing solutions
  - Elevated ammonia levels can be decreased with neomycin
  - Blood transfusions and replacement of clotting factors should be considered as appropriate
  - AFLP generally resolves within 2 to 3 days postpartum
    ○ Cases of fulminant hepatic failure requiring liver transplantation have been reported

CHAPTER 64 ■ ACUTE ABDOMEN AND TRAUMA DURING PREGNANCY

IMMEDIATE CONCERNS

- About 1 in 500 (0.2%) of pregnant women require surgery for nonobstetric conditions.
  - Appendectomy, cholecystectomy, and adnexal procedures constitute most common surgeries during pregnancy.
  - Pregnancy outcomes after surgery are often good.
    - But fetal loss rates can be as high as 2% to 20%, depending on condition.
  - Trauma an additional important cause for surgical intervention during pregnancy.
    - Incidence of trauma is approximately 8%, or 1 in 12 pregnancies.
    - Leading cause of nonobstetric maternal death
    - Fetal losses can be significant.
    - Always consider the possibility of pregnancy in any female between 12 and 44 years of age presenting with abdominal pain or trauma.
- Evaluation
  - First task is to ensure that airway, breathing, and circulation (ABCs) are adequate.
  - Adequate maternal oxygenation and uteroplacental perfusion are the means by which the fetus is also resuscitated.
  - Achieve hemodynamic stability in the mother before evaluation and treatment of pregnancy issues.
  - Physiologic adaptations of pregnancy affect the clinician's ability to address the ABCs (Table 64.1).
  - Once assured that the patient is hemodynamically stable, attention is turned to detailed secondary assessment.
    - Centered on evaluation of specific injuries or organ systems and pregnancy
    - Focused patient history is central to the evaluation of abdominal pain or trauma during pregnancy.

- Abdominal symptoms can be nonspecific during pregnancy.
  ○ Clarify the location, intensity, and quality of pain, including associated symptoms and aggravating or alleviating factors.
  ○ Obstetric symptoms, such as contractions, cramps, bleeding, or fluid leakage, should be noted.

TABLE 64.1

KEY POINTS IN THE ABCS OF THE RESUSCITATION OF PREGNANT WOMEN

Airway	Weight gain
	Breast enlargement
	Short time to establish airway before desaturation
	Edema of airway
	Difficulty in positioning neck
	Delayed gastric emptying—aspiration risk
Breathing	Elevated diaphragm
	Decreased fetal heart rate—rapid desaturation
	Respiratory alkalosis
	Limited chest wall expansion
	Limited accessory muscle use
	Normal large and small airway function
Circulation	Aortocaval compression at >20 weeks gravid
	Increased cardiac output
	Increased resting heart rate
	Decreased peripheral vascular resistance
	Decreased systolic and diastolic blood pressure
	Large shunt due to placental blood flow
	Hypercoagulable state

○ In trauma, important details of the incident should be elicited, including vehicle speed, position seated in the vehicle, use of restraints, airbag deployment, and injuries to the head, abdomen, or extremities.

○ Understanding normal physical changes and common complaints associated with pregnancy will help the clinician determine which symptoms are benign and pregnancy-related versus pathologic.

– Many patients report nausea and vomiting in early pregnancy, but not typical in the later two trimesters.

– Pyrosis due to acid reflux is reported by many gravidas, but is often easily relieved with antacids.

– Constipation is a common complaint, due to the increased transit time of the gastrointestinal tract.

– Transient discomfort or intermittent contractions are not rare, but persistent, rhythmic, or severe abdominal pain merits evaluation.

– In all trimesters, right lower quadrant pain may signal appendicitis.

– Colicky right upper quadrant pain is suggestive of cholelithiasis, and the symptom profile for biliary tract disease in pregnant women is similar to that of their nonpregnant counterparts.

○ In the third trimester, it is important to evaluate and exclude the possibility of obstetric complications such as:

– Preterm labor (PTL)
– Premature rupture of membranes
– Placental abruption
– Intrauterine infection

- Basic obstetric (OB) triage evaluation includes external fetal heart rate monitoring, assessment of contractions, palpation of the uterine fundus, speculum examination for pooling, Nitrazine and fern tests, and digital cervical examination.

- Suggested approach to the initial evaluation of the pregnant patient with surgical diseases or trauma is shown in Table 64.2.

DIAGNOSTIC STUDIES

Laboratory Values

- During pregnancy, results can be misinterpreted or confusing unless pregnancy-specific norms are considered.
- Physiologic changes of pregnancy, including increased blood and plasma volumes, hormone production, and altered metabolic clearance, cause changes in the plasma concentration of many analytes.
- Selected laboratory values are displayed in Table 64.3.

OB Tests of Interest

- **Fetal fibronectin (fFN):** fFN is a protein produced by fetal membranes involved in adhesion of the placenta and membranes to maternal tissues.
  - Between 24 to 34 weeks, fFN is not normally detectable in cervicovaginal secretions
  - Presence of fFN may indicate a disruption of the membranes and decidua.
    - Due to inflammation or other causes

TABLE 64.2

KEY STEPS IN THE APPROACH TO THE PREGNANT PATIENT WITH SURGICAL DISEASES OR TRAUMA

1. Consider pregnancy in any woman of reproductive age presenting after trauma or with abdominal complaints—check urine or serum HCG
2. Perform a primary assessment of airway/breathing/circulation (ABCs)
   a. Use a 15-degree left lateral tilt
   b. IV hydration with isotonic crystalloid solution
   c. Supplemental oxygen as necessary
3. Primary assessment of maternal status should be done prior to evaluation and treatment of fetal issues—should be focused and brief
4. Perform a secondary assessment once patient is hemodynamically stable
   a. Investigate specific injuries or organ systems
   b. Evaluate pregnancy viability and gestational age
   c. Assess for pregnancy complications such as preterm labor (PTL), intrauterine infection, placental abruption, or fetomaternal hemorrhage
   d. Perform cardiotocography for patients over 24 weeks' gestation
5. Do not withhold necessary diagnostic procedures
   a. Consider using modalities that do not use ionizing radiation when possible
   b. Limit ionizing radiation exposure to less than a total dose of 5 rad, as doses less than this amount are not associated with fetal loss or anomalies
6. Obstetric consult for all cases of severe abdominal pain or injury in pregnant patients
   a. Determine if intervention for fetal indications is appropriate
   b. Manage pregnancy complications as necessary
   c. Develop contingency plans for route and timing of delivery where appropriate
   d. Consider neonatal, anesthesiology consultations
   e. Ensure equipment and staff available to effect emergency delivery if indicated

HCG, human chorionic gonadotropin; IV, intravenous.

- In symptomatic patient, a negative test is associated with >95% likelihood of not delivering within 14 days.
- Useful in the management of patients with preterm contractions, not uncommon in the setting of surgical diseases complicating pregnancy
- **Amniocentesis:** In selected cases, evaluation important to exclude intrauterine infection as a cause of abdominal pain
- Abnormal findings in amniotic fluid suggestive of bacterial infection include:
  - Bacteria seen on Gram stain and/or positive culture
  - Low glucose, typically <15 mg/dL
  - High white cell count
  - Inflammatory markers such as high granulocyte colony-stimulating factor (G-CSF), tumor necrosis factor-α (TNF-α), and interleukin-1 (IL-1) and IL-6 are strongly suggestive of amnionitis
  - There is a risk of preterm contractions, premature rupture of the membranes, or fetal loss due to the procedure
    ○ Thus should be done on a selective basis
    ○ Data can be extremely useful when the clinical picture is unclear.

TABLE 64.3

NORMAL LABORATORY VALUES DURING
PREGNANCY

WBC	Increased	5,000–15,000 cells/mm^3
Hemoglobin	Decreased	10.5–13.5 g/dL
Hematocrit	Decreased	30.5%–39%
Platelet	Decreased	150–380 × 10^3 cells/µL
Fibrinogen	Increased	265–615 mg/dL
D-dimer	Frequently positive	—
HCO$_3^-$	Mild acidosis	19–25 mEq/L
BUN	Decreased	3–4 mg/dL
Creatinine	Decreased	0.4–0.7 mg/dL
Albumin	Decreased	2.7–3.7 g/dL
AST, ALT	Unchanged	12–38 U/L
Bilirubin	Unchanged	0.2–0.6 mg/dL
Alkaline phosphatase	Increased	60–140 IU/L

ALT, alanine aminotransferase; AST, aspartate aminotransferase;
BUN, blood urea nitrogen; HCO$_3^-$, bicarbonate; WBC, white blood
cell count.
From Lockitch G. The effect of normal pregnancy on common
biochemistry and hematology tests. In: Barron WM, Lindheimer MD,
eds. *Medical Disorders during Pregnancy.* 3rd ed. St. Louis, MO:
Mosby; 2000.

Diagnostic Imaging Studies

- Medically necessary diagnostic tests should not be withheld solely on the basis of pregnancy.
  - Consider the potential advantages/disadvantages when selecting a particular testing method.
  - Ultrasonography uses sound waves (no ionizing radiation).
    - No known adverse fetal outcomes associated with use of prenatal diagnostic ultrasound under current clinical guidelines for energy exposure.
  - Magnetic resonance imaging (MRI) makes use of the altered energy state of protons to enhance imaging.
    - Chief clinical uses have been to evaluate placental abnormalities and characterize fetal central nervous system (CNS) malformations
    - May also be a valuable tool for assessing for intra-abdominal pathology
    - To date, MRI has been used safely during pregnancy.
  - X-ray studies and computed tomography (CT) involve ionizing radiation and need to be used judiciously in gravid women.

Obstetric Ultrasound

- Serves to confirm fetal viability
- Offers opportunity to assess fetal size, anatomy, amniotic fluid volume, and placental location
- Basic study can be completed quickly at the bedside and can be done at the time of sonographic evaluation for other indications, such as right upper quadrant ultrasound.

Sonography for Trauma

- Focused assessment sonography for trauma (FAST)-US:
  - Done to detect intra-abdominal bleeding after trauma

- Similar sensitivity and specificity among pregnant and nonpregnant patients
  - In 127 pregnant trauma patients, FAST examination identified intraperitoneal fluid in 5 of 6 patients and was negative in 117 of 120 patients without intra-abdominal injury.
  - False-positive scans had serous fluid.
  - In reproductive-age women with blunt abdominal trauma, free fluid in the cul de sac has been associated with a higher injury rate compared to no free fluid in both pregnant and nonpregnant women.
- Of limited value in the diagnosis of placental abruption after trauma.
  - May miss up to 50% to 58% of cases
  - Echotexture may be very similar to that of placental tissue, so identification of retroplacental bleeding is not always possible.
- Graded compression ultrasonography is the initial test of choice in assessment of appendicitis during pregnancy.
  - Imaging focused on the self-reported area of maximal pain
  - Overall accuracy of this technique in diagnosing appendicitis is 86%.
    - May be limited in the setting of a retrocecal appendix or perforated appendicitis
    - Color Doppler sonography can be used as an adjunct for improving the sensitivity of the test.
    - In a series of 42 women with suspected appendicitis during pregnancy, ultrasound was found to be 100% sensitive, 96% specific, and 98% accurate in diagnosing appendicitis.
- Diagnosis of cholelithiasis during pregnancy similar to that in nonpregnant
  - Visualization of stones in gallbladder reported to be as high as 95% using sonography
  - Detection of gallstones in a patient with right upper quadrant pain is suggestive of acute cholelithiasis, other features should be considered
    - Gallbladder wall edema or thickening >4 to 5 mm
    - Murphy sign can also be elicited
      - As patient experiences pain from pressing the transducer over gallbladder

Computed Tomography

- May be considered for abdominal evaluation if initial examination or other studies are equivocal
  - Most common indication for CT is blunt abdominal trauma after motor vehicle crash
  - Other indications include appendicitis and renal colic.
  - Helical CT has good success in detecting injuries after trauma during pregnancy.
    - Abnormal placental enhancement and when uterine rupture occurred, nonuterine injuries, and both uterine and other maternal injuries
    - Estimated radiation exposure was 8.7 to 17.5 mGy, depending on technique.
    - Limited data regarding the accuracy of CT for the diagnosis of appendicitis during pregnancy, one series of seven patients correctly identified all cases
    - Depending on the protocol, pelvic CT can deliver a dose of radiation to the fetus as high as 2 to 5 rad.
      - Threshold for teratogenesis may not be reached with this level.
      - But relative risk of childhood cancer may be increased.

– Odds of dying of childhood cancer increase from a baseline of 1 in 2,000 to approximately 2 in 2,000 after exposure of 5 rads.
  ○ Potential risks and benefits of CT during pregnancy should be discussed with patients.
  ○ CT contrast safe to use in pregnancy and is administered as usual.

Magnetic Resonance Imaging

- MRI used as a tool to identify the cause of abdominal pain during pregnancy
- MRI was able to correctly identify the appendix in 10 of 12 cases where sonography was uninformative.
- 29 pregnant women were evaluated with MRI for abdominal or pelvic pain, and correct prospective diagnoses were made in all but one patient.
- MRI compares favorably with sonography—the overall sensitivity was 100%, specificity 93.5%, and accuracy 94% for detecting appendicitis.
- Gadolinium contrast is not recommended for use in pregnancy.
  - Crosses the placenta and enters the fetal circulation
  - Enters the amniotic fluid, where it is swallowed by the fetus and absorbed
  - A pregnancy category C drug
    ○ Animal studies have revealed adverse effects, but no controlled studies have been performed in humans.

SPECIFIC MANAGEMENT

Specific Conditions: Trauma

- Complicates 1 in 12 pregnancies
- Two-thirds of trauma cases in pregnant women are due to motor vehicle crashes.
- Other common causes are falls, burns, and penetrating wounds.
- Blunt abdominal trauma is the most frequent mechanism of injury.
- 1% to 20% of gravidas experience domestic abuse.
  - Up to 60% of women affected report two or more assaults during pregnancy.
- At one center, nearly 3% of all trauma patients were pregnant.
  - 11% of these pregnancies diagnosed during trauma evaluation.
- Severe trauma requiring admission to intensive care unit infrequent—3 in 1,000 pregnancies
- Maternal death due to trauma is estimated to be 1.9 per 100,000 live births.
  - Representing the leading cause of nonobstetric maternal death
  - Estimated that 1,300 to 3,900 pregnancies lost due to maternal trauma yearly
    ○ Mild maternal injuries carry a 1% to 5% fetal loss rate.
    ○ Life-threatening trauma is associated with loss rates up to 40% to 50%.
    ○ Population-based data indicate that motor vehicle crashes account for 82% of fetal deaths after trauma.
      – Overall rate of 3.7 per 100,000 live births

– Highest rate of fetal death due to trauma seen in patients 15 to 19 years of age
- Fetal death was associated with:
  - Ejection from vehicle
  - Motorcycle crash
  - Pedestrian collision
  - Maternal death
  - Maternal tachycardia
  - Abnormal fetal heart rate (FHR)
  - Lack of restraints
  - An injury severity score (ISS) >9
- Preterm labor was associated with:
  - Gestational age over 35 weeks
  - Assault
  - Pedestrian collisions
- Up to 20% of injured pregnant patients test positive for drugs or alcohol, and one in three do not report using seat belts.
- Worst outcomes take place among those who deliver during their hospital stay for trauma.
  - Odds ratios (OR) are strikingly high for maternal death (OR 69).
  - Fetal death (OR 4.7)
  - Uterine rupture (OR 43)
  - Abruption (OR 9.2)
  - Even minor maternal injury places fetuses at risk.
- Other complications that can contribute to fetal morbidity and mortality include:
  - Abruptio placentae
  - Preterm labor
  - Fetomaternal hemorrhage
  - The diagnosis of abruption is based on signs and symptoms.
    - One of the best indicators of placental abruption is cardiotocography.
    - In patients with a normal study, the risk of abruption after trauma is approximately 1% to 5%.
    - In patients with more than six contractions per hour or abnormal fetal heart rate patterns, the risk of abruption can be 20% or higher.
- All women over 24 weeks' gestation should undergo an initial evaluation with cardiotocographic monitoring for 4 to 6 hours after trauma.
  - Four to six hours of observation is sufficient for patients who have experienced minor trauma and are hemodynamically stable, with a negative primary evaluation, FAST-US, and reassuring cardiotocography.
  - Extended period of observation for 24 hours or more is indicated for women with six or more contractions per hour, nonreassuring FHR patterns, vaginal bleeding, uterine pain or tenderness, premature rupture of membrane (PROM), or serious maternal injury.
  - Consideration for prolonged monitoring is advised if laboratory data are abnormal, such as decreased fibrinogen or a positive Kleihauer-Betke (KB) test, as patients with these characteristics are more likely to experience abruption or other complications.
- Pregnant women occasionally present with other types of injuries due to trauma to the head, pelvis, or chest.
  - Pelvic fractures, especially those involving the acetabulum, are associated with high maternal and fetal mortality rates.
  - Penetrating injury is less common during pregnancy than other forms of trauma.

- Severity of maternal abdominal or vascular injuries may be less than that of nongravid women, but rate of placental injury and fetal loss tends to be high.
- Management is similar to that of nonpregnant persons.
  - With careful and prompt evaluation of the placenta and fetus

Specific Conditions: Appendicitis

- Acute appendicitis complicates approximately 1 in 1,500 pregnancies.
  - Occurs in all trimesters, the second trimester is most typical.
  - More than 80% of patients with appendicitis report right lower quadrant pain, irrespective of the trimester.
    - Difficult to diagnose during pregnancy because signs and symptoms can be easily confused with physiologic changes of pregnancy.
      - Nausea and vomiting are common during pregnancy, but not typically associated with pain.
      - Constipation and bowel irregularity, frequent bothersome symptoms of gestation, can be difficult to interpret.
      - Mild leukocytosis is a normal laboratory finding in pregnant women, rendering it of limited value in making the diagnosis of appendicitis.
        – White blood cell (WBC) count ranges from 5,000 to 15,000 cells/mm^3 in the first two trimesters and can be as high as 20,000 cells/mm^3 in labor.
        – Classic triad of obturator, psoas, and Rovsing sign are present in less than one in three pregnant patients.
        – Imaging plays an important role in the diagnosis of appendicitis during pregnancy.
  - Complications may be increased when appendicitis occurs during pregnancy.
    - Delay in diagnosis and treatment over 24 hours associated with perforation in 14% to 43% of cases, and up to 69% in the third trimester.
    - Fetal loss rates as high as 33% and preterm delivery rates of 14% reported in women undergoing appendectomy
  - When strongly suspected, surgery performed as per usual clinical indications
    - An incision over the point of maximal tenderness is most often recommended.
    - Laparoscopy may be considered as an alternative in patients under 24 weeks' gestation.

Specific Conditions: Gallstones

- Cholelithiasis is common among pregnant women.
  - Seen in 3% to 4% of OB ultrasounds
  - Symptomatic gallstones occur less frequently, in approximately 1 in 1,000 cases
    - Half or more of patients experience recurrent bouts of biliary colic.
    - Traditional management consists of intravenous hydration, nothing orally or a low-fat diet, analgesics, and antibiotics.
    - Cholecystectomy required in 1 to 6 per 10,000 pregnancies.
    - Typical indications for surgery include:
      - Acute cholecystitis (38%)

      - Gallstone pancreatitis (28%)
      - Common bile duct stone (20%)
      - Refractory pain (18%)
  - Laparoscopy has been used successfully during pregnancy.
  - Traditional management emphasized deferring surgery for symptomatic cholelithiasis until after delivery.
    - More recent data suggest that relapse of symptoms seen in 38%.
    - Labor induction due to refractory symptoms results in preterm delivery in some cases.

Specific Conditions: Adnexal Surgery

- True incidence of adnexal masses during pregnancy unclear
  - Estimated to be approximately 1 in 200
  - Simple ovarian cysts compose the vast majority of cases.
  - Adnexal surgery is necessary in 1 in 1,300 pregnancies.
    - Typically due to masses >6 to 8 cm, complex masses, and ovarian torsion
    - Malignancy is uncommon, seen in <10% of cases
    - Care should be taken to avoid removal of the corpus luteum in the first trimester prior to 10 weeks' gestation, as this can result in disruption of the ongoing pregnancy unless progesterone supplementation is provided.

FETAL ASSESSMENT

Risk of Fetal Loss and Recommended Fetal Assessment

- Total fetal loss rate is low, at 2.5%.
  - Birth defects after first trimester surgeries occurred in 3.9%.
  - The miscarriage rate was 5.8%, likely not increased above background rates, but not proven due to lack of controls for comparison.
  - Premature labor after nonobstetric surgery was seen in 3.5%.
  - The overall rate of preterm birth was 8.2%.
  - The highest risk for preterm birth and fetal loss was seen with appendectomy.
    - Preterm delivery rate was 4.6%.
    - Losses occurred in 10.9% of cases.
  - No consensus on optimal fetal monitoring in the perioperative period
    - During first trimester, no specific fetal evaluation is necessary.
      - Documentation of a live intrauterine pregnancy prior to surgery is prudent in those patients who present with abdominal complaints, primarily to exclude the possibility of ectopic pregnancy or nonviable gestation.
    - From 14 to 24 weeks, assessment of fetal heart tones is advised preoperatively and postoperatively.
      - Perioperative assessment of contractions may be considered after 20 to 24 weeks.
    - At 24 weeks or beyond, cardiotocography should be performed before and after completion of surgery.

PRETERM LABOR AND TOCOLYSIS

- In one series of 77 patients undergoing nonobstetric surgery
  - Preterm labor was seen in 26% of patients in the second trimester.
  - 82% of those in the third trimester.
  - Most common after appendicitis and adnexal surgery
    - Actual preterm birth was seen in 16%.
    - Only in 5%, however, was a clear link to the surgical procedure established.
- Tocolytic medications are given to reduce uterine contractions in many cases, because it is difficult to predict accurately which women will go on to deliver prematurely.
  - Most commonly used tocolytic agents include nifedipine, magnesium sulfate, and indomethacin.
  - Selection drug based on gestational age, maternal health conditions, and possible side effects
  - Tocolytic drugs prolong pregnancy for only 2 to 7 days; their chief utility is to allow for administration of steroids to improve fetal lung maturity.
  - Clinical assessment includes physical examination with palpation of the fundus, cervical examination, and cardiotocography.
    - Adjunctive tests to aid in predicting preterm birth include cervical length measurement, fetal fibronectin testing, and possibly amniocentesis.
    - Tocolysis should be undertaken with caution in the surgical patient, and obstetric consultation is recommended in the event of preterm contractions after surgery.

Corticosteroids for Fetal Lung Maturity Enhancement

- All pregnant women 24 and 34 weeks of gestation at risk of preterm delivery within 7 days:
  - Should be given a single course of corticosteroids for fetal lung maturity enhancement
    - Betamethasone, 12 mg intramuscularly every 24 hours for two doses, *or*
    - Dexamethasone, 6 mg intramuscularly every 12 hours for four doses
  - Corticosteroids for fetal lung maturity enhancement reduce the incidence and severity of respiratory distress syndrome in preterm infants.
    - Betamethasone has been shown to decrease neonatal mortality.
    - Intraventricular hemorrhage and necrotizing enterocolitis are decreased with steroid use.

Venous Thromboembolism (VTE) Prevention

- Pregnancy is a prothrombotic state
  - Risk of VTE increased among women who undergo cesarean delivery as compared with vaginal birth.
  - In the gravid trauma patient, pneumatic compression is reasonable and low-molecular-weight heparin (LMWH) prophylaxis can be considered.
- With additional risk factors for thromboembolism beyond pregnancy itself, pharmacologic methods should be combined with use of mechanical approaches

PERIOPERATIVE MANAGEMENT

Anesthesia

- Regional or local anesthetics thought to be safer than general anesthesia
  - For abdominal surgery, has advantage of minimal fetal local anesthetic drug exposure
  - Less likely to be associated with airway complications
  - Local anesthetics are not known to be teratogenic when used in this clinical setting
- Risk of aspiration from gastroesophageal (GE) reflux and delayed gastric emptying
  - Customary to administer a nonparticulate antacid or H_2 blocker
  - And medication to improve GE sphincter tone preoperatively
  - For general anesthesia, preoxygenation and rapid-sequence intubation typical
  - Avoid hyperventilation, as uterine blood flow is impaired.
  - Inhalational agents decrease uterine tone and effectively inhibit labor during surgery
  - Agents for general anesthesia, including a single dose of benzodiazepines, nitrous oxide, and inhalational agents, not shown to be teratogenic
  - Fetal loss, low birth weight, and perinatal mortality increase after nonobstetric surgery appear not to be influenced by the choice of anesthetic
- Guidelines for laparoscopic surgery during pregnancy are displayed in Table 64.4.

TABLE 64.4

SOCIETY FOR AMERICAN GASTROINTESTINAL ENDOSCOPIC SURGEONS GUIDELINES FOR LAPAROSCOPIC SURGERY DURING PREGNANCY (2000)

1. Preoperative obstetric consultation
2. If possible, defer operation until second trimester, when fetal risk is lowest
3. Use pneumatic compression devices whenever possible, as pneumoperitoneum enhances lower extremity venous stasis and pregnancy induced a hypercoagulable state
4. Monitor fetal and uterine status, and use maternal end-tidal CO_2 and/or arterial blood gas (ABG)
5. Protect uterus with a lead shield if intraoperative cholangiography is possible. Use fluoroscopy selectively.
6. Attain abdominal access using an open technique, as the gravid uterus is enlarged
7. Shift the uterus off the inferior vena cava by using dependent positioning/lateral tilt
8. Minimize pneumoperitoneum pressures (8–12 mm Hg) and do not exceed 15 mm Hg

From Lu E, Curet M, El-Sayed Y, et al. Medical versus surgical management of biliary tract disease in pregnancy. *Am J Surg.* 2004;188:755–759, with permission.

Delivery Considerations

- Optimal maternal and infant outcome depends on planning for contingencies.
- Action items that might impact care when managing pregnant trauma or surgery patients are:
  - Admit the mother to a facility able to provide appropriate specialty care, including neonatology and neonatal intensive care unit (NICU) care.
  - Provide level I trauma center care for any gravid trauma patient whenever possible.
  - Ensure immediate availability of equipment for emergency delivery.
    - This includes all items for infant resuscitation, such as warmer bed, oxygen, endotracheal tubes, suction, other supplies, and emergency medications.
  - Plan for adequate staff to address obstetric issues, including fetal monitoring and/or emergency delivery.
  - Plan for adequate nursing care for perioperative needs on labor and delivery ward.
  - Ensure that clear instructions designate which providers or specialty services are responsible for various aspects of patient care.
  - Display contact information for the various providers prominently in patient medical record, in case emergency evaluation and treatment is necessary.
  - Encourage impeccable communication among specialists.
  - Obtain consultations early, and document recommendations or treatment plans.
  - Clearly indicate plans for fetal assessment and whether or not intervention is planned for indications, such as emergent cesarean in the event of nonreassuring fetal heart rate patterns.
  - Delivery timing and route may be individualized.
    - In general, delivery at full term (≥37 weeks) is the goal.
    - Cesarean reserved for usual clinical indications, with the notable exception of the perimortem patient (Table 64.5)
  - Typical trauma care team for a gravid patient includes:
    - Emergency room physician
    - Emergency room nurse
    - Trauma surgeon
    - Obstetrician
    - OB nurse
    - Anesthesiology
    - Pediatrician available
    - NICU or nursery nurse available
    - Operating room team on standby

Perimortem Cesarean

- Intact survival of a fetus is most likely when cesarean delivery is accomplished within 5 minutes of cardiac arrest.
- In 38 cases of perimortem cesarean, there were 34 surviving infants.
  - Time of delivery was available for 25 cases.
  - 12 of 25 (48%) were delivered within 5 minutes, and 9 of these 12 infants had no neurologic deficits on follow-up.
  - Of 20 perimortem cesareans with resuscitable causes, 13 mothers were revived and discharged from the hospital in good condition.

Maternal Brain Death

- Rarely maternal brain death is identified in a pregnant woman while somatic support has been maintained and the fetus remains alive.
  - Determination must be made as to whether to deliver the fetus immediately, to initiate supportive care to allow further fetal maturation, or to allow the fetus to die as the mother is removed from mechanical ventilation.
  - Immediate delivery when gestational age is consistent with neonatal survival is preferred.
  - It is possible to support the mother and previable fetus until fetal maturation allows for neonatal survival.
  - Somatic support can be provided for extended periods with no apparent neonatal or pediatric sequelae.

Ethical Decision Making

- According to the American College of Obstetricians and Gynecologists (ACOG) Ethical Guidelines, "Every reasonable effort should be made to protect the fetus, but the pregnant woman's autonomy should be respected. . . . Intervention against the wishes of a pregnant woman is rarely if ever acceptable."
- In a patient who is incapacitated, state laws vary with respect to who may serve as a surrogate decision maker.
  - Designees should base their decisions on the values and wishes of the patient, which may or may not have previously been stated in writing.
  - If there is no consensus about who should be designated, the advice of an ethics committee should be considered.

DOMESTIC VIOLENCE AWARENESS

- Women who experience physical violence are at higher risk for pregnancy loss and low-birth-weight infants

---

TABLE 64.5

INDICATIONS FOR EMERGENT CESAREAN

Emergent cesarean may be warranted in the following circumstances:
  Fetal heart tones are present (there is a living fetus)
  The fetus is at a viable gestational age (≥23 to 24 weeks)
  Adequate equipment and personnel are available to perform cesarean
  Adequate equipment and personnel are available for neonatal resuscitation
  Lack of response to maternal cardiopulmonary resuscitation (CPR) within 4 minutes (discussed in text)
  Persistent nonreassuring fetal heart rate (FHR) pattern is present—examples include fetal bradycardia, prolonged decelerations, or repetitive late decelerations
  Deteriorating maternal condition—cardiovascular instability
  Direct uterine or fetal injury

- Among 949 women surveyed, low birth weight was increased in those reporting verbal abuse (7.6% vs. 5.1%).
- Neonatal deaths more common among those with physical abuse (1.5% vs. 0.2%).
- 94 women who declined interview had higher rates of low-birth-weight infants (12.8%), preterm birth (5.3% vs. 1.2%), abruption (7.4% vs. 2.2%), and NICU admission (7.4% vs. 2.2%) than those reporting no abuse.

- Battered women are commonly reported to seek medical services at eight times the rate of other women, but they are rarely identified or referred for services.
- Should a patient indicate that domestic violence is a concern, assistance is available from the National Domestic Violence Hotline, 1-800-799-SAFE. This 24-hour, toll-free hotline provides information and referrals from anywhere in the United States.

CHAPTER 65 ■ FETAL MONITORING CONCERNS

IMMEDIATE CONCERNS

- Immediate issues to be evaluated when caring for a pregnant woman include:
  - Viability of the fetus
  - Gestational age of the fetus
  - Assessment of the fetal condition
- Determination of fetal viability is the first priority in the initial assessment
  - Diagnosis of fetal demise eliminates it as a confounding factor in decisions regarding maternal treatment.
  - Confirmation of a live fetus indicates a need to avoid teratogenic agents and optimize oxygen delivery to the placenta.
- Estimation of gestational age is an important factor to establish early.
  - If pregnancy is near term and nonobstetric surgical treatment is indicated, delivery of the fetus prior to such treatment may be warranted.
  - Earliest gestational age at which neonatal survival may occur is around 23 weeks.
    - Survival without significant morbidity becomes more likely at later gestational ages.
- Fetal assessment is dependent on the current gestational age.
  - Early gestational ages, assessment includes only documentation of fetal cardiac activity
  - Later gestational ages, the goal of fetal assessment and monitoring is:
    - Determination of adequacy of fetal oxygenation
    - Alerting the physician to potential hypoxia and/or fetal compromise

FETAL OXYGENATION

- The intervillous space is where maternal blood bathes the fetal chorionic villi and where fetal-[MB1]maternal and maternal-fetal exchange occurs.
  - Characterized by low pressure, but a pressure differential exists and ensures adequate circulation

- Placenta a low-resistance organ, and, accordingly, the pressure differential across the intervillous space is small
- The vascular resistance of the maternal arteries governs the rate of flow into and across the intervillous space.
- During uterine contractions venous pressure increases and causes cessation of flow into the intervillous space.
- Placenta serves as main organ of gas and nutrient exchange for the fetus
  - Oxygen extracted at the fetal–maternal interface serves fetus and placenta
  - Highly metabolic organ uses as much, and possibly more, of the total oxygen and nutrients as the fetus to maintain its own growth and metabolism
- Oxygen consumption remains constant over a wide range of changes in oxygen delivery and decreases only when extraction is maximal and delivery is further reduced.
  - 50% reduction in uterine blood flow is compensated by an increase in umbilical blood flow and an increase in oxygen extraction to maintain oxygen delivery with no change in fetal oxygen consumption
  - Compensatory mechanism adequate only with short-term reductions in uterine blood flow
  - Critical point exists below which oxygen uptake becomes dependent on oxygen delivery
  - Long-term reductions result in decreased consumption secondary to the decrease in delivery.
  - Chronic decrease in oxygen consumption leads to decreases in both fetal growth and fetal activity in an effort to conserve oxygen for cellular homeostasis
  - Where fetal oxygen consumption is decreased, maternal administration of oxygen will increase fetal oxygen consumption to near-normal range.
  - Placenta carries oxygenated blood to the fetus via the umbilical vein.
  - Deoxygenated blood is carried back to the placenta via the two umbilical arteries.
  - Human fetal umbilical venous PO_2 is around 30 mm Hg.
    - Adequate oxygen delivered to fetal tissues
      - Facilitated by the high fetal cardiac output, relative to its body size, and the affinity of fetal hemoglobin for oxygen

- Transfer of carbon dioxide across the placenta is limited by the diffusion capacity.
  - Placenta is highly permeable to carbon dioxide.
  - Alterations in maternal PCO_2 content can lead to disturbances in the fetal PCO_2 content.
    - If maternal PCO_2 is abnormally elevated, fetal transfer is hindered and will result in elevations of fetal PCO_2 and fetal acidosis.
- Glucose is a major energy source for the fetus.
  - Primarily obtains glucose from maternal blood
  - Supplemented by its own glycogenolysis
  - Fetal glucose deprivation causes fetal hypoglycemia, which results in an increase in the maternal–fetal glucose gradient and thus increased glucose transport across the placenta.
    - Glucose transport is limited by the availability of transport proteins in the placenta as well as maternal blood glucose levels.
    - This is facilitated transport, different from simple diffusion
    - Severe glucose deprivation and the resultant decrease in placental uptake may result in fetal growth abnormalities.
    - Chronic glucose deprivation will decrease glucose utilization and increase glycogenolysis and gluconeogenesis by the breakdown of fetal protein.
      - Net protein loss results in fetal growth disturbances and ultimately may lead to growth restriction.
  - Transport of waste includes lactate
- With a drop in oxygen supply and a change to anaerobic metabolism, the fetus begins to produce large amounts of lactate.
  - In this situation, the placenta becomes a major source of lactate clearance from the fetal circulation.
- The placenta, in response to decreased glucose supply, will decrease its consumption of glucose and increase its consumption of lactate to account for the glucose deficit.

FETAL MONITORING

- Electronic fetal monitoring, introduced in the 1960s, has become ubiquitous in labor and delivery units in economically developed countries.
  - Typically used at any gestational age at which *ex utero* survival is possible
  - Requires very little except for an experienced interpreter
    - Results in continuous tracing of the fetal heart rate (FHR), coupled with a tracing of uterine activity
  - Regulation of the fetal heart rate is governed by a complex interplay of the sympathetic and parasympathetic nervous systems.
  - Fetal heart rate variability results from the constant push-pull of these two systems.
  - FHR tracing reactivity is defined by the presence of FHR accelerations.
    - Transient increases in baseline fetal heart rate due to fetal movement
    - Absence of FHR variability for periods of more than 1 hour, especially in the presence of FHR decelerations, is associated with fetal academia.
  - Decelerations occur when the FHR falls below the baseline heart rate and are classified according to their location in relation to uterine contractions and their appearance.
    - Different types of decelerations caused by different mechanisms
    - **Early Decelerations:** Begin at the onset of uterine contractions and appear to mirror the contraction (Fig. 65.1)
      - Caused by pressure on the fetal head, resulting in alteration in cerebral blood flow and stimulation of the vagal center

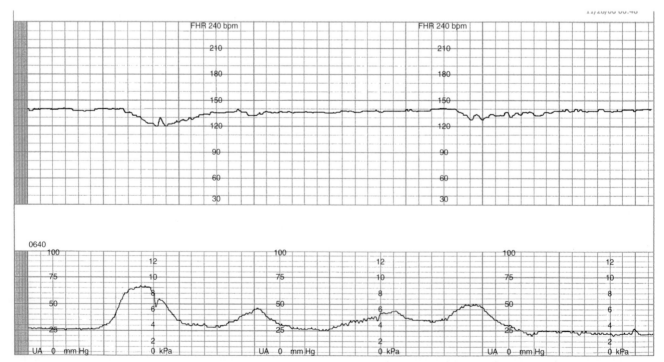

FIGURE 65.1. Early decelerations mirror the contraction and are not associated with fetal compromise.

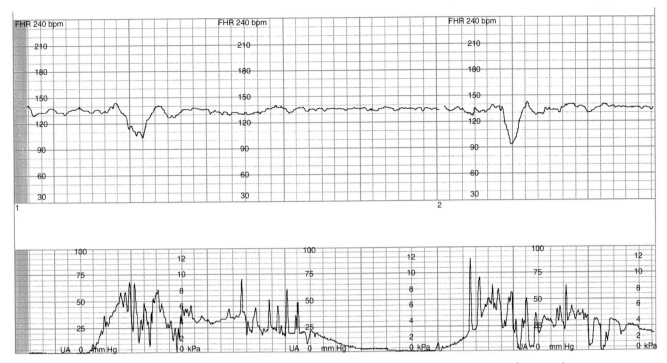

FIGURE 65.2. Variable decelerations occur at various times in relation to the contraction and are a result of transient umbilical cord compression.

○ Generally are not associated with other ominous findings and are not associated with fetal hypoxia, acidosis, or low Apgar scores
- **Variable Decelerations:** Caused by intermittent umbilical cord compression
  ○ Occur most often during uterine contractions, but are seen at variable times in relation to uterine contractions and even in absence of contractions (Fig. 65.2)
  ○ Physiologic basis for decelerations results in either a chemoreceptor or a baroreceptor response due to:
    – Fetal hypertension and stimulation of the baroreceptors
    – Fall in fetal PO_2, leading to chemoreceptor activation and stimulation of vagal activity
  ○ Repetitive moderate or severe variable decelerations may indicate fetal compromise (Table 65.1)
- **Late Decelerations:** Occur late in relation to the uterine contraction. Their onset begins after contraction begins, and they resolve after contraction resolution (Fig. 65.3)
  ○ Occur as a result of decreased uteroplacental oxygen delivery to the fetus

– Intermittent hypoxia, sometimes associated with fetal acidemia, results in fetal hypertension, leading to chemoreceptor and baroreceptor response
– In the presence of fetal acidemia, response may also be mediated by direct myocardial depression
  ○ Many clinical causes of late decelerations:
    – Maternal hypotension
    – Decreased uterine blood flow
  ○ Persistence of late decelerations, especially without fetal variability, is an ominous sign of fetal compromise.
- Other fetal heart rate patterns seen in presence of fetal central nervous system (CNS) dysfunction
- Normal fetus may have episodes of decreased heart rate variability of 30 to 40 minutes due to sleep
  - In CNS dysfunction, may see persistently diminished variability or sinusoidal pattern
    - Patterns resemble a sine wave, with a frequency of 3 to 5 cycles per minute and an absence of fetal heart rate variability
    - Severe fetal anemia another potential cause of sinusoidal fetal heart rate tracing
    - Unstable, or wandering, baseline heart rates also may be seen

TABLE 65.1

CLASSIFICATION OF VARIABLE DECELERATIONS

Classification	Nadir	Duration
Mild variable	100 bpm	<30 seconds
Moderate variable	60 bpm	<60 seconds
Severe variable	<60 bpm or drop of >60 bpm from baseline	60 seconds

ANTENATAL TESTING

- Certain situations indicate periodic assessments of fetal well-being in antepartum period
  - Several methods require only electronic fetal monitoring
  - Some involve use of ultrasound

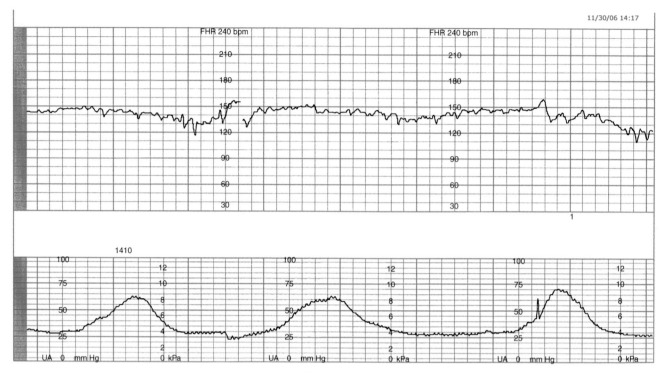

FIGURE 65.3. Late decelerations occur late in relation to the contraction and may be a sign of fetal compromise.

- Primary indication for most aspects of fetal surveillance is the need to evaluate a potentially viable fetus where there is a concern for:
  - Fetal hypoxia
  - Death
  - To assess likelihood of stillbirth during subsequent week
- The goal of fetal surveillance is to identify early fetal hypoxia and prevent perinatal asphyxia
- Most tests of fetal well-being lack specificity and have a low positive-predictive value
  - Used because of their high negative-predictive value

Nonstress Test

- Nonstress testing involves fetal heart rate monitoring for a period of 20 to 40 minutes
  - Underlying premise for this test relates to the fact that a nonacidotic, neurologically intact fetus will have fetal heart rate accelerations in response to fetal movement.
    - Presence within a 20-minute window of two fetal heart rate accelerations lasting at least 15 seconds, peaking at least 15 beats per minute above the baseline, characterizes a reactive nonstress test and is reassuring
    - Absence of these accelerations requires further testing or delivery, depending on the gestational age
      - Less than 32 weeks gestational age may not have reactive nonstress tests despite the absence of compromise
- Nonstress test is simple to perform and generally is required on admission for initial evaluation of fetal well-being.
- A reactive test is highly reassuring, with a false-negative rate of 1.9/1,000.

Contraction Stress Test

- Can be used as a follow-up test to a nonreactive nonstress test or used alone for fetal evaluation
  - Requires at least three spontaneous or elicited contractions during a 10-minute window
  - Evaluates the fetal heart response to these contractions
  - Contraindicated in significantly preterm gestations and those in whom labor is contraindicated
  - Underlying premise involves idea that fetal oxygenation will transiently worsen in presence of uterine contractions
    - In compromised fetus, this will result in late decelerations
    - Interpreted based on the presence or absence of late decelerations
      - Positive contraction stress test is one in which late decelerations occur with at least 50% of contractions and generally indicates that delivery is warranted
      - Negative test result with no late decelerations is highly reassuring, with a false-negative rate of only 0.3/1,000.

Biophysical Profile

- Consists of a nonstress test and an ultrasound evaluation of several parameters
- Performed as a follow-up test to a nonreactive, nonstress test
- Can be used as a form of surveillance on its own
- Attempts to evaluate the fetus in terms of acute and chronic compromise
  - Nonstress test is one of the parameters used for evaluation.

TABLE 65.2

COMPONENTS AND SCORING OF THE BIOPHYSICAL PROFILE

Parameter	Score (= 2)[a]	Score (= 0)[a]
Nonstress test	Reactive with more than 2 accelerations in 20-minute time period	Nonreactive
Fetal breathing	At least one episode of fetal breathing for >30 sec	<30 sec of breathing
Fetal tone	At least one episode of active extension and flexion	No flexion/extension
Gross movement	Three or more limb or body movements in 30 min	Less than three movements in 30 min
Amniotic fluid	Single vertical pocket >2 cm	Largest fluid pocket <2 cm

[a]Score is 2 or 0 for each parameter.

- Ultrasound examination seeks to evaluate the amount of amniotic fluid, fetal tone, gross body movements, and fetal breathing movements (Table 65.2).
  - Final score derived from these various assessments
  - Intervention based on both score and gestational age
  - No contraindications to its use
  - Entire evaluation takes <1 hour to complete
  - High correlation with low scores and fetal compromise
  - Best predictor of perinatal mortality appears to be the absence of fetal tone
  - Normal biophysical profile score of 8 or 10 is very reassuring—the false-negative rate is 0.8/1,000.

Doppler Velocimetry

- Accomplished with the use of color Doppler during an ultrasound examination
- Umbilical artery most widely interrogated vessel for fetal surveillance
- Normal fetuses, the umbilical artery has a high diastolic velocity due to low placental resistance
  - With placental injury or pathology, the umbilical artery resistance may be increased.
    - As resistance rises, diastolic flow decreases.
    - With high levels of resistance, diastolic flow may cease or become reversed.
    - Reversed end diastolic flow in the umbilical artery is associated with significant perinatal morbidity and mortality.
- Doppler interrogation of the middle cerebral artery also has been shown to be of benefit in certain situations.
  - Setting of significant fetal anemia, the blood is thinner and the cardiac ejection fraction increases.
    - Results in an increase in the velocity of blood through the middle cerebral artery
    - Periodic middle cerebral artery interrogation is replacing the assessment of amniotic fluid for monitoring fetuses at risk of anemia

ADJUNCTS TO INTRAPARTUM FETAL HEART RATE MONITORING

Fetal Scalp Sampling

- To delineate fetuses with decelerations and acidemia from those with normal pH, fetal scalp sampling may be performed.
  - Accomplished by taking a blood sample from the fetal scalp
  - Normal fetal scalp pH is 7.25 to 7.35.
    - Values below 7.20 considered acidotic
    - Can be performed only in the presence of labor with ruptured membranes
    - Invaluable tool in the assessment of fetal acidosis
  - Evaluated fetal scalp stimulation and its relation to fetal pH
    - Fetal heart rate acceleration in response to digital stimulation of the scalp reliably have a pH >7.20.
    - Of fetuses without accelerations, 50% have a normal pH, whereas the remaining 50% are noted to be acidotic.
    - Digital stimulation of the fetal scalp can be performed when the membranes are intact, requiring a cervix that is dilated.

ST Segment Analysis

- One of newest advancements is the ability to combine standard fetal heart rate assessment with an automated analysis of the fetal electrocardiogram, ST waveform analysis.
- Fetal ST segment analysis is based on the observation that fetal hypoxia results in characteristic changes in the ST segment as well as the T wave on the fetal electrocardiogram.
  - There is a reduction in neonates born with metabolic acidosis when using ST segment analysis.

CHAPTER 66 ■ THE OBESE SURGICAL PATIENT

- In the economically developed world, the incidence of obesity is rising at epidemic proportions.
  - University medical centers report 25% of routine surgical patients are obese.
  - At least 10% of all patients are morbidly obese (MO).
  - Estimates that incidence rate of morbidly obese patients requiring nonsurgical intensive care treatment approaches 14 cases per 1,000 intensive care unit (ICU) admissions annually
  - Bariatric surgical procedures in the United States increased from 37,000 cases in 2000 up to 200,000 in 2006.
  - The critically ill morbidly obese surgical patient presents the critical care team with many unique problems.
    - Eightfold higher mortality rate after blunt trauma than nonobese patients presenting with the same diagnosis
    - Significant increases in length of ICU stay, mortality, and duration of mechanical ventilation
    - Pathophysiologic consequences of obesity involve all major organ systems
  - Diabetes mellitus and hyperlipidemia contribute to chronic morbidity in the obese.
    - Main concerns for the intensivist, anesthesiologist, and surgeon have been the same for over three decades: the derangements of the cardiopulmonary system

CARDIOVASCULAR (CV) CONSIDERATIONS IN THE MO

- CV disease reported in:
  - 37% of adults with a body mass index (BMI) >30 kg/m^2
  - 21% with a BMI of 25 to 30 kg/m^2
  - 10% in those with a BMI <25 kg/m^2
  - *Obesity*—a BMI ≥30 kg/m^2—an independent risk factor for the development of hypertension.
  - Framingham Heart Study suggests that 65% of the risk for hypertension in women and 78% of the risk in men related to obesity.
  - Mortality rates were reported to be 3.9 times greater in the overweight group versus the normal weight group participating in the Framingham study.
  - Chances of myocardial infarction, heart failure, stroke, and kidney disease are all greater as a patient's blood pressure increases.
  - Many obese individuals also suffer from metabolic syndrome.
    - With strong association as precursor in development of diabetes, cardiovascular disease, and increased mortality rates from cardiovascular disorders
  - Also a 5% increased risk of heart failure for men and 7% for women associated with each unit of increase in body mass.

Preoperative Considerations

Pathophysiology

- In MO patients
  - Blood volume, cardiac output, systemic and pulmonary artery pressures, and left and right ventricular pressures all elevated.
  - Manifest clinically as arterial hypertension
  - With advancing age, may note ischemic heart disease and right–left heart failure.
    - Incidence of severe pre-existing CV disease in MO patients scheduled for elective bariatric surgery reported to be as great as 20%.
    - The complex interaction of hypertension, ischemic heart disease, and pulmonary hypertension contribute to development of global cardiac dysfunction and exacerbates congestive heart failure.
    - Clinical situation is referred to as *obesity cardiomyopathy*.

Arterial Hypertension

- Pathogenesis of obesity-related hypertension complex
  - A continuous relationship between BMI and systolic/diastolic blood pressures
  - Blood pressure is normally regulated by a series of feedback loops:
    - Baroreceptors
    - Vasoactive hormones
      - Renin, angiotensin, aldosterone
      - Catecholamines
  - Derangement in any of these feedback loops may lead to hypertension.
  - Many factors act together to promote vasoconstriction, sodium retention, and volume overload in obesity (Table 66.1).
    - Changes cause glomerular injury, ultimately leading to glomerulosclerosis.
    - Prolonged obesity may lead to a gradual loss of nephron function that worsens with time and exacerbates hypertension.
    - Hypertension contributes to a pressure overload of the heart and expansion of extracellular and blood volume combining to create a volume overload.
  - Other variables that may also lead to hypertension in obese patients by stimulating sympathetic activity and vasoconstriction include:
    - Leptin
    - Free fatty acids
    - Insulin
  - Obesity-induced insulin resistance and endothelial dysfunction may act as amplifiers of the vasoconstrictor response.
  - Obstructive sleep apnea (OSA) is more prevalent in obese patients.

TABLE 66.1

FACTORS THAT ACT TOGETHER TO PROMOTE VASOCONSTRICTION, SODIUM RETENTION, AND VOLUME OVERLOAD IN THE OBESE PATIENT

- Elevated glomerular filtration rate, an elevated renal blood flow, and exhibiting delayed urinary sodium excretion in response to the saline load[a]
- Increased renal sympathetic nervous activity, which directly promotes tubular reabsorption of sodium at the proximal and distal tubules[b]
- The renin–angiotensin–aldosterone system is activated, which contributes to sodium retention and an increase in extracellular volume, despite an elevated blood pressure[c]
- Natriuretic peptide levels are low, both at basal levels and also in response to salt loading[d]
- Hyperinsulinemia directly promotes the tubular absorption of sodium.[e] *Compensatory mechanisms in the obese for overcoming increased sodium reabsorption include renal vasodilation, an increased glomerular filtration rate, and a higher blood pressure.*

[a]Data from Montani JP, Antic V, Yang Z, et al. Pathways from obesity to hypertension: from the perspective of a vicious triangle. *Int J Obes Relat Metab Disord.* 2002;26(Suppl 2):S28–S38.
[b]DiBona GF, Kopp UC. Neural control of renal function. *Physiol Rev.* 1997;77:75–197.
[c]Engeli S, Sharma AM. The renin-angiotensin system and natriuretic peptides in obesity-associated hypertension. *J Mol Med.* 2001;79:21–29.
[d]Dessi-Fulgheri P, Sarzani R, Tamburrini P, et al. Plasma atrial natriuretic peptide and natriuretic peptide receptor gene expression in adipose tissue of normotensive and hypertensive obese patients. *J Hypertens.* 1997;15:1695–1699.
[e]Endre T, Mattiasson I, Berglund G, et al. Insulin and renal sodium retention in hypertension-prone men. *Hypertension.* 1994;23:313–319.

- Leads to periods of apnea and hypoxia, triggering a chemoreceptor response, which causes sympathetic activation

Ischemic Heart Disease (IHD)
- Obesity a recognized risk factor for IHD
  - Risk proportional to duration of obesity and distribution of fat
  - Habitually overweight individual less likely to be at risk than individuals who exhibit continuous weight gain
  - Central distribution of fat more at risk than individuals with a peripheral distribution
  - Hypertension, diabetes, hypercholesterolemia, and increased levels of low-density lipoproteins (LDLs) further increase the risk of coronary stenosis.
  - Nevertheless, more than 40% of obese patients with angina do not have significant coronary artery disease.
  - Angina would then be attributable to the oxygen supply/demand imbalance due to cardiac hypertrophy and other factors.
  - In MO, myocardial oxygen consumption is higher than in normal-weight adults.
    - Ventricular cavity dimension is enlarged due to a chronically augmented preload.
    - Enhanced sympathetic activity and subsequent arterial hypertension and/or increased heart rate promote higher wall tension and ventricular systolic stress.

- In addition, the ventricular wall is commonly hypertrophic.
- With chronic hypoxemia (pickwickian syndrome, obesity hypoventilation syndrome, and obstructive sleep apnea syndrome) secondary polycythemia and, subsequently, elevated blood viscosity develop.
- Due to the higher blood viscosity, contractility is augmented, which consequently increases myocardial oxygen requirements.

Cardiac Failure
- Risk of heart failure of 5% for men and 7% for women per each unit of increase in body mass
  - Linear relationship between body weight and cardiac weight gain attributed to concentric and eccentric hypertrophy
    - Secondary to pressure overload, due to arterial hypertension and possibly increased blood viscosity
  - Circulating blood volume, plasma volume, and cardiac output increase proportionately with rising weight.
  - With a fat mass of 50 kg, blood flow to this fat mass accounts for an extra cardiac output of 1.5 to 2.0 L/minute.
    - Resulting in both ventricular enlargement and an increase in stroke volume
  - Hypertrophy contributes to a reduction in cardiac compliance and left ventricular diastolic function, which leads to increased left ventricular end-diastolic pressure and possible pulmonary edema.
  - Decrease in midwall fiber shortening and a decrease in ejection fraction may become evident in developing obesity cardiomyopathy.
  - Right ventricle can also exhibit hypertrophy secondary to pulmonary hypertension due to obstructive sleep apnea and subsequent chronic hypoxemia and hypercapnia.

Preoperative Evaluation and Optimization for Surgery

Arterial Hypertension
- Urgent and emergent surgeries should be evaluated on a case-by-case basis, and aggressive control of blood pressure in the perioperative period is vital.
- Acute hypertensive episodes and hypertensive emergencies approached as in the nonobese
- Meticulous and adequate monitoring
- Careful drug titration required due to the particular hemodynamic lability of this population
- Pharmacokinetics and dynamics might be altered
- Measurement of blood pressure may be difficult, even to the point of deciding where to make the measurement.
  - Obese individuals—especially women—tend to have a conical shape of the upper arm, termed *gynoid obesity.*
    - Accurate measurement of blood pressure is difficult
    - Alternative is to place the cuff around the forearm for more predictable cuff pressures
    - Increasing arm circumference associated with miscalculation of blood pressure if standard-length cuffs used
- Appropriate-sized cuff that encompasses at least 80% of the arm should be used
- If these maneuvers fail to result in adequate and reliable measurements, invasive blood pressure monitoring should be considered.

Ischemic Heart Disease and Cardiac Failure

- No specific cardiac risk index has been proposed for obese patients.
- Preoperative cardiac assessment of obese patients follows same sequence as for lean patients
  - Careful appraisal of arterial hypertension and its consequences
  - Focus on assessing both cardiac function and the presence and severity of ischemic heart disease
    - Evaluation of cardiac function by clinical signs can be extremely difficult in the obese so objective evaluation of ejection fraction and cardiac function by echocardiography and/or left ventriculography usually necessary
    - The American College of Cardiology/American Heart Association (ACC/AHA) recommendation for preoperative noninvasive evaluation of LV function includes patients with:
      - Current or poorly controlled heart failure
      - History of heart failure
      - Dyspnea of unknown origin—an extremely frequent finding in this population
    - Evaluation for ischemic heart disease requires stress testing
      - No consensus on which type of stress test is optimal
      - Whether or not patients can exercise sufficiently to obtain 85% of predicted maximal heart rate
        - If they cannot, then a pharmacologic stress test is better indicated (e.g., stress echocardiography after dobutamine or atropine administration [DSE] or a dipyridamole thallium nuclear imaging study [DTS])
      - Positive stress test results will require coronary angiography
  - If cardiac catheterization is indicated, patient weight has to be taken into account due to some tables weight limits as low as 300 lb (136.4 kg)
    - Cardiac catheterization is considered safe in these patients
    - 55% of the time, cardiac catheterization results in negative findings
    - When positive, medical management, interventional cardiology therapy, or even cardiac bypass surgery may be indicated
  - When ischemic heart disease identified and severity quantified, three therapeutic options are available prior to elective noncardiac surgery:
    - Revascularization by surgery (coronary artery bypass graft [CABG])
    - Revascularization by percutaneous coronary intervention (PCI)
    - Optimized medical management (typically with β-blockers or α_2-agonists)
- No irrefutable evidence that indications for preoperative cardiac revascularization are any different for obese patients than for nonobese patients

Coronary Artery Bypass Grafting

- Still a controversial topic
- Moderately and morbidly obese patients have a higher rate of deep sternal wound infection, renal failure, prolonged postoperative hospital stay, and operative mortality after CABG.
- Guided by the patient's cardiac condition:
  - Unstable angina
  - Left main coronary artery disease
    - Three-vessel disease
    - Decreased left ventricle (LV) function
    - Left anterior descending artery disease
    - And by added risk of the coronary intervention and the potential consequences of delaying the noncardiac surgery for recovery after the cardiac intervention
- When indicated, patients undergoing coronary revascularization prior to major-risk noncardiac surgery do better postoperatively
  - Comparing this population of preoperatively revascularized patients with those medically managed suggests that the latter patient group had a mortality rate two times higher than the former.

Percutaneous Coronary Intervention

- Evidence suggests that patients who underwent angioplasty prior to elective noncardiac surgery had better outcomes.
- Strongly suggested that elective noncardiac surgery should be delayed for 4 to 6 weeks after PCI with stenting to allow for complete endothelialization of stent and completion of aggressive GP IIb/IIIa inhibitor antiplatelet therapy
- Drug-eluting stents may obviate the need for such prolonged systemic anticoagulation, thus allowing patients to undergo noncardiac surgery sooner.
- Complication rate of PCI in obese patients not reported different from that of nonobese individuals

Medical Management

- Perioperative use of β-blockers efficacious in reducing perioperative morbidity and mortality
- ACC/AHA guidelines recommend initiating β-blockers as early as possible prior to high-risk surgery and titrating the patient's heart rate to 60 bpm.
- Perioperative β-blocker use is recommended for patients with one or more Revised Cardiac Index risk factors despite a negative stress test and for patients with two minor risk factors, even with a good functional status and/or a negative noninvasive stress test.
- Prophylactic role may decrease intraoperative ischemia
- General consensus appears to be that if β-blockers are indicated perioperatively, they should be given not only intraoperatively but, more appropriately, they should be initiated during the preoperative period and—except in the presence of significant contraindications—should be continued through the postoperative period.
- Pharmacokinetics of β-blockers are affected by obesity, and there exists significant pharmacodynamic variability.
  - Dosage of β-blockers should be initiated based on lean body mass and then titrated until the desired clinical effect is achieved.

Intraoperative Considerations

Mechanics

- Surgical beds available that accommodate patients weighing as much as 500 kg
  - These patients require tremendous preparation on behalf of the operative staff
  - Even with appropriate beds, at high risk for falling during sudden motion

- Extremely dangerous to the patient and the supporting staff alike
  - Institution of a lift team
  - Availability of both "bean" bags and bed extensions in order to keep the folds of pannus stable are of the utmost importance to the surgical team
  - Finally, institutional investments in lifting equipment such as ceiling-mounted lifts and beds that oscillate and/or transform into chairs may be necessary to fully deploy the necessary mechanical advantage to care for the obese patient.

Rhabdomyolysis

- Rhabdomyolysis often described in obese patients
  - Generally follows prolonged operations
  - Presents as dark urine, representing muscle necrosis from groups on the flanks or buttock
    - Also termed *pressure-induced myoglobinuria*
    - More commonly noted among patients with diabetes mellitus
    - Generally attributed to lying on a hard surface
    - Frequently associated with an exaggerated lithotomy position in the operating room (OR)
    - Treatment:
      ○ Initiate aggressive hydration
      ○ Monitor creatine phosphokinase (CPK)
        – If CPK exceeds 5,000 IU/L, staff must initiate diuresis with mannitol and alkalinize the urine with sodium bicarbonate
      ○ Acute renal failure may develop, but recovery is generally expected

Anesthetic Technique

- No unquestionable evidence that one or another anesthetic technique is best for MO
  - Total intravenous anesthesia (TIVA) and inhalational, regional, and combined general/epidural or general/spinal anesthetics have been used safely
- Selecting one technique over another will depend on:
  - Patient's clinical status
  - Type of surgery the patient requires
  - Expertise of the senior anesthesiologist
  - Availability of institutional resources
  - Patient's verbal and/or written requests and consent
- The most frequent and prominent risks of MO patient undergoing surgery listed are in Table 66.2.

TABLE 66.2

MOST FREQUENT AND PROMINENT RISKS OF THE MORBIDLY OBESE PATIENT UNDERGOING SURGERY

- Pulmonary aspiration of gastric contents
- Difficult mask ventilation and tracheal intubation
- Rapid development of hypoxemia after apnea
- Pulmonary atelectasis
- Hemodynamic instability
- Decreased ability to deal with the physiologic responses to stressful situations (i.e., hyperglycemia, hypertension, cardiac failure, arrhythmias, and myocardial ischemia)
- Delayed recovery
- Postoperative respiratory dysfunction
- Deep venous thrombosis

- Basic anesthetic goals should be:
  - Hemodynamically smooth and rapid induction
  - Rapid access and securing of the airway
  - Prominent attention paid to hemodynamic stability
  - A high level of analgesia to avoid increments in catecholamine activity
  - Rapid recovery and early ambulation

Postoperative Considerations

Pathophysiologic Principles for a Rational Therapeutic Approach

- Obesity has been likened to "exercise," that is, a *constant* state of "exercise"
- MO patient's cardiovascular system continuously overdemanded, even at rest, mainly because of chronic intravascular volume overload, blood hyperviscosity, and sympathetic hyperactivity.
- These are components of a "dysfunctional compensating mechanism"
  - Tries to satisfy the increased metabolic rate imposed by the excessive adipose tissue
  - Additional increase in CO promoted by any perioperative stress may markedly increase LV filling pressure, often exceeding threshold for pulmonary edema
- Obstructive sleep apnea syndrome (OSAS) and obesity hypoventilation syndrome (OHS) may affect the right heart cavities.
  ○ Heart of MO patient may have less tolerance to any kind of cardiovascular stress:
    – Hypovolemia
    – Hypervolemia
    – Hypertension
    – Hypotension
  ○ At a higher risk of organ failure

Importance of Coupled Cardiorespiratory Function

- Ventilation/perfusion (V/Q) mismatch is a prominent mechanism that can trigger respiratory and subsequent cardiac dysfunction in MO surgical patient.
- In mechanically ventilated MO patients, airway pressure may be elevated.
- MO associated with volume and pressure overload
  - Volume load conditions may fluctuate according to patient positioning
  - Changing position from the "physiologically ideal" reverse Trendelenburg to the supine position can significantly increase venous blood return to the heart
    - Resultant augmentation of cardiac output, pulmonary capillary wedge pressure, and mean pulmonary artery pressure potentially increases the risk of acute heart failure.
    - Maneuver will increase airway pressure as well due to the increased weight of the chest
  - Compression of inferior vena cava (IVC) may reduce venous return to the heart
    - Thus a possible mechanism of hypotension
    - Can be avoided by lateral tilting OR table or ICU bed with a wedge under the patient
      ○ Similar to that during caesarean section to reduce the pressure of the gravid uterus on IVC

- Reverse Trendelenburg position significantly improves cardiac and respiratory performance
  - Should be maintained during the entire perioperative period unless there is a particular contraindication

Drug Dosing

- Distribution, metabolism, protein binding, and clearance of many drugs are altered by the physiologic changes associated with obesity.
  - Additionally patient's underlying disease may substantially influence the pharmacokinetic properties of drugs
  - Net pharmacologic alteration in a patient is often uncertain, especially in the MO
    - Nevertheless, for a number of drugs used in the ICU, toxicity may occur if the patients are dosed based on their actual, rather than ideal or adjusted, body weight:
      ○ Digoxin
      ○ Aminophylline
      ○ Aminoglycosides
      ○ Cyclosporine
    - For drug dosing, base drug calculations on ideal body weight (IBW) and adjust doses through meticulous monitoring

RESPIRATORY CONSIDERATIONS IN THE MORBIDLY OBESE

- Higher morbidity and mortality of hospitalized obese patients may be related to the increased pulmonary complications such as:
  - Atelectasis
  - Aspiration
  - Ventilatory failure
  - Pulmonary embolism
- There are significant physiologic changes associated with obesity:
  - Reduced lung volumes
  - Increased work of breathing
  - Alterations in control of breathing and gas exchange
- Factors involved include, but not limited to:
  - BMI
  - Patient's age
  - Duration of obesity
  - Fat distribution (central or peripheral)
  - Strong association of certain disorders such as OSAS, OHS, and pickwickian syndrome
- Obesity itself has a major detrimental impact on the respiratory system

Preoperative Considerations

Respiratory Disorders

- **Obstructive Sleep Apnea Syndrome:** MO the most common and major risk factor for OSAS
- Prevalence in general U.S. population is 2% to 4%
- Increases to 40% to 78% in MO
- 80% to 90% of U.S. sleep apnea sufferers are undiagnosed
- Detection of OSAS among obese surgical patients is vital for several reasons:

- Obese patients more sensitive to depressant effects of hypnotics and opioids
- Perioperative administration may lead to life-threatening respiratory complications in face of preexisting OSAS
- OSAS associated with difficult laryngoscopy and mask ventilation
- Obese patients have diminished expiratory reserve volume (ERV) with, consequently, reduced oxygen stores
  ○ Promotes faster development of desaturation after apnea
- If OSAS is present, these effects become exaggerated
- **Obesity Hypoventilation Syndrome:** Some obese patients suffer from a disorder characterized by chronic daytime hypoventilation
- Individuals typically extremely obese, with a BMI >40 kg/m^2
- Likelihood of OHS increases as the BMI increases
- OHS is associated with chronic daytime hypoxemia and hypercapnia
  - PaO_2 <65 mm Hg
  - Essential to find out if the obese patient suffers from chronic daytime hypoxemia
    ○ This is a better predictor of pulmonary hypertension and cor pulmonale than the presence and/or severity of OSAS
- **Pickwickian Syndrome:** Patients suffering from OHS who additionally have signs and symptoms of cor pulmonale are termed *pickwickian*—from the Charles Dickens novel, *The Pickwick Papers*
  - They have an increased perioperative morbidity and mortality
- **Respiratory Insufficiency:** Obesity per se not a common cause for chronic respiratory insufficiency
  - Significant respiratory dysfunction more common when chronic obstructive pulmonary disease (COPD) and obesity coexist
  - When respiratory insufficiency is present, impairment of gas exchange greater than expected from a simple summation of the alterations caused by each pathophysiologic process

Simple Obesity

- Obese patients with minimal or no coexisting pulmonary conditions classified as "simple" obesity patients
- Pathophysiology of simple obesity consists of:
  - Alterations in daytime gas exchange and pulmonary function
  - May result from compression and restriction of the chest wall and diaphragm by excess adipose tissue
  - ERV and functional residual capacity (FRC) are particularly affected, being reduced to 60% and 80% of normal, respectively
  - If ERV decreases below the alveolar closing volume:
    ○ Airway closure occurs during normal tidal breathing
    ○ Dependent alveoli are relatively or completely underventilated
    ○ Consequently, V/Q mismatch, pulmonary shunt, and daytime hypoxemia results
    ○ May see, in formerly obese patients after massive weight loss, a marked improvement in the PaO_2 and alveolar–arterial oxygen gradient; improvement directly proportional to increase in ERV
- Other mechanisms may further impair respiratory function
  - Sleep apnea in the obese is usually obstructive, secondary to airway narrowing from abundant peripharyngeal

adipose tissue, and an abnormal decrease of upper airway muscle tone during rapid eye movement (REM) sleep
- Hypopneic and apneic events lead to arousal from REM sleep, oxyhemoglobin desaturation, and sympathetic nervous system activation in response to hypoxemia
- May explain the strong association between OSA and systemic hypertension
- The precise pathophysiologic mechanism of OHS unclear
  - Of most importance is that vital capacity, reduced to 90% of normal in simple obesity, decreases to 60% of normal in OHS
  - Reflects profound and important decrement in lung volumes in OHS, as compared with simple obesity patients
  - One may see:
    – Marked increase in distal airway resistance
    – More profound abnormality in V/Q matching
    – More significant impact on the PaO_2
    – Larger A–a gradient in patients with OHS
  - Supine positioning further reduces lung volume and, as a result, increases the magnitude of all these alterations
  - Diaphragmatic function is also affected due to over-stretching and cephalad displacement, resulting from increased intra-abdominal pressure
  - All of these factors combined may lead to chronic respiratory muscle fatigue and the chronic hypoventilation characteristic of OHS

Venous Thromboembolism

- Perioperative venous thromboembolism (VTE) occurs in 0.2% to 2.4% of bariatric patients receiving thromboprophylaxis
  - American College of Chest Physicians Consensus Statement, obese patients in the ICU will generally fall into high or highest risk categories
    - Left untreated, risk of deep venous thrombosis (DVT) ranges from 20% to 80%
    - Risk of clinical pulmonary embolus (PE) ranges from 2% to 10%
    - Fatal PE occurs in 0.4% to 5% of patients
  - The obese population in surgical ICU requires thromboprophylaxis
    - Best regimen is not clear
    - Multiple variables are worthy of mention in regard to this matter:
      - Venous stasis ulcers are more common in the obese, and in turn, are associated with DVT
      - Prophylactic inferior vena cava filters can be considered, but may also be technically difficult in the heaviest patients
      - Sequential compression devices (SCDs) generally recognized as useful adjunct but may be limited by patient size
      - Adequacy of pedal pumps not clear
      - Unfractionated or low-molecular-weight heparins both viable options
        - Precise dosing regimens and duration of dosage have emerged largely from uncontrolled trials
        - Reports in the bariatric literature that 40 mg of enoxaparin every 12 hours may provide better thromboprophylaxis than 30 mg every 12 hours

Evaluation and Optimization for Surgery

- In simple obesity, preoperative assessment of respiratory function similar to that indicated in lean and healthy patients
- More extensive pulmonary function tests and preoperative treatment may be necessary for the obese patient who smokes or has pulmonary symptoms
- Elements of the history and physical examination can be more important than preoperative testing
- Obese patients who habitually snore and report daytime somnolence and/or have suffered breath interruptions during sleep should be evaluated with polysomnography, the definitive diagnostic test for OSAS
- MO and symptoms of OSA are not, per se, indications for preoperative pulmonary function testing and room air arterial blood gas (ABG) analyses
  - Have failed to demonstrate predictive values and/or lead to optimization of postoperative management or outcomes of bariatric surgery patients, and are not routinely indicated
- Room air pulse oximetry in both the upright and supine positions may be a useful, noninvasive method for screening patients for daytime hypoxemia
  - Supine room air SpO_2 <96% may merit further investigation.
- An elevated hematocrit may also be a clue of chronic hypoxemia
- If clinical evidence of OHS present, ABG analyses indicated because:
  - Chronic daytime hypoxemia—PaO_2 <65 mm Hg
  - Sustained hypercapnia—$PaCO_2$ >45 mm Hg
- The morbidly obese patient without significant obstructive pulmonary disease is diagnostic for this syndrome
- Must differentiate whether MO coexists with either OHS *or* COPD
  - Combinations often result in chronic daytime hypoxemia and increase the chances for pulmonary hypertension, right ventricular hypertrophy, and/or right ventricular failure
  - Assessment of these pickwickian patients may require extensive testing to guide preoperative medical optimization and postoperative management as their morbidity and mortality rate is increased.
- Unclear if appropriate to delay bariatric surgery for aggressive optimization of airway status and oxygenation with continuous positive airway pressure (CPAP) or bilevel positive airway pressure (BiPAP) therapy
  - Two to 3 weeks may be necessary not only to maximize medical benefits
  - Three weeks of nightly CPAP treatment prior to bariatric surgery improved left ventricular ejection fraction and afterload in obese patients with coexisting heart failure.
  - Eight weeks of preoperative nasal CPAP therapy may be required to treat hypertension secondary to OSA.

Intraoperative Considerations

Airway Management

- In some circles it is still debatable whether MO should be considered a risk factor for difficult airway management.
  - Neither absolute obesity nor BMI is associated with problematic intubation in MO

- Only a large neck circumference and a Mallampati score of 3 or more were significantly correlated with a high probability of problematic intubation.
- Preoperative airway assessments similar in both morbidly obese and lean patients
- Whether or not morbid obesity is considered a risk factor for intubation, issues related specifically to the patient's BMI that impact airway management include:
  - Preoxygenation
  - Positioning
  - Immediate availability to adequate resources, both technical and human
    - Technical: special laryngoscopes, blades, tracheal tubes, oro- and nasopharyngeal cannulae, intubating laryngeal airway [ILA], laryngeal mask airway (LMA) Fastrach, Combitube
    - Human: personnel sufficient in both number and expertise
- In perioperative setting, one never knows when an emergent tracheal intubation or reintubation may be necessary or when an unpredicted difficult mask ventilation and difficult tracheal intubation combination may appear.
  - Latter is a common situation in MO patients suffering from OSAS or OHS
  - Presence of any of these urgent/emergent events will likely result in a life-threatening, although preventable/treatable, respiratory misadventure.
  - American Society of Anesthesiologists algorithm for difficult airway management and indications for conscious tracheal intubation should be considered for both obese and lean patients.
  - If conscious intubation is indicated, remember that most episodes of gastroesophageal reflux, and the greatest potential for pulmonary aspiration of gastric contents, occur from and during "bucking" on an endotracheal tube.
    - Appropriate preparation of the patient is crucial.
  - Meticulous patient explanation, a low infusion rate of remifentanil (0.05 μg/kg IBW/minute) to avoid loss of response to verbally required active ventilation, and/or local anesthesia—such as bilateral blockade of the internal branch of the glossopharyngeal nerve—are most effective and safest induction alternative.
  - Prudent to treat morbidly obese patients with prophylactic measures against gastric aspiration, such as cimetidine, ranitidine, Bicitra, and/or metoclopramide
    - Timing of administration of these agents is of great significance

Preoxygenation and Position

- Hypoxemia during induction of general anesthesia in obese individuals is a concern for anesthesiologist and/or intensivist
  - Patients may experience rapid arterial oxygen desaturation after apnea
  - Compared with supine-positioned, preoxygenation in the 25- to 30-degree head-up position with 100% oxygen for 3 minutes achieves higher oxygen tensions—more time and better oxygenation for intubation and airway control
  - Preoxygenation in the 30-degree reverse Trendelenburg position provides a longer, safer apnea period than the 30-degree semi-Fowler and supine positions
    - Recommended as the optimal position for induction of general anesthesia in obese patients

- The head-up position results in an unloading of the intra-abdominal contents from the diaphragm
- Pulmonary compliance and FRC increase, and oxygenation returns toward baseline values, as compared to same patients who were placed supine
- Prior to induction of general anesthesia in any setting—OR, ICU, or in hospital ward—obese patient should be positioned with pillows under the shoulders
  - With the head and upper body elevated in a semirecumbent or reverse Trendelenburg position
  - "Ramped" position strongly recommended in MO, to improve pulmonary function, oxygenation, cardiovascular function, conditions for mask ventilation, laryngoscopic view, and tracheal intubation
  - Extremely obese patients should not lie completely flat
    - Upper body constantly elevated at 25 to 30 degrees in perioperative period

Atelectasis

- In perioperative setting, reduction of chest wall and diaphragmatic muscle tone following the induction of general anesthesia and skeletal muscle relaxation impairs oxygenation.
- In simple obesity, net effect may reduce ERV and FRC to <50% of preinduction values
- Reduction of ERV and FRC increases exponentially with increasing BMI
  - The combination of these factors predisposes MO patient to suffer atelectasis during anesthesia and surgery and in the postoperative period.

Mechanical Ventilation: Invasive Positive Pressure Ventilation

- Initial tidal volume based on ideal body weight rather than actual body weight
  - Adjustments made according to airway pressures and appropriate respiratory monitoring
  - Lung-protective strategy of smaller tidal volumes (6 to 8 mL/kg IBW) and adequate positive end-expiratory pressure (PEEP)/CPAP to prevent airway closure and shear trauma important
  - Technique may result in decreased cardiac output, fluid loading will correct the problem
  - To improve ventilator–patient synchrony and reduce airway pressure, patient's spontaneous respiratory effort should be maintained and assisted with pressure support ventilation

Tracheal Extubation and Intrahospital Transfer

- MO associated with prolonged mechanical ventilation, extended weaning periods, and longer ICU and hospital lengths of stay
  - Strategies suggested for facilitating the weaning process include:
    - Positioning of the patient in a 45-degree reverse Trendelenburg position to optimize lung mechanics, increase tidal volume, and reduce respiratory rate
    - BiPAP postextubation
    - If hemodynamic stability achieved, trachea should be extubated with patient's upper body elevated between 30 and 45 degrees

- Transfer from OR while in a semirecumbent or tilted reverse Trendelenburg position
- Recovering patient should be kept in a head-up position in order to minimize intrapulmonary shunting
- On days 1 and 2 postoperatively, a change from the semirecumbent to the supine position may result in significant decreases in PaO_2
- Obese patients should convalesce in the semirecumbent position while receiving supplemental oxygen if possible
- Intrahospital transfer of a morbidly obese patient is best and most safely accomplished if the patient remains in his or her own hospital bed

Ideal FiO₂ (Supplemental Oxygen)

- One uses the highest concentration of oxygen necessary to maintain life
- But high oxygen concentrations have often been associated with atelectasis formation and recurrence
- Using as low an oxygen concentration as possible has been recommended
- Supplemental oxygen carries clear benefits for patients, especially the MO
  - Evidence suggests that an FiO_2 of 0.8:
    - Ensures appropriate oxygenation without increasing the risk of absorptive atelectasis
    - Reduces the incidence of postoperative nausea and vomiting (PONV) in patients with an increased risk of gastric aspiration
    - Improves the host's defense mechanisms against infection
    - Improvement seen in wound site and in respiratory system
      - Not proven in MO surgical patients, but possible benefit should not be ignored
      - Ideal FiO_2 should, then, result from a balance between a supplemental quantity of oxygen that is sufficient enough to avoid hypoxemia, reduce postoperative infections, and reduce PONV, but not so high as to facilitate the development and maintenance of atelectasis
- Our recommendation is:
  - Deliver 100% oxygen before induction of anesthesia to retard the development of hypoxemia after apnea
  - Once tracheal intubation is confirmed, reduce FiO_2 to 0.8, if possible, according to respiratory monitoring

Monitoring

- FRC is reduced in the morbidly obese patient
  - If it drops below closing capacity dependent airways will collapse, promoting deterioration of gas exchange due to:
    - V/Q mismatch
    - An increase in the shunt fraction
    - An increase in the alveolar–arterial oxygen gradient
  - The more obese the patient, the greater the alveolar–arterial gas difference
    - MO patient will not be able to reach the same PaO_2/FiO_2 ratio as the normal-weight patient
    - MO leaves $PaCO_2$ values unaffected if the patient does not suffer from either OHS or pickwickian syndrome
      - ABG analysis increasingly important as it reflects the respiratory status more accurately than expiratory gas measurements

- MO, comorbidities, and the type of surgery should influence decision of which monitoring devices need be used
  - Routine noninvasive monitoring sufficient in simple cases
  - Presence of OSAS, OHS, pickwickian syndrome, daytime hypoxemia, and/or associated COPD should alert the anesthesiologist or intensivist to modify intra- and postoperative respiratory monitoring and narcotic use
  - Good practice demands obtaining SpO_2 or ABG analysis in the awake obese patient prior to any premedication for a reference
- Anesthesia and CMV will almost always have a negative impact on oxygenation and alveolar ventilation
  - Inadequate oxygen delivery may be reflected in increased, and sometimes unexplained, postoperative complications
  - Monitoring includes SpO_2, respiratory rate, cardiac rhythm monitoring, and blood pressure measurement in the immediate postoperative period
  - With decreasing SpO_2, ABG analysis and a chest x-ray may be useful
    - Sudden onset of respiratory distress, chest pain, and dyspnea may indicate cardiac event or PE
    - PE is major cause of mortality in 30-day postoperative period after bariatric surgery
- Increased risk of respiratory-related complications in postoperative period:
  - Can be as high as 3% for critical respiratory events in obese patients
    - Suggests importance of anesthetic and analgesic management on the speed and quality of recovery of CNS function
    - Combined thoracic epidural/general anesthesia techniques may be quite suitable in these major cases
    - Patients with confirmed or suspected OSAS, OHS, and pickwickian syndrome require more stringent observation
    - Postoperatively, this warrants prolonged surveillance in pulmonary acute care unit or admission to the ICU, especially for surgery lasting more than 4 hours and/or with critical comorbidities
    - Main reasons for ICU admission in MO patients are disturbances in pulmonary gas exchange
      - Preventable with prolonged one-on-one surveillance combined with meticulous medical care

Postoperative Considerations

Hypoxemia and Associated Postoperative Respiratory Disorders

- After major open abdominal surgery without postoperative oxygen supplementation, even normal patients experience hypoxemia (SpO_2 <90%)
- POD # 1 following open bariatric surgery, 75% of MO had PaO_2 <60 mm Hg
  - Usually persisted and worsened in the following days
  - Explanation most frequently utilized is atelectasis
    - Pulmonary aspiration of oral or gastric secretions, pneumonia, acute lung injury, and acute respiratory distress syndrome should also be considered

○ Tracheal tube displacement is mechanism of perioperative hypoxemia
  – Abdominal insufflation and OR table position to Trendelenburg position cause cephalad movement of the diaphragm, and can lead to migration of an initially correctly positioned endotracheal tube
  – In MO patients undergoing laparoscopy can result in right endobronchial intubation and intraoperative hypoxemia
  – Should be considered in intubated ICU patient because of frequent, necessary changes in patient's position

Atelectasis

- Atelectasis is a major cause of gas exchange impairment under anesthesia
  - Alterations in respiratory mechanics promote atelectasis, such as:
    - Decreased chest wall and lung compliance
    - Reduction in functional residual capacity
  - Conscious MO patients have alterations of their respiratory mechanics
    - They are particularly prone to intra- and postoperative atelectasis
    - During general anesthesia and in the immediate postoperative period MO likely to have significant impairment of pulmonary gas exchange and respiratory mechanics
  - Even before induction of anesthesia the MO had more atelectasis than nonobese patients
    - After tracheal decannulation, atelectasis increased in both groups
    - Significantly more severe in MO
    - Finally, 24 hours postoperatively, complete reexpansion of lung occurred in nonobese patients, while amount of atelectasis remained unchanged in MO
    - All possible measures to prevent/reduce severity and duration of atelectasis in this patient population are vital (Table 66.3)
- Some use non-invasive positive pressure ventilation (NIPPV) routinely in postoperative care of MO patients after extubation
  - Others reluctant because of fear of anastomotic disruption
  - There are no data to support this concern
  - MO patients use some form of NIPPV—CPAP or BiPAP—chronically for treatment of OSA
  - Postoperatively these patients at risk for prolonged depressant effects of drugs administered during surgery
  - May promote airway collapse not only in MO patients with diagnosed OSAS
    - But also in previously undiagnosed MO patients
    - Airway collapse most frequent during REM sleep
      ○ Brief in initial postoperative period
      ○ Significantly longer on third to fifth postoperative nights
      ○ Risk increases even days after surgery
      ○ Means that SpO_2 monitoring and O_2 must be administered during this dangerous period
- Prospective study of 1,067 bariatric patients evaluating risk of developing anastomotic leaks and pulmonary complications after gastric bypass
  - 420 had OSAS and 159 were dependent on CPAP
  - Were 15 major anastomotic leaks
    - Two occurred in CPAP-treated patients

TABLE 66.3

VITAL MEASURES TO PREVENT OR REDUCE THE SEVERITY AND DURATION OF ATELECTASIS IN THE OBESE PATIENT

- Place patients in the semirecumbent position and, if possible, out of bed in a chair as tolerated, as this maneuver may increase functional residual capacity.
- Provide effective analgesia, which will allow early and effective mobilization, cough, and excellent tolerance to physiotherapy.
- Institute aggressive incentive spirometry.
- During the first 3 postoperative days, deliver humidified supplemental oxygen, but avoid inspired fractions higher than 0.8. Supplemental humidified oxygen will not reduce atelectasis, but will facilitate respiratory secretion clearance, and will prevent hypoxemic episodes in efforts to improve the host's defenses against bacterial infections.
- During surgery or postoperatively in intubated patients, instituting positive end-expiratory pressure is probably effective in increasing functional residual capacity via recruitment of atelectatic regions of the lung. Applying vital capacity maneuvers (also known as recruitment maneuvers) may also reduce the incidence and/or severity of atelectasis while improving the quality and effective time of alveoli recruitment.[a]
- Noninvasive positive pressure ventilation can be used to avoid intubation in selected patients.

[a]Data from Magnusson L, Spahn DR. New concepts of atelectasis during general anaesthesia. *Br J Anaesth.* 2003;91:61–72.

- No correlation between CPAP utilization and incidence of major anastomotic leakage demonstrated
- No episodes of pneumonia diagnosed in either group
- Conclude that CPAP is useful modality for treating hypoventilation after gastric bypass surgery without increasing the risk of developing postoperative anastomotic leaks
- BiPAP used prophylactically during first 24 hours postoperatively
  ○ Significantly reduces pulmonary dysfunction after gastroplasty in morbidly obese patients
  ○ Accelerates reestablishment of preoperative pulmonary function

Pulmonary Aspiration

- Topic remains controversial
  - Still recommended taking precautions against acid aspiration
  - Massive pulmonary aspiration in MO patients a rare event in current anesthesia practice
  - Occurrence of unwitnessed microaspirations in the postoperative period difficult to assess because of diagnostic problems observed within this population
  - While massive aspiration uncommon, following cautionary list should be noted:
    - While in bed, patient must be adequately positioned in a semirecumbent or reverse Trendelenburg position at all times.
    - The care team must be ready for bag-valve-mask ventilation and tracheal intubation in a ramped position and have technical and adequate human resources.

- Drug dosing must be meticulously titrated to clinical response, based on IBW.

Radiographic Evaluation and Complications

- Radiographic evaluation of the obese patient is complicated
  - Made difficult by weight limitations of modern scanners
  - Patient's inability to cooperate with transfer
  - Tomographic tables now routinely handle patients weighing 400 lb (182 kg)
  - In absence of excellent radiographic capabilities, MO patients may require surgical exploration
    - Both patients and surgical team members must assume those additional risks

Venous, Arterial, and Nutritional Access

- When peripheral access is inadequate, the point of choice may be the internal jugular vein
  - Has fewer complications and requires fewer conversions to different locations
  - Arterial access generally recommended as noninvasive blood pressure cuffs can give inaccurate measurements in this patient population
  - Nutritional access in critically ill obese patients is imperative
    - Despite their weight, these patients can be relatively malnourished.
    - Obese patients preferentially mobilize protein instead of fats compared to lean patients.
    - If the patient requires reoperative interventions, a feeding gastrostomy or jejunostomy can be placed.
    - Percutaneous gastric access can be extremely difficult, especially in a patient following a gastric bypass procedure.

Analgesia

- **Overview:** Acute pain can result in reduced:
  - Tidal volume
  - Vital capacity
  - Functional residual capacity
  - Alveolar ventilation
  - These factors contribute to:
    - Atelectasis
    - V/Q mismatch
    - Hypoxemia
    - Hypercapnia
- Pain-related muscle splinting interferes with the patient's ability to:
  - Cough
  - Clear secretions
  - Efficiently participate in chest physiotherapy

- Efficacy of analgesia must be measured by the ability to cough and move without pain or discomfort, and not only by the absence of pain while in a resting state
- All the potential consequences of poor pain control are of outstanding importance in the MO surgical patient.
- Early mobilization without discomfort considered a major anesthetic target
  - DVT and PE are some of the most frequent causes of mortality during the first 30 postoperative days
- Sufficient and safe postoperative pain control would result in a more effective and tolerable respiratory physiotherapy.
- **Analgesic Strategies (IV, Thoracic Epidural, Multimodal Approach):** Uncertainty remains as to the superiority of one pain treatment modality versus another
  - Open versus laparoscopic surgical techniques
  - Personal skills and experience may influence the patient's and anesthesiologist's choice of pain treatment
  - Postoperative epidural analgesia, using either local anesthetics or opioids
    - May be the route of choice for postoperative analgesia in MO patients as it:
      ○ Allows a more vigorous cough and chest physiotherapy
      ○ Better diaphragmatic function
      ○ More powerful leg exercise
      ○ Earlier ambulation and discharge from hospital
        - These advantages may lead to a more benign postoperative course
        - Other populations who had earlier walking, earlier feeding, had a lower incidence of pulmonary alveolar collapse, and fewer thromboembolic complications
  - Thoracic epidural analgesia (TEA) improved by adding opioids, possibly epinephrine, to epidural solution
  - TEA may be particularly beneficial in the pathophysiologic context of MO:
    ○ LV work conditions (both preload and afterload) may be improved by the sympathetic blockade
      - Reducing the chances for developing heart failure
    ○ Myocardial oxygen balance may be improved
      - Due to a decrease in oxygen demand and augmented myocardial perfusion induced by coronary vasodilation, both secondary to sympathetic block
      - Reducing the risk of ischemia
- Improved efficacy and safety have been shown when IV patient-controlled anesthesia management includes:
  - Adjunct analgesics such as nonsteroidal anti-inflammatory medications
  - Local anesthetic wound infiltration in a multimodal approach

CHAPTER 67 ■ THE GERIATRIC PATIENT

GENERAL

- In 2000 U.S. census, those 62 years of age and older represented 14.7% of the population
  - Those 85 years of age and older numbered 4,239,587, or 1.5% of U.S. population
    - Increase of 1.2 million more than found within the similar population range 10 years earlier
  - In 2000, life expectancy beyond the age of 65 years was:
    - Nearly 19 years for a woman
    - 16 years for a man
    - Predictions for those 85 years old were 7 and 6 years, respectively
  - At dawn of the 20th century
    - Elderly population in United States was 4%, or 3.1 million people
    - Presently it is 35 million people
  - Based on advances in public health and medications and techniques of acute medical care provided to those born in the 20 years after World War II, 70 million individuals will be in "elderly" subgroup by 2030
    - At that time, those 65 years and older will compose 26% of the population of Florida
  - In 2005, spending by Medicare for those older than 65 years totaled $342 billion
    - Representing 17.1% of the total of $2 trillion spent nationwide for health care
    - Intensive care consumes 4% of national health care expenditures
    - During last 6 months of their lives, 11% of Medicare recipients spend 8 or more days in the intensive care unit (ICU)
    - Various studies documenting ICU occupancy by those older than 65 years old note that this ranges from one-quarter to one-half of the available beds

CARDIOVASCULAR (CV) DISEASE IN THE ELDERLY

- Approximately 35% of all deaths in the United States attributable to one of several manifestations of CV disease:
  - Coronary artery disease and other conditions that involve the myocardium
  - Hypertension
  - Arteriosclerosis of the central and peripheral arterial tree and cerebral vascular system
  - Three-fourths of these deaths are directly attributable to cardiac cause
    - Proportion is higher in more aged population
    - CV disease manifests itself as a complicating cofactor in the management of *any* older person's serious illness

- Although only 6% of the U.S. population is 75 years of age or older
- Such individuals account for 30% of all myocardial infarctions and 60% of the infarction-related deaths

Acute Coronary Syndrome in the Elderly

- One of the underpinnings of any strategy is that of expeditious implementation
  - The more quickly the intervention is begun, the greater the mass of myocardial tissue preserved and the greater number of lives saved.
  - Rapid restoration of coronary blood flow is the major goal of treatment for STEMI (ST-segment elevation myocardial infarction)
  - Decrease in mortality of 25% with reperfusion therapy has been demonstrated
  - From identification of STEMI, recommended that the infusion of thrombolytics begin within 30 minutes, or that the dilating balloon be inflated within 90 minutes
    - Percutaneous coronary intervention (PCI) is the preferred mode of treatment for STEMI, as long as the time constraints are met.
      - PCI yields lower mortality in the elderly population than thrombolysis
      - More benefit found as age progressively advanced, although possibly at the risk of a slightly increased rate of major bleeding events
  - In the management of non–ST-segment elevation MI (N-STEMI)
    - Early invasive strategy with catheterization and revascularization (when warranted) significantly benefits those older than 65 years of age
    - Early invasive strategy led to a significant increase in in-hospital major bleeding (16.6% vs. 6.5%; $p = 0.009$) and blood transfusion (20.9% vs. 7.9%; $p = 0.002$) in the patients older than 75 years.

Cardiomyopathy

- Decompensated heart failure (HF) is frequently encountered in management of critically ill elderly
- In the United States, 5 million persons suffer from heart failure
- More than 50,000 new cases diagnosed yearly
- Over 80% of the individuals with heart failure are older than 65 years of age
- Symptomatic heart failure *by itself* carries a dismal prognosis, with a median survival of 1.7 years for men and 3.2 years for women

- Common causes for HF in the elderly include:
  - Coronary artery disease and hypertension
  - Diabetes mellitus
  - Valvular disease (especially aortic stenosis and mitral regurgitation)
  - Cardiomyopathies other than ischemic

Dysrhythmias

- Dysrhythmias are frequent in the elderly patient, including those who manifest no other overt cardiovascular abnormalities.
  - For example, the so-called *lone atrial fibrillation*
    - With advancing age, sinus node and conduction system integrity deteriorate, with gradual replacement of cardiac pacemaker cells by collagen and elastic tissue
    - The occurrence of atrial fibrillation (AF) increases with age, carrying an increased risk of stroke and death in those older than 60 years, even in the absence of other cardiac abnormalities.
      - No clear survival advantage to either rate or rhythm control in AF
      - But rate control strategy did appear to manifest some advantages in the area of medication side effects
      - Choices for immediate rate control include β-blockers and calcium channel blockers
        - Amiodarone or digoxin may be used in those with heart failure in the absence of an accessory pathway
        - Digoxin is not recommended in such patients, as it may precipitate *profound* tachycardia via the accessory pathway, with heart rate nearing 300 bpm, leading to rapid cardiovascular collapse
        - In acute hemodynamic instability, recovery of sinus rhythm with biphasic DC cardioversion after sedation is appropriate
  - No one-size-fits-all solution to the question of anticoagulation
    - Well demonstrated to reduce the incidence of stroke related to AF
    - Equally well demonstrated is the extent to which anticoagulation is *under*used in the elderly, presumably because of concern for bleeding risk in this accident- and fall-prone population, and inadequate awareness of the extent to which AF warrants anticoagulation to minimize the risk of AF-associated stroke.
      - For the long-term patient, anticoagulation is best accomplished by using vitamin K antagonists for those at highest risk of severe stroke (>75 years), and aspirin for those elderly (<65) with less stroke risk.
      - In the 65 to 75 age range, either will suffice.
      - Target international normalization ratio (INR) of 2.0 to 3.0 is recommended for those receiving vitamin K antagonists
      - Maintenance of long-term anticoagulant regimens have limited applicability to the patient who suffers a critical injury or illness, and rapid normalization of INR may be warranted.
      - Quickly reversible heparin may be a better choice.
      - AF that persists beyond 48 hours mandates anticoagulation for 2 weeks

- Complex ventricular dysrhythmias and ventricular tachycardia (VT) are difficult management problems.
  - Sudden cardiac death a product of untreated VT degenerating into ventricular fibrillation (VF), followed by asystole
  - Defibrillation for VF provides the optimal chance of survival if provided within 3 minutes
- With advancing age comes increase in conduction system disease, often mandating permanent pacemaker (PPM)
- In 1990, implantation rate for cardiac pacemakers was 329 devices per million patients
- In 2002, the rate had risen to 612 per million
- Mean age of implanted patients was 75.1 years

PULMONARY DISEASE

- Healthy elderly individuals said to have significantly lower PaO_2 for a given FiO_2, compared to equally healthy younger counterparts
  - Traditional teaching has proposed the following formulae:
    - PaO_2 (mm Hg) = 104.2 − (0.27 × age)
    - PaO_2 = 100.1 − 0.325 × age (years)
    - PaO_2 = 109 − 0.43 (age)
  - More recent studies have yielded varying results

NUTRITIONAL ISSUES

- Malnutrition/undernutrition a common companion of elderly individuals
  - Frequent complicating factor in efficient and successful management of elderly ICU patient
  - The natural decline in energy expenditure with age begins at about age 30
    - Accompanies age-related increase in body fat–to–protein ratio
      - In elderly nursing home patients incidence of undernutrition can approach 85%
        - Mortality considerably higher in malnourished elderly patient, compared to the nutritionally replete
- Undernutrition imposes considerable burden on marginally compensated geriatric patient
  - Conditions known as protein-energy malnutrition (PEM) and micronutrient deficiency complicate treatment of several conditions seen in ICU:
  - The contribution of gastrointestinal tract nonintegrity to multiorgan system failure
- Other common cardiovascular, pulmonary, and infectious issues
  - Wound healing is impeded by a poor nutritional state
  - Development of decubitus ulcers more common in malnourished elderly
    - Successful management is decidedly more difficult
  - PEM patients are at increased risk for serious complications while in hospital:
    - Slower recovery
    - Poorer functional status at discharge
    - Higher rates of mortality after discharge
- Obtaining patient's weight *immediately on admission* an obvious step in assessing nutritional condition

- Calculation of the Quetelet body-mass index (BMI) is helpful to standardize weight to height, providing a relatively standardized estimate of body fat:
  - BMI = weight (in kg) divided by height (in m²)
  - Department of Health and Human Services defines:
    - Normal BMI within the range of 18 to 24.9
    - BMIs <8 being underweight
    - Overweight range being 25 to 29.5
    - BMI >30 being obese
  - In the geriatric population:
    - BMI <20 is predictive of nearly 50% 1-year mortality
      - A stronger predictor of mortality than is diagnosis
      - In general, use of BMI in elderly is suspect, regardless of the height measurement used
      - There are few normal BMI data that specifically describe those older than 65 years
- Several easily measured laboratory parameters reflective of nutritional status on admission:
- Albumin
  - A product of hepatic metabolism
  - Synthesized ultimately from ingested or infused nitrogenous precursors in the presence of adequate caloric support
  - Held that the serum albumin level is reflective of the nutritional state
    - Various factors influencing serum albumin levels make it only vaguely reflective of overall nutritional status
    - ROC (receiver operating characteristic) curve rating of 0.58 compared to the clinical subjective global assessment tool
    - Substantial decline in serum albumin concentration is accurately predictive of mortality and worse outcome among the elderly
    - Half-life of albumin is 18 to 19 days, making it less than optimal in monitoring metabolic and synthetic functions
  - Alternatives include prealbumin and retinol binding protein
  - Former has half-time of 2 days
    - Not affected by age but is elevated with steroid use
  - Latter has a half-time of 12 hours
    - Decreases slightly with age
    - Elevated in the setting of acute liver injury
- Critical illness induces substantial catabolism and resting energy expenditure (REE) rises during the first 2 weeks of this state
  - Mobilization of nitrogen stores a component of associated inflammatory response to physiologic insult
  - Total energy expenditure (TEE) may rise to 40 to 50 kcal/kg/day in critically ill, septic, or trauma patients
    - Repletion most difficult without correcting the underlying inciting process
  - Traditional guidance recommends 25 kcal/kg/day of nutritional support
    - With additional protein supply of 1.2 to 1.5 g/kg/day based on *usual* body weight
    - Obese individuals warrant feeding based on *ideal* (IBW), rather than usual, body weight:
      - **Men:** IBW (kg) = 50 + 2.3 kg per inch over 5 ft
      - **Women:** IBW (kg) = 45.5 + 2.3 kg per inch over 5 ft
    - Greater accuracy achieved using Harris-Benedict equations to determine REE as a guide to calculation of nutritional needs:
      - **Men:** REE = 66.5 + (13.75 × weight in kg) + (5.003 × height in cm) – (6.775 × age in years)

- **Women:** REE = 655.1 + (9.563 × weight in kg) + (1.850 × height in cm) – (4.676 × age in years)
- May be insufficient in the critically ill geriatric patient in the throes of the inflammatory response
- Protein supplementation at a rate of 2 g/kg recommended for the most critically ill, catabolic patients
- Enthusiastic overprovision of macronutrients in a misguided and vain attempt to thwart and correct inflammatory catabolism
  - Leads to a host of complications and considerable morbidity for which geriatric patient may be unable to compensate
  - Measurements of energy expenditure performed at frequent intervals are even more strongly advisable, since energy requirements fluctuate with time and medical condition
- Most studies show that enteral nutrition preferred because of:
  - Purported preservative effects on intestinal mucosal integrity
  - Cost issues
  - Risk exposure to the patient, both infectious and mechanical, associated with placement of flexible nasointestinal feeding tube versus central venous line (CVL) for parenteral nutrition
- Statement is the source of endless controversy

RENAL CONSIDERATIONS

- Deterioration of renal function in a critically ill patient has a dramatic impact on survival.
  - Acute renal failure (ARF) carries mortality of nearly 30% in general ICU population
  - Decline of renal function of lesser severity impacts mortality significantly and more so in geriatric population
  - Chance for at least partial renal functional recovery after critical illness-related ARF is >90% among those alive a year after illness
- A gradual deterioration of renal function, beginning at age 30 years
  - When sixth decade reached deterioration *generally* continues with a very wide bell curve of distribution
    - Decrease in glomerular filtration rate (GFR) of 30% to 40% by age 80
      - Individualize each assessment of GFR by using the Cockcroft-Gault formula to generate more accurate estimate of function based on weight, age, and serum creatinine (S$_{cr}$):
        - Creatinine clearance = [(140 – age) (weight in kg)]/(72 × S$_{cr}$) (arithmetic result × 0.85 = clearance for female patients)
      - Formula provides a snapshot of function at a given time
        - Most useful if calculated on ICU arrival and daily thereafter
        - S$_{cr}$ may be increased by excessive muscle breakdown due to rhabdomyolysis, critical illness, or medications
        - Other laboratory surrogates of GFR are:
          - Measurement of cystatin C
          - MDRD (modification of diet in renal disease) equations

– If GFR remains uncertain, urine collection for measurement of creatinine clearance can be done with fair accuracy using at least an 8-hour urine collection period
   – 24-hour collection is preferred in critically ill patients
- Sodium excretion and reabsorption declines in efficiency, with those older than 60 years requiring considerably more time to achieve homeostasis in the face of sodium overload or deprivation
- Rectification of acid-base perturbations similarly deficient
- Management of deteriorating renal function requires accurate diagnosis of the inciting cause, while addressing complicating or resultant metabolic derangements and preventing further insult:
  ○ Acute kidney injury occurs in as many as 67% of ICU admissions as identified by RIFLE (risk, injury, failure, loss, end-stage) criteria
  ○ Initial evaluation must include:
    – Performance of a physical examination that may reveal an occluded urinary catheter causing an enlarged bladder
    – Hypovolemia, both absolute, as in severe dehydration, and relative, as in sepsis, must be aggressively corrected with appropriate fluid and blood products.
    – Invasive monitoring is warranted in this population of patients with compromised reserve.
    – Dosage adjustment of potentially nephrotoxic medications is mandatory.
    – Loop diuretics, mannitol, and natriuretic peptides have largely been demonstrated **to be of no use in preventing incipient acute renal failure.**
    – Role of *N*-acetylcysteine and bicarbonate to minimize deleterious effect of radiocontrast medium on renal function in critically ill individuals remains controversial.
      • Should generally be used in any elderly patient receiving contrast

ASSESSMENT AND MANAGEMENT OF TRAUMATIC INJURIES

- In 55 to 64 age group, unintentional injury the sixth leading cause of death in 2003
  - In those older than 65 years, nearly 35,000 deaths were attributed to trauma
  - Most serious injuries caused by falls
    - Occurrence rising dramatically as age advances into 60s and beyond
    - From a standing or even sitting position, imparting an apparently trivial amount of kinetic energy to frail tissue may result in fatal injury, disproportionately accounting for half the trauma-related deaths when compared to those of younger people.
    - Most remaining significant traumatic injuries to elderly involve motor vehicles, either as vehicle occupants or as pedestrians
    - Small but persistent incidence of injury and death from penetrating trauma in elderly, <1% in those older than 75 years
- Sequential measurement of routine hematology tests, even in stable patient, may show unsuspected hemorrhage.

- Arterial blood gas analysis a convenient tool
- Quickly performed
- Allows frequent measurement of hemoglobin, base deficit, and lactate
  ○ Latter two values are powerful indicators of resuscitation status and, when elevated, predict increased mortality in the elderly population
  ○ In elderly trauma patients mortality is decreased from 54% to 34% ($p < 0.003$) by:
    – Institution of a protocol of trauma team activation
    – Early noninvasive and subsequently invasive monitoring for resuscitation of all patients older than age 70 years with an injury severity score (ISS) >15, even with nonworrisome initial vital signs and fairly minor injuries
- Certain patterns of injury are found in geriatric patients.
- Traumatic brain injury (TBI) afflicts the elderly with extraordinary severity.
  - High mortality leaves fewer survivors, most of whom suffer debilitating sequelae.
  - In 2003, there were 90,000 emergency department visits involving TBI in those older than 65 years, of whom 38.4% died.
  - Some series document mortality rates for severe TBI in those older than 55 years of age as high as 80%.
    ○ Initial neurologic examination of an elder with significant intracranial injury may be deceptively normal.
  - Cornerstone of TBI treatment is:
    ○ Maintenance of cerebral oxygenation by ensuring adequate oxygen content and cerebral perfusion pressure (CPP)
    ○ Guided by data derived via invasive intracranial monitoring devices that are inserted based on specific indications
    ○ CPP of 70 mm Hg is considered the standard but has not been rigorously tested specifically in the elderly as it affects outcome
    ○ Cerebral autoregulation in the elderly is subject to the same influences as those that affect the younger individual
    ○ Abundance of comorbidities, such as untreated hypertension, may have acclimated the cerebral vasculature to a new baseline, making invasive cerebral monitoring even more critical in ensuring adequate perfusion for the aging brain
- Cervical spine injury common in geriatric trauma patient
  - Plain radiographs may be unrevealing of fracture or difficult to interpret because of age-related boney changes obscuring acute pathology
  - Fracture of upper cervical spine more common in elderly than in younger individuals
    ○ More likely to be unstable
  - Helical computed tomography (CT) is superior to plain radiographs to identify cervical spine injury in this population
  - One must be mindful of the greater likelihood that cervical injuries in elderly often occur in arthritis-prone superior vertebrae--notoriously difficult to depict on plain films--and consider CT evaluation of virtually all geriatric trauma patients in whom even subtle symptoms, history, or mechanism of injury suggest cervical injury, regardless of the initial examination findings or protocol-based decision-assisting algorithm that suggest the safety of less aggressive investigation.

- Traumatic rib fractures impose substantial morbidity.
  - Those older than 45 years of age with more than four fractures are particularly affected.
  - In patients traditionally defined as *elderly*—those older than 64 years—rib fractures profoundly affected morbidity and mortality.
    - Longer length of stay in the ICU
    - More frequent pneumonia
    - Overall mortality rate of 22% versus 10% (p <0.001) in those less seriously affected
    - Rates of mortality and pneumonia both increased with each additional rib fracture
    - Epidural analgesia would appear to be the ideal technique to alleviate the pain associated with rib fractures to optimize pulmonary status and is successful in nongeriatric adults.
- Management of abdominal trauma follows pathways similar to those for younger patients.
  - Findings on physical examination indicating serious abdominal pathology can be subtle.
    - Especially when complicated by distracting orthopedic or mild head injury
    - Liberal use of CT scanning is strongly recommended if mechanism of injury, external abdominal findings such as a seat belt mark, or laboratory evidence of hypoperfusion (elevated base deficit or serum lactate) suggest visceral injury.
    - Nonoperative management of certain radiologically well-characterized injuries of solid organs—namely the spleen, the liver, and the pancreas—in the hemodynamically stable elderly patient is becoming increasingly accepted as evidence of the success this approach accumulates.
- Serious orthopedic injuries frequently befall older victims of polytrauma
  - Decrease in bone mineral density (BMD) with age older than about 30 years heightens the risk of fracture in general.
  - Observed in varying degrees in both genders and all ethnicities
    - But particularly severe in postmenopausal white women
  - Pelvic fracture in the aged is associated with a greater likelihood of significant blood volume transfusion and mortality (p <0.005)
  - Open pelvic fracture often has substantial associated bleeding, which is seldom treatable, with the exception of arterial bleeding, in any way other than with early stabilization, aggressive transfusion, and correction of coagulopathy
    - Arterial bleeding from lacerated pelvic vessels warrants embolization
    - More typical scenario, however, is that of diffuse venous oozing, which may render patient hemodynamically unstable.
      - Requiring large-volume transfusion of blood products as a temporizing measure until anatomic stabilization can be achieved
      - Hemodynamic consequences of large-volume transfusion and frequent septic complications can drive the mortality in both younger and older adults to nearly 80%.
    - Long-bone fractures warrant early immobilization and stabilization to minimize ongoing hemorrhage and generation of fat emboli.
      - Such fixation improves mortality significantly
      - Optimal timing of surgical stabilization of these quite morbid fractures is a complex issue to resolve when they occur in the larger setting of the patient with severe head, chest, or abdominal injuries.
    - Prolonged immobilization with such a fracture prior to stabilization:
      - Forgoes the profound respiratory benefits of early mobilization
      - Exposing the patient to extended intubation, pulmonary thromboembolus, and infection
- In 38,707 elderly trauma patients with a mean ISS of 11.7 ± 0.05 (SEM)
  - 10.3% died in hospital
  - 52.2% of the survivors went home
    - Percentage of patients returning home after serious traumatic injuries, many requiring prolonged intensive care, varied considerably with age:
      - 66.7% of those 65 to 74 years
      - 30.5% of those 85 years of age or older
- With aggressive rehabilitation, improvement in function and independence can continue for substantial periods of time after discharge, including in those who have suffered TBI

OUTCOME AFTER A CRITICAL ILLNESS IN THE GERIATRIC POPULATION

- Most people die after the age of 65 years
  - Life expectancy is greater at any given age now than it was even 15 years ago
  - Geriatric patients represent between 25% and 50% of all ICU admissions
  - In 2000, ICU costs represented 13.3% of hospital costs
    - 4.2% of health care expenditures
    - 0.56% of the U.S. gross domestic product
  - Family member's "do *everything* for Granddad" dictum is familiar
    - Often represents an unrealistic appraisal of the possible benefit from care
    - Complicated technology and meticulous attention to detail that characterize ICU not the basis for "magical"
    - Nonetheless, death can often skillfully be forestalled with polished and professional ICU care to such a degree that:
      - It may occur immediately after a deescalation of such care
      - Later on the general ward, in a step-down unit or rehabilitation facility
      - After returning home (either early or late) to a life with varying similarity to that prior to the original serious medical occurrence
  - Meaningful discussions with elderly patients and their families about the ICU *must* include accurate outcome data.

DRUG DOSING IN THE ELDERLY

- *Pharmacokinetics,* the study of the action of a drug in the body over a period of time, changes with age.

TABLE 67.1

AGE-RELATED CHANGES RELEVANT TO DRUG PHARMACOLOGY

Pharmacologic process	Physiologic change	Clinical significance
Absorption	Decreased absorptive surface Decreased splanchnic blood flow Increased gastric pH Altered gastrointestinal motility	Little change in absorption with age
Distribution	Decreased total body water Decreased lean body mass Increased body fat Decreased serum albumin Altered protein binding	Higher concentration of drugs that distribute in body fluids; increased distribution and often prolonged elimination half-life of fat-soluble drugs Increased free fraction in plasma of some highly protein-bound acidic drugs
Metabolism	Reduced hepatic mass Reduced hepatic blood flow Decreased phase I metabolism	Often decreased first-pass metabolism and decreased rate of biotransformation of some drugs
Elimination	Reduced renal plasma flow Reduced glomerular filtration rate Decreased tubular secretion function	Decreased renal elimination of drugs and metabolites; marked interindividual variation
Tissue sensitivity	Alterations in receptor number Alterations in receptor affinity Alterations in second-messenger function Alteration in cellular and nuclear responses	Patients are more sensitive or less sensitive to an agent

- Physiologic changes accompanying aging affect the pharmacologic processes of absorption, distribution, metabolism, and excretion (Table 67.1)
- Effects of these age-related changes are variable and difficult to predict
- Absorption of drugs, which occurs mainly by passive diffusion, changes little with advancing age.
- In elderly, relative increase in body fat and decrease in lean body mass alter drug distribution so that fat-soluble drugs are distributed more widely and water-soluble drugs less so (Table 67.2)
- Important pharmacokinetic change occurring in elderly is reduced renal drug elimination
  - Results from age-related decline in both GFR and tubular function
  - Drugs that depend on glomerular function (e.g., gentamicin) and/or on tubular secretion (e.g., penicillin) for elimination both exhibit reduced excretion in elderly

- Average creatinine clearance declines by 50% from age 25 to age 85 despite a serum creatinine level that remains unchanged at approximately 1.0 mg/dL
  - Two clinically relevant consequences:
    - Half-lives of renally excreted drugs are prolonged
    - Serum levels of these drugs are increased
- The biochemical and physiologic effects of drugs and their mechanisms of action—*pharmacodynamics*—and the effects of aging are not clearly known.
- Elderly seem to be more sensitive to the sedative effects of given blood levels of benzodiazepine drugs (e.g., diazepam).
  - But less sensitive to the effects of drugs mediated by β-adrenergic receptors (e.g., isoproterenol, propranolol)
  - An age-related decline in hormone receptor affinity or number (e.g., in β-adrenergic receptors) is suspected, but definitive data demonstrating such an alteration are sparse.
  - Other possible explanations offered are alterations in second-messenger function and alterations in cellular and nuclear responses.

TABLE 67.2

VOLUME OF DISTRIBUTION OF COMMONLY PRESCRIBED DRUGS

Increased volume	Decreased volume[a]
Acetaminophen	Cimetidine
Chlordiazepoxide	Digoxin
Diazepam	Ethanol
Oxazepam	Gentamicin
Prazosin	Meperidine
Salicylates	Phenytoin
Thiopental	Quinine
Tolbutamide	Theophylline

[a]If the volume of distribution is decreased, drug levels tend to be higher.

SPECIAL PROBLEMS OF THE ELDERLY

- Over one-half of all ICU admissions are patients older than 65 years of age
- They account for almost 60% of all ICU days
- Many of these older patients' final days before death are spent in the ICU
- 40% of Medicare patients who die are admitted to an ICU during their terminal illnesses
  - Accounting for 25% of all Medicare expenditures
  - There is a 6-month post-ICU survival of 53% in 116 patients over 70 years of age who had required mechanical ventilation for more than 24 hours.
    - Compared to their younger counterparts, octogenarians have a higher ICU mortality rate (10% vs. 6%, $p < 0.01$)

and higher discharge rate to a subacute care facility (35% vs. 18%, *p* <0.01).
  ○ Those discharged to subacute care facility had a higher mortality rate compared to those discharged home (31% vs. 17%).
  ○ Preadmission comorbidities and severity of illness independent predictors of discharge to subacute care facility:
    – Degenerative brain disease
    – Cerebrovascular disease
    – Chronic heart failure
    – Chronic pulmonary disease
    – Diabetes mellitus
- Malnutrition more commonly associated with care dependency

Neurologic Disorders

Delirium

- **Background and Risk Factors.** Delirium is an acute mental disorder common among elderly patients
- 14% to 56% of the hospitalized elderly develop delirium
- This increases 6-month mortality rate among these patients to 10% to 26%
- Recognition difficult, only 25% of cases diagnosed using standard screening tools
- Delirium-associated morbidity:
  - Complicates the hospitalization of 2.3 million older people annually
  - Adding 17.5 million inpatient days
  - $4 billion to Medicare expenditures to cover:
    ○ Increased lengths of stay
    ○ Greater need for postdischarge institutionalization, rehabilitation, and home care
  - Older adults with multiple comorbidities, particularly preexisting cognitive deficits, are predisposed
    ○ Prevalence rate surpassing 50% during intensive care
- **Pathophysiology.** Specific mechanisms are not well understood
  - Can be viewed as a final pathway of various causes of acute brain dysfunction, including:
    - Direct brain injury from trauma
    - Cerebrovascular disease, or central nervous system (CNS) infection
    - Systemic disturbances such as hypoxemia, hypotension, renal failure, hepatic failure, sepsis, and endocrine dysfunction
    - Effects of toxic or pharmacologic agents such as anticholinergics, narcotics, and sedative hypnotics
    - Consequences of withdrawal of substances to which the brain has developed tolerance (e.g., alcohol or benzodiazepines)
    - Current theory proposes alteration of CNS neurotransmitter levels and metabolism by age, medication, or illness, particularly:
      ○ Acetylcholine and dopamine pathways
      ○ Serotonin
      ○ γ-aminobutyric acid
      ○ Histamine
      ○ Glutamine
      ○ Norepinephrine

- **Diagnosis.** Criteria defining delirium are detailed in the *Diagnostic and Statistical Manual of Mental Disorders* (DSM-IV) of the American Psychiatric Association, specifically:
  - A disturbance of consciousness with impaired ability to focus, sustain, or shift attention
  - A change in cognitive function (in terms of memory, orientation, and language) or a perceptual disturbance that is not better explained by preexisting or evolving dementia
  - Disturbance development over a short period of time in hours or days, fluctuating through the day
  - History, physical examination, or laboratory data suggestive of the abnormalities caused by a general medical condition
  - Additional features include:
    - Alteration of sleep–awake cycle and psychomotor activities
    - Patterns of psychomotor symptoms are termed hyperactive and hypoactive
      ○ *Hyperactive* patients are agitated and combative, with loud, inappropriately boisterous outbursts and motor activity that can be harmful to self or a caregiver.
      ○ *Hypoactive* alternate between calm, appropriate behavior and a minimally interactive, withdrawn state, making this variant easy to overlook.
      ○ Delirium may erroneously be attributed to such conditions as dementia or depression (these three may coexist) or simply not be recognized, delaying diagnosis.
      ○ Delays may be explained by:
        – Fluctuating nature of signs and symptoms
        – Inadequate or insufficiently detailed scheduled neurologic and cognitive assessments of patients at risk for delirium
        – Avoidance of interactions with patients displaying altered mental status
        – Misperception of mental status changes "expected" in critically ill patients
      ○ Altered mental status in any patient suggests delirium
        – An organized approach to its investigation focusing on known risk factors is paramount to avoid overlooking the condition
- Of particular interest are alterations of mental status temporally related to surgical procedure
  - Specifically delirium developing within the immediate (minutes to days) postoperative time
  - More indolent neurocognitive decline that may appear days to weeks to months later, termed *postoperative cognitive dysfunction* (POCD)
    ○ Uniqueness of these conditions lies in their association with the postoperative period
    ○ Emergence delirium, the transitory restlessness and disorientation often apparent in the postanesthesia care unit or an ICU that receives patients directly from the operating room, often resolves within a brief period of time.
    ○ More worrisome is interval delirium, appearing 2 to 7 days after operation
      – Patient manifesting disorientation and agitation and being at risk for suboptimal outcome by virtue of its appearance
      – Risk factors for postoperative delirium are additive to those menacing the nonoperated elderly patient, including:
        • Perioperative hypoxemia and hypotension

- Exposure to medications that are used in the operating room—anticholinergics such as atropine, volatile inhalational anesthetics, neuromuscular blocking agents, and potent opioids
  - High-volume blood transfusion and rapid fluid shifts associated with surgery
- Procedures using cardiopulmonary bypass raise the possibility of microscopic atheromatous or air emboli as contributors
- Incidence of postoperative delirium ranges from 0% to 74%, varying with age group, type of surgery, variability of diagnostic criteria, and preoperative and postoperative cognitive status
  - Most cardiac surgery patients suffer various concurrent confounding medical conditions that make the specific effects solely of cardiac surgery on subsequent mental status difficult to isolate
    - Attention to statistical and study control issues allows identification of a substantial incidence (53%) of coronary artery bypass graft (CABG) patients (average age, 60.9 years ± 10.6 years) showing cognitive deterioration consistent with POCD at time of discharge, and 42% at 5 years
    - Age being a univariate predictor of decline
  - Specific cause of POCD is obscure.
    - Suggested causes those noted above as well as more abstract considerations such as brain inflammation, genetic factors, cerebral edema, and blood–brain barrier dysfunction
- Symptomatic treatment uses both pharmacologic and nonpharmacologic strategies:
  - Use of repeated reorientation, cognitive stimulating activities, promotion of adequate sleep on a normal sleep–wake cycle, physical therapy and mobilization
  - Early removal of catheters and physical restraints
  - Provision of eyeglasses and hearing aids
  - Judicious use of medications particularly targeted at calming agitation
    - All neuroactive medications such as benzodiazepines, opioids, or those with anticholinergic effects that are not absolutely fundamental to the patient's treatment plan and improvement should be discontinued.
    - The butyrophenone haloperidol is often used in the management of delirium-induced agitation, having few active metabolites and minimal anticholinergic, sedative, and hypotensive effects.
      - Retrospective analysis suggested haloperidol use was independently associated with lower mortality in 989 critically ill patients.
      - For POCD, there is no management other than prevention.

Stroke

- **Incidence and Risk Factors.** Stroke is the third leading cause of death and the *leading cause of disability* in the elderly.
- About 500,000 individuals in this age group suffer strokes annually in the United States.
  - Corresponding to one event every 45 seconds
  - Leads to one death every 3 minutes
- Among those 55 years and older, the incidence of stroke doubles with each additional decade of life.

- Despite a decline in the United States, Canada, and Western Europe through the later part of the 20th century to the present, attributable to improved management of modifiable risk factors
  - Hypertension is by far the most powerful
  - Aggressive blood pressure control reduces risk of stroke by 40%
  - Coronary atherosclerosis, left ventricular hypertrophy, and atrial fibrillation contribute to stroke risk
  - Diabetes mellitus may increase likelihood of stroke by a factor of 2 to 4
    - Tight glucose control significantly reduces this risk and may postpone such vascular complications as retinopathy and nephropathy.
  - Modifiable factors also include cigarette smoking, hyperlipidemia, and excessive alcohol consumption.
- **Location.** Approximately two-thirds of ischemic strokes occur in middle cerebral artery (MCA) distribution.
- Findings include contralateral hemiplegia and hemianesthesia
  - Proximal MCA occlusion produces profound symptoms: homonymous hemianopsia or deviation of the head and eyes toward the side of the lesion
  - Involvement of dominant MCA distribution may cause aphasia, expressive or receptive
  - Dominant hemisphere MCA lesions may induce depression in the elderly.
  - Those in the nondominant hemisphere produce visuospatial deficits, unilateral neglect, and emotional lability that can mimic depression, sometimes delaying correct diagnosis.
- Anterior cerebral artery (ACA) stroke is least common, accounting for about 2% of ischemic infarcts.
  - Most profoundly affects the contralateral leg and foot, generally with lesser impact on the arm and little involvement of the face.
  - Very proximal ACA occlusion, however, may affect the entire contralateral side
    - Abundant collateral flow in ACA territory yields various symptoms associated with anterior circulation stroke
    - May see frontal lobe features such as emotional lability, mood impairment, personality changes, and intellectual deficits
    - Aphasia uncommon
- Stroke-related paraplegia and incontinence may leave the elderly victim wheelchair bound and unable to control critical body functions, greatly complicating rehabilitation and subsequent independent living.
- Posterior cerebral artery (PCA) strokes manifest a diversity of findings due to the variability of anatomic origin
  - Partial or complete origin from the basilar artery or internal carotid arteries
  - Neurologic consequences of PCA stroke include:
    - Contralateral hemianesthesia and hemianopsia with sparing of central macular vision
    - Difficulty with reading and calculations
    - Hemiballismus from subthalamic involvement
    - With vertebrobasilar atherothrombotic disease, cerebellar dysfunction predominates
      - Common symptoms include vomiting, dizziness, ataxia, nystagmus, and double vision

- Vertigo can be profound, causing an already tenuously balanced elderly person to sustain a fatal fall
- Other symptoms include weakness of the face and the opposite side of the body, with dysarthria or dysphasia
- Facial numbness may occur
- Brainstem involvement may be revealed by altered mental status or quadriplegia
- Lacunar strokes—small occlusions of the penetrating and subcortical arteries—tend to occur in the basal ganglia, internal capsule, thalamus, or pons.
- Depending on specific sites of lesions, a wide variety of presentation may occur, including:
  - Pure motor or sensory findings
  - Symptoms that appear parkinsonian
  - A mixture of presenting abnormalities
- **Cause.** Strokes are either ischemic or hemorrhagic
- Ischemic, about 85% of the total, involve occlusion of the cerebral vessel by embolus or thrombosis
- Remaining 15% include hemorrhage into the brain parenchyma or its surrounding spaces
- Rapid identification of the specific cause of the stroke is fundamental to its management, since modalities of treatment vary with cause
  - Embolic phenomena most often originate from the heart, commonly associated with atrial fibrillation
  - Atherosclerotic disease of the aortic arch is emerging as an increasingly important and recognized risk factor for recurrent stroke when the wall thickness exceeds 4 mm.
    - Atheroma-associated clot formation may produce neurologic syndromes known as *thrombotic stroke*
    - Subintimal vascular disease is the ultimate inciting event, inducing arterial narrowing with ulcerated plaque formation in areas of more turbulent flow, such as the carotid bifurcation, leading ultimately to symptoms ranging from a temporary deficit (i.e., a transient ischemic attack, or TIA) to complete arterial occlusion caused by clot formation
- **Time Course.** Stroke phases are termed acute, subacute, and chronic, each with its unique needs and goals of care. Time spans are generally said to be:
- *Acute phase of stroke (admission to 48 hours):* Management of the acute phase involves, first and foremost, ensuring airway and hemodynamic stability
- Thereafter, the goals of care are:
  - Identification of the stroke as ischemic or hemorrhagic
  - Initiation of thrombolytic therapy when indicated
  - Recognition and therapy of medical or neurologic complications
- First goal is most easily achieved by obtaining a noncontrast-enhanced CT scan of the brain as quickly as possible when stroke is suspected.
  - Hemorrhage is usually obvious on this scan, although early in the course of ischemic stroke there may be no visible abnormality.
  - May reveal one of the many mimics of stroke: subarachnoid hemorrhage, subdural hematoma, neoplasm, or hydrocephalus
  - Contrast enhancement may improve yield if tumor or infection is likely.
  - If decided that ischemic stroke is present, the risks and benefits of thrombolytic therapy must be weighed:

- Current recommendations for management include initiation of intravenous thrombolytic therapy with recombinant tissue plasminogen activator (rt-PA) within 180 minutes of onset of stroke, in the absence of contraindications
- Intra-arterial thrombolysis an option for those with occlusion of MCA
- Use of rt-PA appears to improve outcome from stroke at 3 months
- *Subacute and Chronic Phases:*
  - Acute events and aggressive treatment often stabilize within 48 hours
    - Close attention to complications or neurologic decompensation warranted
    - Early extubation advisable
    - Meticulous attention to the return of intact airway reflexes and sufficient recovery of mental status
    - Otherwise, tracheostomy for airway protection allows withdrawal of sedation, early mobilization, and more robust participation in physical and occupational therapy
    - Common companions of those with compromised mental status:
      - Pulmonary aspiration
      - Skin breakdown
      - Infections
      - Limitation of extremity range of movement
    - Ameliorated by aggressive rehabilitation efforts
    - Early nutritional support via feeding tube must be initiated early
    - General goals of rehabilitation include restoration of motor and sensory function and strengthening of intact functions to facilitate compensation for residual deficits.
    - Stroke recurrence rate of 30% within 10 years warrants continued attention to chronic medical conditions.
    - Framingham study data documents survival in stroke victims of 50% in 5 years
    - Preservation of functional gains, avoidance of complications, and aggressive management of contributing comorbid conditions may well forestall the decline that often follows a stroke in an elderly patient

Sleep Disorders

- **Background.** Insomnia afflicts nearly 50% of older adults
- Genders are generally equally affected, but sleeplessness in men predominates after 85 years
- Prevalence increases in the elderly with the number of coincident medical conditions
- Common sleep complaints among the community-dwelling elderly are:
  - Difficulty in initiation of sleep
  - Nighttime and early morning awakening
  - Sequelae of insomnia include:
    - Physical and mental fatigue
    - Anxiety
    - Irritability
    - All of which worsen as bedtime approaches and personal worries reemerge without the protective diversion of normal daytime activities
- Chronic dysfunctional sleep induces a state of endless fatigue, affecting memory and concentration

- Elderly are particularly affected, with steepened cognitive decline and risk of falls, with associated morbidity and mortality
  - Hospitalization amplifies the morbidity of sleep disturbances
    - ICU admission likely subverts any semblance of a normal sleep pattern
    - Sedation to facilitate mechanical ventilation subdues consciousness but disrupts normal variation in sleep stages, preventing rest
    - Circadian rhythms are disrupted, with dyssynchrony with anticipated light/dark time cycles and adequate daily morning exposure to sufficient bright light
    - Many elderly patients become disoriented at night, exhausted and confused by constant alarms, noises, dressing changes, unscheduled diagnostic procedures, and the impact of acute severe illness, producing delirium in nearly two-thirds of elderly ICU patients.
      - Dementia contributes to this phenomenon.
- **Identification and Management of Sleep Disorders.** Sleep–wake cycle is regulated by a complex neurochemical interaction subserved by the brainstem, hypothalamus, pons, and preoptic areas of brain.
  - Aberrations of sleep patterns produce dysfunctional sleep
  - Normal sleep architecture displays three segments:
    - Light sleep (stages one and two)
    - Deep (delta or slow wave) sleep (stages three and four)
      - The most restorative segment
    - Rapid eye movement, or REM, sleep (stages one and four)
      - In nonelderly adults, typical cycle time between REM and non-REM sleep is 90 to 120 minutes.
  - Advanced age alters sleep by shortening sleep latency and total sleep time, preserving REM sleep, decreasing the delta segment, and advancing the natural onset of sleepiness to an earlier time in the evening.
  - Nocturnal sleep fragmentation worsens
  - Daytime somnolence and frequent napping being commonplace, sometimes causing reversal of the sleep–wake cycle
  - Acute insomnia in the geriatric patient may be precipitated by a host of issues, including the critical illness itself.
  - Effective treatment obviously requires an accurate diagnosis.
    - All possible accommodations should be made to minimize interruption of the older patient's restful nighttime sleep periods.
      - Minimizing noise, procedures, and cycling of lights on and off
      - Daily exposure to bright sunlight through nearby windows is beneficial
      - Various medications are available but each may provoke delirium in elderly patients

CHAPTER 68 ■ UNIVERSAL PRECAUTIONS: PROTECTING THE PRACTITIONER

PRECAUTIONS

- There are several types of precautions used in patient care settings that have been described
  - Implementation of standard precautions (previously termed *universal*) does not negate the need for further specialized infection control precautions if necessary, such as droplet precautions for influenza, airborne isolation for pulmonary tuberculosis, or contact isolation for methicillin-resistant *Staphylococcus aureus* (MRSA)
  - There are four types of precautions recommended in the Centers for Disease Control and Prevention (CDC) guidelines (Table 68.1):
    - Standard (previously termed *universal*)
    - Contact
    - Droplet
    - Airborne

Standard Precautions

- Those that are applied to anyone whom the practitioner comes into contact, regardless of diagnosis
  - Include handwashing before and after contact with every patient, and between anatomic sites on same patients
  - Additional precautions may be required to care for patients who do not have a diagnosis requiring other specific categories of isolation
    - Blood and body fluids (including secretions and excretions, excluding sweat)
    - Broken skin
    - Mucous membranes

TABLE 68.1

RECOMMENDED ISOLATION PRECAUTIONS FOR SELECTED PATHOGENS

Organism	Recommended precaution/isolation
Methicillin-resistant *Staphylococcus aureus*	Contact
Vancomycin-resistant enterococcus	Contact
Clostridium difficile	Contact
Multidrug-resistant Gram-negative infections	Consider contact
Varicella-zoster virus	Contact/airborne
Influenza	Droplet
Tuberculosis	Airborne
Neisseria meningitides	Droplet

- Health care workers (HCWs) may also require use of
  - Gloves
  - Mask
  - Eye protection
  - Face shield
  - Gowning
- Other considerations include special handling of patient care equipment, including sharps and other instruments, and environmental control with correct disposal and cleaning of linen and other contaminated items

Handwashing

- Hands must be washed before and after every patient contact
  - Even where there has been no visual contamination with blood, body fluids, secretions, excretions, and contaminated items
  - Hands must be washed immediately after gloves are removed if they were worn
  - Washing of hands should be done whenever indicated to avoid transfer of micro-organisms to other patients and the environment
    - As after contact with intravenous (IV) tubing or a monitor even when there has been no direct patient contact
  - Plain, nonantimicrobial soap could be used for routine handwashing
    - Antimicrobial soap or a waterless antiseptic agent can be used for specific circumstances
  - Alcohol-based hand sanitizers have been shown to be more convenient, faster, and more efficient than handwashing

Gloves

- Clean, nonsterile gloves are appropriate when contact with blood, body fluids, secretions, excretions, and contaminated items is expected.
  - Clean gloves should be used if expected contact with broken skin or mucous membranes
  - Recommendations also include changing of gloves between tasks and procedures on the same patient if contact with material containing a high concentration of micro-organisms is made.
  - Recommended that gloves be changed between contact with different anatomic sites on the same patient
  - Handwashing or use of a hand sanitizer should always be performed after removal of gloves and prior to seeing the next patient.
    - Use of gloves does not replace the need for handwashing
      - Gloves may have small, inapparent defects or may be torn during use
      - Hands can become contaminated during removal of gloves

Mask, Eye Protection, and Face Shield

- Mucous membranes of HCW, including those of the eyes, nose, and mouth, at risk for exposure when performing procedures or patient care tasks that may generate aerosols or droplets
- Masks, eye protection, or face shields should be worn to protect mucous membranes

Gown

- Gown should be worn if expected direct contact with an infected patient or environment during procedures or routine patient care
  - Clean, nonsterile gown is adequate for protecting skin and preventing soiling of clothing during such procedures and patient care activities
  - Remove immediately after patient contact
  - Hands should be washed after removal of gowns

Patient Care Equipment

- Equipment soiled with blood, body fluids, secretions, and excretions should be handled in a manner that prevents skin and mucous membrane exposures, contamination of clothing, and transfer of micro-organisms to other patients and environments.
- Multiuse equipment should be appropriately cleaned or processed prior to being used for the care of another patient.
- Single-use items should be disposed of in the appropriate manner, including use of a puncture-resistant sharps container if indicated.

Environmental Control and Linen

- Procedures for routine care, cleaning, and disinfection of environmental surfaces, beds, bedrails, bedside equipment, and other frequently touched surfaces should be used.
- Soiled linen should be handled and transported in a manner that prevents skin and mucous membrane exposure and contamination of clothing.

Patient Placement

- Patients who may contaminate an environment, who do not or cannot assist in maintaining appropriate hygiene or environmental control should be placed in private room.

Occupational Health and Bloodborne Pathogens

- Handling of sharps during use, cleaning, or disposal should be done with extreme care.
  - Never recap used needles; avoid manipulation using both hands or a technique that involves the point of a needle being directed toward any part of user's body.
  - Used needles should not be removed from disposable syringes by hand.
  - Bending or breaking, or otherwise manipulating used needles by hand should not be done.
  - Used disposable syringes and needles, scalpel blades, and other sharp items should be placed in an appropriate puncture-resistant container.
    - Located as close as practical to the area in which the items are used
  - Reusable sharps placed in a puncture-resistant container for transport

Contact Precautions

- Designed to reduce the risk of transmission of epidemiologically important micro-organisms
  - Such as antibiotic-resistant Gram-positive or Gram-negative organisms
- Transmission of these organisms may take place either by direct or indirect contact
  - Direct contact transmission from patient to staff includes:
    - Physical transfer of micro-organisms to the HCW from an infected or colonized patient
    - Activities that are a risk for direct contact include:
      ○ Turning and bathing patients
      ○ Assisting patients with personal hygiene
      ○ Performing patient transfers, dressing changes, or other patient care activities that require physical contact
      ○ Can also occur between two patients sharing common areas in same room
  - Indirect contact transmission involves contact of a susceptible host or HCW with a contaminated intermediate object
    - Referred to as *fomites*
    - Described as sources of MRSA, vancomycin-resistant enterococcus (VRE), and Gram-negative organisms such as *Pseudomonas* and *Acinetobacter* because these organisms can potentially survive for months
- Applied to patients with known or suspected infection or colonization with epidemiologically important micro-organisms that can be transmitted by direct or indirect contact
  - Involve patient placement
  - Gloves and handwashing
  - Gowning
  - Precautions with patient transport and patient care equipment
  - Patients should be placed in a private room if possible
    - Door to the room may be left open
  - If private room not available
    - Patient can be placed in a room with a patient who has colonization or active infection with the same micro-organism (*cohorting*)
  - If private room not available and cohorting not achievable
    - Epidemiology of the micro-organism should be considered and patient population taken into consideration when determining placement
      ○ Example includes avoidance of placing immunocompromised patient in same room as one with resistant organism
- Gloves and handwashing used as with standard precautions
  - Gowns used if substantial contact with the patient, environmental surfaces, or items in patient's room
  - Gown also worn if patient is incontinent, has diarrhea, or has an ileostomy, colostomy, or wound drainage not covered or contained by a dressing
- Transport limited to essential purposes
- Patient care equipment such as stethoscopes, thermometers, and IV pumps dedicated to a single patient (or cohort) to avoid transfer of organisms

Droplet Precautions

- Aim to reduce risk of spreading infectious agents by droplet transmission

- Transmission involves contact between conjunctiva and other mucous membranes (nose, mouth) of either a patient or HCW with large droplets (>5 μm in size) containing micro-organisms generated from a person who is either infected or colonized
- Droplets generated by coughing, sneezing, or talking and during procedures such as suctioning or bronchoscopy
- Requires close contact between source and recipient persons
  - Droplets do not remain suspended in the air and generally travel only short distances, usually <3 ft
  - Special air handling and ventilation not required to prevent transmission
  - Door to the patient's room may remain open
- Apply to any patient known or suspected to be infected with epidemiologically important pathogens that can be transmitted by infectious droplets:
  - MRSA
  - Meningococcal infection
  - *Acinetobacter* pneumonia
  - Invasive *Hemophilus influenza* type B
  - Influenza
  - Mycoplasma pneumonia
  - Parvovirus B19
- In addition to standard precautions
  - Patients should be placed in a private room or cohorted
  - If cohorting is not possible, spatial separation of at least 3 ft between other patients and visitors should be maintained
  - Mask should be worn if working within 3 ft of the patient
  - Transport should be limited to essential purposes
    - When transported, patient should be masked

Airborne Precautions

- Designed to reduce the risk of airborne transmission of infectious agents
  - Occurs by dissemination of either airborne droplet nuclei 5 microns or smaller in size, or dust particles containing the infectious agent
  - Micro-organisms carried in this manner dispersed widely by air currents travel long distances through ventilation systems
  - May be inhaled by susceptible host in the same room or by a patient several rooms or floors away
  - Special air handling and ventilation are required
- Airborne precautions apply to patients known or suspected to be infected with epidemiologically important pathogens such as:
  - Tuberculosis
  - Varicella zoster virus
- Patient should be placed in a private room that has:
  - Monitored negative air pressure in relation to surrounding areas
  - 6 to 12 air exchanges per hour
  - Appropriate discharge of air outdoors or monitored high-efficiency filtration of room air before recirculation
  - Room door should be kept closed and the patient should be kept in the room
    - If private room is not available, patient should be cohorted
    - If private room is not available and cohorting is not possible
      - Consultation with infection control professionals

- Respiratory protection should be worn: N95 respiratory mask
  - Susceptible persons should not enter the room of patients known or suspected to have rubeola (measles) or varicella (chickenpox) if other immune caregivers are available
    - If susceptible persons must enter room, must wear N95 respirator
    - Persons immune to measles or chickenpox need not wear respiratory protection
- Patient transport should be limited to essential purposes only
- If transport or movement necessary place N95 mask on patient

VIRUSES

- Major viruses of concern in the health care setting are human immunodeficiency virus (HIV), influenza virus, and the hepatitis B and C (HBV, HCV)
- Nosocomial outbreaks of herpes simplex virus I (HSV type I), pneumonia (13), and varicella zoster virus reported but generally rare
- Application of standard (universal) precautions recommended in all patients

Human Immunodeficiency Syndrome

- HIV causes acquired immunodeficiency syndrome (AIDS)
  - Two species of HIV—HIV-1 and HIV-2—infect humans
  - Thought to have originated in southern Cameroon as a species-jumping event from wild chimpanzees (HIV-1) and an old-world monkey, the Sooty Magabey (HIV-2)
  - Virus was first discovered in France in 1983
    - Named lymphadenopathy-associated virus
    - Confirmed in United States
      - Named human T-cell lymphotropic virus 3 (HTLV-3)
      - In 1986, the name was changed to HIV
    - Virus is a single-stranded RNA virus classified in the genus Lentivirus of the family Retroviridae
      - Upon entry into the cell, the virus uses reverse transcriptase to convert its genome into a double-stranded DNA that then integrates itself into host nuclear DNA for transcription of its genome using host cellular machinery
      - Transcribed virus then enters the cytoplasm where it undergoes translation
      - Later, under the influence of the enzyme protease, becomes cleaved to be incorporated into mature virions
- HIV is transmitted primarily by exposure to blood and other body fluids
  - Three primary methods of transmission are:
    - Via unprotected sexual intercourse
    - Vertical transmission (mother to child)
    - Through contaminated needles (either occupational exposure or with the use of IV drugs)
  - Blood products screened routinely for HIV, and transfusion-associated transmission has been, for the most part, eliminated
  - After initial exposure, HIV replicates within dendritic cells of the skin and mucosa
    - Later spreads via lymphatics, infecting CD4+ cells
    - Process ultimately becomes a chronic disseminated infection

- Delay in systemic spread leaves window of opportunity for postexposure prophylaxis (PEP) using antiretroviral drugs
- Nurses are at highest risk for occupational exposure
  - Most common exposure was via percutaneous injury
  - Other types of exposures among HCWs include:
    – Mucous membrane exposure
    – Nonintact skin exposure
    – Bites resulting in blood exposure
- Average risk of HIV transmission to HCWs:
  - After a percutaneous injury estimated to be approximately 0.3% (95% confidence interval [CI], 0.2%–0.5%)
  - After mucous membrane exposure to be 0.09% (95% CI, 0.006%–0.5%)
  - Transmission of HIV via nonintact skin exposure has been documented but is much less than for mucous membrane exposures
  - Risk for transmission after exposure to fluids or tissues other than HIV-infected blood also has not been quantified but is considerably lower than for blood exposures.
- Several factors may increase risk of HIV transmission after an occupational exposure:
  - Larger quantity of blood from the source
  - Procedure that involves placing a needle directly into a vein or artery
  - Deep tissue injury
  - Blood exposure from a patient with terminal disease, as there is usually a higher viral load in AIDS
  - More blood is transferred by deeper injuries and hollow-bore needles

Postexposure Management

- Administration of antiretroviral medications only active outcome of postexposure evaluation
  - Initial step is prompt treatment of exposure site including:
    - Washing wounds and skin sites with soap and water
    - Flushing mucous membranes with water
  - Followed by immediate reporting to facilitate rapid evaluation of the HCW
    - Including testing for HIV and hepatitis B and C
    - Evaluation of source patient
    - Initiation of medications for HCW if indicated
  - Potentially infectious fluids include:
- Blood and blood-containing fluids
- Fluids from other sites such as semen, vaginal secretions, and cerebrospinal fluid (CSF)
- Synovial, pleural, peritoneal, pericardial, and amniotic fluids
  - Source patient also needs to be evaluated, including:
    - Serologic studies for HIV using antibody testing
    - Hepatitis B surface antigen
    - Hepatitis C antibody
    - If the source patient not found to be infected with a blood-borne pathogen, further testing of the HCW may not be warranted
    - If the infection status of the source remains unknown, the comorbidities, clinical symptoms, and high-risk behaviors of the source patient should be considered
    - If source patient is considered high risk, PEP should be initiated
      - PEP regimens should be started within hours of exposure.
      - Exact course duration of PEP has not been determined. However, 4 weeks is recommended for HCWs and

other occupational exposures, such as law enforcement encounters.
  - PEP has been shown to be protective in animal studies.
    – Basic regimen consists of two nucleoside reverse transcriptase inhibitors (NRTIs)
      - Examples of basic regimens include a combination of lamivudine or emtricitabine with either stavudine or tenofovir; Combivir (zidovudine and lamivudine) or Truvada (tenofovir and emtricitabine)
    – Expanded regimens include the addition of another drug class such as protease inhibitors (PIs) or nonnucleoside reverse transcriptase inhibitors (NNRTIs)
      - Preferred expanded regimen is one that includes the PI lopinavir/ritonavir (Kaletra) with two NRTIs

Influenza Virus

- RNA viruses belonging to the family Orthomyxoviridae
- Infection causes an acute febrile illness usually occurring during the winter months and characterized by:
- Sudden onset of high fever
- Headache
- Myalgia
- Arthralgia
- Cough
- At risk for more severe disease include:
- Young children
- Elderly
- Immunocompromised patients
- Infection can be self-limited
  - May also result in severe prostration in elderly patients
  - Primary influenza pneumonia
  - Secondary bacterial pneumonia
- Transmission occurs person to person via large virus-laden droplets
  - Droplet precautions are used for patients admitted with active or suspected influenza
  - Mainstay of disease prevention is annual immunization of both:
    - HCWs
    - At-risk patient population, which is defined as:
      - Age older than 65
      - Residents of nursing homes or long-term care facilities
      - Pregnant women in the second or third trimester
      - Patients with a chronic pulmonary or cardiac disease
      - Patients with diabetes
      - Individuals on dialysis
      - Immunosuppressed patients
      - Patients on long-term aspirin therapy
      - Children aged 6 to 23 months
- Vaccination done with a live, attenuated influenza vaccine resulting in virus replication in the respiratory epithelium
  - Can result in active viral shedding
  - Inactivated influenza vaccine is recommended for HCWs with direct patient contact

Hepatitides

- Several hepatitis viruses described, including hepatitis A, B, C, D, E, and G

- Hepatitis A is caused by a picornavirus and is transmitted by the oral–fecal route, usually by contaminated food.
  - Causes only an acute form of hepatitis that is generally self-limited and confers immunity to future infections
  - Not usually a concern in the health care setting
- Hepatitis D is caused by a delta virus and can only replicate in the presence of hepatitis B.
- Hepatitis E is like hepatitis A in that it causes an acute, usually self-limited hepatitis and is also transmitted via the oral–fecal route.
  - In a small percentage of cases, hepatitis E can develop into an acute severe liver disease that is often fatal.
  - Pregnant women can develop severe disease with fulminant hepatic failure due to hepatitis E.
- **Hepatitis B.** A hepadnavirus endemic in certain parts of the world
  - Causes both an acute and chronic hepatitis, often with cirrhosis, and still remains a major cause of hepatocellular carcinoma, especially in Asia
  - Transmitted through exposure to blood and body fluids
    - Unprotected sexual contact—16% to 40% of unimmunized partners become infected
    - Blood transfusions
    - Use of contaminated needles and syringes
    - Vertical transmission—20% risk of transmission from mother to child without intervention in a hepatitis B surface antigen (HBsAg)-positive mother
    - Occupational exposure including needlesticks
  - Risk of transmission from a bloodborne exposure closely related to:
    - Volume of blood exposure
    - Number of copies of virus present in the blood of the source
    - Also related to the hepatitis B envelope antigen (HBeAg) status of the source patient
      - Patients both HBsAg and HBeAg positive, risk of developing clinical hepatitis from a needle injury was 22% to 31%; risk of developing serologic evidence of infection was 36% to 62%
      - If the source patient HBsAg positive HBeAg negative, risk of developing clinical hepatitis from a needle injury was 1% to 6%, and the risk of developing serologic evidence of hepatitis B infection was 23% to 37%
      - Hepatitis B survives in dried blood at room temperature for at least 1 week
        - Possible that contact with environmental surfaces is a potential risk for hepatitis B transmission
          - Shown in patients and staff of hemodialysis units
  - Key factor in preventing hepatitis B infection in the health care setting is vaccination
    - As with childhood vaccination, the protocol for adult immunization consists of three doses of the vaccine.
- In event that HCW is not immunized, postexposure prophylaxis available in the form of hepatitis B immune globulin (HBIG)
  - When indicated, HBIG should be given as soon as possible, preferably within 24 hours
  - Data on efficacy when HBIG was given after 7 days are not available

- Multiple doses of HBIG within 1 week of exposure are 75% effective in preventing hepatitis B infection.
- Postexposure hepatitis B vaccination is recommended in addition to HBIG because unimmunized HCWs continue to be at risk for exposure.
  - Data derived from vertical transmission regarding concurrent vaccination and HBIG administration show a better rate of prevention—85% to 95% with combined therapy as opposed to either therapy alone—70% to 75%.
- **Hepatitis C.** Hepatitis C is an RNA virus in the family Flaviviridae.
  - Replicates mainly in the hepatocytes after binding to specific receptors and entering the cells
  - Causes both acute and chronic hepatitis
  - Is a risk factor for development of hepatocellular carcinoma
  - Transmitted by direct contact with blood and body fluids containing blood
    - IV drug abusers seem to have highest incidence of hepatitis C
      - Due to the sharing of contaminated needles
    - Sexual transmission is possible but is largely due to blood contact.
      - Not other body fluids such as semen or vaginal secretions
    - Low incidence after accidental percutaneous exposure
    - Mucous membrane or skin exposures, both intact and nonintact, rarely result in transmission of hepatitis C.
  - No available vaccine for hepatitis C
  - No beneficial effect of giving immune globulin
    - Postexposure management aimed at early detection of hepatitis C infection and the development of chronic disease for which treatment can be given
  - Risk of acquiring hepatitis C varies depending on nature of exposure
    - Accidental percutaneous exposure from known HCV-positive source:
      - Incidence of seroconversion is 1.8%
      - Data limited on survival of HCV in environment
        - HCV-RNA is resistant to drying at room temperature for at least 48 hours

Herpes Viruses (HHV)

- DNA viruses that cause a variety of diseases in humans
- Several HHVs described including:
  - HHV-1 (also known as herpes simplex virus [HSV-1])
  - HHV-2 (herpes simplex virus [HSV-2])
  - HHV-3 (varicella-zoster virus [VZV])
  - HHV-4 (Epstein-Barr virus [EBV])
  - HHV-5 (cytomegalovirus [CMV])
  - HHV-6 (Roseolovirus)
  - HHV-7, and HHV-8 (Kaposi sarcoma–associated virus)
- Importance of these agents:
  - Seroprevalence of CMV documented to be up to 60% to 90% in adult populations
  - EBV generally self-limited mild disease
    - Can cause infectious mononucleosis in teenagers and young adults
  - HHVs of most importance in the health care setting are HSV-1, HSV-2, and VZV

- HSV-1 and HSV-2 cause blisters or sores either in the oral or genital area
  - Transmitted to HCW by direct contact with lesions, when present, and when appropriate use of precautions is forgone
- VZV the causative agent of chickenpox and shingles
  - Like other herpes viruses, VZV lies dormant in the dorsal root ganglia of the nervous system
  - Reactivates to produce zoster ("shingles")
  - Transmitted both by direct contact with a patient who has active skin lesions (vesicles) as well as via respiratory secretions in which the virus is shed during active infection, such as disseminated zoster
    - Recommended approach to patients with varicella-zoster disease includes both contact and airborne isolation
- Exposure of nonimmune pregnant HCW to patients with CMV or VZV disease problematic
  - Primary infection with either virus during pregnancy can be devastating to both mother and child.
  - Up to 50% of pregnant women are seropositive for CMV.
  - Incidence of primary CMV during pregnancy is 1% to 4%.
  - Transmission of CMV requires prolonged or recurrent close contact and can also be transmitted sexually.
  - There are no effective therapies for treatment of CMV in pregnancy.
    - Prevention is best method to avoid complications of disease
    - Any patient can actively shed CMV without clinical signs or symptoms
      - This is the foundation for the CDC's strong recommendation of meticulous adherence to handwashing before and after patient care as the best way to prevent disease transmission in *all* settings. In patients with proven or suspected CMV pneumonitis, mask and eye protection may be a consideration in the nonimmune or seronegative pregnant HCW.
  - Vaccine available for VZV
    - Live, attenuated, and given in two doses spaced 4 to 8 weeks apart
    - 70% to 90% effective in preventing infection
    - 95% effective in preventing severe disease up to 10 years after administration
    - Recommended for nonpregnant women of childbearing age and is not recommended for pregnant women
      - Further stipulation being that women should not become pregnant for at least 1 month after each dose of the vaccine
      - If pregnant HCW who is nonimmune becomes exposed to VZV, postexposure prophylaxis is available.
        - VZV immunoglobulin recommended within 96 hours of exposure and has been reported to be up to 90% effective in preventing severe disease.
        - Recommended that nonimmune HCWs be vaccinated, especially female HCWs of childbearing age
        - If a pregnant HCW is not immune and has had exposure to VZV, prophylaxis should be instituted.
        - Contact and airborne precautions should be used at all times in patients with VZV disease.

Bacteria

- Standard precautions recommended for all patients
- Additional precautions include contact precautions (MRSA, *C. difficile*, VRE) and airborne precautions (tuberculosis)

Methicillin-Resistant *Staphylococcus Aureus*

- A major problem both in hospital-acquired (HA-MRSA) infections as well as community-acquired (CA-MRSA) infections
- Associated with both longer stays and higher costs
- MRSA accounts for 55% of *S. aureus*–related infections in U.S. ICUs
  - CA-MRSA is microbiologically distinct isolate with a specific sensitivity pattern and the presence of the Panton-Valentine leukocidin (PVL) exotoxin
  - Factor responsible for the virulence of CA-MRSA remains uncharacterized
  - Methicillin resistance related to acquisition of a staphylococcal cassette chromosome (SCC) that is known as the *mecA* gene
    - CA-MRSA distinguished from hospital-acquired MRSA by the presence of type 4 SCC
    - Expression of the *mecA* gene leads to an altered penicillin-binding protein, PBP2a, which has a reduced affinity for β-lactam rings
  - CA-MRSA associated with significant skin and soft tissue infections
    - Often requiring emergency room surgical drainage
    - More severe infections, such as necrotizing pneumonia, necessitating hospital admission
  - Nosocomial infections with HA-MRSA include:
    - Catheter-related bacteremia, postsurgical wound infections
    - Postoperative neurosurgical meningitis
    - Ventilator-associated pneumonia
    - Device and graft infections
  - Risk factors for MRSA infection include:
    - Patients with open wounds or pressure ulcers
    - Invasive devices such as catheter, tracheostomy, gastrostomy, nasogastric tube, and indwelling bladder catheter
    - Recent antibiotic therapy
    - Hospitalization or significant health care contact within the past 6 months
    - Increased age
    - Male gender
  - Knowing the MRSA infection status of patients is helpful in determining who should be isolated or cohorted.
    - Nasal swabs for MRSA culture are a way to identify those who are colonized, but time delay in identifying these patients based on cultures makes this option less useful.
    - Polymerase chain reaction (PCR) has been proposed as a means of rapid identification of MRSA-colonized patients; however, this may not be cost effective.
  - There are differences in the ways that hospitals approach the issue of screening patients for MRSA.
    - But once isolated from culture patient should be immediately placed on contact precautions

- There are antibiotic options available to treat MRSA infections, as well as to decolonize carriers of MRSA.
  - Prevention of spread is the most important method in combating MRSA infections.
    ○ The hospital should be placed on contact precautions.
    ○ Handwashing remains a critical factor in preventing spread.
    ○ HCWs must wash their hands before and after any contact with a patient.
      – Even when gloves are worn as part of MRSA contact precautions
      – Recommendations for preventing the spread of MRSA also include cohorting of patients if isolation in a single room is not possible.
      – Contact precautions should be observed meticulously.
      – Mask and eye protection are indicated if exposure to aerosols generated by the coughing patient is likely or when irrigating wounds.
      – Precautions for MRSA-infected or -colonized patients the same regardless of strain (HA-MRSA or CA-MRSA)
- Fomites implicated in transmission of MRSA
  - Environmental surfaces described as vectors of MRSA transmission include:
    ○ Plastic patient chart (survived 11 days)
    ○ Laminated tabletop (survived 12 days)
    ○ Cloth curtain (survived 9 days)
  - In the outpatient setting, environmental surfaces are important sources of transmission including:
    ○ Patient examination table
    ○ Computer keyboard
    ○ Pulse oximeter
    ○ Multiple patient chairs located in the triage station, the waiting room, and the examination room
  - Daily routine cleaning should be done with a disinfectant and performed in a sanitary manner as is done in all rooms regardless of the presence of MRSA.
  - Equipment should be routinely cleaned, disinfected, or sterilized per institution policy.

Clostridium Difficile

- *Clostridium* are Gram-positive rods that are anaerobic and spore forming.
  - *C. difficile* is the causative organism of:
  - Pseudomembranous colitis
  - *C. difficile*–associated diarrhea (CDAD)
    ○ Occurs with the use of antibiotics that eradicate normal gut flora
  - Organism produces two toxins, enterotoxin (toxin A) and cytotoxin (toxin B), which are responsible for diarrhea and inflammation
    ○ Growing *C. difficile* in culture the gold standard for diagnosis
      – Enzyme-linked immunosorbent assay (ELISA) testing for toxin A or B has a high sensitivity and specificity when performed on three separate stool specimens
  - In addition to watery diarrhea, computed tomography (CT) scan of the abdomen demonstrating colonic wall thickening is a key finding.
  - Complications of untreated infection include toxic megacolon and bowel perforation.

- Major risk factor for the development of *C. difficile* diarrhea is the use of antibiotics.
  ○ Especially penicillins, clindamycin, and cephalosporins, particularly third-generation cephalosporins
  ○ Repeated enemas, prolonged nasogastric tube insertion, and gastrointestinal surgery increase the risk of developing a disease.
- The disease is spread from person to person by spores that are shed in stool.
- Spores can survive up to 70 days in the environment
- Can be carried on hands of HCW
  - Have direct contact with uninfected patients or with environmental surfaces—floors, bedpans, toilets—thus contaminating them with *C. difficile*
- Treatment of *C. difficile* colitis includes oral metronidazole or oral vancomycin
  - Newer agent, nitazoxanide, has not received U.S. Food and Drug Administration (FDA) approval for this indication, but shows promise in small clinical trials
  - Longer hospital stays and increased costs have been directly related to infection with *C. difficile*
    ○ Recommendations for preventing spread include:
      – Standard precautions and contact precautions if soiling of clothes is likely
      – Handwashing is the only method to be used in preventing spread of *C. difficile*.
        ● The alcohol substitutes do not kill the spores
        ● Mechanical action of applying the hand sanitizer may eliminate some spores from the hand of the HCW
        ● Limiting the use of inappropriate antibiotics is central to lowering risk of developing *C. difficile*–associated diarrhea.

Vancomycin-Resistant Enterococcus

- Enterococci are Gram-positive, facultatively anaerobic organisms that colonize the gastrointestinal tract
- Two species commensal in the intestines of humans:
  - *Enterococcus faecalis* (90% to 95%)
  - *Enterococcus faecium* (5% to 10%)
- Organism not highly invasive, infections caused by enterococci include:
  - Catheter-related bacteremia
  - Urinary tract infections
  - Diverticular abscess
  - Cholangitis
  - Endocarditis
- Many strains of enterococci remain susceptible to ampicillin, penicillin, and vancomycin
  - An alarming increase in the incidence of VRE
  - Concern regarding resistance in other bacteria, such as *S. aureus*, as VRE appears to have an enhanced ability to pass resistant genes (such as vanA) to other Gram-positive organisms
  - Risk factors for VRE colonization and infection not clearly identified
    ○ Higher incidence in transplant and chemotherapy patients in ICU setting who have renal insufficiency
    ○ Higher risk of colonization and infection is logically associated with intra-abdominal surgery or gastrointestinal tract manipulation such as:
      – Endoscopic retrograde cholangiopancreatography (ERCP)

– Indwelling urinary catheters
– Enteral feeding tubes
– Central venous catheters
○ Patients on broad-spectrum antibiotics
– Especially oral vancomycin, at higher risk for colonization or infection
• Use of intravenous vancomycin is associated to a lesser extent with VRE colonization and infection
• Transmission occurs from a colonized or infected patient to the HCW via direct contact with either the patient or contaminated environmental surfaces (fomites)
• Lack of proper hand hygiene appears to be the major factor in the spread of VRE from patient to HCW and back to other patients
○ Dramatic decrease in incidence of VRE with enforcement of proper hand hygiene
– Either with alcohol-based solutions or with routine handwashing
○ Proper environmental cleaning decreases transmission of VRE
○ Colonized or infected VRE patients should be placed in contact isolation to prevent spread.
• Screening for VRE has been addressed
• Advantage in a clinical active surveillance strategy (culture of a rectal swab on admission, weekly while patient in ICU, and at discharge)
○ Cost savings ranging from $56,258 to $303,334 per month
• Decision should be made at the institutional level regarding the cost effectiveness of a screening program
• Available data support strong consideration for a routine screening program with preventive measures (contact isolation) to help control spread of VRE

Tuberculosis

• *Mycobacterium tuberculosis* (MTb) the causative agent of all forms of tuberculosis—pulmonary, central nervous system (CNS), and disseminated
• Spread by aerosol droplets from persons with active infection when they cough, sneeze, speak, or spit
• Infectious droplets are 0.5 to 5 μm in diameter
• About 40,000 can be produced in a single sneeze
• 3,000 in a single cough
• Transmission from person to person depends on several factors, including:
○ Quantity of infectious droplets expelled
○ Effectiveness of ventilation
○ Duration of exposure
○ Virulence of mycobacterial strain
○ Persons who are in direct contact with an infected patient, either frequently or for a prolonged time, have the highest risk of developing tuberculosis.
– Estimated infection rate of 22%
– Person with untreated, active tuberculosis can infect 10 to 15 people per year.
○ Others at risk for infection include:
– Persons living in endemic areas—some parts of Asia, Haiti, and South America
– Immunocompromised patients—those with HIV/AIDS and those on immunosuppressive medications
– HCWs serving high-risk patients
– IV drug abusers

– Single males, alcoholics, the urban poor—especially the homeless—migrant farm workers, and prison inmates have been associated with a higher frequency of tuberculosis
• Rate of tuberculosis in United States has steadily declined since a resurgence between 1985 and 1992 that correlated with the AIDS epidemic prior to the development of highly active antiretroviral therapy (HAART)
• Now majority of MTb cases in United States diagnosed in persons who are immigrants from endemic areas
• A recent deceleration in the yearly percentage of decline
○ From average of 7.1% per year (1993 through 2000)
○ To 3.8% per year (2001 through 2005)
○ Raised concerns regarding the progress toward the goal of eliminating MTb in United States
○ CDC has noted racial/ethnic disparities, as well as a disparity between U.S.-born and foreign-born MTb rates
– 2005, Hispanics, African Americans, and Asians were respectively 7.3, 8.3, and 19.6 times more likely than whites to become infected with the disease
– MTb rates were 8.7 times higher for foreign-born individuals compared U.S. counterparts
– More than half of foreign-born cases were reported in patients from Mexico, the Philippines, Vietnam, India, and China
– More alarming data from the most recent CDC report is the finding of higher rates of multidrug- and extended drug-resistant tuberculosis
• Most effective way to prevent the spread of tuberculosis to HCW:
• Identify patients at high risk of active infection
○ Includes an assessment of symptoms
– Fever, night sweats, shortness of breath, hemoptysis, and weight loss
○ Demographic factors including questioning about:
– Immigration from an endemic area
– Recent incarceration
– Contact with patients known to have tuberculosis
○ Identified patients must be placed in a negative pressure isolation room with airborne precautions
– Should have three expectorated or induced sputum specimens sent for acid-fast staining and culture for acid-fast bacilli (AFB)
• Patients with suspected MTb infection cannot be removed from isolation until three adequate sputum specimens—or an equivalent, such as specimens obtained by bronchoscopy or bronchoalveolar lavage—have been obtained and are negative for AFB by smear.
• AFB culture may take up to 6 weeks to grow organisms, and is therefore not used to decide on discontinuation of isolation unless there is a very high index of suspicion.
– MTb DNA PCR can be used on a variety of AFB-negative body fluids or can be used to determine if early growth of AFB in liquid media is MTb or a nontuberculosus mycobacteria

Gram-Negative Organisms

• Incidence of multidrug-resistant, Gram-negative infections has stirred debate as to whether isolation precautions as in place for resistant Gram positives should be instituted

- National Nosocomial Infections Surveillance System has reported increases in the prevalence of multidrug-resistant Gram-negative infections including:
  - *Pseudomonas*
  - *Enterobacter*
  - *Klebsiella*
  - Extended-spectrum β-lactamase (ESBL)–producing organisms
- Some institutions have reported outbreaks of highly resistant Acinetobacter *baumannii infections*
  - Interest in *Acinetobacter* is growing now that the organism has been found in soldiers returning from Iraq and Afghanistan
- Not sufficient evidence to determine that infection control measures would be effective in controlling the spread of multidrug-resistant Gram-negative bacteria
- Outbreaks of resistant Gram-negative infections associated with catheters and other intravascular devices including one report of *Stenotrophomonas* prosthetic valve endocarditis
  - Fatalities have been reported
  - Control of outbreaks has included both antibiotic restriction as well as institution of contact isolation
  - When dealing with multidrug-resistant, virulent, Gram-negative organisms, especially in such settings as the ICU
    - Contact isolation should be strongly considered for use in colonized and infected patients as suggested by CDC guidelines

CHAPTER 69 ■ AN APPROACH TO THE FEBRILE INTENSIVE CARE UNIT PATIENT

- Fever is a common problem in the intensive care unit (ICU).
  - Approximately 70% of patients developing a fever at some point during their hospital stays.
  - Infectious and noninfectious etiologies contribute almost equally to causation.
  - Discovery of fever in ICU patient has significant impact on health care costs due to:
    - Blood cultures
    - Radiologic imaging
    - Antibiotics that routinely follow
- Important to have a good understanding of the mechanisms and etiology of fever in ICU patients, how and when to initiate a diagnostic workup, and when initiation of antibiotics is indicated
- Temperature of 38.3°C or greater (101°F) in an ICU patient warrants further evaluation
  - Temperature below 38.3°C (101°F) may also require further investigation
    - Many variables determine a patient's febrile response to an insult
    - Daily fluctuation of temperature by 0.5°C to 1.0°C
      - Women having wider variations in temperature than men
      - With aging, the maximal febrile response decreases by about 0.15°C per decade
- Accurate and reproducible measurement of body temperature important in detecting disease and in monitoring patients with an elevated temperature
  - Methods are used to measure body temperature:
    - Mixed venous blood in pulmonary artery optimal site for core temperature measurement
    - Infrared ear thermometry provides values a few tenths of a degree below temperatures in pulmonary artery and brain

- Rectal temperatures obtained with a mercury thermometer or electronic probe often a few tenths of a degree higher than core
  - Patients perceive having rectal temperatures taken as unpleasant and intrusive
  - Access to rectum may be limited by patient position, with an associated risk of rectal trauma
- Oral measurements influenced by events such as:
  - Eating and drinking
  - Presence of respiratory devices delivering warmed gases
  - Many tachypneic patients are unable to keep their mouth closed to obtain accurate temperature
- Axillary measurements substantially underestimate core temperature and lack reproducibility
- Body temperature therefore most accurately measured with an intravascular thermistor
  - Measurement by infrared ear thermometry or with an electronic probe in the rectum is an acceptable alternative

PATHOGENESIS OF FEVER

- Cytokines released by monocytic cells play a central role in the genesis of fever
- Interleukin-1 (IL-1)
- Interleukin-6 (IL-6)
- Tumor necrosis factor-α (TNF-α)
- Interaction between these cytokines is complex
  - Each able to up-regulate and down-regulate their own expression as well as that of the other cytokines
  - Cytokines bind to specific receptors located in close proximity to preoptic region of the anterior hypothalamus
    - Cytokine receptor interaction activates phospholipase A_2

- Resulting in the liberation of plasma membrane arachidonic acid as substrate for the cyclo-oxygenase pathway
- Some cytokines appear to increase cyclo-oxygenase expression directly, leading to the liberation of prostaglandin E$_2$ (PGE$_2$)
- Is fever good or bad?
  - If fever of hospitalized patients admitted to a trauma ICU treated, a strong trend toward increased mortality
    - All patients who died in aggressive treatment group had an infectious etiology as cause of fever
  - Children with varicella treated with acetaminophen had a more prolonged illness
  - Patients with spontaneous bacterial peritonitis had improved survival if they had a temperature >38°C.
  - Thus, fever from an infectious cause should not be treated unless the patient has limited cardiorespiratory reserve.
  - In contrast, patients with cerebral ischemia or head trauma have worse outcomes with increased temperature.
    - Current recommendation to maintain patient's temperature in normothermic range
- Antipyresis must always include an antipyretic agent, as external cooling alone increases heat generations and catecholamine production
  - Acute hepatitis may occur in ICU patients with reduced glutathione reserves (alcoholics, malnourished, etc.) who have received regular therapeutic doses of acetaminophen

FEVER PATTERNS

- Evaluation of patient's fever pattern fraught with uncertainty and not likely to be helpful diagnostically:
  - Most patients have remittent or intermittent fever
    - When due to infection, usually follows a diurnal variation
    - Sustained fevers have been reported in patients with Gram-negative pneumonia or central nervous system (CNS) damage
  - Appearance of fever at different time points in course of patient's illness may provide some diagnostic clues
    - Fevers that arise more than 48 hours after institution of mechanical ventilation may be secondary to a developing pneumonia
    - Fevers arising 5 to 7 days postoperatively may be related to abscess formation
    - Fevers arising 10 to 14 days after institution of antibiotics for intra-abdominal abscess may be due to fungal infections

CAUSES OF FEVER IN THE INTENSIVE CARE UNIT

- Any disease process releasing IL-1, IL-6, and TNF-α will result in fever.
- Infections are common causes of fever in ICU patients.
  - But noninfectious inflammatory conditions cause release of proinflammatory cytokines and induce a febrile response
  - Not all patients with infections are febrile.
    - Approximately 10% of septic patients are hypothermic, 35% normothermic at presentation
    - Septic patients who fail to develop a fever have a significantly higher mortality than febrile septic patients.

- Important ICU fever be evaluated in a systematic, prudent, clinically appropriate, and cost-effective manner

Infectious Causes of Fever in the Intensive Care Unit

- Prevalence of nosocomial infection in ICUs reported to vary from 3% to 31%
- The most common infectious causes of fever in ICU patients are listed in Table 69.1.

Catheter-Related Bloodstream Infection (CRBI)

- Intravenous (IV) catheters are a major source of infection in the ICU.
- Mean incidence of CRBI in United States is 5.3 per 1,000 catheter-days
  - Coagulase-negative staphylococci account for up to 40% of cases
  - Other common causes of CRBI include:
    - Enterococci
    - *Staphylococcus aureus*
    - *Candida* species
    - Aerobic Gram-negative bacilli
    - Methicillin-resistant *Staphylococcus aureus* (MRSA) and vancomycin-resistant enterococci (VRE) are becoming important causes of CRBI.
- Different mechanisms lead to CRBI:
  - Skin pathogens can infect the catheter exit site and then migrate down the tract along the external catheter surface.
  - Pathogens can also contaminate the catheter hub, leading to intraluminal catheter colonization and infection.
  - Hematogenous seeding of the external surface of the catheter may also occur.
    - Despite rigorous skin disinfection, viable micro-organisms can be impacted during insertion of the distal tip of the catheter, causing infection.
    - A number of factors increase the risk of CRBI:
      - Number of lumens in the central venous catheter
      - Number of stopcocks
      - Transfusion of blood and blood products
      - Parenteral nutrition
      - An open infusion system

TABLE 69.1

MOST COMMON INFECTIOUS CAUSES OF FEVER IN THE INTENSIVE CARE UNIT

Catheter-related bloodstream infection
Ventilator-associated pneumonia
Primary septicemia
Sinusitis
Surgical site/wound infection
Clostridia difficile colitis
Cellulitis/infected decubitus ulcer
Urinary tract infection
Suppurative thrombophlebitis
Endocarditis
Diverticulitis
Septic arthritis
Abscess/empyema

○ Catheter-related thrombosis is associated with an increased risk of catheter infection.
   – Thrombocytopenia has been suggested to be protective against CRBI.
○ AIDS and hematologic malignancies are independent risk factors for CRBI.
- Site of central venous catheter (CVC) placement and length of time it can be left indwelling a controversial topic
  - Generally subclavian catheters have been found to have a lower risk of infection than femoral catheters.
  - No difference in risk of CRBI between subclavian, internal jugular, and femoral catheter placement
  - Risk of CRBI increases with the time the catheter remains *in situ.*
    - Changing catheters at regularly scheduled intervals not shown to reduce risk of CRBI
- Diagnosis of CRBI can be challenging.
  - Routine culture of blood withdrawn from catheter not recommended
  - Catheter exit site should be inspected daily for evidence of erythema or pus
    - Absence of local infection does not exclude CRBI
  - In patient with indwelling CVC developing a fever
    - Two sets of blood cultures should be drawn:
    ○ One from the catheter
    ○ One from a peripheral source
    - If patient has systemic signs of infection and no other identifiable source of infection, catheter should be removed and empiric antibiotics commenced pending culture results
    - In patients with limited venous access, CVC may be replaced with a new catheter over a guidewire.
    ○ Both catheter tip and the intracutaneous portion of the catheter should be sent for culture
    - If catheter culture returns positive (>15 colony-forming units [CFU]), or the blood cultures are consistent with a CRBI, the catheter that was changed over a guidewire must be removed and replaced with a new catheter at a clean site.
    - Follow-up blood cultures should be obtained in patients with CRBI:
    ○ If positive, thorough investigation for septic thrombosis, infective endocarditis, and other metastatic infections should be pursued
- Methods have been investigated for the diagnosis of CRBI that do not require removal of CVC.
  - Comparison of blood cultured from the central catheter with that from a peripheral venous site is a most useful technique.
    ○ In CRBI quantitative culture counts are greater and time to positivity shorter with blood withdrawn from the catheter as opposed to the peripheral site
  - Acridine-orange leukocyte cytospin testing, available in some countries, is a rapid, inexpensive test that can also be used to prevent unnecessary removal of catheters.
  - Endoluminal brushing, in which the CVC is sampled within 3 to 5 cm of the catheter tip, has also been demonstrated to be useful in the diagnosis of CRBI.

Ventilator-Associated Pneumonia (VAP)

- Common source of fever in intubated patient
- Intubation increases the risk of developing pneumonia from 6- to 21-fold

- Between 10% and 25% of patients on mechanical ventilation will develop VAP during ICU stay
- VAP is associated with significant costs and has an attributable mortality of about 25%
- Risk of acquiring VAP is highest in the first week, at 3% a day
  - Thereafter decreasing to 2% a day in the second week
  - Down to 1% a day in the third and subsequent weeks
- Risk of VAP is higher in trauma, burn, and neurosurgical units compared to medical ICUs
- VAP is usually categorized as either:
  - Early: occurring <48 hours after intubation
  - Late onset: occurring after 5 to 7 days of intubation
  - Distinction between these two phases of VAP is vitally important, as they are associated with different pathogens
    - Early-onset VAP is associated with bacteria that are normally sensitive to antibiotics:
    ○ Methicillin-sensitive *S. aureus*
    ○ *Haemophilus influenzae*
    ○ *Streptococcus pneumoniae*
  - Late onset is typically associated with antibiotic-resistant bacteria:
    ○ MRSA
    ○ *Pseudomonas aeruginosa*
    ○ *Acinetobacter* species
    ○ *Enterobacter* species
- Major risk factors for VAP include:
  - Age over 60 years
  - Male gender
  - Chronic lung disease
  - Acute respiratory distress syndrome
  - Aspiration
  - Sinusitis
  - Nasogastric tube
  - Transport in and out of the ICU
  - Failure to elevate the head of the bed
  - Endotracheal cuff pressures <20 cm of H_2O
  - Increased severity of illness
  - Delayed extubation
  - Continuous sedation
  - Cardiopulmonary resuscitation
  - Medications including H_2 blockers and paralytic agents
- Diagnosis of VAP:
  - VAP suspected when a patient on mechanical ventilation develops a new infiltrate on a chest radiograph (CXR) along with:
    - Leukocytosis
    - Fever
    - Purulent tracheobronchial secretions
  - Presence of new infiltrate on CXR, together with two of above-cited clinical findings:
    - Has sensitivity of 69% with a specificity of 75% for diagnosis of VAP
  - Decision to treat a suspected VAP on clinical grounds alone will frequently overdiagnose the condition and lead to treatment that fails to cover the correct pathogen in patients with true VAP
  - Quantitative cultures of secretions obtained from lower respiratory tract can facilitate making VAP diagnosis.
    - Two most common techniques include:
    ○ Protected specimen brush (PSB) sampling
    ○ Bronchoalveolar lavage (BAL)

- These techniques can be performed bronchoscopically or blindly
  - Blind bronchial suctioning and mini-bronchoalveolar lavage are gaining popularity
  - Shown to be as effective as a protected specimen brush
- These are generally safe, inexpensive tests that can be performed by respiratory therapists without a physician present
  - We are aware of significant complications caused by mini-BAL and recommend great care and thought before initiating its use
    - The threshold for positivity is 1,000 CFU/mL for PSB
    - 10,000 CFU/mL for BAL
    - A threshold of 500 and 5,000 CFU/mL, respectively, will increase the sensitivity of the tests, but this is controversial.
    - Microscopic examination of BAL fluid is used to facilitate the diagnosis of VAP.
      - With <50% neutrophils, pneumonia can be excluded.
    - Role of quantitative culture of tracheal aspirates (as opposed to lower respiratory tract sampling) is unclear at this time.
    - Effect of quantitative culture techniques on patient outcome is unclear.
      - However, these techniques result in a significant reduction in the use of antibiotics.

Urinary Tract Infection (UTI)

- Most ICU patients require an indwelling urinary catheter for monitoring fluid balance and renal function.
- UTIs are the third most common infection found in the ICU.
  - In patients admitted to the ICU for at least 48 hours:
    - 6.5% developed a UTI
    - Overall incidence of 9.6 cases per 1,000 ICU days
    - Incidence of bacteremia and fungemia was only 0.1 case per 1,000 catheter-days
    - UTIs more common in medical ICU and least likely in cardiothoracic patients
  - Reported risk factors for UTIs include:
    - Female gender
    - Age over 60 years
    - Antimicrobial therapy use
    - Severity of illness
    - Duration of urinary catheterization
    - Presence of urinary catheter for longer than 4 to 5 days increases risk of UTI
      - Gram-negative bacteria, especially *Escherichia coli* and *Pseudomonas aeruginosa*, account for more than half of pathogens
      - Gram-positive organisms, especially *Enterococcus* and *Candida*, account for remaining cases
  - Risk factors for funguria include:
    - Immunosuppression
    - Diabetes
    - Renal failure
    - Structural or functional abnormalities of the urinary tract
    - Recent surgery
    - Chronic illness
    - Broad-spectrum antibiotics
- Examination of the urine with "dipsticks" for leukocyte esterase and nitrate is insensitive and not a substitute for quantitative culture.

- Significance of UTIs in catheterized ICU patients unclear
- Appear unlikely to lead to increased morbidity or mortality
- Most patients have asymptomatic bacteriuria rather than true infections of the urinary tract.
  - Treatment of patients with asymptomatic bacteriuria is based on a single study performed in the early 1980s that may not be applicable today.
    - In hospitalized patients, bacteriuria $\geq 10^5$ CFU of bacteria per mL urine during bladder catheterization was associated with a 2.8-fold increase in mortality.
      - Based on this study, thousands of ICU patients with urinary tract colonization have been, and continue to be, treated with antibiotics. Recent studies suggest that this approach may not be optimal.
- In patients with indwelling urinary catheters, colonic flora rapidly colonizes the urinary tract.
  - In catheterized patients, bacteria rapidly proliferate in the urinary system to exceed 10^5 CFU/mL over a short period of time
  - Bacteriuria-quantitative culture $\geq 10^5$ CFU/mL reported in up to 30% of catheterized hospitalized patients
    - Bacteriuria implies colonization of the urinary tract without bacterial invasion and an acute inflammatory response
    - Urinary tract infection implies an infection of the urinary tract
    - Criteria have not been developed for differentiating asymptomatic colonization of the urinary tract from symptomatic infection.
    - Presence of white cells in urine is useful for differentiating colonization from infection
      - Most catheter-associated bacteriuria have accompanying pyuria
      - Unclear how many catheterized patients with $\geq 10^5$ CFU/mL actually have UTI
  - Catheter-associated bacteriuria common in ICU patients
    - Less than 3% of catheter-associated bacteriuric patients will develop bacteremia caused by organisms in the urine
      - Surveillance for, and treatment of, isolated bacteriuria in most ICU patients is currently not recommended.
      - Bacteriuria should be treated following:
        - Urinary tract manipulation
        - Surgery in patients with kidney stones
        - Urinary tract obstruction
      - With systemic signs of infection together with bacteriuria and no other obvious source of infection:
        - Prudent to treat this patient with a short course of antibiotics
        - Ultrasonography to exclude urinary tract obstruction and repeat urine culture is recommended
      - Treatment clearly indicated in patients with bacteriuria who develop bloodstream infection
      - Isolated *Candida* lower UTI exceedingly uncommon
        - When diagnosis entertained, *Candida* infection of kidney should be excluded

Sinusitis

- An underappreciated cause of fever in the ICU
  - Diagnosis is usually not considered or made until other, more common infectious causes of fever excluded
  - If not diagnosed and treated in a timely fashion, can lead to nosocomial pneumonia and severe sepsis

- Risk factors of acquiring nosocomial sinusitis:
  - Nasal colonization with enteric Gram-negative rods
  - Nasoenteric tubes
  - Glasgow Coma Scale score <7
  - Patients who are orally intubated are less prone to develop sinusitis than those who are nasotracheally intubated
    – Up to 85% of nasally intubated patients will develop sinusitis within a week
- In patients with radiologic evidence of sinusitis:
  - Aspiration of the sinuses is required to confirm the diagnosis and to identify the causative pathogen.
  - Radiologic tests employed to identify problem
    - Computed tomography (CT) scan of sinuses is considered gold standard study
    - If patient too ill to be transported from ICU, plain films of sinuses may be obtained
      – To maximize chances of making diagnosis, multiple views required
    - Bedside ultrasound gaining popularity in European countries over the past decade
      – May be at least equivalent to CT scanning
- Once sinusitis diagnosed:
  - All nasal tubes should immediately removed
  - Early sinus drainage performed
  - Broad-spectrum antibiotics should be commenced
    - Coverage will includes *Pseudomonas* and MRSA
    - Antibiotics should then be deescalated once culture data are available
    - Topical decongestants and vasoconstrictors, alone or combined with systemic decongestants and antihistamines, are also recommended

Clostridium Difficile Colitis

- See above
- Crucial to diagnose this disease early, as it can lead to severe sepsis, multiorgan system failure, and death
  - Often present with a leukemoid reaction, with white blood cell (WBC) counts reaching >35,000 cells/μL
    - Leukemoid reaction or unexplained leukocytosis may be presenting sign of *C. difficile*
    - Even in the absence of diarrheal symptoms
    - *C. difficile* presenting with a leukemoid reaction associated with worse prognosis and higher mortality
  - Concurrent or prior antibiotic use a strong risk factor
    - Clindamycin
    - β-lactams (especially cephalosporins)
    - Quinolones
  - Proton pump Inhibitors associated with a higher risk of *C. difficile* infection
  - Epidemics of extremely virulent strain of *C. difficile* reported in United States and Canada
    - Suggested that increasing use of fluoroquinolones has played a role
    - Strain associated with higher morbidity and mortality
    - Produces significantly more toxins than do the other strains
  - The diagnosis of *C. difficile* colitis:
    - Usually made by immunoassays of stool against both toxin A and toxin B
    - Presence of *C. difficile* antigen in absence of toxin suggests colonization

- Low sensitivity of the toxin assay results in two stool specimens being examined
- Cytotoxic assay more sensitive and specific but not readily available and takes longer to perform
- Where diagnosis is in doubt, colonoscopy performed to look for pseudomembranes
- CT scan may be helpful
  - 50% of patients will have changes that can be seen on imaging
  - Positive CT scans are associated with leukocytosis, abdominal pain, and diarrhea
- If *C. difficile* colitis is suspected:
  - Empiric treatment should be started until diagnosis excluded
  - Alcohol-based hand hygiene does not kill spore-forming organisms such as *C. difficile*
    - Should not replace handwashing with soap

Skin Infections

- Especially infected pressure ulcers, may be a source of infection in ICU patients
- Several factors increase the risk of ICU patients developing pressure ulcers, including:
  - Emergent admissions
  - Severity of illness
  - Extended ICU length of stay
  - Malnutrition
  - Age
  - Diabetes
  - Infusion of vasopressor agents
  - Anemia
  - Fecal incontinence
- Protocols for prevention of pressure ulcers should be routine in ICU
  - Physicians and nurses should routinely examine their patient's skin
    - Particularly high-pressure areas such as sacrum and heels to detect early signs of skin breakdown

Other Infections

- Nosocomial meningitis exceedingly uncommon in hospitalized patients who have not undergone a neurosurgical procedure
  - Lumbar puncture does not need to be performed routinely in nonneurosurgical ICU patients who develop a fever
    - Unless they have meningeal signs or contiguous infection
- Patients who have undergone abdominal surgery and develop a fever, intra-abdominal infection must always be excluded
  - Evaluation includes CT scanning of the abdomen
  - In patients who have undergone other operative procedures, wound infection must be excluded

Noninfectious Causes of Fever in the Intensive Care Unit

- Many noninfectious conditions result in tissue injury with inflammation and fever Table 69.2.
- Most noninfectious disorders usually do not lead to a fever in excess of 38.9°C (102°F)
  - Reason is unclear

TABLE 69.2

NONINFECTIOUS CAUSES OF FEVER IN THE
INTENSIVE CARE UNIT

Drug-related
Drug fever
Neuroleptic malignant syndrome
Malignant hyperthermia
Serotonin syndrome
Drug withdrawal (including alcohol and recreational drugs)
Intravenous contrast reaction

Posttransfusion Fever
Neurologic
Intracranial hemorrhage
Cerebral infarction
Subarachnoid hemorrhage
Seizures
Endocrine
Hyperthyroidism
Pheochromocytoma
Adrenal insufficiency
Rheumatologic
Crystal arthropathies
Vasculitis
Collagen vascular diseases
Hematologic
Phlebitis
Hematoma
Gastrointestinal/Hepatic
Acalculous cholecystitis
Ischemic bowel
Cirrhosis
Hepatitis
Gastrointestinal bleed
Pancreatitis
Pulmonary
Aspiration pneumonitis
Acute respiratory distress syndrome
Thromboembolic disease
Fat embolism syndrome
Cardiac
Myocardial infarction
Dressler syndrome
Pericarditis
Oncologic
Neoplastic syndromes

- Generally, if the temperature increases above this threshold, the patient should be considered to have an infectious etiology
  - Patients with drug fever may have a temperature >102°F
  - Fever secondary to blood transfusion may exceed 102°F
  - With a temperature >40°C (104°F), must consider:
    ○ Neuroleptic malignant syndrome
    ○ Malignant hyperthermia
    ○ "Serotonin syndrome"
    ○ Subarachnoid hemorrhage

Drug-Induced Fever

- Estimated that about 10% of inpatients develop drug fever during their hospital stay
  - Patients with human immunodeficiency syndrome (HIV) at a particularly high risk of developing a drug fever

- Diagnosis of drug fever in ICU patients is challenging
  - Onset of fever can occur immediately after administration of the drug or it can occur days, weeks, months, or even years after the patient has been on the offending medication.
  - Once implicated medication is discontinued, fever can take 3 to 4 days to resolve.
  - Associated rashes and leukocytosis occur in <20% of cases.
  - Penicillins, cephalosporins, anticonvulsants, heparin, and H_2 blockers commonly used medications in ICU associated with drug fevers
- Five mechanisms have been described that give rise to drug fevers:
  - Most common mechanism is a hypersensitivity reaction to the drug
  - Medications can cause fever by disrupting normal thermoregulatory mechanisms of the body
  - Drugs can cause fever directly related to administration of the drug
    - From contamination of the solution with endotoxin or other exogenous pyrogens
    - Can also cause a chemical phlebitis or inflammation at the site of injection
  - Due to the direct extension of the pharmacologic action of the drug
    - Chemotherapy with cell necrosis, lysis, and the release of various pyrogenic substances
    - Antimicrobial therapy with the release of bacterial products into the circulation, known as the Jarisch-Herxheimer reaction
  - Idiosyncratic reactions including:
    - Malignant hyperthermia
    - Neuroleptic malignant syndrome
    - Serotonin syndrome
    - Glucose-6-phosphate dehydrogenase deficiency
- **Malignant Hyperthermia.** A rare genetic disorder of the muscle membrane causing an increase of calcium ions in the muscle cells
  - Can cause a variety of clinical problems, most commonly a dangerous hypermetabolic state after the use of agents such as succinylcholine and the potent inhaled anesthetic agents
  - Typically occurs within 1 hour of anesthesia but can be delayed for up to 10 hours
  - Patients present with continually increasing fevers, muscle stiffness, and tachycardia.
  - Can rapidly develop hemodynamic instability with progression to multiorgan failure
  - With dantrolene, mortality of malignant hyperthermia has decreased from 80% in the 1960s to <10%
- **Neuroleptic Malignant Syndrome.** Characterized by high fevers, a change in mental status, muscle rigidity, extrapyramidal symptoms, autonomic nervous system disturbances, and altered levels of consciousness
  - Symptoms usually begin within days to weeks of starting the offending drug
  - Typically see very high creatinine kinase levels
  - Caused by excessive dopaminergic blockade causing CNS dopamine deficiency
  - Agents most commonly implicated include:
    ○ Neuroleptic medications
    ○ Certain antiemetics

- Treatment includes discontinuing the offending drug, aggressive supportive care, and close hemodynamic monitoring
- Drug treatment controversial
  - Case control analysis and a retrospective analysis of published cases suggested that dantrolene, bromocriptine, and amantadine may be beneficial.
- **Serotonin Syndrome.** Shares many of the clinical features found in neuroleptic malignant syndrome
  - Typically have lower fevers than those with neuroleptic malignant syndrome, but have more gastrointestinal dysfunction
  - Neuromuscular findings are more consistent with hyperreactivity
    - Tremors
    - Clonus
    - Muscular hypertonicity
  - Presentation is much more rapid than that of neuroleptic malignant syndrome
    - 74.3% of patients presented within 24 hours of medication initiation, overdose, or change in dosage
    - 61.5% presented within the first 6 hours
    - Hunter Serotonin Toxicity Criteria commonly used to evaluate likelihood of serotonin syndrome
      - Criteria include the following features in a patient recently administered a serotonergic agent:
        - Spontaneous clonus
        - Inducible clonus
        - Ocular clonus
        - Agitation or diaphoresis
        - Tremor and hyperreflexia
        - Hypertonicity
        - Fever >38°C
  - Benzodiazepines used for control of agitation
    - Physical restraints should be avoided
    - Cyproheptadine, an H_1-receptor antagonist with nonspecific 5-HT1A and 5-HT2A antagonistic properties, has been used in patients who respond poorly to benzodiazepines alone.
  - Paralysis with nondepolarizing agents, endotracheal intubation, and mechanical ventilation may be needed in severely agitated and hyperthermic patients

Alcohol and Drug Withdrawal

- Withdrawal from alcohol and medications is a common cause of noninfectious fever in hospitalized patients.
- Usually presents within the first few days of hospital admission
- Can present in a variety of ways including:
  - Fever alone
  - Neuroleptic malignant-like syndromes
  - Fever with hemodynamic instability
- Important to get an accurate list of current medications at the time of admission
- Drug withdrawal syndromes have been described with the use of:
  - Baclofen
  - Selective serotonin reuptake inhibitors (SSRI)
  - Antidepressants
  - Levodopa
  - Narcotics

- Certain street drugs
- Some herbal remedies

Crystal-Associated Arthritis

- Patients in the ICU at increased risk of developing gout or pseudogout
  - Thorough physical examination focusing on joints and an arthrocentesis to examine the synovial fluid are essential in making this diagnosis
- Gout will typically present as a monoarthritis
  - Patients at increased risk for gout have:
    - Increased body mass index
    - Hypertension
    - Alcohol consumption
    - Renal disease
  - Trauma, surgery, and severe infection are associated with an abrupt drop in uric acid level, which can trigger acute gout.
  - Loop diuretics, iodinated contrast dye, and total parenteral nutrition may also precipitate gout.
- Calcium pyrophosphate dehydrate crystal deposition disease (pseudogout)
  - Most commonly affects the knee
  - Can be triggered by trauma, surgery, or severe medical illness
  - Increased risk with electrolyte disorders:
    - Hypomagnesemia
    - Hypophosphatemia
  - Also associated with endocrine and metabolic disorders:
    - Hyperparathyroidism
    - Hemochromatosis
    - Wilson disease
    - Hypothyroidism

Acalculous Cholecystitis

- Condition of inflammation of the gallbladder in the absence of calculi
  - Carries significant morbidity and mortality
    - Can lead to:
      - Empyema
      - Gallbladder gangrene
      - Gallbladder perforation
- High index of suspicion required as a difficult diagnosis to make
  - Especially in intubated and sedated patient
  - Initially patients present with very few symptoms
  - Clinical features include:
    - Fever
    - Leukocytosis
    - Abnormal liver function tests
    - Palpable right upper quadrant mass
    - Vague abdominal discomfort
    - Jaundice
  - Untreated, bacterial superinfection may occur
    - Can progress to empyema, peritonitis, and septic shock
- Pathophysiology complex and involves hypoperfusion and biliary stasis
  - Risk factors include everything seen in the ICU:
    - Trauma
    - Surgery
    - Intermittent positive pressure ventilation
    - Coronary heart disease

○ Cholesterol emboli
○ Fasting
○ Total parental nutrition
○ Immunosuppression
○ Transfusions of blood products
○ Hypotension
○ Multiorgan dysfunction
○ Sedation/opiates
○ Diabetes
○ Infections
○ Childbirth
○ Renal failure
- Ultrasound usually first diagnostic test performed, as it may be performed at bedside
  - Ultrasound inferior to morphine cholescintigraphy and CT
  - Ultrasound has sensitivity of 29% to 50% compared to 67% to 90% for morphine cholescintigraphy with specificity of 94% and 100%, respectively
  - Abnormal ultrasound can be seen in 50% of ICU patients, even if they are not suspected of having acalculous cholecystitis
  - As soon as the diagnosis is suspected:
    ○ Blood cultures should be drawn
    ○ Broad-spectrum antibiotics initiated
    ○ Surgical consult requested
    ○ Percutaneous drainage preferable to surgical intervention in unstable patient

Postoperative Fever

- Surgery alone can cause self-limited fever
  - Early postoperative period patient's temperature may increase up to 1.4°C
    - Peak occurs approximately 11 hours after surgery
  - 50% of postoperative patients develop a fever ≥38°C
    - 25% reaching 38.5°C or higher
  - Fever typically lasts for 2 to 3 days
- Postoperative fever believed to be caused by tissue injury and inflammation with associated cytokine release
  - Invasiveness of procedure and genetic factors influences degree of cytokine release and febrile response
  - Physical examination, history of timing, and sequence of events crucial to help differentiate this from other causes of infectious and noninfectious fever
    - Reactions to medications, especially anesthesia, blood products, and infections that might have existed prior to the surgery, should be considered during early postoperative course.
    - Nosocomial and surgical site infections usually develop 3 to 5 days postoperatively.

Atelectasis

- Commonly implicated as a cause of fever even in standard ICU texts
  - No primary reference source to support this assertion
  - Medical students and house-staff have been taught that atelectasis is one of the five main causes of postoperative fever
    - Little data to support this widely held belief
  - In 100 postoperative cardiac surgery patients no relationship between atelectasis and fever
  - Atelectasis induced in experimental animals by ligation of a main stem bronchus shows no fever

- IL-1 and TNF-α levels in macrophage cultures from atelectatic lungs were significantly increased compared with control lungs.
- Thus, atelectasis probably does not cause fever absent pulmonary infection.

Blood Transfusions

- Many patients in the ICU will receive transfusions of blood products.
  - 44% of 4,892 ICU patients received blood transfusion
  - 85% of patients in ICU for longer than 1 week reported to receive a blood transfusion
- Febrile, nonhemolytic transfusion reactions exceedingly common following transfusion
  - Likely mediated by the transfusion of cytokines such as IL-1, IL-6, IL-8, and TNF-α, which accumulate with increasing length of blood storage
  - Normally manifest within first 6 hours after transfusion
  - Are self-limiting
  - Can present with chills and rigors in addition to fever
  - Crucial to differentiate from febrile acute hemolytic transfusion reactions
    - These can be life threatening
  - Leukoreduction shown to reduce risk of febrile nonhemolytic transfusion reactions

Thromboembolic Disease

- Fever reported in 14% to 18% of patients with thromboembolic disease
  - Generally uncommon cause of fever in hospitalized patients
  - If present, the fever is typically low grade (37.5°C–38°C)

AN APPROACH TO THE CRITICALLY ILL PATIENT WITH FEVER

- Following approach is suggested in ICU patients who develop a fever (Fig. 69.1)
- Due to frequency, excess morbidity and mortality associated with bacteremia:
  - Blood cultures are recommended in all ICU patients who develop fever
  - Comprehensive physical examination and review of chest radiograph essential
  - Noninfectious causes of fever should be excluded
  - With an obvious focus of infection:
    - Purulent nasal discharge
    - Abdominal tenderness
    - Profuse green diarrhea
  - Focused diagnostic workup is required
  - If no clinically obvious source of infection:
    - Unless the patient is clinically deteriorating
      ○ Falling blood pressure
      ○ Decreased urine output
      ○ Increasing confusion
      ○ Rising serum lactate concentration
      ○ Falling platelet count
      ○ Worsening coagulopathy
      ○ Temperature in excess of 39°C (102°F)

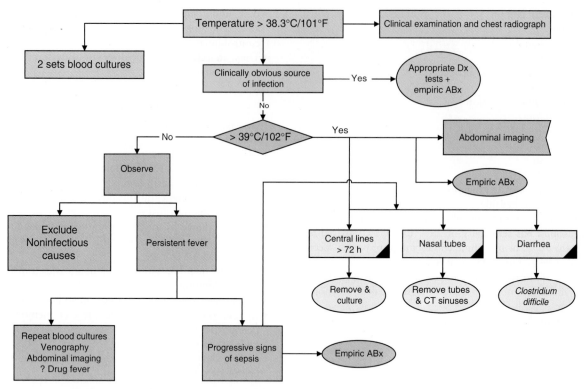

FIGURE 69.1. Suggested diagnostic algorithm for intensive care unit patients who develop a fever. ABx, antibiotics; CT, computed tomography; Dx, diagnostic.

- May be prudent to perform blood cultures and observe before embarking on the further diagnostic tests and commencing empiric antibiotics
  - *ALL neutropenic* patients with fever and patients with severe or progressive signs of sepsis:
    - Should be started on broad-spectrum antimicrobial therapy immediately after obtaining appropriate cultures
- In clinical picture consistent with infection
  - With no clinically obvious source documented
  - Removal of all central catheters more than 48 hours old recommended
    - With semiquantitative or quantitative cultures performed on the intracutaneous segments
  - Stool culture for *C. difficile* toxin in those patients with loose stools
  - CT scan of sinuses with removal of all nasal tubes
  - Urine culture is indicated only in patients with abnormalities of the renal system or following urinary tract manipulation.
    - Bacteriuria common

- If patient at risk of abdominal sepsis or has abdominal signs:
  - Tenderness
  - Distention
  - Inability to tolerate enteral feeds
- CT scan of the abdomen is indicated
- Patients with right upper quadrant tenderness require an abdominal ultrasound or CT examination.
- Reevaluation of status after 48 hours essential:
  - Using all available results
  - Evolution of the patient's clinical condition
  - If fever persists despite empiric antibiotics and no source of infection has been identified
    - Empiric antifungal therapy may be indicated in patients with risk factors
    - Additional diagnostic tests may be appropriate at this time, including:
      - Venography
      - Differential blood count for eosinophils to assist in the diagnosis of drug fever
      - Abdominal imaging

CHAPTER 70 ■ THE ROLE OF ANTIBIOTICS IN THE MANAGEMENT OF SERIOUS HOSPITAL-ACQUIRED INFECTIONS

- ICUs are an important area for emergence of antimicrobial resistance due to:
  - Frequent use of broad-spectrum agents
  - Physical crowding of patients with high-acuity diseases within relatively small specialized areas
  - Reductions in nursing and other support staff due to economic pressures, which increase the likelihood of person-to-person transmission of microorganisms
  - Presence of more chronically and acutely ill patients who require prolonged hospitalizations and often harbor antibiotic-resistant bacteria
- Treatment strategy described is the approach of antibiotic de-escalation
  - Strategy attempts to provide appropriate initial antimicrobial therapy to optimize patient outcomes
  - While avoiding consequences of excessive or unnecessary antibiotic administration

ESSENTIAL DIAGNOSTIC TESTS AND PROCEDURES

- For patients with septic shock:
  - Establish adequate intravenous access and assess intravascular volume status (e.g., measure central venous pressure).
  - Perform a directed medical history and physical examination to identify potential sources and sites of infection.
  - Obtain specimens for microbiologic testing including blood, urine, and lower respiratory tract secretions.
    - Other specimens should be directed by initial history/physical examination (e.g., ascites, pleural fluid, cerebral spinal fluid).
  - Perform radiographic evaluation to identify infection sites requiring expeditious surgical or percutaneous drainage (intra-abdominal abscess, thoracic empyema, necrotizing skin, or visceral infection)

INITIAL THERAPY

- Administer intravenous fluids to patient with septic shock to achieve predetermined goals:
  - Ventral venous pressure >8 mm Hg
  - Oxygen saturation of central venous blood ($S_{svc}O_2$) >70%
- Initial appropriate antibiotic regimen should be prescribed with adequate activity against all pathogens likely to be responsible for the infection

- Dosing and interval of administration should be pharmacokinetically based to ensure that drug concentrations at site of infection are adequate to achieve therapeutic drug levels.
- Antibiotic treatment should be reassessed as soon as microbiologic test results become available.
- Failure of initial antimicrobial therapy should prompt a thorough re-evaluation to identify the reason for failure.
  - Inadequate fluid resuscitation
  - Inappropriate initial antimicrobial therapy
  - Unidentified collection of infected fluid needing drainage
- Drainage of amenable infection sites should occur once the patient has received adequate intravascular fluid replacement and appropriate initial antibiotic therapy.

ANTIMICROBIAL RESISTANCE

Risk Factors and Influence on Outcome

- Antimicrobial use is the key driver for the emergence of antibiotic resistance.
  - Close association between the prior use of antibiotics and the emergence of subsequent antibiotic resistance in both gram-negative and gram-positive bacteria.
  - Other factors promoting antimicrobial resistance include:
    - Prolonged hospitalization
    - Presence of invasive devices such as endotracheal tubes and intravascular catheters (possibly due to the formation of biofilms on the surfaces of these devices)
    - Residence in long-term treatment facilities
    - Inadequate infection control practices
- Antimicrobial regimens that lack action against identified microorganisms causing serious infections (i.e., inappropriate initial antimicrobial therapy) are associated with greater hospital mortality.
  - Changing antibiotic therapy to an appropriate regimen after antimicrobial susceptibility data become available is not demonstrated to improve clinical outcomes.
  - Infectious Disease Society of America/American Thoracic Society (IDSA/ATS) guidelines for the treatment of nosocomial pneumonia emphasize the importance of inappropriate initial antimicrobial therapy as a determinant of hospital mortality.
    - Guideline also stresses importance of maintaining local, frequently updated antibiograms within individual hospitals and ICUs.

- Antimicrobial resistance is associated with excess costs.
  - Most of these costs are simply associated with the acquisition of a nosocomial infection.
  - Presence of antibiotic resistance may also confer added morbidity and costs.

CLINICAL FACTORS THAT AFFECT INITIAL ANTIMICROBIAL SELECTION

- To provide empirical antimicrobial regimen with appropriate spectrum of activity, one must appreciate:
  - Likely pathogens causing various infections
  - Local pathogen distribution and resistance patterns
  - Patient-specific risk factors for resistance
- Recent publication of the NNIS data reported pathogen distribution by site of infection and compared data from 1975 and 2003 as demonstrated in Table 70.1.
  - Occurrence of hospital-acquired infections attributed to potentially antibiotic-resistant bacteria—*Staphylococcus aureus, Pseudomonas aeruginosa*—is increasing
- Gram-negative aerobes remain the most frequently reported pathogen associated with pneumonia (65.9%).
- *Staphylococcus aureus* (27.8%) is the most frequently reported *single* species.
- In patients with primary bloodstream infections:
  - Coagulase-negative staphylococci (42.9%) is the most common pathogen.
  - *Staphylococcus aureus* (14.3%) has been reported as frequently as enterococci (14.5%).
- In patients with urinary tract infections:
  - *Escherichia coli* (26%) is the most frequently reported isolate.
  - *Pseudomonas aeruginosa* constituted 16.3%.
- Surgical site infections:
  - Proportion of gram-negative isolates decreased significantly during past two decades.
  - Gram-positive pathogens are now more commonly associated with both bloodstream infections and skin and skin structure infections.

- Gram-negative aerobes predominate in pneumonia and urinary tract infections.
- Concerning trend reported in NNIS data is increasing isolation of *Acinetobacter* species in urinary tract infections, pneumonia, and surgical site infections.
  - Overall numbers of isolates of *Acinetobacter* are still relatively small (approximately 2.0%); percentage increase is significant.
  - More concerning is community-acquired pneumonia attributed to *Acinetobacter* species, suggesting that this pathogen is extending its area of influence outside of the health care setting.
- For each antibiotic–pathogen combinations tested:
  - Significant increase in resistance between study periods
  - Most impressive were trends in carbapenem- and cephalosporin-resistant *Pseudomonas aeruginosa* and *Acinetobacter* species.
  - Rates of imipenem- and amikacin-resistant *Acinetobacter* isolates are approaching 20%.
    - Organism is intrinsically multidrug-resistant (MDR), which makes these trends particularly worrisome.
      - Many isolates lack effective treatment options and represent a serious public health concern.
- 2003 rates of third-generation cephalosporin-resistance in *Escherichia coli* (6.4%) and *Klebsiella pneumoniae* (14.2%) provide estimates of presence of extended-spectrum β-lactamase (ESBL) producing often MDR bacteria, again with very limited treatment options.
- Prevalence of MDR pathogens varies by patient population, hospital, and type of floor or unit in which the patient resides (Table 70.2).

ANTIBIOTICS, THEIR MODE OF ACTION, CLINICAL INDICATIONS FOR THEIR USE, AND ASSOCIATED TOXICITIES

- Most antimicrobial agents used for treatment of infections are categorized according to principal mechanism of action.

TABLE 70.1

RELATIVE PERCENTAGE BY SITE OF INFECTION OF PATHOGENS ASSOCIATED WITH NOSOCOMIAL INFECTION

Pathogen	PNEU			BSI			SSI			UTI		
Year	1975	1989–1998	2003	1975	1989–1998	2003	1975	1989–1998	2003	1975	1989–1998	2003
Number	4,018	65,056	4,365	1,054	50,091	2,351	7,848	22,043	2,984	16,434	47,502	4,109
Staphylococcus aureus	13.4	16.8	27.8	16.5	10.7	14.3	18.5	12.6	22.5	1.9	1.6	3.6
Pseudomonas aeruginosa	9.6	16.1	18.1	4.8	3	3.4	4.7	9.2	9.5	9.3	10.6	16.3
Enterococcus subspecies	3	1.9	1.3	8.1	10.3	14.5	11.9	14.5	13.9	14.2	13.8	17.4
Enterobacter subspecies	9.6	10.7	10	6	4.2	4.4	4.6	8.8	9	4.7	5.7	6.9
Escherichia coli	11.8	4.4	5	15	2.9	3.3	17.6	7.1	6.5	33.5	18.2	26
Klebsiella pneumoniae	8.4	6.5	7.2	4.5	2.9	4.2	2.7	3.5	3	4.6	6.1	9.8
Serratia marcescens	2.2	—	4.7	2.6	—	2.3	0.5	—	2	1.4	—	1.6
Acinetobacter species	1.5	—	6.9	1.8	—	2.4	0.5	—	2.1	0.6	—	1.6

PNEU, pneumonia; BSI, bloodstream infection; SSI, surgical site infection; UTI, urinary tract infection; —, not reported.
From: Gaynes R, Edwards JR. National Nosocomial Infections Surveillance System. Overview of nosocomial infections caused by gram-negative bacilli. *Clin Infect Dis.* 2005;41:848–854.

TABLE 70.2

DEFINITIONS OF INFECTION CATEGORIES (WITH FOCUS ON BACTERIAL PATHOGENS)

Infection category	Definition
Community-acquired infection	Patients with a first positive bacterial culture obtained within 48 hours of hospital admission lacking risk factors for health care-associated infection
Hospital-acquired infection	Patients with a first positive bacterial culture >48 hours after hospital admission
Health care-associated infection	Patients with a first positive bacterial culture within 48 hours of admission and any of the following: • Admission source indicates a transfer from another health care facility (e.g., hospital, nursing home) • Receiving hemodialysis, wound, or infusion therapy as an outpatient • Prior hospitalization for ≥3 days within 90 days • Immunocompromised state due to underlying disease or therapy (human immunodeficiency virus, chemotherapy)

- For antibacterial agents, the major modes of action include the following:
  - Interference with cell wall synthesis
  - Disruption of the bacterial cell membrane
  - Inhibition of protein synthesis
  - Interference with nucleic acid synthesis
  - Inhibition of a metabolic pathway
- Tables 70.3 through 70.5 review major pathogens, antimicrobials of choice by pathogen, and major toxicities of specific agents.

Cell Wall Active Antibiotics

- Antibacterial drugs that work by inhibiting bacterial cell wall synthesis include:
  - β-lactams, such as the penicillins, cephalosporins, carbapenems, and monobactams
    - Inhibit the synthesis of bacterial cell wall by interfering with enzymes required for the synthesis of peptidoglycan layer
  - Glycopeptides, including vancomycin and teicoplanin
    - Vancomycin and teicoplanin interfere with cell wall synthesis by preventing the cross-linking steps required for stable cell wall synthesis.

Disruption of Bacterial Cell Membrane

- Disruption of the bacterial membrane a less well characterized mechanism of action
  - Polymyxin antibiotics appear to exert their inhibitory effects by increasing bacterial membrane permeability, causing leakage of bacterial contents.
  - Cyclic lipopeptide, daptomycin, appears to insert its lipid tail into the bacterial cell membrane, causing membrane depolarization and eventual death of the bacterium.

Inhibition of Bacterial Protein Synthesis

- Inhibiting protein synthesis:
  - Macrolides
  - Aminoglycosides

  - Tetracyclines
  - Chloramphenicol
  - Streptogramins
  - Oxazolidinones
- Mechanism
  - Macrolides, aminoglycosides, and tetracyclines bind to the 30S subunit of ribosome.
  - Chloramphenicol binds to the 50S subunit.
  - Linezolid is a gram-positive antibacterial oxazolidinone.
    - Binds to the 50S ribosome subunit on a site not shown to interact with other classes of antibiotics.

Inhibition of Nucleic Acid Synthesis

- Fluoroquinolones
  - Disrupt DNA synthesis and cause lethal double-strand DNA breaks during DNA replication

Inhibition of a Metabolic Pathway

- Sulfonamides and trimethoprim block pathway for folic acid synthesis
  - Ultimately inhibits DNA synthesis
  - Antibacterial drug combination of trimethoprim, a folic acid analogue, plus sulfamethoxazole (a sulfonamide) inhibits two steps in the enzymatic pathway for bacterial folate synthesis.

Mechanisms of Resistance to Antibacterial Agents

- Most antimicrobial agents exert their effect by influencing a single step in bacterial reproduction or bacterial cell function.
  - Resistance can emerge with a single point mutation aimed at bypassing or eliminating the action of the antibiotic.
- Some species of bacteria are innately resistant to at least one class of antimicrobial agents.
  - With resulting resistance to all the members of those antibacterial classes
- Several mechanisms of antimicrobial resistance are readily transferred to various bacteria.

TABLE 70.3

MOST COMMON PATHOGENS ASSOCIATED WITH SITES OF SERIOUS INFECTION COMMONLY SEEN IN THE
ADULT INTENSIVE CARE UNIT SETTING

Infection site	Pathogens	
I. Pneumonia		
1. Community-acquired pneumonia (non-immunocompromised host)	*Streptococcus pneumoniae*	
	Haemophilus influenzae	
	Moraxella catarrhalis	
	Mycoplasma pneumoniae	
	Legionella pneumophila	
	Chlamydia pneumoniae	
	Methicillin-resistant *Staphylococcus aureus* (MRSA)	
	Influenza virus	
2. Health care-associated pneumonia	MRSA	
	Pseudomonas aeruginosa	
	Klebsiella pneumoniae	
	Acinetobacter species	
	Stenotrophomonas species	
	Legionella pneumophila	
3. Pneumonia (immunocompromised host)		
a. Neutropenia	Any pathogen listed above	
	Aspergillus species	
	Candida species	
b. Human immunodeficiency virus	Any pathogen listed above	
	Pneumocystis carinii	
	Mycobacterium tuberculosis	
	Histoplasma capsulatum	
	Other fungi	
	Cytomegalovirus	
c. Solid organ transplant or bone marrow transplant	Any pathogen listed above (Can vary depending on timing of infection to transplant)	
d. Cystic fibrosis	*Haemophilus influenzae* (early)	
	Staphylococcus aureus	
	Pseudomonas aeruginosa	
	Burkholderia cepacia	
4. Lung abscess	*Bacteroides* species	
	Peptostreptococcus species	
	Fusobacterium species	
	Nocardia (in immunocompromised patients)	
	Amebic (when suggestive by exposure)	
5. Empyema	*Staphylococcus aureus*	
	Streptococcus pneumoniae	Usually acute
	Group A *Streptococci*	
	Haemophilus influenzae	
	Anaerobic bacteria	Usually subacute or chronic
	Enterobacteriaceae	
	Mycobacterium tuberculosis	
II. Meningitis	*Streptococcus pneumoniae*	
	Neisseria meningitidis	
	Listeria monocytogenes	
	Haemophilus influenzae	
	Escherichia coli	Neonates
	Group B streptococci	
	Staphylococcus aureus	
	Enterobacteriaceae	Postsurgical or post-trauma
	Pseudomonas aeruginosa	
III. Brain abscess	Streptococci	
	Bacteroides species	
	Enterobacteriaceae	Postsurgical or posttrauma
	Staphylococcus aureus	
	Nocardia	Immunocompromised or HIV infected
	Toxoplasma gondii	

(continued)

TABLE 70.3

CONTINUED

Infection site	Pathogens	
IV. Encephalitis	West Nile	
	Herpes simplex	
	Arbovirus	
	Rabies	
	Catscratch disease	
V. Endocarditis	*Streptococcus viridans*	
	Enterococcus species	
	Staphylococcus aureus	
	Streptococcus bovis	
	MRSA	Intravenous drug user, prosthetic value
	Candida species	Prosthetic value
VI. Catheter-associated bacteremia	*Candida* species	
	Staphylococcus aureus	
	Enterococcus species	
	Enterobacteriaceae	
	Pseudomonas aeruginosa	
VII. Pyelonephritis	*Enterobacteriaceae*	
	Escherichia coli	
	Enterococcus species	
	Pseudomonas aeruginosa	Catheter-associated, postsurgical
	Acinetobacter species	
VIII. Peritonitis		
1. Primary or spontaneous	*Enterobacteriaceae*	
	Streptococcus pneumoniae	
	Enterococcus species	
	Anaerobic bacteria (rare)	
2. Secondary (bowel perforation)	*Enterobacteriaceae*	
	Bacteroides species	
	Enterococcus species	
	Pseudomonas aeruginosa (uncommon)	
3. Tertiary (bowel surgery, hospitalized on antibiotics)	*Pseudomonas aeruginosa*	
	MRSA	
	Acinetobacter species	
	Candida species	
IX. Skin structure infections		
1. Cellulitis	Group A streptococci	
	Staphylococcus aureus	
	Enterobacteriaceae	Diabetics
2. Decubitus ulcer	Polymicrobial	
	Streptococcus pyogenes	
	Enterococcus species	
	Enterobacteriaceae	
	Anaerobic streptococci	
	Pseudomonas aeruginosa	
	Staphylococcus aureus	
	Bacteroides species	
3. Necrotizing fasciitis	*Streptococcus* species	
	Clostridia species	
	Mixed aerobic/anaerobic bacteria	
X. Muscle infection		
1. Myonecrosis (gas gangrene)	*Clostridium perfringens*	
	Other *Clostridia* species	
2. Pyomyositis	*Staphylococcus aureus*	
	Group A streptococci	
	Anaerobic bacteria	
	Gram-negative bacteria (rare)	

(continued)

TABLE 70.3

CONTINUED

Infection site	Pathogens
XI. Septic shock	
1. Community-acquired	*Streptococcus pneumoniae*
	Neisseria meningitidis
	Haemophilus influenzae
	Escherichia coli
	Capnocytophaga (DF-2 with splenectomy)
2. Health care-associated	MRSA
	Pseudomonas aeruginosa
	Acinetobacter species
	Candida species
3. Toxic shock syndrome	*Staphylococcus aureus*
	Streptococci species
4. Regional illness or special circumstances	Rickettsial species
	Ehrlichiosis
	Babesiosis
	Catscratch disease (immunocompromised hosts)
	Yersinia pestis
	Francisella tularensis
	Leptospira
	Salmonella enteritidis
	Salmonella typhi

- Organism may acquire genes encoding enzymes, such as β-lactamases, that destroy the antibacterial agent before it can have an effect.
- Bacteria may acquire efflux pumps that extrude the antibacterial agent from the cell before it can reach its target site and exert its effect.
- Bacteria may acquire several genes for a metabolic pathway.
  - Ultimately produces altered bacterial cell walls that no longer contain binding site of antimicrobial agent
  - Bacteria may acquire mutations that limit access of antimicrobial agents to intracellular target site *by* down-regulation of porin genes.
  - Susceptible bacteria can also acquire resistance to an antimicrobial agent by new mutations such as those noted above.

STRATEGIES THAT OPTIMIZE THE EFFICACY OF ANTIBIOTICS WHILE MINIMIZING ANTIBIOTIC RESISTANCE

Formal Protocols and Guidelines

- Antibiotic practice guidelines or protocols:
  - Emerged as potentially effective means of avoiding unnecessary antibiotic administration and increasing effectiveness of prescribed antibiotics
- Automated antimicrobial utilization guidelines:
  - Successfully used to identify and minimize the occurrence of adverse drug effects due to antibiotic administration and to improve antibiotic selection
  - Use also associated with stable antibiotic susceptibility patterns for both gram-positive and gram-negative bacteria

- Possibly as a result of promoting antimicrobial heterogeneity and specific end points for antibiotic discontinuation
- Automated and nonautomated antimicrobial guidelines:
  - Also employed to reduce overall use of antibiotics and limit use of inappropriate antimicrobial treatment
  - Both of which could affect the development of antibiotic resistance
  - Limit unnecessary use of antimicrobial agents by:
    ○ Therapy modification when initial empiric broad-spectrum antibiotics are prescribed
    ○ Culture results reveal that narrow-spectrum antibiotics can be used

Hospital Formulary Restrictions

- Restricted use of specific antibiotics or antibiotic classes from hospital formulary used:
  - Strategy to reduce occurrence of antibiotic resistance and antimicrobial costs
  - Approach shown to achieve reductions in pharmacy expenses and adverse drug reactions from restricted drugs
  - Not all experiences uniformly successful
    - Homogenous use of a single or limited number of drug classes may actually promote the emergence of resistance.
  - Restricted use of specific antibiotics has generally been applied to those drugs with:
    - Broad spectrum of action (e.g., carbapenems)
    - Rapid emergence of antibiotic resistance (e.g., cephalosporins)
    - Readily identified toxicity (e.g., aminoglycosides)
  - Difficult to demonstrate that restricted hospital formularies effective in curbing overall emergence of antibiotic resistance among bacterial species

TABLE 70.4

DRUGS OF CHOICE IN SERIOUS INFECTIONS[a]

Organism	Drug of choice	Alternative drugs
GRAM-POSITIVE COCCI		
Staphylococcus aureus[b] or *Staphylococcus epidermidis*		
Penicillin-sensitive	Penicillin G	Cephalosporin, vancomycin, or clindamycin[c]
Penicillinase-producing[d]	Oxacillin or nafcillin	Cephalosporin, vancomycin, or clindamycin
Methicillin-resistant[e]	Vancomycin (linezolid for pneumonia)	Quinolone, TMP/SMX, minocycline, clindamycin
Non-enterococcal streptococci	Penicillin G	Cephalosporin, vancomycin, or clindamycin
Enterococcus	Penicillin or ampicillin + gentamicin	Vancomycin + gentamicin
Streptococcus pneumoniae [f]	Penicillin G	Cephalosporin, vancomycin, macrolide, or clindamycin
GRAM-POSITIVE BACILLI		
Actinomyces israelii	Penicillin G	Tetracycline
Bacillus anthracis	Penicillin G	Tetracycline, macrolide
Clostridium difficile	Metronidazole	Oral vancomycin
Clostridium perfringens	Penicillin[g]	Clindamycin, metronidazole, tetracycline, imipenem
Clostridium tetani	Penicillin[h]	Tetracycline
Corynebacterium diphtheriae	Macrolide[g]	Penicillin
Corynebacterium JK	Vancomycin	Penicillin G + gentamicin, erythromycin
Listeria monocytogenes	Ampicillin gentamicin	TMP/SMX
Nocardia asteroides	TMP/SMX	carbapenem + amikacin
Proprionobacterium spp.	Penicillin	Clindamycin, erythromycin
GRAM-NEGATIVE COCCI		
Moraxella catarrhalis	TMP/SMX	Amoxicillin-clavulanic acid, ceftriaxone, macrolide, tetracycline
Neisseria gonorrhea	Ceftriaxone	Penicillin G, quinolones
Neisseria meningitidis	Penicillin G	Ceftriaxone
ENTERIC GRAM-NEGATIVE BACILLI		
Bacteroides		
Oral source	Penicillin	Clindamycin, cefoxitin, metronidazole, cefotetan
Bowel source	Metronidazole	Cefoxitin, cefotetan, imipenem, ampicillin-sulbactam ticar-clavulanate, pip-tazobactam, clindamycin
Citrobacter	Cefepime or imipenem/meropenem	Aminoglycoside, quinolone, piperacillin, aztreonam
Enterobacter spp.[i]	Cefepime or imipenem/meropenem	Ciprofloxacin, aminoglycoside, aztreonam
Escherichia coli[j]	Third-generation cephalosporin	Aminoglycoside, carbapenem, cefepime, β-lactam/β-lactamase inhibitor, ciprofloxacin, TMP/SMX
Klebsiella[j]	Third-generation cephalosporin	As for *E. coli*
Proteus mirabilis	Ampicillin	Aminoglycoside, quinolone, cephalosporin, piperacillin, ticarcillin, TMP/SMX
Proteus, non-mirabilis	Third-generation cephalosporin	Aminoglycoside, quinolone, piperacillin, aztreonam, imipenem
Providencia	Second- or third-generation cephalosporin	Gentamicin, amikacin, piperacillin, aztreonam, imipenem, ticarcillin, mezlocillin, TMP/SMX
Salmonella typhi	Ceftriaxone or quinolone	Ampicillin, TMP/SMX
Salmonella, non-typhi[k]	Cefotaxime, ceftriaxone, or quinolone	Ampicillin, TMP/SMX
Serratia	Cefepime or imipenem/meropenem	Aminoglycoside, aztreonam piperacillin, TMP/SMX, quinolone
Shigella	Quinolone	Ampicillin, TMP/SMX, ceftriaxone, cefixime
Yersinia enterocolitica	TMP/SMX	Aminoglycoside, tetracycline, 3rd-generation cephalosporin, quinolone
OTHER GRAM–NEGATIVE BACILLI		
Acinetobacter	Imipenem	Cefepime, aminoglycoside, TMP/SMX, colistin, sulbactam
Eikenella corrodens	Ampicillin	Penicillin G, erythromycin, tetracycline, ceftriaxone
Francisella tularensis	Streptomycin, gentamicin	Tetracycline
Fusobacterium	Penicillin	Clindamycin, metronidazole, cefoxitin
Haemophilus influenzae	3rd-generation cephalosporin	Ampicillin, imipenem, quinolone, cefuroxime[l], quinolone, macrolide, TMP/SMX

(continued)

TABLE 70.4

CONTINUED

Organism	Drug of choice	Alternative drugs
Legionella	Erythromycin (1 g q6h) + rifampin	
Pasteurella multocida	Penicillin G	Tetracycline, cephalosporin, amps-sulbactam
Pseudomonas aeruginosa	Antipseudomonal penicillin[m] + aminoglycoside	Aztreonam, cefepime, imipenem, quinolone
Pseudomonas cepacia	TMP/SMX	Ceftazidime
Spirillum minus	Penicillin G	Tetracycline, streptomycin
Streptobacillus moniliforms	Penicillin G	Tetracycline, streptomycin
Vibrio cholerae[n]	Tetracycline	TMP/SMX, quinolone
Vibrio vulnificus	Tetracycline	Cefotaxime
Xanthomonas maltophilia	TMP/SMX	Quinolone, minocycline, ceftazidime
Yersinia pestis	Streptomycin	Tetracycline, gentamicin
CHLAMYDIAE		
Chlamydia pneumoniae (TWAR)	Macrolide	Tetracycline
Chlamydia psittaci	Tetracycline	Chloramphenicol
Chlamydia trachomatis	Macrolide	Sulfonamide, tetracycline
MYCOPLASMA sp.	Macrolide	Tetracycline
	Tetracycline	Quinolone
SPIROCHETES		
Borrelia burgdorferi	Doxycycline, amoxicillin	Penicillin G, macrolide, cefuroxime, ceftriaxone, cefotaxime
Borrelia spp.	Tetracycline	Penicillin G
Treponema pallidum	Penicillin	Tetracycline, ceftriaxone
VIRUSES		
Cytomegalovirus	Ganciclovir[o]	Foscarnet, cidofovir
Herpes simplex	Acyclovir	Foscarnet, ganciclovir
HIV	See Centers for Disease Control Web site	
Influenza	Amantadine	Rimantadine, oseltamivir, zanamivir
Respiratory syncytial	Ribavirin	
Varicella zoster	Acyclovir	Famciclovir[p]
FUNGI		
Aspergillus	Voriconazole	Amphotericin B, echinocandin, Itraconazole
Blastomyces	Amphotericin B or itraconazole	Ketoconazole
Candida[q]		
Mucosal	Fluconazole, echinocandin[r]	Ketoconazole, itraconazole
Systemic	Fluconazole, echinocandin	Amphotericin B
Coccidioides	Amphotericin B or fluconazole	Itraconazole, ketoconazole
Cryptococcus	Amphotericin	Fluconazole, itraconazole
Histoplasma	Itraconazole or Amphotericin B	
Pseudallescheria	Ketoconazole or itraconazole	
Zygomycosis ("mucor")	Amphotericin B	Posaconazole

[a]This table does not consider minor infections that may be treated with oral agents, single-agent therapy, or less toxic drugs. Sensitivity testing must be done on bacterial isolates to confirm the sensitivity pattern.

[b]Some authorities recommend clindamycin as the first choice for susceptible toxin-producing staphylococci, streptococci, or clostridia.

[c]First-generation cephalosporins are most active. If endocarditis is suspected, do not use clindamycin. Some authorities recommend the addition of gentamicin for endocarditis caused by non-enterococcal streptococci or tolerant staphylococci.

[d]Penicillinase-producing staphylococci are also resistant to ampicillin, amoxicillin, carbenicillin, ticarcillin, mezlocillin, and piperacillin

[e]Methicillin-resistant staphylococci should be assumed to be resistant to all cephalosporins and penicillins, even if disk testing suggests sensitivity. Tigecycline, ceftobiprole, daptomycin, telavancin, and dalbavancin may be alternatives for specific types of methicillin-resistant infection pending future studies and indications.

[f]Some stains show intermediate- or high-level penicillin resistance. Highly resistant strains are treated with vancomycin, or rifampin, or both. In regions with high prevalence of resistant pneumococcus, ceftriaxone or vancomycin should be considered until sensitivity is known.

[g]Use as an adjunct to debridement of infected tissues.

[h]Use as an adjunct to active and passive immunization.

[i]Because of rapid development of resistance, cephalosporins not recommended even if initial tests indicate susceptibility.

[j]*Klebsiella spp.* and *E. coli* producing extended-spectrum beta-lactamase (ESBL) should be preferentially managed with a carbapenem.

[k]Uncomplicated *Salmonella* enteritis should not be treated with antibiotics.

[l]Should not be used in meningitis because of poor CNS penetration.

[m]Antipseudomonal penicillins include ticarcillin, mezlocillin, and piperacillin.

[n]Primary therapy is fluid and electrolyte repletion.

[o]Oral form should be used only in maintenance therapy of retinal cytomegalovirus.

[p]Approved only for mild herpes zoster in immunocompetent hosts.

[q]*Candida kruseii* and *Torulopsis glabrata* may be resistant to azole therapy, *Candida parapsilosis* may be resistant to echinocandins.

[r]Echinocandins include caspofungin, micafungin, and anidulafungin.

TABLE 70.5

TOXICITIES ASSOCIATED WITH ANTIMICROBIALS

Antimicrobial	Serious toxicities, uncommon	Common toxicities[a]
Penicillins Ampicillin Penicillin	Anaphylaxis, seizures, hemolytic anemia, neutropenia, thrombocytopenia, drug fever	Diarrhea, nausea, vomiting, rash
Antistaphylococcal penicillins Nafcillin Oxacillin	Anaphylaxis, neutropenia, thrombocytopenia, acute interstitial nephritis, hepatotoxicity	Diarrhea, nausea, vomiting, rash
B-lactam/B-lactamase inhibitors Amoxicillin/clavulanate Ampicillin/sulbactam Piperacillin/tazolbactam*	Anaphylaxis, seizures, hemolytic anemia, neutropenia, thrombocytopenia C. difficile colitis, cholestatic jaundice,* drug fever	Diarrhea, nausea, vomiting, rash
Ticarcillin/clavulanate Cephalosporins	Anaphylaxis, seizures, neutropenia, thrombocytopenia, drug fever	Diarrhea, nausea, vomiting, rash
Carbapenems Imipenem Meropenem	Anaphylaxis, seizures (imipenem > meropenem, ertapenem) C. difficile colitis, drug fever	Diarrhea, nausea, vomiting
Ertapenem Glycopeptides Vancomycin	Ototoxicity, nephrotoxicity (unlikely without concomitant nephrotoxins), thrombocytopenia	Red-man syndrome
Oxazolidinones Linezolid	*More common with long-term use:* Peripheral and optic neuropathy, myelosuppression *Possible with short-term use:* Lactic acidosis, myopathy anemia	Diarrhea
Lipopeptides Daptomycin		Diarrhea, constipation, vomiting
Streptogramin Quinupristin/dalfopristin		Arthralgia, myalgia, inflammation, pain, edema at infusion site, hyperbilirubinemia
Aminoglycosides Amikacin Gentamicin Tobramycin		Nephrotoxicity, ototoxicity
Fluoroquinolones Second generation	Anaphylaxis, dysglycemia* QTc prolongation, joint toxicity in children, tendon rupture	Nausea, vomiting, diarrhea, photosensitivity, rash
Ciprofloxacin		CNS stimulation, dizziness, somnolence
Third generation Levofloxacin Fourth generation Gatifloxacin* Moxifloxacin Gemifloxacin		
Macrolides Erythromycin* Azithromycin	QTc prolongation (erythromycin > clarithromycin > azithromycin), cholestasis*	Nausea, vomiting, diarrhea, abnormal taste
Clarithromycin Ketolides Telithromycin	Acute hepatic failure QTc prolongation	Nausea, vomiting, diarrhea
Clindamycin	C. difficile colitis	Nausea, vomiting, diarrhea, abdominal pain, rash
Tetracyclines Tetracycline*	Tooth discoloration and retardation of bone growth (in children), renal tubular necrosis,* dizziness, vertigo,[†]	Photosensitivity, diarrhea
Doxycycline		
Minocycline[†] pseudotumor cerebri Glycylcyclines		Nausea, vomiting, diarrhea

(continued)

TABLE 70.5

CONTINUED

Antimicrobial	Serious toxicities, uncommon	Common toxicities[a]
Tigecycline		
Trimethoprim/sulfamethoxazole	Myelosuppression Stevens–Johnson syndrome, hyperkalemia, aseptic meningitis, hepatic necrosis	Rash, nausea, vomiting, diarrhea
Metronidazole	Seizures, peripheral neuropathy	Nausea, vomiting, metallic taste, disulfiram-like reaction
Nitrofurantoin	Pulmonary toxicity, peripheral neuropathy	Urine discoloration, photosensitivity
Antifungal Agents		
Azoles Fluconazole Itraconazole Voriconazole	Hepatic failure, increased AST/ALT, cardiovascular toxicity, hypertension, edema	Nausea, vomiting, diarrhea, rash, visual disturbances, phototoxicity
Amphotericin B products Amphotericin B deoxycholate ABLC ABCD	Acute liver failure, myelosuppression	Nephrotoxicity (less common with lipid formulations), acute infusion-related reactions, hypokalemia, hypomagnesemia
Liposomal amphotericin B Echinocandins Caspofungin	Hepatotoxicity, infusion-related rash, flushing, itching	
Micafungin		
Anidulafungin Flucytosine	Myelosuppression, hepatotoxicity, confusion, hallucinations, sedation	Nausea, vomiting, diarrhea, rash
Antiviral Agents		
Nucleoside analogues Acyclovir	Nephrotoxicity, rash, encephalopathy, inflammation at injection site, phlebitis	Bone marrow suppression, headache, nausea, vomiting, diarrhea (with oral forms)
Valacyclovir		
Ganciclovir		
Valganciclovir Amantadine	CNS disturbances (amantadine > rimantadine)	Nausea, vomiting, anorexia, xerostomia
Rimantadine Neuraminidase inhibitors Oseltamivir Zanamivir	Anaphylaxis, bronchospasm	Nausea, vomiting, cough, local discomfort
Cidofovir	Anemia, neutropenia, fever, rash	Nephrotoxicity, uveitis/iritis, nausea, vomiting
Foscarnet	Seizures, anemia, fever	Nephrotoxicity, electrolyte abnormalities (hypocalcemia, hypomagnesemia, hypokalemia, hypophosphatemia), nausea, vomiting, diarrhea, headache

[a]Toxicities were classified as "common" relative to the other toxicities that agent is known to cause. Because toxicities are classified as "common", it does not imply they are not serious.

- However, use has been successful in specific outbreaks of infection with antibiotic-resistant bacteria, particularly in conjunction with infection control practices and antibiotic educational activities.

Use of Narrow-Spectrum Antibiotics

- Another proposed strategy to curtail development of antimicrobial resistance
  - In addition to the judicious overall use of antibiotics

- Use drugs with a narrow antimicrobial spectrum
- Several lines of evidence suggest infections such as community-acquired pneumonia can be successfully treated with narrow-spectrum antibiotic agents.
  - Especially if infections are not life-threatening.
- Avoidance of broad-spectrum antibiotics...
  - Especially those associated with rapid emergence of resistance (cephalosporins, quinolones)
  - Reintroduction of narrow-spectrum agents (penicillin, trimethoprim, gentamicin)
  - Infection control practices

- Successful in reducing the occurrence of specific infections in hospital setting

Quantitative Cultures and Assessment of Infection Risk

- Pneumonia is the most common hospital-acquired infection in mechanically ventilated patients.
  - Use of quantitative bacterial cultures obtained from the lower respiratory tract may facilitate de-escalation of empiric broad-spectrum antibiotics and reduce drug-specific antibiotic days of treatment
  - Patients with a clinical suspicion for VAP and culture-negative bronchoalveolar lavage (BAL) results for a major pathogen can have antimicrobial therapy safely discontinued within 72 hours.
  - Regardless of whether quantitative culture methods are used
    - Results of microbiologic testing should be used to routinely modify or discontinue antibiotic treatment in the appropriate clinical setting.

Combination Antibiotic Therapy

- No definitive evidence that emergence of antibiotic resistance is reduced by the use of combination antimicrobial therapy.
- Empiric combination therapy directed against high-risk pathogens:
  - Such as *Pseudomonas aeruginosa*
  - Should be encouraged until the results of antimicrobial susceptibility become available
  - Approach to empiric treatment can increase the likelihood of providing appropriate initial antimicrobial therapy with improved outcomes.

Antibiotic Cycling and Scheduled Antibiotic Changes

- Concept of antibiotic class cycling suggested as strategy for reducing emergence of antimicrobial resistance
  - Class of antibiotics or a specific antibiotic drug:
    - Withdrawn from use for a defined time period
    - Reintroduced at a later time in attempt to limit bacterial resistance to cycled antimicrobial agents
  - Mathematical modeling suggests that use of antibiotic cycling inferior to "mixing" of antibiotics as a strategy to reduce emergence of antimicrobial resistance
    - Beneficial outcomes in terms of antibiotic resistance, with benefits extending outside of the ICU setting, have not been confirmed.
    - Antimicrobial heterogeneity or mixing seems to be a logical policy.
  - Simple cycling of antibiotics combined with prolonged treatment exposures:
    - A strategy that will only promote further antibiotic resistance

Antimicrobial Decolonization Strategies

- Topical antibiotic administration (i.e., selective digestive decontamination), with or without concomitant parenteral antibiotics
- Shown to be effective at reducing nosocomial infections
- Routine use of selective digestive decontamination linked to emergence of antimicrobial resistance
- Antimicrobial and nonantimicrobial agents should be considered for oral decontamination only in *appropriate high-risk ICU* patients.
  - Or to assist in the containment of outbreaks of MDR bacterial infections in conjunction with established infection control practices

Shorter Courses of Antibiotic Treatment

- Prolonged administration of antibiotics to hospitalized patients is an important risk factor for the emergence of colonization and infection with antibiotic-resistant bacteria.
  - 7 to 8 days of antibiotic treatment (short course):
    - Acceptable for most *nonbacteremic* patients with VAP
    - Successfully used in patients at low risk for VAP with pyelonephritis
    - For community-acquired pneumonia
    - Associated with a significantly lower risk for the emergence of antimicrobial resistance compared to more traditional durations of antibiotic treatment ranging from 14 to 21 days
- More specific markers for the presence of bacterial infection:
- Procalcitonin
- Soluble triggering receptor on myeloid cells (sTREM1)
- May allow shorter courses of empiric antibiotic administration in patients without identified bacterial infection
- Published guidelines for the antibiotic management of nosocomial pneumonia and severe sepsis currently recommend discontinuation of empiric antibiotic therapy after 48 to 72 hours if cultures negative or signs of infection resolved.

Optimizing Pharmacokinetic/Pharmacodynamic (Pk/Pd) Principles

- Antibiotic concentrations that are sublethal:
- Can promote the emergence of resistant pathogens
- Duration of time the serum drug concentration remains above minimum inhibitory concentration of the antibiotic ($T > MIC$) enhances bacterial eradication with β-lactams, carbapenems, monobactams, glycopeptides, and oxazolidinones.
- See increased $T > MIC$ and improve clinical and microbiologic cure rates with:
  - Frequent dosing
  - Prolonged infusion times
  - Continuous infusions
- To maximize the bactericidal effects of aminoglycosides:
  - Must optimize maximum drug concentration (C_{max})-to-MIC ratio

○ C_{max}:MIC ratio of ≥10:1 using once-daily aminoglycoside dosing (5–7 mg/kg) associated with:
  – Preventing emergence of resistant organisms
  – Improving clinical response to treatment
  – Avoiding toxicity
- 24-hour area under antibiotic concentration curve-to-MIC ratio (AUIC) is correlated with fluoroquinolone efficacy and prevention of resistance development
  - AUIC value of >100 associated with significant reduction in risk of resistance development while on therapy
  - Generally, should use the *maximum approved dose* of an antibiotic for a potentially life-threatening infection to optimize tissue concentrations of the drug and killing of pathogens

New Antimicrobial Agents

- In 1996, the first clinical isolate of *Staphylococcus aureus* with reduced susceptibility to vancomycin (vancomycin-intermediate *Staphylococcus aureus,* or VISA) was reported in Japan.
  - Similar cases have been reported around the world.
  - Now clinical isolates of *Staphylococcus aureus* that are fully resistant to vancomycin have been reported in South Africa and Michigan.
  - Emergence of methicillin-resistant *Staphylococcus aureus* (MRSA) strains with reduced vancomycin susceptibility has limited the treatment options and increased the incidence of treatment failure.
  - Infection with one of these strains may be an independent predictor of mortality.
  - More concerning are observations that upward drift in the minimum inhibitory concentrations for vancomycin in MRSA are associated with an increased risk of clinical treatment failures.

Linezolid

- First licensed member of a new class of antibiotics
  - Oxazolidinones
  - Binds to the ribosome and inhibits microbial protein synthesis
    - Novel mechanism of action provides an antimicrobial activity independent of resistance status toward other antibiotics
  - Linezolid may be associated with improved survival and clinical cure rates compared to vancomycin in patients with nosocomial pneumonia.
  - Linezolid a suitable alternative to vancomycin in nosocomial infections caused by MRSA, particularly in pneumonia
  - General agreement on the superiority of linezolid to vancomycin and teicoplanin is lacking
    - Does not require adjustment for renal function at a dosage of 600 mg every 12 hours.
    - Close monitoring of blood cell count should be done in case of pre-existing myelosuppression and during prolonged treatment.

Daptomycin

- A cyclic lipopeptide active only against gram-positive organisms

- Recently approved for the treatment of complicated skin and soft tissue infections
- Activity against resistant and susceptible isolates of *Staphylococcus aureus*
- Once-daily dosing (4 mg/kg IV) and safety profile (except for some concerns for rhabdomyolysis) make daptomycin an attractive option for the treatment of staphylococcal infections
  - May not be a useful agent for deep-seated tissue infections
  - In 740 patients with pneumonia, treatment terminated early due to a lower level of efficacy compared to ceftriaxone
  - May be related to:
    ○ Molecular size of this drug
    ○ Protein-binding characteristics
    ○ Inhibition by pulmonary surfactant
- Current use limited to skin infections and bacteremia and/or endocarditis

Quinupristin-Dalfopristin

- A semisynthetic, parenteral streptogramin
- Activity against most of the gram-positive pathogens
- Comparing quinupristin-dalfopristin and vancomycin in treatment of nosocomial pneumonia by gram-positive pathogens, similar clinical success rates were observed, including in MRSA subgroup.
- Quinupristin-dalfopristin probably not a better option than vancomycin
- Side effect profile of quinupristin-dalfopristin (myalgia, arthralgia, and thrombophlebitis) and its lack of proven efficacy over vancomycin have limited its overall use

Tigecycline

- The first glycylcycline to be launched
  - One of the very few antimicrobials with activity against gram-negative bacteria and MRSA
  - In contrast to classic tetracyclines, tigecycline can be administered only parenterally.
  - Major side effect appears to be dose-related nausea and emesis
  - Dosing regimen for tigecycline has been validated in clinical trials that involved a 100-mg loading dose
    ○ Followed by 50 mg twice daily in patients with complicated infections of the skin and skin structure, as well as intra-abdominal infections
    ○ Evades acquired efflux and target-mediated resistance to classical tetracyclines but not chromosomal efflux
    ○ C_{max} is low, but tissue penetration is excellent.
    ○ Compound has shown equivalence to imipenem/cilastatin in intra-abdominal infection and to vancomycin plus aztreonam in skin and skin structure infection.
    ○ Tigecycline may prove particularly useful for the treatment of surgical wound infections, where both gram-negative bacteria and MRSA are likely pathogens.
    ○ May also have a role in the treatment of infections due to multiresistant pathogens, including *Acinetobacter* species and extended-spectrum β-lactamase producing gram-negatives

Ceftobiprole

- Ceftobiprole (BAL5788) is the water-soluble prodrug of BAL9141.
  - Novel broad-spectrum cephalosporin
  - Potent bactericidal activities against MRSA and penicillin-resistant *Streptococcus pneumoniae*
  - BAL9141, a novel pyrrolidinone-3-ylidenemethyl cephalosporin:
    - Specifically designed to have strong affinity for penicillin-binding protein (PBP) 2a
    - Known to confer resistance in staphylococci and pneumococci
    - BAL9141 also binds strongly to the relevant PBPs of most gram-positive and gram-negative pathogens and is resistant to many β-lactamases.
  - Ceftobiprole is currently being investigated in patients with pneumonia and complicated skin infections.

Dalbavancin

- A lipoglycopeptide antimicrobial:
  - Studied in phase two trials for complicated skin and skin structure infections and catheter-related bloodstream infection
  - A bactericidal agent
    - Long terminal plasma half-life (9–12 days)
  - Allows for the unique dosing of 1,000 mg given on day 1 and 500 mg given on day 8

Telavancin

- Telavancin is another lipoglycopeptide in development.
  - Exerts concentration-dependent bactericidal activity against gram-positive bacteria, including MRSA
  - Rapid bactericidal activity arises from two mechanisms:
    - Inhibition of peptidoglycan synthesis
    - Interaction with bacterial membrane
  - Effective for treatment of complicated skin and skin structure infections given as a once-daily dosing

Doripenem

- A novel broad-spectrum parenteral carbapenem antimicrobial
  - Chemical formula for doripenem confers β-lactamase stability
  - Resistance to inactivation by renal dehydropeptidases
- Doripenem has spectrum and potency against:
  - Gram-positive cocci most similar to imipenem or ertapenem
  - Gram-negative activity most like meropenem (twofold or fourfold superiority to imipenem)

CHAPTER 71 ■ SURGICAL INFECTIONS

- Surgical patients are at particular risk of infection for many reasons.
  - Surgery is inherently invasive.
    - Creates portals of entry in natural epithelial barriers for pathogens to invade the host
  - Surgical illness is immunosuppressive (e.g., trauma, burns, malignant tumors).
    - As is therapeutic immunosuppression following solid organ transplantation
  - General anesthesia almost always means a period of mechanical ventilation.
    - Period of reduced consciousness during emergence
    - Risk of pulmonary aspiration of gastric contents
    - Nosocomial pneumonia occurs more frequently among surgical patients than comparably ill medical patients.
  - Surgical patients are also uniquely afflicted by infections of incisions.
- Surgical infections traditionally considered to be infections that require surgical therapy
  - Complicated intra-abdominal and soft tissue infections
  - Surgical patients are especially vulnerable to nosocomial infection.
  - Definition includes any infection that affects surgical patients

RISK FACTORS FOR POSTOPERATIVE INFECTION

- General principles of surgical care, critical care, and infection control cannot be overemphasized
  - Resuscitation must be rapid, yet precise
  - Pathology must be identified and treated as soon as possible.
  - Infection control sometimes sacrificed under chaotic conditions of resuscitation
    - Central venous catheters inserted under suboptimal barrier precautions
      - Lack of cap, mask, sterile gown, and sterile gloves for the operator and a full-bed drape for the patient
      - These must be removed and replaced (if necessary) by a new puncture at a new site as soon as patient's condition permits

CONTROL OF BLOOD SUGAR

- Hyperglycemia is deleterious to host immune function.
- May also reflect catabolism and insulin resistance associated with surgical stress response

- Poor perioperative control of blood glucose increases the risk of infection and worsens outcome from sepsis.
  - Diabetic patients undergoing cardiopulmonary bypass surgery have a higher risk of infection of both sternal incision and vein harvest incisions on lower extremities.
  - Moderate hyperglycemia (>200 mg/dL) any time on first postoperative day:
    - Increases risk of surgical site infection (SSI) fourfold after cardiac and noncardiac surgery
  - Insulin infusion to keep blood glucose concentrations <110 mg/dL associated with:
    - 40% decrease in mortality among critically ill postoperative patients
    - Fewer nosocomial infections and less organ dysfunction
    - Meta-analysis of 35 trials of control of blood glucose indicates:
      - Risk of mortality is decreased significantly (risk ratio [RR] 0.85, 95% confidence interval [CI] 0.75–0.97) by tight glucose control
      - Especially so for critically ill surgical patients (RR 0.58, 95% CI 0.22–0.62)
      - Regardless of whether the patients had diabetes mellitus (RR 0.71, 95% CI 0.54–0.93) or stress-induced hyperglycemia (RR 0.73, 95% CI 0.58–0.90)
- Nutritional support is crucial.
  - Surgical stress causes catabolism
  - Restoration of anabolism requires the provision of calories and nitrogen far in excess of basal requirements of 25 to 30 kcal and 1 g nitrogen/kg per day
  - Parenteral nutrition appears to convey no advantage over not feeding the patient at all
    - Perhaps because of inherent morbidity of central intravenous feeding
      - Risk of catheter-related bloodstream infection (CR-BSI)
      - Hyperglycemia
  - Early enteral feeding
    - Within the first 48 hours or immediately if the gut is functional
    - Clearly beneficial, with the possible exception of pneumonia prevention
    - Risk of infection was reduced by 55% (odds ratio [OR] 0.45, 95% CI 0.30–0.66) in a meta-analysis of 15 randomized trials of early enteral feeding following surgery, trauma, or burns

Blood Transfusion

- Blood transfusion can be life saving after trauma or hemorrhage.
  - An increased risk of infection is the consequence.
  - Transfusions exert immunosuppressive effects through:
    - Presentation of leukocyte antigens
    - Induction of shift to T-helper 2 (immunosuppressive) phenotype
    - Mechanism remains somewhat controversial
      - Transfusion of leukocyte-depleted red blood cell concentrates does not reduce the risk of infection
  - Exponential relationship between transfusion risk and infection risk among trauma patients

- Detectable with even 1 unit of transfusion
- A virtual certainty after more than 15 units of transfused blood (RR 1.084, 95% CI 1.028–1.142)
- By meta-analysis risk of infection related to blood transfusion increased for trauma patients by more than fivefold (OR 5.26, 95% CI 5.03–5.43)
  - For surgical patients by more than threefold
  - Increased risk for infection by transfusion has also been identified for critically ill patients in general
    - For CR-BSI and ventilator-associated pneumonia (VAP) specifically
- Banked blood is affected by a "storage lesion" characterized by:
- Loss of membrane 2-3-diphosphoglycerate and adenosine triphosphate
- Leading to loss of membrane deformability
  - Erythrocytes cannot deform as they must transit to the microcirculation
  - Causing disruption of nutrient blood flow and impaired oxygen offloading
  - Thus, blood transfusion does not increase oxygen consumption for critically ill patients with sepsis
    - May actually increase the risk of organ dysfunction
    - Storage lesion becomes fully manifest after about 14 days of storage
    - Transfusion of older blood is an independent risk factor for the development of infection.
    - **It is safe to be conservative in the administration of red blood cell concentrates to stable patients in the intensive care unit (ICU).**

INFECTION CONTROL

- Infection control is an individual and collective responsibility of the critical care team and unit.
  - Hand hygiene is most effective and underutilized means to reduce spread of infection
    - Hand cleansing with soap and water requires a minimum of 30 to 45 seconds to be effective.
    - Alcohol gel hand cleansers are equally effective.
      - Except against the spores of *Clostridium difficile*
      - Compliance with use is higher
      - When used prevalence of multidrug resistant (MDR) bacteria is reduced
      - Universal precautions must be observed whenever there is a risk of splashing of body fluids.
  - Source of most bacterial pathogens is patient's endogenous flora
    - Skin surfaces
    - Artificial airways
    - Gut lumen
    - Wounds
    - Catheters
    - Inanimate surfaces (e.g., bed rails, computer terminals) may become colonized
    - Any break in natural epithelial barriers
      - Incisions
      - Percutaneous catheters
      - Airway or urinary catheters
      - A portal of entry for invasion of pathogens

– Fecal–oral route the most common manner by which pathogens reach the portal
– But health care workers definitely facilitate the transmission of pathogens around a unit
- Contact isolation an important part of infection control
  - Should be used selectively to prevent the spread of pathogens:
    ○ Methicillin-resistant *Staphylococcus aureus* (MRSA)
    ○ Vancomycin-resistant enterococci (VRE)
    ○ MDR Gram-negative bacilli
- Contact isolation may decrease the amount of direct patient contact.
  ○ Appropriate balance must be struck
  ○ Reduced nurse staffing of ICUs has been independently associated with an increased risk of a number of nosocomial infections.

CATHETER CARE

- Optimal catheter care includes:
- Avoidance of use when unnecessary
- Appropriate skin cleansing and barrier protection during insertion
- Proper catheter selection
- Proper dressing of indwelling catheters
- Removal as soon as possible when no longer needed
  - Or after insertion under less than ideal circumstances (e.g., trauma bay, cardiac resuscitation)
- Benefit of information gained by catheterization must always be weighed against the risk of infection (Table 71.1)
- All indwelling catheters carry a risk of infection.
  - Nontunneled central venous catheters and pulmonary artery catheters highest risk
    - Including local site infections and CR-BSIs (see below)
  - Other catheters that pose increased infection risk include:
    - Intercostal thoracostomy catheters (if inserted as an emergency)
    - Ventriculostomy catheters for intracranial pressure monitoring
    - Urinary bladder catheters
  - Each day of endotracheal intubation and mechanical ventilation increases the risk of pneumonia by 1% to 3%.
    - Controversial whether tracheostomy decreases that risk

- Chlorhexidine (bactericidal, viricidal, and fungicidal)
  - Used preferentially for skin preparation for vascular catheter insertion
  - Shown to be superior to povidone-iodine solution
    ○ If povidone-iodine solution is used (of which use is discouraged), it must be allowed to dry, as it is not bactericidal when wet
- Full barrier precautions are mandatory for all bedside catheterization procedures
  - Except arterial and urinary bladder catheterization, for which sterile gloves and a sterile field suffice
  - A central venous line (CVL) inserted under suboptimal conditions must be removed (and replaced at a different site if still needed) as soon as permitted by patient's hemodynamic status, but no more than 24 hours after insertion.
  - Single dose of a first-generation cephalosporin (e.g., cefazolin) only may prevent some infections following emergency tube thoracostomy or ventriculostomy
    ○ Not indicated for vascular or bladder catheterizations
    ○ Topical antiseptics placed postprocedure at insertion site of no benefit for any type of indwelling catheter, and may actually increase the risk of infection
- Dressings must be maintained carefully
  - Challenging if the patient is agitated or the body surface is irregular
    ○ The neck (intrajugular vein catheterization) versus the chest wall (subclavian vein catheterization)
    ○ Importance is crucial
    ○ Marking the dressing clearly with the date and time of each change is a simple and effective way to manage dressing changes
    ○ Dressing carts or similar apparatus should not be brought from patient to patient; rather, sufficient supplies should be kept in each patient's room
    ○ Possibility for inanimate objects (e.g., scissors) to be transmission vectors if not cleansed thoroughly after contact with each patient
    ○ Dedicated catheter care teams reduce the risk of CR-BSI substantially
    ○ Choice of catheter may play a role in decreasing the risk of infection related to endotracheal tubes, central venous catheters, and urinary catheters

TABLE 71.1

RATES OF HEALTH CARE-ASSOCIATED PNEUMONIA AND CATHETER-RELATED BLOODSTREAM INFECTION AMONG VARIOUS ICU TYPES

ICU type	CVC use	CR-BSI rate mean/median	TT use	VAP rate mean/median
Medical	0.52	5.0/3.9	0.46	4.9/3.7
Pediatric	0.46	6.6/5.2	0.39	2.9/2.3
Surgical	0.61	4.6/3.4	0.44	9.3/8.3
Cardiovascular	0.79	2.7/1.8	0.43	7.2/6.3
Neurosurgical	0.48	4.6/3.1	0.39	11.2/6.2
Trauma	0.61	7.4/5.2	0.56	15.2/11.4

CVC use, number of days of catheter placement per 1,000 patient-days in ICU; CR-BSI, catheter-related bloodstream infection; TT use, number of days of indwelling endotracheal tube or tracheostomy per 1,000 patient-days in ICU; VAP, ventilator-associated pneumonia.
Infection rates are indexed per 1,000 patient-days.
From the National Nosocomial Infection Surveillance System, U.S. Centers for Disease Control and Prevention.
Data available at www.cdc.gov, and are in the public domain.

- Continuous aspiration of subglottic secretions (CASS), via an endotracheal tube with an extra lumen that opens to the airway just above the balloon, facilitates the removal of secretions that accumulate below the vocal cords but above the endotracheal tube balloon
  - Incidence of VAP is decreased by one-half by CASS
  - Silver-impregnated endotracheal tubes are effective in reducing airway colonization, but whether VAP incidence is reduced not yet known
- Antibiotic- (e.g., minocycline/rifampin) or antiseptic-coated central venous catheters (e.g., Chlorhexidine/silver sulfadiazine) can reduce the incidence of CR-BSI
  - Especially in high-prevalence units
  - Minocycline/rifampin-coated catheters may be more effective
- Urinary bladder catheters coated with ionic silver reduce the incidence of catheter-related bacterial cystitis by a similar amount
- Ventilator weaning by protocol, combined with daily sedation holidays and spontaneous breathing trials
  - Allows earlier endotracheal extubation and decreases the risk of VAP (see below)
  - Better strategy may be avoidance of endotracheal intubation entirely
    - Noninvasive positive pressure ventilation delivered by mask (e.g., continuous positive airway pressure [CPAP])
    - Improved resuscitation techniques and noninvasive monitoring techniques have decreased the utilization of pulmonary artery catheters, which pose a particularly high risk of infection
  - Most drains do not decrease the risk of infection
    - Risk is probably increased because the catheters hold a portal open for invasion by bacteria.

RISK FACTORS FOR SURGICAL SITE INFECTION

- Clean surgical procedures affect only integumentary and musculoskeletal soft tissues
- Clean-contaminated procedures open a hollow viscus (e.g., alimentary, biliary, genitourinary, respiratory tract) under controlled circumstances.
  - For example, elective colon surgery
- Contaminated procedures involve extensive introduction of bacteria into a normally sterile body cavity, but too briefly to allow infection to become established during surgery
  - For example, penetrating abdominal trauma, enterotomy during adhesiolysis for mechanical bowel obstruction
- Dirty procedures are performed to control established infection
  - For example, colon resection for perforated diverticulitis
- Numerous factors determine whether a patient will develop an SSI, including (Table 71.2):
  - Factors related to patient
  - Environment
  - Therapy
- Most recognized factors are:
  - The wound classification
  - American Society of Anesthesiologists class 3 or higher (class 3: chronic active medical illness)

TABLE 71.2

RISK FACTORS FOR THE DEVELOPMENT OF SURGICAL SITE INFECTIONS

Patient Factors
Ascites (for abdominal surgery)
Chronic inflammation
Corticosteroid therapy (controversial)
Obesity
Diabetes
Extremes of age
Hypocholesterolemia
Hypoxemia
Peripheral vascular disease (for lower extremity surgery)
Postoperative anemia
Prior site irradiation
Recent operation
Remote infection
Skin carriage of staphylococci
Skin disease in the area of infection (e.g., psoriasis)
Undernutrition

Environmental Factors
Contaminated medications
Inadequate disinfection/sterilization
Inadequate skin antisepsis
Inadequate ventilation

Treatment Factors
Drains
Emergency procedure
Hypothermia
Inadequate antibiotic prophylaxis
Oxygenation (controversial)
Prolonged preoperative hospitalization
Prolonged operative time

- Prolonged operative time, where time is longer than the 75th percentile for each such procedure
- Risk of SSI increases with an increasing number of risk factors present, irrespective of the type of operation
- Laparoscopic surgery decreases incidence of SSI under most circumstances
  - Reasons possibly several, including:
    - Decreased wound size
    - Limited use of cautery in the abdominal wall
    - Diminished stress response to tissue injury
- Host-derived factors contribute importantly to the risk of SSI, including:
  - Increased age
  - Obesity
  - Malnutrition
  - Diabetes mellitus
  - Hypocholesterolemia
- Numerous other factors that are not accounted for specifically by the National Nosocomial Infections Surveillance System (NNIS) system
  - In one 6-year study of 5,031 patients undergoing noncardiac surgery, the overall incidence of SSI was 3.2%.
  - In another prospective study of 9,016 patients, 12.5% of patients developed an infection of some type within 28 days after surgery.
- Lapses in the modern operating room can result in increased rates of SSI

- Proper sterilization
- Ventilation
- Skin preparation techniques
  - Operating team must be attentive to personal hygiene (e.g., hand scrubbing, hair)
  - Recent data indicate that a brief rinse with soap and water followed by use of an alcohol gel hand rub is equivalent to the prolonged (and ritualized) session at the scrub sink
- Hypothermia during surgery is common if patients are not warmed actively, owing to:
  - Evaporative water losses
  - Administration of room temperature fluids
- Maintenance of normal core body temperature is unequivocally important for decreasing the incidence of SSI.
  - Mild intraoperative hypothermia is associated with an increased rate of SSI following elective colon surgery and diverse operations.
- Intuitive that oxygen administration in postoperative period beneficial for wound healing
  - Ischemic milieu of the fresh surgical incision is vulnerable to bacterial invasion
  - Oxygen has been postulated to have a direct antibacterial effect
  - Clinical trials have had conflicting results
    - Supplemental oxygenation administration specifically to reduce the incidence of SSI remains plausible, and further studies are needed
- Closure of a contaminated or dirty incision is widely believed to increase the risk of SSI
  - Few good studies exist to help sort out the multiplicity of wound closure techniques available to surgeons
  - "Open abdomen" techniques of temporary abdominal closure for management of trauma or severe peritonitis are utilized increasingly.
  - Retrospective studies indicate that antibiotics are not indicated for prophylaxis of the open abdomen.
    - But infection of the abdominal wall is highly morbid
    - Inability to achieve primary abdominal closure is associated with infectious complications:
      - Pneumonia
      - Bloodstream infection
      - SSI
    - Infectious complications significantly increased costs from prolonged length of stay, but not mortality
- Drains placed in incisions probably cause more infections than they prevent
  - Epithelialization of the wound is prevented and the drain becomes a conduit, holding open a portal for invasion by pathogens colonizing the skin
  - Several studies of drains placed into clean or clean-contaminated incisions show that the rate of SSI is not reduced.
    - Rate is increased
  - Considering that drains pose a risk and accomplish little of what is expected of them, they should be used as little as possible and removed as soon as possible.
  - Under no circumstances should prolonged antibiotic prophylaxis be administered to "cover" indwelling drains.
- Wound irrigation is a controversial means to reduce the risk of SSI.

- Routine low-pressure saline irrigation of an incision does not reduce the risk of SSI.
- High pressure irrigation (i.e., pulse irrigation) may be beneficial.
- Intraoperative topical antibiotics can minimize the risk of SSI.
  - But use of antiseptics rather than antibiotics might minimize possibility of development of resistance

Risk Factors for Pneumonia

- Surgical patients susceptible to pneumonia, particularly if they require mechanical ventilation
- Ventilator-associated pneumonia, defined as pneumonia occurring 48 to 72 hours after endotracheal intubation, is the most common ICU infection among surgical and trauma patients.
  - VAP is partially iatrogenic
  - Nonspecific diagnostic criteria, indiscriminate antibiotic use, and unclear therapeutic end points have all contributed to increased episodes of VAP caused by MDR pathogens.
  - MDR pathogens increase the likelihood of inadequate initial antimicrobial therapy, which exerts further selection pressure for these pathogens and results in higher mortality.
- Distinction is sometimes made between:
  - Early-onset VAP (occurring <5 days after intubation)
  - Late-onset VAP (occurring ≥5 days after intubation)
    - Early-onset VAP, to which trauma patients are particularly prone, is often a result of aspiration of gastric contents and is usually caused by antibiotic-sensitive bacteria such as methicillin-sensitive *S. aureus*, *Streptococcus pneumoniae*, and *Haemophilus influenzae*.
    - Late-onset VAP is at increased risk for infection with MDR pathogens (e.g., MRSA, *Pseudomonas aeruginosa*, or *Acinetobacter* spp.)
- The incidence of VAP depends upon the diagnostic criteria utilized and thus varies in published reports
  - Clinical criteria alone overestimate the incidence of VAP as compared with either microbiologic or histologic data
  - Systematic review of 89 studies of VAP among mechanically ventilated patients reported a pooled incidence of VAP of 22.8% (95% CI 18.8–26.9).
  - NNIS system reported recently that VAP occurred at a rate of 4.9 cases per 1,000 ventilator-days in medical ICUs and 9.3 per 1,000 ventilator-days in surgical ICUs (see Table 71.1).
    - Risk for trauma patients, especially those with traumatic brain injury, is especially high.
    - Incidence of VAP increases with the duration of mechanical ventilation:
      - 3% per day during the first 5 days
      - 2% per day during days 5 to 10
      - 1% per day after that
    - Risk factors for VAP are summarized in Table 71.3.
    - Perhaps most important is airway intubation itself.
      - Risk of VAP increases six- to 20-fold in mechanically ventilated patients.
    - VAP is also especially common in patients with acute respiratory distress syndrome (ARDS), owing to prolonged mechanical ventilation and devastated local airway host defenses.

TABLE 71.3

RISK FACTORS FOR VENTILATOR-ASSOCIATED
PNEUMONIA

Age ≥60 years
Acute respiratory distress syndrome
Chronic obstructive pulmonary disease or other underlying
  pulmonary disease
Coma or impaired consciousness
Serum albumin <2.2 g/dL
Burns, trauma
Blood transfusion
Organ failure
Supine position
Large-volume gastric aspiration
Sinusitis
Immunosuppression

- Several evidence-based strategies can prevent VAP, but to
  be used effectively a thorough understanding of modifiable
  risk factors is required (Table 71.4).
  - Prevention of VAP begins with minimization of endotra-
    cheal intubation and the duration of mechanical ventila-
    tion.
  - Noninvasive positive pressure ventilation (NIPPV) should
    be considered in lieu of intubation, as management of res-
    piratory failure with NIPPV leads to a lower incidence of
    VAP.
  - If endotracheal intubation is required:
    - Orotracheal route is preferred to nasotracheal intubation
      to decrease the risk of VAP by as much as one-half by
      decreasing the risk of nosocomial sinusitis.
    - Evidence-based strategies to decrease the duration of
      mechanical ventilation include:
      - Daily interruption of sedation

TABLE 71.4

STRATEGIES TO PREVENT VENTILATOR-
ASSOCIATED PNEUMONIA

Strategy	Recommended	Insufficient evidence
Universal infection control precautions	+	
Orotracheal intubation	+	
Maintenance of endotracheal cuff pressure >20 cm H_2O	+	
Continuous aspiration of subglottic secretions	+	
Semirecumbent positioning	+	
Postpyloric feeding		+
Postponement of enteral feeding for at least 48 hours following intubation	+	
Selective decontamination of the digestive tract		+
Topical chlorhexidine	+	
Transfusion restriction	+	
Antibiotic cycling		+

- Standardized weaning protocols
- Adequate ICU staffing
- Both maintenance of endotracheal cuff pressure
  >20 cm H_2O and continuous subglottic suction reduce
  the incidence of VAP significantly
- Semirecumbent positioning (30- to 45-degree head-up)
  is also protective as compared to supine positioning,
  especially during enteral feeding.
- Compared to postpyloric feeding, intragastric feeding
  increases both gastroesophageal reflux and aspiration.
  - A meta-analysis of 11 randomized trials reported a
    RR of 0.77 (95% CI 0.60–1.00, $p = 0.05$) for VAP
    with postpyloric as compared to gastric feedings.
  - Promotility agents such as erythromycin may facil-
    itate safe intragastric feeding, should this route be
    used.
  - Early enteral feedings may increase the risk of VAP.
    - Enteral nutrition begun ≤48 hours after the initi-
      ation of mechanical ventilation was independently
      associated with the development of VAP (OR 2.65,
      95% CI 1.93–3.63, p <0.0001).
  - Pharmacologic strategies to minimize the risk of aspira-
    tion include:
    - Minimization of stress ulcer prophylaxis
    - Use of self-decontamination of the digestive tract is cur-
      rently not recommended for the routine prevention of
      VAP
      - Meta-analysis of studies of oropharyngeal decontam-
        ination with topical chlorhexidine provides sufficient
        evidence to recommend the practice especially for car-
        diac surgical patients.
    - Stress ulcer prophylaxis is a known risk factor for VAP.
      - Its use should be reserved for patients at high risk for
        gastrointestinal mucosal hemorrhage (e.g., mechani-
        cal ventilation more than 2 days, intracranial hemor-
        rhage, coagulopathy, glucocorticoid therapy).
      - Results of randomized trials comparing histamine
        type 2 antagonists, sucralfate, and antacids are con-
        flicting for prevention of VAP.
  - Red blood cell transfusion can be an independent risk
    factor for VAP (OR 1.89, 95% CI 1.33–2.68, $p =
    0.0004$).
    - 90% decreased incidence of VAP in a surgical ICU fol-
      lowing implementation of an anemia management pro-
      tocol that resulted in fewer blood transfusions

Risk Factors for Catheter-Related Bloodstream Infection

- Critically ill patients often require reliable large-bore central
  venous access (e.g., femoral, internal jugular, or subclavian
  vein), but the catheters are highly prone to infection (see Table
  71.1).
- Strict adherence to infection control and proper insertion
  technique crucial
  - Under elective (controlled) circumstances, optimal inser-
    tion technique includes:
    - Chlorhexidine skin preparation (not povidone-iodine)
    - Draping the entire bed into the sterile field
    - Donning a cap, a mask, and sterile gown and gloves

○ If technique is breached, the risk of infection increases exponentially, and the catheter should be removed and replaced (if still needed) at a different site using strict asepsis and antisepsis as soon as the patient's condition permits, but certainly within 24 hours.

○ Infection risk for femoral vein catheters is highest, and is lowest for catheters placed via the subclavian route

○ Peripheral vein catheters, peripherally inserted central catheters (PICCs), and tunneled central venous catheters (e.g., Hickman, Broviac) pose less risk of infection than percutaneous central venous catheters.

Risk Factors for Sinusitis

- Nosocomial sinusitis an uncommon closed-space infection that may be clinically occult but can have serious consequences
  - Sinusitis often part of the differential diagnosis of fever
    - Incidence is low in comparison to other nosocomial infections in the ICU, and the diagnosis can be difficult to document convincingly
    - Likely pathogenesis of sinusitis is anatomic obstruction of the ostia draining the facial sinuses, especially the maxillary sinuses
    - Transnasal endotracheal intubation is the leading risk factor
      ○ Incidence of sinusitis estimated to be one-third after 7 days of intubation
    - Maxillofacial trauma, with obstruction of drainage by retained blood clots, is another clear risk factor.
    - Nasogastric intubation, nasal packing for epistaxis, and corticosteroid therapy have also been implicated, but the evidence is less convincing.

ANTIBIOTIC PROPHYLAXIS

- Prophylactic antibiotics are used most often to prevent infection of a surgical incision.
- Does not prevent postoperative nosocomial infections
- Actually occur at an increased rate after prolonged prophylaxis, selecting for more resistant pathogens when infection does develop
- Preoperative antibiotic prophylaxis has been proven to reduce the risk of postoperative SSI in many circumstances.
  - Only the incision is protected, but only while it is open and vulnerable to inoculation
  - Indicated for most clean-contaminated and contaminated (or potentially contaminated) operations
  - Current Surgical Care Improvement Project (SCIP) guidelines for antibiotic prophylaxis of elective colon surgery give equal weighting to oral prophylaxis alone, parenteral prophylaxis alone, or the combination (Table 71.5).
  - Antibiotic prophylaxis of clean surgery is controversial.
    - Where bone is incised (e.g., craniotomy, sternotomy) or a prosthesis is inserted, antibiotic prophylaxis generally indicated
    - Meta-analysis of randomized controlled trials shows some benefit of antibiotic prophylaxis of breast cancer surgery without immediate reconstruction but no decrease of SSI rate for groin hernia surgery even when a nonabsorbable mesh prosthesis is implanted.
    - Arterial reconstruction with prosthetic graft material is an example of clean surgery where the susceptibility to infection is high, owing to the presence of ischemic tissue and the infrainguinal location of many such operations.
      ○ Meta-analysis identified 23 randomized, controlled trials of prophylactic systemic antibiotics for peripheral arterial reconstruction (Table 71.6).
      ○ Prophylactic systemic antibiotics reduced the risk of SSI by approximately 75%, and early graft infection by about 69%.
      ○ No benefit to prophylaxis for more than 24 hours, antibiotic bonding to the graft material itself, or preoperative bathing with an antiseptic agent compared with unmedicated bathing
  - Four principles guide the administration of antimicrobial agents for prophylaxis:
  - Safety

TABLE 71.5

SURGICAL CARE IMPROVEMENT PROGRAM: APPROVED ANTIBIOTIC PROPHYLACTIC REGIMENS FOR ELECTIVE SURGERY

Type of operation	Antibiotic(s)
Cardiac (including CABG)[a], vascular[b]	Cefazolin, cefuroxime, or vancomycin[f]
Hip/knee arthroplasty[b]	Cefazolin, cefuroxime, or vancomycin[f]
Colon[c,d]	Oral: Neomycin sulfate plus either erythromycin base or metronidazole, administered for 18 hours before surgery Parenteral: cefoxitin, cefotetan, or cefazolin plus metronidazole or ampicillin-sulbactam or ertapenem
Hysterectomy[e]	Cefazolin, cefoxitin, cefotetan, cefuroxime, or ampicillin-sulbactam

[a]Prophylaxis may be administered for up to 48 hours for cardiac surgery; for all other cases, the limit is 24 hours.
[b]For β-lactam allergy, clindamycin or vancomycin is an acceptable substitute for cardiac, vascular, and orthopedic surgery.
[c]For β-lactam allergy, clindamycin plus gentamicin, a fluoroquinolone, or aztreonam; or metronidazole plus gentamicin or a fluoroquinolone is an acceptable choice.
[d]For colon surgery, either oral or parenteral prophylaxis alone, or both combined, is acceptable.
[e]For β-lactam allergy, clindamycin plus gentamicin, a fluoroquinolone, or aztreonam; or metronidazole plus gentamicin or a fluoroquinolone or clindamycin monotherapy is an acceptable choice.
[f]Vancomycin is acceptable with a physician-documented justification for use in the patient's medical record.

TABLE 71.6

META-ANALYSIS OF MEASURES TO PREVENT INFECTION FOLLOWING
ARTERIAL RECONSTRUCTION

Intervention	No. of trials	Odds ratio	95% CI
Systemic antibiotic prophylaxis			
Surgical site infection	10	0.25	0.17–0.38
>24 h prophylaxis	3	1.28	0.82–1.98
Early graft infection	5	0.31	0.11–0.85
Rifampicin bonding of polyester grafts			
Graft infection—1 month	3	0.63	0.27–1.49
Graft infection—2 years	2	1.05	0.46–2.40
Suction wound drainage—groin	2		
Surgical site infection		0.96	0.50–1.86
Preoperative antiseptic bath	3		
Surgical site infection		0.97	0.70–1.36
In situ surgical technique	2		
Surgical site infection		0.48	0.31–0.74

Data from Stewart A, Evers PS, Earnshaw JJ. Prevention of infection in arterial reconstruction. *Cochrane Database Syst Rev.* 2006;3:CD003073.

- Appropriate narrow spectrum of coverage of relevant pathogens
- Little or no reliance upon the agent for therapy of infection (owing to the possible induction of resistance with heavy usage)
- Administration within 1 hour before surgery and for a defined, brief period of time thereafter (no more than 24 hours [48 hours for cardiac surgery]; ideally, a single dose)
  ○ According to these principles, quinolones or carbapenems are undesirable agents for surgical prophylaxis.
    – Ertapenem and quinolone prophylaxes have been endorsed by the SCIP for prophylaxis of colon surgery (the latter with metronidazole for penicillin-allergic patients) (see Table 71.5).
- Most SSIs are caused by Gram-positive cocci.
- Prophylaxis should be directed primarily against staphylococci for clean cases and high-risk clean-contaminated elective biliary and gastric surgery.
  ○ First-generation cephalosporin is preferred in almost all circumstances (Table 71.7), with clindamycin used for penicillin-allergic patients.
  ○ If Gram-negative or anaerobic coverage is required, a second-generation cephalosporin or the combination of a first-generation agent plus metronidazole is most experts' regimens of first choice.
  ○ Vancomycin prophylaxis is generally appropriate only in institutions where the incidence of MRSA infection is high (>20% of all SSIs caused by MRSA).
- Optimal time to give parenteral antibiotic prophylaxis is within 1 hour prior to incision.
  ○ Given sooner they are ineffective, as are agents given after the incision is closed.
  ○ In 2001 only 56% of patients who received prophylactic antibiotics did so within 1 hour prior to the skin incision.
  ○ Timeliness was documented in only 76% of cases in a 2005 audit in Veterans Affairs hospitals
    – Most inappropriately timed first doses of prophylactic antibiotic occur too early

– Antibiotics with short half-lives (<2 hours, e.g., cefazolin or cefoxitin) should be redosed every 3 to 4 hours during surgery if the operation is prolonged or bloody.
– SCIP specifies a 24-hour limit for prophylaxis (Table 71.8).
  - Excessively prolonged antibiotic prophylaxis is both pervasive and potentially harmful.
  - Recent U.S. data show that only 40% of patients who receive antibiotic prophylaxis do so for <24 hours.
  - As a result of ischemia caused by surgical hemostasis, antibiotic penetration into the incision immediately after surgery is questionable until neovascularization occurs (24–48 hours).
  - Antibiotics should not be given to "cover" indwelling drains or catheters, in lavage or irrigation fluid, or as a substitute for poor surgical technique.
- Prolongation of antibiotic prophylaxis beyond 24 hours is not only nonbeneficial, but also may be harmful.
- *Clostridium difficile*–associated disease (CDAD) follows disruption of the normal balance of gut flora, resulting in overgrowth of the enterotoxin-producing *C. difficile*.
- Virtually any antibiotic may cause CDAD (even a single dose).
- Prolonged antibiotic prophylaxis increases risk.
- Prolonged prophylaxis also increases the risk of nosocomial infections unrelated to the surgical site, and the emergence of MDR pathogens.
- Pneumonia and vascular catheter-related infections have been associated with prolonged prophylaxis as has the emergence of SSI caused by MRSA.

EVALUATION OF POSSIBLE POSTOPERATIVE INFECTION

- Some infected patients do not become febrile and may even become hypothermic.

TABLE 71.7

APPROPRIATE CEPHALOSPORIN PROPHYLAXIS FOR SELECTED OPERATIONS[a]

Operation First-generation cephalosporin (i.e., cefazolin, cefuroxime)	Alternative prophylaxis in serious penicillin allergy Clindamycin (for all cases herein except amputation)[b]
Cardiovascular and thoracic	
Median sternotomy	Vancomycin
Pacemaker insertion	
Vascular reconstruction involving the abdominal aorta, insertion of a prosthesis, or a groin incision (except carotid endarterectomy, which requires no prophylaxis)	
Implantable defibrillator	
Pulmonary resection	
Lower limb amputation	Gentamicin and metronidazole
General	
Cholecystectomy (High risk only)	Gentamicin
Gastrectomy (High risk only: Not uncomplicated chronic duodenal ulcer)	Gentamicin and metronidazole
Hepatobiliary	Gentamicin and metronidazole
Major debridement of traumatic wound	Gentamicin
Genitourinary (Ampicillin plus gentamicin a reasonable alternative)	Ciprofloxacin
Appendectomy	Metronidazole with/without gentamicin (all cases herein) Second generation (i.e., cefoxitin)[c]
Colon surgery	
Surgery for penetrating abdominal trauma	
Gynecologic	
Cesarean section (stat)	Metronidazole (after cord clamping)
Hysterectomy (cefoxitin a reasonable alternative)	Doxycycline
Head and neck/oral cavity	Gentamicin and clindamycin or metronidazole
Major procedures entering oral cavity or pharynx	
Neurosurgery	
Craniotomy	Clindamycin, vancomycin
Orthopedics	
Major joint arthroplasty	Vancomycin[b]
Open reduction of closed fracture	Vancomycin[b]

[a]Should be given as a single intravenous dose just before the operation. Consider an additional dose if the operation is prolonged longer than 3–4 h.
[b]Primary prophylaxis with vancomycin (i.e., for the non–penicillin-allergic patient) may be appropriate for cardiac valve replacement, placement of a nontissue peripheral vascular prosthesis, or total joint replacement in institutions where a high rate of infections with methicillin-resistant *Staphylococcus aureus* or *Staphylococcus epidermidis* has occurred. The precise definition of "high rate" is debated. A single dose administered immediately before surgery is sufficient unless operation lasts for more than 6 h, in which case the dose should be repeated. Prophylaxis should be discontinued after a maximum of two doses, but may be continued for up to 48 h.
[c]An intraoperative dose should be given if cefoxitin is used and the duration of surgery exceeds 3–4 h, because of the short half-life of the drug. A postoperative dose is not necessary, but is permissible for up to 24 h.

TABLE 71.8

COMPARISON OF ANTIBIOTIC UTILIZATION (MEDIAN DEFINED DAILY DOSES) FOR SURGICAL INTENSIVE CARE UNITS (SICUs) AND INPATIENT UNITS, 1998–2002

Agent	Inpatient	SICU
First-generation cephalosporins	76	168
Third-generation cephalosporins	81	142
Vancomycin		104
Fluoroquinolones	62	87
Ampicillins	63	83
Second-generation cephalosporins	34	NR

NR, not reported.
From the National Nosocomial Infections Surveillance System, U.S. Centers for Disease Control and Prevention. Data abstracted from www.cdc.gov. Data are in the public domain.

- Elderly patients
- Those with open abdominal wounds or large burns
- Patients on extracorporeal support (e.g., continuous renal replacement therapy)
- Patients with end-stage liver disease or chronic renal failure
- Patients taking anti-inflammatory or antipyretic drugs
- Absent a fever, hypotension, tachycardia, tachypnea, confusion, rigors, skin lesions, respiratory manifestations, oliguria, lactic acidosis, leukocytosis, leukopenia, immature neutrophils (i.e., bands >10%), or thrombocytopenia may indicate a workup for infection and immediate empiric therapy.
- Definition of fever is arbitrary, and depends on how and when temperature was measured
  - In addition to host biology, a variety of environmental forces in an ICU can also alter body temperature:
    - Specialized mattresses
    - Lighting, heating, or air conditioning
    - Peritoneal lavage

- Renal replacement therapy
- Thermoregulatory mechanisms can be disrupted by drugs or by injury to the central nervous system (CNS).
- Often difficult to determine if an abnormal temperature is a reflection of a physiologic process, a drug, or an environmental influence
- In surgical patients, the substantial possibility ($\sim$50%) that a fever is due to a noninfectious cause must be considered
- Many ICUs consider any patient with a core temperature $\geq38.3°C$ ($\geq101°F$) to be febrile and to warrant evaluation to determine if infection is present.
  - Lower threshold may be decided upon for immunocompromised patients
  - Laboratory tests or imaging studies to search for infection should be performed only after a clinical assessment (history and physical examination) indicates that infection might be present.

Blood Cultures

- Should be obtained with a new fever when clinical evaluation does not strongly suggest a noninfectious cause
  - Site of venipuncture should be cleaned with either 2% chlorhexidine gluconate in 70% isopropyl alcohol or 1% to 2% tincture of iodine
  - Povidone-iodine (10%), while acceptable, is not bactericidal until dry
  - One blood culture is defined as a 20- to 30-mL sample of blood drawn at a single time from a single site
    - Regardless of how many bottles or tubes are filled for processing
  - Sensitivity of blood culturing for detection of true bacteremia or fungemia is related to many factors:
  - Most importantly the volume of blood drawn
  - Obtaining the cultures before initiation of anti-infective therapy
  - Cumulative yield of pathogens is optimized when three blood cultures with adequate volume (20- to 30-mL each) are drawn.
    - Ideally drawn by separate venipuncture or through a separate intravascular device
      ○ Not through multiple ports of the same intravascular catheter
      ○ No evidence that the yield of cultures drawn from an artery or vein is different
      ○ Drawing two to three blood cultures with appropriate volume from separate sites of access at the onset of fever is the most effective way to discern whether an organism found in blood culture represents:
      – True pathogen (multiple cultures are often positive)
      – Contaminant (only one of multiple blood cultures is positive for an organism commonly found on skin and clinical correlation does not support infection)
      – Bacteremia/fungemia from an infected catheter (one culture from the source catheter is positive, often with a positive catheter tip, and other cultures are not)

Intravascular Devices

- **All intravascular devices and insertion sites must be assessed daily:**

- As part of a comprehensive physical examination
- To determine if they are still needed
- Whether signs of infection are present locally (e.g., inflammation or purulence at the exit site or along the tunnel) or systemically
- Contaminated catheter hubs are common portals of entry for organisms colonizing the catheter's endoluminal surface
- Infusate (i.e., parenteral fluid, blood products, or intravenous medications) can become contaminated and produce bacteremia or fungemia, which is especially likely to result in septic shock.
  - Abrupt onset of signs and symptoms of sepsis or shock in patients with an indwelling vascular catheter should prompt suspicion of infection of an intravascular device.
  - Recovery in multiple blood cultures of staphylococci or *Candida* spp. strongly suggests infection of an intravascular device.
- Removal and culture of the catheter historically the gold standard for diagnosis of CR-BSI particularly with short-term catheters
  - Demonstrated the reliability of semiquantitative or quantitative catheter tip culture methods for the diagnosis of CR-BSI
  - Confirmed when a colonized catheter is associated with concomitant bloodstream infection with the identical organism, with no other plausible source
  - Some ICU clinicians culture central venous catheters routinely on removal, regardless of whether infection is suspected
    ○ Approximately 20% of central venous catheters are colonized at removal, most unassociated with local or systemic infection, so this practice is expensive and can lead to unnecessary therapy.
    ○ Predictive value of a positive catheter culture is very low when there is a low pretest probability of line sepsis.
    ○ Catheters removed from ICU patients should only be cultured if there is strong clinical suspicion of CR-BSI.
- For patients with fever alone without systemic inflammatory response syndrome (SIRS):
  - Usually no need to remove or change all indwelling catheters immediately
    - Although such an approach would be prudent in a patient with a prosthetic heart valve or a fresh arterial graft
- If patients have severe sepsis or septic shock, peripheral embolization, disseminated intravascular coagulation, or ARDS:
  - Removal of all intravascular catheters is indicated, even if the catheters are cuffed or tunneled devices.
- Infected phlebitis (suppurative phlebitis) of central vein due to a CVL is unusual.
  - With suppurative phlebitis, bloodstream infection characteristically persists
  - Originates from a peripheral vein catheter site with infected intravascular thrombus
  - Producing a picture of overwhelming sepsis with high-grade bacteremia or fungemia
  - Syndrome is most often encountered in burn patients or other ICU patients who develop unrecognized catheter-related infection
  - In patients with persistent *S. aureus* bacteremia or fungemia, echocardiography is appropriate to assess for endocarditis and guide further therapy.

INTRACRANIAL DEVICE–RELATED FEVER

- When a patient with an intracranial device such as an extraventricular drain (EVD) (ventriculostomy catheter) or a ventriculoperitoneal shunt becomes febrile, cerebrospinal fluid (CSF) should be analyzed.
  - Access to CSF in the patient with an EVD is straightforward.
  - Patient with a shunt or Ommaya reservoir should have the reservoir aspirated.
  - Patients with EVDs who develop stupor or signs of meningitis should have the catheter removed and the tip cultured.
- Basic tests of CSF for suspected CNS infection include:
  - Cell counts and differential
  - Glucose and protein concentrations
  - Gram stain
  - Bacterial cultures
- Patients with bacterial meningitis typically have:
  - CSF glucose concentration <35 mg/dL
  - CSF:blood glucose ratio <0.23
  - CSF protein concentration >220 mg/dL
  - >2,000 total white blood cells/μL, or >1,180 neutrophils/μL
    - Conversely, the presence of a normal opening pressure, <5 white blood cells/μL, and a normal CSF protein concentration essentially exclude meningitis.
    - Measurement of CSF lactate concentration may be useful in neurosurgical patients to distinguish infection from postoperative aseptic meningitis.

NONINFECTIOUS CAUSES OF FEVER IN THE INTENSIVE CARE UNIT

Postoperative Fever

- Fever is common during the initial 72 hours following surgery and is usually noninfectious in origin.
  - Presuming that unusual breaks in sterile technique or pulmonary aspiration did not occur
  - Once a patient is more than 96 hours postoperative, fever is more likely to represent infection.
  - Chest radiograph:
    - Not mandatory for evaluation of postoperative fever unless:
      - Respiratory rate
      - Auscultation
      - Abnormal blood gases
      - Pulmonary secretions suggest a high yield
    - Atelectasis often considered to be a cause of postoperative fever, but is not
      - Patient could have aspirated during the perioperative period
      - Patient could have been incubating a community-acquired pneumonia prior to the operation caused, for example, by pneumococci or influenza A
  - Urinary tract infection is common postoperatively in non-trauma patients because of the use of urinary drainage catheters.
    - Duration of catheterization increases the risk of bacteriuria by about 5% per day

      - Increases the risk of nosocomial cystitis or pyelonephritis
    - A urinalysis or culture is not mandatory to evaluate fever during the initial 3 days postoperatively unless there is reason by history or examination to suspect an infection at this site.
    - After trauma, urinary tract infection is common only after injury to the urinary tract.
- Fever can be related to hematoma or infection of the surgical field.
  - Surgical site infection is rare in the first few days after operation, except for group A streptococcal infections and clostridial infections.
    - Can develop within hours to 1 to 3 days after surgery
    - These causes should be suspected on the basis of inspection of the incision
  - Many emergency abdominal operations are performed for control of an infection (e.g., perforated diverticulitis).
    - Even under optimal circumstances (definitive surgical source control and timely administration of appropriate broad-spectrum antibiotics), it may take $\geq$72 hours for such patients to defervesce.
    - New or persistent fever more than 4 days after surgery should raise suspicion of persistent pathology or a new complication.
    - Mandatory to remove the surgical dressing to inspect the incision
    - Swabbing an open wound or collecting fluid from drains (if present) for culture rarely helpful because the likelihood of colonization is high
    - **Muscle compression injury** (either direct trauma or as a result of compartment syndrome) and **tetanus** are two rare complications of traumatic wounds that may cause fever.
    - Toxic shock may accompany infection with group A streptococci or *S. aureus*.
    - Other potentially serious noninfectious causes of postoperative fever include:
      - Deep venous thrombosis or pulmonary embolus
      - Tissue ischemia or necrosis
      - Adrenal insufficiency
      - Drug-induced fever
      - Anesthesia-induced malignant hyperthermia
      - Acute allograft rejection

Drug-Related Fever

- "Drug fever" is decidedly unusual in surgical patients.
- Must be considered a diagnosis of exclusion
- Some drugs cause fever by producing local inflammation at the site of administration (phlebitis, sterile abscesses, or soft tissue reaction), such as:
  - Amphotericin B
  - Erythromycin
  - Potassium chloride
- Drugs or their delivery systems (diluent, intravenous fluid, or intravascular delivery devices) may also contain pyrogens or, rarely, microbial contaminants
- Some drugs may also stimulate heat production (e.g., thyroxine), limit heat dissipation (e.g., atropine or epinephrine), or alter thermoregulation (e.g., butyrophenone tranquilizers, phenothiazines, antihistamines, or antiparkinson drugs)

- Among drug categories, drug fever in surgical ICUs is most often attributed to antimicrobial agents (e.g., vancomycin, β-lactams) and anticonvulsants (especially phenytoin).
- Two important syndromes, malignant hyperthermia (MH) and neuroleptic malignant syndrome, deserve consideration when fever is especially high because the results can be devastating if left untreated:
  - MH more often identified in the operating room than the ICU, but onset can be delayed for as long as 24 hours, especially if the patient is on steroids.
    - MH believed to be genetically determined response mediated by a dysregulation of cytoplasmic calcium flux in skeletal muscle, resulting in intense muscle contraction, fever, and increased creatinine phosphokinase concentration.
    - Can be caused by succinylcholine and inhalational anesthetics.
  - The neuroleptic malignant syndrome is slightly more common and more often identified in the ICU than malignant hyperthermia.
    - Strongly associated with the neuroleptic medications:
      - Phenothiazines
      - Thioxanthenes
      - Butyrophenones
        - Most frequently haloperidol in the ICU
    - Also manifests as muscle rigidity, fever, and increasing creatinine phosphokinase concentration.
    - Unlike MH, the initiator of muscle contraction is central, the syndrome is often less intense, and mortality is less.
- Drug withdrawal from alcohol, opioids, barbiturates, and benzodiazepines may be associated with:
  - Fever
  - Tachycardia
  - Diaphoresis
  - Hyperreflexia
    - History of use of these drugs may not be available when the patient is admitted to the ICU.
    - Withdrawal and related fever may therefore occur several hours or days after admission.
- Other noninfectious causes of fever are listed in Table 71.9.

CLINICAL INFECTION SYNDROMES

Biliary Tract Infections

- Biliary tract infections remain an important cause of critical illness.
  - Difficult to diagnose in critically ill patients, owing to their relative rarity and the nonspecificity of symptoms noncommunicative patients may manifest
  - Unless diagnosed and treated aggressively, organ dysfunction and death may ensue rapidly.
  - Signs and symptoms of hepatobiliary infection commonly include:
    - Abdominal pain
    - Fever
    - Nausea and vomiting
  - Clinical presentation may range in severity from the appearance of a chronic disease state to overt septic shock.
    - Leukocytosis is common.

TABLE 71.9

CAUSES OF FEVER RELATED TO NONINFECTIOUS STATES

Acalculous cholecystitis
Acute myocardial infarction
Acute respiratory distress syndrome (fibroproliferative phase)
Adrenal insufficiency
Cytokine release syndrome
Fat embolism
Gout
Hematoma
Heterotopic ossification
Immune reconstitution inflammatory syndrome (IRIS)
Intracranial hemorrhage
Pancreatitis
Pericarditis
Pulmonary infarction
Thyroid storm
Transfusion of blood or blood products
Transplant rejection
Tumor lysis syndrome
Venous thromboembolic disease
Withdrawal syndromes (drug, alcohol)

- Patterns of liver enzyme abnormalities overlap to such a degree that it may be difficult to make a definitive diagnosis based on history, physical examination, and laboratory values alone.
- May be difficult to distinguish liver dysfunction caused by primary infection from that caused by multiple organ dysfunction syndrome
- Imaging of the biliary tree is often of paramount importance.

Acute Cholecystitis

- In outpatients, acute cholecystitis usually occurs when gallstones migrate into the cystic duct, causing outflow obstruction.
  - Obstruction causes sterile inflammation and edema of the gallbladder wall initially, followed by bacterial superinfection.
  - Acute calculous cholecystitis presents with:
    - Fever
    - Right upper quadrant pain
    - Nausea and vomiting
  - Physical examination may range from:
    - Arrest of inspiration due to tenderness on palpation in the right upper quadrant (Murphy sign)
    - To signs of peritonitis in advanced cases
    - Concomitant jaundice suggests the presence of choledocholithiasis
  - Ultrasound highly sensitive and specific test (95% and 97%, respectively)
    - Diagnostic findings include:
      - Presence of stones in the gallbladder
      - Thickening of the gallbladder wall (>3.5 mm)
      - Pericholecystic fluid
      - Tenderness with application of the ultrasound probe (sonographic Murphy sign)

- Most cases (~80%) of acute calculous cholecystitis resolve with bowel rest, fluid resuscitation, and intravenous antibiotics and are treated ultimately by cholecystectomy.
- Patients ill enough to require ICU care generally have gallbladder gangrene that progresses to perforation, resulting in either subhepatic abscess or free perforation with bile peritonitis.
  - Associated with a 30% mortality rate
  - Tends to occur in older patients
- Emphysematous cholecystitis, a severe manifestation of acute cholecystitis with predilection for elderly patients and patients with diabetes mellitus
  - Defined by the presence of gas in the gallbladder wall as visualized on ultrasound or computed tomography (CT)
  - Characterized by polymicrobial infection including *Clostriduim* spp., *Escherichia coli, Klebsiella* spp., and *Streptococcus* spp.
  - Roughly one-half of all cases of emphysematous cholecystitis are acalculous.
  - Reported mortality ranges from 15% to 25%
- Acalculous cholecystitis has been reported in all age groups.
  - Most often occurs in the setting of severe illness or injury
  - May also occur in the postoperative setting, particularly in males after emergency surgery complicated by large-volume blood loss
  - Review of 31,710 cases of cardiac surgery found a 0.05% incidence
  - After open abdominal aortic aneurysm repair incidence has been reported to be between 0.7% and 0.9%
  - A grave condition of insidious onset in patients who are often already critically ill with mortality approaching 30%
  - Diagnosis of acalculous cholecystitis must always be entertained in a patient with sepsis for whom no clear source of infection can be determined.
  - Pathogenesis of acalculous cholecystitis most likely splanchnic ischemia-reperfusion injury
    - Alternatively, bile stasis associated with critical illness may lead to distention of the gallbladder, which, in combination with hypoperfusion, may cause ischemia and ultimately necrosis.
    - Factors such as mechanical ventilation, total parenteral nutrition, cytokine activation, and endotoxemia have also been implicated.
  - Diagnosis of acalculous cholecystitis difficult to make in the ICU
    - Patients who communicate may report abdominal pain localizing to the right upper quadrant or diffuse pain in the case of peritonitis
    - Fever usually present
    - Physical examination may reveal signs ranging from localized tenderness in the right upper quadrant to frank peritonitis.
    - Right upper quadrant abdominal phlegmon may be palpable.
    - Altered mental status that often accompanies critical illness may obscure any useful information that might be obtained from the history and physical examination.
    - Laboratory values are nonspecific but usually include:
      - Leukocytosis

      - Elevated liver enzymes, particularly of bilirubin, transaminases, and alkaline phosphatase
      - Hyperbilirubinemia is typical and occurs more often in acalculous than calculous cholecystitis
    - Ultrasound is perhaps the ideal radiologic study to investigate the diagnosis of acalculous cholecystitis in the ICU.
      - May reveal hydrops of the gallbladder
      - Pericholecystic fluid
      - Gallbladder wall thickening
        - If thickness ≥3.5 mm, ultrasound is 98.5% sensitive and 80% specific for the diagnosis of acalculous cholecystitis
  - Upon making diagnosis:
    - Decision about method of source control must be made
    - Empiric antibiotic therapy started:
      - Up to one-half of cases of acute acalculous cholecystitis are associated with culture-negative bile at least initially
      - Empiric antibiotics needed because distinguishing sterile from infected cases can be clinically impossible
      - Organisms most frequently cultured from the bile in acalculous cholecystitis are *E. coli, Klebsiella*, and *Enterococcus faecalis*
    - Source control for cholecystitis, whether calculous or acalculous, traditionally cholecystectomy:
      - Percutaneous cholecystostomy tube placement is a minimally invasive alternative to cholecystectomy that is favored increasingly
      - Complications of percutaneous cholecystostomy include bacteremia, hemorrhage, bile peritonitis, and tube dislodgement
      - With uncomplicated cholecystitis should improve rapidly after gallbladder decompression
      - Failure to improve should raise suspicions of an incorrect diagnosis or inadequate source control and surgical exploration mandated

Cholangitis

- An acute infection of the main biliary ductal system
- Pathogenesis of cholangitis requires both obstruction and bacterial superinfection
- Most common cause of intrinsic obstruction in the Western world is choledocholithiasis
  - Both primary and metastatic malignant disease of the abdominal viscera may cause extrinsic obstruction, among other causes
  - Obstruction from calculi more likely to cause cholangitis than malignant obstruction
  - May also occur in the postoperative setting, particularly after a biliary-enteric anastomosis
- Bile is sterile in the normal biliary tree and naturally bacteriostatic
  - Antegrade flow of bile from liver to duodenum serves as a flushing mechanism
  - Sphincter of Oddi is an anatomic barrier, preventing reflux of enteric flora
  - Bile salts absorb intraluminal endotoxins and may also exhibit a trophic effect on small bowel mucosa
- Charcot triad of fever, right upper quadrant pain, and jaundice

- Observed in 50% to 70% of patients who present with cholangitis
- Fever present most consistently (90%)
- Hypotension and altered mental status (i.e., severe sepsis or septic shock) in addition constitute the Reynolds pentad
- Typically have leukocytosis, direct hyperbilirubinemia (88%–100%), and elevated alkaline phosphatase (80%)
- Transaminitis is usually mild
- Common duct bile cultures positive 80% to 100% of the time in cholangitis
  - Positive blood cultures found in up to two-thirds of patients
  - Concordance rate between bile and blood cultures is 33% to 84%
    - Bile cultures being polymicrobial in roughly one-half of cases
  - Typical florae are *Klebsiella*, *E. coli*, and *Enterococcus*
- Imaging of patients with cholangitis is possible using ultrasound, CT, or magnetic resonance imaging (MRI)
  - Ultrasound detects cholelithiasis and bile duct dilation reliably, but is only 50% sensitive for detecting choledocholithiasis
  - CT detects ductal dilation with 98% accuracy and is superior to ultrasound in defining the level of obstruction, but may fail to visualize the 85% of biliary calculi that are radiolucent
  - Stones can be visualized on MRI
    - Magnetic resonance cholangiopancreatography (MRCP) provides the most complete imaging as to the etiology of biliary obstruction
  - Endoscopic retrograde cholangiopancreatography (ERCP) and Percutaneous transhepatic cholangiopancreatography (PTC) are both 90% to 100% sensitive for defining the site and nature of biliary obstruction.
    - Either can be used diagnostically or therapeutically to decompress the biliary tree.
    - Both ERCP and PTC have rare potential complications (e.g., bile leak, bleeding) that may precipitate ICU admission.
- Treatment of cholangitis consists of:
  - Immediate fluid resuscitation and broad-spectrum antibiotics
  - Followed by urgent or emergent biliary decompression
  - Many authorities prefer a single broad-spectrum agent such as piperacillin/tazobactam or a carbapenem
  - 10% to 15% will require emergent decompression
    - ERCP is the safest and most efficacious treatment for acute cholangitis with a success rate of 90% and a mortality rate of 10%, considerably lower than that of emergency surgical decompression of the common bile duct.
    - Other complications of ERCP include pancreatitis, perforation, aspiration, systemic sepsis, and failure to decompress the bile duct.
    - Percutaneous transhepatic biliary drainage carries 30% morbidity.
      - Complications such as hemorrhage, pneumothorax, subphrenic abscess, and bile peritonitis
      - Mortality for PTC is estimated to be between 5% and 10%, similar to that seen with ERCP.
    - Surgery is now infrequent in the primary management of acute cholangitis

- In situations that require surgery (e.g., resectable malignant obstruction), patients may be temporized by ERCP or PTC
  - Also indicated in patients who fail less invasive treatment methods
  - Standard emergency surgical therapy includes cholecystectomy, choledochotomy, and T-tube placement

Liver Abscess

- Most common cause (50% to 65%) of liver abscesses is now ascending biliary tract infection (e.g., cholangitis, direct extension of acute suppurative cholecystitis).
- Seeding from the portal vein accounts for 10% to 25% of abscesses and is typically a result of intra-abdominal sources of infection such as diverticulitis.
- Systemic seeding via the hepatic artery occurs in 1% to 10% of cases from processes such as bacterial endocarditis, dental abscesses, or interventions such as hepatic artery chemoembolization, intraoperative cryoablation, or radiofrequency ablation.
- Liver abscess complicates fewer than 1% of blunt liver injuries managed nonoperatively and is more common in patients requiring damage-control laparotomy and perihepatic packing to control hemorrhage.
- Patients with pyogenic hepatic abscess usually present with fever and chills, abdominal pain, and weight loss.
  - Nonspecific abdominal complaints and constitutional symptoms are common, and presentation can range from the appearance of a chronic disease state to overt septic shock.
  - Laboratory workup demonstrates leukocytosis in most patients, with liver enzymes being moderately abnormal as well.
  - Due to the protean manifestations of liver abscess and the mimicry of a number of disease processes, radiographic imaging is crucial.
    - Ultrasound and CT both have >95% sensitivity for the diagnosis.
    - One-half of patients will present with more than one abscess, and approximately 75% of all liver abscesses will be found in the right lobe of the liver.
- Pyogenic liver abscesses are equally likely to be polymicrobial as monomicrobial.
  - Approximately 5% to 27% show no growth in culture.
  - Failure to speciate bacteria in culture may reflect prior antibiotic treatment.
    - Flora found in liver abscesses reflects the underlying source of the infection.
    - Overall the most common Gram-negative aerobes found in pyogenic liver abscesses are *E. coli* and *Klebsiella* spp.
    - Most common Gram-positive aerobes are *Enterococcus* spp., viridans streptococci, and *S. aureus*. Among cultured anaerobes, *Bacteroides* spp. predominate.
    - Medical management carried a mortality rate of 60% to 100%.
      - Recent case series demonstrate success rates for antibiotics alone of up to 80% when multiple (military) abscesses are too small or too numerous for percutaneous drainage.
      - Preferred method of treatment is broad-spectrum antibiotics in conjunction with drainage of all abscesses.

- Most can be drained successfully by image-guided percutaneous techniques, with a success rate of 70% to 93%.
- Surgical drainage is indicated in patients who:
  - Fail percutaneous drainage
  - Require surgical management of the underlying problem (e.g., diverticulitis)
  - Have abscesses that are not amenable to minimally invasive techniques because of their location
- Contemporary series quote a mortality rate for hepatic abscess between 6% and 31%.
- Factors associated with a worse prognosis include:
  - Underlying diagnosis of malignant disease
  - Multiple abscesses
  - High presenting APACHE II score

Postoperative Infections after Biliary Tract Operations

- Perihepatic infections may occur as a result of commonly performed hepatobiliary surgical procedures.
- Postoperative bile leaks may occur after any operation in which a bile duct is opened
  - Hepatectomy
  - Hepaticoenterostomy
  - Hepatic transplant
  - Cholecystectomy
- Leaking bile may induce chemical peritonitis or cause infection with microbial flora present in or introduced into tissue at the time of operation, or by translocation from the gut.
  - Leading to an infected intrahepatic or perihepatic collection, known as a biloma
- After cholecystectomy, bile leaks occur in up to 1% of patients.
  - Present with right upper quadrant pain, fever, nausea, vomiting, or jaundice
  - Discrimination between sterile bile peritonitis and infection may be difficult without culture of the collection
  - Postoperative fluid collections may be imaged with ultrasound, CT, or nuclear scintigraphy
- Diagnosis of bile leak can also be made by image-guided aspiration of the collection
- Treatment of postoperative bile leakage hinges first upon drainage and then definitive treatment of the underlying problem.
- Perihepatic or intra-abdominal abscess complicates 8% to 30% of major liver resections.
  - Associated with preoperative biliary stenting, hepaticoenterostomy, increased operative time, greater extent of resection, and the need for blood transfusion
- Preoperative hyperbilirubinemia as a result of biliary obstruction occurs frequently in patients with malignant biliary tract obstruction.
  - Such patients are at increased risk for complications of surgical resection.
  - Preoperative stent placement to alleviate biliary obstruction leads to increased rates of postoperative infectious complications.
- Resection of hepatic parenchyma leaves dead space in the abdomen that collects bile and blood and is in proximity to ischemic tissue at the resection margin.
  - Bacterial superinfection may occur, leading to the formation of an abscess

- Infected bilomas are heralded by fever, right upper quadrant pain, leukocytosis, and elevated liver enzymes.
- Imaging modalities for posthepatectomy abscesses include CT, ultrasound, and MRI
- Cultures reveal that 50% to 75% of postoperative perihepatic abscesses are polymicrobial.
  - Bacteria of enteric origin (e.g., *E. coli*, *Enterococcus*) predominate
  - Image-guided percutaneous drainage is the treatment of choice where feasible, with reoperation reserved for those patients in whom percutaneous drainage is not possible or unsuccessful.
- Liver transplantation is plagued by complication rates ranging from 24% to 64%.
- Incidence of bile leak after orthotopic liver transplantation is between 10% and 40%.
  - Leaks arise most commonly from hepatic resection lines, T-tube sites, and biliary anastomoses.
  - Patients may present up to 6 months after transplantation.
  - CT is used to image the collection, which may be intrahepatic in up to two-thirds of cases.
  - ERCP, PTC, or cholangiogram through a preexisting T tube may be used to delineate the origin of the leak.
  - Most collections can be drained percutaneously, and in the event of direct communication with the biliary tree, ERCP can be used to reestablish preferential enteric drainage.
  - Blood supply to the biliary tree is provided by the hepatic artery; anastomotic leaks after liver transplantation may occur as a result of ischemia from hepatic artery thrombosis.
    - Assessment of the patency of the graft hepatic artery must be determined.
    - Some cases of biloma associated with hepatic artery thrombosis may respond to conservative measures, up to two-thirds will require retransplantation.

SURGICAL SITE INFECTION

- SSIs among the most frequently encountered complications in surgical patients regardless of specialty
- Simply opening and draining the incision in cases of superficial incisional SSI
- Infections extending below the superficial fascia (deep incisional SSIs) invariably require formal surgical debridement and open wound care to resolve the infection.
- Vacuum-assisted closure (VAC) and antimicrobial therapy also improved outcomes.
  - MDR pathogens may complicate resolution of ostensibly simple infections in the postoperative period particularly if they required antimicrobial therapy
- Surgical site infection remains a clinical diagnosis
  - Presenting signs and symptoms depend on the depth of infection
    - Typically as early as postoperative day 4 or 5
    - Clinical signs range from local induration only to the hallmarks of infection (e.g., erythema, edema, tenderness, warm skin, and pain-related immobility).
      - May manifest before wound drainage

- In deep incisional SSIs, tenderness may extend beyond the margin of erythema, and crepitus, cutaneous vesicles, or bullae may be present.
- With ongoing infection, signs of SIRS herald the development of sepsis
- Cultures are not mandatory for management of superficial incisional SSIs.
  - In cases of deeper infection or infection that has arisen in the hospital, exudates or drainage specimens should be sent for analysis.
  - Culturing surgically opened wound (as opposed to the already opened wound, which becomes colonized) by the swab method shown experimentally to be reliable
  - CT and MRI are more sensitive in detecting small amounts of gas in soft tissues.
  - CT-guided aspiration or drainage often facilitates treatment and may serve as definitive source control for an organ/space SSI.
- More severe SSIs, especially the dangerous forms of necrotizing soft tissue infection (NSTI)
  - True emergencies that need immediate surgical attention
  - Even modest delays can increase patient mortality substantially
    - Mortality increased from 32% to 70% when therapy was delayed more than 24 hours.
    - With an established diagnosis of NSTI, immediate and widespread operative debridement is indicated without waiting for precise determination of the causative pathogen or the identification of a specific clinical symptom.
      - Often require planned, sequential, repetitive surgical debridement sessions to control the infection
- When faced with a potential SSI, the first steps in management are:
  - Remove the appropriate sutures
  - Open and examine the suspicious portion of the incision
  - Decide about further surgical treatment
  - If infection is not confined to the skin and superficial underlying subcutaneous tissue:
    - Urgent surgical exploration and debridement is essential to obtain local control of the infection, remove necrotic tissue, and restore aerobic conditions to prevent further spread of the infection.
    - Surgical site infection must also be considered the cause of delayed or failed wound healing and prompt the same decisions as described above.
- Superficial SSIs:
  - Functionally are subcutaneous abscesses, rarely lead to systemic infection
  - Usually do not make patients seriously ill
  - Antibiotic therapy is not indicated for patients who do not have systemic signs of infection
  - Formal surgical intervention is limited to complications such as loculated abscesses or necrosis of the skin or underlying tissue
- Deep incisional SSIs typically present with extensive discomfort in more seriously ill patients.
  - Extend to superficial fascia or beneath
  - May cause extensive tissue necrosis and liquefaction beyond the obvious limits of the cutaneous signs, making it necessary to explore the wound formally in the operating room

- Broad-spectrum antimicrobial therapy should be given empirically
- Organ or space SSIs occur within a body cavity
  - Directly related to a surgical procedure, and may manifest as intra-abdominal, intrapleural, or intracranial infections
  - May remain occult or present with few symptoms, mimicking incisional SSIs and leading to inadequate initial treatment, becoming apparent only when a major complication ensues
  - Diagnosis of organ or space SSI usually requires imaging to confirm the site and extent of infection.
    - Adequate source control requires a drainage procedure, whether open or percutaneous.
- VAC optimizes blood flow, decreases tissue edema, and removes fluid from the wound bed, thereby facilitating the removal of bacteria from the wound.
  - Mechanical deformation of the wound promotes tissue expansion to cover the defect, and subatmospheric pressure in the milieu may trigger a cascade of intracellular signals that increases the rate of cell division and formation of granulation tissue.
  - Clinical value of VAC systems has been described only in small case series and cohort studies, mostly for sternal infections following cardiac surgery, abdominal wall dehiscence, and the management of complex perineal wounds, or as a method to secure skin grafts.
  - A lack of well-designed randomized, controlled trials precludes more specific recommendations.

PERITONITIS

- Only about 15% of patients with secondary peritonitis are ill enough to require ICU care.
  - Severe secondary peritonitis may follow penetrating intestinal injury that is not recognized or treated promptly (>12-hour delay).
  - Other causes include dehiscence of a bowel anastomosis with leakage and development of an intra-abdominal abscess.
- Secondary peritonitis is polymicrobial.
  - Anaerobic Gram-negative bacilli (e.g., *Bacteroides fragilis*) predominating
  - *E. coli* and *Klebsiella* spp. isolated commonly from community-onset infections
- When secondary peritonitis develops in a hospitalized patient as a complication of disease or therapy, the flora are more likely to reflect MDR pathogens encountered in the hospital.
  - Outcomes are worsened if empiric therapy is not appropriate.
- Failure of two source control procedures with persistent intra-abdominal collections is referred to as tertiary peritonitis.
  - Tertiary peritonitis is characterized by complete failure of intra-abdominal host defenses.
  - Controversy whether tertiary peritonitis is a true invasive infection, or rather peritoneal colonization with incompetent local host defenses, and thus, whether antibiotics should be prescribed and if so, for how long
  - Bacteria isolated in tertiary peritonitis are avirulent opportunists such as Methicillin-related *S. epidermis* (MRSE),

enterococci, *Pseudomonas,* and *Candida albicans,* supporting the incompetent host defense hypothesis.

- Some authorities recommend management with an open-abdomen technique, so that peritoneal toilet can be provided manually.
- May be no alternative to open-abdomen management if the infection extends to involve the abdominal wall and extensive debridement is required

Empiric Antibiotic Therapy

- Strategies have been promulgated to optimize antibiotic administration, including:
  - Reliance upon physician prescribing patterns
  - Computerized decision support
  - Administration by protocol
  - Formulary restriction programs
- Crucial for initial empiric antibiotic therapy to be targeted appropriately, administered in sufficient dosage to ensure bacterial killing, narrowed in spectrum (*deescalation*) as soon as possible based on microbiology data and clinical response, and continued only as long as necessary

Choice of Antibiotic

- Antibiotic choice is based on several interrelated factors (Table 71.10).
- Paramount is activity against identified or likely (for empiric therapy) pathogens, presuming infecting and colonizing organisms can be distinguished, and that narrow-spectrum coverage is always desired
- Local knowledge of antimicrobial resistance patterns is essential, even at the unit-specific level
- Patient-specific factors of importance include:
  - Age
  - Debility
  - Immunosuppression
  - Intrinsic organ function
  - Prior allergy or other adverse reaction
  - Recent antibiotic therapy
- Institutional factors of importance include:
  - Guidelines that may specify a particular therapy
  - Formulary availability of specific agents
  - Outbreaks of infections caused by MDR pathogens
  - Antibiotic control programs

TABLE 71.10

FACTORS INFLUENCING ANTIBIOTIC CHOICE

Activity against known or suspected pathogens
Disease believed responsible
Distinguish infection from colonization
Narrow-spectrum coverage most desirable
Antimicrobial resistance patterns
Patient-specific factors
Severity of illness
Age
Immunosuppression
Organ dysfunction
Allergy
Institutional guidelines or restrictions

TABLE 71.11

ANTIBACTERIAL AGENTS FOR EMPIRIC USE

ANTIPSEUDOMONAL
Piperacillin-tazobactam
Cefepime, ceftazidime
Imipenem, meropenem
Ciprofloxacin, levofloxacin (depending on local susceptibility patterns)
Aminoglycoside

TARGETED SPECTRUM
Gram positive
Glycopeptide
Lipopeptide (not for known/suspected pneumonia)
Oxazolidinone
Gram negative
Third-generation cephalosporin (not ceftriaxone)
Monobactam
Antianaerobic
Metronidazole

BROAD SPECTRUM
Piperacillin-tazobactam
Carbapenems
Fluoroquinolones
Tigecycline (plus an antipseudomonal agent)

ANTIANAEROBIC
Metronidazole
Carbapenems
β-Lactam/β-lactamase combination agents
Tigecycline

- Numerous agents are available for therapy (Table 71.11).
  - Agents may be chosen based on spectrum, whether broad or targeted (e.g., antipseudomonal, antianaerobic), in addition to the above factors.
  - Nosocomial Gram-positive pathogen is suspected (e.g., wound or surgical site infection, CR-BSI, pneumonia) or MRSA is endemic, empiric vancomycin (or linezolid) is appropriate
  - Some authorities recommend dual-agent therapy for serious *Pseudomonas* infections (i.e., an antipseudomonal β-lactam drug plus an aminoglycoside), but evidence of efficacy is lacking.
  - It is important to use at least two antibiotics for empiric therapy of any infection that may be caused by either a Gram-positive or Gram-negative infection (e.g., nosocomial pneumonia).

Antifungal Prophylaxis and Therapy

- Incidence of invasive fungal infections is increasing among critically ill surgical patients
- Several conditions are predictors for invasive fungal infection complicating critical illness, including:
  - Intensive care unit length of stay
  - Altered immune responsiveness
  - Number of medical devices placed
  - Neutropenia, diabetes mellitus, new-onset hemodialysis, total parenteral nutrition, broad-spectrum antibiotic administration, bladder catheterization, azotemia, diarrhea, and corticosteroid therapy are also associated with invasive fungal infection.

Duration of Therapy

- End point of therapy is largely undefined, in part because quality data are few
  - If cultures are negative, empiric antibiotic therapy should be stopped in most cases.
    - Unnecessary antibiotic therapy in the absence of infection clearly increases the risk of MDR infection.
    - Therapy beyond 48 to 72 hours with negative cultures usually is unjustifiable.
    - Morbidity of antibiotic therapy includes allergic reactions, development of nosocomial superinfections (e.g., fungal, enterococcal, and *C. difficile*–related infections), organ toxicity, promotion of antibiotic resistance, reduced yield from subsequent cultures, and induced vitamin K deficiency with coagulopathy or accentuation of warfarin effect.
  - If *bona fide* evidence of infection is evident, then treatment is continued as indicated clinically.
    - Some infections can be treated with therapy lasting 5 days or less.
    - Every decision to start antibiotics must be accompanied by a decision regarding the duration of therapy.
    - A reason to continue therapy beyond the predetermined end point must be compelling. Bacterial killing is rapid in response to effective agents, but the host response may not subside immediately.
    - Seldom should antibacterial therapy continue for more than 7 to 10 days.
    - Examples of bacterial infections that require more than 14 days of therapy include:
      - Tuberculosis of any site
      - Endocarditis
      - Osteomyelitis
      - Selected cases of brain abscess, liver abscess, lung abscess, postoperative meningitis, and endophthalmitis

ABBREVIATIONS

ARDS	Acute respiratory distress syndrome
CASS	Continuous aspiration of subglottic secretions
CDAD	*Clostridium difficile*–associated disease
CI	Confidence interval
CNS	Central nervous system
CPAP	Continuous positive airway pressure
CR-BSI	Catheter-related bloodstream infection
CSF	Cerebrospinal fluid
CT	Computerized tomography
ERCP	Endoscopic retrograde cholangiopancreatography
EVD	Extraventricular drain
ICU	Intensive care unit
MDR	Multidrug resistant
MRCP	Magnetic resonance cholangiopancreatography
MRI	Magnetic resonance imaging
MRSA	Methicillin-resistant *Staphylococcus aureus*
MRSE	Methicillin-related *S. epidermis*
NIPPV	Noninvasive positive pressure ventilation
NNIS	National Nosocomial Infections Surveillance System
NSTI	Necrotizing soft tissue infection
OR	Odds ratio
PICC	Peripherally inserted central catheters
PTC	Percutaneous transhepatic cholangiopancreatography
RR	Relative risk
SCIP	Surgical Care Improvement Project
SIRS	Systemic inflammatory response syndrome
SSI	Surgical site infections
VAC	Vacuum-assisted closure
VAP	Ventilator-associated pneumonia
VRE	Vancomycin-resistant enterococci

CHAPTER 72 ■ SKIN WOUNDS AND MUSCULOSKELETAL INFECTION

WOUND CLASSIFICATION

Surgical Site Infections

- In the United States an estimated 27 million surgical procedures are performed annually.
  - Surgical site infections (SSIs) are third most common nosocomial infection in most hospitalized patients, accounting for 14% to 16%

- Among surgical patients, SSIs were most common nosocomial infection
  - Accounting for 38% of infections
  - 66% of SSIs remained confined to the incision site
    - Remainder involved organs or spaces accessed during the surgical procedure
  - 1980 estimated that SSI increased hospital stay by 10 days and cost an additional $2,000 per patient
  - 1992 that number had decreased to 7.5 days' increased stay; however, the cost had increased to $3,152 per patient

- SSI contribution to the cost of health care in United States is calculated at $130 to $180 million per year
- Effects of SSIs are not only felt locally, such as tissue destruction, pain, scar formation, septic thrombophlebitis
  ○ Extend systemically to septicemia, shock, organ dysfunction, and death

Center for Disease Control (CDC) Classification of Surgical Site Infections

- **Superficial Incisional SSIs:** Infection occurs within 30 days of surgery and involves only skin or subcutaneous tissue with the following:
  - Purulent drainage
  - Presence of organisms in drainage
  - Pain or tenderness, swelling, redness
- **Deep Incisional SSIs:** Infection within 30 days of surgery, or within 1 year if implant is present. Infection involves deep soft tissues with the following:
  - Purulence from deep incision, not the organ space of operation
  - Dehiscence of deep incision or opened wound by surgeon due to symptoms of fever, pain, tenderness
  - Abscess found on direct examination or reoperation
- **Organ/Space SSIs:** Infection within 30 days of surgery, or within 1 year if implant is present. Infection involves any part of the anatomy other than the incision opened during operation with the following:
  - Purulence from a surgically placed drain in the organ space
  - Positive cultures from that organ space
  - Abscess found on direct examination or reoperation
  - Purulence alone not hallmark of infected wound
    - If present, however, a wound can be considered infected, even if confirmatory cultures are negative.
    - Absence of confirmatory pathogens can be a result of inadequate techniques of culture, the patient's current antimicrobial therapy, or a particularly fastidious organism.
    - Patients with immunologic dysfunction or those who are granulocytopenic may not always produce purulent material.
- Surgical wounds are grouped into four classes, each with its infection risk (Table 72.1):
  - Class I (clean): Uninfected operative wound in which no inflammation is encountered and the respiratory, alimentary, genital, or uninfected urinary tract is not entered.
    - Clean wounds are primarily closed and, if necessary, drained with closed drainage.
    - Operative incisional wounds that follow nonpenetrating (blunt) trauma should be included in this category if they meet the criteria.

- Class II (clean to contaminated): Operative wound in which respiratory, alimentary, genital, or urinary tracts are entered under controlled conditions and without unusual contamination.
  - Operations involving the biliary tract, appendix, vagina, and oropharynx are included in this category, provided no evidence of infection or major break in technique is encountered.
- Class III (contaminated): Include open, fresh, accidental wounds
  - Operations with major breaks in sterile techniques (e.g., open cardiac massage) or gross spillage from the gastrointestinal tract, and incisions in which acute nonpurulent inflammation is encountered
- Class IV (dirty to infected): Old traumatic wounds with retained devitalized tissue and those that involve existing clinical infection or perforated viscera
  - Organisms causing postoperative infection were present in the operative field before the operation

Risk Factors

- All surgical wounds are at risk for infection.
- National Nosocomial Infection Surveillance (NNIS) system was developed in the early 1970s to monitor the incidence of health care-associated infections (HAIs) and their associated risk factors and pathogens. NNIS has identified wound infection risk factors as the following:
  - Wound classified as contaminated or dirty
  - A patient with an ASA (American Society of Anesthesiologists) score of 3, 4, or 5 prior to operation
  - A procedure lasting longer than T hours, where T represents the 75th percentile of duration of time expected for that surgery
- To identify a patient's risk index category (RIC), each factor, if present, receives a score of 1, with a range between 0 and 3
- NNIS also publishes recommendations for reducing the risk of SSIs. The weight of these recommendations is based on the scientific evidence used to support the conclusions:
  - Category IA recommendations for SSI prevention:
    ○ Treat remote infection before performing an elective operation
    ○ Do not remove hair from operative sites unless it interferes with surgery and then only use electric clippers just prior to surgery
    ○ Select an agent with efficacy against the suspected organism, making sure the therapeutic serum levels exist from the beginning of the operation
    ○ Mechanical preparation of the colon with enemas and cathartics before elective colorectal operations and the use of nonabsorbable oral antimicrobials the day before operation have been beneficial
  - Category IB recommendations for SSI prevention:
    ○ Control serum glucose prior to operation
    ○ Cease tobacco use 30 days prior to operation
    ○ Shower night before surgery
    ○ Prepare operative site with an antiseptic skin agent
    ○ Do not routinely use vancomycin for antimicrobial prophylaxis

TABLE 72.1

SURGICAL WOUND CLASSIFICATION AND RISK OF INFECTION (IF NO ANTIBIOTICS USED)

Classification	Description	Infection risk (%)
Class I	Clean	<2
Class II	Clean to contaminated	<10
Class III	Contaminated	20
Class IV	Dirty	40

○ The operative team should keep nails short and not wear artificial nails

○ A 2- to 5-minute preoperative surgical scrub for the surgical team should occur

• Category II recommendations for SSI prevention:

○ Prepare skin in concentric circles from the incision site outward

○ Keep preoperative stay in the hospital as short as possible

○ Clean underneath each fingernail prior to performing first scrub of the day

○ Do not wear hand or arm jewelry

○ Limit the number of personnel entering the operating room

• No recommendation or unresolved issue:

○ Restriction of scrub suits to the operating suite, or coverage of scrub suits outside of theater

Pressure/Decubitus Ulcers

• Term *decubitus* has been applied to any area that develops an ulcer secondary to prolonged pressure between a bony prominence and an unyielding surface.

• Term *pressure ulcer* is a more accurate description.

• To overcome arterial and capillary hydrostatic pressure and develop subsequent tissue necrosis with ulceration, an individual must be subjected to 32 mm Hg pressure at the level of the ischium, sacrum, or heels for a prolonged period of time, usually exceeding 2 hours.

• Points of greatest pressure with a supine patient are seen over the sacrum, heel, and occiput at 40 to 60 mm Hg.

• In a prone position, the chest and knees absorb the greatest pressure, which may be 50 mm Hg.

• When the patient is sitting, the ischial tuberosities are under the most pressure, measured at near 100 mm Hg.

• If sensation is intact, ulceration usually will not occur as the incipient pain would lead to a change in position.

○ This occurs during the sleep cycle

• Risk factors associated with pressure ulcer development can be divided into external and internal causes.

• Externally, the patient might be subjected to a constant pressure for a period of time, or friction exists between exposed skin and a surface that remains static, or a region remains moist and may have desquamation, leading to a loss of the epithelial protective mechanism.

○ Placement of splints can also alter a patient's ability to change position.

○ Administration of sedatives or paralytics can also remove the normal feedback pathways that exist to prevent pressure ulcer formation.

• Internally, factors responsible for pressure ulceration include:

• Malnutrition (serum albumin levels <3.0 g/dL preoperatively)

• Anemia

• Endothelial dysfunction

• Diabetes, peripheral vascular disease, and episodes of hypotension also increase the risk as do sensory deficits in patients with plegia or paresis

• Patients with dementia may also not be sensitive to the importance of changing position frequently and may also be more prone to pressure ulceration.

• Most patients with pressure ulcers (66%) are older than 70 years old, with a prevalence rate in nursing homes of 17% to 28%.

• In contrast, patients admitted with an acute illness have an incidence rate of 3% to 11%.

• In both subsets of patients, recurrence rates as high as 90% may be seen.

• In the operating room, where patients are immobile, there is a report that up to 25% of all pressure ulcers are instigated there.

• Anatomic sites affected are:

• Hip and buttocks (67% of the cases involve ischial, trochanteric, and sacral tuberosity)

• 25% in malleolar, heel, patellar, or pretibial area

• Remainder occurring on the nose, chin, occiput, chest, back, or elbow

• In paraplegic patients, pressure ulcers are a leading cause of death, responsible for an 8% mortality rate.

• Overall an estimated 60,000 people die each year from a pressure ulcer complication.

• The health care cost in the United States alone per year is in excess of $1 billion.

• Several scoring systems are used to grade the risk for ulceration:

• Braden scale is a summation rating scale made up of six subscores consisting of sensory perception, moisture, activity, mobility, nutrition, and friction/shear, each ranging from 1 to 3 or 4 points, with total scores ranging from 6 to 23.

○ Subscores measure functional capabilities of patient that contribute to either higher intensity and duration of pressure or lower tissue tolerance for pressure.

○ Lower Braden score indicates lower levels of functioning with a higher risk for pressure ulcer development.

• Daniels classification looks at muscle and subcutaneous tissue breakdown, which occurs before dermal and epidermal changes are observed.

○ Epidermal necrosis occurs later because epidermal cells are able to better withstand prolonged absence of oxygen than cells in the deeper tissues both *in vivo* and *in vitro*.

○ Once skin damage is visible, irreversible internal damage may have already occurred.

• Shea staging describes ulcers that start superficially and progress to deeper structures:

○ Grade I: Limited to superficial epidermis and dermis

○ Grade II: Involving the epidermis and dermis and extending to the adipose tissue

○ Grade III: Extending through the superficial structures and adipose tissue down to muscle

○ Grade IV: Complete soft tissue destruction down to bone

• Currently the most widely accepted classification system for pressure ulcers is that produced by the National Pressure Ulcer Advisory Panel (NPUAP).

○ Considered to be a modification of the Shea system, it is used only to determine initial depth and is not a system to follow the natural history of the ulcer.

○ Limited by the presence of eschar, which will mask the underlying damage

○ Stage I represents intact skin with signs of impending ulceration

– Clinically, this may consist of blanchable erythema from reactive hyperemia that should resolve within 24 hours of relief of pressure
– Warmth and induration may also be present
– Continued pressure creates erythema that does not blanch
– Skin may appear white from ischemia. With proper treatment, resolution should be expected in 5 to 10 days.
○ Stage II represents a partial-thickness loss of skin involving epidermis and possibly dermis. This lesion may present as an abrasion, blister, or superficial ulceration, with pigmentation changes. These too represent a reversible condition.
○ Stage III represents a full-thickness loss of skin with extension into subcutaneous tissue but not through the underlying fascia.
– Lesion presents as a crater with or without undermining of adjacent tissue.
– On examination this will appear as a necrotic, foul-smelling crater with altered light and dark pigmentation.
○ Stage IV represents full-thickness loss of skin and subcutaneous tissue and extension into muscle, bone, tendon, or joint capsule.
– Osteomyelitis with bone destruction, dislocations, or pathologic fractures may be present.
– Sinus tracts and severe undermining commonly are present.

Treatment

• All modalities of care for pressure ulcers fall along four paths:
• Pressure reduction:
  • Frequent turning and repositioning the patient at least every 2 hours
  • Adopted because of nursing issues (it took 2 hours for the nurse to rotate all ward patients)
  • Debate in the literature as to this being an adequate amount of time
  • Mattresses that reduce pressure, such as low-air-loss and air-fluidized beds should be used for patients with stage III and IV ulcers.
  • For stage I and II ulcers, the use of static mattresses such as air, foam, or water overlays are the most beneficial.
• Wound management:
  • Removal of dead tissue and debris, drainage, and protecting the surrounding healthy tissue are the goals.
  • Pressure needed to clean wounds with no necrotic material is 2 to 5 psi
  • If necrotic debris is present, the pressure required increases by a factor of 2 to 3
  • The old wound dictum—if it is dry, wet it; if it is wet, dry it—has some validity.
    ○ A draining wound needs either a hydrocolloid or alginate
    ○ A wound without drainage will respond to simple moist gauze; the surrounding skin of both need to be kept lubricated, but not wet, to reduce friction.
  • Negative pressure therapy enhances wound healing by reducing edema, increasing the rate of granulation tissue formation, and stimulating circulation.

TABLE 72.2

DRESSING CATEGORIES

Category	Properties/Uses
Alginates	Absorption of drainage, dead space obliteration, autolysis of necrotic material
Foams	Absorption of drainage, dead space obliteration, mechanical debridement, moisture retention
Gauzes	Absorption of drainage, dead space obliteration, mechanical debridement, moisture retention
Hydrocolloids	Dead space obliteration, autolysis of necrotic material, moisture retention
Vacuum-assisted closure	Dead space obliteration, induction of granulation
Ostomy appliances	Drainage diversion

• Increased blood flow translates into a reduction in the bacterial load and delivery of infection-fighting leukocytes.
• Significant contraindications for the use of vacuum-assisted or negative pressure therapy include:
  ○ Malignancy of the wound
  ○ Untreated osteomyelitis
  ○ Nonenteric fistulas
  ○ Exposed vessels, organs, or nerves
• Various dressing categories are presented in Table 72.2.
• Surgical intervention:
  • Debridement is the process of removing devitalized tissue.
  • Stages III and IV ulcers will require some form of debridement, whether it is from surgical, autolytic, mechanical, or via enzymatic means
  • The patient's wound and overall status will dictate the means of debridement, a more stable patient receiving a more aggressive means of removing the necrotic material.
  • Larger wounds may respond only to the placement of flaps, either fasciocutaneous or musculocutaneous.
    ○ Flap failure can be seen after insufficient excision of soft tissue and bone and if systemic factors such as nutritional status are suboptimal.
• Nutritional support:
  • Malnourished patients have a higher susceptibility for ulcer formation
  • Once formed these patients also have a diminished ability to heal or to prevent further ulcer formation in other sites.
  • Serum albumin levels <3 mg/dL may be candidates for supplemental feedings via enteral or parenteral routes.

PRIMARY BACTERIOLOGIC INFECTIONS

• Skin and soft tissue infections are usually easily treated but have the potential of being lethal.
• Tender, firm, painful, and rapidly expanding area of redness on the skin surrounding violation of the skin barrier should be a cause for concern.
• Red streaks between lymph node–bearing areas may be visible, and this is indicative of a potentially spreading infection.

- Certain areas are more prone in becoming infected depending on age group:
  - Facial cellulitis occurring more commonly in adults older than 50 years and in children 6 months to 3 years of age
- Most common causative organisms in skin infections are:
  - Group A β-hemolytic streptococci
  - *Staphylococcus aureus*
  - Depending on the source of contamination and whether the patient is immunocompromised, Gram-negative rods and fungus can be seen.
  - If the insult occurs during exposure to fresh water, the causative organism may be *Aeromonas*, a Gram-negative rod.
- Predisposing states where minor break in the skin barrier leads to significant infection include:
  - Diabetes
  - Immunodeficiency
  - Varicella
  - Venous, arterial, or lymphatic insufficiency, such as that seen after lymphatic removal during mastectomy
  - Vein stripping for varicosities
- Treatment of uncomplicated cellulitis:
  - Begins with removing the nidus of infection
  - Cleansing the wound with an antiseptic agent
  - Dressing wound with an antiseptic ointment if indicated
  - Considering a course of oral antibiotics
  - Dicloxacillin, 500 mg orally four times a day for 7 days
  - Cephalexin, 500 mg orally four times a day for 7 days
  - With a suspected or known penicillin allergy, clindamycin, 400 mg, is given orally four times a day

Erysipelas

- A form of cellulitis that affects the epidermis primarily extending into cutaneous lymphatics
  - During Middle Ages referred to as St. Anthony's fire after Egyptian healer who was successful in treating condition
  - Shares the same underlying cause as cellulitis with bacterial inoculation into an area of skin violation
  - More commonly seen in children and elderly
  - Differs from cellulitis in that inflamed area is distinct from surrounding skin, being raised and demarcated
  - Often found on face; however, it can also develop on the arms and legs
    - Sometimes skin will have what is called a *peau d'orange*, or orange peel, look to it
  - As with cellulitis, streptococcus is the primary organism identified with its toxin responsible for the brisk inflammation associated with this condition.
  - Treatment:
    - Elevation of affected extremity
    - Penicillin, 250 to 500 mg orally or 0.6 to 1.2 million units intramuscularly, given every 4 to 6 hours for a 10- to 20-day course
    - In penicillin allergy, a macrolide or cephalosporin usually suffices
    - If the area affected becomes ulcerated, saline dressings changed every 12 hours will assist with wound closure

Impetigo

- Also known as pyoderma, it is the most common bacterial infection of the skin seen.
- Contagious and occurs at any age, but is more common in young children
- Patients report skin lesions, often with associated adenopathy, with minimal systemic signs and symptoms
- Presents in two forms:
  - Small vesicles with a honey-colored crust known as *impetigo contagiosa*
  - Purulent-appearing bullae, known as *bullous impetigo*
- Most commonly caused by *S. aureus*
- Group A beta-hemolytic strep is also commonly seen in the over-2-year-old population.
- Warm temperatures, humidity, poor hygiene, and crowded living conditions exacerbate spread.
- When associated with lymphadenitis in deeper infections, the term *ecthyma* is given
- Topical mupirocin (Bactroban) applied three times a day for 5 days is successful in treating >90% of cases
  - More effective than oral erythromycin
  - Lesions usually resolve completely within 7 to 10 days

CUTANEOUS FUNGAL INFECTIONS

- The most common important fungal infections that occur in the intensive care unit (ICU) setting are for the most part due to *Candida*, especially *albicans, glabrata,* and *tropicalis*.
- In immunocompromised or morbidly obese patients
  - Usually manifests itself as cutaneous moniliasis
  - Can be treated with topical powders or ointments
  - Vaginitis treated with suppositories
  - Funguria is addressed by removing or replacing the urinary catheter, which will be successful in about one-third of patients.

MUSCULOSKELETAL INFECTIONS

- First described in 1848
- Deep soft tissue infection a disease of unknown cause until 1920 when Meleney identified 20 patients in China in whom a hemolytic streptococcus was identified in the wounds
- In Meleney gangrene, there is extensive necrosis of the skin and subcutaneous tissue caused by synergistic infection between microaerobic staphylococcal and hemolytic streptococcal infection.
- Term *necrotizing fasciitis* (NF) first coined in 1952 and involves the underlying fascia and subcutaneous tissue and spares muscle
- Myositis results in muscle involvement, which becomes exquisitely tender and indurated
  - Muscle involvement leads to elevation of the creatine phosphokinase and can spread over several hours to contiguous muscle groups, thus heightening the need for early diagnosis and treatment.
- Fournier's gangrene listed as a separate entity due to its predilection for the perineum

The main provisions in the Bill provide for :

- the recognition of schools for the purposes of funding by public funds
- the establishment of the schools Inspectorate on a statutory basis
- the establishment of boards of management of schools on a statutory basis
- the establishment and role of parents' associations
- the functions of Principals and teachers
- appeals by students or their parents
- the making of regulations by the Minister
- the establishment of the National Council for Curriculum and Assessment
- regulation of the State examination system.

13.12   Funding

In 1996, the cost of the education system was £2.2 billion.[8]

The table below is based on research carried out by the Organisation for Economic Co-operation and Development in 1995 and shows that, while investment in Ireland in third-level education is on a par with that in other countries, spending per pupil in first and second-level schools is considerably less in Ireland than the European Union or OECD averages. The table shows a disparity between spending at different levels of the education system, a disparity which is likely to be wider at present following the abolition of fees for third-level education (which effectively means that the State pays all undergraduate fees) from 1996.

Table No. 1

Education spending per pupil in US dollars 1992[9]

	Primary	Second level	Third level
Ireland[10]	1,770	2,770	7,270
EU average	3,413	4,773	8,096
OECD average	2,902	4,193	6,872

Source : OECD (1995) Education at a glance (OECD indicators)

13.13   Changes in demographic structures

Changes are taking place in Ireland's demographic structures which have important implications for education provision.

The number of pupils at primary level is projected to fall by some 31,000 by the year 2001, while at second level the number will fall by some 14,000.

---

8   Revised Estimates for Public Services, 1996.

9   Reproduced from submission of the Combat Poverty Agency to the Review Committee on Third Level Education.

10   For 1994, figures for Ireland are: 2,090, 3,400 and 7,600 respectively.

Table No. 2

Changes in the school population over the coming years

Primary School year	Total No. of pupils
1997/1998	458,000
1998/1999	446,000
1999/2000	435,000
2000/2001	427,000

Post Primary School year	Total No. of pupils
1997/1998	368,000
1998/1999	364,000
1999/2000	358,000
2000/2001	354,000

The projected fall in enrolments will have enormous implications for the future of Ireland's education system. The number of teachers required to maintain a set pupil-teacher ratio will steadily decline in proportion to the decline in enrolments. It has been suggested to the Commission that this development, together with the continued favourable forecasts for economic growth, presents opportunities to make progress, in particular in relation to redressing educational disadvantage :

- Resources can be targeted at specific problems within the education system; for example, providing for the additional needs of pupils with a disability and providing new responses for students whose needs are not being met by the system or who are leaving school early without qualifications.
- New lower targets can be set for the pupil-teacher ratio, allowing for smaller classes on a nation-wide basis, particularly at primary level.

13.14 Provision for pre-school children

As pointed out in Chapter 12 while compulsory school age is six years in Ireland, in practice most children start school on 1 September, following their fourth birthday and consequently half of all four-year-olds and almost all five-year-olds attend primary school, so in comparative terms, Ireland provides well for a significant number of four-year-olds and almost all five-year-olds within the formal education system.[11]

The Department of Education and Science has introduced a pilot pre-school programme, the Early Start programme, with a specific education focus, aimed particularly at children who,

11   The ESRI survey carried out on behalf of the Commission showed that 28,900 four-year-olds and 59,900 five-year-olds surveyed were at school.

Education has a central role to play in determining the life chances of young people today. Those who leave school without qualifications are more likely to face unemployment, with a consequent lack of financial independence and fewer choices in relation to their lives.[14] Thus, while the majority of young people (90 per cent), successfully make the transition to adulthood, independence and parenthood, and go on to raise their own families, there is a need for special interventions to address the needs of the 10 per cent of children who are at risk of losing out on educational attainment.

13.16 The priorities for the years ahead

The Commission is of the view that the economic progress which Ireland is now experiencing, together with the demographic picture presented by the falling school population, presents an unique opportunity for a major investment in children through the education system. Social commentators have called for a major investment in all aspects of our children's environment. The Commission concurs with this view and would like to single out priority matters within the education system.

The *first priority relates* to investment in children who are not yet at school. The Commission considers that there is a need for investment in children in these important years and in the development of services for young children of pre-school age.

The *second priority* relates to the need to balance investment in the different levels of education in favour of the early years at school and throughout primary level.

Investment at these levels should be seen as a primary preventive measure to give every child a positive start in formal schooling and to tackle educational disadvantage for the 10 per cent of children who face this risk.

These priorities must be matched by a targeted approach to prevent early school-leaving and to compensate those children whose needs are not being met by the system.

Provision for adults is also important by way of second-chance education and training opportunities for those who have left school early without qualifications.

The strategy to combat educational disadvantage while prioritising preventive measures provides for a continuum of interventions which begin at pre-school level and continues through to adulthood. This approach is essential to break the inter-generational cycle of disadvantage, and it must be accompanied by a national certification framework with alternative routes of progression to higher levels of training and education.

The importance of alternative routes to further education and training has been stressed to the Commission as a key factor in promoting equality of opportunity in education. This requires a flexibility on the part of educational institutions to recognise forms of learning other than the traditional Leaving Certificate. In this context, the Commission notes the negotiation by the National Council for Vocational Awards of a formal pathway to RTC/DIT courses for holders of NCVA Level 2 awards having completed post leaving certificate courses.

because of disadvantage, are most at risk of not succeeding in education. The programme is in place in 40 centres in Dublin, Cork, Limerick, Waterford, Wicklow, Galway, Drogheda and Dundalk. Enrolment in Early Start classes totalled 1,566 children in September 1996.

The pilot phase of the programme is currently being evaluated and the result of the evaluation will inform the future policy approach on early education. The Department of Education and Science also provides a number of pre-school classes for Traveller children and a specific pre-school programme in an inner city Dublin area (Rutland Street).

Outside Early Start and the specific programmes aimed at compensating for educational and social disadvantage, there is no State education provision for the general population of pre-school children who have not reached their fourth birthday and, therefore, are not eligible for primary school.

The Commission notes the recent convention of a National Forum on Early Education by the Minister for Education and Science and the proposals for a White Paper on early childhood education. [12]

13.15   The success arising from investment in education

Irish investment in education since the 1960s is the success story of Europe. Two out of three people who are now reaching retirement left school with only a primary certificate. Today, 81 per cent of school-leavers have a Leaving Certificate and nearly half go on to third-level education. The influence of improved education levels in the population has been cited as a significant factor in the emergence of the 'so-called Celtic Tiger' and our improved economic well being in recent years. The *ESRI Medium-Term Review 1997-2003* points to the accumulated investment in human capital as one of the main catalysts of the present progress. Thus the case for continued and increased investment in education, in terms of improved economic well-being alone, is most persuasive. Moreover, the long-term effects of rising educational levels are still in the making. The first beneficiaries of free secondary education are still only in their early forties and the products of the education boom of more recent years are still only in early adulthood.[13]

---

12   The National Forum on Early Childhood Education was convened by the Minister for Education and Science from 23 March 1998 to 27 March 1998. The National Forum was representative of all groups involved in providing early childhood education services throughout the country and brought together service providers and experts in the field for the purpose of advising on a strategy for the future development of early childhood education services. The objective of the Forum was to provide an opportunity for all interested groups to engage in a full exchange of views and for each group to put forward their own particular concerns and objectives, while at the same time, taking account of the objectives and concerns of the other partners in the process. An independent report of the Forum's proceedings and conclusions is now being prepared by the Secretariat and will be published under the authority of the Secretary General of the Forum. This report will be a key contribution to a White Paper on early childhood education to be published before the end of 1998.

13   Draws on *Welfare Implications of Demographic Trends*, Tony Fahey, John Fitz Gerald, Oaktree Press/ Combat Poverty Agency, Dublin, 1997.

- All subgroups have common pathogenicity with organisms spreading from subcutaneous tissues to both superficial and deep fascial planes
- Local effect is vascular occlusion, ischemia, and necrosis
- Systemic effect is sepsis, end organ dysfunction with mortality rate as high as 75% with Fournier's gangrene and up to 100% in patients with multiple organ failure
- Mortality rate varies with age and extent of involvement
  - Survivors younger
  - Male:female ratio of affliction ranges 2 to 3:1

Types of Necrotizing Fasciitis

- See Table 72.3 for types of necrotizing fasciitis.
- Type I (polymicrobial):
  - Usually seen after injury or surgery
  - Can be misdiagnosed as a simple cellulitis
  - As tissue necrosis and hypoxia continue, pain and systemic symptoms of fever, chills, and malaise increase as underlying tissue liquefies while overlying skin may show minimal changes
    - In the late stages, extension into the muscle itself occurs
- Over 2 to 3 days erythema increases, with occasional bullae formation
- Cultures may show combination of aerobic and anaerobic organisms
- Deep soft tissue infection of perineum termed *Fournier's gangrene*
  - Many of these patients have predisposing systemic issues:
    - Diabetes
    - Immunosuppressed states
    - Histologically, thrombosis of blood vessels and abundant bacteria with many polymorphonuclear cells are typically seen
- Type II (group A streptococcal):
  - Also known familiarly as *flesh-eating bacteria* or as Meleney's synergistic gangrene
  - Nearly normal appearing overlying skin may result in a delay in diagnosing underlying ongoing necrosis
  - A simple incision into the region affected can demonstrate drainage or even gas in advanced cases
  - Other predisposing factors include:
    - Varicella infection
    - Use of nonsteroidal anti-inflammatory drugs (NSAIDs)

    – NSAID use an immunomodulator, which may predispose to this condition
  - An association with streptococcal toxic shock syndrome, similar to its staphylococcal counterpart except for the presence of necrosis as precipitant event
- Type III (gas gangrene or clostridial myonecrosis):
  - Rapidly progressive infection coined *necrotizing fasciitis*
    - Most commonly caused by *Clostridium perfringens* and less frequently by *C. septicum*
    - Most cases arise in setting of recent surgery or trauma
    - Less commonly spontaneous as in types I and II
    - *C. perfringens* (formally *C. welchii*) an anaerobic Gram-positive spore-forming organism that produces at least 10 distinct exotoxins
      - Most important exotoxin leading to human pathogenesis is the α-toxin, which hemolyzes red blood cells, hydrolyzes cell membranes, and exerts a direct cardiodepressive effect
      - Within 12 to 24 hours, crepitation of soft tissues may be detected by palpation
    - Variant of type III, known as *anaerobic streptococcal myonecrosis*, has a slower progression and less gas production.
    - *Aeromonas hydrophilia*, a facultatively anaerobic, Gram-negative bacillus most commonly encountered in freshwater, can also yield a type III-like syndrome
- Fournier's gangrene (idiopathic gangrene of the penis and scrotum):
  - First described in 1764 by Baurienne, entity received its name from a French venereologist, Jean-Alfred Fournier
  - In 1883 he presented a case of gangrene of the perineum in an otherwise healthy young man.
  - 95% of cases, an identifiable cause can be found, with the disease process originating from the anorectum, the urogenital tract, or the skin of the genitalia
  - Anorectum causes include:
    - Malignancy
    - Diverticulitis
    - Appendicitis
  - Urethral injury, urethral stricture, urogenital manipulation, or infection can initiate Fournier's gangrene
  - Cutaneous conditions like hidradenitis suppurativa or trauma can be precursors
  - Systemic factors may predispose, such as:
    - Leukemia

TABLE 72.3

SUBTYPES OF NECROTIZING FASCIITIS (NF)

Subtype	Organisms present	Treatment	Mortality
Type I	Gram-negative, Gram-positive, aerobes and anaerobes	Antibiotics, penicillin, clindamycin, debridement	Without organ dysfunction, 25%; with organ dysfunction, 75%; dependent on age
Type II	Streptococcus	Antibiotic, cessation of non-steroidal anti-inflammatory drug use, debridement	Same as above
Type III	*Clostridium perfringens, Clostridium septicum*	Wide local debridement, hyperbaric oxygen, immunoglobulin, antibiotics	75%
Fournier's	Polymicrobial, same as type III	Wide local debridement, hyperbaric oxygen, antibiotics	75%

○ Systemic lupus erythematosus
○ Crohn disease
○ Human immunodeficiency virus (HIV) or other conditions of immunodeficiency
- Other predisposing comorbidities associated with Fournier's include:
  ○ Obesity
  ○ Cirrhosis
  ○ Vasculitides of the perineum
  ○ Steroid use
  ○ Diabetes
- On examination the typical Fournier's patient will be an elderly male in his sixth or seventh decade of life with one or more of the above comorbidities.
- Clinically, patient may have a history of fever and lethargy for approximately 1 week.
  ○ Pain, tenderness, and erythema of the genitalia and overlying skin will progress to a dusky appearance, ultimately with purulent-appearing drainage.
- No predictive tests as to when a superficial infection will develop into a deep infection nor is there a chemistry test for identifying a soft tissue infection
- Investigation has focused on polymerase chain reaction tests specific for streptococcal pyrogenic exotoxin (SPE) genes, variants A, B, and C along with streptococcal superantigens
  ○ Superantigens cause the release of cytokines through binding to a specific segment of the T-cell receptor, resulting in an overwhelming production of tumor necrosis factor-α (TNF-α), interleukin-1 (IL-1), and IL-6 with subsequent systemic effects of sepsis and septic shock.
  ○ Work has also centered on the filamentous M protein, which is anchored to the cell membrane and has antiphagocytic properties.

Imaging Studies for Necrotizing Fasciitis

- Summary of different imaging studies is presented in Table 72.4
- Computerized tomography shown with great sensitivity the presence and extent of gas or subcutaneous air
- Magnetic resonance imaging (MRI) T2-weighted images can show well-defined areas of high signal intensity significant for tissue necrosis, and absence of gadolinium contrast enhancement on T1 images reliably detects fascial necrosis in those who might require operative debridement.

- Ultrasound, although able to detect fluid or gas within soft tissues, requires the probe to be applied directly on the involved tissues.
- Patients with NF, especially those with Fournier's, may not tolerate this, plus there may be a limitation of the anatomic site, causing difficulty in visualizing deep tissues.
  ○ Ultrasound has a sensitivity of 88% and a specificity of 93% (positive predictive value of 83%)
  ○ Diagnostic criteria include diffuse thickening of the subcutaneous tissue accompanied by fluid accumulation more than 4 mm in depth along the fascial layer.
- Additionally diagnosis can be made with culture and biopsy of the affected tissue
  - Gram stain to identify single or multiple organisms would be helpful in distinguishing type I from type II NF.
  - Once diagnosis is made, either on physical examination or through other diagnostic means, including culture, biopsy, or excision, multimodality therapy should be used early due to the rapidity of progression.

Therapy

- Until the organism is identified, broad-spectrum antibiotics should be administered.
- For aerobic organisms, one regimen might be ampicillin, 8 to 14 g per day intravenous (IV) administered every 6 hours in divided dosages, and gentamicin, 3 mg/kg per day IV divided every 8 hours
- Penicillin G, 8 to 24 million units per day IV in divided dosages every 4 to 6 hours should be given for presumed necrotizing fasciitis
- If concern of anaerobic organisms clindamycin, 600 mg IV every 6 hours, or metronidazole, not to exceed 4 g per day, can be given
- In the presence of group A streptococcal infection, use of clindamycin may be advantageous as it is not affected by inoculum size or stage of growth.
  - Clindamycin suppresses toxin production, facilitates phagocytosis of streptococcus pyogenes by inhibiting M-protein synthesis, and suppresses production of regulatory elements controlling cell wall synthesis.
- Other nonsurgical modalities include hyperbaric oxygen (HBO).
- No prospective study exists to justify its value.
- HBO can increase the oxygen saturation in infected wounds by a thousandfold, is bacteriocidal, improves

---

TABLE 72.4

IMAGING STUDIES

Type	Role of study	Limitations	Advantages
Ultrasound	Detection of fluid and gas within soft tissues	Requires direct contact, painful	Fast, reproducible, portable to bedside
Magnetic resonance imaging	T2-weighted images. T1-weighted images	Unstable patients unable to tolerate time required for study	High sensitivity for extent of involvement
Plain radiographs	Identification of air in subcutaneous location	Seen in <50% of cases	Fast, reproducible
Computerized tomography	Detection of extent of fluid/gas in soft tissues	Requires transport, dye is nephrotoxic	High sensitivity for extent of involvement

TABLE 72.5

CLINICAL INDICATORS PROMPTING WIDE SURGICAL INTERVENTION IN NECROTIZING FASCIITIS

Indicator	Remarks
Failure of improvement	After hours of parenteral antibiotics for presumed cellulitis, no decrease in signs and symptoms is detected or if there is progression
Profound toxic effects occurring at the onset of infection	These include malaise, weakness, generalized aching, loss of appetite/concentration
Extensive necrosis	Necrosis or gas is noted in the wound or is evident on radiographs
Compartment syndrome suspected	Edema within muscle group resulting in ischemic injury

polymorphonuclear leukocytes (PMN) function, and enhances wound healing.

- There may be higher oxygenation and saturation in infected necrotic tissue secondary to HBO-induced vasodilation.
- HBO has been reported by some to improve patient survival by as much as 50% and decrease number of debridements required to achieve wound control, whereas others have failed to show any beneficial effect.
- Typical treatment protocol involves HBO given aggressively after first surgical debridement.
  - Three treatment sessions, in a multiplace chamber at 3 atmospheres absolute (ATA) at 100% oxygen for 90 minutes each, can be given in the first 24 hours; in a monoplace chamber, 2.5 to 2.8 ATA, 100% oxygen for 90 minutes per session can be given.
  - Beginning the second day, twice-daily treatments are given until granulation tissue is seen, usually requiring a total of 10 to 15 treatments.
  - Since clostridial myonecrosis is a monobacterial anaerobic infection, HBO therapy has a greater logistic role in inhibiting clostridial growth and alpha toxin production.
- IV immunoglobulin (IVIG) has also been used with necrotizing soft tissue infections, although there are no prospective randomized trials to support its use,
  - 21 consecutive patients with group A streptococcal toxic shock syndrome were administered IVIG and had a survival benefit rate of 33%
  - Several adverse side effects occurred in <5% of patients, which can mimic a worsening course of NF.
  - Adverse effects include pallor, flushing, fever, muscle aches, hypotension, anaphylaxis, erythema multiforme, and blood-borne pathogen transmission
- Wide local debridement is the classical therapy for cases of necrotizing soft tissue infections (Table 72.5).
  - Series of small incisions under local anesthesia can be performed to delineate the extent and presence of muscle or facial necrosis.

- Frozen sections of tissue specimens obtained can establish diagnosis
- Once diagnosis confirmed no role for conservative debridement or incision and drainage
  - Two most common pitfalls with a necrotizing soft tissue infection are diagnostic delay and inadequate debridement
  - Excision of nonviable areas should be early and aggressive
  - Repeat debridements performed until the local process has been controlled
  - Use of electrocautery will aid in reducing the considerable operative blood loss if area of involvement is extensive
  - With perineal involvement, fecal diversion via colostomy allows for less contamination of wound site
  - With urogenital involvement, continued use of a urethral catheter is safe
    - Occasionally suprapubic cystostomy necessary
    - In Fournier's gangrene testicles are usually spared
    - To prevent desiccation usually placed in surgically made subcutaneous pocket
      - If not viable, orchiectomy performed
      - In all cases of NF, vacuum-assisted closure devices have shown great promise in decreasing time to grafting and closure of the debrided area

Factors Associated with Poor Outcome

- Factors associated with poor outcome are:
- Older age
- Female gender
- Elevated creatinine and lactate
- Extent of tissue involved
- Inadequate debridement
- Truncal involvement
- Chest wall involvement
- Presence of diabetes when in conjunction with renal dysfunction or peripheral vascular disease

CHAPTER 73 ■ NEUROLOGIC INFECTIONS

- Central nervous system (CNS) infections often rapidly progressive and fatal if left undiagnosed and/or treatment delayed
  - Prompt diagnosis and treatment crucial to decreasing morbidity and mortality
- Patients with CNS infections commonly require intensive care unit (ICU) support, particularly for airway protection and mechanical ventilation in the presence of an altered mental status
  - Patients with undiagnosed CNS infections may be admitted to ICU, offering intensivists opportunity to make challenging diagnoses and alter patient outcomes with early and effective therapy
- Presence or absence of focal neurologic findings the most important distinction to be made in patients with suspected neurologic infections
  - Helps to focus differential diagnosis and identifies patients in whom lumbar puncture may be contraindicated—at least until neuroimaging is completed
  - Major neurologic infections encountered in critically ill include:
    - Acute bacterial meningitis
    - Encephalitis
    - Brain abscess
    - Subdural empyema
    - Epidural abscess
    - Suppurative intracranial thrombophlebitis
- CNS normally protected by various host defenses
  - Most important is blood–brain barrier
  - Once micro-organisms gain entry, they are able to proliferate rapidly due to low concentration of immunoglobulins and leukocytes in CNS.
  - CNS infections can be caused by:
    - Viral
    - Bacterial
    - Mycobacterial
    - Fungal
    - Parasitic agents
  - Important risk factors for acquiring specific types of infections or pathogens:
    - Patient age
    - Underlying host factors
    - Epidemiologic exposures including:
      - Travel
      - Animal or vector exposures
      - Contacts with infectious cases
  - Prompt physical examination to identify patients in need of urgent interventions—including endotracheal intubation—needed, followed by lumbar puncture and/or imaging

MENINGITIS

Key Points

- Untreated acute bacterial meningitis universally fatal
  - Early recognition, rapid diagnostic testing, and emergent administration of antimicrobials crucial
  - Classic triad of fever, nuchal rigidity, and change in mental status occurs in <66% of patients with bacterial meningitis
    - Absence of all three findings excludes diagnosis with 99% to 100% sensitivity
  - Lumbar puncture (LP) should be performed urgently in all patients with suspected meningitis.
  - Neuroimaging with computed tomography (CT) or magnetic resonance imaging (MRI) to rule out mass lesions should precede LP in those with:
    - Abnormal level of consciousness
    - Focal neurologic deficits
    - Papilledema
    - History of CNS disease
    - Immune compromise
    - Seizure within 1 week of presentation
- Empiric antimicrobial agents administered as soon as possible after blood cultures collected if neuroimaging to be performed prior to LP or immediately following CSF collection
  - Specific microbiology and choice of empiric therapy depend on:
    - Patient risk factors, especially age
    - Underlying host immune status
    - History of preceding infections or neurosurgical procedures
  - Dexamethasone shown to decrease mortality in adults with *Streptococcus pneumoniae* meningitis and children with *Haemophilus influenzae*
    - Should be administered before or concomitant with first dose of antimicrobial in all cases pending Gram stain and culture results
- Neurologic complications of bacterial meningitis include:
  - Seizure
  - Cerebral edema
  - Cerebral infarction
  - Cranial nerve involvement
  - Venous sinus thrombosis
  - Brain abscess
  - Subdural empyema
  - Coma
- Intracranial pressure monitoring and/or other surgical interventions may be required.

TABLE 73.1

CAUSES OF ACUTE MENINGITIS

	Common	Uncommon
Viruses	Enteroviruses nonpolio Human immunodeficiency virus (HIV) Arboviruses (including West Nile virus, St. Louis encephalitis virus) Herpes simplex virus types 1 and 2 (HSV-2)	Influenza Parainfluenza Lymphocytic choriomeningitis virus (LCM) Varicella-zoster virus (VZV) Polio Mumps Cytomegalovirus (CMV) Epstein-Barr virus (EBV) Adenovirus
Bacteria	*Streptococcus pneumoniae* *Neisseria meningitides* *Haemophilus influenzae* *Listeria monocytogenes* Enterobacteriaceae *Staphylococcus aureus* *Mycobacterium tuberculosis* *Borrelia burgdorferi* (Lyme disease) *Streptococcus agalactiae*	*Treponema pallidum* (syphilis) *Rickettsiae* *Mycoplasma* *Brucella* *Chlamydia* *Leptospira*
Fungi	*Cryptococcus neoformans* *Histoplasma capsulatum* *Coccidioides immitis*	*Candida* *Aspergillus* *Blastomyces dermatitidis* *Sporothrix schenckii*
Parasites		*Toxoplasma gondii* *Naegleria fowleri* (free-living amoeba) *Angiostrongylus cantonensis* (eosinophilic meningitis) *Strongyloides stercoralis* (hyperinfection syndrome)
Other infectious syndromes	Parameningeal focus (brain abscess, subdural empyema, epidural abscess) Infective endocarditis	
Noninfectious causes	Medications Intracranial tumor Stroke Lymphoma/leukemia Meningeal carcinomatosis Post procedure (neurosurgery) Seizure	Autoimmune diseases (SLE, sarcoid, Behçet) Migraine syndromes

SLE, systemic lupus erythematosus.

- Chemoprophylaxis and/or immunoprophylaxis are available for *Neisseria meningitidis, Haemophilus influenzae,* and infections in specific circumstances.
  - In suspected meningococcal or *Haemophilus influenzae* meningitis, droplet isolation should be strictly enforced **until 24 hours of effective antimicrobial therapy** has been completed or alternate diagnosis reached.
  - Isolation in other cases of meningitis, including pneumococcal meningitis, not required
- Aseptic meningitis refers to inflammation of meninges not attributed to bacterial infection.
  - Cerebrospinal fluid (CSF) analysis usually reveals:
    - Normal glucose
    - Elevated protein
    - Elevated white blood cell (WBC) count with lymphocytic predominance
  - Negative Gram stain and bacterial cultures
  - Differential diagnosis of aseptic meningitis includes:
    - Viral infection
    - Mycobacterial infection
    - Syphilitic infection
    - Fungal infection
    - Amoebic infection
    - Parameningeal infection
- Meningitis, or inflammation of the meninges, may be caused by a wide variety of micro-organisms (Table 73.1).
  - Infectious agents gain entry to CSF via hematogenous, transdural, or transparenchymal routes.
  - Important to consider noninfectious syndromes in the differential diagnosis of meningitis, including:
    - Meningeal carcinomatosis
    - Vasculitic syndromes

- Drug effect (e.g., nonsteroidal anti-inflammatories, anti-microbials, immunosuppressants, anticonvulsants)
  - Identification of such noninfectious conditions is essential, as therapies differ from those used in the treatment of infectious syndromes.
  - Specifically, high dose corticosteroid therapy may be indicated in some of these cases.
  - Aseptic meningitis, inflammation of meninges not attributed to bacterial infection
- Critically ill patients, however, present much more commonly with bacterial meningitis by virtue of the more rapid and fulminant presentation of bacterial as opposed to aseptic meningitis.

Bacterial Meningitis

- Acute bacterial meningitis (ABM) accounts for approximately 1.2 million cases annually worldwide.
  - Most common meningeal pathogens include *Streptococcus pneumoniae* and *Neisseria meningitides*
  - Specific etiologic agents and frequencies vary with underlying host factors such as age, immune status, and route of acquisition.
  - Case fatality rate for adults with ABM approximately 25%
    - Transient or permanent neurologic sequelae in 21% to 28% of survivors
- ABM develops as a result of several mechanisms:
  - Micro-organisms colonizing nasopharynx may invade local tissues and spread to bloodstream and CNS
  - Bacteremia and subsequent CNS invasion may also develop from localized sources such as pneumonia or urinary tract infection
  - Direct entry from contiguous infection (such as via the sinuses or mastoids), trauma, neurosurgery, or prosthetic devices such as CSF shunts or cochlear implants also occurs
- Host factors predispose to bacterial meningitis (Table 73.2)
  - Other risk factors for development of meningitis include:
    - Recent exposure to a patient with ABM
    - Recent travel to areas with endemic meningococcal disease
    - Injection drug use
    - Recent neurotrauma or CSF leak, and otorrhea

TABLE 73.2

PREDISPOSING HOST FACTORS TO SPECIFIC
ETIOLOGIC AGENTS OF MENINGITIS

Immunoglobulin deficiency	*S. pneumoniae*
Asplenia	*S. pneumoniae*
Complement deficiency	*N. meningitides*
Corticosteroid excess	*L. monocytogenes, Cryptococcus*
HIV infection	*Cryptococcus, L. monocytogenes, S. pneumoniae*
Bacteremia	*S. aureus,* Enterobacteriaceae
Fracture of cribriform plate	*S. pneumoniae*
Basal skull fracture	*S. pneumoniae, H. influenzae, S. pyogenes*
Neurotrauma, postneurosurgery	*S. aureus, S. epidermidis,* Gram-negative bacilli including *P. aeruginosa*

HIV, human immunodeficiency virus.

- Median duration of symptoms prior to admission in ABM averages approximately 24 hours
- Classic triad of fever, nuchal rigidity, and change in mental status occurs in <66% of cases
  - Almost all patients have at least one of these findings
  - Absence of these findings excludes diagnosis with 99% to 100% sensitivity
- Nuchal rigidity can be detected with passive or active flexion of the neck
  - Kernig and Brudzinski signs are well-described physical examination techniques but are neither sensitive nor specific
- In addition to severe headache, patients often note:
  - Photophobia
  - Seizures
- Focal neurologic deficits and papilledema may be seen on physical examination
- Some patients may not manifest classic signs and symptoms of ABM particularly:
  - Neonates
  - Those with underlying immunosuppressive conditions including:
    - Diabetes
    - Chronic organ failure
    - Neutropenia
    - Chronic corticosteroid use
    - Transplantation
    - Human immunodeficiency virus (HIV) infection
- Certain micro-organisms may present with specific physical findings:
  - Meningococcal meningitis may present with characteristic skin manifestations consisting of diffuse petechiae and purpura on distal extremities
    - Skin findings occur in approximately one-fourth of bacterial meningitis cases, over 90% of which are due to *Neisseria meningitidis* infection
  - Resultant to widespread use of conjugate vaccine for *H. influenzae* type b in infants, *Streptococcus pneumoniae* the most frequently observed cause of ABM
    - Accounts for 47% of total cases
    - *S. pneumoniae* serotypes causing bacteremic disease those commonly responsible for meningitis
    - Focal infection common with contiguous or distant sites, including sinusitis, mastoiditis, pneumonia, otitis media, and endocarditis
    - Major risk factors for pneumococcal meningitis include:
      - Asplenia
      - Hypogammaglobulinemia
      - Alcoholism
      - Chronic renal or hepatic disease
      - Malignancy
      - Diabetes mellitus
      - Basal skull fracture with CSF leak
      - Presence of a cochlear implant
    - Mortality rate range from 19% to 30%
  - *Neisseria meningitidis* commonly causes meningitis in children and young adults.
    - Serogroups B, C, and Y responsible for most endemic disease in North America, accounting for 32%, 35%, and 26% of cases, respectively.
    - Epidemic disease most commonly caused by serogroup C, with fewer outbreaks due to serogroup A.

TABLE 73.3

INCIDENCE BY CAUSE OF BACTERIAL MENINGITIS
IN THE UNITED STATES, 1995

Micro-organism	Rate per 100,000
Streptococcus pneumoniae	1.1
Neisseria meningitidis	0.6
Streptococcus agalactiae (group B streptococcus)	0.3
Listeria monocytogenes	0.2
Haemophilus influenzae type b	0.2

From Schuchat A, Robinson K, Wenger JD, et al. Bacterial meningitis
in the United States in 1995. Active Surveillance Team. *N Engl J Med.*
1997;337(14):970–976, with permission.

- Risk factors for invasive meningococcal disease include:
  - Nasopharyngeal carriage
  - Terminal complement deficiency
  - Properdin deficiency
- Characteristic rapidly evolving petechial or purpuric rash strongly suggests *N. meningitides*
  - Similar rash may be seen in splenectomized patients with overwhelming *S. pneumoniae* or *H. influenzae* type b infection
- *H. influenzae* previously accounted for a large proportion of cases of bacterial meningitis
  - Widespread vaccination against *H. influenzae* type b has markedly decreased incidence (Table 73.3)
  - Isolation of *H. influenzae* type b in adults suggests presence of an underlying condition such as:
    - Sinusitis
    - Otitis media
    - Pneumonia
    - Diabetes mellitus
    - Alcoholism
    - CSF leak
    - Asplenia
    - Immune deficiency
- *Listeria monocytogenes* meningitis:
  - Carries a mortality rate of 15% to 29%
  - Occurs in neonates, adults older than 50 years of age, and in those with risk factors including:
    - Alcoholism
    - Malignancy
    - Pregnancy
    - Immune suppression secondary to corticosteroid therapy or transplantation
  - Infection seen infrequently in HIV-infected patients for unknown reasons
  - Pregnant women may be asymptomatic carriers and transmit infection to infants
  - *L. monocytogenes* commonly makes up part of the fecal flora of farm animals and can be isolated from soil, water, or contaminated vegetables
    - Outbreaks associated with unpasteurized dairy products such as milk and cheeses, vegetables, and processed meats
- Aerobic Gram-negative bacilli can cause meningitis in specific groups of patients

- Predisposing risk factors include:
  - Neurosurgical procedures
  - Neonatal status
  - Advanced age
  - Immune suppression
  - Gram-negative bacteremia
  - Disseminated *Strongyloides stercoralis* infection with hyperinfection syndrome
- *Escherichia coli* a common cause of meningitis in neonates
- *Staphylococcus aureus* or *Staphylococcus epidermidis* can both cause meningitis
  - Less common than previously described micro-organisms
  - Both staphylococcal species exist as part of normal skin flora
  - Predominantly causing infections following neurosurgery or neurotrauma or when prosthetic material is present
    - Particularly external ventricular drains or ventriculoperitoneal shunts
    - Some patients with staphylococcal bacterial meningitis have underlying infective endocarditis, paraspinal or epidural infection, sinusitis, osteomyelitis, or pneumonia
- Other less common causes of bacterial meningitis include:
  - Enterococci
  - Viridans group streptococci
  - Beta-hemolytic streptococci
  - Diphtheroids
  - *Propionibacterium acne*
    - Generally only in the setting of prosthetic material
  - Anaerobic species

Viral Meningitis

- The most commonly isolated pathogens in aseptic meningitis
  - Nonpolio enteroviruses, especially Coxsackie viruses A and B, and echoviruses common
  - Account for 85% to 95% of cases with identified pathogen
  - Enteroviruses:
    - Occur worldwide
    - Transmitted by fecal–oral or respiratory droplet spread
    - Exhibit summer and fall seasonality in temperate climates
  - Infants, children, and young adults commonly affected
  - Clinical manifestations depend on host age and immune status but generally include:
    - Abrupt onset of severe headache, fever, nausea, vomiting, photophobia, nuchal rigidity, and malaise
    - Rash and upper respiratory symptoms common
    - Only rarely is illness severe enough to require critical care
- Arboviruses more commonly cause encephalitis but also isolated in cases of aseptic meningitis
  - Arboviruses endemic to North America include:
    - The flaviviruses
      - St. Louis encephalitis virus
      - Colorado tick fever
      - Japanese encephalitis virus
      - West Nile virus
    - California encephalitis viruses
  - Arboviruses occur predominantly in summer and early fall when vector exposure most likely
    - St. Louis encephalitis virus is mosquito borne and causes epidemic disease in the Mississippi River area

○ Japanese encephalitis virus less commonly causes meningitis, is endemic in Asia, and requires prolonged stays in rural settings for acquisition so is uncommon even in returned travelers

○ West Nile virus (WNV) came to widespread attention in 1999 when first North American cases identified
  – Virus has spread extensively across North America and should be considered in all patients with meningitis
  – Particularly in late summer or early fall
  – Infection asymptomatic in 80% of cases
  – Remaining patients present with:
    • West Nile nonneurologic syndrome (approximately 20%; formerly named West Nile fever)
    • West Nile neurologic syndrome (WNNS; <1%)
  – West Nile nonneurologic syndrome is a self-limited febrile illness characterized by:
    • Fever
    • Headache
    • Malaise
    • Myalgias
    • Often a rash (50%)
  – WNNS may present as encephalitis, meningitis, or flaccid paralysis
    • Meningitis the least common presentation of WNNS

• Lymphocytic choriomeningitis (LCM) virus:
  • A zoonotic disease
  • Transmitted by contact with infected rodents or their feces
    ○ House mice
    ○ Rats
    ○ Hamsters
  • Now rare, LCM virus was one of first viruses associated with aseptic meningitis
  • Infection more common in winter months
  • Presenting manifestations include an influenza-like syndrome and meningismus, with occasional rash, orchitis, arthritis, myopericarditis, and transient alopecia

• Six of the eight recognized human herpesviruses can cause meningitis
  • Herpes simplex viruses (HSV) most commonly associated with aseptic meningitis during primary genital infection
    ○ Affects 36% of women and 13% of men with primary genital herpes
    ○ HSV-2 infection responsible for most infections
    ○ HSV-1 genital infection and concomitant meningitis can also occur
    ○ Meningitis much less likely in setting of genital herpes recurrences
    ○ Presenting symptoms:
      – Headache
      – Photophobia
      – Meningismus
    ○ Genital lesions are present in 85% of patients with primary HSV-2 meningitis and generally precede meningeal symptoms by several days.
  • Herpes zoster aseptic meningitis, with or without typical skin lesions also reported
    ○ Particularly in older patients
  • Cytomegalovirus (CMV), Epstein-Barr virus (EBV), and human herpes virus 6 (HHV-6) all capable of causing aseptic meningitis
    ○ Occur very rarely, predominantly in immune-suppressed populations

• HIV-associated aseptic meningitis can occur with primary infection in approximately 5% to 10% of patients
  • Cranial neuropathies may be present along with headache, fever, and meningismus
  • Symptoms usually self-limited
• Mumps, now rare as a result of universal vaccination programs, once relatively common cause of aseptic meningitis
  • Clinical manifestations include fever, vomiting, headache, and parotitis in approximately 50% of patients
  • Meningismus, lethargy, and abdominal pain may also be present.

Other Less Common Infectious Causes

• Spirochetal meningitis may be caused by *Treponema pallidum* or *Borrelia burgdorferi*
  • *T. pallidum,* etiologic agent of syphilis, is acquired by:
    • Sexual contact
    • Placental transfer
    • Direct contact with active lesions
      ○ These include condyloma lata, mucous patches, or the rash of secondary syphilis
  • Syphilitic meningitis usually occurs during primary or secondary infection, complicating 0.3% to 2.4% of untreated infections during the first 2 years
  • *B. burgdorferi* is transmitted by the *Ixodes* tick and causes Lyme disease
    • The most common vector-borne disease in the United States
    • Meningitis can occur during the first stage of disease
      ○ Concurrently with erythema migrans at tick bite site
    • Dissemination of the micro-organism in second stage of disease, 2 to 10 weeks following exposure, may also result in aseptic meningitis
    • Late or chronic disease may include subacute encephalopathy but not meningitis

• *Mycobacterium tuberculosis* may cause a subacute or chronic form of meningitis.
  • Infection of meninges results from rupture of a tuberculous focus into subarachnoid space
  • In very young patients, concomitant disseminated systemic infection is common.
  • Epidemiologic risk factors include:
    • Known prior history of tuberculosis (TB) exposure
    • Residence in an endemic area
    • Contact with an active case
    • Incarceration
    • Homelessness
    • HIV infection
  • Tuberculin skin testing is negative in over half of patients with tuberculous meningitis
    • Negative skin test cannot be used to exclude tuberculous meningitis
    • Newer tests, such as the QuantiFERON-TB Gold test, may be available in some centers

• Fungal meningitis, although uncommon, should be considered, particularly given the high mortality associated with untreated infection.
  • *Cryptococcus neoformans* predominantly affects immunocompromised hosts but can also infect the immunocompetent.
    • Encapsulated yeast distributed worldwide
    • Prefers wet forested regions with decaying wood

- Found in particularly high concentrations in pigeon guano
- Risk factors for cryptococcal infection include:
  - HIV/acquired immunodeficiency syndrome (AIDS)
  - Prolonged corticosteroid therapy
  - Immunosuppression posttransplantation
  - Malignancy
  - Sarcoidosis
- Clinical presentation is typically indolent, occurring over 1 to 2 weeks
  - Characterized by fever, malaise, and headache
    - Meningismus, photophobia, and vomiting occur in <33% of patients.
- *Cryptococcus gattii*, a serotype usually restricted to tropical climates, emerged on Vancouver Island, British Columbia (BC), Canada in 1999.
  - Since been responsible for numerous cases of CNS infection in predominantly immunocompetent hosts in BC and the U.S. Pacific Northwest
- *Coccidioides immitis*, a dimorphic fungus, is found in soil in the dry desert regions of the southwest United States, Mexico, and Central and South America
- Infection results after inhalation of arthroconidia, usually following a dust storm or during building construction.
- Infection usually confined to respiratory system in those with competent immune systems.
  - Extrapulmonary dissemination to the meninges can occur in patients with immune compromise or during pregnancy.
  - Patients present with headache, vomiting, and altered level of consciousness.
- Risk factors for the development of disease include:
  - Travel to or residence in an endemic region
  - Immune deficiency
- Coccidioidal meningitis is universally fatal if untreated
- Less common fungal causes of meningitis include:
  - *Blastomyces dermatitidis*
  - *Histoplasma capsulatum*
  - *Sporothrix schenckii*
  - Rarely, *Candida* species
  - *B. dermatitis*, *H. capsulatum*, and *S. schenckii* are all dimorphic fungi with similar presentations to coccidioidal meningitis:
    - Primary infection occurs via inhalation
    - Disseminated infection occurs predominantly in immune compromised populations
    - *B. dermatitidis* and *H. capsulatum* endemic in Mississippi and Ohio River valleys
    - *S. schenckii* reported worldwide, with most cases in the tropical regions of the Americas
  - *Candida* exists only in yeast form:
    - Part of the normal flora of skin and gastrointestinal tract
    - CNS involvement most commonly due to candidemia with subsequent meningeal seeding
    - Predisposing risk factors for candidemia include:
      - Use of broad-spectrum antibiotics
      - Presence of indwelling devices such as vascular or urinary catheters
      - Parenteral nutrition
      - ICU admission
      - Prolonged hospital stay
      - Immune compromise

- Specific risk factors for *Candida* CNS infection include:
  - Ventricular shunts
  - Trauma
  - Neurosurgery
  - Lumbar puncture
  - *C. albicans* the most commonly isolated species
  - Non-*albicans* species becoming more prevalent, particularly in ICU populations
- Meningitis caused by protozoa or helminths is extremely rare.
  - Free-living amoebas *Acanthamoeba*, *Balamuthia*, and *Naegleria fowleri* are associated with fresh water exposure.
    - Usually acquired by individuals diving into contaminated lakes or swimming pools
    - CNS invasion occurs via penetration of nasal mucosa and cribriform plate
  - *N. fowleri* can cause a primary amoebic meningoencephalitis
  - *Acanthamoeba* and *Balamuthia* rarely cause meningitis; they commonly present as encephalitis.
  - *Angiostrongylus cantonensis*, the rat lungworm, is the classic infectious cause of eosinophilic meningitis (>10% eosinophils in the CSF) (Table 73.4).
    - Humans are incidental hosts and develop neurologic symptoms as a result of larval migration through the CNS.
    - Endemic in Southeast Asia and the Pacific Islands
    - Acquired by ingesting raw mollusks such as snails or slugs
  - *Gnathostoma spinigerum*, acquired by ingestion of raw and undercooked fish and poultry, is not primarily neurotropic.
    - May also cause eosinophilic meningitis as a result of migration of larvae up nerve tracts to CNS

TABLE 73.4

CEREBROSPINAL FLUID TESTS IN SUSPECTED CNS INFECTION

Routine tests	Further testing
Cell count and differential	Lactate
	Viral studies: Viral culture PCR for enteroviruses, HSV, WNV, VZV, influenza
Protein	AFB stain and mycobacterial culture
Glucose (preferably with simultaneous serum glucose)	Cryptococcal antigen test (can send serum as well, sensitivity comparable to CSF)
Gram stain	Fungal culture
Bacterial culture and sensitivity	VDRL, FTA-Abs, *T. pallidum* PCR[a]
	Cytology
	Cytospin and flow cytometry if available
	Wet mount if PAM suspected
	Lyme-specific Ab and PCR[a]

CNS, central nervous system; PCR, polymerase chain reaction; HSV, herpes simplex virus; WNV, West Nile virus; VZV, varicella-zoster virus; AFB, acid-fast bacillus; CSF, cerebrospinal fluid; VDRL, Venereal Diseases Research Laboratory; FTA-Abs, fluorescent treponemal antibody absorption; PAM, primary amoebic meningoencephalitis.
[a]Experimental, available only in research laboratories

- Gnathostomiasis is endemic in Asia, especially Thailand and Japan, and more recently in Mexico.
- *Baylisascaris procyonis,* a roundworm infection of raccoons
  - Rarely causes human eosinophilic meningoencephalitis following accidental ingestion of ova from raccoon feces in contaminated water, soil, or foods

Diagnosis

- LP should be performed emergently in all patients suspected of having bacterial meningitis unless contraindicated.
  - Commonly unnecessarily delayed while neuroimaging is performed to exclude mass lesions
  - Complications associated with LP uncommon
    - Incidence of life-threatening brain herniation has been reported to range from <1% to 6%
    - Clinical features at baseline associated with abnormal findings on CT scan, and thus, increased risk of brain herniation are:
      - Age ≥60 years
      - History of CNS disease such as a mass lesion, stroke, and focal infection
      - Immune compromise such as HIV or immunosuppressive therapy
      - History of seizure ≤1 week before presentation
      - Specific abnormal neurologic findings
    - Guidelines for which adult patients should undergo CT prior to LP have been recommended (Table 73.5).
- Nosocomial meningitis rare in nonneurosurgical patients
  - Nevertheless, LP often performed in hospitalized patients with unexplained fever and/or decreased level of consciousness
  - Yield of performing an LP in the nonneurosurgical population is extremely low and of questionable utility
- CSF analysis is extremely important in the diagnosis of meningitis.
  - Basic laboratory analyses, including cell count and differential, protein, glucose, Gram stain, and bacterial cultures, most useful in distinguishing between viral, bacterial, tuberculous, and fungal infection (see Table 73.4)

Bacterial Meningitis

- Usually presents with an elevated systemic WBC count and left shift (immature forms such as bands and myeloids)

TABLE 73.5

INDICATIONS FOR IMAGING PRIOR TO LP IN ADULTS WITH SUSPECTED BACTERIAL MENINGITIS

Immunocompromised state (HIV/AIDS, immunosuppressive therapy)
History of CNS disease (mass lesion, stroke, or focal infection)
New-onset seizure (≤1 week of presentation)
Papilledema
Abnormal level of consciousness
Focal neurologic deficit (dilated nonreactive pupil, abnormalities of ocular motility, abnormal visual fields, arm or leg drift)

LB, lumbar puncture; HIV, human immunodeficiency virus; AIDS, acquired immunodeficiency syndrome; CNS, central nervous system.

- Leukopenia may occasionally present in severe infection.
- Thrombocytopenia may be a result of sepsis, disseminated intravascular coagulation, or meningococcemia alone.
- Renal and hepatic dysfunction may occur as part of multi-organ failure in severe disease.
- Blood cultures are often positive and should always be drawn prior to administration of antimicrobials, particularly if LP cannot be performed immediately.
  - Approximately 66% of patients with bacterial meningitis have positive blood cultures.
- CSF analysis in bacterial meningitis classically shows:
  - Neutrophilic pleocytosis with hundreds to thousands of cells and >80% neutrophils
  - Low CSF WBC count is usually a marker of poor prognosis in this setting
- CSF glucose concentration is usually low and should be compared with a simultaneous serum glucose measurement.
  - Abnormal CSF-to–serum glucose ratio (<0.5) common in bacterial meningitis
    - Often much lower than 0.5
    - Acute illness in diabetics may increase serum glucose levels markedly, making the CSF-to–serum glucose ratio inaccurate
- In postoperative neurosurgical patient, CSF lactate concentrations ≥4.0 mmol/L shown to be superior to CSF-to-blood glucose ratios
- Initiation of empirical antimicrobial therapy in this setting should be considered pending the results of additional studies.
- CSF protein and opening pressure usually elevated in bacterial meningitis (Table 73.6)
- Gram staining permits rapid identification of bacterial species
  - Positive in approximately 50% to 60% of patients with bacterial meningitis
  - Presence of bacteria is virtually 100% specific, but sensitivity is variable
  - Gram stain more likely to be positive in patients with high bacterial loads
    - Gram-positive diplococci suggest *S. pneumoniae* infection
    - Gram-negative diplococci suggest *N. meningitidis* infection
    - Gram-positive rods suggest *L. monocytogenes* infection
    - Small pleomorphic coccobacilli suggest *H. influenzae* infection
- CSF bacterial cultures are positive in approximately 70% to 85% of cases
  - Yield decreases significantly in patients treated with antimicrobials prior to CSF collection
  - Antigen assays (latex agglutination tests) have been used in these cases, but due to their low sensitivity are no longer routinely offered by many laboratories
  - Broad-based polymerase chain reaction (PCR) may be useful for excluding the diagnosis of bacterial meningitis but is unavailable in many centers

Viral Meningitis

- In acute viral meningitis, CSF cell count is usually in the low hundreds with lymphocytic predominance.
  - Predominance of neutrophils may be seen in the first 24 hours of disease, occasionally confusing the diagnosis.

TABLE 73.6

TYPICAL CSF PARAMETERS IN PATIENTS WITH MENINGITIS

Etiology	WBC count (cells/mm³)	Predominant cell type	Protein (mg/dL)	Glucose (mg/dL)	Opening pressure (cm H₂O)
Normal	0–5	Lymphocyte	15–40	50–75	8–20
Viral	10–500	Lymphocyte[a]	Normal	Normal	9–20
Bacterial	100–5,000	Neutrophil	>100	<40	20–30
Tuberculous	50–300	Lymphocyte	>100	<40	18–30
Cryptococcal	20–500	Lymphocyte	50–200	<40	18–30

CSF, cerebrospinal fluid; WBC, white blood cell.
[a]Neutrophils may predominate in the first 24 hours.

- CSF glucose concentration is usually within normal range.
- CSF protein is usually mildly elevated.
- Opening pressure is usually normal.
- Viral cultures and nucleic acid amplification tests are most commonly used in the diagnosis of viral meningitis.
  - Enteroviruses may be cultured from CSF, throat, or rectal swabs.
    - Sensitivity of 65% to 70%
  - Or identified by nucleic acid amplification testing
    - PCR is both sensitive and specific
  - PCR for HSV is also widely available
    - In studies of HSV-1 encephalitis, HSV PCR demonstrated a specificity of approximately 100% and sensitivity of 75% to 98%
    - False negatives occur mostly within the first 72 hours of infection.
  - Diagnosis of WNV can be made by detection of serum immunoglobulin-M (IgM) or a fourfold rise in IgG between acute and convalescent titers
  - WNV PCR of serum and CSF are also available
    - Sensitivity higher in CSF specimens due to short-lived viremia in humans

Other Less Common Causes

- CSF analysis in syphilitic meningitis characterized by:
- Mild lymphocytic pleocytosis
- Decreased glucose
- Elevated protein
- *T. pallidum* cannot be cultured.
- Diagnosis made using alternate methods, predominantly serology.
- Direct visualization by darkfield microscopy or direct fluorescent antibody testing possible if primary chancre or skin lesion of secondary syphilis—condyloma latum or mucous patch—is present.
- Serologic testing should include:
  - Nontreponemal (RPR, rapid plasma reagin; VDRL, Venereal Diseases Research Laboratory)
  - And treponemal (TPPA, *Treponema pallidum* particle agglutination; FTA-Abs, fluorescent treponemal antibody absorption) tests for the diagnosis of active syphilis infection
  - *Treponema*-specific enzyme immunoassays (EIA) for IgM and IgG, replacing above traditional serologic tests as initial laboratory diagnostic test
  - CSF VDRL used in diagnosis of syphilitic meningitis
    - Specificity is high, but false positives occur in bloody specimens

  - Major limitation of CSF VDRL is low sensitivity (30% to 70%), so a negative result should not be used to rule out infection in setting of high clinical suspicion
  - CSF FTA-Abs more sensitive
    - False positives common due to serum antibody leak into the CSF
  - PCR recently used to detect *T. pallidum* DNA in CSF
- Lyme meningitis is characterized by:
  - Mild lymphocytic pleocytosis
  - Low glucose
  - Elevated protein
  - CSF concentration of *B. burgdorferi* antibody
    - Compared to serum levels, is a sensitive and specific diagnostic method
    - PCR is currently available only in research laboratories
    - CSF oligoclonal bands and *B. burgdorferi* culture also available
      - But neither is sensitive or specific
- CSF analysis in tuberculosis meningitis demonstrates:
  - Lymphocytic pleocytosis
  - Low glucose
  - Markedly elevated protein
  - Markedly elevated opening pressure
  - Elevation in protein particularly marked in setting of CSF block
  - Acid-fast bacillus (AFB) smears are very low yield
    - Only 10% to 22% of cases positive
    - Mycobacterial cultures, although slow growing—taking several weeks—become positive in up to 88% of cases
    - DNA probes and nucleic acid amplification techniques (mainly PCR) recently available with great improvements in sensitivity and specificity
  - Meningeal biopsy is rarely performed but may show caseating granulomata
  - Skin testing and QuantiFERON-TB Gold testing have been discussed in the previous section
  - Sputum and urine AFB and mycobacterial blood cultures are part of the TB workup in these patients.
- Cryptococcal meningitis characterized by:
  - Lymphocytic pleocytosis
  - Decreased glucose
  - Elevated protein
  - Opening pressures may be markedly elevated
  - Culture of *C. neoformans* or *C. gattii* from the CSF diagnostic
  - Detection of serum or CSF cryptococcal antigen (CrAg) >90% sensitive
    - India ink previously regarded as standard diagnostic test

- Due to low sensitivity (50%) largely replaced by antigen testing
- Fungal blood cultures may also be useful, as cryptococcal meningitis occasionally occurs in the setting of disseminated cryptococcal infection with cryptococcemia, especially in HIV-infected patients
- Other fungal meningitides similarly characterized by:
  - Lymphocytic pleocytosis
  - Low to normal glucose
  - Elevated protein
  - Coccidioidal meningitis may present with eosinophilic pleocytosis and peripheral eosinophilia
  - Fungal cultures diagnostic and most useful in *Candida* or *Aspergillus* infection
  - Dimorphic fungal infection diagnosed serologically, as isolating these organisms from the CSF is challenging and of low yield
    - Detection of complement-fixing (CF) IgG antibodies or immunodiffusion tests for IgM and IgG in CSF currently standard diagnostic tests
    - Low-titer false positives may occur in setting of parameningeal foci
    - False negatives may occur in early disease
- Primary amoebic meningoencephalitis due to *N. fowleri* results in:
  - Neutrophilic pleocytosis
  - Increased red blood cells
  - Low glucose
  - Elevated protein
  - Demonstration of motile trophozoites on wet mount of CSF or biopsy specimens diagnostic
- Diagnosis of *A. cantonensis*, *G. spinigerum*, or *B. procyonis* requires:
  - Appropriate epidemiologic exposure
  - Peripheral blood eosinophilia
  - Characteristic eosinophilic pleocytosis
  - Serologic tests helpful but performed only in reference laboratories

Treatment

- Initial management of patient with suspected meningitis primarily guided by epidemiologic risk factors and lumbar puncture results.
  - CSF cell count, glucose, and Gram stain crucial in guiding empiric therapy
  - If LP delayed for any reason, empiric antimicrobial therapy should not be withheld (Table 73.7)
    - Delays in therapy associated with adverse clinical outcomes and increased mortality
    - Administration of antimicrobials should immediately follow blood culture collection and should not be delayed by neuroimaging or other tests performed prior to LP.

Bacterial Meningitis

- LP should be performed urgently in those with suspected meningitis.
  - Imaging should be performed prior to LP in specific populations (see Table 73.5)
    - Should not result in a delay in initiation of antimicrobial therapy
    - Empiric therapy based on age, underlying host factors, and initial CSF Gram stain results (see Table 73.7)
- Choice of antimicrobial therapy in bacterial meningitis influenced by:

TABLE 73.7

EMPIRIC THERAPY OF BACTERIAL MENINGITIS BASED ON AGE AND HOST FACTORS

	Most common causes	Recommended therapy
Age: Preterm to <1 month	*Streptococcus agalactiae* *Escherichia coli* *Listeria monocytogenes*	Ampicillin + cefotaxime or ceftriaxone
Age: 1 month to 50 years	*Streptococcus pneumoniae* *Neisseria meningitidis* *Haemophilus influenzae*	Cefotaxime or ceftriaxone + vancomycin[a] + dexamethasone[b]
Age: >50 years or alcoholism or other debilitating diseases or impaired cellular immunity	*Streptococcus pneumoniae* *Listeria monocytogenes* Coliform Gram-negative bacilli	Ampicillin + cefotaxime or ceftriaxone + vancomycin[a] + dexamethasone[b]
Postneurosurgery, neurotrauma, or cochlear implant	*Streptococcus pneumoniae* *Staphylococcus aureus* Coliform Gram-negative bacilli *Pseudomonas aeruginosa*	Vancomycin + ceftazidime or meropenem
Ventriculitis/meningitis due to infected shunt	*Staphylococcus epidermidis* *Staphylococcus aureus* Coliform Gram-negative bacilli Diphtheroids *Propionibacterium acnes*	Vancomycin + ceftazidime or meropenem

[a]Vancomycin should be added in centers where *S. pneumoniae* may be resistant to third-generation cephalosporins.
[b]Dexamethasone is efficacious in children with *H. influenzae* and in adults with *S. pneumoniae*. The first dose is to be given 15 to 20 minutes prior to or concomitant with first dose of antibiotic. Dose, 0.15 mg/kg IV every 6 hours for 2 to 4 days; discontinue if micro-organism isolated other than listed above.

- Blood–CSF barrier penetration
- Effect of meningeal inflammation on penetration
- Bactericidal efficacy
- CSF penetration is enhanced in meningeal inflammation due to increased permeability
- High lipid solubility, low molecular weight, and low protein binding increase CSF drug levels
- Bactericidal efficacy may be decreased in purulent CSF, particularly with aminoglycosides, due to low pH
- Penicillins, third-generation cephalosporins, carbapenems, fluoroquinolones, and rifampin achieve high CSF levels and are all bactericidal
- Should be adjusted based on renal and hepatic function
- Therapeutic drug monitoring may be required to ensure adequate levels and prevent toxicity (e.g., vancomycin, aminoglycosides).
- Should be adjusted based on culture and susceptibility results as soon as possible (Table 73.8)
- In suspected meningococcal or *H. influenzae* meningitis, droplet isolation strictly enforced until 24 hours of effective antimicrobial therapy completed or alternate diagnosis reached
  - Single room
  - Gowns
  - Gloves
  - Surgical masks
  - Dedicated patient care equipment

TABLE 73.9

MORTALITY RATES IN BACTERIAL MENINGITIS BY PATHOGEN

Cause	Mortality
Neisseria meningitidis	3%–13%
Streptococcus pneumoniae	19%–30%
Haemophilus influenzae	3%–6%
Listeria monocytogenes	15%–29%
Streptococcus agalactiae	7%–27%
Staphylococcus aureus	14%–77%

- Isolation in other cases of meningitis, including pneumococcal meningitis, not required (Table 73.9)
- *Streptococcus pneumoniae.* Empiric therapy guidelines for pneumococcal meningitis recently modified due to increasing incidence of penicillin resistance
- Once uniformly susceptible to penicillin, mutations in penicillin-binding proteins have resulted in varying levels of resistance
- Empiric therapy consists of:
  - Third-generation cephalosporin until susceptibility available
  - Once minimum inhibitory concentration (MIC) available, adjust therapy accordingly

TABLE 73.8

SPECIFIC THERAPY OF BACTERIAL MENINGITIS

Bacterium	Recommended therapy
Haemophilus influenzae	
Ampicillin susceptible	Ampicillin
Ampicillin resistant	Cefotaxime or ceftriaxone
Neisseria meningitidis	
Penicillin MIC <0.1 μg/mL	Penicillin G or ampicillin
Penicillin MIC 0.1–1.0 μg/mL	Cefotaxime or ceftriaxone
Streptococcus pneumoniae	
Penicillin MIC <0.1 μg/mL	Penicillin G or ampicillin
Penicillin MIC $\geq$0.1 μg/mL	Cefotaxime or ceftriaxone
Ceftriaxone MIC $\geq$1.0 μg/mL	Vancomycin plus cefotaxime or ceftriaxone
Enterobacteriaceae	Cefotaxime or ceftriaxone unless member of SPICEM group[a]
Pseudomonas aeruginosa	Meropenem or ceftazidime or cefepime or aztreonam or ciprofloxacin PLUS tobramycin
Listeria monocytogenes	Ampicillin or penicillin G
Staphylococcus aureus	
Methicillin susceptible	Nafcillin or oxacillin
Methicillin resistant	Vancomycin
Prosthesis associated	Consider adding rifampin to above choices
Staphylococcus epidermidis	Vancomycin
Prosthesis associated	Consider adding rifampin
Streptococcus agalactiae	Ampicillin or penicillin G

MIC, minimum inhibitory concentration.
[a]SPICEM group includes *Serratia marcescens*, *Providencia*, indole-positive *Proteus* (*P. vulgaris*), *Citrobacter freundii* group, *Enterobacter* spp., and *Morganella morganii*). These micro-organisms carry chromosomal, inducible β-lactamases (ampC), which are capable of inactivating third-generation cephalosporin even if reported to be susceptible. Carbapenems (meropenem has greatest cerebrospinal fluid penetration), fluoroquinolones, or trimethoprim/sulfamethoxazole may be used to treat these micro-organisms, if susceptible.

- Isolates with penicillin MIC <0.1 μg/mL, penicillin G (4 million units intravenous [IV] every 4 hours) or ampicillin (2 g IV every 4 hours) should be used
- Isolates with a MIC $\geq$0.1 μg/mL, treatment with a third-generation cephalosporin should be continued
  ○ Either cefotaxime (2 g IV every 6 hours) or ceftriaxone (2 g IV every 12 hours)
  ○ Isolates with ceftriaxone MIC $\geq$1 μg/mL, vancomycin and a third-generation cephalosporin are recommended therapy
    – Vancomycin dosed 1 g IV every 12 hours, or 500 to 750 mg IV every 6 hours, to maximum of 2 to 3 g per day
    – Adjusted based on therapeutic drug monitoring to maintain a trough serum concentration of between 15 and 20 μg/mL
    – Meropenem a reasonable alternative
      • Does not carry the theoretical risk of decreasing seizure threshold seen with imipenem
    – Efficacy of newer antimicrobials, such as linezolid and daptomycin, not established
    – Dexamethasone **should be administered** prior to or with the first dose of antimicrobial
    – Treatment duration is 10 to 14 days
- *Neisseria meningitides.* Initial treatment of meningococcal meningitis is with a third-generation cephalosporin
  - Cefotaxime (2 g IV every 6 hours) or ceftriaxone (2 g IV every 12 hours)
  - Should be stepped down to penicillin if susceptibility confirmed
  - Duration of treatment is 7 days
  - Chloramphenicol (25 mg / kg, to a maximum of 1 g IV every 6 hours) a reasonable alternative in the beta-lactam–allergic patient
  - Meropenem (2 g IV every 8 hours) is another alternative
    • A high degree of cross-reaction in penicillin-allergic patients
    • Dexamethasone **not indicated** in confirmed meningococcal meningitis
- *Haemophilus influenzae.* Therapy for *H. influenzae* meningitis initially a third-generation cephalosporin
  - Can be changed to ampicillin, 2 g IV every 4 hours if susceptibility confirmed
  - Total of 7 days of therapy recommended
  - Dexamethasone **should be administered** as adjunctive therapy **in children**
- *Listeria monocytogenes.* *L. monocytogenes* meningitis should be treated with ampicillin, 2 g IV every 4 hours
  - Gentamicin may be added for antimicrobial synergy, but aminoglycosides have poor penetration into CSF.
    • Gentamicin administered as a 2 mg/kg loading dose, followed by 1.7 mg/kg every 8 hours
  - Trimethoprim/sulfamethoxazole (TMP/SMX), 20 mg/kg per day of the trimethoprim component, divided into 6 to 12 hourly doses, can be used in penicillin-allergic patients
  - Alternate therapies include meropenem and, potentially, linezolid and rifampin
  - Third-generation cephalosporins have no activity against *L. monocytogenes*
  - Treatment duration is 14 to 21 days

- **Aerobic Gram-negative bacilli:** Aerobic Gram-negative bacilli treated empirically with a third-generation cephalosporin or meropenem
  - Susceptibility results should be obtained to guide therapy in consultation with an infectious diseases specialist
  - For *Pseudomonas aeruginosa* infections, ceftazidime or cefepime, 2 g IV every 8 hours, or meropenem, 2 g IV every 8 hours, with tobramycin 2 mg/kg IV every 8 hours, should be used
    • Cefotaxime and ceftriaxone not used; no antipseudomonal activity
  - Ciprofloxacin or aztreonam is acceptable alternative if the isolate is susceptible
  - Duration of therapy is prolonged, generally 21 days
- **Staphylococcus:** Staphylococcal meningitis therapy depends on methicillin susceptibility
  - Methicillin-susceptible strains should be treated with nafcillin or oxacillin, 2 g IV every 4 hours
  - Methicillin-resistant strains should be treated with vancomycin, 1 g IV every 12 hours or 500 to 750 mg IV every 6 hours, to a maximum of 2 to 3 g per day
    • Ensure adequate serum levels of 15 to 20 μg/mL
  - Vancomycin is recommended in patients with penicillin allergy
  - Infected prosthetic material should be removed if possible
  - Antimicrobial therapy continued for 10 to 14 days after removal
    • If removal not possible, rifampin may be added
    • Cure rates are poor with hardware retention
  - Linezolid and daptomycin may become alternate therapies, but data are lacking
- Adjunctive therapies in bacterial meningitis include:
  - Corticosteroids
  - Procedures to reduce intracranial pressure
  - Surgery
  - Corticosteroid therapy decreases inflammatory response while allowing antimicrobial therapy to eradicate infection
    • Administration may decrease CSF penetration and bactericidal activity of antimicrobials but randomized controlled trials suggest benefit
    • In children, administration of dexamethasone has demonstrated reduction in incidence of hearing impairment and severe neurologic complications in *H. influenzae* meningitis
    • Adjunctive corticosteroid therapy has also been evaluated in adults, showing a mortality benefit in patients with pneumococcal meningitis
    • Treatment recommendations suggest dexamethasone, 0.15 mg/kg 10 to 20 minutes before, or at least concomitant with, the first dose of antimicrobial therapy and continued every 6 hours
    • Should be continued for 2 to 4 days only if the Gram stain or cultures demonstrate *H. influenzae* in children or *S. pneumoniae* in adults
- Intracranial pressure monitoring may be beneficial for patients with bacterial meningitis and elevated intracranial pressure (ICP)
- Complications of bacterial meningitis divided into neurologic and nonneurologic
  • Neurologic complications include seizures, cerebral edema, cerebral infarction, cranial nerve palsies, venous

sinus thrombosis, brain abscess, subdural empyema, and coma.
  ○ Late complications include hearing impairment, obstructive hydrocephalus, learning disabilities, sensory and motor deficits, mental retardation, cortical blindness, and seizures.
- Nonneurologic complications include septic shock, coagulopathy, and the syndrome of inappropriate antidiuretic hormone secretion (SIADH).

Viral Meningitis

- Treatment for viral meningitis is supportive, given its benign and self-limited course.
  - IV immunoglobulin[MB2] has been used in agammaglobulinemic patients with chronic enteroviral meningitis.
  - No specific therapy exists for arboviruses, mumps, or LCM.
  - HIV-associated meningitis should be treated with combination antiretroviral therapy.
  - Not clear whether antiviral treatment alters course of HSV meningitis
    - Nevertheless, primary episodes of genital herpes treated as per guidelines
    - Some extend therapy to 14 days with concomitant meningitis
    - Intravenous acyclovir, 5 mg/kg every 8 hours, used in severe disease
  - Ganciclovir the treatment of choice for CMV meningitis in immunocompromised hosts

Other Less Common Causes

- Syphilitic meningitis does not respond to benzathine penicillin.
  - Used to treat most forms of syphilis
  - Requires a 2-week course of high-dose IV penicillin G (4 million units every 4 hours)
  - RPR titers should be monitored after therapy.
  - Repeat CSF examination should be performed if titers do not decline fourfold at 6 months after therapy.
  - All HIV patients with syphilitic meningitis should have a LP repeated 6 months following therapy.
  - Patients with penicillin allergy should undergo desensitization, as there are no proven effective alternative therapies for syphilitic meningitis.
- Treatment of Lyme meningitis achieved with ceftriaxone, 2 g daily, or cefotaxime, 2 g IV every 8 hours for 14 to 28 days
  - Alternate therapy is penicillin (4 million units every 4 hours) for 14 to 28 days
- Treatment of tuberculous meningitis depends on resistance pattern in community and results of susceptibility testing
  - Consultation with an ID[MB3] specialist recommended
  - In general, standard combination therapy includes isoniazid (INH), rifampin (RIF), ethambutol (ETB), and pyrazinamide (PZA)
    - ETB may be discontinued once INH and RIF susceptibilities confirmed
    - Treatment continued for minimum of 12 to 24 months
  - Adjunctive therapy with dexamethasone for the first month has been shown to decrease complications and is recommended
  - Pyridoxine, 25 to 50 mg daily, administered to prevent INH-related neuropathy

- Therapy for fungal meningitis is complicated by the lack of standardized susceptibility testing and interpretation for many fungi.
- Area of antifungal therapy is an evolving area with an increasing number of antifungal agents from which to choose.
- Cryptococcal meningitis treated with:
  - 14-day induction phase of amphotericin B, 0.7 to 1 mg/kg per day IV, with or without flucytosine, 100 mg/kg per day orally dosed every 6 hours
  - Consolidation therapy with fluconazole, 400 mg daily, should be continued for 8 weeks following induction
  - Maintenance (or suppressive) therapy with fluconazole, 200 mg per day, continued in patients with HIV/AIDS until immune reconstitution achieved
  - May require:
    ○ Daily therapeutic lumbar punctures
    ○ An external ventricular drain
    ○ Ventriculoperitoneal shunt to relieve increased intracranial pressure
    ○ Therapy is identical in non-HIV/AIDS patients, with the exception that consolidation therapy is continued for 10 weeks
    ○ Further prolongation may be required in transplant patients
    ○ Echinocandins, such as caspofungin and micafungin, are not active in cryptococcosis
- Treatment for coccidioidal meningitis is oral fluconazole, 400 mg daily
  - Some initiate therapy with dose of 800 mg per day or may add intrathecal amphotericin B
  - Treatment must be continued lifelong, as relapses are frequently lethal
- Therapy for *H. capsulatum* meningitis consists of amphotericin B, 0.7 to 1 mg/kg per day to complete a total dose of 35 mg/kg
  - Fluconazole, 800 mg per day, for an additional 9 to 12 months, may be used to prevent relapse
  - If relapse occurs, long-term therapy with fluconazole or intraventricular amphotericin B recommended
  - Itraconazole avoided due to poor CSF penetration
- Although very rare, *S. schenckii* meningitis treated with amphotericin B
  - Itraconazole, despite its poor CSF penetration, may be tried after initial therapy for lifelong suppression.
- For candidal meningitis preferred initial therapy is amphotericin B, 0.7 mg/kg per day
  - With flucytosine, 25 mg/kg dosed every 6 hours and adjusted to maintain serum levels of 40 to 60 μg/mL
  - Fluconazole therapy, in susceptible species, may be used for follow-up or suppressive therapy.
  - Therapy should continue for at least 4 weeks after resolution of symptoms.
  - All prosthetic material must be removed to achieve cure.
- Primary amoebic meningoencephalitis caused by *N. fowleri* usually fatal
  - A few cases successfully treated with early diagnosis and treatment with high-dose intravenous and intrathecal amphotericin B or miconazole and rifampin
- Eosinophilic meningitis caused by *A. cantonensis* and *G. spinigerum* treated supportively

- Corticosteroids recommended to decrease inflammatory response to intracranial larvae
  - Antihelminthic therapy relatively contraindicated
    - Clinical deterioration and death may occur following severe inflammatory reactions to dying larvae

Prevention

- Chemoprophylaxis (medications) and immunoprophylaxis (vaccines) available to prevent infection in contacts of cases or in times of epidemic spread
  - Prophylaxis indicated for cases of *H. influenzae* type b in household contacts
    - Those residing with index case or with more than 4 hours of close contact
  - And day care contacts
    - Same day care as index case for 5 to 7 days before onset of disease
  - If there is unvaccinated contact at 4 years of age or younger in the household, chemoprophylaxis recommended for all household contacts except pregnant women
    - Rifampin, 20 mg/kg, with a usual adult dose of 600 mg daily, for four doses, recommended therapy
  - Prophylaxis for *N. meningitidis* is recommended for close contacts of cases
    - Includes intimate contacts (e.g., kissing)
    - Close contacts with ≥4 hours contact 1 week prior to the onset of illness
      - Close contacts include roommates, day care center contacts, cellmates, and/or military recruits
      - Medical personnel exposed to oropharyngeal secretions during intubation, nasotracheal suctioning, or mouth-to-mouth resuscitation should also receive chemoprophylaxis.
    - Rifampin, 600 mg orally every 12 hours for a total of four doses, or single doses of ciprofloxacin (500 mg orally) or ceftriaxone (250 mg intramuscularly) all efficacious
      - Avoid ciprofloxacin in children younger than 16 years and pregnant women, based on joint cartilage injury demonstrated in animal studies
- Vaccination available for prevention of *H. influenzae*, *N. meningitidis*, and *S. pneumoniae*
  - *H. influenzae* type b vaccination is part of routine childhood immunization
  - Unvaccinated children 2 years or younger exposed to index case should receive chemoprophylaxis and vaccination.
  - *S. pneumoniae* vaccination available in two preparations:
    - Not indicated as postexposure prophylaxis
    - 23-valent polysaccharide vaccine
      - Recommended for all individuals >65 years and those >5 years old with high-risk conditions (see below)
      - Of limited immunogenicity and efficacy
    - 7-valent conjugate vaccine
      - Recommended routinely in all children 23 months and younger and in those at high risk of invasive disease older than 23 months
        - Sickle cell disease and other hemoglobinopathies
        - Functional or anatomic asplenia
        - HIV infection
        - Immunocompromising conditions
        - Chronic medical conditions

- *N. meningitidis* vaccine available in two forms:
  - Conjugate and polysaccharide
    - Available conjugate vaccines include a quadrivalent (MCV4) vaccine, as well as the monovalent serogroup C (Men-C) vaccine
    - Available polysaccharide vaccines include a quadrivalent vaccine containing A, C, Y, and W-135 and a bivalent vaccine with serogroups A and C.
  - Vaccination indicated in:
    - High-risk populations, including those with specific immune deficiencies (see Table 73.2)
    - Those traveling to endemic and epidemic regions
    - Laboratory workers routinely exposed to *N. meningitides*
    - First-year college students living in dormitories
    - Military recruits

ENCEPHALITIS

Key Points

- Distinguishing encephalitis from meningitis, most useful finding is altered mental status
- Encephalitis most commonly viral or postinfectious in etiology
- Herpes simplex encephalitis the most common cause of sporadic encephalitis in Western countries
  - Accounts for 10% to 20% of cases
  - Temporal lobe involvement on MRI and electroencephalographic (EEG) characteristic
  - PCR 75% to 98% sensitive
    - False negatives occur predominantly during first 72 hours of illness
  - Mortality approaches 70% without therapy
    - Significantly reduced with early antiviral therapy
- Defined as inflammation of brain parenchyma
  - Encephalitis and meningitis may present with similar clinical findings
  - Two syndromes are pathophysiologically distinct
    - Major distinguishing feature is presence or absence of normal brain function
    - Patients with meningitis may be drowsy or lethargic but should have normal cerebral function
    - Those with encephalitis generally have altered mental status
    - Occasionally patients may present with combination of findings in overlap syndrome of meningoencephalitis
    - Important to distinguish between syndromes, as etiologic agents and treatments may differ
- Encephalitis most commonly viral or postinfectious (Table 73.10)
  - Viral encephalitis caused by direct viral invasion of the CNS
  - Postinfectious encephalitis an immune-mediated process
  - May be difficult to differentiate the two
    - Encephalitis with resolving infectious symptoms suggests a postviral cause
  - Most common viruses causing postinfectious encephalitis include mumps, measles, varicella-zoster virus, rubella, and influenza
  - Access to the CNS highly virus specific

TABLE 73.10

MOST COMMON VIRAL CAUSES OF ENCEPHALITIS, THEIR VECTORS OR ANIMAL HOSTS, AND GEOGRAPHIC DISTRIBUTIONS

Viral cause	Vector or animal host	Geographic distribution
Alpha viruses	Mosquitoes	
Eastern equine (EEE)	*Culiseta melanura*	New England
Western equine (WEE)	*Culex tarsalis*	West of Mississippi River
Venezuelan equine (VEE)	*Culex* spp.	South and Central America
Flaviviruses	Mosquitoes or ticks	
St. Louis	*Culex* spp.	Throughout the United States
West Nile (WNV)	*Culex pipiens* and *tarsalis*	Americas, Africa, Asia, Middle East, Europe
Japanese	*Culex tritaeniorhyunchus*	Asia and SE Asia
Murray Valley	*Culex* and *Aedes* spp.	Western Australia
Tick-borne	*Ixodes ricinus* and *persulcatus* ticks	Russia, Central Europe, China, North America, British Isles
Powassan virus		
Louping ill virus		
Herpes viruses	N/A	Worldwide
Herpes simplex virus (HSV-1)		
Varicella-zoster virus (VZV)		
Cytomegalovirus (CMV)		
Epstein-Barr virus (EBV)		
Human herpesviruses 6, 7		
Enteroviruses	N/A	Worldwide
Polioviruses		
Coxsackieviruses		
Echoviruses		
Adenoviruses	N/A	Worldwide
Human immunodeficiency virus (HIV)	N/A	Worldwide; particularly high prevalence in sub-Saharan Africa, Central and Southeast Asia, Eastern Europe
Rabies	Dogs, cats, raccoons, wolves, foxes, bats	Worldwide
Colorado tick fever	*Dermacentor andersoni* tick	Western United States and Canada
Mumps	N/A	Unvaccinated populations worldwide
Measles	N/A	Unvaccinated populations worldwide

N/A, not applicable.

- Occurs via hematogenous or neuronal routes
- After CNS entry, viruses enter neural cells, causing inflammation and cell dysfunction
- Clinical manifestations the result of specific cell-type invasion
  - Oligodendroglial cell invasion causes demyelination
  - Cortical invasion results in altered mental status
  - Neuronal invasion may result in focal or generalized seizures
- Focal pathology is the result of specific neural tropism
- Muscle weakness and flaccid paralysis may present concurrently in patients with encephalitis
- Arboviruses are acquired via vector exposure, mainly mosquitoes and ticks, and are most prevalent during summer and early fall months when vectors most active
  - Eastern equine encephalitis (EEE)
  - Western equine encephalitis (WEE)
  - St. Louis encephalitis
  - Venezuelan equine encephalitis (VEE)
  - California encephalitis (caused by La Crosse virus)
  - Japanese encephalitis
  - Yellow fever
  - WNV

- EEE has a high mortality rate, whereas WEE is a much milder illness
- WNV, identified in North America in 1999, causes WNNS in <1% of exposed individuals
  - WNNS most commonly manifests as encephalitis and occurs in those with diabetes mellitus, alcoholism, and of older age
- Japanese virus encephalitis, occurring principally in Southeast Asia, China, India, and Japan, the most common viral encephalitis outside the United States
- Colorado tick fever prevalent in western United States
  - Most affected individuals have history of camping and hiking in wooded endemic areas
- Malaria, in those with an appropriate travel history, should also be considered in the differential diagnosis of encephalitis
- Rabies, a zoonotic disease that requires contact with infected animals, should be considered in all cases of encephalitis.
  - Once CNS infection is established, the mortality is essentially 100%.
  - Can be acquired from many sources including dogs, cats, raccoons, bats, and foxes

- History of animal bite, useful if present, is absent in most cases of rabies
- Herpes viruses cause disease by primary infection or reactivation
  - Herpes simplex encephalitis (HSE), the most common cause of sporadic encephalitis in Western countries, accounting for 10% to 20% of cases
  - Caused by type 1 virus in >90% of cases, occurs year-round, and affects all age groups
  - Two-thirds of cases due to reactivation of virus in trigeminal ganglion, with retrograde transport along the olfactory tract to the orbitofrontal and mediotemporal lobes
  - Untreated HSE has mortality rate of 50% to 75%
    - All survivors suffer neurologic sequelae
  - Outcomes correlate strongly with severity of disease at presentation, as well as time to initiation of antiviral therapy
  - Varicella-zoster encephalitis generally affects immune-compromised patients and may occur with or without concomitant cutaneous lesions.
- Nonviral causes of encephalitis include bacterial, rickettsial, fungal, and parasitic infections.
  - Bacterial causes include *Mycoplasma, Listeria monocytogenes, Borrelia burgdorferi* (Lyme disease), *Leptospira* spp., *Brucella, Legionella, Nocardia, Treponema pallidum* (syphilis), *Salmonella typhi,* and mycobacterial species, *Coxiella burnetii* (Q-fever), and Ehrlichia.
  - Most common rickettsial species include *R. rickettsii* (Rocky Mountain spotted fever) and *R. typhi* (endemic typhus)
  - Fungal causes include *Cryptococcus* spp., *Aspergillus* spp., *Candida, Coccidioides immitis, Histoplasma capsulatum,* and *Blastomyces dermatitidis*
  - *Trypanosoma brucei* complex (African sleeping sickness), malaria, *Toxoplasma gondii, Echinococcus granulosus,* and *Schistosoma* spp. can cause encephalitis but require epidemiologic exposures or specific risk factors
    - For example, toxoplasma encephalitis most common in advanced HIV
- Clinical findings of encephalitis include:
- Classic triad of fever, headache, and altered mental status
- Onset of symptoms may be acute, subacute, or chronic
- Acuity and severity of symptoms at presentation correlate with prognosis
  - Symptoms may be preceded by a viral prodrome consisting of fever, headache, nausea, vomiting, lethargy, and myalgias.
- Disorientation, amnesia, behavioral and speech changes, movement disorders, and focal or diffuse neurologic abnormalities such as hemiparesis, cranial nerve palsies, or seizures are common presenting.
  - Neck stiffness and photophobia may also be noted.
- Varicella-zoster virus (VZV), EBV, CMV, measles, and mumps may present with rash, lymphadenopathy, and hepatosplenomegaly.
- HSE incidence is unrelated to a history of oral or genital lesions.
- Laboratory findings may include:
- Peripheral leukocytosis or leucopenia
- CSF examination usually reveals a pleocytosis with lymphocytic predominance
  - Neutrophilic predominance may be present early in infection.

- Red blood cells, in the absence of a traumatic tap, are suggestive of HSV but may be seen in other necrotizing viral encephalitides.
- Protein levels usually elevated, and glucose may be normal or slightly decreased
- Viral cultures are rarely positive, molecular methods have become the diagnostic tests of choice
  - Demonstration of HSV DNA in the CSF by PCR is both sensitive and specific (75%–98% and 100%, respectively)
    - May miss cases in first 72 hours of illness
  - PCR testing available for WNV, VZV, enteroviruses, adenoviruses, rabies, CMV, EBV, HHV-6, and HHV-7 in most reference laboratories
  - Serology may be diagnostic if IgM is detected or a fourfold rise in acute and convalescent IgG titers is demonstrated
  - Corneal or neck (posterior, at the hairline) biopsies and saliva PCR can be diagnostic for rabies
  - Brain biopsy may be considered if all other tests are non-diagnostic
- Other investigations that may aid in diagnosis include EEG, CT, or MRI
- EEG particularly helpful in HSE, showing characteristic focal changes (spiked and slow wave patterns) from temporal regions in 80% of patients
- MRI the most sensitive imaging modality at detecting early viral encephalitis and may show virus-specific changes
- CT scans are more available on an urgent basis and are useful in ruling out space-occupying lesions.
  - Rarely able to visualize encephalitic changes
- There are few specific therapies for viral encephalitis
- Treatment of HSE with acyclovir, 10 mg/kg IV every 8 hours the main exception
  - Treatment should be initiated as soon as possible, delays correlate with mortality
  - Therapy should be started empirically in all patients with encephalitis until confirmatory testing is available, given the dramatic effect on outcome
  - Acyclovir should also be considered in VZV encephalitis even though data regarding efficacy in this form of VZV disease are only anecdotal.
- Supportive therapy, including ICU admission with intubation and mechanical ventilation, may be required.
- Ganciclovir or foscarnet for ganciclovir-resistant strains used to treat CMV encephalitis
- Role of antivirals for EBV and HHV-6 encephalitides unproven
  - International Herpes Management Forum recommends use of ganciclovir or foscarnet for HHV-6 encephalitis*
- Outcomes related to multiple factors include:
- Host age and immune response
- Organism virulence
- Time to effective therapy
- Poor outcomes more common in younger (<1 year) and older (>55 years) populations
- HSE, Japanese encephalitis, and EEE have highest mortality rates

---

*Data on CMV encephalitis come from several papers related to HIV patients, including International Herpes Management Forum (IHMF) recommendations (*Herpes.* 2004;11(Suppl 2):95A–104A). Data on HHV-6 are more limited, but antivirals are still suggested by the IHMF (*Herpes.* 2004;11(Suppl 2):105A–111A).

- HSE mortality approaches 70% without therapy but can be reduced to 28% with early antiviral treatment.
- 62% of HSE patients recover with significant neurologic deficits
  - Paresis, seizures, cognitive and memory deficits

BRAIN ABSCESS

Key Points

- Brain abscess results from focal infection, trauma, or surgery.
- Solitary abscess usually result of contiguous infection from otitis, mastoiditis, sinusitis, or dental infection
- Multiple abscesses commonly result from hematogenous spread from chronic pulmonary, endocardial, skin, intra-abdominal, or pelvic infections
- Microbiology of brain abscess depends on primary site of infection, patient age, and underlying host factors. Infections commonly polymicrobial, and empiric therapy should include targeted anaerobic activity.
- Clinical manifestations nonspecific and depend on size and location of abscess. Headache is the most common presenting feature.
- MRI more sensitive than CT scanning and is neuroimaging test of choice
- Blood and abscess culture results should be used to tailor antimicrobial therapy, which is generally prolonged (6 to 8 weeks) and guided by serial imaging
- Surgical excision may be indicated in patients with traumatic brain abscesses, fungal abscesses, and multiloculated or large (>2.5 cm) abscesses.
- Brain abscess uncommon but potentially life-threatening infection
  - Characterized by localized intracranial suppurative collections
  - Usually the result of:
    - Extension of focal infection (45%)
    - Trauma (10%)
    - Surgery
    - Bacteria may gain entry to CNS by hematogenous seeding in 25% of cases
  - Mortality rates with treatment range from 4.5% to 13%
    - Even with new imaging techniques, antimicrobials, and surgical therapies
    - Infection begins as a localized area of cerebritis, with subsequent central necrosis, suppuration, and fibrous capsule formation (Table 73.11)
  - Solitary abscesses
    - Usually result of contiguous infection including otitis, mastoiditis, frontal or ethmoid sinusitis, or dental infection
    - Bullet fragments or other foreign bodies may serve as nidus of infection and develop into abscesses even years after initial injury.
    - Postneurosurgical brain abscesses may also present in a delayed fashion.
  - Multiple abscesses
    - More commonly result of hematogenous seeding from chronic pulmonary, endocardial, skin, intra-abdominal, or pelvic infections

TABLE 73.11

RISK FACTORS FOR BRAIN ABSCESS

Otic infection (otitis media, mastoiditis)
Sinusitis (frontal, ethmoid, sphenoid)
Dental infection
Neurosurgical intervention or neurotrauma
Bacterial endocarditis
Neutropenia
Immune compromise (HIV infection, immunosuppressive therapy)
Chronic lung infection (abscess, bronchiectasis, empyema)
Congenital heart disease

HIV, human immunodeficiency virus.

  - Patients with hereditary hemorrhagic telangiectasia (Osler-Weber-Rendu syndrome) and children with coronary heart disease predisposed to brain abscesses
- Primary site or underlying condition cannot be identified in 20% to 40% of patients with brain abscess.
- Location of brain abscess may be suggestive of source
  - Temporal lobe or cerebellar abscesses commonly result from otic infections
  - Frontal lobe abscesses from sinusitis or dental infection
  - Abscesses in the distribution of the middle cerebral artery from hematogenous seeding
- Microbiology of brain abscesses diverse and depends on primary site of infection, age of patient, underlying host factors:
  - Common aerobic species include:
    - Streptococci (viridans, anginosus group, and microaerophilic species) isolated in up to 70% of cases
    - Aerobic Gram-negative bacilli—*Klebsiella pneumoniae, Pseudomonas* spp., *Escherichia coli,* and *Proteus* spp.—and *S. aureus* are common pathogens with contiguous infection
    - Less common pathogens, *Rhodococcus, Listeria, Nocardia,* mycobacteria, and fungi—*Candida, Cryptococcus, Aspergillus,* agents of zygomycosis, *Pseudoallescheria boydii,* and the dimorphic fungi such as *Histoplasma, Coccidioides,* and *Blastomyces*—cause disease in immunocompromised hosts.
    - Postsurgical or posttraumatic abscesses usually due to *S. aureus* and aerobic Gram-negative bacilli
    - Advanced HIV-infected patients commonly present with *Toxoplasma gondii* infection
  - Anaerobes present in 40% to 100% of brain abscesses
    - Although anaerobic cultures not routinely performed in all laboratories and may be falsely negative
    - May originate from the oropharynx with contiguous head and neck infections, or from the abdomen or pelvis when infection is due to hematogenous seeding
    - Commonly isolated anaerobes include *Peptococcus, Peptostreptococcus, Bacteroides* spp., *Prevotella* spp., *Propionibacterium, Fusobacterium, Eubacterium, Veillonella,* and *Actinomyces.*
  - Helminths occasionally cause localized brain infection in immigrant populations.
    - Neurocysticercosis, intracranial infection with the larval cyst of *T. solium* or pork tapeworm, most common and results from the ingestion of *T. solium* ova

TABLE 73.12

COMMON PRESENTING FEATURES IN BRAIN ABSCESS

Headache
Mental status changes
Fever
Focal neurologic deficits
Neck stiffness
Papilledema, nausea, or vomiting with increased intracranial pressure
Seizures

- *Entamoeba histolytica, Schistosoma japonicum* and *mekongi* species, *Paragonimus,* and *Toxocara* also described as causes of brain abscess
- Clinical manifestations of brain abscess are relatively nonspecific, resulting in delays in presentation and diagnosis (Table 73.12)
- Onset may be acute or chronic
  - Most of presenting features related to size and location of abscess
  - Systemic toxicity uncommon
  - Headache is most common presenting symptom, usually localized to side of abscess
    - Sudden worsening of headache may be due to rupture of abscess into ventricular space
    - Fever present in only half of patients and not a reliable sign
    - Seizure a common presenting feature
    - Focal neurologic findings relatively uncommon
    - Neck stiffness occurs in 15% of patients most commonly seen with occipital abscesses
    - Altered mental status and vomiting are late signs, indicating the development of elevated intracranial pressure.
  - Specific presenting features correlate with abscess location
    - Frontal lobe abscesses often present with changes in personality or mental status, hemiparesis, motor speech difficulties, and seizures.
    - Temporal lobe abscesses may cause visual field defects or dysphasia if located in the dominant hemisphere.
    - Cerebellar abscesses may present with ataxia, nystagmus, and dysmetria.
    - Brainstem abscesses usually extend longitudinally, with minimal compressive effect, and therefore present with few classic features.
    - Papilledema occurs late with increased intracranial pressure.
- Imaging of the brain parenchyma diagnostic test of choice
  - LP contraindicated in patients with focal findings or papilledema
    - Should be avoided in patients with suspected brain abscess
  - CT scanning or MRI should be performed, with choice of test depending on stability of the patient and availability of imaging technique
  - Contrast CT scanning not as sensitive as MRI but more easily obtained urgently
  - MRI with gadolinium enhancement more sensitive than CT in detecting early cerebritis
    - Can more accurately estimate extent of central necrosis, ring enhancement, and cerebral edema

- MRI also better able to visualize the brainstem, cerebellum, and spinal cord and can detect lesions 1.5 cm or smaller, which the CT scan may miss
- Blood cultures should be drawn in all patients with suspected or confirmed brain abscess
- Abscess specimens obtained by stereotactic CT-guided aspiration or surgery to confirm diagnosis and guide antimicrobial therapy
- Bacterial, mycobacterial, and fungal cultures should be requested
  - Serology may be helpful for specific causes, such as *Toxoplasma gondii* and neurocysticercosis
  - In toxoplasma brain abscesses, IgG should be positive, as most infections are reactivation, not primary infection
  - Positive IgG antibody, however, does not prove *T. gondii* is the cause of a brain abscess
  - Brain biopsy may establish diagnosis but not routinely recommended
- Empiric therapy without aspiration for microbiologic samples not generally advised except in specific situations where a high likelihood of specific pathogen
  - If clinical and radiologic responses not evident within 7 and 14 days, respectively, microbiologic specimen should be obtained
- Therapy for brain abscess requires combination medical and surgical therapy for cure
- Antimicrobial therapy alone rarely effective
- Empiric therapy should be initiated after imaging confirms the presence of an intraparenchymal lesion, pending aspiration for definitive diagnosis
- Therapy directed by most likely source and respective pathogens
- Presumed otic, mastoid, sinus, or dental sources, or temporal or cerebellar abscesses
  - Third-generation cephalosporin (cefotaxime, 2 g IV every 4 hours, or ceftriaxone, 2 g IV every 12 hours) and metronidazole (15 mg/kg IV load, followed by 7.5 mg/kg IV every 8 hours)
- Suspected hematogenous spread
  - Antimicrobial with activity against *S. aureus* should be used
  - Nafcillin or oxacillin, 2 g IV every 4 hours appropriate in settings with low prevalence of methicillin resistance
  - Vancomycin, 15 mg/kg IV every 12 hours—adjusted for renal function and monitored with therapeutic drug levels—used where methicillin resistance common or in penicillin-allergic patients
  - Vancomycin penetrates CNS poorly
    ○ Need a trough level of 15 to 20 μg/mL
  - Metronidazole and/or a third-generation cephalosporin may be added, depending on the clinical setting
- For postneurosurgical or posttrauma patients with brain abscess:
  - Nafcillin, oxacillin, or vancomycin plus meropenem, a third-generation cephalosporin, preferably one with antipseudomonal activity such as ceftazidime, should be used
- Therapy adjusted once pathogen identification and susceptibility results are available and continued intravenously for 6 to 8 weeks
  - Guided by clinical response and serial imaging
  - Oral antimicrobial therapy for 2 to 6 months often administered

○ Efficacy of this approach has not been established
- Therapy continued until complete resolution of symptoms and CT/MRI findings
- Antifungal therapy guided by fungal cultures and used in combination with surgical therapy
  - Candidal brain abscesses treated with amphotericin B and flucytosine
    ○ Efficacy of fluconazole not sufficiently evaluated to recommend use
  - Aspergillus brain abscesses historically treated with amphotericin B
    ○ Voriconazole has become treatment of choice
    ○ Combination antifungal therapy with voriconazole, plus either an echinocandin or an amphotericin B formulation, increasingly used
  - Cerebral zygomycosis almost invariably fatal, although amphotericin B the treatment of choice
    ○ Posaconazole may be alternative for zygomycoses
    ○ Voriconazole inactive in these cases
  - *P. boydii* demonstrates *in vitro* resistance to amphotericin B
    ○ Voriconazole recommended as antifungal of choice in these cases
- Neurosurgical consultation should be sought at time of diagnosis
  - Aspiration through burr hole or complete excision following craniotomy both appropriate treatment options
  - Therapeutic aspiration may be performed with CT/MRI guidance
  - Surgical excision indicated with traumatic brain abscesses, fungal abscesses, and large (>2.5 cm) or multiloculated abscesses
  - If no clinical improvement within 1 week of initiation of treatment and aspiration, mental status declines, or intracranial pressure or abscess size increases despite therapy:
    - Surgical excision also indicated
    - Antibiotic therapy may be shortened to 2 to 4 weeks following surgical excision
- Dexamethasone should be initiated with significant edema and mass effect
- Prophylactic antiseizure medications frequently administered
- Poor prognostic factors in brain abscess include:
  - Rapid progression
  - Mental status or neurologic impairment on presentation
  - Rupture into a ventricle
  - Neurologic sequelae, usually seizures, occur in 30% to 60% of patients

CRANIAL SUBDURAL EMPYEMA (CSE)

Key Points

- CSE and brain abscess share epidemiologic risk factors and microbiology
  - Presenting symptoms include:
  - High fever
  - Unilateral headache
  - Recent history of contiguous otic, mastoid, sinus, or meningeal infection

- MRI is the diagnostic test of choice
- Therapy should include prolonged antimicrobials and surgical drainage for cure
- CSE is an intracranial collection of pus in subdural space
  - Potentially life-threatening condition
  - Accounts for 15% to 20% of all intracranial infections
  - Universally fatal prior to antimicrobial therapy
    - Mortality with combined medical and surgical therapy now approximates 12%
    - Usually complete recovery in survivors
  - Spread of infection to subdural space occurs via emissary veins or by direct extension of cranial osteomyelitis with accompanying epidural abscess
    - Subdural space lacks septations, infection spreads rapidly and progressively
    - Most CSEs involve frontal lobe
      ○ But area of involvement generally related to contiguous infection
    - Cerebral edema and hydrocephalus may develop when blood or cerebrospinal flow is disrupted by increased ICP
    - Cerebral infarction may also result from septic venous thrombosis
  - Common predisposing infections include:
    - Otic and sinus infections in up to 50% to 80% of cases
      ○ With chronic otitis media, the middle ear and mastoids are commonly predisposing sites of infection
    - Traumatic brain injury with skull fracture
    - Neurosurgical procedures
    - Infection of a preexisting hematoma
    - Chronic pulmonary infection
    - Preceding meningitis
  - CSE invariably polymicrobial, including:
    - Streptococci, staphylococci, aerobic Gram-negative bacilli, and anaerobes
    - *S. aureus*, Enterobacteriaceae, and *Pseudomonas* more common following neurosurgical procedures or neurotrauma
- Clinical presentation of CSE rapidly progressive; early diagnosis and treatment crucial
  - Presenting symptoms generally include:
    - High fever and unilateral headache
    - History of sinusitis, otitis media, mastoiditis, meningitis, cranial surgery or trauma, sinus surgery, or pulmonary infection within 2 weeks common
    - Altered mental status present in approximately 50% of patients on admission
      ○ Initially characterized by confusion and drowsiness
      ○ Progresses to coma in most untreated cases
      ○ Focal neurologic signs most commonly include:
        – Hemiparesis or hemiplegia
        – Seizures develop in up to 50% of patients
        – Cranial nerve palsies
        – Homonymous hemianopsia
        – Dysarthria or dysphasia
        – Ataxia
        – Fixed, dilated pupil portends imminent cerebral herniation
          - Requires emergent surgical intervention
- Diagnosis of CSE requires high index of suspicion
  - Should be considered in patients presenting with meningeal signs and focal neurologic deficits, with or without systemic toxicity

- LP contraindicated because of risk of cerebral herniation with increased ICP
- Diagnostic imaging tests of choice are contrast CT or MRI
  - Demonstrate typical crescentic collection running parallel to cranial vault
  - Midline shift implies significant mass effect
  - Gadolinium-enhanced MRI the most sensitive, visualizing subdural empyemas too small to be detected by CT
  - MRI can also detect falcine, basal, and posterior fossa empyemas and differentiate between subdural empyemas and cystic hygromas or chronic hematomas, which CT is unable to do
  - Imaging of sinuses, middle ear, and/or mastoids performed in appropriate clinical settings to identify potential sources
- Treatment of CSE requires emergent combined medical and surgical therapy
  - Surgical drainage mandatory, as antimicrobials alone cannot effectively cure
  - Cultures required to guide antimicrobial therapy
  - Antiseizure treatment and/or prophylaxis may be warranted
  - Standard therapy for increased ICP should be instituted
  - Empiric antimicrobial therapy initiated as soon as aspiration of empyema performed or immediately on admission in unstable patients
    - Guided by most likely source of primary infection
    - Recommended therapy includes:
      - Third-generation cephalosporin (cefotaxime, 2 g IV every 4 hours, or ceftriaxone, 2 g IV every 12 hours)
      - Or meropenem, 2 g IV every 8 hours with metronidazole (15 mg/kg IV load, followed by 7.5 mg/kg IV every 12 hours)
      - If *S. aureus* is suspected, nafcillin or oxacillin (2 g IV every 4 hours) should be used
      - Vancomycin, 1 g IV every 12 hours or 500 to 750 mg IV every 6 hours, to maximum of 2 to 3 g per day used in patients with penicillin allergy or in regions with high prevalence of methicillin resistance
        – Want serum trough level of 15 to 20 μg/mL
      - If *Pseudomonas aeruginosa* infection is suspected, ceftazidime, cefepime, or meropenem should be used in place of other third-generation cephalosporins.
      - IV antimicrobials administered for 3 to 6 weeks
        – Depends on clinical response and serial imaging
        – Therapy for 6 to 8 weeks warranted if contiguous osteomyelitis or mastoiditis is present
      - Surgical therapy of CSE includes:
        – Burr hole drainage or craniotomy
        – Debridement of necrotic bone and surgical correction of sinus and otic infections important adjuvant surgical therapies

EPIDURAL ABSCESS (EA)

Key Points

- An EA a localized collection of pus between the dura and overlying skull (cranial epidural abscess) or vertebral column (spinal epidural abscess)
  - Severe symptoms may result due to compression of brain or spinal cord

- Prompt diagnosis and treatment are crucial
- Cranial EA commonly accompanied by CSE
  - Emissary veins may translocate infection across cranial dura
  - Microbiology identical to CSE (see previous section)
- Spinal EA nine times more common than cranial EA
  - Epidural space a potential space extending from foramen magnum down length of spinal canal
  - Space is larger in lumbar area and predominantly posterior
  - Most spinal EAs occur in this area
  - Spinal EA most commonly originate when intervertebral disk (diskitis) or vertebral body (osteomyelitis) become infected via hematogenous seeding
  - As abscess extends may track longitudinally in epidural space, causing damage via direct compression of spinal cord or local vascular damage (thrombosis, thrombophlebitis, vasculitis)
  - Most spinal EAs extend approximately three to five vertebral spaces
    - But can extend entire length of spinal canal
  - Risk factors for development of spinal EA includes:
    - Injection drug use
    - Diabetes mellitus
    - Bacteremia
    - Infective endocarditis
    - Chronic indwelling venous catheterization
    - Epidural catheterization
    - Decubitus ulcers
    - Chronic skin conditions
    - Paraspinal abscess
    - Back surgery
    - Lumbar puncture
    - CT-guided needle biopsies
    - Blunt or penetrating spinal trauma
    - Secondary hematogenous spread occurs in 25% to 50% of cases
- *S. aureus* is most common pathogen isolated from spinal EAs
  - Accounts for approximately 65% of cases
  - Other implicated micro-organisms include:
    - Streptococci
    - Aerobic Gram-negative bacilli, particularly *Escherichia coli* and *Pseudomonas aeruginosa*
    - Coagulase-negative staphylococci, usually with previous spinal instrumentation
    - Anaerobes
    - Less common pathogens include *Actinomyces, Nocardia,* and fungi, predominantly *Candida*
  - Infections polymicrobial in 5% to 10% of cases
  - *M. tuberculosis* makes up approximately 25% of spinal EA and should be suspected in patients with previous history of tuberculosis, residence in a TB-endemic region, or other TB risk factors
- Clinical manifestations in patients with cranial EA usually insidious
- Headache the most common presenting feature
- Once infection spreads to involve meninges, subdural space, and brain parenchyma, focal neurologic signs and symptoms may develop
- If abscess is located near the petrous bone, osteomyelitis of the petrous ridge may result in Gradenigo syndrome—cranial nerve V and VI palsies with unilateral pain or otalgia

- Spinal EA presents classically with:
- Fever
- Back pain
  - Usually first symptom
- Neurologic deficits
- All three symptoms present in only 13%
  - Paresthesias, motor weakness, and sensory changes occurring in affected nerve roots
  - Bladder and bowel dysfunction, as well as paralysis late signs; should prompt urgent surgical consultation
- Diagnosis of EA begins with identification of risk factors and clinical suspicion
- Routine blood work may demonstrate peripheral leukocytosis or elevated erythrocyte sedimentation rate or C-reactive protein
- MRI with gadolinium enhancement imaging modality of choice for both cranial and spinal EAs
  - CT scanning cannot visualize spinal cord adequately and less sensitive at identifying contiguous diskitis or osteomyelitis
- Blood cultures should be collected in all patients
  - Positive in 62% of patients
  - LP relatively contraindicated in setting of EA
    - CSF analysis routinely Gram stain negative
    - Cultures positive in 19% of cases
  - Highest-yield (90%) culture comes from abscess itself
    - Ultrasound- or CT-guided drainage should be performed as soon as possible
    - Bacterial, mycobacterial, and fungal cultures should be requested
    - Additional studies to diagnose active tuberculosis should be performed in patients with suspected spinal TB
      - Sputum AFB smears and cultures
      - Urine AFB culture
      - Tuberculin skin testing or QuantiFERON-TB Gold testing
- Management of EA requires combination of medical and surgical therapy
  - Empiric antimicrobial therapy for cranial EA should include third-generation cephalosporin or meropenem plus metronidazole
  - Nafcillin, oxacillin, or vancomycin may be added if *S. aureus* is strongly suspected
  - Surgical drainage is crucial for cure
  - Management of spinal EA similarly requires empiric antimicrobial therapy and surgical decompression, drainage, and debridement
    - Because of predominance of *S. aureus* infection, empiric therapy fairly targeted
      - Vancomycin if methicillin-resistant *S. aureus* likely or if patient is penicillin allergic
      - Nafcillin or oxacillin if local prevalence of methicillin resistance low
      - Surgical intervention within first 24 hours of presentation results in improved outcomes.
      - Medical therapy alone may be successful when blood or abscess aspirate cultures are available to guide therapy and there are no neurologic deficits on presentation.
      - Serial imaging required in these cases to confirm improvement in abscess size

- Surgery pursued if neurologic deterioration occurs at any time or if resolution of abscess not evident with medical therapy alone
- Therapy with antimicrobials is prolonged:
  - Usually 4 to 8 weeks
  - Guided by serial imaging to ensure complete resolution of the abscess
  - Repeat imaging occurs at approximately 4-week intervals or at any time if neurologic deterioration occurs
  - Prognosis is fair but 37% of patients experience residual neurologic deficits.
  - Degree of residual deficit affected by duration of neurologic deficit prior to surgery and diagnostic delays of >24 hours

SUPPURATIVE INTRACRANIAL THROMBOPHLEBITIS (SIT)

Key Points

- SIT is septic venous thrombosis of the cortical veins
  - Occurs as complication of infections in:
    - Sinus
    - Middle ear
    - Mastoid
    - Oropharynx
    - Face
  - Bacterial meningitis, EA, or subdural abscess may also result in SIT
  - Absence of valves in the cerebral veins and venous sinuses aids spread of infection from proximal sites
- Location of intracranial infection depends on original source of infection
  - Bacterial meningitis, infection spread via drainage of meningeal veins into superior sagittal sinus
  - Superior sagittal sinus may also be involved following facial, scalp, subdural, and epidural space infections
  - Otitis media and mastoiditis are usual causes of lateral sinus and petrosal sinus thromboses
  - Paranasal sinus, facial, or oropharyngeal infections may result in cavernous sinus thrombosis
  - Risk factors for cerebral venous stasis include:
    - Hypercoagulable states—specifically antiphospholipid antibody syndrome
    - Volume depletion
    - Polycythemia
    - Pregnancy or use of oral contraceptives
    - Malignancy
    - Sickle cell disease
    - Traumatic brain injury
- Bacterial pathogens involved in SIT depend on originating source of infection:
- *S. aureus* commonly involved following facial infection
- Otherwise, sinusitis and otitis media pathogens cause most infections; these include:
  - Staphylococci
  - Streptococci
  - Aerobic Gram-negative bacilli
  - Anaerobes such as *Fusobacterium* and *Bacteroides*
  - *Aspergillus* and agents of zygomycosis rarely cause SIT

○ Most often seen in patients with diabetes mellitus or immune deficiencies
- Clinical manifestations of SIT depend on anatomic site(s) involved
  - Septic thrombosis of the superior sagittal sinus presents with:
    - Fever, headache, confusion, nausea, vomiting, and seizures
    - Mental status depression and progression to coma may occur rapidly
    - Upper motor neuron lower extremity weakness or hemiparesis may be present
    - When a complication of bacterial meningitis, nuchal rigidity may be present
  - Compressive cranial nerve palsies may result from increased pressure in cavernous sinus.
    - Cranial nerves III, IV, V-1, V-2, and VI, and the internal carotid artery travel through cavernous sinus
    - Classic symptoms of septic cavernous sinus thrombosis include:
      ○ Fever, headache, diplopia, and retro-orbital pain
      ○ Depending on specific nerves involved, ptosis, proptosis, chemosis, hyperesthesia, and decreased corneal reflexes may be present
      ○ Venous engorgement of retinal veins and papilledema are common
  - Septic transverse sinus thrombosis presents with:
    - Headache and otitis
  - SIT may also be a complication of Gradenigo syndrome, with spread of infection around the carotid sheath and surrounding venous plexus.
  - Patients with sigmoid sinus and internal jugular vein thrombosis may present with neck pain.
- Diagnosis of SIT made by MRI, demonstrating absence of flow within affected veins and venous sinuses
- MR venography or angiography used to confirm diagnosis, and sinus imaging should be concomitantly performed
- Compared to CT scanning, MRI offers additional benefits of detecting cerebritis, intracranial abscess, cerebral infarction, hemorrhage, or edema
- Despite lower sensitivity, CT scanning is commonly performed before MRI, as it is more easily obtained on an urgent basis.
- Treatment of suppurative intracranial thrombophlebitis includes:
  - Antimicrobials
  - Surgical therapy
  - Anticoagulation
  - Choice of antimicrobial therapy depends on:
    - Risk factors
    - Most probable source of infection
    - Culture results, if available
    - In antecedent sinusitis, empiric therapy with cefotaxime or ceftriaxone, and metronidazole reasonable
    - In cavernous sinus thrombosis, an agent active against *S. aureus* should be included
    - Antimicrobial therapy continued for 6 weeks or until radiographic resolution of thrombosis
  - If antimicrobial therapy is ineffective:
    - Surgical therapy may be required for drainage of infected sinuses, ligation of internal jugular vein, or for source control (e.g., oropharyngeal or dental infections)
    - Anticoagulation with heparin is beneficial in cavernous sinus thrombosis, particularly if used early, and should be strongly considered.
      ○ Small intracerebral hemorrhage not an absolute contraindication to heparin therapy
      ○ Efficacy of thrombolysis in SIT not adequately evaluated

CHAPTER 74 ■ INFECTIONS OF THE HEAD AND NECK

OTOLOGIC INFECTIONS

Otitis Externa (OE)

- Acute OE (AOE) is diffuse inflammation of the external ear canal and may also involve the pinna or tympanic membrane.
  - Also known as "swimmer's ear" or "tropical ear" due to a higher prevalence with prolonged water exposure during swimming or living in warm and humid climates
  - Annual incidence of AOE is about 1:100 to 1:250 within general population
- Risk factors for AOE are:
  - Prolonged exposure to water from swimming
  - Dermatologic conditions such as seborrhea, psoriasis, eczema
  - Trauma from ear cleaning and foreign objects
  - Use of assistive devices such as earplugs or hearing aids
  - Anatomic abnormalities such as exostoses and narrow ear canals
  - Immunocompromising systemic conditions such as diabetes or human immunodeficiency virus (HIV)
  - Concomitant ear diseases such as cholesteatoma, suppurative otitis media
  - History of cancer radiotherapy
- Symptoms and signs of ear canal inflammation usually rapid onset
  - Some presenting symptoms may be:
    - Otalgia
    - Itching
    - Aural fullness
    - Decreased hearing
    - Pain with chewing
  - AOE has disproportionately severe pain and significant tenderness when pushed on the tragus or with manipulation of pinna
  - Otoscopic examination usually reveals ear canal cellulitis and edema
    - Depending on severity of ear canal swelling, tympanic membrane may or may not be visualized
    - Ear canal often filled with purulent discharge and debris
    - Regional lymphadenopathy may be present on examination
- Most cases of AOE are bacterial
  - *Pseudomonas aeruginosa* and *Staphylococcus* species the most common pathogens
  - Fungal involvement uncommon in primary AOE
    - More often seen in chronic otitis externa or as secondary overgrowth following treatment of bacterial infection
- Initial treatment of AOE involves:
  - Removal of debris from external ear canal
  - Pain control
  - Use of topical medications
    - If marked edema of ear canal prevents proper penetration of medicated drops into canal, placement of cotton wick directly into ear canal for several days facilitates delivery of medication
  - Acidification of ear canal
  - Control of predisposing factors
  - Recommended topical preparations consist of antibiotics and steroid combinations
    - Quinolone antibiotic preparations may have broader microbial coverage and a low risk of contact dermatitis
    - Neomycin-containing topical preparations have potential for neomycin to cause contact sensitivity and lead to worsening of symptoms
      - Also have low risk of causing permanent sensorineural hearing loss
      - Use with caution in patients with perforated tympanic membranes
    - Acetic acid, boric acid, aluminum acetate, and silver nitrate also effective
  - In immunocompromised patients or if AOE spread beyond ear canal, consider using systemic antibiotics
    - Choice based on antipseudomonal and antistaphylococcal properties

Chronic Otitis Externa (COE)

- Persistent inflammatory disorder of ear canal
  - Usually caused by repeated mechanical debridement or water exposure
  - Other potential causes are allergic, contact dermatitis, or dermatologic disorders
  - Chronic inflammation may lead to development of granulation
- Treatment involves debridement, avoidance of ear canal manipulation, elimination of the offending agent, and topical corticosteroids
  - Regular flushing of canal with mild acidic solution, acetic acid or vinegar and distilled water, can help to eradicate infection and keep canal free of debris

Otomycosis

- A fungal infection of external ear canal
  - Constitutes roughly 10% of all cases of otitis externa
  - More common in geographic locations with a warm and humid climate, in patients following long-term topical

antibiotic therapy, and in patients with diabetes, HIV, or other immunocompromising condition
- Canal will often have cellulitis and edema on otoscopic examination
- Canal debris may have cheeselike or grayish appearance with visualized fungal hyphae
- *Aspergillus* species and *Candida* species most common pathogens
- Treatment consists of debridement, acidification, and drying of the ear canal
  - For candidal infections, topical antifungal therapy may also be effective

Necrotizing/Malignant Otitis Externa (MOE)

- MOE is an aggressive infection that begins as otitis externa but spreads through surrounding tissues toward the skull base.
  - Seen predominantly in the elderly, diabetic, or immunocompromised patient
  - *Pseudomonas aeruginosa* the most common causative pathogen
    - Staphylococcal species also known to cause infection
    - Fungal causes less common, *Aspergillus* species the predominating pathogen
- Initially presents with AOE symptoms and signs
  - Subsequently progresses to temporal bone osteomyelitis and affects adjacent cranial nerves (VII–XII), blood vessels, and soft tissue
  - If not treated aggressively can expand intracranially
  - On otoscopic examination, granulation tissue classically seen at bony-cartilaginous junction
    - Raised erythrocyte sedimentation rate (ESR) and abnormal computed tomography (CT) or magnetic resonation imaging (MRI) helps with confirmation
    - Other imaging techniques that assist in diagnosis include:
      ○ Gallium scan
      ○ Indium-labeled leukocyte scan
      ○ Technetium bone scan
      ○ Single photon emission tomographs
  - Treatment is with systemic antibiotics that cover pseudomonal and staphylococcal infection, including methicillin-resistant *Staphylococcus aureus*

Furunculosis (Ear Canal Abscess)

- A localized infection of ear canal usually caused by infected hair follicle
- May present with otalgia, otorrhea, and localized tenderness
- Tender, often fluctuant nodule within lateral ear canal identified on examination
- Most common pathogen is *S. aureus*
- Treatment includes application of heat, incision and drainage of the infected area, and systemic antibiotic treatment with staphylococcal coverage

Acute Otitis Media (AOM)

- AOM an inflammation of middle ear generally characterized by rapid onset of otalgia, aural fullness, and occasionally fever
  - In pediatrics common signs are irritability, sleeplessness, and pulling at affected ear
  - On pneumatic otoscopy, the tympanic membrane (TM) has red, opaque, and bulging appearance with decreased mobility due to accumulation of purulent fluid in middle ear space
  - Erythema of TM may be noted
    - If TM is ruptured patients will present with otorrhea
- Predominant pathogens in AOM are *Streptococcus pneumoniae, Haemophilus influenzae,* and *Moraxella catarrhalis*
- Observation for 24 to 48 hours in case of nonsevere illness in otherwise healthy individual >6 months old an initial option
  - If symptoms persist, antimicrobial therapy initiated
    - Amoxicillin recommended for initial treatment of AOM, dose of 80 to 90 mg/kg per day
    - In penicillin allergy, azithromycin, clarithromycin, erythromycin-sulfisoxazole, or trimethoprim-sulfamethoxazole used
    - With increased incidence of β-lactamase–producing organisms
      ○ Bacterial coverage expanded if no improvement within 48 to 72 hours
      ○ Rarely if pain or fever is excessive, immediate tympanocentesis or myringotomy required
- Otitis media with effusion is a presence of fluid in middle ear without signs or symptoms of acute ear infection and should be distinguished from AOM.
  - Otitis media with effusion occurs as a result of eustachian tube dysfunction or middle ear inflammation following acute infection.
    - Most common in pediatric population between ages of 6 months and 4 years
    - On pneumatic otoscopy, TM usually retracted, has decreased mobility, and air–fluid level or bubbles often visualized
    - Patients often report a decrease in hearing
  - Often self-limited and likely to resolve spontaneously within 3 months
  - If persistent, hearing testing is recommended, particularly in children with language delay, learning problems, or suspicion of significant hearing loss
  - With persistent middle ear effusion leading to hearing loss or structural damage, myringotomy with tympanostomy tube insertion should be considered
  - Decongestants not shown effective in treatment of middle ear effusion
  - In adult presenting with unilateral middle ear effusion, examination of nasopharynx performed to rule out possibility of nasopharyngeal mass causing obstruction of eustachian tube.

Chronic Otitis Media (COM)

- COM diagnosed when infection persists more than 1 to 3 months
- May present as:

- Chronic suppurative otitis media (CSOM) characterized by persistent bacterial infection and drainage from ear
- Chronic otitis media with effusion (COME) resulting from unresolving inflammation of middle ear and persistent middle ear secretions with intact TM
- COM may be associated with cholesteatoma
- Keratin cyst forming from accumulation of squamous debris in middle ear with potential for growth and erosion of surrounding structures
- CSOM will present with hearing loss, painless purulent otorrhea, and chronic TM perforation
  - Evaluation includes visual examination, bacterial culture, and radiographic imaging
  - Gram-negative and anaerobic organisms usually seen on cultures
    - *Pseudomonas aeruginosa* predominant organism
  - Temporal bone CT scan allows evaluation of extent of disease and reveals potential complications
  - Medical treatment of CSOM is topical debridement, topical and systemic antibiotics
    - Topical drops consist of antibiotic and steroid combinations
    - Ciprofloxacin recommended for systemic use
      - Cannot be given to children younger than 17 years old
  - Surgical treatment used for eradication of infection and middle ear reconstruction
- COME characterized by persistent hearing loss and middle ear space filled with thick mucus
  - Chronic inflammation of middle ear begins with obstruction of eustachian tube
    - Resulting negative pressure in middle ear leads to transudate
    - Secondary to chronic inflammation, middle ear lining becomes hyperplastic and produces further mucus
  - On examination TM intact and has thickened, opaque appearance
    - Pneumatic otoscopy shows TM not moving
    - With progression TM retracts and drapes over ossicles
    - Nasal obstruction and sinus disease may contribute to eustachian tube insufficiency and lead to middle ear fluid accumulation
    - Treatment of COME consists of fluid drainage, which is accomplished by myringotomy with ventilation tube insertion
    - Treating sinus disease and relieving nasal obstruction may improve eustachian tube function
- Untreated acute or chronic OM may lead to complications (Table 74.1).

Labyrinthitis

- Inflammation or infection of vestibular apparatus
- Patients present with vertigo, nausea, vomiting, and malaise
- Cause most often viral or traumatic but can be bacterial
  - Bacterial labyrinthitis often arises as spread of infection from meningitis or OM
  - Can be serous or suppurative
- Viral infections such as mumps, measles, Lassa fever, varicella-zoster, and herpes simplex associated with labyrinthitis

TABLE 74.1

COMPLICATIONS OF OTITIS MEDIA

Intratemporal
Tympanic membrane perforation
Mastoiditis
Petrositis
Facial nerve paralysis
Labyrinthitis
Ossicular discontinuity

Intracranial
Meningitis
Extradural abscess
Subdural empyema
Encephalitis
Brain abscess
Sigmoid sinus thrombosis
Hydrocephalus

- Labyrinthitis may or may not be associated with a sensorineural hearing loss, which can be temporary or permanent depending on cause, patient's age, and severity of loss

Bell's Palsy

- Defined as acute unilateral peripheral facial nerve weakness
- Diagnosis made when other causes of facial nerve paralysis such as systemic diseases, infection, trauma, central nervous system disorders, and neoplasm ruled out
- Usually present with abrupt onset of unilateral facial weakness
  - Other symptoms may include numbness or pain around ear, decreased taste, and increased sensitivity to sounds
- Herpes simplex virus thought to be etiologic factor for disease
- Most commonly occurs in individuals between 10 to 40 years of age
  - Pregnant women and diabetics at higher risk
- Usually spontaneously improves within 6 months
  - Residual facial nerve weakness persists in about 15%
- Treatment consists of early administration of high-dose prednisone and acyclovir
  - Artificial tears and protecting the eyes during sleep prevent corneal abrasion and eye infection
  - Treatment should be initiated within 72 hours of onset of symptoms

Ramsay Hunt Syndrome

- Caused by reactivation of varicella-zoster virus (VZV) in geniculate ganglion
- Associated with eruption of auricular or oropharyngeal vesicular rash, facial paralysis, and otalgia
  - Tinnitus, hearing loss, nausea, vomiting, vertigo, and nystagmus can accompany
- Patients with Ramsay Hunt syndrome present more severe symptoms and have a worse prognosis for recovery of facial nerve function relative to patients with Bell's palsy.

- Timing between onset of facial paralysis and vesicular eruption may vary.
- Some patients present with facial paralysis, have a rise in VZV antibody, but never develop cutaneous manifestations.
  - Termed *Ramsay Hunt sine herpete* and often labeled as Bell's palsy
- Initiation of early treatment with prednisone and acyclovir is currently recommended.

Chondritis/Perichondritis

- Chondritis/perichondritis of the ear is an infection of auricular cartilage/perichondrium
  - Often caused by penetrating injury to ear, particularly piercing of pinna
  - Blunt trauma with auricular hematoma can lead to infection
  - Cartilage involvement can also be seen in spreading otitis externa
  - Due to its relative avascularity, cartilage is more susceptible to infection
  - Infections are more often reported during warm weather, after exposure to water in pools, lakes, or hot tubs
- Patients present with a very tender, erythematous, and indurated auricle
  - Generally doughy on palpation and rarely fluctuant
  - *Pseudomonas aeruginosa* the most likely cause of the infection
- Treatment consists of removing foreign body and drainage of abscess or hematoma
  - Treat aggressively with antibiotics providing coverage for *Pseudomonas*
  - Cartilage necrosis or subperichondrial fibrosis, leading to auricular deformity, may be seen following infectious process.
  - Recurrent auricular chondritis raises suspicion for diagnosis of relapsing polychondritis.

NASAL INFECTIONS

Septal Abscess

- Rare and is defined as collection of pus between cartilaginous (bony) nasal septum and overlying mucoperichondrium or mucoperiosteum
  - Leading cause is trauma that leads to septal hematoma
  - Also shown in association with influenza, sinusitis, nasal furuncle, and dental infection
  - Immunocompromised patients at higher risk of dangerous complications
- Patients complain of nasal congestion, nasal pain, fever, and headache
  - On examination there is evidence of anterior intranasal mass
    - The septum will appear swollen and fluctuant
- Most common causative organisms are *S. aureus* and group A β-hemolytic streptococcus
  - *Staphylococcus epidermidis, S. pneumoniae, H. influenzae,* and anaerobes possible pathogens
- Treatment involves antibiotics and surgical drainage
  - Ischemic necrosis of septal cartilage may lead to saddle nose deformity or septal perforation

- Complications may involve intracranial infections such as meningitis, brain abscess, and subarachnoid empyema.

Rhinoscleroma

- A chronic infectious granulomatous disease originates in nose but can involve any part of respiratory tract
  - More common in the Middle East, parts of Latin America, and Eastern Europe
  - Often diagnosed in young adults
- Three clinical stages are recognized:
  - The catarrhal-atrophic stage: mucosal congestion and suppurative discharge
  - The granulomatous stage: presents with epistaxis and nasal deformity and is associated with granulomatous nodules and infiltration
  - The sclerotic stage: fibrosis and stenosis develop
- Typically patients present with crusting and nodular thickening of the nasal mucosa
- Biopsy and culture of diseased area provides diagnosis
- Presence of *Klebsiella rhinoscleromatis* diagnostic
- Diagnosis is usually made in the proliferation stage
  - Biopsy shows an abundance of Mikulicz cells
  - Surgical debridement, prolonged antibiotic therapy effective against disease
    - Streptomycin, tetracycline, rifampin, second- or third-generation cephalosporins, and fluoroquinolones effective
  - Treatment requires months to years, and relapses are common.
  - Patients require long-term follow-up with repeat cultures and biopsies.

Rhinosinusitis

Acute Bacterial Rhinosinusitis

- Most often develops following a viral upper respiratory infection
  - Presenting diagnostic symptoms include purulent nasal discharge; nasal congestion; maxillary, tooth, or facial pain; and worsening of symptoms following initial improvement
  - Other symptoms include general malaise and a more generalized headache, fever unusual
  - Predisposing physiologic factors include obstruction of sinus ostia, reduction in number or function of sinus cilia, and a change in the quality of secretions
- Most common pathogens are *S. pneumoniae, H. influenzae, Moraxella catarrhalis,* and *S. aureus*
- In immunocompromised, cystic fibrosis, and sinusitis of nosocomial origin (on mechanical ventilation, with nasal tubing) patients, *P. aeruginosa* and other aerobic Gram-negative rods common causative pathogens
  - Anaerobic bacteria usually associated with sinusitis of dental origin
  - Often difficult to distinguish between viral and bacterial sinusitis
- Diagnosis usually based on medical history and clinical findings
  - Bacterial sinusitis symptoms usually present for >7 days

- Sinus puncture with aspiration of sinus contents the most accurate diagnostic technique
- Radiographic imaging may help confirm the presence of sinus disease
  - Plain films difficult to interpret
  - CT the preferred examination and findings will include thickened mucosa, sinus opacification, or air–fluid levels
  - Nasal endoscopy often demonstrates swelling within middle meatus or sphenoethmoidal recess, with purulent discharge
- Antimicrobial treatment of acute sinusitis includes amoxicillin, amoxicillin-clavulanic acid, cephalosporins, trimethoprim-sulfamethoxazole, macrolides, doxycycline, and quinolones.
  - Can be supplemented with nasal saline irrigation, antihistamines, decongestants, and intranasal steroids
  - If not treated, may be complicated by development of several orbital and intracranial complications, particularly when the infection involves the ethmoid, frontal, or sphenoid sinuses (Table 74.2).

Chronic Bacterial Rhinosinusitis

- Diagnosed when symptoms present for at least 12 weeks
  - Symptoms similar to acute infection, with nasal congestion and purulent discharge predominating, sometimes associated with facial pressure, aural fullness, and anosmia
  - Nasal endoscopy may reveal nasal polyps, edema, or purulent discharge
  - CT findings show mucosal thickening, sinus opacification, polyps, or air–fluid levels
  - Predisposing factors include smoking, inhalant allergies, obstruction of ostiomeatal complex, immune deficiency, and genetic factors.
  - Pathogens are similar to those found in acute infections, greater predominance of staphylococcus, *Pseudomonas*, and possibly anaerobes.
    - Most common anaerobic bacteria include *Peptostreptococcus* species, *Fusobacterium* species, *Prevotella* and *Porphyromonas* species
- In cases of *P. aeruginosa*, aminoglycosides, fourth-generation cephalosporins, or fluoroquinolones used

TABLE 74.2

POTENTIAL COMPLICATIONS OF SINUSITIS

Acute sinusitis
  Orbital
    Periorbital cellulitis
    Orbital cellulitis
    Subperiosteal abscess
    Orbital abscess
    Optic neuritis
    Cavernous sinus thrombosis
  Intracranial
    Meningitis
    Epidural abscess
    Subdural empyema
    Brain abscess
Chronic sinusitis
  Mucocele
  Osteitis/osteomyelitis

- More prolonged course of antibiotic therapy may be required, from 3 to 6 weeks
- Adjunctive therapy including decongestants, mucolytics, and steroids may be helpful
- Nonresponders to medical therapy are considered for surgical drainage

Viral Rhinosinusitis

- Viral rhinosinusitis more common than bacterial
- Most common pathogens are rhinovirus, influenza viruses, adenoviruses, parainfluenza viruses, and respiratory syncytial virus
- Inflammatory symptoms of viral rhinosinusitis thought due to host response to virus
- Present with symptoms of common cold such as nasal congestion, nasal discharge, sneezing, cough, fever, malaise, and muscle ache
- Usually self-limited
- Antiviral therapy may be used for specific viruses
- Nasal saline irrigation and anti-inflammatories may aid with symptomatic relief

Fungal Rhinosinusitis

- **Acute Necrotizing Fungal Rhinosinusitis.** A fulminant invasive infection often life threatening
- Usually affects immunocompromised patients
  - Diabetics, immunodeficiency disorders, undergoing chemotherapy, or requiring prolonged stays in intensive care unit
- Present with acute onset of fever, headache, cough, mucosal ulcerations, and epistaxis
- Examination shows nasal eschar spreading through mucosa, soft tissue, and bone
- Histopathology shows necrosis and inflammatory infiltrate with giant cells, lymphocytes, and neutrophils
  - Gomori methenamine silver or periodic acid-Schiff histologic fungal stains demonstrate tissue and vascular invasion by fungal hyphae
- Common pathogens are *Aspergillus*, *Rhizopus*, and *Mucor* species
- Treatment involves emergent surgical debridement, intravenous antifungals such as amphotericin B, and treatment of the underlying immunocompromising disorder.
- If not treated may lead to rapid dissemination and death
- **Chronic Invasive Fungal Rhinosinusitis.** A chronic, more indolent, and slowly invasive fungal infection
- Usually affects immunocompromised patients
  - Also been reported in otherwise healthy individuals
- Present with orbital apex syndrome due to the extension of the infection into orbit
  - Decreased vision, ocular immobility, and proptosis
  - Erosion may also occur into infratemporal fossa, anterior cranial fossa, or premaxillary region
  - Histopathology reveals a dense accumulation of hyphae, with a chronic inflammatory infiltrate of lymphocytes, giant cells, and necrotizing granulomas
- Untreated may invade cerebral blood vessels, leading to ischemic injury or directly invade the brain
- Treatment involves repeated surgical debridement and antifungal drugs

ORAL CAVITY

Gingivitis

- Affects 50% to 90% of adult population
  - Caused by oral microflora in accumulating dental plaque
    - Usually contains both aerobic and anaerobic bacteria
  - A reversible disease
    - Chronic gingivitis leads to bleeding of gums during tooth brushing
    - May progress to periodontitis, leading to loss of supporting connective tissue and alveolar bone
      - This is nonreversible and may lead to loss of involved teeth
- Treatment involves good oral hygiene and mechanical removal of plaque and calculus

Acute Necrotizing Ulcerative Gingivitis (Trench Mouth)

- A rare periodontal disease characterized by gingival necrosis, ulceration, pain, and bleeding
  - Most commonly seen in young adults with sudden onset of gingival inflammation
  - Gingival lacerations covered with gray membranes and gingival bleeding noted
  - Causative organisms are fusospirochetal bacteria, pathogenic with compromised immune system function
    - *Bacteroides* and *Selenomonas* species also implicated
  - Diagnosis is based on clinical findings
  - Risk factors include dental crowding, physical fatigue, increased stress, low socioeconomic status, immunosuppression, smoking, and poor oral hygiene
- Treatment includes eliminating precipitating factors, treatment of underlying immunosuppression, oral hygiene, mechanical debridement of affected areas, and antibiotics
  - Penicillin or metronidazole is recommended for antibiotic treatment

Herpetic Gingival Stomatitis

- An infection due to herpes simplex virus
  - Most commonly manifests in children between the ages of 2 and 5 years
  - Present with fever and irritability, oropharyngeal pain, mucosal edema, and erythema
  - Vesicular lesions appear on mobile or nonkeratinized mucosal surfaces (buccal, labial) and attached or keratinized surfaces (gingiva, hard palate).
    - Usually rupture within 24 hours, leaving small ulcers with an elevated margin
  - Diagnosis confirmed by viral studies and biopsy
  - Treatment usually supportive, although acyclovir may shorten severity and duration

Herpangina

- Disease that commonly occurs in children
  - Coxsackie A virus most common causative organism
  - Present with fever, malaise, and sore throat
  - On examination oropharyngeal erythema noted
  - Vesicles and small ulcers present on the posterior pharynx, often on the uvula and soft palate
  - Course usually self-limiting

Candidiasis

- Caused by overgrowth of *Candida albicans*
- Often patient predisposed, with a history of immunosuppression, radiation, or altered microflora following long-term broad-spectrum antibiotic use
  - Pseudomembranous form, yellow-white plaques are present likened to milk curds
  - Erythematous form, these plaques have disappeared
  - Diagnosis confirmed with potassium hydroxide staining revealing fungal hyphae
  - Initial therapy usually consists of oral hygiene and topical treatment
    - Oral nystatin preparations, amphotericin lozenges, and clotrimazole troches
    - Ketoconazole, fluconazole, or itraconazole used for systemic treatment if indicated

Odontogenic Infections

- Originate from infected pulp and may spread to fascial spaces of head and neck where abscess may form
  - Most common causative organisms *S. aureus*, group A streptococci, and anaerobic bacteria
  - Treatment with broad-spectrum antibiotics recommended

Ludwig's Angina

- Infection involving left and right sublingual and submandibular spaces
  - Most often seen in adults with poor dentition, usually from infection involving second or third molar
  - Other sources include inflammation of tongue or floor of mouth and lingual tonsillitis
  - Present with submandibular swelling but not fluctuance
    - Swelling of floor of mouth pushing tongue upward/backward toward palate
    - In advanced disease, may present in acute distress with fever, difficulty handling secretions, and dyspnea that favors a seated and head forward position
  - Can be rapidly progressive, leading to airway compromise
  - Anaerobic organisms and streptococci most common causes
  - Treatment requires close airway monitoring with prophylactic tracheotomy in most cases for airway protection, administration of antibiotics, and surgical drainage

PHARYNX

Tonsillitis/Pharyngitis

- Common disease characterized by infection of the nasopharynx and oropharynx and associated lymphoid tissue
  - Acute tonsillopharyngitis caused by viral or bacterial infection; virus most common
  - Often difficult to distinguish between a bacterial and viral cause

- Present with fever, malaise, odynophagia, and lymphadenitis
- Examination shows tonsillar enlargement, erythema, and exudate
- Upper respiratory viruses such as rhinovirus, coronavirus, and adenovirus most common
- Most common cause is group A β-hemolytic streptococci (GABHS)
  - Diagnosed by performing a group A streptococcus test
  - Other pathogens associated with disease such as *M. catarrhalis, H. influenzae, S. aureus,* and *S. pneumoniae*
  - Diphtheria and gonococcal infections should also be considered
- Penicillin, amoxicillin, erythromycin, or first-generation cephalosporins recommended for treatment
  - Recommended to perform group A streptococcus test prior to initiation of antimicrobials
  - Untreated may lead to complications that can be suppurative and nonsuppurative
    - Nonsuppurative include scarlet fever, acute rheumatic fever, and poststreptococcal glomerulonephritis
    - Suppurative complications include peritonsillar, parapharyngeal, and retropharyngeal cellulites and/or abscess
  - Recurrent infections unresponsive to antimicrobials might require tonsillectomy

Peritonsillar Abscess

- The most common deep infection of the head and neck
  - Occurs as complication of bacterial tonsillitis or infrequently infectious mononucleosis
  - Most commonly diagnosed in adults or adolescents
    - Present with increasing pharyngeal pain, dysphagia, trismus, dysarthria, drooling, and muffled voice
    - Clinical examination reveals trismus, peritonsillar bulging that displaces the soft palate medially, and uvular deviation toward opposite side
    - Often see tonsillar exudates and tender cervical lymphadenopathy
  - Usually polymicrobial, with group A streptococci and anaerobes the most common pathogens
  - Diagnosis usually made on physical examination
    - CT scan may help if diagnosis uncertain
  - Treatment involves aspiration or incision and drainage of the abscess along with antibiotic therapy
  - If recurrent, a tonsillectomy indicated
  - Peritonsillar space infection has potential for spreading to parapharyngeal space, manifestations of which may be delayed

Lemierre Syndrome

- Described as presence of oropharyngeal infection, sepsis, internal jugular vein thrombosis, and septic emboli caused by *Fusobacterium necrophorum*
  - A Gram-negative anaerobic organism part of normal human oropharyngeal, gastrointestinal, or genitourinary flora
  - Disease rather uncommon due to the availability of antibiotics

- Most often affects young adults with recent history of oropharyngeal, tonsillar, or peritonsillar infection
- Present with tenderness and swelling of the lateral neck, secondary to thrombophlebitis of the internal jugular vein
- Septic emboli may spread and affect other organs, especially the lungs
- Requires immediate antibiotic treatment with clindamycin, metronidazole, ampicillin-sulbactam, or ticarcillin-clavulanate for period of at least 6 weeks
  - In case of abscess formation, surgical drainage might be required
  - Rarely ligation or excision of the jugular vein might be indicated

Infectious Mononucleosis

- A systemic disease caused by Epstein-Barr virus (EBV)
- Most commonly occurs in teenagers and young adults
- Transmitted through saliva
- Present with fever, fatigue, malaise, sore throat, generalized nontender lymphadenopathy
- On examination see inflamed tonsils with exudate
  - Hepatosplenomegaly may also be present
  - Diagnosis confirmed by the presence of atypical lymphocytes on peripheral smear, a positive monospot test, and positive EBV titers
- Treatment of mononucleosis supportive
  - Corticosteroids used to decrease inflammation, particularly where airway obstruction a concern
  - In severe cases of airway obstruction, a secure airway indicated
  - Patients develop a rash if treated with amoxicillin for presumed bacterial tonsillitis; thus administration of amoxicillin should be avoided

LARYNX/AIRWAY

Supraglottitis/Epiglottitis

- An infectious disease of epiglottis and supraglottis, most commonly bacterial in origin
  - Usually sudden onset, with high fever, pain with swallowing, drooling due to difficulty handling secretions, and respiratory distress
  - On presentation patient often found sitting in hunched-forward position with extended neck and open mouth (sniffing position)
  - Lateral neck film, edema of epiglottis and a ballooning of the hypopharynx (thumb sign) noted (Fig. 74.1)
  - Epiglottis will appear erythematous (cherry-red) and swollen on direct examination
  - Airway manipulation may quickly precipitate complete airway obstruction
- *H. influenzae* type b used to be most common causative agent
  - With the vaccine incidence of *H. influenzae*-related epiglottitis significantly decreased
  - Currently *S. pneumoniae*, group A β-hemolytic streptococci the most common causative agents

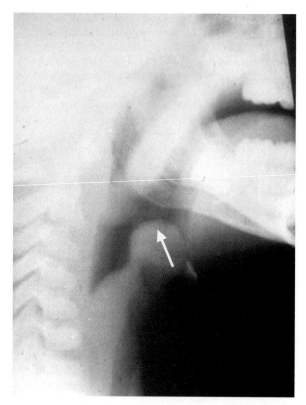

FIGURE 74.1. Lateral plain neck radiograph demonstrating edema of the epiglottis associated with epiglottitis.

- Considered emergency as it has potential for rapid complete airway obstruction, particularly in children
  - When diagnosed, a secure airway should be established via endotracheal intubation or tracheostomy.
  - Decision to extubate or decannulate based on clinical improvement
  - Treatment with intravenous ceftriaxone or ampicillin/ sulbactam, and steroids
  - Adults may present with supraglottitis where epiglottitis not involved
    - Here the airway can be managed conservatively, although close in-hospital observation required

Laryngitis

- Acutely most often occurs as part of upper respiratory infection, usually caused by rhinovirus
  - Laryngoscopy reveals diffuse laryngeal erythema and edema
  - Treatment often supportive: voice rest, humidification, and anti-inflammatory medications

Croup

- An inflammatory disease of subglottic airway
  - Almost always associated with parainfluenza and influenza viruses
  - Most commonly occurs in pediatric population between the ages of 1 and 3 years
  - Present with fever, tachypnea, inspiratory stridor, hoarseness, and a barking cough
  - History often includes a preceding upper respiratory infection

- Patients require close observation and sometimes establishment of a secure airway
  - Glucocorticoids recommended to decrease airway inflammation
    - Racemic epinephrine treatments often helpful
  - When recurrent, airway evaluation with laryngoscopy and bronchoscopy recommended to assess for anatomic abnormalities

Diphtheria

- An infectious disease of the upper airway
  - Caused by *Corynebacterium diphtheriae*
  - Rather rare due to widespread immunization
  - Present with fever and malaise
    - Bloody nasal discharge and pseudomembranes in nose, oropharynx, and larynx noted on examination
    - Membranes may lead to airway obstruction and respiratory failure
  - Exotoxins produced by bacteria may affect heart, liver, kidney, and brain
  - Diagnosis confirmed by bacterial smear and cultures on Löffler or tellurite media
  - Treatment consists of ensuring secure airway, administration of antitoxin, and antibiotics
    - Penicillin or erythromycin recommended

Bacterial Tracheitis

- A rare, potentially life-threatening respiratory infection
  - Characterized by presence of thick membranous tracheal secretions that do not readily clear with coughing and may lead to occlusion of airway
  - Present with fever, cough, stridor, and generalized malaise
  - Does not respond to racemic epinephrine treatment
  - Radiographically irregular tracheal margins with a normal-appearing epiglottis
  - Diagnosis made with direct visualization of thick membranous tracheal secretions or the presence of purulent tracheal secretions in glottis and subglottis
  - Most commonly isolated pathogen is *S. aureus*
    - Other pathogens include *H. influenzae*, *S. pneumoniae*, *Streptococcus pyogenes*, *M. catarrhalis*, *Klebsiella*, and *Pseudomonas* species
  - Treatment consists of securing airway, endoscopically removing tracheal membranes, and administration of antibiotics

NECK

Salivary Gland Infections

Viral Infections

- **Mumps.** A viral infection caused by paramyxovirus; the most common viral infection involving salivary glands
  - Other viruses that infect salivary glands are coxsackie A, echovirus, choriomeningitis, parainfluenza type 1 and 3, and cytomegalovirus
- Patients display signs of fever and malaise

- Painful parotid swelling occurs within 24 hours; is often bilateral
  - May experience pain with salivation
- 10% of patients have submandibular gland involvement
- 25% of affected adolescent or adult males develop orchitis
  - 5% of females present with oophoritis
- Mastitis, pancreatitis, and central nervous system involvement may also occur in affected individuals.
- Mumps infection can also lead to sensorineural hearing loss.
- Treatment usually supportive
- In children the disease has a less severe course than in adults

Bacterial Infections

- Often develop following salivary stasis, secondary to ductal obstruction by a stone or mass, or a decrease of salivary flow secondary to dehydration
- Most common causative pathogens are *S. aureus* and *Streptococcus viridans*
- Parotid gland affected more often, likely due to lower bacteriostatic activity of saliva from this gland compared to submandibular or sublingual glands
- Present with pain, swelling, and erythema in the region of the salivary gland
  - Exacerbated by eating
- Also have fever, malaise, and an elevated white blood cell count
- Treatment involves hydration to increase salivary flow, massaging affected gland, sialogogues, and administration of antistaphylococcal antibiotics
  - Chronic/recurrent disease, removal of obstruction or excision of gland recommended

Lymphadenitis

- An inflammatory process involving lymph nodes
- Pediatric group more commonly affected
  - Upper respiratory viral infections the most common cause of cervical lymphadenopathy
  - Condition is self-limited and usually does not require treatment
  - Bacterial lymphadenitis occurs as complication of skin or respiratory infection
    - Most common causative organisms are *S. aureus* and group A streptococci
    - Present with tender lymphadenopathy, may progress to abscess formation
    - Treatment with β-lactamase–resistant antibiotics is recommended
    - With progression to abscess formation, incision and drainage indicated

Catscratch Disease

- Usually presents with subacute solitary or regional lymphadenopathy in patients with a previous contact with a kitten or cat
  - Primarily caused by *Bartonella henselae*
    - Cases of *Bartonella clarridgeiae* and *Bartonella elizabethae* reported
  - Lymphadenopathy occurs 1 to 3 weeks after a scratch, bite, or other contact
    - Small red-brown nontender papules develop at inoculation site 3 to 30 days after contact

- Lymph nodes draining affected site gradually enlarge; are moderately tender
  - Overlying skin appearing warm and erythematous
- Up to 10% of lesions may require surgical drainage
- Indirect fluorescent antibody test and enzyme immunoassay are used for detection of specific serum antibody to *B. henselae*

Mycobacterium

- Nontuberculous mycobacterial infection a rare cause of lymphadenitis
  - Presents as a slowly enlarging, nontender cervical mass
  - Can affect adults; most commonly found in children younger than 5 years of age
  - Often diagnosed after failure to respond to treatment with antibiotics
  - Most common causative pathogen is *Mycobacterium avium-intracellulare*
    - Other reported pathogens are *M. scrofulaceum*, *M. kanasasaii*, *M. fortuitum*, and *M. malmoense*
  - Intradermal purified protein derivative (PPD) test aids in diagnosis of nontuberculous lymphadenitis
    - Positive cultures more definitive
    - Complete surgical resection of infected tissues the gold standard for treatment
    - Treatment with antituberculous medications, such as macrolides (clarithromycin), shown to be effective in some cases
    - Antibiotic therapeutic trial prior to surgical excision or as an adjunct to surgical excision appropriate

Actinomycosis

- Infection caused by *Actinomyces israelii*, a Gram-positive anaerobic bacterium
  - Has multiple presentations and often misdiagnosed
  - Most infections occur in head and neck region (>50%)
    - Most often entering the tissue through an area of prior trauma
    - As infection develops, patients noted to have a woody induration
      - Eventually leads to central abscess formation
      - Abscess generally tracks to mucosal surface or externally to skin, forming sinus or fistulous tract
      - Suppurative drainage contains so-called sulfur granules, yellow flecks containing the bacterial colonies
      - Diagnosis best made by culture
        - But may have to rely on the clinical picture and histology
        - Organisms stain best with Gram and Gomori methenamine silver stains
        - Treatment is drainage and debridement of infected area with administration of penicillin.

Deep Neck Space Infections

Retropharyngeal Space Abscess

- Infection usually develops from infected retropharyngeal lymph nodes
  - More common in children
  - Trauma is another common cause

- Present with fever, pain with swallowing, decreased oral intake, drooling, malaise, and torticollis
- Trismus and neck swelling often present
- Most common causative organisms are *S. pyogenes* and anaerobic bacteria
- Lateral radiographic images of neck in extension show thickened prevertebral soft tissue
- CT aids in determining presence of an abscess
- Therapy involves administration of intravenous antibiotics and drainage of abscess
- Transoral drainage recommended unless extension lateral to great vessels (i.e., the carotid artery)
- Untreated, spontaneous rupture of abscess may lead to aspiration of infectious material
  - Spreading to parapharyngeal and prevertebral spaces, leading to mediastinitis, or involve the great vessels

Parapharyngeal Space Abscess

- Pharyngeal infections, molar tooth infections, gingivitis, mastoiditis may spread to parapharyngeal space
- Untreated, infection may spread to retropharyngeal space, mediastinum, and involve great vessels causing internal jugular thrombosis and erosion of internal carotid artery
- Present with a prior history of a sore throat or tooth infection
- Initial symptoms are fever and pain with swallowing
- Tender, erythematous swelling at angle of mandible and parotid typically found
  - Does not appear fluctuant even if abscess present
- Examination of pharynx often shows medial displacement of ipsilateral tonsil
- Trismus may develop; torticollis toward opposite side often results from inflammation of lymph nodes under sternocleidomastoid muscle
- Patients may also complain of otalgia; airway compromise may occur
- Most common causative pathogens are *S. aureus, S. pyogenes,* and anaerobic bacteria
- CT aids in evaluation of site and extent of infection, distinguishing between cellulitis and abscess
- Require immediate treatment with intravenous antibiotics and surgical drainage if abscess present

CHAPTER 75 ■ CATHETER-RELATED BLOODSTREAM INFECTIONS (CRBSI)

- Intravascular devices are a ready conduit for bacterial and fungal invasion, resulting in catheter-related bloodstream infections (CRBSI). (Table 75.1)
- Can be complicated by:
  - Septic thrombophlebitis
  - Infective endocarditis
  - Other metastatic infections, such as lung abscess, brain abscess, and endophthalmitis
- The most common cause of hospital-acquired infections in the critically ill.
  - \>80,000 CRBSIs are estimated to occur annually in ICUs in the United States.
  - Attributable mortality ranging from 12% to 25%
    - 9,600 to 20,000 patients die from CRBSI in ICUs annually.
  - Added cost ranges from $28,690 to $56,167 per individual episode in ICU patients.
  - Immunocompromised hosts with central venous catheters (CVCs) in place are also at significant risk.

PATHOGENESIS

- First step in primary infection is the colonization of the CVC.
- For short-term, nontunneled, noncuffed, multilumen catheters—which make up 90% of CRBSIs—the skin insertion site is the source of the colonization.
- Organisms migrate along catheter's external surface, through the subcutaneous layers, and infect the catheter tip.
- For long-term catheters—the cuffed, tunneled, silicone catheters, Hickman or Broviac—or implantable devices
  - Lumen of the hub or belt of the port is primary source of entry.
- Microorganisms are introduced via the hands of medical personnel while manipulating the hub during, for example, flushing and drawing of blood.
- Colonization is universal after insertion of a CVC, can occur as early as 1 day after insertion, **and is quantitatively independent of a catheter-related infection.**
- These sources explain the prevalence of primary organisms causing CRBSI:
  - *Staphylococcus aureus*
  - Coagulase-negative *Staphylococcus* (CNS)
  - Enterococci
  - Nonenteric hospital-acquired gram-negative bacilli
    - *Stenotrophomonas maltophilia*
    - *Pseudomonas aeruginosa*
    - *Acinetobacter* spp.
  - Mycobacteria
  - *Candida* spp.
- Secondary seeding of the CVC
  - Whereby organisms become bloodborne and colonize the catheter, has been suggested

TABLE 75.1

DEFINITIONS OF CATHETER-RELATED
BLOODSTREAM INFECTIONS

PROBABLE CRBSI
- Clinical manifestations of infection (fever >38°C, chills/rigors, or hypotension)
- No apparent source of the sepsis/bloodstream infection other than the catheter
- Common skin organisms (e.g., coagulase-negative staphylococci) isolated from two blood cultures from patients with intravascular device or a known pathogen (*Staphylococcus aureus* or *Candida*) isolated from a single blood culture

DEFINITE CRBSI
Probable CRBSI criteria outlined above with any of the following:
- Differential quantitative blood cultures with 5:1 ratio of the same organism isolated from blood drawn simultaneously from the central venous catheter (CVC) and peripheral vein

OR
- Differential positivity time (positive result of culture from a CVC is obtained at least 2 h earlier than positive result of culture from peripheral blood)

OR
- Positive quantitative skin culture whereby the organism isolated from an infected insertion site is identical to that isolated from blood

OR
- Isolation of the same organisms from the peripheral blood and from a quantitative or semiquantitative culture of a catheter segment or tip

- To the point of recommending treatment of urinary tract infections *prior* to CVC insertion to prevent a potential CRBSI
- Role in CRBSI has not been documented.
- Contamination of the infusate or additives, such as contaminated heparin flush, is a rare cause of colonization and infection of the vascular devices.
  - Nationwide outbreaks of *Enterobacter agglomerans* and *Enterobacter cloacae* in 1971 led to widespread changes and surveillance.
  - Nutritional components present in the total parenteral nutrition promote the growth of certain fungi such as *Candida parapsilosis* and *Malassezia furfur*, as well as bacteria such as *Klebsiella pneumoniae* and *E. cloacae*
- Second step in the pathogenesis of CRBSI
  - Ability of some microbes to form a biofilm of extracellular, polysaccharide-rich, slimy material
    - Promotes adhesiveness of bacteria to the surface of CVC
    - Form on the external surface of short-term catheters and the internal surface of long-term catheters—that is, those with a dwell time of at least 30 days
    - Enables bacteria not only to adhere to the surface of the catheter, but also to resist antibiotics, such that "chronic" biofilm eradication becomes a difficult task
    - Another factor promoting adherence is thrombin layer that covers both surfaces of a catheter during its insertion.

- Composition of the host's blood components enables *S. aureus*, for example, to adhere to fibrinogen, coagulase-negative *Staphylococcus* (CNS) to fibronectin, and *Candida* spp. to fibrin
- Other factors could also potentiate the risk for a CRBSI, including:
- Femoral catheterization
  - Associated with a higher rate of infections and thrombotic complications when compared to subclavian catheterization in a prospective randomized, controlled trial involving ICU patients
- Transparent occlusive dressings associated with significantly increased rates of insertion site colonization ($p < 0.001$) in patients having CVCs for more than 3 days when compared to gauze dressing
  - Explained by the warm atmosphere created by occlusive dressings, which promoted microbial growth

CLINICAL MANIFESTATIONS

- Clinical manifestations of CRBSIs can be divided into two categories: local and systemic.
- Local manifestations include:
  - Erythema
  - Edema
  - Tenderness
  - Purulent discharge
  - These are neither sensitive nor specific, and cannot be relied on to identify catheter colonization or CVC-related bloodstream infection
    - Peripherally inserted central catheters (inserted in the basilic or cephalic veins) are associated with a 26% rate of sterile local exit site inflammation secondary to irritation of small veins
    - CNS, the most frequent pathogen involved, incites little local or systemic inflammation
  - The Centers for Disease Control and Prevention suggested the following definitions:
    - *Exit-site infection*: Purulent drainage from the catheter exit site, or erythema, tenderness, and swelling within 2 cm of the catheter exit site, and colonization of the catheter if removed
    - *Port-pocket infection*: Erythema and/or necrosis of the skin or subcutaneous tissues either over or around the reservoir of an implanted catheter, and colonization of the catheter if removed
    - *Tunnel infection*: Erythema, tenderness, and induration of the tissues above the catheter and more than 2 cm from the exit site, and colonization of the catheter if removed
- The systemic features of CRBSIs:
  - Generally indistinguishable from those of secondary bloodstream infections arising from other foci of infection
  - Include
    - Fever and chills
    - May be accompanied by:
    - Hypotension
    - Hyperventilation
    - Altered mental status
    - Nonspecific gastrointestinal manifestations such as:
      - Nausea
      - Vomiting

– Abdominal pain
– Diarrhea
- Deep-seated infections such as endocarditis, osteomyelitis, retinitis, and organ abscess may complicate CRBSIs
  ○ Caused by some virulent organisms such as *S. aureus*, *P. aeruginosa*, and *Candida albicans*.

DIAGNOSIS

- Clinical diagnosis of CRBSI is frequently inaccurate
  - Removal of the CVC had previously been mandatory to prove the CRBSI
  - Microbiologic methods requiring removal of the CVC were studied with semiquantitative roll plate catheter cultures
    - Considered the gold standard
  - Majority of the catheters were removed unnecessarily
    - There are different methods used for the microbiologic diagnosis of CRBSI (Table 75.2)

Catheter-sparing Diagnostic Methods

Simultaneous Quantitative Blood Cultures

- Consists of obtaining paired quantitative blood cultures (QBCs) simultaneously from the CVL and peripheral vein
  - Both samples drawn <10 minutes apart **with the same volume of blood**
  - Hypothesis is that higher load of organisms on the internal lumen of CVL signifying CRBSI would translate into a colony count from CVL greater by manyfold than the peripheral stick.

TABLE 75.2

SENSITIVITY AND SPECIFICITY OF TESTS USED IN THE DIAGNOSIS OF CRBSI[a]

Diagnostic tests	Sensitivity	Specificity
Paired quantitative blood cultures	75%–93%	97%–100%
Differential time to positivity		
Short-term CVCs	89%	87%
Long-term CVCs	90%	72%
Acridine orange leukocyte cytospin technique	87%	94%
Semiquantitative culture of catheter tip (roll-plate technique)		
Short-term CVCs	84%	85%
Long-term CVCs	45%	75%
Quantitative catheter culture		
Short-term CVCs	82%	89%
Long-term CVCs	83%	97%

CRBSI, catheter-related bloodstream infection; CVC, central venous catheter.
[a]The data on the sensitivities and specificities are based on a meta-analysis of diagnostic methods by Safdar N, Fine JP, Maki DG. Meta-analysis: methods for diagnosing intravascular device-related bloodstream infection. *Ann Intern Med.* 2005;142[6]:451–466.

- CVL/peripheral ratio of CFU/mL of 5:1 has been chosen by the Infectious Diseases Society of America to represent true infection—this is what we use.
- Multiple cutoffs have been used, including 2:1, 3:1, 4:1, 5:1, and 10:1.
- Meta-analysis found that quantitative blood culture is the most accurate.
- Sensitivity of 75% to 93%
- Specificity of 97% to 100%
- Recommended culturing *only* if CRBSI is suspected clinically
- Method is limited by the fact that it is expensive and labor intensive, in addition to the difficulty in obtaining samples through the catheter in some cases.

Differential Time to Positivity

- Differential time to positivity (DTP) of qualitative paired CVC and peripheral blood culture is a more practical test for centers that lack the logistics for QBCs.
- Hypothesis suggests that time to positivity of a culture is closely related to the inoculum size of microorganisms.
- Technique involves measuring the difference between the time required for culture positivity in simultaneously drawn samples of catheter blood and peripheral blood.
- DTP of 120 minutes was associated with:
  - 81% sensitivity and 92% specificity for short-term catheters
  - 93% sensitivity and 75% specificity for long-term catheters
  - Meta-analysis showed that the DTP of 120 minutes predicts CRBSI
    - Sensitivity and specificity of 89% and 87% for short-term catheters
    - Sensitivity and specificity of 90% and 72% for long-term catheters
- Technique also demands a simultaneous blood draw (within 10 minutes) from CVL and peripheral vein **with the same amount of blood.**
- Limitation is that sensitivity could be compromised when antibiotics are given intraluminally at the time of drawing the blood cultures through the catheters.

Acridine Orange Cytospin Technique

- Test involves 1 mL of ethylenediaminetetraacetic acid (EDTA) blood aspirated through CVL.
  - The sample is added to 10% formalin saline solution for 2 minutes.
  - Then centrifuged, supernatant decanted, and the cellular deposit homogenized and cytocentrifuged
  - Monolayer is stained with 1 in 10,000 acridine orange staining and viewed by ultraviolet light.
  - Positive test is indicated by the presence of any bacteria.
- Method is expensive but takes 30 minutes.
  - Sensitivity of 87% and specificity of 94%
  - Technique only tested by a small group of investigators and is not easy to perform

Catheter-drawn Quantitative Blood Culture

- Method includes a single quantitative blood culture drawn through CVL.
  - Cutoff of 100 CFU/mL establishes the diagnosis.
  - Sensitivity of 81% to 86%, specificity of 85% to 96%
  - In pediatric cancer population, the technique showed a sensitivity of 75% and a specificity of 69%.

- Positive predictive value of 79%
- Likelihood ratio of 2.44
  - Odds of having a true CRBSI with the >100 CFU/mL cutoff increase by 2.44 when compared to <100 CFU/mL.
- Major drawback to technique is that it cannot distinguish between CRBSI and high-grade bacteremia, especially in immunocompromised patients.

Diagnostic Methods Requiring Catheter Removal

Semiquantitative Roll-plate Catheter Culture

- Described by Maki in 1977 and remains the international reference diagnostic method
  - Consists of rolling a 3- to 5-cm section of the distal tip of the CVL at least four times back and forth over an agar plate surface and leaving it to incubate overnight
  - Cutoff of ≥15 CFU defines catheter colonization.
  - If at the same time a peripheral culture grows with same organism, CRBSI is diagnosed.
  - Method does not sample the internal lumen of CVL.
    - Source of the infection in long-term catheters
  - Nevertheless, pooled sensitivity and specificity in 14 trials involving short-term catheters was 84% and 85%, respectively.
    - Decreased to 45% and 75%, respectively, with long-term CVLs
      - Those with more than 30 days of dwell time

Quantitative Catheter Cultures

- Involves flushing or sonicating a catheter segment in broth with the target of retrieving organisms from both surfaces of CVL
  - Threshold of ≥1,000 CFU correlated best with colonization.
  - CRBSI defined by same cutoff
    - Accompanied by high clinical suspicion and absence of evidence of other sites of infection
  - Sonication method had a higher sensitivity than the roll-plate method for long-term CVLs
  - Both sonication and vortexing had the same sensitivity and specificity of the roll-plate method for short-term CVLs.
    - Meta-analysis revealed:
      - Sensitivity and specificity of 82% and 89% for short-term catheters
      - Sensitivity and specificity of 83% and 97% for long-term catheters

Stain and Microscopy Rapid Diagnostic Techniques

- Method suggests staining of the removed catheter segments and subsequent microscopy testing.
  - Cutoff value of 1 organism per 20 oil immersion fields indicates catheter is colonized.
  - Reported 100% sensitivity, 97% specificity
  - Positive predictive value of 84%, and a negative predictive value of 100%
    - Not reproduced in another study
- In a similar technique, acridine orange staining has been used for diagnosis, in which fluorescence is indicative of positivity.
  - Sensitivity of 84% and a specificity of 99%

- Acridine orange staining is more easily performed than Gram staining.

PREVENTIVE STRATEGIES

- CVLs should only be used when medically necessary, and they should be removed as soon as possible to prevent potential complications.
- Reviewing 1,981 ICU months of data, collective antiseptic measures consisting of:
  - Hand washing
  - Maximal sterile barriers during insertion
  - Cutaneous antisepsis with Chlorhexidine
  - Avoidance of femoral site
  - Removal of CVCs determined to be unnecessary were associated with a significant decrease in CRBSI rate
    - From 7.7 per 1,000 catheter-days to 1.4 per 1,000 catheter-days ($p < 0.001$) over 18 months of follow-up
- When CVLs or pulmonary artery catheters were changed/exchanged over guidewire every 3 days
  - Former procedure resulted actually in an increase in the risk of mechanical complications
  - Latter technique increased the risk of bloodstream infection
- Preventive strategies to decrease colonization risk of CVLs are noted in Table 75.3.
- Novel strategies aiming at controlling all factors that could lead to colonization of CVL, and hence decreasing the rate of CRBSI have been reviewed and are noted in the following text.

Cutaneous Antiseptics

- Guidelines recommend with level 1A evidence usage of 2% chlorhexidine (CHX)-based preparation
  - Prospectively randomized study of 68 ICU patients to 10% povidone-iodine, 70% alcohol, or 2% aqueous chlorhexidine to disinfect the site before insertion of CVCs and for site care every other day thereafter
  - 2% aqueous chlorhexidine preparation tended to decrease rate of CRBSI.

TABLE 75.3

PREVENTIVE MEASURES TO DECREASE THE RISK OF COLONIZATION OF CENTRAL VENOUS LINES

- Hand hygiene
- Avoiding femoral site insertion if possible
- Removing unnecessary catheters
- Cutaneous antiseptic agents (2% chlorhexidine-based preparation)
- Maximal sterile barrier (handwashing, sterile gloves, large drape, and sterile gown, mask, and cap)
- Antimicrobial catheter lock solutions (a combination of an anticoagulant like heparin or ethylenediaminetetraacetic acid plus an antimicrobial agent, such as vancomycin, minocycline, or ciprofloxacin)
- Antimicrobial coating of catheter (with minocycline/rifampin or chlorhexidine/silver sulfadiazine)

- Lower concentrations of CHX decreased the effectiveness of this method.
  - Tincture of chlorhexidine gluconate 0.5% no more effective in preventing CRBSI or CVL colonization than 10% povidone-iodine,
- Meta-analysis of eight randomized trials found overall reduction of 49% in CRBSIs when disinfectant containing chlorhexidine was used.

Maximal Sterile Barrier

- Involves wearing a sterile gown, gloves, and a cap and using a large drape similar to those used in the operating room during catheter insertion
  - As opposed to the regular precautions consisting of sterile gloves and a small drape only
  - Healthcare Infection Control Practices Advisory Committee/Centers for Disease Control and Infection guidelines recommend this technique while inserting CVLs, PICC lines, and pulmonary artery catheters (category 1A).
  - Prospective study with long-term, nontunneled silicone CVLs and PICC lines in a cancer patient population demonstrated:
    - Reduction of CRBSIs ($p = 0.03$)
    - Practice was cost effective
  - Another prospective study with pulmonary artery catheters found less stringent barrier precautions associated with significantly increased risk of CRBSI (relative risk = 2.1, $p = 0.03$).
  - Technique failed to reduce arterial catheter-related colonization.

Antimicrobial Catheter Lock Solutions

- Antimicrobial catheter lock involves flushing catheter lumen and then filling with 2 to 3 mL of a combination of an anticoagulant plus an antimicrobial agent.
  - Dwell (lock) time varies between clinicians, but 20 to 24 hours is the most preferred.
    - Might not be possible if catheter has to be used
- Intervention often used in CVLs that remain in place longer than 30 days
  - Combination of vancomycin and heparin, with or without ciprofloxacin, was equivalent
  - Each was superior to heparin alone.
    - Heparin prevents formation of fibrin sheath on inner surface of line
- Four of six studies revealed a significant reduction in CRBSI with the above lock solution; two demonstrated no benefit.
- Vancomycin-heparin lock solutions did not promote vancomycin resistance.
  - Risk of superinfection with gram-negative bacilli and *Candida* is present because vancomycin spectrum is limited to gram-positive bacteria.
  - Meta-analysis concluded that the use of vancomycin lock solution in high-risk patient populations being treated with long-term central intravascular devices (IVDs) reduces the risk of bloodstream infection with a risk ratio of 0.34 (95% confidence interval [CI], 0.12–0.98; $p = 0.04$).

- Minocycline and EDTA (M-EDTA) was reported in a prospective randomized trial to significantly reduce the risk of catheter colonization and infection when compared with heparin in long-term hemodialysis CVLs,
  - Solution superior in an *in vitro* biofilm model and in an animal model to vancomycin-heparin lock solution
  - Study of pediatric cancer populations showed M-EDTA significantly reduces risk of catheter infection and colonization when compared to heparin
- Prospective nonrandomized study of tunneled CVLs in pediatric cancer population:
  - Ethanol used as a lock solution and reduced risk of relapse of CRBSI and was well tolerated
    - Symptoms of fatigue, nausea, dizziness, and headache were reported,
  - Involved filling catheter lumen with 2.3 mL of a 74% ethanol solution for 20 to 24 hours
  - Solution then flushed through to prevent clotting inside the catheter
  - Each port was alternately blocked for 3 days, allowing the unblocked port to be used.
  - Recent study showed M-EDTA in 25% ethanol highly effective in eradicating organisms embedded in biofilm.
    - Even after a short exposure of 15 to 60 minutes
- Prolonged dwell time of more than 8 hours often required for nonalcohol-based antibiotic lock solutions.
  - Makes use limited, particularly in critically ill patients those requiring total parenteral nutrition

Antimicrobial Impregnation of Catheters

- Consists of impregnation of external and/or internal surface of the catheter with antiseptic or antibiotics
  - Slow release of antimicrobials would prevent initial bacterial adherence and biofilm formation, with virtually undetectable serum levels.
  - Healthcare Infection Control Practices Advisory Committee/Centers for Disease Control and Infection, with a category 1B, recommends use of the coated CVLs.
    - First-generation catheters were impregnated on the external surface with CHX and silver sulfadiazine (CHX/SSD).
    - Technique lowered the rate of CRBSI from 7.6 to 1.6 cases per 1,000 catheter-days ($p = 0.03$)
      - With a decrease in the rate of colonization (relative risk, 0.56 [95% CI, 0.36–0.89]; $p = 0.005$)
      - Estimated cost savings per CVL was $196.
      - Other studies failed to show that difference.
      - Explained by the fact that short-term catheter infection is due to external colonization
      - Long-term CRBSIs due to internal colonization not prevented by external coating
      - Catheters do not protect if the CVL dwell time is more than 3 weeks, secondary to wearing off of the antimicrobial activity.
    - Second-generation CHX/SSD-coated catheters impregnated on both surfaces
      - Multicenter, randomized double-blind prospective study from 14 French ICUs: Second-generation catheters failed to decrease the rate of CRBSI when compared to noncoated catheters.

– They significantly decreased the rate of colonization (from 11 to 3.6/1,000 catheter-days, $p = 0.01$).
- 1997 polyurethane catheter impregnated on both surfaces with minocycline-rifampin (M/R)
  ○ Prospective trial comparing M/R catheters with first-generation CHX/SSD-impregnated catheters found that:
    – Former was three times less likely to be colonized ($p <0.001$).
    – CRBSI was 12-fold more likely to occur in the CHX/SSD catheters ($p <0.002$).
  ○ The use of antibiotic-impregnated CVCs in medical and surgical units was associated with a significant decrease in nosocomial bloodstream infections, including vancomycin-resistant enterococci (VRE) bacteremia, catheter-related infections, and length of hospital and ICU stay.
  ○ M/R-coated catheters saved $9,600 per each CRBSI and $81 per each catheter placed when compared to first-generation CHX/SSD.
- Concern for emergence of antibiotic-resistant organisms raised with M/R coated catheters
  ○ Four prospective studies evaluated skin at catheter insertion site before and after the insertion of antibiotic-coated catheters.
    – Failed to detect any emergence of resistance
  ○ Retrospective review of M/R-coated CVL experience in bone marrow transplant patients also detected no emergence of resistance of *Staphylococci* to either component
- M/R-coated CVLs are shown to bring risk of CRBSI to a level ≤0.3 per 1,000 catheter-days in nontunneled, non-cuffed CVLs.
  ○ Lower than the 1.4 per 1,000 catheter-days achieved with multiple other aseptic measures applied collectively

Silver-impregnated Catheters

- Other catheters incorporate silver, platinum, and carbon (SPC) into the polyurethane, allowing topical silver ion release.
- A prospective randomized study compared these catheters to the M/R-coated type.
  - The latter was more efficacious in reducing, to a significant degree, CVL colonization with gram-positive and gram-negative bacteria ($p = 0.039$).
  - CRBSI rates were low and similar between the two groups.
- Another prospective, randomized, controlled, open-label, multicenter clinical trial resulted in SPC CVLs failing to show any benefit in reducing CRBSI or colonization.

MANAGEMENT

- Management of CRBSIs involves:
- Confirming the source of infection
- Determining the choice of antimicrobials
- Determining the duration of therapy
- Deciding whether to remove the catheters
- Confirmation of the infection is dependent on the diagnostic measures outlined above

- Duration of therapy depends on whether the infection is complicated (i.e., by a septic phlebitis or endocarditis) or uncomplicated

Coagulase-negative *Staphylococcus*

- CNS are the primary organisms involved in CRBSIs, as they are the most common skin organisms.
- For the same reason, they are most frequent blood contaminants.
- QBC collected through CVL, with a cutoff point of 15 CFU/mL, could be a useful laboratory criterion, together with positive clinical findings for differentiating true bacteremia from false-positive contaminated blood cultures.
- Sensitivity of 96%, specificity of 94%, positive predictive value of 86%, and negative predictive value of 98%
- The Infectious Disease Society of America (IDSA) guidelines recommend removing CVL and treating for 5 to 7 days.
  - If CVL is to be retained, duration of treatment should be 10 to 14 days.
    ○ Antibiotic lock therapy should be considered.
  - Leaving CVL in place carries a risk of recurrence of 20%.
- Lock solutions used included vancomycin plus heparin.
  - Limited activity of vancomycin against *Staphylococcus* embedded in biofilms led other alternatives.
    ○ M-EDTA, ethanol, or the triple combination was used as an alternative.
- Systemically, vancomycin is the most frequently used glycopeptides.
  - Dalbavancin, a new, long-acting glycopeptide that is dosed weekly
    ○ Noted to be superior to vancomycin for adult patients with CRBSIs caused by CNS and *S. aureus*, including methicillin-resistant *S. aureus* (MRSA) in a phase 2, open-label, randomized, multicenter study
    ○ Side effect profile was comparable.
  - Linezolid and daptomycin were also used successfully.

Staphylococcus Aureus

- *S. aureus* CRBSI is associated with high rates of deep-seated infection:
- Osteomyelitis
- Septic phlebitis
- Endocarditis
- Patients whose intravascular device was not removed were 6.5 times more likely to relapse or die of their infection than were those whose device was removed.
  - IDSA guidelines recommend removing the CVL.
  - Results in a more rapid response and lower relapse rate
  - Might keep it and initiating systemic and lock solutions in case of thrombocytopenia or lack of other vascular access
  - In 40 CRBSIs—including all 12 cases reported to involve *S. aureus*—the antibiotic lock technique in addition to standard parenteral therapy was used for patients with a hemodialysis catheter-related infection
    ○ These were cured and the catheter salvaged.
    ○ Lock solutions most frequently used *in vivo* and *in vitro* are vancomycin plus heparin, or M-EDTA
    ○ Former combination—with or without ceftazidime, depending on the organism—was associated with a 60% failure rate in hemodialysis MRSA catheter infections.

- Ethanol is another appealing component for use in combination lock solutions.
  - Combination of M-EDTA in 25% ethanol was highly efficacious in eradicating *S. aureus* in biofilm within 60 minutes of dwell time.
- For methicillin-sensitive *S. aureus,* nafcillin or first-generation cephalosporins are first-choice agents.
- Vancomycin, linezolid, daptomycin, and dalbavancin are all appropriate options for MRSA.
- Duration of therapy usually consists of 10 to 14 days of IV if CVL removed.
  - And if no deep-seated infection present
  - If fever or bacteremia persists more than 72 hours after catheter removal, transesophageal echocardiography should be considered to rule out infectious endocarditis, and IV therapy duration should be expanded to at least 4 weeks.

Gram-negative Bacilli

- Gram-negative bacilli (GNB) bacteremia rarely due to CVL
  - Generally arises from a visceral source of infection such as:
    - Genitourinary tract
    - Pulmonary system
    - Gastrointestinal tract
    - However, CRBSIs caused by such organisms as *K. pneumoniae, Enterobacter* spp., *P. aeruginosa* spp., *Acinetobacter* spp., and *Stenotrophomonas maltophilia* have been reported.
      - 15-year experience of 149 episodes of septicemia caused by *Xanthomonas maltophilia* and *Pseudomonas* spp. in cancer patients where CVL was the most common source
      - Catheter removal within 72 hours of onset of catheter-related GNB is the only independent protective factor against the relapse of infection (odds ratio, 0.13; 95% confidence interval, 0.02–0.75; $p = 0.02$)
- IDSA guidelines recommend removing nontunneled CVLs and treating for 10 to 14 days.

- No data to guide the use of IV versus oral antibiotics.
- Appropriate to try CVL salvage in certain situations using systemic and lock solution therapies
  - When unable to access other vascular sites due to anatomic challenges
  - If there is a high risk of hemorrhagic complications because of thrombocytopenia or elevated prothrombin time
  - However, lock therapy for GNB CRBSIs is anecdotal.
    - Successful cases salvaged using gentamicin, amikacin, or ceftazidime.

Candida

- Five large prospective studies of *Candida* CRBSI proved catheter retention associated with:
  - Increased mortality
  - Increase in the mean duration of candidemia
  - Higher severity scores, nonremoval of the catheter, persistent candidemia, and lack of antifungal therapy adversely affect outcome
- Retrospective study of 404 patients with candidemia and indwelling CVL, using a multivariate analysis:
  - Demonstrated that catheter removal 72 hours or sooner after onset of candidemia improved the response to antifungal therapy exclusively in patients with catheter-related candidemia ($p = 0.04$)
- IDSA guidelines recommend removing CVL and treating for 14 days after last positive blood culture in uncomplicated cases.
  - Endophthalmitis merits 6 weeks of therapy.
  - Further studies are needed to define the role of antifungal lock solution in these cases.
  - Fluconazole and caspofungin were equivalent to amphotericin B in candidemia, but with a better safety profile
    - Therefore, fluconazole or caspofungin should be considered in documented cases of catheter-related candidemia.
  - If rates of fluconazole-resistant *Candida glabrata* and *Candida krusei* in hospital are high
    - An echinocandin—caspofungin, micafungin, or anidulafungin—the best alternative to amphotericin B

CHAPTER 76 ■ RESPIRATORY INFECTIONS IN THE ICU

PNEUMONIA

- Pneumonia is differentiated as being either community or hospital acquired.
  - *Community-acquired pneumonia* (CAP) begins while the patient is in an outpatient setting.
  - *Hospital-acquired pneumonia* (HAP) occurs while the patient is in an inpatient setting.

- Pneumonia is defined as hospital acquired when it occurs 48 hours or more after admission.
- This dichotomous classification scheme insufficient to characterize all patients suffering from pneumonia
  - Among HAPs, those occurring during mechanical ventilation (VAP) must be distinguished from others.
    - Significant number of VAPs occur within 48 hours of hospital admission.

- Consequently, the 48-hour HAP threshold no longer appropriate.
  - It does remain adequate for HAP occurring apart from mechanical ventilation.
  ○ Outpatients benefit from health care services such as dialysis, chemotherapy, or ambulatory surgery.
    - Pneumonia developing in such patients is now defined as a *health care–associated pneumonia*.
- Thus, four classes of pneumonia can be distinguished:
  - Community-acquired pneumonia (CAP)
  - Ventilator-associated pneumonia (VAP)
  - Hospital-acquired pneumonia (HAP)
  - Health care–associated pneumonia (HCAP)

Severe CAP

Immediate Concerns

- CAP is a common infectious disease affecting about 1 per 1,000 of the adult population per year.
- ICU admission for severe CAP is required for 2% of patients.
- Most frequent pathogen is *Streptococcus pneumoniae*
- Despite progress in antibiotic therapy and ICU management, the mortality of pneumococcal pneumonia remains elevated.

Diagnosis of CAP

- CAP suspected on the basis of clinical symptoms:
  - Cough
  - Dyspnea
  - Sputum production
  - Pleuritic chest pain
  - Elevated body temperature
- Symptoms can be absent or moderated in older patients.
- Signs are not specific of pneumonia.
  - Chest radiograph (CXR) or computed tomography (CT) scan revealing a new infiltrate is required to document a pneumonia diagnosis.
  - CXR might offer insights into the etiologic diagnosis
    - Intracellular pathogens typically presenting with interstitial pneumonia
    - *S. pneumoniae* resulting in lobar pneumonia
    - However, none of these findings is specific.
  - CXR allows for staging of severity according to localization and number of involved lobes.
  - Helpful to detect complications:
    ○ Pleural effusion
    ○ Cavitation
    ○ Acute respiratory distress syndrome (ARDS)
  - CT scan used to show evocative patterns, particularly in immunosuppressed patients:
    ○ Halo or crescent signs in pulmonary aspergillosis of neutropenic patients
    ○ Cavitation in tuberculosis

Definition of Severe CAP and Decision for Admission to the ICU

- No gold standard to define severe CAP; criteria do exist.
- According American Thoracic Society (ATS) guidelines, CAP is considered severe when any one of the following criteria present:

- Respiratory frequency >30 breaths/minute on admission
- Severe respiratory failure (PaO_2/FiO_2 <250 mm Hg)
- Requirement for mechanical ventilation
- Bilateral or multilobar or extensive (≥50% within 48 hours of admission) involvement of the CXR
- Shock (SBP <90 mm Hg or DBP <60 mm Hg)
- Requirement for vasopressors for more than 4 hours
- Low urine output (<20 mL/hour or 80 mL/4 hours) or acute renal failure requiring dialysis
- New definition of severe CAP adopted by the ATS in 2001
- Diagnosis of CAP is considered severe and requiring ICU admission for patients exhibiting either:
  - One of two major criteria (need for mechanical ventilation, septic shock) or
  - Two of three minor criteria (SBP ≤90 mm Hg, multilobar involvement on CXR, or PaO_2/FiO_2 <250 mm Hg)
- In 2001, the British Thoracic Society (BTS) proposed assessing the severity of CAP utilizing three groups of adverse prognostic features:
- Four "core" factors (**CURB** score):
  - **C**onfusion
  - Blood **U**rea nitrogen >19 mg/dL [7 mmol/L]
  - **R**espiratory rate ≥30 breaths/minute
  - Low **B**lood pressure—SBP <90 mm Hg and/or DBP ≤60 mm Hg)
- Two "additional" factors:
  - Hypoxemia—SpO_2 <92% or PaO_2 <60 mm Hg (8 kPa)
  - Bilateral or multilobar involvement on chest radiograph
  - Two "pre-existing" factors:
    ○ Age 50 years or older
    ○ Presence of coexisting disease
  - CAP was considered and treated as severe in patients having two or more core adverse prognostic features.
    ○ Patients exhibiting only one of these core factors had decision based on clinical judgment.
      - Assisted by taking into account pre-existing and additional factors

Diagnostic Studies

- Evaluation for etiologic diagnosis is helpful to confirm infectious origin of pneumonia and allow adequate antimicrobial therapy (including secondary deescalation therapy).
- Methods available for microbiologic diagnosis of pneumonia:
  - Sputum stains and cultures necessitate rigorous interpretation criteria.
    - Presence of >25 PMNs and <10 squamous epithelial cells per HPF required to interpret sample
    - A single predominant organism on Gram stain suggests etiology.
    - Other stains can be used according to particular clinical context and may allow for a positive diagnosis without any sample validation (*Mycobacterium tuberculosis, Legionella pneumophila, Pneumocystis jiroveci*).
  - More invasive sampling methods (endotracheal aspiration, protected specimen brush, bronchoalveolar lavage, transtracheal aspiration) are discussed in the VAP section but can also be used to diagnose CAP.
  - Blood cultures drawn before antibiotic therapy rarely positive (6%–20% of cases)
    - When positive, are most often for *S. pneumoniae, Staphylococcus aureus,* and gram-negative bacilli

MICROORGANISMS CAUSING SEVERE CAP REQUIRING ADMISSION TO AN ICU[a]

References	Yoshimoto et al.[b]	Leroy et al.[c]	Shorr et al.[d]
Number of patients	72	308	199
Unknown pathogen	55.6%	45%–45.9%	43.7%
Streptococcus pneumoniae	13.9%	38.7%–41%	44.7%
Haemophilus influenzae	2.8%	15.8%–24.5%	10.6%
Legionella pneumophila	2.8%	3.2%–3.8%	8.9%
Staphylococcus aureus	2.8%	2.8%–7.4%	8.9%
Pseudomonas aeruginosa	8.3%	ND	4.9%
Other gram-positive	2.8%	17%–17.9%	ND
Enterobacteriaceae	11.1%	7.5%–8.4%	6.5%
Chlamydia spp.	ND	1.9%–3.2%	ND
Mycobacterium tuberculosis	2.8%	ND	2.4%
Other	1.4%	3.2%–3.8%	13%

ND, no data.
[a]Data presented as number or percentage.
[b]Yoshimoto A, Nakamura H, Fujimura M, et al. Severe community-acquired pneumonia in an intensive care unit: risk factors for mortality. *Intern Med.* 2005;44:710.
[c]Leroy O, Saux P, Bedos JP, et al. Comparison of levofloxacin and cefotaxime combined with ofloxacin for ICU patients with community-acquired pneumonia who do not require vasopressors. *Chest.* 2005;128:172.
[d]Shorr AF, Bodi M, Rodriguez A, et al. Impact of antibiotic guideline compliance on duration of mechanical ventilation in critically ill patients with community-acquired pneumonia. *Chest.* 2006;130:93.

- Rapid diagnostic tests recently introduced
  - Urinary antigen test highly sensitive for diagnosis of *L. pneumophila* type 1
  - Urinary antigen test has been introduced for the diagnosis of pneumococcal pneumonia
    - In the ICU, patients with severe CAP displayed sensitivity, specificity, and positive and negative predictive values of 72%, 90%, 68%, and 92%, respectively.
  - Rapid diagnosis is available for influenza A.
    - Available tests can detect influenza viruses in 30 minutes.
    - Types of specimens acceptable for use (i.e., throat, nasopharyngeal, or nasal; and aspirates, swabs, or washes) vary by test.
    - Specificity and, in particular, the sensitivity of rapid tests are lower than for viral culture and vary by test.
- Serologic testing is less useful for rapid diagnosis.
  - Presence of IgM with a titer ≥6 generally indicates recent infection.
  - Rarely observed in the initial phase of infection when antibiotic therapy must be chosen.
    - Fourfold rise in antibody titer requiring samples drawn 2 weeks apart indicates, retrospectively, infection.
  - Serologic diagnosis can be useful for some pathogens:
    - *Mycoplasma pneumoniae*
    - *Chlamydia pneumoniae* and *Chlamydophila psittaci*
    - *Legionella* spp.
    - *Coxiella burnetii*
    - Adenovirus, parainfluenza viruses, and influenza A virus
- Polymerase chain reaction (PCR) testing is a promising future field.
  - Cannot be recommended routinely, as questions concerning sensitivity, specificity, and clinical relevance remain

Etiology of Severe CAP

- Despite intensive microbiologic testing, definitive diagnosis obtained in about 50% of cases.

- **Organisms causing CAP in hospitalized patients requiring ICU admission:**
  - The epidemiology of CAP patients admitted to the ICU does not appear to be different from other hospitalized individuals with CAP.
  - Most frequent pathogen isolated in ICU-hospitalized CAP patients is *S. pneumoniae* (Table 76.1).
    - Other pathogens responsible for severe CAP include:
      - *L. pneumophila*
      - *S. aureus*
      - *Pseudomonas aeruginosa*
      - *Aspergillus* spp.
      - Influenza
- **Drug-resistant pathogens**
  - Major challenge is emergence and dissemination of drug-resistant microorganisms
  - Major concerns are caused by penicillin-resistant pneumococci (PRP) and methicillin-resistant staphylococci
    - For *S. pneumoniae,* macrolide resistance is above 20% in the United States and higher than 50% in some European or Asian-Pacific countries.
    - Decreased susceptibility or resistance to penicillin was observed in 30% to 50% of strains.
  - Fluoroquinolone resistance is increasing, and fluoroquinolone-prescribing habits may affect resistance rates.
    - Resistance reaches 5.6% in Italy.
  - Community-acquired MRSA is a new challenge.
    - MRSA strain carrying Panton-Valentine leukocidin (PVL) genes was recently described in the community.
    - Primarily causes skin and soft tissue infections but can be responsible for rapidly progressing necrotizing pneumonia.
  - *P. aeruginosa* are naturally resistant to numerous antibiotics and can elevate to a high-level resistance under treatment.
    - Risk of *P. aeruginosa* is increased in patients presenting with a previous chronic pulmonary disease such as chronic obstructive pulmonary disorder (COPD) or cystic fibrosis,

recent antibiotic therapy, or a stay in the hospital, especially the ICU.
- **Specific etiologies in immunosuppressed patients**
  - Immunosuppressed patients have an increased risk of severe CAP.
  - All have more frequent bacterial pneumonia, particularly due to *S. pneumoniae* or *P. aeruginosa*.
    - Different types of immunodeficiency can also result in different epidemiology.
      - HIV-infected patients used to have a 25-fold higher risk of developing bacterial pneumonia.
        - In developed countries, risk has been tremendously decreased with the use of newer antiretroviral drugs.
        - Incidence of bacterial pneumonia in a French cohort was 0.8 per 100 patient-years, little difference from the general population.
        - *P. jiroveci* pneumonia remains a frequent AIDS-defining diagnosis.
        - Less frequent causes of severe pneumonias include cytomegalovirus (CMV), toxoplasma, and mycobacteria.
      - Patients with severe, prolonged chemotherapy-induced neutropenia (<500 neutrophils/μL and >10 days)
        - Have an increased risk of invasive pulmonary aspergillosis and severe bacterial pneumonia
        - Risk also exists with targeted monoclonal antibody therapies, which increase the risk of CMV and *P. jiroveci* pneumonia.
      - Patients with solid organ transplant have increased risk of severe CAP.
        - Usual bacterial pathogens, as well as *P. jiroveci* and *Aspergillus*, have been described.
      - Patients treated by anti–tumor necrosis factor (TNF)-α monoclonal antibodies have an increased risk of infection, including severe pneumonia.
        - Bacterial, viral, and fungal pneumonia have been described.

Treatment of Severe CAP

- **Antibiotic therapy**
  - Ideal antibiotic
    - Should have a "kill spectrum" to cover all pathogens responsible for severe CAP
    - Factors such as cost-effectiveness and selective pressure need to be assessed, so the choice of antimicrobial regimen usually results in a compromise.
    - Most frequent and/or most severe pathogens (*S. pneumoniae, Haemophilus influenzae, L. pneumophila*) should be covered by initial antimicrobial regimen.
    - Initial coverage of other pathogens (i.e., *S. aureus, P. aeruginosa*, opportunistic agents) evaluated on case-by-case basis according to patient history and presentation.
  - Timing of initial therapy
    - IDSA guidelines recommend initial antibiotics administration within 4 hours of admission.
    - Reduced mortality (adjusted odds ratio, 0.85, 95% confidence interval [CI] 0.76–0.95) observed in patients with early therapy.
    - However, time to first antibiotic dose may be a marker of disease severity rather than an indicator of prognosis.
  - Antimicrobial choices
    - Drug choice depends on numerous factors:
      - Pharmacodynamics/pharmacokinetics
      - Spectrum
      - Dosing schedule
      - Adverse events
      - Costs
      - Availability
    - Antimicrobial should have sufficient diffusion in pulmonary tissues
      - β-Lactam antibiotics have a good extracellular diffusion but are ineffective on intracellular organisms.
      - Concentration in the alveolar lining fluid (ALF) reached 10% to 20% of the serum concentration after a single administration.
      - Macrolides, on the other hand, have a variable intracellular distribution—low for erythromycin and elevated for the newer macrolides (clarithromycin, azithromycin).
      - Fluoroquinolones have an excellent intracellular and ALF diffusion.
    - Little data are available on best antimicrobial regimen for CAP.
      - Retrospective studies suggested combination regimen, including a macrolide, might be superior to β-lactam monotherapy for CAP.
        - Particularly for bacteremic pneumococcal pneumonia
        - Similar results were reported with a β-lactam–fluoroquinolone combination.
      - Impact of combination therapy on prognosis of pneumococcal bacteremia confirmed
        - Lower mortality associated with combination therapy for **critically ill patients** (14-day mortality, 23.4% vs. 55.3%; $p = 0.0015$), but **not for all patients** receiving combination versus monotherapy (10.4% vs. 11.5%, $p = $ NS)
        - All combinations using a β-lactam had enhanced response
- Recommendations
  - Guidelines published by North American and European medical societies mostly recommend the utilization of a β-lactam with a macrolide or a fluoroquinolone (Table 76.2).
- **Duration of therapy**
  - Usually based on the pathogen, response to treatment, comorbid illness, and complications
  - For pneumonia caused by *S. pneumoniae* should continue, at least, until patient has been afebrile for 72 hours
  - Bacteria causing necrosis of the pulmonary parenchyma (e.g., *S. aureus, P. aeruginosa, Klebsiella*, and anaerobes) should probably be treated for no less than 2 weeks.
  - Pneumonia caused by intracellular organisms should probably be treated for at least 2 weeks.
- **Nonantimicrobial therapy**
  - Activated protein C
    - Severe sepsis is associated with a generalized inflammation and procoagulant response to infection.
    - Activated protein C is an important endogenous modulator of response.
      - Activation of protein C impaired during sepsis
      - Reduced levels of activated protein C in most patients with severe sepsis
    - Drotrecogin-α an activated, recombinant form of human activated protein C (r-aPC)

TABLE 76.2

INITIAL EMPIRIC ANTIBIOTIC THERAPY IN PATIENTS ADMITTED TO AN ICU FOR SEVERE CAP

Clinical characteristics	Recommended antibiotics
No *Pseudomonas* or methicillin-resistant *Staphylococcus aureus* (MRSA) or penicillin allergy	A β-lactam (cefotaxime, ceftriaxone, ampicillin/sulbactam) **plus** azithromycin or a respiratory fluoroquinolone[a]
Patients with penicillin allergy	A respiratory fluoroquinolone, with azithromycin
Suspected *Pseudomonas* infection	An antipseudomonal β-lactam[b] Plus ciprofloxacin or levofloxacin[a] Or plus an aminoglycoside and an antipneumococcal fluoroquinolone[a]
Suspected community-acquired MRSA	Addition of vancomycin or linezolid

[a]Dosage of levofloxacin should be 750 mg daily.
[b]Antipseudomonal agents include piperacillin-tazobactam, imipenem, meropenem, or cefepime. Azithromycin can be substituted for penicillin allergy.
Adapted from Mandell LA, Wunderink RG, Anzueto A, et al. Infectious Diseases Society of America/American Thoracic Society consensus guidelines on the management of community-acquired pneumonia in adults. *Clin Infect Dis.* 2007;44(Suppl 2):S27.

- Exhibits profibrinolytic, antithrombotic, and anti-inflammatory characteristics
- Randomized, double-blind, placebo-controlled, multicenter study (PROWESS) composed of 1,690 patients demonstrated that treatment with r-aPC significantly decreased 28-day and hospital discharge mortality rates in patients with severe sepsis
  - Retrospective analysis of these 1,690 patients included in the PROWESS trial identified 602 patients (r-aPC, $n = 324$; placebo, $n = 278$) classified as exhibiting severe CAP
  - Compared with placebo, r-aPC provided a relative risk reduction in a 28-day mortality of 28%.
  - Survival benefit even more pronounced in patients with severe pneumococcal CAP and in patients with a high risk of death assessed by an Acute Physiology and Chronic Health Evaluation (APACHE) II score of at least 25, or a Pneumonia Severity Index score ≥ 4
- Conversely, in patients with severe sepsis but a low risk of death defined by an APACHE II score <25 or a single organ failure, r-aPC compared with placebo provided no beneficial effect and was associated with an increased incidence of bleeding events.
- Use of r-aPC should be limited in severe CAP, as in other severe infections, to patients at high risk of death.
  - APACHE II score ≥ 25 or multiple organ failure must be present
- Corticosteroids
  - Preliminary randomized trial, hydrocortisone (200 mg IV bolus followed by infusion at a rate of 10 mg/hour for 7 days) compared with placebo in 46 patients
    - On day 8, hydrocortisone treatment was associated with a significant improvement in PaO_2/FiO_2 and chest radiograph score, as well as a significant decrease in C-reactive protein levels and Multiple Organ Dysfunction Syndrome score, and a lower incidence of delayed septic shock.
    - Moreover, length of hospital stay and mortality were decreased.
    - Results as yet insufficient to propose the systematic use of hydrocortisone in severe CAP

- **Expected clinical course**
  - Evaluation on day 3
    - Generally, a decrease in fever and oxygenation requirements is not observed in responding patients prior to day 3 or 4.
    - Absent rapid clinical deterioration, initial therapy should not be changed prior to completion of 48 to 72 hours of the initial therapy.
    - Day 3 usually sees the return of microbiologic exams, including cultures and antimicrobial sensitivity.
      - Can allow for treatment adaptation (de-escalation or treatment for a pathogen not covered by first-line therapy)
      - For example, negative results of urinary antigen test combined with blood cultures positive for *S. pneumoniae* make it possible to simplify therapy to target *S. pneumoniae* with an aminopenicillin.
  - Complications and failure to improve
    - Poor clinical response by day 3 is usually a sign of treatment failure.
    - In the ICU, other diagnoses such as pulmonary embolism or cardiac failure should be considered.
    - Treatment failure can be due to an organism not covered by the first-line antimicrobial therapy, thus demanding a change or addition to the previous treatment regimen.
    - Other causes of treatment failure can include complications despite adequate antimicrobial therapy, including:
      - Lung abscess
      - Necrosis
      - Meningitis
      - Endocarditis
      - Superinfection

Prognosis of Severe CAP

- Mortality in patients with severe CAP requiring admission to the ICU remains high, ranging in the literature from 18% to 46%.
- A meta-analysis of 788 evaluable ICU patients found a mean mortality rate of 36.5%.
- 11 independent prognostic factors associated with a mortality of CAP:

- Male gender (odds ratio [OR] = 1.3)
- Pleuritic chest pain (OR = 0.5)
- Hypothermia (OR = 5.0)
- Systolic hypotension (OR = 4.8)
- Tachypnea (OR = 2.9)
- Diabetes mellitus (OR = 1.3)
- Neoplastic disease (OR = 2.8)
- Neurologic disease (OR = 4.6)
- Bacteremia (OR = 2.8)
- Leukopenia (OR = 2.5)
- Multilobar pulmonary involvement (OR = 3.1)
- Prognosis of patients admitted to the ICU for severe CAP depends on preadmission health status of patient, the initial severity of illness, and the evolution during ICU stay (Table 76.3).

TABLE 76.3

INDEPENDENT PROGNOSTIC FACTORS ASSOCIATED WITH MORTALITY OF PATIENTS WITH SEVERE CAP

Preadmission Health Status
- Age older than 70 yr
- Immunosuppression
- Comorbidities with anticipated death within 5 yr

Initial Severity of Illness
- Antibiotic administration prior to hospital presentation
- Simplified Acute Physiologic Score (SAPS) I >12 or SAPS II >45
- Septic shock
- Requirement for mechanical ventilation
- Acute renal failure
- Bilateral or multilobar pulmonary involvement
- *K. pneumonia* or *P. aeruginosa* as etiologic agent
- Bacteremia
- Nonaspiration pneumonia

Evolution during ICU Stay
- Radiographic spread of pneumonia
- Number of nonpulmonary organs that failed
- Increase in Logistic Organ Dysfunction score from D1 to D3
- Delay in hospital antibiotic administration of more than 4 h
- Ineffective initial antimicrobial therapy
- Occurrence of non–pneumonia-related complications
- Increase of procalcitonin level in serum from D1 to D3

Data from Pachon J, Prados MD, Capote F, et al. Severe community-acquired pneumonia. Etiology, prognosis, and treatment *Am Rev Respir Dis.* 1990;142:369; Almirall J, Mesalles E, Klamburg J, et al. Prognostic factors of pneumonia requiring admission to the intensive care unit. *Chest.* 1995;107:511; Leroy O, Santré C, Beuscart C, et al. A five-year study of severe community-acquired pneumonia with emphasis on prognosis in patients admitted to an intensive care unit. *Intensive Care Med.* 1995;21:24; Paganin F, Lilienthal F, Bourdin A, et al. Severe community-acquired pneumonia: assessment of microbial aetiology as mortality factor. *Eur Respir J.* 2004;24:779; Tejerina E, Frutos-Vivar F, Restrepo MI, et al. Prognosis factors and outcome of community-acquired pneumonia needing mechanical ventilation. *J Crit Care.* 2005;20:230; Boussekey N, Leroy O, Alfandari S, et al. Procalcitonin kinetics in the prognosis of severe community-acquired pneumonia. *Intensive Care Med.* 2006;32:469; Torres A, Serra-Batlles J, Ferrer A, et al. Severe community-acquired pneumonia. Epidemiology and prognostic factors. *Am Rev Respir Dis.* 1991;144:312; Leroy O, Devos P, Guery B, et al. Simplified prediction rule for prognosis of patients with severe community-acquired pneumonia in ICUs. *Chest.* 1999;116:157; Wilson PA, Ferguson J. Severe community-acquired pneumonia: an Australian perspective. *Intern Med J.* 2005;35:699.

- Initial empiric treatment must be instituted as soon as possible (<4 hours after hospital admission) and must be adequate to be as effective as possible.
- Non–pneumonia-related complications—such as upper gastrointestinal bleeding, catheter-related infection, deep venous thrombosis, and pulmonary embolism—and complications attributed only to underlying medical conditions must be prevented during the ICU stay.
- Mortality risk scores specific to CAP have been elaborated.
  - Pneumonia Severity Index (PSI) and stratifies risk using a two-step approach
    - First, patients with a low risk (class I) are identified by age younger than 50 years and the absence of comorbidities and vital sign abnormalities.
    - For remaining patients, the score is determined by adding points assigned to age and different variables, taking into account comorbid conditions, physical examination findings, and laboratory and radiographic abnormalities (Table 76.4).
      - According to the value of this score, patients are classified into:
        - Class II (≤70 points)
        - Class III (71–90 points)
        - Class IV (91–130 points)
        - Class V (>130 points)
        - From class I to class V, mortality rates observed in the validation cohort were 0.1%, 0.6%, 2.8%, 8.2%, and 29.2%, respectively.
  - A specific prediction rule for mortality of patients with severe CAP admitted to an ICU has been proposed.
    - Rule takes into account data on prognostic factors, emphasizing that the prognosis of severe CAP depends on both *initial* baseline characteristics of the patient and *evolution* during the ICU stay, and is based on two successive steps.
    - On ICU admission, an initial risk score based on six independent variables associated with the prognosis is established. These variables and their respective point value are:
      - Age 40 years or older (+1 point)
      - Anticipated death within 5 years (+1 point)
      - Nonaspiration pneumonia (+1 point)
      - Chest radiograph involvement greater than one lobe (+1 point)
      - Acute respiratory failure requiring mechanical ventilation (+1 point)
      - Septic shock (+3 points)
        - The initial risk score, obtained by summing up these points, allows inclusion of each patient into one of the three risk classes of increasing mortality
          □ Class I (0–2 points) mortality risk is low (<5%)
          □ Class II (3–5 points), mortality risk is intermediate (25%)
          □ Class III (6–8 points), mortality risk is high (>50%)
      - Risk score based on three independent factors identified **during** ICU stay allows definite evaluation of final prognosis
        □ These three independent factors and their point scoring are:
        □ Hospital-acquired, lower respiratory tract superinfections (+1 point)

TABLE 76.4

CRITERIA AND POINT SCORING SYSTEM USED IN THE PNEUMONIA SEVERITY
INDEX (STEP 2; CLASSES II–V)

Variables	Points	Variables	Points
Age	Age (yr)	**Vital sign abnormality**	
Female gender	−10	Altered mental status	+20
Nursing home resident	+10	Respiratory rate >30 breaths/min	+20
		Systolic blood pressure <90 mm Hg	+20
		Temperature <35°C or ≥40°C	+15
		Tachycardia >125 breaths/min	+10
Comorbidity		**Laboratory and radiographic data**	
Neoplastic disease	+30	Arterial pH <7.35	+30
Liver disease	+20	Blood urea nitrogen ≥30 mg/dL	+20
Congestive heart failure	+10	Sodium <130 mmol/L	+20
Cerebrovascular disease	+10	Glucose ≥250 mg/dL	+10
Renal disease	+10	Hematocrit <30%	+10
		PaO_2 <60 mm Hg	+10
		Pleural effusion	+10

Adapted from Fine MJ, Auble TE, Yealy DM, et al. A prediction rule to identify low-risk patients with
community-acquired pneumonia. *N Engl J Med.* 1997;336:243.

□ Nonspecific CAP-related complications (+2 points)
□ Sepsis-related complications (+4 points) occurring during the ICU stay
□ This risk score appears particularly useful for patients in the intermediate-risk class II on ICU admission

Prevention of CAP

- Many factors associated with increase in CAP risk (tobacco use, malnutrition, chronic pulmonary disease, diabetes, liver disease, older age, confinement to a nursing home) are not amenable to prevention.
- Immunization remains the most significant method of prevention.
  - Two vaccines are available for preventing pneumococcal disease.
    - Pneumococcal polysaccharide vaccine is recommended for persons 65 or more years of age, and for persons 2 or more years of age who are immunocompetent but at increased risk for illness and death associated with pneumococcal disease because of chronic illness, with functional or anatomic asplenia, who live in environments in which the risk for disease is high, or are immunosuppressed and at high risk for infection.
    - Pneumococcal conjugate vaccine is recommended only for children
  - The Advisory Committee on Immunization Practices (ACIP) recommends the inactivated influenza A vaccine for all persons older than 50 years of age, those at risk for influenza complications, and household contacts of high-risk persons (including health care workers).

VAP

- VAP defined as pneumonia occurring in intubated or tracheotomized patients undergoing mechanical ventilation (MV).

- Usual guidelines suggest a delay of 48 to 72 hours between the beginning of MV and occurrence of pneumonia to qualify for this diagnosis; recent data suggest that a pneumonia acquired earlier than the 48th hour of mechanical ventilation could also be considered a VAP.
- VAP represents 80% of pneumonia acquired during hospitalization.
- VAP is the most frequent hospital-acquired infection in ICUs.

Immediate Concerns

- The major dilemmas regarding VAP at present are following:
  - Prevention remains a challenge.
  - No gold standard for diagnosis.
  - Rate of multidrug-resistant causative pathogens has dramatically increased during recent years.
  - Prompt initiation of an adequate antibiotic therapy essential.

Incidence

- The exact incidence of VAP is difficult to assess for a number of reasons:
  - Study populations vary greatly from one study to another.
  - Criteria used to diagnose VAP can be quite different (i.e., clinical vs. bacteriologic diagnosis).
  - Overlap between VAP and other hospital-acquired lower respiratory tract infections such as nosocomial tracheobronchitis exists.
  - With this in mind, one must carefully analyze the extant studies, which show an incidence varying from 5.6% to 82.4% (Table 76.5).
- In a U.S. inpatient database composed of 9,080 patients mechanically ventilated for more than 24 hours, the incidence of VAP was 9.3%.
  - The percentages of episodes of VAP occurring during the first 2 days of hospitalization, between days 3 and 6, and after hospital day 6 were 45.2%, 29.1%, and 25.7%, respectively.

TABLE 76.5

INCIDENCE OF VAP IN THE ICU

References	No. of patients	Characteristics of patients	Diagnostic criteria	Incidence of VAP
Torres et al.[a]	322	Medicosurgical patients	Clinical and Rx	24%
Chevret et al.[b]	540	Medicosurgical patients	Clinical and Rx	12.6%
Baker et al.[c]	514	Trauma patients	Clinical, Rx, and Q. bacteriologic cultures	5.6%
Chastre et al.[d]	56	Patients with ARDS	Clinical, Rx, and Q. bacteriologic cultures	55%
Tejada Artigas et al.[e]	103	Trauma patients	Clinical, Rx, and Q. bacteriologic cultures	22.3%
Ibrahim et al.[f]	880	Medicosurgical patients	Clinical and Rx	15%
Bouza et al.[g]	356	Heart surgical patients	Clinical, Rx, and Q. bacteriologic cultures	7.9%
Hilker et al.[h]	17	Patients with acute stroke	Clinical and Rx	82.4%

Rx, radiologic; ARDS, acute respiratory distress syndrome; Q., quantitative.

[a]Torres A, Aznar R, Gatell JM, et al. Incidence, risk, and prognosis factors of nosocomial pneumonia in mechanically ventilated patients. *Am Rev Respir Dis.* 1990;142:523.
[b]Chevret S, Hemmer M, Carlet J, et al. Incidence and risk factors of pneumonia acquired in intensive care units. Results from a multicenter prospective study on 996 patients. European Cooperative Group on Nosocomial Pneumonia. *Intensive Care Med.* 1993;19:256.
[c]Baker AM, Meredith JW, Haponik EF. Pneumonia in intubated trauma patients. Microbiology and outcomes. *Am J Respir Crit Care Med.* 1996;153:343.
[d]Chastre J, Trouillet JL, Vuagnat A, et al. Nosocomial pneumonia in patients with acute respiratory distress syndrome. *Am J Respir Crit Care Med.* 1998;157:1165.
[e]Tejada Artigas A, Bello Dronda S, Chacon Valles E, et al. Risk factors for nosocomial pneumonia in critically ill trauma patients. *Crit Care Med.* 2001;29:304.
[f]Ibrahim EH, Tracy L, Hill C, et al. The occurrence of ventilator-associated pneumonia in a community hospital: risk factors and clinical outcomes. *Chest.* 2001;120:555.
[g]Bouza E, Perez A, Munoz P, et al. Ventilator-associated pneumonia after heart surgery: a prospective analysis and the value of surveillance. *Crit Care Med.* 2003;31:1964.
[h]Hilker R, Poetter C, Findeisen N, et al. Nosocomial pneumonia after acute stroke: implications for neurological intensive care medicine. *Stroke.* 2003;34:975.

- Most episodes of VAP (63.2%) developed within 48 hours of mechanical ventilation.
  - Thereafter, 16% occurred between 48 hours and 96 hours of mechanical ventilation, and 20.8% after 96 hours of mechanical ventilation.
- In a cohort of 1,014 patients ventilated for 48 hours or more, the overall incidence of VAP was 14.8 cases per 1,000 ventilator-days.
- The daily risk for developing VAP is highest in the early course of hospital stay.
  - Estimated to be 3% per day at day 5
  - 2% at day 10
  - 1% at day 15

Pathogenesis

- Pneumonia occurs resultant to the entry of bacteria into the normally sterile lower respiratory tract.
  - Leading to colonization and subsequently to infection when bacteria overwhelm host defenses secondary to a large bacterial inoculum, a virulent pathogen, or a defect in the local host defenses
- Bacteria can reach the lower respiratory tract by four different pathogenic mechanisms:
  - Contiguous spread
  - Hematogenous spread
  - Inhalation
  - Aspiration
- First two mechanisms of invasion are infrequent.
  - Inhalation of gastric material or direct inoculation of bacteria into the lower respiratory tract through contami-

nated "devices" (aerosol, bronchoscopes, ventilator circuit, nebulizer, tracheal suctioning) is rarely associated with VAP.
- Aspiration of bacteria colonizing the oropharynx is the main route of entry into the lower respiratory tract.
  - Colonization of oropharyngeal airways by pathogenic microorganisms occurs during first hospital week in most critically ill patients.
  - Microorganisms that replace normal microflora of oropharynx can be either endogenous (enteric gram-negative bacteria) or exogenous *via* a cross-contamination from other ICU patients.
  - Stomach, sinuses, and dental plaque may be potential reservoirs for pathogens colonizing oropharynx.
    - Exact contribution still remains controversial.
    - The endotracheal tube (ETT) compromises the natural barrier between the oropharynx and lower respiratory tract.
    - Leakage of contaminated secretions around ETT cuff allows bacterial entry into trachea.

Risk Factors

- Many risk factors for VAP are host related and, thus, not accessible to intervention.
- Patient-related risk factors include:
  - Male gender
  - Pre-existing pulmonary disease
  - Coma
  - AIDS
  - Head trauma

TABLE 76.6

MICRO-ORGANISMS CAUSING VAP[a]

References	Trouillet et al.[b]	Leroy et al.[c]	Rello et al.[d]
Number of episodes of VAP	135	124	290
Number of bacteria identified	245	154	321
Pseudomonas aeruginosa	39 (15.9%)	48 (31.1%)	102 (31.7%)
Acinetobacter baumannii	22 (9%)	9 (5.8%)	38 (11.8%)
Stenotrophomonas maltophilia	6 (2.4%)	8 (5.2%)	8 (2.5%)
Klebsiella species	9 (3.7%)	5 (3.2%)	ND
Escherichia coli	8 (3.3%)	8 (5.2%)	ND
Proteus species	7 (2.9%)	5 (3.2%)	ND
Enterobacter species	5 (2.0%)	7 (4.5%)	ND
Morganella species	4 (1.6%)	—	ND
Serratia species	4 (1.6%)	7 (4.5%)	ND
Haemophilus species	15 (6.1%)	10 (6.5%)	26 (8.1%)
Methicillin-resistant *Staphylococcus aureus*	32 (13.1%)	10 (6.5%)	10 (4.0%)
Methicillin-sensitive *S. aureus*	20 (8.2%)	19 (12.4%)	38 (11.8%)
Streptococcus pneumoniae	3 (1.2%)	9 (5.8%)	25 (7.8%)
Streptococcus species	33 (13.5%)	2 (1.3%)	10 (3.1%)
Enterococcus species	5 (2.0%)	—	ND
Coagulase-negative staphylococcus	4 (1.6%)	1 (0.6%)	ND
Anaerobic pathogens	6 (2.4%)	—	ND

ND, no data.
[a]Data are presented as number and (percentage).
[b]Trouillet JL, Chastre J, Vuagnat A, et al. Ventilator-associated pneumonia caused by potentially drug-resistant bacteria. *Am J Respir Crit Care Med.* 1998;157:531.
[c]Leroy O, Girardie P, Yazdanpanah Y, et al. Hospital-acquired pneumonia: microbiological data and potential adequacy of antimicrobial regimens. *Eur Respir J.* 2002;20:432.
[d]Rello J, Sa-Borges M, Correa H, et al. Variations in etiology of ventilator-associated pneumonia across four treatment sites: implications for antimicrobial prescribing practices. *Am J Respir Crit Care Med.* 1999;160:608.

- Age older than 60 years
- Neurosurgical procedures
- Multiorgan system failure
- Among accessible risk factors, most important is the presence of MV, which associated with a 3- to 21-fold risk.
- ETT:
  - Limits draining of secretions that leak around the cuff
  - Favors bacterial multiplication
  - Offers a focus for bacterial adherence and colonization
  - Impairs ciliary clearance and cough
- MV patient requires other devices such as nebulizers or humidifiers, which can be a source of microorganisms.
- Risk of infection is highest during the first 8 to 10 days of MV and increases with MV duration.
- Accidental extubation, rather than reintubation, increases the risk of VAP.
  - Likely due to nonexistent preparation for extubation
  - Enteral nutrition administered *via* NG—rather than a postpyloric—tube also increases risk of VAP.
    - NG tube might increase the risk of reflux and subsequent colonization of the airways.
  - Use of H_2 blockers or antacids favors gastric colonization and may contribute to VAP.
  - Other factors facilitating inhalation of oropharyngeal secretions favor VAP:
    - Supine position
    - Patient transportation out of the ICU
    - Sedation
    - Failed subglottic aspiration

  - Intracuff pressure <20 cm H_2O
  - Tracheostomy
  - Aerosol treatment

Etiology

- VAP may be caused by a wide spectrum of bacteria and is often polymicrobial (Table 76.6).
  - Gram-negative enteric bacilli, *P. aeruginosa,* and *S. aureus* are the leading etiologies.
  - However, microorganisms responsible for VAP may differ according to patient groups, unit types, hospitals, and countries.
  - Main epidemiologic patterns—principally the susceptibility patterns of causative pathogens—may also vary in a given unit over the course of time.
- Presence of altered level of consciousness, admission into a medical ICU, and a high Simplified Acute Physiologic Score are independent factors associated with the development of VAP caused by anaerobes.
- In trauma patients, VAP due to *Stenotrophomonas maltophilia* are independently associated with prior exposure to cefepime and tracheostomy.
- Cytotoxic chemotherapy and use of corticosteroids are independent factors predisposing to the development of nosocomial pneumonia due to *L. pneumophila.*
- Neurosurgery, ARDS, head trauma, and large-volume pulmonary aspiration are independent risk factors for VAP due to *Acinetobacter baumannii.*

- COPD, prior use of antibiotics, and duration of mechanical ventilation longer than 8 days are independently associated with VAP due to *P. aeruginosa*.
- Coma is an independent risk factor for VAP caused by *S. aureus*.
- Even if such factors are important to consider, there is major overlap between these different factors and, consequently, they are not sufficiently discriminant.
- The time of onset of VAP influences the etiology of VAP, making it useful to distinguish early-onset VAP from late-onset VAP.
  - Early-onset VAP, the main causative pathogens are:
    - *S. pneumoniae*
    - Methicillin-susceptible *S. aureus*
    - *H. influenzae*
    - Susceptible gram-negative enteric bacilli
  - In late-onset VAP the main causative organisms are:
    - MRSA
    - *P. aeruginosa*
    - *A. baumannii*
    - *S. maltophilia*
- Distinction between early- and late-onset VAP useful, but no consensus on number of days considered that separate VAP types
  - According to the literature, threshold varies from 3 to 7 days.
  - Unclear whether threshold refers to number of days in hospital or to number of days of mechanical ventilation.
  - Recent ATS/IDSA guidelines note the duration of hospitalization fewer than, or more than, 5 days, respectively, separates early- from late-onset VAP.
- Rate of multidrug-resistant (MDR) pathogens dramatically increased recently.
  - Numerous factors associated with emergence of resistant strains (Table 76.7)
- VAP due to fungi such as *Candida* species and *Aspergillus* species or to viruses such as influenza, parainfluenza, measles, adenovirus, and respiratory syncytial virus is uncommon in immunocompetent patients.

Diagnostic Strategies and Diagnostic Testing

- In the ICU, the diagnosis of VAP remains a challenge.
  - No gold standard for diagnosis
  - Usually, the diagnostic approach is based on two successive steps:
    - Diagnosis of pneumonia must be established.
    - Etiologic pathogen(s) of pulmonary parenchymal infection must be identified.
  - Pneumonia is suspected when current signs of infection present:
    - Fever or hypothermia
    - Leukocytosis or leucopenia
    - Tachycardia
    - Purulent sputum, a decline in oxygenation, and pulmonary infiltrates on CXR suggestive of pulmonary involvement
    - Among these signs and symptoms, none is specific for pneumonia.
  - Presence of a new or progressive radiographic infiltrate associated with at least two of three major clinical findings (fever >38°C, purulent tracheal secretions, and leukocytosis or leucopenia) considered most accurate combination.

TABLE 76.7

RISK FACTORS FOR MDR PATHOGENS AS CAUSATIVE ORGANISMS IN VAP

- Admission from a nursing home or an extended-care facility
- History of regular visits to an infusion or dialysis center
- Prior antimicrobial treatment in the preceding 90 days
- Prior use of broad-spectrum antibiotics
- Prior hospitalization in the preceding 90 days
- Current hospitalization for ≥5 days
- Duration of mechanical ventilation ≥7 days
- Immunosuppression
- High level of antibiotic resistance in the community or in local intensive care unit

Data from American Thoracic Society, Infectious Diseases Society of America. Guidelines for the management of adults with hospital-acquired, ventilator-associated, and healthcare-associated pneumonia. *Am J Respir Crit Care Med.* 2005;171:388; Trouillet JL, Chastre J, Vuagnat A, et al. Ventilator-associated pneumonia caused by potentially drug-resistant bacteria. *Am J Respir Crit Care Med.* 1998;157:531; Leroy O, Girardie P, Yazdanpanah Y, et al. Hospital-acquired pneumonia: microbiological data and potential adequacy of antimicrobial regimens. *Eur Respir J.* 2002;20:432; Porzecanski I, Bowton DL. Diagnosis and treatment of ventilator-associated pneumonia. *Chest.* 2006;130:597; Rello J, Torres A, Ricart M, et al. Ventilator-associated pneumonia by *Staphylococcus aureus.* Comparison of methicillin-resistant and methicillin-sensitive episodes. *Am J Respir Crit Care Med.* 1994;150:1545; Trouillet JL, Vuagnat A, Combes A, et al. *Pseudomonas aeruginosa* ventilator-associated pneumonia: comparison of episodes due to piperacillin-resistant versus piperacillin-susceptible organisms. *Clin Infect Dis.* 2002;34:1047; Leroy O, Jaffre S, D'Escrivan, et al. Hospital-acquired pneumonia: risk factors for antimicrobial-resistant causative pathogens in critically ill patients. *Chest.* 2003;123:2034.

- Numerous techniques have been proposed to identify causative organism(s) of VAP:
- Blood cultures are rarely positive.
- Positive pleural effusion culture is generally considered as a specific result.
  - However, spread of infection to pleural space is a rare event.
- Analysis of lower respiratory secretions the most frequently used technique to identify causative organism(s) of VAP.
  - Microscopy and qualitative culture of expectorated sputum or endotracheal aspirates associated with a high percentage of false-positive results because of colonization of the upper respiratory tract and/or tracheobronchial tree.
  - However, initial empiric antimicrobial treatment of VAP could be guided by a reliable tracheal aspirate Gram stain.
  - Quantitative cultures with a threshold of 10^6 colony-forming units (CFU)/mL to differentiate colonization from lung infection provide a diagnostic accuracy nearly similar to that of quantitative cultures from samples obtained by bronchoscopic techniques.
  - When culture of endotracheal secretions is sterile in a patient with no recent (<72 hours) change in antimicrobial therapy, diagnosis of VAP can be ruled out with a high probability
    - Negative predictive value is >90%.
    - Extrapulmonary infectious process must be investigated.

○ Protected specimen brush (PSB) allows uncontaminated specimens from the infected pulmonary area to be collected.
  – Threshold set at 10^3 CFU/mL is the most adequate for quantitative cultures.
  – False-positive results are infrequent.
  – False-negative results are observed when sampling is performed at an early stage of infection, in a technically incorrect (unaffected pulmonary area) manner, in a patient where a new antimicrobial treatment has been initiated, and/or if specimens are incorrectly processed.
○ Bronchoalveolar lavage (BAL) explores larger lung area than PSB.
  – Quantitative cultures of BAL fluid, with a threshold set at 10^4 CFU/mL seem to provide results similar to those obtained by PSB.
  – Possible microscopic examination of BAL fluid immediately after the procedure a clear advantage
  – The detection with Gram or Giemsa staining of BAL cells containing intracellular bacteria allows for a rapid diagnosis and guides initial antibiotic treatment.
○ Arguments favoring these bronchoscopic techniques are:
  – Ability to confirm diagnosis of VAP by identifying causative organism(s) and guide antimicrobial treatment
  – When cultures are negative, they can point to an alternative diagnosis.
  – When cultures are positive, a more targeted antimicrobial treatment plan is possible, and selective pressure for antibiotic resistance may be reduced.
  – Having accurate microbiologic diagnosis may reduce VAP mortality.
○ Major limitations of bronchoscopic techniques are:
  – Questionable accuracy in patients in whom a new antimicrobial treatment has been introduced before sampling
  – Significant cost
  – Possible occurrence of complications (i.e., hypoxemia)
  – Low impact on therapeutic decisions since physicians are often reluctant to modify (or discontinue) an effective treatment
○ ATS/IDSA guidelines propose a "mixed" diagnostic strategy as follows:
  – Diagnosis of VAP suspected in presence of a new or progressive pulmonary infiltrate associated with at least two of the following three infectious signs:
    • Fever >38°C
    • Leukocytosis or leucopenia
    • And/or purulent secretions
    • For patients with ARDS, radiographic changes are difficult to analyze; consequently, hemodynamic instability and/or deterioration of blood gases could be considered sufficient to suspect VAP.
  – When diagnosis suspected, lower respiratory tract samples are obtained for microscopy, and quantitative or semiquantitative cultures and empiric antimicrobial therapy are started unless there is both a low-clinical suspicion for VAP and a negative microscopy of the respiratory sample.
  – On days 2 and 3, the results of cultures should be available, and the clinical response is assessed.

  – According to whether the clinical picture is improving or worsening and the results of cultures:
    • Antimicrobial therapy will be stopped, de-escalated, or adjusted, and an investigation for other pathogens, other diagnoses, other sites of infection, or complications is performed.
  – Quantitative cultures of respiratory samples appear more accurate than qualitative or semiquantitative cultures for diagnosis of VAP.

Antibiotic Treatment

• **Principles of initial empiric treatment**
  • Prompt initiation of adequate antimicrobial treatment is a cornerstone of therapy, as inadequate initial antibiotic treatment is associated with significantly increased VAP mortality.
  • Timing of adequate antibiotic treatment is an important determinant of outcome.
  • Delayed appropriate antibiotic treatment—defined as a period ≥24 hours between time VAP was suspected and administration of adequate treatment—resulted in significantly higher mortality than those receiving nondelayed treatment (69.7% vs. 28.4%; p <0.001).
    ○ Patients with delayed treatment received antibiotics, on average, only 16 hours later than patients without delay.
    ○ Once bacteriologic and susceptibility data become available, it does not reduce the excess mortality induced by inadequate treatment given initially.
      – Adequate antibiotic therapy could be defined as the administration, at an appropriate dose, of at least one antibiotic with good penetration into lung tissues and to which all causative pathogens are susceptible *in vitro*.
      – Although inappropriate doses and/or choice of agents with poor lung penetration could explain inadequacy of treatment, the most common reason is resistance of causative pathogen(s).
      – Consequently, antibiotics must be selected according to presence or absence of risk factors for MDR pathogens (see Table 76.7) and the local microbiologic patterns of VAP.
• **Guidelines for initial empiric antibiotic therapy**
  • On basis of time of onset of VAP and presence or absence of risks for MDR pathogens, ATS/IDSA guidelines propose two different schemes for initial empiric antibiotic therapy
  • With no risk factors for MDR pathogens and an early-onset VAP (duration of hospitalization <5 days), limited-spectrum antibiotic therapy based on monotherapy seems appropriate (Table 76.8).
  • In patients with late-onset VAP (≥5 days) or exhibiting risk factors for MDR pathogens, a broad-spectrum antibiotic regimen based on two or three combined antibiotics is usually required (see Table 76.8).
• Initial choice should take into account:
  • Patient characteristics (underlying diseases associated with contraindications to specific antibiotic agents or classes)
  • Class of antibiotic to which the patient was recently exposed
  • Local microbiologic data (resistance patterns)
    ○ Recent exposure to one antibiotic could lead to resistance to entire class.

TABLE 76.8

INITIAL EMPIRIC ANTIBIOTIC THERAPY IN PATIENTS WITH VAP

Characteristics of patient	Recommended antibiotics and recommended dosages[a]
Early-onset VAP and no risk factors for MDR pathogens	• Ceftriaxone (1–2 g/24 h) • *or* • Levofloxacin (750 mg/24 h), moxifloxacin (400 mg/24 h), or ciprofloxacin (400 mg/8 h) *Or* • Ampicillin (1–2 g) plus sulbactam (0.5–1 g)/6 h • *or* • Ertapenem (1 g/24 h)
Late-onset VAP or risk factors for MDR pathogens	• Antipseudomonal cephalosporin: Cefepime (1–2 g/8–12 h) or ceftazidime (2 g/8 h) *Or* • Antipseudomonal carbapenem: Imipenem (500 mg/6 h or 1 g/8 h) or meropenem (1 g/8 h) *Or* • β-Lactam/β-lactamase inhibitor: Piperacillin-tazobactam (4.5 g/6 h) *plus* • Antipseudomonal fluoroquinolone: Levofloxacin (750 mg/24 h) or ciprofloxacin (400 mg/8 h) *Or* • Aminoglycoside[b]: Gentamicin (7 mg/kg/24 h) or tobramycin (7 mg/kg/24 h) or amikacin (20 mg/kg/24 h) *Plus* • Vancomycin (15 mg/kg/12 h)[c] *Or* • Linezolid (600 mg/12 h)

Adapted from American Thoracic Society, Infectious Diseases Society of America. Guidelines for the management of adults with hospital-acquired, ventilator-associated, and health care–associated pneumonia. *Am J Respir Crit Care Med.* 2005;171:388.
[a]Dosages are based on normal hepatic and renal function.
[b]Trough levels for gentamicin and tobramycin should be <1 mg/L and for amikacin should be <4–5 mg/L.
[c]Trough levels for vancomycin should be <15–20 mg/L.

○ If patients develop VAP shortly after, or during, antibiotic treatment, it is recommended that an antibiotic be chosen from a different antimicrobial class for empiric treatment.

○ Local epidemiologic patterns (predominant pathogens and local antibiotic susceptibility) must lead to the implementation of specific institutional guidelines for the treatment of VAP, which are of particular importance.

○ In 95% of cases, routine quantitative cultures of endotracheal aspirates obtained twice a week in mechanically ventilated patients before onset of VAP identified the same microorganisms as BAL cultures are obtained when VAP was suspected.

○ Thus, antibiotic choice based on the results of last available quantitative culture of endotracheal aspirate could increase adequacy of initial empiric treatment.

○ Although prospective comparative studies are required to validate these results, it is possible to imagine routine cultures of ETT aspirates could also help clinician to choose most appropriate antibiotic(s) among all proposed agents.

• **De-escalation strategy**

• A therapeutic strategy based on narrow-spectrum initial therapy, followed by a broadened-spectrum therapy once culture results are available, must be avoided.

  • Most patients suffering from VAP exhibited either a late-onset VAP or risk factors for multidrug-resistant pathogens.

• Most patients with VAP are treated with a broad-spectrum antibiotic therapy that combines two or three agents.

• The widespread use of broad-spectrum empiric therapy in the ICU may result in the emergence of MDR pathogens.

○ To preempt this vicious circle, a de-escalating strategy has been proposed.

○ Once the results of blood or respiratory tract cultures become available, strategy recommends change from a broad- to a narrow-spectrum antibiotic to which the isolated organism is sensitive as well as removing an antibiotic from an initial combination when the anticipated organism is not recovered.

○ De-escalation is possible in 31.4% of 115 patients in one study.

  – Strategy was applied to 40.7% of patients with early-onset and 12.5% of patients with late-onset VAP.

  – Obviously, a de-escalation strategy is not possible in patients without cultures.

• **Duration of therapy**

• Prospective, multicenter, randomized, double-blind trial performed to determine whether 8 versus 15 days of antibiotic treatment equally effective

• Patients receiving appropriate antimicrobial treatment during 8 days had neither excess mortality nor more recurrent infection than patients treated for 15 days.

• In patients suffering from VAP due to nonfermenting gram-negative bacilli (mainly *P. aeruginosa* and *A. baumannii*), the outcome was similar in two groups, but there was a trend to greater rates of pulmonary infection recurrences (relapses and/or superinfection) in short duration of treatment group.

- ATS/IDSA guidelines suggest shortening duration of therapy to 7 days, providing that causative pathogen is neither *P. aeruginosa* nor *A. baumannii*, and patient exhibits a good clinical response.
- Whatever treatment duration, when aminoglycosides are used in combination with other agents, they may be stopped after no more than 5 to 7 days.
- Prompt initiation of empiric antibiotic therapy is a cornerstone of VAP treatment.
- In absence of gold standard, diagnosis of VAP remains difficult.
  - Among all empirically treated patients, some will not have VAP.
  - Empiric antibiotic therapy may be safely discontinued after 72 hours when a noninfectious etiology for the pulmonary infiltrates is discovered or when signs and symptoms of active infections resolve.
  - Sterile culture of lower respiratory tract secretions rules out, absent a new antibiotic in past 72 hours, presence of bacterial pneumonia.
  - In a case such as this, withholding antibiotics is justified.
- **Specific antibiotic regimens**
- *P. aeruginosa*, *A. baumannii*, and MRSA are the main causative pathogens of VAP.
- Combination of antibiotics for *P. aeruginosa* VAP commonly used
  - Aim of combination is to achieve antibiotic synergy and prevent the emergence of resistant strains during therapy
  - While two recent meta-analyses showed that, for septic patients, combination β-lactam plus aminoglycoside compared with β-lactam monotherapy provides no clinical benefit and has no beneficial effect on development of antimicrobial resistance among initially antimicrobial-susceptible isolates, these analyses suffer from limitations that weaken the interpretation.
    - Low number of studies included in analysis
    - Heterogeneity of those studies
    - Outdated aminoglycoside administration schedules
  - These results are not sufficiently strong to justify discontinuing the use of short-term aminoglycoside–β-lactam combination therapy for *P. aeruginosa* VAP.
- Vancomycin remains standard therapy for treatment of serious infections due to MRSA.
  - Linezolid is a recent agent proposed for treatment of these infections.
  - Two multicenter studies demonstrated equivalence between linezolid and vancomycin for treatment of hospital-acquired pneumonia due to MRSA.
    - Linezolid may provide better outcome and a lower mortality than vancomycin.
    - However, results appear conflicting, and a prospective validation of the superiority of linezolid required.
    - Nevertheless, linezolid may be preferred to vancomycin in patients with or at risk for renal insufficiency.
- *A. baumannii* exhibits native resistance to many classes of antimicrobial agents and has seen the emergence of resistance to carbapenems.
  - Despite reported nephrotoxicity of polymyxins, they may be safely used.

- Safety and efficacy of intravenous colistin in patients with VAP due to *A. baumannii* resistant to carbapenems has been shown.
- **Local instillation and aerosolized antibiotics**
  - Aminoglycosides and polymyxin B have been used for local instillation or aerosolization to treat VAP due to pathogens that are "resistant" to systemic antimicrobial agents.
  - There is a lack of large or randomized prospective studies evaluating the value of these administration routes.
  - Routine use of local instillation/aerosolized antibiotics not recommended.

Response to Therapy

- **Normal pattern of resolution**
- Improvement usually apparent only after 48 to 72 hours of adequate antibiotic therapy.
  - Unless rapid clinical deterioration, antimicrobial therapy should not be changed during this period following initiation of therapy.
- Fever and hypoxemia appear to be the best indicators to monitor response to treatment.
  - In patients without ARDS, most respond with a resolution of fever to <38°C and resolution of hypoxemia with a PaO$_2$/FiO$_2$ improving to >250 within first 72 hours of adequate treatment.
  - For responding patients with ARDS, hypoxemia resolves more slowly and, consequently, this parameter should not be used to define the resolution of VAP.
    - Although fever takes twice as long to resolve, core temperature appears as most useful indicator of clinical response.
  - Monitoring of white blood cell count not accurate to evaluate the response to therapy.
  - Similarly, chest radiographs are of limited value for defining clinical improvement in VAP.
    - Initial radiograph deterioration is common.
    - However, quick radiographic resolution suggests that initial diagnosis of VAP could be erroneous.
- **Reasons for deterioration or nonresolution**
  - When a patient fails to improve or exhibits rapid deterioration, several causes may be considered (Table 76.9).
  - When possible, antimicrobial spectrum should be broadened.
  - Careful clinical evaluation to rule out diagnostic possibilities based on differential diagnosis must be performed.
  - Sampling of respiratory tract secretions must be repeated.
    - If cultures reveal a resistant pathogen (inadequate initial empiric choice, development of resistance or superinfection with a resistant strain), an adequate antibiotic therapy must be rapidly instituted, even if such a change has a low prognostic impact.
    - If cultures do not yield a resistant pathogen, one must consider a noninfectious process, another site of infection, or occurrence of complications.
      - Vascular catheters must be removed and cultured, and blood and urine samples must be drawn for culture.
      - Radiographic procedures such as CT scanning of the thorax and, possibly, of extrathoracic sites (sinuses, abdomen) may reveal complications (e.g., lung abscess, empyema) or other infectious sites (e.g., sinusitis).
  - Finally, when entire workup remains negative—including the microbiologic and radiographic evaluations for VAP,

TABLE 76.9

CAUSES OF NONRESOLUTION OR DETERIORATION IN PATIENTS WITH VAP

Factors	Comments
Wrong initial diagnosis of VAP	Many noninfectious processes can mimic VAP: • Pulmonary embolism • Congestive heart failure • Lung contusion • Atelectasis • Chemical pneumonitis from aspiration • ARDS • Pulmonary hemorrhage
Host factors	Despite adequate treatment, many conditions are known to be associated with failure: • Underlying fatal condition • Age older than 60 yr • Prior pneumonia • Prior antibiotic treatment • Chronic lung diseases

Bacterial factors	• Infecting bacteria can be resistant and can acquire resistance during treatment (*Pseudomonas aeruginosa*)
	• Infecting pathogen can be a nonbacterial pathogen:
	  • Mycobacteria
	  • Virus
	  • Fungus
	• Some pathogens, even with effective treatment, are difficult to eradicate (*P. aeruginosa*)

Occurrence of complications	• Complications of initial pneumonia:
	  • Empyema
	  • Lung abscess
	• Other sites of infection:
	  • Urinary tract infection
	  • Catheter-related infection
	  • Sinusitis
	  • Pseudomembranous enterocolitis
	• Drug fever, pulmonary embolism, and sepsis with multiple system organ failure

ARDS, acute respiratory distress syndrome.
Adapted from American Thoracic Society, Infectious Diseases Society of America. Guidelines for the management of adults with hospital-acquired, ventilator-associated, and healthcare-associated pneumonia. *Am J Respir Crit Care Med.* 2005;171:388.

with or without resistant pathogens, noninfectious processes mimicking VAP, VAP complications, or an extrapulmonary site of infection, physicians must consider the following:
- ○ Coverage for unusual pathogens (i.e., mycobacteria, fungi)
- ○ Need for an open-lung biopsy
- ○ Initiation of anti-inflammatory therapy such as corticosteroids

- In one review, the main causes of nonresponsiveness were:
  - ○ Inappropriate initial treatment (23%)
  - ○ Superinfections (14%)
  - ○ Another site of infection (27%)
  - ○ Noninfectious process (16%)
  - ○ In 36% of nonresponding patients, no cause of failure was identified.

Prognosis of VAP

- Crude mortality rates associated with VAP vary from 24% to 76%.
- Widely diverging crude mortality rates can be explained by differences both in studied populations and diagnostic criteria used.
- One of the most important concerns about VAP is to know whether it is associated with significant attributable mortality.
  - In some studies, VAP was not associated with any significant attributable mortality.
  - In others, VAP was associated with a significant attributable mortality set around 25%.
- Numerous independent prognostic factors associated with hospital mortality of patients suffering from VAP were identified.
  - Patients' underlying illnesses (malignancy, immunosuppression, anticipated death within 5 years, American Society of Anesthesiology grade 3 or more)
  - Age older than 64 years
  - Severity of disease justifying ICU admission (high APACHE II score, Simplify Acute Physiology Score >37)
  - Initial severity of VAP (chest radiographic involvement of more than one lobe, platelet count <150,000 cells/μL, Logistic Organ Dysfunction score >4, time of onset of VAP >3 days, surgery, or hypotension)
  - Initial therapeutic approach (delayed initial appropriate antibiotic treatment)

Prevention of Ventilator-Associated Pneumonia

- Basic infection control techniques are necessary to limit cross-contamination of resistant organisms through health care workers, such as:
- Hand washing
- Glove use
- Sterile equipment
- Adequate staffing
- Primary intervention to reduce VAP is to minimize intubation frequency and duration.
  - Noninvasive positive pressure ventilation (NIPPV) using a face mask as an alternative ventilation mode in ICU patients.
  - Associated with a relative risk reduction for VAP ranging from 0.67 to 0.87
  - When intubation is necessary, orotracheal route is preferred.
  - Strategies to reduce duration of MV, such as optimized sedation and weaning protocols, are also effective.
  - Continuous aspiration of subglottic secretions associated with relative risk reduction for VAP of 0.45
  - Semirecumbent (45-degree) patient position also reduces VAP, particularly compared to the supine position with enteral nutrition.
- Stress ulcer prophylaxis has controversial impact on VAP.
  - Benefit offered by decreasing risks of gastric hemorrhage might outweigh increased risk of VAP.

TABLE 76.10

MEASURES RECOMMENDED BY THE CDC TO
REDUCE THE INCIDENCE OF VAP

- Changing the breathing circuits of ventilators only when
  they malfunction or are visibly contaminated
- Preferential use of orotracheal rather than nasotracheal
  tubes
- Use of noninvasive ventilation
- Use of an endotracheal tube with a dorsal lumen to allow
  drainage of respiratory secretions

Data from Tablan OC, Anderson LJ, Besser R, et al. Healthcare
Infection Control Practices Advisory Committee, Centers for Disease
Control and Prevention. Guidelines for preventing
health-care–associated pneumonia, 2003: recommendations of the
CDC and the Healthcare Infection Control Practices Advisory
Committee. *MMWR Recomm Rep.* 2004;53(RR-3):1.

- Enteral nutrition is associated with VAP, but the alternative—parenteral nutrition—carries the risk of catheter-related bacteremia.
  - Postpyloric feeding reported to reduce VAP.
- Ventilator circuit management, transfusion practices, and glycemic control are also issues that may be addressed to reduce VAP.
- The CDC published 2004 guidelines on the prevention of VAP (Table 76.10).
- ICU providers caring for immunosuppressed patients with severe neutropenia and/or allogeneic hematopoietic stem cell transplant recipients must take measures to prevent legionellosis or aspergillosis.
  - Legionellosis prevention based on control of hot water system.
  - Aspergillosis prevention necessitates rooms with high-efficiency particulate air filters and the use of high-efficiency respiratory protection devices (e.g., N95 respirators) by patients when they leave their rooms and/or when dust-generating activities are ongoing in the facility.
- One last highly controversial issue is use of selective digestive decontamination (SDD).
  - The subject of multiple trials using application and ingestion of topical nonabsorbed antimicrobials (usually combining polymyxin, aminoglycoside, and amphotericin B) with or without the addition of a short-duration systemic broad-spectrum antibiotic.
  - Theory is topical agents will eradicate potential pathogens (gram-negative aerobic intestinal bacteria, *S. aureus,* and fungi) but not anaerobic flora.
  - Impressive results have been recently published, with a 20% decrease in ICU mortality.
  - However, methodologic flaws (ward, no patient randomization, and unblinded trials) and an extremely low rate of drug-resistant organisms, including zero MRSA colonization, make generalization of results difficult.
    - Preventive effects of SDD for VAP are lower in ICUs with high endemic levels of antibiotic resistance, and, in such cases, SDD increases the selective antibiotic pressure and can increase incidence of drug-resistant microorganisms.
  - To date, generalized routine use of SDD in ICUs not recommended.
    - Should be decided according to patient population and ICU characteristics

HAP

- HAP defined as pneumonia occurring <2 days from hospital admission, but without any criteria defining VAP.
  - Data about HAP acquired outside the ICU, treated outside the ICU, or requiring ICU admission for treatment are scarce.
  - Information suggests most patients who acquired HAP in medical wards exhibited severe underlying diseases (i.e., chronic pulmonary diseases, immunosuppression) and developed HAP late during hospital stay.
  - Microbiologic data demonstrate major role played by Enterobacteriaceae, *P. aeruginosa,* and MRSA, and variations in local epidemiology (Table 76.11)
  - Mortality rate varies from one study to another between 18.8% and 53%.
  - ATS/IDSA guidelines suggest that all patients with HAP be managed as if they were VAP cases.

HCAP and Nursing Home Pneumonia

- HCAP includes any patient:
  - Hospitalized in an acute care hospital for 2 or more days within 90 days of infection
  - Resides in nursing home or long-term care facility (LTCF)
  - Received recent intravenous antibiotic therapy, chemotherapy, or wound care within 30 days of current infection
  - Attends a hospital or hemodialysis clinic
- Most pneumonia occurring in hosts with therapeutic immunodeficiency are now classified as HCAP.
- In nursing homes. pneumonia is the leading cause of mortality, morbidity, and transfers to acute care facilities among residents.
- Pneumonia is second most common infection in LTCFs.
- Incidence of 0.3 to 4.7 cases per 1,000 resident-days
- An independent risk factor for death in LTCF patients
- Mortality in these patients ranges from 5% to 40%.
  - Coincides with mortality seen in community-dwelling patients diagnosed with pneumonia and admitted to an ICU
  - These differ in presentation due to modified host response seen in elderly.
- In older individuals, fever and respiratory signs may be minimal.
  - An altered mental status might be only evident symptom.
- Pneumonia risk factors in nursing home residents include:
  - Decreased functional status
  - Diminished ability to clear airways
  - Underlying comorbidities (such as COPD and heart disease)
  - Swallowing disorders
  - Use of sedatives
- Etiology of nursing home–acquired pneumonia remains controversial.
  - Using strict criteria, *S. pneumoniae* and *H. influenzae* are the major pathogens.
  - Gram-negative bacilli account for 0% to 12% of cases.
- The ATS/IDSA guidelines recommend that, when hospitalized, these patients be managed like those with HAP until an etiologic diagnosis is made.
- Recommendations are summarized in Tables 76.8 and 76.9.

TABLE 76.11

MICROORGANISMS THAT CAUSE HAP[a]

References	Valles et al.[b]	Sopena et al.[c]	Kollef et al.[d]
Number of episodes of HAP	96	165	835
Number of bacteria identified	75	60	ND
Pseudomonas aeruginosa	18 (24%)	7 (11.7%)	18.4%
Acinetobacter baumannii	1	5 (8.3%)	2.0%
Stenotrophomonas maltophilia	ND	ND	ND
Enterobacteriaceae	7 (9.3%)	8 (13.3%)	16.1%
Haemophilus species	2	2 (3.3%)	5.6%
Legionella pneumophila	9 (12%)	7 (11.7%)	ND
Methicillin-resistant *Staphylococcus aureus*	} 9 (12%)	1 (1.6%)	22.9%
Methicillin-sensitive *S. aureus*		3 (5%)	26.2%
Streptococcus pneumoniae	11 (15%)	16 (26.7%)	3.1%
Streptococcus species	2	ND	13.9%
Enterococcus species	ND	ND	ND
Coagulase-negative staphylococcus	ND	ND	ND
Anaerobic pathogens	ND	ND	ND
Aspergillus species	13 (17%)	7 (11.7%)	ND

ND, no data.
[a]Data are presented as number and/or (percentage).
[b]Valles J, Mesalles E, Mariscal D, et al. A 7-year study of severe hospital-acquired pneumonia requiring ICU admission. *Intensive Care Med.* 2003;29:1981.
[c]Sopena N, Sabria M, Neunos 2000 Study Group. Multicenter study of hospital-acquired pneumonia in non-ICU patients. *Chest.* 2005;127:213.
[d]Kollef MH, Shorr A, Tabak YP, et al. Epidemiology and outcomes of health-care-associated pneumonia: results from a large US database of culture-positive pneumonia. *Chest.* 2005;128:3854.

TRACHEOBRONCHITIS

Acute Exacerbations of Chronic Obstructive Pulmonary Disease

- Acute exacerbation of COPD defined by impairment in patient's baseline dyspnea, cough, and/or sputum
- Need for ICU or special care unit admission based on severity of respiratory failure and/or presence of associated organ dysfunction (i.e., shock, hemodynamic instability, neurologic disturbances)
- Therapy in the ICU is based on supplemental oxygen, ventilatory support, bronchodilators, corticosteroids, and antibiotics.
- Role of bacterial infection in acute exacerbation of COPD remains controversial.
  - Even in the absence of symptoms of exacerbation, numerous bacteria colonize lower respiratory tract of COPD patients.
  - Bacteria colonizing lower respiratory tract vary from one patient to another, as COPD patients are heterogeneous.
  - Information provided by sputum culture does not really reflect conditions in distal airways.
  - Only half of episodes of acute exacerbations of COPD are linked to bacterial infection.
  - Animal models are limited by the fact that the most often isolated bacteria (*S. pneumoniae, H. influenzae, Moraxella catarrhalis*) are exclusively human pathogens.
  - Clinical studies addressing impact of antibiotic therapy during acute exacerbation of COPD suggest that such a treatment provides only a small improvement in the most severely ill patients.

- Despite uncertainties ATS/European Respiratory Society Task Force proposed to institute antibiotic treatment in all patients suffering from a severe acute exacerbation of COPD requiring ICU admission.
- Prospective, randomized, double-blind, placebo-controlled trial assessing effects of ofloxacin.
  - Antibiotic treatment reduced mortality rate, need for additional antibiotics in preventing occurrence of nosocomial pneumonia, and duration of mechanical ventilation and hospital stay.
- An inadequate initial antibiotic treatment increased hospital mortality and was significantly associated with failure of noninvasive ventilation, leading to secondary intubation and invasive MV.
  - Inadequacy of initial empiric treatment mainly occurred when colonizing pathogens not the usual community-acquired pathogens (*S. pneumoniae, H. influenzae, M. catarrhalis*) but were instead nonfermenting (*P. aeruginosa*) or enteric gram-negative bacilli
- Current recommendations propose an antibiotic therapy based on amoxicillin/clavulanate or respiratory fluoroquinolones (gatifloxacin, levofloxacin, moxifloxacin).
  - If *Pseudomonas* spp. or *Enterobacteriaceae* spp. are suspected, combination therapy should be considered.
  - A wide-spectrum β-lactam combined with an antipseudomonal fluoroquinolone or an aminoglycoside may be of use.
  - Finally, an ongoing study of local microbiology and susceptibility patterns by routine bacteriologic investigation in COPD patients appears the best means to provide initial adequate antibiotic treatment for acute exacerbations of COPD.

Nosocomial Tracheobronchitis

- Only a few studies have addressed nosocomial tracheobronchitis acquired during MV
  - Most recent data has potentially major limitation that studies performed in a single ICU
    - Consequently, the results may not be applicable to other units.
    - Retrospective analysis of 2,128 mechanically ventilated patients more than 48 hours
    - Incidence of nosocomial tracheobronchitis was 10.6%.
      - No significant difference between medical (9.9%; 165 of 1,655) and surgical patients (15.3%; 36 of 234)
  - In patients without underlying chronic respiratory insufficiency, incidence was 8%.
  - Delay between initiation of MV and occurrence of tracheobronchitis was up to 10 days.
  - In medical patients, nosocomial tracheobronchitis significantly associated with:
    - Age younger than 60 years (OR = 1.8)
    - COPD (OR = 1.57)
    - Receiving prior antibiotics within the 2 weeks preceding ICU admission (OR = 1.52)
  - Main pathogens identified in culture of tracheal aspirates were *P. aeruginosa*, *A. baumannii*, and MRSA.
- Impact of nosocomial tracheobronchitis on patient outcome is difficult to assess.
  - Two case-control studies comparing patients with and without nosocomial tracheobronchitis
    - In both COPD patients and in patients without chronic respiratory insufficiency, nosocomial tracheobronchitis was significantly associated with longer durations of mechanical ventilation and ICU stay.
    - Conversely, occurrence of tracheobronchitis had no significant influence on mortality rates.
  - Indications for antibiotic treatment in these patients are still debated.
    - Some physicians consider that antibiotic treatment is not justified, whereas others consider antibiotics to be useful in patients with tracheobronchitis and weaning difficulties.
    - Despite results suggesting that appropriate antibiotic treatment might reduce duration of mechanical ventilation only well-designed prospective studies will answer the question.

LUNG ABSCESS

- Can be associated with aspiration pneumonia, poor dental hygiene, alcohol consumption, or chronic lung disease
- Relatively uncommon in developed countries
  - Where it occurs mostly in immunosuppressed patients or as a postobstructive complication
  - Risk factors and underlying diseases are presented in (Table 76.12).

Bacteriology of Lung Abscesses

- Predominant pathogens are considered to be anaerobes
  - Account for 60% to 80% of cases

TABLE 76.12

RISK FACTORS AND UNDERLYING DISEASES OF ADULT PATIENTS WITH COMMUNITY-ACQUIRED LUNG ABSCESS[a]

References	Hammond et al.[b]	Wang et al.[c]
Number of patients	34	90
Characteristic (%)		
Smoking	ND	57%
Chronic lung disease	29%	37%
Diabetes mellitus	ND	31%
Previous aspiration pneumonia	29%	32%
Malignancy	3%	19%
Alcohol abuse	38%	14%
Dental caries	26%	ND
CNS disease	9%	11%
Chronic liver disease	ND	11%
Steroid use/SLE	9%	6%
None	12%	18%

ND, no data; CNS, central nervous system; SLE, systemic lupus erythematosus.
[a]Data are presented as number or percentage.
[b]Hammond JM, Potgieter PD, Hanslo D, et al. Etiology and antimicrobial susceptibility patterns of micro organisms in acute community-acquired lung abscess. *Chest*. 1995;108:937.
[c]Wang JL, Chen KY, Fang CT, et al. Changing bacteriology of adult community-acquired lung abscess in Taiwan: *Klebsiella pneumoniae* versus anaerobes. *Clin Infect Dis*. 2005;40:915.

- In a study of 34 patients with community-acquired lung abscess
  - 2.3 bacterial species per episode
  - Anaerobes were identified in 75% of cases.
  - Infection due to an aerobe observed in only 19% of cases.
- More recent studies reveal a more mixed pattern
  - Study of 90 patients with lung abscesses in Taiwan observed polymicrobial infection in only 20% of cases.
  - Gram-negative bacilli, mostly *Klebsiella pneumoniae* the most frequently isolated microorganisms (47%)
  - Anaerobes were only isolated in 31%.
  - Main bacteriologic data are reported in (Table 76.13).

Diagnosis

- Blood cultures and sputum examination are rarely positive.
- Methods to obtain a specimen uncontaminated with colonizing bacteria from upper airway preferred.
  - Percutaneous aspiration, transtracheal aspiration, or thoracocentesis from empyema fluid make isolation of both aerobic and anaerobic bacteria possible.

Treatment

- A severe disease
- Historically, death in one-third of cases when surgical resection or drainage was only available tool.

Antimicrobial Therapy

- Generally treated successfully with prolonged systemic antibiotic therapy

TABLE 76.13

PATHOGENS ISOLATED FROM ADULT PATIENTS
WITH COMMUNITY-ACQUIRED LUNG ABSCESS[a]

References	Hammond et al.[b]	Wang et al.[c]
Number of patients	34	90
Number of bacteria identified	79	118
Anaerobes	59 (75%)	40 (34%)
Microaerophilic streptococci	7 (20%)	11 (12%)
Prevotella	17 (50%)	8 (9%)
Bacteroides	4 (12%)	6 (7%)
Fusobacterium	4 (12%)	3 (3%)
Porphyromonas	7 (20%)	1 (1%)
Gram-negative bacilli	3 (9%)	42 (47%)
Klebsiella pneumoniae	2 (6%)	30 (33%)
Gram-positive cocci	12 (35%)	30 (33%)
Streptococcus milleri	ND	19 (21%)
Staphylococcus aureus	5 (15%)	2 (2%)
Viridans streptococci	7 (20%)	5 (5%)
Other	5 (15%)	5 (5%)

ND, no data.
[a]Data are presented as number and (percentage).
[b]Hammond JM, Potgieter PD, Hanslo D, et al. Etiology and
antimicrobial susceptibility patterns of micro organisms in acute
community-acquired lung abscess. *Chest.* 1995;108:937.
[c]Wang JL, Chen KY, Fang CT, et al. Changing bacteriology of adult
community-acquired lung abscess in Taiwan: *Klebsiella pneumoniae*
versus anaerobes. *Clin Infect Dis.* 2005;40:915.

- Preferred antimicrobial therapy, based on high frequency of
  anaerobes was clindamycin
  - β-lactamase inhibitor/aminopenicillin also effective
  - Both regimens obtain cure rates between 60% and 70%
    with a 3-week course.

Other Therapies

- Lack of improvement may necessitate drainage procedures
  in 10% to 20% of patients who remain symptomatic and
  eventually require other therapy.
  - Percutaneous radiographic-guided drainage is effective in
    only a selected subgroup of patients.
  - Reported catheter drainage times averaged 9.8 to 20.1 days.
  - With range of 4 to 59 days
    - Procedure may be difficult in patients with hemostatic
      abnormalities.
    - Risk of soiling pleural space with abscess contents
    - Surgical resection of the diseased lung and abscess might
      be necessary.
    - Endoscopic drainage could be useful in patients who have
      an airway connection to the abscess or an endobronchial
      obstruction preventing drainage.

PLEURAL EMPYEMA

Pathophysiology of Pleural Infection

- Pleural space is normally sterile.
  - Pleural effusion favored by an increase in hydrostatic pres-
    sure, a decrease of oncotic pressure, or alterations of pleural
    permeability.

- Infection follows colonization of pleural fluid.
- Formation of an empyema arbitrarily divided into three
  phases:
  - An exudative phase with accumulation of pus
  - A fibropurulent phase with fibrin deposition and locula-
    tion of pleural exudate,
  - An organization phase with fibroblast proliferation lead-
    ing to scar formation and lung entrapment
- In up to half of cases, empyema is a complication of pneu-
  monia.
  - Approximately one-fourth of empyemas are due to a trau-
    matic or iatrogenic injury (surgery, thoracocentesis, chest
    tube placement).
  - In remaining cases, pleural infection is due to a contiguous
    infection (i.e., mediastinum, esophagus, subdiaphragmatic
    areas) extending to the pleura.

Bacteriology of Pleural Infection

- Bacterial etiology of empyema depends on underlying mech-
  anism leading to pleural colonization.
- Three-fourths of empyemas develop as complication of pneu-
  monia or traumatic or iatrogenic injury.
  - The most isolated aerobic organisms are:
    - *Streptococcus* species
    - *S. pneumoniae*
    - *S. aureus*
  - The main isolated aerobic gram-negative organisms are:
    - *Klebsiella* species
    - *P. Aeruginosa*
    - *H. Influenzae*
    - *Escherichia coli*
      - These are commonly part of mixed growths with anaer-
        obes.
      - Anaerobic isolates are identified in 12% to 34% of cul-
        tures.
      - Can cause empyema without aerobic copathogens in
        about 15% of cases

Management of Patients with Pleural Infection

Identification of Pleural Effusion

- In empyema, clinical symptoms may be nonspecific.
  - Fever
  - Chills
  - Chest pain
  - Night sweats
- Physical examination alterations may be limited to:
  - Diminished breath sounds
  - Basilar dullness to percussion
  - Pleural friction rub
  - In mechanically ventilated patients, these signs and symp-
    toms may be less relevant.
- CXR remains the most important clue for diagnosis of pleural
  effusion.
  - With a volume of pleural fluid exceeding 200 mL, blunting
    of posterior costodiaphragmatic sulcus occurs.

- CXR can reveal a pulmonary infiltrate, which suggests possibility of a parapneumonic collection.
- Ultrasonography is particularly useful in unstable or critically ill patients, since devices are at bedside.
  - Precisely locates fluid collection and allows for a guided diagnostic aspiration
  - Some ultrasonographic characteristics (i.e., echogenicity, septations) may help distinguish empyema from transudative pleural effusion and solid mass, and may detect the presence of loculated collections.
- When diagnosis difficult, contrast-enhanced CT scan is useful to:
  - Differentiate pleural empyema from a lung abscess.
  - Detect complications of pleural infection.
  - Identify an intra- or extrathoracic focus of infection that extends to the pleura.

Indication of Pleural Fluid Sampling

- Management of pleural effusion guided by biologic characteristics of pleural fluid
  - Diagnostic pleural fluid sampling is recommended in all patients exhibiting pleural effusion in association with pneumonia, recent chest surgery or trauma, or an infectious process contiguous to pleura.
  - In the ICU, numerous patients develop pleural effusion without any relationship to pleural infection (i.e., hypoalbuminemia, heart failure, and atelectasis).
    - In patients at low risk of infection, pleural fluid sampling is not immediately useful in the absence of sepsis.
  - Gross appearance and chemical, physical, and microscopic characteristics of pleural fluid must be determined.
    - pH, lactic dehydrogenase (LDH) and glucose levels, and white blood cell count must be measured.
    - An appropriate microscopic examination of stained smears and cultures of pleural fluid must be performed.
    - Empyema usually has:
      - A pH value <7.0
      - An LDH level >1,000 IU/L
      - A glucose level <40 mg/dL
      - Positive Gram stain and/or culture
- In patients with parapneumonic pleural effusions, gross appearance and biologic characteristics of pleural fluid can differentiate simple parapneumonic from complicated parapneumonic effusion and empyema, and guide management
  - In simple parapneumonic effusion:
    - Macroscopic appearance reveals a clear fluid
    - pH is >7.2.
    - LDH level is <1,000 IU/L.
    - Glucose level is >40 mg/dL.
    - No organism is identified on Gram stain and culture.
  - In complicated parapneumonic effusion:
    - Pleural fluid is clear, cloudy, or turbid.
    - pH is <7.2.
    - LDH level is >1,000 IU/L.
    - Glucose level is >40 mg/dL.
    - Gram stain and/or culture are positive
  - In empyema, macroscopic examination reveals frank pus exhibiting biologic characteristics described earlier.

Treatment

- Treatment of empyema requires adequate antimicrobial therapy, drainage of pus, and re-expansion of the lung.

- **Antibiotics:** As soon as pleural infection is diagnosed, antibiotic treatment must be started.
  - When pleural fluid cultures are positive, antibiotics must be chosen according to organisms identified and sensitivities.
  - Penicillins and cephalosporins exhibit good penetration into pleural space.
    - Drugs of choice for treating empyemas due to *Streptococcus* sp. and *S. pneumoniae*.
    - Nafcillin is the drug of choice for MRSA infection.
    - Third-generation cephalosporins and carbapenems are preferred choices in case of empyema due to gram-negative aerobic bacilli.
    - Infections due to MRSA and penicillin- and cephalosporin-resistant *S. pneumoniae* are treated with vancomycin.
    - Aminoglycosides are avoided, as penetration into pleural space is poor and they lose their activity in acid pleural fluid.
    - When anaerobic organisms are causative pathogens, a β-lactam combined with a β-lactamase inhibitor, imipenem, metronidazole, and clindamycin are drugs of choice.
  - When cultures are negative, antibiotics must be chosen according to likely causative organisms.
    - Choice depends on mechanism of empyema.
    - Origin of infection (community acquired *versus* hospital acquired)
    - Local hospital policy
    - BTS guidelines suggest following empirical antibiotic regimens:
      - In community-acquired infection, second- and third-generation cephalosporins, amoxicillin, β-lactam–β-lactamase inhibitor combination, meropenem, clindamycin, and benzyl penicillin combined with quinolone may be proposed.
      - In hospital-acquired infection, such as empyema following a nosocomial pneumonia or recent chest surgery, antibiotics should cover both gram-positive and gram-negative aerobes and anaerobes.
        - Antipseudomonal penicillins (piperacillin-tazobactam, ticarcillin-clavulanic acid), carbapenems, and third-generation cephalosporins combined with vancomycin may be used.
  - Duration of antibiotic treatment remains controversial because specific clinical trials are absent.
    - Recent BTS guidelines suggest duration of 3 weeks is probably appropriate.
- **Chest tube drainage:** Prompt chest tube drainage is indicated in patients with frankly purulent or turbid/cloudy pleural fluid on sampling.
  - Pleural fluid pH <7.2 and the presence of pathogens identified by Gram stain or culture of nonpurulent pleural fluid require prompt chest tube drainage.
  - If despite appropriate antibiotic treatment, clinical improvement is poor or when radiologic investigations demonstrate the presence of a loculated pleural collection, chest tube drainage may be suggested.
  - No consensus about the optimal size of chest tube or about efficacy of intrapleural fibrinolytic drugs
    - Randomized, double-blind trial compared intrapleural streptokinase (250,000 IU twice daily for 3 days) to placebo among 427 patients.

○ Streptokinase did not reduce mortality, need for drainage surgery, or duration of hospital stay, and it did not improve radiographic and spirometric outcomes.
- Meta-analysis does not support routine use of fibrinolytic treatment for patients requiring chest tube drainage for empyema or complicated parapneumonic effusion.
- **Surgical treatment:** Must be considered in all patients exhibiting persisting sepsis associated with continuous pleural collection despite being appropriately treated with antibiotics and chest tube drainage
- Choice between video-assisted thoracoscopic surgery, open thoracic drainage, or thoracotomy with decortication depends on:
  - Patient status (age, comorbidity)
  - Surgical preferences
  - Anatomy of pleural effusion assessed by recent thoracic CT scanning

CHAPTER 77 ■ ADULT GASTROINTESTINAL INFECTIONS IN THE ICU

- Diarrhea occurs in close to one occurrence per person per year in the United States.
  - Varies from short-lasting mild illness to various more serious enteric syndromes
    - Include watery diarrhea with dehydration, febrile dysentery, and gastroenteritis with sepsis
  - Usually acquired by exposure to contaminated food, water, or the environment
    - Foodborne enteric diseases estimated to cause:
      ○ Approximately 76 million cases of illness
      ○ 325,000 hospitalizations
      ○ 5,000 deaths in the United States
    - Known pathogens account for:
      ○ Estimated 14 million cases of illnesses
      ○ 60,000 hospitalizations
      ○ 1,800 deaths
- Diarrhea has two important definitions:
  - Increase in normal frequency of stools associated with decrease in form
  - Progressing from formed stools to those showing a watery or loose (soft) consistency
  - Passage of more than 200 g/day of unformed stool in an adult on standard Western diet
- Divided into three stages based on duration:
  - *Acute* ($\leq$14 days)
  - *Persistent* ($\geq$14 days)
  - *Chronic* ($\geq$30 days)
  - Cause of the illness is different in the three groups
    - Viruses, bacteria, and toxins explain most acute episodes (Table 77.1)
    - Parasitic agents more involved in persistent cases (Table 77.1)
    - Noninfectious causes characteristically associated with chronic diarrhea
- Severity of diarrhea determined according to a functional definition:
  - Mild—requires no change in activities
  - Moderate—requires a change in activities but doesn't disable
  - Severe—disables, usually confining affected person to bed; usually leads to hospitalization

ETIOLOGY OF ACUTE DIARRHEA IN THE UNITED STATES

- Community-acquired, acute infectious diarrhea is caused by various organisms (see Table 77.1).
- Bacterial causes include various *Escherichia coli* species.
  - Enterotoxigenic (ETEC)
  - Enteroaggregative (EAEC)
  - Shigatoxin-producing (STEC) including *E. coli* O157:H7
  - Enteropathogenic (EPEC)
  - Enteroinvasive (EIEC)
- In the community, most common causes of diarrhea are viral.
  - Noroviruses being most important
  - Usually mild and require no specific treatment
  - Varies with season
    ○ More viral cases in spring and winter
    ○ More bacterial cases in summer and spring
- Etiology of diarrheal cases presenting to a hospital and hospital-acquired diarrhea different from community-based diarrhea
  - More severe compared to community diarrhea
  - Causative agent may be a bacterial (most common), parasitic, or viral (rarely)
  - May be due to bacteria (*Clostridium difficile* or *Salmonella*), viruses (rotavirus, noroviruses), or fungi (*Candida albicans*), or most commonly to noninfectious agents

TABLE 77.1

POTENTIAL ETIOLOGIC AGENTS IN PATIENTS WITH ACUTE DIARRHEA

Viral	Bacterial	Protozoal
Noroviruses	*Shigella* sp.	*Entamoeba histolytica*
Rotavirus	*Salmonella* sp.	*Giardia lamblia*
Cytomegalovirus	*Vibrio cholerae*	*Cryptosporidium*
	Clostridium difficile	*Cyclospora*
	Campylobacter jejuni	*Isospora*
	Staphylococcus aureus	*Microsporidia*
	Bacillus cereus	
	Shigatoxin-producing *E. coli* (STEC)	
	Enteropathogenic *E. coli* (EPEC)	
	Enteroaggregative *E. coli* (EAEC)	
	Enterotoxigenic *E. coli* (ETEC)	
	Aeromonas	
	Plesiomonas	
	Yersinia sp.	
	Clostridium perfringens	
	Non-cholera *Vibrio*	

EVALUATION OF THE PATIENT WITH SEVERE DIARRHEA

Emergency Department

- First priority is to evaluate vital signs and hydration status of patient.
- Second, electrolyte disturbances need to be sought and corrected.
- Primary concern to immediately reverse circulatory or organ failure resulting from loss of fluid and salt
- Diagnostic investigations for identifying causative agent done simultaneously or after stabilization of patient.
  - Epidemiologic history and clinical features may provide clues to diagnosis.
  - Travel to an economically developing country suggests a bacterial cause.
  - A person receiving antibacterial or chemotherapeutic drugs may have *C. difficile.*
  - Proctitis in a male with history of having gay sex suggests sexually transmitted pathogens including *Neisseria gonorrhoeae, Chlamydia trachomatis,* herpes simplex, or *Treponema pallidum.*
  - Figure 77.1 provides an algorithm to identify steps in patient workup.
- Laboratory studies will help establish the diagnosis.
  - Fecal leukocytes indicates patient has diffuse colonic inflammation.
  - Occult blood in stool supports inflammatory type of diarrhea.
  - Gross blood passed in stool may indicate dysenteric pathogen including:
    - *Shigella*
    - *Campylobacter*
    - Shigatoxin-producing *E. coli* (often *E. coli* O157:H7)
    - *C. difficile*
    - Stool cultures, parasite examination, or toxin test for *C. difficile* may help define cause of illness.

- Characteristics requiring aggressive and thorough laboratory workup are fever >102°F with systemic findings suggesting presence of sepsis.
- Useful to categorize diarrhea into one of two physiologic classifications
  - Noninflammatory and inflammatory (Table 77.2)
    - Subcategory of inflammatory is hemorrhagic or dysenteric diarrhea

Hospital-Acquired Diarrhea

- Diarrhea developing 3 days or longer after admission considered health care associated.
- Between 10% and 30% of nosocomial diarrhea due to *C. difficile*
- Other important causes of nosocomial diarrhea include antibiotics, chemotherapeutic agents, proton pump inhibitors, tube feedings, laxatives, other drugs, and various iatrogenic and idiopathic conditions.
- Always appropriate in hospital-associated diarrheas, when patient receiving antibacterial treatment, to consider *C. difficile* as causative agent.
  - Empiric treatment advisable in more severe cases while laboratory tests pending
- Other pathogens rarely found in hospital-associated diarrhea.
  - Including rotaviruses in pediatric wards, noroviruses, and *Salmonella* spp.

The International Traveler

- Incidence of traveler's diarrhea (TD) ranges from 13.6% to 54.6% in high-risk regions and approximately 4% in low-risk regions.
- Various parts of world classified into three different groups: low, intermediate, and high risk, based on the frequency of TD in the traveling public

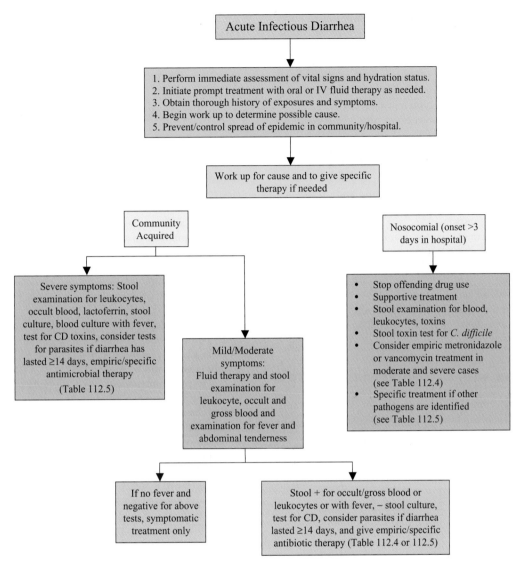

FIGURE 77.1. Flow chart showing approach to a patient with acute infectious diarrhea.

- Important causes of TD are ETEC, EAEC, noroviruses, *Campylobacter, Shigella,* and *Salmonella*
  - Less commonly, parasitic agents cause TD and should be suspected in persistent illness.
    - Important parasitic pathogens in persistent TD include *Giardia, Cryptosporidium,* and *Cyclospora.*

The Immunosuppressed Patient

- Patient with congenital or acquired immunodeficiency, HIV/AIDS, or receiving immunosuppressive or cancer chemotherapy drugs will have increased susceptibility to diarrhea.

TABLE 77.2

CLASSIFICATION OF ACUTE DIARRHEA BASED ON FINDINGS OF FECAL MARKERS OF INFLAMMATION (LEUKOCYTES OR LACTOFERRIN) OR PRESENCE OF GROSS FECAL BLOOD

Types of diarrhea	Possible causes	Measures to be taken
Noninflammatory (negative for inflammatory markers or dysentery)	Toxin-mediated, viral, noninvasive pathogens like *Vibrio cholerae,* ETEC *Shigella, Salmonella,* STEC, *Entamoeba histolytica, Giardia, Campylobacter, Clostridium difficile*	Oral/IV fluid replacement and empiric therapy if required
Invasive, cytotoxic, or enterohemorrhagic (positive for inflammatory markers or presence of dysentery)		Oral/IV fluid therapy based on hydration status and thorough laboratory investigations with specific antibiotic therapy if indicated[a]

ETEC, enterotoxigenic *E. coli;* STEC, Shigatoxin-producing *E. coli.*
[a]Specific therapies are listed in Table 77.5.

- Etiology of diarrheal diseases in immunocompromised hosts different from other populations in that they are at risk of developing infections from various opportunistic organisms in addition to routine diarrheal pathogens
  - Use of various chemotherapy drugs or immunomodulators such as cyclosporine, mycophenolate mofetil, tacrolimus, or sirolimus results in drug-induced diarrhea
  - Diarrhea in transplant recipients can also be due to graft-versus-host disease (GVHD)
  - Various organisms to consider as causes of diarrhea in this group of patients include *Clostridium difficile, Salmonella* enterica, noroviruses, *Cryptosporidium, Isospora, Cyclospora,* cytomegalovirus, and *Mycobacterium avium intracellulare* complex.
  - Rapid diagnostic tests include:
    - Direct stool examination for ova, cysts, and parasites
    - Stool test for *C. difficile* toxin
    - Polymerase chain reaction (PCR) for cytomegalovirus or herpesvirus
    - Stool and blood cultures
  - If aforementioned tests do not provide specific diagnosis, endoscopy and mucosal biopsy are pursued to establish etiologic diagnosis.

The Patient with Extraintestinal Disease

- Blood cultures, computed tomography of abdomen, and serology (for *Entamoeba histolytica*) may help determine primary cause of disease.
- In sepsis, blood cultures and stool studies may provide diagnosis.
- Systemic complications often seen with invasive bacterial and parasitic infections
  - Systemic complications of enteric infection include:
    - Hemolytic uremic syndrome (HUS) or thrombotic thrombocytopenic purpura (TTP)
    - Guillain-Barré syndrome
    - Sepsis
    - Infective endocarditis
    - Abdominal abscesses or localized abscess elsewhere
    - Pyogenic arthritis
  - In immunocompromised patients with diarrhea, systemic complications can occur with any etiologic agent

- Antimotility drugs **should not** be used in inflammatory diarrhea.
- Amoebiasis—uncommon in the United States—shows extended spectrum of extraintestinal complications including liver abscess and disseminated infection.

MANAGEMENT OF ACUTE DIARRHEA

Dehydration

- Defined as excess loss of body fluids resulting in fluid and electrolyte abnormalities
- Classifications of dehydration are provided in Table 77.3.
- Dry skin and mucous membranes, sunken eyes, decreased urine output, loss of skin turgor, dizziness/light-headedness all manifestations of moderate to severe dehydration
- The most common serious complication of diarrhea and should be promptly recognized and managed
- Routine testing of electrolytes in patients with severe diarrhea of proven value
- Rehydration done, depending on severity of dehydration, either by oral or IV route
  - Oral rehydration salt (ORS) solution used in mild or moderate dehydration
    - Also for maintenance of hydration after IV fluid administration in severe dehydration
  - Standard or reduced osmolarity (low-salt) ORS formulations preferable where available
  - When due to cholera, reduced-osmolarity ORS may lead to subclinical reduction of body electrolytes, making standard ORS preferable here
  - In the United States, ORS is not readily available, but Pedialyte or Ricelyte is used to maintain hydration and treat minor degrees of dehydration.
  - Specific fluid replacement strategies based on severity are described in Table 77.3.

Dysentery

- Diagnosis when subjects are passing grossly bloody stools
  - Historically classified as bacillary dysentery (shigellosis) versus amoebic dysentery

---

TABLE 77.3

CLASSIFICATION OF DEHYDRATION IN A PATIENT WITH ACUTE DIARRHEA

Dehydration		Symptoms	Suggested management
Mild dehydration	3%–5% loss in body weight	Increased thirst and slightly dry mucous membranes	Oral rehydration solution (ORS) 50 mL/kg over first 2–4 h
Moderate dehydration	6%–9% loss in body weight	Loss of skin turgor, dry mucous membranes, tenting of skin	ORS 100 mL/kg over first 2–4 h
Severe dehydration	≥10% loss in body weight	Lethargy, altered consciousness, prolonged skin retraction time, cool extremities, decreased capillary refill	Immediate IV fluid replacement with 20 mL/kg of lactated Ringer solution to restore perfusion and mental status. Continue with 100 mL/kg ORS or IV 5% dextrose and 0.45% saline solution at two times the maintenance rate.

From Duggan C, Santosham M, Glass RI. The management of acute diarrhea in children: oral rehydration, maintenance, and nutritional therapy. Centers for Disease Control and Prevention. *MMWR Recomm Rep.* 1992;41(RR-16):1–20; and King CK, Glass R, Bresee JS, et al. Managing acute gastroenteritis among children: oral rehydration, maintenance, and nutritional therapy. *MMWR Recomm Rep.* 2003;52(RR-16):1–16, with permission.

TABLE 77.4

EMPIRIC ANTIMICROBIAL THERAPY OF ACUTE DIARRHEA

Indication	Recommended therapy
Febrile dysentery: Fever (temperature >100.2°F [>38°C]) plus dysentery (passage of grossly bloody stools)	Azithromycin, 500 mg PO daily for 3 days
Moderate to severe traveler's diarrhea with fever and dysentery	Azithromycin, 500 mg PO daily for 3 days
Moderate to severe traveler's diarrhea without fever and dysentery	Rifaximin, 200 mg tid for 3 days; ciprofloxacin, 500 mg bid for 3 days; or levofloxacin, 500 mg once a day for 3 days; or azithromycin, 500 mg once a day for 3 days
Severe hospital-acquired diarrhea in a patient with comorbidity and prior receipt of antibacterial therapy	Oral metronidazole, 500 mg tid for 10 days; or vancomycin, 125–500 mg qid for 10 days

bid, twice a day; PO, orally; qid, four times a day; tid, three times a day.

- Bacillary dysentery is also caused by several invasive pathogens in addition to *Shigella* spp. including *Campylobacter, Clostridium difficile,* STEC, and *Salmonella.*
- Specific cause should be established followed by specific treatment.
  - Empiric and specific antibiotic treatments are provided in Tables 77.4 and 77.5.

Clostridium difficile (CD) Diarrhea and Colitis
- CD first identified as causative agent of antibiotic-associated diarrhea in early 1970s
- Then was associated with clindamycin use
- A gram-positive, spore-forming anaerobic bacteria producing enterotoxin known as toxin A and a cytotoxin called toxin B

TABLE 77.5

SPECIFIC THERAPY FOR PATHOGEN-SPECIFIC DIARRHEA, ONCE ETIOLOGIC DIAGNOSIS IS ESTABLISHED

Identified pathogen	Suggested antimicrobial therapy
Clostridium difficile	Oral metronidazole, 500 mg tid for 10 days; or vancomycin, 125–500 mg qid for 10 days (newer therapies being evaluated including nitazoxanide, rifaximin, and *Saccharomyces*)
Salmonella sp. (treat only for suspected sepsis based on presence of high-risk host*)	For high-risk host[a]: Fluoroquinolones: ciprofloxacin, 500 mg bid; or levofloxacin, 500 mg once a day for 7 to 10 days
Shigella	Fluoroquinolones, dose as in *Salmonella* above, give for 3 days
Campylobacter	Azithromycin, 500 mg once a day for 3 days; or erythromycin, 500 mg bid for 5 days
Shigatoxin-producing *E. coli* (STEC)	No antimotility drugs, antibiotic treatment not usually given as they may increase the risk of occurrence of hemolytic uremic syndrome (HUS)
Enterotoxigenic *E. coli* (ETEC)	Rifaximin, 200 mg tid for 3 days; fluoroquinolone in above dose for 3 days; or azithromycin, 500 mg once a day for 3 days.
Enteropathogenic *E. coli* (EPEC)	Same as *Shigella*
Enteroaggregative *E. coli* (EAEC)	Same as ETEC
Enteroinvasive *E. coli* (EIEC)	Same as *Shigella*
Vibrio spp. (*Vibrio cholerae* or noncholera *Vibrios*)	Tetracycline, 500 mg qid for 3 days; or 300 mg doxycycline, single 100 mg dose for adults
Aeromonas/Plesiomonas	Same as *Shigella*
Yersinia	Same as *Shigella*
Entamoeba histolytica	Metronidazole, 750 mg tid for 5–10 days and diloxanide furoate, 500 mg tid for 10 days; or paromomycin, 500 mg tid for 10 days
Giardia	Metronidazole, 250–750 mg tid for 7–10 days; tinidazole, 2 g as a single dose
Cryptosporidium	Nitazoxanide, 500 mg bid for 3 days; in HIV/AIDS or immunosuppressed patients nitazoxanide, 500/1,000 mg bid for 14 days or more. Paromomycin, 500 mg qid for 7–14 days; or spiramycin, 3 g/day for up to 1 week
Cyclospora	TMP–SMX, 160 and 800 mg, respectively, bid for 7 days; in AIDS patients, TMP–SMX treatment is given for 14 days followed by 3 times weekly for up to 10 weeks
Isospora	TMP–SMX, 160 and 800 mg, respectively, bid for 7 days; in AIDS patients, treatment is followed by thrice weekly TMP–SMX for up to 10 weeks
Microsporidium	Albendazole, 400 mg bid for 7 days and for 4 weeks in immunocompromised patients
Cytomegalovirus	In immunocompromised patient, ganciclovir, 5 mg/kg bid for 14 days

bid, twice a day; ETEC, enterotoxigenic *E. coli*; qid, four times a day; tid, three times a day; TMP-SMZ, trimethoprim-sulfamethoxazole.
[a]High-risk patients for *Salmonella* enterica species (nontyphoid *Salmonella*): Any subject who is toxic with fever >102°F (39°C), age <3 months or 65 years of age or greater, and subjects with malignancy or AIDS, on steroids, with inflammatory bowel disease or renal failure, or undergoing hemodialysis, with hemoglobinopathy such as sickle cell disease. Patients with simple gastroenteritis are best not given antibacterial drugs.

- A third type of toxin produced, called binary toxin, which is an actin-specific ADP ribosylating toxin
- Toxin A causes necrosis, increased intestinal permeability, and inhibition of protein synthesis
- Toxin B thought to become effective once gut wall damaged
- Increased virulence of CD strains presumably associated with higher levels of toxin production by a fluoroquinolone-resistant CD strain variably classified as PCR ribotype 027, pulsed-field gel electrophoresis (PFGE) type NAP1, restriction endonuclease analysis (REA) type BI, and toxin type III
- Incidence of CD acute diarrhea (CDAD) rising due to excess use of antibiotics and emergence of resistant and more virulent strains
  - Nosocomial CDAD increasing in ICUs of large and hospital-wide in smaller hospitals
  - Rise nearly doubled from the years 1996 to 2003.
  - Disproportionately increased in elderly population
  - Conservative estimate of cost of disease in the United States is $1.1 billion per year.
    - With 54% increase in individual adjusted hospital costs
    - Extension of hospital stay by 3.6 days for each affected person
    - Normal hospital surveillance of CDAD identifies half of affected patients.
      - Real burden of CDAD seems to be much more than estimated.
- Major risk factors for CDAD include:
  - Antimicrobial use
  - Age older than 65 years
  - Severity of existing health condition
  - Use of other drugs such as chemotherapeutic agents and proton pump inhibitors
  - Renal insufficiency
  - Gastrointestinal surgery
  - In CDAD, advanced age and comorbidity, plus severity of underlying impairment, predict frequency of infection and outcome
- Associated risk factors for CDAD should be considered
  - Low albumin level (<2.5 g/dL)
  - Recent admission to a health care institution
  - Use of proton pump inhibitors
  - In nonhospitalized patients with other predisposing conditions such as cancer, prolonged antibiotic use is a recognized risk factor for CDAD.
    - Especially with first-generation cephalosporins, fluoroquinolones, or clindamycin
- Recurrence very common in CDAD
  - Estimated that 15% to 30% of patients have recurrent illness after initial treatment
    - Include both reinfections with new strains and relapse of original infecting strain
    - 56% of recurrences due to reinfection
    - Risk factors for early recurrence of CDAD are:
      - Renal failure
      - White blood cell counts >15,000 cells/μL with the initial episode
      - Community-acquired CDAD with first episode
      - Failure to mount a serum antibody response to toxin A during an initial episode of CDAD
- Diagnosis of CDAD based on clinical and laboratory findings
  - Customary way to make diagnosis is to recover a toxigenic strain of CD through microbiologic culture or to detect one or both of the known CD toxins, A and B, in stool samples
  - Stool toxin studies include commercial tissue culture cytotoxin assay for toxin B or an enzyme immunoassay (EIA) for one or both of toxins
  - In a highly probable clinical case with severe disease or fragile clinical picture often advisable to initiate prompt empiric treatment
  - Colonoscopy considered in patients in whom diagnosis not obvious, after initial screening, when there are extraintestinal complications, and in those not responding to empiric treatment

Treatment

- Prompt diagnosis and treatment important to management of CDAD (see Table 77.5)
- Cessation of causative antibiotic use if possible
- Initiation of either oral metronidazole (first-line therapy) or oral vancomycin for 10 days is standard practice.
  - Vancomycin may be slightly more effective than metronidazole.
- Both metronidazole and vancomycin used in treatment of recurrent CD diarrhea
  - Independent predictors of second recurrence are age and duration of hospitalization after first recurrence.
  - Strategies for treating recurrent CD diarrhea or colitis include:
    - Repeating antibiotics either with metronidazole or vancomycin, with tapering of antibiotic dose after a 10-day standard and administering the drug for 2 months or longer
    - Use of probiotics (*Saccharomyces boulardii*) along with high-dose (500 mg four times a day) vancomycin
      - *Saccharomyces* reduces risk of recurrence by 50%
    - Use of IVIG
- If more than one recurrence, various drugs used for prolonged therapy including:
  - Vancomycin
  - Rifaximin
  - *Saccharomyces*
  - Other useful approaches include the restoration of normal colonic flora by fecal enema or by nasogastric tube administration
- Surgical management of CDAD done after failure of medical therapy or if life-threatening complications occur, including colonic perforation, peritonitis, or bowel infarction

Diarrhea Epidemics in the Hospital

- Early identification and controlling spread of rare hospital epidemics of enteric disease keys to successful management
- Universal protocols of isolation and personal hygiene measures important
- Putting infected persons in contiguous areas away from uninfected persons
- Using dedicated hospital personnel for their care an important strategy
- Judicious use of antibiotics in hospital and prompt discontinuation of possible inciting drugs also helpful
- Agents showing potential for epidemics in hospitals are:
  - *C. difficile*
  - *Salmonella* spp.

- *Shigella*
- *Campylobacter*
- *Vibrio*
- *Aeromonas*
- *Yersinia*
- Noroviruses, and rotavirus
- Early therapy of treatable enteric pathogens should occur (see Table 77.5).

Prevention of Diarrhea in the Hospital

- Appropriate use of antibiotics in hospitalized patients
  - With use of narrowest-spectrum antibiotics safely possible to minimize disruption of gut flora should prevent cases of CDAD

- Additionally *Saccharomyces* has been used to prevent CDAD
- Enteric isolation practices for patients with enteric infection in hospital helps prevent spread of diarrhea and lowers incidence
- Effective and widespread hand washing with soap and water
  - Note that alcohol-based hand cleaners not effective against *C. difficile.*
- Meticulous environmental cleaning with chlorine-based bleach products in clinical settings where *C. difficile*–infected patients have been housed proven to prevent spread of infections in hospital

CHAPTER 78 ■ CATHETER-ASSOCIATED URINARY TRACT INFECTIONS IN THE ICU: IMPLICATIONS FOR CLINICAL PRACTICE

- ICUs represent a meeting point between:
  - Most seriously ill patients receiving aggressive therapy
  - Most resistant pathogens that are selected by the use of broad-spectrum antimicrobial therapy
  - Most patients in ICUs receive an indwelling urinary catheter to monitor urine output
  - Urinary tract infection (UTI) remains a leading cause of nosocomial infections with significant morbidity, mortality, and, hence, additional hospital costs.
- UTIs represents 30% to 40% of nosocomial infections.
  - Prevalence in patients admitted to the ICU is approximately 20%.
  - UTIs are the third most common cause of nosocomial infections in the ICU.
  - Incidence of urosepsis:
    - Defined as an inflammation of upper urinary tract that causes sepsis
    - Occurs in approximately 16% of the ICU patient population

DEFINITIONS

- CDC definitions of symptomatic UTIs and asymptomatic UTIs are collected in Tables 78.1 through 78.3
- In the ICU, UTI is consequence of placement of an indwelling catheter.
  - This results in the concept of *catheter-associated UTI.*
    - Definition of which is restricted to the presence of bacteria in the bladder of a patient with an indwelling catheter

- Bacteriuria is defined as the detection of $\geq 10^5$ microorganisms per milliliter of urine with no more than two species of organisms.
- Contrary to non–ICU-acquired UTIs, this definition does not take into account the clinical symptoms.

PATHOPHYSIOLOGY

- Except for the distal urethra, the urinary tract is normally sterile.
- Resistance to UTI is influenced by:
  - Exposure to uropathogenic bacteria
  - Age
  - Hormonal status
  - Urine flow
- Insertion of a catheter allows organisms to gain access to bladder.
  - Catheter induces an inflammation of the urethra.
  - Allows bacteria to ascend into bladder in space between urethral mucosa and catheter
  - Catheter-associated UTI usually follows the formation of biofilm.
    - Consists of adherent microorganisms, their extracellular products, and host components deposited on both the internal and external catheter surfaces
    - Biofilm protects organisms from antimicrobials and host immune response.
    - Ascending route of infection is predominant in women.
      - Owing to their short urethra and contamination with anal flora

TABLE 78.1

DEFINITIONS FOR SYMPTOMATIC UTIs

At least one of the following criteria:

Criterion 1
Patient has at least one of the following signs or symptoms with no other recognized cause: fever ($>38°C$), urgency, frequency, dysuria, or suprapubic tenderness, *and* patient has a positive urine culture with $\geq 10^5$ microorganisms/mL of urine with no more than two species of microorganisms.

Criterion 2
Patient has at least one of the following signs or symptoms with no other recognized cause: fever ($>38°C$), urgency, frequency, dysuria, or suprapubic tenderness *and at least one of the following:* (a) positive dipstick for leukocyte esterase and/or nitrate; (b) pyuria (urine specimen with 10 white blood cells (WBC)/μL or ≥ 3 WBC/ high-power field of unspun urine); (c) organisms seen on Gram stain of unspun urine; (d) at least two urine cultures with repeated isolation of the same uropathogen (gram-negative bacteria or *Staphylococcus saprophyticus*) with $\geq 10^2$ colonies/mL in nonvoided specimens; (e) $\leq 10^5$ colonies/mL of a single uropathogen (gram-negative bacteria or *S. saprophyticus*) in a patient being treated with an effective antimicrobial agent for a urinary tract infection; (f) physician diagnosis of a urinary tract infection; or (g) physician institutes appropriate therapy for a urinary tract infection.

Criterion 3
Patient ≤ 1 year of age with *at least one of the following signs or symptoms with no other recognized cause:* fever ($>38°C$), hypothermia ($<37°C$), apnea, bradycardia, dysuria, lethargy, or vomiting *and* positive urine culture with $\geq 10^5$ microorganisms/mL of urine with no more than two species of microorganisms.

Criterion 4
Patient ≤ 1 year of age with *at least one of the following signs or symptoms with no other recognized cause:* fever ($>38°C$), hypothermia ($<37°C$), apnea, bradycardia, dysuria, lethargy, or vomiting *and* (a) positive dipstick for leukocyte esterase and/or nitrate; (b) pyuria (urine specimen with 10 WBC/μL or ≥ 3 WBC/high-power field of unspun urine); (c) organisms seen on Gram stain of unspun urine; (d) at least two urine cultures with repeated isolation of the same uropathogen (gram-negative bacteria or *S. saprophyticus*) with $\geq 10^2$ colonies/mL in nonvoided specimens; (e) $\leq 10^5$ colonies/mL of a single uropathogen (gram-negative bacteria or *S. saprophyticus*) in a patient being treated with an effective antimicrobial agent for a urinary tract infection; (f) physician diagnosis of a urinary tract infection; or (g) physician institutes appropriate therapy for a urinary tract infection.

From Garner JS, Jarvis WR, Emori TG, et al. CDC definitions for nosocomial infections, 1988. *Am J Infect Control.* 1988;16:128.

- Internal route of contamination (i.e., through lumen of catheter) less frequent
  - Related to reflux of pathogens from drainage system into bladder
  - Occurs when the drainage system fails to close or with contamination of urine in the collection bag

MICROBIOLOGY

- Isolated pathogens in ICU patients with bacteriuria are essentially relatively few (Table 78.4):

- *Escherichia coli*
- *Pseudomonas aeruginosa*
- *Enterococcus* species
- Polymicrobial infections represent a relatively small percentage—5% to 12%—of total infections.
- In nosocomial infections in ICU patients:
  - Gram-negative bacteria caused 71% of UTIs.
    - With stability over a 17-year period of surveillance
    - Resistance to antimicrobials increased during this period.
      - With rates of resistance to third-generation cephalosporins up to 20% for *E. coli*
  - Cross-transmission probably plays a much greater role than suggested at present.

TABLE 78.2

DEFINITIONS FOR ASYMPTOMATIC UTIs

One of the following criteria:

Criterion 1
Patient has had an indwelling urinary catheter within 7 d before the culture *and* patient has a positive urine culture with $\geq 10^5$ microorganisms/mL of urine with no more than two species of microorganisms and patient has no fever ($>38°C$), urgency, frequency, dysuria, or suprapubic tenderness.

Criterion 2
Patient has not had an indwelling urinary catheter within 7 d before the first positive culture and patient has had at least two positive urine cultures with $\geq 10^5$ microorganisms/mL with repeated isolation of the same microorganism and no more than two species of microorganisms and patient has no fever ($>38°C$), urgency, frequency, dysuria, or suprapubic tenderness.

From Garner JS, Jarvis WR, Emori TG, et al. CDC definitions for nosocomial infections, 1988. *Am J Infect Control.* 1988;16:128.

TABLE 78.3

OTHER UTIs

One of the following criteria:

Criterion 1
Patient has organisms isolated from culture of fluid (other than urine) or tissue from affected site.

Criterion 2
Patient has an abscess or other evidence of infection seen on direct examination, during surgical operation, or during a histopathologic examination.

Criterion 3
Patient has at least two of the following signs or symptoms with no other recognized cause: fever (>38°C), localized pain, or tenderness at the involved site *and at least one of the following:* (a) purulent drainage from affected site; (b) organisms cultured from blood that are compatible with suspected site of infection; (c) radiographic evidence of infection (e.g., abnormal ultrasound, computed tomography [CT] scan, magnetic resonance imaging [MRI], or radiolabel scan); (d) physician diagnosis of infection of the kidney, ureter, bladder, urethra, or tissues surrounding the retroperitoneal or perinephric space; or (e) physician institutes appropriate therapy for an infection of the kidney, ureter, bladder, urethra, or tissues surrounding the retroperitoneal or perinephric space.

Criterion 4
Patient ≤1 year of age with at least one of the following signs or symptoms with no other recognized cause: fever (>38°C), hypothermia (<37°C), apnea, bradycardia, dysuria, lethargy, or vomiting *and at least one of the following:* (a) purulent drainage from affected site; (b) organisms cultured from blood that are compatible with suspected site of infection; (c) radiographic evidence of infection (e.g., abnormal ultrasound, CT scan, MRI, or radiolabel scan); (d) physician diagnosis of infection of the kidney, ureter, bladder, urethra, or tissues surrounding the retroperitoneal or perinephric space; or (e) physician institutes appropriate therapy for an infection of the kidney, ureter, bladder, urethra, or tissues surrounding the retroperitoneal or perinephric space.

From Garner JS, Jarvis WR, Emori TG, et al. CDC definitions for nosocomial infections, 1988. *Am J Infect Control.* 1988;16:128.

RISK FACTORS

- In ICU patients, UTIs are associated with the presence of indwelling catheters.
- The first step of prevention is to highlight the risk factors of catheter-associated UTI in this specific population.

- In assessing risk factors for bacteriuria in 553 patients with a urinary catheter for more than 48 hours and hospitalized in an ICU, independent risk factors were:
  - Female gender
  - Length of ICU stay
  - Prior use of antibiotics

TABLE 78.4

PERCENTAGE OF PATHOGENS ASSOCIATED WITH NOSOCOMIAL UTIs

	Percentage of isolates		
Pathogens	Leone et al.[a] (*n* = 53)	Laupland et al.[b] (*n* = 290)	Gaynes et al.[c] (*n* = 4,109)
Gram negative			
Escherichia coli	39	23	26
Pseudomonas aeruginosa	22	10	16.3
Enterobacter species	15	3	6.9
Acinetobacter acinus	11	—	1.6
Proteus species	11	5	—
Klebsiella species	11	5	9.8
Citrobacter species	2	1	
Gram positive			
Enterococcus species	4	15	17.4
Staphylococcus aureus	2	1	3.6
Coagulase-negative *Staphylococcus*	2	5	4.9
Yeast			
Candida albicans	2	20	—
Candida non-*albicans*		8	—

[a]Leone M, Albanese J, Garnier F, et al. Risk factors of nosocomial catheter-associated urinary tract infection in a polyvalent intensive care unit. *Intensive Care Med.* 2003;29:1077.
[b]Laupland KB, Bagshaw SM, Gregson DB, et al. Intensive care unit-acquired urinary tract infections in a regional critical care system. *Crit Care.* 2005;9:R60.
[c]Gaynes R, Edwards JR, National Nosocomial Infections Surveillance System. Overview of nosocomial infections caused by gram-negative bacilli. *Clin Infect Dis.* 2005;41:848.

- Severity score on admission
- Duration of catheterization
- Reducing duration of catheterization the most important clinical step identified for prevention
  - In 21% of 202 patients, the initial indication for the placement of a urinary catheter was unjustified.
  - In a medical ICU, excessive duration of urinary catheter use for monitoring urine output resulted in 64% of the total of unjustified patient-days.

IMPACT OF UTIs in the ICU

- The real impact of ICU-acquired UTIs on outcome remains unclear.
  - In a general hospital population, nosocomial UTIs were associated with significant attributable mortality.
  - Picture probably different in a specific ICU population
    - Even after controlling for many risk factors, UTIs have a higher incidence in ICUs as compared to other wards.
    - Though the urinary tract is source of sepsis in only 10% to 14% of the cases
      ○ Far less than the lung—44% to 68% (Table 78.5)
    - Development of ICU-acquired UTIs associated with:
      ○ Increase in the length of ICU stay
      ○ Increased crude rate of mortality
      ○ Adequately powered studies demonstrate that UTIs are not dependent factors for mortality
- *Urosepsis* is defined as inflammation of the upper urinary tract that causes seeding of the blood with bacteria, resulting in local and distant destruction of tissue.
- 126 trauma patients with a urinary catheter were evaluated for sepsis.
  - Twenty (16%) were diagnosed with urosepsis.
  - Correlated with:
    - Age older than 60 years
    - Extended length of stay in the ICU and/or hospital
    - Duration of catheterization
- Mortality rates (15%) of the patients without urosepsis and with urosepsis did not differ.
- A prospective, cohort study of 235 catheter-acquired infections among 1,497 patients, 90% of whom were asymptomatic, reported only one (0.42%) secondary bloodstream infection.

TABLE 78.5

RATES OF SEPSIS ACCORDING TO EACH SITE

Sites	Percentages of patients	
	Vincent et al.[a] (*n* = 1,177)	Angus et al.[b] (*n* = 192,980)
Lung	68%	44.0%
Abdomen	22%	8.6%
Blood	20%	17.3%
Urine	14%	9.1%

[a]Vincent JL, Sakr Y, Sprung CL, et al. Sepsis in European intensive care units: results of the SOAP study. *Crit Care Med.* 2006;34:344.
[b]Angus DC, Linde-Zwirble WT, Lidicker J, et al. Epidemiology of severe sepsis in the United States: analysis of incidence, outcome, and associated costs of care. *Crit Care Med.* 2001;29:1303.

- Finally, UTIs can incur significant additional cost.
  - Episode of symptomatic nosocomial UTI in a hospitalized patient is expected to result in an average of $676 in additional cost.
  - In a study calculating the daily antibiotic costs per infected ICU patient, UTIs had the lowest daily antibiotic cost per infected patient ($52).

DIAGNOSTIC TOOLS IN THE ICU

- Urosepsis should be suspected any time a patient has a febrile episode.
  - Routine daily bacteriologic monitoring of urine from all catheterized patients is not an effective way to decrease the incidence of symptomatic, catheter-associated UTI and is not recommended.
  - Three clinical trials have assessed the effectiveness of urinary dipsticks (leukocyte esterase and nitrite) for screening patients instead of quantitative urine culture in the ICU (Table 78.6).
  - Leukocyte esterase activity is an indicator of pyuria.
  - Urinary nitrite production is an indicator of bacteriuria.
  - Our best sense of these data is that the use of dipsticks—instead of quantitative urine culture—cannot be recommended for symptomatic UTIs in ICU patients.
  - The Infectious Diseases Society of America guidelines recommend that asymptomatic bacteriuria or funguria not be screened in patients with an indwelling urethral catheter.
    ○ In symptomatic patients, quantitative urine culture with Gram stain examination is recommended to obtain rapid identification of the pathogen.

PREVENTION

- The best prevention of ICU-acquired UTIs is to reduce the use of indwelling urethral catheters.
  - In a medical ICU, 64% of the total unjustified patient-days with urethral catheter resulted from its prolonged use for monitoring urine output.

TABLE 78.6

ASSESSING URINARY REAGENT STRIPS IN THE ICU

	Tissot et al.[a]	Mimoz et al.[b]	Legras et al.[c]
Prevalence (%)	31	38	42
Sensitivity (%)	87	84	90
Specificity (%)	61	41	65
Positive predictive value (%)	31	46	61
Negative predictive value (%)	96	81	91

[a]Tissot E, Woronoff-Lemsi MC, Cornette C, et al. Cost-effectiveness of urinary dipsticks to screen asymptomatic catheter-associated urinary infections in an intensive care unit. *Intensive Care Med.* 2001;27:1842.
[b]Mimoz O, Bouchet E, Edouard A, et al. Limited usefulness of urinary dipsticks to screen out catheter-associated bacteriuria in ICU patients. *Anaesth Intens Care.* 1995;23:706.
[c]Legras A, Cattier B, Perrotin D. Dépistage des infections urinaires dans un service de rintérêt des bandelettes réactives. *Med Mal Infect.* 1993;23:34.

TABLE 78.7

COMPARATIVE STUDIES PERFORMED IN THE ICU ON THE PREVENTION OF CATHETER-ASSOCIATED UTI

	Leone et al.[a]	Leone et al.[b]	Thibon et al.[c]	Bologna et al.[d]
Method (number of patients)	Prospective Not randomized ($n = 311$)	Prospective Randomized ($n = 224$)	Prospective Randomized Multicenter ($n = 199$)	Prospective Not randomized Multicenter ($n = 108$)
Rate of bacteriuria (%)	8	12	11	8.1 vs. 4.9
Study group	Two-chamber simple closed drainage system	Two-chamber simple closed drainage system	Catheter coated with hydrogel and silver salts	Hydrogel latex Foley catheter with silver metal
Control group	Complex closed system	Complex closed system	Standard catheter	Standard catheter
Conclusion	No difference	No difference	No difference	No difference

[a]Leone M, Garnier F, Dubuc M, et al. Prevention of nosocomial urinary tract infection in ICU patients. Comparison of effectiveness of two urinary drainage systems. *Chest.* 2001;120:220.
[b]Leone M, Garnier F, Antonini F, et al. Comparison of effectiveness of two urinary drainage systems in intensive care unit: a prospective, randomized clinical trial. *Intensive Care Med.* 2003;29:410.
[c]Thibon P, Le Coutour X, Leroyer R, et al. Randomized multi-centre trial of the effects of a catheter coated with hydrogel and silver salts on the incidence of hospital-acquired urinary tract infections. *J Hosp Infect.* 2000;45:117.
[d]Bologna RA, Tu LM, Polansky M, et al. Hydrogel/silver ion-coated urinary catheter reduces nosocomial urinary tract infection rates in intensive care unit patients: a multicenter study. *Urology.* 1999;54:982.

- Each member of the critical care medicine team should attempt to reduce the length of urethral catheterization.
- This evaluation should occur during daily rounds.
- Other measures can be useful only in units with a restrictive policy of catheterization (Table 78.7).

Urinary Drainage System

- To prevent infection, maintenance of a closed sterile drainage system is recommended as the most successful method.
- Closed drainage system described for the first time in 1928
  - Subgroup analysis of a randomized study, in which analyzed patients did not receive antibiotic treatment, showed a reduction in mortality in the group using the closed system.
  - "Open systems" were large, uncapped glass bottles.
    - Drainage catheters were inserted into the glass bottles, often below the level of urine.
    - Urine was stagnant, and bacteria could easily grow and ascend through the drainage catheter.
    - Introduction of closed drainage systems was a major improvement, and use has greatly reduced the rate of bacteriuria.
    - In the modern era, several studies have failed to confirm the benefit of complex closed systems compared with simple devices.
- Two studies in the literature specifically focused on ICU patients and comparing a two-chamber, open drainage system with a complex closed drainage system.
  - Performed by the same team of investigators
  - Found similar results, although one of these studies was not randomized
  - In randomized and prospective trial, 311 patients requiring an indwelling urinary catheter for longer than 48 hours

were assigned to the two-chamber drainage system group or to the complex closed drainage system group to compare the rates of bacteriuria.
  - Rates of UTIs were 12.1 and 12.8 episodes per 1,000 days of catheterization, respectively.
  - Data extracted from recent literature do not support use of complex closed drainage systems in ICU patients in view of the increased cost.
- Owing to the lack of specific ICU studies, the guidelines for the management of drainage systems should be viewed as recommendations at best. The following are reasonable suggestions:
- Only those with the proper technique of aseptic insertion and maintenance of catheter should handle catheters.
- Hospital personnel should be given periodic in-service training stressing the proper techniques and potential complications of urinary catheterization.
- Hand washing should be performed immediately before and after any manipulation of the catheter site or apparatus.
- If small volumes of fresh urine are needed for examination, the distal end of the catheter, or preferably the sampling port if present, should be cleansed with a disinfectant, and urine then aspirated with a sterile needle and syringe.
- Larger volumes of urine for special analyses should be obtained aseptically from the drainage bag.
- Unobstructed flow should be maintained.
  - In order to achieve free flow of urine:
    - Catheter and collection tube should be kept from kinking.
    - Collection bag should be emptied regularly using a separate collecting container for each patient (the draining spigot and nonsterile collection container should never come into contact).
    - Poorly functioning or obstructed catheters should be irrigated or, if necessary, replaced.

○ Collection bags should always be kept below the level of the bladder.

○ Indwelling catheters should not be changed at arbitrary fixed intervals.

Types of Urethral Catheters

- A large number of articles in the literature stress that the efficacy of antiseptic-impregnated catheters, including silver oxide or silver alloy, and antibiotic-impregnated catheters in hospitalized patients.
- Two meta-analyses clarify some points related to these devices.
  - Silver oxide catheters are not associated with a reduction in bacteriuria in short-term catheterized adults.
    - Silver alloy catheters reduce the incidence of asymptomatic bacteriuria and the risk of symptomatic UTI in catheterized adults.
    - Economic evaluation is required to confirm that the reduction of infection compensates for their increased cost.
  - Catheters coated with a combination of minocycline and rifampin or nitrofurazone may also be beneficial in reducing bacteriuria in hospitalized men catheterized <1 week, but this requires further testing.
    - No trials directly compare nitrofurazone-coated and silver alloy–coated catheters.
- A randomized, prospective, double-blind multicenter trial compared catheters coated with hydrogel and silver salt with classic urinary tract catheters in 199 patients requiring urethral catheterization for more than 3 days.
  - Cumulative incidence of UTIs associated with catheterization was 11.1% overall, 11.9% for the control group, and 10% for the coated catheter group.
    - Odds ratio was 0.82 (95% confidence interval [CI] 0.3–2.2).
    - Differences between the two groups were not significant, although the power of the study was more than 90%.
- Prior trial, which included five hospitals selected to participate in a blinded prospective study, exchanged the standard latex Foley catheter for a hydrogel latex Foley catheter with a monolayer of silver metal applied to the inner and outer surfaces of the device.
  - Adjusted catheter-associated infection rate during the baseline and intervention periods was 8.1 and 4.9 infections per 1,000 catheter-days ($p = 0.13$), respectively.

Meatal Care

- Twice-daily cleansing of the urethral meatus with povidone-iodine solution and daily cleansing with soap and water have failed to reduce catheter-associated UTIs.
  - Daily meatal care with either of these two regimens cannot be endorsed.
- A randomized, controlled, prospective clinical trial involving 696 patients hospitalized in medical and surgical units undertaken to determine effectiveness of 1% silver sulfadiazine cream applied twice daily to urethral meatus in preventing transurethral catheter-associated bacteriuria.
  - Overall incidence of bacteriuria was approximately 13% in both groups ($p = 0.56$).

- Absent data from an ICU-specific patient population, the aforementioned guidelines should be followed.
- No data available on the level of sterility required to insert a urinary catheter
  - Experts recommend that catheters should be inserted using an aseptic technique and sterile equipment, including gloves, drapes, and sponges.
  - In a prospective study conducted in the operating room, 156 patients underwent preoperative urethral catheterization, randomly allocated to "sterile" or "clean/nonsterile" technique groups.
  - No statistical difference between the two groups with respect to the incidence of UTI, but the cost differed considerably between the two groups.

Vesical Irrigation and Antiseptic in the Drainage System

- Objective of antibiotic irrigation is to clear bacteria from urinary tract.
  - Randomized study compared 89 patients receiving a neomycin-polymyxin irrigation administered through a closed urinary catheter to 98 patients not so irrigated
    - Number of ICU patients was not specified in this clinical study
    - 19 of the 98 (18%) patients not irrigated became infected as compared with 14 out of the 89 (16%) of those who were irrigated.
    - Organisms from the irrigated patients were more resistant.
  - Another study was conducted in 264 urology patients, evaluating the effect of povidone-iodine bladder irrigation prior to catheter removal on subsequent bacteriuria.
    - Of 264 patients, 138 received irrigation and 126 were controls.
    - Urine cultures were positive in 22% in the control group and 18% in the study group.
    - Irrigation methods failed to demonstrate efficacy in surgical patients, and its use is not recommended in ICU patients.
  - Addition of antimicrobial agents to drainage device has not been studied in the ICU
    - Largest reported clinical trial evaluating the effect of H_2O_2 insertion into the drainage device of 353 patients, and comparing this to 315 control patients, failed to show a benefit in the treatment group.
    - 68% of these patients required an indwelling catheter for hemodynamic monitoring and antimicrobial therapy was prescribed in 75% of the patients, suggesting that these results may apply to ICU patients.
    - Expert opinion recommends that we not use irrigation unless obstruction is anticipated, as might occur with bleeding after prostatic or bladder surgery.

Alternatives to a Urinary Catheter

- For selected patients, other methods of urinary drainage should be considered as alternatives to indwelling urethral catheterization.
  - Condom catheters

- Suprapubic catheterization
- Intermittent urethral catheterization
- Limited ICU data available to assess these alternative devices
  - There is evidence that suprapubic catheterization is advantageous, as compared to indwelling catheters, with respect to bacteriuria, recatheterization, and discomfort.
- Use of a condom connected to a collection bag has been evaluated in a study comparing 167 patients over two periods of 6 months.
  - Occurrence of bacteriuria was significantly decreased for the period using the condom catheters (26.7 vs. 2.4%).
  - Issue merits further study to determine whether or not this alternative method may actually reduce bacteriuria rates.
- Use of intermittent catheterization is also associated with a lower risk of bacteriuria than indwelling urethral catheter.
  - Procedure has never been investigated in ICU patients.

Miscellaneous Measures

- Although low risk of bacteremia during urinary catheterization, administration of antimicrobial therapy at the time the device is placed leads to a reduction in bacteriuria.
  - Efficacy of antibiotic treatment has been assessed as optimal for catheterization lasting <14 days.
  - Prophylactic use of antibiotics in the ICU can be detrimental to the bacterial ecology by increasing the pressure for antimicrobial resistance among bacteria.
  - Thus, practice of administration of prophylactic antimicrobials in this manner must be discouraged in our ICUs.
  - In most ICU studies, 75% of the patients with an indwelling catheter require antibiotics for reasons unrelated to the urinary catheter.
    - All measures aimed at reducing the burden of nosocomial infections can reduce the rate of UTIs.

TREATMENT AND MANAGEMENT

- Management of catheter-associated UTI has not been evaluated in ICU patients.
- Several nonspecific measures, including hydration, have been advocated in the therapy of UTI.
  - Adequate hydration appears to be important.
  - No evidence that it improves the effectiveness of an appropriate antimicrobial therapy
- Management of complicated UTIs in the ICU may include mechanical intervention.
  - Consequently, appropriate diagnostic tests and urologic consultation should be included in the algorithm of the management of these patients.

Management of Asymptomatic Bacteriuria

- Asymptomatic catheter-associated UTI does not require treatment.
  - Antimicrobial treatment may be considered for asymptomatic women with a catheter-acquired UTI that persists 48 hours after catheter removal.

- In an ICU population, 60 patients with an indwelling urethral catheter for longer than 48 hours who developed an asymptomatic positive urine culture were randomized to receive either a 3-day course of antibiotics associated with the replacement of the indwelling urethral catheter 4 hours after the first antibiotic administration or no antibiotics and no catheter replacement.
  - Six patients equally distributed in the two groups developed urosepsis.
  - Profile of bacterial resistance was similar in the two groups.
  - Treating a positive urine culture in an asymptomatic patient with an indwelling urethral catheter does not reduce the occurrence of urosepsis.

Management of Symptomatic UTIs

Choice of Antimicrobial Agents

- Optimal characteristics of agents to treat UTI must include:
  - Activity against the major pathogens involved in these infections
  - Good tissue penetration
  - Minimal side effects
  - High urinary levels should be present for an adequate period to eliminate the organisms
    - Disappearance of bacteriuria correlates with the sensitivity of the pathogen to the concentration of antimicrobial agent achieved in urine.
    - Inhibitory urinary concentrations are achieved after administration of essentially all commonly used antibiotics.
    - An antibiotic that achieves active concentrations in renal tissue is required for infection of renal tissue.
    - Antibiotic concentration in serum or plasma can be used as surrogate markers for the antibiotic concentrations in the renal tissue.
- Most clinical studies have shown that renal concentrations of cephalosporins remained higher than minimal inhibitory concentration for the most common bacteria during the time interval between the administration of two doses.
- By contrast, β-lactam antibiotics, which have a low pKa and poor lipid solubility, penetrate poorly into the prostate.
  - Except for some cephalosporins
- Good to excellent penetration into the prostatic tissue has been demonstrated with many antimicrobial agents:
  - Aminoglycosides
  - Fluoroquinolones
  - Sulfonamides
  - Nitrofurantoin
- Many patients develop renal failure, which is associated with the inability to concentrate antimicrobial agents in the urine.
  - Administration of drugs with potential renal toxicity may worsen renal insufficiency.
  - There is significant literature demonstrating that the use of fluoroquinolone is associated with the emergence of resistant pathogens.

Cystitis

- Acute uncomplicated cystitis is infrequent in ICU patients.
  - *E. coli* is the evident target pathogen.

- IDSA guidelines recommend treatment with trimethoprim-sulfamethoxazole for 3 days as standard therapy for acute uncomplicated cystitis.
- A meta-analysis determined that 3 days of antibiotic therapy is similar to 5 to 10 days in achieving symptomatic cure during uncomplicated UTI treatment, while the longer treatment is more effective in obtaining bacteriologic cure.
- Quinolones are recommended for acute cystitis in regions where the level of resistance to trimethoprim-sulfamethoxazole is high.
- Antibiotic treatment of UTI depends on ability of antibiotic to inhibit growth or kill the bacteria present in urinary tract.
  - This is related to the concentration of antibiotics at the site of infection.
  - Very high concentrations of antibiotics with renal clearance are obtained in urine.
  - Consequently, even in the presence of pathogens exhibiting *in vitro* resistance, the high concentrations of antibiotics in urine inhibit the growth of pathogens, rendering them effective to treat a UTI.

Prostatitis

- For outpatients, bacterial prostatitis is a common diagnosis and a frequent indication for antibiotics.
  - Urethral instrumentation and prostatic surgery are known causes of prostatitis.
  - Incidence of prostatitis among ICU patients has never been assessed.
  - There is only a weak relation between acute and chronic prostatitis.
  - Acute prostatitis is an acute infection producing:
    - Local heat
    - Tenderness
    - Fever
    - With the presence of IgA and IgG bacteria-specific immunoglobulins in the prostatic secretions
    - Few symptoms, usually perineal discomfort, are exhibited with prostatitis.
    - Most patients with chronic prostatitis have no history of positive urine or urethral cultures.
- In ICU patients, acute bacterial prostatitis is probably a common infection.
  - The patient presents septic, but without an evident source of infection.
  - There may be a history of urine retention due to bladder outlet obstruction.
  - Rectal examination, a crucial step in the diagnosis, reveals a warm, swollen, and tender prostate.
  - Prostatic fluid contains leukocytes and the pathogen responsible for the infection.
  - Fluoroquinolones are the drugs of choice to treat acute prostatitis because of their excellent penetration in the tissue and excretions.
  - Targeted pathogens are:
    - *E. coli*
    - *Proteus* sp.
    - *Klebsiella* sp.
    - *Enterococcus* sp.
    - *Staphylococcus aureus*
    - *Neisseria gonorrhoeae*
    - *Chlamydia trachomatis*

- For acute prostatitis occurring without bacteremia:
  - Antimicrobial treatment consists of oral ofloxacin 200 mg twice per day for 28 days.
  - Ceftriaxone 2 g/day has good prostatic tissue penetration and represents an alternative to ofloxacin.
  - Gentamicin 3 mg/kg/day is added in the presence of positive blood cultures (Table 78.8).
  - Of importance, urethral instrumentation should be discouraged.
    - If acute retention occurs, suprapubic drainage of urine is required.
  - Treatment of chronic prostatitis is based on the oral administration of ofloxacin 200 mg twice per day, or trimethoprim 160 mg–sulfamethoxazole 800 mg twice per day for at least 28 days.

Acute Pyelonephritis

- No specific data available on management of acute pyelonephritis in the ICU.
  - The urine of all patients with suspicion of complicated pyelonephritis should be cultured and a Gram stain of the spun urine performed.
  - Blood cultures, which are positive in 36% of women not admitted to the ICU, are also required.
  - All patients with acute pyelonephritis should have an ultrasound examination or a renal computed tomography scan to evaluate for obstruction and stones.
- For uncomplicated acute pyelonephritis, the IDSA, in 1999, derived two conclusions from the analysis of randomized clinical trials.
  - Trimethoprim-sulfamethoxazole is preferred over ampicillin.
  - There is a relatively high prevalence of organisms causing acute pyelonephritis that are resistant to ampicillin.
  - Second conclusion is that 10 to 14 days of therapy appears to be adequate for the majority of women.
  - 255 outpatients were randomized to oral ciprofloxacin, 500 mg twice per day for 7 days, followed by placebo for 7 days versus trimethoprim-sulfamethoxazole, 160/800 mg twice per day for 14 days.
    - A 7-day ciprofloxacin regimen was associated with greater bacteriologic and clinical cure rates than a 14-day trimethoprim-sulfamethoxazole regimen
    - Gatifloxacin appears to be equivalent to ciprofloxacin for this indication.
- Patients with complicated acute pyelonephritis should be hospitalized and initial administration of broad-spectrum intravenous (IV) antibiotics begun.
  - Targeted bacteria are:
    - *Enterobacter* sp.
    - *E. coli*
    - *Proteus* sp.
    - *Enterococcus* sp
  - Ciprofloxacin, 500 mg twice daily, is administered orally for 14 to 21 days.
  - Gentamicin, 3 mg/kg/day IV, is added during the first 3 days.
  - Oral ciprofloxacin is as effective as the IV regimen in the initial empirical management of complicated pyelonephritis.
  - Gatifloxacin is as effective as ciprofloxacin.
  - Ceftriaxone, 2 g/day IV, is an alternative choice to ciprofloxacin.

TABLE 78.8

ANTIMICROBIAL TREATMENT OF UTIs[a]

Source of infection	Pathogens	Treatment	Duration
Acute prostatitis (without bacteremia)	Escherichia coli, Proteus sp., Klebsiella sp., Enterococcus sp., Staphylococcus aureus, Neisseria gonorrhoeae, Chlamydia trachomatis	Ofloxacin 200 mg twice daily (oral)	28 d
Acute prostatitis (with bacteremia)	E. coli, Proteus sp., Klebsiella sp., Enterococcus sp., S. aureus, N. gonorrhoeae, C. trachomatis	Ofloxacin 200 mg twice daily (oral) or Ceftriaxone 2 g/d And gentamicin 3 mg/kg/d IV	28 d 3 d
Chronic bacterial prostatitis	E. coli, Proteus sp., Klebsiella sp., Enterococcus sp., S. aureus, N. gonorrhoeae, C. trachomatis	Ofloxacin 200 mg twice daily (oral) or Trimethoprim 160 mg/sulfamethoxazole 800 mg twice daily (oral)	28 d
Acute pyelonephritis (uncomplicated)	Enterobacteriaceae, E. coli, Proteus sp., Enterococcus sp.	Ciprofloxacin 500 mg twice daily (oral) If oral route not possible: Ceftriaxone 2 g/d IV	14 d
Acute pyelonephritis (complicated)	Enterobacteriaceae, E. coli, Proteus sp., Enterococcus sp.	Ciprofloxacin 500 mg twice daily (oral) Or Ceftriaxone 2 g/d IV And Gentamicin 3 mg/kg/d	14–21 d 3 d

[a]Each empirical treatment must be adapted to the susceptibility testing results.

- Drainage of urine must be urgently performed using bladder catheterization, percutaneous nephrostomy drainage, or definitive surgery.
  - Antimicrobial treatment is administered after urine and blood specimen collection.
- Antibiotic selection is based on the result of the Gram stain of the urine and knowledge of local ecology.
- Antimicrobial treatment should be adapted to the susceptibility testing results as soon as possible.
- De-escalation should be performed in favor of a narrow-spectrum antibiotic.

Specificities of Complicated UTIs in the ICU

- Little in the literature on the treatment of UTIs in the ICU.
  - One presumes the need for IV antibiotics for these patients because of the possibility of bacteremia or sepsis.
  - Guidelines from the Surviving Sepsis Campaign state that:
    - Antibiotic therapy should be started within the first hour of recognition of severe sepsis, after appropriate cultures have been obtained.
    - Initial empirical anti-infective therapy should include one or more drugs that have activity against the likely pathogens and that penetrate the presumed source of sepsis.
    - Monotherapy is as effective as combination therapy with a β-lactam and an aminoglycoside as empiric therapy of patients with severe sepsis or septic shock.
    - For the septic shock patients whose presumed source is urine, we recommend, empirically:

    - Combination of a β-lactam antibiotic with antipseudomonal activity and a fluoroquinolone

Management of Candiduria

- Candiduria represents from 3% to 15% of catheter-associated UTI in the ICU.
  - Candida albicans and Candida (Torulopsis) glabrata found in 46% and 31% of cases, respectively
  - According to the International Conference for the Development of a Consensus on the Management and Prevention of Severe Candidal Infections, colonized patients without evidence of infection do not require treatment.
    - But contributing cause should be addressed, such as changing or removing the indwelling catheter and discontinuing inappropriate antibiotic therapy
    - Fluconazole may be the best option for treating a candiduria only if the species is C. albicans.
    - Voriconazole may be more effective against non-albicans species.
- A prospective, randomized trial compared fungal eradication rates among 316 hospitalized patients with candiduria treated with fluconazole (200 mg) or placebo daily for 14 days.
  - Candiduria cleared by day 14 in 50% of the patients receiving fluconazole and 29% of those receiving placebo.
  - Higher eradication rates among patients completing 14 days of therapy
  - Fluconazole initially produced high eradication rates, but cultures at 2 weeks revealed similar candiduria rates among treated and untreated patients.
  - In 41% of the catheterized subjects, candiduria was resolved as the result of catheter removal only.
  - Outcomes of patients were not provided in the results.

- Bladder irrigation using amphotericin B has been proposed as an alternative technique to clear *Candida* from the urine.
- Comparative and randomized study of 109 elderly patients showed that funguria was eradicated in 96% of the patients treated with amphotericin B and 73% of those treated with fluconazole (*p* <0.05).
  - One month after study enrollment, the mortality rate associated with all causes was greater among patients who

were treated with amphotericin B bladder irrigation than among those who received oral fluconazole therapy (41% vs. 22%, respectively; *p* <0.05).
- This finding suggests that irrigation therapy could be associated with poorer survival.
- There has only been one study performed in ICU patients developing candiduria, which reached the same conclusions.
  - Methodologic issues restrict the interest of this study.

CHAPTER 79 ■ FUNGAL AND VIRAL INFECTIONS

FUNGAL INFECTIONS

Fungal Pathogens

- Medically relevant fungi are classically considered as one of three types of organism:
  - **Yeasts**
    - Grow as smooth colonies on culture plates
    - Microscopically, they are oval or spherical, and they reproduce by budding
    - Most common human yeast pathogens are *Candida* spp. and *Cryptococcus* spp.
  - **Molds**
    - Appear as fuzzy colonies on agar plates
    - Microscopically, they have hyphae.
      - Tubular or filamentous morphologies that grow by branching and longitudinal extension
      - Hyphae can be septated (i.e., with cross walls perpendicular to hyphal cell wall) or aseptated (no cross walls)
    - Most common human pathogens are *Aspergillus* spp. and *Rhizopus* spp.
  - **Dimorphic agents**
    - *Dimorphic fungi* used to describe the endemic fungi
      - Found in distinct geographic locations
      - Grow as filaments in the environment at ambient temperatures and as yeasts at higher body temperatures
      - Three most common pathogens are:
        - *Histoplasma capsulatum*
        - *Coccidioides immitis*
        - *Blastomyces dermatitidis*
      - Term, dimorphic fungi, as commonly used in the medical literature is misleading
        - *Candida albicans*
          - Not grouped with the endemic dimorphic fungi
          - Frequently assumes filamentous morphologies in tissue (pseudohyphae and hyphae)
- Most fungal pathogens, except for *Candida* spp., are widespread in nature
  - Acquired by inhalation into the lungs

- In immunocompetent hosts, inhaled fungi are generally arrested in lungs by host immune system.
- *Candida* spp., with the exception of *Candida parapsilosis*, are part of the human gastrointestinal flora.
  - Infections with these organisms are usually endogenous in origin.
- Diagnosis of infection (i.e., fungal disease):
  - Often difficult to distinguish from colonization
  - Definitive diagnoses generally require either the presence of the organism at sterile sites or histopathology demonstrating tissue-invasive disease.
  - Many fungi show morphologies that are indistinguishable by histopathology (e.g., *Aspergillus* spp. vs. *Fusarium* spp. and other acute-angle branching, septated molds).
    - Identification of organism from culture is the only means to ascertain etiologic agent.
  - In ICU settings, *Candida* spp. and, to a much lesser extent, *Aspergillus* are the major fungal pathogens.

Infections Caused by *Candida* Species (Candidiasis)

- *Candida* spp. cause a wide range of clinical syndromes.
  - Benign cutaneous to fatal deep-seated infections (Table 79.1)
  - Can affect otherwise healthy patients, as well as those with defective immune systems
  - In the ICU, the most common and serious form of disease is invasive candidiasis.
- Invasive candidiasis typically refers to:
  - Candidemia and deep-organ infections resulting from bloodborne dissemination
    - Candidemia is not always detected.
    - Deep-seated organ involvement is frequently the first evidence of candidiasis.

Epidemiology

- In the ICU, *Candida* spp. is the third most common cause of blood stream infections.

TABLE 79.1

MAJOR CLINICAL CANDIDAL SYNDROMES

Type of candidiasis	Specific clinical syndromes	Frequency	Risk factors	Types of hosts	Treatment
Cutaneous: skin, nails		Most common form of candidiasis; Self-limited	Prolonged exposure of skin to moisture	Immunocompetent Immunocompromised	Topical antifungals
Mucocutaneous: Mucous membranes of the mouth, esophagus, vagina	Oropharyngeal	About 25% in patients with solid tumors and 60% in patients with hematologic malignancies and/or following bone marrow transplantation; up to 90% in AIDS	Extremes of age, broad-spectrum antibiotics, inhaled or systemic steroids, radiation to the head and neck	Immunocompetent Immunocompromised, especially patients receiving cytotoxic chemotherapy or systemic immunosuppressive therapy, those with AIDS, malignancy, or chronic mucocutaneous candidiasis	Topical or systemic azole agents
	Esophagitis	15%–20% in AIDS	Broad-spectrum antibiotics, acid-suppressive therapy, prior gastric surgery, mucosal barrier injury, inhaled or systemic steroids, esophageal motility disorders	Mostly immunocompromised, especially patients receiving cytotoxic chemotherapy or systemic immunosuppressive therapy, those with AIDS or malignancy	Systemic antifungal agents: oral azole (preferred treatment), parenteral echinocandin or AmB
	Vaginitis	70%–75% of healthy adult women	Pregnancy, diabetes mellitus, and broad-spectrum antibiotics	Immunocompetent Immunocompromised	Topical or systemic azole agents
Disseminated candidiasis			Colonization with *Candida*, broad-spectrum antibiotics, end-stage renal disease, central venous catheters, critically ill patients, hyperalimentation, GI surgery, burn patients, neonates	Immunocompromised, especially granulocytopenia, bone marrow or solid organ transplant, chemotherapy, mucositis	Systemic antifungal agents

AIDS, acquired immunodeficiency syndrome; AmB, amphotericin B; GI, gastrointestinal.

- Account for approximately 10% of cases
- Crude mortality rates range from 40% to 75%.
- Candidemia associated with excess ICU and hospital stays and increased costs of care
- Postmortem studies suggest that mortality rates due to invasive candidiasis may be higher than generally realized because of undiagnosed infections.

Risk Factors

- Leading predisposing factors for invasive candidiasis include:
  - Prolonged ICU stay
  - Previous surgery (especially solid organ transplant and gastrointestinal surgery)
    - Solid organ transplant recipients at highest risk among the surgical patients
    - Small bowel, liver, and pancreas recipients have prevalence of from 9% to 59%
  - Acute renal failure
  - Receipt of antibacterial agents or hyperalimentation
  - Presence of a central venous catheter
  - Although risk factors are well defined
    - Diversity of factors and underlying diseases associated with invasive candidiasis make it difficult to reliably identify large subgroups of patients within the ICU who might merit particular attention or targeted interventions.

Microbiology

- *C. albicans* the most common *Candida* species involved in invasive candidiasis
  - Followed by *C. glabrata*, *C. tropicalis*, and *C. parapsilosis*
  - Other species less common and often associated with underlying malignancy or chemotherapy
  - *C. tropicalis* and *C. glabrata* are found largely in adults
  - *C. parapsilosis* the leading pathogen in neonatal population

- In many tertiary care centers, *C glabrata* has surpassed *C. albicans* to become the most common *Candida* sp. in invasive candidiasis.
  - Accounting for up to 35% of all candidemias
  - Among non-*albicans Candida* species, *C. krusei* and *C. glabrata* are particularly important because of their resistance and decreased susceptibility to fluconazole, respectively.

Clinical Manifestations

- Clinical manifestations are often nonspecific
  - Fever is frequently the first and only sign of invasive candidiasis
  - Other signs that should raise concern for candidemia are:
    - Papulopustular or macronodular skin lesions
    - Ocular involvement such as chorioretinitis or endophthalmitis
    - Deep-seated infections often present, with findings localized to the particular tissue site
- Invasive candidiasis can be divided into four major clinical entities:
  - Catheter-related candidemia
  - Acute disseminated candidiasis
  - Chronic disseminated candidiasis
  - Deep-organ candidiasis (Table 79.2)

Diagnosis

- A challenge due to nonspecific clinical manifestations and the low sensitivity of microbiologic culture techniques
  - Blood cultures should be routinely obtained in patients with suggestive signs and symptoms, as well as those at high risk for invasive candidiasis.
  - Candidemia is the most common manifestation of invasive candidiasis.
    - Other forms of invasive candidiasis generally originate from bloodborne dissemination.

TABLE 79.2

FORMS OF INVASIVE CANDIDIASIS

Forms	Portal of entry	Characteristics	Blood cultures	Management
Catheter-related candidemia	Intravascular catheter	Frequently self-limited, but can rarely spread to deep-seated organs	Positive for *Candida* sp.	Systemic antifungal agents and removal of the catheter
Acute disseminated candidiasis	Intravascular catheter or GI tract is most common	Frequently involves deep-seated organ(s)	Can be positive or negative	Systemic antifungal
Chronic disseminated candidiasis (or hepatosplenic candidiasis)	GI tract is the most common portal; intravascular catheter	Almost exclusively seen in neutropenic patients or bone marrow transplant recipients. Typical presentation: Persistent fever, right upper quadrant pain, elevated alkaline phosphatase, lucencies on CT or ultrasound of the liver	Typically negative at the time of the diagnosis	Systemic antifungal
Deep-organ candidiasis	Intravascular catheter or GI tract is most common	Frequently follows an episode of undiagnosed candidemia	Typically negative at the time of the diagnosis	Systemic antifungal

GI, gastrointestinal; CT, computed tomography.

- Deep-seated candidiasis can occur without a positive blood culture.
  - Blood cultures are positive in <50% of patients.
  - Autopsy data demonstrate as few as 15% to 40% of patients with invasive candidiasis have an antemortem diagnosis of the disease.
  - Diagnosis, therefore, should also rely on histopathology and/or fungal cultures obtained by biopsy of sterile sites.
  - *Candida* spp. are common colonizers of humans.
    - Difficult to differentiate between colonization or true infections when organisms are isolated from the urine and nonsterile sites
- Given the potential for antifungal resistance among the non-*albicans Candida* spp.
  - Isolates recovered from blood or sterile sites should be identified to the species level
  - Availability of special fungal media (such as CHROMagar) and rapid *in situ* hybridization techniques have significantly shortened the time to speciation
- Nonculture-based diagnostic methods for invasive candidiasis
  - Antibody-based assays have not been useful.
  - Beta D-glucan assay, an antigen test, has recently been approved for the diagnosis of invasive fungal infections.
    - Assay measures [1, 3]-beta-D-glucan levels released from cell wall of most fungi
    - Sensitivity in diagnosing invasive candidiasis 81%
    - Specificity 84%
    - Positive and negative predictive values (PPV and NPV) are 84%, and 75%, respectively.
    - Test is able to detect various *Candida* spp.
      - Potential drawback is its nonspecificity for *Candida*
      - It also detects *Aspergillus, Fusarium,* and *Trichosporon*
    - Other factors that can contribute to false-positive tests results include dialysis filters, gauze, and sponges.
- Azole MICs correlate with likelihood of success in treating patients.
  - Antifungal susceptibility testing of *Candida* is currently performed in relatively few clinical laboratories.
  - Not considered the standard of care, unlike antibacterial susceptibility testing
  - Antifungal susceptibility patterns are predictable in most cases based on species and prior exposure to antifungal agents.
  - For this reason, identification of isolates to the species level is usually more important than MIC data in the management of individual patients.
    - *C. krusei* is intrinsically resistant to fluconazole.
    - Significant minority of *C. glabrata* strains develop resistance to fluconazole
    - For other species, the vast majority of bloodstream isolates remain susceptible to fluconazole.
    - Cross-resistance to other azoles is often seen, which limits the utility of this class against fluconazole-resistant isolates.
- Reports of resistance to echinocandin class of antifungals are beginning to appear.
  - MICs of echinocandins against *C. parapsilosis* are generally higher than against other species, and breakthrough infections among patients receiving these agents have been described.

- Amphotericin B resistance is difficult to document using current testing methods.
  - Resistance among *C. lusitaniae* and *C. guilliermondii* isolates is well described but not seen with all isolates.
  - Avoid amphotericin B if elevated MICs are documented.
- At centers where candidiasis is a particular problem and antifungal use is widespread, it is useful to conduct periodic susceptibility testing to generate an institutional antibiogram.
- Clinicians should be aware if such reports exist at their institution, as susceptibility patterns against different species can be used to guide empiric antifungal therapy.

Management

- **Invasive Candidiasis:** The major antifungal agents and their activity are summarized in Table 79.3.
  - Current guidelines for management of invasive candidiasis are summarized in Table 79.4.
    - Amphotericin B (conventional or lipid formulations) or caspofungin should be the first-line treatment of critically ill patients with invasive candidiasis.
    - Caspofungin, an echinocandin agent, is better tolerated and has fewer side effects than amphotericin B.
    - Fluconazole can also be considered when resistant species such as *C. krusei* are ruled out.
    - Anidulafungin and micafungin, two newly approved echinocandin agents, are as effective as caspofungin in management.
  - All patients with candidemia should have an ophthalmologic exam to rule out retinal involvement.
    - All vascular catheters should be removed if possible.
    - *Candida* spp. tend to form biofilms on catheters, which can render otherwise susceptible isolates resistant to antifungal agents.
- ***Candida* Recovered from Urine or Sputum/Bronchoalveolar Lavage (BAL):** As mentioned earlier, *Candida* spp. are part of endogenous flora and frequent colonizers of mucosal surfaces.
  - In the ICU setting, urine and sputum are two most common sites of colonization
  - *Candida in the Urine. Candida* spp. the most common organisms recovered from urine of surgical ICU patients
    - Risk factors include:
      - Urinary catheters
      - Old age
      - Receipt of antibacterial agents
    - Colony counts and urine analysis are not helpful in deciding whether candiduria is of clinical importance.
      - Asymptomatic candiduria in the low-risk patient is of little clinical relevance and should not be treated.
      - In a small subset of patients, candiduria is a marker for invasive candidiasis.
        - Treatment indicated for:
          - Symptomatic patients
          - Those who are neutropenic
          - Have undergone a urologic manipulation
          - Received a kidney transplant
      - Treatment entails removal of the urinary catheter and therapy with a systemic antifungal agent.
        - Fluconazole or amphotericin B for 7 to 14 days
        - In the event that catheter removal is not possible, changing the catheter might be of benefit and should be performed.

TABLE 79.3

CURRENTLY AVAILABLE SYSTEMIC ANTIFUNGAL AGENTS

Class of antifungal	Mechanisms of actions of specific drugs	Routes of administration and daily doses	Spectrum of activity	Side effects and toxicity
Polyene	Potent antifungal agents that act by binding to ergosterol in the fungal cell membrane, leading to leakage and cell death Amphotericin B (AmB), available in 4 formulations: • AmB deoxycholate (dAmB; often called conventional AmB) • AmB colloidal dispersion (ABCD) • AmB lipid complex (ABLC) • Liposomal AmB (L-AmB)	IV for invasive candidiasis Usual daily dosages: dAmB, 0.3–1.5 mg/kg ABCD, 3–6 mg/kg ABLC, 5 mg/kg L-AmB, 3–5 mg/kg	AmB is active (fungicidal) against most pathogenic fungi, except the following: Trichosporon beigelii, Aspergillus terreus, Pseudallescheria boydii, Malassezia furfur, Fusarium spp. Some Candida lusitaniae and C. guilliermondii isolates are resistant.	Infusion-related (fever, chills, and myalgia). Nephrotoxicity: Azotemia, electrolyte wasting (potassium, magnesium), renal tubular acidosis. Overall, the lipid formulations of AmB are less nephrotoxic.
Azoles	Inhibition of cytochrome P450 14α-demethylase, an enzyme involved in the sterol biosynthesis pathway Fluconazole	PO and IV Usual daily dosage: 6 mg/kg. Doses of 12 mg/kg are increasingly used to overcome intermediately susceptible (i.e., dose-dependent) organisms.	Fungistatic agent, active against Candida spp., Cryptococcus spp., and Coccidioides immitis. Candida krusei is intrinsically resistant, and resistance has been reported among isolates of several other Candida spp., especially C. glabrata. No activity against molds. Limited activity against Histoplasma capsulatum, Blastomyces dermatitidis, and Sporothrix schenckii.	In general, well-tolerated. Hepatotoxicity is rare.
	Itraconazole	PO and IV Daily dosage: PO: 100–400 mg (at 400 mg/d doses, better levels are achieved with bid dosing) IV: 200 mg bid for 2 days, followed by 200 mg/d	Active against yeasts, molds, and dimorphic fungi.	Generally benign. Hepatotoxicity is rare.
	Voriconazole	PO and IV Daily dosage: PO: 200 mg bid IV: 3–6 mg/kg every 12 h	Limited activity against Fusarium and Zygomycetes. Resistance has been reported among Candida and Aspergillus spp.	Dose-related, transient visual disturbances, skin rash, and elevated hepatic enzyme levels have been reported.
	Posaconazole	PO Daily dosage: 600–800 mg/d in divided doses with food	Active against yeasts, molds, and dimorphic fungi. Variable activity against Fusarium. Limited activity against Zygomycetes. Resistance has been reported among Candida and Aspergillus spp. Active against yeasts, molds (including Zygomycetes) and dimorphic fungi. Variable activity against Fusarium.	Nausea and headache. Rash, dry skin, nausea, taste disturbance, abdominal pain, dizziness, and flushing can occur. Posaconazole can cause abnormalities in liver function.
Glucan synthesis inhibitors (echinocandins)	Block the synthesis of a major fungal cell wall component, 1–3-beta-D-glucan Caspofungin Anidulafungin Micafungin	IV Caspofungin: 70 mg load, then 50 mg daily Anidulafungin: 200 mg, then 100 mg/d Micafungin: 100 mg/kg	Activity is mainly against Candida spp. and Aspergillus spp. No activity against Cryptococcus or Zygomycetes.	Side-effects are limited Liver toxicity

564

TABLE 79.4

RECOMMENDED ANTIFUNGAL AGENTS AGAINST INVASIVE CANDIDIASIS

Host	Primary therapy	Alternative therapy	Comments
Nonneutropenic	AmB, 0.6–1 mg/kg/d IV *or* Fluconazole, 400–800 mg/d IV or PO *or* Caspofungin, 70 mg IV once, then 50 mg/d IV *or* Voriconazole, 6 mg/kg IV every 12 h for 2 doses, then 3 mg/kg/d IV every 12 h (can be switched to 200 mg bid PO after 3 days) *or* Anidulafungin, 200 mg IV for 1 dose, then 100 mg/d IV *or* Micafungin, 100 mg/d IV	AmB, 0.7 mg/kg IV plus fluconazole, 800 mg IV or PO for 4–7 d, then fluconazole, 800 mg/d	Duration: 14 days after the last positive blood culture and resolution of signs and symptoms Removal of all vascular catheters
Neutropenic	AmB, 0.7–1 mg/kg/d IV *or* Lipid formulations of AmB, 3–5 mg/kg/d IV *or* Caspofungin, 70 mg IV for 1 dose, then 50 mg/d IV	Fluconazole, 6 to 12 mg/kg/d	Duration: 14 days after the last positive blood culture, resolution of signs and symptoms, and of neutropenia Removal of vascular catheters if possible (controversial issue)

- *Candida in the Sputum:* Specimens from the airways—sputum, tracheal aspirates, and BAL—are frequently contaminated with oropharyngeal flora, including *Candida* spp.
- *Candida* spp. frequently isolated from the respiratory tree of ICU patients
- Primary *Candida* pneumonia is extremely rare.
  - Diagnosis of *Candida* pneumonia requires evidence of parenchymal invasion by hyphae on a biopsy specimen.
  - Antifungal therapy should not be instituted in response to *Candida* isolates recovered from respiratory samples.
    - Strategies of not identifying or reporting *Candida* spp. in respiratory samples:
      - Decrease length of stay

- Hospital costs
- Unnecessary antifungal therapy
- Without any negative effects on accurate diagnosis of *Candida* pneumonia or patient outcome

Prevention

- Given the nonspecific clinical manifestations, low yield of blood cultures, and high mortality rates of invasive candidiasis, investigators have studied three treatment strategies in the absence of a definitive diagnosis:
- Prophylactic strategy: Administration of an antifungal agent at a period of high risk to prevent candidiasis
- Controversial
- See Table 79.5.

TABLE 79.5

CLINICAL TRIALS DEMONSTRATING A POSITIVE IMPACT OF ANTIFUNGAL PROPHYLAXIS IN NONNEUTROPENIC ICU PATIENTS

Patient population	Intervention	Impact on fungal infections
Surgical patients with recurrent gastrointestinal perforations or anastomotic leakage	Randomized prospective double-blind, placebo-controlled study: fluconazole (400 mg/day IV) ($N = 25$) or placebo ($N = 22$) continued until resolution of the underlying surgical condition	Fluconazole reduced candida colonization by 47% (15% vs. 62%; $p = 0.04$) and *Candida* peritonitis by 31% (4% vs. 35%; $p = 0.02$) No impact on survival
Medical and surgical adult ICU patients with mechanical ventilation for at least 48 h	Randomized double-blind, placebo-controlled study: fluconazole, 100 mg daily ($N = 103$) or placebo ($N = 101$)	Fluconazole reduced *Candida* infections by about 10% (5.8% vs. 16%). No impact on survival (mortality rate 39% vs. 41%)
Medical and surgical adult ICU patients in septic shock	Randomized double-blind study: fluconazole, 200 mg IV daily ($N = 32$) or placebo ($N = 39$) during the course of their septic shock	Fluconazole improved 30-day survival by 32% (78% vs. 46%) in patients with intra-abdominal sepsis. No impact on survival in patients with septic shock due to nosocomial pneumonia
Surgical ICU patients with a length of ICU stay of at least 3 days	Randomized placebo-controlled study: fluconazole, 400 mg orally or placebo (total $N = 260$)	Fluconazole reduced the risk of fungal infection by 55%. No impact on survival

- Preemptive strategy: Administration of an antifungal agent to treat suspected invasive candidiasis based on particular warning signs.
  - Based on specific findings on computed tomography (CT) scan or laboratory markers such as galactomannan
  - Popular approach in patients undergoing bone marrow transplantation or those with neutropenia from a hematologic malignancy
  - No good indicators for preemptive approaches in nonneutropenic ICU patients
- Empiric therapy: Administration of an antifungal agent in persistently febrile patients without a known source or with no response to appropriate antibacterial agents
  - Widely used but not validated by clinical trials
  - Mathematical models suggest strategy might be proven effective.
    - Theoretical cost-effectiveness analysis was performed on a target population of ICU patients with fever, hypothermia, or unexplained hypotension who had not responded to 3 days of antibacterial therapy.
    - Assuming that 10% of the target population would have invasive candidiasis, the authors concluded that empiric fluconazole was the most reasonable strategy.
      - Cost: $12,593 per discounted life-year saved
      - One life saved for 71 patients treated
      - Empiric fluconazole:
        - Estimated to decrease mortality from 44% to 30.4% in patients with invasive candidiasis
        - From 22.4% to 21.0% in the overall target cohort
        - Strategy justifiable if likelihood of invasive candidiasis at least 2.5%
        - Until clinical trials validate empiric strategies within well defined at-risk populations, however, they cannot be broadly recommended

Infections Caused by *Aspergillus* Species (Aspergillosis)

- Less common human pathogens in the ICU than *Candida* spp. but cause greater morbidity and mortality
- These molds are ubiquitous in the environment.
- In normal hosts, generally saprophytes that colonize the bronchopulmonary tree
- Four classical clinical syndromes of pulmonary aspergillosis are discussed in Table 79.6.
- Focus here on two syndromes most commonly encountered in ICU setting:
  - Chronic necrotizing pulmonary aspergillosis (CNPA)
  - Invasive pulmonary aspergillosis (IPA)
  - In both of these diseases, *Aspergillus* spp. invade tissue and blood vessels, causing necrosis and possibly disseminating to the brain and elsewhere.
  - Entities similar to allergic bronchopulmonary aspergillosis, CNPA, and IPA are also found in the sinuses.

Epidemiology

- IPA is estimated to occur in:
  - 5% to 13% of patients who have undergone bone marrow transplantation

- 5% to 25% of patients who have received heart or lung transplants
- 10% to 20% of patients receiving intensive chemotherapy for leukemia
- Mortality rates are 50% to 90%
- Not as common in patients with less profound immunosuppression and exceedingly uncommon in immunocompetent hosts
  - In immunocompetent hosts, the rare cases of IPA often follow influenza or other infectious respiratory processes.
- CNPA is generally a disease of patients with underlying lung disease.

Risk Factors

- Major risk factors predisposing to invasive aspergillosis are summarized in Table 79.7.
- There are increasing reports of disease among debilitated patients in the ICU.

Microbiology

- Over 100 species of *Aspergillus*
  - Only a few cause diseases in humans.
    - *A. fumigatus* is most common, followed by *A. flavus*
    - Less common pathogens include *A. terreus, A. niger,* and *A. clavatus.*
  - Antifungal susceptibility testing against molds not recommended routinely
    - Reproducible testing methodologies have been developed, but interpretive criteria have not been established
    - Nevertheless, elevated MICs to amphotericin B have been documented against a number of *A. terreus* isolates.
      - Elevated MICs of itraconazole against a small percentage of *A. fumigatus* isolates

Clinical Manifestations

- Most *Aspergillus* spp. infections originate from the inhalation of fungal spores into lungs.
  - Cases of direct skin inoculation of *Aspergillus* have been described.
    - Associated with insertion of intravenous (IV) devices or the taping of arm boards to the extremities
    - Patients with severe burns can also develop local burn wound infections, especially if they are rolled in the dirt to extinguish flames.
    - Regardless of the portal of entry, any local form of aspergillosis can disseminate to various sites if host immune function is impaired.
- Almost any organ may be involved in disseminated aspergillosis, including:
  - Integument (onychomycosis, cutaneous aspergillosis)
  - Ear (otomycosis)
  - Respiratory tract (sinusitis, pneumonia, empyema)
  - Heart (endocarditis, myocarditis)
  - Gastrointestinal (GI, hepatosplenic aspergillosis)
  - Central nervous system (cerebral aspergillosis, meningitis)
  - Eye (endophthalmitis)
  - Bone (osteomyelitis, mediastinitis)
  - Lungs and sinuses are the two most common primary sites of aspergillosis
  - CNS is the most common secondary site.

TABLE 79.6

CLINICAL SPECTRUM OF ASPERGILLOSIS

Clinical syndromes	Description and epidemiology	Predisposing factors	Clinical characteristics	Outcome
Aspergilloma	Fungus ball (a mass of fungal mycelia, inflammatory cells, tissue debris) within a pre-existing lung cavity. Usually, the fungus does not invade the surrounding lung parenchyma or blood vessels. 17% of patients with pre-existing lung cavity have aspergilloma.	Pre-existing lung cavity.	Often asymptomatic. Some develop hemoptysis. Chest radiograph shows a mobile intracavitary mass with an air crescent in the periphery.	Asymptomatic patients: No treatment. Symptomatic patients: Intracavitary AmB or antimold azole agents. Surgical resection: Reserved for patients with massive hemoptysis; carries significant morbidity and mortality.
Allergic Broncho-pulmonary aspergillosis (ABPA)	Hypersensitivity reaction to *Aspergillus* colonization of the tracheobronchial tree. This can occur by itself or in conjunction with aspergillus sinusitis. 7%–10% of patients with steroid-dependent asthma and 7% of patients with cystic fibrosis have ABPA. The incidence is much less among all patients with asthma (<1%).	Patients with asthma or cystic fibrosis.	Typical presentations: fever and pulmonary infiltrates unresponsive to antibacterial therapy; cough with mucous plugs. Suggestive findings: asthma, eosinophilia, a positive skin test result for *A. fumigatus*, serum IgE level >1,000 IU/dL, fleeting pulmonary infiltrates, central bronchiectasis, mucoid impaction, and positive test results for *Aspergillus* precipitins.	Systemic corticosteroids (inhaled steroids have no effect). For recurrent ABPA, itraconazole in conjunction with systemic steroids speeds the resolution of symptoms and facilitates steroid taper.
Chronic necrotizing aspergillosis	Chronic, indolent destructive process of the lung due to invasion by *Aspergillus*. The rate of disease is not known.	Underlying lung disease. Patients with mild immunosuppression, diabetes, poor nutrition, chronic lung diseases (such as COPD, inactive tuberculosis, previous radiation therapy, pneumoconiosis, cystic fibrosis), lung infarction, sarcoidosis. This syndrome can also follow aspergilloma.	Typical presentations: fever, cough, sputum production, and weight loss for several months. Chest radiographs show an infiltrative process with or without a fungal ball. The diagnosis requires confirmation by demonstration of fungal tissue invasion and the growth of *Aspergillus* species on culture.	Systemic antifungal therapy with voriconazole (or itraconazole) or lipid formulations of AmB. Caspofungin might also be considered. Surgical resection is considered if the disease is focal and refractory to antifungal therapy.
Invasive aspergillosis	Rapidly progressive, often fatal infection. Characterized by fungal invasion of blood vessels. Infection can disseminate to various organs. Epidemiology: refer to discussion in text.	Patients with profound immunosuppression: prolonged neutropenia; recipients of bone marrow transplant or solid organ transplant; advanced AIDS or chronic granulomatous disease; severe burn.	Typical presentations: fever refractory to antibacterial agents, cough, pleuritic chest pain, or hemoptysis. Suggestive chest radiograph findings: pulmonary nodules with or without surrounding halo sign, crescent sign (indicative of cavitation), wedge-shaped or pleural-based nodules or infiltrates.	Systemic antifungal therapy with voriconazole. Itraconazole, lipid formulations of amphotericin B, and caspofungin are alternative treatments.

COPD, chronic obstructive pulmonary disease; AIDS, acquired immunodeficiency syndrome.

PREDISPOSING FACTORS TO INVASIVE ASPERGILLOSIS

Underlying conditions	Notes	Predisposing factors
Allogeneic bone marrow transplant (BMT) recipients	Risk highest for transplantation from an unrelated donor >HLA-mismatched related donor >HLA-matched related donor	Early after BMT: receipt of T-cell-depleted or CD34-selected stem cell products; neutropenia; use of steroids; CMV disease; respiratory viral infections 1–6 mo: defective cellular immunity; use of steroids >6 mo: use of steroids for GVHD; CMV disease
Cord blood transplant	Higher risk of fungal infections than other allograft recipients during the early and late transplant period	Early: slower myeloid engraftment >6 mo: use of steroids for GVHD
Autologous bone marrow transplant	Lowest risk of infections among the bone marrow transplants	Use of CD34-enriched autografts Use of previous potent immunosuppression for treatment of refractory malignancy
Solid organ transplant	Lung transplant has the highest risk	Immunosuppression to treat allograft rejection
Neutropenia	Highest risk among patients treated with chemotherapy for acute leukemia or aplastic anemia	Intensity (absolute neutrophil count <200 cells/μL) and duration of neutropenia (>10 d)
Receipt of immunosuppressive therapy	Therapy for autoimmune diseases	Receipt of high-dose steroids (dose equivalent to prednisone more than 20 mg for >3 wks), antilymphocyte immunoglobulin, anti-TNFα agents, and other immunosuppressive drugs
AIDS	Advanced HIV infection with CD4$^+$ <100 cells/μL	

CMV, cytomegalovirus; GVHD, graft versus host disease; TNF, tumor necrosis factor.

Diagnosis

- Diagnosis of invasive aspergillosis is problematic.
  - *Aspergillus* spores are ubiquitous, common colonizers of the bronchopulmonary tree.
  - Definitive diagnosis, therefore, requires histologic evidence of tissue invasion by hyphal elements, as well as culture of the organism.
  - Sensitivity of tissue biopsy in diagnosing invasive aspergillosis is low (e.g., 30% for lung biopsies).
  - Recovery of *Aspergillus* from the blood is extremely rare, with a recovery rate approximating 5% in cases of *Aspergillus*.
  - In immunocompromised hosts
    - Positive culture from a respiratory sample (sputum or BAL) is highly associated with invasive pulmonary disease.
    - Sensitivity of culture of sputum or BAL is only 50%.
- **Radiography:** In neutropenic patients and bone marrow transplant recipients, high-resolution CT scan of the chest has become an important adjunct to the diagnosis of IPA.
  - One or more nodules surrounded by halo signs (ground glass opacity or haziness) are early findings of angioinvasive mold infections.
  - Cavitation is a late finding.
  - These lesions are highly suggestive of IPA in high-risk patients.
    - Other infections (other fungi, *Nocardia*, and so forth) can also present with halo signs.
    - Classic CT scan findings lead to earlier diagnosis of IPA, more timely administration of antifungal therapy, and improved outcome.
- **Serologic Detection:** A double-sandwich enzyme-linked immunosorbent assay (ELISA) for the detection of galactomannan (GM) in serum has been used as a marker for aspergillosis.
- GM is a cell wall polysaccharide of most *Aspergillus* and *Penicillium* species that is released in serum during growth in tissue.
  - Sensitivity of the test in different reports has ranged from 30% to 100%, with the wide range explained in part by various definitions of positive tests (e.g., different cutoff values and number of values above a cutoff) and different patient populations.
- In adult neutropenic patients, a single serum GM level of ≥0.8 ng/mL is equivalent to two consecutive serum GM levels of ≥0.5 ng/mL.
- Sensitivity using these cutoffs (0.8 *vs.* 0.5 ng/mL) 96.5% and 93.3%
- Specificity 96.5% and 98.6%
- Positive predictive values (PPV) 97.3%, and 98.6%, respectively
- Negative predictive value (NPV) 93.3% and 98.4%, respectively
- Major limitation of this assay is false-positive results
  - Drugs such as piperacillin-tazobactam or cyclophosphamide and certain foods can result in falsely high serum GMs
- In 27 studies encompassing about 4,000 patients
  - Overall sensitivity of the serum ELISA was 61% to 71%
  - Specificity of 89% to 93%
  - PPV of 26% to 53%

TABLE 79.8

RECOMMENDED ANTIFUNGAL AGENTS AGAINST ASPERGILLOSIS

Antifungal agents	Primary therapy	Alternative therapy
Monotherapy		
Voriconazole	More effective and yields better outcome than conventional AmB. There have not been head-to-head comparisons between voriconazole and lipid formulations of AmB.	
Posaconazole	Has not been evaluated as initial monotherapy for invasive aspergillosis.	Yields favorable response (42%) when used as salvage therapy
Caspofungin	Has not been evaluated as initial monotherapy for invasive aspergillosis.	Yields favorable response (45%) when used as salvage therapy. To date only caspofungin has been evaluated for invasive aspergillosis among echinocandins
Lipid formulations of AmB	Have not been evaluated in controlled trials.	Anecdotal reports demonstrating efficacy as salvage therapy
Combination Therapy		
Liposomal formulations of AmB and caspofungin	Have not been evaluated in controlled trials.	Yield favorable outcome in 40%–60% of patients
Voriconazole and caspofungin	Has not been evaluated in controlled trials.	Superior to voriconazole alone in salvage therapy of invasive aspergillosis

- NPV of 95% to 98%
- Test performed best among bone marrow transplant recipients and patients with hematologic malignancies
- Serial testing strategies in these populations are widely accepted.
- Experience among solid organ transplantation is much more limited.
  - In lung and liver transplant recipients
    ○ Sensitivities of the assay were 30% and 56%, respectively
    ○ Specificities of 93% to 95% and 87% to 94%, respectively
    ○ Not clear at present whether serial GM testing of serum plays a useful role in surveillance for IPA among solid organ transplant recipients
    ○ Moderate sensitivity and relatively low positive predictive value of the serum GM in diagnosing IPA might be improved by applying the assay to BAL samples
      – Among bone marrow transplant recipients and patients with hematologic malignances, detection of GM within BAL samples reported to add to sensitivity of both BAL culture and serum GM detection.
      – Specificity of BAL GM detection has generally been good
        • High rates of false-positive results were reported.
        • BAL testing is likely to be influenced by the collection techniques of individual bronchoscopists.

Management

- Voriconazole the first-line therapy against invasive aspergillosis.
  - Proven superior to conventional amphotericin B
  - There have not been head-to-head comparisons of voriconazole versus lipid formulations of amphotericin B.
  - Therapy is generally prolonged for at least 6 weeks or until the primary infection is resolved.

- Role of other systemic antifungal agents is summarized in Table 79.8.
- Debridement of the involved sinuses or primary cutaneous aspergillosis should be performed in conjunction with systemic antifungal therapy.
- Combined antifungal therapy and surgical resection of single lesions from the lungs or central nervous system (CNS) might clear the infection faster than antifungal therapy alone, improve outcome, and prevent reactivation during consecutive chemotherapy courses.
- Procedures are generally well tolerated and associated with low rates of complications and mortality.
- Patients who recover from an episode of invasive aspergillosis are at risk for recurrence of disease during subsequent chemotherapy or transplantation.
  - Should be treated with a systemic antifungal agent for at least 6 weeks or until the primary infection resolves, whichever is longer, before further immunosuppressive therapy is considered
  - Secondary prophylaxis is advised during any subsequent periods of immunosuppression.

VIRAL INFECTIONS

- Recent years have seen the emergence of unexpected viral diseases with high case fatality rates, including:
  - Hantavirus pulmonary syndrome
  - West Nile virus encephalitis
  - Severe adult respiratory syndrome
  - Avian influenza
- Several reasons for critical care physicians to be familiar with a range of viral infections and to consider viral causes in their differential diagnosis
  - There is a small window of time to effectively intervene with antiviral agents in many of these diseases.

- Timely identification of persons with potentially infectious viral diseases has significant public health implications and may reduce the risk of transmission to other persons.
- In the era of long-distance travel, clinicians must recognize previously unfamiliar diseases.
- Viruses such as those causing hemorrhagic fevers are possible agents of bioterrorism.
- In general, viral infections can be diagnosed by several means:
  - Serologic tests: The antibody response to viral antigens can be detected in the serum of patients with viral infections
    - IgM response usually indicates recent exposure to a virus.
    - Presence of IgG reflects past exposure
  - Culture: Several types of cells are available for growing viruses, and no single cell line is appropriate for all of them.
  - Pathology: Histologic examination of biopsy and autopsy tissues may demonstrate changes that are typical of certain viruses (e.g., DNA viruses usually produce inclusions in the cytoplasm).
  - Detection of viral antigens: Viral antigens can be detected in tissues by direct or indirect immunofluorescence using appropriate antibodies.
  - Amplification of viral nucleic acids: Small copy numbers of viral DNA and RNA can be detected by polymerase chain reaction (PCR) and reverse transcription-PCR (RT-PCR), respectively. Real-time amplification methods permit simultaneous detection and quantification of viral nucleic acids.
- Table 79.9 lists leading viruses that might be encountered in the ICU.

Viral Infections on Admission to the Intensive Care Unit

Viral Pneumonitis

- Severe community acquired pneumonia is caused by bacteria in approximately 60% of cases.
  - In a French ICU, bronchoscopy of 41 patients with severe pneumonia revealed that 30% of all BALs and 63% of bacteria-negative BALs were positive for a respiratory virus.
  - Influenza A and B are the most common causes of viral pneumonia in immunocompetent adults.
  - CMV and other herpes viruses are more important in immunocompromised patients.
- Frequently difficult to differentiate bacterial from viral pneumonia
  - Viral pneumonia often less severe
  - Patients may complain of a dry hacking cough.
  - Cultures often necessary to make definitive diagnosis
  - Radiographic findings of viral pneumonia generally nonspecific
    - Ranging from minimal changes on chest radiograph to hyperinflation or bilateral reticular opacities that are diffuse in distribution
    - Uncommonly, viral pneumonias can be associated with thickened interlobular septae that result in Kerley B lines.
    - Viral pneumonias are rarely associated with pleural effusions, unless complicated by secondary bacterial pneumonia.
    - CT scan of the chest may show poorly defined air space nodules, patchy areas of peribronchial ground glass opacity, and consolidation.

Influenza Virus

- Epidemics of influenza typically occur during the winter.
  - Approximately 66% of patients hospitalized with influenza are older than 64 years of age.
  - Morbidity and mortality are highest among:
    - The elderly
    - Children younger than 2 years of age
    - Persons of any age who have comorbid illnesses such as cardiac, pulmonary, or renal diseases, diabetes mellitus, and/or immunosuppression
- **Microbiology:** Human infections are caused by influenza A, B, or C viruses.
  - Wild birds are the natural host for influenza A.
    - Virus infects humans, birds, pigs, and other animals.
  - Influenza B and C viruses are usually found only in humans.
  - Influenza A and B can cause severe disease and occur in epidemics.
    - Influenza A can also be responsible for pandemics.
    - Influenza C causes only mild illness in humans.
      - Does not result in epidemics or pandemics
  - Influenza A viruses are divided into subtypes on the basis of the two main surface glycoproteins, hemagglutinin (HA) and neuraminidase (NA).
    - 16 known HA and 9 known NA subtypes of influenza A
    - New influenza virus variants result from frequent antigenic change, termed *antigenic drift.*
      - Resulting from point mutations that occur during viral replication
  - Influenza B viruses undergo antigenic drift less rapidly than influenza A viruses.
    - In 2006–2007, H5N1 virus (avian influenza) was the circulating virus in Asia and Europe.
    - Caused severe respiratory diseases, life-threatening complications, and death
  - Immunity to the surface antigens, particularly HA, reduces the likelihood of infection and severity of disease
    - Antibody against one influenza virus type or subtype confers limited or no protection against another type or subtype of influenza.
    - Furthermore, antibody to one antigenic variant of influenza virus might not completely protect against a new antigenic variant of the same type or subtype.
    - Antigenic drift is the basis for seasonal epidemics and the reason for the incorporation of one or more new strains in each year's influenza vaccine.
    - More dramatic antigenic changes, or shifts:
      - Occur less frequently
      - Can result in the emergence of a novel influenza virus with potential to cause a pandemic
- **Clinical Manifestations:** The classic influenza symptoms in healthy adults include:
  - Abrupt fever
  - Myalgia
  - Headaches
  - Upper respiratory symptoms
  - In the elderly or immunocompromised hosts, these classic symptoms might be absent, and patients might present only with fever and altered mental status.
  - Influenza-associated lower respiratory tract infections can be classified into four general forms:

TABLE 79.9

VIRAL PATHOGENS MOST LIKELY TO BE ENCOUNTERED IN THE ICU

DNA Viruses

Family	Viruses	Acute critical illness
Adenoviridae	Adenovirus	Myocarditis
Hepadnaviridae	Hepatitis B	Fulminant liver failure, myocarditis
	Hepatitis delta virus	Fulminant liver failure
Herpesviridae	Herpes simplex	Myocarditis
	Varicella zoster	Pneumonitis
	Cytomegalovirus	Opportunistic infection in immunosuppressed hosts
	EBV	Fulminant liver failure
	HHV8 (Kaposi sarcoma virus)	Pulmonary or GI bleeding in HIV
Papovaviridae	JC, BK, other polyomavirus	Renal failure, encephalitis
Parvoviridae	Parvovirus B19	Myocarditis
Poxviridae	Vaccinia	Postvaccinia vaccine complication

RNA Viruses

Family	Viruses	Acute critical illness
Arenaviridae	Lymphocytic choriomeningitis virus	Encephalitis
	South American hemorrhagic fever	Hemorrhagic fever
Bunyaviridae	California encephalitis	Encephalitis
	Hantavirus pulmonary syndrome	Pneumonitis
	Bunyavirid hemorrhagic fever	Hemorrhagic fever
Coronaviridae	Coronavirus (including SARS associated)	Pneumonitis
Filoviridae	Marburg	Hemorrhagic fever
	Ebola	Hemorrhagic fever
Flaviviruses	Yellow fever	Encephalitis
	Dengue, dengue hemorrhagic fever	Hemorrhagic fever
	Japanese encephalitis	Encephalitis
	West Nile encephalitis	Encephalitis
	St. Louis encephalitis	Encephalitis
	Tick-borne encephalitis	Encephalitis
	Hepatitis C	Myocarditis
Orthomyxoviridae	Influenza virus	Pneumonitis, myocarditis
	Avian influenza	Pneumonitis
Paramyxoviridae	Parainfluenza	Pneumonitis
	Mumps	Myocarditis
	Respiratory syncytial virus	Pneumonitis in children, IC
	Human meta-pneumovirus	
	Measles virus (rubeola)	Encephalitis, myocarditis
Picornaviridae	Enterovirus	Myocarditis
	Hepatitis A	Fulminant hepatic failure
	Poliovirus	Myocarditis
	Coxsackievirus, echovirus, and newer enteroviruses	Myocarditis
	Rhinovirus	
Retroviridae	Human T-cell lymphotropic virus I and II	Acute adult T cell leukemia
	Human immunodeficiency virus	Refer to Chapter 81
Rhabdoviridae	Vesicular stomatitis virus and related virus	Encephalitis
	Rhabdovirus	
Togaviridae	Rubella virus (German measles)	Myocarditis

EBV, Epstein-Barr virus; HHV8, human herpes virus 8; GI, gastrointestinal; SARS, severe acute respiratory syndrome; IC, intensive care.

- Influenza without radiographic evidence of pneumonia—up to 30% of hospitalized patients with influenza have no evidence of pulmonary infiltrates
- Viral pneumonia followed by bacterial pneumonia—true incidence is unknown
  ○ Most common bacteria:
    - *Staphylococcus aureus*
    - *Streptococcus pneumoniae*
    - *Haemophilus influenzae*
- Rapidly progressive diffuse viral pneumonia—may be decreasing due to increased rate of influenza vaccination in the elderly
- Concomitant viral and bacterial pneumonia—*S. aureus*, *S. pneumoniae*, and *Haemophilus influenzae*
  ○ Generally more ill than other groups
    - Higher rate of ICU admission
    - Greater morbidity
    - Poor outcomes result from:

- Worsening of underlying heart or lung conditions
- Secondary bacterial pneumonia
- Toxic shock syndrome
- Endotoxemia
- Myopericarditis
- Cytokine-induced shock syndrome
- Encephalitis
- Transverse myelitis

- **Diagnosis:** Several tests can be performed to diagnose influenza. Nasopharyngeal swabs, nasal washes, and aspirates obtained within the first 4 days of illness are preferred respiratory samples.
  - *Rapid influenza tests:* provide results within 30 minutes, and some distinguish between influenza A and B
    - Overall sensitivity is 70% to 75%
    - Specificity of 90% to 95%
    - Useful in the diagnosis of individual patients and in detecting outbreaks
  - *Direct immunofluorescent antibody (DFA) staining:* Requires 2 to 4 hours for results
    - Distinguishes influenza A and B
    - Often performed in a panel that also detects parainfluenza and respiratory syncytial viruses
  - *RT-PCR:* Detects and distinguishes both influenza A and B in 1 to 2 days
  - *Viral culture:* Takes up to 10 days
    - Essential for determining influenza A subtypes and influenza A or B strains
    - Information needed for following year's vaccine
  - *Serology:* Used mainly for research or public health investigations
    - Results not helpful for clinical decision making
- **Treatment:** Two classes of antiviral drugs are available for the prevention and treatment of influenza (Table 79.10):
  - *Amantadine* and *rimantadine:*
    - Target the M2 protein of influenza A
    - Not effective against other influenza viruses
    - Both are generally well tolerated
      - CNS side effects are more common in the elderly.
      - Dosing modification is based on renal function.
  - *Zanamivir* and *oseltamivir:*
    - Neuraminidase inhibitors active for prevention and therapy against both influenza A and influenza B
    - Work best if initiated within 48 hours of clinical symptoms
    - Only oseltamivir has been shown to reduce lower respiratory tract complications requiring antibiotics
    - Patients with asthma or COPD are advised to have a fast-acting inhaled bronchodilator available when inhaling zanamivir.
      - Zanamivir should be stopped if patients develop difficulty breathing.
- **Prevention:** Yearly vaccination is the best means to prevent influenza.
  - Particularly important in people who are at high-risk of having serious complications:
    - Those 65 years of age or older
    - Those with:
      - Cardiac or pulmonary diseases
      - Diabetes or other metabolic diseases
      - Renal dysfunction
      - Hemoglobinopathies
      - Immunosuppression

- People (physicians, nurses) caring for those at high risk for serious complications
- During influenza outbreaks within institution/community:
  - Public health practice is to:
    - Combine influenza vaccine and antiviral medications.
    - Vaccine is given to the exposed patients and staff.
    - Antiviral agent is also given for about 2 weeks until the vaccine takes effect.

Respiratory Syncytial Virus (RSV)

- RSV causes acute respiratory illness in persons of all ages
  - Annual frequency of RSV infection in the elderly and high-risk adults is about 5.5%.
  - Among patients admitted to a hospital for community-acquired pneumonia
    - RSV is second to influenza among viral causes.
    - RSV and influenza A result in comparable lengths of stay, admissions to ICUs, and mortality (8% and 7%, respectively).
- **Transmission:** RSV is transmitted:
  - Person-to-person through close contact
  - By inhalation of large droplets following sneezing or coughing
  - By contact with infected fomites
  - In the United States, RSV outbreaks occur in the winter.
    - In tropical regions, outbreaks occur usually in the rainy season.
- **Clinical Manifestations:** The clinical presentation varies depending on the patient's age and health status.
  - Older children and young adults typically present with upper respiratory symptoms or tracheobronchitis.
  - Elderly and immunocompromised may develop pneumonia.
    - Wheezing occurs in 35% of elderly patients with RSV infection.
  - Presentations can be difficult to differentiate from other causes of viral illnesses, including influenza.
    - In general, URI symptoms tend to last longer than those caused by other respiratory viruses.
      - Associated with a bronchitic cough and wheezing
  - Findings on chest radiograph range from focal interstitial or lobar consolidations to diffuse alveolar interstitial infiltrates
  - Infections are particularly severe in compromised hosts.
    - Mortality of 30% to 100% in bone marrow transplant recipients
- **Diagnosis:** The diagnosis is made by viral detection (by culture or immunofluorescence) or by detection of viral antigens, RNA, or serology.
  - Cultures are performed on respiratory secretions and require 4 to14 days for results.
  - Rapid assays using *antigen capture technology:*
    - Can be performed in <30 minutes
    - Sensitivity and specificity approach 90%
  - Multiplex PCR ELISA is being developed to allow simultaneous diagnosis of multiple respiratory pathogens.
  - In general, diagnosis is more difficult to establish in adults than in children due to low titers of viral shedding.
- **Treatment:** Therapy is mainly supportive.
  - Bronchodilators may help to relieve bronchospasm in some patients.
  - Early use of inhaled ribavirin has been shown to reduce morbidity and mortality in adult bone marrow transplant patients who develop RSV infections.

TABLE 79.10

ANTIVIRAL AGENTS (EXCLUDING ANTI-HIV DRUGS)

Drugs	Description	Viral agents	Infection and sites	Dose in patients with normal renal function	Toxicities	Viral resistance	Mechanism of resistance
Acyclovir	Acyclic guanosine nucleoside analogue	HSV1, HSV2, and VZV	Mucocutaneous HSV infection HSV or VZV encephalitis or VZV pneumonitis	400 mg tid PO or 5 mg/kg q8h IV (also available as topical agent) 10 mg/kg q8h IV	Headache, nausea Renal, neurologic toxicities	> 1% in immuno-competent hosts 6%–8% in immuno-compromised hosts 11%–17% in patients with AIDS and transplant recipients	Most common: no or low production of viral thymidine-kinase (TK) → cross-resistant to penciclovir and ganciclovir Altered TK substrate specificity Altered viral DNA polymerase
Valacyclovir	L-valine ester prodrug of acyclovir	HSV1, HSV2, and VZV	Mucocutaneous HSV Cutaneous HZV	1 g bid PO 1 g tid PO	Similar to acyclovir		Same as acyclovir
Famciclovir	Ester prodrug of penciclovir	HSV1, HSV2, and VZV	Mucocutaneous HSV Cutaneous VZV	125–500 mg bid PO 500–750 mg bid to tid PO	Headache, nausea, and diarrhea		Inactive against TK-deficient strains of HSV and VZV
Ganciclovir	Acyclic guanosine nucleoside analogue	HSV1, HSV2, VZV, CMV, EBV	CMV retinitis, pneumonitis, or other organ disease	5 mg/kg q12h IV	Hematologic	About 8% of isolates in AIDS patients are resistant to ganciclovir after a course of therapy; resistance also documented among transplant recipients	Mutation of UL97 gene or of viral DNA polymerase Some ganciclovir-resistant strains with DNA polymerase mutations are cross-resistant to foscarnet and cidofovir
Valganciclovir	Ester prodrug of ganciclovir	CMV	CMV retinitis	900 mg bid po	Hematologic	Same as ganciclovir	Same as ganciclovir
Foscarnet	Pyrophosphate analogue	HSV1, HSV2, VZV, CMV, HIV	CMV	60 mg/kg q8h IV or 90 mg/kg IV q12h IV	Renal (azotemia, acute tubular necrosis)	<5% of patients on foscarnet therapy	Point mutations in DNA polymerase of HSV and CMV, and reverse transcriptase of HIV. In general, no cross-resistance with ganciclovir or cidofovir, although some ganciclovir-resistant strains with DNA polymerase mutations are cross-resistant to foscarnet and cidofovir
			HSV	40 mg/kg q8h or 60 mg/kg q12h IV	Metabolic and electrolyte imbalance		
			VZV	60–90 mg/kg q12h IV	Neurotoxicity (tremor, headache)		

(continued)

TABLE 79.10

CONTINUED

Drugs	Description	Viral agents	Infection and sites	Dose in patients with normal renal function	Toxicities	Viral resistance	Mechanism of resistance
Cidofovir	Nucleotide analogue	HSV1, HSV2, VZV, HHV-6, HHV-8, CMV, EBV, DNA viruses (papilloma, poyloma, pox viruses)	CMV retinitis	5 mg/kg once a week IV	Renal (proximal tubular dysfunction), Ocular (anterior uveitis or ocular hypotony)	Uncommon	Ganciclovir-resistant CMV (due to DNA polymerase mutations plus UL97 mutations) and some foscarnet-resistant CMV strains are cross-resistant to cidofovir
Amantadine Rimantadine	Tricyclic amine	Influenza A	Influenza A within 48 h of symptoms	100 mg bid po	Gastrointestinal complaints and neurologic toxicities (rimantadine has lower neuro effects)	Up to 30% of patients treated shed-resistant viruses by the 5th day	Cross-resistance between amantadine and rimantadine Resistant viruses remain susceptible to neuraminidase inhibitors
Zanamivir	Neuraminidase inhibitor	Influenza A, B	Influenza within 48 h of symptoms	10 mg bid via inhalation	Bronchospasm		
Oseltamivir	Neuraminidase inhibitor	Influenza A, B	Influenza within 48 h of symptoms	75 mg bid po	Neuropsych, nausea		
Ribavirin	Nucleoside analogue	RSV	RSV in infants	6 g/300 mL over 12–18 h/d via aerosol	Teratogenic, embryotoxic Anemia Reversible hyperbili-rubinemia	No viral resistance has been detected (except for Sindbis virus)	
		Hepatitis C	Hepatitis C	500–600 bid po (together with IFN)			
		Lassa fever or Hantavirus		IV, may be obtained from CDC			
Interferon alpha		Hepatitis C virus	Hepatitis C (with ribavirin)	Peg IFN alfa-2a 180 mg/wk SC (in combination with ribavirin)	Depression Flulike symptoms Bone marrow toxicity		
		Hepatitis B virus	Hepatitis B	Peg IFN alfa-2a 180 mg/wk SC			
Lamivudine	Nucleoside analogue	Hepatitis B HIV	Hepatitis B	100 mg daily po	Benign	16%–31% resistance after 6 mo to 1 y. Rate is higher in transplant recipients	Mutations in HBV DNA polymerase
Entecavir	Nucleoside analogue	Hepatitis B	Hepatitis B	0.5–1 mg PO daily	Headache, Abdominal pain Pharyngitis	Rare in nucleoside-naïve patients	
Adefovir	Nucleotide analogue	Hepatitis B	Hepatitis B	10 mg PO daily		9%, 18%, and 28% resistance after 3, 4, and 5 y, respectively	Mutations in HBV reverse transcriptase domain

- More aggressive therapy with combined ribavirin, IV immunoglobulin with high titers of neutralizing RSV antibody, and/or steroids can be considered in immunosuppressed patients with severe RSV pneumonia.

Varicella-Zoster Virus (VZV)

- VZV causes chickenpox or shingles.
  - Primary infection usually occurs in childhood.
  - Generally a benign self-limited illness in immunocompetent hosts
  - Pneumonia is uncommon complication of varicella in healthy children.
    - The most frequent complication in healthy adults
    - Reported incidence rate is about 2.3 in 400 cases in the United States.
    - Overall mortality between 10% and 30%.
      - With respiratory failure due to VZV pneumonia requiring mechanical ventilation
        - Mortality rates approach 50% despite institution of aggressive therapy and supportive measures.
    - Risk factors for VZV pneumonia:
      - Cigarette smoking
      - Pregnancy
      - Immunosuppression
      - Male gender
- **Clinical Manifestations:** VZV pneumonia develops insidiously 1 to 6 days after onset of:
  - Vesicular rash
  - With symptoms of cough, shortness of breath, fever, and occasionally pleuritic chest pain or hemoptysis
  - Examination of the chest may reveal rhonchi or wheezes.
  - Chest radiograph typically reveals diffuse or patchy nodular infiltrates with a prominent peribronchial distribution.
    - Reticular markings, pleural effusions, and hilar adenopathy may be seen as well.
- **Treatment:** Prompt treatment with IV acyclovir
  - Dose of 10 mg/kg every 8 hours associated with clinical improvement and resolution of pneumonia
  - Addition of steroids for treatment of life-threatening varicella pneumonia is controversial
    - In one series, patients who received steroids as adjunctive therapy had shorter hospitalizations and ICU stays and no mortality.
    - Rapid institution of extracorporeal life support has been reported to improve outcome in patients with severe life-threatening varicella pneumonia.

Hantavirus Pulmonary Syndrome (HPS)

- Among agents causing HPS, the *Sin Nombre* (Spanish for "nameless" or "without a name") virus that caused the 1993 Four Corners outbreak in the southwestern United States was the most severe.
  - Many hantaviruses are shed in the urine, feces, or saliva of infected rodents.
    - Transmission to humans occurs via aerosols
    - Deer mouse *Peromyscus maniculatus* the predominant reservoir
    - CDC reported an increase in human cases of HPS during January through March of 2006 in Arizona, Texas, North Dakota, New Mexico, and Washington
- **Clinical Manifestations:** Incubation period is 1 to 3 weeks.
  - After which patients experience:

- Fever
- Muscle pain
- Fatigue
- Some also experience headache, dizziness, vomiting, or diarrhea
- Four to 10 days later patients develop:
  - Cough
  - Respiratory distress
- No defined sets of symptoms and signs that reliably distinguish HPS from other forms of noncardiogenic pulmonary edema or ARDS
- Features associated with HPS are:
  - Thrombocytopenia
  - Hemoconcentration
  - Leukocytosis with increased band forms on differential
  - Hypoalbuminemia
  - Lactic acidosis
- Classic diagnostic triad includes thrombocytopenia, neutrophilia, and an immunoblast count of >10% of the total lymphocytes.
  - Shock and lactic acidosis associated with poor prognosis
  - Case fatality ratio is 30% to 40%.
- **Diagnosis:** Consider HPS in the differential diagnosis of previously healthy patients from endemic areas who present with fever >101°F and develop bilateral diffuse interstitial edema of the lungs within 72 hours of hospitalization.
  - Edema can resemble ARDS on chest radiograph.
  - Serologic tests are the main method of diagnosing HPS.
    - High levels of IgM antibodies present by the time symptoms are evident.
  - In the United States, states that offer hantavirus diagnostic testing use IgG and mu capture IgM ELISA assays developed and distributed by the Centers for Disease Control and Prevention.
- **Treatment:** No specific antiviral therapy for HPS, and treatment is mainly supportive, with early initiation of mechanical ventilation to treat respiratory failure.
  - Use of extracorporeal membrane oxygenation (ECMO) should be considered in patients with a cardiac index of <2.5 L/minute/m² despite inotropes.
  - Placebo-controlled double-blind trial of IV ribavirin for the treatment of hantavirus cardiopulmonary syndrome in North America was terminated early due to the drug's probable ineffectiveness.

Severe Acute Respiratory Syndrome (SARS)

- SARS a serious pulmonary illness caused by a coronavirus that jumped species from semidomesticated animals to humans and spread from China to Hong Kong in late 2002.
- Infection spread by close person-to-person contact via respiratory droplets
- Incubation period is 2 to 10 days.
- Patients first experience:
  - High fever associated with chills, headache, and myalgia
  - Diarrhea is seen in approximately 10% to 20%.
  - Two to 7 days later a dry nonproductive cough develops.
    - Hypoxia that progresses to ARDS and multiple organ dysfunction maybe seen.
    - Ten percent to 20% require mechanical ventilation.
- RT-PCR, serology, and cultures of blood, stool, and nasal secretions possible diagnostic tools.
  - Routine clinical use difficult

TABLE 79.11

COMMON CAUSES OF VIRAL MENINGITIS AND ENCEPHALITIS

Types of infection	Viral pathogen	Comments
Viral meningitis	Enterovirus	Most common cause of viral meningitis
		More than 50 serotypes of enteroviruses
		Can cause meningitis or meningoencephalitis
	Herpes simplex type 2	Associated with genital herpes infection
	HIV	Generally develops at the time of HIV seroconversion
	Lymphocytic choriomeningitis (LCM)	Sporadic cause of meningitis
		Can cause meningitis or meningoencephalitis
	Adenovirus	Rare cause of viral meningitis
		Can cause severe meningoencephalitis in children
Encephalitis	Japanese encephalitis	Most common cause worldwide
	Herpes simplex type 1	Most common cause of sporadic viral encephalitis
		Associated with focal symptoms
	Arboviruses	Transmitted by mosquitoes or ticks.
	CMV, VZV	Causes disease in immunocompromised patients only

HIV, human immunodeficiency virus; CMV, cytomegalovirus; VZV, varicella-zoster virus.

- No specific treatment against SARS-associated coronavirus
  - Supportive care remains principal therapeutic alternative
  - Ribavirin and corticosteroids have been used.
    - Efficacy has not been established.
  - Mortality approximates 11%.
  - Infection control practices are extremely important in halting progression of an outbreak.

Other Viruses

- Although uncommon in adults
  - Adenovirus pneumonia outbreaks have been described among military recruits and among adults in chronic care facilities.
  - Diagnosis is established by culture of a nasopharyngeal aspirate or swab, throat swab, or sputum.
  - Other viruses associated with acute pneumonias in adults include:
    - Measles
    - Parainfluenza
    - Parvovirus

Viral Meningitis and Encephalitis

- Refer to infections of the leptomeninges and brain parenchyma, respectively.
  - Important differentiating feature between viral meningitis and encephalitis is presence or absence of altered sensorium
    - With viral meningitis, one sees lethargy and severe headache, but cerebral function remains normal.
    - In encephalitis, cerebral functions are abnormal, including altered mental status, altered behavior and personality changes, speech or movement disorder, and focal neurologic deficits.
  - Reported incidences:
    - Viral meningitis 11 per 100,000 person years
    - Encephalitis 7 per 100,000 person-years
  - Patients may have both a parenchymal and meningeal process called *meningoencephalitis*

Viral (Aseptic) Meningitis

- Common causes of viral meningitis are summarized in Table 79.11.
- Other viruses are even rarer causes, such as:
  - Epstein-Barr virus (EBV)
  - Cytomegalovirus (CMV)
  - Human herpes virus 6 (HHV-6)
  - Herpes zoster (reactivation of VZV infection) of aseptic meningitis
- Arboviruses such as St. Louis encephalitis and California encephalitis (SLE and CE, respectively)
  - More commonly cause encephalitis or meningoencephalitis
  - But can also cause aseptic meningitis
- Clinical presentations of viral meningitis are nonspecific:
  - Fever
  - Headache
  - Photophobia
  - Nuchal rigidity
  - Helpful clues to the diagnosis include:
    - Travel to arbovirus endemic areas
    - Exposure history (rodents, ticks)
    - Sexual activity (HSV-2)
    - Contact with other people with similar symptoms (enteroviruses)
  - Clinicians should look for:
    - Pharyngitis and pleurodynia (enteroviruses)
    - Rash (zosteriform rash of VZV, vesicular rash of HSV, maculopapular rash measles or enteroviruses)
    - Adenopathy (primary HIV or EBV)
  - Cerebrospinal fluid (CSF) findings include:
    - White blood cells (WBC) <500 cells/μL
      - Of which >50% are lymphocytes
    - Protein <80 mg/dL
    - Normal glucose
    - Negative Gram stain
    - CSF should be sent for:
      - Bacterial and viral cultures
      - HSV PCR

- HIV viral load
- Other tests that can be sent if indicated include:
  - Enterovirus PCR
  - Acute/convalescent serologic testing for specific viruses
- If patient is neither immunocompromised nor toxic appearing
- One can observe without giving antibiotic therapy.
- Treatment for enteroviral meningitis is mostly supportive (pain management and hydration).
- Pleconaril
  - Inhibits viral attachment to host cells and viral uncoating
  - Has shown disappointing results in the treatment of enteroviral meningitis
- If the patient is immunosuppressed, elderly, or toxic appearing, or has received antibiotics before presentation
  - May consider empiric antibiotics for 48 hours while waiting for culture results

Viral Encephalitis

- In the United States, most common cause of sporadic encephalitis is HSV-1
- Arboviruses account for approximately 5% of viral encephalitis.
  - SLE virus the most common.
  - Clues to arboviral infection include:
    - Season (arboviruses cause disease when mosquitoes are active, whereas HSV-1 can occur at any time)
    - Location (woody or marshy areas would suggest viruses such as the cause of Colorado tick fever or nonviral illness such as Lyme disease or Rocky Mountain spotted fever)
    - Geographic region (SLE occurs in the midwest and southern United States, whereas West Nile virus [WNV] occurs in multiple continents)
    - History of animal exposure (rabies)
  - Clues on physical exam include:
    - Parotitis (mumps)
    - Flaccid paralysis (WNV)
    - Tremors of the eyelids, tongue, lips, and extremities (SLE)
    - Findings of hydrophobia, aerophobia, and hyperactivity (rabies)
- CSF findings can be similar to those of viral meningitis.
  - Depending on clinical suspicion, the CSF can also be sent for:
    - PCR for enteroviruses, HSV, or CMV
    - Acute and convalescent sera against specific viral pathogens such as arboviruses, and lymphocytic choriomeningitis virus (LCMV) might also be useful in determining a cause
    - CT scan with IV contrast or MRI should be obtained:
      - To exclude an intracranial process (cerebritis, abscess, subdural empyema, mass occupying lesions)
      - To detect findings suggestive of a viral cause
        - Temporal and basal frontal lobe involvement suggests HSV encephalitis.
        - Basal ganglia and thalamic involvement suggest Eastern equine encephalitis.
  - Until HSV encephalitis is ruled out
    - Acyclovir at 10 mg/kg IV every 8 hours should be considered in patients with suspected viral encephalitis

- **HSV encephalitis:** A fulminant hemorrhagic and necrotizing meningoencephalitis that involves primarily the temporal and basal frontal cortices and the limbic system
- HSV-1 accounts for most fatal cases of sporadic encephalitis in adults.
  - HSV-1 encephalitis can arise either from:
    - Primary infections, or
    - Reactivation of a latent infection
  - No difference in outcome from patients suffering encephalitis from a primary or reactivation HSV infection
- Herpes simplex virus type 2 (HSV-2) accounts for herpes encephalitis in 80% to 90% of neonates and children.
- *Clinical Manifestations:* Most common early symptoms are fever and headache.
  - Additional symptoms include:
    - Meningeal irritation
    - Nausea
    - Vomiting
    - Altered consciousness
    - Generalized seizures
    - Other changes are referable to involved brain areas, including:
      - Anosmia
      - Memory loss
      - Abnormal behavior
      - Speech defects
      - Olfactory and gustatory hallucinations
      - Focal seizures
  - Can be rapid progression of the disease in some patients with the development of focal paralysis, hemiparesis, and coma
- *Diagnosis:* Diagnosis of HSV encephalitis can be strongly suggested if:
  - Typical clinical presentations associated with specific findings on EEG and MRI
  - Typical EEG findings are:
    - Focal temporal abnormalities
      - Found in about 80% of patients
    - Periodic lateralized epileptiform discharges also suggest HSV encephalitis
      - Although not as specific
    - In HSV encephalitis, a normal EEG essentially excludes the diagnosis.
    - Typical MRI appearance is:
      - Medial temporal abnormalities that do not respect hippocampal borders
    - CSF findings are similar to other cases of viral meningoencephalitis.
    - Isolation of HSV from CSF is rare
      - Occurring in <5% of cases
    - Definitive diagnosis is made by detection of HSV DNA in CSF by PCR.
      - Which is very sensitive and specific
      - Availability of PCR has largely obviated the need for brain biopsy, the previous gold standard diagnostic test
- *Treatment:* Morbidity and mortality are reduced by early antiviral therapy.
  - IV acyclovir, 10 mg/kg every 8 hours
  - Continued for 14 to 21 days
  - A 5% relapse rate after the discontinuation of antiviral therapy

- **Rabies:** Caused by neurotropic RNA viruses
  - In addition to classic rabies virus, at least 10 other rabies-related viruses can cause clinically indistinguishable fatal encephalitis.
  - Has a worldwide distribution
    - Found throughout the United States except Hawaii
    - In developing countries, dogs are major reservoir.
    - Wild animals remain most important reservoir in the United States
      - Most reported cases occur in carnivores
        - Raccoons in the northeast
        - Skunks in the south and southwest
        - Foxes in the southwest and Alaska
      - And insectivorous bats
  - In the United States, an average of three fatal human cases per year since 1980
  - Acquisition of rabies usually occurs after:
    - Bite from an infected animal
    - Scratching and licking by a rabid animal
    - Cases have also been reported after solid organ, cornea, or vascular tissue transplantation from unsuspected rabies-infected individuals
  - *Clinical Manifestations:* Human rabies assumes two forms: furious (encephalitic) and paralytic (dumb).
    - Furious form—observed in 80% of patients—manifests as:
      - Hyperactivity
      - Hydrophobia
      - Pharyngeal spasms
      - Aerophobia
    - Paralytic form can mimic Guillain-Barré syndrome with quadriparesis, sphincter involvement, and late cerebral involvement
    - Some bat-associated rabies may present atypically with:
      - Neuropathic pain
      - Sensory or motor deficits
      - Choreiform movements of the bitten limb
      - Focal brainstem signs
      - Myoclonus
      - Seizures
  - Regardless of presentation, the disease is almost always fatal.
  - *Diagnosis:* Confirmed in several ways:
    - Detection of viral RNA in saliva by RT-PCR
    - Biopsy of the nape of the neck for detection of RNA or viral antigen within hair follicles by RT-PCR or immunofluorescence staining, respectively
    - Antibodies in serum and CSF
    - Presence of pathognomonic Negri bodies (eosinophilic neuronal cytoplasmic inclusions) in brain biopsy
  - *Treatment:* There is no proven effective treatment for rabies after the onset of illness.
    - Only six survivors have been reported.
    - Five of whom received postexposure vaccination
    - The sixth patient survived after induction of coma and treatment with ribavirin and amantadine.
      - Clinicians who wish to consider this protocol should contact Dr. Rodney Willoughby at Children's Hospital of Wisconsin (414-266-2000).
    - Rabies vaccination after onset of illness is not recommended and may be detrimental.
    - After definitive diagnosis, the primary focus is comfort care.
  - Management of patients with rabies poses no greater risk to health care providers than caring for patients with more common infections.
    - Adherence to standard precautions should be maintained:
      - Gloves
      - Gowns
      - Masks
      - Eye protection
      - Face shield (particularly during intubation or suctioning)
  - Because of the lack of effective treatment:
    - Postexposure prophylaxis should be initiated as soon as possible after exposure to rabid or unknown animals.
    - Includes the administration of:
      - Human rabies immunoglobulin (HRIG: HyperRab Tm S/D or Imogam Rabies-HT)
      - Rabies vaccination (purified chick embryo cell vaccine (PCECV; 1-800-244-7668; www.rabavert.com)
- **West Nile virus:** WNV a single-stranded RNA virus that can infect humans, mosquitoes, and animals such as birds and horses.
  - In temperate climates, WNV is transmitted primarily in the summer or early fall.
  - Transmission can occur year round in warmer climates.
  - Most human WNV infections result from mosquito bites.
  - Infection can also be transmitted via:
    - Transfusion of WNV-infected blood products
    - Transplacental fetal infection
    - Transplantation of infected organs
  - *Clinical Manifestations:* Patients infected with WNV can be asymptomatic (80%), develop West Nile fever (WNF, 20%) or West Nile neuroinvasive disease (WNND, <1%).
    - WNND includes:
      - Meningitis, encephalitis, and acute flaccid paralysis
      - WNV encephalitis is more common in the elderly or immunocompromised patients.
    - Incubation period ranges from 3 to 14 days.
    - Symptoms generally last 3 to 6 days.
    - Patients with WNF or WNND present with an abrupt onset of:
      - Fever
      - Headache
      - Fatigue
      - Anorexia
      - Gastrointestinal complaints
      - Myalgia
      - Lymphadenopathy
      - Generalized nonpruritic maculopapular rash
    - Patients with WNND also present with:
      - Altered mental status (46% to 74%)
      - Tremor (12% to 80%)
      - Extrapyramidal features such as rigidity or bradykinesia (67%)
      - Cerebellar abnormalities (11% to 57%)
      - Myoclonus—present in 33% of cases—a clue to WN infection
        - Rare in other causes of viral encephalitis
      - Seizures are unusual (1% to 16%)
  - *Diagnosis:* Diagnosis of WNV infection is based on a high index of suspicion and obtaining specific laboratory tests.

- IgM antibody capture ELISA (MAC-ELISA) can detect WNV in nearly all CSF and serum specimens from WNV-infected patients.
- IgM antibody does not cross blood–brain barrier.
  - IgM antibody in the CSF strongly suggests acute CNS infection.
  - WNV testing of patients with encephalitis, meningitis, or other serious CNS infections can be obtained through local or state health departments.
- *Treatment:* Treatment is supportive, with hospitalization, IV fluids, respiratory support, and prevention of secondary infections for patients with severe disease.
  - Ribavirin and interferon alpha 2b have some activity against WNV *in vitro.*
    - No controlled studies have been completed.
    - Role of corticosteroids has not been assessed.

Viral Infections Acquired during Intensive Care Unit Stay

- Herpes family viruses recognized as pathogens in immunosuppressed transplant patients and HIV/AIDS patients.
  - Increasingly reported as pathogens in nonimmunosuppressed critically ill
- At least 14% of chronic critically ill surgical patients had occult CMV or HSV infection/reactivation.

CMV Infection

- Infects about 60% to 70% of people during their lifetimes
  - Like other members of the herpes family, becomes latent or persistent after primary infection
  - Infection can reactivate at a later time
    - Especially in the settings of immunodeficiency or significant stress from operations or injuries
- **Transmission:** CMV can be found in body secretions:
  - Urine
  - Saliva
  - Sputum
  - Breast milk
  - Semen
  - Cervical fluid
  - In circulating mononuclear and polymorphonuclear cells, vascular endothelium, and renal epithelium
  - CMV spreads from person to person by contact with body fluids.
    - Transmission is particularly high among toddlers in day care.
    - Day care employees are also at significant risk for CMV exposure and/or infection.
    - So are health care personnel with direct patient contact
    - Congenital transmission from a mother with acute infection during pregnancy is a significant cause of neurologic abnormalities and deafness in newborns.
    - Can also be transmitted by:
      - Breastfeeding
      - Blood transfusion
      - Receipt of an organ transplant
      - Major risk factors for CMV disease in solid organ transplant recipients are CMV mismatch...

- Transplantation of a CMV-positive organ into a CMV-seronegative recipient
- ...and the degree of immunosuppression
- **Clinical manifestations:** Most immunocompetent children and adults who are infected with CMV do not develop symptoms.
- Some may experience an illness resembling infectious mononucleosis with fever, swollen glands, and mild hepatitis.
- Rare complications of primary CMV infection include:
  - Hepatitis
  - Interstitial pneumonia
  - Guillain-Barré syndrome
  - Meningoencephalitis
  - Pericarditis
  - Myocarditis
  - Thrombocytopenia
  - Hemolytic anemia
- In immunocompromised patients, primary CMV infection is life threatening. Most common manifestations:
  - Myelosuppression
  - Encephalitis
  - Hepatitis
  - Pneumonitis
  - Retinitis
  - GI infection
- Reactivation of latent CMV causes disease in immunocompromised hosts, although typically milder than primary infection.
  - In general, the severity of CMV disease is related to the degree of immunosuppression.
  - CMV appears to target allografts in particular.
    - Hepatitis common in liver transplant recipients
    - Pancreatitis in pancreatic transplant
    - Pneumonitis in lung and heart-lung transplant
    - CMV pneumonia highest among bone marrow transplant recipients
    - In solid organ transplant recipients, CMV infections predispose to other opportunistic infections, especially fungal or *Pneumocystis* infections
- CMV infection can also affect graft survival.
  - Causing early allograft rejection in renal transplant recipients
  - Chronic allograft rejection in cardiac transplant recipients (allograft atherosclerosis)
  - Vanishing bile duct syndrome in liver transplant recipients
- **Diagnosis:** CMV can be shed in biologic fluids from patients with no evidence of disease.
  - Gold standard for diagnosis remains finding intranuclear inclusion bodies in histologically examined tissue.
  - Infection may be confirmed by *in situ* hybridization or direct or indirect staining of intranuclear inclusions using specific antibodies linked to an indicator system.
  - Histopathology is limited by poor sensitivity.
  - Tests that can detect and quantify CMV or its products in blood, leukocytes, or tissues are reviewed in Table 79.12
  - CMV excretion in saliva and urine is common in immunocompromised patients.
    - Generally of little consequence
    - Viremia in organ transplant patients identifies those at greatest risk for CMV disease.

TABLE 79.12

DIAGNOSTIC TESTS FOR CMV INFECTION

Test	Concept	Advantages/disadvantages	Interpretation of positive tests in the immunocompromised host	Interpretation of tests in the immunocompetent host
SEROLOGY				
CMV-specific IgG	Detect IgG seroconversion.	Disadvantage: Need acute and convalescent sera (or known baseline negative IgG).	Documented seroconversion implies primary CMV infection. Primary infection.	Documented seroconversion implies primary CMV infection. Primary infection.
CMV-specific IgM	Acute phase of primary CMV infection should have positive CMV-specific IgM and negative IgG antibodies.	Advantage: Depending on assays used, sensitivity and specificity can be as high as 100% and 98%, respectively. Disadvantage: Interference due to presence of rheumatoid factor and antinuclear antibody.	Since IgM can also be elevated in reactivation, positive IgM alone does not indicate primary CMV infection. In this setting, should interpret in conjunction with CMV-specific IgG. In the immunocompromised host, IgM might persist for a long time after primary infection.	Problems with false-positive and persistent IgM due to reactivation are less than with the immunocompromised hosts.
Detection of virus	Recovery of CMV from the biologic sites signifies either primary infection, reactivation, or asymptomatic shedding without infection.			
Shell-vial assay	Detection and quantitation of viremia.	Disadvantage: 1. Tissue culture is time-consuming. Shell-vial assay can provide results within 24 h. 2. Low sensitivity. 3. Loss of CMV viability in stored clinical samples.	High risk of developing CMV disease. Marker for initiation of antiviral therapy and monitoring the efficacy of therapy.	Specific for primary CMV infection. Sensitivity of 26.3%, highest within 1 mo of primary infection. Test positivity can last up to 4–6 mo. Low false-positive rate.
Antigenemia	Detection and quantitation of leukocytes that are positive for CMV phosphoprotein pp65.	Advantages: 1. Rapid test with turnover time of a few hours. 2. In transplant recipients, antigenemia becomes positive before viremia detection, but later than DNA-emia at the onset of CMV infection. Disadvantages: 1. Subjective slide reading. 2. Levels of antigenemia might lag behind clinical response to antiviral therapy.	Associated with CMV disease.	Specific for primary CMV infection. Sensitivity of 57.1%, highest within 1 mo of primary infection. Test positivity can last 4–6 mo. Negligible false-positive rate.
CMV DNA in blood (DNA-emia)	Detection and quantitation of CMV DNA in whole blood and leukocytes: PCR and hybridization techniques.	Advantages: 1. Useful for diagnosis of systemic or local CMV infections (CNS, eye, central nervous system, amniotic fluid). 2. Useful for evaluation of efficacy of antiviral therapy	1. Systemic and local site CMV infections.	Marker for primary CMV infection. Leukocyte DNA-emia has sensitivity of 100%, highest within 1 month of primary infection. Test positivity can last 4–6 mo.
Immediate-early and late CMV mRNA (RNA-emia)	Detection of immediate-early and late CMV mRNA transcripts in blood	Advantage: slightly more sensitive than DNA-emia in diagnosing early phase of primary CMV infection. Disadvantage: Slightly less sensitive than DNA-emia in the late phase of primary CMV infection.	1. RNA-emia in blood is a marker of CMV replication 2. Late viral transcripts are markers for active CMV replication and dissemination.	Immediate-early mRNA in the blood is a marker for primary infection.

- Bone marrow transplant recipients, the sensitivity of viremia as a marker for CMV pneumonia is 60% to 70%
  - Lack of viremia also has a high negative predictive value
- Detection of CMV or its products in the blood of transplant recipients is a basis for starting antiviral therapy.
- Value of positive CMV tests in the nontransplant ICU patient less clear.
- Viremia does not necessarily signify CMV disease in ICU patients.
- Data needed to elucidate impact of CMV infection/reactivation in critically ill patients and to clarify the effects of CMV treatment on morbidity and mortality
- **Management:** Ganciclovir, foscarnet, and cidofovir are antiviral agents active against CMV (Table 79.10).
- Efficacy of anti-CMV therapy evaluated primarily in immunocompromised hosts
- CMV disease in transplant recipients is typically treated with a 3-week course of ganciclovir.
  - Foscarnet is an alternative for patients who cannot tolerate, or fail to respond to, ganciclovir.
    - Foscarnet is associated with high rates of nephrotoxicity.
    - CMV retinitis requires a longer course of systemic therapy.
      - Intravitreal administration of ganciclovir or fomivirsen, an antisense inhibitor of CMV, frequently used in addition to systemic therapy
      - Long-term maintenance therapy is required for AIDS patients who do not undergo immune reconstitution; this strategy is generally not required for transplant recipients.
    - Recurrence of CMV disease seen in up to 25% of transplant recipients.
      - Appears to respond to ganciclovir as well as the initial episode

HSV Infection

- HSV-1 and HSV-2 are closely related, but the epidemiology of infections by the viruses is distinct.
  - HSV-1 is transmitted mainly by contact with infected saliva.
  - HSV-2 is transmitted by contact with the genital tract.
  - HSV-1 is acquired more commonly and at an earlier age than HSV-2.
  - By age 50 years, over 90% of people have antibodies against HSV-1.
    - HSV-1 is also more common among ICU patients.
- **Clinical manifestations:** HSV encephalitis and meningitis are discussed above.
  - HSV-1 can infect virtually any mucocutaneous or visceral site.
  - Primary infections associated with:
    - Systemic signs and symptoms

- Mucosal and extramucosal involvement
- Longer duration of symptoms
- Viral shedding
- Higher complication rates
- Gingivostomatitis and pharyngitis are the most common clinical syndromes of HSV-1 infection.
  - Lesions are ulcerative with or without exudates and can be difficult to differentiate from bacterial pharyngitis.
  - HSV-1 has predilection for regenerating epithelium.
    - Healing partial-thickness skin burns
    - Skin donor sites
    - Skin diseases (e.g., eczema, pemphigus, Darier disease)
    - Areas of cutaneous trauma are common sites of infection
  - HSV-1 keratitis is the most frequent cause of corneal blindness.
    - Can also cause chorioretinitis—a sign of disseminated infection—and acute necrotizing retinitis, affecting both immunocompetent and immunocompromised hosts
- In immunocompromised hosts and patients with atopic eczema or burns
  - Severe orofacial HSV lesions can rapidly spread and disseminate infection.
  - Bone marrow and solid organ transplant recipients are at highest risk for HSV reactivation during the pre-engraftment period or within the first month posttransplant.
  - Complications include pneumonitis, tracheobronchitis, esophagitis, hepatitis, and disseminated viral infection.
- HSV-1 shedding is observed in immunocompetent but critically ill patients.
  - Significance unclear
  - HSV-1 may predispose to subsequent bacterial or fungal infection.
- **Diagnosis:** The diagnosis of HSV-1 infection can be made using a direct immunofluorescence test or by culture of tissue or aspirated fluid.
  - Serology is helpful in diagnosing primary HSV infection.
  - Improved testing methods have led to increased detection of HSV-1 in ICU patients.
    - As with CMV, it is often unclear whether HIV-1 is an active pathogen or merely a marker of immune dysfunction.
- **Management:** For mucocutaneous and visceral infections
  - Acyclovir or related agents (famciclovir and valacyclovir) the standard therapy
  - For disseminated disease or encephalitis due to HSV-1
    - IV acyclovir is recommended
  - For HSV keratitis
    - Debridement along with topical therapy with idoxuridine or vidarabine is the treatment of choice.
    - Other ophthalmologic disease such as chorioretinitis or retinal necrosis requires systemic antiviral therapy.

CHAPTER 80 ■ INFECTIONS IN THE IMMUNOCOMPROMISED HOST

- Consider when evaluating immunocompromised patient presenting with suspected infection
  - Due to impaired inflammatory response, signs and symptoms of infection may be absent.
    - Organ transplant recipient with perforated viscus presents with fever but no clinical evidence of peritonitis.
    - Neutropenic patient with pneumonia has cough but no infiltrate on chest radiograph (CXR).
  - Thorough repeated history and physical examination basis for investigations and management
    - Subtle signs often basis for fruitful investigation
  - Assessment of immune deficits based on underlying condition and immunosuppressive therapies, and other therapeutic interventions suggest probable pathogens.
- Aggressive initial approach to diagnosis is generally warranted.
  - Cultures of blood, urine, and sputum; CXR; and so forth should be performed.
  - Invasive procedures such as biopsy and bronchoscopy should be considered early.
  - Delay in arriving at a diagnosis results in delays of appropriate therapy or exposure to toxicities of unneeded therapies.
    - Will compromise treatment outcomes
- When tissue or body fluids are collected, specimens are evaluated for both infectious and noninfectious syndromes.
  - Such as malignancy, drug toxicity, rejection, and graft-versus-host disease (GVHD)
- Initial empiric antimicrobial therapy warranted due to severity of presentation and/or potential for rapid clinical deterioration.
  - Microbiologic specimens obtained prior to antimicrobial therapy facilitate diagnosis and directed therapy to limit toxicities and improve patient outcome.

THE IMMUNOCOMPROMISED HOST WITH SUSPECTED INFECTION

- Infection risk in immunocompromised host determined by interaction of two factors:
  - Epidemiologic exposures including timing, intensity, and virulence of organisms to which individual is exposed
  - Patient's "net state of immunosuppression"
    - Measure of host factors potentially contributing to infection risk (Table 80.1)
      - Including anatomic defects and exogenous immunosuppression
    - Specific immunosuppressive therapies and deficits predispose to specific types of infection (Table 80.2).

- Consideration of these factors allows development of differential diagnosis.
- Aggressive approach to making microbiologic diagnosis undertaken
  - Delays in appropriate therapy may compromise outcome.
    - Initiate empiric therapy while awaiting results of investigations.
    - Infections often due to organisms with antimicrobial resistance patterns that make selection of empiric therapy more difficult
  - Perform appropriate histologic and microbiologic investigations of fluids and tissues
  - Diagnosis may require special stains:
    - Modified acid-fast stain for *Nocardia*

TABLE 80.1

FACTORS CONTRIBUTING TO THE NET STATE OF IMMUNOSUPPRESSION

IMMUNOSUPPRESSIVE THERAPY
- Type
- Temporal sequence
- Intensity
- Cumulative dose

PRIOR THERAPIES
- Chemotherapy or antimicrobials

MUCOCUTANEOUS BARRIER INTEGRITY
- Surgery
- Catheters
- Lines
- Drains
- Fluid collections

NEUTROPENIA/LYMPHOPENIA
- Often drug induced

UNDERLYING IMMUNE DEFICIENCY
- Hypogammaglobulinemia (e.g., from proteinuria)
- Complement deficiencies
- Autoimmune diseases (e.g., systemic lupus erythematosus)
- Other disease states:
  - HIV
  - Lymphoma/leukemia

METABOLIC CONDITIONS
- Uremia
- Malnutrition
- Diabetes mellitus
- Cirrhosis

IMMUNOMODULATORY VIRAL INFECTIONS
- Cytomegalovirus
- Hepatitis B and C
- Respiratory viruses

TABLE 80.2

INFECTIONS ASSOCIATED WITH SPECIFIC IMMUNE DEFECTS

Defect	Common causes	Associated infections
Granulocytopenia	Leukemia, cytotoxic chemotherapy, AIDS, drug toxicity, Felty syndrome	Enteric gram negatives, *Pseudomonas*, *Staphylococcus aureus*, *Staphylococcus epidermidis*, streptococci, *Aspergillus*, *Candida*, and other fungi
Neutrophil chemotaxis	Diabetes, alcoholism, uremia, Hodgkin disease, trauma (burns), Lazy leukocyte syndrome, connective tissue disease	*S. aureus*, *Candida*, streptococci
Neutrophil killing	Chronic granulomatous disease, myeloperoxidase deficiency	*S. aureus*, *Escherichia coli*, *Candida*, *Aspergillus*, *Torulopsis*
T-cell defects	AIDS, congenital lymphoma, sarcoidosis, viral infection, connective tissue disease, organ transplants, steroids	Intracellular bacteria (*Legionella*, *Listeria*, *Mycobacteria*), herpes simplex virus, varicella-zoster virus, cytomegalovirus, Epstein-Barr virus, parasites (*Strongyloides*, *Toxoplasma*), fungi (*Candida*, *Cryptococcus*) *Pneumocystis carinii (jiroveci)*
B-cell defects	Congenital/acquired agammaglobulinemia, burns, enteropathies, splenic dysfunction, myeloma, acute lymphocytic leukemia	*Streptococcus pneumoniae*, *Haemophilus influenzae*, *Salmonella* and *Campylobacter* spp., *Giardia lamblia*
Splenectomy	Surgery, sickle cell, cirrhosis	*S. pneumoniae*, *H. influenzae*, *Salmonella* spp., *Capnocytophaga*
Complement	Congenital/acquired defects	*S. aureus*, *Neisseria* spp., *H. influenzae*, *S. pneumoniae*
Anatomic	Vascular/Foley catheters, incisions, anastomotic leaks, mucosal ulceration, vascular insufficiency	Colonizing organisms, resistant nosocomial organisms

- ○ Silver stain for *Pneumocystis carinii (jiroveci)*
- ○ Or culture media for *Mycobacteria* species
- ○ Since noninfectious etiologies such as organ rejection, drug toxicity, and GVHD are often in differential diagnosis, histology is integral to making definitive diagnosis.

THE NEUTROPENIC PATIENT

- Neutropenic patients from cytotoxic chemotherapy for hematologic or solid tumors commonly encountered immunocompromised hosts
  - With absolute neutrophil count <500 cells/μL, risk of infection increases.
    - Reduction in absolute neutrophil count impairs innate host immune response of phagocytosis.
    - Predisposing neutropenic patient to array of bacterial and fungal infections
      - ○ Usually from endogenous colonization

Presentation, Common Pathogens, and Infectious Disease Syndromes

- Fever is defined as:
  - Single oral temperature ≥38.3°C (101°F) or
  - A temperature ≥38°C (100.4°F) for ≥1 hour
  - It is often the only predictor of infection.
    - About 50% of neutropenic patients with fever have documented infection.
    - About 20% of those with neutrophil counts <100 cells/μL have bacteremia.

- Gastrointestinal tract including oropharynx and periodontium
- Where chemotherapeutic agents induce mucosal damage
- The most common source of infection in febrile neutropenic patients
- Often difficult to document:
  - Pulmonary infections and bacteremia—especially related to central venous lines (CVLs)—more commonly documented
- Historically, gram-negative (GN) organisms are seen in most bloodstream infections:
  - *Escherichia coli*
  - *Klebsiella* species
  - *Pseudomonas aeruginosa*
- Gram-positive (GP) organisms now isolated in almost 66% of bloodstream infections:
  - *Streptococcus* species and coagulase-negative *Staphylococcus*
- Shift from GN to GP bacteremia related to placement of CVLs
  - Also reduction in risk of GN infections with fluoroquinolone prophylaxis
- Skin, especially CVL sites, and lower respiratory and urinary tracts other common infection sites
- Risk of opportunistic fungal infection increases with the duration and severity of neutropenia.
  - Up to 33% of febrile neutropenic patients failing to respond to 1-week course of empiric antibacterial therapy have systemic fungal infections.
  - Most commonly (>80%) due to *Candida* or *Aspergillus* species

- Epidemiology of invasive fungal infections evolved with growing "at-risk" population and increased use of azole prophylaxis.
  - Over 50% of bloodstream isolates seen are due to non-*albicans Candida*.
    - With increasing intrinsic (*Candida krusei*) or acquired (*Candida glabrata*) fluconazole resistance
  - Neutropenic patients become infected with highly resistant non-*Aspergillus* molds in addition to *Aspergillus*.

Approach to Diagnosis

- Signs and symptoms of inflammation may be minimal or absent in neutropenic host.
- Cutaneous infection often occurs at former sites of intravenous (IV) catheters or drains.
  - May be tender or edematous, without the usual signs of cellulitis
- Urinary tract infection may present without pyuria, often with viral pathogens.
- CXR often normal despite rapidly progressive pneumonia.
  - Up to 50% of neutropenic patients with a normal CXR and fever lasting 2 days, despite empiric antibiotic therapy, will have findings on chest CT suggestive of pneumonia.
- Daily search for subtle signs and symptoms of infection should be performed:
  - Periodontium
  - Oropharynx
  - Perianal
  - Skin
  - Vascular access sites
- Basic investigations include:
  - CBC with differential
  - Serum creatinine, liver enzymes, and liver function tests
  - Cultures of blood, urine, and sputum
  - CXR
    - If CXR is normal but the patient has pulmonary symptoms or no identified source of infection, a CT scan should be performed.
- Collection of additional specimens guided by clinical presentation and preliminary investigations
  - Oral ulcerations should be swabbed for viral (herpes simplex virus [HSV]) studies.
  - Skin lesions should be biopsied for culture and histology.
  - Unexplained pulmonary infiltrates should be assessed with bronchoscopy and bronchoalveolar lavage (BAL), and/or transbronchial biopsy, or open lung biopsy.
- In those recovering from neutropenia with persistent fever:
  - Liver function tests and chest and abdominal imaging performed to look for:
    - Hepatosplenic candidiasis
    - Typhlitis
    - Invasive mold infection
  - Many infections asymptomatic during neutropenic event
    - Becoming apparent with recovery

Management

- Identification of best candidates for empiric therapy and avoiding excessive use of prophylactic antimicrobial agents and toxicities associated with many therapies are central goals

- After obtaining microbiologic studies, empiric antimicrobial therapy indicated in neutropenic patients with or without fever.
- Selection of initial empiric antibiotic regimen takes into consideration:
  - General trend of increasing GP infections
  - Local hospital epidemiology
  - Susceptibility patterns of isolates from neutropenic patients
  - Clinical presentation, epidemiologic exposures, and antimicrobial use history
- Options include monotherapy with:
  - Third- or fourth-generation cephalosporin (e.g., ceftazidime or cefepime)
  - Carbapenem such as imipenem or meropenem
  - Piperacillin-tazobactam
  - Dual therapy may be used without a glycopeptides.
    - Antipseudomonal β-lactam plus aminoglycoside or fluoroquinolone
    - For inpatients with recent surgery or vascular access catheters, a glycopeptides, vancomycin, can be combined with one- or two-drug therapy.
- Empiric addition of vancomycin therapy in febrile neutropenia is not shown to alter outcomes in patients without pulmonary infiltrates, septic shock, CVL or skin and soft tissue infections, or documented GP infections resistant to primary empiric therapy
  - Vancomycin use is associated with the emergence of vancomycin-resistant *Enterococcus*.
- Controversy exists regarding optimal timing of adding antifungal therapy.
- Patients in the ICU >5 to 7 days, hypotensive or otherwise critically ill, anti-*Candida* therapy added after cultures obtained (Table 80.3)
- Those failing to defervesce on empiric antibiotic therapy after 5 to 7 days
  - In whom no source of infection identified
  - High risk of systemic fungal infection, and empiric therapy should be added
    - Amphotericin B the historical gold standard for empiric therapy
    - Lipid products of amphotericin B (e.g., liposomal amphotericin B [AmBisome, Astellas, Deerfield, IL] and amphotericin B lipid complex [Abelcet, Elan, Dublin, Ireland]) have similar efficacy with less toxicity
    - Voriconazole, caspofungin, other echinocandins (e.g., anidulafungin and micafungin), and posaconazole are effective in persistently febrile patients with neutropenia.
    - Renal and hepatic function, potential drug interactions, cost, and suspected source of fungal infection are all considerations in choosing initial empiric antifungal agent.

THE CORTICOSTEROID-TREATED PATIENT

- Treatment with corticosteroids results in:
  - Reduced proliferation of B and T lymphocytes
  - Inhibition of neutrophil adhesion to endothelial cells
  - Inhibition of macrophage differentiation

TABLE 80.3

RISK FACTORS FOR CANDIDEMIA IN THE ICU
SETTING[a]

- Prolonged length of stay (≥10 d)
- Immunosuppression
- High acuity of illness
- Cancer and chemotherapy
- Acute renal failure
- Severe acute pancreatitis
- Hemodialysis
- Surgery (gastrointestinal)
- Broad-spectrum antibiotics
- Transplantation
- Central venous catheter (≥3 d)
- Prematurity/low Apgar/congenital malformations
- Parenteral nutrition
- *Candida* colonization at multiple sites (longer than about 8 d)
- Burns
- Mechanical ventilation
- Diabetes

d, days.
[a]Reviewed in Rex JH, Sobel JD. Prophylactic antifungal therapy in the
intensive care unit. *Clin Infect Dis.* 2001;32(8):1191; and
Ostrosky-Zeichner L, Pappas PG. Invasive candidiasis in the intensive
care unit. *Crit Care Med.* 2006;34(3):857.

- Reduced recruitment of mononuclear cells, including monocytes, into sites of immune inflammation
- Suppress cellular (Th1) immunity and promote humoral (Th2) immunity
- Risk of infection in corticosteroid-treated patients related to dose and duration of therapy
  - Treated with more than 10 to 20 mg/day of prednisone for more than a month at risk for infectious complications
  - Corticosteroids have a broad effect on immune system, but primary immune deficit is cell-mediated immunity.
    ○ Placing host at risk for fungal, viral, protozoal, and intracellular bacterial infections.
    ○ Common pathogens to be considered include:
       – *P. carinii (jiroveci)*
       – *Listeria monocytogenes*
       – *Legionella*
       – *Nocardia* species

Pneumocystis carinii (jiroveci)

- Has a worldwide distribution and is an important cause of pneumonia in immunocompromised patients
- Most notably those with HIV infection
- Also those immunosuppressed due to malnutrition, organ transplantation, and prolonged corticosteroid use
  - Usually at a dose >15 to 20 mg/day
  - Those requiring prolonged steroid therapy are appropriate candidates for prophylaxis with trimethoprim-sulfamethoxazole (TMP–SMX).

Presentation

- Onset of symptoms is often associated with recent dose reduction or discontinuation of steroids and/or with intensification of overall immunosuppressive regimen.

- Generally presents as subacute illness with history of weeks of progressive dyspnea and nonproductive cough in HIV-infected individuals
- But non-HIV immunocompromised patients with *Pneumocystis carinii* pneumonia (PCP) have a more acute presentation.
- PCP patients are generally hypoxemic with few physical or radiographic findings
  - Nonproductive cough, dyspnea, and low-grade fever frequently present.
  - Physical examination findings nonspecific, inspiratory crackles on auscultation, with or without other signs of respiratory distress
  - May progress to respiratory failure requiring intubation and mechanical ventilation.

Diagnosis

- Classic CXR appearance of PCP: bilateral interstitial infiltrates with perihilar predominance
  - Can be highly variable, including patchy airspace disease and small pulmonary nodules
- Elevated lactate dehydrogenase level is a nonspecific finding associated with PCP.
- Definitive diagnosis relies on identification of organism by staining from pulmonary secretions or tissue.
  - Diagnosis may be made by staining secretions obtained through sputum induction with hypertonic saline.
    - 97% negative predictive value
  - If diagnosis remains uncertain, bronchoscopy with transbronchial tissue biopsy is the gold standard for diagnosis of PCP.
    - Yielding better results than BAL
  - Examination done quickly by staining with Gomori methenamine silver or calcofluor white
    - Diagnosis improved with immunofluorescent staining with monoclonal antibodies

Treatment

- Treatment for PCP is outlined in Table 80.4.

Listeria monocytogenes

- A GP bacillus capable of intracellular survival after phagocytosis by macrophages
  - Capable of infecting normal hosts
  - Invasive disease seen predominantly in those with cell-mediated immune deficits due to such factors as extremes of age (neonates and the elderly), pregnancy, malignancy, organ transplantation, or other immunosuppressive therapy

Presentation

- Infection presents as meningitis or primary bacteremia in 80% to 90% of cases.
  - Gastrointestinal symptoms present in a minority of cases.
- Onset of symptoms may be acute or subacute.
  - Fever nearly universal
  - Central nervous system (CNS) involvement may present as meningitis with headache and neck stiffness, focal parenchymal involvement with cerebritis and/or abscess, or meningoencephalitis with impaired level of consciousness.

TABLE 80.4

TREATMENT MODALITIES FOR THE COMMONEST INFECTIONS

Infectious agent	Primary therapy	Secondary therapy	Other considerations
Pneumocystis jiroveci (PCP)	Trimethoprim-sulfamethoxazole (TMP–SMX), dosed as 15–20 mg/kg/d of TMP component, divided every 6–8 h × 21 days	• Atovaquone 750–1,500 mg orally bid • Pentamidine 4 mg/kg/d, to max of 300 mg • Dapsone 100 mg orally plus TMP as above • Clindamycin 600 mg IV every 6 h plus primaquine 15–30 mg/d (as base)	Adjunctive use of corticosteroids common but not evidence based in non-HIV patients
Listeria monocytogenes	***Empiric or confirmed:*** Ampicillin 2 g IV every 4 h × 21 d or more ***For synergy:*** Ampicillin plus TMP–SMX 20 mg/kg/d divided every 6 h	Ampicillin plus gentamicin 2 mg/kg IV load, then 1.7 mg/kg IV every 8 h	
Legionella pneumophila and other species	Levofloxacin 250–750 mg IV every 24 h × 7–14 d	Azithromycin 500 mg daily for 7–14 d	
Nocardia asteroides complex	TMP–SMX, dosed as 15 mg/kg/d of TMP component, divided every 6–12 h, PO or IV	• Imipenem 500 mg IV every 6 h plus amikacin 7.5 mg/kg IV every 12 h, both × 3–4 wk, then switch to PO regimen • Linezolid 300–600 mg orally bid × 3–24 mo	• Surgical resection of necrotic material often necessary • Therapy duration is 6–12 mo; for central nervous system infection 9–12 mo

Diagnosis

- Generally made through culture of blood or cerebrospinal fluid (CSF)
- Approximately 75% of cases of CNS listeriosis are associated with bacteremia.
  - Positive blood culture for *Listeria* should prompt a CSF examination.
  - CSF parameters are variable.
    - Common presentation is pleocytosis with neutrophil predominance, elevated protein, and normal glucose
    - Gram stain is frequently negative.

Treatment

- See Table 80.4.
- In patients at risk for *Listeria* presenting with meningitis of uncertain etiology
- Empiric therapy should include ampicillin, 2 g IV every 4 hours initially.
- If confirmed, ampicillin is the drug of choice.
- *In vitro* data suggest bactericidal synergy of combination of ampicillin and gentamicin.
  - Also demonstrated between ampicillin and TMP–SMX
  - This combination is superior to ampicillin and gentamicin in treatment of *Listeria* meningoencephalitis.
  - May be indicated in those with severe disease
  - Minimum duration of therapy recommended is 3 weeks.
    - May be extended based on clinical response and radiographic resolution of CNS parenchymal disease if present

Legionella

- Small GN bacilli widely distributed in aqueous environment
  - Both community and hospital outbreaks have occurred in association with contaminated water sources such as air conditioners, cooling towers, and whirlpools
- Capable of causing disease in normal hosts
  - Patients with impaired cell-mediated immunity are at highest risk.

Presentation

- Most commonly presents as pneumonia
  - Extrapulmonary disease and a self-limited febrile illness, *Pontiac fever,* may occur.
  - Physical and laboratory findings and radiographic appearance are not specific.
  - Fever with pulse-temperature dissociation, diarrhea, hyponatremia, and elevated liver enzymes may occur, but are not distinctive enough.
  - In patients at risk, must be considered in differential diagnosis of pneumonia
    - Empiric therapy administered when appropriate

Diagnosis

- A fastidious organism
  - Culture of respiratory secretions for diagnosis is insensitive and time-consuming.
  - Immunofluorescent microscopy improves sensitivity of culture techniques.

- More rapid diagnosis with urinary antigen test and nucleic acid detection
- Urinary antigen tests sensitive for *Legionella pneumophila* serogroup 1
  - Perform less well in other serogroups of *L. pneumophila*, or other *Legionella* species
- Combination culture, urinary antigen detection, and serology may optimize diagnosis.

Treatment

- See Table 80.4.
- Macrolides and fluoroquinolones have *in vitro* activity against *Legionella* sp.
  - Quinolones may be superior to macrolides.
    - Fewer complications and shorter hospital stays in those receiving quinolones
    - No comparison of newer macrolides (e.g., azithromycin) to new quinolones

Nocardia

- Part of aerobic actinomycetes genus, ubiquitous environmental saprophytes
- There are several species
  - *Nocardia asteroides* complex—*Nocardia asteroides senso strictu*, *Nocardia farcinica*, and *Nocardia nova*—most common cause of disease
- Immunosuppression the major risk factor for nocardial infections
  - Solid organ transplant recipients, advanced HIV patients (CD4$^+$ counts <100 cells/μL), patients with lymphoreticular malignancy, patients on chronic corticosteroid therapy

Presentation

- Predominantly causes pneumonia
  - Initial presentation includes respiratory symptoms generally in association with fever
  - CXR demonstrates nodular lesions, may progress to cavitation
    - Diffuse infiltrates or consolidation may also occur
- Has high propensity to disseminate to CNS
  - Immunocompromised patients with nocardiosis may present with CNS symptoms.
    - With or without concomitant pulmonary symptoms
- Usual route of infection is inhalational.
  - Direct cutaneous inoculation with resultant skin disease, subcutaneous nodules, seen

Diagnosis

- Definitive diagnosis with special stain and culture from suspected site of infection
  - Modified acid-fast stain (Kinyoun) demonstrates branching and beading GP bacilli.
  - Grows on nonselective media; lab should be notified if diagnosis suspected.
    - Selective media can be used to avoid overgrowth by other organisms.
    - When diagnosis of pulmonary nocardiosis made, neuroimaging to exclude CNS dissemination is performed.

Treatment

- See Table 80.4.
- Antimicrobial therapy the foundation of treatment, although adjunctive surgical resection of necrotic tissue necessary on occasion
- Duration of therapy individualized based on clinical response.
  - Pulmonary and cutaneous disease is treated for at least 6 to 12 months.
  - CNS disease is treated for at least 9 to 12 months.
  - Immunosuppression is reduced as much as possible to aid in treatment.

PATIENTS TREATED WITH IMMUNOMODULATORY AGENTS

- A number of monoclonal antibody therapies have revolutionized treatment of rheumatologic as well as other systemic inflammatory and autoimmune conditions (Table 80.5).
- Immune modulation results in selected immune deficits, and infectious complications have been recognized with several of these agents.

Tumor Necrosis Factor–α Antagonists

- Three tumor necrosis factor (TNF)–α antagonists are currently marketed in the United States:
  - Infliximab (Remicade, Centocor Inc., Horsham, PA)
  - Etanercept (Enbrel, Amgen and Wyeth Pharmaceuticals, Thousand Oaks, CA)
  - Adalimumab (Humira, Abbott Laboratories, Abbott Park, IL)
  - Effective for rheumatoid arthritis, active Crohn disease, and ankylosing spondylitis

TABLE 80.5

SELECTED THERAPEUTIC ANTIBODIES

Antibody	Trade name	Target	Indication
Antithymocyte globulin	Thymoglobulin (others)	T cells (polyclonal rabbit IgG)	Transplant induction, rejection
Muromonab OKT3	Orthoclone OKT3	CD3$^+$	Transplant induction, rejection
Alemtuzumab	Campath-1H	CD52$^+$	B-cell chronic lymphoid leukemia
Daclizumab	Zenapax	Interleukin (IL)-2 receptor a chain (CD25$^+$)	Transplant induction
Basiliximab	Simulect	IL-2 receptor a chain (CD25$^+$)	Transplant induction
Efalizumab	Raptiva	CD11a$^+$	Psoriasis
Natalizumab	Tysabri	α_4-integrin	Multiple sclerosis, Crohn disease

- Blockade of TNF-α results in improvement in systemic inflammatory conditions.
  - However, TNF-α, and interferon-γ and other cytokines are an important component in maintaining cellular immunity.
- Tuberculosis (TB) associated with TNF-α antagonists
  - Probably resultant from cell-mediated immune deficits
  - Majority of cases occurred with infliximab
  - Cases also described with etanercept and adalimumab
  - Occurred in those with risk factors for latent TB infection
    - TB skin testing is recommended prior to initiation of a TNF-α antagonist.
    - Regardless of TB skin testing results, TB in differential diagnosis in patient presenting on TNF-α antagonist with compatible symptoms
  - Other infections including histoplasmosis, listeriosis, aspergillosis, coccidiomycosis, and candidiasis associated with use of TNF-α antagonists

Rituximab

- Rituxan (Genentech Inc., San Francisco, CA; and Biogen Idec, Boston, MA) a chimeric murine/human monoclonal antibody
- Binds CD20$^+$ marker, expressed on B lymphocytes
- Results in rapid depletion of circulating CD20$^+$ B cells
- Approved for treatment of CD20$^+$ B-cell lymphoma
- In combination with methotrexate for rheumatoid arthritis
- Used for treatment of posttransplant lymphoproliferative disease, idiopathic thrombocytopenia (ITP), autoimmune hemolytic anemia, systemic lupus erythematosus, multiple sclerosis, GVHD, treatment of antibody-mediated graft rejection
- Following rituximab therapy, antibody production is maintained by plasma cells.
  - CD20$^-$
- Peripheral B-cell recovery takes 3 to 12 months.
- Despite B-cell deficiency and use of rituximab for treatment of malignant and autoimmune conditions
  - No evidence of an increased risk of infection in patients treated

Natalizumab

- Tysabri (Biogen Idec, Boston, MA, and Elan Pharmaceuticals, Dublin, Ireland) a recombinant humanized monoclonal antibody that binds to α_4-integrin
  - Inhibiting α_4-integrin–mediated leukocyte adhesion
  - Prevents transmigration of leukocytes across the endothelium into inflamed tissue
- Monotherapy for treatment of patients with relapsing multiple sclerosis and in those with inadequate response to, or who are unable to tolerate, alternate therapies
  - Increases remission rate and improves quality of life in patients with active Crohn disease
- Progressive multifocal leukoencephalopathy
  - Demyelinating disease of CNS caused by human polyomavirus John Cunningham virus
  - Reported in three patients who received natalizumab
  - U.S. FDA-approved application for resumed marketing in June of 2006

- Given mechanism of action, it is possible that further opportunistic infections may be associated with the use of this agent.

THE SOLID ORGAN TRANSPLANT RECIPIENT

Timeline of Posttransplant Infections

- Three overlapping periods of risk for infection after transplantation, each most often associated with unique groups of pathogens:
  - Perioperative period to approximately 4 weeks after transplantation, reflecting surgical and technical complications
  - Period 1 to 6 months after transplantation, depending on the rapidity of tapering immunosuppression and the use of antilymphocyte "induction" therapy, reflecting intensive immunosuppression with viral activation and opportunistic infections
  - Period beyond 6 to 12 months after transplantation, reflecting community-acquired exposures and some unusual pathogens based on the level of maintenance immunosuppression
- First month after transplantation
  - Infections related to surgery, similar to those in complex general surgical population
    - Include pneumonia and surgical site, urinary tract, and CVL–associated infections caused by typical bacterial and fungal pathogens such as *Candida*
    - Exposure to nosocomial pathogens and colonization alter use of empiric antimicrobial therapy, including those for:
      - Methicillin-resistant *S. aureus* (MRSA)
      - Vancomycin-resistant *Enterococcus*
      - Fluconazole-resistant *Candida* species
      - *Clostridium difficile*
      - *P. aeruginosa*
  - Opportunistic infections rarely occur the first month posttransplant unless there has been pretransplant immunosuppression.
    - Absent prophylaxis 24% to 34% of recipients will have HSV disease
      - Most occurring as orolabial or genital disease due to reactivation of latent infection in the recipient during first posttransplant month
    - Rarely, infections are transmitted from bacteremic or fungemic donor with potentially serious complications.
      - Including seeding of vascular suture line
      - Use of prophylactic antibiotics in recipient, directed by donor culture results, allows organs from donors with bacteremia and/or meningitis to be safely used without compromising transplant outcomes.
- First through sixth month posttransplant are the highest-risk period for opportunistic infections.
  - Effects of immunosuppression greatest during this period
  - Infections may include:
    - Viral (cytomegalovirus [CMV], varicella-zoster virus [VZV], Epstein-Barr virus [EBV], and hepatitis B)
    - Bacterial (*Nocardia, Listeria,* and TB)
    - Fungal (*Aspergillus* and *Cryptococcus*)

- Parasitic (*Pneumocystis, Toxoplasma* and *Strongyloides*) infections
- Beyond 6 months, most recipients are on reduced levels of maintenance immunosuppression with good graft function and are at low risk for opportunistic infections.
  - Most infectious complications here due to conventional community-acquired pathogens occurring in the general population.
  - These include:
    - Viral respiratory infections
    - Pneumococcal pneumonia
    - Gastroenteritis
  - Intense exposure to opportunistic pathogen may result in disease
    - Transplant recipients should be counseled regarding strategies to avoid high-risk exposures
    - If augmentation of immunosuppression needed for management of acute chronic rejection, and for those with chronic or recurrent CMV infection, increased risk for other opportunistic infections, particularly:
      ○ *P. carinii* (*jiroveci*)
      ○ Invasive fungal infection
      ○ EBV-associated, posttransplant lymphoproliferative disease

Disease-specific Prevention and Management

Cytomegalovirus
- Remains significant cause of morbidity in organ transplant recipients
  - Strategies for prevention have decreased the morbidity and mortality.
  - Risk of CMV disease depends on a number of factors, including:
    - Donor and recipient serostatus
    - Immunosuppression
      ○ Particularly the use of antilymphocyte antibody preparations for induction or treatment of rejection
- The American Society of Transplantation Guidelines on CMV prevention and management are used to guide institutional approaches to CMV prevention in conjunction with local CMV epidemiology, available laboratory support, and infrastructure.
- If both donor and recipient are CMV negative:
  - Antiherpes virus prophylaxis (for HSV and VZV) are generally used for the first 3 to 12 months posttransplantation.
  - 5% to 10% of such patients may develop community-acquired CMV at some point after transplant
- CMV-seronegative recipients who receive seropositive organ are at greatest risk of primary CMV infection.
  - Receive prophylaxis with valganciclovir (900 mg/day) for 100 days
- CMV-seropositive recipients receive either prophylaxis with valganciclovir or preemptive therapy based on results of sensitive monitoring assay (e.g., CMV antigenemia or polymerase chain reaction [PCR]) used.
- Given the high risk of CMV infection and disease in seropositive lung and heart–lung recipients, prophylaxis is generally preferred.
- All patients are at risk for CMV receiving lymphocyte-depleting agents for induction or treatment of rejection should receive antiviral prophylaxis.

- CMV disease refers to the presence of symptoms attributable to CMV in face of viral replication:
  - "CMV syndrome"
    - Defined by constellation of fever >38°C, neutropenia or thrombocytopenia, and detection of CMV in blood by antigenemia, PCR, or shell vial culture
  - Tissue-invasive disease
    - Requires biopsy for confirmation, except in case of retinitis
    - Defined by presence of signs or symptoms of organ dysfunction in association with histologic evidence of CMV in affected tissue
- Established CMV syndrome or tissue-invasive disease treated with:
  - IV ganciclovir, 5 mg/kg every 12 hours
    - No data to support oral ganciclovir/valganciclovir use in treatment of CMV disease
  - Therapy continued a minimum of 14 days until symptoms resolved and viremia cleared (until CMV PCR/antigenemia undetectable)
  - Ganciclovir-resistant CMV an emerging problem; risk factors include:
    - Donor–recipient mismatch, donor is seropositive and recipient seronegative
    - Prolonged use of ganciclovir
    - Suboptimal ganciclovir levels
    - Intense immunosuppression
    - High CMV viral load
  - Ganciclovir-resistant CMV suspected in setting of:
    - Stable, or rising, viral load in patients treated with ganciclovir
    - No decrease in antigenemia after 7 days of therapy
    - Lack of clinical improvement after 14 days of full-dose IV ganciclovir
    - CMV infection developing shortly after prolonged course of low-dose ganciclovir
    - If resistance suspected, ID/microbiology consulted for consideration of molecular resistance testing and alternative (e.g., foscarnet, cidofovir) or adjunctive (CMV-Ig) therapies

Epstein-Barr Virus and Posttransplant Lymphoproliferative Disease
- Primary EBV infection after transplantation is the most important risk factor for posttransplant lymphoproliferative Disease (PTLD).
  - Complications with mortality ranging as high as 40% to 60%.
  - Risk exacerbated by occurrence of CMV disease and treatment with polyclonal or monoclonal antilymphocyte antibody.
  - Some benefit of antiviral prophylaxis.
  - Quantitative EBV viral load monitoring shown to decrease the risk of PTLD.
- For patients at high risk of PTLD (EBV donor seropositive/recipient seronegative)
  - Preventative strategies with antiviral prophylaxis
  - EBV viral load monitoring may be considered
  - If EBV viremia is detected, immunosuppression reduction is considered.
- PTLD represents highly diverse spectrum of disease with variable clinical presentation:
  - Benign B-cell proliferation (mononucleosis)

- To true monoclonal malignancy
  - May be nodal or extranodal and localized or disseminated, and commonly involves allograft
  - Diagnosis of PTLD requires histologic confirmation and staging of disease.
- Options for treatment of PTLD depend on histology and stage of disease.
  - In all cases, attempts are made to reduce or withdraw immunosuppression.
  - Additional considerations for treatment depend on clinical presentation and previously mentioned criteria
  - In addition to immunosuppression reduction or withdrawal, potential options include:
    - Antiviral agents
    - IVIG
    - Surgical resection
    - Local radiation
    - Use of rituximab, anti-CD20 monoclonal antibody, a second-line option if reduction in immunosuppression alone fails given its low toxicity and response rates, which range from 61% to 76%.
    - Cytotoxic chemotherapy is generally considered third-line option due to high incidence of toxicity in this population.

Pneumocystis carinii (jiroveci)
- Absent prophylaxis, *P. pneumoniae* occurs in 5% to 15% of solid organ transplant recipients.
  - TMP–SMX prophylaxis, one single-strength tablet daily, eliminates risk.
    - Indicated in all nonallergic transplant recipients for minimum of 6 months following transplantation
    - Also acts as prophylaxis for a number of other infections:
      - *Nocardia*
      - *Listeria*
      - Community-acquired pneumonia
- In sulfa-allergic patients, dapsone 100 mg daily, aerosolized pentamidine 300 mg monthly, or atovaquone 1,500 mg daily are alternatives.

Toxoplasmosis
- Of particular concern among cardiac transplant recipients given the site of latency is cardiac muscle
  - Seronegative recipients of a seropositive heart are at risk and require prophylaxis.
  - TMP–SMX is used effectively for prophylaxis as one double-strength tablet daily.
    - Lifelong prophylaxis is recommended.

Diagnosis and Treatment of Infectious Syndromes
- Initial approach to transplant patient with suspected infection includes:
  - Thorough history and physical examination to assess overall state of immune function and exposure history and localize potential site of infection
  - Basic testing includes CBC, creatinine, liver enzyme and function studies, blood cultures, and CXR.
  - Additional specimens for microbiologic testing are obtained as directed by history and physical examination (e.g., urine cultures, stool for bacterial culture, *Clostridium difficile* toxin, ova and parasites, blood for CMV antigenemia, or PCR).

TABLE 80.6

DIFFERENTIAL DIAGNOSIS OF FEVER AND PULMONARY INFILTRATE IN ORGAN TRANSPLANT RECIPIENTS

Chest radiograph finding	Acute onset	Subacute/chronic onset
Consolidation	Bacteria	Fungal
	Pulmonary embolism	*Nocardia*
	Hemorrhage	Tuberculosis
	Pulmonary edema	Viral (adenovirus)
Reticulonodular	Pulmonary edema	*Pneumocystis carinii (jiroveci)*
	Viral	Drug reaction (including sirolimus)
	P. carinii (jiroveci)	
	Bacterial	Viral
Nodular	Bacterial	Fungal
		Nocardia
		Tuberculosis
		Tumor (including PTLD)

PTLD, posttransplant lymphoproliferative disease.

Fever and Pulmonary Infiltrate
- Transplant patients presenting with fever and pulmonary infiltrate, differential diagnosis broad
  - Includes infectious and noninfectious etiologies
  - Infection is ultimately identified in 75% to 90% of cases.
  - Dual or sequential infections are common.
- Pneumonia may rapidly progress in immunocompromised hosts with high mortality
  - Initial empiric therapy is directed at likely pathogens following collection of blood and sputum cultures, viral respiratory studies, a complete blood count, and serum creatinine.
  - Consultation with pulmonary and infectious diseases specialists is recommended.
  - Identification of pathogen is key to directing appropriate therapy
    - Consider early invasive diagnostic tests (bronchoscopy, lung biopsy).
  - CXR, clinical presentation, rate of progression, exposure history, and assessment of net state of immunosuppression help narrow differential diagnosis (Table 80.6).
  - Chest CT will delineate extent of pulmonary disease and guide invasive diagnostic tests.

CNS Infections
- Presentation of CNS infection in transplant patients may differ from general population due to immunosuppression.
  - Fever may or may not be present, and presentation can be subtle.
    - Headache or minor changes in mental status
  - Differential diagnosis in transplant patients presenting with neurologic symptoms with or without fever (Table 80.7)

TABLE 80.7

COMMON CNS INFECTIONS IN TRANSPLANT
RECIPIENTS

Community-Acquired Pathogens
- Pneumococcus
- Meningococcus
- *Listeria monocytogenes*
- Herpes simplex virus
- *Cryptococcus neoformans*
- Lyme disease

Metastatic Infection
- Bacteremia (endocarditis)
- *Mycobacterium tuberculosis*
- *Aspergillus*
- *Nocardia* species
- *Strongyloides stercoralis* (gram-negative meningitis)
- Mucoraceae (sinuses)
- Dematiaceae—cerebral phaeohyphomycosis (skin)
- *Histoplasma* and *Pseudoallescheria/Scedosporium,
  Fusarium*

Other CNS Processes
- Cytomegalovirus (nodular angiitis)
- Varicella – zoster virus
- Human herpesvirus 6
- *Toxoplasma gondii*
- JC virus (progressive multifocal leukoencephalopathy)
- West Nile virus, lymphocytic choriomeningitis virus
- Lymphoma (PTLD)
- *Naegleria/Acanthamoeba*

- Consultation with ID/microbiology is recommended to assist in diagnosis and to ensure appropriate samples collected for diagnostic testing
- CSF analysis after neuroimaging with CT and/or MRI should be obtained in such individuals

HEMATOPOIETIC STEM CELL TRANSPLANT RECIPIENT

- Despite advances, severe infectious complications are common.
  - Up to 40% of hematopoietic stem cell transplant (HSCT) recipients requiring ICU admission
  - 60% of these require mechanical ventilation.
    - Associated with high mortality rate
  - Outcomes of HSCT recipients admitted to the ICU are improving with advances in infection prevention, diagnosis and management, and ICU care.
- In attempt to eliminate malignant cells and decrease risk of GVHD, positively selected CD34$^+$ progenitor cells may be used for transplantation.
  - Results in significant T-lymphocyte and monocyte depletion of graft
  - Increased risk of opportunistic infection
- Resultant from pretransplant conditioning chemotherapy, with or without total body irradiation, humoral- and cell-mediated immunity are diminished.
  - Natural host barrier defenses are impaired by mucositis and use of CVLs.

- Risk of infectious complications in HSCT recipient divided into three phases:
  - Period from conditioning therapy to engraftment when patients are neutropenic—the pre-engraftment phase—carries high risk of bacterial and fungal infections.
  - Second phase, from engraftment to day 100—or during period of treatment for acute GVHD—viral and filamentous fungal infections predominate.
  - Beyond day 100—late phase or with chronic GVHD—incidence of infections is reduced.
    - Determined by level of immunosuppression needed for chronic GVHD

Phase 1: Pre-engraftment Infections

- Early pre-engraftment, neutropenic phase lasts 10 to 15 days in most current nonmyeloablative HSCT patients, and longer with ablative regimens
- Predominant infections seen to time of engraftment similar to those in association with neutropenia
  - Shift from predominantly GN to GP—coagulase-negative *Staphylococci, Streptococci, Enterococci*—bacterial infections with use of fluoroquinolone prophylaxis
- Azole prophylaxis has reduced incidence of candidemia.
  - But continues to be early cause of bloodstream infection with increase in risk of azole-resistant *Candida*
  - HSV may reactivate during this phase.
    - Prevented with prophylactic acyclovir in seropositive HSCT recipients

Phase 2: Engraftment to Day 100 (Acute GVHD)

- Characterized by deficits in cellular immunity
  - Most important infectious complications are viral, particularly CMV, and invasive mold infections.
  - Most common manifestations of CMV disease in HSCT recipients are pneumonia and gastrointestinal disease
  - Highest risk of disease occurs in seropositive recipients of seronegative transplants
  - CD34$^+$ selected PBSC transplantation associated with increased risk of CMV infection due to T-lymphocyte depletion
  - Use of ganciclovir prophylaxis or preemptive therapy resulted in decreased risk of CMV infection during this period.
    - Most infections now occurring after ganciclovir are discontinued.
- Interstitial pneumonitis, an important clinical syndrome, presents during the postengraftment phase.
  - Etiologies include CMV, respiratory viruses, *Pneumocystis*, or idiopathic pneumonia syndrome.
  - Diagnosis of CMV pneumonitis requires histology for definitive diagnosis.
    - Often impractical, and presumptive diagnosis made on basis of presence of interstitial pneumonia, detection of CMV antigen/nucleic acid in peripheral blood and/or respiratory secretions, combined with negative investigations for other etiologies of pneumonitis

- Despite treatment with IV ganciclovir and CMV hyperimmunoglobulin or IVIG, mortality from CMV pneumonitis remains ≥50%.
- *P. carinii (jiroveci)* essentially eliminated as cause of pneumonitis with TMP–SMX prophylaxis.
- Respiratory viral infections such as RSV, parainfluenza virus, and human metapneumovirus are increasingly recognized as etiology of pneumonia in HSCT.
- Noninfectious etiologies of pneumonia also exist, including idiopathic pneumonia syndrome and diffuse alveolar hemorrhage, which must also be considered in differential diagnosis of HSCT recipients with pneumonitis.
- Majority of invasive mold infections occur during the postengraftment phase and are associated with treatment of acute GVHD.
  - *Aspergillus* the is predominant pathogen.
  - Non-*Aspergillus* molds, including Zygomycetes, are emerging pathogens.
  - Present as pulmonary nodules, but invasive sinus disease and disseminated disease including CNS involvement also common
  - Given high mortality associated with invasive mold infections, empiric antifungal therapy is initiated while definitive diagnosis is aggressively pursued.
    - Empiric liposomal amphotericin is preferred to voriconazole in HSCT patients with fever or pulmonary infiltrates.
    - It has the broadest spectrum of activity.
    - Treatment of choice for documented invasive aspergillosis is voriconazole.
      - Has survival benefit over amphotericin B deoxycholate therapy and is associated with less toxicity, particularly nephrotoxicity
      - Despite appropriate therapy, mortality of invasive mold infections remains high.
        - In those with disseminated or CNS disease, mortality reaches 80% to 100%.
        - Newer antifungal agents, such as posaconazole, and combination therapies are not fully studied for therapy.

Phase 3: Late Infections beyond 100 Days

- Beyond 100 days posttransplant, a gradual recovery of humoral and cellular immune function occurs.
- Infection risk is driven by extra immunosuppression induced by chronic GVHD and treatment.
  - Up to 40% of HSCT recipients develop varicella–zoster virus infection.
    - Generally as result of reactivation of latent infection
    - Most cases occurring during first year
    - Disseminated disease associated with high mortality rate
    - Should be treated with IV acyclovir, 10 mg/kg every 8 hours
  - Late CMV disease occurs and is associated with history of early CMV disease and GVHD.
    - Late CMV disease is treated same as that occurring early.
    - Outcome of late disease is poor, particularly for CMV pneumonia.
  - Late invasive mold infections occur, particularly in GVHD and preceding viral (CMV) infection.
    - Management of late mold infections mimics that of early infections.
      - Attempt to decrease immunosuppression to assist in treatment of infection.
- About 33% of patients with chronic GVHD may develop recurrent infection with encapsulated bacteria (sinopulmonary, bacteremia).
  - Predominant pathogen is *Streptococcus pneumoniae*.
  - *Haemophilus influenzae* and *S. aureus* are also common.
  - Risk is related to deficit in opsonizing antibody.
  - HSCT recipients respond poorly to pneumococcal vaccine within the first 1 to 2 years posttransplant.
    - Antibiotic prophylaxis with penicillin or TMP–SMX is recommended in those with chronic GVHD.
    - In patients with chronic GVHD admitted with sepsis, broad-spectrum empiric antibiotic therapy is recommended pending microbiologic identification.

CHAPTER 81 ■ HUMAN IMMUNODEFICIENCY VIRUS IN THE ICU

EPIDEMIOLOGY OF HIV-INFECTED PATIENTS IN THE ICU

ICU Admission Rates and Outcomes

- The first cases of HIV/AIDS were reported in 1981.
- Many developments in HIV treatment and associated diseases
  - Most notably introduction of HAART in 1996

- ICU admission rates/-related mortality for HIV-infected patients have shifted multiply during AIDS epidemic.
  - Analysis of ICU admissions during early 1980s reported mortality rates of nearly 70% for HIV-infected patients, with most patients admitted for *Pneumocystis carinii* pneumonia (PCP).
  - Despite increasing hospital admissions of HIV-infected patients after 1984, rates of ICU admission declined.

TABLE 81.1

MORTALITY ASSOCIATED WITH ICU ADMISSION AMONG HIV-INFECTED PATIENTS IN THE HAART ERA

Setting	ICU patients (N)	Time period	HIV unknown at admission	HAART at admission	HIV or AIDS-related illness	Overall ICU mortality	Independent predictors of ICU or in-hospital mortality[a]
University hospital, Jacksonville, FL, USA	141	1995–1999	—	—	—	30%[b]	Transfer from another hospital ward, APACHE II score
University hospital, Paris, France	230	1997–1999	40%	28%	37%	20%	SAPS II score, mechanical ventilation, Omega score
University hospital, Paris, France	236	1998–2000	28%	50%	50%	25%	PCP with pneumothorax; mechanical ventilation; Kaposi sarcoma; inotropic support; $CD4^+$ count <50 cells; SAPS II score
Urban hospital, New York, NY, USA	259	1997–1999	—	48%	60%	30%	Mechanical ventilation; admission with HIV-related illness
Urban hospital, New York, NY, USA	53	2001	—	52%	33%	29%[b]	No multivariate analysis provided; low albumin associated with increased mortality on univariate analysis
Urban hospital, San Francisco, CA, USA	295	1996–1999	7%	25%	37%	29%[b]	Mechanical ventilation; PCP; APACHE II scores >13; albumin <2.6 g/dL; AIDS-associated diagnosis
Hospital Virgen de la Victoria, Malaga, Spain	49	1997–2003	31%	31%	61%	57%	Not reported

ICU, intensive care unit; HIV, human immunodeficiency virus; HAART, highly active antiretroviral therapy; AIDS, acquired immunodeficiency syndrome; APACHE, Acute Physiology and Chronic Health Evaluation; SAPS, Simplified Acute Physiology Score; PCP, *Pneumocystis* pneumonia.
[a]In order of descending magnitude of association.
[b]Data given as in-hospital rather than ICU mortality.

- Likely result of both physicians' and patients' views of ICU care as futile
- In the late 1980s, mortality rates decreased coincident with introduction of adjunctive corticosteroids to treat PCP.
- In the early 1990s, ICU mortality increased in setting of increased rates of ICU use, possibly because of renewed optimism in outcomes.
- Data from immediate pre-HAART period of 1992 through 1995 showed overall improvement in mortality rate to 37% compared to early days of AIDS epidemic.
- In studies from San Francisco General Hospital, ICU mortality decreased significantly from 37% in 1992 through 1995 to 29% in 1996 through 1999.
- Likewise, studies comparing the mortality rate between 1991 and 1992 and 2001 from Beth Israel Medical Center in New York showed a decrease in mortality from 51% to 29%.
  - Analyses of ICU admissions in a Paris hospital found ICU mortality was unchanged comparing before and during the HAART era.
- Overall average reported in-hospital mortality for HIV-infected patients admitted to the ICU ranged between 25%

and 40%, with median ICU length of stay of 5 to 11 days (Table 81.1).
- Despite decreasing hospitalization rates for HIV-infected patients, ICU admission rates have not changed substantially in the HAART era.
- Approximately 5% to 12% of hospital admissions for HIV-infected patients involve ICU care.
  - A large proportion of HIV-infected patients continue to be admitted to the ICU without prior known HIV infection (range 28% to 40%)
  - Approximately 50% of patients are not on HAART at the time of admission.
- Overall survival has improved in HIV-infected patients on HAART.
  - Number of persons living with HIV has increased.

Indications for ICU Admission

- Spectrum of diseases requiring ICU admission is changing in setting of HAART.

- Early in the epidemic, most patients were admitted with AIDS-associated condition, usually PCP.
- Now HIV patients are admitted with a non–AIDS-associated condition.
  - Non–HIV-related disease increased substantially from 12% of all admissions in 1991 through 1992 to 67% in 2001.
- Acute respiratory failure (ARF) is the most common indication for ICU care.
  - Accounts for approximately 25% to 50% of ICU admissions in HIV-infected patients
  - *Pneumocystis jiroveci* is the responsible pathogen in 25% to 50% of patients in earlier investigations.
    - Remains significant cause of respiratory failure in recent studies, accounting for 14% to nearly 50% of cases
  - Bacterial pneumonia is a frequent ARF cause and is as common as or more common than PCP.
- Sepsis is an increasingly frequent indication for ICU admission.
  - Increasing from 3% to 23% of admissions for HIV-infected patients recently
- Other commonly reported causes of ICU admission include:
  - Central nervous system dysfunction (11% to 27%)
  - Gastrointestinal bleeding (6% to 15%)
  - Cardiovascular disease (8% to 13%)
  - Other reasons for ICU admission unrelated to immunodeficiency include:
    - Trauma, routine postoperative care, noninfectious pulmonary diseases such as asthma and pulmonary embolism, renal failure, metabolic disturbances, and drug overdose
    - Given frequent coinfection with hepatitis C among patients with HIV, liver disease may be increasing as a cause of death.
    - Solid organ transplantation (liver, kidney) is currently being studied in HIV-infected patients.

Predictors of Mortality during ICU Admission

- Mortality in the ICU is related to reason for ICU admission.
  - Highest ICU mortality rates for HIV-infected patients are associated with sepsis and respiratory failure.
  - Mortality rates of 50% to 68% reported for sepsis
  - Respiratory failure due to PCP mortality remains nearly 50%.
    - Increased if complicated by PCP-associated pneumothorax
  - AIDS patients admitted to the ICU for other HIV-related reasons reported lower mortality.
    - Reported mortality for central nervous system dysfunction is 20% to 48%.
    - For gastrointestinal disease, 30% to 35%
- Patients admitted with non–HIV-related conditions may have better outcomes.
  - Patients admitted with non–AIDS-associated diagnosis are significantly more likely to survive than patients admitted with an AIDS-associated condition (odds ratio [OR] 2.9, 95% confidence interval [CI] 1.5–5.8, $p = 0.002$).
- Mortality during hospitalization is related to severity of acute illness (see Table 81.1).

- Predictors of increased hospital mortality include:
  - Need for mechanical ventilation
  - Disease severity (as assessed by scoring systems such as the Simplified Acute Physiology Score I [SAPS I], and the Acute Physiology and Chronic Health Evaluation II [APACHE II] score)
  - Decreased serum albumin level or history of weight loss
  - CD4+ T-cell count and the plasma HIV RNA level are generally not independent predictors of short-term mortality during ICU stay.
    - Long-term mortality after ICU admission is related to underlying severity of HIV disease.
    - Long-term survival following ICU discharge improved in HAART era.

PULMONARY MANIFESTATIONS OF HIV

Spectrum of Respiratory Diseases and Approach to Diagnosis

- ARF is still most common cause of ICU admission for HIV-infected patients.
  - Can occur from a multitude of causes including:
    - Infections
    - Neoplasms
    - Drug overdose
    - Neurologic conditions that may be both HIV- and non–HIV-related
  - Appropriate workup includes chest radiograph and occasionally computed tomography of the chest. Blood and sputum cultures should be obtained.
  - Bronchoscopy with BAL strongly considered for definitive diagnosis.
  - Biopsy of other sites such as lymph nodes or bone marrow can be useful.
  - Diagnoses such as pulmonary embolism, asthma, chronic obstructive pulmonary disease, and cardiogenic pulmonary edema also present with respiratory failure, and appropriate testing should be performed.

Pneumocystis carinii Pneumonia

- PCP is historically the most common cause of respiratory failure in AIDS patients.
  - **Treatment and Corticosteroids:** Duration of PCP treatment is 21 days.
  - First-line therapy for moderate to severe PCP is intravenous (IV) trimethoprim-sulfamethoxazole (Table 81.2).
  - Adjunctive corticosteroids are shown to decrease mortality in patients with moderate to severe PCP.
    - Administration of corticosteroids is associated with a risk ratio of 0.56 for mortality and 0.38 for requiring mechanical ventilation.
    - Patients with a room air arterial oxygen pressure < 70 mm Hg or with an alveolar-arterial gradient >35 mm Hg should receive corticosteroids.

TABLE 81.2

SUMMARY OF TREATMENT REGIMENS FOR PCP IN THE ICU IN DECREASING ORDER OF PREFERENCE

Agent	Dose	Side effects
Trimethoprim-sulfamethoxazole	15–20 mg/kg/d trimethoprim with 75–100 mg/kg/d sulfamethoxazole IV, divided every 6–8 h	Bone marrow suppression, hyponatremia, hyperkalemia, nausea, nephrotoxicity, rash, transaminitis
Pentamidine isethionate	3–4 mg/kg/d IV	Bone marrow suppression, hypoglycemia or hyperglycemia, hypotension, nausea, pancreatitis, nephrotoxicity
Clindamycin-primaquine	900 mg IV every 8 h (clindamycin) 30 mg PO daily (primaquine)	Diarrhea, hemolytic anemia, leukopenia, methemoglobinemia, nausea, rash
Adjunctive therapy: Prednisone if PaO_2 <70 mm Hg or A-a gradient >35 mm Hg	40 mg PO every 12 h for 5 d, 40 mg PO daily for 5 d, 20 mg PO daily for 11 d	Psychosis, hyperglycemia

PCP, *Pneumocystis* pneumonia; ICU, intensive care unit; IV, intravenously; PO, by mouth; PaO_2, arterial oxygen tension; A-a, alveolar-arterial; d, day; h, hour.

- Therapy should be started within 24 to 72 hours of initiation of PCP treatment, regardless of whether diagnosis is confirmed or only suspected.
- Corticosteroids reduce inflammatory response seen during first few days of treatment.
- Recommended regimen is 40 mg of oral prednisone given twice daily for 5 days, then 40 mg once daily for 5 days, and 20 mg daily for 11 days.
- If unable to tolerate oral medications, IV methylprednisolone or dexamethasone can be substituted.
- **Ventilatory Support:** Physiology of PCP is very similar to that of acute respiratory distress syndrome (ARDS).
  - Principles of ventilatory management the same
  - Barotrauma is of particular concern in ventilated patients with PCP.
    - Development of pneumothorax heralds a poor prognosis.
    - Should probably be ventilated with tidal volumes of 6 mL/kg and levels of positive end-expiratory pressure as needed to maintain oxygenation according to the ARDSnet guidelines.
    - Noninvasive positive pressure ventilation with continuous positive airway pressure or bilevel positive airway pressure may be useful.
      - Noninvasive positive pressure ventilation may decrease rate of intubation, lower the number of pneumothoraces, and improve survival.

Bacterial Pneumonia

- Absolute numbers of cases of bacterial pneumonia (BP) have declined since the introduction of HAART.
- Clinical risk factors for BP include:
  - IV drug use
  - Cigarette smoking
  - Older age
  - Lower $CD4^+$ cell count
- One study found that 83% of HIV-infected patients admitted to the ICU with BP survived.

- $CD4^+$ cell count <100 cells/μL shock, and radiographic progression associated with mortality from BP in HIV-infected patients
- **Clinical Presentation:** Clinical presentation of BP in the HIV-infected patient is similar to that in the non–HIV-infected population.
- Typically present with an acute onset of fever, cough, shortness of breath, and purulent sputum
- Chest radiographs frequently reveal lobar infiltrates that may progress to an ARDS-like picture in severe cases.
- Most common causes of BP in HIV include *Streptococcus pneumoniae, Haemophilus influenzae, Pseudomonas aeruginosa,* and *Staphylococcus aureus.*
- Atypical pneumonia with *Mycoplasma pneumoniae* reported in 20% to 30% of HIV-infected patients with community-acquired pneumonia (CAP).
  - Less commonly a cause of ICU admission
- HIV-infected patients more likely to be bacteremic, particularly those with *Streptococcus pneumoniae* infection.

Other Respiratory Diseases

- Other respiratory diseases that occur in HIV-infected ICU patients include:
- *Mycobacteria tuberculosis* pneumonia
- Fungal pneumonias such as *Cryptococcus neoformans, Histoplasma capsulatum, Coccidioides immitis,* and *Aspergillus fumigatus*
- Cytomegalovirus (CMV) pneumonia
- *Toxoplasma gondii* pneumonitis
- Malignancies such as Kaposi sarcoma and non-Hodgkin lymphoma also lead to respiratory failure but are less common than infections.

IMMUNE RECONSTITUTION INFLAMMATORY SYNDROME

- Immune reconstitution inflammatory syndrome (IRIS) is a life-threatening syndrome occurring in HIV-infected patients started on HAART.

- In days to months following initiation of HAART, patients experience paradoxical worsening or new onset of infectious signs or symptoms.
- Results from an improvement in immune system with increased inflammatory response against infectious agents that can occur before CD4$^+$ cell count has risen
- IRIS most often seen in infection with *Mycobacterium tuberculosis*, CMV, *Pneumocystis*, *Mycobacterium avium* complex, and endemic fungi
- Manifestations of IRIS resulting in the need for ICU care include pneumonitis, meningitis, hepatitis, and pericarditis.
- Respiratory failure secondary to IRIS most common in tuberculosis and PCP.
  - Paradoxical worsening in these cases presents with fever, hypoxemia, and new or increased radiographic infiltrates.
  - Care is supportive, and corticosteroids are generally advocated, particularly in PCP.
  - Antiretroviral regimens should be continued whenever possible.
  - Syndrome is difficult to distinguish from acute opportunistic infections or other causes of respiratory deterioration.
    - Imperative that other causes of respiratory failure are sought before assigning a diagnosis of IRIS

FEVER OF UNKNOWN ORIGIN

- Fever is common in all ICU patients.
- Differential for fever is broad in the HIV-infected patient and includes:
  - Infections
  - Neoplasms
  - Medications
  - Collagen vascular diseases
- Etiology of fevers of unknown origin in those with HIV infection found to be infectious
  - Mycobacterial diseases are most commonly diagnosed.
  - PCP and bacterial infections are also seen.
  - The most common neoplastic cause of prolonged fever is lymphoma.
- Common infectious causes of fever in the ICU include:
  - Hospital-acquired pneumonia
  - Catheter-related infections
  - Sinusitis
  - Pseudomembranous colitis
- Noninfectious causes include:
  - Drug reactions (which are particularly common in those with HIV)
  - Pancreatitis
  - Venous thromboembolism
  - Acalculous cholecystitis
  - Adrenal insufficiency
  - Thyroid storm
- Diagnostic workup should include standard evaluation for infections such as blood, sputum, and urine cultures.
  - Bronchoscopy with BAL performed in patients who demonstrate a new infiltrate on chest radiograph or have a worsening respiratory status
  - Testing performed for mycobacterial and fungal pathogens
  - Other testing performed as would be done in the non–HIV-infected population

ANTIRETROVIRAL THERAPY IN THE ICU

Treatment Strategies

- Use of antiretroviral therapy in critically ill patients presents distinct issues related to drug delivery, dosing, drug interactions, and antiretroviral-associated toxicities.
- No randomized clinical trials and no consensus guidelines to assist in decisions regarding HAART use in the ICU
- Patients receiving HAART prior to ICU admission with evidence of virologic suppression (plasma HIV RNA below the limit of detection) should continue HAART.
  - Prompt placement of a feeding tube is critical in these patients.
  - Lapses in therapy create potential for subtherapeutic antiretroviral drug levels and the emergence of HIV drug resistance.

Drug Delivery, Dosing, and Interactions

- All currently approved antiretroviral medications are dispensed orally.
  - Either as tablets or capsules
  - With sole exception of enfuvirtide, a fusion inhibitor that is delivered subcutaneously (Table 81.3)
- Critical illness may complicate absorption of antiretroviral medications.
- Decreased gastric motility, continuous feeding, nasogastric suctioning, and gastric alkalinization recommended for stress ulcer prophylaxis may contribute to variations in absorption of enterally administered drugs.
  - H$_2$-blockers and proton pump inhibitors for stress ulcer prophylaxis are contraindicated with certain antiretroviral medications, necessitating the use of alternative prophylaxis agents or antiretroviral medications (Table 81.4).
- Presence of renal insufficiency or hepatic impairment will affect antiretroviral dosing.
  - Renal insufficiency will reduce the clearance of all nucleoside reverse transcriptase inhibitors (NRTIs) except abacavir and will require dose adjustment of these NRTIs (see Table 81.3).
  - Patients with renal insufficiency cannot use most fixed-dose NRTI combinations.
    - Each antiretroviral medication must be used individually and dosed accordingly.
    - Liver impairment will reduce the hepatic metabolism of many protease inhibitors and nonnucleoside reverse transcriptase inhibitors and will require dose adjustment of these medications (see Table 81.3).
    - Finally, as the patient's renal and hepatic functions change, the dose of these medications must be readjusted accordingly.
- Antiretroviral medications, especially nonnucleoside reverse transcriptase inhibitors and ritonavir-boosted protease inhibitor regimens, have several important drug interactions with other medications (see Table 81.4).

TABLE 81.3

ANTIRETROVIRAL MEDICATION FORMULATIONS AND DOSING

Medication	Available formulation(s) Tablet/capsule	Other	Daily dose	Dosing in renal insufficiency			Dosing in hepatic impairment
Nucleoside/Nucleotide Reverse Transcriptase Inhibitors							
Abacavir, ABC (Ziagen)	300-mg tablets	20 mg/mL oral solution	300 mg BID or 600 mg QD	No dosage adjustment			No dosage recommendation
Didanosine, ddI (Videx EC)[a]	125-, 200-, 250-, 400-mg enteric coated (EC) capsules		More than 60 kg 400 mg QD _With tenofovir_ 250 mg QD <60 kg 250 mg QD _With tenofovir_ 200 mg QD	(EC capsules) CrCl (mL/min) 30–59 10–29 <10* 75 mg *Includes patients receiving CAPD and HD; administer dose after dialysis.	Dose/d >60 kg 200 mg 125 mg	<60 kg 125 mg 100 mg 125 mg	No dosage recommendation
Emtricitabine, FTC (Emtriva)	200-mg hard gelatin capsule	10 mg/mL oral solution	200 mg QD or 240 mg (240 mL) oral solution QD	CrCl (mL/min) 30–49 15–29 <15* CrCl (mL/min) 30–49 15–29 <15* *Includes patients receiving HD; administer dose after dialysis.	Capsule dose 200 mg q48h 200 mg q72h 200 mg q96h Oral solution dose 120 mg q24h 80 mg q24h 60 mg q24h		No dosage recommendation
Lamivudine, 3TC (Epivir)	150-, 300-mg tablets	10 mg/mL oral solution	150 mg BID or 300 mg QD	CrCl (mL/min) 30–49 15–29 5–14 <5* *Includes patients receiving HD; administer dose after dialysis.	Dose 150 mg QD 150 mg once, then 100 mg QD 150 mg once, then 50 mg QD 50 mg once, then 25 mg QD		No dosage recommendation

(continued)

597

TABLE 81.3

CONTINUED

Medication	Available formulation(s) Tablet/capsule	Available formulation(s) Other	Daily dose	Dosing in renal insufficiency	Dosing in hepatic impairment
Stavudine, d4T (Zerit)	15-, 20-, 30-, 40-mg capsules	1 mg/mL oral solution	$\underline{60\text{ kg}}$ 40 mg BID $\underline{<60\text{ kg}}$ 30 mg BID	CrCl (mL/min) — Dose/d: >60 kg / <60 kg 26–50: 20 mg q12h / 15 mg q12h 10–25*: 20 mg q24h / 15 mg q24h *Includes patients receiving CAPD and HD; administer dose after dialysis.	No dosage recommendation
Tenofovir disoproxil fumarate, TDF (Viread)	300-mg tablet		300 mg QD	CrCl (mL/min) — Dose 30–49: 300 mg q48h 10–29: 300 mg twice weekly ESRD*: 300 mg q7d *Includes patients receiving HD; administer dose after dialysis.	No dosage recommendation
Zidovudine, AZT, ZDV (Retrovir)	100-mg capsules 300-mg tablets	10 mg/mL oral solution 10 mg/mL IV solution	300 mg BID 200 mg TID	Severe renal impairment or HD: 100 mg TID	No dosage recommendation
Combination					
Zidovudine + lamivudine (Combivir)	300- + 150-mg tablets		300/150 mg BID	Use individual antiretroviral medications dosed accordingly	No dosage recommendation
Zidovudine + lamivudine + abacavir (Trizivir) [2]	300- + 150- + 300-mg tablets		300/150/300 mg BID	Use individual antiretroviral medications dosed accordingly	No dosage recommendation
Abacavir + lamivudine (Epzicom)	600- + 300-mg tablets		600/300 mg QD	Use individual antiretroviral medications dosed accordingly	No dosage recommendation
Tenofovir + emtricitabine (Truvada)	300- + 200-mg tablets		300/200 mg QD	CrCl (mL/min) — Dose 30–49: 300/200 mg q48h <30: Not recommended	No dosage recommendation
Tenofovir + emtricitabine + efavirenz (Atripla)	300- + 200- + 600-mg tablets		300 + 200 + 600 mg QD	Use individual antiretroviral medications dosed accordingly CrCl <50 mL/min Not recommended	No dosage recommendation

Nonnucleoside Reverse Transcriptase Inhibitors						
Delavirdine, DLV (Rescriptor)[b]	100-, 200-mg tablets		400 mg TID	No dosage adjustment		No dosage recommendation; use with caution
Efavirenz, EFV (Sustiva)[a]	50-, 100-, 200-mg capsules, 600-mg tablets		600 mg QD on an empty stomach	No dosage adjustment		No dosage recommendation; use with caution
Nevirapine, NVP (Viramune)	200-mg tablets	50 mg/5 mL oral suspension	200 mg QD for 14 d, then 200 mg BID	No dosage adjustment		No data available; avoid use in patients with moderate to severe impairment
Atazanavir, ATV (Reyataz)[c]	100-, 150-, 200-mg capsules		400 mg QD *With tenofovir or efavirenz* RTV 100 mg QD must be added to ATV 300 mg QD	No dosage adjustment		C–P Score / Dose 7–9: 300 mg QD >9: Not recommended
Darunavir, DRV Prezista[c,d,f]	300-mg tablet		*With ritonavir* 600 mg BID (RTV 100 mg BID)	No dosage adjustment		No dosage recommendation; use with caution
Fosamprenavir, f-AP (Lexiva)	700-mg tablet		ARV naïve 1,400 mg BID *With ritonavir* 1,400 mg QD (RTV 200 mg QD) or 700 mg BID (RTV 100 mg BID) *With efavirenz* (RTV 100 mg BID must be added to f-APV 700 mg BID or RTV 300 mg QD added to f-APV 1,400 mg QD)	No dosage adjustment		C–P Score / Dose 5–8: 700 mg BID >9: Not recommended RTV boosting should not be used
Indinavir, IDV (Crixivan)[b,d]	200-, 333-, 400-mg capsules		800 mg q8h[a] *With ritonavir* 800 mg q12h (RTV 100 or 200 mg q12h)		No dosage adjustment	Mild to moderate insufficiency due to cirrhosis: 600 mg q8h
Lopinavir/ritonavir, LPV/r (Kaletra)	200/50-mg capsule	400/100 mg/5 mL oral solution Oral solution contains 42% alcohol	400/100 mg BID or 800/200 mg QD (only if ARV naïve) *With efavirenz or nevirapine* 600/150 mg BID	No dosage adjustment		No dosage recommendation; use with caution

(continued)

TABLE 81.3

CONTINUED

Medication	Available formulation(s)		Daily dose	Dosing in renal insufficiency	Dosing in hepatic impairment
	Tablet/capsule	Other			
Nelfinavir, NFV (Viracept)[b,c]	250-, 625-mg tablets	50 mg/g oral powder	1,250 mg BID or 750 mg TID	No dosage adjustment	No dosage recommendation; use with caution
Ritonavir, RTV (Norvir)[b,e]	100-mg capsules	600 mg/7.5 mL oral solution	600 mg q12h (when used as sole protease inhibitor) 100–400 mg daily in 1 to 2 divided doses (when used as pharmacokinetic booster)	No dosage adjustment	No dosage adjustment in mild impairment; no data for moderate to severe impairment, use with caution
Saquinavir hard gel capsule, SQV HGC (Invirase)[b,d]	200-mg capsules		*With ritonavir* 1,000 mg BID (RTV 100 mg BID)	No dosage adjustment	No dosage recommendation; use with caution
Tipranavir, TPV (Aptivus)[c,d,f]	250-mg capsules		*With ritonavir* 500 mg BID (RTV 200 mg BID)	No dosage adjustment	No dosage recommendation; use with caution; contraindicated in C-P Class B and C
Enfuvirtide, T20 (Fuzeon)[b,f]		108 mg/1.1 mL sterile H$_2$O (90 mg/1 mL)	90 mg SQ BID	No dosage adjustment	No dosage recommendation

BID, twice a day; QD, once daily; CAPD, continuous ambulatory peritoneal dialysis; HD, hemodialysis; ESRD, end-stage renal disease; TID, three times a day; C-P, Child-Pugh; SQ, subcutaneously.

[a] Hold enteral nutrition 2 h before and 1 h after administration.
[b] Generally not recommended as initial therapy if alternatives are available due to inferior virologic activity, inconvenient dosing, high pill burden, and/or increased toxicity and adverse events.
[c] Administration with food increases bioavailability. Take with food. For atazanavir, avoid taking with antacids.
[d] Generally not recommended unless accompanied by ritonavir as a pharmacokinetic booster.
[e] Generally not recommended as the sole protease inhibitor but used in combination with other protease inhibitors as a pharmacokinetic booster.
[f] No clinical trial data in antiretroviral therapy-naïve patients.
Adapted from Guidelines for the Use of Antiretroviral Agents in HIV-1-Infected Adults and Adolescents. These guidelines are updated frequently, and the most recent information is available on the AIDS*info* Web site: http://AIDSinfo.nih.gov. Accessed October 10, 2006.

COMMON ICU MEDICATIONS AND POTENTIALLY SERIOUS
LIFE-THREATENING INTERACTIONS WITH ANTIRETROVIRALS

Drug	Antiretroviral	Interaction
NEUROLOGIC AGENTS		
Anticonvulsants	Darunavir	May decrease ARV levels
Phenytoin, phenobarbital, carbamazepine	Delavirdine Efavirenz	May decrease anticonvulsant levels
SEDATIVES/ANALGESICS		
Midazolam/triazolam[a]	Most PIs, NNRTIs	Increased sedative effects
Methadone	Most PIs, NNRTIs, NRTIs	Narcotic withdrawal
Meperidine	Ritonavir	Increased normeperidine levels
ANTIMICROBIALS		
Metronidazole	Amprenavir Ritonavir Tipranavir	Disulfiram-like reaction
Rifampin	Most PIs Delavirdine Efavirenz Nevirapine	Decreased ARV levels Increased hepatotoxicity
Voriconazole	Efavirenz Ritonavir	Decreased voriconazole levels Increased ARV levels
RESPIRATORY AGENTS		
Fluticasone	Most PIs	Increased plasma fluticasone levels and adrenal suppression
CARDIAC AGENTS		
Amiodarone	Most PIs	Increased cardiac effects
Diltiazem	Amprenavir Atazanavir Indinavir	Increased cardiac effects
Nifedipine	Amprenavir Darunavir Delavirdine Lopinavir/ritonavir	Increased cardiac effects
Simvastatin/lovastatin	PIs Delavirdine Efavirenz	Increased statin levels
Sildenafil	Most PIs	Increased sildenafil effects
GASTROINTESTINAL AGENTS		
Proton pump inhibitors/H_2 blockers	Atazanavir Delavirdine	Decreased ARV levels

ICU, intensive care unit; ARV, antiretroviral; PI, protease inhibitor; NNRTI, nonnucleoside reverse transcriptase inhibitor; NRTI, nucleoside reverse transcriptase inhibitor.
[a]Midazolam can be used with caution as a single dose and given in a monitored situation for procedural sedation.

Drug Toxicity

- Newer antiretroviral medications possess better safety profiles compared to their predecessors.
  - Several antiretroviral medications are associated with potentially life-threatening and serious adverse effects (Table 81.5).
    - Abacavir associated with a hypersensitivity syndrome rarely can lead to death if patient is rechallenged

- Rash associated with nevirapine can be severe, presenting with systemic symptoms and, in rare cases, progressing to Stevens-Johnson syndrome and toxic epidermal necrosis.
- Efavirenz is associated with mental status alterations that may be attributed erroneously to analgesics, sedatives, or the sleep-disrupted schedule in the ICU.

TABLE 81.5

POTENTIALLY LIFE-THREATENING AND SERIOUS ADVERSE EFFECTS OF ANTIRETROVIRAL AGENTS

Life-threatening and adverse effect	Principal antiretroviral agent	Estimated frequency, onset	Prevention/monitoring and management
Dermatologic-Hypersensitivity reaction (HSR)—fever, diffuse rash; may progress to hypotension, respiratory distress, and vascular collapse	Abacavir (ABC)	Approximately 5%–8% Onset, 9 d (median); approximately 90% within first 6 wk	• Discontinue ABC and other ARVs. Most signs and symptoms resolve 48 h after discontinuation • Rule out other causes of symptoms • Discontinue other potential agent(s) • Do not rechallenge patients with ABC after suspected HSR
Dermatologic-Stevens-Johnson syndrome/toxic epidermal necrolysis (TEN)	Chiefly NNRTIs: Nevirapine (NVP) more than efavirenz (EFV), delavirdine (DLV)	NVP: 0.3%–1%, EFV and DLV: 0.1%; case reports for other ARVs Onset within first few days to weeks	• NVP: 2-week lead in period with 200 mg QD dosing, then increase to 200 mg BID. Avoid use of corticosteroids during lead-in period—may increase incidence of rash • Discontinue NNRTI and other ARVs • Rule out other causes of symptoms • Discontinue other potential agent(s) • Do not rechallenge patients with NNRTI
Neurologic-Central nervous system (CNS) effects including drowsiness, somnolence, insomnia, hallucination, psychosis, suicidal ideation, exacerbation of psychiatric illness	Efavirenz (EFV)	More than 50% may have some symptoms Onset within first few days; most symptoms subside or diminish after 2–4 wk	• Administer at bedtime or 2–3 h before bedtime for nonintubated, nonsedated patients • Take on an empty stomach to reduce drug concentration and CNS effects • Consider discontinuing EFV if symptoms persist and cause significant impairment or exacerbation of psychiatric illness
Gastrointestinal-Hepatotoxicity	All ARVs, especially nevirapine (NVP)	Frequency varies with ARV Onset (NRTIs), months to years; PIs generally weeks to months; NVP, 2/3 within first 12 wk	• Monitor liver enzymes • Rule out other causes of hepatotoxicity • For symptomatic patients, discontinue all ARVs • Discontinue other potential agent(s)
Gastrointestinal-Pancreatitis	Didanosine (ddI), also stavudine (d4T) plus ddI	ddI: 1%–7%, d4T plus ddI: increased frequency Onset usually weeks to months	• ddI should not be used in patients with a history of pancreatitis • Avoid concomitant use of ddI with d4T • Monitoring of serum amylase/lipase in asymptomatic patients is generally not recommended • Discontinue offending agent
Hematologic-Bone marrow suppression	Zidovudine (AZT, ZDV)	Anemia: 1.1%–4%; neutropenia: 1.8%–8% Onset, weeks to months	• Avoid use in patients at risk • Avoid other bone marrow suppressants if possible • Monitor CBC with differential • Switch to another NRTI if there is an alternative • Discontinue concomitant bone marrow suppressants if there are alternatives • Identify and treat other causes for anemia and neutropenia • Blood transfusion if indicated • Consider erythropoietin therapy for anemia • Consider filgrastim for neutropenia

(*continued*)

TABLE 81.5
CONTINUED

Life-threatening and adverse effect	Principal antiretroviral agent	Estimated frequency, onset	Prevention/monitoring and management
Lactic acidosis, hepatic steatosis ± pancreatitis (severe mitochondrial toxicities)	NRTIs, especially stavudine (d4T), didanosine (ddI), and zidovudine (AZT, ZDV)	Rare, but mortality up to 50% in some case series. Onset, months	• Discontinue ARV if this syndrome is highly suspected • Routine monitoring of lactic acid is generally not recommended • Some patients may require IV bicarbonate infusion, hemodialysis, or hemofiltration • Thiamine, riboflavin, and/or L-carnitine resulted in rapid resolution of hyperlactatemia in some case reports
Lactic acidosis, rapidly progressive ascending neuromuscular weakness	Stavudine (d4T), most frequent	Rare. Onset, months; then dramatic motor weakness may occur within days to weeks	• Discontinue ARV. Symptoms may be irreversible • Do not rechallenge patients with suspected ARV • Plasmapheresis, high dose corticosteroids, intravenous immunoglobulin, carnitine, acetylcarnitine attempted with varying success
Renal-Nephrolithiasis/ urolithiasis/crystalluria	Indinavir (IDV) most frequent	Approximately 12%. Onset is any time after beginning of therapy, especially at times of decreased fluid intake	• Maintain hydration, increase hydration at first sign of darkened urine • Monitor serum creatinine, urinalysis • Consider switching to alternative agent or therapeutic drug monitoring • Stent placement may be required
Renal-Nephrotoxicity	Indinavir (IDV), potentially tenofovir (TDF)	Frequency unknown. Onset-(IDV): months; (TDV): weeks to months	• Avoid use of other nephrotoxic medications • IDV: Maintain hydration, increase hydration at first sign of darkened urine • Monitor serum creatinine, urinalysis, serum potassium and phosphorus • Stop offending agent (generally reversible)

ARV, antiretroviral; NNRTI, nonnucleoside reverse transcriptase inhibitor; QD, daily; BID, twice a day; NRTI, nucleoside reverse transcriptase inhibitor; PI, protease inhibitor; CBC, complete blood count.
This table only lists potential life-threatening and serious adverse effects with an onset starting from initial dose up to months after initiation of therapy. However, there are several important adverse effects including cardiovascular effects, hyperlipidemia, insulin resistance or diabetes mellitus, and osteonecrosis that may result from antiretroviral therapy.
Adapted from Guidelines for the Use of Antiretroviral Agents in HIV-1-Infected Adults and Adolescents. These guidelines are updated frequently, and the most recent information is available on the AIDSinfo Web site: http://AIDSinfo.nih.gov. Accessed October 10, 2006.

HIV TESTING IN THE ICU

• In the current era, up to 40% of patients are unaware of HIV infection at time of ICU admission.
• Current guidelines recommend HIV testing whenever HIV infection is suspected.
• However, prompt recognition of previously undiagnosed HIV infection and HIV testing and disclosure requirements present challenges to critical care physicians.
• In general, HIV testing requires consent from the patient.
• If the patient is incapacitated, some states permit a surrogate to consent.

• HIV testing cannot be performed if a patient or their surrogate refuses.
• In cases where HIV testing cannot be performed, well-intentioned physicians may wish to order plasma HIV RNA assays or CD4+ cell counts to infer HIV status.
• This practice is ill advised and may be in violation of legal statutes in some states.
• Normal CD4+ cell count argues strongly against the presence of an HIV-associated opportunistic infection such as PCP; low CD4+ counts characteristic of advanced HIV disease are often seen in critically ill patients without HIV.

CHAPTER 82 ■ UNUSUAL INFECTIONS

- This chapter describes the epidemiology, clinical presentation, diagnosis, therapy, and prevention of relatively unusual infections.
- The incidence of these is low in the United States, they have potential to cause rapidly progressive disease, and, in some cases, they present unique problems in management and infection control in critical care.
- Prompt diagnosis and rapid treatment are critical.
- Many organisms causing these infectious diseases have gained new relevance as potential biologic warfare agents.
  - Epidemiology, clinical presentation, and management of infections resulting from intentional release may differ significantly from disease resulting from traditional modes of spread.
  - An intentional bioterrorist attack will result in large social disruptions affecting housing, public hygiene, and mass migration.
    - This may allow epidemic transmission of some agents.
- Globalization with increased travel of humans, and transport of animals and plant materials all increase likelihood that unusual infections will become more prevalent in the United States.

TULAREMIA

- A multisystem zoonotic infection caused by gram-negative coccobacillus, *Francisella tularensis*
- Tularemia has been recognized since the 1800s.
- Primarily transmitted through contact with infected animals, contaminated food and water, or arthropod bites
- Tularemia is listed as a category A bioterrorism agent and defined as follows:
  - Can be easily disseminated or transmitted from person to person
  - Results in high mortality rates and has the potential for major public health impact
  - Might cause public panic and social disruption
  - Requires special action for public health preparedness

Epidemiology

- Incidence in the United States has declined since 1950s and is currently <200 per year
  - In the United States, most cases occur in the western and southwestern states in small sporadic clusters.
  - Primarily occurs during summer months, likely due to increased exposure to biting arthropods
  - Cases during the fall and winter linked to hunting and handling infected animals.
  - A 3-to-1 preponderance of male-to-female cases.

- Inhalational exposures occurred in Martha's Vineyard in Massachusetts.
  - Were associated with mowing grass and cutting brush
- In the United States, ticks and biting flies are the most important arthropod vectors.
  - Major animal reservoirs are lagomorphs (rabbits and hares) and rodents including prairie dogs, squirrels, and rats.
  - Mosquitoes were implicated as primary vector in Scandinavia in one large outbreak.
  - Direct contact with infected animals is another significant mode of transmission.
  - Hunting, trapping, butchering animal carcasses, and handling meat are all risk factors.
  - Contamination of food and water by rodents and other carriers is also linked to human infection.
  - Organism survives well in cold, moist conditions and can withstand freezing.
  - Cats and other carnivores transiently carry organisms in mouths or claws.
    - Can thereby transmit infection to humans
    - Pets increase likelihood of tick-borne transmission to humans.
- Inhalational exposure may occur in laboratory or as consequence of deliberate release of weaponized *Francisella* cultures.
- Human-to-human transmission of tularemia is not known to occur.

Clinical Presentation

- Classically described as presenting one of six syndromes:
  - Ulceroglandular
  - Oculoglandular
  - Glandular
  - Pharyngeal
  - Typhoidal
  - Pneumonic
- Individual patients may have symptoms of several of these types simultaneously.
- After initial entry into host, through cutaneous inoculation, ingestion, or inhalation
  - Organisms multiply at site of infection.
  - Vigorous inflammatory response ensues, leading to subsequent necrosis
  - Organism multiplies within macrophages and travels to regional lymph nodes, kidney, liver, lung, and spleen.
  - Meninges and pericardium are occasionally involved secondarily in untreated tularemia.
  - Inhalation/cutaneous inoculation of 10 to 50 organisms is sufficient for infection.
  - Symptoms begin 3 to 5 days after infection.
    - Although longer incubation periods are possible

- Differences in clinical presentation are partly attributable to type and route of infection.
- Tick-borne infection is more likely to result in skin lesions on head and neck, trunk, and perineum.
- Animal-associated infections more commonly result in upper extremity lesions.
- Ingestion of contaminated water or food is more likely to cause pharyngeal infection.
- Inoculation into mucous membranes of eye results in oculoglandular syndrome.
  - Ocular lesion with local lymphadenopathy
- Inhalation of organism leads to pneumonic form of tularemia.
  - Other forms of tularemia can also cause pulmonary involvement through hematogenous dissemination.
- Typhoidal form of tularemia occurs in <30% of cases, in which there are no characteristic localized mucocutaneous or glandular signs or symptoms.
- Onset of systemic symptoms in tularemia is abrupt and includes:
  - Fever, headache, myalgia, coryza, cough, malaise, and chest pain or tightness
  - Mucocutaneous infection, presenting complaint is usually painful lymphadenopathy
    - May precede or follow skin lesion
    - Purely glandular form, there is no apparent skin lesion
    - Skin lesions usually begin as erythematous painful papules.
      ○ Progress to necrotic ulcers that are slow to heal
      ○ Enlarged lymph nodes slow to resolve and may suppurate.
  - Ocular infection, a painful conjunctivitis occurs
- Pharyngeal tularemia presents as exudative pharyngitis with adenopathy unresponsive to standard therapy.
- Tularemic pneumonia is characterized by fever, cough, and pleuritic pain.
  - Sputum production and hemoptysis are unusual.
  - Relative bradycardia, with normal pulse despite elevated temperature, is common (40%) in tularemia and may be a useful diagnostic finding.
  - Chest radiograph (CXR) findings include hilar adenopathy, patchy or less commonly lobar infiltrates, and pleural effusions.
- There has not been a documented biologic attack with weaponized tularemia organisms.
  - An aerosolized release of organisms would likely cause pneumonic disease.
    - Would also likely result in ocular and cutaneous forms
  - Tularemia in urban settings and among healthy individuals should prompt suspicion of a biologic attack.
  - Onset of symptoms is expected to be rapid.
    - Closely resemble acute onset of influenza
    - Differential diagnosis of pneumonia due to an aerosolized biologic weapon attack would include anthrax, plague, and Q fever.
  - Important distinguishing characteristics between these causes would include:
    ○ More rapid and fulminant course in both anthrax and plague
    ○ Pneumonic anthrax would not cause bronchopneumonia but would result in mediastinal widening.
    ○ Pneumonic plague results in frankly purulent sputum with hemoptysis and rapid progression.

    ○ Laboratory testing is important in distinguishing between these various causes
    ○ Initial empiric treatment will require diagnosis based primarily on clinical and epidemiologic data.

Diagnosis

- Cultures require incubation on special supportive media.
  - Cultures of pharyngeal washings, sputum, and fasting gastric aspirates most likely to yield positive results.
  - Blood samples are usually negative.
- Direct fluorescent staining of specimens performed by specialized laboratories for a relatively rapid diagnosis.
- Serology is positive approximately 10 days after infection.
- Serology is useful for confirmation of suspected cases.
- It is important to promptly contact the hospital epidemiologist or infection control department.

Treatment

- Treatment regimens for most of the select agents are devised for either a contained or a mass casualty setting (Table 82.1).

PLAGUE

- Caused by the gram-negative bacillus *Yersinia pestis*
  - One of oldest and most feared illnesses known to man
  - Developed by various groups and nations as a biologic weapon since the 1950s
  - Listed as an important potential agent of bioterrorism.

Epidemiology

- Primarily a rural disease that occurs in all continents except Australia.
- Most common in rural settings in developing nations
  - Most cases occur between spring and autumn in the western United States where disease is enzootic in wild rodents.
  - Humans are infected via bites from infected rodent fleas or by handling infected animals, either domestic pets or wild animals.
  - Worldwide, the most important reservoir is the domestic rat.
    - But, as in the United States, sylvatic foci (in wild animals) also exist.
  - Human-to-human transmission can occur in pneumonic plague.
    - Requires close contact
    - In the United States, the last known case acquired in this manner was reported in 1925.

Clinical Manifestations

- Three main types of plague are:
- Bubonic
- Septicemic
- Pneumonic

TABLE 82.1

TREATMENT RECOMMENDATIONS FOR TULAREMIA

Contained casualty setting

Adults	*Preferred choices:* Streptomycin, 1 g IM BID Gentamicin, 5 mg/kg IM or IV once daily *Alternative choices:* Doxycycline, 100 mg IV BID Chloramphenicol, 15 mg/kg IV QID Ciprofloxacin, 400 mg IV BID
Children	*Preferred choices:* Streptomycin, 15 mg/kg IM BID (not to exceed 2 g/d) Gentamicin, 2.5 mg/kg IM or IV TID *Alternative choices:* Doxycycline If weight 45 kg or more, 100 mg IV BID If weight <45 kg, 2.2 mg/kg IV BID Chloramphenicol, 15 mg/kg IV QID Ciprofloxacin, 15 mg/kg IV BID
Pregnant women	Same as adults above except chloramphenicol is not recommended.

Mass casualty setting

Adults, including pregnant women	*Preferred choices:* Doxycycline, 100 mg PO BID Ciprofloxacin, 500 mg PO BID
Children	*Preferred choices:* Doxycycline If ≥45 kg, 100 mg PO BID If <45 kg, 2.2 mg/kg PO BID Ciprofloxacin, 15 mg/kg PO BID[a]

BID, twice daily; IM, intramuscularly; IV, intravenously; PO, orally; TID, three times daily; QID, four times daily.
For full details and most current treatment recommendations, the reader is referred to the CDC Web site: Centers for Disease Control and Prevention. Consensus statement: tularemia as a biological weapon: medical and public health management. http://www.bt.cdc.gov/agent/tularemia/tularemia-biological-weapon-abstract.asp#4. Accessed February 6, 2007.
[a]Ciprofloxacin dosage should not exceed 1 g/d in children.

- No current experience with pneumonic plague acquired from biologic attack
  - But clinical presentation expected to differ from natural infection

Bubonic Plague

- The most common type of plague
  - Occurring in 76% of cases reported in the United States between 1990 and 2005
  - Large numbers of bacteria inoculated at site of flea bite and multiply locally.
    - Followed by rapid replication in nearby lymph nodes
  - Incubation period is between 2 and 7 days.
  - Abrupt onset of fever, chills, and headache
  - Characteristic bubo typically develops as an extremely tender smooth, firm oval mass.
  - Overlying skin is warm and erythematous, but suppuration is rare.
  - Primary lesion is often inapparent but can develop into an ulcer.

- Most common site of buboes is in femoral lymph nodes.
  - Also seen in inguinal, cervical, and axillary locations depending on location of inoculation
- Bacteremia occurs in about 25% of cases.
- In untreated cases, mortality is approximately 50%.
  - Deterioration is usually rapid, with progression of typical signs of shock and death occurring as early as 2 to 3 days.

Septicemic Plague

- Defined as plague absent an apparent bubo
- Diagnosis of septicemic plague is often delayed and prognosis is poorer than other forms of plague.
- In the United States, from 1990 to 2005, 18% of reported plague cases were septicemic.
  - 38% of the cases in 2006 were of this variety.
- Useful clue to diagnosis of septicemic plague is that gastrointestinal symptoms (nausea and vomiting, diarrhea, and abdominal pain) were prominent in several recent cases.
- Disseminated intravascular coagulation (DIC) may develop with cutaneous and visceral hemorrhage.
  - Rapidly progressive gangrene may also develop.
- Septicemic plague and pneumonic plague are fatal if untreated.
  - Even with treatment, mortality rates of 33% in septicemic plague were reported from New Mexico in the 1980s.

Pneumonic Plague

- May develop secondary to either bubonic or septicemic plague
  - Incidence of secondary pulmonary involvement approximates 12%.
  - In the United States, recent cases of primary pneumonic plague occurred from laboratory accidents or cat exposure.
- Similar to other acute pneumonia with abrupt onset of fever and dyspnea
  - Bloody, watery or purulent sputum is produced.
  - Is HIGHLY infectious
- Transmission *via* respiratory droplets
  - Simple respiratory isolation with droplet precautions is sufficient.
- Chest radiograph usually reveals bronchopneumonia and multilobar consolidation, or cavitation may be seen
- Clues to plague arising as result of biologic attack include:
- Cases outside areas of known enzootic infection
- Occurrences in area without associated rodent die-offs
- Numerous cases of pneumonia in otherwise healthy patients
- Routine laboratory tests are not markedly different from those in fulminant pneumonia and sepsis.
  - White blood cell count is often markedly elevated.
  - Fibrin degradation products are detectable in cases where DIC present.

Diagnosis

- Specialized laboratory tests to definitively/rapidly identify *Y. pestis* are not widely available.
  - When suspected, coordination with state public health officials and the Centers for Disease Control and Prevention (CDC) allows more specialized tests and susceptibility testing to be performed.

• Blood, sputum, lymph node aspirates, and lesion swabs examined by Gram or Wright-Giemsa stain for presence of bipolar-staining gram-negative bacilli
  • Have appearance of safety pins
  • Laboratory alerted to possibility of plague so appropriate biosafety procedures followed

Treatment

• Recommendations for therapy of plague provided were derived from recommendations of Working Group on Civilian Biodefense and CDC.
• Treatment recommendations are complicated by lack of clinical efficacy trials, lack of experience with widespread pneumonic plague, and potentially unpredictable clinical responses in infections due to a biologic attack.
  • Historically, the proven, effective antibiotic therapy for plague has been streptomycin.
  • Because of limited availability of streptomycin, gentamicin is the recommended alternative.
  • Tetracycline and doxycycline are effective and recommended for the treatment of plague.
  • Recommended duration of therapy for plague (Table 82.2) is 10 days.
    • Oral therapy is substituted when condition improves.
  • Duration of postexposure prophylaxis to prevent plague infection is 7 days.

ANTHRAX

• Extremely rare disease in the United States until bioterrorism attacks of 2001
  • Caused by the gram-positive, spore-forming bacillus *Bacillus anthracis*
  • Anthrax was tested as a biologic weapon by the United States in the 1960s and other countries until the 1970s.
  • Technology to produce highly infectious anthrax spores and disseminate as aerosol exists and is known to have been developed for use as a biologic warfare agent.

Epidemiology

• Three major modes of infection with anthrax:
  • Inhalational
  • Cutaneous
  • Gastrointestinal
• *Cutaneous anthrax* is the most common type.
  • Extremely rare in the United States, with 224 cases reported from 1944 to 1994.
• Barring exposure to intentionally produced anthrax, *inhalational anthrax* is less common.
  • Occurs primarily in those with occupational or laboratory exposure
  • Prior to 2001, only 18 cases of inhalational anthrax were reported from 1900 to 1978.
• *Gastrointestinal anthrax* is most commonly reported.
  • Improperly cooked meat contaminated with large numbers of anthrax bacilli is consumed.

TABLE 82.2

RECOMMENDATIONS FOR TREATMENT OF PATIENTS WITH PNEUMONIC PLAGUE IN CONTAINED AND MASS CASUALTY SETTINGS AND FOR POSTEXPOSURE PROPHYLAXIS

CONTAINED CASUALTY SETTING

Adults — *Preferred choices:*
Streptomycin, 1 g IM BID
Gentamicin, 5 mg/kg IM or IV once daily or
2 mg/kg loading dose followed by 1.7 mg/kg IM or IV TID
Alternative choices:
Doxycycline, 100 mg IV BID or 200 mg IV once daily
Ciprofloxacin, 400 mg IV BID
Chloramphenicol, 25 mg/kg IV QID

Children — *Preferred choices:*
Streptomycin, 15 mg/kg IM BID (maximum daily dose, 2 g)
Gentamicin, 2.5 mg/kg IM or IV TID†
Alternative choices:
Doxycycline
If 45 kg or more, give adult dosage
If <45 kg, give 2.2 mg/kg IV BID (maximum, 200 mg/d)
Ciprofloxacin, 15 mg/kg IV BID
Chloramphenicol, 25 mg/kg IV QID
In children, ciprofloxacin dose should not exceed 1 g/d, and chloramphenicol should not exceed 4 g/d. Children younger than 2 y should not receive chloramphenicol.

Pregnant Women — Same as adults above except chloramphenicol is not recommended.

MASS CASUALTY SETTING AND POSTEXPOSURE PROPHYLAXIS

Adults, including pregnant women — *Preferred choices:*
Doxycycline, 100 mg PO BID
Ciprofloxacin, 500 mg PO BID
Alternative choice:
Chloramphenicol, 25 mg/kg PO QID

Children — *Preferred choices:*
Doxycycline
If ≥45 kg, give adult dosage.
If <45 kg, give 2.2 mg/kg PO BID
Ciprofloxacin, 20 mg/kg PO BID
Alternative choice:
Chloramphenicol, 25 mg/kg PO QID (maximum 200 mg/dL)

BID, twice daily; IM, intramuscularly; IV, intravenously; PO, orally; TID, three times daily; QID, four times daily.

Clinical Manifestations

• Presentation of anthrax due to a biologic attack is still incompletely characterized.
• Most information relevant to inhalational anthrax from anthrax manufactured as a biologic weapon is from the

2001 U.S. attacks and an unintentional release in Sverdlovsk, Russia, in 1979.

- There were 11 cases of inhalational anthrax resulting from exposures in 2001.
- Aspects of pathophysiology of inhalational anthrax are highly relevant to clinician.
  - Infection occurs after spores are inhaled and deposited in alveoli.
  - Spores are phagocytosed by macrophages and transported to regional lymph nodes to germinate and replicate vegetatively.
  - There may be a period of extended latency in lymph node because spores remain dormant.
    - Although usual, incubation period is 2 to 6 days.
    - Cases have occurred as late as 6 weeks after exposure to aerosolized anthrax.
    - When replication occurs, toxin production leads to edema, necrosis, and hemorrhage.
- Typical symptoms are:
  - Fever and chills
  - Chest discomfort and dyspnea
  - Severe fatigue
  - Vomiting
- Two stages may occur, with an initial period of improvement followed by rapid deterioration.
  - Initial finding on CXR is widened mediastinum due to mediastinal lymph node involvement.
  - Hemorrhagic mediastinal lymphadenitis ensues, often accompanied by bloody pleural effusions.
    - 8 of 11 patients in 2001 developed bloody pleural effusions.
    - 10 of 11 had radiologic evidence of mediastinal adenopathy.
    - Anthrax does not cause typical bronchopneumonia.
    - Pulmonary infiltrates or consolidation were observed in 8 of 11 cases.
    - In an autopsy series from the Sverdlovsk outbreak, primary focal hemorrhagic necrotizing pneumonia was described in 11 of 42 cases.
- Anthrax may present as meningitis, which was the initial presentation of index case in 2001.
  - As many as 50% of inhalational anthrax cases may develop meningitis.
  - Causes rapidly progressive hemorrhagic meningitis with characteristic large gram-positive bacilli in cerebrospinal fluid (CSF)
- Although portal of infection is lung, hemorrhagic submucosal lesions may develop in gastrointestinal tract along with mesenteric infection.
  - Such lesions were seen in 39 of 42 of autopsy cases reported in the Sverdlovsk outbreak and in one 2001 case.
    - Latter patient presented with primarily gastrointestinal symptoms.
- Diagnosis of inhalational anthrax is difficult, especially in early stages.
  - Tachycardia and severe diaphoresis may be present.
  - Rhinorrhea or sore throat are common in viral respiratory infections but were uncommon in inhalational anthrax.
  - High index of clinical suspicion should be maintained.
  - Blood cultures are invariably positive if obtained prior to antibiotics.

- Cutaneous anthrax is expected to occur as a result of a biologic anthrax attack.
  - Cutaneous cases occurred up to 12 days after exposure in the Sverdlovsk outbreak.
  - Initial lesion is papule or macule.
  - Leads to ulceration at site of inoculation within 2 days, followed by vesiculation
  - Lesion is painless, although it may be highly pruritic.
  - Vesicular fluid contains large amounts of bacteria.
  - Characteristic depressed black eschar that subsequently develops is painless.
  - Surrounding edema is often a prominent feature of cutaneous anthrax lesions.
  - In the 2001 case, cutaneous anthrax developed in a 7-month-old infant, and microangiopathic hemolytic anemia and renal insufficiency occurred.

Diagnosis

- Blood cultures obtained when anthrax suspected
  - Blood smears examined for presence of organisms
- CXR and chest CT scans are obtained to look for evidence of mediastinal widening, pleural effusions, and parenchymal abnormalities.
- Thoracentesis of pleural effusions should be performed.
- Lumbar puncture (LP) should be done as indicated.
- Clinical microbiology laboratory and state public health department should be notified.
  - Specimens can be sent to specialized laboratories (Laboratory Response Network) for specific testing such as immunohistochemical staining or polymerase chain reaction (PCR).
  - Cutaneous lesions, especially vesicle fluid, should be swabbed for stain and culture.
  - Punch biopsy of the periphery of lesions may also be performed and analyzed by immunohistochemistry or PCR if Gram stain is negative.
  - Nasal swabs are not sensitive indicators of exposure or infection and should not be used to diagnose or rule out infection in individual patients.
  - Sputum culture generally negative in inhalational anthrax.

Treatment

- Current recommendations for anthrax therapy provided here are derived from the Working Group on Civilian Biodefense and CDC guidelines (Table 82.3).
- Treatment summary guidelines are as follows:
  - For a mass exposure setting
    - Both treatment and prophylaxis, where parenteral or multidrug therapy problematic
    - Consist of oral ciprofloxacin, 500 mg every 12 hours or 10 to 15 mg/kg twice daily for children
  - Gastrointestinal and oropharyngeal anthrax: use regimens recommended for inhalational anthrax
  - Cutaneous anthrax: recommendations are ciprofloxacin or doxycycline alone at same doses as inhalational anthrax
  - Recommended duration of treatment is a minimum of 60 days after exposure because of the risk of latent spores that may cause reactivation

TABLE 82.3

INHALATIONAL ANTHRAX TREATMENT PROTOCOL IN THE CONTAINED CASUALTY SETTING

Adults (including pregnant women)	Ciprofloxacin, 400 mg every 12 h *or* Doxycycline[a] 100 mg every 12 h *and* one or two additional antimicrobials[b]	IV treatment initially. Switch to oral antimicrobial therapy when clinically appropriate. Continue for 60 days (IV and PO combined)
Children	Ciprofloxacin[c], 10–15 mg/kg every 12 h *Or* Doxycycline[a] Older than 8 y and >45 kg: 100 mg every 12 h Younger than 8 y or ≤45 kg: 2.2 mg/kg every 12 h *And* One or two additional antimicrobials[b]	Same as adult

[a]If meningitis is suspected, doxycycline may be less optimal because of poor central nervous system penetration.
[b]Other agents with *in vitro* activity include rifampin, vancomycin, penicillin, ampicillin, chloramphenicol, imipenem, clindamycin, and clarithromycin. Because of concerns of constitutive and inducible beta-lactamases in *Bacillus anthracis,* penicillin and ampicillin should not be used alone.
[c]The ciprofloxacin dosage in children should not exceed 1 g/d.

- Use of adjunctive steroids may be considered in anthrax meningitis.
- Initial therapy may be altered based on clinical course of patient.
  - One or two first-line antimicrobials—ciprofloxacin or doxycycline—may be adequate as patient improves.

VIRAL HEMORRHAGIC FEVER

- Major diseases considered here are Marburg, Ebola, and Lassa fevers
- Marburg and Ebola viruses are filoviruses.
- Lassa virus is an arenavirus with different clinical characteristics.
- All have the potential to create similar problems in hospital management because of the sometimes dramatic nature of illness and potential for human-to-human transmission.

Epidemiology

- Since 1976, approximately a dozen outbreaks of Ebola in Africa
- Mortality ranging from 53% to 88%
- In the United States, eight cases of documented human infection occurred from contact with imported monkeys from Philippines.
  - Infections with this Reston strain of Ebola virus are subclinical.
- Marburg virus is associated with six outbreaks since the disease was recognized in 1976 in German and Yugoslav laboratory workers infected by African green monkeys of Ugandan origin.
- Six other infection clusters in Africa, most recently in Angola and Democratic Republic of Congo
  - Involving more than 400 people
  - Mortality was 83% and 90%, respectively, in last two outbreaks.

- Infections transmitted by exposure to infected primate blood or cell culture.
- Secondary transmission occurs from exposure to blood and body fluids and by intimate contact.
- Ebola transmission ranged from 3% to 17% in household contacts.
- Droplet and small-particle aerosol transmission thought to have occurred in Reston outbreak, but not documented in human-to-human transmission.
- Nosocomial transmission associated with
  - Percutaneous exposure and mucous membrane
  - Cutaneous exposure to infected body fluids
  - Skin of patients also infected and serves as source of secondary transmission
- Lassa virus chronic infection of rodents and is endemic throughout West Africa
  - Human transmission is through infected rodents, primarily through contact with urine.
  - Person-to-person transmission primarily via contact with infected body fluids.
    - Aerosol transmission may also occur.
    - Incubation is between 3 and 16 days.
  - Other arenaviruses present worldwide in rodent reservoirs and are potential source of new clinical syndromes.

Clinical Manifestations

- Clinical pictures of Ebola and Marburg infection similar
- Incubation period ranges between 5 and 10 days.
- Abrupt onset of fever, myalgias, and headache is typical.
- Nausea/vomiting, abdominal pain, diarrhea, chest pain, and pharyngitis are common.
- Photophobia, lymph node enlargement, jaundice, and pancreatitis are all manifestations of widespread organ involvement.
- Central nervous system involvement manifests as obtundation or coma.
- Bleeding diathesis is seen in at least 50% of patients.
- Characteristic maculopapular rash described by day 5 of illness.

- By the second week, either a period of defervescence and improvement, or further deterioration with multiorgan system failure
  - DIC as well as hepatic and renal failure may ensue.
- Convalescence often protracted
- Mortality is estimated at:
  - 25% for Marburg
  - 50% for Ebola-Sudan
  - 90% for Ebola-Zaire
  - Ebola-Reston has not led to any known human deaths.
  - There is viremia with infection of all organs
    - Leading to necrosis in areas of viral replication
  - Pathogenesis thought also due to cytokine release
    - With increased vascular permeability and hemodynamic instability
- Lassa fever presents with relatively nonspecific signs and symptoms
  - Makes recognition of cases in initial stages difficult
  - Combination of fever, retrosternal pain, pharyngitis, and proteinuria indicative of Lassa fever
  - Diffuse capillary leak syndrome in second week of illness is a cardinal manifestation.
  - Mortality of hospitalized cases ranges from 15% to 25%.
  - Seventh cranial nerve deafness is a common sequela of Lassa infection.
    - Occurs in approximately one-third of cases.
    - Persistent vertigo is another reported side effect.
  - Pathogenic mechanism of Lassa fever is not well understood.
    - Variable necrosis in affected organs
    - Systemic manifestations of vascular dysfunction perhaps due to soluble macrophage-derived factors

Diagnosis

- History of travel to endemic areas and clinical syndrome compatible with viral hemorrhagic fever (VHF) are key elements.
- Cluster of cases with signs and symptoms of VHF may be the first clue of biologic attack.
- Specialized testing for Marburg and Ebola is available through reference laboratories.
  - Includes PCR and direct antigen visualization in clinical samples
  - Local public health authorities and CDC involvement allows testing *via* mobile laboratory facilities.
    - BSL-4 level containment facilities are required for attempts to isolate virus and BSL-3 facilities for routine testing.
  - Lassa virus is easily cultured, as levels of viremia are usually high.
  - Reverse transcription-PCR (RT-PCR) may also be used to identify Lassa virus.

Treatment

- Treatment of Marburg and Ebola virus primarily supportive
- No effective specific therapy
- Interferon is felt to not be useful.
- Unnecessary movement/manipulation of patient avoided
- Contact and respiratory isolation of the patient necessary, including:

- Use of goggles and face shields to prevent exposure to body fluids
- Thorough disinfection of all materials coming into contact with patient performed
  - Containers of biologic waste should be externally disinfected.
- In Lassa fever, where aspartate transaminase levels exceed 150 IU/L
  - Early treatment with IV ribavirin reported to be beneficial in tapering doses over 12 days.

SMALLPOX

- Caused by infection with variola, a double-stranded DNA orthopoxvirus
- One of the most feared and lethal diseases known
- Was virtually eliminated as natural threat by vaccination
- In 1980, the World Health Organization declared it to be eradicated worldwide.
  - Last know naturally occurring case was in 1977.
- In the United States, the universal childhood vaccination ended in 1972.
  - Most people in the United States today susceptible to smallpox infection.
- The 2001 Anthrax attacks raised the possibility of smallpox being used as biologic weapon.
  - Classified as a category A bioterrorism agent
  - High-priority organism that poses a risk to national security
  - Considered one of most dangerous agents because of high infectiousness, capability for rapid spread, lack of effective treatment, and capacity to induce mass social disruption and overburden the public health system

Epidemiology

- Spread by direct close contact *via* large droplet inhalation
  - No known animal reservoirs
  - Spread can also occur by contact with lesions or infected fomites
- Household spread is reported to range from 30% to 80%.
- Outbreaks were most common during winter and early spring.
- All ages susceptible
- Patients are most contagious when they have rash.
  - May be infectious during symptomatic prodrome prior to development of skin lesions
  - Incubation is from 7 to 17 days, during which period the patient is not infectious.

Clinical Manifestations

- Prodromal phase: patient experiences high fever with back pain and prostration
- Rash follows within a 1 or 2 days
- With more lesions on face, oral mucosa, and extremities than on the trunk
  - Termed *centrifugal pattern*

- Lesions begin as macules, progress to vesicles, and become pustules over first week
- Fever is usually persistent throughout period of rash development.
- Lesions are deep seated, firm, and painful.
- Important for diagnosis: **All lesions at same stage of development at each phase.**
  - These characteristics of rash serve to differentiate it from rash of chickenpox.
    - Superficial, appears in crops, is centripetal in distribution, and is associated with relatively mild prodrome
- Extent of smallpox rash correlates with mortality, which ranges from 10% to 75%.
- In fatal cases, death usually occurs by second week.
- Lesions begin to crust over after 7 to 9 days.
- Patient is noninfectious only after all scabs have fallen off.
- Scarring and pitting result in characteristic pock-marked appearance of survivors.
- Pathologic damage in smallpox is generally confined to skin and mucous membranes.
  - Although virus present throughout internal organs
  - Systemic manifestations and fatalities are attributed to toxinemia and antigenemia.
- Vaccine-modified smallpox presents as milder illness with fewer lesions, mortality <10%.
- Hemorrhagic form of smallpox may occur:
  - There is diffuse erythema
  - Followed by petechial hemorrhages
  - Reported to have mortality approaching 100%
- In malignant or "flat" smallpox, discrete lesions do not develop, but confluent rubbery lesions present.
- Form of smallpox known as variola minor, with much milder symptoms and mortality <10%, now known due to genetically distinct strain of virus.

Diagnosis

- Specimens of vesicular or pustular fluid obtained for culture and electron microscopic examination
  - Transported in double-sealed, leakproof containers designed for transport of body fluids
  - Specimens handled only in BSL-4 laboratories
  - Public health authorities notified to assist with specimen handling if case of smallpox suspected
  - Diagnosis of orthopoxvirus infection is made by electron microscopic examination.
    - Speciation performed by molecular techniques such as PCR and DNA sequencing

Treatment and Prevention

- The following principles should be followed:
- Patient is isolated.
- Contact and airborne precautions are instituted when case of smallpox suspected.
- All personnel with face-to-face contact with patient are vaccinated.
  - As are all personnel with patient contact while the latter was febrile

- Local health authorities are contacted immediately.
- CDC will provide assistance with prioritizing contacts for vaccination and monitoring.
- Contraindications to vaccinations do not apply to high-risk exposures.
- Treatment is primarily supportive.
  - Maintaining hemodynamic stability and treating secondary infections

MONKEYPOX

- Clinically similar to smallpox
- Sporadically reported in Africa since 1960
- Pronounced lymphadenopathy is an additional sign that may help differentiate it from smallpox.
- Monkeypox thought endemic in rodents and transmitted to humans *via* direct animal contact
- Occasional human-to-human transmission
- Vaccination against smallpox is thought to ameliorate symptoms and lessen likelihood of infection.
- Cidofovir has activity against monkeypox *in vitro*
  - Used in severe infection
  - No clinical data regarding its effectiveness

MALARIA

- The fourth largest killer of children younger than 5 years of age
- Causes over 350 million clinical episodes and one million deaths per year
- *Plasmodium falciparum* is strain of parasite is most likely to cause high-level parasitemia and severe life-threatening malaria.

Epidemiology

- Endemic throughout much of world
- Greatest number of cases in Africa and Asia
- Officially eradicated in the United States since 1970
  - About 1,200 cases are reported annually, mostly in travelers from endemic areas.
  - Other cases are due to:
    - Local transmission from infected mosquitoes (so-called airport malaria)
    - Congenital malaria
    - Malaria acquired from blood transfusion
    - Local transmission of malaria in the United States has occurred at least 11 times since 1970, with 20 probable cases.
    - In recent outbreak in Florida, seven cases were verified as being caused by the same strain of *P. vivax*.
- In endemic areas, adults are partially immune to malaria and, although infected, may be asymptomatic.
  - Children are particularly prone to infection and to developing severe disease.
  - Other high-risk groups include pregnant women, asplenic individuals, and other immunocompromised hosts.

Clinical Manifestations

- Typically has an incubation period of 1 to 3 weeks
- May be extended by partial immunity or chemoprophylaxis
  - Suggested that any traveler returning from endemic area be considered at risk for as long as 3 months
- Clinical presentation usually nonspecific:
  - Fever and headache universally present.
  - Myalgia, sweats, and weakness are common.
  - Paroxysmal and cyclical fever classically associated with malaria not consistently present
  - In case of falciparum malaria, fever is often continuous.
  - Other infections are common in malaria-endemic areas, but malaria is considered one of most likely diagnoses in a patient with a consistent clinical picture and travel history.
    - If is suspected, ID consultation indicated to help with management and assess likelihood of alternate diagnoses.
- Pathogenesis of malaria complex and related to both:
  - Direct effects of parasite on erythrocytes and vasculature
  - Indirect effects on cytokine production, tissue oxygen consumption, and other systemic effect
  - Several aspects of biology of *Plasmodium falciparum* relevant to development of severe malaria
    - *P. falciparum* sequesters itself in venous microcirculation of virtually all tissues, including brain
    - Hypoglycemia common during *P. falciparum* infection
      - Thought to be due to oxygen consumption by replicating parasites
      - As well as result of increased tissue metabolism
  - Severe anemia may occur due to lysis of infected erythrocytes and clearance of uninfected erythrocytes and decreased erythrocyte production.
    - Anemia in severe malaria is often normochromic and normocytic.
  - A combination of factors aggravate tissue hypoxia and lead to metabolic acidosis.
  - Capillary leak syndrome due to parasite sequestration and cytokine production leads to pulmonary edema.
  - Renal failure is multifactorial and more common in adults than children.
  - Hemoglobinuria may be severe enough to cause dark urine.
    - Termed, when present, *blackwater fever*

Diagnosis

- Gold standard for diagnosis remains microscopic identification of parasites on blood smear.
  - Examination of thick and thin blood smears performed immediately by trained personnel.
  - If initial examination is negative, repeat every 12 to 24 hours for total of 48 to 72 hours.
  - When parasites are detected, the percentage of parasitemia can be calculated by:
    - Counting number of infected and noninfected RBCs
    - Number of white blood cells in microscopic field used as internal standard to aid in estimated parasite density and percentage when thick smears are examined
- Malaria is a nationally notifiable disease.

- State health authorities are notified when diagnosis of malaria made.
- The CDC maintains a 24-hour malaria hotline to assist clinicians with the management of suspected and confirmed malaria cases
  - The numbers to call are: 770-488-7788 Monday to Friday, 8:00 a.m. to 4:30 p.m.
  - Off-hours, weekends, federal holidays: 770-488-7100 and ask to have the malaria clinician on call to be paged

Treatment

- Patients, particularly nonimmune, may deteriorate rapidly.
- Hospitalization of patients during initial phase of treatment is prudent.
  - May have severe illness before manifesting high degrees of parasitemia
  - Patients who manifest any of symptoms or signs of severe malaria and have any degree of parasitemia on blood smear should be treated as case of severe malaria.
- The World Health Organization promulgated criteria for diagnosis of severe malaria (Table 82.4).
  - Cases meeting these criteria are treated with IV therapy.
  - IV quinidine gluconate is currently only available parenteral drug recommended for severe malaria in the United States.
    - Administered as a loading dose of 6.25 mg base/kg (= 10 mg salt/kg), over 1 to 2 hours
    - Followed by continuous infusion administered at 0.0125 mg/kg/minute base (= 0.02 mg salt/kg/minute)
    - Quinidine levels maintained in range of 3 to 8 mg/L
    - After 24 hours of IV therapy, if patient is able to take oral drugs
      - Treatment can be switched to oral quinine/
      - 10 mg salt/kg every 8 hours for a total of 7 days of therapy
  - All patients with severe malaria are also treated with IV doxycycline (100 mg every 12 hours) or clindamycin (5 mg base/kg every 8 hours).
    - In addition to quinidine until oral therapy tolerated

TABLE 82.4

WORLD HEALTH ORGANIZATION CRITERIA FOR SEVERE MALARIA

Criteria for severe malaria requiring parenteral therapy:
- Impaired consciousness/coma
- Severe normocytic anemia
- Renal failure
- Pulmonary edema
- Acute respiratory distress syndrome
- Circulatory shock
- Disseminated intravascular coagulation
- Spontaneous bleeding
- Acidosis
- Hemoglobinuria
- Jaundice
- Repeated generalized convulsions
- Parasitemia of more than 5%

- ○ If hospital pharmacy unable to obtain IV quinidine quickly
  - – Contact Eli Lilly at 1-800-821-0538
  - – Assistance from company to arrange rapid shipment of drug available between hours of 6 a.m. and 6 p.m.
- The CDC may also be contacted for advice at malaria hotline.
- Two aspects of quinidine therapy in this setting are very important to remember.
  - First is the possibility of ventricular arrhythmias.
  - Prolongation of the Q-T$_C$ interval is commonly seen during quinidine therapy
  - Careful monitoring of ECG and electrolytes is mandatory
  - Avoid combining with other drugs that prolong Q-T$_C$ interval.
  - Second is propensity of quinidine and quinine to cause hypoglycemia
    - Given likelihood of hypoglycemia in severe malaria due to the disease itself, serum glucose must be carefully monitored and supplemented as necessary
    - Quinidine is administered in the ICU, with the assistance of a cardiologist if needed.
- Recommended by the CDC that exchange transfusion be considered where parasitemia exceeds 10% or when severe complications present.
  - Benefits have not been proven in randomized trial; exchange transfusion has potential benefit of both reducing parasite burden and circulating cytokines and toxins.
  - Exchange transfusion is recommended until parasitemia is below 1%.

ROCKY MOUNTAIN SPOTTED FEVER (RMSF)

- A disease that presents with nonspecific signs and symptoms
- For which there is no specific rapid diagnostic test
- When not treated appropriately has high mortality
- Important for practicing clinician to have a high index of suspicion for RMSF and to be familiar with its epidemiology, clinical manifestations, and treatment

Epidemiology

- RMSF is caused by *Rickettsia rickettsii.*
- In the United States, intracellular bacterium is primarily transmitted by:
  - Dog tick, *Dermacentor variabilis*, in eastern states
  - Wood tick *Dermacentor andersoni*, in Rocky Mountain States
- Ticks are also primary reservoir for *R. rickettsii.*
- Most cases of RMSF occur in the southeastern United States.
  - More than half of all reported cases are from North Carolina, South Carolina, Tennessee, Oklahoma, and Arkansas.
  - Cases have been reported in all 48 continental states except Vermont and Maine.
- Most cases occur between April and September.
- Children are at highest risk of RMSF.
  - Peak incidence is between 5 and 9 years of age.

- Males are reported to be at higher risk.
  - ○ More cases among girls than boys
- Most bites are unnoticed.
  - ○ Tick must be attached for 6 to 10 hours for feeding and infection to take place.

Clinical Manifestations and Pathogenesis

- Rickettsial organisms primarily target and infect endothelial cells.
- Primary pathology consists of diffuse cell injury and increased vascular permeability caused by cell-to-cell spread of organisms after initial hematogenous and lymphatic seeding.
- Infection occurs in virtually all internal organs.
- Vascular injury occurs in lung, heart, brain, gastrointestinal tract, skin, and elsewhere.
- Symptoms typically begin 2 to 14 days after tick bite.
- Virtually all experience classical triad of fever, headache, and rash.
- Rash is present in only about 50% of cases within first 3 days.
  - Rash usually appears by second to fifth day but is absent in about 10%.
  - Rash is often faint in initial stages and more difficult to detect in patients with dark skin.
  - Begins as blanching, pink maculopapular exanthema
  - Most commonly beginning at wrists and ankles
  - Develops into palpable lesions that spread centrally
  - Often becomes petechial and may involve the palms and soles
  - Associated symptoms occurring in more than 50% of patients are:
    - ○ Myalgias
    - ○ Nausea/vomiting
    - ○ Abdominal pain
      - – Serum AST often elevated
      - – Thrombocytopenia and hyponatremia in up to 50% of cases
- Central nervous system abnormalities occur in about 25% and carry poor prognosis.
  - CSF abnormalities are observed in one-third of patients and consist of:
    - ○ Pleocytosis
    - ○ Elevated protein levels
    - ○ CSF glucose usually normal
- Fulminant form of disease, with death occurring in the first 5 days, described
  - Glucose-6-phosphate dehydrogenase deficiency linked to this form of disease
  - Neurologic deficits and limb loss most serious sequelae observed in survivors

Diagnosis

- Delay in diagnosis and seeking medical attention is associated with poor outcome.
- Factors likely to lead to delay in diagnosis include:
  - Absence of rash or delayed appearance of rash

- No history of tick bite
- Presentation early in course of disease
- *R. rickettsii* isolated in culture or demonstrated by immuno-histochemistry in tissue specimens
  - Methods not routinely available
  - Empiric therapy should not await result of laboratory testing
  - Serology likewise useful for confirmation of diagnosis
  - Diagnosis made on basis of epidemiologic and clinical findings described above

Treatment

- Recommended therapy for RMSF is doxycycline
- Administered at a dose of 100 mg twice daily
  - Continued for 7 days and a minimum of 3 days after patient has defervesced
  - Treatment of suspected RMSF instituted promptly with doxycycline either IV or orally
  - Doxycycline for RMSF is not contraindicated in children.

CHAPTER 83 ■ NON-ST ELEVATION ACUTE CORONARY SYNDROME: CONTEMPORARY MANAGEMENT STRATEGIES

OVERVIEW

Definition of Terms

- Acute coronary syndrome (ACS) ranges from ST-segment elevation myocardial infarction (STEMI) to non–ST-segment elevation MI (N-STEMI) and unstable angina (UA). Acute myocardial ischemia may revert to the presymptomatic state or evolve into a non–Q-wave (nontransmural) or Q-wave (transmural) MI (Fig. 83.1).
- The boundaries between UA, N-STEMI, and STEMI are not always well defined. These are different and dynamic clinical manifestations of a continuous pathogenetic spectrum.
- N-STE-ACS is represented by UA and N-STEMI.

Unstable Angina

- Anginal pain is the pivotal symptom; its intensity, duration, and exercise-related threshold are graded according to the Canadian Cardiovascular Society (CCS) classification (Table 83.1). UA may have three clinical presentations (Table 83.2).

- A low threshold for angina (CCS III and IV) is an essential feature of UA. The presence of angina at rest is associated with a worse prognosis and a higher rate of events.
- Extracardiac conditions that intensify or precipitate myocardial ischemia (secondary UA) such as anemia, fever, infection, hypotension, uncontrolled hypertension, hypoxemia, and thyrotoxicosis must be excluded.
- The resting ECG may show transient ST-segment depression and/or T-wave inversion, ST-segment elevation or, rarely, may remain normal. The serum markers (troponin I, troponin T, and CK-MB) may remain between normal biological ranges and levels diagnostic of MI (twice the upper normal limit).
- Prinzmetal variant angina is an atypical ischemic coronary syndrome characterized by sudden onset angina occurring almost exclusively at rest, particularly in the first hours of the day, associated with ST-segment elevation on the ECG. Caused by a focal spasm of a coronary artery, it may be associated with subendocardial and/or transmural myocardial ischemia, acute MI, or severe cardiac arrhythmias—including ventricular tachycardia and fibrillation, and sudden death.

Non–ST-Segment Elevation Myocardial Infarction

- N-STEMI may have symptoms and a clinical pattern indistinguishable from UA. Resting ECG more frequently shows ST-segment depression or T-wave inversion (Fig. 83.2) that may be persistent. ST-segment elevation is sometimes observed but, by definition, never sustained. The serum biomarkers

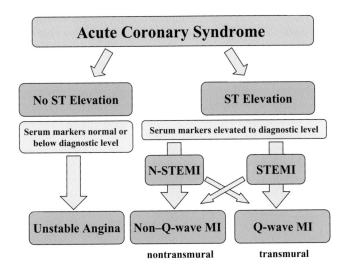

FIGURE 83.1. The interrelationship of the components of ACS on presentation, during evolution and at final outcome [Adapted from Braunwald E, Antman EM, Beasley JW, et al. ACC/AHA 2002 guideline update for the management of patients with unstable angina and non–ST-segment elevation myocardial infarction–summary article: a report of the American College of Cardiology/American Heart Association task force on practice guidelines (Committee on the Management of Patients With Unstable Angina). *J Am Coll Cardiol.* 2002; 40(7):1366–1374].

TABLE 83.1

PRINCIPAL PRESENTATIONS OF UNSTABLE ANGINA

New-Onset Angina	New-onset angina of at least CCS Class III severity.
Increasing Angina	Previously diagnosed angina that has become distinctly more frequent, longer in duration, or lower in threshold (i.e., increased by ≥1 CCS class to at least CCS Class III severity).
Postinfarction Angina	Patients with recent myocardial infarction (within 2 wk) in whom biomarkers of myocardial necrosis have returned within normal range.

From Myler RK, Shaw RE, Stertzer SH, et al. Unstable angina and coronary angioplasty. *Circulation.* 1990;82(3 Suppl):II88–II95.

TABLE 83.2

GRADING OF ANGINA PECTORIS ACCORDING TO THE CANADIAN CARDIOVASCULAR SOCIETY CLASSIFICATION

I	Ordinary physical activity does not cause angina, such as walking 2 blocks or climbing stairs. Angina occurs with strenuous, rapid, or prolonged exertion at work or recreation.
II	"Slight limitation of ordinary activity." Angina occurs on walking or climbing stairs rapidly; walking uphill; walking or stair climbing after meals; in cold, in wind, or under emotional stress; or only during the few hours after awakening. Angina occurs on walking more than 2 blocks on level ground and climbing more than 1 flight of ordinary stairs at a normal pace and under normal conditions.
III	"Marked limitations of ordinary physical activity." Angina occurs on walking 1–2 blocks on the level and climbing 1 flight of stairs under normal conditions and at a normal pace.
IV	"Inability to carry on any physical activity without discomfort—anginal symptoms may be present at rest."

Modified from Braunwald E, Antman EM, Beasley JW, et al.; American College of Cardiology; American Heart Association. Committee on the Management of Patients with Unstable Angina. ACC/AHA 2002 guideline update for the management of patients with unstable angina and non–ST-segment elevation myocardial infarction–summary article: a report of the American College of Cardiology/American Heart Association task force on practice guidelines (Committee on the Management of Patients with Unstable Angina). *J Am Coll Cardiol.* 2002;40(7):1366–1374.

always rise to levels diagnostic for MI, which is the essential difference between UA and N-STEMI.

- **Epidemiology of N-STEMI.** Among those who reach the hospital alive: 13% will die, 8% are left with UA, 1.5% to 3% have new strokes, and 17% to 20% are rehospitalized for a further episode of ACS over the next 6 months. The risk is greatest during the first 15 to 30 days from symptom presentation.

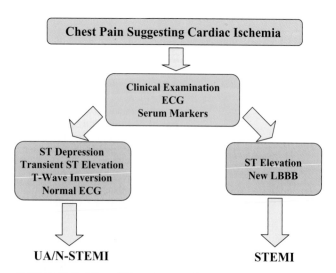

FIGURE 83.2. The differentiation of unstable angina/non–ST-segment elevation myocardial infarction from ST-segment elevation myocardial infarction.

- Pathogenesis of N-STE-ACS:
  - N-STE-ACSs are usually caused by a sudden reduction of myocardial perfusion resulting from a nonocclusive thrombus, a consequence of disruption or erosion of an atherosclerotic plaque. Distal microembolization of thrombus and disrupted plaque components may further reduce perfusion of the distal microvasculature.
  - The vulnerable plaque, more prone to rupture, has a necrotic lipid core infiltrated by inflammatory cells, with intraplaque hemorrhage and abundant vasa vasorum on the adventitial site, surrounded by a thin fibrous cap. Expression of proteases and proteolytic inhibitors that weaken the fibrous cap may play a critical role in plaque rupture.
  - The severity of obstruction and volume of affected myocardium determine the pattern of clinical presentation. Complete occlusion may manifest with a STEMI if a substantial volume of myocardium is involved, although the same occlusion in the presence of extensive collateralization may manifest as an N-STEMI or UA.
  - After clinical stabilization of low-risk ACS patients, exercise stress testing may be appropriate. Early-onset symptoms during exercise, a short exercise time, a fall in blood pressure during exertion, ST-segment elevation, new postexercise ST-segment depression and/or prolonged ST-segment depression are the characteristics of a strongly positive test. Angiography defines the nature and extent of the coronary disease and enables the planning of appropriate revascularization.

EARLY EVALUATION AND RISK STRATIFICATION

Immediate Concerns

- ACS constitutes a clinical emergency, early recognition and initiation of treatment is mandatory. Every patient with chest pain should be comprehensively evaluated, including a history and clinical examination of the cardiovascular system, the immediate recording of a resting ECG, and urgent evaluation of the serum markers of myocardial injury.
- Particular attention must be paid to the factors that influence the patient's risk stratification. These factors are found among the clinical features, the magnitude of ECG change, and the elevation of serum markers of myocardial necrosis. Among those without ST elevation on the ECG, an ACS is diagnosed by the presence of a clinical syndrome of acute ischemia with either pain at rest or a crescendo pattern of ischemic pain with minimal exertion, plus electrocardiographic and/or marker evidence of acute ischemic injury. The predictive accuracy of ST elevation for a final diagnosis of MI is very high, but for N-STEMI, <50% are suspected as infarction on initial presentation.

Symptoms and Physical Examination

- Usually well recognized, the pain varies from mild compressive discomfort to sharp, severe pain located in the anterior chest, particularly substernal, or predominantly involve the mandible, neck, shoulders, either or both arms, the back, or epigastrium.

- Generally of short duration, pain may last >30 minutes without resulting in MI. Spontaneous in onset and unrelated to the usual stressors, it may occur with no—or less than the usual amount of—provocation and may be more severe or more prolonged. Repeated attacks of chest pain, ongoing chest pain before admission, or pain that recurs on treatment is associated with a worse outcome.
- Less frequently, ACS may present with atypical pain or features of an acute transient reduction in cardiac output—tachycardia, hypotension, and poor peripheral circulation, pulmonary venous congestion, breathlessness or pulmonary edema, or rarely a potentially lethal ventricular tachyarrhythmia.
- Shortness of breath, perspiration, palpitations, nausea or vomiting may be present but do not predict the severity of coronary involvement.
- Male gender, age >50 years, early menopause in women, as well as a history of smoking, dyslipidemia, hypertension, diabetes mellitus, and/or a family history of coronary disease all increase the likelihood of ACS.
- There may be no abnormal findings on physical examination; however, a fourth heart sound, mitral regurgitant murmur, or signs of pulmonary congestion are suggestive of transient ischemic myocardial dysfunction.
- Heart failure (HF) is a frequent complication that significantly worsens prognosis; with three to four times the 6 month mortality, longer hospital stays and higher readmission rates. The development of HF during hospitalization—as opposed to HF at admission—is associated with worse outcome and increased frequency of percutaneous coronary intervention (PCI). Those who undergo revascularization have lower cumulative 6-month mortality rates than those who do not.

Electrocardiogram

- The presence of ECG changes, especially when occurring at rest and associated with angina, are a powerful indicator of higher risk. When the other elements of baseline risk are under control, ST deviation conveys the same risk for death whether this deviation is upwards or downwards (Fig. 83.3). New-onset T-wave changes—especially T-wave inversion, although less specific—are also important markers of subendocardial ischemia.

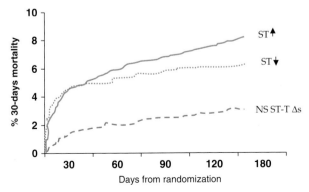

FIGURE 83.3. Probability of 30-day mortality among patients with ACS and different ECG patterns at admission [From Savonitto S, Ardissino D, Granger CB, et al. Prognostic value of the admission electrocardiogram in acute coronary syndromes. *JAMA.* 1999;281: 707–713].

- The normalization of ECG alterations and anginal relief are very important within minutes after sublingual nitrate administration; persistence of pain and ECG alterations for >20 minutes despite repeated nitrates is a marker of increased risk for MI.

Biochemical Markers

- Not all N-STE-ACS patients have elevated serum markers; especially when obtained very shortly after onset, these markers may be within normal limits. All patients with normal serum marker results on presentation must have a second assessment 4 to 6 hours later, or 8 to 12 hours after the onset of symptoms, whichever is longer. Elevated levels of creatine kinase (CK), creatine kinase MB iso-enzyme (CK-MB), troponin T or I, and myoglobin are indicators of myocardial injury (Table 83.3).
- Myoglobin, a very sensitive indicator of infarction, is the earliest to appear in the serum. Its clinical usefulness is limited by the high incidence of false-positive results. CK in conjunction with CK-MB, CK-MB alone, and the troponins are all sensitive and specific markers of myocardial injury/infarction that appear from about 4 hours after the onset of the ischemic event. Whereas CK and CK-MB are cleared within 2 to 3 days, elevated troponin may persist up to 14 days, making them poor markers of early reinfarction.
- A "multimarker strategy" that evaluated CK-MB, troponin I or T, and myoglobin is much superior to any "single-marker" strategy or evaluation without myoglobin in reaching an earlier diagnosis and identifying those at higher risk of death or MI by 30 days. Elevated levels of troponin T or I or CK-MB on admission indicate a poorer outcome (Fig. 83.4). The later appearance of an elevated troponin level, suggesting ongoing ischemia, is also associated with higher risk. In all instances, the risk predictors should complete, not replace, clinical judgment.
- Elevated troponin is a powerful and independent predictor of thrombotic complications, including MI and death. They can be used as part of the measures to identify higher risk and the potential for gain from PCI. Newer-generation assays have higher sensitivity and diagnostic accuracy; even very minor increases predict a higher risk of cardiac complications and death.
- Certain biomarkers reflect an upregulation of the inflammatory/thrombotic systems—for example, high-sensitivity C reactive protein (hsCRP), interleukin 6 (IL-6), CD40 ligand, and platelet–monocyte complexes. The acute phase reactant biomarkers are also elevated as a consequence of myocyte injury. hsCRP is a powerful predictor of death in the following 1 to 2 years. Elevation of both hsCRP and troponin signifies a substantially higher risk of death than either marker alone; the patient is at very low risk of future cardiac events in the absence of both markers. A single B-type natriuretic peptide measured after presentation with an ACS has associations with short-term and long-term risk of death and HF; changes over time also predict long-term outcomes.

Imaging Modalities

- Echocardiographic ultrasounds may be extremely useful in evaluation of left ventricular function, especially with

TABLE 83.3

ADVANTAGES AND DISADVANTAGES OF BIOCHEMICAL CARDIAC MARKERS FOR THE EVALUATION AND MANAGEMENT OF PATIENTS WITH SUSPECTED ACS

Marker	Advantages	Disadvantages
CK-MB	1. Rapid, cost-efficient, accurate assays 2. Ability to detect early reinfarction	1. Loss of specificity in setting of skeletal muscle disease or injury, including surgery 2. Low sensitivity during very early MI (<6 h after symptom onset) or later after symptom onset (>36 h) and for minor myocardial damage (detectable with troponins)
CK-MB Isoforms	1. Early detection of MI	1. Specificity profile similar to that of CK-MB 2. Current assays require special expertise
Myoglobin	1. High sensitivity 2. Useful in early detection of MI 3. Detection of reperfusion 4. Most useful in ruling out MI	1. Very low specificity in setting of skeletal muscle injury or disease 2. Rapid return to normal range limits sensitivity for later presentations
Cardiac Troponins	1. Powerful tool for risk stratification 2. Greater sensitivity and specificity than CK-MB 3. Detection of recent MI up to 2 wk after onset 4. Useful for selection of therapy 5. Detection of reperfusion	1. Low sensitivity in very early phase of MI (<6 h after symptom onset) and requires repeat measurement at 8 to 12 h, if negative 2. Limited ability to detect late minor reinfarction

Modified from Braunwald E, Antman EM, Beasley JW, et al.; American College of Cardiology; American Heart Association. Committee on the Management of Patients with Unstable Angina. ACC/AHA 2002 guideline update for the management of patients with unstable angina and non–ST-segment elevation myocardial infarction–summary article: a report of the American College of Cardiology/American Heart Association task force on practice guidelines (Committee on the Management of Patients with Unstable Angina). *J Am Coll Cardiol.* 2002;40(7):1366–1374.

increasing emphasis on early reperfusion and prevention of left ventricular remodeling. It also excludes nonischemic causes of chest pain, ECG alterations, and elevated biomarker levels. It is noninvasive, cheap, and portable; myocardial contrast echocardiography to assess perfusion also holds promise.

• Single-photon emission computed tomography or magnetic resonance imaging can detect wall motion abnormalities in patients with recent or established infarction, but their role remains to be determined.

• Stress echocardiography and/or myocardial perfusion imaging should be reserved for the patient with a particular clinical problem, when such specialized facilities are available locally. Coronary angiography is advised if the functional test demonstrates ischemia.

ESTIMATION OF THE LEVEL OF RISK AND RISK SCORES

• The patient with N-STE-ACS is at risk of major cardiovascular complications and death, the extent of this risk is dependent on acute and pre-existing risk factors (Table 83.4). These risk factors also predict future cerebrovascular and peripheral vascular complications. Early risk stratification plays a central

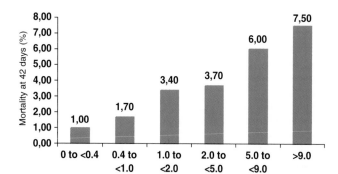

FIGURE 83.4. Relationship between cardiac troponin levels and risk of mortality in patients with ACS. [From Antman EM, Tanasijevic MJ, Thompson B, et al. Cardiac specific troponin I levels to predict the risk of mortality in patients with acute coronary syndromes. *N Engl J Med.* 1996;335:1342–1349].

TABLE 83.4

RISK INDICATORS OF A POOR OUTCOME IN ACS

Event-Related	• Ongoing or recurring chest pain • ST-segment depression/new ischemia on ECG • Elevated serum biomarkers of cardiac injury/infarction • Hemodynamic instability
Preexisting	• Age over 65 y • Three or more risk factors for CAD, especially diabetes mellitus • Aspirin use within 7 d • Known CAD • Prior left ventricular dysfunction

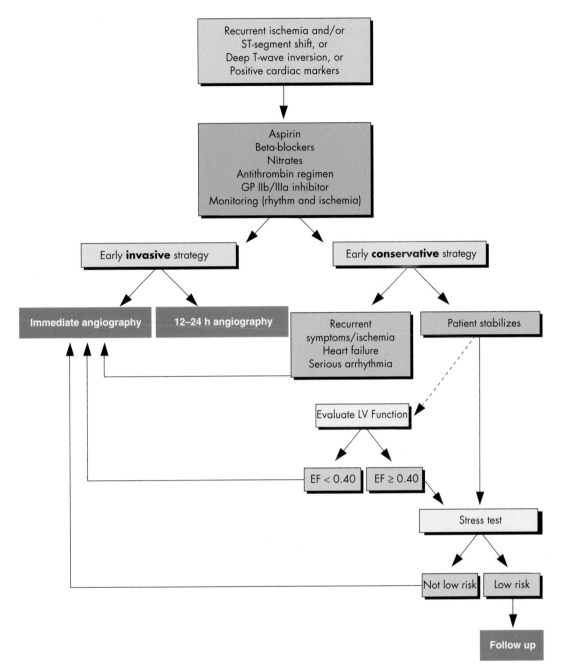

FIGURE 83.5. Acute ischemia pathway [From Braunwald E, Antman EM, Beasley JW, et al. ACC/AHA 2002 guideline update for the management of patients with unstable angina and non-ST-segment elevation myocardial infarction–summary article: a report of the American College of Cardiology/American Heart Association task force on practice guidelines (Committee on the Management of Patients With Unstable Angina). *J Am Coll Cardiol.* 2002;40(7):1366–1374].

role, as the benefit of newer, more aggressive, and costly treatment strategies seem to be proportional to the risk of adverse clinical events (Figs. 83.5 to 83.7).

• Different scores are now available based on initial clinical history, ECG, and laboratory tests that enable early risk stratification on admission (Table 83.5). All these scores were developed for short-term prognosis; however, a significant proportion of adverse events in N-STE-ACS patients occur after the first 30 days, and it is not known whether these risk scores can also predict their occurrence.

HOSPITAL CARE AND MANAGEMENT STRATEGIES: EARLY PHARMACOLOGIC TREATMENT

Control of Pain

• Although analgesics have no influence on the pathophysiological process, narcotic analgesia with IV morphine sulphate and/or sedation with oral benzodiazepines assist in alleviating

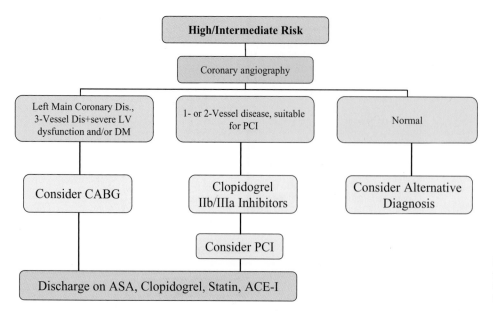

FIGURE 83.6. Algorithm for the management of NSTE-ACS patients at high-intermediate risk undergoing coronary angiography.

pain and anxiety. Morphine may induce nausea and vomiting, it is advisable to premedicate with IV metoclopramide.

- It is important to be aware of other analgesic treatments such as tramadol, a synthetic analogue of codeine, which may have been administered by paramedical staff during transport to the hospital. Intramuscular injection may perturb certain serum markers of cardiac injury/infarction, have variable absorption, and are, in general, more painful and less humane than IV injections.

Anti-ischemic Drugs

- Nitrates act by reducing preload and afterload, promoting coronary vasodilation, relieving coronary vasospasm or vasoconstriction, and by putative effects upon platelet aggregability. These effects combine to improve myocardial blood flow, relieve ischemia and cardiac ischemic pain but do not improve the outcome in ACS. They may be administered sublingually, orally, or intravenously in standard doses (Table 83.6).
- Beta-blockers reduce myocardial oxygen demand and diminish ischemia. Although large trials demonstrate the benefit of β-blockade following acute MI, there is limited evaluation in N-STE-ACS. The dose should be titrated to a resting heart rate of 50 to 60 beats/minute, while maintaining an adequate blood pressure and peripheral perfusion.

- Calcium channel blockers are a diverse group of compounds that cause smooth muscle relaxation by blocking cellular calcium entry, this results in coronary vasodilation and afterload reduction. They should be reserved for the control of intractable chest pain or hypertension that cannot be alleviated by other means. Furthermore, the use of any calcium channel blocker is contraindicated when there is left ventricular dysfunction.
- The dihydropyridine group of calcium channel blockers may increase the resting heart rate and should be used only in combination with β-blockade. Short-acting dihydropyridine calcium channel blockers are detrimental in UA and should not be used at all.
- The nondihydropyridine group—diltiazem and verapamil—reduce the resting heart rate, and thus tend to diminish myocardial oxygen demand. Diltiazem reduces reinfarction and postinfarction angina in non–Q-wave MI, but does not improve mortality. Although β-blockers are preferred in all other patients, diltiazem may be used alone as an alternative therapy if β-blockade is not possible. Although verapamil

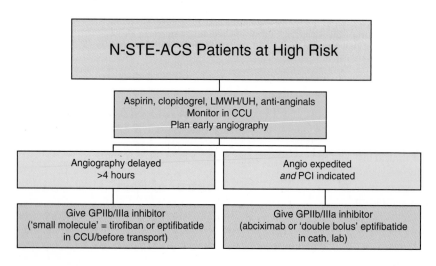

FIGURE 83.7. Algorithm for the treatment of high-risk patients with unstable angina/non–ST-segment elevation myocardial infarction.

TABLE 83.5

RISK SCORES FOR N-STE-ACS

TIMI (0–7)	Age ≥65 y	1
	3 or more risk factors for CAD	1
	Use of ASA (last 7 d)	1
	Known CAD (stenosis ≥50%)	1
	More than 1 episode rest angina in <24 h	1
	ST-segment deviation	1
	Elevated cardiac markers	1
PURSUIT (0–18)	Age, separate points for enrollment diagnosis	
	Decade (UA [MI])	
	50	8 (11)
	60	9 (12)
	70	11 (13)
	80	12 (14)
	Sex	
	Male	1
	Female	0
	Worst CCS-class in previous 6 wk	
	No angina or CCS I/II	0
	CCS III/IV	2
	Signs of heart failure	2
	ST-depression on presenting ECG	1
GRACE (0–258)	Age (y)	
	<40	0
	40–49	18
	50–59	36
	60–69	55
	70–79	73
	≥80	91
	Heart rate (bpm)	
	<70	0
	70–89	7
	90–109	13
	110–149	23
	150–199	36
	≥200	46
	Systolic BP (mm Hg)	
	<80	63
	80–99	58
	100–119	47
	120–139	37
	140–159	26
	160–199	11
	≥200	0
	Creatinine (mg/dL)	
	0–0.39	2
	0.4–0.79	5
	0.8–1.19	8
	1.2–1.59	11
	1.6–1.99	14
	2–3.99	23
	≥4	31
	Killip class	
	Class I	0
	Class II	21
	Class III	43
	Class IV	64
	Cardiac arrest at admission	43
	Elevated cardiac markers	15
	ST-segment deviation	30

has similar effects to diltiazem, its effects in ACS have not been evaluated.

Antiplatelet Therapy (see Table 83.7)

- Aspirin irreversibly inhibits cyclooxygenase-1, thus reducing the generation of thromboxane A2, a potent mediator of platelet aggregation. The most recent update of the Antithrombotic Trialists' Collaboration, based on 287 studies in 13,500 patients, demonstrates a highly significant reduction in the risk of MI/stroke/vascular death as a result of antiplatelet treatment versus control. Overall, the event rates were 13.2% in control patients and 10.7% with antiplatelet therapy, a 22% relative risk reduction. In acute MI, and in other high-risk patients, the absolute and relative risk reductions were greater: 23 per 1,000 fewer vascular deaths and 13 per 1,000 fewer MIs. The bleeding risk doubles for aspirin doses above 160 mg daily, with no improved efficacy. Without specific contraindications—intolerance or allergy; active bleeding; hemophilia; severe hypertension; retinal, genitourinary, or gastrointestinal bleeding; active peptic ulcer—aspirin should be given to all patients with N-STE-ACS as soon as possible and continued indefinitely. Additional antiplatelet treatment requires evidence of benefit on top of aspirin, rather than as an alternative to aspirin.

- Thienopyridines (ticlopidine and clopidogrel) inhibit adenosine diphosphate–mediated platelet aggregation, clopidogrel has superseded ticlopidine due to superior safety and more rapid onset of action. The blockade of adenosine diphosphate receptors is irreversible but relatively slow to manifest, several days for ticlopidine, and a substantial number of individuals appear to be resistant to the antiplatelet action of thienopyridines. For this reason, a high loading dose of 300 to 600 mg of clopidogrel or 500 mg of ticlopidine can be used to obtain a rapid onset of action. In N-STE-ACS, the AHA/ACC guidelines recommend approximately 9 months of treatment with clopidogrel.

- Thienopyridines reduce the risk of stent thrombotic occlusion and are now part of standard treatment for at least 4 weeks in all patients undergoing elective PCI. With drug eluting stents, at least 6 months and perhaps 12 months of clopidogrel and aspirin are required.

- As the antiaggregation effects of aspirin and thienopyridines are mediated by different mechanisms, an additive benefit may exist. The CURE trial tested clopidogrel in 12,562 N-STE-ACS patients on top of background treatment and aspirin, A 2.1% absolute risk reduction (20% relative risk reduction) occurred in the frequency of nonfatal MI, stroke, or cardiovascular death. Although the absolute benefits were greatest in the first 3 months of treatment, the relative risk reduction was the same beyond 3 months. Approximately 1% more patients experienced major bleeding.

- The association of aspirin and clopidogrel increases the risk of bleeding during major surgery and coronary surgery (CABG), thus clopidogrel should be interrupted 5 to 7 days before elective surgery. If early diagnostic catheterization is scheduled within 24 to 36 hours, clopidogrel can be initiated after coronary angiography when it is clear that CABG will not be undertaken; in the case of immediate percutaneous revascularization, the therapy can be initiated with a loading dose immediately. In candidates for very urgent CABG, a small molecule Gp IIb/IIIa inhibitor—eptifibatide or tirofiban—can be used before surgery.

TABLE 83.6

DOSAGES OF NITROGLYCERIN AND NITRATES IN ANGINA

Agent	Route	Dosage
Nitroglycerin	• Sublingual tablets • Spray • Transdermal • Intravenous	• 0.3–0.6 mg up to 1.5 mg • 0.4 mg as needed • 0.2–0.8 mg/h every 12 h • 5–200 mcg/min
Isosorbide dinitrate	• Oral • Oral, slow release	• 5–80 mg, 2 or 3 times daily • 40 mg 1 or 2 times daily
Isosorbide mononitrate	• Oral • Oral, slow release	• 20 mg twice daily • 60–240 mg once daily
Pentaerythritol tetranitrate	• Sublingual	• 10 mg as needed
Erythritol tetranitrate	• Sublingual • Oral	• 5–10 mg as needed • 10–30 mg 3 times daily

Modified from Braunwald E, Antman EM, Beasley JW, et al.; American College of Cardiology; American Heart Association. Committee on the Management of Patients with Unstable Angina. ACC/AHA 2002 guideline update for the management of patients with unstable angina and non–ST-segment elevation myocardial infarction–summary article: a report of the American College of Cardiology/American Heart Association task force on practice guidelines (Committee on the Management of Patients with Unstable Angina). *J Am Coll Cardiol.* 2002;40(7):1366–1374.

TABLE 83.7

COMMONLY USED ANTIPLATELET AND ANTICOAGULANT AGENTS IN UNSTABLE ANGINA AND N-STEMI—DRUG DOSES AND SPECIAL PRECAUTIONS

Agent	Dose	Precautions
Oral antiplatelet agent		
Aspirin	Initially 300 mg p.o.; then 75–150 mg daily	• GI bleeding
Clopidogrel (Plavix/Iscover)	Initial loading dose of 300 mg (or 600 mg); then 75 mg daily	• Peptic ulceration • Aspirin allergy • Increased bleeding risk • Antiplatelet therapy contraindicated
Heparins		
Unfractionated heparin	60 U/kg IV bolus to a maximum of 4,000 units; then 12 units/kg/h infusion to a maximum of 1,000 units/h	• Monitor PTT: keep at 50–70 s
Low-molecular-weight heparin	120 IU/kg subcutaneously every 12 h	• Any abnormal bleeding
Dalteparin (Fragmin)	1 mg/kg subcutaneously every 12 h	• Any major surgery <30 d
Enoxaparin (Clexane)		• Thrombocytopenia • Risk of bleeding • As above
Glycoprotein IIb/IIIa inhibitors		
Eptifibatide (Integrilin)	180 μg/kg IV over 1–2 min; then 2 μg/kg/min infusion over 72 h or until hospital discharge, whichever occurs first	• Bleeding disorder
	When initiating immediately before PCI, as above but repeat 180 μg/kg IV bolus 10 min after the first bolus	• Thrombocytopenia • Surgery <6 wk • Abnormal bleed <30 d • Active GI ulceration • Puncture of a noncompressible vessel • Prior stroke, organic CNS pathology • Any systolic BP >180 mm Hg during the acute event • As above • 1/2 dose in renal insufficiency
Tirofiban (Aggrastat)	0.4 μg/kg/min IV over 30 min; then 0.1 μg/kg/min infusion for 48–108 h	• As above
Abciximab (ReoPro)	0.25 mg/kg IV bolus 10–60 min before PCI, then 10 μg/min IV infusion for 12 h	

- Glycoprotein IIb/IIIa Receptor Antagonists. Platelet aggregation involves the GP IIb/IIIa receptor linked to fibrinogen or von Willebrand factor. IV GP IIb/IIIa receptor antagonists have been extensively tested in patients with ACS and, in a meta-analysis of all the major randomized trials, the absolute risk reduction for death or MI at 30 days was 1% (11.8% control vs. 10.8% with Gp IIb/IIIa). The absolute treatment benefit was largest in high-risk patients—in particular, those with evidence of troponin release or those undergoing acute PCI. Among those without troponin elevation or PCI, no significant benefits were observed.
  - Abciximab may reduce the composite of death, MI, or urgent target vessel revascularization within 30 days in patients with N-STEMI treated with PCI and clopidogrel.
  - Tirofiban given several hours before coronary angiography may improve myocardial perfusion, a higher myocardial contrast echocardiographic score, and lower rates of post-procedure troponin elevation in high-risk ACS patients.
  - Upstream GPI therapy may be more effective than downstream use in moderate- to high-risk patients managed with an invasive strategy in whom immediate catheterization is not planned.

Anticoagulation Therapy

- Thrombin (factor IIa) is a highly potent stimulus fibrin generation and platelet activation. In addition, it leads to monocyte chemotaxis, mitogenesis, increased permeability of the vascular wall, and secretion of cytokines and growth factors from smooth muscle cells. Effective antithrombotic treatment requires the inhibition of both platelet function and thrombin.
- Unfractionated heparin has been widely used but suffers from practical difficulties in maintaining antithrombin activity within the therapeutic range, which are influenced by acute-phase proteins and binding to antithrombins. Heparin, either unfractionated or low-molecular-weight heparin (LMWH), reduces absolute rates of death or MI.
- Direct antithrombins may provide significant advantages over the indirect inhibitors (unfractionated and LMWH), though hirudins are only approved for treatment of heparin-induced thrombocytopenia and not licensed for ACS. LMWHs partially inhibit factor Xa, but newer specific inhibitors of Xa have been developed—for example, bivalirudin and fondaparinux. Bivalirudin reduces bleeding compared to treatment with GP IIb/IIIa inhibitors. Fondaparinux may substantially reduce major bleeding and improve long-term mortality and morbidity compared to LMWH.
- Ximelagatran is an orally administered, direct thrombin antagonist. It does not require anticoagulation monitoring, and is administered as a fixed dose and may reduce the frequency of death, nonfatal MI, and severe recurrent ischemia. As an alternative to warfarin in the management of atrial fibrillation, it demonstrates similar efficacy but less bleeding. A potential hazard involves alterations in liver enzymes to at least three times the upper limit of normal, which appears to resolve with or without cessation of drug treatment.

HMG-CoA Reductase Inhibitors

- Intensive therapy with atorvastatin, 80 mg, compared with pravastatin, 40 mg, should begin in the early post-ACS phase.

This reduces risk of death, MI, stroke, or rehospitalization for recurrent ACS; consistent with greater early pleiotropic effects. A number of potential early benefits of statins independent of LDL have been postulated and include favorable effects on inflammation, endothelial function (including flow-mediated dilation), and the coagulation cascade. This early benefit may be associated with the more profound reduction in CRP achieved.

- To achieve goals of LDL <70 mg/dL and CRP <2 mg/L associated with relatively lower rates of death and recurrent ischemic complications, better control of traditional risk factors and even more potent pharmacologic therapy are necessary. Dose adjustment is not required in patients who achieve very low LDL concentrations, <40 mg/dL. Statins may be of greatest benefit when combined with aspirin and clopidogrel.

HOSPITAL CARE AND MANAGEMENT STRATEGIES: INVASIVE STRATEGIES

The Role of Coronary Angiography

- Presently, coronary angiography represents the only reliable tool for the assessment of coronary anatomy in patients with N-STE-ACS. Patients with high-risk coronary lesions—left main disease, three vessel disease, and proximal left anterior descending coronary artery disease—represent about 50% of all patients with N-STE-ACS.
- Despite the use of risk scores and biomarkers of myocardial damage, it is frequently impossible identify these high-risk patients who are most likely to benefit from revascularization both in terms of survival and symptom improvement (Table 83.8).
- Thus, the concept of low- and high-risk patients suggested by the various scores derived by investigational studies and registry is rather relative. According to the TIMI risk score, about 50% of patients with N-STE-ACS are in the low risk subgroup (score <3); nevertheless about 25% of these patients develop a major event—death, non-fatal MI, or urgent revascularization—within 14 days from

TABLE 83.8

HIGH-RISK FEATURES FAVORING AN EARLY INVASIVE STRATEGY

- Recurrent angina/ischemia at rest or with low-level activities despite intensive anti-ischemic therapy
- Elevated troponin level
- New or presumably new ST-segment depression
- Recurrent angina/ischemia with symptoms of heart failure, an S_3 gallop, pulmonary edema, worsening rales, or new or worsening mitral regurgitation
- High-risk findings on noninvasive stress testing
- Left ventricular systolic dysfunction (ejection fraction <40% on a noninvasive study)
- Hemodynamic instability
- Sustained ventricular tachycardia
- Percutaneous coronary intervention within

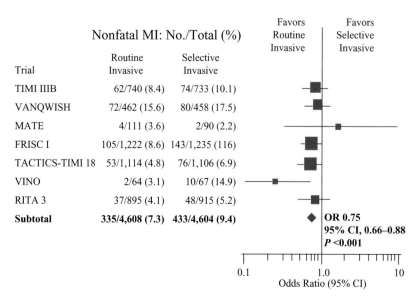

Trial	Nonfatal MI: No./Total (%)		
	Routine Invasive	Selective Invasive	
TIMI IIIB	62/740 (8.4)	74/733 (10.1)	
VANQWISH	72/462 (15.6)	80/458 (17.5)	
MATE	4/111 (3.6)	2/90 (2.2)	
FRISC I	105/1,222 (8.6)	143/1,235 (116)	
TACTICS-TIMI 18	53/1,114 (4.8)	76/1,106 (6.9)	
VINO	2/64 (3.1)	10/67 (14.9)	
RITA 3	37/895 (4.1)	48/915 (5.2)	
Subtotal	**335/4,608 (7.3)**	**433/4,604 (9.4)**	OR 0.75 95% CI, 0.66–0.88 *P* <0.001

FIGURE 83.8. Odds of nonfatal myocardial infarction (MI) from randomization to end of follow-up in a meta-analysis of 7 trials of routine versus selective invasive management of acute coronary syndromes. *P* = 0.51 for heterogeneity across the trials. CI,confidence interval; OR,odds ratio. [From Bavry AA, Kumbhani DJ, Rassi AN, et al. Benefit of early invasive therapy in acute coronary syndromes: a meta-analysis of contemporary randomized clinical trials. *J Am Coll Cardiol.* 2006;48:1319–1325].

hospitalization. Thus, all patients with N-STE-ACS should be regarded at risk to develop major coronary events.

Early Conservative versus Invasive Strategies

- An early invasive approach appears to improve long-term survival and reduce late nonfatal MI and rehospitalization for symptom recurrence versus conservative strategies. The issue is not whether but when a patient with N-STE-ACS should undergo coronary angiography and eventually revascularization.
- The goal in N-STE-ACS should be to perform early invasive therapy within 48 hours from hospital admission (Fig. 83.8). Obviously, coronary angiography should be anticipated if clinical instability occurs.
- The best revascularization strategy (PCI or CABG) should be evaluated for each case according to coronary anatomy, clinical symptoms, and associated diseases.

CHAPTER 84 ■ ST ELEVATION MYOCARDIAL INFARCTION (STEMI): CONTEMPORARY MANAGEMENT STRATEGIES

OVERVIEW OF ST ELEVATION MYOCARDIAL INFARCTION

Definition of Terms

- The definition of acute myocardial infarction (MI) is **death of cardiac myocytes** caused by prolonged ischemia. Electrocardiographic (ECG) changes are associated with elevation of the biomarkers of myocardial damage. The standard biomarker for myocardial damage is cardiac troponin (I or T), which has high specificity and sensitivity, and creatine kinin (CK)-MB mass, which is less tissue-specific but more specific for irreversible injury.

- Acute evolving MI in the presence of clinically appropriate symptoms:
  - **ST elevation MI (STEMI),** new ST-segment elevation at the J-point with the cutoff points ≥0.2 mV in V_1 through V_3 and ≥0.1 mV in other leads, usually indicates transmural MI.
  - **Non-ST elevation MI (N-STEMI),** ST-segment depression or T-wave abnormalities with elevated biomarkers, usually indicates subendocardial MI.
- Clinically established MI defined by any Q wave in leads V_1 through V_3, or a Q wave ≥0.03 s in leads I, II, aVL, aVF, V_4, V_5, or V_6.
- Recently, a global task force redefined the ESC/ACC criteria for the diagnosis of MI from various perspectives

TABLE 84.1

NEW DEFINITION OF MYOCARDIAL INFARCTION

Criteria for acute MI

The term *MI* should be used when there is evidence of myocardial necrosis in a clinical setting consistent with myocardial ischemia. Under these conditions, any of the following criteria meets the diagnosis for MI:

- Detection of rise and/or fall of cardiac biomarkers (preferably troponin) with at least one value above the 99th percentile of the URL together with evidence of myocardial ischemia with at least one of the following:
  - Symptoms of ischemia
  - ECG changes indicative of new ischemia (new ST-T changes or new LBBB)
  - Development of pathological Q waves in the ECG
  - Imaging evidence of new loss of viable myocardium or new regional wall motion abnormality
  - Sudden, unexpected cardiac death, involving cardiac arrest, often with symptoms suggestive of myocardial ischemia and accompanied by presumably new ST elevation, or new LBBB, and/or evidence of fresh thrombus by coronary angiography and/or at autopsy, but death occurring before blood samples could be obtained, or at a time before appearance of cardiac biomarkers in the blood
- For PCI and CABG in patients with normal baseline troponin values, elevation of cardiac biomarkers above the 99th percentile URL are indicative of periprocedural myocardial necrosis. By convention, increases of biomarkers $>3 \times$ 99th percentile URL has been designated as defining PCI-related MI and elevations of biomarkers $>5 \times$ 99th percentile URL plus either new pathological Q waves or new LBBB or angiographically documented new graft or native coronary artery occlusion, or imaging evidence of new loss of viable myocardium, have been designated as defining CABG-related MI.
- Pathological findings of an acute MI

Criteria for prior MI

Any one of the following criteria meets the diagnosis for prior MI:

- Development of new pathological Q waves with or without symptoms
- Imaging evidence of a region of loss of viable myocardium that is thinned and fails to contract, in the absence of a nonischemic cause
- Pathological findings of a healed or healing MI

MI, myocardial infarction; URL, upper reference limit; ECG, electrocardiogram; LBBB, left bundle branch block; PCI, percutaneous coronary intervention;. CABG, coronary artery bypass grafting.

(Table 84.1). Clinically, the various types of MI, according to this new definition, can be classified as shown in Table 84.2.

Pathogenesis of ST Elevation Myocardial Infarction and Its Complications

- ST elevation represents transmural ischemia in response to total and prolonged occlusion (less frequently spasm) of a major coronary artery.
- Dysfunction or disruption of critical myocardial structures may require an immediate combination of pharmacologic, catheter-based, and surgical treatments.
- This may lead to **ventricular remodeling,** referring to changes in size, shape, and thickness of the left ventricle involving both infarcted and noninfarcted segments. An extra load is placed on the residual functioning myocardium, which results in compensatory hypertrophy. Additionally, cardiac dysrhythmias may result from electrical instability, pump failure/excessive sympathetic stimulation, and conduction disturbances.

Early Evaluation

Immediate Concerns and Questions to be Addressed at the Initial Evaluation

- Rapid diagnosis and early risk stratification can improve outcomes (Table 84.3). A working diagnosis of acute MI is usually based on the history of severe **chest pain** lasting for

TABLE 84.2

CLINICAL CLASSIFICATION OF DIFFERENT TYPES OF MYOCARDIAL INFARCTION

Type 1
Spontaneous MI related to ischemia due to a primary coronary event such as plaque erosion and/or rupture, fissuring, or dissection

Type 2
MI secondary to ischemia due to either increased oxygen demand or decreased supply (e.g., coronary spasm, coronary embolism, anemia, arrhythmias, hypertension, or hypotension)

Type 3
Sudden unexpected cardiac death, including cardiac arrest, often with symptoms suggestive of myocardial ischemia, accompanied by presumably new ST elevation, or new LBBB, or evidence of fresh thrombus in a coronary artery by angiography and/or autopsy, but death occurring before blood samples could be obtained, or at a time before the appearance of cardiac biomarkers in the blood

Type 4a
MI associated with PCI

Type 4b
MI associated with stent thrombosis as documented by angiography or at autopsy

Type 5
MI associated with CABG

MI, myocardial infarction; LBBB, left bundle branch block; PCI, percutaneous coronary intervention; CABG, coronary artery bypass grafting.

AIMS OF ACUTE MANAGEMENT OF ST ELEVATION MYOCARDIAL INFARCTION

- Rapidly establish a working diagnosis after presentation.
- Treat acute dysrhythmic and hemodynamic complications, including cardiac arrest.
- Provide prompt pain relief and adequate arterial oxygen concentration.
- Initiate reperfusion therapy to limit the extent of infarction and minimize the complications of pump failure and dysrhythmias.
- Treat complications of acute myocardial infarction.
- Provide risk assessment for longer-term management and to initiate secondary prevention.

20 minutes or more, not responding to nitroglycerin (Fig. 84.1). Important clues are a previous history of coronary artery disease and radiation of the pain to the neck, lower jaw, or left arm. The pain may not be severe and, particularly in the elderly, other presentations such as **fatigue, dyspnea, syncope,** and feeling faint or "poorly" are common.
- Physical signs may include hypotension or a narrow pulse pressure, irregularities of the pulse, bradycardia or tachycardia, and a third heart sound. The presence and severity of basal pulmonary rales is a pivotal tool for an early risk stratification of STEMI patients (Table 84.4).

- Certain patients, including the elderly and diabetics, may present **without typical symptoms.**
- Perform immediate **ECG;** if ST-segment elevations or new or presumed new left bundle branch block are present, reperfusion therapy should be initiated as soon as possible. During the early evolution of infarction, the ECG may be without significant ST elevation. It is important to institute continuous ST monitoring or perform repeat ECGs to ensure that such evolution is detected promptly. However, even in proven infarction, it may never demonstrate the classic features of ST-segment elevation and new Q waves.
- **Alternative diagnoses** are presented in Table 84.5. Myocardial perfusion scintigraphy or magnetic resonance imaging may be used to detect the presence of ischemia or infarction, and a normal result also effectively excludes significant MI.
- First blood sample for **biomarkers** may be negative. It is not reasonable to wait for the next results before initiating a reperfusion regimen. Elevated biomarkers are sometimes helpful in deciding to initiate reperfusion therapy (e.g., left bundle branch block). When the history, ECG, and serum biomarkers are not diagnostic of acute MI, the patient can proceed safely to stress testing for underlying coronary artery disease.

Hemodynamic Compromise and Cardiac Arrest

- Resuscitation may be required for ventricular fibrillation (VF) or ventricular tachycardia (VT) with diminished cardiac output. With extensive MI and/or heart failure, additional

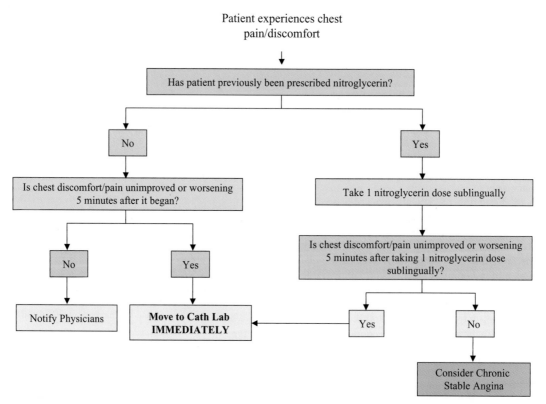

FIGURE 84.1. Patient (advance) instructions for nitroglycerin use and emergency medical service (EMS) contact in the setting of non–trauma-related chest discomfort/pain. (Modified from Antman EM, Anbe DT, Armstrong PW, et al. American College of Cardiology; American Heart Association Task Force on Practice Guidelines; Canadian Cardiovascular Society. ACC/AHA guidelines for the management of patients with ST elevation myocardial infarction: a report of the American College of Cardiology/American Heart Association Task Force on Practice Guidelines [committee to revise the 1999 Guidelines for the Management of Patients with Acute Myocardial Infarction]. *Circulation.* 2004;110[9]:e82–e292.)

TABLE 84.4

PERCENT MORTALITY BY KILLIP CLASS[a]

Killip class	Killip and Kimball (in-hospital)	Fibrinolytic trials (30 d)			
		GISSI-1		International Study Group: Fibrinolytic	ASSENT-2: Fibrinolytic
		Placebo	Fibrinolytic		
I = no rales	6	7	6	5	5
II = rales <50%	17	20	16	18	13
III = pulmonary edema	38	39	33	32	26
IV = cardiogenic shock	81	70	70	72	56[b]

[a]Values cited are subject to survivor bias.
[b]Highly selected group of patients.

circulatory support may be necessary, including an intra-aortic balloon pump, as a bridge to revascularization.

Early In-Hospital Care and Management Strategies

Pharmacologic Treatment in the Acute Phase of ST Elevation Myocardial Infarction

- **Pain management** is a key element, directed toward relief of myocardial ischemia and necrosis symptoms, heart's metabolic demands, anxiety, and apprehension. **Morphine**

TABLE 84.5

DIFFERENTIAL DIAGNOSIS OF ST ELEVATION MYOCARDIAL INFARCTION

Life threatening
- Aortic dissection
- Pulmonary embolus
- Perforating ulcer
- Tension pneumothorax
- Boerhaave syndrome (esophageal rupture with mediastinitis)

Other cardiovascular and nonischemic entities
- Pericarditis
- Atypical angina
- Early repolarization
- Wolff-Parkinson-White syndrome
- Deeply inverted T waves suggestive of a central nervous system lesion or apical hypertrophic cardiomyopathy
- Left ventricular hypertrophy with strain
- Brugada syndrome
- Myocarditis
- Hyperkalemia
- Bundle branch blocks
- Vasospastic angina
- Hypertrophic cardiomyopathy

Other noncardiac entities
- Gastroesophageal reflux and spasm
- Chest wall pain
- Pleurisy
- Peptic ulcer disease
- Panic attack
- Biliary or pancreatic pain
- Cervical disc or neuropathic pain
- Somatization and psychogenic pain disorder

sulfate remains the analgesic agent of choice for pain for patients with pulmonary edema and promotes peripheral arterial and venous dilation.
- **Fibrinolysis**
  - Prompt and effective reperfusion by pharmacologic therapy is the cornerstone of treatment for STEMI and can diminish infarct size and major cardiac complications (Table 84.6).
  - Limitations of fibrinolysis: The major limitation is that reperfusion is gradual and incomplete or inadequate in a significant proportion of patients. This ranges from about 40% showing failure to achieve thrombolysis in myocardial infarction (TIMI) 3 flow within the first 3 hours of reperfusion therapy when streptokinase is used, to 20% to 30% with tissue plasminogen activator (tPA) or tenecteplase (TNK) (Table 84.7).
  - The principal hazards are **stroke and intracranial hemorrhage**; about four extra strokes, two fatal, occur per 1,000 patients treated. Accelerated tPA (alteplase) results in fewer deaths than streptokinase but at the risk of additional strokes. Single-bolus agents provide logistic advantages and

TABLE 84.6

CONTRAINDICATIONS TO FIBRINOLYTIC THERAPY

Absolute contraindications
- Hemorrhagic stroke or stroke of unknown origin at any time
- Ischemic stroke in preceding 6 mo
- Central nervous system damage or neoplasms
- Recent major trauma/surgery/head injury (within preceding 3 wk)
- Gastrointestinal bleeding within the last month
- Known bleeding disorder
- Aortic dissection

Relative contraindications
- Transient ischemic attack in preceding 6 mo
- Oral anticoagulant therapy
- Pregnancy or within 1 wk postpartum
- Noncompressible punctures
- Traumatic resuscitation
- Refractory hypertension (systolic blood pressure >180 mmHg)
- Advanced liver disease
- Infective endocarditis
- Active peptic ulcer

TABLE 84.7

COMPARISON OF APPROVED FIBRINOLYTIC AGENTS

	Streptokinase	Alteplase	Reteplase	Tenecteplase-tPA
Dose	1.5 MU over 30–60 min	Up to 100 mg in 90 min based on weight[a]	10 U × 2 each over 2 min	30–50 mg based on weight[b]
Bolus administration	No	No	Yes	Yes
Antigenic	Yes	No	No	No
Allergic reactions	Yes	No	No	No
Systemic fibrinogen depletion	Marked	Mild	Moderate	Minimal
90-min patency rates (approximate %)	50	75	7	75
TIMI grade 3 flow (%)	32	54	60	63
Cost per dose (US $)	613	2,974	2,750	2,833 for 50 mg

MU, mega units; TIMI, thrombolysis in myocardial infarction.
[a]Bolus 15 mg, infusion 0.75 mg/kg × 30 min (maximum 50 mg);, then 0.5 mg/kg, not to exceed 35 mg over the next 60 min to an overall maximum of 100 mg.
[b]Thirty milligrams for weight <60 kg; 35 mg for 60–69 kg; 40 mg for 70–79 mg; 45 mg for 80–89 kg; and 50 mg for 90 kg or more.

minimize delay in the prehospital and emergency room settings; both reteplase-PA or weight-adjusted TNK have equivalent efficacy to accelerated tPA. TNK has a lower rate of noncerebral bleeds and a lesser need for blood transfusion.

- Prehospital fibrinolysis: Myocardial salvage is highly dependent on the time from the beginning of symptoms to reperfusion. Efficacy of thrombolysis decreases exponentially in patients treated >3 hours after the onset of chest pain. Prehospital thrombolysis results in decreased mortality and likely superior myocardial salvage compared with in-hospital thrombolysis and possibly also primary percutaneous coronary intervention (PCI).
- Fibrinolysis combined with newer antithrombotic agents: To improve the rates of TIMI 3 flow by pharmacologic reperfusion therapy, glycoprotein (GP) IIb/IIIa inhibitor and antithrombin (bivalirudin) have been tried with thrombolytics. Neither combination has been shown to offer any advantage; in patients older than 70 years, the combination increased the risk of intracranial hemorrhage and extracranial bleeding.
- Anti-ischemic drugs
  - Oxygen: Even with uncomplicated MI, some patients are modestly hypoxemic initially, presumably from ventilation/perfusion mismatch and excessive lung water. Nitrates reduce preload and afterload through peripheral arterial and venous dilation, improve coronary flow by relaxation of epicardial coronary arteries, and dilate collateral vessels, potentially creating a more favorable subendocardial-to-epicardial flow ratio. Nitrates in all forms should be avoided in patients with initial systolic blood pressures <90 mmHg or ≥30 mmHg below baseline, marked bradycardia or tachycardia, or known or suspected right ventricular (RV) infarction.
  - β-Adrenergic blockers within 24 hours of suspected STEMI onset are associated with reduced risk of reinfarction and VF but increased risk of cardiogenic shock. In general, consider starting β-blocker therapy in hospital only when the hemodynamic condition after STEMI has been stabilized.
- Antiplatelet therapy
  - Aspirin should be given to the patient with suspected STEMI as early as possible and continued indefinitely, regard-

less of the strategy for reperfusion or whether additional antiplatelet agents are administered; known true aspirin allergy is the only exception.
- Thienopyridine: A thienopyridine (e.g., ticlopidine or clopidogrel) should be substituted when aspirin is contraindicated because of hypersensitivity or major gastrointestinal intolerance. Combination therapy, clopidogrel and low-dose aspirin, improves infarct-related coronary artery patency after fibrinolytic therapy in STEMI, safely reduces in-hospital mortality and major vascular events, and is recommended for all patients after stent implantation. Prasugrel, a new thienopyridine derivative, is 10 times more potent but results in low and similar rates of bleeding when compared with clopidogrel.
- Platelet glycoprotein IIb/IIIa receptor antagonists: Adjunctive treatment with GP IIb/IIIa (abciximab, tirofiban, and eptifibatide) blockade reduces the incidence of acute ischemic events by 35% to 50% among the broad population of patients undergoing primary PCI. GP IIb/IIIa inhibitors decrease coronary thrombus, improve TIMI flow grade, enhance epicardial reperfusion when combined with thrombolysis, improve 30-day clinical outcomes after MI (Fig. 84.2) including reinfarction, speed resolution of ST-segment elevation, and improve coronary artery flow reserve and myocardial blush grade. Abciximab in STEMI is associated with a significant reduction in 30-day and long-term mortality in patients treated with primary PCI but not fibrinolysis where a higher risk of major bleeding complications is observed.
- Antithrombotic therapy
  - Unfractionated heparin (UFH): In fibrinolytic therapy, recommendations for UFH therapy depend on the agent chosen. The nonspecific fibrinolytic agents (streptokinase, anistreplase, and urokinase) produce a systemic coagulopathy, including production of fibrinogen degradation products and depletion of factors V and VIII; the need for adjunctive systemic anticoagulation is less compelling. When primary PCI is chosen as the route of reperfusion, weight-adjusted boluses of heparin in the range of 70 to 100 U/kg are recommended based on angioplasty observations that an activated clotting time of at least 250 to 350 seconds is associated with a lower rate of complications. When

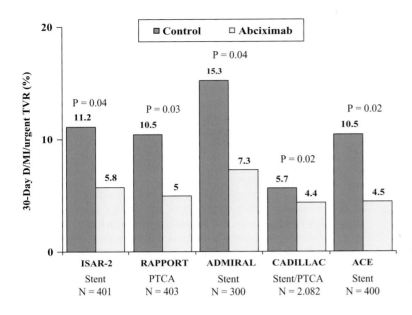

FIGURE 84.2. Randomized trials demonstrating the clinical benefits of abciximab in the setting of ST elevation myocardial infarction (STEMI). D, death; MI, myocardial infarction; TVR, target vessel revascularization; PTCA, percutaneous transluminal coronary angioplasty.

GP IIb/IIIa antagonists are used, the UFH bolus should be reduced to 50 to 70 U/kg to achieve a target activated clotting time of 200 seconds.

- Low-molecular-weight heparin (LMWH). In the setting of STEMI, LMWH may be an attractive alternative to UFH as ancillary therapy to patients with and without fibrinolysis. The two LMWHs studied most extensively are enoxaparin and dalteparin.
- Direct antithrombin agents: Compared to UFH, a 25% reduction in reinfarction results with either hirudin or bivalirudin treatment in STEMI, but univalent thrombin inhibitors such as argatroban, efegatran, and inogatran are less efficacious. Bivalirudin alone is as safe and effective long term as heparin or heparin and GP IIb/IIIa in STEMI.
- **Fondaparinux** binds antithrombin III, inducing a conformational change that increases its anti-Xa activity more than 300 times, resulting in dose-dependent inhibition of factor Xa. In STEMI, particularly those not undergoing primary PCI, fondaparinux seems to reduce mortality and reinfarction without increasing bleeding and strokes.
- Other pharmacologic agents
- Angiotensin-converting enzyme inhibitors should be given to patients with impaired left ventricular (LV) function or congestive heart failure (CHF) in the early phase of an MI and should be started in the first 24 hours after STEMI.
- Calcium antagonists: Immediate-release nifedipine does not reduce the incidence of reinfarction or mortality and may be particularly detrimental in patients with hypotension or tachycardia. Immediate-release verapamil initiated several days after STEMI, in noncandidates for β-blockade, may reduce reinfarction and death, provided LV function was well preserved. Verapamil is detrimental to patients with CHF or bradyarrhythmias during the first 24 to 48 hours after STEMI. Patients with non–Q-wave MI or with Q-wave MI, preserved LV function, and no evidence of CHF may benefit from immediate-release diltiazem.
- Inodilators may be used when severe hypotension occurs. Positive inotropic agents, especially **phosphodiesterase inhibitors** and adrenergic agonists such as dobutamine, are associated with increasing myocardial oxygen demand and the potential to induce malignant dysrhythmias and myocar-

dial ischemia, contributing to further cell death or necrosis. **Levosimendan** is a calcium sensitizer that, by virtue of its unique mechanism of action and its negligible effect on myocardial oxygen demand, is the only inodilator that has been associated with favorable short-term outcomes in patients with acute MI.

- Magnesium: Magnesium can continue to be administered for repletion of documented electrolyte deficits and life-threatening ventricular arrhythmias such as torsades de pointes.
- Lidocaine: Although it has been demonstrated that lidocaine can reduce the incidence of VF in the acute phase of MI, this drug significantly increases the risk of asystole. The routine prophylactic use of this drug is therefore not justified.
- Glucose-insulin-potassium, administered routinely, may favorably influence metabolism in the ischemic myocardium and therefore confer a clinical benefit.

Early In-Hospital Care and Management Strategies: Invasive Strategies

Primary Percutaneous Coronary Intervention

- Percutaneous coronary intervention (PCI) without prior thrombolytic therapy is associated with several potential advantages and disadvantages (Table 84.8). Primary PCI results in better acute arterial patency compared to lytics, further improving survival and reducing the hazards of excess cerebral and systemic bleeding and recurrent ischemia, especially in high-risk patients (Fig. 84.3).
- Primary PCI improves LV function with less reperfusion injury, cardiogenic shock, and myocardial rupture than fibrinolytic therapy.

Facilitated Percutaneous Coronary Intervention

- Facilitated PCI refers to treatment with low-dose thrombolytic therapy, platelet GP IIb/IIIa inhibitors, or both, **before PCI** to provide the earliest possible pharmacologic reperfusion before an attempt at definitive mechanical revascularization. Primary PCI is superior to facilitated PCI with lower

TABLE 84.8

ADVANTAGES AND DISADVANTAGES OF PRIMARY
PERCUTANEOUS CORONARY INTERVENTION
VERSUS THROMBOLYSIS

Advantages of primary PCI versus thrombolysis
- Immediate definition of coronary anatomy
- Early risk stratification
- Superior acute vessel patency and TIMI flow grade
- Less reocclusion, recurrent ischemia, and reinfarction
- Better survival in high-risk patients
- Less reperfusion injury and myocardial rupture
- Lower risk of intracranial hemorrhage
- Useful in thrombolytic ineligible patients
- Shorter length of hospital stay

Disadvantages of primary PCI versus thrombolysis
- Skilled interventional cardiologists and catheterization laboratory must be available
- Logistic delays

PCI, percutaneous coronary intervention; TIMI, thrombolysis in myocardial infarction.

rates of death, stroke, cardiogenic shock, or CHF within 90 days and less bleeding.
- Conversely, thrombolytics (half-dose reteplase and abciximab) given to high-risk patients with STEMI in **noninterventional centers** prior to immediate transfer for PCI improves outcomes.

Rescue Percutaneous Coronary Intervention

- Rescue PCI is performed in patients without response to thrombolytic treatment within 90 minutes after therapy (<50% ST-segment resolution and/or symptom regression). Current guidelines recommend it only for certain high-risk subgroups of patients. Rescue PCI has better event-free survival than repeated thrombolysis or conservative treatment.

Transport for Primary Percutaneous Coronary Intervention

- For hospitals without on-site PCI facilities, patient transfer needs to be considered. Several trials compare immediate transfer to on-site thrombolytic therapy in STEMI patients at community hospitals without PCI capability (Fig. 84.4); complications during transfer (death, ventricular dysrhythmias, and second- or third-degree heart block) were rare.
- For transfer times of 2 hours or less from a community hospital to the start of PCI, there is a significant reduction in death, reinfarction, and stroke compared with thrombolysis. This benefit may not apply to transfer for primary PCI in low-volume centers or to situations in which transfer delays exceed 2 to 3 hours. The time from symptom onset to first balloon inflation must be minimized, requiring that the transferred patient is delivered directly to an experienced "ready and waiting" catheterization laboratory.

The Crucial Role of Time in Reperfusion Therapies

- The shorter the time is from symptom onset to treatment, the greater the survival benefit with either reperfusion therapy. The choice between therapies should take into account reperfusion treatment times (Figs. 84.5 and 84.6). Within the **first 2 hours,** the reduction in mortality is twice as large as beyond 2 hours (Fig. 84.7).
- The European guidelines for the management of acute MI recommend that for those patients with clear-cut changes of acute infarction, no more than **20 minutes** should elapse between hospital arrival and the administration of thrombolytic therapy (or prehospital administration) or no more than **60 minutes** between hospital arrival and balloon inflation for primary PCI.
- A second and critically important reason for minimizing prehospital delay is to treat early VF. At least as many deaths may be saved by prompt resuscitation therapy in early acute MI as are saved by reperfusion therapy.

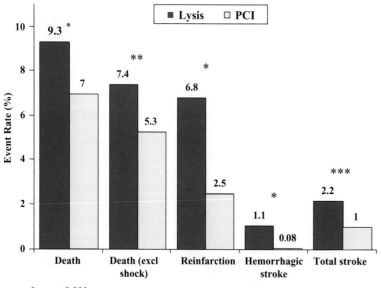

    *   : p <0.001
   **   : p = 0.003
  ***: p = 0.002

FIGURE 84.3. Meta-analysis of 23 randomized trials of primary percutaneous coronary intervention (PCI) versus thrombolysis. (Modified from Keeley EC, Grines CL. Primary coronary intervention for acute myocardial infarction. *JAMA.* 2004;291[6]:736–739.)

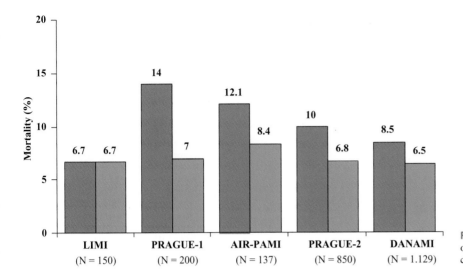

FIGURE 84.4. Randomized trials comparing on-site fibrinolysis and transfer for primary percutaneous coronary intervention (PCI).

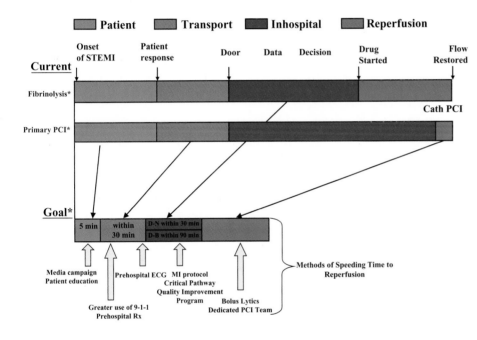

FIGURE 84.5. Major components of time delay between onset of symptoms from ST elevation myocardial infarction (STEMI) and restoration of flow in the infarct-related artery. PCI, percutaneous coronary intervention. (Modified from Antman EM, Anbe DT, Armstrong PW, et al. American College of Cardiology; American Heart Association Task Force on Practice Guidelines; Canadian Cardiovascular Society. ACC/AHA guidelines for the management of patients with ST-elevation myocardial infarction: a report of the American College of Cardiology/American Heart Association Task Force on Practice Guidelines [committee to revise the 1999 Guidelines for the Management of Patients with Acute Myocardial Infarction]. *Circulation.* 2004;110[9]:e82–e292.)

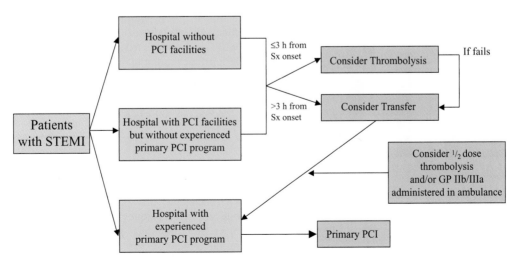

FIGURE 84.6. Possible strategies for the acute management of ST elevation myocardial infarction (STEMI) patients based on the hospital availability of an experienced primary percutaneous coronary intervention (PCI) program. GP, glycoprotein.

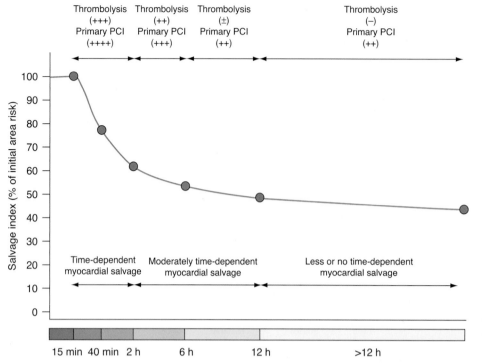

FIGURE 84.7. Time dependency of myocardial salvage expressed as percentage of initial area at risk. The initial parts of the curve up to 2 hours were reconstructed based on the experimental studies. The other parts of the curve showing myocardial salvage from 2 to 12 hours from the symptom onset are reconstructed according to the data of scintigraphic studies. Efficacy of reperfusion is expressed as follows: ++++, very effective; +++, effective; ++, moderately effective; ±, uncertainly effective; −, not effective. PCI, percutaneous coronary intervention. (From Schomig A, Ndrepepa G, Kastrati A. Late myocardial salvage: time to recognize its reality in the reperfusion therapy of acute myocardial infarction. *Eur Heart J.* 2006;27: 1900–1907.)

- The relationship between **mortality and time delay** from symptom onset to treatment is stringent with thrombolytic therapy in STEMI. It is much weaker with primary PCI (Fig. 84.8); however, the benefits of primary PCI may diminish with excessive delays in opening the infarct-related artery

(Fig. 84.9). With thrombolytic therapy, there is an inverse relationship between the rate of achieving normal blood flow and the time-to-treatment interval and an increased risk for mechanical complications, such as myocardial rupture. Therapy is more often complicated by reocclusion of the infarct-related artery, reinfarction, and worse long-term survival as compared to primary PCI. With primary PCI, mechanical complications are rare.

Coronary Artery Bypass Surgery

- Coronary artery bypass surgery (CABG) may be indicated when PCI has failed or is not feasible, with sudden occlusion of a coronary artery during catheterization, in cardiogenic shock, or in association with surgery for a ventricular septal defect or mitral regurgitation due to papillary muscle dysfunction and rupture.
- CABG is also indicated if coronary angiography demonstrates lesions, such as left main stenosis or three-vessel disease with poor LV function, for which surgery improves prognosis.

LONG-TERM POST-MYOCARDIAL INFARCTION

Pharmacologic Treatment

- Pharmacologic therapies aimed at limiting risk factors and coronary plaque instability with lipid-lowering therapies and inhibiting post-MI remodeling with neurohumoral antagonists can significantly improve long-term outcomes including death, reinfarction, and worsening CHF (Table 84.9). Clinical trials have also shown the benefits of antiplatelet, anticoagulant, and newer platelet inhibitors in

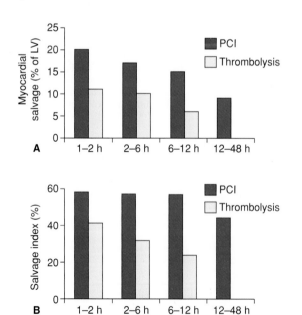

FIGURE 84.8. Time dependence of myocardial salvage according to time-to-treatment interval in patients with ST elevation myocardial infarction (STEMI) treated by percutaneous coronary intervention (PCI) or thrombolysis. **A:** Myocardial salvage expressed as percentage of the left ventricle (LV). **B:** Myocardial salvage expressed as proportion of the initial area at risk salvaged by reperfusion therapy. (From Schomig A, Ndrepepa G, Kastrati A. Late myocardial salvage: time to recognize its reality in the reperfusion therapy of acute myocardial infarction. *Eur Heart J.* 2006;27:1900–1907).

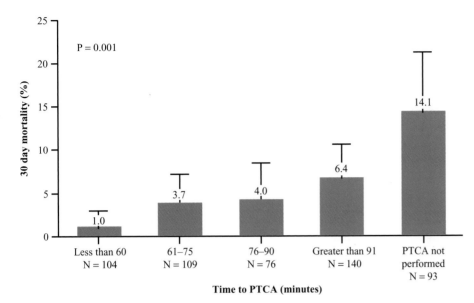

FIGURE 84.9. Relationship between 30-day mortality and time from study enrollment to first balloon inflation. PTCA, percutaneous transluminal coronary angioplasty. (Modified from Berger PB, Ellis SG, Holmes DR Jr, et al. Relationship between delay in performing direct coronary angioplasty and early clinical outcome in patients with acute myocardial infarction: results from the Global Use of Strategies to Open Occluded Arteries in Acute Coronary Syndromes [GUSTO-IIb] trial. *Circulation.* 1999;100:14–20.)

limiting recurrent myocardial ischemia and its consequences (Table 84.10).

Special Issues

Acute Congestive Heart Failure and Cardiogenic Shock

• Acute CHF arises from a sudden injury or structural failure and constitutes approximately 10% of CHF admissions. Etiologies include acute coronary syndromes (ACSs), acute valvular dysfunction, pericardial disease, new arrhythmia, myocarditis, and malignant hypertension.

TABLE 84.9

AMERICAN COLLEGE OF CARDIOLOGY/AMERICAN HEART ASSOCIATION GUIDELINES FOR MANAGEMENT OF ST ELEVATION MYOCARDIAL INFARCTION

Acute therapy	Discharge therapy
Aspirin	Aspirin
Clopidogrel	Clopidogrel
β-Blocker	β-Blocker
ACE inhibitor	ACE inhibitor
Heparin (UFH or LMWH)	Aldosterone antagonist
GP IIb/IIIa Inhibitor (if receiving PCI)	Statin
	Smoking cessation
	Cardiac rehabilitation

ACE, angiotensin-converting enzyme; UFH, unfractionated heparin; LMHW, low-molecular-weight heparin; GP, glycoprotein; PCI, percutaneous coronary intervention.
Table made with data from Antman EM, Anbe DT, Armstrong PW, et al. American College of Cardiology; American Heart Association Task Force on Practice Guidelines; Canadian Cardiovascular Society. ACC/AHA guidelines for the management of patients with ST-elevation myocardial infarction: a report of the American College of Cardiology/American Heart Association Task Force on Practice Guidelines (committee to revise the 1999 Guidelines for the Management of Patients with Acute Myocardial Infarction). *Circulation.* 2004;110(9):e82–e292.

• Patients with ACS accompanied by CHF have **considerable mortality** and clearly benefit from emergent revascularization (Fig. 84.10). Medical management includes the standard therapies for ACS (antiplatelet therapy and anticoagulation); β-blockers are contraindicated in the presence of systolic CHF but are probably helpful in diastolic CHF.

• For patients with hypotension or hypoperfusion, serious consideration should be given to placement of a **pulmonary artery catheter**. An **intra-aortic balloon pump** is the most physiologic for improving cardiac output in the setting of ACS as it improves coronary perfusion while increasing blood pressure and decreasing afterload (Fig. 84.11). All currently available inotropes may worsen ischemia and are proarrhythmic.

• Cardiogenic shock remains the leading cause of death in patients hospitalized with acute MI. **Early mechanical revascularization** for cardiogenic shock in acute MI is a class I recommendation by the American College of Cardiology and the American Heart Association for patients younger than 75 years with ST elevation left bundle branch block acute MI due to a significant mortality benefit over initial medical stabilization followed by late or no revascularization (Fig. 84.12).

Other Possible In-Hospital Complications

• Mitral regurgitation may be present in 50% of patients within 30 days of MI, with a graded positive association between the severity of mitral regurgitation, including mild cases, and CHF or death.

• Deep vein thrombosis and pulmonary embolism: These complications are now relatively uncommon after MI, except in patients kept in bed for comorbidities or complications of MI. When they occur, they should be treated with therapeutic doses of LMWH followed by oral anticoagulation for 3 to 6 months.

• Intraventricular thrombus and systemic emboli: Echocardiography may reveal intraventricular thrombi, especially in patients with a large anterior MI. If the thrombi are mobile or protuberant, they should be treated initially with intravenous UFH or LMWH and subsequently with oral anticoagulants for at least 3 to 6 months.

TABLE 84.10

LARGE-SCALE CLINICAL TRIALS OF THERAPY FOR AMI SURVIVORS

Study	Reference	Patient population (n)	Treatment	Background therapy	Average duration	All-cause mortality risk reduction	Re-infarction
Antiplatelet							
ATC	BMJ. 1994; 308:81–106	AMI (20,000)	Aspirin	None	4.5 y	25% p <0.02	34% p <0.02
ACEIs/ARBs							
SMILE	N Engl J Med. 1995;332: 80–85	AMI (1,556)	Zofenopril	Aspirin (53%), β-blockers (18%), CCBs (10%)	6 wk	29%[a] p = 0.01	37% p = N/A
ISIS-4	Lancet. 1995; 345:669–685	AMI (58,050)	Captopril	Nitrates/diuretics	15 mo	7% at 1 mo p = 0.02	No difference
GISSI-3	Lancet. 1987;2: 871–874	AMI (18,895)	Lisinopril	IV β-blockers (31%), fibrinolytic therapy (72%), aspirin (84%), antiplatelets (4%)	6 wk	11% p = 0.03	No difference
Including patients with LVD or HF							
SAVE	N Engl J Med. 1992;327: 669–77	AMI with LVD (2,231)	Captopril	Aspirin (59%), β-blockers (75%), thrombolytics (32%), PCI (17%), CCBs (42%)	3.5 y	19% p = 0.019	25% p = 0.015
AIRE	Lancet. 1993; 342:821–828	AMI with HF (2,006)	Ramipril	Aspirin (77%), β-blockers (24%), thrombolytics (59%), CCBs (15%)	15 mo	27% p = 0.002	p = NS
TRACE	N Engl J Med. 1995;333: 1670–1676	AMI with LVD (1,749)	Trandolapril	Aspirin (92%), β-blockers (17%), thrombolytics (45%), CCBs (28%)	2–4 y	22% p = 0.0001	14% p = NS
OPTIMAAL	Lancet. 2002; 360:752–760	AMI with HF (5,477)	Losartan vs Captopril	Aspirin (96%), β-blockers (79%), thrombolytics (55%) PCI (17%), CCBs (22%), statins (31%)	2.7 y	13% Increase in risk p = 0.07	3% increase in risk p = NS
VALIANT	N Engl J Med. 2003;349: 1893–1906	AMI with HF/LVD (14,703)	Valsartan vs. Valsartan plus Captopril	Aspirin (91%), β-blockers (70%), ACEIs (40%), antiplatelets (25%), PCI (20%), thrombolytics (35%)	24.7 mo	No difference p = NS	No difference p = NS
Statins							
CARE	N Engl J Med. 1996;335: 1001–1009	AMI (4,159)	Pravastatin	Aspirin (83%), β-blockers (41%), ACEIs (15%), CCBs (40%)	5 y	No difference	24%[b] p = 0.003
HPS	Lancet. 2002; 360:7–22	History of MI (8,510)	Simvastatin	Aspirin (21%), β-blockers (19.5%), ACEIs (25%)	5 y		24%[b]
MIRACL	JAMA. 2001;285:1711–1718	ACS (3,086)	Atorvastatin	Aspirin (91%), β-blockers (78%), ACEIs/ARBs (49%), antiplatelets (11%), CCBs (48%)	16 wk	16%[c] p = 0.048	10% p = NS

Trial	Citation	Population (n)	Drug	Concomitant therapy	Follow-up		
PROVE IT-TIMI	N Engl J Med. 2004;3: 1495–1504	ACS (4,162)	Pravastatin or Atorvastatin	Aspirin (93%), β-blockers (85%), ACEIs/ARBs (83%), antiplatelets (72%), PCI (69%)	2 y	28% p = 0.07	18% p = 0.06
A to Z trial	JAMA. 2004; 292:1307–1316	ACS (4,497)	Simvastatin 40 mg for 30 d, then 80 mg vs. placebo for 4 mo, then 20 mg	Aspirin (98%), β-blockers (90%), ACEIs/ARBs (71%)	6–24 mo	11%[d] p = NS	4% p = NS
Aldosterone antagonists							
EPHESUS	Cardiovasc Drugs Ther. 2001;15: 79–87	AMI with LVD or HF (6,642)	Eplerenone	Aspirin (88%), β-blockers (87%), ACEIs/ARBs (47%), statin (47%), thrombolysis or PCI (45%)	16 mo	15% p = 0.008	N/A
β-Blockers							
Goteborg	Lancet. 1981;2: 823–827	AMI (1,395)	Metoprolol tartrate	None	3 mo	36% p = 0.03	p = NS
MIAMI	Am J Cardiol. 1985;56: 15G–22G	AMI (5,778)	Metoprolol tartrate	Antihypertensives (5%), anticoagulants (2%)	15 d	p = NS	p = NS
ISIS-1	Lancet. 1986;2: 57–66	AMI (16,027)	Atenolol	Antiplatelets (5%), anticoagulants (6%)	1 wk	15% p < 0.04	p = NS
TIMI II-B	Circulation. 1991;83: 422–437	AMI (1,434)	Immediate vs. late Metoprolol tartrate	N/A	12 mo	NS	p = NS
Lopressor Intervention Trial	Eur Heart J. 1987;8: 1056–1064	AMI (2,395)	Metoprolol tartrate	None	12 mo	Increase risk 4% NS	p = NS
Norwegian	N Engl J Med. 1985;313: 1055–1058	AMI (1,884)	Timolol	None	17 mo	39% p = 0.0003	28% p = 0.0006
BHAT	JAMA. 1981; 246:2073–2074	AMI (3,837)	Propranolol	Aspirin (21%)	25 mo	26% p < 0.005	16% p = NS
Including Patients with LVD or HF							
CAPRICORN	Lancet. 2001; 357:1385–1390	AMI with LVD or HF (1,959)	Carvedilol	ACEIs (98%), aspirin (86%), lipid-lowering (24%), thrombolytics (36%), PCI (12%)	15 mo	23% p = 0.031	41% p = 0.014

AMI, acute myocardial infarction; ACEI, angiotensin-converting enzyme inhibitor; ARB, angiotensin-II receptor blocker; CCB, calcium channel blockers; IV, intravenous; LVD, left ventricular dysfunction; HF, heart failure; PCI, percutaneous coronary intervention ACS, acute coronary syndrome; .
[a]Risk reduction at one year.
[b]Cardiac death or reinfarction.
[c]Primary end-point event defined as death, nonfatal AMI, cardiac arrest with resuscitation, or recurrent symptomatic myocardial ischemia with objective evidence and requiring emergency rehospitalization.
[d]Composite of cardiovascular death, nonfatal myocardial infarction, readmission for ACS, and stroke.

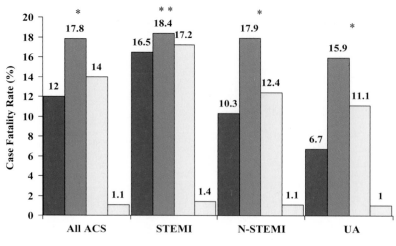

FIGURE 84.10. Impact of presence of heart failure (HF) at admission or development of HF during hospitalization (H) in all patients with acute coronary syndromes (ACSs). STEMI, ST elevation myocardial infarction; N-STEMI, non–ST elevation myocardial infarction; UA, unstable angina. (Modified from Steg PG, Dabbous OH, Feldman LJ, et al.; Global Registry of Acute Coronary Events Investigators. Determinants and prognostic impact of heart failure complicating acute coronary syndromes: observations from the Global Registry of Acute Coronary Events [GRACE]. *Circulation.* 2004;109:494–499.)

- Pericarditis: Acute pericarditis is associated with a worse outcome, giving rise to chest pain that may be misinterpreted as recurrent MI or angina. The pain is distinguished by its sharp nature and relationship to posture and respiration, and may be confirmed by a pericardial rub. It may be treated by high-dose oral or intravenous aspirin, nonsteroidal **anti-inflammatory** agents, or steroids. A hemorrhagic effusion with tamponade is uncommon but especially associated with anticoagulant treatment. Recognized echocardiographically, it may be treated by pericardiocentesis if needed.

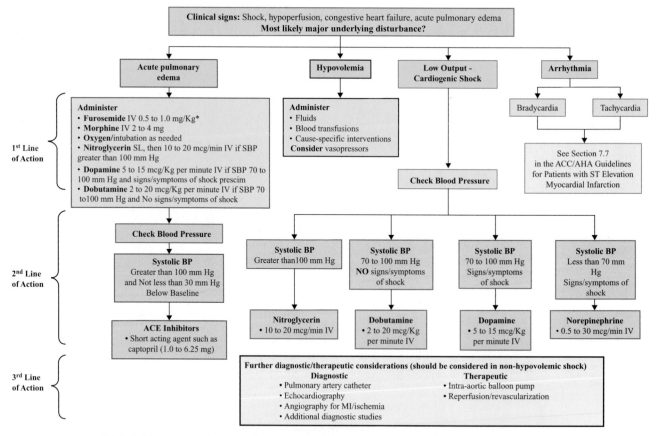

FIGURE 84.11. Emergency management of complicated ST elevation myocardial infarction (STEMI). The emergency management of patients with cardiogenic shock, acute pulmonary edema, or both is outlined. HF, heart failure; IV, intravenous; SL, sublingual; SBP, systolic blood pressure; BP, blood pressure; ACE, angiotensin-converting enzyme; MI, myocardial infarction. (Modified from Antman EM, Anbe DT, Armstrong PW, et al. American College of Cardiology; American Heart Association Task Force on Practice Guidelines; Canadian Cardiovascular Society. ACC/AHA guidelines for the management of patients with ST-elevation myocardial infarction: a report of the American College of Cardiology/American Heart Association Task Force on Practice Guidelines [committee to revise the 1999 Guidelines for the Management of Patients with Acute Myocardial Infarction]. *Circulation.* 2004;110[9]:e82—292.)

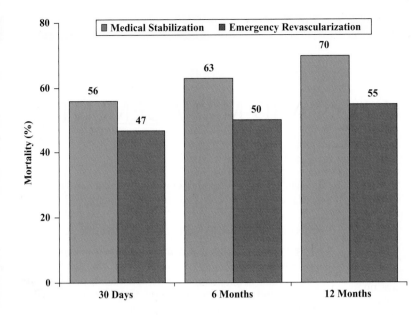

FIGURE 84.12. Mortality of medical stabilization vs. emergency revascularization by percutaneous coronary intervention (PCI) in ST-elevation myocardial infarction (STEMI) patients with shock. (Modified from Hochman JS, Sleeper LA, Webb JG, et al.; SHOCK Investigators. Early revascularization in acute myocardial infarction complicated by cardiogenic shock. *N Engl J Med.* 1999;341:625–634.)

- Late ventricular dysrhythmias: VT and VF occurring on the first day have a low predictive value for recurring dysrhythmias. Dysrhythmias developing later are liable to recur and are associated with a high risk of death. VT or VF during the first week postinfarction is associated with more extensive myocardial damage; a careful assessment of coronary anatomy and ventricular function should always be undertaken. If induced by ischemia, revascularization by PCI or surgery should be considered; otherwise a variety of therapeutic approaches are available including the use of β-blockers, amiodarone, electrophysiologically guided antidysrhythmic therapy, and/or insertion of an implantable converter defibrillator.
- Postinfarction angina and ischemia: The routine use of elective PCI after fibrinolytic therapy in the absence of spontaneous or provocable ischemia does not improve LV function or survival. In treating angina or recurrent or inducible ischemia, however, revascularization by PCI or CABG has a definite role. It may also be of value in managing dysrhythmias associated with persistent ischemia.
- Right ventricular (RV) infarction encompasses a spectrum of disease states ranging from asymptomatic mild RV dysfunction through cardiogenic shock. Most patients demonstrate a return of normal RV function over a period of weeks to months, which suggests that RV stunning, rather than irreversible necrosis, has occurred. Only 10% to 15% of patients show classic hemodynamic abnormalities. A common clinical presentation is profound hypotension after administration of sublingual nitroglycerin, with the **degree of hypotension often out of proportion** to the ECG severity of the infarct.
- RV infarction with hemodynamic abnormalities accompanying inferior STEMI is associated with a significantly higher mortality and should be considered in high-priority candidates for reperfusion. The high mortality rate is similar to that for patients with LV shock.
- The treatment of patients with RV ischemic dysfunction is different compared to management of LV dysfunction. It includes maintenance of **RV preload**, reduction of RV afterload, **inotropic support** of the dysfunctional RV, and early reperfusion. Because of their influence on preload, drugs routinely used in management of LV infarctions, such as nitrates and diuretics, may reduce cardiac output and produce severe hypotension when the RV is ischemic.
- Although **volume loading** is a critical first step in the management of hypotension associated with RV ischemia/infarction, inotropic support—in particular, with **dobutamine**—should be initiated promptly if cardiac output fails to improve after 0.5 to 1 L of fluid has been administered. Excessive volume loading may further complicate the right-sided filling pressure increase and RV dilatation, resulting in decreased LV output secondary to shift of the interventricular septum toward the LV.

Indications for Hemodynamic Monitoring

- It is important to accurately **assess the severity of LV dysfunction** because maneuvers performed in the coronary care unit may worsen this state. More than half of the patients with a moderate reduction in resting cardiac output and an increase in LV filling pressure have no clinical signs of LV dysfunction.
- Correlation of the chest radiograph and clinical evaluation with hemodynamic measurements have demonstrated that the presence of **cardiomegaly, gallop rhythms, and pulmonary edema** may help predict which patients with MI will develop shock.
- There is an unfortunate tendency to institute potent therapeutic measures in patients with MI before precise hemodynamic indices are known. Intravenous furosemide, for example, may create a decline in pulmonary artery occlusion pressure without compromising the cardiac output if ventricular filling pressures are elevated and there is pulmonary congestion. However, if the clinical diagnosis of CHF is incorrect and the pulmonary artery occlusion pressure is normal, diuretic therapy may actually decrease the cardiac output and cause deterioration of an already compromised myocardial flow reserve. This can be particularly detrimental in patients who present with RV infarction.

CHAPTER 85 ■ EVALUATION AND MANAGEMENT OF HEART FAILURE

- The World Health Organization developed classification nomenclature for the cardiomyopathies based on anatomic and physiologic findings: restrictive, hypertrophic, and dilated. This chapter focuses on the dilated cardiomyopathies (DCM); nearly half are secondary to ischemic heart disease, and all remaining etiologies are primary muscle diseases. The hallmark findings of DCM are a dilated left ventricle (LV) and a low LV ejection fraction (EF). Nearly 25% have no pre-existing risk factors. A small number of DCMs are secondary to toxins such as alcohol, anthracyclines, and cocaine; endocrine diseases such as diabetes mellitus and thyroid disease; human immunodeficiency virus and Lyme disease infections; sarcoidosis; thiamine deficiency; peripartum cardiomyopathy; hemochromatosis; and underlying collagen vascular diseases.

CELLULAR DETERMINANTS OF MYOCARDIAL CONTRACTION

The Contractile Proteins

- The interaction of the proteins actin, myosin, and the troponin complex is responsible for myocardial contraction. Engagement of actin and myosin occurs when calcium (Ca^{2+}) levels in the cytosol increase in the presence of adenosine triphosphate (ATP), as regulated by a complex that consists of troponin C and other proteins (Fig. 85.1).
- Removal of Ca^{2+} from the cytosol results in dissociation from troponin C, with subsequent cessation of actin–myosin cross-linkage, signaling the end of contractile activity and the start of relaxation—a process known as *inactivation*.

Calcium and Cyclic Adenosine Monophosphate

- Alterations in the delivery, use, myofibrillar sensitivity to Ca^{2+} and removal of Ca^{2+} from the myofibril and the myocyte cytosol constitutes the basis for abnormalities in both contractility and relaxation. Entry of Ca^{2+} from extracellular locations occurs through either voltage-dependent, gated "slow channels" activated by membrane depolarization or via sodium–calcium ($Na^+–Ca^{2+}$) exchange across the sarcolemma.
- Calcium and cyclic adenosine monophosphate-mediated (cAMP-mediated) transfer of phosphates to phospholamban increases Ca^{2+} influx by additional voltage-dependent channels which triggers Ca^{2+} release from the sarcoplasmic reticulum (SR), termed Ca^2 -dependent Ca^{2+} release for contractile activity (Fig. 85.2).
- Altered Ca^{2+} kinetics are responsible for the increases in contractility observed in other circumstances. The increased contractility of postextrasystolic beats, increased heart rate, and during manipulation with cardiac glycosides, phosphodiesterase inhibitors, sympathomimetic amines, and caffeine are dependent on changes in intracellular Ca^{2+} and/or cAMP levels.
- Absolute Ca^{2+} levels and hormonal changes such as hyperthyroidism increase contractility via increased troponin C affinity for Ca^{2+}, increased ATPase activity with concomitant increased cAMP levels, and changes in intracellular Ca^{2+} handling.

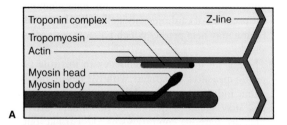

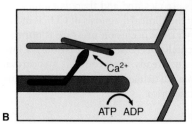

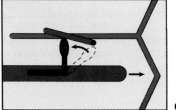

FIGURE 85.1. A schematic representation of tropomyosin, troponin complex, actin, myosin, and calcium during relaxation (**A**), activation (**B**), and contraction (**C**). During relaxation, the myosin is prevented from interacting with actin by tropomyosin. Activation by the interaction of calcium with troponin C confers a configurational change in tropomyosin, allowing the interaction of myosin and actin.

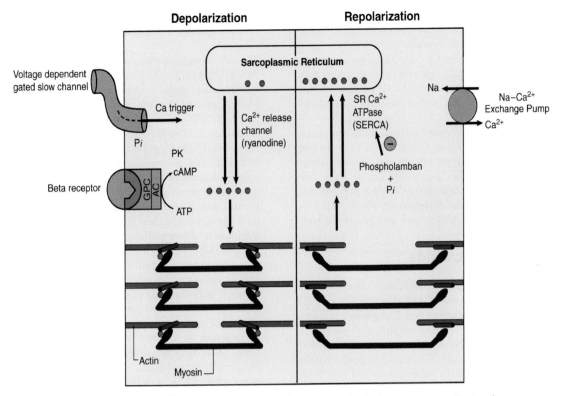

FIGURE 85.2. The role of calcium in excitation and contraction in the human myocyte. During depolarization, Ca^{2+} enters from the extracellular space through the voltage-dependent, gated slow channel, the so-called L-type channel. This entry is facilitated by β-receptor stimulation of a protein receptor, which in turn stimulates adenyl cyclase (AC), producing cyclic adenosine monophosphate (cAMP) and phosphorylation of the calcium channel. However, this intrusion of calcium into the cell does not moderate the interaction of actin and myosin. Rather, it acts as a trigger for the release of calcium from the sarcoplasmic reticulum through the Ca^{2+} release or ryanodine receptor channel. During repolarization, the sarcoplasmic reticulum (SR) Ca^{2+} ATPase (SERCA) mediates the uptake of cytosolic calcium into the SR. cAMP-mediated phosphorylation of phospholamban prevents the inhibition by phospholamban of SERCA activity. The Na–Ca^{2+} exchange pump is the dominant mechanism of Ca^{2+} extrusion out of the cytosol into the extracellular space.

- Individual muscle units in the failing and hypertrophied ventricle have depressed function. The myocardial depression accompanying anoxia, acidosis, hypothyroidism, barbiturate use, administration of local and general anesthetics, Ca^{2+} antagonists, and ischemia all result from abnormalities in the Ca^{2+}-dependent mechanisms described here.

and hypertrophic cardiomyopathy. Impairment of relaxation occurs secondary to increased levels of Ca^{2+} within the myocyte in diastole, owing to diminished genetic expression of the SR uptake pump, decreased phospholamban activity and transcription, down-regulation or uncoupling of β-receptors, and G-protein inhibition of β-receptor function.

CELLULAR DETERMINANTS OF RELAXATION

- Inactivation signals the end of actin–myosin interaction with the rate and extent of Ca^{2+} removal affecting the rate and extent of relaxation. SR Ca^{2+} ATPase (SERCA) mediates the uptake of cytosolic Ca^{2+} into the SR. Primarily after adrenergic stimuli, cAMP-dependent phosphorylated phospholamban increases SR uptake of Ca^{2+}.
- In addition, the Na^+–Ca^{2+} exchange pump—also requiring ATP—allows the efflux of Ca^{2+} into the extracellular space from the cytosol (see Fig. 85.2). As the myofibril shortens, its affinity for Ca^{2+} decreases, limiting Ca^{2+} effects and affecting relaxation. All of these mechanisms can be facilitated or inhibited by drugs or neurohumoral factors.
- The process of relaxation has been extensively studied in DCM, left ventricular hypertrophy (LVH), ischemia,

MEDIATORS OF CONTRACTILITY

β-Receptors and Guanine Nucleotide Regulatory Proteins

- Adrenergic stimulation of cardiac myocytes is an important regulator of both Ca^{2+} influx and cAMP levels within the cell (seeFig. 85.2). β-receptor stimulation activates adenylate cyclase (AC) which increases cAMP resulting in increased Ca^{2+} influx and increased contractile force. These Ca^{2+} channels are known as "receptor-operated channels."
- The coupling between β-receptors and AC occurs through guanine cyclic nucleotides, also known as G proteins, which have both stimulatory and inhibitory influences on AC. The G-protein complex (GPC) in its active form contains guanosine triphosphate. G proteins also stimulate cardiac contractility by α-receptor stimulation via a cAMP-independent

mechanism. cAMP-dependent mechanisms have delays in response of 2 to 20 seconds, as opposed to G-protein pathway delays in response of 150 milliseconds.

- Inhibitory G proteins, activated by acetylcholine receptors, inhibit Ca^{2+} influx via cyclic guanosine monophosphate (cGMP). A cGMP system activates cGMP protein kinase, which inhibits calcium inward currents previously stimulated by cAMP.
- In addition to changes in receptor function, molecular alterations in β-receptor production occurs in various disease states. In DCM, both β_1-receptor mRNA and absolute receptor levels are depressed; also β-receptor kinase levels are elevated, evidence of dysfunctional (uncoupled) β receptors. This may explain catecholamine insensitivity observed in failing hearts after cardiopulmonary bypass and possibly sepsis.

Nitric Oxide

- Nitric oxide (NO) has cholinergic depressant effects on cardiac contractility mediated via cGMP. Antagonists of NO (methylene blue, oxyhemoglobin, and L-arginine) enhance the positive inotropic action of the β agonist isoproterenol.
- Tumor necrosis factor-α (TNF-α) may cause the myocardial depression seen in septic shock. N-methyl-L-arginine blocks the myocardial effect of TNF by inhibition of NO synthesis. Methylene blue, an inhibitor of guanylate cyclase, also blocks TNF-induced cardiomyocyte depression.

Endothelin

- Endothelins and the closely related vasoactive intestinal contractor are potent vasoconstrictors and positive inotropes, acting via a yet incompletely defined mechanism. Endothelins may sensitize the myofibrils to calcium; high-affinity receptors have been isolated in mammalian atria and ventricles. Found ubiquitously in mammalian tissues, their intracardiac site of genesis is unknown but believed to be the endothelium of the coronary arteries and microvasculature.
- Endothelin causes an increase in intracellular pH that increases myofibrillar sensitivity for Ca^{2+}, and subsequently increases contraction. This effect is completely inhibited by pretreatment with amiloride, blocking Na^+–H^+ exchange across the sarcolemmal membrane and prevents increase in intracellular pH. The effect of endothelin may be mediated via G proteins participating in signal transduction after binding of endothelin to its sarcolemmal receptor.

THE CELLULAR BASIS OF HEART FAILURE

- Heart failure, either acute or chronic, results from loss of myocytes or loss of intrinsic contractility within individual myocytes. Several functional abnormalities involving excitation–contraction coupling of contractile proteins within myocytes and myocardial energetics have been identified.
- The importance of Ca^{2+} in the regulation of myocardial contraction cannot be overstated. In heart failure, there is a blunted rise of depolarization, causing slower activation and a slower rate of fall during repolarization. This is likely mediated by impaired reuptake of Ca^{2+} into the SR because Ca^{2+}–adenosine triphosphatase activity (SERCA2) is reduced. The

activity of SERCA2 activity is inhibited by phosphorylation of phospholamban through cAMP stimulated by β-adrenergic receptors.

- The calcium release channel (CRC) of the SR mediates release of Ca^{2+} into the cytosol during contraction and is critical for activation of the contractile elements. The CRC is hyperphosphorylated by protein kinase A in heart failure, resulting in a high rate of Ca^{2+} leakage from the SR throughout the cardiac cycle. The Na^+–Ca^{2+} exchanger has increased activity in heart failure, perhaps as a compensation for reduced SERCA2, and decreased mRNA and protein levels of the voltage-dependent Ca^{2+} channel.
- **Contractile protein alteration in the failure heart:** Both troponin I and T, and myosin heavy and light chains revert to fetal phenotypes in chronic heart failure.
- **Regulation of interstitial collagen:** Collagen provides stents along which myocytes are aligned. The quantity and nature of the collagen are determined by the balance between synthesis and degradation; the latter is regulated by matrix metalloproteinases. In heart failure, there is a maladaptation of collagen stents, perhaps mediated by increased activity of matrix metalloproteinases.
- **Adaptations to changes in load or myocardial injury:** In these situations, the ventricle can maintain cardiac output by increasing ventricular preload (so-called Frank–Starling effect) (Fig. 85.3), activation of neurohumeral systems such as the renin-angiotensin–aldosterone system, release of norepinephrine, or myocardial remodeling via chamber dilatation, and augmentation of myocardial mass.
- At the cellular level, there are increases in number of mitochondria, cell size, and amount of collagen within the extracellular matrix. When the injury or stress exceeds the ability of these adaptive mechanisms to compensate, myocardial contractility decreases. The transition to failure involves inadequate hypertrophy to maintain contractility, re-expression of fetal genes and decreased expression of adult genes, alteration in proteins involved in excitation–contraction coupling, myocardial death by necrosis or apoptosis, and changes in myocardial energetics.

Frank Starling Relationship

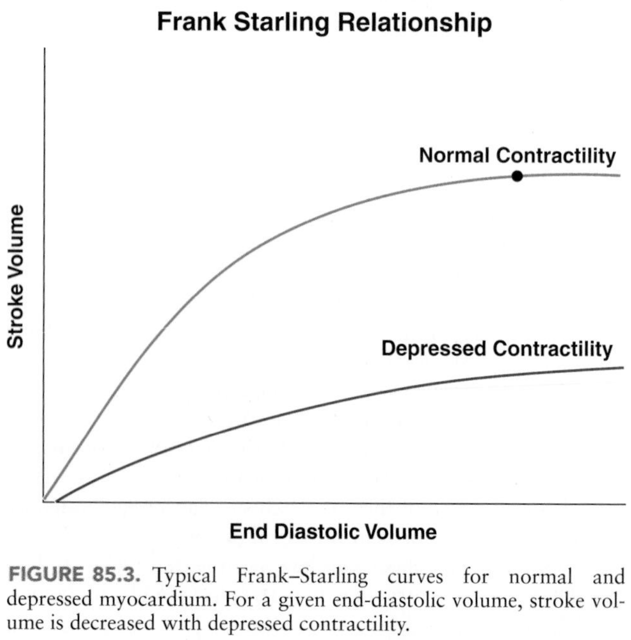

FIGURE 85.3. Typical Frank–Starling curves for normal and depressed myocardium. For a given end-diastolic volume, stroke volume is decreased with depressed contractility.

- **Neurohormonal abnormalities in heart failure:** Low cardiac output decreases renal perfusion pressure and stimulates the renin-angiotensin system. Angiotensin II is a potent vasoconstrictor; the discovery of angiotensin-converting enzyme (ACE) inhibitors to interrupt this pathway was a major breakthrough in heart failure therapy. Another was the realization that chymase, CAGE, and cathepsin G, enzymes located in the myocardium, could also cleave angiotensin I into angiotensin II. This discovery cemented the idea that the heart was a neuroendocrine organ.
- Elevated levels of aldosterone are also seen in patients with LV systolic dysfunction. Mechanisms of increased aldosterone are renin-angiotensin stimulation, decreased hepatic clearance, and sodium-restricted diets. Elevated aldosterone leads to sodium and water retention; plasma volume is increased. Low cardiac output also causes the adrenal gland to produce more norepinephrine. Higher levels of circulating catecholamines in heart failure predict a higher mortality.
- Elevated levels of norepinephrine, angiotensin II, and aldosterone result in maladaptive changes in LV structure. These neurohormones lead to dilatation of the LV and changes in cardiocyte architecture, collagen type and content, and β-adrenergic receptor abnormalities. Collectively, these changes in LV architecture are known as remodeling.
- Eccentric hypertrophy results from expression of embryonic genes with contractile protein units assembled in series, rather than in parallel, as seen in concentric hypertrophy. Factors that lead to the hypertrophic response include growth factors, peptides, and cytokines, with the most comprehensively studied substances being insulin growth factor I, angiotensin II, endothelin, and those that activate a form of guanosine triphosphate–binding protein (ras) signaling pathways, cytokines including interleukin-6, and heteromeric (G_q).
- Abnormal amounts of neurohormones are produced in heart failure as part of compensatory mechanisms to alleviate the adverse effects of low cardiac output.
  - Vasoconstrictors, including endothelin and angiotensin II, keep perfusion pressure up. Aldosterone stimulates renal retention of sodium and water but at the cost of potassium secretion, vascular and myocardial fibrosis, baroreceptor dysfunction, and prevention of myocardial norepinephrine uptake.
  - Activated arterial baroreceptors causes nonosmotic stimulation of arginine vasopressin from the supraoptic nucleus of the hypothalamus stimulating both V_{1a} vascular smooth muscle receptors and V_2 receptors on the collecting duct. V_2 receptor stimulation increases aquaporin-2 water channel trafficking in the collecting duct; causing increased water reabsorption and hyponatremia.
  - The adrenal gland also produces more norepinephrine to increase heart rate; however, prolonged exposure leads to intracellular migration and down-regulation of β-adrenergic receptors; remaining β receptors are less responsive to isoproterenol.
- Neurohormones beneficial in heart failure include the natriuretic peptides made in response to LV dilatation, especially brain natriuretic peptide (BNP). This hormone has natriuretic and vasodilatory properties to counteract the deleterious effects of aldosterone and angiotensin II. BNP levels are elevated in heart failure and become more elevated as they become more symptomatic (New York Heart Association Functional Class increases). Levels may be more elevated

in decompensated heart failure compared to the compensated state. Other substances with vasodilatory properties include bradykinin, nitric oxide, and prostaglandins; ACE inhibitors have a secondary effect of blocking bradykinin degradation.
- Once LV dysfunction is present, cytokine over-expression of interleukins and TNF-α promote LV dilatation and remodeling; contributing to the progression of heart failure. Elevated TNF-α levels are found in advanced heart failure, and a trend toward higher mortality with higher TNF-α levels has been observed.
- **Remodeling** is a complex process in response to either acute or chronic injury to cardiocytes. Myocardial remodeling takes longer to develop with different patterns of gene activation for several peptide growth factors. There are two distinct patterns, concentric (increased mass without ventricular dilatation) in pressure overload and eccentric hypertrophy (increased mass and ventricular dilatation) in volume overload. In both cases, wall stress is returned toward normal, at least initially.
- **Concentric hypertrophy,** seen with aortic stenosis or chronic untreated hypertension, is characterized by increased elastic stiffness and an elevated end diastolic pressure (EDP) for a given volume. Pressure overload is characterized by parallel replication of myofibrils and thickening of individual myocytes
- **Eccentric hypertrophy,** as seen with mitral or aortic insufficiency, is characterized by increased ventricular volume but little or no change in elasticity; this results in little increase in pressure at increased volumes. Volume overload results in increased diastolic stress with a series replication of sarcomeres, elongation of myocytes, and ventricular dilatation.
- The term *remodeling* encompasses LV dilatation, eccentric hypertrophy, apoptosis, changes in valvular structure, and arrhythmias.
- With increase in chamber size, geometry is altered; the LV loses its elliptical shape and develops a more spherical shape. The spherical LV has been associated with higher end-systolic wall stress and abnormal distribution of fiber shortening.
- Mitral regurgitation, due to misalignment of papillary muscles and subvalvular structures and distortion at the mitral annulus secondary to LV enlargement, frequently accompanies LV remodeling. Left atrial enlargement and pulmonary venous hypertension are frequent sequelae of mitral regurgitation.
- Electrocardiographic abnormalities and arrhythmias are also common problems in heart failure, including left bundle branch block, P-R interval prolongation, atrial flutter and atrial fibrillation, and ventricular tachycardia (VT). Syncope, an ominous predictor for sudden cardiac death, may be secondary to VT or atrial arrhythmias, with rapid ventricular response.

DIASTOLIC DYSFUNCTION IN HEART FAILURE

- LV diastolic function is dependent on many intrinsic and extrinsic factors. Relaxation can be further divided into the *extent of relaxation* and the *rate of relaxation*. Alterations in the extent, rate, or both characterize the abnormalities of relaxation and result in characteristic hemodynamic patterns.

- **LV compliance and the diastolic left ventricular pressure–volume relationship:** A nonlinear relationship normally exists between pressure and volume during ventricular diastole. Shifts are reflected by a change in slope (LV stiffness) or intercept of the relationship resulting from various disease states.
- **Extent of relaxation** reflects LV compliance and is the major determinant of end-diastolic volume and end-diastolic pressure (EDP). Abnormalities in extent of relaxation affect the end-diastolic pressure–volume (EDP–V) relationship to the greatest extent.
- LV geometry (i.e., thickness, size, and chamber dimension) in large part determines the LV EDP–V relationship, as determined by mathematic approximations based on Laplace's law. *Coronary vascular turgor* decreases LV diastolic compliance through its erectile effect on LV stiffness by increasing LV wall volume, resulting in a higher EDP for a given volume. This effect seems to be independent of pericardial influences and predominates in the late diastolic filling period.
- *Load-dependent relaxation* phenomena are alterations in elastic properties and the rate of relaxation of the myocardium, mediated via changes in the load sensed by the LV during relaxation. These cause instantaneous changes in LV compliance and the rate of relaxation independent of heart rate when LV muscle is abruptly stretched.
- Manifestations of viscosity: The clinical importance of viscoelasticity has been disputed.
  - *Stress relaxation*—a decrease in the distending pressure of the ventricle over time
  - Creep—a rightward shift in the diastolic P–V relationship
- LV hypertrophy results in abnormalities of relaxation that are characteristic of the manner in which the hypertrophy developed and of the type of hypertrophy formed. Elevated EDP is seen in chronic pressure overload hypertrophy.
- Ischemia affects the extent of relaxation as evidenced by upward shift in the EDP–V relationship. These effects are independent of pericardial, right ventricular (RV), or lung interactions, implying a change in the intrinsic myocardial elastic properties. As previously discussed, changes in diastolic properties secondary to changes in myocardial Ca^{2+} handling and in hydrogen ion accumulation and repeated systolic stretch of the ischemia segment interact to produce the observed changes.
  - The changes in compliance appear restricted to the region of active ischemia.
  - The remaining normal areas of myocardium appear to utilize the Frank–Starling mechanism to maintain stroke volume (SV) in compensation for the effects of abnormal contractility or an upward shift of the regional diastolic P–V relationship within the ischemic areas.
- In addition, the constraining effect of the pericardium and the degree of ventricular interaction affect the extent of relaxation.
- **Rate of relaxation:** Abnormalities occur early in diastole and therefore do not alter EDP and EDV and tend to have minimal effect on the EDP–V relationship.
  - Changes in the diastolic P–V relationship that depend on the rate at which the LV deforms are known as viscoelasticity, a property that the myocardium shares with most biomaterials. This property is manifest when filling rates are highest, occurring during the first half of diastole or after atrial contraction.

- The determinants of relaxation rate are many, and their interactions complicated. Increases in heart rate and inotropy result in increased rates of relaxation. Alterations in end-diastolic loading conditions result in changes in the rate of relaxation during experimental conditions. Nonuniformity of relaxation refers to distribution of load and electric inactivation during diastole in space and time. Ventricular suction, or the ability of the ventricle to generate pressures below equilibrium diastolic pressures, may alter the rate and extent of LV filling. Ischemia can alter the rate and the extent of relaxation.

Extrinsic Influences on the Diastolic Pressure–Volume Relationship

- External loads can also profoundly influence ventricular compliance properties. Specifically, the RV, the pericardium, and the lungs all may acutely induce shifts of the LV diastolic P–V relationship. It is likely that each of these influences may be exerted when both ventricles are dilated and when the lungs are hyperinflated during ventilator therapy.
- The influence of the pericardium in the diastolic P–V relationship is a function of both its stiffness and its ability to constrain the entire heart. An increase in size of one ventricle therefore causes an increase in the EDP for a given volume (i.e., a shift upward in the P–V relationship) (Fig. 85.4). Although this effect is present with the pericardium open, the coupling is much stronger when it is closed.
  - Little normal pericardial effect is observed at normal filling pressures. The constraining effect is dependent on its intrinsic compliance and how it affects LV pressures; dilatation of the LV (i.e., a high LV filling pressure) amplifies the pericardium's influence.
  - The intact pericardium allows interaction between the atria and the LV and between the RV and LV. The effect of left atrial pressure is approximately one-fourth that of the RV pressure in determining the LV diastolic pressure. Ventricular interaction is an important mechanism underlying acute reductions in LV compliance; this may be why improved LV compliance is observed with vasoactive medications that reduce volume return to the RV, such as nitrates.
- Acute pulmonary hypertension alters LV geometry and upward shifts the LV diastolic P–V relationship with changes in RV afterload, largely mediated via a reduction in the LV septum to the free wall dimension and an increase in intrapericardial pressure. The LV septal/free wall axis appears disproportionately reduced when compared with either the base-to-apex or the anteroposterior axis.
- The special case of acute right ventricular failure: The established mechanisms for acute RV failure are shown in Table 85.1. An inverse relationship between RV stroke volume and pulmonary input resistance, vascular load, has been demonstrated. The RV tolerates up to triple the normal pulmonary artery pressure (PAP) by both the heart rate (chronotropic) response and the Frank–Starling mechanism (preload reserve) to maintain cardiac output. ATP and creatine phosphate levels are normal up to this point (Table 85.2); further increases in PAP create afterload mismatch with a disproportionate increase in end-systolic volume compared with end-diastolic volume (i.e., stroke volume and ejection fraction decrease as

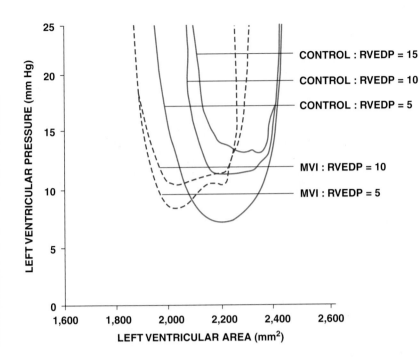

FIGURE 85.4. Diastolic portions of left ventricular pressure-area loops. Representative loops are depicted during both control and a microvascular injury (MVI) of the lungs at different right ventricular preloads or right ventricular end-diastolic pressures of 5, 10, and 15 mm Hg. The loops during both control and MVI are shifted upward by increasing right ventricular end-diastolic pressure (RVEDP), although left ventricular end-diastolic area is reduced at a given RVEDP during MVI.

a result). At this particular point, the RV is performing largely pressure work and very little flow work.

- As the RV dilates within an intact pericardium, RV end-diastolic pressure increases the intrapericardial pressure. This external pressure is exerted on the LV and affects its distensibility; this effect is independent of any change in heart rate.

- The transeptal pressure gradient decreases or, in fact, reverses with leftward shift of the septum further impairing LV filling. There is an inverse relationship between the transeptal pressure gradient and the LV septal–free wall dimension.

Evaluation and Treatment

- Growing public health and economic concerns have led to publication of guidelines by the Heart Failure Society of America, joint guidelines by the American Heart Association and the American College of Cardiology, with endorsement of the latter by the Heart Rhythm Society (Fig. 85.5).
- Treatment goals are set for Stage A (at risk), Stage B (asymptomatic abnormalities in cardiac structure and function), and Stages C and D with overt heart failure.
- The guidelines also give recommendations for initial evaluation of patients with both systolic and diastolic heart

---

TABLE 85.1

CAUSES OF RIGHT VENTRICULAR FAILURE

Increased pressure load
Pulmonary embolism
    Pulmonary disease (hypoxic pulmonary vasoconstriction, destruction of pulmonary vascular bed)
    Chronic airflow obstruction (emphysema, chronic bronchitis)
    Interstitial lung disease
    Neuromuscular chest wall restriction
Primary pulmonary hypertension
Elevated pulmonary venous pressure
    Left ventricular failure
    Mitral stenosis and insufficiency
Adult respiratory distress syndrome
Positive-pressure ventilation
Pulmonic valve stenosis

Increased volume load
Atrial septal defect
Ventricular septal defect
Tricuspid valve insufficiency

Decreased contractility
Ischemia
    Right coronary artery occlusion
    Systemic hypotension (poor right coronary perfusion)
    Right ventricular contusion (chest trauma)
    Mediastinal radiation
    β-Blockade

TABLE 85.2

MYOCARDIAL ADENOSINE TRIPHOSPHATE AND CREATINE PHOSPHATE IN OPEN PERICARDIA EXPERIMENTS ($N = 8^a$)

	ATP (μmol/g wet weight)	CP (μmol/g wet weight)
Baseline	5.52 ± 1.33	9.49 ± 3.24
Doubling of mean PAP	5.41 ± 1.28	8.78 ± 3.28
Tripling of mean PAP	5.12 ± 0.60	9.19 ± 1.20
RVF	3.63 ± 1.73^b	3.11 ± 3.22^b

ATP, adenosine triphosphate; CP, creatine phosphate; PAP, pulmonary artery pressure; RVF, right ventricular failure.
[a]$p < 0.05$, compared with baseline and doubling and tripling of mean PAP.
[b]Values are expressed as mean $\pm$ standard deviation.

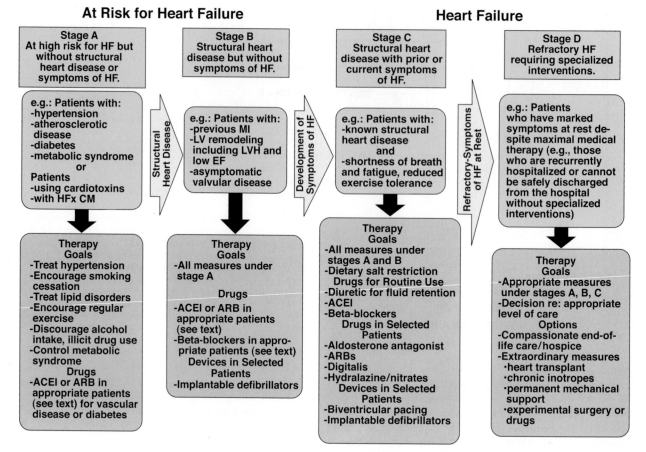

FIGURE 85.5. American College of Cardiology/American Heart Association 2005 guideline update for the diagnosis and management of chronic heart failure in the adult—summary article. A report of the American College of Cardiology Heart Association, Task Force in Practice Guidelines. (Writing Committee to Update the 2001 Guidelines for the Evaluation and Management of Heart Failure. *J Am Coll Cardiol.* 2005;46:1116–1143.)

failure, chronic outpatient management for the wide range of New York Heart Association (NYHA) classes, and inpatient management of acute decompensated heart failure (ADHF).

- Initial evaluation—patients presenting with new-onset heart failure—should have a thorough history and physical examination, with special attention to risk factors and noncardiac disorders that may aggravate their condition. Behaviors or therapies that may cause heart failure or exacerbate LV dysfunction should also be sought.
- Twelve-lead electrocardiogram, complete blood count, blood urea nitrogen, creatinine, electrolytes, fasting lipid panel and glucose, hemoglobin A_{1C} in diabetics, and thyroid-stimulating hormone, should be obtained; baseline BNP may be useful.
- If common etiologies are not present, test for HIV, hemochromatosis, sleep apnea, amyloidosis, pheochromocytoma, and rheumatologic disorders. Endomyocardial biopsy should be considered only if the results would influence therapy.
- Posteroanterior and lateral chest radiographs and echocardiography assess for pulmonary congestion, LV dimensions, LVEF, LVH, and valvular and wall motion abnormalities. Radionuclide ventriculography may also be performed to assess LVEF, LV volumes, and RV ejection fraction.

- In patients with angina pectoris or ischemia, coronary angiography should be performed unless contraindicated to evaluate for revascularization. Noninvasive imaging to determine myocardial viability is reasonable in patients with known coronary disease but without angina.

Prognosis in Heart Failure

- The overall 5-year survival is 50%, whereas the 1-year survival for end-stage heart failure is 75%. Negative prognostic factors include the presence of an S_3, low pulse pressure, elevated jugular venous pulse, and high NYHA class. Other important comorbidities include diabetes mellitus, renal insufficiency, and depression.
- Cardiac testing plays an important role in prognostication:
  - EF is a very important marker for prognosis and as a target for new therapies such as implantable cardioverter defibrillator (ICD) and biventricular pacing.
  - Peak oxygen consumption is an objective prognostic measurement (Fig. 85.6); mortality rates vary from 20% per year if peak VO_2 is ≥ 14 but <18 mL/kg/minute to 60% per year if peak VO_2 is ≤ 10 mL/kg/minute.
  - Distance covered in the 6-minute walk is predictive of morbidity and mortality.

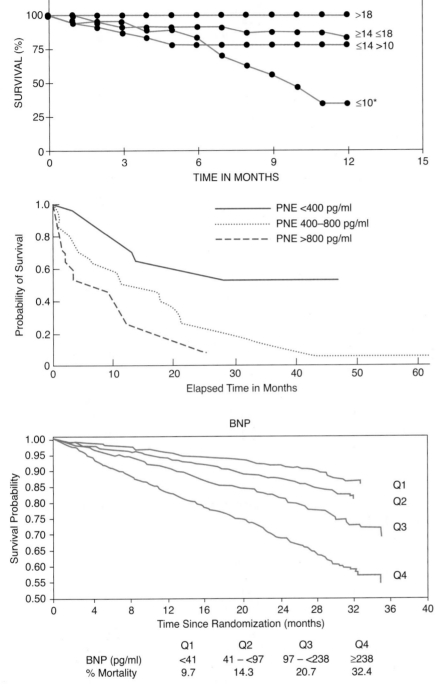

FIGURE 85.6. Survival curves for heart failure patients by peak VO$_2$ (**upper panel**), plasma norepinephrine (**middle**), and brain natriuretic peptide (BNP, **lower panel**). Survival is best with peak VO$_2$ >18 mL/kg/min, plasma norepinephrine <400 pg/mL, and BNP <100 pg/mL. (Reproduced from Mancin DM, Eisen H, Kausmaul W, et al. *Circulation.* 1991;83:778–786; Cohn JN, Levin B, Olivari MT, et al. *N Engl J Med.* 1984;311:819–823; and Anand IS, Fisher LD, Chiang Y, et al. Changes in brain natriuretic peptide and norepinephrine over time and mortality and morbidity in the Valsartan Heart Failure Trial (Val-HeFT) *Circulation.* 2003;107:1278–1283.)

	Q1	Q2	Q3	Q4
BNP (pg/ml)	<41	41 – <97	97 – <238	≥238
% Mortality	9.7	14.3	20.7	32.4

- Hemodynamic variables measured at catheterization, such as cardiac index, systemic and pulmonary vascular resistances, PAP, and pulmonary capillary wedge pressures, are important indicators of prognosis and aid diagnosis. Stroke work index is an especially important predictor, as it incorporates both flow and pressure work.
- Inverse relationships exist between survival and plasma norepinephrine, renin, vasopressin, aldosterone, atrial and B-type natriuretic peptides, and endothelin-1 (seeFig. 85.6). Plasma norepinephrine, pro-BNP, and BNP are independent factors affecting prognosis, but only BNP has become a routine laboratory test in suspected heart failure patients

- Multivariate models can be used in critically ill patients to assess the severity of acute decompensated heart failure.
- Acute Physiology and Chronic Health Evaluation (APACHE) II score predicts mortality in acute heart failure and after ventricular assist device implantation (Fig. 85.7); survivors had lower APACHE II scores than nonsurvivors.
- The Acute Decompensated Heart Failure Registry acuity model for heart failure identifies three predictors: blood urea nitrogen ≥43 mg/dL, serum creatinine >2.5 mg/dL, and systolic blood pressure (SBP) <115 mm Hg to partition patients into one high-risk group (three factors present,

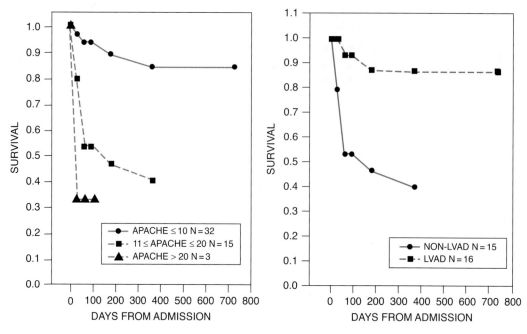

FIGURE 85.7. Kaplan-Meier survival curves for non–left ventricular assist device (LVAD)-treated heart failure patients demonstrates a strong relationship between survival and APACHE II scores (**left panel**) and survival curves for heart failure patients with APACHE II scores between 11 and 20 for both LVAD and non–LVAD-treated patients (**right panel**). (Right panel from Gracin N, Johnson MR, Spokes D, et al. The use of Apache II scores to select candidates for left ventricular assist device placement. *J Heart Lung Transplant.* 1998;17:1017–1023.)

crude mortality 21.9%), three intermediate-risk groups (varying combinations of risk factors present, crude mortality 5.5%–12.4%), and one low-risk group (no risk factors present, crude mortality 2.14%).

THERAPEUTIC TRIALS AND FINDINGS

Angiotensin-converting Enzyme Inhibitors

- ACE inhibitors are the foundation therapy for heart failure as they delay development of both heart failure symptoms and hospitalizations and increase survival. ACE inhibitors should be prescribed for all patients with asymptomatic LV systolic dysfunction and asymptomatic valvular heart disease (stage B) and in patients with symptomatic and/or refractory heart failure (stages C and D) unless the patient is intolerant to ACE inhibitors. In stage A patients, ACE inhibitors are indicated for those with diabetes mellitus and LVH. Patients experiencing angioedema, intolerable cough, or other untoward effects of ACE inhibitors should be prescribed angiotensin II receptor blockers (ARBs).
- ACE inhibitors increase survival in patients with LV systolic dysfunction (LVEF ≤35%) and symptoms of heart failure, especially NYHA class IV, by reducing progression of disease. They also improve NYHA functional class with treatment.
- Asymptomatic patients with LV dysfunction have a reduced risk in the combined end point of death plus development of heart failure with ACE inhibitors and fewer hospitalizations for heart failure or death.
- In acute myocardial infarction (MI) with LV systolic dysfunction (LVEF <40%), ACE inhibitors decrease all-cause mortality, the development of severe heart failure, fatal and

nonfatal major cardiovascular events, congestive heart failure end points requiring hospitalization, and recurrent MIs.
- Trials of ACE inhibitors in survivors of MI showing improved survival with the ACE inhibitors and less development of LV systolic dysfunction.

Angiotensin II Receptor Blockers

- ARBs are better tolerated with less cough but have no difference on all-cause mortality, sudden death, or increases in serum creatinine compared to ACE inhibitors. ARBs decrease cardiovascular death or admission to hospital for heart failure in patients intolerant to ACE inhibitors. Combination therapy with ACE inhibitors has the most drug-related adverse events.
- In chronic heart failure and in heart failure after MI (LVEF <40% and NYHA classes II through IV heart failure), ARBs may decrease the combined end point of mortality and morbidity in addition to ACE inhibitors or β-blockers. For those already on ACE inhibitors but still experiencing heart failure symptoms, ARBs decrease the combined outcome of cardiovascular death or hospitalization for heart failure.
- With preserved LV systolic dysfunction (NYHA classes II through IV and baseline LVEF >40%) there is no benefit of ARB therapy in terms of cardiovascular death or admission to hospital for heart failure.

β-Adrenergic Receptor Antagonists

- β-Blockers, in addition to ACE inhibitors, decrease LV size and improve EF. However, not just any β-blocker can be used in heart failure patients.

- Carvedilol, a nonselective β-blocker and an α-blocker, decreases hospitalization and improves quality of life in patients with NYHA classes II and III heart failure. In patients with severe heart failure (LVEF of <25% and NYHA classes IIIB to IV) already receiving standard heart failure therapy (ACE inhibitors or ARBs plus diuretic), carvedilol reduces mortality and the combined end point of death or hospitalization. After acute MI with LV dysfunction, it reduces all-cause mortality, cardiovascular mortality, and recurrent, nonfatal MIs.
- Selective β_1 antagonists, bisoprolol and extended-release metoprolol, decrease all-cause mortality and sudden death in symptomatic heart failure patients. Short-acting metoprolol does not have the same affect on survival.
- Bucindolol, a nonselective β-blocker and a weak α-blocker, does not improve survival. This is possibly due to its sympatholytic activity, which decreases norepinephrine levels. Bucindolol appears to worsen mortality in African Americans and those with NYHA class IV versus class III heart failure.

Aldosterone Receptor Antagonists

- ACE inhibitors may only transiently suppress aldosterone production. As aldosterone promotes retention of sodium, sympathetic activation, inhibition of the parasympathetic nervous system, myocardial and vascular fibrosis, and loss of magnesium and potassium, blockade of aldosterone receptors may alter progression of LV dysfunction. Spironolactone in addition to standard therapy decreases mortality, though use is limited by hyperkalemia and renal insufficiency.

Other Vasodilators

- When digoxin and diuretics were the standard of care, vasodilators were explored as therapeutic options in heart failure. Prazosin 20 mg/day was equivalent to placebo; however, the combination of hydralazine (300 mg/day) and isosorbide dinitrate (160 mg/day) reduced mortality.
- This combination was later compared to and found inferior to ACE inhibitor therapy, especially in Caucasians.
- African Americans have similar survival with ACE inhibitors and combination vasodilator therapy, possibly due to a less active renin–angiotensin system and lower NO bioavailability than other racial groups. Combination therapy—hydralazine plus isosorbide dinitrate—improves survival in NYHA classes III and IV African Americans who remain symptomatic with heart failure despite standard therapy, including ACE inhibitors or ARBs in ACE-intolerant patients, β-blockers, digoxin, spironolactone, and diuretics.

Digoxin

- After acceptance of ACE inhibitors for heart failure, the efficacy of digoxin became controversial. However, in the era prior to β-blockers, digoxin was shown to be efficacious for treatment of heart failure.
- When digoxin is withdrawn from patients managed with either diuretics or diuretics and ACE inhibitors, however, maximal exercise and functional capacity worsens, treatment failure increases, time-to-treatment failure

decreases, LV EF decreases, and both weight and heart rate increase.
- In patients with LV EF <45% on diuretics and ACE inhibitors, the addition of digoxin has no effect on mortality but decreases total hospitalizations and hospitalizations for worsening heart failure.

ACUTE DECOMPENSATED HEART FAILURE

- ADHF has a variety of presentations; common symptoms include fatigue, shortness of breath, and congestion of the lungs and abdominal organs that can mimic other disease states. Patients with preserved systolic function and systemic hypertension comprise the majority of hospitalized patients; a minority have poor end-organ perfusion, low EF, and hypotension. Despite advances in therapeutics, both pharmacologic and devices, risk of death, and rehospitalization remain high.
  - Hospitalization constitutes the bulk of the cost in caring for patients with heart failure.
  - BNP is a useful diagnostic test as values over 400 (normal range: 0–100 pg/mL) have a high probability for heart failure, whether systolic or diastolic in origin.
- The Heart Failure Society of America guidelines recommend hospitalization for altered mentation, worsening renal function, hypotension, resting dyspnea, hemodynamically significant arrhythmias, and acute coronary syndromes. Hospitalization should be considered when congestion has worsened with evidence of weight gain of ≥ 5 kg, and when there are signs and symptoms of abdominal or pulmonary congestion, even in the absence of weight gain. Other considerations include major electrolyte abnormalities, repeated ICD discharges, and associated comorbid conditions.
  - Blood urea nitrogen level >43 mg/dL at admission is the best single discriminator between survivors and nonsurvivors of hospitalization for ADHF. The second best predictor is SBP <115 mm Hg.
  - Use of pulmonary artery catheters to help guide clinical management may not improve hospital mortality or length of stay in either the intensive care unit or in hospital and are associated with complications including hematoma at the insertion site, arrhythmias, and infection. When used, nesiritide is more effective than nitroglycerin to lower pulmonary capillary wedge pressure from baseline.
- Current guidelines for inpatient management of ADHF include identification of precipitating factors and etiology, optimizing volume status, treating with recommended vasodilator therapy, and minimizing side effects. Educating patients about lifestyle changes, including sodium and fluid restriction, and self-management techniques are recommended general measures. Precipitating factors include development of arrhythmias, acute infections, and nonadherence with medications and dietary restrictions.
- Optimization of medical therapy involves daily weights and accurate recordings of intake and output. Intravenous (IV) loop diuretics are recommended; with inadequate diuresis continuous IV infusion of loop diuretics or addition of other diuretics, such as metolazone, should be considered. In those not responding to the foregoing measures and without symptomatic hypotension, IV nitroglycerin, nitroprusside, or nesiritide may be used additionally.

- IV inotropes should be reserved for those with advanced heart failure and evidence of end-organ dysfunction and/or decreased peripheral perfusion, especially if SBP is <90 mm Hg.
- Ultrafiltration is an alternative to diuretics for volume removal, does not require central venous access, and can be performed through a 16-gauge 35-cm peripheral catheter. It is well tolerated and can also be used in conjunction with diuretics.

NONPHARMACOLOGIC AND NONSURGICAL THERAPY FOR CHRONIC HEART FAILURE

- Electrophysiologic therapy is a new addition to the heart failure management arsenal and is having enormous impact. Combination therapy with defibrillators and biventricular pacing reduces mortality to a greater degree in ischemic versus nonischemic cardiomyopathy.
- Automatic implantable cardioverter defibrillators were first shown to be effective at improving long-term survival after symptomatic VT or cardiac arrest, in ischemic cardiomyopathy with EF <30%, and asymptomatic inducible VT. Other indications include nonischemic cardiomyopathy patients with QRS duration >120 msec, with LVEF <35%, and having had an admission for heart failure in the previous year.
- Indications for automatic implantable cardioverter defibrillators for primary prevention of sudden cardiac death in heart failure are:
  - Prior MI ≥40 days old, with EF 30% to 40%, and NYHA class II or III on optimal therapy.
  - Prior MI ≥40 days old, with EF 30% to 35%, and NYHA class I on optimal therapy.
  - Nonischemic cardiomyopathy, with EF 30% to 35%, and NYHA class II or III on optimal therapy.
- Biventricular pacing is achieved by implantation of a LV lead, generally via the coronary sinus to the great cardiac vein, in addition to a RV lead. This strategy is based on the fact that most patients with intraventricular conduction delay have dyssynchronous LV contraction, which reduces cardiac efficiency (decreased contractile force and impaired myocardial energetics).
  - It improves NYHA class, exercise tolerance, dp/dt, EF, cardiac index, and mortality.
  - Cardiac resynchronization reverses remodeling the LV.

CARDIAC TRANSPLANTATION AND LEFT VENTRICULAR ASSIST DEVICES

- When patients continue to experience advanced heart failure symptoms despite maximization of medical therapy, cardiac transplantation and left ventricular assist devices (LVADs) may be considered.
- There are currently three LVADs available for use in the United States.
  - The Abiomed system is available for temporary use as either right, left, or biventricular assist systems. It is most commonly used after high-risk coronary artery bypass surgery in patients who fail to wean from the cardiopulmonary bypass machine. Cannulae are placed in the atria, and the pumps

are external to the body. Because the cannulae are implanted in the atria, removal is feasible should the patient recover. Additionally, one ventricular system may be removed at a time; this system requires full anticoagulation.
  - The Thoratec Heart Mate device is approved for use as a bridge to transplantation and as destination therapy in those not considered transplant candidates. The outflow cannula is placed in the proximal ascending aorta, and the inflow cannula is placed in the LV apex. Cannulae are named with respect to the pump that is commonly implanted in the left upper abdominal quadrant preperitoneally. This device does not require anticoagulation, although antiplatelet therapy with aspirin is recommended.
  - The World Heart LVAD is implanted in a fashion similar to that of the Heart Mate device and is currently approved by the Food and Drug Administration as a bridge to transplantation. Currently, a clinical trial is under way for its potential use as destination therapy. This device requires full anticoagulation with warfarin, aspirin, and clopidogrel.
- There have been 40,192 cardiac transplantation procedures between 1988 and August 31, 2006; 2,125 of these procedures were performed in 2005. Kaplan–Meier survival rates for heart transplantation procedures performed between 1997 and 2004 ranged from 85.7% to 90.6% at 1 year; 75.2% to 81.8% at 3 years; and 68.8% to 72.6% at 5 years. Ranges are given as the data were based on the United Network of Organ Sharing status at the time of transplantation.
- Criteria to be considered for transplantation include advanced symptoms despite maximization of medical therapy—including tailoring therapy via hemodynamic monitoring with pulmonary artery catheterization—and a peak oxygen consumption <15.0 mL/kg/minute during exercise testing.
- Exclusion criteria include fixed pulmonary hypertension with >4 Wood units not responsive to vasodilator therapy; tobacco, alcohol, or illicit drug use; other life-threatening illnesses such as cancer or advanced peripheral arterial disease; noncompliance with physician visits, diet, and medications; psychiatric or personality disorders likely to become exacerbated by, or that would interfere with, posttransplant care; and lack of social support.

THERAPEUTIC GUIDELINES FOR SYMPTOMATIC LEFT VENTRICULAR SYSTOLIC DYSFUNCTION

- Polypharmacy has become standard therapy for patients with symptomatic systolic dysfunction.
- ACE inhibitors are recommended for all patients; those with contraindications (other than renal insufficiency or hyperkalemia) or intolerable side effects should be treated with ARBs. After the introduction of ACE inhibitor or ARB therapy, β-adrenergic receptor blockade should be started consisting of either carvedilol or long-acting metoprolol (Toprol XL).
- β-Blockers should be instituted in patients with euvolemia, starting with low doses and titrating the dose up every 2 weeks as tolerated, to doses achieved in clinical trials; achievement of these doses may take 8 to 12 weeks. For patients being discharged from the hospital with ADHF,

low-dose β-blockers may be instituted in-hospital once euvolemia has been achieved. In patients on stable doses of β-blockers who then experience an acute decompensation requiring hospitalization, continuation of β-blocker therapy is recommended.

- Aldosterone antagonists are recommended for patients with NYHA class III or IV symptoms in addition to standard therapy, including diuretics. They are not recommended in patients with creatinine clearance <30 mL/minute, serum potassium >5.0 mmol/L, or serum creatinine >2.5 mg/dL. Guidelines recommend frequent monitoring of serum potassium levels after initiation of or change in dose of aldosterone antagonists.
- Hydralazine and oral nitrate combination may be considered in those not tolerating ACE inhibitors or ARBs. The combination of hydralazine and oral nitrates is recommended for African American patients—in addition to ACE inhibitors and β-blockers—who remain NYHA class III or IV despite these drugs.

- Loop and distal tubule diuretics should be viewed as necessary adjuncts to relieve sodium and water retention.
- Guidelines recommend that digoxin should be considered for symptomatic patients receiving standard therapy and that the dose should be 0.125 mg in the majority of patients. Serum digoxin level should be <1.0 ng/mL.
- Amiodarone and other antiarrhythmic medications should not be used for primary prevention of sudden death, but amiodarone may be considered in those with ICDs to decrease the frequency of repetitive ICD discharges should this become an issue.
- Patients with mild heart failure symptoms (NYHA class II) should restrict their sodium intake to 2 to 3 g daily. Those with more advanced symptoms (NYHA classes III to IV) should restrict their sodium intake to 2 g daily. Patients with severe hyponatremia—serum sodium <130 mEq/L—should restrict their fluid intake to <2 L/day, as should individuals in whom fluid balance is difficult to maintain despite sodium restriction and high-dose diuretics.

CHAPTER 86 ■ CARDIAC MECHANICAL ASSIST DEVICES

Cardiac mechanical assist devices are used during periods of hemodynamic instability and persistent low cardiac output in an attempt to restore normal hemodynamic parameters and preserve vital organs. There is a stepwise progression of therapy with respect to cardiac assist interventions beginning with inotropic and vasodilator drugs, then intra-aortic balloon pump, and ultimately mechanical ventricular assist device (VAD) placement. In this chapter, we briefly discuss these devices with special emphasis on their indications, contraindications, placement, complications, and potential pitfalls.

INTRA-AORTIC BALLOON PUMP

- Indications: 10% to 15% of acute myocardial infarctions have shock that may require temporary hemodynamic support with an intra-aortic balloon pump (Fig. 86.1). Other indications include unstable angina, prophylaxis for high-risk surgery or percutaneous coronary intervention, acute mitral insufficiency, ventricular septal rupture after an ischemic event, postcardiotomy failure: inability to separate patient from cardiopulmonary bypass after cardiac surgical procedure, and traumatic myocardial contusion with low cardiac output.
- Contraindications:
  - *Aortic insufficiency:* Leaking of the aortic valve makes the use of an intra-aortic balloon pump potentially detrimental. During periods of diastolic augmentation, enhanced reversal of flow actually exacerbates the aortic insufficiency.
  - *Atheromatous aorta:* Patients who are known to have severe atheromatous disease of the aorta are poor candidates for balloon pump therapy. There is the risk of atheroembolization, either distally or retrograde into the cerebral vasculature, during pump use or manipulation.
  - *Severe peripheral vascular disease or aortic dissection:* The balloon pump is typically inserted in a retrograde fashion from the groin. This relative contraindication of peripheral vascular disease can be overcome by the use of alternate insertion techniques.

Techniques of Insertion

- The most commonly used method of intra-aortic balloon pump insertion is via the retrograde approach from percutaneous access to the femoral artery (Fig. 86.2) with or without a vascular sheath. When a groin incision is present related to coronary artery bypass cannulation or some other intervention, it is possible to insert the balloon pump via direct arterial access.
- For patients who have their balloon pump for an extended period of time or need to ambulate during balloon pump use, the balloon pump may be placed directly through the axillary artery. A sheath is not routinely used for placement. In more extreme circumstances, such as coexisting peripheral vascular disease and postcardiotomy failure, placement may require an antegrade approach either directly into the arch or through a small graft sewn onto the ascending aorta or arch and tunneled to the chest wall.

FIGURE 86.1. Intra-aortic balloon pulsation (IABP). Example of standard 7.5 French 40-mL IABP.

Verification of Location

- The balloon pump should be positioned just distal to the left subclavian artery in the descending thoracic aorta (Fig. 86.3). The location may be verified by fluoroscopy, chest roentgenogram, or transesophageal echocardiography if performed concurrently with balloon pump insertion. The tip should be high in the left chest in appropriate relation to the aortic arch.
- Also important is selecting the appropriate-sized balloon pump for the patient. They range in size from those appropriate for a small infant to those used in large adults (Fig. 86.4). The standard adult size is 40 mL; the manufacturer's labeling, recommendations, and the patient's habitus should be considered.

Mechanism of Action

- There are two complementary effects of an intra-aortic balloon pump. Both of these mechanisms augment left ventricular function and serve in complementary fashion to help those patients with right ventricular dysfunction.

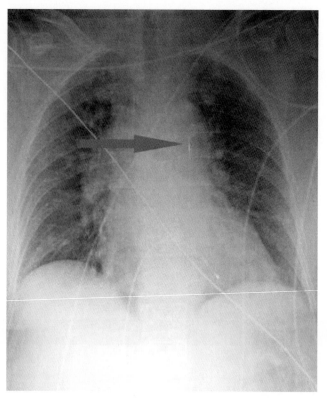

FIGURE 86.3. Chest radiograph showing intra-aortic balloon pulsation (IABP) device in place. Marked distal tip of IABP.

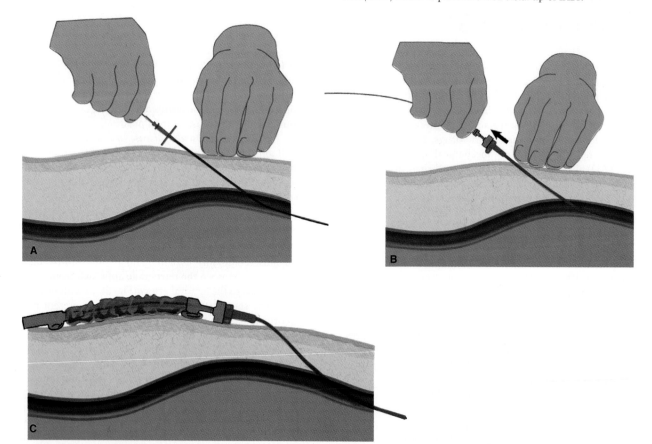

FIGURE 86.2. Intra-aortic balloon pulsation (IABP). Insertion from femoral approach. **A:** Artery is accessed and wire advanced. **B:** Sheath inserted over wire. **C:** IABP advanced over wire and through sheath to appropriate level.

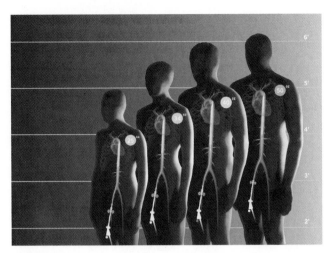

FIGURE 86.4. Different sizes of intra-aortic balloon pulsation (IABP) devices.

- The first is the diastolic augmentation of coronary blood flow. The balloon pump is carefully timed to the cardiac cycle so that the pump inflates during aortic valve closure and thus enhances the diastolic pressure in the proximal aorta. This allows increased coronary blood flow and enhanced myocardial oxygen delivery.
- The second action involves the afterload reduction at the time of cardiac systole, thereby allowing enhanced runoff for the failing ventricle. The balloon should be properly timed to deflate during aortic valve opening, thereby creating a pocket of reduced afterload and thus enhancing the ability of the heart to eject the blood during systole. This action serves to lower the left ventricular end systolic volume.
- It is a common misperception that a balloon pump is not beneficial or indicated, for right ventricular dysfunction. In clinical practice, patients with right ventricular dysfunction benefit from the diastolic augmentation of coronary blood flow in the right coronary artery. Additional benefit is derived from the reduced left ventricular end-diastolic pressure and left atrial pressure, thereby allowing increased forward flow and decreased afterload for the failing right ventricle.

Complications

- Although complications related to balloon pump insertion and use are relatively infrequent, they can be quite serious.
- During insertion of the balloon pump, direct trauma to the arterial insertion site may occur. It is important that insertion occurs relatively high in the thigh in the femoral artery, near the inferior edge of the inguinal ligament. A misplaced balloon may shear off a major arterial branch, and placement through a smaller-caliber artery may cause complete occlusion and ischemia. In arteries that are not particularly calcified, the balloon pump may be placed without a vascular sheath, which reduces the maximal diameter of obstruction in the artery and perhaps reduces the potential for thrombus.
- Improper proximal location of the balloon pump risks impingement of the arch vessels, causing cerebral ischemia from atheroembolization or thromboembolism from micro-

thrombi forming on the balloon pump itself. When too distal, the pump may impede the visceral arteries.
- When it is placed as part of a cardiopulmonary bypass procedure, blood is equally oxygenated in the arterial and venous vessels, and there is no pulsatile flow at the time of insertion. This makes differentiating artery from vein difficult and has led to inadvertent placement of balloon pumps via the femoral vein into the right atrium. Hemodynamic instability at the time of insertion may also lead to suboptimal confirmation of balloon pump location.
- In more chronic management of the balloon pump, ranging from several days to weeks or months, infectious complications become more predominant. In addition to meticulous sterile insertion techniques, balloon pumps also require daily attention from the nursing staff. Attention to the insertion site for signs of erythema or purulence and close monitoring of the patient's temperature are mandatory. When a patient's hemodynamic status fails to stabilize with balloon pump therapy, a VAD is the next course of progressive therapy.

VENTRICULAR ASSIST DEVICES

Preoperative Considerations

- Indications for VADs include unstable hemodynamic measurements and failure to stabilize measurements with other less-invasive therapies. Common hemodynamic parameters for device placement are listed in Table 86.1.
- In the preoperative assessment, determine the likelihood that right ventricular support will be needed as a course of therapy. Several scoring systems are commonly used; most center on the calculation of right ventricular stroke work and other hemodynamic indices.
  - Use caution if the central venous pressure is greater than the pulmonary capillary wedge pressure or if the patient's central venous pressure is >20 mm Hg after optimization.
  - Dependence on the right ventricle to support a left-sided device in such instances may prove to be difficult. Patients who are very debilitated at the time of implantation, with organ deterioration (elevated liver enzymes, abnormal coagulation parameters, and renal dysfunction) caused by right heart dysfunction, are more likely to require right-sided support devices.
- Select the device based on the goal of therapy; devices may be implanted as a *bridge to recovery,* a *bridge to transplantation,* or as a *destination therapy.*

TABLE 86.1

HEMODYNAMIC PARAMETERS SUGGESTING NEED FOR MECHANICAL SUPPORT

Hemodynamic parameters	Values
Pulmonary capillary wedge pressure	>20 mm Hg
Central venous pressure	>20 mm Hg
Cardiac index	<2.0 L/m^2
Mean arterial pressure	<60 mm Hg

- The lines between bridge to recovery and bridge to transplantation can sometimes become blurred when the neurologic status of patients cannot be defined prior to implantation. These patients have been termed *bridge to decision*, where a short-term device may be appropriate to stabilize hemodynamics until the neurologic status and overall candidacy for transplantation are better elucidated.
- Destination therapy refers to permanent device implantation, intended to remain in use for the duration of the patient's lifetime for patients who are not transplant candidates because of age or end organ dysfunction.

Preparation of the Patient

- Before the operative implantation of the VAD, it is often useful to have a period of volume optimization, or a preoperative "tune-up." This is done to ensure that right ventricular function is as well preserved as possible for placement of a left VAD.
- This may include diuretic and inotropic therapy. In cases where the decision for biventricular support is difficult, a 24- to 48-hour period of intra-aortic balloon pumping may be a useful prognostic indicator. This helps to demonstrate the response of the right ventricular function to a reduced left ventricular end-diastolic pressure.
- During this period of optimization, it is ideal to use an arterial pressure monitor and a pulmonary artery catheter to allow fine tuning of medications and volume status.
- Antimicrobial prophylaxis is essential during the period of preoperative optimization. This usually involves selective skin decontamination with Hibiclens scrub; additionally, Bactroban (mupirocin) is often used to reduce the number of pathogens in the nasal passages.
- Red cell augmentation may be performed in semielective implants, as frequently there is a 5- to 7-day delay before implantation. Erythropoiesis-stimulating drugs, such as erythropoietin, can be combined with iron supplementation to achieve a significant increase of hematocrit.

Classification of Ventricular Assist Devices

- Flow type
  - **Pulsatile:** In these devices, the intermittent relocation of a pusher plate or blood sack emits a pulsatile wave similar to that of the natural heart (Fig. 86.5).
  - **Axial flow:** The term *nonpulsatile* is frequently applied to these devices, although this is a misnomer. These pumps actually have a central blade that rotates at a rapid rate, similar to a jet engine in an airplane (Fig. 86.6). The native function of the left ventricle does intermittently augment the inflow to the pump, which generates a pulsatile output at appropriate speeds.
  - **Centripetal flow:** These pumps have a continuous spinning impeller that generates a flow similar to axial pumps. However, the more advanced pumps, currently in development, may be magnetically levitated to function without bearings (Fig. 86.7).
- Mechanism
  - **Pneumatic:** These pumps are operated by air, where intermittent external application of compressed gas through a tube to a blood sac emits the pulse of the pump (Fig. 86.8).

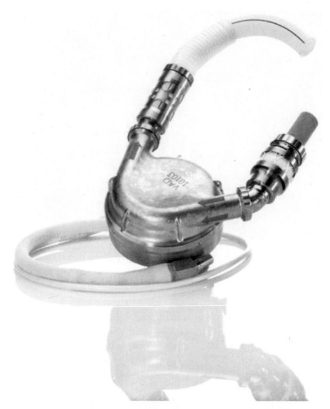

FIGURE 86.5. HeartMate XVE, an example of a pulsatile pusher plate device. (Thoratec Corp, Pleasanton, CA, with permission.)

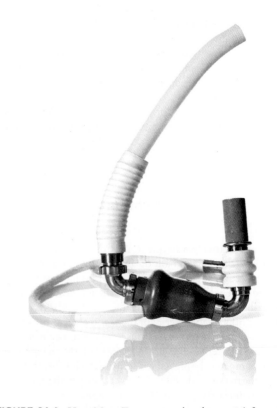

FIGURE 86.6. HeartMate II, an example of an axial flow device. (Thoratec Corp, Pleasanton, CA, with permission.)

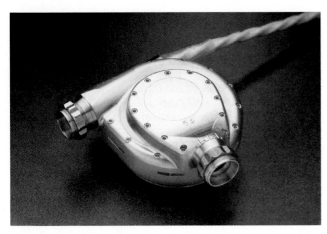

FIGURE 86.7. WorldHeart Levacor, magnetically levitated, centripetal pump (in development).

- **Electric:** Electric pumps are driven by batteries or alternating current via an adapter. They may have the axial flow motor or the pusher plate-driven motor.
- Location
  - **Paracorporeal:** These pumps are placed outside of, but in continuity with, the body, usually connected via transcutaneous cannulas that are surgically implanted into the heart (Figs. 86.8 and 86.9).
  - **Intracorporeal.** This term typically refers to those pumps that are placed completely within the body with only a drive line exiting the skin (Fig. 86.10). The main pumping mechanism is within the body, rather than external to it.

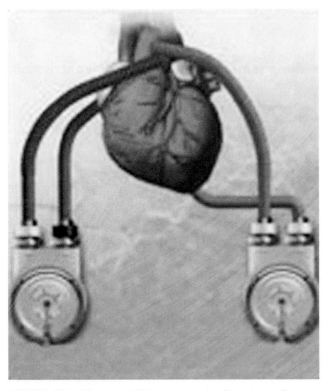

FIGURE 86.8. Thoratec pVAD., an example of pneumatically actuated ventricular assist device as biventricular support.

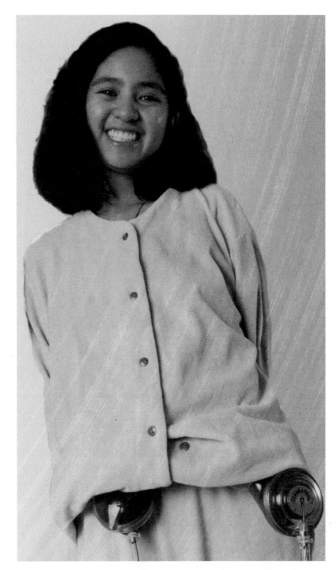

FIGURE 86.9. Thoratec pVAD, a paracorporeal device.

- **Percutaneous:** *Percutaneous* refers to a small group of pumps that are indicated for extremely short-term use and are inserted transcutaneously, either via the femoral vein and then transseptally into the left atrium or retrograde across the aortic valve (Fig. 86.11).
- Potential duration of support based on device type
  - **Short term:** These devices are placed to resolve immediate hemodynamic instability as either a bridge to recovery, a bridge to decision, or for use during a short-term procedure. Their use is intended for hours to weeks.
  - **Medium term:** These devices are inserted with the intention of being used to allow recovery of the native heart function or as a short-term bridge to transplantation. They are indicated for weeks to months.
  - **Long term:** These devices are intended to be used for either long-term bridge patients who will require an extended period of time to acquire donor hearts or for those patients who may potentially have the device as destination therapy.

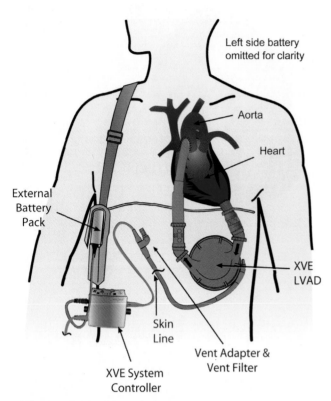

Left side battery omitted for clarity

Aorta

Heart

External Battery Pack

XVE LVAD

Skin Line

Vent Adapter & Vent Filter

XVE System Controller

FIGURE 86.10. Implanted HeartMate XVE, an intracorporeal left ventricular assist device. (Thoratec Corp, Pleasanton, CA, with permission.)

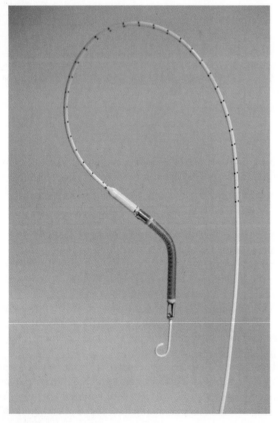

FIGURE 86.11. Impella (Abiomed), a temporary percutaneous ventricular assist device. (Courtesy of Abiomed, Danvers, MA.)

Important Implications for Potential Emergency Situations while the Patient is Supported by Ventricular Assist Devices

- It is important to understand the physiologic implications of each VAD, not only while they are in use but during periods of unintended pump arrest. One of the critical differentiations between the various types of pumps is the presence or absence of valves and the potential for retrograde flow during periods of pump stoppage.
  - The presence of valves should prevent retrograde flow; pump arrest merely means that the augmented flow no longer exists. This is a key point to consider during emergency management.
  - The pumps with no valves, such as the axial flow devices, will allow volumes in excess of 1.5 L/minute of retrograde flow during periods of pump arrest. This degree of acute aortic insufficiency will frequently lead to ventricular arrhythmias and cardiovascular collapse.
- Knowledge of these internal components and working mechanisms leads to proper decision making during emergencies. Health care providers must know whether the pump can be temporally actuated via an external mechanism (blood sac pumps) by an individual (as opposed to the driver) and whether the pump electronics are defibrillation-compatible.
- Future devices: Most future generations will be designed to have a longer life span so they are better suited for destination therapy. Enhanced battery life will allow for greater independence, and a reduced need for transcutaneous attachment to the device, thus reducing infectious complications. They will focus on total elimination of bearings and metal-to-metal contact through magnetically levitated bearingless designs to resolve issues of anticoagulation and thromboembolic events.

Management of the Post-left Ventricular Assist Device Patient

- Most VAD centers strive to support patients with left-sided devices only and limit the number of patients who require right VADs whenever possible. Patients on single ventricular support are more mobile and more rapidly rehabilitated. A major focus of post–left VAD management is the stabilization of right heart function and prevention of right heart failure.
- To accomplish this goal, the most important factor is the selection of patients who have sustainable right ventricular hemodynamic parameters preoperatively. The previously discussed period of optimization is crucial and ranks just under the requirement that the right heart can support the function of the left VAD.
  - Additionally, right heart function is frequently supported for some period of time with inotropic therapy. The most commonly used drugs are dobutamine or milrinone.
  - Aggressive attempts are made to lower the pulmonary artery resistance by using nitroso-dilators, such as sodium nitroprusside, nitroglycerin, and inhaled nitric oxide. Inhaled prostacyclin may be a less expensive alternative to inhaled nitric oxide.
  - Other more novel options in evolution include the use of orally available, direct-acting drugs on the pulmonary

vasculature, such as the use of sildenafil, a phosphodiesterase type 5 inhibitor.

- After placement of a left VAD, meticulous care of the drive line site is important to reduce the risk of ascending infection. This typically involves diligent immobilization of the drive line and the use of topical treatments, initially several times a day. In cases where infection is noted at the drive line site despite all efforts, topical treatments can be used with success.

Dysfunction and Complications of Left Ventricular Assist Devices

- **Cannula kinking:** In the paracorporeal devices, this is particularly problematic. Shifting of patient position or rolling in the bed can lead to either dislodgement or, more frequently, kinking of the transcutaneous cannula. This will lead to flow alarms and sudden dysfunction of the device and can usually be addressed by simply removing the kink in the cannula. Often, centers have found it beneficial to keep a folded towel under the device to keep it off the patient's skin and to keep the cannulas straight. With the intracorporeal devices, this problem is usually secondary to device migration, either from chest closure in the operating room or from postoperative ambulation. With intracorporeal devices, this frequently requires reoperation for adjustment of the device.
- **Thrombosis and embolism:** The Achilles heel of all device therapy remains the poorly understood human coagulation system and the effects of foreign bodies in the bloodstream. Depending on the specific device selected and the type of valves within the device, variable amounts of anticoagulation are recommended by the manufacturer. Regardless of the anticoagulation therapy used, thrombosis, embolism, and bleeding events are a concern with all devices. It is important to treat patients with any new symptom, such as abdominal pain or a cold leg, as if it were a thromboembolic event. With appropriate management of anticoagulation and diligent patient care, these events are relatively infrequent.
- **Mechanical device issues:** The devices themselves may have mechanical issues related to valve dysfunction or problems with either bearings or motor wear. These are addressed in the materials supplied by the manufacturers. All of the devices require some type of ongoing surveillance and assessment for wear and potential mechanical failure.
- **Patent foramen ovale and hypoxemia after left ventricular assist placement:** Patients need to be carefully screened in the operating room with transesophageal echocardiography and provocation maneuvers during a bubble test to identify a patent foramen ovale. With the altered hemodynamics after left VAD placement, the left atrial pressure is suddenly dramatically lower than the right atrial pressure. This allows even the smallest patent foramen ovale to become clinically significant, with right-to-left shunting resulting in hypoxemia.
  - Partial digital occlusion of the main pulmonary artery is a provocative maneuver that may be used during the bubble study to enhance intraoperative detection of patent foramen ovale during device placement.
  - A patent foramen ovale discovered in the operating room prior to placement of the VAD and those discovered after the device is activated in the operating room should be closed at that time.

- **Right heart failure and the potential need for a right VAD:** Despite best efforts, a small percentage of patients will develop refractory right heart failure necessitating device therapy.
  - If this occurs in the operating room while the cardiopulmonary bypass cannulas are still in place, a circuit is set up where blood is drawn from the right atrium, oxygenated by the cardiopulmonary bypass circuit, and then returned to the pulmonary artery. Often referred to as a *Berlin bridge,* it may be a beneficial intermediate step as the effect of superoxygenated blood on the pulmonary artery may result in a reduction in pulmonary resistance over several minutes and obviate the need for a right VAD.
  - When right heart dysfunction and failure develop several days after a left VAD placement, some type of short-term device support may be required if the heart remains refractory to initial interventions including pharmacotherapy.
- **Bleeding** is most common during the perioperative period but can also occur with anticoagulation during device use. Individual institutions must make the decision regarding the appropriateness of aprotinin therapy. It has been our standard practice to use a full dose of aprotinin (full Hammersmith protocol; see package insert) at the time of device implantation and with subsequent transplantation because of the tremendous importance of hemostasis.
  - The administration of blood products, especially plasma and platelets, increases pulmonary resistance that, in combination with their volume, can precipitate right heart failure. This outcome should always be considered when using blood product therapy.
  - At the time of the second exposure, a test dose is administered only when cardiopulmonary bypass is immediately available because of the risk of a hypersensitivity reaction.
- **Patient factors** include accidental disconnects, where a patient, in spite of optimal education from physicians and VAD staff, simultaneously disconnects all power sources to his or her device, resulting in pump stoppage. Additionally, traction injuries are common. Particular attention should be given to entering and exiting vehicles and traversing through narrow doorways, as these seem to be particularly problematic for the drive lines of VADs.

TRANSITION FROM INTENSIVE CARE UNIT TO THE FLOOR AND OUTPATIENT MANAGEMENT

- It is beyond the scope of this chapter to discuss personnel management. However, dedicated staff members are essential and must be thoroughly trained to deal with outpatient management of VADs.
- Communication and current knowledge of the device are paramount to the success of the VAD program. This requires the establishment of community resources and alternate caregiver training so that there is redundancy at every level of the system.
- Although minor problems with these patients and their devices are not uncommon, most are easily handled if the support staff are prepared and adequately trained. Mechanical assist devices can enhance not only the quantity but the quality of life for these patients.

CHAPTER 87 ■ VALVULAR HEART DISEASE

IMMEDIATE CONCERNS

- Critically ill patients with valvular heart disease (VHD) presenting to the intensive care unit (ICU) fall into three primary categories:
  - **Acute**-onset, newly acquired VHD
  - **Exacerbation** or complications of pre-existing VHD
  - **Concomitant** VHD critically ill from other causes
- Most patients present with instability secondary to left heart valvular disease, including diminished cardiac output (CO) with tissue hypoperfusion, and pulmonary venous hypertension with pulmonary edema that, if severe, leads to pulmonary hypertension (PHT) and right heart failure. Isolated right-sided valvular lesions present with reduced CO and systemic venous congestion.
- Life-threatening valvular disease generally presents manifestations of congestive heart failure (CHF) that require immediate stabilization. Initial interventions are aimed at controlling circulatory shock and respiratory failure; then 2 levels of diagnosis must be established.
  - Define the type and severity of valvular heart disease.
  - Determine acute precipitating events including cardiac problems such as acute changes in the valvular lesion, endocarditis, myocardial infarction, and cardiac dysrhythmias to systemic problems impacting cardiac performance such as uncontrolled hypertension, noncompliance with diet or medication regimens, infection, pulmonary embolism, endocrine abnormalities—particularly diabetic ketoacidosis or hyperthyroid crisis—and acute renal failure.
- Once both levels of diagnosis have been made, an estimate of the reversibility of the hemodynamic defect is possible, and plans for management can be developed. Specific management decisions depend on the lesion, its inherent physiology, and the presence of complicating factors.
- Invasive measurements such as arterial blood pressure, cardiac filling pressures, CO, mixed venous oxygen saturation, and calculated cardiovascular variables such as left ventricular (LV) stroke work index, systemic vascular resistance, and pulmonary vascular resistance are particularly useful for guiding and assessing the results of management.

CRITICAL ILLNESS CAUSED BY VALVULAR HEART DISEASE

- Detection by physical examination may be made difficult by environmental noise, pulmonary rhonchi, or other factors. With severe aortic or mitral stenosis and a failing LV, cardiac murmurs may be unimpressive or even absent. Clinical signs of common valve lesions are noted in Table 87.1.
- Electrocardiography frequently reveals concomitant ischemic heart disease, left ventricular hypertrophy (LVH), atrial abnormalities, arrhythmias, or right ventricular (RV) hypertrophy.
- Plain chest film can reveale pulmonary venous or arterial hypertension, pulmonary edema, pleural effusions, and lung parenchymal abnormalities and can evaluate cardiac contour.
- Early echocardiography is imperative in unexplained heart failure; if transthoracic echocardiogram (TTE) is not optimal, transesophageal echocardiography (TEE) should be performed.

CRITICAL ILLNESS IN PATIENTS WITH UNDERLYING VALVULAR HEART DISEASE

- When patients are critically ill from noncardiac causes, VHD is often discovered as murmurs on physical examination, valve calcification or cardiac contour abnormalities on chest radiograph (CXR), or unexplained LVH or atrial abnormality on electrocardiogram (ECG).
- Echocardiography is the most useful diagnostic tool for defining the type and extent of the valvular abnormality. Its impact on the management plan can then be determined by consideration of its severity and specific hemodynamic characteristics. All valve lesions share several common considerations.
  - Antibiotic prophylaxis for endocarditis is important as infections are common in critically ill patients, particularly with invasive procedures or indwelling catheters.
  - Fever and increased work of breathing may increase oxygen demand to a degree not well tolerated and should be treated vigorously.
  - Sinus tachycardia, atrial fibrillation (AF) with rapid ventricular response, and paroxysmal atrial tachycardia reduce LV filling time and may lead to hemodynamic deterioration. Treat aggressively, particularly in severely stenotic lesions.
  - Treatment of dysrhythmias includes correction of electrolyte abnormalities, judicious use of digoxin, and intermittent or constant infusion of β-adrenergic blockers, calcium channel blockers, amiodarone, or other antidysrhythmic drugs. Hemodynamically compromised patients who do not promptly respond may need urgent cardioversion.

CRITICAL ILLNESSES WITH SPECIFIC VALVULAR ABNORMALITIES

Aortic Stenosis

- Etiology: Aortic stenosis (AS) is the most common primary valvular heart disease. Stenosis of the normal tricuspid valve is caused by pathology similar to coronary artery disease. A

TABLE 87.1

CLINICAL SIGNS IN VALVULAR HEART DISEASE

	Aortic stenosis	Aortic regurgitation	Acute mitral regurgitation	Chronic mitral regurgitation	Mitral stenosis
General signs	Nothing remarkable	Look for Marfan syndrome, ankylosing spondylitis, or seronegative arthropathies	Tachypnea, circulatory shock	Tachypnea	Mitral facies (malar flush), tachypnea, peripheral cyanosis
Pulse	Small volume (parvus) and late peaking (tardus)	Water-hammer pulse, wide pulse pressure	Sinus tachycardia	Irregularly irregular in AF	Reduced or normal volume, irregularly irregular in AF
Neck and JVP	Prominent a wave	Prominent carotid pulsations (Corrigan sign)	Prominent a wave	Absent a wave in AF	Prominent a wave in PHT, absent a wave in AF
Precordium	Sustained, nondisplaced or slightly displaced apical impulse, palpable S4, systolic thrill at the base and at carotids	Diffuse, hyperdynamic and displaced apical impulse	Nondisplaced hyperdynamic apical impulse, systolic thrill	Hyperdynamic, inferolateral displaced apical impulse, parasternal heave (LAE)	Tapping apical impulse (palpable S1), palpable P2, and parasternal heave in PHT, diastolic thrill rarely
AUSCULTATION					
S1	Soft		Normal/soft	Soft	Loud
S2	Narrow split or reverse split S2, absent A2 in severe AS	Soft in acute AR; P2 loud in acute AR	Accentuated P2/wide paradoxical split	Normal P2/wide paradoxical split	P2 loud in PHT
S3/S4	Prominent S4	S3 heard	Present/present	Present/absent	
Clicks and added sounds	Systolic ejection click indicates mobile valve			Midsystolic click in MVP	Opening snap
Murmur	Systolic soft musical murmur, decreasing intensity in advanced disease	High-pitched, long diastolic murmur in chronic versus low-pitched short diastolic murmur in acute AR along left sternal border, diastolic murmur of early mitral diastolic closure	Early systolic loud radiating toward base (anterior directed jet) or axilla (posterior directed jet)	Holosystolic, soft or harsh and radiating toward axilla/back, late systolic murmur in MVP	Mid-diastolic murmur with late diastolic accentuation best heard at apex

AF, atrial fibrillation; JVP, jugular venous pulse; PHT, pulmonary hypertension; LAE, left atrial enlargement; AR, aortic regurgitation; AS, aortic stenosis; MVP, mitral valve prolapse.

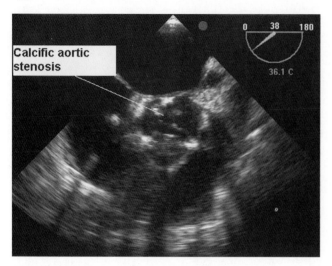

FIGURE 87.1. Transesophageal echocardiographic appearance of severe calcific aortic stenosis.

fibrocalcific process may involve the bicuspid valve, though the process is slower. Rheumatic aortic valve disease, rare in industrialized societies, may be seen with mitral valve disease.

- Hemodynamics: Obstruction causes **concentric hypertrophy** of the LV, which decreases wall stress but increases oxygen demand and dependence on left atrial (LA) contraction for ventricular filling. Subendocardial ischemia in LVH predisposes to ventricular dysrhythmias. Decreased forward flow and associated peripheral vasodilatation with exercise can cause syncope or sudden death. Later, the ventricles dilate and cardiac function is maintained by Frank–Starling mechanisms.
- Diagnosis: ECG features include LVH with strain pattern, left bundle branch block, and LA hypertrophy (biphasic P waves in precordial lead V_1). CXR may reveal a boot-shaped heart, calcification of the aortic valve, poststenotic dilatation of the aorta, and pulmonary venous congestion. Echocardiography is the principal modality for confirming AS (Fig. 87.1) and evaluating LV function. Severity is determined by peak gradients and valve area (Table 87.2). Gradients will be lower with severe AS if the flow across the valve is reduced by hypovolemia or by poor LV function. Systolic function may be preserved, but significant diastolic dysfunction, which predisposes patients to pulmonary edema, may be present.
- Therapeutic considerations: The triad of syncope, angina, and dyspnea indicate severe AS and require surgical intervention. Coronary angiography is indicated before surgery to rule

TABLE 87.2

ECHOCARDIOGRAPHIC ASSESSMENT OF AORTIC STENOSIS (AS)

	Mild AS	Moderate AS	Severe AS
Valve area (cm²)	>1.5	1–1.5	<1
Mean transvalvular gradient (mm Hg)	<25	25–40	>40
Jet velocity of blood flow across the valve (m/s)	<3	3–4	>4

out associated coronary artery disease. ICU admission may be required for acute cardiogenic shock, pulmonary edema, severe angina, ventricular dysrhythmias or, less commonly, AF and systemic embolization.

- Drugs: Commonly used drugs carry significant risks in AS. β-Blockers, calcium channel blockers, and other antidysrhythmics should be used with caution as patients are sensitive to myocardial depression.
  - Treat pulmonary congestion with careful administration of diuretics and nitroglycerin; may cause inadequate preload; digitalis carries the risk of dysrhythmias.
  - Increased LV mass and intracavitary systolic pressure decrease tolerance to vasodilatation and tachycardia. Angiotensin-converting enzyme inhibitors and other vasodilators can cause syncope or sudden death and are relatively contraindicated.
  - Undesirable hemodynamic effects of sedative drugs should be considered in patients with fixed CO. Narcotics can blunt the hypertensive sympathetic responses without significant myocardial depression and are usually the agents of choice.
  - Patients with diastolic dysfunction are extremely sensitive to fluids and can develop pulmonary edema, even when systolic function and ejection fraction are preserved.
- Monitoring: Hemodynamic stabilization with drugs and fluids should be carried out with careful monitoring of arterial and cardiac filling pressures. Normal central venous pressure does not ensure adequate filling with a stiff LV. Placement of a pulmonary artery catheter (PAC) provides useful information about LV filling pressures, CO, and mixed venous oxygenation and can be used for transvenous pacing but may precipitate malignant dysrhythmias. Pulmonary capillary wedge pressure can underestimate LV end-diastolic pressure (LVEDP) in patients with markedly reduced ventricular compliance; echocardiography can be useful in such situations. Monitor for ischemia with continuous ECG leads V_5 and II; however the ECG manifestations of LVH may make detection more difficult.
- Hemodynamic goals: LVH renders the atrial contraction—and thus sinus rhythm and preload—more crucial for diastolic filling. Severe bradycardia should be avoided as severe AS results in a fixed stroke volume and CO.
  - AF should be reversed with prompt cardioversion and initiation of antidysrhythmic therapy with amiodarone and/or β-blocking drugs. Procainamide has an increased risk of myocardial depression and hypotension. If cardioversion is unsuccessful, control of the ventricular rate is essential as decreased diastole increases the risk of ischemia.
  - Maintain adequate preload. Severe myocardial dysfunction with low blood pressure and ischemia may require administration of inotropes. Afterload reduction can impair coronary perfusion pressure; vasopressors may be necessary in patients with optimized volume and myocardial contractile status.
  - Patients who are refractory to medical management may benefit from insertion of an intra-aortic balloon counterpulsation pump (IABP).
- Definitive therapy: Any patient with severe AS who continues to deteriorate despite medical therapy should be seen by a cardiologist and cardiac surgeon for possible balloon valvotomy or open-valve replacement. Balloon valvotomy affords temporary improvement in transvalvular gradient and may

relieve symptoms, thus serving as a bridge to surgery. It is often very effective for young adults and adolescents with bicuspid valves but carries a mortality of 10% in patients with calcific AS.

Aortic Regurgitation

- Etiology: Acute aortic regurgitation (AR) results from infective endocarditis, aortic dissection extending into the aortic annulus or aortic root, and trauma. Severe, acute hypertension may also cause sudden-onset AR that often reverses after control of hypertension. Chronic AR causes are diverse and may involve the valve or the aortic root. Primary valvular diseases include congenital bicuspid valve, prolapse of aortic cusp, rheumatic heart disease, calcific degenerative disease, connective tissue diseases, and subacute bacterial endocarditis. Diseases associated with aortic root dilatation include systemic hypertension, Marfan disease (see Fig. 87.2), Ehlers–Danlos disease, granulomatous diseases of the aorta, senile and cystic medial degeneration, annuloaortic ectasia, and syphilis.
- Hemodynamics: In chronic AR, the LV dilates and hypertrophies when subjected to volume overload but, as the compensatory limit is reached, the wall stress begins to rise, and systolic function deteriorates. Severe decompensated AR results with decreasing forward-stroke volume and increasing LV end-diastolic volume and LV end-diastolic pressure, and symptoms of heart failure. In acute AR, there is no opportunity for compensation; increased end-diastolic pressures cause pulmonary venous congestion and pulmonary edema. The severity is dependent on the regurgitant orifice size, duration of diastole—as the degree of AR increases with bradycardia—and the diastolic pressure gradient between aorta and LV.
- Diagnosis: An ECG is performed to rule out ischemic heart disease in acute AR. The CXR will reveal cardiomegaly in chronic AR or pulmonary congestion with a normal-size heart in acute AR. TTE is performed to define the mechanism and severity of AR. TEE is useful, as TTE windows are limited; it defines the nature of perivalvular pathology and diagnoses an acute aortic dissection with high sensitivity and specificity. TEE is superior to magnetic resonance imaging and computed

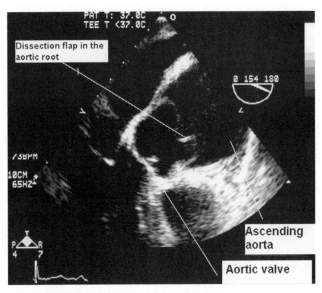

FIGURE 87.3. Aortic dissection intimal flap involving aortic root.

tomography scan to characterize the valve pathology in cases of acute dissection, and obviates the need for aortography (Fig. 87.3). Coronary angiography can rule out ischemic heart disease before surgery in chronic AR but is rarely indicated before emergency surgery in acute AR.

- Therapeutic considerations: Though medical therapy may allow mild acute AR to reach a chronic compensated state, emergency aortic valve replacement (AVR) is almost always indicated with severe acute AR after medical stabilization. The principle of therapy is to optimize CO and systemic perfusion, reduce pulmonary venous congestion, and initiate therapy for any underlying disorder. β-Blockers are avoided as tachycardia is beneficial in maintaining CO and decreases the regurgitant fraction by decreasing the duration of diastole. Hypertension and increased afterload are to be avoided. Inotropic therapy is advised only with depressed systolic function. An IABP is absolutely contraindicated, as it will increase the regurgitant fraction.
- In contrast to other causes of AR, inotropic therapy is avoided with aortic dissection. A result of long-standing, poorly controlled hypertension or trauma, LV contractility is preserved, and inotropes are not indicated. β-Adrenergic blockade may be initiated to reduce the velocity of LV ejection and aortic wall stress, therefore preventing extension of the aortic dissection or aortic rupture.
- In chronic AR with an acute decompensation, search for the precipitating cause, and pay particular attention to possible endocarditis. Most patients stabilize with medical therapy, and early elective surgery should be considered. Patients who do not improve with aggressive medical therapy should undergo emergency AVR.

Mitral Regurgitation

- The mitral valve apparatus is composed of the valve leaflets, mitral annulus, chorda tendineae, papillary muscles, and adjacent cardiac chambers, namely the LA and LV. Any disruption in the integrity of the mitral valve apparatus may

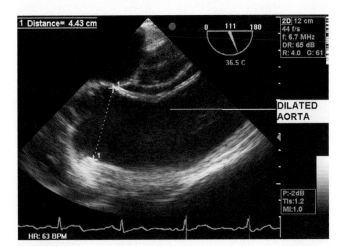

FIGURE 87.2. Dilatation of aortic root and ascending aorta by transesophageal echocardiography in a patient with Marfan disease.

TABLE 87.3

FUNCTIONAL CLASSIFICATION OF MITRAL REGURGITATION

Type of MR	Pathology	Disease
Type I	Normal motion of leaflets	Endocarditis (leaflet perforation) or various etiologies causing left ventricular dysfunction (annular dilatation)
Type II	Increased leaflet motion with free edge of the leaflet traveling above the plane of the annulus; due to chordal elongation or rupture, papillary muscle rupture	Degenerative myxomatous valve disease
Type IIIA	Restricted leaflet motion during diastole and systole	Rheumatic heart disease
Type IIIB	Restricted leaflet motion during systole, papillary muscle displacement	Ischemic or dilated cardiomyopathy

result in regurgitation. One of the major breakthroughs in the management of mitral regurgitation (MR) was the functional classification by Carpentier in the early 1980s (Table 87.3).

- Etiology: Acute MR usually results from infective endocarditis, connective tissue or myxomatous disorders; or ischemic heart disease. Acute rheumatic mitral valvulitis is less common today.
- Hemodynamics: Chronic MR leads to adaptation of the LV by dilatation and eccentric hypertrophy. Over many years, systolic function may fail, resulting in decreased ejection fraction and PHT; LA dilatation leads to AF. In the absence of a precipitating event, patients with chronic MR are rarely critically ill on presentation. In acute MR, however, increased LA pressure is transmitted to the pulmonary venous system, resulting in pulmonary edema. Sudden volume overload causes LV failure; CO falls, and systemic vascular resistance rises, which further increases the regurgitant fraction.
- Diagnosis: Patients may present with acute onset of fatigue, dyspnea, and chest pain or have pulmonary edema and circulatory shock. The ECG may show AF, LVH, and RV strain or suggest ischemia; the CXR may show cardiomegaly, indicating pre-existing heart disease. Pulmonary venous congestion and/or edema with a normal-sized heart indicate acute MR. Echocardiography remains the standard; TTE is easy and safe and can be performed at the bedside. TEE has superior resolution, definition of the mitral valve apparatus, and assessment of the severity of MR (Fig. 87.4). The mechanism and type of MR should be defined. Qualitative and quantitative assessment of MR can be done by color and spectral Doppler methods.
- The suitability for repair and LV function is assessed. EF is unreliable as it is increased when contractility is normal. Normal EF indicates significant loss of myocardial function; with **EF, ≤50%** advanced myocardial dysfunction is generally present.
- The American Heart Association/American College of Cardiology guidelines recommend medical treatment when EF is <30% and surgical treatment, even in asymptomatic patients, with EF <60% to prevent progression of disease.
- Urgent coronary angiography is indicated if myocardial ischemia or infarction is a real consideration and may delineate a culprit lesion amenable to catheter-based interventions. Severe triple-vessel disease should be referred for surgery. In

the case of chordal rupture or infective endocarditis without risk factors for CAD, angiography may be deferred.

- Therapeutic considerations: In acute, severe MR, medical therapy has a limited role and is aimed at stabilizing hemodynamics in preparation for surgery. Early valve surgery is life saving and should not be delayed. Often with a complication of myocardial infarction, therapy should maintain coronary perfusion pressure and reduce myocardial oxygen consumption. Use of a PAC and invasive arterial pressure monitoring is recommended. Sinus tachycardia maintains the forward flow and should not be suppressed. Hypertension and vasopressors should be avoided as increased afterload will increase the regurgitant fraction. Diuretics may be needed to reduce pulmonary venous congestion. If normotensive, vasodilators can increase forward flow and decrease the regurgitant fraction but should not be used except in combination with inotropes if hypotensive. With failure of medical management, IABP may be life saving.
- The surgical intervention is determined by the nature of the lesion. **Chordal rupture** or prolapse of the posterior leaflet can be repaired. Revascularization alone may improve

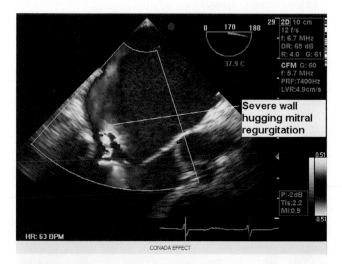

FIGURE 87.4. Transesophageal echocardiographic diagnosis of mitral regurgitation (MR) severity. Left atrial wall hugging eccentric regurgitant jet indicates severe MR.

transient papillary muscle ischemia without rupture. The standard of care for acute ischemic MR refractory to medical management and nonsurgical revascularization is a combination of revascularization with mitral valve repair or replacement with posterior chordal sparing. Mitral valve annuloplasty is the best approach for ischemic MR due to annular dilatation, diminished systolic contraction of the annulus, or papillary muscle malalignment; valve replacement should be considered if the repair is unsatisfactory. Papillary muscle rupture carries a high mortality without surgical intervention.

- **Infective endocarditis** should be treated with antibiotics. Indications for surgery include CHF refractory to medical treatment, uncontrolled infection despite antibiotics, recurrent systemic embolism, perivalvular or pericardial extension of infection, fungal endocarditis, and prosthetic valve endocarditis. Surgery should not be delayed for microbiologic clearance.
- **Mitral valve prolapse** deserves special mention because it is the most prevalent valvular heart disease and the most common cause of MR. Presentation includes severe MR, AF with transient ischemic attacks, long QT syndrome and tachyarrhythmias, PHT, cerebral embolism, infective endocarditis, or even sudden death. Medical stabilization and elective surgical repair of the mitral valve are recommended therapies.

Mitral Stenosis

- Etiology: Mitral stenosis (MS) is mostly related to rheumatic heart disease; degenerative calcific stenosis, congenital stenosis, and connective tissue disorders are other causes. Atrial myxomas and LA ball-valve thrombus can cause intermittent mitral obstruction and mimic MS.
- Hemodynamics: In rheumatic MS, inflammation of the connective tissue leaves patients with a funnel-shaped mitral apparatus. As the condition progresses, LA pressure and the transmitral gradient increase to maintain flow. The subsequent rise in pulmonary venous pressure leads to hydrostatic pulmonary edema, pulmonary vasoconstriction, and increased RV afterload. Persistently elevated pulmonary artery (PA) pressure leads to permanent structural changes, intimal hyperplasia, and medial hypertrophy, resulting in fixed PHT. RV dilatation and failure result in tricuspid insufficiency and systemic venous congestion.
- The impact of MS on CO is initially determined by the severity of the stenosis. As the disease progresses, severe **RV failure** may limit CO. Similarly, progression of rheumatic disease may impair LV function, important after surgical repair as increase in transmitral flow may expose the LV to a sudden increase in preload, causing failure.
- Presentation: MS often presents with acute cardiogenic pulmonary edema. Precipitating factors such as infective endocarditis, fever, anxiety, pain, AF, and pregnancy should be identified. Occlusion from an enlarging atrial myxoma should be ruled out. Right-sided heart failure with hepatic dysfunction, acute hemoptysis, systemic embolism, and hoarseness of voice may also be present.
- Diagnosis: The ECG may show LA enlargement, RV hypertrophy (RVH), and AF. CXR shows straightening of the left heart border, indicating LA and PA enlargement. **Kerley A and B lines** indicate pulmonary venous hypertension. TTE findings include doming of the anterior leaflet, decreased

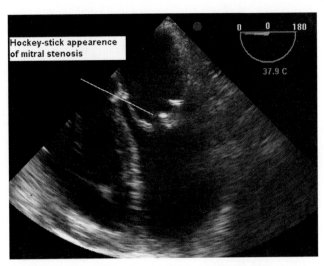

FIGURE 87.5. Typical appearance of rheumatic mitral stenosis.

leaflet mobility, increased leaflet calcification and thickness, commissural fusion, calcification of the subvalvular apparatus, increased LA size, and the presence of an LA thrombus (Fig. 87.5). Color flow will show associated MR. Doppler echocardiography allows calculation of pressure gradients, mitral valve area, and estimation of PA systolic pressure. Cardiac magnetic resonance imaging is increasingly used in the evaluation of stenotic valvular lesions; it measures valve area by planimetry. Its advantage over echocardiography is the lack of dependence upon good echocardiographic windows.

- Therapeutic considerations: New-onset AF with hemodynamic instability should be treated with cardioversion. Cardioversion in AF of >48 hours or an unknown duration must be preceded by 3 weeks of anticoagulation or TEE to exclude LA thrombus. Anticoagulation should be continued for 4 weeks after cardioversion because the enlarged LA remains "stunned" and does not immediately recover a normal contractile state. Anticoagulants should also be used with a prior embolic event and LA diameter >55 mm by echocardiography. Antidysrhythmics may be used to maintain sinus rhythm but should not be expected to provide indefinite success.
- **Pulmonary edema** should be stabilized with oxygen, morphine, anxiolytics, diuretics, and digoxin; the latter is especially useful in atrial dysrhythmias and CHF. Sympathetic nervous system activity is increased with MS, and overactivity worsens the symptom complex; β-blockers are very useful in this situation.
- Intravenous nesiritide, a synthetic human natriuretic peptide, is used with acute decompensated cardiac failure and PHT; it does not appear to have proarrhythmic effects. Nesiritide also appears to be effective and well tolerated in patients receiving concomitant β-blocker therapy and those with renal insufficiency.
- Inotropes to improve LV function may cause tachycardia and pulmonary edema. Inodilators may be useful in improving RV dysfunction and reducing PHT. Systemic blood pressure may need support with vasopressors but may adversely impact pulmonary vascular resistance.
- Assessment of volume status is difficult as the pulmonary capillary wedge pressure does not correlate with LV end-diastolic pressure but does give useful information about the propensity to develop pulmonary edema.

- Emergency invasive intervention is rarely required. If the precipitating events are controlled, surgery or balloon valvotomy can be scheduled electively after medical optimization. Balloon valvotomy is indicated in patients with suitable anatomy: pliable leaflets, no commissural fusion, and minimal subvalvular calcification. LA thrombus and significant (3+ to 4+) MR should be excluded by echocardiography. Patients who are not candidates should be referred for surgery. Because of extensive calcifications and marked anatomic distortion, mitral valve repair often is not possible in rheumatic mitral disease, and replacement is necessary.

Tricuspid Stenosis

- Etiology: Tricuspid valve obstruction can be due to anatomic disease or functional, causes secondary to right atrial (RA) tumors and thrombus. Anatomic disease is usually related to rheumatic heart disease; other causes are carcinoid syndrome, infective endocarditis, congenital stenosis or atresia, and methysergide toxicity.
- Hemodynamics: Obstruction to RV inflow results in systemic venous congestion: elevated jugular venous pulse (JVP), congestive hepatomegaly, and peripheral edema. Diastole is shortened by increasing heart rate, thus causing dramatic increases in transvalvular gradients. Most patients are symptomatic from coexisting MS. The presence of systemic venous congestion out of proportion to pulmonary venous congestion should raise the suspicion for involvement of the tricuspid valve.
- Clinical signs: Physical exam will reveal an elevated JVP, a prominent a wave, and distention of veins of the upper arm and dorsum of extended hand. A diastolic thrill may be palpated at the lower left sternal border; the S_1 is increased, and an opening snap and diastolic murmur may be heard at the lower left sternal border. Assigning the murmur to the tricuspid valve is based on its location; the higher, shorter, and softer nature of tricuspid stenosis (TS) in comparison to MS; and the absence of crackles that commonly accompany the murmur of MS. Right-sided murmurs are increased during inspiration.
- Diagnosis: The ECG may show evidence of RA enlargement: a P wave exceeding 2.5 mm in lead II and 1.5 mm in V_1. RA enlargement may cause first-degree heart block or AF in advanced disease. The CXR may show cardiomegaly, RA enlargement, and calcification of the valve. Echocardiography shows thickened leaflets, limited mobility, and a dome-shaped structure in diastole; RV function and the presence of tumor, thrombus, or vegetations can also be assessed. Spectral and color Doppler methods allow calculation of pressure gradients to grade the stenosis (mild <5 mm Hg, moderate 5 to 10 mm Hg, and severe >10 mm Hg) and valve area. Catheterization is unnecessary with good echocardiographic windows.
- Therapeutic interventions: Complete obstruction of the tricuspid valve by vegetations, thrombus, and/or tumors is an indication for emergency valve surgery (Fig. 87.6). Sodium restriction, careful diuresis, rate control, and anticoagulation are helpful, but surgical correction is required when the transvalvular gradient exceeds 5 mm Hg and the valve area falls below 2 cm². Percutaneous valvotomy or, more often, a bioprosthetic valve replacement is necessary. Mechanical valves are avoided because of the very high risk of thromboembolism in this position.

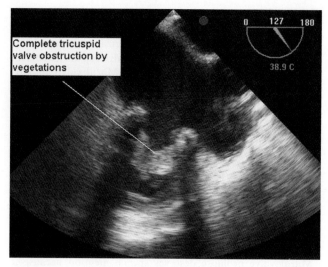

FIGURE 87.6. Complete obstruction of prosthetic tricuspid valve by vegetations, requiring emergency surgery.

Tricuspid Regurgitation

- Etiology: Tricuspid regurgitation (TR) can be classified as structural or functional. Most cases are chronic, but acute presentation may follow penetrating trauma, RV infarction, infective endocarditis, or repeated endomyocardial biopsies to diagnose allograft rejection.
  - Structural TR is caused by rheumatic disease, infective endocarditis, carcinoid syndrome, radiation therapy, Marfan syndrome, congenital heart disease, or tricuspid valve prolapse.
  - Functional TR is usually secondary to left-sided pathology, such as LV failure, mitral or aortic (less frequent) valve disease, primary PHT, pulmonic stenosis, RV infarction, and dilated cardiomyopathy; a small number are idiopathic.
- Hemodynamics: Elevated RA pressure from TR gives rise to the signs and symptoms of systemic venous congestion; RA dilatation may lead to AF and thrombus formation. An RA thrombus may lead to pulmonary or systemic (with patent foramen ovale [PFO]) emboli. RV volume overload leads to eccentric hypertrophy and dilatation. RV systolic dysfunction develops, leading to further decompensation and annular dilatation that increase the severity of TR. The left heart also suffers from low CO because the RV fails to deliver enough blood to the LV. Ventricular interdependence and paradoxical septal motion also decrease LV output with RV volume overload.
- Clinical symptoms and signs: Shock and hypotension may develop with acute TR after RV infarction or papillary muscle rupture. Signs of right-sided failure are present: distended neck veins with a prominent c-v wave, pulsatile hepatomegaly, a precordial bulge, and parasternal heave from RVH; soft S_1, prominent P_2, and right-sided S_3 from RV dilatation; pansystolic thrill; and a murmur heard at the left lower sternal border.
- Isolated tricuspid valve endocarditis may disseminate emboli to the lungs, resulting in multiple septic emboli and abscess formation. Peripheral stigmata of infective emboli are usually absent but may indicate paradoxical embolism or left-sided lesions.

- Diagnosis: The ECG may show AF, right axis deviation, RVH, and a right bundle branch block. Right-sided leads will show ST elevation in RV infarction and may be associated with LV inferior wall infarction. Enlarged RV and cardiomegaly are seen on CXR.
- Echocardiography can yield structural issues—prolapse, vegetations, annular diameter, and rheumatic disease—and rules out thrombus and PFO. With PFO, elevated RA pressure frequently exceeds LA pressure, causing right-to-left shunt and possible refractory hypoxemia.
- Severity of TR can be assessed by hepatic venous systolic flow reversal and estimation of regurgitant orifice area (>40 mm^2 is severe). Also, pulmonary systolic pressure can be estimated by continuous wave Doppler signal of tricuspid regurgitation. Augmenting ultrasound signal with 10% air, 10% patient's blood, and 80% saline, and estimation of PA systolic pressures correlate well with PAC-measured PA systolic pressures. Right heart catheterization shows RV pressure >60 mm Hg in functional TR compared to <40 mm Hg in structural TR.
- Therapeutic considerations: In general, acute TR can be effectively managed with diuretics and inotropes; rare instances may require valvular surgery when refractory to medical therapy. Once stabilized, long-term prognosis depends on the etiology and severity. Mild and moderate degrees of chronic TR are tolerated in the presence of normal LV function; correction of left-sided heart lesions and treatment of left-sided failure and PHT take priority.
  - If functional TR is severe, ring annuloplasty can improve survival. Cardiac resynchronization therapy with biventricular pacemakers and the Dor procedure (endoventricular circular patch plasty) help patients with functional TR due to systolic heart failure.
  - Rheumatic TR may be treated with open valvotomy or valve replacement. Valves compromised by infective endocarditis can simply be removed after an aggressive course of antibiotics; valve replacement can be performed later if there is no recurrence of drug abuse. When acute TR is the result of RV infarction, the usual management of acute coronary insufficiency must be observed, including β-blockers, aspirin, fluids, thrombolysis, coronary angiography, angioplasty, and stenting and, in suitable patients, coronary artery bypass grafting.

Pulmonic Stenosis

- Etiology: Pulmonic stenosis (PS) is usually congenital. Though it does occur in isolation, subvalvular and supravalvular stenosis usually comprise part of a larger syndrome. Severe forms, or those associated with other cardiac anomalies, are generally identified and treated in childhood. Acquired forms of PS include rheumatic, carcinoid disease; infundibular stenosis from PHT; extrinsic compression from aneurysm of the sinus of Valsalva; tumors; and scarring from previous surgery.
- Pathophysiology: PS causes obstruction to RV outflow resulting in RVH and subsequent RV failure or TR. The degree of stenosis, once established, tends to be stable; if decompensation does not occur in childhood, subsequent deterioration is unlikely. Occasionally, RV obstruction increases, possibly by secondary infundibular hypertrophy.

- Presentation: Mild PS is often asymptomatic. Patients with more severe stenosis commonly develop fatigue, atypical chest pain, and syncope. When RV failure or TR occurs, systemic venous hypertension may be present. Elevated RA pressures in the presence of a PFO or atrial septal defect can result in a **right-to-left shunt**. Physical examination reveals a large venous a wave; in the absence of RV failure or TR, JVP remains normal. A left parasternal systolic lift is common with significant PS. The murmur is best heard at the left upper sternal border and radiates to the left clavicle; a thrill and ejection click may be present. Increasing duration, late systolic peaking, and wide splitting of the second sound (as P$_2$ is increasingly delayed) are indicators of significant stenosis; intensity of the murmur is not.
- Diagnostic studies: The ECG is normal in mild PS; with increasing severity, RVH and RA enlargement are common. The CXR may reveal poststenotic dilatation of the main and left PA. Echocardiography is particularly useful in assessing the valve morphology, calculating pressure gradients, grading the severity of stenosis, and evaluating RV function. The presence of other congenital abnormalities, TR, and RA enlargement can also be ruled out by echocardiography. Cardiac catheterization provides confirmation of pressure gradients, full hemodynamic assessment, and identification of associated PA branch stenosis. Pulmonary stenosis is graded based on the peak pressure gradient: **mild,** with a **gradient** of 25 to 49 mm Hg; **moderate,** 50 to 75 mm Hg; and **severe,** >75 mm Hg.
- Currently, balloon valvuloplasty is recommended for symptomatic patients and those with a peak gradient >50 mm Hg. Surgical valvuloplasty is reserved for severe calcification, dysplasia, endocarditis, and previous valvuloplasty failure. Medical management includes infective endocarditis prophylaxis, treatment of right heart failure and AF, and anticoagulation to prevent thromboembolic complications.

Pulmonic Insufficiency

- Etiology: Pulmonic insufficiency (PI) may be secondary to PHT or, rarely, leaflet damage caused by infectious endocarditis, rheumatic fever, or carcinoid syndrome. Occasionally, PI is congenital.
- Pathophysiology: In the absence of PHT, volume overload of the RV is well tolerated; RV failure can occur when PHT develops from other causes.
- Presentation: Generally an isolated abnormality with a benign course, the natural history is that of the associated lesions. PI is usually an incidental auscultatory finding: decrescendo diastolic murmur along the upper left sternal border. The intensity of the murmur does not correlate well with the severity of regurgitation.
- Diagnostic studies: The ECG is usually normal; RVH suggests PHT. The CXR is normal in mild insufficiency; the pulmonary trunk may be prominent when moderate to severe. Echocardiography can be useful for differentiating pulmonic from aortic insufficiency and establishing right heart chamber sizes and associated abnormalities.
- Therapeutic considerations: Specific treatment is rarely required, but PHT should be controlled when present. When the right heart fails, diuretics, sodium restriction, and possibly cardiac glycosides are helpful. Surgical treatment

(bioprosthetic valve replacement) is reserved for advanced right heart failure. In patients with a remote repair of tetralogy of Fallot and chronic PI, RV dilatation has been linked to sudden death and may warrant valve replacement.

Mixed Valve Lesions

- **Mitral stenosis with regurgitation:** The combination of pressure and volume overload on LA favors early development of symptoms, AF, and CHF. Because transvalvular gradients may overestimate the degree of stenosis, Doppler measurement of valve area should be considered. Decision making is complex, and intervention is often required before either of the lesions reaches a severe degree. Moderate MR is a contraindication for balloon valvotomy.
- **AS and regurgitation:** This combination causes both pressure and volume overload on the LV. The predominant lesion is indicated by the size of the LV: a normal-sized but hypertrophied LV signifies predominant AS; a dilated LV suggests dominant AR. Transvalvular gradients may overestimate AS, so planimetry or the continuity equation method should be considered. The threshold for surgery is lowered as compared to single valve–defect patients. Surgery in patients with predominant AR can be delayed until symptoms develop or asymptomatic LV dysfunction becomes apparent on echocardiography.
- **MS and AS:** This combination causes serial obstructions resulting in reduced CO and early development of pulmonary venous congestion and hypertension. Low transvalvular gradients characterize this AS because of low CO. Mitral valvotomy is done first, followed by AVR as indicated.
- **MS and AR:** This combination creates a challenge for the physician attempting to make a diagnosis. MS decreases the volume overload of AR, and AR attenuates antegrade mitral valve flow by increasing LV diastolic pressure, thereby decreasing transmitral gradients. Balloon mitral valvotomy followed by AVR, as indicated, is a reasonable approach.
- **MR and AS:** AS aggravates MR by increasing the afterload. MR, by its pressure release effect, obscures even severe AS. Systolic function remains normal with low transaortic gradients. If both lesions are severe, AVR with mitral valve repair or replacement is necessary. Moderate or mild MR may improve after AVR for AS, especially if there is no anatomic lesion in the mitral valve. Intraoperative TEE plays an important role in this decision.
- **MR and AR:** These lesions create additive volume loads on the LV; the sequelae of dyspnea and LV dysfunction appear sooner.

Prosthetic Valve Dysfunction

- Prosthetic valves are broadly divided into mechanical, bioprosthetic, and homograft valves. St. Jude bileaflet valves are commonly used mechanical valves that need lifelong anticoagulation. Carpentier-Edwards and Hancock bioprosthetic valves are common tissue valves; they do not require long-term anticoagulation but have a short life span and are prone to degenerative changes and failure. Acute valvular complications may result from infective endocarditis, paravalvular leak, valve ring abscess, thrombosis, pannus formation,

degenerative calcification, lipid infiltration, dehiscence of the valve, and strut fracture.
- Progressive congestive cardiac failure is a common presentation with stenosis and regurgitation. Acute, complete valvular obstruction may lead to sudden death in the absence of surgical intervention. Embolic phenomenon, hemolytic anemia (indicating a paravalvular leak), and a new atrioventricular block (indicating a valve ring abscess) may be other presenting symptoms. Prosthetic valve thrombosis may present with nonspecific cardiac symptoms. Normally functioning prosthetic valves are associated with clicks and murmurs.
- Echocardiography is essential to make a diagnosis and has replaced cardiac catheterization. Fluoroscopy may be needed to identify the nature of the disease and assess the effects of thrombolysis. Excessive rocking motion of the valve ring or limited motion of the valve components due to thrombus or vegetation; calcification; thickening around the valve due to an abscess; and a pseudoaneurysm can be identified with two-dimensional echocardiography. The color Doppler technique may show a paravalvular leak, pseudoaneurysms, and/or fistula formation.
- Calculation of transvalvular gradients helps to diagnose prosthetic valve stenosis. Gradients depend on the valve type and size and dynamic conditions such as CO, blood volume, heart rate, and contractility. Measurements should be compared to values obtained immediately after valve replacement. It has also been suggested that it may be more appropriate to calculate the prosthetic valve area using the continuity equation:

$$Area_1 \times velocity\ time\ integral_1 = Area_2 \times velocity\ time\ integral_2$$

- Medical therapy is directed toward treatment of CHF: diuretics, vasodilators, and inotropes; initiation of antibiotics for infective endocarditis after obtaining blood cultures; and thrombolysis for certain cases of prosthetic valve thrombosis. Staphylococcal organisms predominate in early (<60 days after placement) prosthetic valve endocarditis, whereas in late (>60 days after placement) endocarditis, there are equal percentages of streptococcal and staphylococcal organisms. Empiric antibiotics are started until culture results and sensitivities are available. Fibrinolytic therapy is recommended for right-sided thrombosis with a large clot burden or New York Heart Association classes III to IV symptoms. Fibrinolysis for left-sided lesions is associated with a 12% to 15% risk of cerebral embolism and thus reserved for patients in whom emergency surgery is high risk or contraindicated. Ultimately, all prosthetic valve lesions require valve replacement surgery; reoperative mortality is high.

IMPORTANT CONSIDERATIONS IN THE TREATMENT OF RIGHT VENTRICULAR FAILURE SECONDARY TO VALVULAR HEART DISEASE

- Patients with chronic RV failure secondary to valvular heart disease (VHD) are usually debilitated, with low CO and pulmonary, hepatic, and renal dysfunction. Ascites, malnutrition, reduced systemic vascular resistance, jaundice, coagulopathy, and renal failure—the hepatorenal syndrome— are the manifestations of hepatic dysfunction. Hepatorenal

syndrome is challenging and often requires renal replacement therapy.
- Treatment of PHT in the critically ill patient with VHD decreases RV afterload and helps prevent or decrease RV failure. This approach, combined with maintenance of adequate coronary perfusion pressure, forms the mainstay of treatment of acute RV failure. Exacerbating factors of PHT, such as hypoxemia, hypercarbia, acidosis, hypothermia, hyperv-

olemia, and increased intrathoracic pressure, should be corrected aggressively.
- Recent advances in pharmacology provide intensivists with a wide variety of options for selective pulmonary vasodilatation including inhaled prostaglandins and nitric oxide. Inhaled pulmonary vasodilators are preferred because they do not decrease systemic blood pressure or increase shunt fraction.

CHAPTER 88 ■ CARDIAC DYSRHYTHMIAS

BRADYARRHYTHMIAS

- Bradycardia is a common finding in hospitalized patients, especially during sleep. An increase in vagal tone may result in sinus bradycardia, sinus pauses, or atrioventricular (AV) nodal block—all physiologic findings that may have no clinical significance.

Sinoatrial Abnormalities

- Sinoatrial (SA) conduction block occurs when impulses generated by the sinus node are not conducted to the atrial myocardium.
  - First-degree SA block is not manifested on electrocardiogram (ECG), as it is merely the delay between the sinus impulse formation and atrial activation.
  - Second-degree type I SA block (Wenckebach) is manifested by group beating, with progressive shortening of PP intervals until a P wave is absent; this PP interval is usually less than twice the shortest cycle.
  - Second-degree type II SA block has fixed PP intervals, followed by a pause without a P wave that is twice the PP interval (Fig. 88.1).
  - Third-degree SA block is not visible on ECG, as no sinus impulse can escape the SA node. This disorder cannot be differentiated from sinus arrest.
- Sinus arrest is the failure of automaticity in which no impulses are generated by the sinus node (Fig. 88.2). Sick sinus syndrome is dysfunction of the sinus node or SA conduction in which no adequate escape mechanism is present, and the patient becomes symptomatic because of bradycardia. There are intrinsic and extrinsic causes of SA abnormalities.
  - The most prevalent intrinsic cause of sinus node dysfunction is aging, with replacement of the sinus node and the surrounding atrium by fibrotic degeneration.
  - Extrinsic causes of sinus node dysfunction include drugs (Table 88.1), electrolyte abnormalities (hyperkalemia), endocrine disorders (hypothyroidism), neurally mediated

conditions (vasovagal syncope), and intracranial hypertension.
- Diagnosis and treatment of SA abnormalities
  - Record a 12-lead ECG. Evaluate for myocardial infarction (MI), mechanism of bradycardia, P-wave regularity (sinus or an atrial rhythm). Abrupt pauses or group beating in the sinus rhythm suggests SA block. P waves without QRS complexes suggest AV block. Evaluate also for QRS axis and width for coexistent bundle branch block.
  - If hypotension, dizziness, and presyncope are absent, no immediate treatment is required. Symptoms dictate the treatment plan. Asymptomatic bradycardia due to sinus node dysfunction is not an emergency!
  - In sinus bradycardia, give intravenous (IV) atropine; 0.04 mg/kg, if hypotensive.
  - With SA block or sinus arrest, give no treatment unless hypotension is present or the rhythm is digitalis-induced (stop drug).
  - For sick sinus syndrome, treatment depends on symptoms such as dizziness, presyncope, and congestive heart failure.
  - Acute inferoposterior MI with SA block, coronary reperfusion is indicated.

TABLE 88.1

DRUGS AFFECTING SINUS NODE FUNCTION

Drug types	
Antiarrhythmics	Class IA (quinidine, procainamide, disopyramide)
	Class IC (flecainide, propafenone)
	Class III (sotalol, amiodarone)
Beta-blocking agents	
Calcium channel blockers	Verapamil
	Diltiazem
Cardiac glycosides	
Miscellaneous	Lithium
	Cimetidine
	Diphenylhydantoin
	Clonidine and dexmedetomidine

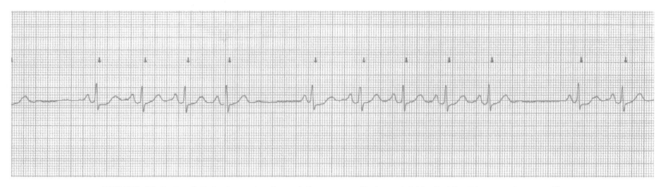

FIGURE 88.1. Lead II rhythm strip. Second-degree type II sinoatrial block. The PP interval is initially 720 ms and appears to prolong to 1,440 ms.

Atrioventricular Conduction Abnormalities

- Noninvasive methods for determining site of block
  - In AV block, the conduction abnormality may be located within the AV node, the His bundle, or the bundle branches. Determining the location of block is important, as this will affect immediate and long-term treatment.
  - On ECG, baseline PR interval, QRS duration, and axis are important.
  - Bedside responses to noninvasive interventions, including IV atropine administration, exercise, or vagal maneuvers, may differentiate between AV nodal and infranodal block (Table 88.2). Specifically, interventions that slow AV nodal conduction, such as carotid sinus massage, will worsen AV nodal block but, because of sinus slowing, will seem to improve infranodal block. Conversely, interventions that improve AV nodal conduction, such as exercise and atropine, may worsen infranodal conduction because of acceleration of sinus rate.
- **First-degree AV block or prolonged PR interval:** The PR interval is a reflection of AV conduction time and is measured from the onset of the P wave to the beginning of the QRS complex. Conduction delay in the atrium, AV node, bundle of His, or bundle branches all may result in a prolonged PR interval; ≥280 ms usually indicates abnormal AV nodal conduction.

- **Second-degree type I AV block (AV Wenckebach):** There is progressive lengthening of the PR interval before there is a blocked P wave (Fig. 88.3). The QRS duration may be narrow or wide, depending on the presence of bundle branch block. When the QRS is narrow, it is most likely a block occurring at the level of the AV node; it is seen in young healthy individuals with increased vagal tone. Patients with an acute inferior MI can have AV nodal block (≥20%), indicating a proximal right coronary occlusion.
- **Second-degree type II AV block (Mobitz II):** The PR intervals are normal or slightly prolonged and are exactly the same length before and after the nonconducted P waves (Fig. 88.4). Type II AV block is most likely infranodal in the His bundle if there is a narrow QRS duration (rare) or in the bundle branches if there is wide QRS duration (common). These patients are often symptomatic, with shortness of breath, fatigue, and syncope, and sudden progression to complete AV block.
- **Two-to-one AV block:** Every other P wave conducts to the ventricle and the conducted PR interval may be either normal or prolonged (Fig. 88.5). The level of block—AV nodal versus infranodal—cannot be determined with certainty without an electrophysiology study. A narrow QRS duration suggests that the block is in the AV node or the His bundle, whereas a wide QRS suggests block in the bundle branches.

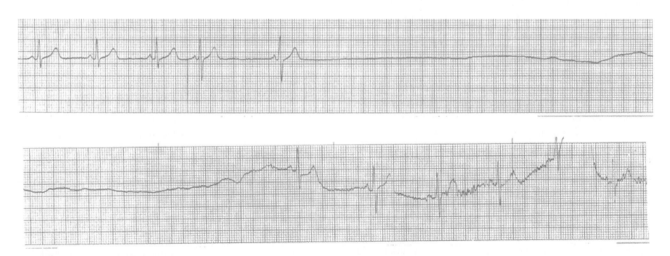

FIGURE 88.2. Lead II rhythm strip. Sinus arrest with no ventricular escape.

TABLE 88.2

NONINVASIVE INTERVENTIONS TO DETERMINE SITE OF
ATRIOVENTRICULAR (AV) BLOCK

Intervention	AV nodal site of block	Infranodal site of block
Atropine	AV block improves	AV block worsens
Exercise	AV block improves	AV block worsens
Carotid sinus massage	AV block worsens	AV block improves

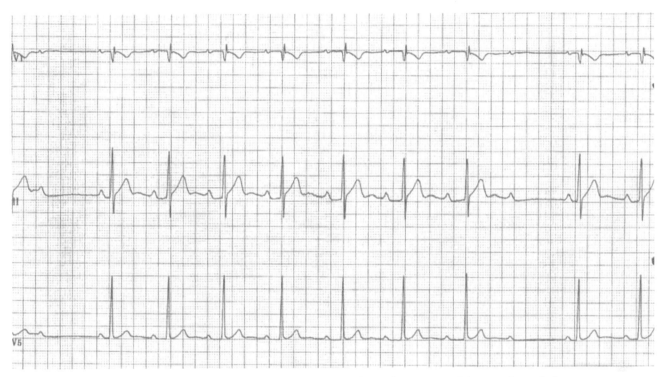

FIGURE 88.3. A 12-lead electrocardiogram. Sinus rhythm with type I second-degree atrioventricular conduction block.

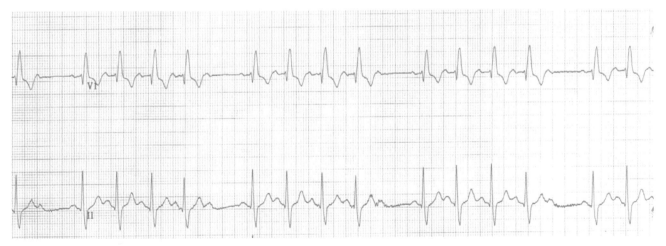

FIGURE 88.4. A 12-lead electrocardiogram. Sinus rhythm with second-degree type II atrioventricular conduction block.

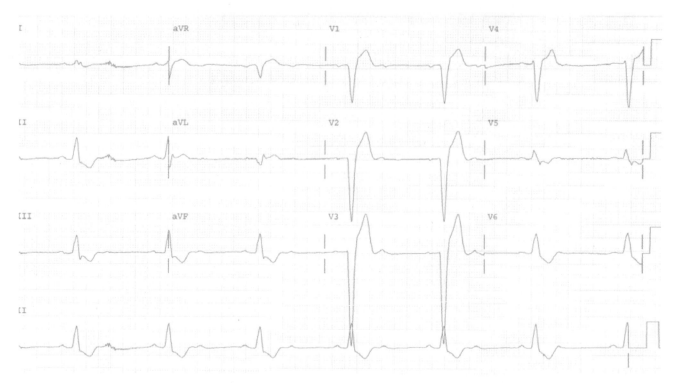

FIGURE 88.5. A 12-lead electrocardiogram. Sinus rhythm with 2:1 atrioventricular conduction block with left bundle branch block suggesting block below the His bundle.

• **Third-degree AV block or complete AV block:** There is no P wave-to-QRS relationship. Sinus rate (PP intervals) is usually faster than the escape rate. The escape rate is usually <50 beats per minute (bpm), with the exception of a congenital AV block (Fig. 88.6). If the escape rhythm has a narrow QRS complex, it originates in the AV junction and the site of block is either AV nodal or, less likely, bundle of His. If the QRS is wide, the site of block is likely within the bundle branches.

• Diagnosis and treatment of AV conduction abnormalities
  • Record a 12-lead ECG and try to determine site of block by noninvasive methods.

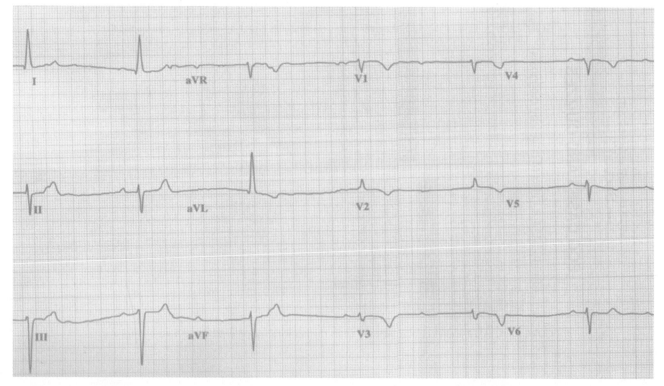

FIGURE 88.6. A 12-lead electrocardiogram. Sinus bradycardia with third-degree AV conduction block.

- In the setting of an acute inferior MI, the site of block is usually the AV node and transient with successful reperfusion. Insert a temporary pacemaker if there is cardiogenic shock secondary to heart block. Use permanent pacing only if there is chronic, symptomatic second- or third-degree AV nodal block.
- Type II AV block: If there is no PR prolongation prior to block, it is most likely in the His–Purkinje system. Temporary pacemaker is required when associated with syncope; permanent pacemaker can be used in most cases.
- Two-to-one AV block: PR interval ≥160 ms suggests His bundle or below. Temporary pacemaker is indicated in patients with acute MI, wide QRS, and/or if symptomatic.
- Third-degree AV block: Temporary pacemaker required in acute anterior MI, wide QRS, and/or if symptomatic

NARROW QRS TACHYCARDIA

- *Narrow QRS tachycardia* is defined as an arrhythmia with a rate faster than 100 bpm and QRS duration of <120 ms. Patients are usually symptomatic, complaining of palpitations, lightheadedness, shortness of breath, or anxiety. 12-lead ECG features during tachycardia and sinus rhythm in the same leads and tachycardia response to carotid sinus massage will facilitate the correct diagnosis of the tachycardia. Pulsations in the neck may often reveal the mechanism of the tachycardia (Table 88.3) Sinus tachycardia can be differentiated from other narrow QRS tachycardias by the sinus

TABLE 88.3

JUGULAR PULSATION AND SUPRAVENTRICULAR TACHYCARDIA

Diagnosis of SVT	Jugular pulsation
Sinus tachycardia	Normal pulsation
Atrial tachycardia	Normal pulsation
Atrial flutter	Flutter waves
Atrial fibrillation	Irregular pulse
AV nodal re-entrant tachycardia	Large "A" waves
AV re-entry tachycardia	Large "A" waves
Junctional tachycardia	Large "A" waves

SVT, supraventricular tachycardia; AV, atrioventricular.

morphology of the P wave on a 12-lead ECG. The three most common causes of regular narrow QRS tachycardia are AV nodal re-entry tachycardia (AVNRT), AV re-entrant tachycardia (AVRT), and atrial tachycardia, respectively.

Atrial Tachycardia

- An ectopic (nonsinus) P wave precedes the QRS complex and can often be localized using the ECG morphology of the P wave (Fig. 88.7). The atrial rate is regular, with PP intervals ranging between 120 and 250 bpm; AV block may be present. Atrial tachycardias may be paroxysmal or persistent (inces-

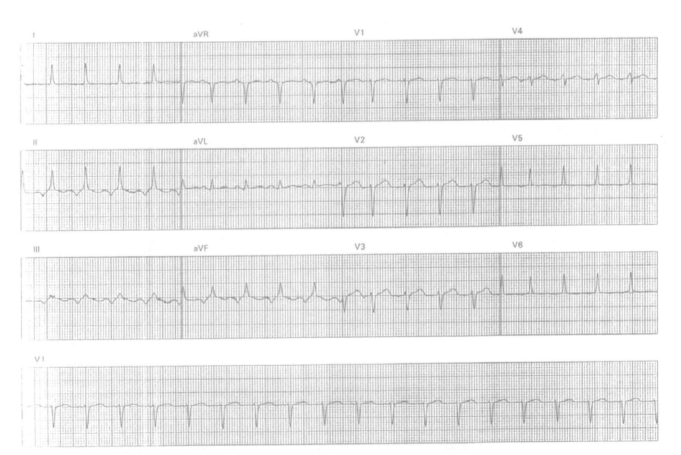

FIGURE 88.7. A 12-lead electrocardiogram. Atrial tachycardia with a P wave preceding each QRS complex. The origin of the P wave is low atrial septal.

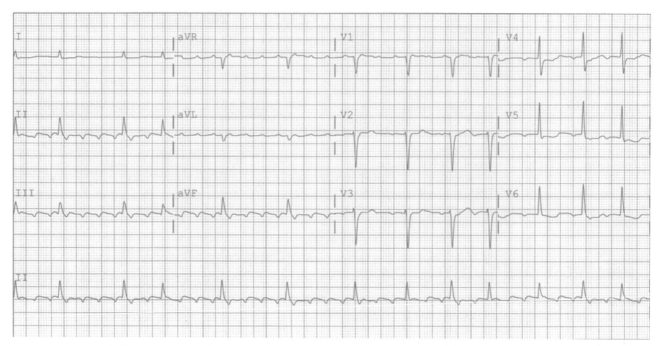

FIGURE 88.8. A 12-lead electrocardiogram. Atrial flutter with variable atrioventricular conduction.

sant). Paroxysmal tachycardias can originate from a focal area of the myocardium or may be due to re-entry within a macro-re-entrant circuit. Persistent or incessant atrial tachycardia is rare but important to recognize; patients who are in tachycardia >50% of the time may develop tachycardia-induced dilated cardiomyopathy.

Atrial Flutter

- Typical atrial flutter has a classic saw-tooth pattern of atrial activation in the inferior leads of the ECG (Fig. 88.8) with an atrial rate of 250 to 350 bpm; the ventricular response can

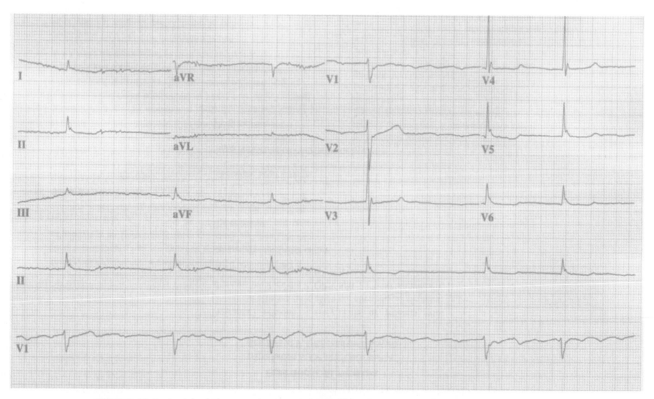

FIGURE 88.9. A 12-lead electrocardiogram. Atrial fibrillation with slow ventricular response. Note that there are no discernible P waves and that the rhythm is irregular.

be regular or irregular. The most common form of atrial flutter uses a right atrial macrore-entrant circuit, including the cavotricuspid isthmus. Flutter waves can be better appreciated during rapid tachycardia with slowing of the ventricular response by carotid sinus massage.

Atrial Fibrillation

- The atrial rhythm in atrial fibrillation (AF) is irregular, a rate of 350 to 500 bpm (Fig. 88.9), with variable AV conduction resulting in narrow QRS tachycardia and varying RR intervals. It is the most common supraventricular tachyarrhythmia (SVT) in the United States, and a major cause of cardiovascular morbidity and mortality, with an increased risk of death, congestive heart failure, and stroke.
  - The incidence increases with age, with a lifetime risk of one in four men and women older than the age of 40. Similarly, the risk of embolic stroke from AF increases with age (>65 years) and other risk factors including hypertension, prior history of strokes, heart failure, left ventricular function of $\geq 35\%$, mitral stenosis, prosthetic heart valve, and diabetes.
  - Stroke prevention is the key focus in the management of AF. Anticoagulation with warfarin, with an international normalized ratio (INR) between 2.0 and 3.0, is recommended in patients with AF and one or two of the afborementioned risk factors.
  - AF can be divided into four categories: (a) new onset; (b) paroxysmal (spontaneous termination); (c) persistent (terminates only by pharmacologic or electrical conversion); and (d) permanent.

AV Nodal Re-entry Tachycardia

- AVNRT is the most common form of a regular SVT and is due to re-entry within AV nodal and perinodal tissue. The heart rhythm is regular, usually between 130 and 250 bpm. Different forms of AVNRT are classified based on the direction of the circuit and the electrophysiologic properties of the circuit. Typically, there is simultaneous activation of the atria and ventricles, with P waves either hidden or partially visible at the end of the QRS (Fig. 88.10A), producing a pseudo-r' in V1 and pseudo-s in inferior leads during tachycardia that is not present in sinus rhythm (Fig. 88.10B and C).

AV Re-entrant Tachycardia

- AVRT occurs due to re-entry involving an accessory pathway, an abnormal electrical connection between the atria and ventricle.
  - If the accessory pathway conducts anterogradely, certain characteristics, such as a short PR interval, broad QRS, and a delta wave typical of Wolff–Parkinson–White syndrome, may be present on surface 12-lead ECG during sinus rhythm (Fig. 88.11A).
  - Orthodromic AV re-entry (seeFig. 88.11B) is a narrow QRS tachycardia that conducts anterogradely down the AV node to activate the ventricles and then conducts retrogradely up the accessory pathway to activate the atria; both the atria

and ventricles are essential parts of the circuit. This is a regular paroxysmal tachycardia, usually with the RP interval less than the PR interval (seeFig. 88.11C).
  - If AF occurs in a patient with an anterograde-conducting accessory pathway, the impulse can conduct rapidly down the accessory pathway anterogradely, resulting in variable QRS morphologies (seeFig. 88.11D). This rhythm can degenerate into ventricular fibrillation and sudden death. Treatment with IV ibutilide or procainamide should be first-line medical therapy as other drug therapies can cause hypotension and further hemodynamic compromise without affecting the properties of the accessory pathway or converting to sinus rhythm.

Treatment of Regular Narrow-complex Tachycardia

- Record a 12-lead ECG during tachycardia and in sinus rhythm; record the termination of the tachycardia. On physical examination, evaluate the jugular pulse.
- Vagal maneuver: If no success, then 6 mg of rapid IV adenosine and repeat with 12 mg of IV adenosine. If tachycardia continues, consider beta-blockers, calcium channel blockers (verapamil 5–10 mg IV, if normal left ventricular function), or digoxin.
- If tachycardia persists, use antiarrhythmic medications such as IV amiodarone, IV procainamide (10 mg/kg, no faster than 50 mg/minute), or sotalol.
- If tachycardia persists and/or patient is hemodynamically unstable, cardiovert.

Treatment of Atrial Fibrillation

- Recent onset (<48 hours) without significant heart disease and stable
- Pharmacologic cardioversion with flecainide (300 mg PO once), propafenone (600 mg po), procainamide (5–10 mg/kg IV over 20 minutes), ibutilide (1 mg IV over 10 minutes, then repeat), or amiodarone (1,000 mg IV over first 24 hours).
- Electrical cardioversion with sedation
- Recent onset (<48 hours) and unstable: Proceed with immediate cardioversion.
- More than 48 hours and stable:
  - Control ventricular rate with beta-blockers, calcium channel blockers, and/or digoxin.
  - Aspirin can be used in patients with lone AF (no risk factors of heart failure, history of thromboembolism, hypertension, or diabetes).
  - Patients with risk factors should be on oral anticoagulation with warfarin, with a goal of INR of 2.0 to 3.0.
  - If plan to cardiovert or treat with antiarrhythmic medications, either anticoagulate for ≥ 3 weeks prior to cardioversion with therapeutic INR or use transesophageal echocardiography with cardioversion if no thrombus is identified, followed by warfarin anticoagulation.
- More than 48 hours and difficulty in obtaining adequate rate control:
  - Proceed with transesophageal echocardiogram and, if no thrombus is present, cardiovert and anticoagulate.

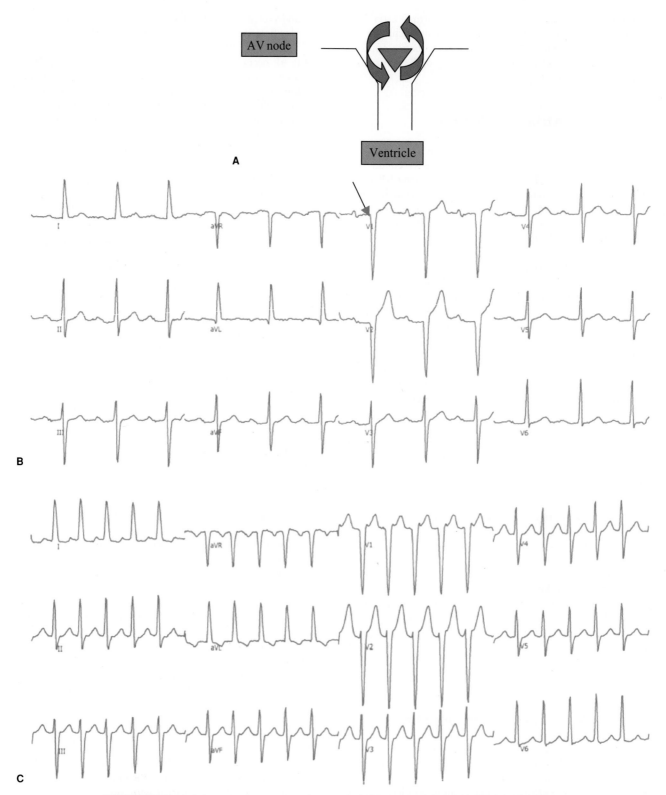

FIGURE 88.10. **A:** Schematic of atrioventricular (AV) nodal re-entrant tachycardia (AVNRT) where the ventricle is passively activated. The most common form is anterograde conduction down the slow pathway and retrograde conduction up the fast pathway. **B:** A 12-lead electrocardiogram. Sinus rhythm of a patient with AVNRT; there is no r′ in lead V1. **C:** A 12-lead electrocardiogram. AVNRT with pseudo r′ in lead V1 denoted by the *arrow.*

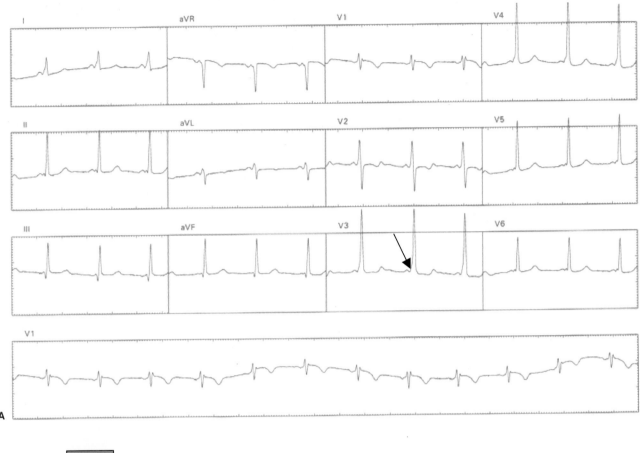

A

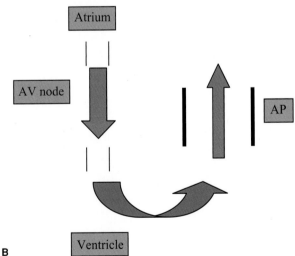

B

FIGURE 88.11. A: A 12-lead electrocardiogram. Sinus rhythm with ventricular pre-excitation manifested as a delta wave (*arrow*), consistent with Wolff–Parkinson–White syndrome. **B:** Schematic of orthodromic atrioventricular (AV) re-entrant tachycardia (AVRT) with anterograde ventricular activation from the AV node and retrograde activation through an accessory pathway (AP). Next page. (*continued*)

• If thrombus is present, anticoagulate and control rate until thrombus has resolved

WIDE QRS TACHYCARDIA

Ventricular Tachycardia

• Independent atrial and ventricular activity (AV dissociation) is an important ECG finding that is present in 60% of patients with ventricular tachycardia (Fig. 88.12). Physical examina-

tion findings of an irregular jugular pulse, known as cannon "A" waves, varying intensity of the first heart sound, and beat-to-beat changes in systolic blood pressure all are consistent with AV dissociation.

• Presence of supraventricular capture beats (sinus beats that are conducted to the ventricle with a narrow QRS during a wide-complex tachycardia) or fusion beats (sinus beats that fuse with the wide-complex beat, resulting in a QRS that is narrower than the tachycardia) would be consistent with a diagnosis of ventricular tachycardia (Fig. 88.13).

• The wide QRS of ventricular tachycardia does not usually mimic a true bundle branch block, as in ventricular

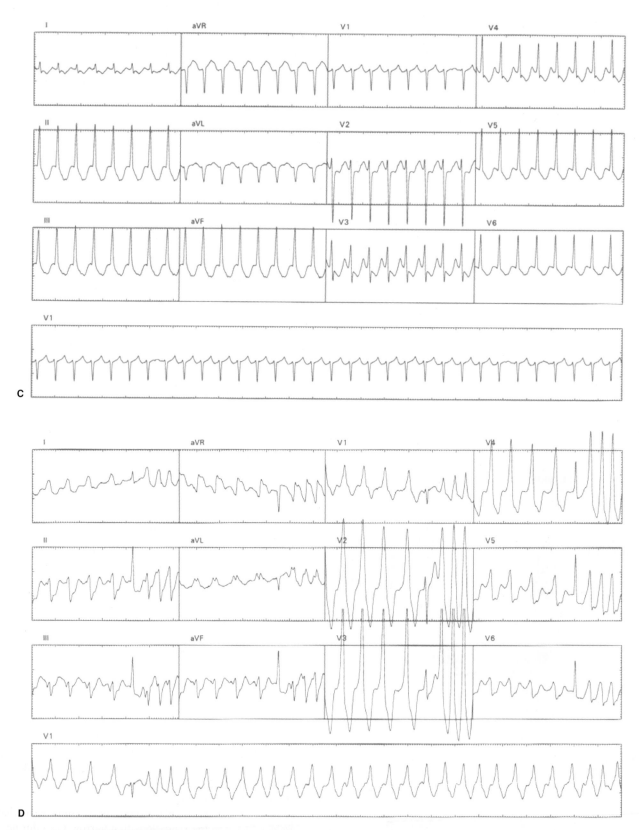

FIGURE 88.11. (*Continued*) **C:** A 12-lead electrocardiogram. Narrow-complex tachycardia in the same patient was found to be AVRT with anterograde conduction down the AV node and retrograde conduction up the accessory pathway. **D:** A 12-lead electrocardiogram. Atrial fibrillation in a patient with anterograde-conducting accessory pathway. There are various QRS widths as there is conduction simultaneously down both the AV node and the accessory pathway. This patient is at risk for ventricular fibrillation and sudden cardiac death.

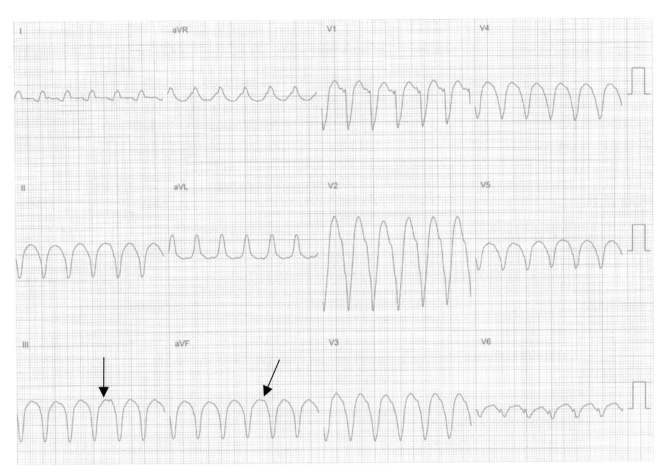

FIGURE 88.12. A 12-lead electrocardiogram. Ventricular tachycardia with atrioventricular dissociation (*arrows* indicate P waves) and negative concordance. There is an atypical left bundle branch block pattern.

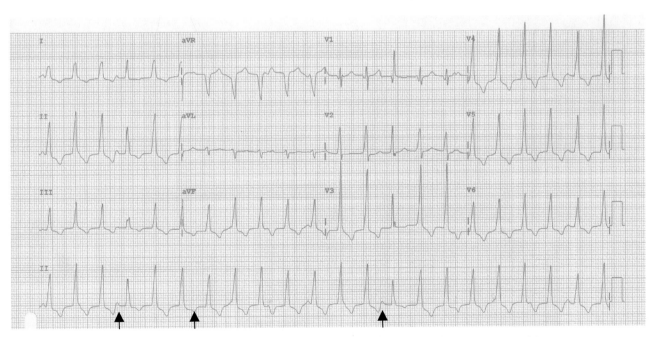

FIGURE 88.13. A 12-lead electrocardiogram. Ventricular tachycardia with AV dissociation and fusion beats (*first* and *second arrows*) and supraventricular capture beats (*third arrow*) confirming the diagnosis of ventricular tachycardia.

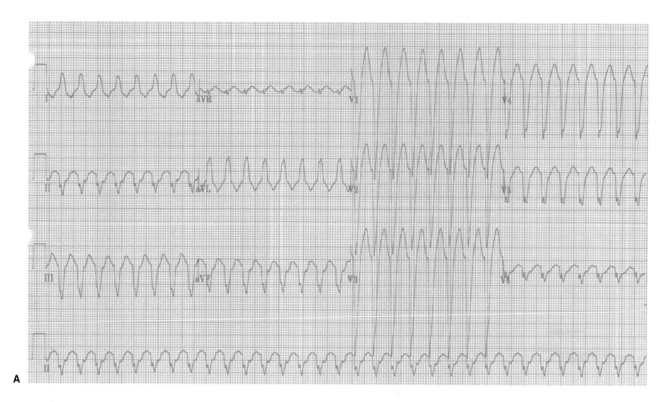

A

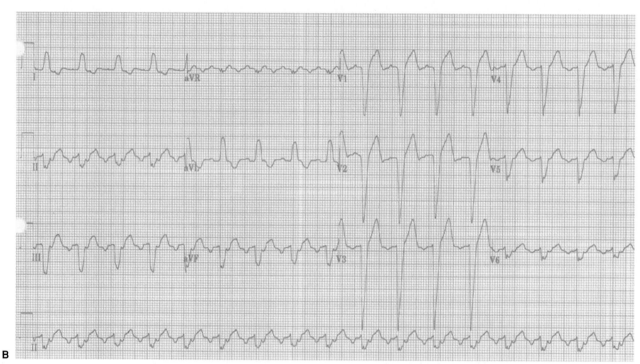

B

FIGURE 88.14. A: A 12-lead electrocardiogram. Atrial flutter with 1:1 conduction and typical left bundle branch block aberrancy. **B:** A 12-lead electrocardiogram. Atrial flutter with 2:1 conduction and typical left bundle branch block aberrancy in the same patient as in Figure 88.12A.

tachycardia, the impulse is generated in the ventricles; therefore, careful examination of the QRS morphology can usually differentiate ventricular tachycardia from right or left bundle branch block aberrancy.

• In addition, if all the QRS complexes in the precordial leads V1 to V6 are negative (negative concordance), this is con-

sistent with the diagnosis of ventricular tachycardia (see Fig. 88.12).

• The wider the QRS, the more likely that tachycardia is ventricular in origin.

• Hemodynamic stability, age of the patient, and ventricular rate or regularity should never be used to distinguish between supraventricular or ventricular tachycardia, as they can be misleading.

Supraventricular Tachycardia with Aberrancy

- Supraventricular tachycardia with aberrancy still conducts down the AV node to the ventricle and can either present with a functional (intermittent) aberrancy or a fixed bundle branch block. The pattern of aberrancy is either typical left or right bundle branch block, and a baseline 12-lead ECG can determine the presence of underlying bundle branch block (Fig. 88.14A and B).

Pre-excited Tachycardia

- In patients with AV accessory pathways or Wolff–Parkinson–White syndrome, wide-complex (pre-excited) tachycardias can be seen. In the antidromic AV re-entrant variety, the atrial impulse activates the ventricle anterogradely via the accessory pathway, and retrograde conduction to the atrium is through either the AV node or another accessory pathway (Fig. 88.15). Atrial tachycardias or atrial flutter can conduct via the accessory pathway to produce pre-excited tachycardias.

Treatment of Wide QRS Tachycardia

- A correct and rapid diagnosis is essential, as incorrect treatment may result in hemodynamic decompensation and death.

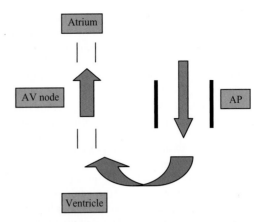

FIGURE 88.15. Schematic of antidromic atrioventricular (AV) re-entry, a pre-excited tachycardia with anterograde conduction down the accessory pathway (AP) and retrograde conduction up the AV node.

- Monomorphic wide-complex tachycardia that is thought to be ventricular in origin in a stable patient can be treated with amiodarone (150 mg IV over 10 minutes; repeat as needed to a maximum dose of 2.2 g IV per 24 hours). If amiodarone is not successful or the patient develops hemodynamic instability or symptoms, electrical cardioversion is appropriate.
- If the wide-complex tachycardia is thought to be SVT with aberrancy, adenosine administration is recommended (6 mg rapid IV push; if no effect, 12 mg IV push can be tried). Adenosine may be therapeutic (terminating the tachycardia by blocking the AV node) if the patient has a re-entrant SVT or diagnostic (causing transient increase in AV block) if the patient has AF or flutter. In the latter case, if patient

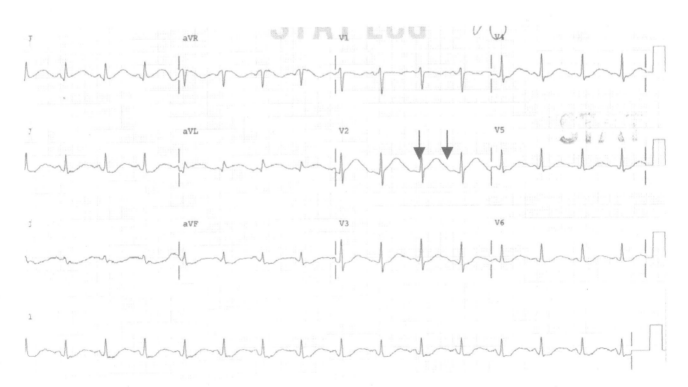

FIGURE 88.16. A 12-lead electrocardiogram. Sinus rhythm with a long QT interval (*arrows* indicate QT measured at approximately 520 ms).

remains stable, rate-controlling IV drugs that have longer-lasting effects, such as beta-blockers or diltiazem, may be administered. Avoid the administration of IV verapamil if the patient has left ventricular dysfunction, heart failure, and/or if there is a possibility that the rhythm could be ventricular in origin, as verapamil has been shown to cause clinical deterioration and death. If the patient is hemodynamically unstable, synchronized cardioversion is appropriate.

- In a patient with Wolff–Parkinson–White and in AF with anterograde conduction down the accessory pathway, first-line medical therapy should be IV procainamide, 100 mg every 5 minutes (maximum 25–50 mg/minute or 17 mg/kg maximum if normal renal function) or IV ibutilide, 1 mg over 10 minutes (may be repeated). These drugs block the rapid conduction over the accessory pathway and may also terminate the AF. If there is no effect or the patient is unstable, immediate cardioversion is indicated.

DRUG-INDUCED ARRHYTHMIAS

- Many antiarrhythmic agents, noncardiac drugs, and nonprescription medications can cause QT prolongation (Fig. 88.16) and, subsequently, torsade de pointes.

Torsade de Pointes

- Polymorphic VT with beat-to-beat changes in the QRS axis (Fig. 88.17); there is QT prolongation, often with a pause or bradycardia-dependent initiation of the arrhythmia. The mechanism is thought to be related to reaching the threshold potential for the slow calcium channel, resulting in early afterdepolarizations and ectopic impulse formation, triggering reentrant excitation. If a drug is responsible for prolonging the QT duration, it should be discontinued. The administration

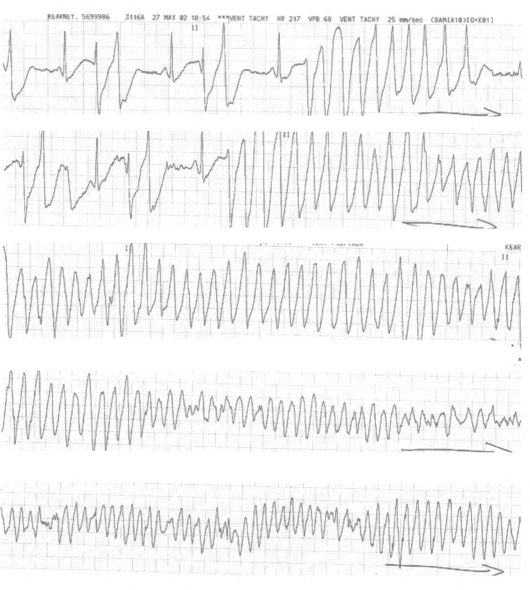

FIGURE 88.17. Lead II rhythm strip. Long QT interval with torsade de pointes.

of IV magnesium is effective for treatment, even when serum magnesium is normal; hypokalemia should also be corrected. Close monitoring is essential, and if bradycardia persists, give atropine or institute temporary pacing. Isoproterenol infusion, between 1 and 4 μg/minute, can be used transiently to increase the heart rate.

Digitalis-induced Arrhythmias

- Digitalis, frequently used in heart failure and AF, is a positive inotrope. It slows the ventricular rate during AF, increases vagal tone, causes diuresis, and has vasodilatory effects. It has a narrow therapeutic window, with women requiring a lower dose than men, and unrecognized digitalis intoxication is a common problem. Often missed by clinicians, the symptoms are nonspecific (gastrointestinal symptoms, visual changes, neuropsychiatric problems, and weakness) and serum drug levels do not correlate well with toxicity. It is important for any health care professional caring for patients who take digitalis to be familiar with ECG findings consistent with digitalis toxicity.

- Diagnosis: Arrhythmias due to digitalis toxicity include atrial tachycardia, junctional tachycardia, ventricular tachycardia, and bradyarrhythmias, including AV block. Many other comorbidities and conditions can potentiate digitalis toxicity, including sympathetic stimulation, hypokalemia, hypercalcemia, hypomagnesemia, diuretics, ischemia and reperfusion, and heart failure.

- Digitalis toxicity can manifest as four ECG features: (a) bradycardia when the heart rate was previously normal or fast; (b) tachycardia when the heart rate was previously normal; (c) unexpected regular rhythm when the patient previously had an irregular rhythm; and (d) an irregular rhythm that regularly repeats itself.

- The treatment of digitalis toxicity depends on the clinical condition and not the drug level. The first step when suspecting digitalis toxicity is to discontinue the medication. Rest, continuous ECG monitoring, and correction of electrolyte abnormalities will often help. If the arrhythmia is life threatening, administering digitalis antibodies or phenytoin may be indicated. The patient's kidney function must be determined to estimate the severity of the suspected intoxication.

CHAPTER 89 ■ PERICARDIAL DISEASE

THE NORMAL PERICARDIUM

- The normal pericardium forms a sac around the heart and proximal large arteries and veins. It has a thin visceral mesothelial layer that closely adheres to the epicardial surface of the heart. The parietal layer consists of the same thin mesothelium and a thicker (up to 2 mm), fairly nonelastic fibrous layer on the outside. Physiologically, the space between both mesothelial layers contains 20 to 30 mL of fluid.

- The fibrous part of the pericardium is attached to the surrounding mediastinal structures and holds the heart in its position within the chest. It limits cardiac dilatation, contributes to the interventricular interaction, and primarily affects diastolic function. The smooth mesothelial surfaces and the pericardial fluid between them reduce friction and act as a barrier to inflammation from surrounding structures. The pericardium is well innervated, and pathologic processes can cause severe episodic or continuous pain.

- The intrapericardial pressure is usually negative; it is approximately equal to and varies with the pleural pressure at the same hydrostatic level. Pericardial pressure affects myocardial transmural pressure by the following relationship:

$$\text{Transmural pressure} = \text{cavitary pressure} - \text{adjacent intrapericardial pressure}$$

Because the intrapericardial pressure is normally negative, this usually adds to the normal transmural pressure gradient.

- The relationship between intrapericardial and pleural pressures causes a simultaneous fall of pressures in both spaces during inspiration and leads to an increased venous return into the right chambers (increased preload), with a subsequent increase in cardiac output. Inspiration influences filling and cardiac output of the left heart only indirectly and very little.

ACUTE PERICARDITIS

Etiology

- Inflammation of the pericardial sac is either an isolated problem or part of a systemic process. Depending on the frequency and time course, pericarditis can be acute, recurrent, or chronic. Common causes of acute pericarditis are shown in Table 89.1. Most often, clinically recognizable pericarditis in the adult is idiopathic, though various viruses are often suspected.

- The most commonly demonstrated virus is the Coxsackie B group, which causes myopericarditis in children and pleuropericarditis in adults (also called Bornholm disease). Enteric cytopathic human orphan (ECHO), influenza, Epstein-Barr, varicella, hepatitis, mumps, and human immunodeficiency viruses can also cause pericarditis.

- Up to one-third of patients with end-stage renal disease will develop uremic pericarditis, and the symptoms usually

TABLE 89.1
COMMON CAUSES OF PERICARDITIS

Idiopathic
Viral
Uremic
Neoplastic
  Metastatic
  Contiguous spread
  Primary
Autoimmune
  Systemic lupus erythematosus
  Postpericardiotomy syndrome (Dressler)
  Rheumatoid arthritis
  Scleroderma
Postmyocardial infarction
Bacterial
Parasitic
Mycotic
Trauma with contusion of the heart
Aortic dissection or ventricular rupture
Radiation induced
Myxedema
Drug-induced
  Procainamide
  Hydralazine
  Quinidine
  Isoniazid
  Methysergide
  Daunorubicin
  Penicillin
  Streptomycin
  Phenylbutazone
  Minoxidil
Sarcoid
Amyloidosis
Acute pancreatitis
Chylopericardium

disappear after beginning or increasing the frequency of dialysis. Increased toxin levels from declining renal function are suspected causes of the inflammatory process, but there is no direct association with serum blood urea nitrogen level or serum creatinine and the acute illness. Note that uremic patients are susceptible to infections that may cause pericarditis, and the underlying disease process leading to the renal insufficiency may also be the cause for the pericardial inflammation.

- Acute pericarditis after myocardial injury is thought to be due to direct irritation of the visceral mesothelium. Historically affecting up to 20% after transmural myocardial infarction; the frequency has decreased due to reperfusion therapy. Symptoms typically occur after 1 to 3 days and can mimic recurrent angina pectoris. If receiving anticoagulants, the inflammation can lead to hemorrhagic intrapericardial effusion and possibly cardiac tamponade.
- Acute pericardial inflammation is also found after open heart surgery, implantation of cardiac pacemakers, percutaneous coronary interventions, or external cardiac trauma. The **postpericardiotomy syndrome** was originally described as postmyocardial infarction pericarditis but later seen in children and adults after opening of the pericardium. The syndrome occurs in 10% to 30% after pericardiotomy and is thought

to be an immune complex reaction. In contrast to pericarditis caused by myocardial injury, chest pain and fever begin after several weeks to months.

- Neoplastic pericarditis is most often caused by cancer of the lung, breast, or esophagus and lymphoma and melanoma. The tumor directly invades the pericardial space or metastasizes through lymphatics or blood vessels; primary pericardial tumors such as mesothelioma are rare. The likelihood of finding previously undiagnosed cancer in a patient presenting with pericarditis is about 6% to 7%. In known malignancy, only 50% to 60% are neoplastic pericarditis; idiopathic and radiation-induced pericarditis are the most common benign causes. The prognosis of neoplastic pericarditis and effusion is poor.
- Pericarditis is also seen in patients with systemic lupus erythematosus, rheumatoid arthritis, and scleroderma. Inflammation of the pericardium is often the first manifestation of lupus in female patients; this diagnosis should be ruled out during the workup for a first episode of idiopathic pericarditis. Radiation pericarditis often follows a mediastinal dose of 4,000 rad or more and can lead to pericardial effusion and acute cardiac tamponade. The long-term effects of radiation also can lead to constrictive pericarditis.
- Pericarditis caused by infectious organisms other than viruses is less frequent now than it was in the preantibiotic era. Pneumonia is still the most common cause; others include sepsis or direct spread from mediastinitis or necrotizing fasciitis of the head or neck. Immunocompromised and elderly patients are more prone to infectious pericarditis than the general population. In adults, *Staphylococcus aureus* is still the most common organism, and there is an apparent decline in infections with *Streptococcus* spp., *Pneumococcus* spp., and *Haemophilus influenzae*.
- Tuberculous pericarditis was once a common cause of acute and constrictive pericarditis but, with the overall decline of tuberculosis, it has become a rare entity in the United States. States with a high percentage of immigrants have reported rising numbers, as 1% to 2% of patients with pulmonary tuberculosis will develop tuberculous pericarditis. Mycobacterial infection must be ruled out in any case of suspected purulent pericarditis.
- The most common fungal organism to cause pericarditis is *Histoplasma capsulatum*. Histoplasmosis in the United States is most common in the Mississippi and Ohio River valleys. Diagnosis is usually delayed and made by positive fungal culture of the pericardial fluid and/or a significant rise of serologic antibody titers (>1:32) against *Histoplasma capsulatum*.

Clinical Presentation

- The typical patient is young and was previously healthy. Symptoms of acute pericarditis include sharp and, usually, persistent chest pain that is generally increased with respiration and motion. It is worse in the supine position and usually improves sitting up and/or with shallow breathing. The pain can radiate to the neck, and dyspnea may also be present. Other common findings preceding or accompanying pericarditis are fever, myalgia, malaise, and tachycardia.
- The characteristic and pathognomonic three-component friction rub is best heard at the left sternal border or the

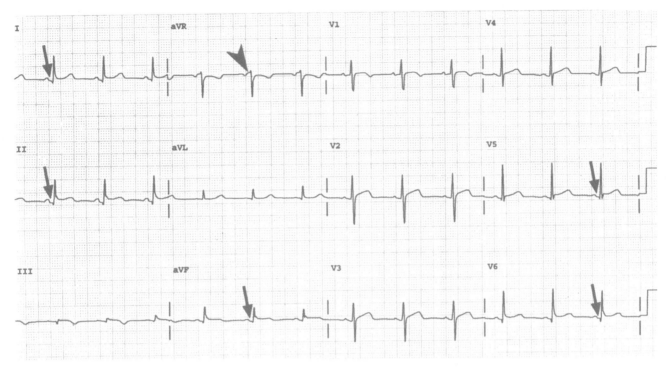

FIGURE 89.1. Electrocardiogram of a patient with acute pericarditis. Note the PR-segment depressions (*arrows*) and convex ST-segment elevations in the inferolateral leads and PR-segment elevation (*arrowhead*) and ST-segment depression in lead aVR, consistent with stage I of electrocardiogram findings in acute pericarditis.

cardiac apex and described as coarse, leathery, superficial—like "pulling Velcro." The rub is only intermittently heard; auscultate frequently in a quiet setting with an upright position leaning forward.

- An electrocardiogram (ECG) should be obtained in every patient presenting with chest pain. Four ECG stages, evolving over hours to days and weeks, have been described:
  - Stage I includes classic and diffuse ST elevations with a concave ST segment and significant PR-segment depression (Fig. 89.1).
  - Stage II is normalization of the ECG.
  - Stage III is development of diffuse T-wave inversion that may persist or normalize.
  - Stage IV is final normalization of the ECG.
- The ECG may show all, several, or none of the stages during an episode of acute pericarditis. The key to the ECG diagnosis is the diffuse nature of the changes, the absence of localization to a particular ECG anatomic area, PR-segment depression, and the absence of ST depression except in lead aVR. Variant angina, hypertrophic cardiomyopathy, and the benign finding of early repolarization can mimic the ECG changes described.
- Atrial arrhythmias are rare but do occur and can be the first manifestation of acute pericarditis. Sustained atrial or ventricular arrhythmias are suggestive of concomitant myocarditis.
- A chest radiograph will be normal in most cases of pericarditis; an enlarged cardiac silhouette is suggestive of a pericardial effusion (>200 mL) and should be further evaluated.
- The laboratory may report positive acute-phase reactants (especially the erythrocyte sedimentation rate) and an elevated white blood cell count; however, these are nonspecific findings. Cardiac troponin T or I and CK-MB isoenzymes are often minimally elevated. Viral studies may confirm the

cause of the pericarditis but are low yield and do not change management. In cases of suspected infectious etiology, cultures from blood and pericardial fluid, if available, should be examined for bacterial and mycobacterial pathogens.

- Echocardiography should be performed in every patient with the suspected diagnosis of pericarditis to evaluate for and follow pericardial effusion (Fig. 89.2) and to help diagnose cardiac tamponade.
- The triad of typical chest pain, pericardial friction rub, and the aforementioned ECG changes confirms the diagnosis of

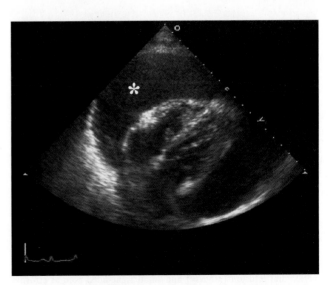

FIGURE 89.2. Subcostal echocardiogram showing a giant pericardial effusion (*asterisk*) in a patient with neoplastic pericarditis.

TABLE 89.2

LIFE-THREATENING DIFFERENTIAL DIAGNOSIS OF ACUTE PERICARDITIS

Acute coronary syndrome
Pulmonary embolism
Aortic dissection
Pericardial tamponade

TABLE 89.3

PRESENTING FACTORS PREDICTING COMPLICATED COURSE

Fever >38°C
Symptoms developing over weeks in immunocompromised
  patient
Traumatic pericarditis
Patient on oral anticoagulants
Large effusion (>20 mm) or tamponade
Failure to respond to nonsteroidal anti-inflammatory drugs

acute pericarditis. However, this diagnosis should be made only after life-threatening conditions with similar presentation have been ruled out (Table 89.2). Computed tomography (CT) of the chest may be necessary to rule out pulmonary embolism or aortic dissection (Fig. 89.3); with newer scanners, a *triple rule-out* scan can evaluate the pulmonary artery tree, thoracic aorta, and coronary arteries on a single breath-hold, contrasted, ECG-gated exam.

Treatment

- Acute pericarditis has a high likelihood of uncomplicated recovery; however, several factors are described as being associated with a complicated course and should prompt hospitalization for their initial treatment (Table 89.3).
- Acute idiopathic or viral pericarditis usually responds to nonsteroidal anti-inflammatory drugs (NSAIDs). The drug regimen consists of high-dose aspirin (325–975 mg three to four times daily for 4 weeks), with a proton pump inhibitor to lessen gastrointestinal effects.
  - Alternatively, indomethacin (25–50 mg four times daily) or ibuprofen (400–600 mg four times daily) can be given.
  - Colchicine has been shown to be effective as a second-line treatment for patients who do not respond to NSAIDs or who have recurrence of their acute pericarditis. Routine initial use of colchicine (1–2 mg on day 1 followed by

0.5–1 mg/day for 3 months) in addition to aspirin may significantly reduce symptoms at 72 hours and recurrence at 18 months compared to aspirin alone. Diarrhea is a known side effect of colchicine and may cause discontinuation of drug therapy in about 5% of patients.

- Symptoms of acute pericarditis respond rapidly to systemic steroids, but there seems to be an increase in relapse after tapering. Corticosteroid therapy should be reserved for recurrent pericarditis not responding to NSAIDs and colchicine. The recommended regimen is 1 to 1.5 mg/kg of prednisone for at least 1 month before slowly tapering the dose by 5 mg/week until the drug is withdrawn. The possible side effects include peptic ulcer disease, sodium retention, hypokalemia, hyperglycemia, Cushing syndrome, and suppression of the adrenal axis. Treatment with corticosteroids also requires the exclusion of infection or an appropriate antibiotic regimen before initiation of therapy.
- The treatment of choice for uremic pericarditis consists of intensive, initially daily dialysis therapy. Heparin should be used sparingly during dialysis to reduce the risk of intrapericardial hemorrhage and possible tamponade.
- The presence of acute pericarditis in acute myocardial infarction also requires caution with the use of intravenous anticoagulants. These drugs are not, however, absolutely contraindicated. Thrombolytic agents have been reported to lead to cardiac tamponade and should be used with caution in the patient with acute myocardial infarction and acute pericarditis.
- The postpericardiotomy syndrome is usually self-limited if left untreated; however, it may increase the risk of early coronary artery bypass graft closure so aggressive treatment with NSAIDs has been recommended. Refractory cases may occur but usually respond rapidly to systemic corticosteroids. Advocates of corticosteroid therapy claim that this treatment reduces the incidence of late constrictive pericarditis.
- Nonviral infectious etiology of pericarditis requires prompt evacuation of pus from the pericardium, usually by operative intervention, because of the need to establish a definitive diagnosis, eradicate the infection, and prevent constrictive pericarditis.
- Recurrence of acute pericarditis is quite common and often requires long-term drug therapy as noted earlier. In a few selected cases refractory to medical therapy, radical pericardectomy may need to be considered.
- In general, acute pericarditis symptoms subside within several days to weeks. The major immediate complication is cardiac tamponade, which occurs in fewer than 5% of patients. For diagnostic and treatment approach in patients with

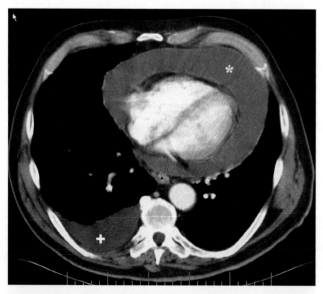

FIGURE 89.3. Computed tomography (CT) of the chest with large pericardial effusion (*asterisk*) and small right-sided pleural effusion (*plus sign*). The dark rim between the pericardial effusion and the right heart represents epicardial fat.

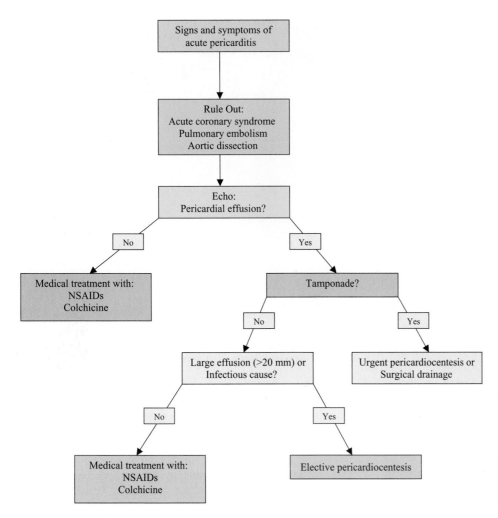

FIGURE 89.4. Diagnostic and treatment algorithm for patients presenting with signs and symptoms of acute pericarditis.

suspected acute uncomplicated or complicated pericarditis, see Figure 89.4.

PERICARDIAL EFFUSION AND CARDIAC TAMPONADE

Etiology

- With acute pericarditis, exudation of fluid and occlusion of the normal drainage through epicardial venous and lymphatic systems by the inflammatory process result in pericardial effusion. The most common causes of tamponade include idiopathic pericarditis, cancer of the lung and breast, lymphoma, renal failure, and tuberculosis.
- Pericardial effusion may also occur in the absence of pericardial inflammation as in hemorrhagic effusion from internal sources such as a pacemaker, angioplasty, coronary artery bypass grafting surgery, aortic dissection, ventricular rupture, or external cardiac trauma.
- Regardless of their size, pericardial effusions can either be clinically silent or cause hemodynamic compromise; the latter situation is called **cardiac tamponade.** The pericardium resists sudden stretching but can gradually expand in response to a chronic distending force. The factor most important to the

development of cardiac tamponade is not the total amount of pericardial fluid but the rate at which it accumulates. A small (<200 mL) but rapidly developing effusion can cause tamponade, whereas a very large pericardial effusion (1,000 mL) developing over weeks or months may be completely asymptomatic.

- The pericardial pressure–volume curve is generally flat until the limits of distention are reached. The pressure–volume curve then becomes curvilinear, and very small volumes of additional fluid raise the intrapericardial pressure significantly. Once the intrapericardial pressure exceeds the filling pressures of the right atrium and/or the right ventricle, central venous pressure rises, cardiac output drops, and cardiac tamponade—and consequently cardiogenic shock—occur.
- Physiologically, the total cardiac volume is limited, and volume in one chamber can increase only if volume in another chamber decreases. This physiologic interdependence of the ventricles is accentuated in cardiac tamponade when right ventricular filling during inspiration causes a significant decrease in left ventricular filling and a significant decrease in stroke volume.
- Cardiac tamponade, if not treated aggressively and rapidly, may be fatal. If diagnosed in a timely fashion, treatment may be successful so cardiac tamponade needs be included in the initial differential diagnosis of cardiogenic shock or pulseless electrical activity.

Clinical Presentation

- The patient with early pericardial tamponade is often confused, agitated, pale, and diaphoretic and complains of chest pain and dyspnea. Initially, compensatory catecholamine release, caused by a decreased cardiac output, leads to sinus tachycardia and often to peripheral vasoconstriction. Later, bradycardia occurs, indicating imminent pulseless electrical activity and cardiorespiratory arrest unless the effusion is immediately decompressed.

- Classic clinical signs include jugular venous distension, demonstrating a rapid x-descent but no y-descent because of right atrial and ventricular compression throughout the entire diastolic cycle. In this situation, the central venous pressure is usually >15 mm Hg, but jugular venous distention may be missing in trauma patients with rapidly developing hemorrhagic tamponade or in patients with uremic pericarditis due to volume depletion from blood loss or dialysis, respectively (*low-pressure tamponade*).

- A drop in systolic blood pressure of >10 mm Hg with inspiration, termed **pulsus paradoxus,** is very suggestive of cardiac tamponade in a patient with hypotension and tachycardia. It can be ascertained through invasive arterial pressure tracing, by palpation or with a sphygmomanometer. Paradoxical pulse is absent in patients with severe aortic insufficiency or atrial septal defect and is difficult to assess in acute cardiac tamponade with hypotension, as the pulse may be unobtainable or disappear completely with inspiration. It is not specific and can also present in other conditions such as chronic obstructive pulmonary disease, pulmonary embolism, pneumothorax, acute asthma, and hypovolemic shock. Patients with tamponade physiology often drop their systolic blood pressure more than 20 mm Hg with inspiration.

- Other clinical signs of cardiac tamponade are distant and muffled heart sounds and clear lungs. The patient with chronic tamponade may present with a low-output state, right-upper quadrant pain caused by swelling of the hepatic capsule, or even ascites and lower-extremity edema. The two main differential diagnoses for cardiac tamponade are tension pneumothorax and pulmonary edema; both conditions can present with tachycardia, hypotension, and jugular venous distension.

- The ECG usually shows signs of acute pericarditis, including sinus tachycardia, PR depression, and abnormal T-wave changes. Electrical alternans of the ECG is almost pathognomonic of pericardial tamponade; it represents a change of direction and amplitude of the P, QRS, and T vectors with every other heart beat and probably results from the "swinging" movement of the heart in a large volume of fluid. A change of the electrical QRS alternans alone is the most common finding. Its absence does not rule out large effusion or tamponade, particularly if they develop rapidly.

- The chest radiograph may show a globular heart hanging down in the mediastinum—*the water bottle heart* (Fig. 89.5). It is also helpful to rule out diagnoses presenting similarly to tamponade, such as tension pneumothorax and pulmonary edema.

- **Echocardiography** is a very useful tool to assess pericardial effusion and determine its hemodynamic significance. It can detect very small pericardial effusions (<20 mL), helps estimate amount and distribution, and visualizes clot or tumor

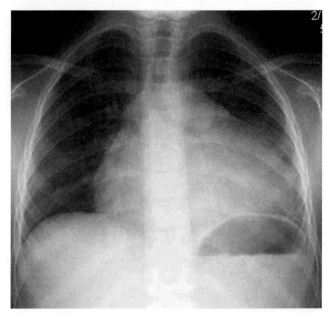

FIGURE 89.5. Anteroposterior chest radiograph in patient with a very large pericardial effusion. The extensive widening of the cardiac silhouette resembles a water bottle.

in the fluid if present. Small effusions (<1 cm) are seen only inferolaterally and around the right atrium (Fig. 89.6). Pericardial effusion tracks between the inferolateral wall and the descending thoracic aorta in the parasternal long-axis view and separates both structures (Fig. 89.7), whereas pleural effusion is found only posterior to the aorta in this view. Effusions causing tamponade are mostly large (>2 cm) and circumferential; in acute tamponade, they are usually smaller.

- Once a pericardial effusion begins to compromise the hemodynamics, there are several characteristic echocardiographic findings. There is diastolic collapse, first of the right atrium,

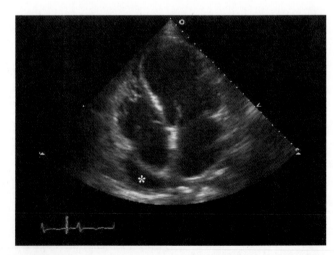

FIGURE 89.6. Apical four-chamber view echocardiogram in patient presenting with acute pericarditis. The very small pericardial effusion is seen only around the right atrial wall (*asterisk*). The right atrium is not compressed by the effusion. This location may be the only one in which an early or small pericardial effusion can be seen in a patient with poor subcostal windows.

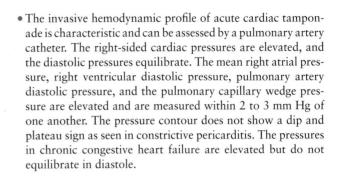

- The invasive hemodynamic profile of acute cardiac tamponade is characteristic and can be assessed by a pulmonary artery catheter. The right-sided cardiac pressures are elevated, and the diastolic pressures equilibrate. The mean right atrial pressure, right ventricular diastolic pressure, pulmonary artery diastolic pressure, and the pulmonary capillary wedge pressure are elevated and are measured within 2 to 3 mm Hg of one another. The pressure contour does not show a dip and plateau sign as seen in constrictive pericarditis. The pressures in chronic congestive heart failure are elevated but do not equilibrate in diastole.

Treatment

- Patients with newly diagnosed pericardial effusion, without tamponade physiology, should be monitored in the hospital for 24 to 48 hours, with at least one repeat echocardiogram prior to discharge. A follow-up echocardiogram should be performed for large pericardial effusions 4 to 6 weeks after the initial presentation or with change in symptoms suggestive of early hemodynamic significance.
- Hemodynamically significant cardiac tamponade, defined as systolic blood pressure <110 mm Hg or pulsus paradoxus >10 mm Hg, should receive immediate aggressive fluid resuscitation with normal saline to increase right-sided filling pressures to at least temporarily stabilize hemodynamics. Inotropic support with dobutamine, dopamine, isoproterenol, or norepinephrine may be needed to further stabilize the blood pressure. More definitive treatment with percutaneous pericardiocentesis or surgically created pericardial window should follow promptly. Any patient presenting with traumatic hemopericardium should be treated surgically.
- Pericardiocentesis should be performed in any patient with acute tamponade and hemodynamic compromise or when an infectious or malignant cause of the pericardial effusion is

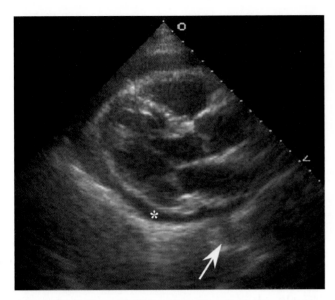

FIGURE 89.7. Parasternal long-axis echocardiographic view in a patient presenting with clinical symptoms of acute pericarditis. There is a small to moderate-sized concentric effusion (*asterisk*). It tracks between the inferolateral wall and the descending thoracic aorta (*arrow*) and thereby confirms the diagnosis of pericardial effusion. A pleural effusion may be seen in the same inferolateral location but would not separate the heart from the aorta.

and then right ventricle, both of which worsen during expiration when right-sided filling is reduced. Diastolic collapse lasting more than one-third of diastole is considered indicative for tamponade (Fig. 89.8). Reciprocal respiratory variation of >20% to 25% of the peak transmitral and transtricuspid Doppler velocities is another very specific indicator (Fig. 89.9). Lifesaving treatments for an unstable or deteriorating patient suffering from cardiac tamponade should not be delayed by waiting for an echocardiogram to be performed.

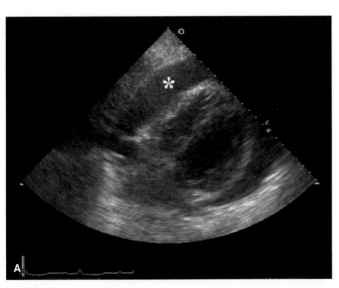
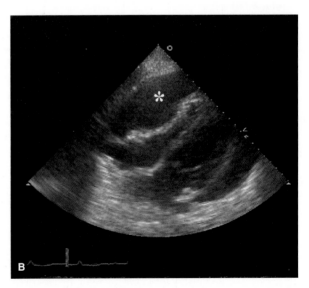

FIGURE 89.8. Subcostal echocardiogram in a patient with cardiogenic shock. Compared to early systole (**A**), there is significant collapse of the right ventricular free wall until very late into the diastolic filling phase (**B**), consistent with pericardial tamponade. The treatment of choice is immediate decompression of the effusion (*) by percutaneous or surgical drainage.

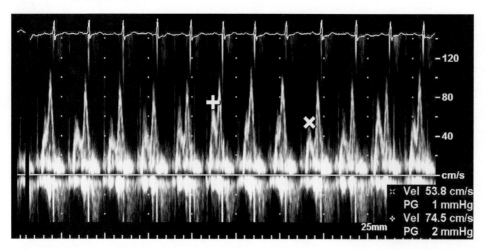

FIGURE 89.9. Transmitral pulse-wave Doppler tracing with significant (>20%) decrease of E-wave velocity during inspiration (x) when compared to velocity during expiration (+). This finding indicates hemodynamic significance if found in conjunction with a pericardial effusion, and immediate drainage of the effusion via percutaneous or surgical route should be considered.

suspected. The procedure is usually performed in the cardiac catheterization laboratory but, in an emergency, may be done at the bedside if clinically necessary.

- Position the patient supine at a 45-degree angle. The area between the xiphoid and the left costal arch should be sterilely prepped using a chlorhexidine–alcohol solution and draped, then anesthetized with a 1% or 2% lidocaine solution. A 7.6-cm (3-inch) aspiratory needle (16–18 gauge) with a short bevel, attached to a three-way stopcock and a 50-mL syringe, is advanced with negative pressure at an angle of 30 to 45 degrees to the abdominal wall and oriented in a posterocephalad direction toward the left shoulder. Once in the pericardial space, fluid can be easily removed. Removal of a small amount of fluid may provide significant clinical improvement. A temporary catheter is then placed into the pericardial space via the Seldinger technique and connected to a bag draining to gravity for several days. This approach provides more complete drainage and reduces the risk for reaccumulation of the effusion. The first sample of fluid retrieved should be sent for microbiologic studies and several other diagnostic tests (Table 89.4).
- Echocardiography can be used to locate the ideal spot for percutaneous puncture, determine distance from the surface to the effusion, demonstrate liver or lung tissue in the projected path, and confirm position within the pericardial effusion. Alternatively, the needle is connected to a V lead of the ECG via an alligator clamp to detect needle contact with the epicardium by sudden demonstration of ST-segment elevation. Complications of this procedure include pneumothorax, myocardial and coronary artery laceration, dysrhythmias, and death.

TABLE 89.4

DIAGNOSTIC TESTS ON PERICARDIAL FLUID

- Complete blood count (CBC) and differential
- Microbiology (Gram stain, culture, acid-fast bacillus smear)
- Chemistry (glucose, protein, albumin, LDH, amylase)
- Cytology

LDH, lactate dehydrogenase.

- If the patient with acute cardiac tamponade can be stabilized by volume expansion and vasopressor support, a safer and equally effective drainage of pericardial fluid can be accomplished by surgical subxiphoid pericardial resection and drainage. Subxiphoid resection can be performed in a sterile environment under local anesthesia; pericardial fluid can be removed and pericardial tissue obtained for biopsy and culture.
- Malignant recurrent pericardial effusions often require a pericardial window to allow fluid to drain into the adjacent pleural space. More recently, percutaneous balloon pericardiotomy has been developed as a nonsurgical approach to create such a window and to drain large pericardial effusions.

CONSTRICTIVE PERICARDITIS

Etiology

- Constrictive pericarditis occurs when chronic inflammation leads to scarring and, in some cases, calcification of the pericardium. Tuberculosis is the most common cause worldwide; the leading causes in the United States are idiopathic pericarditis, previous mediastinal radiation, or cardiac surgery. The thickened (>2 to 3 mm) and shrunken pericardium leads to compromise of diastolic filling and elevation and equalization of end-diastolic pressures in all four cardiac chambers. Up to 20% of patients with surgically proven constriction may present without any pericardial thickening (Fig. 89.10).
- Contrary to pericardial tamponade, the initial diastolic ventricular filling is very rapid; filling abruptly ceases once ventricular volume has reached the limits allowed by the constricted pericardium. Together, these two findings compose the dip and plateau or square root sign of constrictive pericarditis seen during pulmonary artery catheterization (Fig. 89.11).
- The signs and symptoms of constrictive pericarditis generally develop over a prolonged period and are similar to those of biventricular congestive heart failure, restrictive cardiomyopathy, cor pulmonale, cirrhosis, and pericardial tamponade.

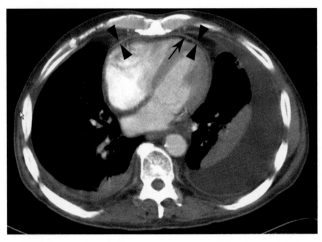

FIGURE 89.10. Axial slice of chest computed tomography in a patient with clinical findings of severe right heart failure. The pericardium is well seen (*arrowheads*) due to the separation from the myocardium by a very small pericardial effusion (*arrow*). Of note is that the pericardium is neither thickened (maximally 3 mm in thickness) nor calcified; however, preoperative cardiac catheterization results and the intraoperative findings during surgical pericardial stripping confirmed the diagnosis of constrictive pericarditis.

Features of cardiac tamponade and constrictive pericarditis can occur simultaneously, referred to as *effusive-constrictive pericarditis*. This likely represents a transitional state from effusive to constrictive pericarditis and is commonly seen with malignant pericardial effusion from thoracic neoplasm and constrictive pericarditis after radiation to the chest.

Clinical Presentation

- Patients often complain of fatigue, increasing dyspnea on exertion, abdominal discomfort, and abdominal and lower-extremity swelling. Physical findings include increased jugular venous pressure with a prominent x- and y-descent. A loud early diastolic sound, a "pericardial knock," caused by the sudden cessation of ventricular filling is heard in up to 50% of patients and pathognomonic for pericardial constriction. The lungs remain clear initially and later develop left-sided or bilateral pleural effusions. The liver is enlarged secondary to congestion; ascites, splenomegaly, and significant lower-extremity edema are also present.
- Unlike in cardiac tamponade, blood pressure is maintained, and fewer than 20% of patients have a significant pulsus paradoxus. A lateral chest radiograph may show pericardial calcium in up to 50% (Fig. 89.12).
- The ECG findings are nonspecific and include T-wave inversions, low voltage, and atrial fibrillation. Echocardiography is helpful to distinguish right heart failure from pericardial constriction; however, echocardiographic findings are not specific for the diagnosis. They include paradoxical septal motion, rapid deceleration of the early diastolic mitral inflow velocity (E wave), significant respiratory variation of mitral inflow velocity (>25%), and normal mitral valve annular tissue Doppler velocity. In the absence of a pericardial effusion, a thickened pericardium is often hard to distinguish from the myocardium.
- Cardiac CT and cardiac magnetic resonance imaging (MRI) are very useful to precisely determine the pericardial

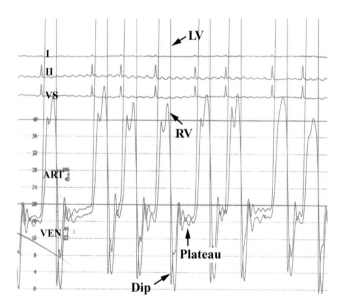

FIGURE 89.11. Right (RV) and left ventricular (LV) pressure tracings in a patient with clinical findings consistent with constrictive pericarditis. The early diastolic dip is followed by plateau, with elevation and equalization of right and left ventricular pressures. Note that contrary to ventricular discordance, the dip and plateau sign is classic but not specific for constrictive pericarditis and can be found in several other medical conditions (see text for details). The electrocardiographic tracing shows atrial fibrillation seen often in constrictive pericarditis.

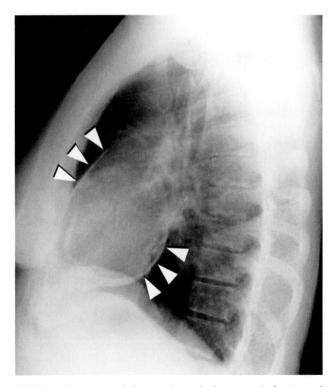

FIGURE 89.12. Lateral chest radiograph showing calcifications of the anterior and inferolateral pericardium in a patient with constrictive pericarditis (*arrowheads*).

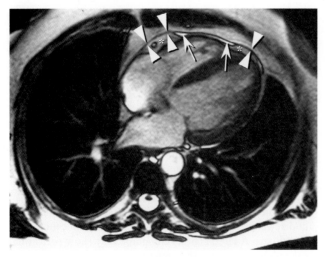

FIGURE 89.13. Four-chamber view of electrocardiogram-gated cardiac magnetic resonance imaging (MRI) in a patient with suspected pericardial constriction. The normal-appearing pericardium (*arrowheads*) is very precisely visualized in areas with pericardial effusion (*arrows*) and with pericardial fat (*asterisk*) only. The outstanding soft-tissue imaging capabilities of MRI make it preferable over cardiac computed tomography (CT) to evaluate the pericardium in patients with no or very little pericardial effusion. ECG, electrocardiogram.

thickness. Cardiac MRI is better suited to image soft tissues and can, in contrast to CT, show normal pericardium, even in the absence of pericardial effusion (Fig. 89.13). Furthermore, tagged cine MRI is able to demonstrate adhesions between the pericardium and myocardium.

- Cardiac catheterization pressure tracings are still the gold standard to diagnose constrictive pericarditis and to differentiate it from restrictive cardiomyopathy. The hemodynamic findings of elevated and equalized diastolic pressures in all four chambers and the dip and plateau sign are classic, although not very specific for constriction. In contrast, respiratory variation of ventricular pressures (right ventricular pressure rises and left ventricular pressure falls during inspiration and vice versa during expiration, causing ventricular discordance) has been shown to be highly sensitive and specific for the diagnosis of constrictive pericarditis (Fig. 89.14). Hemodynamically silent constrictive pericarditis can be evaluated by performing volume loading during catheterization; the initially normal right and left heart pressures may elevate and equilibrate in diastole.

Treatment

- Patients with acute onset of constrictive symptoms may improve significantly with medical treatment that includes NSAIDs, colchicine, and steroids. Chronic constrictive pericarditis can be treated initially with diuretics and with sodium and fluid restriction, if symptoms are mild.
- Moderate to severe disease requires definitive treatment with complete removal of the pericardium by surgical stripping. This major procedure is associated with a perioperative mortality of >6%; it can be life-saving and improves symptoms drastically in most patients; however, poor outcome is likely if the constriction is radiation induced.

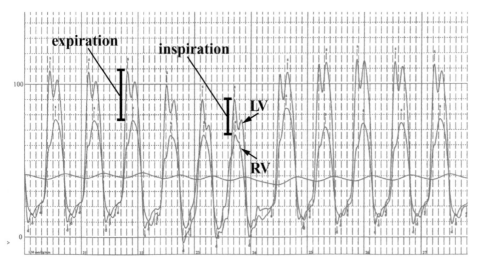

FIGURE 89.14. Simultaneous invasive left (LV) and right ventricular (RV) pressure tracings. Note the ventricular discordance with respiration: RV pressure rises and LV pressure falls during inspiration and vice versa during expiration. This finding is highly sensitive and specific for the diagnosis of constrictive pericarditis; its presence rules out the differential diagnosis of restrictive cardiomyopathy.

CHAPTER 90 ■ ACUTE HYPERTENSION MANAGEMENT IN THE ICU

DEFINITIONS

- Acute hypertension is a common issue in the intensive care unit (ICU). The settings in which blood pressure (BP) elevation occur are highly variable, and optimal care must be tailored to the pathophysiology of the specific circumstances in which it is encountered.
- The terminology used in the literature to classify this heterogeneous group of disorders has been somewhat inconsistent and confusing (Table 90.1).
  - The terms *hypertensive emergency* or *hypertensive crisis* are commonly defined as a marked increase in BP associated with target-organ damage. We define a hypertensive emergency broadly—as any condition in which BP should be lowered immediately. Although the term *malignant hypertension* has been discouraged, it is still widely used to describe the syndrome where organ dysfunction is a direct consequence of the elevated BP rather than an epiphenomenon. The presence of papilledema is not necessarily required for this diagnosis to be made.
  - In contrast, a hypertensive urgency is a condition with severe BP elevation and no target-organ damage, such that the BP can be decreased more gradually over the course of several hours, often with oral medications.
- It is the presence or absence of organ dysfunction, rather than the absolute degree of BP elevation, that determines whether a patient is classified as having a hypertensive emergency or urgency.
  - It is not always clear how clinicians distinguish between hypertensive urgencies and severe, poorly controlled, chronic hypertension.
  - The most recent Joint National Committee Guidelines classify patients with hypertension into stage 1 (systolic blood pressure [SBP] 140–159 mm Hg or diastolic blood pressure [DBP] 90–99 mm Hg) and stage 2 (SBP ≥160 mm Hg or DBP ≥100 mm Hg). The previously used category of "stage 3 hypertension" (SBP ≥180 mm Hg or DBP ≥110 mm Hg) has been combined with stage 2.

EPIDEMIOLOGY AND ETIOLOGY

- Hypertension is extraordinarily common, with only a minority having adequate BP control. The incidence of hypertensive emergencies and urgencies has not been assessed in population-based studies but <1% with chronic hypertension ever present in this fashion. Nevertheless, because hypertension is so common and a wide variety of conditions other than malignant hypertension can be categorized as hypertensive emergencies, acutely elevated BP is still a factor in a substantial number of medical visits to emergency departments and a frequent problem in the ICU (Table 90.2).

TABLE 90.1

DEFINITIONS

1. *Hypertensive emergency:* Any condition in which hypertension is causing or potentially exacerbating organ dysfunction and should be lowered emergently
2. *Hypertensive urgency:* Severe hypertension that is not associated with acute organ dysfunction and requires gradual reduction in blood pressure over several hours
3. *Malignant hypertension:* A syndrome in which uncontrolled hypertension directly causes organ dysfunction (note that this is a subtype of 1). Although previous definitions have sometimes mandated the presence of retinopathy with papilledema, this is only one of several possible clinical manifestations and should not necessarily be required.

TABLE 90.2

TYPES OF HYPERTENSIVE EMERGENCIES

Malignant hypertension
- Hypertensive encephalopathy/RPLS
- Retinopathy and papilledema
- Acute heart failure
- Myocardial ischemia
- Malignant nephrosclerosis and acute renal failure
- Microangiopathy

Neurocritical care emergencies
- Acute ischemic stroke requiring thrombolysis
- Acute intracerebral hemorrhage
- Subarachnoid hemorrhage
- Severe hypertension following craniotomy
- Cerebral hyperperfusion syndrome (postendarterectomy or stenting)
- Normal perfusion pressure breakthrough (after AVM resection)

Cardiovascular emergencies
- Acute myocardial infarction
- Acute heart failure
- Aortic dissection
- Severe hypertension following cardiovascular surgery

Preeclampsia/eclampsia

RPLS, reversible posterior leukoencephalopathy syndrome; AVM, arteriovenous malformation.

Malignant Hypertension

- Peak incidence occurs between the ages of 40 and 50; risk factors include poor long-term BP control, lack of a primary care physician, noncompliance with antihypertensive medications, male gender, African American ethnicity, illicit drug use, and lower socioeconomic class. Prior to effective antihypertensive therapy, the mortality very high, with approximately 80% of patients dying within a year (hence, the term *malignant*).
- At least 90% to 95% of patients with chronically elevated BP can be classified as having "essential" hypertension, meaning that the underlying cause is multifactorial and not specifically known.
- A small proportion have **"secondary" hypertension,** where there is an identifiable and sometimes treatable condition. Among patients who present with malignant hypertension, as many as 50% to 80% may have a secondary etiology. Other clues are a history of BP resistant to medical therapy, sudden worsening in a previously well-controlled patient, and the onset of hypertension at an unusually young or old age. A careful history, physical examination, and appropriate diagnostic testing to exclude causes of secondary hypertension are indicated during the hypertensive emergency and after it has resolved (Table 90.3).
- **Renovascular** disease, the most common cause, may be present in up to 45% with severe or malignant hypertension, although the proportion is higher in Caucasians than African Americans. Features that suggest renovascular hypertension include atherosclerotic vascular disease in other organ systems, systolic-diastolic abdominal bruits, a history of deterioration in renal function with exposure to angiotensin-converting enzyme (ACE) inhibitors, or angiotensin II receptor blockers, recurrent flash pulmonary edema, and small kidneys (determined by ultrasound or other imaging).

TABLE 90.3

ETIOLOGIES OF MALIGNANT HYPERTENSION

Essential hypertension
Secondary hypertension
  Renovascular disease
    Atherosclerosis, thrombosis
    Fibromuscular dysplasia
    Medium- and large-vessel vasculitis
  Glomerular disease
    Glomerulonephritis
    Small-vessel vasculitis
    Microangiopathies
    Scleroderma
  Renal parenchymal disease
    Polycystic kidney disease (and others)
    Renin-producing tumors
  Endocrine causes
    Pheochromocytoma
    Primary hyperaldosteronism
    Cushing syndrome
    Hypercalcemia
Aortic coarctation
Medications (e.g., cyclosporine, tacrolimus, erythropoietin)
Sympathomimetic drugs (e.g., cocaine, amphetamines)

- Hypertension is almost universally present in patients with acute or chronic kidney disease, especially when the etiology is a glomerulonephropathy. A common manifestation of obstructive sleep apnea, hypertension can be improved by use of noninvasive positive airway pressure.
- Various rare **endocrine** causes, including primary aldosteronism, Cushing syndrome, hypercalcemia, hypothyroidism, and pheochromocytoma, are responsible for a small proportion of cases.
- Several **illicit drugs** can cause malignant hypertension in addition to other hypertensive emergencies. Sympathomimetics, such as cocaine and methamphetamine, have been implicated in causing intracerebral hemorrhage (ICH) and subarachnoid hemorrhage (SAH), ischemic stroke, and aortic dissection.
- Various drugs used in clinical practice can cause severe hypertension, or even hypertensive emergencies. The most commonly implicated are **erythropoietin** and various **immunosuppressants,** most notably cyclosporine, tacrolimus, interferon, and high-dose corticosteroids, although it is sometimes difficult to separate the hypertension-inducing effects of these drugs from the complications of the diseases they are intended to treat.

Neurologic Hypertensive Emergencies

- **Acute stroke** is one of the most common indications for which emergent BP control may be necessary and often the most frequent form of end-organ damage. Stroke is the second leading cause of death worldwide and is also a major reason for long-term disability. Cerebral ischemia is responsible for 70% to 80% of strokes, whereas ICH and SAH account for 5% to 20% and 1% to 7%, respectively.
- Overall, >80% of patients with ischemic or hemorrhagic strokes are initially hypertensive to some degree. Even without treatment, the BP usually declines gradually over the first several hours or days in hospital. An even larger proportion of patients with ICH develop, and are treated for, acute hypertension. The incidence of hypertension with SAH is somewhat lower, but aggressive treatment is sometimes advocated to minimize the initial risk of rebleeding from the aneurysm.

Perioperative Hypertension

- Depending on the patient population, type of surgery (especially neurosurgical and cardiovascular), and how hypertension is defined, 3% to 34% of operations are complicated by postoperative hypertension in the recovery room or ICU, with the most important risk factors being inadequately controlled pain and a history of hypertension, especially if antihypertensives were withdrawn preoperatively.
- Elevations in BP occur most often during the initial 30 to 60 minutes after surgery, may last for several hours, and have been associated with higher rates of postoperative hemorrhage and myocardial ischemia in certain patient populations.
- Preoperative hypertension is predictive of intra- and postoperative BP fluctuations, and has been associated with the occurrence of complications and worse outcomes. The American Heart Association recommends that nonemergent surgery be deferred if the BP exceeds 180/110 mm Hg; it remains

controversial whether delaying surgery ultimately modifies perioperative risks.

Pregnancy-induced Hypertension

- Hypertension complicates approximately 12% of pregnancies and is responsible for 18% of maternal deaths in the United States. When BP elevation occurs prior to 20 weeks' gestation, it is considered chronic hypertension. If it occurs without complication after 20 weeks, it is referred to as gestational hypertension.
- **Preeclampsia** is a form of pregnancy-induced hypertension that is associated with vasoconstriction, endothelial dysfunction, platelet aggregation, and increased coagulation.
  - Usually defined by the concomitant presence of hypertension and proteinuria (>300 mg of protein per 24 hours), some develop severe symptoms without proteinuria.
  - Preeclampsia occurs in 2% to 10% of pregnancies, with important risk factors including nulliparity, antiphospholipid antibodies, diabetes mellitus, obesity, family history, multiple (twin) pregnancies, maternal age beyond 40, and a previous history during other pregnancies.
  - Maternal complications can include progression to eclampsia, pulmonary edema, microangiopathy, and renal failure. The most common neonatal complications are prematurity and growth restriction. **Eclampsia** is defined as the development of severe neurologic manifestations, including seizures and a depressed level of consciousness, in women with preeclampsia.

Cardiovascular Hypertensive Emergencies

- Acute heart failure is responsible for 5% to 10% of hospital admissions. Hospital mortality is about 4% but increases to >50% by 1 year. In patients presenting with flash pulmonary edema, acute hypertension is particularly common and is likely to be both a consequence and contributing cause.
- A history of chronic hypertension exists in about 40% to 70% of patients with acute coronary syndromes, and about 30%

have an elevated BP when initially assessed. Severe uncontrolled hypertension at admission (>180/110 mm Hg) is a relative contraindication to thrombolysis for ST elevation myocardial infarction (STEMI).
- **Aortic dissection** is a relatively rare condition; mortality has decreased from as high as 90% to about 20% to 35% with modern medical and surgical therapy. More than 70% have chronic hypertension, but BP can be highly variable at presentation. Most type B dissections (descending aorta) have an admission systolic pressure of >150 mm Hg compared with just more than a third of type A dissections (ascending aorta).

PATHOPHYSIOLOGY OF HYPERTENSION-INDUCED END-ORGAN DYSFUNCTION

- Autoregulation keeps blood flow to organs relatively constant despite variations in BP; its limits are usually between mean arterial pressure of 60 and 150 mm Hg. Extreme hypertension exceeding the upper range of autoregulation causes edema, hemorrhage, and organ dysfunction, whereas reductions in BP beyond the lower limits of autoregulation result in tissue hypoperfusion and ischemia (Fig. 90.1).
- In addition to the systemic myogenic response, there are also organ-specific vascular regulatory mechanisms to protect against the effects of acute hypertension. The likelihood of end-organ damage increases not only with the absolute degree of BP elevation but also with the rate at which this occurs.
- With chronic hypertension, the walls of small arteries and arterioles hypertrophy, shifting the autoregulation curve toward the right to maintain blood flow even at unusually high BPs. Conversely, ischemia may occur when BP falls to levels that would otherwise be well tolerated. In the setting of neurologic injury, autoregulation is often impaired, and cerebral blood flow becomes directly dependent on BP (see Fig. 90.1).
- Normal endothelial function is necessary for the regulation of vascular tone, BP, and regional blood flow. The endothelium

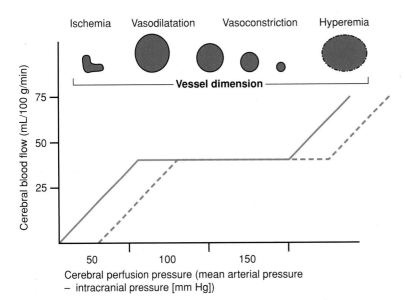

FIGURE 90.1. Cerebral blood flow autoregulation: effect of changes in cerebral perfusion pressure on cerebral blood flow and vascular caliber in normal and hypertensive patients (*dashed line*).

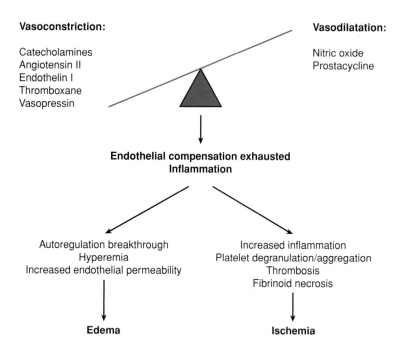

FIGURE 90.2. Simplified pathophysiology of acute hypertension-induced organ dysfunction. (Adapted from Vaughan CJ, Delanty N. Hypertensive emergencies. *Lancet.* 2000;356:411–417.)

is involved in maintaining a delicate balance between vasodilating substances (e.g., nitric oxide, bradykinin, prostacyclin) and vasoconstrictors (e.g., endothelin), as well as between coagulation and fibrinolysis.

- When BP is elevated, **natriuretic peptides** are released from the endothelium, which in turn induce sodium and water loss, with decreased intravascular volume.
- Excessive activation of the **renin-angiotensin** system causes vasoconstriction and inflammation, leading to hypertensive emergencies, an effect that can be blocked by ACE inhibitors.
- **Angiotensin II** levels are elevated in most cases of malignant hypertension, particularly when the etiology is a renal condition. Increased wall stress and prolonged vasoconstriction in the face of severe hypertension eventually causes endothelial compensatory mechanisms to fail, such that a vicious cycle ensues, with consequent hyperemia, increased permeability, inflammation (endarteritis), platelet aggregation, coagulation, and thrombosis.
- Transmural necrosis and the entry of blood components into the vessel wall lead to obliteration of the lumen and replacement of smooth muscle with fibrous tissue, a process called **fibrinoid necrosis.** Patients with malignant hypertension may therefore paradoxically develop both hyperemia (due to endothelial dysfunction and loss of autoregulation) and ischemia (due to thrombosis and fibrinoid necrosis) (Fig. 90.2).

MANIFESTATIONS

Hypertensive Encephalopathy and Reversible Posterior Leukoencephalopathy Syndrome

- Severe elevations in BP eventually cause a breakdown of the blood–brain barrier, with subsequent development of vaso-genic cerebral edema. White matter is less tightly packed than the overlying cerebral cortex, making it more vulnerable to the spread of edema.

- Swelling occurs predominantly, but not exclusively, in the **posterior regions of the brain.** Possibly it is due to a larger concentration of sympathetic fibers around arterioles in the anterior brain, resulting in a greater degree of vasoconstriction and relative protection against the effects of severe hypertension.
- Characteristic clinical features and magnetic resonance imaging (MRI) findings of vasogenic edema in posterior white matter led to the description of a clinical radiologic syndrome, now most commonly termed *reversible posterior leukoencephalopathy syndrome* (RPLS) or posterior reversible encephalopathy syndrome.
- Although occurring most commonly in association with severe hypertension, other conditions may at least predispose to, if not directly cause, the development of RPLS, perhaps by inducing endothelial toxicity. RPLS has been described in association with certain medications and immunosuppressive agents (most notably cyclosporine), and in the setting of microangiopathies, connective tissue diseases, vasculitis, and preeclampsia.
- RPLS is best visualized using T_2 and fluid-attenuated inversion recovery MRI sequences. Diffusion-weighted MRI has confirmed that vasogenic edema is much more prominent than cytotoxic edema and, although RPLS is usually "reversible," some patients do develop ischemic strokes.
- Many patients do not adhere perfectly to the typical patterns of RPLS: gray-matter involvement of the cerebral cortex and basal ganglia and edema occurring in the frontal lobes, posterior fossa, and brainstem have all been described. It is rare for only one vascular territory to be involved (Fig. 90.3).
- The clinical manifestations of RPLS in the setting of acute BP elevation are collectively described by the term *hypertensive encephalopathy,* which is characterized by the subacute development of neurologic signs and symptoms and may

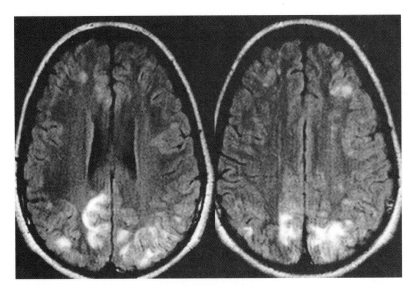

FIGURE 90.3. Fluid-attenuated inversion recovery magnetic resonance imaging sequences of a 15-year-old patient with a history of Wegener granulomatosis presenting with seizures and altered mental status. The findings are consistent with reversible posterior leukoencephalopathy syndrome (RPLS). Although vasogenic edema is seen predominantly posteriorly, anterior changes are also present.

include headache, altered mental status, seizures, and visual disturbances.

- **Headaches** are usually generalized, severe, and poorly responsive to analgesics and improve rapidly with treatment of hypertension.
- **Altered mental status** can range from lethargy and confusion to stupor and coma, although the latter is unusual.
- The posterior predominance of RPLS is reflected by the frequent occurrence of unilateral or bilateral visual disturbances, including hemianopsia, visual neglect, cortical blindness, Anton syndrome (patient is not aware of blindness), and visual hallucinations.
- **Focal seizures** originating in the occipital regions have also been described, although they most often generalize, and may be recurrent.

Retinopathy

- Endothelial damage and leakage of plasma proteins into the retina lead to edema and the formation of hard exudates (Fig. 90.4). Focal areas of ischemia and infarction within the nerve fiber layer cause white areas, called cotton-wool spots, to appear. Breakdown of the blood–retinal barrier results in flame-shaped hemorrhages within the retina.
- The development of papilledema has historically been used to differentiate "accelerated" from "malignant" hypertension. However, the presence or absence of papilledema has little impact on the natural history and prognosis of hypertensive emergencies, nor should it significantly alter management. The mechanism of papilledema may include raised intracranial pressure (ICP), present in some patients with hypertensive encephalopathy and ischemia of the optic nerve head.

Nephropathy and Microangiopathy

- Certain conditions causing acute renal failure may cause hypertensive emergencies, but severely elevated BP can also cause renal dysfunction, a condition called malignant nephrosclerosis. Renal biopsies reveal fibrinoid necrosis,

hyperplastic arteriolitis, neutrophilic infiltration, and thrombosis of glomerular capillaries. The histologic appearance can be difficult to distinguish from other microangiopathies, such as hemolytic uremic syndrome and thrombotic thrombocytopenic purpura.

- More than a fourth of patients with malignant hypertension, especially those with acute renal failure, have typical clinical features of microangiopathy, including thrombocytopenia, elevated lactate dehydrogenase, and schistocytes on blood smear.
- Impaired renal perfusion leads to greater activation of the renin-angiotensin system, which further augments vasoconstriction, fluid retention, and BP elevation. The earliest evidence of renal involvement is the presence of abnormal urine sediment, with proteinuria, hematuria, and the appearance of red and white blood cell casts.
- Acute renal failure follows, which is sometimes severe enough to require dialysis and occasionally results in end-stage renal disease. This is more common when the etiology is secondary

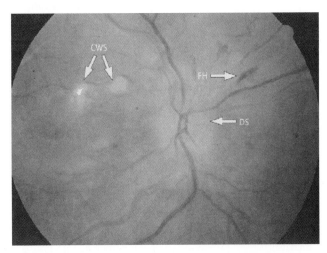

FIGURE 90.4. Severe hypertensive retinopathy with evidence of disc swelling (DS, papilledema), cotton wools spots (CWS), and flame-shaped hemorrhage (FH). (From Wong T, Mitchell P. The eye in hypertension, *Lancet.* 2007;369:425–435, used with permission.)

rather than essential hypertension, particularly with renal causes. The degree of renal dysfunction is an important prognostic variable.

Cardiovascular Complications

- Approximately 20% of patients with malignant hypertension present with cardiac complications, which may include myocardial ischemia or pulmonary edema. Many have chronic hypertension, left ventricular hypertrophy, and diastolic dysfunction; a smaller subset also have impaired systolic function. Left ventricular hypertrophy increases myocardial oxygen requirements while also outstripping vascular supply and compressing coronary arterioles.
- The increased afterload associated with severe hypertension further increases myocardial wall stress and oxygen demand, such that ischemia occurs, especially with concomitant coronary artery disease.
- Increased wall thickness and changes to the extramyocardial collagen network impair myocardial relaxation and compliance. As a result, even small increases in intravascular volume and afterload can produce pulmonary edema.

TREATMENT: PHARMACOLOGIC AGENTS

- An ideal pharmacologic agent (Table 90.4) for treatment of hypertensive emergencies should have a rapid onset but also be short-acting and easy to titrate to avoid excessively lowering the BP for long periods of time.
- Sodium nitroprusside (NTP) is considered first-line therapy, largely because of its rapid onset, short duration of action, affordability, familiarity, and efficacy. NTP is a parenterally administered, potent arterial and venous vasodilator, which has an onset within <30 seconds and a duration of action of only 2 to 3 minutes, such that cessation of the infusion allows BP to rise back to previous levels within 1 to 10 minutes.
  - Cardiac output is either preserved or increased, and cardiac filling pressures decrease. The mechanism of action involves the release of nitric oxide into the bloodstream, activation of guanylate cyclase, and subsequent conversion of guanosine triphosphate to cyclic guanosine monophosphate in vascular smooth muscle, which in turn inhibits the intracellular movement of calcium.
- The usual starting dose of NTP is 0.25 to 0.5 μg/kg/minute, and it is increased in increments of 0.5 μg/kg/minute every 5 to 10 minutes until the goal BP is achieved.
- NTP has the potential for several serious, life-threatening complications.
  - Despite lowering preload and afterload, NTP may induce **coronary steal,** whereby excessive vasodilatation of coronary arterioles shunts blood away from ischemic regions.
  - Vasodilation of cerebral vasculature increases **cerebral blood volume** and ICP. This phenomenon is not entirely consistent and may be avoided with a somewhat slower administration.
  - Each NTP molecule has five **cyanide** moieties, such that cyanide makes up 44% of its molecular weight. Cyanide is metabolized by transsulfuration in the liver to thiocyanate, which is 100 times less toxic than cyanide, and is cleared in the urine and stool. When this pathway is overwhelmed, cyanide accumulates and causes toxicity. Patients are particularly vulnerable when treated with prolonged, high-dose infusions, especially if hepatic and renal function are impaired or if sulfur stores are depleted because of malnutrition.
  - Cyanide blocks oxidative phosphorylation and essentially causes tissue anoxia and lactic acidosis despite adequate oxygen delivery and high venous oxygen saturation levels. Manifestations of cyanide poisoning include depressed mental status, seizures and, eventually, bradycardia and hemodynamic collapse. Cyanide levels are not easily monitored, and the development of lactic acidosis is a late finding. The development of tachyphylaxis to nitroprusside, with consequent increasing dose requirements, may be a harbinger of toxicity.
  - Treatment of cyanide poisoning consists of discontinuation of nitroprusside, supportive care with the delivery of 100% oxygen, and the administration of **sodium nitrite** (300 mg IV), followed by **sodium thiosulfate** (12.5 g IV). The use of sodium nitrite is controversial, as it actually causes the production of methemoglobin, which, although

TABLE 90.4

INTRAVENOUS PHARMACOLOGIC AGENTS FOR MANAGEMENT OF HYPERTENSIVE EMERGENCIES

Drug	Dose	Onset	Duration	Precautions
Nitroprusside	0.25–10 μg/kg/min (ideally <2 μg/kg/min)	Immediate	1–10 min	Cyanide toxicity with prolonged infusions; coronary steal; ↑ ICP
Nitroglycerin	10–200 μg/min	Immediate	3–10 min	Severe hypotension in hypovolemic patients; ↑ ICP; contraindicated if on PDE-5 inhibitors
Labetalol	10–40-mg boluses 1–4 mg/min infusion	5–15 min	2–4 h	Bradycardia, heart block; LV dysfunction; asthma
Esmolol	0.5 mg/kg load, 50–200 μg/kg/min	5 min	10–30 min	Bradycardia, heart block; LV dysfunction; asthma
Nicardipine	3–15 mg/min	5–15 min	30–60 min	Rebound tachycardia; ICP effects require more study
Fenoldopam	0.1–1.6 μg/kg/min	5–15 min	20–60 min	Glaucoma
Enalaprilat	0.625–2.5-mg bolus every 6 h	15 min	4–6 h	Renal failure; hyperkalemia
Hydralazine	10–20 mg every 4–6 h	5–20 min	2–6 h	Reflex tachycardia; ischemic heart disease

ICP, intracranial pressure; PDE-5, phosphodiesterase-5; LV, left ventricular.

also potentially toxic, binds avidly to cyanide. Sodium thiosulfate acts as a sulfur donor to promote the formation of thiocyanate and has been used effectively as monotherapy. Hydroxycobalamin combines with cyanide to form cyanocobalamin and may provide synergy with sodium thiosulfate. Accumulation of thiocyanate, although far less toxic than cyanide, may also cause complications.

- Despite these concerns, NTP has an extensive track record, and many prospective studies have not found evidence of clinical toxicity even after using it for several days. Still, NTP should be administered at as low a dose as possible and for as short a duration as possible.
- Nitroglycerin: Because nitroglycerin produces more venous than arterial vasodilatation, it is usually not used as first-line therapy for hypertensive emergencies unless there is concurrent pulmonary edema or myocardial ischemia. Usually started at 5 to 10 μg/minute, it can be titrated up every 5 to 10 minutes to doses as high as 200 to 300 μg/minute.
- Particular caution must be exercised in the setting of hypovolemia.
- Patients using drugs for erectile dysfunction should not be given nitroglycerin or nitroprusside, as this may induce profound hypotension.
- It may increase ICP and should be used with caution in brain-injured patients.
- β-Blockers: Labetalol is the most commonly used IV β-blocker for the management of hypertensive emergencies. One of its unique properties is that it blocks both α and β receptors, although the β-blocking effect is more prominent. Usually administered as 10- to 20-mg boluses, it can be repeated every 15 minutes until the desired effect is achieved. BP lowering begins within 2 to 5 minutes, with maximal effect after about 10 to 15 minutes. It can also be delivered as an infusion, beginning at a dose of 1 to 2 mg/minute.
- Labetalol has been demonstrated to be safe and effective in the management of severe hypertension, with advantages including that it does not cause reflex tachycardia, and has little effect on cerebral blood flow or ICP.
- Labetalol does not cross the placenta well, and there is extensive experience using it in pregnancy, making it one of the preferred agents in preeclampsia and eclampsia.
- **Esmolol** is an extremely short-acting, relatively cardioselective β-blocker, has an onset within less than a minute, and is uniquely metabolized by red blood cell esterases, such that its duration of action is only 10 to 20 minutes. A loading dose of 0.5 mg/kg is administered over 1 minute, followed by an infusion of 50 μg/kg/minute, which can be adjusted as often as every 5 minutes to a maximum dose of 200 μg/kg/minute. It is a useful agent when BP is elevated and cardiac output is preserved, especially when there are concerns about myocardial ischemia.
- Nicardipine is a dihydropyridine calcium channel blocker that inhibits calcium influx through L-type channels, thereby preventing smooth-muscle contraction, particularly in vascular smooth muscle, rather than cardiac myocytes. This causes arterial vasodilatation, with minimal venodilatation or change in cardiac output. It is most often administered as an IV infusion, beginning at 3 to 5 mg/hour, to a maximum of 15 mg/hour, but can also be given as 0.5- to 3-mg boluses. Because of a distribution half-life of <3 minutes and an intermediate elimination half-life of <45 minutes, nicardipine has a relatively rapid onset and offset.

- It has compared favorably with NTP, as therapeutic targets are achieved in a similar amount of time but with fewer episodes of severe hypotension and less frequent dose adjustment.
- Nicardipine has been used in a variety of settings, including malignant hypertension, perioperative hypertension, preeclampsia, and acute heart failure. It is generally well tolerated, with few adverse effects when used with caution.
- Given that nicardipine increases cerebral blood flow, one might expect that it would raise ICP, but this does not appear to be a major concern.
- Fenoldopam is a selective dopamine-1 (DA-1)-receptor agonist, which produces peripheral, renal, splanchnic and, to a lesser degree, coronary vasodilatation. Stimulation of DA-1 receptors also promotes natriuresis. It is typically administered in doses of 0.025 to 1 μg/kg/minute and begins to lower BP after as little as 2 minutes, although the maximal effect is not seen for at least 20 to 30 minutes or more. With discontinuation of an infusion, the elimination half-life is <10 minutes. Reflex tachycardia, thought to be related to activation of the baroreflex, may occur and can be attenuated with concomitant use of a β-blocker.
- Unlike dopamine, fenoldopam does not have any effect on DA-2 receptors, nor does it act at the α- or β-adrenergic receptor level. It does not cross the blood–brain barrier, and therefore has little effect on cerebral blood flow and ICP.
- A theoretical advantage of fenoldopam is improved renal blood flow but, despite a slight increase in creatinine clearance, it remains unclear that this will translate into clinically important prevention of renal failure.
- Fenoldopam has been demonstrated to be effective at controlling BP in hypertensive emergencies, with similar efficacy to NTP, but has shown no clear improvement in outcomes and is considerably more expensive.
- Overall, fenoldopam seems to have few adverse effects. It **does raise intraocular pressure** and should therefore probably be avoided in patients with a known history of glaucoma.

TREATMENT FOR SPECIFIC HYPERTENSIVE EMERGENCIES

Malignant Hypertension

- Because of the shift in the autoregulatory curve that occurs with prolonged hypertension, rapid reductions in BP may cause organ ischemia.
- With hypertensive urgencies, the BP should be reduced carefully and gradually with oral medications over the course of several days. It is not certain how long it takes for the autoregulatory curve to recover and shift back toward the left; the initial goal should never be a normal BP.
- With hypertensive emergencies, the BP must be reduced immediately, with an initial goal of no more than a **15% reduction**. Specific treatment goals should be individualized to ensure that the pressure is reduced sufficiently for organ failure to resolve without compromising perfusion. To facilitate keeping BP within a narrow range, placement of an arterial catheter and careful observation in the ICU are recommended.

Neurologic Hypertensive Emergencies

- Acute ischemic stroke: Although acute hypertension is common, optimal treatment remains uncertain. The greatest priority is to preserve as much of the ischemic penumbra as possible. Because autoregulation is usually impaired within the penumbra, pressure reductions may cause blood flow to fall, which in turn may increase infarct size.
  - Transcranial Doppler middle cerebral artery flow velocities, cerebral perfusion as determined by MRI, and neurologic examination may improve with supranormal augmentation of BP using a vasopressor.
  - The best outcomes occur in patients with a presenting systolic BP of about 150 mm Hg. The American Stroke Association guidelines currently recommend not treating hypertension unless the systolic pressure **exceeds 220 mm Hg or the diastolic pressure exceeds 120 mm Hg.**
  - The exception to this rule is if the patient is a candidate for IV, or possibly intra-arterial, thrombolysis. Of patients who receive IV rt-PA, approximately 5% to 6% will develop ICH; whether lowering BP helps to limit this risk is not certain.
- Intracerebral hemorrhage: Good neurologic recovery is very uncommon if the volume of ICH exceeds 30 to 60 mL. Hematoma growth is a dynamic process that occurs over several hours, with a significant proportion having detectable expansion even within the first few hours after presentation to the emergency department or ICU. Patients with early hematoma enlargement have substantially worse outcomes, and it is likely that therapy that can limit this early growth will improve outcomes.
  - Patients with higher BP at presentation are more likely to develop hematoma expansion and have a higher mortality, though a randomized controlled trial of lowering BP for acute ICH has not yet been performed.
  - The American Heart Association guidelines are conservative and recommend the following goals: mean arterial pressure <130 mm Hg, SBP <180 mm Hg, and DBP <105 mm Hg. The main reason for concern has been the observation that there is reduced blood flow around areas of ICH and the belief that this represents an ischemic penumbra that could be compromised with lower BP.
  - Positron emission tomography and MRI have suggested that decreased flow surrounding ICH is appropriate for the corresponding reduction in cerebral metabolic rate, and CBF autoregulation in this region appears to be preserved.
- SAH: Nontraumatic SAH results from a ruptured intracranial aneurysm in >80% of cases. The risk of recurrent hemorrhage from the aneurysm is about 4% on the first day, followed by 1% to 2% per day for the next 2 to 3 weeks. Although the risk of rebleeding has decreased with early surgical clipping or endovascular coil embolization, the incidence of this devastating complication remains approximately 7%, with a mortality of >50%. Many centers attempt to decrease the risk of recurrent hemorrhage by reducing BP prior to the aneurysm being secured, with a goal SBP <140 to 180 mm Hg.
  - The efficacy of this practice remains uncertain, with conflicting results from observational studies. Particular caution should be exercised when treating patients with high-grade SAH who are stuporous or comatose, because these patients may have a raised ICP, and excessive reduction in BP may compromise cerebral perfusion and promote ischemia.
  - After the aneurysm has been treated, the most concerning complication is cerebral vasospasm and delayed ischemic neurologic deficits, which occur in 20% to 30% of patients, with maximum risk between days 4 and 12 after the event. Hypertension should not routinely be treated during this time, even at relatively high levels, as this increases the risk of delayed infarction. If clinical vasospasm develops, first-line therapy actually involves hemodynamic augmentation, using vasopressors to raise BP to increase CBF and improve cerebral perfusion.
- Perioperative neurosurgery: Hypertension occurs in the setting of craniotomy more often than any other type of surgery. Neurosurgery results in the release of large amounts of vasoactive substances that raise BP, including catecholamines, endothelin, and renin. Important is that severe hypertension occurring intraoperatively or during the first 12 postoperative hours has been associated with a higher risk of ICH.
  - In certain procedures, tight postoperative BP control is particularly important. With carotid stenting or endarterectomy, the sudden resolution of carotid stenosis results in a sudden, asymptomatic, 20% to 40% increase in ipsilateral CBF.
  - In some patients, the increase can be much more profound, to the degree that it overcomes the autoregulatory capacity of the corresponding, previously hypoperfused territory. The resulting cerebral hyperperfusion syndrome is characterized by the presence of vasogenic edema, which resembles RPLS in that there is a posterior predilection.
  - Patients who are most vulnerable are those with relatively severe carotid stenosis and poor collateral circulation, but postoperative hypertension is also an important risk factor. Cerebral hyperperfusion syndrome is treated with tight BP control, but agents that cause cerebral vasodilatation, including nitroprusside and perhaps calcium channel blockers, ideally should be avoided.
  - Mild intraoperative hypotension is sometimes used for vascular neurosurgical procedures, such as microsurgical excision or endovascular obliteration of arteriovenous malformations to reduce the risk of hemorrhage. With arteriovenous malformations, the sudden "repressurization" of previously hypotensive arterioles may contribute to the development of regional hyperemia, edema, and bleeding, a condition sometimes referred to as "normal perfusion pressure breakthrough." Consequently, hypertension should be avoided in the immediate postoperative period. Conversely, the sacrifice of vascular branches during the procedure, or vasospasm from surgical manipulation and retraction, may also create areas of relative underperfusion, such that hypotension would also be deleterious.

Cardiovascular Hypertensive Emergencies

- Aortic dissection: The purpose of emergently lowering BP in aortic dissection is to decrease shear stress in the aorta and limit propagation of the intimal tear and false lumen. To concomitantly reduce both BP and the force of left ventricular contraction, first-line therapy consists of a β-blocker or, if contraindicated, a calcium channel blocker with

negative inotropic and chronotropic properties (e.g., diltiazem or verapamil).
- If the BP remains elevated despite adequate β-blockade, a vasodilator can be added. Pure vasodilators should not be used in isolation.
- If possible, the heart rate should be <60 beats/minute, and the BP reduced as much as can be tolerated, ideally below a SBP 120 mm Hg.
- Use of opiates for the substantial chest discomfort may greatly reduce antihypertensive requirements.
- Acute pulmonary edema: Acute hypertension exists in the majority of patients presenting with flash pulmonary edema and is likely to be both a consequence and contributing cause. The venodilating properties of **nitroglycerin** make it an excellent initial choice as an antihypertensive in both normotensive and hypertensive patients, especially if there is failure to improve after administration of a loop diuretic.
  - In titrating the dose of IV nitroglycerin, clinicians should be aware that relatively large doses, often in excess of 100 μg/minute, may be required to significantly lower cardiac filling pressures and improve symptoms.
  - Patients who benefit from aggressive **afterload reduction,** such as those with acute aortic or mitral regurgitation (if not hypotensive), may require a more potent arterial vasodilator than nitroglycerin, such as NTP or nicardipine.
  - Although ACE inhibitors are standard care for chronic heart failure, there is little evidence of benefit for acute decompensated heart failure. The only IV preparation, enalaprilat, was potentially harmful when routinely administered to patients within the first 24 hours following STEMI and is therefore not recommended.
  - Considerable caution must be exercised when intubating hypertensive patients with acute pulmonary edema, as it is very common for BP to drop precipitously with sedation and positive pressure ventilation.
  - **Nesiritide** (recombinant human brain natriuretic peptide) has been proposed for use in acute heart failure. However, it has not demonstrated improved clinically important outcomes when compared with standard therapy, may worsen renal function, and has been linked to a possible increased risk of short-term death.
- Acute coronary syndrome (ACS): Although definitive therapy for ACS involves revascularization, tachycardia and hypertension increase myocardial oxygen requirements and can potentially worsen ischemia and increase infarct size. β-Blockers are recommended for all ACS patients without a contraindication.
  - An IV β-blocker is therefore a good initial choice as an antihypertensive but must be used with caution with reduced

left ventricular systolic function and in those in whom there is concern about impaired cardiac conduction (e.g. inferior myocardial infarction).
- Early β-blockade in patients with STEMI has an increased risk of cardiogenic shock. If the BP remains significantly elevated, especially with ongoing chest pain or pulmonary edema, nitroglycerin should be used. In addition to reducing preload and afterload, nitrates also vasodilate coronary arteries, especially at the site of plaque disruption. If three sublingual tablets (0.4 mg over 5 minutes) are ineffective, an IV infusion should be started and adjusted to alleviate chest pain and reduce BP (10% reduction in normotensive patients, 30% reduction in hypertensive patients).

Preeclampsia and Eclampsia

- Although hypertensive encephalopathy and eclampsia have largely been considered separate entities, they have a similar pathophysiology and essentially the same MRI findings (RPLS). Definitive treatment for severe preeclampsia and eclampsia is delivery, but careful IV BP control is frequently also necessary.
- Treatment of hypertension in severe preeclampsia has not been shown to improve perinatal outcomes and may actually contribute to a decrease in neonatal birth weight. Pharmacologic therapy is not recommended unless the degree of BP elevation is severe (defined as SBP exceeding 160 mm Hg or DBP exceeding 105 to 110 mm Hg) or there are end-organ complications.
- Oral medications, with a goal pressure of 140 to 155/90 to 105 mm Hg, may be sufficient in the absence of organ dysfunction, but more rapid and tighter control is necessary for severe preeclampsia and eclampsia.
- Although there has been extensive experience with IV hydralazine (5–10 mg every 15–20 minutes to a maximum dose of 30 mg), this agent has a relatively slow onset, has not commonly been used as an infusion, may overshoot BP goals, and has recently been linked to worse outcomes, including more placental abruption, adverse effects on fetal heart rate, lower Apgar scores, and a greater need for cesarean section.
- Other IV agents that have been successfully and safely used include labetalol and nicardipine.
- In addition to the foregoing, magnesium sulfate should be given to prevent the development of seizures in patients with severe preeclampsia, and should be used to treat acute seizures when eclampsia occurs.

CHAPTER 91 ■ NONINVASIVE VENTILATORY SUPPORT MODES

- Noninvasive ventilation (NIV) refers to the provision of ventilatory assistance using techniques that do not bypass the upper airway. The theoretical advantages of NIV include avoiding the complications associated with endotracheal intubation, improving patient comfort, and preserving airway defense mechanisms. NIV may be delivered through various devices including negative and positive-pressure ventilators.
- The following sections deal with the history and epidemiology of NIV and currently available equipment and techniques, practical applications, appropriate indications, and possible adverse effects. In this chapter, continuous positive airway pressure delivered noninvasively is referred to as *CPAP*, and NIV using intermittent positive-pressure ventilation with or without positive end-expiratory pressure (PEEP) is referred to as noninvasive positive-pressure ventilation (NPPV). The term *NIV* is considered to include either CPAP or NPPV.

EQUIPMENT AND TECHNIQUES

- The following paragraphs discuss various interfaces and ventilatory modes available for administration of NIV. Cough-enhancing techniques are also described.

Interfaces

- Interfaces are devices that connect ventilator tubing to the face, allowing the delivery of pressurized gas into the airway during NIV. Currently available interfaces include nasal and oronasal masks, helmets, and mouthpieces. Selection of a comfortable interface that fits properly is a key issue for the success of NIV.

Nasal Masks

- The standard nasal mask is a triangular or cone-shaped clear plastic device that fits over the nose and uses a soft cushion or flange to seal over the skin. Because of the pressure exerted over the bridge of the nose, the mask may cause skin irritation and redness and occasionally ulceration For occasional patients who cannot tolerate commercially available masks, custom-molded, individualized masks that conform to facial contours of the patient can be constructed. Several types of strap systems have been used to hold the mask in place.

Nasal Pillows

- Nasal pillows or seals consist of soft rubber or silicone plugs that are inserted directly into the nostrils As they exert no pressure over the bridge of the nose, nasal pillows may be useful in patients who develop irritation or ulceration on the nasal bridge while using nasal or oronasal masks.

Oronasal Masks

- Oronasal or face masks cover both the nose and the mouth The oronasal mask is largely used in patients with copious air leaking through the mouth during nasal mask ventilation. Interference with speech, eating, and expectoration and the likelihood of claustrophobic reactions are greater with oronasal than with nasal masks. In the acute setting, however, oronasal masks are preferable to nasal masks because dyspneic patients are mouth breathers, predisposing to greater air leakage during nasal mask ventilation.
- A type of oronasal mask is the "total" face mask, which is made of clear plastic and uses a soft silicone flange that seals around the perimeter of the face like a hockey goalie's mask, avoiding direct pressure on facial structures.

Helmet

- The helmet is made of transparent latex-free polyvinyl chloride and is secured by two armpit braces at two hooks (one anterior and the other posterior) of the plastic ring that joins the helmet with a seal connection soft collar adherent to the neck. The pressure increase during ventilation makes the soft collar sealing comfortable to the neck and shoulders, avoiding air leakage.
- The entire apparatus is connected to an intensive care unit (ICU) ventilator by a standard respiratory circuit. The two ports of the helmet act as inlet and outlet for inspiratory and expiratory gas flows. The inspiratory and expiratory valves are those of the mechanical ventilator. The main advantages of the helmet include a good tolerability in both adult and pediatric populations, with a satisfactory interaction of the patients with the environment; a lower risk of dermal lesions; and, compared with the mask, easier applicability to any patient regardless of the face contour.

Mouthpieces

- Mouthpieces are simple and inexpensive devices used to provide NPPV for as long as 24 hours a day to patients with chronic respiratory failure If nasal air leaking reduces efficacy; ventilator tidal volume may be increased; or cotton plugs or nose clips may be used for occluding the nostrils. NPPV via mouthpieces has proved to be a valid alternative to tracheostomy in some patients with chronic respiratory muscle insufficiency.

Noninvasive Ventilatory Modes

Continuous Positive Airway Pressure

- CPAP delivers a constant pressure throughout spontaneous inspiration and exhalation *without* assisting inspiration.

Because spontaneous breathing is not assisted, this technique requires an intact respiratory drive and adequate alveolar ventilation. CPAP increases functional residual capacity and opens underventilated alveoli, thus decreasing right-to-left intrapulmonary shunt and improving oxygenation and lung mechanics. Moreover, CPAP may reduce the work of breathing and dyspnea in COPD patients by counterbalancing the inspiratory threshold load imposed by intrinsic PEEP.

- Effects on hemodynamics during CPAP have been widely described. By lowering left ventricular transmural pressure in patients with left congestive heart failure, CPAP may reduce left ventricular afterload without compromising cardiac index. CPAP can be applied by various devices including low-flow generators with an inspiratory reservoir, high-flow jet venturi circuits (both of them with an expiratory mechanical or water valve), and bilevel and critical care ventilators.
- Continuous positive pressure may be administered using the demand flow (DF) or the gold standard continuous flow (CF) system. With DF CPAP, the patient has to trigger a preset pressure to open the demand valve, whereas with CF CPAP, no valves are present. The work of breathing is significantly greater with the DF system than with the CF one. It is crucial to provide an adequate air flow rate for maintaining a continuous positive pressure, especially in dyspneic patients who breathe at high flow rates.

Pressure Support Ventilation

- Pressure support ventilation (PSV) is a pressure-triggered, pressure-targeted, flow-cycled mode of ventilation. It delivers a preset inspiratory pressure to assist spontaneous breathing, augmenting spontaneous breaths and offsetting the work imposed by the breathing apparatus. A sensitive patient-initiated trigger causes the delivery of inspiratory pressure support that is maintained throughout inspiration, and a reduction in inspiratory flow drives the ventilator to cycle into expiration. Therefore, the patient can control either inspiratory duration or breathing rate. Typical starting pressures are a PEEP of 3 to 5 cm H_2O and an inspiratory airway pressure of 8 to 12 cm H_2O

Bilevel Positive Airway Ventilation

- In bilevel positive airway pressure, a valve sets two pressure levels, the expiratory positive airway pressure (EPAP) level and the inspiratory positive airway pressure (IPAP) level, even in the presence of rapidly changing flows. With this technique, ventilation is produced by the cyclic delta pressure between IPAP and EPAP. EPAP also recruits underventilated lung and offsets eventual intrinsic PEEP.

Controlled Mechanical Ventilation

- In the mandatory controlled mechanical ventilation mode, no patient effort is required, as full ventilatory support is provided. In this mode, ventilator settings include inflation pressure or tidal volume, frequency, and the timing of each breath. Controlled mechanical ventilation can be delivered noninvasively as a volume control or pressure control mode.

Proportional Assist Ventilation

- Proportional assist ventilation is an alternative technique in which both flow and volume are independently adjusted. In

this technique, the ventilator generates volume and pressure in proportion to the patient's effort, increasing comfort and so improving success and compliance with NPPV. Despite the promising concept, there is a substantial lack of large clinical studies.

Ventilatory Mode Selection

- All ventilatory modes of NPPV have been used to achieve physiologic or clinical benefit, with theoretical advantages and limitations. Spontaneously breathing patients with respiratory failure of various causes may benefit from CPAP to correct hypoxemia. In acute cardiogenic pulmonary edema (CPE), mask CPAP can result in early physiologic improvement and reduce the need for intubation
- Pressure-targeted modes maintain delivered tidal volume in patients with air leaking better than volume-targeted modes. Therefore, pressure-targeted ventilators are preferred over volume-targeted ventilators to deliver NPPV in the presence of substantial leaks. To best compensate for air leaks, pressure-targeted ventilators should have high and sustained maximal inspiratory flow capabilities (>3 L/sec); adjustable I:E ratios and other mechanisms to limit inspiratory duration so that inversion of the I:E ratio is avoided; and adjustable trigger sensitivities or algorithms to prevent autocycling. Ventilatory systems for air leak detection, calculation, and compensation are now largely available.
- When PSV is used as a noninvasive ventilatory assistance mode, some forms of patient–ventilator asynchrony might be intensified, causing breathing discomfort. In acute hypercapnic exacerbations of chronic obstructive pulmonary disease (COPD), NPPV performed by different ventilatory modes including PSV, assist control ventilation (ACV), and proportional assist ventilation is able to provide respiratory muscle rest and improve respiratory physiologic parameters. As in the intubated mechanically ventilated COPD patients, application of external PEEP is effective in counterbalancing the effects of auto-PEEP and dynamic hyperinflation. The use of noninvasive ventilatory modes in patients with hypoxemic acute respiratory failure (ARF) of various causes can improve arterial blood gases, respiratory rate, and dyspnea, and unload the accessory muscles of respiration.
- Triggering systems are critical to the success of NPPV in both assist and control modes. During assisted ventilation, flow triggering reduces breathing effort more effectively as compared with pressure triggering, obtaining a better patient–ventilator interaction.

PRACTICAL APPLICATION OF NONINVASIVE VENTILATION

- NIV should be considered early when patients first develop signs of incipient respiratory failure needing ventilatory assistance. It is crucial that caregivers can identify patients who are likely to benefit from NIV and exclude those for whom NIV would be unsafe. Once the decision to institute NIV has been taken, an interface and ventilatory mode must be chosen, and a close monitoring in an appropriate hospital location must be provided. The initial approach should consist in fitting the interface and familiarizing the patient with the apparatus,

TABLE 91.1

CRITERIA FOR NONINVASIVE VENTILATION
DISCONTINUATION AND ENDOTRACHEAL
INTUBATION

Technique intolerance (pain, discomfort, or claustrophobia)
Inability to improve gas exchanges and/or dyspnea
Hemodynamic instability or evidence of shock, cardiac
  ischemia, or ventricular dysrhythmia
Inability to improve mental status within 30 min after the
  application of NIV in hypercapnic, lethargic COPD patients
  or agitated hypoxemic patients

NIV, noninvasive ventilation; COPD, chronic obstructive pulmonary
disease.

TABLE 91.2

CONTRAINDICATIONS TO NONINVASIVE
VENTILATION

Unconsciousness or mental obtundation (chronic obstructive
  pulmonary disease [COPD] patient may be an exception)
Inability to protect the airway
Inability to clear respiratory secretions
Severe upper gastrointestinal bleeding
Life-threatening hypoxemia
Unstable hemodynamic conditions (blood pressure or rhythm
  instability)
Recent gastroesophageal surgery
Fixed obstruction of the upper airway
Vomiting
Recent facial surgery, trauma, burns, or deformity
Undrained pneumothorax

explaining the purpose of each piece of equipment. Patients should be motivated and reassured by the clinician, instructed to coordinate their breathing with the ventilator, and encouraged to communicate any discomfort or fears. Collaboration among medical practitioners including physicians, respiratory therapists, and nurses is critical to the success of NIV during the early phase of milder respiratory failure and after an initial period to 20 minutes' interruption. For patients with more severe failure, NIV application has to be continuous for at least 12 to 24 hours, and discontinuation is allowed for short periods only when the clinical situation improves. Aggressive physiotherapy is crucial during the periods of NIV discontinuation. Endotracheal intubation must be rapidly accessible, when indicated (Table 91.1).

Patient Selection

- The criteria for selecting appropriate patients to receive NIV for ARF include clinical indicators of acute respiratory distress, such as moderate-to-severe dyspnea, tachypnea, accessory muscle use and paradoxical abdominal breathing, and gas exchange deterioration. Blood gas parameters aid in identifying patients with acute or acute superimposed on chronic CO_2 retention. A conscious and cooperative patient is crucial for initiating NIV (Table 91.2), although hypercapnic patients with narcosis who are otherwise good candidates for NIV may represent an exception.
- NIV should be avoided in patients with hemodynamic instability and in those who are unable to protect the airways (coma, impaired swallowing, and so on) (see Table 91.2). Patients with severe hypoxemia (PaO_2/FiO_2 <100) or morbid obesity (>200% of ideal body weight) should be closely managed only by experienced personnel and with a low threshold for intubation. In the presence of a pneumothorax, NIV can be initiated provided an intercostal drain is inserted. Criteria for NIV discontinuation and endotracheal intubation must be thoroughly considered to avoid dangerous delays (see Table 91.1).
- Identification of predictors of success or failure may help in recognizing patients who are appropriate candidates for NIV and those in whom NIV is not likely to be effective, thereby avoiding its application and unnecessary delays before invasive ventilation is given. The severity of acidosis at baseline

is a logical starting point for identifying patients who might benefit from NPPV. Patients affected by acute respiratory distress syndrome with a Simplified Acute Physiology Score II >34, and whose PaO_2/FiO_2 does not improve over 175 after 1 hour of NPPV should be carefully treated under strict monitoring within the ICU where endotracheal intubation and invasive ventilation are promptly available. It is still unclear whether the higher mortality observed in patients who failed NPPV and are eventually intubated might be due to a delayed intubation.

Machine Settings

- Pressures commonly used to administer CPAP in patients with ARF range from 5 to 12 cm H_2O. For pressure-cycled ventilation, it is suggested to start at low pressures to facilitate patient tolerance (appropriate initial pressures are a CPAP of 3 to 5 cm H_2O and an inspiratory pressure of 8 to 12 cm H_2O) and, if necessary, gradually increase pressure settings as tolerated to obtain alleviation of dyspnea, decreased respiratory rate, adequate exhaled tidal volume, and good patient–ventilator interaction (Table 91.3). In the presence of air leaks, adequate inspiratory flows and durations should be set, triggering sensitivity should be adjusted to prevent autocycling, and a mechanism to limit inspiratory time and avoid I:E ratio inversion should be considered when available. A backup rate should be applied in patients with inadequate triggering.

Monitoring

- In the acute setting, patients can initiate NIV anywhere; at the onset of the acute respiratory distress, but after initiation, they should be transferred to an ICU or a step-down unit for continuous monitoring until they are sufficiently stable to be moved to a medical ward. During transfers, NIV and monitoring should not be discontinued. The early use of NIV for less acutely ill patients with COPD on a medical ward seems to be effective, but if pH is <7.30, admission to an

TABLE 91.3

PROPOSED VENTILATOR SETTINGS FOR PRESSURE SUPPORT VENTILATION MODE

	Initial setting	Treatment setting
PEEP	3–5 cm H_2O	Slowly increased to up to 8–12 cm H_2O in hypoxemic patients
PSV	8–12 cm H_2O	Increased as tolerated to 20 cm H_2O to obtain an exhaled tidal volume of about 7 mL/kg and respiratory rate <25 breaths/min
FiO_2	Titrated to achieve an arterial saturation >90% or 85%–90% in patients at risk of worsening hypercapnia	Titrated to achieve an arterial saturation >90% or 85%–90% in patients at risk of worsening hypercapnia

PEEP, positive end-expiratory pressure; PSV, pressure support ventilation.

environment with intensive care monitoring is highly recommended (Table 91.4).
- If a poor response to NIV occurs and the specific measures used to correct the situation fail to address an adequate improvement within a few hours, NIV should be considered a failure, and invasive ventilation should be promptly considered.

CLINICAL APPLICATION OF NONINVASIVE VENTILATION

- The following sections review the available evidence on the efficacy of NIV for various applications in the acute care setting.

Acute Exacerbations of Chronic Obstructive Pulmonary Disease

- In patients with ARF resulting from acute exacerbations of COPD, the use of NPPV has been proven to be effec-

TABLE 91.4

MONITORING OF PATIENTS RECEIVING NONINVASIVE VENTILATION IN THE ACUTE CARE SETTING

Bedside observation
- Conscious level
- Comfort
- Chest wall motion
- Accessory muscle recruitment
- Patient–ventilator synchrony

Vital signs
- Respiratory rate
- Exhaled tidal volume (and flow, volume, and pressure waveform for poor synchrony problems)
- Heart rate
- Blood pressure
- Continuous electrocardiography

Gas exchange
- Continuous oximetry
- Arterial blood gas at baseline, after 1–2 h, and as clinically indicated

tive in ameliorating dyspnea, improving vital signs and gas exchange, preventing endotracheal intubation, and improving hospital survival. Consequently, there is a general agreement concerning the early use of NPPV in such patients.
- During NPPV, the combination of external PEEP and PSV offsets the auto-PEEP level and reduces the work of breathing that the inspiratory muscles must generate to produce the tidal volume.
- In general, NPPV should be considered the first-line therapeutic option to prevent endotracheal intubation and improve outcome in patients with exacerbations of COPD who have no contraindication to NPPV (see Table 91.2).

Asthma

- NPPV is considered an option in asthmatic patients at risk for endotracheal intubation. However, to date, guidelines for NPPV in severe asthma are not supported by strong data.

Hypoxemic Respiratory Failure

- Trials of NPPV in patients with hypoxemic respiratory failure, defined as those with ARF not related to COPD, have yielded conflicting results.
- NPPV can be initially used to treat hypoxemic patients without hypercapnia as long as there are no clear contraindications. However, an extremely prudent approach is needed, limiting the application of NPPV to hemodynamically stable patients who can be closely monitored in the ICU where endotracheal intubation is promptly available. A decisional flow chart may be adopted in applying NPPV to patients with acute respiratory distress syndrome (Fig. 91.1).

Cardiogenic Pulmonary Edema

- Applying positive air pressure has been shown to decrease the work of breathing and left ventricular afterload while maintaining cardiac index, thereby benefiting patients with cardiac dysfunction and ARF.
- In the comparison of NIV modalities, bilevel positive airway pressure has the potential advantage over CPAP of assisting the respiratory muscles during inspiration, which would result in faster alleviation of dyspnea and exhaustion.

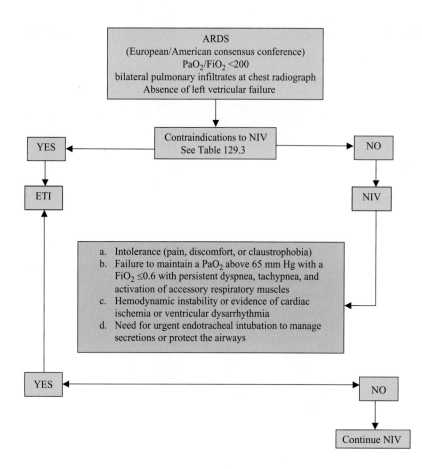

FIGURE 91.1. Decisional flow chart for the application of noninvasive ventilation to acute respiratory distress syndrome (ARDS). ETI, endotracheal intubation; NIV, noninvasive ventilation.

Pneumonia

- The application of NIV to treat pneumonia has yielded no definitive conclusions. NPPV's best application here is in COPD patients with community-acquired pneumonia, but caution should be applied in pneumonia patients without COPD, as the benefit of NPPV in such patients is currently unclear.

Immunocompromised Patients

- Immunocompromised patients in whom respiratory failure develops often require mechanical ventilatory assistance. Endotracheal intubation is associated with numerous complications and, in immunosuppressed patients, invasive mechanical ventilation is associated with a significant risk of death. A decreased mortality by the application of NPPV in selected cases of immunosuppressed patients has been reported in several studies.

Facilitation of Weaning and Extubation

- NPPV has been used to permit early extubation in patients who fail to meet standard extubation criteria, thus reducing the complications related to endotracheal tube.
- Besides weaning facilitation, another potential application of NIV in the weaning process is to avert the need for reintubation in patients with extubation failure, thereby avoiding

the risk of increased morbidity and mortality associated with failed extubation.

Do-Not-Intubate Orders

- Applying NPPV has been described in patients with ARF who are poor candidates for endotracheal intubation or who are reluctant to undergo invasive ventilation. NPPV offered an effective, comfortable, and dignified method for these patients in providing symptomatic relief of dyspnea and maintaining continuous verbal communication with loved ones, allowing a more aggressive pain and discomfort control therapeutic plan.

Postoperative Patients

- Thoracic and upper-abdominal surgery are associated with a prolonged postoperative gas exchange deterioration and reduction in functional residual capacity, PaO_2, and forced vital capacity. Applying mask CPAP or NPPV can improve oxygenation and pulmonary function. Furthermore, accumulating evidence supports the use of NIV to improve gas exchange and avoid reintubation.

Obstructive Sleep Apnea

- CPAP is recognized to be effective in correcting the respiratory and arousal abnormalities and improving sleep quality in obstructive sleep apnea syndrome. CPAP is believed to act by pneumatically "splinting" the pharyngeal airway, thus preventing its collapse during sleep. Also, nasal NPPV has been used in patients with ARF after obstructive sleep apnea syndrome, with improvements in clinical status and arterial blood gas values.

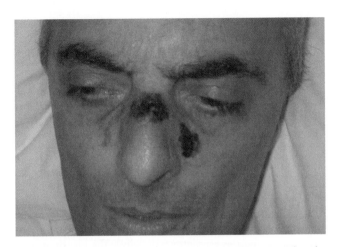

FIGURE 91.2. Skin lesions caused by a mask. Please note that the point at major risk to develop skin necrosis is the bridge of the nose. (Photograph printed with the permission of the patient.)

Trauma

- ARF in trauma patients is generally associated with reduced pulmonary compliance and functional residual capacity and with subsequent restrictive defects. NIV in association with aggressive use of regional and neuraxial anesthetic block can be used in patients with respiratory insufficiency secondary to chest trauma, but caution should be used to avoid unnecessary delay of intubation in patients with flail chest. Despite the favorable results obtained, large randomized studies are needed before definitive recommendations on the use of NIV in posttraumatic ARF can be made.

Restrictive Diseases

- NPPV has a role in the treatment of respiratory failure caused by some types of restrictive thoracic diseases. Aggressive respiratory physiotherapy is also crucial in all patients with thoracic restriction.

Bronchoscopy

- In nonintubated patients, severe hypoxemia is an accepted contraindication to fiberoptic bronchoscopy. Specific seal connectors have been applied with success to maintain adequate O_2 saturation while performing a fiberoptic bronchoscopy, with or without alveolar lavage.

ADVERSE EFFECTS AND COMPLICATIONS OF NONINVASIVE VENTILATION

- Major adverse effects of NIV seldom occur in appropriately selected patients and are minimized when the technique is applied by experienced caregivers. The most frequently encountered complications are related to the interface, ventilator airflow or pressure, or patient–ventilator interaction (Fig. 91.2).

CHAPTER 92 ■ INVASIVE VENTILATORY SUPPORT MODES

PHYSICS OF VENTILATION: THE EQUATION OF MOTION

- During spontaneous breathing, air flows into the lungs as the result of the pressure generated by the respiratory muscles. Exhalation normally occurs passively due to the elastic recoil pressure of the respiratory system.
- The pressure generated by the respiratory muscles during inspiration is opposed by the elastic forces of the lungs and chest wall, and by the resistance to gas flow that occurs in the airways:

$$P_{MUS} = P_E + P_R,$$

where P_{MUS} is the pressure generated by the respiratory muscles, P_E is the pressure required to overcome the elastic properties of the respiratory system, and P_R is the pressure required to overcome the resistive properties of the respiratory system.

- During positive pressure ventilation, the driving pressure for air to flow is applied by the ventilator and, depending on the mode, the respiratory muscles. Hence:

$$P_{APPL} = P_{MUS} + P_{VENT} = P_E + P_R,$$

where P_{APPL} is the pressure applied across the respiratory system to inflate the lungs, and is the combination of contributions from the respiratory muscles (P_{MUS}) and the ventilator (P_{VENT}).
- P_E is the result of elastance (E) and tidal volume (V_T):

$$P_E = elastance \times V_T.$$

Because elastance is the reciprocal of compliance (C), a more familiar version is

$$P_E = V_T/C.$$

P_R is determined by the resistance of the airways:

$$P_R = \dot{V} \times R,$$

where $\dot{V}$ is gas flow and R is resistance.

- These physiologic relationships are described by the equation of motion of the respiratory system for both spontaneous breathing and mechanical ventilation:

$$P_{APPL} = P_{MUS} + P_{VENT} = V_T/C + \dot{V} \times R$$

- This states that a pressure applied to the respiratory system—whether it is from the respiratory muscles, the ventilator, or both—generates gas flow through the airways and volume change in the lungs that is opposed by the airway's resistance and respiratory system elastance. From the equation of motion, we can derive three important principles to guide the delivery of positive pressure ventilation:
  - The result of any ventilator setting depends not only on what is set on the ventilator but on the physiologic characteristics of the patient—compliance and resistance—and any active inspiratory effort of the respiratory muscles. Hence, for the appropriate application of mechanical ventilation, we must understand the ventilator operation and the patient's respiratory mechanics and the interaction between the ventilator and any active breathing efforts of the patient.
  - For any independent variable set on the ventilator (e.g., P_{VENT}), physiologic variables (compliance and resistance) in the patient, and respiratory muscle pressure generated by the patient (P_{MUS}), there is only one possible result for the dependent variables (e.g., flow and tidal volume). The ventilator typically controls the independent variables of flow (volume-controlled ventilation [VCV]) or pressure (pressure-controlled [PCV] or pressure support ventilation [PSV]). The ventilator cannot regulate both pressure and volume (i.e., flow) during mechanical ventilation.
  - If we know the volume and flow during VCV, we can calculate resistance and compliance from the pressures required. Similarly, if we know the resistance and compliance during PCV, we can calculate the flow and tidal volume. This is relatively straightforward if the patient is being passively ven-

tilated ($P_{MUS} = 0$) but becomes more difficult if the patient is actively breathing. Hence, it is difficult to predict respiratory mechanics in the actively breathing patient receiving PCV or PSV.

NOMENCLATURE: DESCRIPTION OF A VENTILATOR BREATH

The Trigger

- The trigger starts inspiration. Breaths are triggered either by the patient or by the ventilator. If the ventilator initiates the breath, the trigger is time (i.e., the operator sets a respiratory rate), and the ventilator will deliver the breath at time intervals to achieve that rate. If the breath is initiated by the patient, inspiration starts when the ventilator detects a pressure or flow change at the airway (pressure trigger and flow trigger).
- With a pressure trigger (Fig. 92.1), a decrease of pressure at the airway relative to positive end-expiratory pressure (PEEP; adjustable sensitivity, but generally set at 0.5–2 cm H_2O) results in closure of the expiratory valve, opening of the inspiratory valve, and delivery of gas to the airway. With a flow trigger (see Fig. 92.1), a flow increase at the airway (adjustable sensitivity but generally set at 1–3 L/min) results in initiation of the inspiratory phase. In modern ventilators, both flow triggers and pressure triggers are very sensitive. If the trigger sensitivity is set correctly, either flow triggering or pressure triggering is acceptable

The Limit

- The limit determines the size of a breath. When volume is the preset variable (VCV), flow and volume delivery by the ventilator are limited, but the pressure applied to the airway can vary. When pressure is the preset limit variable (PCV or PSV), the pressure applied at the airway is limited, but the flow and tidal volume are variable.

Pressure Trigger

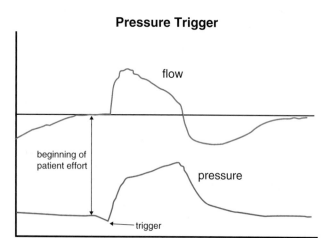

Flow Trigger

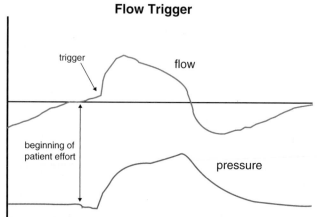

FIGURE 92.1. Pressure triggering and flow triggering. With pressure triggering, the ventilator responds to a decrease in airway pressure. With flow triggering, the ventilator responds to a change in flow.

The Cycle

• The cycle is what ends the breath. This can be volume, time, flow, or pressure. In modern ventilators, time is the cycle criteria with VCV or PCV. Note that for VCV, the ventilator actually controls the flow during inspiration, and inspiration is time-cycled. With PSV, the cycle is usually flow; inspiration ends when the flow rate reaches a fraction of the peak flow (adjustable on some ventilators) or a fixed flow. During VCV or PCV, pressure cycle is an alarm condition that avoids application of unsafe high pressure to the airway.

VENTILATOR MODES

• Modern ventilators are equipped to provide various modes. For all modes, the ventilator delivers one of two types of breath: mandatory or spontaneous (Fig. 92.2). A mandatory breath is triggered by the ventilator or the patient and cycled by the ventilator. A set volume (VCV) or pressure (PCV) is delivered regardless of the contribution from the patient and regardless of whether the breath is triggered by the patient or the ventilator. A spontaneous breath is triggered and cycled by the patient.

• A ventilator mode describes the pattern of breath delivery from the ventilator. With continuous mandatory ventilation (CMV), also called assist/control ventilation, every breath is a mandatory breath type. With continuous spontaneous ventilation, every breath is a spontaneous breath type. With synchronized intermittent mandatory ventilation (SIMV), the ventilator delivers a mix of mandatory and spontaneous breaths. With CMV or SIMV, a minimum backup rate is set on the ventilator, but the patient can trigger at a more rapid rate. With continuous spontaneous ventilation, there is no backup

rate other than the alarm parameter set on the ventilator. The taxonomy of ventilator modes is shown in Figure 92.2.

Continuous Mandatory Ventilation

• The main feature of CMV (or assist/control ventilation) is that it supplies full support of the patient's respiratory muscles, provided that the level of support is set appropriately.

Volume-controlled Ventilation

• With VCV, the ventilator controls the flow and the inspiratory time to deliver the resultant tidal volume. In some cases (e.g., Draeger ventilators), tidal volume, flow, and inspiratory time are each set. In this case, an inspiratory breath hold occurs if the inspiratory time setting is greater than that required to deliver the tidal volume at the flow selected. For example, for a tidal volume of 0.5 L, flow 60 L/minute, and inspiratory time 1 second, a 0.5-second inspiratory breath hold will result.

• On other ventilators (e.g., Puritan-Bennett 840), an inspiratory hold (pause) is set separately, which prolongs the inspiratory time. For VCV, tidal volume, flow, and inspiratory time are the independent variables. The dependent variable is the inflating pressure applied to the lungs, which is affected by the ventilator settings, the patient's lung mechanics, and the inspiratory effort of the patient, as explained by the *equation of motion* (see earlier). Hence, during VCV, the pressure applied by the ventilator will increase with a higher tidal volume, higher flow, lower compliance, and higher resistance.

• Also, the pressure applied by the ventilator will decrease if the patient generates a vigorous inspiratory effort (i.e., a higher P_{MUS}). This explains the deformation of the airway pressure waveform during VCV in patients who are generating vigorous inspiratory efforts and are dyssynchronous with the

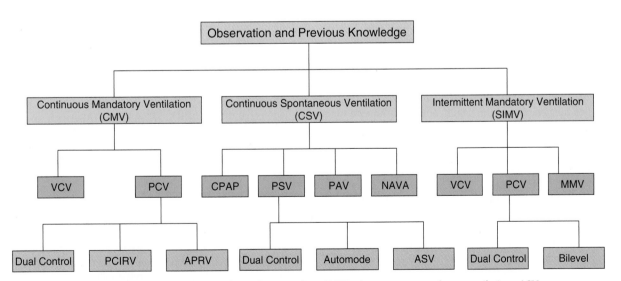

FIGURE 92.2. The taxonomy of ventilator modes. APRV, airway pressure release ventilation; ASV, adaptive support ventilation; CPAP, continuous positive airway pressure; MMV, mandatory minute ventilation; NAVA, neurally adjusted ventilatory assist; PAV, proportional assist ventilation; PCIRV, pressure-controlled inverse ratio ventilation; PCV, pressure-controlled ventilation; PSV, pressure support ventilation; VCV, volume-controlled ventilation.

ventilator. Inspiratory flow should be set to meet the demand of patients in respiratory failure.

- The main advantage of VCV is the ability to control the tidal volume. This may be important when the $PaCO_2$ must be closely controlled, such as in patients with head trauma or when a low tidal volume is used in patients with acute lung injury/acute respiratory distress syndrome as part of a lung-protective ventilation strategy. Limitations of VCV are related to the fixed tidal volume and flow pattern. This can result in patient–ventilator dyssynchrony in actively breathing patients if efforts are not made to set the inspiratory flow appropriately or to provide adequate sedation. With VCV, a high peak inspiratory pressure may occur with changes in lung mechanics. However, this increases the risk of lung injury only if the high peak inspiratory pressure is associated with an increase in plateau pressure. Accordingly, it is important to monitor plateau pressure on a regular basis when VCV is used.

Pressure-controlled Ventilation

- With PCV, airway pressure and inspiratory time are set on the ventilator. In some cases (e.g., Draeger ventilators), the inspiratory pressure setting is the peak pressure but, more commonly, the pressure control setting is the pressure applied above PEEP. For PCV, pressure and inspiratory time are the independent variables. The dependent variables are flow and volume, which are affected by the ventilator settings, the patient's lung mechanics, and the inspiratory effort of the patient as described by the *equation of motion* (see earlier). Hence, during PCV, the flow and tidal volume will increase with a higher pressure control setting, higher compliance, and lower airways resistance.
- Also, the flow and tidal volume will increase if the patient generates a vigorous inspiratory effort (i.e., an increase in P_{MUS}). In other words, during PCV, the distending pressure (P_{VENT} + P_{MUS}) and tidal volume increase if the patient makes an active inspiratory effort. Compared to VCV, this may improve patient–ventilator synchrony but with an increased risk of overdistension lung injury. An understanding of the equation of motion as it applies to PCV prevents errors when assessing lung mechanics or risk of overdistension when PCV is used.
- A potential advantage of PCV is that it limits the pressure applied to the alveoli and the risk of ventilator-induced lung injury. However, it is important to note that this benefit occurs only if the patient is making no inspiratory effort, because any inspiratory efforts of the patient will increase the transpulmonary distending pressure during PCV. The variable inspiratory flow pattern may improve patient–ventilator synchrony during active breathing efforts, although this has not been tested in the setting of a low lung volume, lung-protective ventilation strategy.
- The pressure waveform with PCV produces a higher mean airway (and alveolar) pressure than the pressure waveform associated with constant flow volume ventilation.

Dual-controlled Ventilation

- Dual-controlled modes allow the ventilator to control pressure or volume based on a feedback loop. At any given time, the ventilator controls either pressure or volume but cannot

do both at the same time. Pressure-regulated volume control (PRVC) provides PCV and in addition ensures a minimum tidal volume. PRVC (Servo, Viasys), AutoFlow (Draeger), and VC+ (Puritan-Bennett) are trade names that function in a similar manner. The proposed advantage of dual control is the ability of the ventilator to meet patient demand (an advantage of PCV) while maintaining a minute ventilation constant (an advantage of VCV). However, the tidal volume and transpulmonary distending pressure during PRVC can potentially exceed safe limits, as illustrated by the example in Figure 92.3.

- Moreover, if patient effort increases, the level of support decreases, which could result in dyssynchrony and discomfort. Additionally, as the pressure level is reduced, mean airway pressure will fall, potentially resulting in a fall in PaO_2. Because this mode depends on the measured tidal volume, any errors in tidal volume measurement will result in decision errors.

Pressure-controlled Inverse Ratio Ventilation

- With pressure-controlled Inverse ratio ventilation PCIRV, the inspiratory time is set longer than the expiratory time (Fig. 92.4). The result is a higher mean airway pressure and enhanced lung recruitment but also a higher potential for air trapping and hemodynamic compromise. The likelihood of an improvement in oxygenation using PCIRV is small, and the risk of auto-PEEP and hemodynamic compromise is great. Moreover, the prolonged inspiratory time may not be well tolerated and may require high levels of sedation and, in some cases, paralysis.

Airway Pressure Release Ventilation

- Current-generation ventilators use an active exhalation valve whereby the ventilator controls the inspiratory pressure by allowing the exhalation valve to open if pressure increases and by adding additional flow if the pressure decreases below the pressure control setting. Such a design can also allow spontaneous breathing during the inspiratory phase of the ventilator, which is what happens in airway pressure release ventilation (APRV). The ventilator allows spontaneous breathing at two levels of pressure (Fig. 92.5). Because the low pressure is applied for a short period, generally all of the spontaneous breathing occurs at the high level. In the absence of spontaneous breathing, APRV is exactly the same as PCIRV.
- The potential advantage of APRV is to provide lung recruitment at lower airway pressures than with traditional positive pressure ventilation by taking advantage of the spontaneous breathing efforts.

Continuous Positive Airway Pressure

- For the intubated patient, CPAP is usually applied with a ventilator (Fig. 92.6). Modern ventilators provide efficient CPAP by virtue of having very-low-resistance exhalation valves and minimal time delay for triggering and cycling. CPAP is used to treat hypoxemia by maintaining alveolar recruitment to treat acute cardiogenic pulmonary edema by raising intrathoracic pressure and to counterbalance auto-PEEP in patients with obstructive lung disease.

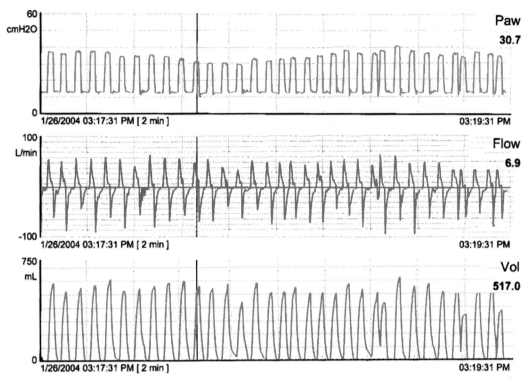

FIGURE 92.3. Airway pressure (P_{aw}), flow, and volume waveforms demonstrating the response of a dual-control algorithm over a 2-minute period with varying patient effort. The tidal volume varies above and below the target (500 mL) by as much as 150 mL. (From Branson RD, Johannigman JA. The role of ventilator graphics when setting dual-control modes. *Respir Care.* 2005;50:187, with permission.)

- Despite an apparent contradiction in terms, CPAP can be set to 0 cm H_2O (although in reality the ventilator often applies a small level of inspiratory pressure support) and is commonly used as a spontaneous breathing trial to test extubation readiness.

Pressure Support Ventilation

- With PSV, the ventilator applies a set inspiratory pressure to support each patient-initiated breath (Fig. 92.7). Tidal volume is determined by the level of inspiratory pressure support,

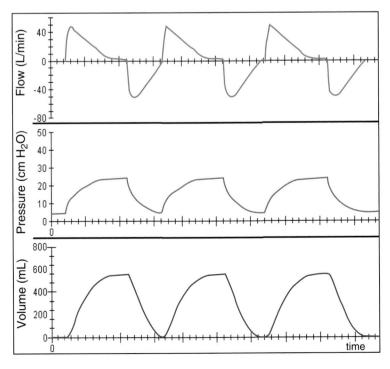

FIGURE 92.4. Flow, pressure, and volume waveforms during pressure-controlled inverse ratio ventilation.

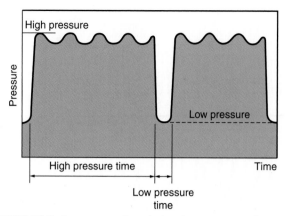

FIGURE 92.5. Pressure waveform during airway pressure release ventilation (APRV).

respiratory mechanics, and the patient's inspiratory effort. The initial part of the breath is delivered in a manner similar to PCV. During inspiration, the flow is delivered at a variable rate. In addition, rise time can be adjusted in a manner similar to that during PCV. When the set pressure is reached, the flow decreases at a rate determined by lung mechanics and the patient's inspiratory effort.

- With PSV, inspiration continues until the inspiratory flow falls to a ventilator preset value—commonly 25% of the peak flow or a fixed flow such as 5 L/minute. In newer-generation ventilators, the flow cycle criteria can be adjusted (expiratory sensitivity, Fig. 92.8).

Dual Control

- Dual-controlled ventilation can also be applied during a PSV breath. Volume-assured pressure support combines the high

initial flow of PSV with the constant flow delivery of a volume-controlled breath (Fig. 92.9). After inspiration is triggered, the ventilator reaches the set airway pressure as occurs with PSV. The ventilator's microprocessor determines the volume that has been delivered and compares this to the set tidal volume. If the set tidal volume is not reached, the ventilator prolongs the inspiratory phase until the set tidal volume is delivered. Volume-assured pressure support is designed to reduce the work of breathing (pressure support) while maintaining a minimum tidal volume (volume control).

- A concern with this mode is that the ventilator takes away support if the patient's respiratory demand increases and tidal volume exceeds the set tidal volume. This results in increased work of breathing for the patient.

AutoMode

- AutoMode is a dual-controlled mode available on the Servo 300 and Servo 300A ventilators. It provides automated weaning from PCV to PSV and automated escalation of support if patient effort diminishes. The ventilator provides PRVC if the patient is making no breathing efforts.

Adaptive Support Ventilation

- Adaptive support ventilation is based on the minimal work-of-breathing concept, which suggests that a patient will breathe at a tidal volume and respiratory frequency that minimize the elastic and resistive loads while maintaining oxygenation and acid-base balance.

- If a patient breathes spontaneously, the ventilator will support breaths. Spontaneous and mandatory breaths can be combined to meet the minute ventilation target. The pressure limit of both the mandatory and spontaneous breaths is

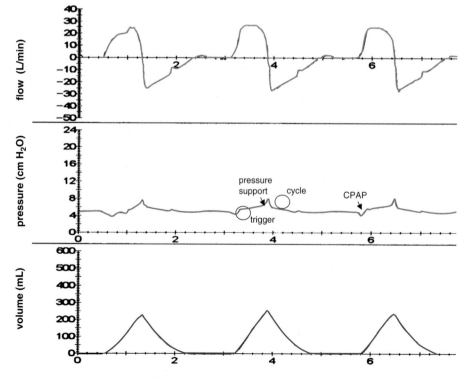

FIGURE 92.6. Flow, pressure, and volume waveforms during continuous positive airway pressure (CPAP). Note that the airway pressure fluctuates above and below the set CPAP level of 5 cm H_2O. There is a pressure decrease below CPAP to trigger the breath, a low level of pressure support is applied during inhalation, and there is a small increase in pressure to cycle the end of inhalation.

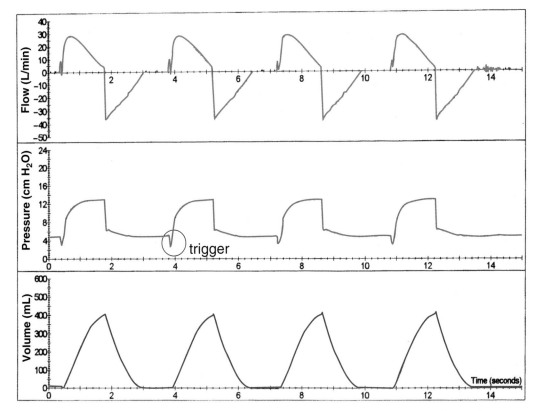

FIGURE 92.7. Flow, pressure, and volume waveforms during pressure support ventilation. (From Gibbons FK, Hess DR. Mechanical ventilation. In: Bigatello LM, ed. *Critical Care Handbook of the Massachusetts General Hospital.* 4th ed. Philadelphia, PA: Lippincott Williams & Wilkins; 2006, with permission.)

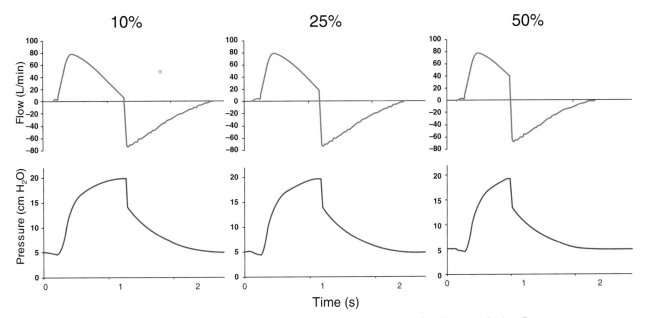

FIGURE 92.8. Examples of flow termination criteria of 10%, 25%, and 50% using a Puritan-Bennett 840 ventilator with pressure support of 15 cm H_2O and PEEP 5 cm H_2O. (From Gibbons FK, Hess DR. Mechanical ventilation. In: Bigatello LM, ed. *Critical Care Handbook of the Massachusetts General Hospital.* 4th ed. Philadelphia, PA: Lippincott Williams & Wilkins; 2006, with permission.)

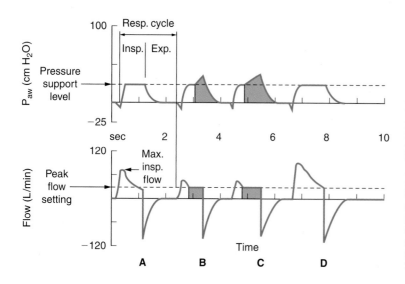

FIGURE 92.9. The possible breath types during volume-assured pressure support ventilation. In breath **A**, the set tidal volume (V_T) and delivered V_T are equal. This is a pressure support breath (patient triggered, pressure limited, and flow cycled). Breath **B** represents a reduction in patient effort. As flow decreases, the ventilator determines that delivered V_T will be less than the minimum set volume. At the *shaded* portion of the waveform, the breath changes from a pressure-limited to a volume-limited (constant flow) breath. Breath **C** demonstrates a worsening of compliance and the possibility of extending inspiratory time to ensure the minimum V_T delivery. Breath **D** represents a pressure support breath in which the V_T is greater than the set V_T. (From Branson RD, Johannigman JA. The role of ventilator graphics when setting dual-control modes. *Respir Care.* 2005;50:187, with permission.)

adjusted continuously. This means that adaptive support ventilation is continuously using dual-control breath-to-breath of mandatory and spontaneous breaths.

Tube Compensation

- Tube compensation (TC) is designed to overcome the flow-resistive work of breathing imposed by the endotracheal or tracheostomy tube. TC uses the known resistive coefficients of the artificial airway (tracheostomy or endotracheal tube) and measurement of instantaneous flow to apply a pressure proportional to resistance throughout the total respiratory cycle. With TC, the ventilator targets the tracheal pressure rather than proximal airway pressure, increasing the proximal airway pressure necessary to overcome the flow-resistive properties of the artificial airway (Fig. 92.10).

Proportional Assist Ventilation

- With proportional assist ventilation (PAV), the ventilator delivers gas as a positive feedback controller, where respiratory elastance and resistance are the feedback signal gains, defined as K_1 (cm H_2O/L) and K_2 (cm $H_2O/L/s$), respectively.
- A potential advantage of PAV is that it should provide optimal patient–ventilator synchrony. By following and amplifying the patient's inspiratory flow and volume on a breath-by-breath basis, the ventilator provides support in proportion to patient demand. This differs from PSV, in which the level of support is constant regardless of demand, and VCV, in which the level of support decreases when demand increases. It is important to note that, like other continuous spontaneous breathing modes, PAV requires the presence of an intact ventilatory drive. A concern with PAV is its dependence on measures of resistance and compliance, often under- or overestimated.

Neurally Adjusted Ventilatory Assist

- Control of the ventilator through direct measurement of the output of the respiratory center is presently not possible. However, it is possible to transform neural drive into ven-

tilatory output (neuroventilatory coupling) by measuring the electrical activation of the diaphragm. This neurally adjusted ventilatory assist will vary on a moment-by-moment basis according to diaphragmatic electrical activity and the gain factor selected on the ventilator. This allows a patient's respiratory center to be in direct control of the mechanical support provided throughout the course of each breath, provided there is a functioning phrenic nerve and neuromuscular junction and also that the diaphragm is the primary inspiratory muscle. Although neurally adjusted ventilatory assist is clinically attractive, it is not yet commercially available.

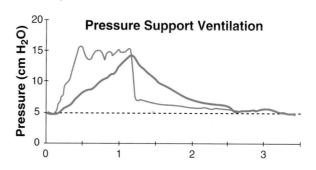

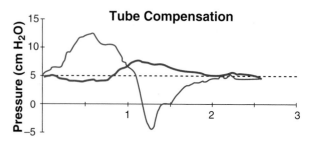

FIGURE 92.10. Tube compensation. Pressure waveforms from the trachea (*heavy lines*) and the proximal airway (*light lines*) during pressure support ventilation and automatic tube compensation. Note that the tracheal pressure fluctuates very little during automatic tube compensation. (From Fabry B, Haberthur C, Zappe D, et al. Breathing pattern and additional work of breathing in spontaneously breathing patients with different ventilatory demands during inspiratory pressure support and automatic tube compensation. *Intensive Care Med.* 1997;23:545, with permission.)

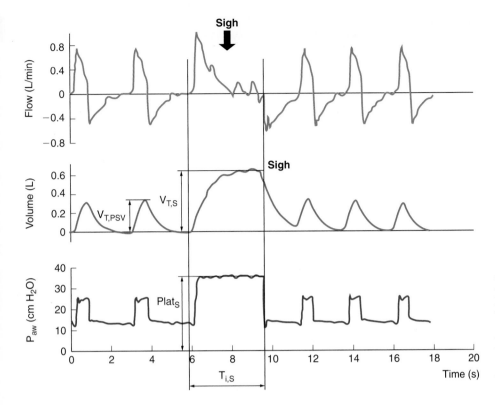

FIGURE 92.11. Using a sigh breath in conjunction with pressure support ventilation. The patient is ventilated with a Draeger Evita 4 (PCV+ mode). P_{aw}, airway pressure. (From Patronati N, Foti G, Cortinovis B, et al. Sigh improves gas exchange and lung volume in patients with acute respiratory distress syndrome undergoing pressure support ventilation. *Anesthesiology.* 2002;96:788, with permission.)

Synchronized Intermittent Mandatory Ventilation

- With synchronized intermittent mandatory ventilation (SIMV), the ventilator provides a mandatory breath rate. If the patient breathes at a more rapid rate, the additional breaths are unsupported. If the patient does not breathe at a rate more rapid than that set on the ventilator, SIMV and CMV are synonymous.

Mandatory Minute Ventilation

- Mandatory minute ventilation is intended to guarantee the minute ventilation that the patient receives. If the patient's spontaneous ventilation does not match the target minute ventilation set by the clinician, the ventilator supplies the difference between the patient's minute ventilation and the set minute ventilation.

Bilevel and PCV+

- This mode is available on the Puritan-Bennett 840 (Bilevel) and the Draeger Evita 4 (PCV+). It is essentially a modification of SIMV that uses PCV for the mandatory breaths and PSV for the spontaneous breaths. This mode can be thought of as PSV with a sigh. The mandatory breath rate is set at 1 to 4 breaths/minute, with the pressure during the sigh set at 25 to 30 cm H_2O and a sigh duration of 2 to 4 seconds (Fig. 92.11). This mode may be more comfortable than the sighs traditionally incorporated into ventilators because it is a pressure-controlled breath using an active exhalation valve.

CHAPTER 93 ■ HIGH-FREQUENCY VENTILATION

- High-frequency ventilation (HFV) has been recognized as a modality that can provide optimal lung protection from iatrogenic complication in patient with acute lung injury (ALI) and acute respiratory distress syndrome (ARDS).

SUBTYPES OF HIGH-FREQUENCY VENTILATION

- HFV is a collection of ventilatory modes grouped together by their common property of employing high respiratory rates, all >60 breaths/minute. In addition to high-frequency oscillation (HFO), other modes in this group include high-frequency jet ventilation (HFJV) and high-frequency percussive ventilation (HFPV).

High-frequency Jet Ventilation

- HFJV is a mode of ventilation in which gas is delivered through a small-bore catheter into the lungs at rates of 100 to 150 breaths/minute. Delivered tidal volume is still small but higher than just the volume exiting the jet, as the jets entrain an additional flow of gas by the *Venturi effect*. Exhalation is passive during HFJV, and gas trapping or dynamic hyperinflation can be an issue. In practice, a conventional ventilator is set up as a "slave" to the jet to provide positive end-expiratory pressure along with basic monitoring and alarms.
- HFJV is a very efficient mode for removing CO_2. Additionally, because of HFJV's very high flow rates and the differing pulmonary time constants in the clinical setting of bronchopleural fistulae, this mode of ventilation is purported to have beneficial effects in the presence of this disorder; however, these benefits have not been verified during objective testing. Concerns with HFJV relate to the delivery of high pressures (10–50 pounds per square inch), unpredictable tidal volumes, and the development of dynamic hyperinflation, all of which may worsen ventilator-induced lung injury (VILI) rather than minimize it. In addition, problems with adequate humidification of inspired gas and the subsequent risks of tracheobronchitis have been noted and documented.

High-frequency Percussive Ventilation

- HFPV is the newest and least well studied of the HFV modes. It combines a high-frequency rate of 200 to 900 breaths/minute superimposed on a conventional pressure mode of ventilation. HFPV is reported to enhance the clearance of respiratory secretions and has been successfully used in this regard in patients with burns and inhalational injury.

High-frequency Oscillation

- High-frequency oscillation (HFO is a mode of mechanical ventilation that delivers very small tidal volumes around a set mean airway pressure at high respiratory rates of 3 to 15 Hz (equivalent to 180–900 breaths/minute, as 1 Hz = 60 breaths/minute). HFO has been widely and effectively used in neonates and children for close to 20 years but only recently has become available in the adult intensive care unit; previous versions of this ventilator were capable of generating only sufficient flow so as to provide adequate CO_2 elimination in patients <35 kg. In contrast to other HFV modes, humidification is less of an issue during HFO, as a continuous bias flow of humidified gas is passed in front of an oscillating membrane (Fig. 93.1). This oscillating membrane pushes the humidified gas into the patient and also provides active expiration, a factor that likely accounts for the lack of important gas trapping that is observed when HFO is employed at adequate airway pressures. The elegance of HFO is that it allows for "decoupling" of oxygenation and ventilation. Alveolar ventilation, and thus carbon dioxide elimination, are dependent on the frequency and tidal volume but are relatively independent of lung volume. In contrast, oxygenation is proportional to mean airway pressure and lung volume.

RATIONALE FOR THE USE OF HIGH-FREQUENCY VENTILATION IN ACUTE LUNG INJURY TO LIMIT VENTILATOR-INDUCED LUNG INJURY WITH CONVENTIONAL VENTILATION

- VILI is histologically indistinguishable from ARDS; three decades of experimental research have shown it to occur through a number of mechanisms, including (a) overdistention injury (*volutrauma*), (b) collapse–reopening injury (*atelectrauma*), and (c) oxygen toxicity. Each of these can lead, in turn, to further injury—termed *biotrauma*—the release of inflammatory mediators that may worsen pulmonary injury and propagate systemically to harm distant organs.
- Numerous studies, performed using both small and large animals, consistently show that ventilatory high end-inspiratory stretch can cause a clinical and histologic picture similar to ARDS even in the absence of any other noxious stimulus. Patients with ARDS are at increased risk of regional lung overdistention because of the patchy nature of ARDS; the small areas of relatively normal lung (the so-called "baby lung") receive the bulk of the tidal volume and are at particular risk of volutrauma. Repeated opening and closing of alveolar units can also cause VILI. In the injured lung, alveolar

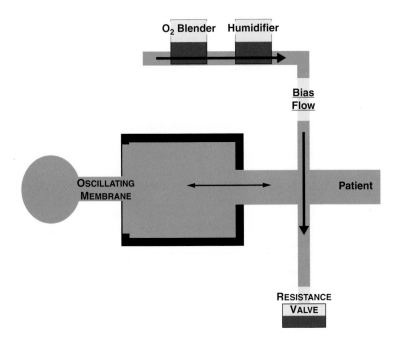

FIGURE 93.1. Schematic overview of the high-frequency oscillation (HFO) circuit. (Reused with permission from Ferguson ND, Stewart TE. New therapies for adults with acute lung injury: high-frequency oscillatory ventilation. *Crit Care Clin.* 2002;18:91–106.)

damage and absolute, or qualitative, deficiencies in alveolar surfactant lead to alveolar instability and localized lung unit collapse. Through each respiratory cycle, these unstable alveoli undergo collapse and reopening, a process that generates injurious mechanical forces and causes further lung injury. There is a substantive body of animal evidence showing that efforts to limit lung unit closing on expiration by maintaining an adequate positive end-expiratory pressure (PEEP) are relatively protective against atelectrauma. Here, the paradigm is one of "opening the lung and keeping it open," thereby avoiding cyclic collapse and recruitment/derecruitment.

- The goals of mechanical ventilation in a patient at risk of VILI, therefore, should be to ventilate and oxygenate the patient while staying within a "safe window," avoiding both overdistention and derecruitment—collapse—as illustrated in the volume–pressure curve of the lung shown in Figure 93.2.

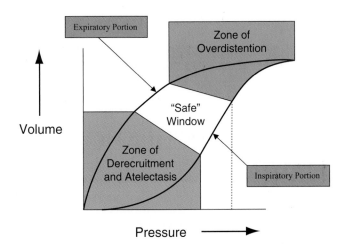

FIGURE 93.2. Volume–pressure curve of the injured lung. (Reused with permission from Froese AB. High-frequency oscillatory ventilation for adult respiratory distress syndrome: let's get it right this time. *Crit Care Med.* 1997;25[6]:906–908.)

- A large, methodologically rigorous, and adequately powered trial conducted by the National Institutes of Health ARDS Network did show important differences in mortality. A low-stretch strategy with a targeted tidal volume of 6 mL/kg predicted body weight (PBW) and a plateau pressure limit of 30 cm H_2O was compared to a higher-stretch strategy using a targeted tidal volume of 12 mL/kg PBW and a plateau pressure limit of up to 50 cm H_2O. The low-stretch strategy was associated with a mortality reduction from 40% in the control group to 31% in the experimental group (relative risk [RR] 0.78; 95% confidence interval [CI] 0.65–0.93). This trial clearly indicates that avoiding volutrauma saves lives in patients with acute lung injury. The trial has subsequently generated significant discussion regarding its mechanisms of benefit and its choice of control strategy but, nevertheless, 6 mL/kg PBW has emerged as a standard for tidal volume limitation against which other strategies are compared.

- Another early randomized controlled trial published in the late 1990s demonstrated dramatic reductions in mortality using a lung-protective strategy whose goal was to limit both volutrauma and atelectrauma using low tidal volumes and higher PEEP compared with traditional ventilation. Though no single trial has definitively shown an incremental mortality benefit with higher PEEP and attempts to limit atelectrauma while already avoiding overdistention injury, when viewed together, these trials suggest that this benefit may well exist. These studies clearly demonstrated that ventilatory strategy is important in patients with ARDS and that lung-protective strategies can minimize VILI and decrease mortality in humans with ARDS. As such, and given the proposed mechanisms of lung protection (see Fig. 93.2), a strategy that minimizes overdistention and allows the use of high PEEP should be the ideal mode in patients with ARDS. This is where HFO may have great clinical benefit.

- The very small delivered tidal volumes are the key to the lung-protective potential of HFO. Because cyclic alveolar stretch is minimal, clinicians are able to set the mean airway pressure

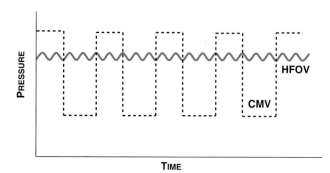

FIGURE 93.3. Pressure–time curve contrasts tidal variations in airway pressure associated with conventional ventilation (*dashed line*) and high-frequency oscillation (*solid line*). HFOV, high-frequency oscillation ventilation; CMV, conventional mechanical ventilation. (Reused with permission from Ferguson ND, Stewart TE. New therapies for adults with acute lung injury: high-frequency oscillatory ventilation. *Crit Care Clin.* 2002;18:91–106.)

(mP_{AW}) on HFO significantly higher than they are able to set PEEP on conventional ventilation, thereby avoiding cyclic collapse and atelectrauma—and yet they are still able to avoid very high peak inspiratory pressures and subsequent volutrauma (Fig. 93.3).

IMPLEMENTING AND OPTIMIZING HIGH-FREQUENCY OSCILLATION IN ADULTS

- Several key messages for HFO can be gleaned from animal studies on the use of HFO in ALI and ARDS models.
  - At adequate mP_{AW}, gas trapping is not an issue despite very high respiratory rates.
  - Increasing mP_{AW} leads to improved oxygenation through lung recruitment.
  - Tidal pressure swings measured in the trachea can be increased with either underrecruitment or overdistention of the lung.

- Recruitment maneuvers (sustained inflations) may be required to adequately recruit severely injured lungs.
- Taken together, and in keeping with the current understanding of VILI mechanisms, these studies suggest that HFO in adults should be employed using an open-lung strategy, facilitated by higher mean airway pressures and lung recruitment maneuvers.
- Most of the clinical information available on HFO is based on its use as rescue therapy for patients with extremely severe disease who were "failing" conventional ventilation. Despite being limited by their uncontrolled nature and by selection bias, consistent messages that arise from these rescue series include the following:
  - HFO is usually effective in improving oxygenation.
  - HFO appears safe, with no obvious increased rates of complications.
  - Both baseline oxygenation index and duration of CMV prior to HFO are associated with increased mortality.
- Despite the very strong physiologic rationale and the encouraging clinical data to date, there are potential detrimental consequences of HFO.
  - First, the physiologic benefit of HFO is likely derived from recruitment of the lung with higher mean airway pressures, though still not overdistending alveoli because of the very small tidal volumes. Hence, patients with mild disease and minimal collapsed or consolidated lung may not be good candidates for HFO.
  - Second, the high mean airway pressures may negatively impact hemodynamics.
  - Third, because the bias flow rate is insufficient to meet the inspiratory flow demands of adults in respiratory distress, all adults on HFO must have their respiratory efforts suppressed with intravenous sedation.
- This means that the majority of adults will be heavily sedated, and many may need transient neuromuscular blockade. Due to these concerns and to target a population in need of recruitment, we believe that future studies should enroll patients with severe ARDS who are likely to have significant lung collapse and who frequently require significant amounts of sedation, with or without paralysis, on conventional ventilators.

CHAPTER 94 ■ EXTRACORPOREAL CIRCULATION FOR RESPIRATORY OR CARDIAC FAILURE

- Extracorporeal life support (ECLS) is the use of an artificial heart (pump) and lung (membrane oxygenator) to replace organ function for days or weeks, to allow time for diagnosis, treatment, and organ recovery or replacement. The indications for ECLS are acute, severe heart or lung failure not improving on conventional management. This review is limited to the adult population.

EXTRACORPOREAL LIFE SUPPORT TECHNIQUE AND PHYSIOLOGY

- ECLS is simply the use of a modified heart/lung machine to provide gas exchange (and systemic perfusion if necessary) to prolong the life of a patient when native heart and lung functions are not adequate to sustain life. The heart–lung machine used for cardiac surgery is modified, both in devices and technology, to be used for days or weeks in the intensive care unit, but the purpose is the same: to keep the body alive during heart or lung failure. The technique is invasive and complex.

- A large catheter (No. 23–30 French) is inserted into the inferior vena cava or right atrium; venous blood is drained, passed through an artificial lung, and pumped back into the patient, either into the aorta (venoarterial [VA] bypass) or into the right atrium (venovenous [VV] bypass). VA bypass puts the artificial lung in parallel with the native lungs and substitutes for both heart and lung function. In VV bypass, the artificial lung is in series with the native lungs, and the patient is reliant on his or her own hemodynamics for pulmonary and systemic perfusion. ECLS allows decreasing the ventilator to nondamaging "rest" settings (typically FiO_2 0.3, pressure 20/10, rate 4), decreasing vasoactive drugs, and optimizing other aspects of treatment.

- Because the surfaces of the extracorporeal devices are plastic, it is necessary to anticoagulate the blood with a continuous infusion of heparin, titrated to a low but constant level of anticoagulation. This level of anticoagulation is measured by whole blood-activated clotting time (ACT). The normal is 120 seconds, and during ECLS, ACT is maintained at approximately 180 seconds. Although this level of heparinization prevents thrombosis in the extracorporeal circuit, circulating platelets still adhere to the plastic surfaces, become activated (which attracts more platelets), grow into platelet aggregates, and eventually break off and recirculate as effete platelets, which are removed by the reticuloendothelial system in the liver and spleen.

- Because heparinization and thrombocytopenia are necessary components of ECLS, the major risk of the procedure is bleeding. As currently practiced, significant bleeding is rarely a serious problem, but this requires the continuous bedside attendance of a specialist whose primary job is to measure the ACT and platelet count at very frequent intervals and titrate heparin dose and platelet infusions accordingly. Properly managed, ECLS can be used for weeks without hemolysis, device failure, clotting, or bleeding, but it is invasive and expensive. The technology not only must be learned and practiced by the intensive care unit team but must be endorsed by the entire hospital. Management of the patient during ECLS includes management of perfusion and gas exchange as earlier but also attention to fluid balance, oxygen consumption and delivery, nutrition, position, and the monitoring and sustaining of function of other organs.

- In *respiratory failure*, VV access is preferred. Gas exchange across the native lungs is usually minimal during the first several days of ECLS; therefore, the patient is totally dependent on the extracorporeal system. As native lung function returns, systemic blood oxygenation and CO_2 clearance improve, improved gas exchange can be measured at the airway, and the extracorporeal blood flow rate is gradually decreased, allowing the native lungs to assume a larger percentage of gas exchange. When the native lungs have improved, the patient is tried off ECLS at nondamaging ventilator settings. When this trial is successful, the cannulas are removed, and recovery continues. Patients who are successfully weaned off ECLS have a 90% likelihood of complete recovery.

- In *cardiac failure*, VA access is required (usually via the femoral vessels). Inotropes and pressors are weaned off,

and systemic perfusion is maintained by extracorporeal flow. Lung function usually returns to normal in a day or two, and the patient can be awakened and extubated. When the patient is stable and the function of other organs can be determined (especially the brain), a decision can be made regarding bridge to recovery or bridge to ventricular assist device (VAD) and transplantation. When ECLS is used for cardiac support, the pulmonary and left ventricular blood flow is decreased in proportion to the extracorporeal flow. This can lead to two problems. First, if the heart stops altogether, the left atrium and the left ventricle will gradually distend with bronchial venous blood, leading to high left atrial pressure and pulmonary edema. This condition is diagnosed by the lack of pulsatility in the systemic arterial system. If left ventricular function is inadequate to maintain emptying of the left heart, the left side of the heart must be drained into the venous line, either by direct catheterization of the left atrium or by creation of an atrial septal defect. The second problem with VA bypass in the totally failing heart is thrombosis in the left atrium or left ventricle. This will occur even in the presence of systemic heparinization. Thrombosis is diagnosed by echocardiography. If a patient has left atrial or left ventricle thrombus, it is important to avoid spontaneous left ventricular function. Usually such patients are candidates for VAD or cardiac replacement, and the clot is removed before embolism could occur.

CLINICAL RESULTS

- The most recent data from the Extracorporeal Life Support Organization registry are shown in Table 94.1. Participation in the Extracorporeal Life Support Organization is voluntary, but almost all cases treated with ECLS in established centers are included in the registry. There are currently more than 30,000 patients who have been managed with ECLS. Although there are extensive data on gas exchange, perfusion, coagulation, and so on, the only important statistic is hospital discharge survival because the technique is a life-support technique, and it is applied only to patients who are not expected to survive otherwise, with a high (80%–100%) risk of dying with continuing conventional treatment. The mortality risk is measured differently in different age groups.

Extracorporeal Life Support for Acute Respiratory Distress Syndrome

- The University of Michigan has reported the largest experience with ECLS for ARDS. In that series, the overall survival rate was 52% and rose to 65% in 2002. The series is large enough to characterize the patient population and identify the likelihood of recovery based on age and days on mechanical ventilation.

- As technology for adult respiratory failure has evolved, ECLS is now practiced using primarily venovenous access, with high blood flow adequate to sustain oxygenation and CO_2 removal, lung rest, diuresis, and prone positioning. This approach leads to 50% to 60% survival. Though the majority of adult patient were treated with ECLS for severe ARDS, this technology can be utilized for severe status asthmaticus, refractory to all conventional therapy.

TABLE 94.1

TABLE 94.1

OVERALL PATIENT OUTCOMES WITH EXTRACORPOREAL LIFE SUPPORT FOR
CARDIAC AND RESPIRATORY FAILURE

	Total	Surv	ECLS	Surv to	DC
Neonatal					
Respiratory	20,993	17,889	85%	16,005	76%
Cardiac	2,898	1,684	58%	1,095	38%
ECPR	274	176	64%	109	40%
Pediatric					
Respiratory	3,390	2,173	64%	1,895	56%
Cardiac	3,658	2,199	60%	1,624	44%
ECPR	523	263	50%	200	38%
Adult					
Respiratory	1,255	740	59%	646	51%
Cardiac	671	300	45%	216	32%
ECPR	189	80	42%	59	31%
	33,851	25,504	75%	21,849	65%

Surv, survival; ECLS, extracorporeal life support; DC, discharge; ECPR, extracorporeal cardiopulmonary
resuscitation.
Extracorporeal Life Support Organization registry data, December 2006. The data for 2006 are incomplete.

Extracorporeal Life Support for Cardiac Failure

- The experience with ECLS for cardiac failure in adults is shown in Table 94.1. The most common indication for ECLS for cardiac support in adults is acute myocardial failure after myocardial infarction or heart failure after cardiac operation. Most of the patients treated with ECLS have failed balloon pumping and full inotropic support. If a balloon pump is in place through one of the femoral arteries, it is best left in place because of the risk of bleeding once the pump has been removed. The opposite femoral artery is used for arterial access.
- Adult patients in acute cardiac failure are candidates for left ventricular assist device placement as a bridge to recovery or a bridge to transplantation. However, in the acute failure situation, it is best to institute ECLS first, to stabilize the circulation and gas exchange and to determine whether other organs are

functioning, specifically the brain. If severe brain injury has occurred during the period of acute cardiac failure, ECLS is discontinued, avoiding the futile thoracotomy and the need for a left ventricular assist device placement. The survival for ECLS in adult cardiac failure is 40% to 50%.

Extracorporeal Life Support for Cardiac Arrest

- ECLS can be used in association with resuscitation to support cardiac and pulmonary function in cardiac arrest or profound shock. In this application, the ECLS circuit must be primed and available within minutes. Therefore, the ECLS for cardiopulmonary resuscitation cases are done primarily in established ECLS centers, which have both the equipment and the team to institute ECLS on a moment's notice. Survival with satisfactory neurological recovery has been described up to 40%.

CHAPTER 95 ■ WEANING FROM MECHANICAL VENTILATION

- A framework of seven stages of weaning has recently been proposed (Fig. 95.1).
- From a pathophysiologic standpoint, factor that affect weaning can be related to gas exchange or to the ventilatory pump. In a third group of patients, psychological factors may contribute to weaning failure.

IMPAIRED GAS EXCHANGE

- Conditions characterized by failure of the lungs as a gas exchange unit include those associated with ventilation–perfusion mismatching and (less often) conditions associated with increased shun.

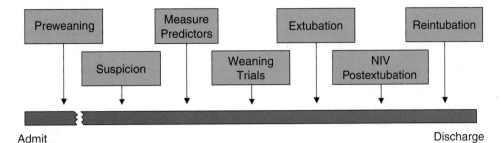

FIGURE 95.1. Seven stages of weaning. Stage 1 is preweaning, a stage that some patients never get beyond. Stage 2 is the period of diagnostic triggering, the time when a physician begins to think that the patient might be ready to come off the ventilator. Stage 3 is the time of measuring and interpreting weaning predictors. Stage 4 is the time of decreasing ventilator support (abruptly or gradually). Stage 5 is either extubation (of a weaning success patient) or reinstitution of mechanical ventilation (in a weaning failure patient). Stage 6 is use of noninvasive ventilation (NIV) after extubation. Stage 7 is reintubation. Failure to appreciate stage 2 probably leads to the greatest delays in weaning. (From Tobin MJ, Jubran A. Weaning from mechanical ventilation. In: Tobin MJ, ed. *Principles and Practice of Mechanical Ventilation*. New York, NY: McGraw-Hill; 2006:1185, with permission.)

- The ratio of dead space to tidal volume—an approximation of impaired gas exchange due to lung units with abnormally high ventilation–perfusion ratios—is normally about 0.30 at rest and less during exercise. In patients requiring prolonged mechanical ventilation, the ratio can increase to 0.74 or more.

- Patients can compensate for such an increase in dead space by increasing minute ventilation by as much as 2.5 times. Such an increase in minute ventilation poses a minor challenge when respiratory mechanics and respiratory muscles are normal; for example, hypercapnia is uncommon with pulmonary vascular disease. Likewise, in the presence of large shunts, increases in minute ventilation can be sufficient to prevent hypercapnia. Accordingly, an increase in dead space ventilation or shunt should not be considered the primary mechanisms responsible for weaning failure unless there is a concurrent abnormality in the mechanical load of the respiratory muscles or in their contractile performance or there are concurrent abnormalities in the control of breathing. For example, increases in dead space ventilation may develop during weaning trials as the result of rapid shallow breathing and dynamic hyperinflation. Finally, an increase in carbon dioxide production can probably only be a contributory factor and not a sole cause of weaning failure.

IMPAIRED VENTILATORY PUMP

Decreased Respiratory Drive

- Specific conditions such as central alveolar hypoventilation secondary to neurologic lesions (trauma, infections, infarction) can contribute to, or cause, weaning failure. In most weaning-failure patients, however, estimations of respiratory drive indicate that drive is increased, not decreased. as suggested by the increased measured airway occlusion pressure at 100 ms ($P_{0.1}$) in patient failure to wean after 3 week of mechanical ventilation.

- The high neuromuscular inspiratory drive, however, is poorly transformed into ventilatory output—the tidal volumes can be lower in weaning failure patients than in weaning success patients—and therefore associated with increased respiratory rate.

- In approximately 10% of patients, however, a decrease in drive relative to the ventilatory demands may still contribute to weaning failure with acute hypercapnia during a trial of spontaneous respiration, primarily because of (relative) respiratory center depression. Whether sleep deprivation decreases respiratory drive remains controversial.

Increased Mechanical Load

- From 30% to 50% of patients who fail a weaning trial usually experience greater inspiratory resistance; 100% of the patients experience greater dynamic elastance with up to a 200% increase of intrinsic positive end-expiratory pressure (PEEP). Abnormal mechanics arise from bronchoconstriction, bronchial edema, pulmonary edema, and lung inflammation. Rapid shallow breathing can aggravate the abnormalities in lung elastance, intrinsic PEEP, and carbon dioxide clearance. Expiratory muscle recruitment can also increase intrinsic PEEP and breathing effort.

- Increased mechanical load contributes to weaning failure by increasing work of breathing. Furthermore, in weaning failure patients, the mean inspiratory flow—or tidal volume to inspiratory time ratio—produced for a given level of neuromuscular inspiratory drive ($P_{0.1}$ to mean inspiratory flow ratio or *effective inspiratory impedance*) is higher than in patients who are successfully weaned (Fig. 95.2). The higher *effective inspiratory impedance* results entirely from a greater neuromuscular drive and not from a reduced mean inspiratory flow. This correlation indicates a worse load-capacity balance in weaning failure patients than in weaning success patients.

Respiratory Muscle Weakness

- In healthy subjects, maximum inspiratory airway pressure is usually more negative than –80 cm H_2O. In mechanically ventilated patients recovering from an episode or acute respiratory failure, maximum inspiratory airway pressure can range from less negative than –20 cm H_2O to about –100 cm H_2O. Values of maximal airway pressure during voluntary maneuvers depend greatly on a level of motivation and comprehension of the maneuver, often not obtainable in

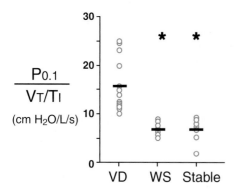

FIGURE 95.2. Effective inspiratory impedance ($P_{0.1}/V_T/T_I$) during periods of unassisted breathing in long-term ventilator-dependent (VD) patients with chronic obstructive pulmonary disease (COPD) ($n = 12$), in patients with COPD who were successfully weaned (WS) from mechanical ventilation after a period of prolonged ventilation ($n = 8$), and in stable patients with COPD ($n = 9$). Effective inspiratory impedance was less in weaning successes and in stable patients than in patients who were ventilator dependent. *Asterisks, $p < 0.05$,* VD versus WS and Stable; *horizontal bars,* average values. (Modified from Purro A, Appendini L, De Gaetano A, et al. Physiologic determinants of ventilator dependence in long-term mechanically ventilated patients. *Am J Respir Crit Care Med.* 2000;161:1115.)

critically ill patients. Thus, it is not surprising that, in patients requiring short-term mechanical ventilation, measurements of maximum inspiratory airway pressure commonly do not differentiate between weaning successes and weaning failure patients.

- Pre-existing conditions that can cause respiratory muscle weakness include disorders such as neuromuscular diseases, malnutrition, endocrine disorders, and hyperinflation. The existence of pre-existing conditions should be clinically recognized before instituting mechanical ventilation, when ventilator support is being delivered, or when the patient fails a weaning trial.

- New-onset respiratory muscle weakness in critically ill patients may result from conditions that are unique to these patients and that include ventilator-associated respiratory muscle dysfunction (a reduction of diaphragmatic force generation that can cause decreases in diaphragmatic endurance), sepsis-associated myopathy, and intensive care unit (ICU) acquired paresis. New-onset respiratory muscle weakness may also result from conditions that are not unique to critically ill patients and that include acid-base disorders, electrolyte disturbances, decreased oxygen delivery, or medications.

Respiratory Muscle Fatigue

- Whether critically ill patients develop short-lasting or long-lasting contractile fatigue of the respiratory muscles has not been clear. Patients who fail a trial of weaning from mechanical ventilation are at particular risk of developing fatigue because they experience marked increases in respiratory load. The addition of a new injury to the respiratory muscles (secondary to the development of contractile fatigue) might be the ultimate determinant of whether some patients are ever successfully weaned.

- The *tension-time index* of the diaphragm—an index of the ability of the diaphragm to sustain a given inspiratory load calculated by multiplying two ratios: the respiratory duty

cycle (inspiratory time divided by the time of a total respiratory cycle) and the mean inspiratory pressure per breath divided by maximum inspiratory pressure—has been shown in research protocols to be a promising tool to predict time to failure before obvious clinical signs of fatigue.

Impaired Cardiovascular Performance

- Spontaneous respiratory efforts decrease intrathoracic pressure and thus increase the pressure gradient for systemic venous return. In addition, decreases in intrathoracic pressure increase left ventricular afterload, causing additional stress on the left ventricle. In patients with coronary artery disease, the increased stress can alter myocardial perfusion and cause transient left ventricular dilation.

- The occurrence of myocardial ischemia during periods of spontaneous respiration has been associated with a greater risk of weaning failure and greater risk of ventilator dependence. In weaning successes, oxygen transport increases, mainly resulting from an increase in cardiac index; in weaning failures, the increase in demand is met by an increase in oxygen extraction, resulting in a decrease in mixed venous oxygen saturation (Fig. 95.3). A decrease in mixed venous oxygen saturation is consistent with a failing cardiovascular response to an increased metabolic demand.

Psychological Factors

- Possible mechanisms for psychological dysfunction in mechanically ventilated patients include respiratory discomfort, severity of illness, sleep deprivation, sensory deprivation (Fig. 95.4), and medication side effects. The delivery of mechanical ventilation itself can cause psychological dysfunction. Mechanical ventilation limits mobility, fosters isolation, impairs communication, and interferes with or blocks patient control of the act of breathing. Anxiety and depression can decrease motivation, interfere with performing simple tasks, and can decrease self-esteem.

- Aggressive treatment of depression may increase the likelihood of weaning. Biofeedback, improving the patients' environment, communication, and mobility, and specialized weaning centers have been used to decrease psychological problems in ventilated patients.

PREDICTION OF WEANING OUTCOME

Respiratory Frequency to Tidal Volume Ratio

- The ratio of respiratory frequency to tidal volume (f/V_T)[†] is measured during 1 minute of spontaneous breathing (Fig. 95.5). Measurements of f/V_T in the presence of pressure support or continuous positive airway pressure will result in

---

[†]For example, for a spontaneous respiratory rate of 25 breaths/minute and a spontaneous tidal volume of 600 mL (0.6 L), the $f/V_T = 25/0.6 = 41.7 = 42$.

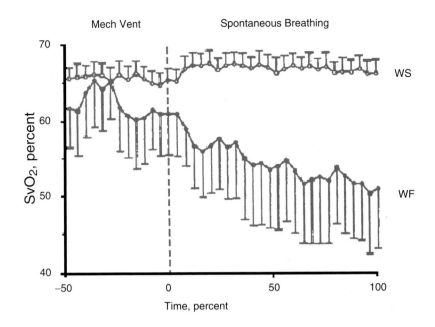

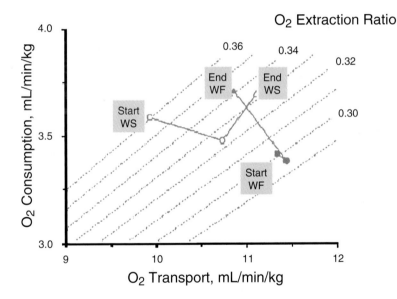

FIGURE 95.3. **Top:** Mixed venous oxygen saturation (SvO_2) during mechanical ventilation and a trial of spontaneous breathing in 11 weaning success (WS) patients (*open symbols*) and in 8 weaning failure (WF) patients (*closed symbols*). During mechanical ventilation, SvO_2 was similar in the two groups ($p = 0.28$). Between the onset (*dashed line*) and the end of the trial, SvO_2 decreased in the failure group ($p < 0.01$) whereas it remained unchanged in the success group ($p = 0.48$). Over the course of the trial, SvO_2 was lower in the failure group than in the success group ($p < 0.02$). *Bars,* standard error (SE). **Bottom:** Oxygen transport, oxygen consumption, and isopleths of oxygen extraction ratio in the success (WS, *open symbols*) and failure (WF, *closed symbols*) groups during mechanical ventilation (*squares*) and at the onset (*circles*) and end (*triangles*) of a spontaneous breathing trial. See text for details. (Modified from Jubran A, Mathru M, Dries D, et al. Continuous recordings of mixed venous oxygen saturation during weaning from mechanical ventilation and the ramifications thereof. *Am J Respir Crit Care Med.* 1998;158:1763.)

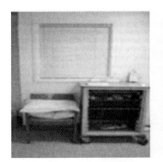
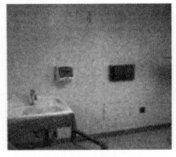
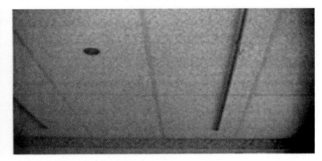

FIGURE 95.4. The environment in which ventilated patients are being cared for can promote sensory deprivation through the lack of windows with a view (**left**), bare walls (**middle**), and tedious ceiling (**right**). (From Martin UJ, Criner GJ. Psychological problems in the ventilated patient. In: Tobin MJ, ed. *Principles and Practice of Mechanical Ventilation.* 2nd ed. New York, NY: McGraw-Hill; 2006:1142, with permission.)

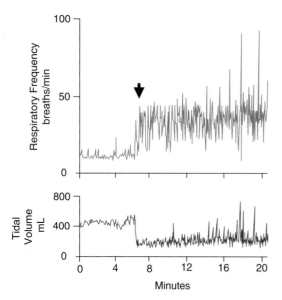

FIGURE 95.5. A time-series, breath-by-breath plot of respiratory frequency and tidal volume in a patient who failed a weaning trial. The *arrow* indicates the point of resuming spontaneous breathing. Rapid, shallow breathing developed almost immediately after discontinuation of the ventilator. (From Tobin MJ, Perez W, Guenther SM, et al. The pattern of breathing during successful and unsuccessful trials of weaning from mechanical ventilation. *Am Rev Respir Dis.* 1986;132:1111, with permission.)

inaccurate predictions of weaning outcome. The higher the f/V_T ratio, the more severe the rapid, shallow breathing and the greater the likelihood of unsuccessful weaning. An f/V_T ratio of 100 best discriminates between successful and unsuccessful attempts at weaning.

- The average sensitivity in all of the studies on f/V_T was 0.89, and 85% of the studies reveal sensitivities above 0.90.

Pulmonary Gas Exchange

- Mechanical ventilation is virtually never discontinued in a patient who has severe hypoxemia, such as arterial oxygen tension (PaO_2) <55 mm Hg with inspired oxygen fraction (FiO_2) >0.40. Arterial-to-inspired oxygen ratio (PaO_2/FiO_2), alveolar-arterial oxygen tension gradient, and arterial/alveolar oxygen tension ratio (PaO_2/PAO_2) are indices derived from arterial blood gas measurements proposed as predictors of weaning outcome. Though threshold values of the efficiency of indices derived from arterial blood gas measurements cannot be recommended for weaning prediction, weaning attempts are not recommended in patients with borderline hypoxemia.

Minute Ventilation

- A minute ventilation of <10 L/minute was a classic index used to predict a successful weaning outcome. When prospectively assessed, however, minute ventilation has a high rate of false-negative and false-positive results and cannot be recommended as a predictor of weaning outcome.

Maximum Inspiratory Pressure

- A maximum inspiratory pressure value more negative than −30 cm H_2O was found to be associated with successfully weaning, whereas all patients with a maximum inspiratory pressure less negative than −20 cm H_2O failed a weaning trial. However, these threshold values have shown poor sensitivity and specificity.

Vital Capacity

- The normal vital capacity is usually between 65 and 75 mL/kg, and a value ≥ 10 mL/kg has been suggested to predict a successful weaning. Patients with a vital capacity <7 mL/kg are unable to tolerate as few as 15 minutes of spontaneous breathing. Vital capacity is rarely used as a weaning predictor, and it is often unreliable.

Airway Occlusion Pressure

- A $P_{0.1}$ values above 3.4 to 6.0 cm H_2O can help discriminating between weaning success and weaning failures. However, other investigators have found $P_{0.1}$ to be quite inaccurate. One mechanism that could contribute to the poor performance of $P_{0.1}$ is the limited reproducibility of the measurement. The within-individual coefficient of variation of $P_{0.1}$ is about 50%, and the interindividual coefficient of variation is as high as 60%.

WEANING TRIALS

Intermittent Mandatory Ventilation

- With intermittent mandatory ventilation (IMV) weaning, the ventilator's mandatory rate is reduced in steps of 1 to 3 breaths/minute, and an arterial blood gas is obtained about 30 minutes after each rate change. Unfortunately, titrating the ventilator's mandatory rate according with the results of arterial blood gases can produce a false sense of security. In difficult-to-wean patients, as the IMV rate is decreased, inspiratory work increases progressively not only for the spontaneous breaths but also for the assisted breaths, largely due to the inability of the respiratory center to adapt its output rapidly to intermittent support.

Pressure Support

- What exactly constitutes a "minimal level of pressure support" has never been defined. For example, pressure support of 6 to 8 cm H_2O is widely used to compensate for the resistance imposed by the endotracheal tube and ventilator circuit. It is reasoned that a patient who can breathe comfortably at this level of pressure support will be able to tolerate extubation.

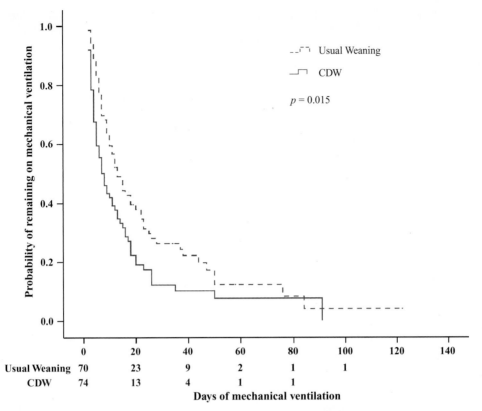

FIGURE 95.6. Kaplan–Meier analysis of weaning time until successful extubation or death in patients undergoing usual weaning ($n = 70$) and in patients undergoing computer-driven weaning (CDW)—that is, computer-driven closed-loop knowledge-based algorithm ($n = 74$). The probability of remaining on mechanical ventilation was less with computer-driven weaning than with usual weaning (log-rank test, $p = 0.015$). (From Lellouche F, Mancebo J, Jolliet P, et al. A multicenter randomized trial of computer-driven protocolized weaning from mechanical ventilation. *Am J Respir Crit Care Med.* 2006;174:894, with permission.)

Computer-driven Weaning Protocol

- A recent computer-driven pressure-supported ventilation weaning has reduced the median duration of weaning, mechanical ventilation, and ICU stay (Fig. 95.6). However, there was no difference from physician-driven weaning in terms of reintubation rate, hospital length of stay, ICU mortality, and hospital mortality.

T-Tube Trials

- Today, it is usual to limit a T-tube trial to once a day. If the trial is successful, the patient is extubated. If the trial is unsuccessful, the patient is given at least 24 hours of respiratory muscle rest with full ventilator support before another trial is performed.
- Tube trials ranging from 30 to 120 minutes have been studied. Whether the patient completes 30 minutes or 120 minutes, there is no difference in percentage of patients who successfully are liberated from mechanical ventilation. However, it is unclear if this holds true in more chronic, difficult to wean patients.
- Patients are judged to have failed a T-tube trial when they develop severe tachypnea, increased accessory muscle activity, diaphoresis, facial signs of respiratory distress, oxygen desaturation, tachycardia, arrhythmias, hypertension, or hypotension.

Noninvasive Ventilation in Weaning

- Noninvasive positive pressure ventilation has been used to facilitate extubation in intubated patients with chronic obstructive pulmonary disease and acute hypercapnic respiratory failure.
- Insufficient data are available on the role of noninvasive ventilation in weaning from hypoxemic respiratory failure. See Chapters 91 and 96 for more detailed information.

CHAPTER 96 ■ ACUTE LUNG INJURY AND ACUTE RESPIRATORY DISTRESS SYNDROME

OVERVIEW

- The acute respiratory distress syndrome (ARDS) is characterized by nonhydrostatic pulmonary edema and hypoxemia associated with a variety of etiologies that cause both direct and indirect insults to the lungs. The process develops acutely (usually within 72 hours of the precipitating event), requires immediate recognition, and often leads to death despite maximal medical support. ARDS is a devastating injury to the lungs, characterized by diffuse pulmonary inflammation, hypoxemia, and respiratory distress. In 1994, the American–European Consensus Committee on ARDS changed the word "adult" back to "acute" because development of ARDS was not restricted to adults. The consensus meeting further defined diagnostic criteria to include (a) acute onset; (b) bilateral radiographic infiltrates; (c) pulmonary artery occlusion pressure (PAOP) ≤ 18 mm Hg, or no evidence of left atrial hypertension; and (d) PaO_2/FiO_2 ratio of ≤ 300 mm Hg for acute lung injury (ALI) and ≤ 200 mm Hg for ARDS.
- This definition is far from perfect. Respiratory distress, characterized by tachypnea, dyspnea, and acute respiratory alkalosis not relieved by correcting hypoxemia, is common to many pulmonary processes. Bilateral radiographic infiltrates may be seen with cardiogenic edema, pneumonitis, and several other entities. The PaO_2/FiO_2 ratio may be influenced by therapy, especially positive end-expiratory pressure (PEEP) and the FiO_2 itself. It seems specious to separate "acute lung injury" from ARDS when the two terms reflect only somewhat different severity of the same processes. Heart failure may be present at a PAOP <18 mm Hg and may coexist with ARDS, but heart failure may not be present with a PAOP of ≥ 18 mm Hg. Nonetheless, although presently undergoing revision, this definition has stood the test of time and forms the basis for all investigation done on ARDS in the past decade.
- The Lung Injury Score (LIS) based on chest radiographic findings, degree of hypoxemia (using PaO_2/FiO_2 values), compliance of the pulmonary system (if ventilated), and PEEP levels attempts to better define the range of lung injury (Table 96.1). A patient was considered to have ARDS if the score was >2.5. The LIS value and the LIS did not add accuracy to the definitions of the consensus statement.
- Multiple risk factors for ALI/ARDS have been identified, with sepsis syndrome having the highest prevalence (30% to 50%). The pathogenesis for pulmonary and extrapulmonary causes for ALI may be different; the Consensus Committee categorized ARDS into direct versus indirect causes (Tables 96.2A and 96.2B). Secondary predisposing factors described in the literature are alcohol abuse, chronic lung disease, and a low systemic pH.
- Although ARDS is usually considered a homogeneous entity, it should be considered the final common pathway of a very heterogeneous group of insults. Although the pulmonary injury is widespread, it does not uniformly affect lung tissue; this nonuniformity has important therapeutic consequences. There are also two broad etiologies of ARDS: In *pulmonary ARDS* (generally corresponding to "direct" disease), there is primary lung injury (e.g., pneumonia) that involves the alveolar epithelium and may be confined to single organ failure. In *extrapulmonary ARDS* (generally corresponding to "indirect" disease), the inflammatory effect of a remote

TABLE 96.1

LUNG INJURY SCORE

Points	
Chest roentgenogram score	
0	No alveolar consolidation
1	Alveolar consolidation in one quadrant
2	Alveolar consolidation in two quadrants
3	Alveolar consolidation in three quadrants
4	Alveolar consolidation in four quadrants
Hypoxemia score	
0	$PaO_2/FiO_2 \geq 300$
1	PaO_2/FiO_2 225–299
2	PaO_2/FiO_2 175–224
3	PaO_2/FiO_2 100–174
4	$PaO_2/FiO_2 <100$
Respiratory system compliance score (mL/cm H_2O)	
0	≥ 80
1	60–79
2	40–59
3	20–39
4	≤ 19
PEEP score (cm H_2O)	
0	≤ 5
1	6–8
2	9–11
3	12–14
4	≥ 15
Final value	
0	No lung injury
1–2.5	Acute lung injury (ALI)
>2.5	Severe lung injury (ARDS)

ARDS, acute respiratory distress syndrome.

TABLE 96.2A

MAJOR CATEGORIES OF ARDS RISK

DIRECT
- Pneumonia
- Aspiration
- Pulmonary contusion
- Fat emboli
- Near-drowning
- Inhalational injury
- Reperfusion after lung transplant or pulmonary embolectomy

INDIRECT
- Sepsis
- Severe trauma with shock
- Multiple transfusions
- Cardiopulmonary bypass
- Drug overdose
- Acute pancreatitis
- Multiple transfusions

ARDS, acute respiratory distress syndrome.
From Bernard GR, Artigas A, Brigham KL, et al. The American-European Consensus Conference on ARDS. *Am J Respir Crit Care Med.* 1994;149:818.

TABLE 96.2B

CONDITIONS ASSOCIATED WITH ARDS

SHOCK

Hemorrhagic	Cardiogenic
Septic	Anaphylactic

TRAUMA

Burns	Nonthoracic trauma
Fat emboli	(especially head trauma)
Lung contusion	Near-drowning

INFECTION

Viral pneumonia	Gram-negative sepsis
Bacterial pneumonia	Tuberculosis
Fungal pneumonia	

INHALATION OF TOXIC GASES

Oxygen	Cadmium
Smoke	Phosgene
NO_2, NH_3, Cl_2	

ASPIRATION OF GASTRIC CONTENTS (ESPECIALLY WITH A pH <2.5)

DRUG INGESTION

Cocaine	Fluorescein
Heroin	Propoxyphene
Methadone	Salicylates
Barbiturates	Chlordiazepoxide
Ethchlorvynol	Colchicine
Thiazides	Dextran 40

METABOLIC

Uremia	Diabetic ketoacidosis

MISCELLANEOUS

Pancreatitis	Leukoagglutinin reaction
Postcardiopulmonary bypass	Eclampsia
Postcardioversion	Air or amniotic fluid emboli
Multiple transfusions	Bowel infarction
DIC	Carcinomatosis

ARDS, acute respiratory distress syndrome; NO_2, nitrogen dioxide; NH_3, ammonia; Cl_2, chlorine; DIC, disseminated intravascular coagulation.
From Taylor RW, Duncan CA. The adult respiratory distress syndrome. *Res Med.* 1983;1:17.

insult—usually sepsis—reaches the capillary endothelium via a systemic inflammatory response syndrome phenomenon, and lung failure becomes one more component of multiorgan dysfunction syndrome (MODS). Although there are important differences in pathophysiology, the outcome between ARDS of pulmonary and extrapulmonary origin does not appear to differ greatly. Although the vast majority of studies reviewed here consider ARDS to be a single entity, questions remain as to whether this is true.
- A recent study reported the incidence of ALI to be 78.8 cases per 100,000 and for ARDS to be 58.7 cases per 100,000.

OUTCOME

- The cause of death in ARDS patients is more often associated with MODS than deficient oxygenation. The overall mortality rate has declined from 68% in the 1980s to 36% in 1993, and presently ranges widely from 30% to 58%, depending on the specific patient group—based on age and etiology of lung injury—being studied. ARDS patients who leave the hospital seem to have no increased risk of subsequent death when matched for comorbidities.
- Patients with ARDS who die within the first several days do so because of the underlying condition and respiratory failure. Many of those who survive the original insult succumb to sepsis or MODS. Of those who survive ARDS, most return to their premorbid state of respiratory function by about 6 months after extubation.

PATHOPHYSIOLOGY

- The inciting process in ALI is the pathologic loss of integrity of the alveolar–capillary membrane complex associated with exuberant inflammation, with increased endothelial and epithelial permeability and leakage of proteinaceous edema and cellular components into the interstitial and alveolar spaces. This occurs in response to some provocative stimulus, which may arise from various disease processes or physical or chemical insults, including primary pulmonary or extrapulmonary events (Fig. 96.1) (see Tables 96.2A and 96.22B). Histopathology changes of the lung are described in Table 96.3. Accumulation of proinflammatory mediators such as tumor necrosis factor-α (TNF-α), interleukin-1β (IL-1β), and IL-8 in the alveolar fluid of ARDS patients portends the amplified production of cytokine and toxic reactive oxygen and nitrogen radical species (Table 96.4). Activated complement components accumulate with fibrin and immunoglobulins to form alveolar hyaline membranes, further worsening compliance. Fibroproliferation and accelerated collagen deposition may begin early in the inflammatory sequence and continue into the proliferative phase (7 to 21 days), with thickening of the alveolar walls already denuded of type 1 pneumocytes.

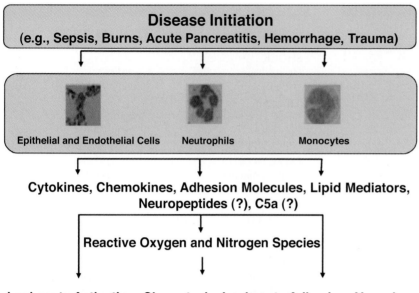

FIGURE 96.1. Pictorial detail of the pathogenesis of acute respiratory distress syndrome. (With permission from Bhatia M, Moochhala S. Role of inflammatory mediators in the pathophysiology of acute respiratory distress syndrome. *J Pathol.* 2004;202[2]:145–156.)

- Although the original inciting event may resolve, judicious correction of persistent metabolic and infectious issues, and meticulous attention to appropriate ventilatory techniques, must continue in order to minimize iatrogenic contributions to self-sustaining inflammation (see Ventilator Associated Lung Injury below). Evolution into the *fibrotic phase* generally occurs after 3 to 4 weeks. Variable degrees of fibrosis and parenchymal tissue loss yield "diffuse alveolar damage," the histologic correlate of advanced ARDS, characterized by widespread and severe damage to the alveolar–capillary unit. Micro- and macrocystic areas abut dilated ectatic bronchi, with fibrotic noncompliant septa and collapsed alveoli—no longer tethered open by healthy surrounding tissue—and interwoven with thrombosed capillaries that provide no capacity for gas exchange (i.e., dead space ventilation). Hypoxemia from tenaciously collapsed, fibrotic, shunt-producing alveoli accompanies the hypercarbia and respiratory acidosis of large dead space fractions from non–gas exchanging overdistended alveoli, dilated cystic areas, and thrombosed non–CO_2-excreting pulmonary capillaries.

Clinical Presentation Physical Examination

- The clinical findings in ARDS may be roughly grouped into four phases (Table 96.5).

TABLE 96.3

HISTOPATHOLOGIC CHANGES IN ARDS

	Exudative phase	Proliferative phase	Fibrotic phase
Macroscopic Microscopic	• Heavy, rigid, dark • Hyaline membranes • Edema • Neutrophils • Epithelial > endothelial damage	• Heavy, gray • Barrier disruption • Edema • Alveolar type II cell proliferation • Myofibroblast infiltration • Neutrophils • Alveolar collapse • Alveoli filled with cells and organizing matrix • Epithelial apoptosis • Fibroproliferation	• Cobblestoned • Fibrosis • Macrophages • Matrix organization • Deranged acinar architecture • Patchy emphysematous change
Vasculature	• Local thrombus	• Loss of capillaries • Pulmonary hypertension	• Myointimal thickening • Tortuous vessels

TABLE 96.4

INFLAMMATORY MEDIATORS IN ARDS

Inflammatory mediator	Function
TNF-α	Proinflammatory; neutrophil activation in ARDS
IL-1β	Proinflammatory; neutrophil activation in ARDS
IL-6	Leukocyte growth/activation; proliferation of myeloid progenitor cells; acute-phase response; pyrexia
IL-10	Anti-inflammatory; inhibits release of proinflammatory cytokines
TGF-β	Resolution of tissue injury; proinflammatory
GM-CSF	Host defense; hematologic growth factor
PAF	Platelet activation; neutrophil activation and chemotaxis
ICAM-I	Neutrophil adhesion
C5a	Leukocyte chemoattractant; dual pro- and anti-inflammatory role
Substance P	Proinflammatory
Chemokines	Leukocyte activation and chemotaxis
VEGF	Endothelial cytokine; plays a role in angiogenesis and vascular permeability
IGF-I	Alveolar macrophage-derived growth factor; profibrotic
KGF	Epithelial-specific growth factor; important for lung development repair
Reactive oxygen and nitrogen species	Regulation of vascular tone, antimicrobial action

- The changes seen on the chest radiograph in ARDS are characteristic but nonspecific, rarely revealing the etiology of the syndrome. Acutely, pulmonary edema is seen. Interstitial infiltrates progress to a diffuse, fluffy, panacinar pattern.
- Whereas a two-dimensional chest radiograph may suggest diffuse homogeneous infiltrates, the chest computed tomography (CT) scan usually demonstrates remarkably inhomogeneous lung involvement. Dependent regions of the lung appear to be much more involved than nondependent regions.

TABLE 96.5

PROGRESSION OF CLINICAL FINDINGS IN ARDS

PHASE 1: ACUTE INJURY
- Normal physical examination and chest radiograph
- Tachycardia, tachypnea, and respiratory alkalosis develop

PHASE 2: LATENT PERIOD
- Lasts approximately 6–48 h after injury
- Patient appears clinically stable
- Hyperventilation and hypocapnia persist
- Mild increase in work of breathing
- Widening of the alveolar-arterial oxygen gradient
- Minor abnormalities on physical examination and chest radiograph

PHASE 3: ACUTE RESPIRATORY FAILURE
- Marked tachypnea and dyspnea
- Decreased lung compliance
- Diffuse infiltrates on chest radiograph
- High-pitched crackles heard throughout all lung fields

PHASE 4: SEVERE ABNORMALITIES
- Severe hypoxemia unresponsive to therapy
- Increased intrapulmonary shunting
- Metabolic and respiratory acidosis

ARDS, acute respiratory distress syndrome.
From Taylor RW. The adult respiratory distress syndrome. In: Kirby RR, Taylor RW, eds. *Respiratory Failure.* Chicago: Year Book Medical Publishers; 1986:208.

TREATMENT

Fluid Management

- Adequate intravascular volume must be maintained to avoid tissue hypoperfusion, although we recommend that the minimal amount of fluid be given and that judicious attempts at diuresis be undertaken in the hemodynamically stable patient. However, a large study conducted by the National Heart, Lung, and Blood Institute (NHLBI) Acute Respiratory Distress Syndrome Clinical Trials Network found no difference in 60-day mortality when comparing liberal and conservative fluid management strategies.

Bronchodilators

- Aerosolized β-agonists can decrease airway resistance, even in patients without underlying chronic obstructive pulmonary disease or asthma. By reducing airway resistance, the work of breathing can be decreased.

Steroids

- Routine use of corticosteroids is not advocated, especially in the acute phase of ARDS. During the late phase, fibroproliferation often occurs in response to tissue injury and is associated with persistent inflammation. In this setting, fever and systemic inflammatory response syndrome are present in the absence of infection. A small uncontrolled trial suggested that improvement in "late" ARDS patients—those mechanically ventilated for approximately 15 days—with progressive fibroproliferation may be seen when corticosteroid treatment begins during that period

Respiratory Support

- The indications for respiratory support are well defined and include hemodynamic instability, protection and maintenance of the airway, inability to maintain PaO_2 >55 mm Hg on a $FiO_2 = 60\%$, need for positive airway pressure, and progressive ventilatory insufficiency with rising respiratory rate and hypercarbia. Lung CT studies have demonstrated the distribution of areas of alveolar collapse and distention characteristic of ARDS to be regional rather than diffuse. The presence of several or all of these features in most individuals with ALI mandates endotracheal intubation and mechanical ventilation to optimize gas exchange and minimize work of breathing. Noninvasive positive pressure ventilation has been employed in some instances for those with less severe pulmonary impairment and preserved mental status, although studies are few with fairly high rates of eventual endotracheal intubation.

- In 1990, a trial of mechanical ventilation, with limited tidal volume and plateau pressures compared to the higher values in common use at the time resulted in a reduction in mortality from 40% to 31% with the experimental protocol parameters. Although the trial has been criticized from a number of standpoints, none is sufficiently compelling to negate the persuasiveness of its results. In our practice, low tidal volume ventilation (V_t = 6 to 8 mL/kg ideal body weight) is considered standard, maintaining a plateau pressure <30 cm H_2O. Tidal volumes exceeding these parameters have been implicated in generating lung injury caused by mechanical ventilation itself. This phenomenon, termed *ventilator-associated lung injury* (VALI), is a by-product of the interaction of mechanical ventilation and the cytokine proliferation that is a fundamental pathophysiologic feature of ARDS. As described below, components of VALI include (a) *barotrauma,* the appearance of air outside the airways and alveoli, attributed to airway pressures that exceed certain thresholds; (b) *volutrauma,* increased alveolar and capillary permeability due to alveolar overdistention and leading to pulmonary edema; and (c) *atelectrauma,* the destructive repetitive opening and closing of stiff, collapsed, surfactant-depleted, fibrotic alveoli with thickened interstitium that are associated with cyclic positive pressure ventilation. Excessive alveolar stretch is associated with inflammatory cytokine proliferation, in particular during excursions into ranges of tidal volume that induce VALI. Of note, this cytokine proliferation can be limited by using a lung-protective ventilation strategy (using a pressure–volume curve to determine tidal volume and PEEP).

- The importance of limitation of tidal volume as a guide to appropriate mechanical ventilation in the acutely injured lung may be more easily understood when viewed within a conceptional framework of patchy, unevenly distributed alveolar injury. When such an injured lung receives a positive pressure breath, the gas distribution is impacted by the variability of compliance and resistance in the injured and healthy areas. Flow preferentially enters unaffected (i.e., low resistance, relatively high compliance) pulmonary tissue, risking unintentional overdistention and injury of these normal areas despite inflation with an "appropriate" tidal volume based on body weight. This is often termed *the baby lung phenomenon*, as the volume of unaffected lung parenchyma within the ARDS patient's thorax more closely approximates that of a child than an adult. Delivered tidal volumes, therefore, must more closely approximate those appropriate for a smaller lung, usually on the order of 6 to 8 mL/kg; exceeding these volumes risks iatrogenic perpetuation of lung injury because a positive pressure breath inflates a smaller volume of lung tissue than would be predicted by ideal body weight.

- The importance of PEEP and recruitment maneuvers in providing efficient ventilator management of ARDS patients warrants further discussion. Although the traditional approach of oxygen supplementation may improve the PaO_2 within the limits of a marginal functional reserve capacity (FRC), such supplementation should be looked upon only as a temporizing measure. Prolonged high FiO_2 use risks toxicity and absorption atelectasis, leaving the underlying cause of hypoxemia neither identified nor corrected. Recovery of FRC by reinflation of atelectatic areas using recruitment maneuvers and PEEP will restore gas flow to previously nonaerated areas of lung. These modalities of treatment are commonly utilized in the modern strategy of ARDS treatment.

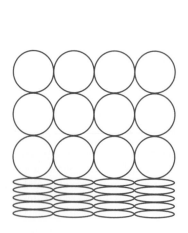
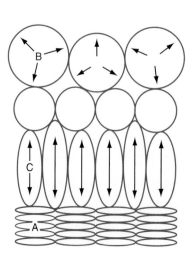

FIGURE 96.2. Atelectrauma and the interdependence of lung units. (With permission from Moloney ED, Griffiths MJ. Protective ventilation of patients with acute respiratory distress syndrome. *Br J Anaesth*. 2004;92[2]:261–270.)

- Areas of particularly tenacious atelectasis will often require an inspiratory time (T_i) equal to several inspiratory time-constants (one "time-constant" equals product of compliance and resistance, both easily measurable by current ventilators) to achieve inflation. Insufficient T_i may leave such areas persistently collapsed, worsening shunt fraction and compromising FRC and oxygenation. Despite the most heroic efforts, a substantial percentage of ARDS patients harbor lung tissue that is only variably "PEEP recruitable." The benefit of recruitment maneuvers and PEEP can be understood within the context of the *Law of LaPlace* (actually the Young-LaPlace equation), which states that the pressure difference across a fluid interface is equal to the surface tension times the mean curvature of the surface.
- In pulmonary physiology and ARDS, this means that the pressure difference between alveolar gas and alveolar epithelium contracts the alveolus inward unless counteracted by surfactant.
- Furthermore, the relationship between surface tension and alveolar radius is inverse. Thus, the smaller the alveolar radius, the greater the force contracting it even further inward (i.e., toward collapse). Because surfactant decreases surface tension, the inward force within a collapsed alveolus is greater than that within its surfactant-replete, healthy, "noncollapsed" neighbor with lower surface tension, resulting in a temporary high-pressure requirement to open a collapsed alveolus. The alveolus may then be maintained open, with PEEP exceeding the alveolar closing pressure. Because low tidal volume (6 mL/kg) followed by PEEP in itself is generally ineffective in expanding collapsed alveoli, a "recruitment maneuver," the temporary application of airway pressure far above any possible alveolar retractive force, may be warranted to open and stabilize collapsed alveoli, preventing exposure to repetitive cyclic collapse and associated destructive shear forces by maintaining an "open lung" (Fig. 96.2).
- Most clinicians feel that utilizing a level of PEEP above the lower inflection point on a pressure–volume curve (see below)

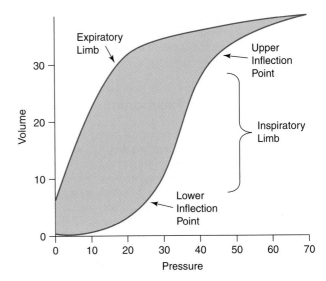

FIGURE 96.3. Pressure–volume curve of an idealized lung, showing both the inspiratory and expiratory limbs as well as the upper and lower inflection points.

improves FRC and oxygenation by inflating recruitable alveoli, and thus decreasing venous admixture.

- The selection of tidal volume is intimately linked to the pressure–volume curve. Optimal gas exchange with minimal alveolar injury is achieved when the lung is positioned on the vertical portion of the pressure–volume curve (Fig. 96.3).
- A not uncommon observation when monitoring gas exchange in ARDS is hypercarbia with mild acidemia, often more uncomfortable for the clinician to observe than the patient to experience. However, "permissive hypercapnia" is safe and acceptable when not contraindicated by underlying medical condition (e.g., elevated intracranial pressure), though it often warrants protocol-delivered sedation.

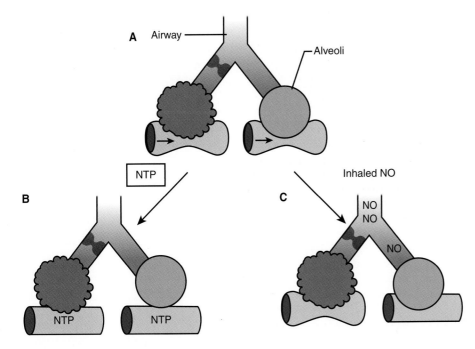

FIGURE 96.4. Intravenous versus inhaled vasodilator effects on pulmonary circulation. **A:** Shows two idealized alveoli, one occluded (left) and the other normal; both have hypoxic pulmonary vasoconstriction (HPV)-induced decreased pulmonary blood flow. **B:** Shows the result of using an intravenous vasodilator: HPV is removed to both the occluded and nonoccluded alveoli, resulting in significant shunt. **C:** Shows the result of utilization of inhaled nitric oxide (NO): HPV is reversed in the area of the ventilated alveolus, but not the obstructed one. NTP, nitroprusside. (With permission from Lunn RJ. Inhaled nitric oxide therapy. *Mayo Clin Proc.* 1995;70[3]:247–255.)

• The mode of mechanical ventilation used in ALI/ARDS has not been standardized. It is likely that the use of mechanical ventilation is more dependent on the comfort level of the practitioner than on "best evidence."

Prone Positioning

• Several large studies have documented improvements in oxygenation without significant improvement in mortality. Considerable skill and experience are needed to pronate and support a critical patient bearing invasive monitoring and therapeutic devices. The risks to potential pressure-bearing ventral body structures—face, eyes, chest, and knees—and of accidental device removal must be weighed against the benefits.

Inhaled Vasodilators

• Aerosolized vasoactive medications, such as nitric oxide or prostaglandin-I, diffuse from ventilated alveoli and result in

relaxation of endothelial smooth muscle within remotely constricted vascular beds, thus improving ventilation/perfusion matching while vessels adjacent to collapsed alveoli remain unaffected. Selective vasodilation in ventilated areas decreases shunt fraction and contributes to alleviation of pulmonary hypertension (Fig. 96.4).

COMPLICATIONS

• Significant morbidity or mortality may occur during supportive therapy for ALI/ARDS, as summarized in Table 96.6.
• The additional inflammatory insult induced by suboptimal mechanical ventilation technique is termed *ventilator-associated lung injury.*
• *Barotrauma* refers to the presence of air outside the alveoli when receiving positive pressure ventilation. Air leaks track along the perivascular sheath to the mediastinum and pleural cavities, or along fascial planes to extrathoracic areas. It seems intuitive that such occurrences are related to pressures exceeding the limits of tissue structural integrity, but the issue is clearly more complicated, as musicians are repeatedly able

---

TABLE 96.6

COMPLICATIONS ASSOCIATED WITH ARDS

PULMONARY Pulmonary emboli Pulmonary barotrauma Pulmonary fibrosis Oxygen toxicity	**COMPLICATIONS ATTRIBUTABLE TO INTUBATION AND EXTUBATION** Prolonged attempt at intubation Intubation of a mainstem bronchus Premature extubation Self-extubation
GASTROINTESTINAL Gastrointestinal hemorrhage Ileus Gastric distention Pneumoperitoneum	**COMPLICATIONS ASSOCIATED WITH ENDOTRACHEAL/TRACHEOSTOMY TUBES** Tube malfunction Nasal necrosis Paranasal sinus infection
RENAL Renal failure Fluid retention	Tracheal stenosis Tracheomalacia Polyps Erosion
CARDIOVASCULAR Invasive catheters Arrhythmia Hypotension Low cardiac output	Fistulae Airway obstruction Hoarseness **COMPLICATIONS ATTRIBUTABLE TO OPERATION OF THE VENTILATOR** Machine failure
INFECTION Sepsis Nosocomial pneumonia	Alarm failure Alarms silenced Inadequate nebulization or humidification
HEMATOLOGIC Anemia Thrombocytopenia DIC	**COMPLICATIONS OCCURRING DURING POSITIVE AIRWAY PRESSURE THERAPY** Alveolar hypoventilation Alveolar hyperventilation Massive gastric distention
OTHER Hepatic Endocrine Neurologic Psychiatric Malnutrition	Barotrauma Atelectasis Pneumonia Hypotension

ARDS, acute respiratory distress syndrome; DIC, disseminated intravascular coagulation.
From Taylor RW. The adult respiratory distress syndrome. In: Kirby RR, Taylor RW, eds. *Respiratory Failure.* Chicago: Year Book Medical Publishers; 1986:208.

to generate 150 cm H_2O airway pressure with no sequelae. It is speculated that barotrauma represents regional overinflation in areas of diseased lung, such areas thereby being particularly at risk for structural failure and air leak. *Volutrauma* occurs when excessive inspiratory volumes induce microvascular edema; the offending agent appears to be excessive *volume*, rather than the excessive *pressure* required to supply that volume.

- Compromised surfactant production and function leads to increased surface tension, provoking alveolar collapse with increased venous admixture and subjecting alveolar epithelium to the tissue-destructive shear stresses of recruitment/derecruitment in the process known as *atelectrauma*.
- Finally, over the last few years, there has been recognition of the inflammatory cytokine release, as well as alveolar and interstitial neutrophil infiltration associated with ventilator-related pulmonary disruption, leading to MODS. While it is indisputable that "excessive" tidal volume ventilation augments systemic cytokine levels, the specific causal relationship with worse outcome has yet to be validated.

CHAPTER 97 ■ DROWNING

THE DROWNING PROCESS

- Drowning is the process resulting from primary respiratory impairment from submersion or immersion in a liquid medium.
- The drowning process is a continuum that begins when the victim's airway is initially below the surface of the water; he or she first will voluntarily hold his or her breath. Some victims will swallow significant quantities of water during this time. This period of voluntary breath holding, lasting a few seconds is followed by an involuntary period of laryngospasm secondary to water in the oropharynx or at the level of the larynx acting as a foreign body. During this period of breath holding and laryngospasm, the patient cannot breathe; therefore, oxygen is depleted and carbon dioxide is not eliminated. This results in the patient becoming hypercarbic, hypoxic, and acidotic.
- As the patient's arterial oxygen tension drops further, laryngospasm abates, and the patient then actively breathes water. Further evidence of the magnitude of negative pressure created during laryngospasm is the fact that the lungs of drowning victims frequently demonstrate significant hyperinflation at autopsy.
- The amount of liquid a drowning victim breathes varies considerably between victims. Studies comparing the biochemical changes occurring in humans after a drowning episode with those in experimental animals suggest that, while the volume of liquid actually inhaled varies considerably from one victim to another, only 15% of persons who die in the water aspirate in excess of 22 mL/kg of water, and the percentage is considerably less in those who survive. Changes occur in the lung, body fluids, and electrolyte concentrations, which are dependent on both the composition and volume of the liquid aspirated.

RESUSCITATION

- Irreversible damage to brain tissue is reported to begin approximately 3 minutes after the PaO_2 falls below 30 mm Hg under normothermic conditions in otherwise normal people. Such data suggest that if the victim is rescued and effective resuscitation efforts are applied within 3 minutes of the cessation of respiration (i.e., submersion in water), the vast majority of such victims should be able to be resuscitated and suffer no permanent brain damage. After the 3-minute time frame has been exceeded, although some normal survivors are reported, it becomes less likely that normal survival will result from resuscitation efforts. This time frame may be prolonged if hypothermia occurs rapidly because it decreases the cerebral requirement for oxygen.
- Persons who become hypothermic due to immersion or submersion in extremely cold water will rapidly develop hypothermia, which protects the brain by decreasing its oxygen requirement and prolongs survival. It should be noted, however, that hypothermia is a two-edged sword; although it can protect the brain from oxygen deprivation, it also can cause death in the water secondary to its effect on the conduction system of the heart, resulting in circulatory arrest either by asystole or ventricular fibrillation.

PATHOPHYSIOLOGY

- It has consistently been shown that, acutely, drowning produces asphyxia (i.e., hypoxia, hypercarbia, and acidosis). The hypercarbia is due to absent or ineffective ventilation and is readily correctable when aggressive mechanical ventilation is instituted. The hypoxia that occurs initially is not as readily correctable and may be persistent for long periods of time. This hypoxia is first due to apnea and then primarily to intrapulmonary shunting from alveoli that are perfused but not being ventilated, or not being ventilated adequately. The acidosis is mixed, and the respiratory component rapidly disappears with effective ventilation. The patient is, however, frequently left with significant metabolic acidosis caused by anaerobic metabolism during the period of time that profound tissue hypoxia secondary to absent or ineffective respiration and cardiac output was present. The hallmark of this high anion gap metabolic acidosis is an increased level of serum lactic acid.

Pulmonary

- In freshwater drowning, the aspirated water alters the surface tension properties of pulmonary surfactant. Thus, the alveoli become unstable and do not maintain their normal shape or patency, resulting in an increase in both absolute and relative intrapulmonary shunt. On the contrary, seawater does not change the surface tension properties of pulmonary surfactant, but, because it is hypertonic, it pulls fluid from the circulation into the alveoli, thus producing obstruction to gas exchange at the alveolar level. Bronchoconstriction also has been reported after aspiration of even small quantities of water.
- Freshwater, being hypotonic, is absorbed very rapidly into the circulation and, because of the transient hypervolemia that occurs and the change in the surface tension properties of pulmonary surfactant, pulmonary edema results. Pulmonary edema also occurs when seawater is aspirated, secondary to a semipermeable membrane effect because the seawater is hypertonic compared to plasma. Even though the etiology of the hypoxia is different between freshwater and seawater aspiration, the result of both is to increase intrapulmonary shunt.
- The treatment of the respiratory lesion requires providing mechanical ventilatory support in a fashion that will restore an adequate functional residual capacity and keep the alveoli open during all phases of the respiratory cycle, thus decreasing the intrapulmonary shunt. Obviously, if foreign material such as sand, silt, or plant life is aspirated into the lung, it may produce obstruction, and it should be removed via bronchoscopy.

Cardiovascular

- The cardiovascular changes that occur during a drowning episode can best be ascribed to inadequate oxygenation. Although fatal arrhythmia such as ventricular fibrillation is rarely documented in human drowning victims, ventricular fibrillation can occur with profound hypoxia, especially if very significant changes in serum potassium and serum sodium result from the movement of fluid and rupture of red blood cells.

Renal

- Detrimental changes in renal function are rarely seen in persons recovering from near-drowning. However, when present, they likely are the result of inadequate perfusion and oxygenation rather than anything specifically related to the drowning episode per se.

INITIAL RESCUE AND RESUSCITATION

- To ensure survival after a drowning episode, it is imperative that one never lose sight of the fact that time is of the essence. The longer a person is without the ability to breathe air, the more profound are the hypoxia and permanent damage to vital tissues.
- While removing the victim from the water, care should be taken to avoid complicating neck injuries when they are suspected. Routine stabilization of the neck is unnecessary unless the circumstances leading to the drowning episode suggest that trauma was likely. These circumstances include a history of diving, use of a water slide, signs of injury, or evidence of alcohol intoxication. If neck injury is suspected, gentle immobilization of the head should be accomplished, securing it in a neutral position. However, if the neck appears to be obviously deformed and the patient has pain with neck movement, the neck should be immobilized in the existing position. Drowning victims in cardiac arrest should receive standard advanced cardiac life support.
- Although the airway should rapidly be inspected for the presence of obstructing material, the abdominal thrust maneuver, which had been advocated by some in the past, has been thoroughly debated and found not to be of value in treating a drowning victim unless solid material is actually blocking the conducting airway
- Drowning episodes in cold water may produce significant hypothermia. There are several methods of rewarming that have been recommended including, but not necessarily limited to, heating blankets, warmed intravenous fluids, warmed humidification of breathing circuits, gastric lavage, and cardiopulmonary bypass. The method used should be tailored to the resources available and the condition of the patient. It must be remembered, however, that rewarming peripheral tissues before the patient's circulation is capable of supplying adequate amounts of oxygenated blood can imbalance oxygen supply ratio and increase the degree of metabolic acidosis by accelerated production of lactic acid.

CHAPTER 98 ■ SEVERE ASTHMA EXACERBATION

DEFINITION AND CHARACTERISTICS OF SEVERE ASTHMA—DIFFERENT PHENOTYPES

- The National Asthma Educational and Prevention Program (NAEEP) and Global Initiative for Asthma (GINA) guidelines both assess disease severity on the basis of nocturnal symptoms, use of short-acting bronchodilators, frequency of exacerbations that affect daily activities, and baseline pulmonary function measurements before treatment (Table 98.1).
- The pathophysiology of asthma consists of three key abnormalities:
  - Bronchoconstriction
  - Airway inflammation
  - Mucous plugging
- Refractory asthma is not meant to describe only patients with "fatal" or "near-fatal" asthma, but it is meant to encompass the asthma subgroups previously described as "severe asthma," "steroid-dependent and/or resistant asthma," "difficult-to-control asthma," "poorly controlled asthma," "brittle asthma," or "irreversible asthma." Clinically, patients with refractory asthma may present with a variety of separate and/or overlapping conditions, including:
  - Widely varying peak flows (brittle asthma)
  - Severe but chronic airflow limitation
  - Rapidly progressive loss of lung function
  - Mucus production ranging from absent to copious
  - Varying responses to corticosteroids
- Whether these groups form distinct clinical, physiologic, and pathologic groups is unclear. The American Thoracic Society Workshop definition required one of two major criteria (see Table 98.1), and two of seven additional minor criteria. Numerous attempts at classifying potential phenotypes of severe asthma have been proposed, as shown in Table 98.2. Although these phenotypes may overlap, there is reasonable supporting evidence for the presence of at least six—and likely more—severe asthma phenotypes as defined by clinical parameters (natural history, clinical presentation, atopy, airflow obstruction), type of inflammation, and treatment-related parameter.
- From a clinical point of view, three categories of severely asthmatic patients seem to be of particular importance:
  - Those with frequent severe asthma exacerbations
  - Those with fixed airway obstruction
  - Those with oral steroid dependency
- Together, these three categories encompass most of the patients referred with difficult-to-control asthma.

Respiratory Mechanics

- The main pathophysiologic mechanism of acute severe asthma is pulmonary hyperinflation caused by a combination of factors (Fig. 98.1). The driving force for expiratory flow is reduced because of an abnormally low pulmonary elastic recoil, the etiology of which is uncertain. Persistent activation of the inspiratory muscles during expiration causes outward recoil of the chest wall, further reducing the driving force for expiration. At the same time, resistance to airflow is greatly augmented because of severely reduced airway caliber and, perhaps, also narrowing of the glottic aperture during expiration. Expiration is prolonged so that the following inspiration starts before static equilibrium is reached. Consequently the end-expiratory alveolar pressure remains positive, a phenomenon known as *auto-PEEP* (positive end-expiratory pressure) or *intrinsic PEEP* (PEEPi) or static PEEPi (PEEPi, st).
- It should be noticed that the lung is extremely inhomogeneous during acute severe asthma. The distribution of bronchial obstruction is uneven because of both anatomic reasons—variable amounts of secretions, edema, bronchospasm—and variable external compression exerted on the distal airways by intrathoracic positive pressure during expiration. Thus, illustratively, four parallel compartments can be recognized (Fig. 98.2):
  - Compartment A represents the portion of the lung with neither bronchial obstruction nor hyperinflation.
  - Compartment B is the part of the lung where the airways are entirely obstructed during the whole respiratory cycle (mucous plugging).
  - In compartment C, obstruction appears only during expiration, inducing alveolar hyperinflation and high PEEPi.
  - In compartment D, partial obstruction of the airways is present throughout the respiratory cycle, causing a lesser extent of alveolar hyperinflation and PEEPi than in compartment C.

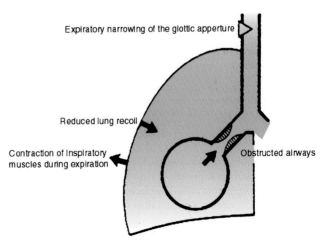

FIGURE 98.1. Mechanisms responsible for dynamic hyperinflation in asthma.

TABLE 98.1

TERMS AND DEFINITIONS IN SEVERE ASTHMA

Severe persistent asthma (2)	Continual symptoms, frequent nocturnal symptoms, limited activity, frequent exacerbations, FEV_1 or PEV<60% predicted, PEF variability >30%
Severe/refractory Asthma (5) Definition requires that at least one major criterion and two minor criteria are met, other disorders have been excluded, exacerbating factors have been treated, and patient is generally compliant.	MAJOR: 1. Treatment requires continuous or nearly continuous (≥50% of year) oral corticosteroids. 2. Treatment requires high-dose (>880 μg/d fluticasone or equivalent) inhaled corticosteroids. MINOR: 1. Asthma symptoms needing short-acting β-agonist use on a daily or near-daily basis. 2. Need for additional daily treatment with a controller medication (e.g., long-acting β-agonist, theophylline, or leukotriene antagonist). 3. Persistent airway obstruction (FEV_1<80% predicted, diurnal peak expiratory flow variability >20%). 4. One or more urgent care visits for asthma per year. 5. Three or more oral steroid bursts per year. 6. Prompt clinical deterioration with ≤25% reduction in oral or intravenous corticosteroid dose. 7. Near-fatal asthma event in the past.
Severe asthma (4)	Diagnosis requires at least three of the following: 1. Seen by a consultant in asthma >2 y. 2. Has persistent symptoms and decreased quality of life 3. Has received maximal asthma therapy (high-dose inhaled corticosteroids [ICS]) with documented adherence 4. History of respiratory failure/intubation 5. Has repeated low FEV_1 <70% predicted
Status asthmaticus:	Severe airway obstruction and asthmatic symptoms persist despite the administration of standard acute asthma therapy.
Difficult-to-treat asthma:	Failure to achieve asthma control when maximally recommended doses of inhaled therapy are prescribed for at least 6–12 mo
Steroid-resistant Asthma[a]	Failure of FEV_1 or PEF to improve >15% after 14-d course of at least 40 mg/d of prednisone
Steroid-dependent Asthma[a]	Asthma that can be controlled only with oral corticosteroids, but in contrast to corticosteroid-resistance, there is a response to this agent, although only when high doses are given.
Irreversible asthma	Persistent airflow obstruction despite maximum controller therapy; presumably related to airway and parenchymal structural alterations
Near-fatal asthma[b]	Attack associated with respiratory failure, intubation, and/or hemodynamic and metabolic compromise; usually requiring intensive care unit admission
Fixed airway obstruction	Persistent airflow obstruction despite maximal controller therapy; presumably related to airway and parenchymal structural alterations
Brittle asthma[a]	Unstable, unpredictable asthmatics with wide variability in PEF; type I—persistent PEF variability (>40%) despite controller therapy; type II—prone to sudden, dramatic falls in PEF
Asthma related to specific triggers or circumstances	*Premenstrual asthma:* Worsening of asthma 7 d premenstrually. *Aspirin-induced asthma.*

FEV_1, forced expiratory volume in 1 s; PEV, peak expiratory velocity; PEF, peak expiratory flow; ICS, inhaled corticosteroids.
[a]Barnes PJ. Difficult asthma. *Eur Respir J.* 1998.
[b]Romagnoli M, Caramori G, Braccioni F, et al. Near-fatal asthma phenotype in the ENFUMOSA Cohort. *Clin Exp Allergy.* 2007;37:552–557.

- Hyperinflation compromises the force-generating capacity of the diaphragm for a variety of reasons (Fig. 98.3).
- The imbalance between the load faced by the respiratory muscles and their capacity to develop force results in dyspnea and predisposes the respiratory muscle to the development of fatigue, which is a terminal event, likely to be present in an asthmatic crisis, necessitating intubation and mechanical ventilation.

Gas Exchange

- Widespread occlusion of the airways leads to development of extensive areas of alveolar units in which ventilation (V) is severely reduced but perfusion (Q) is maintained; that is, areas with very low $\dot{V}/\dot{Q}$ ratios, frequently lower than 0.1. Intrapulmonary shunt appears to be rare in the majority of

TABLE 98.2

PHENOTYPES OF ASTHMA

Parameter	Description
Natural history	• Early-onset (childhood-onset) • Late-onset (adult-onset)
Type of airway inflammation	• Predominantly eosinophilic • Predominantly neutrophilic • Pauci-inflammatory phenotype
Response to treatment	• Steroid-dependent • Steroid-resistant • Steroid-sensitive
Severity	• Mild • Moderate • Severe • Near-fatal asthma • Fatal asthma
Pattern of broncho-constriction	• Brittle • Stable • Fixed obstruction
Presence or absence of atopy	• Atopic • Nonatopic
Major trigger factor	• Gastric asthma • Aspirin-sensitive asthma • Hormonal asthma

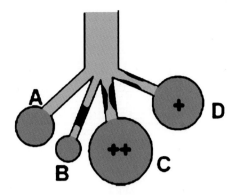

FIGURE 98.2. Effect of varying amounts of airway obstruction on end-expiratory alveolar volumes and pressures. (From Oddo M, Feihl F, Schaller MD, et al. Heliox improves pulsus paradoxus and peak expiratory flow in nonintubated patients with severe asthma. *Intensive Care Med.* 2006;32:501–510, with permission.)

patients because of the collateral ventilation and the effectiveness of the hypoxic pulmonary vasoconstriction. Hypoxemia is, therefore, common in every asthmatic crisis of some severity; mild hypoxia is easily corrected with the administration of relatively low concentrations of supplemental oxygen. More severe hypoxemia and the need for higher concentrations of supplemental oxygen may relate to some contribution of shunt physiology.

• Dead space increases substantially in most severe cases due to alveolar overdistention, that is, areas with very high V̇/Q̇ ratios. This is accompanied by increased CO_2 production from the increased work performed by the respiratory muscles. The respiratory muscles are unable to further increase minute ventilation, and thus hypercapnia ensues.

Cardiovascular System Effects

• Acute severe asthma may also compromise hemodynamics. During expiration, because of the presence of dynamic hyperinflation, increased intrathoracic pressure impedes venous return and increased right ventricular afterload. During the ensuing inspiration, forceful inspiratory muscle contraction

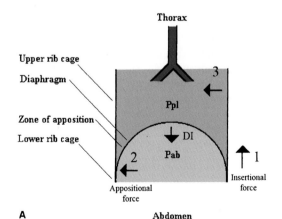

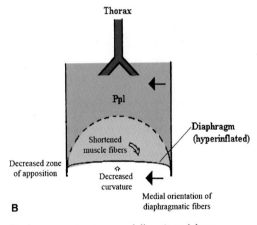

FIGURE 98.3. A: Actions of the diaphragm: When the diaphragm contracts, a caudally oriented force is being applied on the central tendon and the dome of the diaphragm descends (DI). Furthermore, the costal diaphragmatic fibers apply a cranially oriented force to the upper margins of the lower six ribs that has the effect of lifting and rotating them outward (insertional force, *arrow 1*). The zone of apposition makes the lower rib cage part of the abdomen and the changes in pressure in the pleural recess between the apposed diaphragm and the rib cage are almost equal to the changes in abdominal pressure. Pressure in this pleural recess rises rather than falls during inspiration because of diaphragmatic descent, and the rise in abdominal pressure is transmitted through the apposed diaphragm to expand the lower rib cage (*arrow 2*). All these effects result in expansion of the lower rib cage. On the upper rib cage, isolated contraction of the diaphragm causes a decrease in the anteroposterior diameter and this expiratory action is primarily due to the fall in pleural pressure (*arrow 3*). **B:** Deleterious effects of hyperinflation on the diaphragm.

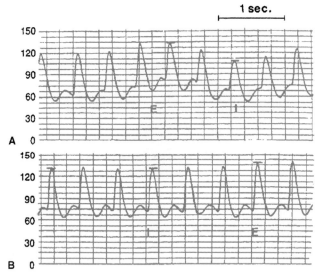

FIGURE 98.4. Arterial pressure of an asthmatic patient when breathing air (**A**) and heliox (**B**). Pulsus paradoxus was lower when the patient was breathing heliox. E, expiration; I, inspiration. (From Manthous CA, Hall JB, Caputo MA, et al. *Am J Respir Crit Care Med.* 1995;151: 310–314, with permission.)

renders intrathoracic pressure negative again, rapidly increasing venous return. Rapid filling of the right ventricle during inspiration shifts the interventricular septum toward the left ventricle, and leads to its incomplete filling during diastole, and thus to left ventricular diastolic dysfunction. The large negative intrathoracic pressure generated during inspiration increases left ventricular afterload and impairs systolic emptying.

- This combined effect leads to the appearance of pulsus paradoxus, defined as a reduction of >10 mm Hg of the arterial systolic pressure during inspiration (Fig. 98.4). A variation >12 mm Hg in systolic blood pressure between inspiration and expiration represents a sign of severity in asthmatic crisis.

TABLE 98.3

PATIENTS AT HIGH RISK OF ASTHMA-RELATED DEATH

- Patients with a history of near-fatal asthma requiring intubation and mechanical ventilation
- Patients who have had a hospitalization or emergency care visit for asthma in the past year
- Patients who are currently using or have recently stopped using oral glucocorticosteroids
- Patients who are not currently using inhaled glucocorticosteroids
- Patients who are overdependent on rapid-acting inhaled β_2-agonists, especially those who use more than one canister of salbutamol (or equivalent) monthly
- Patients with a history of psychiatric disease or psychosocial problems, including the use of sedatives
- Patients with a history of noncompliance with an asthma medication plan

Global Initiative for Asthma. Global strategy for asthma management and prevention. Bethesda, MD: National Institutes of Health, National Heart, Lung, and Blood Institute; 2006.

TABLE 98.4

DIFFERENT PATTERNS OF FATAL ASTHMA

Variable	Scenario of asthma death	
	Type 1	Type 2
Time course	Subacute worsening (days). Slow onset–late arrival	Acute deterioration (hours). Sudden asphyxic asthma
Frequency	≈80%–85%	≈15%–20%
Airways	Extensive mucus plugging	More or less empty bronchi
Inflammation	Eosinophils	Neutrophils
Response to treatment	Slow	Faster
Prevention	Possible	(?)

Clinicopathologic Patterns of Life-threatening Asthmatic Attacks

- Patients at high risk of asthma-related death are described in Table 98.3.
- Two different patterns of fatal asthma are described Table 98.4.

Diagnosis

- There are four parameters that should be investigated before the diagnosis of severe asthma is made for the first time, which are the following:
  - Incorrect diagnosis. The diagnosis of severe asthma is based on a solid confirmation of asthma. In case of doubt, alternative diagnoses should be excluded (Tables 98.5 and 98.6).
  - Continuing exposure to sensitizing agents (see Tables 98.5 and 98.6).
  - Unrecognized aggravating comorbidities (see Tables 98.5 and 98.6).
  - Noncompliance with therapy.
- Clinical evaluation of exacerbations include symptoms, signs, and functional assessment (Table 98.7). In particular, analysis of arterial blood gases is important in the management of patients is useful for decisions regarding hospital admission or tracheal intubation, but it is not predictive of outcome (Table 98.8). Other relevant laboratory data are listed in Table 98.9.

THERAPEUTIC APPROACHES: MANAGEMENT OF ACUTE SEVERE ASTHMA

- The aims of treatment are to relieve airflow obstruction and hypoxemia as quickly as possible, and to plan the prevention of future relapses.
- Schematically, a management plan of acute severe asthma in adults is shown in Table 98.10. These, for acute severe asthma, include the therapies discussed in the following sections.

TABLE 98.5

ALGORITHM OF POSSIBLE STRATEGIES AND RECOMMENDATIONS FOR MANAGING PATIENTS WITH
DIFFICULT-TO-CONTROL ASTHMA DESPITE MAXIMUM COMBINATION TREATMENT

Patients with uncontrolled asthma symptoms with:
1. Persisting refractory symptoms and poor lung function (reduced FEV_1) despite high dose ICS + LABA
2. Frequent use of oral steroids
3. Regular use of health care resources (doctors' consultations, emergency services, hospital admissions)

1. Review inhalation technique	**YES**		
2. Written self-management plan		**POOR COMPLIANCE**	
3. Reassessment at next visit			

NO

	DIAGNOSTIC CONFIRMATION/VERIFICATION FOR		
	DISEASES THAT MIMIC ASTHMA	**CONDITIONS ASSOCIATED WITH ASTHMA**	**UNUSUAL ASTHMA TRIGGER**
	• Bronchiectasis	• Chronic rhinosinusitis	• Occupational exposure
	• Constrictive bronchiolitis	• Gastroesophageal reflux	• Domestic irritants
YES	• COPD	• Anxiety, panic-fear, depression	• Respiratory infections
	• CHF		• Drugs (aspirin, NSAIDs, ACE inhibitors, beta-blockers)
	• Dysfunctional breathlessness	• Dysfunctional breathlessness	
	• Vocal cord dysfunction	• Vocal cord dysfunction	• Food (e.g., sulphite sensitivity)
	• Upper airway obstruction	• Obesity	
	• ABPA	• Obstructive sleep apnea	• Smoking
	• Chung-Strauss syndrome		• Inflamed upper airways
	• Eosinophilic pneumonia		• Acid reflux
	• Thyrotoxicosis		• Stress

SHORT-COURSE ORAL STEROIDS			
NEGATIVE RESPONSE	1. Management of the condition	1. Management of the condition	1. Avoid triggers
	2. Reassess at next visit	2. Reassess at next visit	2. Reassess at next visit

NO
1. Titrate down oral steroids (administer the lowest amount of oral steroid to control/stabilize symptoms).
2. Consider adding a steroid-sparing drug (e.g., azathioprine, methotrexate).
3. Add treatment for steroid-induced adverse effects (e.g., osteoporosis).
4. If uncontrolled, consider alternative therapeutic options (e.g., omalizumab, etanercept, high-dose IVIG).
5. Frequent periodic re-evaluations.

FEV_1, forced expiratory volume in 1 s; ICS, inhaled corticosteroids; LABA, long-acting β-agonists; COPD, chronic obstructive pulmonary disease; CHF, congestive heart failure; ABPA, allergic bronchopulmonary aspergillosis; NSAIDs, nonsteroidal anti-inflammatory drugs; ACE, angiotensin-converting enzyme.
Adapted from Holgate ST, Polosa R. The mechanisms, diagnosis, and management of severe asthma in adults. *Lancet.* 2006;368(9537):780–793.

Oxygen

• High-flow oxygen should be given to all patients with acute severe asthma, as these individuals are hypoxemic. Unlike patients with chronic obstructive pulmonary disease, there is little danger of precipitating hypercapnia with high-flow oxygen. Hypercapnia indicates the development of near-fatal asthma and the need for emergency specialist/anesthetic intervention. Oxygen therapy should be titrated against pulse oximetry (SaO2 92% to 94%) to maintain satisfactory oxygen saturation.

β_2-Agonist Bronchodilators

• Inhaled β_2-agonists are the cornerstone of asthma treatment. Continuous or repetitive nebulization of rapid-acting β_2-agonists is the safest and most effective means of reversing airflow obstruction and should be administered as early as possible.

• Continuous nebulization of β_2-agonists is at least as efficacious as bolus nebulization in relieving acute asthma. In severe asthma, with peak expiratory flow (PEF) <50% of personal best or FEV_1 <50% predicted, and asthma that is poorly responsive to an initial bolus dose of β_2-agonist, continuous nebulization should be considered. However, studies have shown no difference in the effects of continuous versus intermittent administration of nebulized albuterol. Although albuterol has been used occasionally intravenously (IV) for severe asthma attack, its use by this route does not lead to significant clinical improvements when compared with the inhalation route.

• The subcutaneous route of epinephrine (0.01 mg/kg, divided into three doses of approximately 0.3 mg given at 20-minute

TABLE 98.6

HISTORY AND PHYSICAL EXAMINATION OF PATIENTS WITH DIFFICULT-TO-CONTROL ASTHMA

Medical history

History of asthma development
- Age of asthma onset
- Atopic syndrome and family history of asthma
- Management of disease and response to treatment
- Smoking history

Severity of disease
- Severe asthma exacerbations and hospitalization in past year
- Any admissions to asthma centers
- Any number of ICU admissions

Exogenous aggravating factors
- Exposure to allergens, occupational agents, chemicals
- Use of aspirin, NSAIDs, beta-blockers, ACE inhibitors, estrogens
- Influence of foods or food additives (nitrite, sulphate)

Endogenous aggravating factors
- Rhinosinusitis or previous surgery for nasal polyps
- Gastroesophageal reflux
- History of psychiatric disease
- Obstructive sleep apnea

Influence of menstruation

Miscellaneous

Adherence with medications

Adverse effects of treatment

Psychosocial circumstances

Physical examination (specific points of attention)
- Body mass index
- Evidence of comorbidities (e.g., nasal polyps)
- Evidence of alternative diagnoses (e.g., cardiac failure)
- Evidence of adverse effects of treatment

ICU, intensive care unit; NSAID, nonsteroidal anti-inflammatory drugs; ACE, angiotensin-converting enzyme.
Bel EH. Severe asthma. *Breathe*. December 2006;3(2):129–139.

intervals) or terbutaline (0.25 mg, which can be repeated every 20 minutes for three doses) might, however, be useful in several situations and should be considered:
- In children in whom inhaled agents are often difficult to administer. In addition, the pediatric population has a reduced susceptibility to β_1 toxicity, making subcutaneous administration a useful route of drug delivery.
- In seriously ill asthmatic patients with impending respiratory arrest in whom rapid delivery of β-agonists to the airway is desirable.
- In patients unable to cooperate secondary to depression of mental status, apnea, coma.

Steroids

- Systemic corticosteroids in adequate doses should be administered in all cases of acute asthma, especially if:
  - The initial rapid-acting inhaled β_2-agonist therapy fails to achieve lasting improvement
  - The exacerbation develops even though the patient was already taking oral glucocorticosteroids

- Previous exacerbations required oral glucocorticosteroids
- Minimal or no side effects occur with a single large dose of IV steroid. Some enhancement of β-agonist effect may be seen as early as 1 hour; however, 4 to 6 hours are required for anti-inflammatory activity. One common approach is the IV administration of 60 to 125 mg of methylprednisolone every 6 hours during the initial 24 to 48 hours of treatment (Table 98.11), followed by 60 to 80 mg daily in improving patients, with gradual tapering during the next 2 weeks.

Anticholinergics

- Although ipratropium produces less bronchodilatation at peak effect than a β-agonist and is associated with a less predictable clinical response, literature in general supports the use of ipratropium as adjunctive therapy in patients with acute severe asthma. The nebulizer dose is 0.5 mg.

Magnesium

- Magnesium's potential to reverse bronchoconstriction is multifactorial and is based on characteristics of inhibition of the calcium channel and decreased acetylcholine release.
- A single dose of IV magnesium sulphate (2 g) should be considered for patients with:
  - Acute severe asthma, with FEV_1 25% to 30% predicted at presentation
  - Adults and children who fail to respond to initial treatment
  - Life-threatening or near-fatal asthma

Antibiotics

- Routine administration of antibiotics is not indicated and should be reserved for those with evidence of infection such as pneumonia or sinusitis. When an infection precipitates an exacerbation of asthma, it is likely to be viral in nature.

Helium–Oxygen Therapy

- A blended mixture of helium and oxygen (heliox) is available in mixtures of 60:40, 70:30, and 80:20. Heliox is less dense than air and can be delivered through a tight-fitting nonrebreathing mask or, in the intubated patient, through the ventilatory circuit. This less dense gas mixture results in decreased airway resistance. Heliox may have potential benefit in delaying need for intubation while bronchodilators exert their effect, as well as decreasing peak airway pressures and auto PEEP in the mechanically ventilated patient.

Sedatives and Hypnotics

- Sedation should be used with caution during exacerbations of asthma because of the respiratory depressant effect of anxiolytic and hypnotic drugs. An association between the use of these drugs and avoidable asthma deaths has been demonstrated. Ketamine has sedative and analgesic properties that may be useful if intubation is planned.

TABLE 98.7

CLINICAL AND FUNCTIONAL ASSESSMENT OF SEVERE ASTHMA EXACERBATIONS[a]

Variable	Severe exacerbation	Imminent respiratory arrest
SYMPTOMS		
Dyspnea	At rest	
	Hunched forward	
Speech	Single words, not sentences or phrases	
Alertness	Usually agitated	Drowsy or confused
SIGNS		
Respiratory rate	Often >30 breaths/min	
Heart rate	>120 beats/min	Bradycardia
Pulsus paradoxus	Often present >25 mm Hg	Absence suggests respiratory muscle fatigue
Use of accessory muscles and suprasternal reactions	Usually evident	Abdominal paradox (paradoxical thoracoabdominal movement)
Wheeze	Usually loud	Absence of wheeze "Silent chest"
FUNCTIONAL ASSESSMENT		
PEF (after initial bronchodilator, % predicted or% personal best)	<60% of predicted or personal best (<100 L/min adults) Or Response lasts <2 hours	
PaO_2	<60 mm Hg Possible cyanosis	
$PaCO_2$	>42 mm Hg Possible respiratory failure	
SpO_2	<90%	

PEF, peak expiratory flow.
[a]The presence of several parameters, but not necessarily all, indicates the general classification of the exacerbation.
Adapted from Global Initiative for Asthma. Global strategy for asthma management and prevention. Bethesda, MD: National Institutes of Health, National Heart, Lung, and Blood Institute; 2006.

REFERRAL TO THE INTENSIVE CARE UNIT

- All patients transferred to the ICU should be accompanied by a physician suitably equipped and skilled to perform endotracheal intubation, if necessary. Indications for admission to intensive care facilities or a high-dependency unit include patients requiring ventilatory support and those with severe acute or life-threatening asthma who are failing to respond to therapy, as evidenced by:
- Deteriorating PEF
- Persisting or worsening hypoxia
- Hypercapnia
- Worsening acidosis
- Exhaustion, feeble respiration
- Drowsiness, confusion
- Coma or respiratory arrest

Admission Decisions

Criteria for Discharge from the Emergency Department versus Hospitalization

- Criteria for determining whether a patient should be discharged from the emergency department or admitted to the hospital have been succinctly reviewed and stratified based on consensus. Patients with a pretreatment FEV_1 or PEF <25% of predicted/personal best, or those with a posttreatment FEV_1 or PEF <40% of predicted/personal best, require hospitalization.

TABLE 98.8

STAGING SEVERE ASTHMA CRISIS BY ARTERIAL BLOOD GASES

	Stage 1	Stage 2	Stage 3	Stage 4	Stage 5
PaCO	Normal	↓ $PaCO_2$	↓ $PaCO_2$	Normal	↑ $PaCO_2$ (respiratory failure)
PaO_2	Normal	Normal PaO_2 (hyperventilation has led to normalization of PaO_2).	↓ PaO_2 (hyperventilation is now unable to compensate totally for a widened $P(A - a)O_2$.	↓↓↓ PaO_2 (inspiratory fatigue is now prominent).	↓↓↓PaO_2. These findings indicate an impending respiratory arrest.

LABORATORY INVESTIGATIONS AND DIAGNOSTIC
TESTS FOR PATIENTS WITH
DIFFICULT-TO-CONTROL ASTHMA

Diagnostic tests
- Peripheral blood
- Erythrocyte sedimentation rate
- Full blood count (eosinophils)
- Total serum IgE
- Specific IgE to common and less common allergens
- Free-T4, thyroid-stimulating hormone

Lung function
- Spirometry (pre- and postbronchodilator)
- Lung volumes
- Arterial blood gases
- Histamine challenge test

Radiology
- Chest radiography
- Sinus CT scan

Additional tests for comorbidities and alternative diagnoses
- Nasal endoscopy
- 24-hour esophageal pH monitoring or trial with proton pump inhibitors
- Polysomnography
- Bronchoscopy
- High-resolution CT scan of the thorax
- D-dimer
- ANCA
- IgG against Aspergillus fumigatus

Ig, immunoglobulin; CT, computed tomography; ANCA,
antineutrophilic cytoplasmic antibody.
Bel EH. Severe asthma. *Breathe* 2006;3(2):129–139.

Indications for Mechanical Ventilation Support

- Careful and repeat assessment of patients with severe exacerbations is mandatory. Not all patients admitted to the ICU need invasive mechanical ventilation and a trial of 1 to 2 hours of non invasive ventilation (BiPAP) can be scheduled for patients in distress but fully alert. When used, noninvasive positive pressure ventilation should be started with low levels of inspiratory pressure support (5–10 cm H_2O) and PEEP (3–5 cm H_2O). Pressure support should be progressively increased by 2 cm H_2O every 15 minutes, the goal being to reduce respiratory rate <25 breaths/minute, while keeping peak inspiratory pressure <25 cm H_2O. Future prospective randomized controlled trials are required to definitely establish the role of noninvasive positive pressure ventilation in acute severe asthma.
- The exact time to intubate is based mainly on clinical judgment:
  - Patients presenting with apnea or coma should be intubated immediately.
  - Progressive exhaustion, patient fatigue, and worsening hypercapnia despite maximal therapy including noninvasive ventilation, together with altered level of consciousness, are indications for intubation.

Intubation

- A larger endotracheal tube reduces flow-resistive pressure during inspiration, but this is not important during controlled mechanical ventilation. Given the extraordinary high resistance of the patient's airways, the effect of the larger-bore tube on expiratory flow is also trivial. Intubation should be performed by the most skilled operator available to avoid repeated airway manipulation, which may induce laryngospasm and bronchoconstriction. Table 98.12 summarizes drugs used to facilitate intubation of patients with severe asthma.

Invasive Mechanical Ventilation

- The main strategy of ventilatory support is to minimize hyperinflation and avoid excessive airway pressure development (overdistention). Thus, controlled hypoventilation or permissive hypercapnia is often required.
- For any level of minute ventilation and with constant (square wave) inspiratory flow rate, end-inspiratory lung distention is minimized by a combination of low tidal volume (V_T) and high respiratory rate. This is because in the inhomogeneous asthmatic lung, most of the tidal volume delivered by positive-pressure ventilation goes to the parts of lung parenchyma with almost normal mechanical characteristics Because such "mechanically normal" areas represent only a small fraction of the total asthmatic lung, they become overdistended. Thus, the lower tidal volume would cause less end-inspiratory lung overdistention.
- When keeping minute ventilation, tidal volume, and respiratory rate constant, increasing inspiratory flow allows inspiratory time (T_I) to be reduced and thus expiratory time (T_E) to be increased. When minute ventilation is high (>10 L/minute), increasing inspiratory flow and thus reducing T_I allows a decrease in lung hyperinflation. At any given minute ventilation, inspiratory flow should be 60 to 80 L/minute, as further prolonging T_E by greater inspiratory flow will not significantly reduce hyperinflation.
- Four common causes of acute deterioration in any intubated patient are recalled by the mnemonic DOPE (tube **D**isplacement, tube **O**bstruction, **P**neumothorax, **E**quipment failure). Another common cause of deterioration common in asthmatics is the occurrence of dynamic overinflation (auto-PEEP),
- Dynamic hyperinflation can be monitored in two different ways:
  - By measuring the volume passively exhaled from end-inspiration to the static functional residual capacity in the course of a prolonged apnea and subtracting the delivered tidal volume (V_{EI}): Although this is the most accurate way of measuring dynamic hyperinflation and estimating the attendant risks of hypotension and barotrauma, the need for complete muscle relaxation, with its potential complications (see later discussion), and practical aspects of the measurement reduce its clinical applicability. Furthermore, it cannot measure the volume of air trapped behind closed airways (compartment and C).
  - By measuring the average pressure developed in the airways at the end of expiration (PEEPi) after occluding the airways and allowing sufficient time for equilibration (the end-expiratory occlusion technique): This pressure represents the average recoil pressure of the respiratory

TABLE 98.10

MANAGEMENT OF ACUTE SEVERE ASTHMA IN ADULTS IN THE EMERGENCY DEPARTMENT

ALGORITHM OF POSSIBLE STRATEGIES AND RECOMMENDATIONS FOR MANAGING PATIENTS WITH DIFFICULT-TO-CONTROL ASTHMA DESPITE MAXIMUM COMBINATION TREATMENT

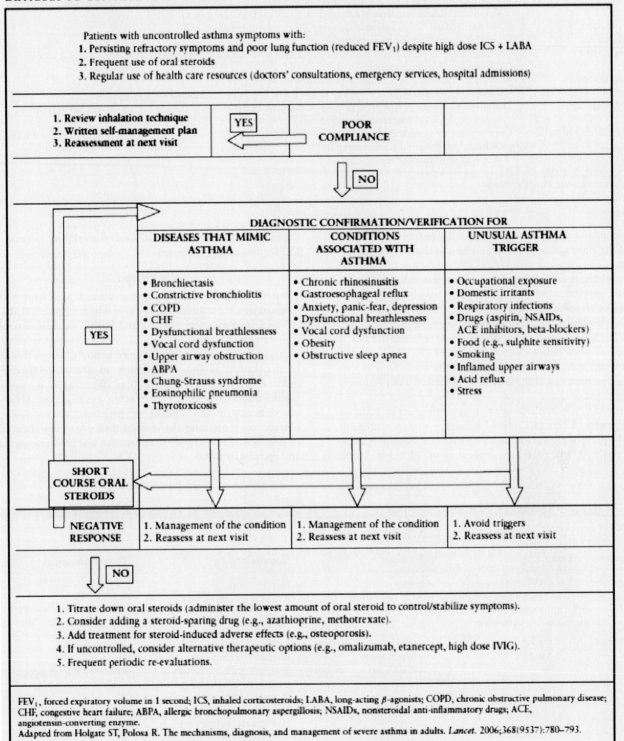

Patients with uncontrolled asthma symptoms with:
1. Persisting refractory symptoms and poor lung function (reduced FEV_1) despite high dose ICS + LABA
2. Frequent use of oral steroids
3. Regular use of health care resources (doctors' consultations, emergency services, hospital admissions)

| 1. Review inhalation technique
2. Written self-management plan
3. Reassessment at next visit | YES ← | POOR COMPLIANCE |

NO

DIAGNOSTIC CONFIRMATION/VERIFICATION FOR

DISEASES THAT MIMIC ASTHMA	CONDITIONS ASSOCIATED WITH ASTHMA	UNUSUAL ASTHMA TRIGGER
• Bronchiectasis • Constrictive bronchiolitis • COPD • CHF • Dysfunctional breathlessness • Vocal cord dysfunction • Upper airway obstruction • ABPA • Chung-Strauss syndrome • Eosinophilic pneumonia • Thyrotoxicosis	• Chronic rhinosinusitis • Gastroesophageal reflux • Anxiety, panic-fear, depression • Dysfunctional breathlessness • Vocal cord dysfunction • Obesity • Obstructive sleep apnea	• Occupational exposure • Domestic irritants • Respiratory infections • Drugs (aspirin, NSAIDs, ACE inhibitors, beta-blockers) • Food (e.g., sulphite sensitivity) • Smoking • Inflamed upper airways • Acid reflux • Stress

YES

| SHORT COURSE ORAL STEROIDS | | |

| NEGATIVE RESPONSE | 1. Management of the condition
2. Reassess at next visit | 1. Management of the condition
2. Reassess at next visit | 1. Avoid triggers
2. Reassess at next visit |

NO

1. Titrate down oral steroids (administer the lowest amount of oral steroid to control/stabilize symptoms).
2. Consider adding a steroid-sparing drug (e.g., azathioprine, methotrexate).
3. Add treatment for steroid-induced adverse effects (e.g., osteoporosis).
4. If uncontrolled, consider alternative therapeutic options (e.g., omalizumab, etanercept, high dose IVIG).
5. Frequent periodic re-evaluations.

FEV_1, forced expiratory volume in 1 second; ICS, inhaled corticosteroids; LABA, long-acting β-agonists; COPD, chronic obstructive pulmonary disease; CHF, congestive heart failure; ABPA, allergic bronchopulmonary aspergillosis; NSAIDs, nonsteroidal anti-inflammatory drugs; ACE, angiotensin-converting enzyme.
Adapted from Holgate ST, Polosa R. The mechanisms, diagnosis, and management of severe asthma in adults. *Lancet.* 2006;368(9537):780–793.

PEF, peak expiratory flow; FEV_1, forced expiratory volume in 1 second; IV, intravenously; CXR, chest x-ray; VM, ventimask.

TABLE 98.11

PHARMACOLOGIC TREATMENT IN THE EMERGENCY DEPARTMENT

Agent	Dose
Salbutamol	2.5 mg (0.5 mL) in 2.5 mL normal saline by nebulization continuously, or every 15–20 min until a significant clinical response is achieved or serious side effects appear
Epinephrine	0.3–0.4 mL of a 1:1,000 solution SC every 20 min for three doses
Terbutaline	Preferable to epinephrine in pregnancy
β-Agonists IV	IV administration should be considered in patients who have not responded to inhaled or SC, in whom respiratory arrest is imminent
Corticosteroids	Methylprednisolone 60–125 mg IV or prednisone 40 mg *per os.*
Anticholinergics	Ipratropium bromide 0.5 mg by nebulization every 1–4 hours, combined with salbutamol
Methylxanthines	Theophylline 5 mg/kg IV over 30 min—loading dose in patients not already taking theophylline, followed by 0.4 mg/kg/h IV maintenance dose. Serum levels should be checked within 6 h.
Magnesium sulfate	Usually given as a single 2-g infusion IV over 20 min, only following consultation with senior medical staff. Nebulized salbutamol administered in isotonic magnesium sulfate provides greater benefit than if it is delivered in normal saline.

SC, subcutaneously; IV, intravenously.

system at the end of expiration and is an indirect measure of the end expiratory lung volume and thus of hyperinflation.

- The addition of PEEP during controlled mechanical ventilation in asthma patients results in a variable and unpredictable response. In some patients, extrinsic PEEP (PEEPe) causes overinflation; in others, functional reserve capacity and PEEPi are decreased; and in still others no response to PEEP is observed until PEEPe exceeds baseline PEEPi. This might be due to the great heterogeneity of the asthmatic lung with various combinations of the previously described compartments in each patient.
- When PEEPe is applied—a stepwise application of PEEP in increments of 2 cm H_2O every 5 minutes—with measurement of the plateau pressure at each step might be a useful bedside approach. If Pplat decreases, application of PEEPe is deflating

the lung and is beneficial; if plateau pressure (Pplat) increases, PEEPe should be withdrawn.

Weaning

- Once dynamic hyperinflation has abated sufficiently, as assessed by a substantial resolution of wheezing on chest auscultation and decrease of Pplat and PEEPi, weaning should be initiated using standard procedures. Suppression of respiratory muscle activity with controlled hypoventilation should be maintained as short as possible to prevent ventilator-induced diaphragmatic dysfunction. Weaning is normally rapidly achieved in patients with acute severe asthma. Weaning difficulty in the absence of persistent severe airway obstruction must raise the suspicion of myopathy induced by previous administration of neuromuscular blocking agents and corticosteroids.

TABLE 98.12

DRUGS USED FOR INTUBATION IN ACUTE SEVERE ASTHMA

Agents	Dose	Advantages	Side effects	Contraindications
Midazolam	1 mg (IV) slowly, every 2–3 min until the patient allows positioning and airways inspection	Amnesia Muscle relaxation	Hypotension Respiratory depression	
Ketamine	1–2 mg/kg (IV) at a rate of 0.5 mg/kg/min	No respiratory depression No hypotension Short-term bronchodilation	Increased laryngeal reflexes Increased laryngeal secretions Sympathomimetic effects (hypertension, tachycardia) Increased intracranial pressure Delirium Hallucinations (prevented by midazolam coadministration)	Atherosclerosis Hypertension Increased intracranial pressure
Propofol	60–80 mg/min initial IV infusion up to 2.0 mg/kg	Rapid onset and resolution of sedation Bronchodilation	Hypotension Respiratory depression	Hemodynamic instability

IV, intravenously.

CHAPTER 99 ■ ACUTE RESPIRATORY FAILURE IN CHRONIC OBSTRUCTIVE PULMONARY DISEASE

- Chronic obstructive pulmonary diseases (COPDs) are a group of disorders characterized by airflow limitation that is not fully reversible. There are several diseases under this designation (Table 99.1), the most common of which are chronic bronchitis and emphysema. These two disorders represent the extremes of the COPD spectrum and usually coexist in COPD patients. Bronchitis is predominantly a disease of the airways and presents as a chronic productive cough for at least 3 months during 2 consecutive years, whereas emphysema is a disease of the parenchyma and consists of permanent airspace enlargement associated with rupture of the alveolar septa.
- The common final pathway leading to COPD is an increased inflammatory response to inhaled particles or gases, of which the most common is cigarette smoke. This inflammatory process involves the airways and the lung parenchyma, leading to mucosal gland hypertrophy and disruption of alveolar septa with loss of elastic recoil. These alterations ultimately lead to the obstructive ventilatory defect that defines COPD. Some patients develop pulmonary hyperinflation caused by the loss of elastic recoil and increased airway resistance. During exacerbations, there might be a secondary dynamic pulmonary hyperinflation caused by the increased ventilatory requirement and shortened expiratory time. The capacity of the respiratory muscles to generate inspiratory pressure is limited by their shortened operating length and impaired geometric arrangement. Long-term steroid use and/or malnutrition also contribute to strength impairment in many patients with severe chronic disease.
- Rarely, the disease results from an inborn imbalance between the proteases and antiproteases present in the lung, as occurs in the autosomal recessive α_1-antitrypsin deficiency.

CLINICAL FINDINGS

- There is initially a slow decline in lung function that goes unnoticed over the years. Cough is the first finding, usually after the patient has been a smoker for many years. The dyspnea worsens slowly over time, although sometimes patients deny the deterioration of lung function because they slowly adapt their level of activity to their exercise capacity. The decrease in lung function might become steeper during exacerbations, with a slow recovery to baseline levels after resolution of the decompensation
- The ratio of the forced expiratory volume in the first second of the exhalation (FEV_1) to the forced vital capacity is diagnostic of an obstructive ventilatory defect if <0.7. The FEV_1 is a useful marker of the disease severity (Table 99.2) and is well suited as a longitudinal monitor of lung function.
- Both total lung capacity and residual volume may be increased because of loss of lung elastic recoil. The carbon monoxide diffusing capacity may be diminished with the progression of the disease, reflecting the loss of the functional parenchyma.

TABLE 99.1

DISEASES ASSOCIATED WITH CHRONIC OBSTRUCTIVE PULMONARY DISEASE

Chronic bronchitis
Emphysema
Bronchiolitis
Bronchiectasis
Tuberculosis
α_1-Trypsin deficiency

TABLE 99.2

CLASSIFICATION OF SEVERITY ACCORDING TO GOLD

Stage	Characteristics
0: At risk	Normal spirometry Chronic symptoms (cough, sputum production)
I: Mild COPD	$FEV_1/FVC <70\%$ $FEV_1 = 80\%$ predicted With or without chronic symptoms (cough, sputum production)
II: Moderate COPD	$FEV_1/FVC <70\%$ $50\% = FEV_1 <80\%$ predicted With or without chronic symptoms (cough, sputum production)
III: Severe COPD	$FEV_1/FVC <70\%$ $30\% = FEV_1 <50\%$ predicted With or without chronic symptoms (cough, sputum production)
IV: Very severe COPD	$FEV_1/FVC <70\%$ $FEV_1 <30\%$ predicted or FEV_1 $<50\%$ predicted plus chronic respiratory failure

GOLD, Global Initiative for Chronic Obstructive Lung Disease; COPD, chronic obstructive pulmonary disease; FEV_1, forced expiratory volume in the first second of the exhalation; FVC, forced vital capacity. From Rabe KF, Hurd S, Anzueto A, et al. Global Strategy for the Diagnosis, Management, and Prevention of Chronic Obstructive Pulmonary Disease: Gold Executive Summary. *Am J Respir Crit Care Med.* 2007;176:532–555.

EXACERBATION

- COPD exacerbation can be defined as an increase in dyspnea, cough, or sputum production that requires therapy. The two most commonly identified precipitating factors are infection—viral, such as *Rhinovirus* spp. or influenza, and bacterial, such as *Haemophilus influenzae, Streptococcus pneumoniae, Moraxella catarrhalis, Enterobacteriaceae* spp., or *Pseudomonas* spp.—as well as environmental exposure to air pollutants. However, in about one-third of cases, no underlying cause is identified. Infectious agents can also be recovered from some patients with stable COPD, indicating that in some instances, their presence in decompensated COPD represents an epiphenomenon.

Treatment of Exacerbations

- Admission criteria according to the American Thoracic Society/European Respiratory Society guidelines include:
  - High-risk comorbidities including pneumonia, cardiac arrhythmia, congestive heart failure, diabetes mellitus, renal failure, or liver failure
  - Inadequate response of symptoms to outpatient management
  - Marked increase in dyspnea
  - Inability to eat or sleep because of symptoms
  - Worsening hypoxemia
  - Worsening hypercapnia
  - Changes in mental status
  - Inability to care for oneself (i.e., lack of home support)
  - Uncertain diagnosis
- The mainstay of pharmacologic treatment is the use of bronchodilators, corticosteroids, and antibiotics, which are discussed in the following sections.

Bronchodilators

- β_2-Agonists: The bronchodilators most commonly used are the inhaled short-acting β_2-agonists because of their rapid onset of action. Same considerations of the section dedicated to severe asthma are applicable here. Long-acting β_2-agonists can also be considered. Subcutaneous or intravenous administration should not be used unless there is contraindication for the inhaled route because of their increased systemic effects.

Corticosteroids

- Steroids are usually recommended for exacerbations of COPD. If feasible, prednisone can be given orally at a dose of 30 to 40 mg/day for 10 to 14 days. If the oral route is not an option, hydrocortisone or methylprednisolone can be substituted in equivalent doses. Some investigators advocate the use of much higher doses (methylprednisolone, 125 mg intravenously four times daily).
- Recently, the combination of salmeterol, 50 μg, and fluticasone, 500 μg, given twice daily, has been compared with placebo and resulted in a reduction in mortality of 3 years ($p = 0.052$), fewer exacerbations, and improved health status and lung function.

Antibiotics

- Antibiotics decrease mortality during exacerbations. These agents are indicated when there is increased production or change in the color of the sputum. For mild exacerbations, amoxicillin, sulfamethoxazole-trimethoprim, or doxycycline for 7 to 10 days is usually adequate. Patients requiring hospitalizations should receive penicillin/penicillinase (e.g., amoxicillin/clavulanate), a respiratory quinolone (levofloxacin, gatifloxacin, moxifloxacin), or a third-generation cephalosporin together with a macrolide (e.g., ceftriaxone plus clarithromycin). In addition to their antimicrobial activity, macrolides possess anti-inflammatory and mucoregulatory properties that may confer beneficial effects to patients with COPD.

Respiratory Support

- The goal of respiratory support in patients with exacerbations of COPD is to correct hypoxemia/acidemia and reduce the respiratory work, thus avoiding respiratory muscle fatigue.

Oxygen Therapy

- To improve the hypoxemia commonly present in exacerbations of COPD, controlled oxygen therapy is the cornerstone of hospital treatment. Long-term oxygen therapy is established as the standard of care for selected patients with advanced chronic stable hypoxemia due to COPD. However, in the acute setting, some patients have an impaired response to hypercapnia when treated with supplementary oxygen, leading to worsening of CO_2 retention. Venturi masks are more accurate sources of oxygen than are nasal prongs, but they are more likely to be removed by the patient.
- Controlled oxygen therapy must be started at a low inspiratory oxygen fraction—0.24 to 0.28—and titrated upward to reach a $PaO_2 \geq 60$ mm Hg or $SaO_2 \geq 90\%$ without significant retention of CO_2. A clinically significant increase in $PaCO_2$ has been arbitrarily defined as a raise in CO_2 of 6.5 mm Hg, especially if clinical mental deterioration occurs.

Noninvasive Mechanical Ventilation

- Noninvasive positive pressure ventilation is an alternative treatment for patients admitted to the hospital with hypercapnic respiratory failure secondary to acute exacerbation of COPD that is associated to a lower rate of complication than invasive ventilation. Many studies have shown that noninvasive positive pressure ventilation increases pH, reduces $PaCO_2$, reduces the severity of breathlessness in the first 4 hours of treatment and decreases the length of hospital stay. More importantly, mortality and the intubation rate are consistently reduced by this intervention. In clinical-physiological terms, the expected elevation of pH after 1 hour of treatment should be around 0.03 (95% CI, 0.02 to 0.04) and the expected reduction in $PaCO_2$ in the same interval around –3.0 mm Hg (95% CI, –5.1 to –0.2).
- Unfortunately, noninvasive ventilation is not appropriate for all patients. Failure rates between 9% and 50% have been reported. One important signal that this procedure is not working for a patient is the progression—even slight—of

hypercapnia or acidosis 30 to 60 minutes after the procedure, and deterioration of the mental status.
- The classic indications for noninvasive mechanical ventilation in exacerbated COPD patients are:
  - Respiratory distress with respiratory rate >30 to 35 breaths/minute
  - Respiratory acidosis with a pH <7.35, and with normal or high standard base excess
  - PaO_2 <45 mm Hg.
- Noninvasive mechanical ventilation is contraindicated for patients with profound bradypnea, defined as a respiratory rate <12 breaths/minute, severe hypercapnic encephalopathy with Glasgow Coma Scale score <10, cardiac and/or respiratory arrest, and hemodynamic instability.
- There are many approaches to set the noninvasive ventilation. An easy way is to set the expiratory pressure at 5 cm H_2O, the inspiratory pressure at 10 cm H_2O—resulting in a "delta P" of 5 cm H_2O—and to increase the delta P in increments of 5 cm H_2O, up to 20 to 25 cm H_2O or the maximum tolerated, over 1 hour. An alternative approach is to adjust the inspiratory pressure in order to obtain a tidal volume of 6 to 8 mL/kg and a respiratory rate of 25 to 30 breaths/minute, setting the end-expiratory pressure to 5 cm H_2O to offset the inspiratory threshold induced by intrinsic PEEP.
- If inspiratory comfort is not achieved, especially when wasted inspiratory efforts are visible without a prompt response from the ventilator, meaning that the patient effort is not enough to easily trigger the assisted breath, trials of 2 cm H_2O elevations in the PEEP/CPAP levels must be performed in order to further reduce the extra load imposed by the intrinsic PEEP. During these trials of augmentation of external PEEP, the minimum inspiratory pressure should be provided that maintains a stable tidal volume. Oxygen should be offered to keep oxygen saturation >85% to 90%.
- The choice for an appropriate mask is an important aspect of noninvasive mechanical ventilation. In general, patients benefit from a facial mask that covers the mouth and the nose; this is more efficient than the nasal type to deliver effective inspiratory pressures. Leaks directed at the eyes, sores in the nasal area, and a dry mouth are frequent causes of extreme discomfort to patients. The total face mask may be better tolerated by some patients, but not all, and greatly reduces the skin sores. However, one has to be aware that the anatomic dead space may increase a bit with this mask, which also imposes some challenges to the mechanical ventilator in terms of synchrony and PEEP maintenance.

Invasive Mechanical Ventilation

- Invasive mechanical ventilation can be either the initial choice in patients with COPD exacerbation or the strategy to be applied after failure of a trial of noninvasive ventilation.
- Assuming that all appropriate measures to improve airflow obstruction have already been taken (see section on asthma), minimization of dynamic hyperinflation is a key objective of the ventilatory support of these COPD patients.
- There is no optimal ventilation modality to support exacerbated COPD patients. The peak airway pressure may reach high values in the volume-controlled mode, but this is of limited clinical relevance because most of this pressure is dissipated in the large airways and, consequently, it does not reflect the alveolar pressure. One limitation of the volume-

controlled mode is the impossibility of continuously monitoring the plateau pressure, as the use of an inspiratory pause every breath may worsen dynamic hyperinflation. On the other hand, in the pressure-controlled mode, conditions of fluctuating airway resistance and auto-PEEP entail the risk of variable tidal volume, with sometimes unacceptably low alveolar ventilation. Furthermore, with this latter mode, severe respiratory alkalosis may develop if airway obstruction subsides rapidly.
- Although there is no clear advantage of one over the other, volume-controlled ventilation is currently the preferred mode by most investigators. The use of decelerating-flow waveform usually minimizes peak pressure, allowing full delivery of the tidal volume, with less interruption by opening of the pop-off safety valve. By forcing a slower flow at the end of inspiration, this flow waveform could result in two theoretical benefits: (i) less overdistention of alveoli distal to the least obstructed airways, and (ii) slightly better CO_2 exchange. When initiating mechanical ventilation in the pressure-controlled mode, one must keep in mind that the inspiratory time should be set in proportion to the inspiratory time constant in order to deliver the desired tidal volume with the lowest possible plateau pressure. Thus, patients with increased airways resistance will need a longer inspiratory time. For a fixed respiratory rate, the increase in inspiratory time always occurs at the expense of a shortening of the expiratory time, which might aggravate pulmonary hyperinflation. Therefore, the ideal inspiratory time would optimize delivery of tidal volume without increasing air trapping. That will occur if, when looking at the flow-volume curve, both end-inspiratory and end-expiratory flows are equal or close to zero.
- After choosing the best respiratory rate and inspiratory and expiratory times, the physician has to decide on how much PEEP to apply. The sequence approach has been described in Chapter 96.
- As soon as possible, the ventilation mode should be switched from controlled to assisted ventilation in order to decrease muscle atrophy. There are no objective indicators of the best moment to start assisted ventilation; therefore, at least daily trials of assisted ventilation should be made, with close monitoring of patient comfort and plateau pressure. Humidification should be achieved with a heated humidifier, not with heat and moisture exchangers. The latter devices are undesirable for three reasons:
  - They increase expiratory airway resistance, which would hardly be of any help to reduce hyperinflation.
  - When inserted between the tracheal tube and the Y-piece of ventilator tubing, they increase dead space and, therefore, contribute unnecessarily to hypercapnia.
  - The efficacy of any inhalational medication will be blunted by the heat and moisture exchanger.
- Weaning from the ventilator should be initiated as soon as possible in order to avoid mechanical ventilator-associated complications. According to recent published experiences of two specialized weaning units, 19% of patients with COPD exacerbation remained partially dependent on the ventilator. The classic rapid shallow breathing criterion (<80 breaths/minute/L) was met by 56% of COPD patients who failed the weaning trial. General patient condition and subjective dyspnea seemed to be more effective predictors of success of extubation than quantifiable indexes. Using

spontaneous breathing trials or progressive reduction in pressure support is equally effective to wean the patient from the ventilator. Automatic algorithms for pressure support reduction are available today, which resulted in a faster weaning process when compared with the physician-driven approach.

- If the spontaneous breathing trial is chosen, it can be applied for at least 30 minutes, up to 2 hours once a day. After tracheal decannulation, the use of intermittent or continuous support with noninvasive mechanical ventilation for at least 24 hours is strongly recommended, using settings similar to those used during conventional ventilation weaning. The last technique is associated with higher rates of extubation success, lower length of stay in the intensive care unit and/or hospital, and a lower mortality at 60 days. A recent alternative strategy of weaning implies early use of PSV and early extubation with support "switched" to noninvasive mechanical ventilation using the same ventilatory settings as before tracheal decannulation. This approach is associated with less ventilator-associated pneumonia, a shorter length of stay in the intensive care unit, and a lower mortality rate.

CHAPTER 100 ■ PULMONARY EMBOLISM (PE)

- PE remains an underrecognized and lethal entity
  - Estimates suggest it affects more than 600,000 patients per year in the United States.
  - PE causes or contributes to 50,000 to 200,000 deaths per year.
  - Incidence of PE causing, contributing to, or accompanying death in hospitalized patients relatively constant at 15% for the past 40 years.
  - Antemortem diagnosis of fatal PE fixed at about 30% over same time period.
  - Observational studies of PE reported unexpectedly high mortality rates.
    - In one study, overall 3-month mortality in patients with PE was 17% with an in-hospital mortality of 31% when PE was associated with hemodynamic instability.
    - In another, 90-day mortality was 14.5% in hemodynamically stable PE patients and 51.9% in those with hemodynamic instability.
      - PE-attributable mortality was 34% and 62.5% in the respective groups.
  - In fatal PE it is long appreciated that two-thirds of PE deaths will occur within 1 hour of presentation.
    - Anatomically massive PE accounts for only one-half of the deaths.
    - Remainder can be attributed to smaller submassive or recurrent emboli.
  - Several important implications of these observations:
    - Evidenced-based approach is nearly impossible to define for hemodynamically unstable PE.
    - Reasonable to propose that outcome from PE is related to embolism size and underlying cardiopulmonary function.
      - Similar hemodynamic and clinical outcomes will manifest from an anatomically massive PE in patients with normal cardiopulmonary function and an anatomically submassive embolism in patients with impaired cardiopulmonary function.

- Understanding of PE physiology will allow for application of physiologic risk stratification used for diagnostic evaluation and therapeutics.
  - Combination of embolism size and underlying cardiopulmonary status that produces cardiac arrest is associated with a predicted mortality of 70%.
    - Implies that 30% of arrested PE patients will survive and warrants continued use of chest compressions to mechanically fracture the embolism and consideration toward thrombolysis or embolectomy even without a definitive diagnosis when PE is highly suspected
  - Combination of embolism size and cardiopulmonary status that fails to produce right ventricle (RV) dilatation is associated with a 0% to 1% mortality.
    - Provided therapeutic anticoagulation is achieved
  - Combination of embolism size and cardiopulmonary status that produces hemodynamic instability or shock is associated with a 30% mortality rate.
  - Presence of shock has traditionally defined the threshold for thrombolysis.
  - Syncope represents an intermediary position between shock and cardiac arrest as failure to recover consciousness results in cardiac arrest, and patients who regain consciousness have a high incidence of hemodynamic instability.
  - Outcomes and mortality associated with emboli in transit and PE patients with a patent foramen ovale (PFO) have not been well reported.
- Spectrum of PE most likely to confront the intensivist is predominantly confined to two situations:
  - Patient presenting with undifferentiated shock or respiratory failure
  - An established hospital or intensive care unit (ICU) patient who develops PE after admission
  - In either situation, the diagnostics and therapeutics are challenging

- Differentiating PE from other life-threatening cardiopulmonary disorders can be exceedingly difficult

PREVENTION OF VENOUS THROMBOEMBOLISM (VTE)

Principles of Prophylaxis

- Prophylaxis is defined as any measure "designed to preserve health and prevent the spread of disease."
- Use of pharmacologic, mechanical, or vena caval interruption as a means for reducing occurrence of VTE qualifies as a measure intended to preserve health
- The Agency for Healthcare Research and Quality (AHRQ) has identified "appropriate use of prophylaxis to prevent venous thromboembolism in patients at risk" as the number one opportunity for improvement of patient safety, supporting more widespread implementation.
- Choice of primary prophylaxis is based on patient's risk of bleeding and thrombosis and is presented in Table 100.1.

Risk Factors

- Virchow's triad of stasis, vessel trauma, and hypercoagulability remain fundamental risk factors for VTE
- Risk factors can be considered:
  - Clinical (i.e., multiple trauma or major abdominal surgery, acute myocardial infarction or stroke, need for mechanical ventilation)
  - Or patient-related (prior history of VTE, malignancy, inherited coagulopathy)
- With respect to lower extremity deep VTE, observational studies of medical-surgical ICU patients have identified these as risk factors:
  - Mechanical ventilation
  - Treatment with neuromuscular blockers
  - Presence of a central venous line (CVL)
    - CVL, in particular, reported to confer an increased relative risk (RR) of 1.04 for each day catheter is in place

TABLE 100.1

VENOUS THROMBOEMBOLISM PROPHYLAXIS OF CRITICAL CARE PATIENT

Bleeding risk	Thrombosis risk	Prophylaxis recommendation
Low	Moderate	LDH 5,000 units sq twice a day
Low	High	LMWH • Dalteparin • Enoxaparin
High	Moderate	GCS or IPC → LMWH when bleeding risk subsides
High	High	GCS or IPC → LMWH when bleeding risk subsides

LDH, low dose heparin; LMWH, low molecular-weight heparin; GCS, graded compression stockings; IPC, intermittent pneumatic compression devices.
Adapted from *Chest.* 2003;124(6)S:357S–363S.

- Among 261 medical-surgical ICU patients, multivariate regression analysis defined as independent risk factors for VTE:
  - Exposure to platelet transfusions
  - Use of vasopressors
- The two most powerful patient-related risk factors are prior history of VTE and malignancy.
  - Malignancy most common acquired hypercoagulable state encountered in the ICU
  - End-stage renal disease identified as an independent risk factor for ICU-acquired deep vein thrombosis (DVT)
  - Activated protein C resistance from factor V Leyden (FVL) is the most common hereditary defect predisposition for DVT.
    - In order of descending prevalence among the general population predisposing development of DVT:
      - Prothrombin gene mutation 20210A
      - Antithrombin, protein C and S deficiency
      - Elevations in homocysteine and coagulation factors VIII, IX, and XI
      - Heparin-induced thrombocytopenia (HIT), an acquired platelet disorder, results in increased risk of both venous and arterial thrombosis
- Cancer and the presence of a CVL are the two most powerful risk factors for upper extremity DVT (UEDVT).
- CVL at the site of the upper extremity DVT present in 60% of patients and 46% were diagnosed with cancer
- Underscoring the possible additive nature of two risk factors:
  - 76% of patients with cancer also had an indwelling CVL
  - A review of cancer patients with an indwelling CVL showed reported prevalence of UEDVT, symptomatic or asymptomatic, from 6.7% to 48%
  - Prospective registry of 592 patients with UEDVT
    - Presence of an indwelling CVL the strongest independent predictor of occurrence (odds ratio, 7.3)
    - Nearly 30% of patients will develop an UEDVT with no apparent cause
      - Inherited thrombophilia (FVL), prothrombin G20210A mutation, anticoagulant protein deficiencies causative
    - Evaluated prospectively for median follow-up of 5.1 years, recurrence of primary UEDVT reported to be 4.4% in those with inherited thrombophilia compared to 1.6% in those without

Prevalence/Incidence

- DVT in the setting of critical illness underappreciated
  - Systematic screening shows 10% of medical-surgical ICU patients have existing proximal lower extremity DVT on admission to ICU
- When no form of prophylaxis is used, incidence of DVT during ICU stay is variable but high
- Patients undergoing major general surgery have an event rate of 25% without DVT prophylaxis:
  - 9% of patients will have clinically detectable DVT
    - 7% will have proximal DVT
  - In trauma patients not receiving prophylaxis, 58% developed a DVT
    - One-third of which were proximal

- Patients undergoing elective hip surgery and not receiving prophylaxis had a 50% incidence of DVT.
  - 23% clinically detectable and 20% proximal
- Pooled incidence of detectable DVT in neurosurgical patients is 22%.
  - Incidence in acute spinal cord injury patients is as high as 90% when prophylaxis was not used.
- Incidence of DVT in critically ill medical patients reported to be 1% to 15%
  - Depends on screening technique used
- No studies specific to critically ill performed regarding upper extremity DVT
  - No prospective studies using systematic screening techniques available to assess prevalence or incidence
  - Has been an increase over the past several decades attributed to the greater use of transvenous pacemakers and CVLs
  - Symptomatic PE reported to occur in 7% to 9% of these patients
  - Using systematic ventilation/perfusion scanning in patients previously diagnosed with upper extremity DVT have reported high-probability scans in 13%.

Pharmacologic Prophylaxis

- Little data available regarding anticoagulant prophylaxis in critical care setting
  - Two published randomized trials of thromboprophylaxis versus placebo in medical-surgical ICU patients:
    - Prospective, double-blind randomized controlled trial (RCT) of unfractionated heparin (UFH), 5,000 U administered subcutaneously (SQ) twice daily versus placebo
      - Rate of objectively confirmed DVT was reduced from 29% to 13%
    - Patients requiring mechanical ventilation (MV) ≥ 48 hours for chronic obstructive pulmonary disease (COPD) exacerbations, treatment with the low-molecular-weight heparin (LMWH) nadroparin once daily versus placebo
      - Decreased DVT rates from 29% to 16%
    - Another prospective trial, only abstracted, demonstrated the efficacy of UFH versus placebo as thromboprophylaxis.
      - Reducing the DVT rates from 31% to 11%
  - In acutely ill hospitalized medical patients and high-risk surgical patient
    - Comparison of enoxaparin, 40 mg or 20 mg, with placebo administered once daily for 6 to 14 days (MEDENOX)
      - Resulted in fewer DVTs in those receiving 40-mg dose
    - Randomized, placebo-controlled trial of dalteparin for the prevention of VTE (PREVENT)
      - Dalteparin, 5,000 IU once daily, halved rate of VTE with low risk of bleeding
    - Does SQ administration of LMWH have sufficient bioavailability to achieve therapeutic plasma levels (≥0.3 IU/mL) in critically ill?
      - Prospective, controlled, open-labeled study of enoxaparin, 40 mg once daily in critically ill patients with normal renal function demonstrated significantly lower anti-Xa levels when compared with medical patients in the normal ward.

- Body weight seems to have negative correlation with anti-Xa levels.
- Calls into question whether once-daily dosing is appropriate for the critically ill
- Fondaparinux, a synthetic factor Xa inhibitor in doses of 2.5 mg SQ daily:
  - Reported to decrease VTE rates by half versus placebo in older acutely ill medical patients (ARTEMIS)
  - More effective than enoxaparin, 30 mg twice daily, for VTE prophylaxis after elective major knee surgery
  - Equivalent to dalteparin, 5,000 IU daily, for the prevention of VTE in high-risk abdominal surgery (PEGASUS)
  - Patients requiring MV and those with severe sepsis and septic shock excluded from these trials and most were not in ICU
- Notion that these are drugs superior to placebo in prevention of VTE is supported.

Mechanical Prophylaxis

- Graded compression stockings (GCS), intermittent pneumatic compression devices (IPC), and venous foot pumps (VFP) attractive and without bleeding risk
  - No RCTs available to guide use in medical-surgical ICU patients
  - In an unblended study of 422 trauma patients, more DVT occurred in patients in whom IPC devices were used than with LMWH (2.7% vs. 0.5%).
- Use of IPC did not appear to have additional benefit when used with either UFH or LMWH in randomized pilot trial for VTE prophylaxis in patients undergoing craniotomy.
- IPC less effective in preventing PE when used in addition to UFH versus LMWH alone in prospective, randomized, multicenter trial involving acute spinal cord injury patients.
- Poor fitting GCS may lead to undue constriction and stasis of the limb on which it is applied, increasing risk of subsequent clot.
- Mechanical prophylaxis in isolation not shown to reduce risk of death or PE
  - Mechanical VTE prophylaxis alone not likely to be effective in ICU and, unless bleeding is of great concern, these devices should be deferred in favor of pharmacologic prophylaxis

Inferior Vena Cava Filters (IVCF)

- Idea of interrupting IVC to prevent transit of lower extremity thromboses to pulmonary circulation attributed to Trousseau in 1868
- IVC interruption most often carried out by percutaneous insertion of a filter or "umbrella" via the femoral or jugular vein
- Performed nearly 50,000 times a year
- Categorical indications for IVCF placement include:
  - Contraindications to anticoagulation (absolute or relative)
  - Complications of previously instituted anticoagulation (failure, bleeding, thrombocytopenia, drug reactions)
  - As prophylactic adjunct to anticoagulation in patients thought to be unable to withstand another embolic event
  - Failure of previous IVCF

- In association with another procedure (thrombectomy, embolectomy, or thrombolysis)
- Methodologically sound literature in support of specific indications for filter placement lacking
- Consequently, recommendations for filter placement largely opinion
- The first and only randomized controlled trial (RCT) of IVCFs for the prevention of PE in patients with documented proximal LEDVT followed patients for 2 years in initial report, and results of a longer-term follow-up in same patients reported after 8 years
  - Initial report, 400 patients were randomized to receive a filter or no filter in addition to anticoagulation with UFH or LMWH
  - At 12 days, fewer patients suffered symptomatic or asymptomatic PE in filter group
    - Bleeding and mortality unaffected
  - At 2 years, number of patients suffering symptomatic PE no longer significantly different
    - As a result of more symptomatic PE between years 1 and 2 in the filter group
    - Recurrence of DVT significantly higher in filter group
    - Placement of an IVCF had no effect on survival
  - At 8-year follow-up patients with filters still had higher DVT rates
    - Symptomatic PE was lower than in patients without filter
    - Mortality still unaffected
  - No differences in edema formation, occurrence of varicose veins, trophic disorders, ulcer formation, or postthrombotic syndrome have been shown between those with and without a filter.
    - Filter placement in SVC may also be considered for prevention of symptomatic PE due to acute upper extremity DVT.
    - IVCF use not systematically studied in critical care outside the setting of major trauma, where the deployment of retrievable IVCFs (R-IVCF) has been favored.
      - Only about one in five of these devices in fact retrieved, suggesting that they have simply become permanent filters
    - A small study of morbidly obese patients undergoing R-IVCF placement prior to gastric bypass surgery reported a 95% success rate when filter retrieval was attempted. Still, 21% developed VTE postoperatively.
- No RCT of IVCF for prevention of PE, generalizable to the critically ill, yet published
  - Use recommended for those in whom anticoagulation is contraindicated or failed altogether

Diagnosis of DVT

- Physical examination unhelpful
- Gold standard for DVT lower limb venography
  - Adequately performed, able to detect all clinically important forms of DVT
    - Including calf thrombosis, thrombosis of the pelvis, and IVC
    - Due to technical nature of test, risk of radiocontrast-induced nephrotoxicity, and need to transport patient from ICU rarely performed outside research settings
- Compression ultrasound (CUS) most commonly reported method of detecting DVT in ICU setting

- For symptomatic patients reported pooled sensitivity for CUS in excluding a proximal DVT is 97%, but only 62% in asymptomatic patients
- CUS lacks sensitivity in detection of distal DVT, yielding pooled sensitivities of 73% and 53% for symptomatic and asymptomatic patients, respectively
- Negative serial CUS over 7- to 10-day period may effectively rule out clinically important DVT.
  - Only validated in symptomatic outpatients
- Alternative to both venography and CUS is computed tomography venography (CTV) of the lower extremities and the pelvic veins as continuation of CT angiography of pulmonary arteries
  - In setting of diagnostic workup for PE, CTV has reported sensitivity and specificity of 70% and 96%, respectively, for all DVT.
    - Comparable to CUS in one study, and superior to CUS for detection of iliofemoral DVT (yielding 100% sensitivity and specificity)
    - PIOPED investigators reported CTV and CUS diagnostically equivalent
      - Reporting 95.5% concordance between CTV and CUS for diagnosis or exclusion of LEDVT
      - Choice of imaging technique can be made on the basis of safety, expense, and time constraints
- In case of upper extremity DVT:
  - First-line diagnostic test is color duplex ultrasound with a three-step protocol involving compression, color, and color Doppler
  - Reported sensitivity and specificity ranging from 78% to 100% and 82% to 100%, respectively
    - With vessel incompressibility but the presence of isolated flow abnormalities in combination with persistent clinical likelihood, contrast venography should be considered.
    - Magnetic resonance venography (MRV) has shown disappointing results.
      - Sensitivities are 50% and 71% for MRV with and without gadolinium enhancement, respectively.

Treatment of DVT

- The mainstay of therapy for all forms of VTE is anticoagulation.
- See section for treatment of PE for further details
- For larger clot burden involving the iliofemoral system, some suggest thrombolytics.
  - A Cochrane review concluded that thrombolysis reduces postthrombotic syndrome and maintains venous patency after DVT when compared to traditional anticoagulation.
  - Optimum drug, dose, and route of administration have to be determined.
  - Endovascular catheter-directed thrombolysis is another promising treatment for acute iliofemoral thrombosis.

PULMONARY EMBOLISM (PE)

- Combination of mechanical obstruction and neurohumoral factors combined with patients underlying cardiopulmonary status results in increased pulmonary vascular impedance and induction of pressure load on the RV.

- Effect of neurohumoral influence is significantly underappreciated
  - Release of factors from platelets in imbedded clot, which include:
    - Serotonin
    - Adenosine diphosphate (ADP)
    - Thrombin
  - All precipitate vasoconstriction in the pulmonary artery system
  - Development of pressure load precipitates RV decompensation and decreases RV output
  - As the heart is two hydraulic pumps linked in series
    - Diminished output of the RV will result in diminished left ventricle (LV) preload
    - Consequence of diminished LV preload is decreased CO and resultant loss of mean arterial pressure (MAP)
      - RV perfusion pressure is the difference between MAP and right ventricular end diastolic pressure (RVEDP)
      - PE increases RVEDP
        - Through induction of a RV pressure load and the development of right ventricular decompensation
      - This increases RV myocardial oxygen demand
        - Because of diminished gradient between MAP and RV subendocardium
        - Induces further RV decompensation and resultant RV ischemia
      - RV compensates through Starling mechanism
        - Increases RV volume
        - Results in left septal shift of the intraventricular septum, further jeopardizing LV filling
        - Pericardial restraint, further limits of LV filling, and further impairments of LV distensibility additionally decrease LV preload
      - Pathophysiologic sequence results in a vicious cycle of ventricular decompensation that manifests as hemodynamic instability and shock
    - PE has a spectrum of presentations and the most extreme form of PE will result in gross hemodynamic instability and cardiac arrest.
- Care of the critically ill patient often proceeds along two parallel pathways:
  - Physiologic resuscitation
  - Generation of a differential diagnosis that eventually leads to a definitive diagnosis and treatment
- Gas exchange abnormalities in PE are exceedingly complex.
  - A function of size and character of embolic material
  - Magnitude of occlusion against background of patients underlying cardiopulmonary status
  - Interval time since embolic event
- Multiple causes of hypoxia have been attributed to:
  - An increase in alveolar dead space
  - Ventilation perfusion abnormalities
  - Right-to-left shunting
  - In the case of cardiogenic shock, a low mixed venous O_2
- Although seemingly counterintuitive, multiple inert gas technique suggests a low V/Q relationship develops and precipitates hypoxia in PE.
  - Consequent to redistribution of blood flow away from embolized area
  - Resulting in excessive perfusion in unembolized lung regions and subsequent reperfusion through atelectatic area of previous clot

- There is significant correlation observed between magnitude of angiographic obstruction and mean pulmonary artery pressure (mPAP), right atrial pressure (RAP), PaO_2, and pulse.
- Pulmonary vascular resistance (PVR) of > 500 dyne. s. cm^{-5} correlative with a degree of obstruction exceeding 50%
- Depression in SpO_2 common
  - May occur with as little as 13% angiographic obstruction
  - Commonly the only clinical manifestation when obstruction is < 25%
  - When pulmonary vascular obstruction is 25% to 30%, pulmonary hypertension begins to develop (normal mPAP, 20 mm Hg)
    - Patients without underlying cardiopulmonary disease are unable to generate a mPAP > 40 mm Hg.
      - Reported maximal pressure healthy RV can generate
    - In patients without underlying cardiopulmonary disease:
      - A large single embolus
      - Or the cumulative incremental effects of multiple recurrent emboli generating obstructions over 50%
    - Needed to precipitate RV failure
    - Consequently mPAP > 40 mm Hg represents either significant underlying cardiopulmonary disease or the effects of multiple embolic events occurring over a prolonged time period, enabling the development of the right ventricular hypertrophy.
- Relationship between PVR and extent of anatomic obstruction is hyperbolic not linear.
  - Direct increases in PVR occur when anatomic obstruction exceeds 60%.
- In population with no underlying cardiopulmonary disease:
  - Increase in pulmonary arterial pressure (PAP) and setting of PE almost uniformly indicative of severe pulmonary vascular obstruction
  - PAP characteristically related to mPAP but generally not elevated until the latter is >30 mm Hg and anatomic obstruction exceeds 35% to 40%
  - PAP can be elevated without decreased cardiac output in patients with PE
  - However, decreased cardiac output without increased PAP suggests alternative non-PE–related diagnosis
- Patients with previous cardiopulmonary disease characteristically manifest significantly greater degrees of cardiovascular impairment with less anatomic vascular obstruction.
  - Best exemplified in European Pulmonary Embolism Trial where 90% of patients presenting in shock had prior cardiopulmonary disease
    - 56% with prior cardiopulmonary disease presented in shock compared to only 2% of patients without cardiopulmonary disease
    - With prior cardiac disease the level of mPAP disproportionately elevated compared to that of anatomic obstruction
      - Strongly suggests underlying cardiopulmonary hemodynamics dominates presentation process
      - With mean angiographic obstruction of only 23%, significant elevations in mPAP reported in population with previous cardiopulmonary disease
        - Increment in mPAP directly related to pulmonary capillary wedge pressure (PCWP)
  - In patients with prior cardiopulmonary disease PAP reported to be unreliable indicator of magnitude of embolic event

○ Limited its usefulness in assessment of extensive vascular obstruction and life-threatening disease
○ No apparent consistent relationship between the extent of embolic obstruction and right ventricular impairment in patients with previous cardiopulmonary disease

Readily Available Diagnostic Studies

- Development of differential diagnosis in the undifferentiated shock patient or existing patients in ICU usually predicated on elements derived from:
  - The history
  - Physical findings
  - Readily available diagnostic studies:
    - Electrocardiogram (ECG)
    - Chest x-ray (CXR)
    - Arterial blood gas (ABG) analysis

Electrocardiogram

- Since description in 1935 of $S_1Q_3T_3$ pattern in a limited number of patients with PE-induced cor pulmonale
- Plethora of ECG manifestation reported
- Several important points from large series regarding ECG findings for PE helpful:
  - Normal ECG distinctly unusual
    ○ Reported in a minority of patients without cardiopulmonary disease (14%–30%)
    ○ Rhythm disturbances uncommon
    – Incidence of atrial fibrillation and flutter as presenting component of PE exceedingly small as are first-, second-, or third-degree heart blocks
    ○ Most common ECG findings related to abnormalities in ST-T wave segment:
    – Occurring in 42% to 49% of patients
    – Anterior T-wave inversion pattern the most common abnormality in PE
    – Occurs in 68% of patients
    – The ECG sign most correlative with severity of underlying embolic event:
      • 90% of patients with anterior T-wave inversion had Miller score >50% (mean 60%), and 81% of those had a mPAP elevation >30 mm Hg
      • Early appearance of T-wave inversion reported to be an even stronger marker of severity of event
        • It is similarly correlative with efficacy of thrombolytic therapy as T-wave normalization occurs in patients with successful thrombolytic therapy

Chest Radiograph

- CXR cannot be used to include or exclude PE.
  - It is helpful in contributing diagnostic assessment by excluding other diseases that may mimic PE and defining abnormalities necessitating further evaluation.
  - May provide a crude assessment of severity
  - Normal CXR in angiographic-proven PE unusual
    ○ Occurs in 16% to 34% of patients without cardiopulmonary disease
    ○ Appears to be association between severity of thromboembolic event and:
    – CXR findings defined by relationships between PAP, oxygen saturation

– CXR findings when normal CXR view compared to those with parenchymal and vascular abnormalities
  • Vascular abnormalities including relative oligemia in the area of embolic event were correlative with the severity of PE.
  • Other findings on CXR suggestive of PE include:
    • Abrupt cutoff of pulmonary artery
    • Relative or focal oligemia
    • Distention of the proximal portion of the pulmonary artery

Arterial Blood Gas

- Hypoxia in PE not uniform
  - PaO_2 readings >80 mm Hg seen in 12% to 19% of patients
- A normal PaO_2 does not exclude PE
  - Occurs in approximately 14% of patients
- In patients without underlying cardiopulmonary disease likely these small changes in oxygen saturation reflect low levels of severity in PE.
  - Appears to be no correlation between arterial oxygen saturation or PaO_2 and magnitude of the embolic event in patients with cardiopulmonary disease
  - Change in oxygen saturation or requirement of escalating levels of inspired oxygen should prompt consideration toward evaluation for PE
  - If capable of measuring dead space (Vd/Vt) or end-tidal CO_2, these should similarly be used given the physiologic imprint of increased dead space with PE

DIAGNOSTIC THERAPEUTIC APPROACH

Risk Stratification

- Contemporary approach to physiologic risk stratification depicted in Figure 100.1
- Combination underlying cardiopulmonary status and embolic size that precipitates cardiac arrest surprisingly associated with mortality of only 70%
  - Underscores necessity of aggressively pursuing patients with suspected underlying PE presenting with cardiac arrest, as about 30% with PE and cardiac arrest survive
- At other extreme, predicted mortality of patients with hemodynamically stable PE and normal RV very low when treated with appropriate anticoagulation
- Combination of embolic size and cardiopulmonary status precipitating decompensation resulting in shock associated with 30% mortality
  - Syncope and emboli in transit have predicted mortalities just below that of shock patient
- An anatomic obstruction of approximately 30% necessary to elevate PAP and precipitate RV dilatation
- Presence of hemodynamic deterioration or shock in PE represents the failure of compensatory mechanisms to maintain forward flow and is associated with significant increases in mortality; shock traditionally used as discriminator to define likelihood of survivorship from PE.
  - Presence of shock in PE associated with three to seven times increase in mortality

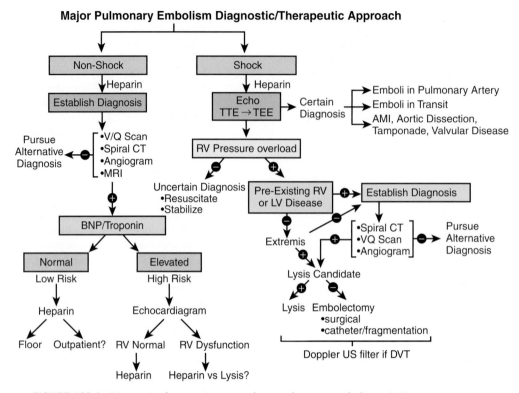

FIGURE 100.1. Diagnostic therapeutic approach to pulmonary embolism. AMI, acute mesenteric ischemia; CT, computed tomography; DVT, deep vein thrombus; LV, left ventricle; RV, right ventricle; TEE, transesophageal echocardiography; TTE, transthoracic echocardiography; US, ultrasound; V/Q, ventilation/perfusion.

- Vast majority of patients with anatomically massive PE do not present in shock
  - Without underlying cardiopulmonary disease, associated anatomically massive PE presents with a normal cardiac output
  - Hemodynamically stable patients not in shock, who have experienced submassive or massive PE, have similar mortality rates
  - Anatomically massive PE unaccompanied by physiologic decompensation resulting in shock and hemodynamic instability does not appear to be associated with increased mortality
- Spiral CT scanning supplanted ventilation/perfusion scanning as diagnostic modality of choice in PE
  - In patients with elevated creatinine or inability to tolerate CT scan, V/Q scanning is a reasonable alternative given the overwhelming experience using this technique
  - Pretest probability characterizations are pivotal in the diagnosis of PE whether CT scanning or ventilation/perfusion scanning is used
- Further risk stratification of hemodynamically stable patients with PE may be undertaken using brain natriuretic peptide (BNP) and troponin levels.
  - Patients with hemodynamic stability and confirmed PE with normal BNP and troponin levels have an excellent predicted outcome.
  - Presence of elevated BNP and troponin define a high-risk population.
    - Warrant admission and close observation
- Patients with suspected PE and hemodynamic instability at high risk for rapid deterioration and sudden death

- Demands expeditious approach to diagnosis, resuscitation, and therapy
- Echocardiography ideal first assessment of hemodynamically unstable patient
  - Findings suggestive of PE include:
    - Right-sided thrombi
    - RV dilatation
    - Hypokinesis
    - Tricuspid regurgitation
    - Paradoxical shifting of ventricular septum
  - Echocardiographic findings of acute myocardial infarction, tamponade, aortic dissection, or valvular disease may be equally useful in confirming the diagnosis and excluding PE.
  - In patients without underlying cardiopulmonary disease
    - Magnitude of abnormalities on echocardiogram correlate with the degree of pulmonary artery outflow obstruction
    - An obstruction of 30% is necessary to produce RV dilatation
    - Presence of RV dysfunction not specific for PE
      - May be seen in spectrum of diseases ranging from RV infarct with cardiomyopathy to cor pulmonale and antecedent pulmonary hypertension
  - Echocardiographic findings reported to be useful in differentiating PE from non-PE events
    - Patients with baseline cor pulmonale or recurrent PE characteristically have evidence of RV hypertrophy with thickness measuring >5 mm and minimal septal shift

– Acute RV failure secondary to PE should not be associated with RV hypertrophy nor accompanied by a septal shift

– In patients with pre-existing cardiopulmonary disease, it is imperative to establish diagnosis of PE

  • Spiral CT scanning has supplanted V/Q scans in the critically ill population

  • In patients with confirmed PE candidacy for either medical thrombectomy with thrombolytic therapy or surgical embolectomy should be undertaken

  • Crucial to recognize that absence of RV pressure overload in unstable patient in whom PE is being considered effectively excludes PE as cause of hemodynamic instability

  • In appropriate clinical context, patients without underlying cardiopulmonary disease who are in extremis and with anticipated arrest, with evidence of RV dilatation and high pretest probability for PE, may be considered as candidates for medical embolectomy with thrombolytic therapy or surgical embolectomy without complete workup

Resuscitation and Stabilization

• Escalating oxygen requirements may necessitate intubation and mechanical ventilation.

• Intubation may precipitate cardiovascular collapse with major PE for several reasons:

  • Sedative hypnotics used for intubation can mitigate the catecholamine surge on which a patient is dependent and similarly produce vasodilatation, which impairs the perfusion pressure gradient to RV subendocardium, provoking further ischemia and cardiac decompensation.

  • Excessive lung ventilation on initial intubation may create air trapping and diminish venous return.

  • Initiation of MV can increase the pulmonary vascular resistance and further jeopardize RV function.

• Volume expansion with 1 to 2 L of crystalloid solution is initial treatment for hypotension in patients with undifferentiated shock

  • In patients with PE-related shock, increases in RV pressure and volume generate significant increases in systolic wall stress, provoking myocardial ischemia.

  • Excessive fluid resuscitation further dilates the RV and produces increased wall stress, resulting in further RV decompensation.

  • In patients with anatomically massive PE and low cardiac output who were normotensive and required vasopressors on presentation, increased cardiac output with a 500-mL fluid challenge was reported.

  • Increase in cardiac output was consistently proportional to baseline RV end diastolic volume index.

  • Therefore, fluid may be used judicially in normotensive patients without evidence of significant RV dysfunction.

  • In patients with echocardiographic evidence of severe RV dysfunction, fluid resuscitation may provoke increased wall stress, ischemia, and RV dysfunction.

    ○ When measured RV pressures are high or there is evidence of severe RV dysfunction, early consideration should be given to vasopressor therapy.

• No controlled human trials related to vasoactive support in PE

  • Extrapolation from animal models suggests that norepinephrine improves RV dysfunction through vasoconstriction that augments MAP and enhances perfusion pressure gradients to RV subendocardium

  • Additionally, norepinephrine possesses modest inotropic properties shown to provide complementary enhancement of RV function

  • May be reasonable to consider use of inhaled nitric oxide to decrease pulmonary vascular afterload in patients with evidence of pressor dependant severe RV dysfunction

  • Small reports suggest that inhaled prostacyclin and nitric oxide will increase cardiac output, decrease PAP, and improve gas exchange in cases of shock-related PE.

• Presence of shock or hemodynamic decompensation with proven PE an indication for either medical embolectomy with thrombolytic therapy or surgical embolectomy

  • Use of thrombolytic therapy controversial in patients hemodynamically stable; it is acknowledged as the therapeutic choice in hemodynamically unstable patient

    • There is greater rapidity in rate of resolution when comparing heparin to thrombolytic therapy in terms of the percentage resolution detected by perfusion scanning and angiography up to day 7 of diagnosis; thereafter there is no difference in the degree of embolic resolution.

    • By 1 year, the extent of angiographic resolution was 77% in the heparin group and 78% in the urokinase group (Tables 100.2 and 100.3).

    • There does not appear to be any difference related to the effectiveness of thrombolytic agents provided they are given in equivalent doses over a similar timeframe.

    • Assessing efficacy of thrombolytic therapy difficult in first several hours

      ○ Mortality in group that underwent successful embolectomy was 0% compared to 30% mortality in group that failed to respond to thrombolytic therapy

      ○ As continuous echocardiography and imaging studies are not available, monitoring of end-tidal CO_2 proposed to monitor the efficacy of thrombolytic therapy

        – End-tidal CO_2 significantly increases in patients who survived with thrombolytic therapy compared to those with no appreciable change in end-tidal CO_2 measurements in patients who did not survive

        – Unsuccessful thrombolysis reported to occur in approximately 8% of patients undergoing therapy

          • In limited literature that compares repeat thrombolysis to surgical thromboembolectomy, there appears to be significant survival benefit in undertaking surgical embolectomy.

          • Mortality in patients undergoing surgical embolectomy after failed thrombolytic therapy was reported to be 7% compared to 38% of patients who underwent repeat thrombolysis.

          • Recurrent PE significantly higher in patients who underwent repeat thrombolysis and was the cause of death in a significant number

          • Patients who underwent surgical thromboembolectomy also had the placement of vena cava filters

• Thrombolytic therapy in hemodynamically stable patients remains a controversial topic.

TABLE 100.2

RATE AND EXTENT OF PERFUSION SCAN RESOLUTION IN UROKINASE PULMONARY EMBOLISM TRIAL (UPET)

	Heparin 25.4%		Urokinase 26.2%	
	Absolute resolution (%)	Resolution (%)	Absolute resolution (%)	Resolution (%)
24 hours	2.7	8.1	6.2	22.1
Day 2	4.9	17	8.0	25.8
Day 5	9.3	35.5	11.3	40.6
Day 14	14.7	58.2	14.9	52.0
1 year		77.2		78.8
No CPD → 90% resolution		91% of patients		88% of patients
CPD → 90% resolution		72% of patients		77% of patients

CPD, cardiopulmonary disease.
From Urokinase pulmonary embolism trial. Phase 1 results: a cooperative study. *JAMA.* 1970;214:2163–2172; and Urokinase pulmonary embolism trial. *Circulation.* 1973;47(Suppl):1–108.

- Long-term outcome of patients with thrombolytic therapy not well described but it appears that most undergo an uneventful course
  - Mortality is approximately 8%
  - Major bleeding reported in 9.6%
  - Recurrent PE reported in 7.6%
  - Mean vascular obstruction diminished from 64% to 29% within 48 hours, and RV function was reversible within 48 hours in 80% of patients
  - Lung scan improved 45% within 6 to 8 days of therapy
  - Predictive indicators of poor hospital course in patients receiving thrombolytic therapy were initial pulmonary vascular obstruction >70% and hemodynamic instability at presentation associated with persistence of paradoxical septal motion on echocardiography.
  - Long-term mortality related to older age, persistence of vascular obstruction >30% after thrombolytic therapy and cancer
- Surgical embolectomy indicated for patients presenting in shock or cardiopulmonary instability and an inability to tolerate thrombolytic therapy
- Ideally, these emboli are large and located centrally and consideration of embolectomy is undertaken prior to cardiac arrest.
  - Requires preoperative localization via CT documentation and ideally echocardiographic of right heart function
  - In the era of modern surgical embolectomy there was a 6% operative mortality and only 12% late deaths from disease other than PE
  - The overall improvement in operative mortality related to surgical thromboembolectomy most likely relates to preoperative selection of patients who had not experienced cardiac arrest and the use of cardiopulmonary bypass.
- Approach to hemodynamically stable patients with PE and RV dysfunction remains controversial and contentious
  - Use of BNP, which is indicative of right ventricular stress, and troponin levels, which are indicative of myocardial ischemia, have been used in the stratification.
  - Biomarkers reported to allow for severity characterization of patients with PE
    - Where there is absence of elevation in BNP or troponin predicted outcome is excellent and these patients do not warrant intensive care evaluation
    - Elevations in BNP and troponin levels are associated with a higher mortality and are evolving as discriminators for use of thrombolytic therapy in patients with PE

TABLE 100.3

RANDOMIZED TRIALS: LYSIS VERSUS HEPARIN

	Early				
Study	Angio	Scan	Hemodyn	Echo	Late
UPET 1970	↑ 24 h	↑ 24 h	↑ 24 h	—	Scan, day 5; pulmonary HTN
Tibbutt 1974	↑ 72 h	—	↑ 72 h	—	Limited
Arnesen 1978	↑ 72 h	—	—	—	—
Ly 1978	↑ 72 h	—	—	—	—
Marini 1988	→ 7 d	→ 24 h	→ 7 d	—	No difference, 1 y
PIOPED 1990	→ 2 h	→ 24, 48 h	↑ PVR 1.5 d	—	No difference
Giuntini 1984	—	↑ 24 h	—	—	Scan, day 3
Levine 1990	—	↑ 24 h	—	—	Scan, day 7
PAIMS 1992	↑ 2 h	→ 7 d	↑ 2 h PAP/CI	—	Scan/angio, day 7
Goldhaber 1993	—	↑ 24 h	—	↑ 3, 24 h	—

HTN, hypertension; PVR, pulmonary vascular resistance; PAP/CI, pulmonary artery pressure/cardiac index.

CHAPTER 101 ■ OTHER EMBOLIC SYNDROMES (AIR, FAT, AMNIOTIC FLUID)

GAS EMBOLISM

- Gas embolism is defined as the entrance of gas into the vascular compartment.
- Air and other gases, CO_2 and nitrogen, may result in gas emboli
- Gas may reach any organ
  - Most significant damage is to the organs with high oxygen consumption rates, such as brain and heart
- Gas embolism can be venous or arterial
- Most frequently, it is an iatrogenic problem that may be fatal (Table 101.1)
  - Highest-risk surgical procedures for venous air embolism (VAE) are: sitting neurosurgical operations, posterior fossa and neck surgery, laparoscopic procedures, total hip arthroplasty, cesarean section, and central venous line procedures—both placement and removal.
  - During a neurosurgical procedure in the sitting position, air usually enters through the noncollapsing veins, including the dural venous sinuses and emissary veins.
  - While true incidence of VAE is unknown, as most cases are asymptomatic and the sensitivity of detection methods differs significantly, incidence is reported to be between 7% and 50% using Doppler detection methodology.
    - One study that used the transesophageal detection method reported an incidence of 76%.

Pathophysiology

- Severity of gas embolism related to volume of gas entering circulation as well as rate of gas accumulation
  - Fatal gas volume in humans is unknown, but in a canine model, it is 7.5 mL/kg
  - Estimated fatal volume for humans is between 200 and 300 mL
    - With underlying impaired cardiac contractility, volume of air needed to cause cardiac arrest is less than in adults with normal cardiac function
- Entry of air into pulmonary venous system acutely increases pulmonary artery pressure, degrades gas exchange, and provokes cardiac dysrhythmias.
  - Mean arterial pressure (MAP) decreases rapidly, perhaps secondary to an immediate decrease in cardiac output or due to a reflex mechanism resulting in the release of vasoactive substances.
  - A "paradoxical" gas embolism can occur with a right-to-left shunt.
    - As in patient with a patent foramen ovale

- Term *paradoxical* used as the right-sided pressures need be higher than those on the left side for passage of the gas from right to left heart
  - These may be increased with the application of positive end-expiratory pressure (PEEP), the Valsalva maneuver, and/or a venous air embolism (VAE), creating a right-to-left shunt
  - Hypoxemia and hypercapnia seen with gas embolism primarily related to V/Q inequality
- Arterial gas embolism (AGE) is caused by entry of gas into the arterial system.
  - Can be caused by venous gas embolism entering arterial circulation via a right-to-left shunt or directly via the pulmonary capillary bed by overloading of the pulmonary filtering capacity
  - In compressed air diving, the cause of AGE is pulmonary overpressurization by failing to exhale or due to regional gas trapping during ascent.
    - Leads to alveolar rupture and entry of gas into pulmonary capillaries
    - Iatrogenic causes include accidental air injection during cardiopulmonary bypass or angiography
    - Can also be caused by pulmonary barotrauma during mechanical ventilation
    - Rarely a complication of thoracic trauma and lung surgery
  - Gas distribution to organs dependent on blood flow
    - Gas entering coronary circulation may result in a typical infarct
    - Gas passing into cerebral circulation may cause ischemic stroke

Diagnosis

- Most important diagnostic tool is patient history
  - If patient has undergone high-risk procedure, a high index of suspicion for gas embolism required
- Most common symptoms and signs are acute dyspnea and hemodynamic instability
- Numerous nonspecific symptoms and signs including nausea, vomiting, respiratory distress, tachypnea, wheezing, chest tightness, pallor, sweating, tachycardia, bradycardia, hypotension, and sudden cardiac arrest
- Neurologic symptoms may include acute dizziness, unconsciousness, paresthesias, paraparesis, paraplegia, and/or seizures
- So-called mill-wheel murmur is auscultated in precordial area
  - Secondary to the presence of air in the cardiac chambers
- Hemodynamic changes may be initial signs of gas embolism
  - Hypotension and acute increase in pulmonary arterial pressure (PAP) observed at early periods of gas embolism

TABLE 101.1

ETIOLOGY OF GAS EMBOLISM

Decompression injury	
Vascular entrance of gas	Central line placement and removal
	Arterial catheterization
	Invasive radiologic procedures
	Intra-aortic balloon rupture
	IV fluid administration
	Rapid IV infusion systems
Gastrointestinal procedures	Gastrointestinal endoscopy
	Laparoscopic surgery
	Endoscopic retrograde cholangiopancreatography
Neurosurgical procedures	Sitting-position craniotomies
	Posterior fossa surgery
	Cervical laminectomy
	Spinal fusion
	Deep brain stimulator placement
	Lumbar puncture
	Epidural catheter placement
Neck procedures	Radical neck dissection
	Thyroidectomy
	Nd:YAG laser surgery
Ophthalmologic procedures	Eye surgery
Cardiac procedures	Extracorporeal bypass
	Coronary angiography
Obstetric and gynecologic procedures	Cesarean section
	Intravaginal, intrauterine gas insufflation during pregnancy
Orthopedic procedures	Hip surgery
	Spinal surgery
	Gas insufflation during arthroscopic surgery
Urologic procedures	Transurethral prostatectomy
	Radical prostatectomy
Thoracic procedures	Lung biopsy
	Lung trauma
	Thoracoscopy
	Chest tube placement

- Central venous pressure (CVP) may increase, along with a right ventricle (RV) pressure increase due to elevated PAP or air in RV
  - Differential diagnosis is noted in (Table 101.2)
- End tidal CO_2 ($PetCO_2$) routinely used in operating room and increasingly available for intubated ICU patients
  - Case reports of sudden and severe drop in $PetCO_2$ values in gas embolism
  - Rapid progressive fall in $PetCO_2$ a sign of gas embolism despite normal blood pressure
  - Sudden or progressive drop in $PetCO_2$ not specific sign of gas embolism
    - May indicate presence of important complication
      - Pulmonary thromboembolism, pneumothorax, or airway obstruction
- Pulse oximetry is standard of care for operating room procedures as well as for ICU patients
  - Sudden drop in pulse oximetric measured oxygen saturation (SpO_2) a common finding of gas embolism
  - Typically indicates a severe disturbance of pulmonary function

TABLE 101.2

DIFFERENTIAL DIAGNOSIS OF GAS EMBOLISM

Pulmonary embolism	Thromboembolism
	Fat embolism
Respiratory failure	Pulmonary edema
	Acute bronchospasm
	Pneumothorax
Stroke	
Cardiac events	Myocardial infarction
	Pericardial tamponade
	Arrhythmias with hemodynamic compromise
Shock	Cardiogenic
	Septic
	Hypovolemic
Hypoglycemia	

- Chest x-ray (CXR) may show air in vascular compartments and heart
- Electrocardiogram (ECG) changes may be observed related to myocardial ischemia.
  - Often, first change noted is peaking of the P wave; S-T segment depression can follow peaking of P wave, depending on the severity of gas embolism
- Hemoconcentration, related to a shift of intravascular fluid to extravascular space, may be observed.
- Precordial Doppler a sensitive indicator that can be used to detect gas embolism
  - Placed on left parasternal border (second or third intercostal space) during a high-risk procedure and appears to be very accurate in diagnosing gas embolism
- Transthoracic echocardiography (TEE) the most sensitive method for detecting gas embolism
  - Considered gold standard, but is costly and more invasive than precordial Doppler
  - TEE increasingly used for routine intraoperative monitoring for detection of VAE during high-risk surgeries such as sitting craniotomies.
    - A patent foramen ovale (PFO) can be detected with TEE
    - May allow identification of patients at high risk for paradoxical gas embolism
- Esophageal Doppler a sensitive indicator of air embolism
  - Optimal position for VAE detection at level of superior vena cava (SVC) above its junction with right atrium (RA)

Prevention and Treatment

- Gas embolism in ICU is mostly iatrogenic and mostly preventable
- Patient positioning after suspected VAE controversial
  - Recent studies that compared different positions in canine models of VAE showed no benefit of left lateral recumbent and LLR head-down over supine positions
  - Claimed that placing patients with suspected VAE in supine position might afford better opportunity to administer supportive therapy, including ventilatory support and oxygen, to establish access for catecholamine delivery and perform CPR
  - Trendelenburg position may not decrease incidence of cerebral microembolism compared to the supine position
- Positioning of patients during central venous line (CVL) placement and removal also a matter of debate
  - Our practice is to place patients who will have a SCV or internal jugular vein (IJ) CVL inserted in head-down position
    - Only situation in which this may not be appropriate is if the patient has elevated intracranial pressure (ICP) or severely compromised pulmonary function
    - Policy also utilized for removal of CVLs
  - Placement or removal of femoral CVLs would indicate that patient be placed in reverse Trendelenburg
  - Placement or removal of CVLs should essentially never be done while patient is sitting
  - If cooperative, patient may be asked to perform Valsalva maneuver (i.e., breath holding during expiration and humming), which can increase venous pressure

- Air embolism after catheter removal through the residual tract reported many times in literature
  - Proper maintenance of entrance site should be performed
- VAE via disconnected line or fractured catheter hub may also occur
- CO_2 embolism can occur during laparoscopic surgery.
  - Most commonly occurs when pneumoperitoneum created through a tear in a vessel in the abdominal wall or peritoneum
  - If CO_2 embolism is suspected, insufflation of gas should be discontinued
- Application of PEEP not helpful in preventing air embolism during sitting-position craniotomies
  - Furthermore, it may be harmful
- Low CVP may increase the negative pressure gradient between the atrium and wound site and, thus, the risk for VAE.
  - Increasing CVP to upper normal limits can decrease the risk for VAE
- Aggressive resuscitation and CPR is started immediately following collapse of patient.
  - Aggressive volume resuscitation recommended to increase right arterial pressure (RAP)
    - Can prevent further air entry into the venous circulation
    - $FiO_2 = 1.0$ maximizes oxygenation of patient
      - Can also decrease volume of embolus via elimination of nitrogen component of embolus
  - Aspiration of air from RA with existing CVL may remove up to 60% of air
    - Our experience with this technique not uniformly positive
    - Catheter type and position very important for successful removal of air
      - Multiorifice catheters are superior to single-lumen catheters

Treatment for Arterial Gas Embolism

- Mechanical ventilation (MV) in intubated patients can decrease the time it takes to eliminate air from cerebral arteries if performed at $FiO_2 = 1.0$.
  - Hyperventilation currently not recommended in MV patients
- Seizures after cerebral embolism may not respond to benzodiazepines.
  - Although barbiturates can suppress seizure activity in these patients
- Hypotension should be avoided, as this can increase bubble entrapment and decrease cerebral blood flow (CBF).
  - Short period of hypertension can facilitate bubble redistribution through the arterioles to the capillaries and veins

Hyperbaric Oxygen Therapy (HBO)

- HBO therapy recommended for cerebral air embolism and is gold standard for AGE
- Patients breathe $FiO_2 = 1.0$ at supra-atmospheric pressures with HBO
  - Pressure in chamber decreases volume of air bubbles and creates hyperoxia

- With HBO, alveolar PO_2 can reach 2,000 mm Hg
  - Hyperoxia creates diffusion gradient for O_2 and N_2 in air bubble
  - Majority of oxygen dissolved in plasma
  - High levels of oxygen carried to tissues can help to reduce cerebral ischemia
  - HBO prevents further brain edema development by reducing vascular permeability
- Optimal time to start HBO unclear
- Immediate treatment has best response
- Delayed therapy, >6 hours after injury, may still have benefits
- Decision for HBO therapy for delayed cases based on patients clinical status and transport risk

FAT EMBOLISM

- Fat embolism in patient with severe crush injury was first described by Zenker in 1862
- Still no single definition for fat embolism syndrome (FES)
- Fat embolus is a pathophysiologic condition, and FES is a clinical condition that occurs with fat embolus
  - Classic presentation of FES is petechial rash, respiratory distress, and confusion, with onset of 24 to 48 hours following pelvic or long bone fracture
  - Clinically most crucial part of FES is respiratory insufficiency
    - Can easily be confused with other concomitant problems such as lung contusion, aspiration, and pulmonary edema
  - Mental status changes may be secondary to cerebral contusion, drugs, and systemic inflammatory response syndrome (SIRS), in addition to FES
  - If petechial rash is delayed or absent, diagnosis may be very difficult
  - FES resulted in a 10% to 20% mortality rate in the 1960s and, although it has declined since then, mortality still remains high
- FES reported to occur most commonly with long bone fractures, it is also associated with:
- Bone marrow transplantation
- Sickle cell disease
- Pancreatitis
- Liposuction
- Soft tissue injuries
- Extracorporeal circulation
- Burns
- Decompression sickness or high altitude
- Osteomyelitis
- Fatty liver
- Epilepsy
- Diagnostic criteria for FES proposed by Gurd are widely used, but not universally accepted.
  - Clinical features of FES divided into major and minor features (Table 101.3)
  - Diagnosis of FES requires presence of one major and four minor criteria according to Gurd
  - Fat embolism index score is defined for predetermined and designated clinical signs and symptoms (Table 101.4)
  - Score of 5 or more is diagnostic of FES, and negative if <5

TABLE 101.3

CLINICAL FEATURES OF FAT EMBOLISM

Major	Petechial rash
	Respiratory symptoms and bilateral infiltrates on chest radiograph
	Altered mental status
Minor	Tachycardia
	Fever
	Retinal fat or petechia
	Anuria, oliguria, fat globules in urine
	Sudden drop in hemoglobin level
	Sudden thrombocytopenia
	High erythrocyte sedimentation rate
	Fat globules in sputum

Epidemiology

- Difficult to estimate the true incidence of fat embolism
  - No universal definition
  - Many cases with fat embolus may not develop FES
  - True incidence of FES probably higher than the reported rates of 19% in patients with major trauma
  - Occurrence of fat embolism in autopsy reports in trauma patients ranges between 52% and 96%
    - Only 1% to 5% of patients develop FES
  - Incidence of FES related to femoral shaft fractures reported as 0.9% to 13.2%
    - Depending on type of fracture and time of stabilization
    - Most recent data suggest an incidence of FES 0.9% to 11% among trauma patients with long bone fractures
- FES seldom occurs with fractures of the upper limb
- Patients with nailing of lower extremity found to have embolic showers in 41% of cases
  - Only 16% defined as severe
- Fat emboli noted by TEE in:
  - 94% of pathologic femur fractures
    - 59% severe, defined as FES with respiratory distress
  - 62% of femur fractures (6% severe)
  - 94% of tibial fractures (none severe)
- Paradoxical embolus may occur in patients with PFO and increases mortality risk
  - Hypoxemia seen in 35% to 74% of these patients
  - An alveolar-arterial gradient above 20 mm Hg observed in nearly all patients with uncomplicated long bone and pelvic fractures

TABLE 101.4

FAT EMBOLISM INDEX SCORE

Symptom or sign	Points*
Petechiae	5
Diffuse alveolar infiltrates	4
Hypoxemia (PaO$_2$ <70 mm Hg)	3
Confusion	1
Fever ≥38.5°C	1
Tachycardia ≥120 beats/min	1
Tachypnea ≥30 breaths/min	1

*A positive fat embolism syndrome score is ≥5 points.

- Incidence of full-blown FES decreased from 22% to 1.4% after implementation of internal fixation in patients with long bone fractures
  - Timing of fracture fixation has important impact on incidence of FES
    - Early surgery resulting in lesser risk by as much as fivefold
    - Reports have shown no difference between plating versus nailing
  - Incidence of FES increases with:
    - Number of fractures
    - In military situations, in those with femoral shaft fractures from high-velocity missile wounds of the thigh
    - Absent in those with low-velocity missile wounds without fracture

Pathophysiology

- Two explanations of pathophysiologic mechanisms of FES are mechanical and biochemical theories, these are likely intimately related.
  - When bones fracture, or medullary channel is manipulated or pressurized
    - Fat cells disrupted and enter venous circulation
    - Large fat globules and spongiosa bone fragments obstruct pulmonary capillaries
    - Smaller fat globules bypass pulmonary circulation and enter systemic circulation
    - Major systemic emboli occur with migration of fat globules through pulmonary capillary circuit
    - As previously mentioned, with an intracardiac defect such as a PFO there can be direct access of fat particles to the systemic circulation.
      - PFO seen in 20% to 30% of population
  - Mechanical obstruction of the pulmonary artery (PA) with fat may be an important reason for immediate death after trauma.
    - Obstruction of cerebral capillaries may be cause of altered mental status observed in FES
    - Petechial hemorrhages may be secondary to the presence of fat emboli in the subcutaneous capillaries
  - Manipulation of the bone medulla during surgery increases intramedullary pressure, normally ranges between 30 and 50 mm Hg
  - In animal models, intramedullary pressure of 300 to 400 mm Hg results in fat emboli in vena cava blood even when bone intact
  - According to biochemical theory, increased levels of free fatty acids (FFAs) after bone fracture or manipulation have a direct toxic effect on pneumocytes.
    - FFAs can be freely moving in circulation or accumulate in pulmonary capillaries
    - Capillary leakage, clot formation, and platelet adhesion resulting from toxic effects of FFAs lead to organ damage
    - Lipase released from pneumocytes breaks down bone marrow fat to glycerol and free fatty acids, the latter in toxic concentrations
    - FFA damage to pulmonary endothelium results in capillary damage and nonhydrostatic pulmonary edema
    - Role of PMNLs in FES not clear
      - IV injection of fat may result in accumulation of PMNLs in pulmonary capillaries
    - Lung tissue damage, as well as neutrophil and platelet activation, leads to the release of vasoactive substances:
      - Histamine, serotonin, and bradykinin
      - Result is inflammation and edema, with resultant respiratory distress and multiorgan system failure
      - Manipulation of bone, with resultant fat embolism, is the reason for the hypercoagulable state seen after orthopedic surgery
        - Includes increased platelet aggregation and tissue factor release
    - NO, phospholipase (PL)-A_2, O_2-free radicals, and proinflammatory cytokines such as tumor necrosis factor (TNF)-α, interleukin (IL)-1β, and IL-10 play a role in pathogenesis of FES-induced acute respiratory distress syndrome (ARDS)
    - Alveolar macrophages are probably the major source of inducible NO synthase, producing NO in the lung
  - Neurologic signs of FES likely occur via several mechanisms:
    - Cerebral blood vessel occlusion by fat emboli
    - Disruption of blood–brain barrier due to toxic FFAs
    - Obstruction due to alteration in the solubility of fat in blood

Clinical Presentation and Diagnosis

- No universal definition for FES
- Diagnosis of FES requires high index of suspicion in proper setting
- Is a diagnosis of exclusion
- Severity of symptoms and signs depends on size of fat embolus
- Classical triad for fat embolism includes respiratory insufficiency, altered mental status, and upper extremity and thoracic petechiae
  - All three are seldom seen together
- Most commonly used criteria for FES defined by Gurd
  - Major and minor signs and symptoms
  - One major and four minor criteria required for FES diagnosis (see Table 101.3)
- Clinical signs do not usually appear within 12 hours after injury
- Major signs appear within 24 hours in 65% and within 48 hours in 85% of patients
- Most common signs and symptoms of FES are:
  - Hypoxia, fever, tachycardia, anemia, and altered mental status
  - Early fever, >38.5°C, a common sign and may be seen at emergency department presentation
  - In trauma patients with fractures, early fever raises suspicion of fat embolism
  - Petechiae important findings, but present in one-third of patients
    - Microscopic examination of petechiae reveal fat droplets obstructing capillaries
- Respiratory involvement the most common feature, with tachypnea, dyspnea, and bilateral diffuse infiltrates evident on CXR
- Cyanosis observed if hypoxia is significant, but anemia along with FES can prevent the occurrence of cyanosis even with significant hypoxia

- The $PaCO_2$ decreases secondary to hyperventilation
  - If pulmonary deterioration continues, it may rise
- CXR shows diffuse bilateral pulmonary infiltrates
  - 70% of patients show CXR changes within 24 and no later than 48 hours after injury
- Early clinical signs of FES are actually signs of SIRS
  - Clinical presentation of FES very similar to ARDS with multiple organ failure
  - Retinal examination may reveal exudates, hemorrhages, and, rarely, fat globules
- High-resolution chest CT scan findings of FES include ground glass opacities, which may be associated with thickened interlobular septa
  - Patchy distribution resulting in a "geographic" appearance, which represents the existence of normal and abnormal lung areas with sharp borders and nodular patterns, also observed
  - Resolution of the abnormalities occurs within 2 weeks
- Cerebral manifestations can occur with a wide range of symptoms ranging from confusion, drowsiness, and lethargy to convulsions and coma
  - Pulmonary contusion along with long bone fractures may increase the risk for cerebral fat embolism
  - Typically cerebral CT scan reveals no abnormalities
  - Cerebral MRI may demonstrate hypointense lesions, disruption of the blood–brain barrier, and multiple diffuse foci of hyperintensity in the white matter of the subcortical, periventricular, and centrum semiovale regions, as well as changes related to vasogenic edema, petechial hemorrhages, or hemorrhagic infarcts involving gray and white matter ranging in size from a few millimeters to several centimeters.
- Transcranial Doppler study in trauma patients with long bone fractures can detect cerebral fat embolism.

Treatment

- No specific treatment for FES
  - Therapy is mostly supportive
  - General goals for hypoxic respiratory failure instituted for presumed FES:
    - Methylprednisolone prophylactically may reduce incidence of FES and can reduce the degree of hypoxemia associated with long bone fractures of the lower extremity.
    - High-dose prophylactic steroids with aspirin can result in significant normalization of blood gases, coagulation proteins, and platelet numbers.
      - Prophylactic steroids did not improve mortality in any of the studies
    - Fluid loading, which dilutes the amount of free fatty acids, or increased glucose intake, which decreases free fatty acid mobilization, not found helpful
    - FES may lead to cerebral edema and increased ICP
      - If there are signs of cerebral edema, ICP monitoring recommended
    - ation and analgesia appropriately titrated to allow for frequent neurologic examinations of patient
    - Ethanol shows no benefit in prevention of fat embolism
- Early fixation of long bone fractures helpful to prevent occurrence of FES

- Long bone fixation may result in additional embolizations and FES
- But delayed stabilization of fracture in patient with multiple injuries increases incidence of pulmonary complications (ARDS, fat embolism, and pneumonia) as well as hospital and ICU stay

AMNIOTIC FLUID EMBOLISM (AFE)

- Ricardo Meyer first described entry of amniotic fluid into the maternal circulation in 1926
  - AFE not recognized as syndrome until 1941 with report of sudden death of woman during labor with fetal mucin, amorphous eosinophilic material, and squamous cells in pulmonary vessels
- AFE an uncommon and catastrophic syndrome that occurs during pregnancy or shortly after delivery
  - Pathophysiology thought to involve embolization of amniotic fluid
  - But syndrome results from biochemical mediators released after embolization occurs
  - Suggested that syndrome be renamed as the "anaphylactoid syndrome of pregnancy" because of similarities among the characteristics of AFE, septic shock, and anaphylactic shock
- AFE an important cause of maternal death in developed countries
  - With high morbidity and mortality rates
  - Associated mortality and morbidity has dramatically decreased to approximately 16% recently
    - May be due to improved recognition of the disorder
      - So that even mild cases are included in the analysis
      - As well as to improvements in resuscitation

Epidemiology

- True incidence is not known
  - AFE thought to account for up to 10% of maternal deaths in United States
  - United Kingdom AFE registry investigated maternal and fetal morbidity and mortality rates between 1997 and 2004
    - Data of 44 women with AFE studied
    - Maternal death rate 29.5% (13 patients)
- Incidence of pulmonary embolism (PE) cases associated with pregnancy and/or delivery 0.8% of total PE cases in Japan
  - AFE found in 73.3% (33 of 45) of the PE cases with vaginal delivery and in 21.2% (7 of 33) of PE cases with cesarean delivery
- AFE identified in 19 patients between 1971 and 1988 in Swedish studies
  - Occurred during labor in 70% of the women
  - After vaginal delivery in 11%
  - During cesarean section in 19%
- In the Maternal Health Study Group of the Canadian Perinatal Surveillance System between 1991 and 2002, total rate of AFE was:
  - 14.8 per 100,000 multiple deliveries
  - 6.0 per 100,000 singleton deliveries
  - Mortality rate was 0.8 per 100,000 singleton deliveries
  - None was fatal in multiple deliveries

- In 1,094,248 deliveries during a 2-year period, 53 single-ton pregnancies had the diagnosis of AFE, for a population frequency of 1 per 20,646 pregnancies
- A series of 10 cases of AFE had a maternal mortality rate of 22%
  - Neonatal survival rate was 95%
  - Routine discharge was reported as 72%

Pathophysiology

- Pathophysiology of AFE remains unclear
  - Uterine contractions during normal labor force amniotic fluid into the maternal venous circulation through small tears in the lower uterine segment or high endocervical canal
  - For AFE to occur, there must be a pressure gradient favoring the entry of amniotic fluid from the uterus into the maternal circulation, as well as ruptured membranes
  - Small tears in lower uterine segment and endocervix common during labor and delivery
    - Now thought to be the most likely entry site
    - Two separate life-threatening processes seem to occur either simultaneously or in sequence: cardiorespiratory collapse and coagulopathy

Cardiorespiratory Collapse

- Conventional explanation states particulate matter such as fetal squamous cells, lanugo, and meconium contained in the amniotic fluid produce pulmonary vascular obstruction, leading to pulmonary hypertension, right- and left-sided heart failure, hypotension, and death.
- Current evidence suggests mechanical origin less likely than immunologic reaction.
  - Pulmonary vasospasm causes physiologic PA obstruction in reaction to abnormal substances such as leukotrienes and metabolites of arachidonic acid in amniotic fluid.
    - Arachidonic acid metabolites implicated in inflammatory response, and may in part be responsible for AFE
    - Presence of these metabolites in AFE suggests a possible humoral mechanism
    - Humoral pathways invoking a proinflammatory response with release of cytokines and arachidonic acid metabolites in AFE, anaphylaxis, and shock may be responsible for the similar clinical presentation
    - Complex inflammatory cascade with mediator release leads to SIRS and development of multiple organ system failure
- Mild to moderate PAP elevations only transiently noted in AFE
  - Biphasic model proposed to explain hemodynamic abnormalities
    - Acute pulmonary hypertension and vasospasm the initial hemodynamic response
    - Resulting right heart failure and accompanying hypoxia could account for the cases of sudden death or severe neurologic impairment
    - Limited hemodynamic data obtained by invasive pulmonary artery monitoring or echocardiography during the hyperacute phase of AFE demonstrated left ventricle (LV), not RV, failure as dominant finding
    - Myocardial dysfunction may be the result of a sudden increase in maternal plasma endothelin levels that occurs with introduction of amniotic fluid, which contains a high concentration of endothelin.

Disseminated Intravascular Coagulation (DIC)

- DIC commonly observed as late sequela of AFE
  - May be attributed to antithrombin- or thromboplastin-type effects of amniotic fluid or even complement activators
  - Amniotic fluid has highly potent, total thromboplastinlike activity
    - Procoagulant activity increases with duration of gestation
  - Amniotic fluid has relatively strong antifibrinolytic activity
    - Also increases during gestation

Clinical Presentation

- Symptoms of AFE commonly occur during labor (80%) and delivery, or in immediate postpartum period
  - AFE can also develop 4 to 48 hours postpartum or after cesarean delivery, amniocentesis, or removal of the placenta, or with first- and second-trimester abortions
- Risk factors associated for AFE are:
  - Older age
  - Multiparity
  - Marked exaggeration of uterine contraction following rupture of the uterine membranes
  - Markedly exaggerated uterine contraction due to the use of oxytocin or other uterine stimulatory agents
  - Prolonged gestation
  - Instrumented vaginal delivery
  - Eclampsia
  - Polyhydramnios
  - Fetal distress
  - Large fetal size
  - Meconium staining of the amniotic fluid
  - Cesarean section
  - Uterine rupture
  - High cervical laceration
  - Premature separation of placenta
  - Intrauterine fetal death
  - Blunt abdominal trauma, surgical intervention, cervical suture removal, and saline amnioinfusion other rare causes of AFE (Table 101.5)
- Classic clinical presentation of AFE is the sudden onset of dyspnea, respiratory failure, and hypotension, followed by cardiovascular collapse and DIC.
  - Cardiorespiratory collapse almost invariably present
  - Presenting symptom in 51% of patients was respiratory distress, hypotension in 27%, coagulopathy in 12%, and seizures in 10%
  - Fetal bradycardia (17%) and hypotension (13%) also common presenting features
- Typically patient in active labor with intact amnion and develops sudden respiratory failure and circulatory collapse, followed by a systemic thrombohemorrhagic disorder
  - In some women, postpartum consumptive coagulopathy appears to be the sole presenting sign
  - Abrupt fetal bradycardia followed by coagulopathy can occur
- Acute hypoxia immediately followed by an initial increase in blood pressure, with subsequent hypotension, suggestive of left atrium (LA) and LV failure, can be observed in AFE

TABLE 101.5

RISK FACTORS OF AMNIOTIC FLUID EMBOLISM

Older age
Multiparity
Physiologic intense uterine contractions
Medical induction of labor
Instrumental vaginal delivery
Prolonged gestation
Cesarean section
Uterine rupture
Polyhydramnios
High cervical tear
Premature placental separation
Intrauterine fetal death
Large fetal size
Meconium staining of the amniotic fluid
Placental abruption
Eclampsia
Fetal distress
Trauma to abdomen
Surgical intervention
Saline amnioinfusion

- Cardiogenic pulmonary edema due to LV failure occurs
- Seizures occur in 10% to 20% of patients
- Profound hypoxia and right-sided heart failure follow pulmonary arterial spasm and may account for the 50% mortality rate within the first hour
- DIC is a common finding, seen in up to 83%
  - Half of these patients develop coagulopathy within 4 hours of initial presentation
- Presenting manifestation of DIC is profound hemorrhage, prompting an extensive search for anatomic causes of bleeding
- There are three identified phases of AFE in humans:
- Phase 1: Pulmonary—Respiratory distress and cyanosis
- Phase 2: Hemodynamic—Pulmonary edema and hemorrhagic shock
- Phase 3: Neurologic—Confusion and coma
- Manifestations occur in combination, separately, and in different magnitudes
  - Of patients surviving initial cardiorespiratory insult, 40% to 50% progress into phase 2
    - Characterized by coagulopathy, hemorrhage, and shock
    - Left-sided heart failure is evident and is the most reported sign in humans
    - Increased pulmonary capillary wedge pressure (PCWP) and CVP are characteristics of pulmonary edema
- In phase 3, acute symptoms disappear, and injury to the brain, lung, and renal systems are noted
  - Phase 3 may last weeks
  - Patients may die as a result of severe brain and lung injury
    - Infection and multiple organ system failure may also cause death

Diagnosis

- AFE is largely a diagnosis of exclusion
  - Differential diagnosis includes:
    - Air or thrombotic pulmonary emboli
    - Septic shock
    - Acute myocardial infarction
    - Cardiomyopathy
    - Anaphylaxis
    - Aspiration
    - Placental abruption
    - Eclampsia
    - Uterine rupture
    - Transfusion reaction
    - Local anesthetic toxicity
- Diagnosis of AFE considered when pregnant woman with one or more risk factors suddenly develops respiratory distress, bleeding, or shock
- Several methods suggested for diagnosing AFE
  - None of these diagnostic tests is reliable
- The initial presenting signs often seen on ECG and the pulse oximeter
  - Former may show tachycardia with a right-heart strain pattern and ST-T–wave changes
  - Pulse oximetry may reveal a sudden drop in oxygen saturation
  - Clinical diagnosis is made most frequently in 65% to 70% of cases during labor and much less frequently in 11% of cases in the postpartum period
- Initial laboratory data should include:
  - Arterial blood gas (ABG) analysis to determine adequacy of ventilation and degree of hypoxemia
  - Diagnostic markers for AFE based on peripheral blood samples introduced
    - Sialyl Tn (STN), mucin-associated disaccharide antigen carried by apomucins, zinc coproporphyrin, and complement factor consumption
      - Significantly higher serum STN levels were found in patients with clinically apparent AFE
    - Monoclonal antibody THK-2, an antibody directed to STN, may be a specific pathologic marker for AFE
    - Fetal megakaryocytes and syncytiotrophoblastic cells can be found in maternal pulmonary circulation by monoclonal antibodies (CD-61—GPIIIa, β-hCG, and factor VIII-vW hPL antibodies) and may be diagnostic.
- Laboratory tests to evaluate the development of DIC are:
  - Anti-thrombin III level
  - Fibrinopeptide A level
  - D-dimer level
  - Prothrombin fragment 1.2 (PF 1.2)
  - Thrombin precursor protein
  - Platelet count
  - Global tests, including the prothrombin time (PT), partial thromboplastin time (PTT), and fibrinogen level, are helpful
- When correlated with clinical signs and symptoms, other diagnostic tools may be employed to support the presumptive diagnosis of AFE.
- Echocardiography may show severe pulmonary hypertension and RV dilatation
  - Displaced intraventricular septum pressing on LV
  - TEE may show RV failure with leftward deviation of the interventricular septum and severe tricuspid regurgitation.
- CXR a helpful diagnostic tool, but it is limited by a lack of specificity
  - In mothers with AFE, 24% to 93% of CXRs show a pulmonary edema pattern

- Multiple patchy, nodular infiltrates and small pleural effusion may also be seen
- Histologic examination demonstrates foreign material in the pulmonary capillaries, arterioles, and arteries.
  - Special stains such as TKH-2, a monoclonal antibody to fetal glycoprotein sialyl Tn antigen, have been applied to pathologic specimens

Treatment

- Treatment is supportive.
  - Despite the decline in mortality, no new therapies have emerged
  - Aggressive resuscitation indicated depending on the clinical presentation
  - Management strategies include:
    - Improving oxygenation, support of circulation, and correcting coagulopathy
    - Arterial and PA catheters should be placed to help guide the therapy when hemodynamic deterioration is severe
  - If fetus is sufficiently mature and undelivered at the time of maternal cardiac arrest, cesarean section should be instituted as soon as possible.
  - Maternal oxygenation to $PaO_2 > 60$ mm Hg achieved by administering oxygen via face mask to all nonintubated patients
    - Tracheal intubation and MV instituted in patients with refractory hypoxemia or seizures, or in the comatose individual
    - Vasoactive drug therapy must be tailored to clinical situation.
      - Dopamine is suggested to enhance cardiac output and support blood pressure.
      - In severe shock, epinephrine or norepinephrine may be required.
  - In <4 hours, half of patients who survive develop DIC, with massive hemorrhage.
    - Therefore, blood products should be prepared ahead of time, and replacement with typed-and-crossed packed red blood cells, or with O-negative blood, is essential.

- Treatment of DIC requires the transfusion of packed red blood cells and blood products.
- Large-bore IV access is essential.
- Platelets, cryoprecipitate, and fresh frozen plasma should be administered as guided by laboratory assessment of the thromboelastogram (TEG) or international normalized ratio (INR)/PT/PTT, fibrinogen, and fibrin and fibrin degradation products.
- Plasma exchange, cardiopulmonary bypass, aprotinin, and recombinant activated factor VII (rVIIa) in the management of the associated coagulopathy are used to treat AFE.
- Successful use of uterine arterial embolization to control massive bleeding in two cases of AFE has been described.
- During CPR and chest compressions, and before delivery, uterus should be displaced to the left to avoid compressing the aorta and inferior vena cava, which would compromise maternal venous return to the heart.
  - Uterus can be displaced manually or by placing a wedge under the patient's right hip.

Prognosis

- AFE remains one of the most feared and lethal complications of pregnancy.
- Prognosis and mortality of AFE have improved significantly with early diagnosis and prompt and early resuscitative measures.
  - Parturient with a known history of atopy or anaphylaxis also at a high risk of AFE
  - In the National Amniotic Fluid Embolism Registry known history of drug allergy and atopy was found in 41% of the 46 patients with AFE
- Mainstay of a successful outcome remains the identification of high-risk patients
- In some cases, death is inevitable despite early and appropriate management
- Neonatal survival is reported as 70%
- Although there are many new developments with respect to knowledge of the diseases, AFE continues to be a catastrophic illness

CHAPTER 102 ■ ELEVATED INTRACRANIAL PRESSURE

DEFINITION OF INTRACRANIAL PRESSURE (ICP)

- ICP is the pressure of compartment inside skull.
  - Brain is almost completely incompressible.
  - Expansion of volume in any component within skull causes an increase in pressure of cranial compartment.
  - Increased ICP can lead to decreased cerebral blood flow (CBF) resulting in:
    - Decreased oxygen delivery to brain
    - Neuronal dysfunction due to:
      ○ Global ischemia
      ○ Herniation of brain with compression of vital structures
      ○ Death
  - Principles of increased ICP defined by Monro-Kellie doctrine

CAUSES OF INCREASED ICP

- Intracranial hypertension complicates many neurologic disorders.
  - Head trauma can result in diffuse brain edema, increased blood flow, and mass lesions such as subdural, epidural, or intraparenchymal hemorrhage.
    - Brain edema following head injury is primarily cellular edema, although vasogenic edema can occur transiently.
  - Ruptured aneurysm can cause subarachnoid hemorrhage, resulting in vasospasm and hydrocephalus.
  - Ischemic or hemorrhagic strokes can result in mass lesion and cellular edema.
  - Obstructive or communicating hydrocephalus from multiple causes can result in increased cerebrospinal fluid (CSF) volume.
  - Fulminant hepatic failure can cause significant cerebral edema.
  - Brain tumors or infection can occupy volume within intracranial space.

PHYSIOLOGY OF THE INTRACRANIAL SPACE

Monro-Kellie Doctrine

- Intracranial compartment partially divided into two compartments by tentorium cerebelli

- Shelf of dura divides skull into the supratentorial compartment
  - Containing cerebral hemispheres
- And infratentorial compartment
  - Containing brainstem and cerebellum
- Increased ICP in supratentorial compartment can cause uncal herniation
  - With temporal lobe herniating through incisura of tentorium and compressing midbrain
- Continued increase in ICP in superior fossa or increased ICP in posterior fossa can cause tonsillar herniation
  - With tonsils of cerebellum herniating through foramen magnum with compression of medulla

CIRCULATION OF CEREBROSPINAL FLUID

- CSF contained within ventricles of brain provides a buffer to changes in other volumes within intracranial space.
  - Choroid plexus, located within lateral and fourth ventricles, secretes CSF
  - CSF drains from lateral ventricles through two foramina of Monro into third ventricle
  - From third ventricle drains via cerebral aqueduct into fourth ventricle
  - From fourth ventricle it drains into subarachnoid space through two lateral foramina of Luschka and median foramen of Magendie and into central canal of the spinal cord
  - In subarachnoid space CSF is resorbed at arachnoid villi
  - Normal total CSF volume in adult is 150 mL
    ○ In a day, 450 mL of CSF is secreted
    ○ Thus CSF volume recirculated three times each day
      – Increased secretion or decreased absorption can cause communicating hydrocephalus
      – Blockage of circulation of CSF can cause obstructive hydrocephalus
      – Absorption of CSF pressure dependent, secretion is not

ICP PRESSURE: VOLUME CURVE

- ICP is a nonlinear function of increasing volume in the intracranial space (Fig. 102.1).
  - Early increases in volume of mass lesion result in CSF displacement from cranial compartment into spinal compartment.
    - Cause little increase in ICP

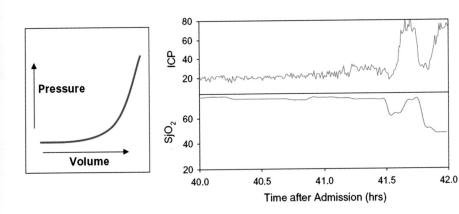

FIGURE 102.1. The **left graph** illustrates the nonlinear nature of the relationship between the volume of intracranial contents and intracranial pressure. The **right graph** shows the actual intracranial pressure (ICP) and jugular venous oxygen saturation (SjO$_2$) tracings in a patient who developed a delayed intracranial hematoma. Initially the rise in ICP was minimal as the brain was able to compensate for the increasing volume from the hematoma. Later when these compensatory mechanisms were exhausted, there was a very rapid increase in ICP associated with compromise of cerebral blood flow and a decrease in SjO$_2$.

- Once maximal amount of CSF is displaced from intracranial compartment, ICP increases rapidly.
  - As ICP increases cerebral perfusion pressure decreases and blood flow to the brain decreases.

CEREBRAL PERFUSION PRESSURE (CPP)

- See above
- Pressure autoregulation is the intrinsic ability of cerebral vasculature to maintain flow constant over a wide range of CPP values.
  - Dynamic pressure autoregulation is commonly dysfunctional in injured brain.
    - When impaired, the lower limit of autoregulation shifted upward from 50 to 60 to 90 mm Hg.
    - When entirely absent, perfusion passively follows CPP.
  - Loss of normal autoregulation requires careful maintenance of sufficient mean arterial pressure (MAP) and adequate control of ICP to avoid brain hypoperfusion.
  - Extremely elevated MAP should also be avoided as it can cause increased ICP.

BRAIN METABOLISM

- See above
- 15% of blood flow goes to brain
  - Normal CBF is 50 to 55 mL per 100 g/minute
  - Each 100 g of brain tissue requires at least 20 mL of blood flow per minute to function normally
  - Between 8 and 20 mL/100 g/minute of blood flow, brain tissue survives for at least a period of time but does not function normally
  - Below 8 mL/100 g/minute brain tissue dies
  - Brain consumes 20% of oxygen used by body
    - Using 3.5 mL of oxygen per 100 g/minute
  - Brain dependent on delivery of glucose in blood as it has almost no intrinsic energy stores
- CBF thresholds determined in normal brain
  - Seem to hold true for brain-injured patients
  - Low CBF, particularly in early postinjury period, highly predictive of a poor outcome
    - Traumatic brain injury (TBI) patients with CBF < 18 mL/100 g/minute had significantly worse outcome compared to patients with higher CBF

- Within 12 hours of injury
  - Every 10 mL/100 g/minute increase in CBF associated with threefold increase in probability of surviving

COMMONLY MONITORED PARAMETERS IN PATIENTS WITH ELEVATED ICP

Intracranial Pressure

- Elevated ICP can be measured and treated
- Normal ICP in adult is <10 mm Hg
- ICP value of 20 to 30 mm Hg is mild intracranial hypertension
- ICP above 40 mm Hg is severe, life-threatening intracranial hypertension
- Goal of treatment should be to maintain ICP below 20 to 25 mm Hg
- TBI patients with elevated ICP have worse outcome than those with ICP below 20 mm Hg
- Gold standard for monitoring ICP is ventriculostomy catheter inserted through burr hole into one of the lateral ventricles.
  - Catheter connected to drainage system and can be used to monitor ICP through fluid-coupled external pressure transducer
  - Most accurate measurement of ICP and stable over time
  - Allows drainage of CSF for control of ICP
  - Problems associated with ventriculostomy catheters include:
    - Blockage of catheter
    - Displacement of catheter from ventricle
    - Infection
      - Antibiotic-impregnated ventriculostomy catheters reduce risk of infection from 9.4% to 1.3%

Cerebral Perfusion Pressure

- See above
- CPP defined as MAP minus the ICP
  - Measured using a combination of ICP monitor and an arterial line or a noninvasive blood pressure monitor
  - The second major parameter monitored and treated in patient with elevated ICP
  - Can be supported by maintaining mean arterial pressure (MAP) with IV fluids and vasopressors and by lowering ICP
  - For most patients, a CPP of at least 60 mm Hg is adequate

Brain Oxygenation

- See above
- Brain tissue oxygenation measured either by:
  - Positron emission tomography (PET) imaging techniques to obtain a single time point sample across entire brain
  - Using probes to continuously monitor:
    - Brain tissue pO_2 ($PbtO_2$)
    - Jugular venous oxygen saturation ($SjvO_2$)

Brain Tissue Oxygen Tension

- Insertion of $PbtO_2$ probe allows continuous monitoring of O_2 tension in local region of brain
- Location of probe is critical and determines nature of pO_2 information obtained (Fig. 102.2)
  - If inserted near focal lesion, O_2 can be monitored in tissue at greatest risk should injury expand
  - Insertion in uninjured brain allows monitoring of local area that should be representative of overall less-injured O_2 status of brain
  - Provides information that is similar to SjO_2 monitoring
- Normal values and critical threshold values for $PbtO_2$ are somewhat less accepted.

- In anesthetized subjects, $PbtO_2$ in normal brain ranges from 20 to 40 mm Hg.
  - Comparing $PbtO_2$ values to PET measurements of O_2 extraction fraction (OEF) shows PbO_2 value associated with OEF of 40% (mean value in normal subjects) was 14 mm Hg.
- Values of $PbtO_2$ indicating tissue hypoxia/ischemia probably <14 mm Hg
  - Serial measurements of both SjO_2 and PbO_2 suggest a $PbtO_2$ of 8.5 mm Hg and indicates a similar level of oxygenation as SjO_2 of 50%
  - $PbtO_2$ <15 mm Hg associated with poor outcome
  - Treatment protocol keeping brain $PbtO_2$ >25 mm Hg may reduce mortality when compared to patients treated similarly with no $PbtO_2$ probe

Jugular Venous Oxygen Saturation

- See above
- Episodes of $SjvO_2$ desaturation associated with worse neurologic outcome
  - Increased $SjvO_2$ may indicate decreased oxygen uptake in brain

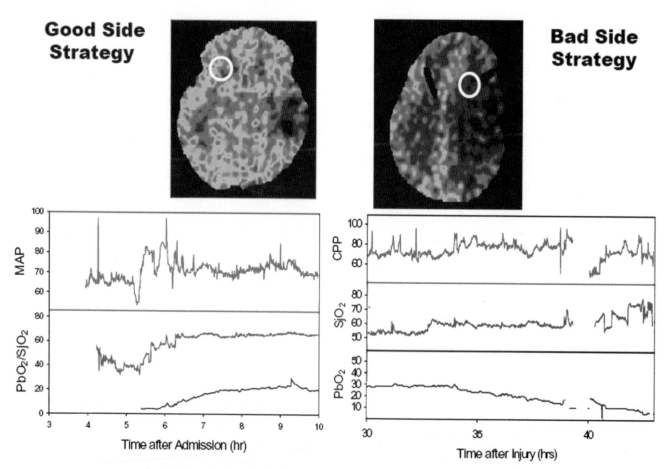

FIGURE 102.2. Location of the brain tissue oxygen tension (PbO_2) catheter relative to the injured brain determines the nature of the pO_2 information that will be obtained. On the **left** is a patient where the PbO_2 catheter was placed in relatively normal brain opposite a temporal contusion. The PbO_2 reflected the global oxygenation of the brain measured with jugular venous oxygen saturation (SjO_2). On the **right** is a patient where the PbO_2 catheter was placed near a contusion. As this contusion evolved, the PbO_2 decreased even though the global measures (SjO_2 and cerebral perfusion pressure [CPP]) remained unchanged. MAP, mean arterial pressure.

- Major limitation of $SjvO_2$ monitoring is it cannot detect local ischemia within brain
- Normal values for $SjvO_2$ better established than for $PbtO_2$
  - In 50 normal young males $SjvO_2$ ranged from 55% to 71% (mean 61.8%)
    - Normal $SjvO_2$ values may be as low as 45%
    - Normal $SjvO_2$ lower than normal SvO_2, indicating that brain normally extracts oxygen more completely from arterial blood than do other organs

WHAT IS THE MOST IMPORTANT PHYSIOLOGIC END POINT (ICP, CPP, OR BRAIN OXYGENATION)?

- Some have advocated ICP is not important as long as CPP is maintained.
  - Led to the use of CPP-directed therapy where induced hypertension was used to drive CPP to high levels, even though ICP was also increased by therapy
  - All these physiologic parameters related to outcome
  - No clear evidence that one parameter is more important than others
  - Table 102.1 presents normal values and treatment thresholds for these parameters
- Best circumstance when ICP, CPP, and $PbtO_2$/$SjvO_2$ are all maintained in normal range
  - This should probably be goal of management
  - When not possible, it is important to understand limitations of each monitor when making therapeutic decisions

IMMEDIATE CONCERNS FOR TREATMENT

Identification of Patients with Increased ICP

- Patient with mildly increased ICP can present with headache and blurred vision.
  - Further increases in ICP associated with decreased level of consciousness and symptoms of herniation
    - Herniation of temporal lobe over edge of tentorium can compress cranial nerve III, causing ipsilateral pupillary dilation and decreased reaction to light

TABLE 102.1

NORMAL VALUES AND TREATMENT THRESHOLDS FOR PHYSIOLOGIC PARAMETERS

	Normal	Treatment threshold
ICP	0–10 mm Hg	20–25 mm Hg
CPP	50 mm Hg	60 mm Hg
$SjvO_2$	55%–71%	50%
$PbtO_2$	20–40 mm Hg	8–10 mm Hg

ICP, intracranial pressure; CPP, cerebral perfusion pressure; $SjvO_2$, jugular venous oxygen saturation; $PbtO_2$, brain tissue oxygen tension.

- Direct compression of brainstem can cause contralateral posturing or hemiparesis
  - If the brainstem is displaced and compressed against opposite side of tentorium, there may be ipsilateral symptoms, called Kernohan notch phenomenon.
- Further symptoms of herniation are hypertension, bradycardia, and widening pulse pressure, the Cushing triad.
- Respiratory abnormalities may include:
  - Cheyne-Stokes respiration
  - Hypoventilation
  - Central neurogenic hyperventilation
- If elevated ICP suspected, noncontrast computed tomography (CT) scan of brain is needed to evaluate for mass lesions, hydrocephalus, subarachnoid hemorrhage, or other treatable causes

Initial Stabilization and Management of Patients with Elevated ICP

- Initial steps in managing elevated ICP defined by ABCs of trauma resuscitation
- Episodes of hypoxemia ($PaO_2 < 60$ mm Hg) or hypotension (systolic blood pressure <90 mm Hg) associated with significantly worse outcome in patients with TBI
- Airway protection essential
  - Patients with Glasgow Coma Scale (GCS) of 8 or less should be intubated to protect airway
  - Patients with GCS above 8 may also need intubation if they cannot adequately protect their airway
  - Supplemental oxygen and mechanical ventilation (MV) may be necessary to avoid hypoxemia
- Blood pressure supported with fluid resuscitation and vasopressors, as necessary
  - Hypotension should not be attributed to brain injury unless all other possible causes excluded
  - Patients with elevated ICP should be cared for in dedicated neurological intensive care unit with a neurosurgeon included in care team
- Immediate aggressive management of elevated ICP initiated in patients with signs and symptoms of herniation include:
- Mild hyperventilation, to a $PaCO_2$ of 30 to 35 mm Hg
  - Can reduce ICP by constricting cerebral blood vessels
- Once fluid resuscitation completed, osmotic therapy with either mannitol or hypertonic saline initiated
- Standard dose for mannitol is IV bolus of 1 g/kg
  - With subdural hematoma and signs of herniation, early preoperative administration of mannitol 1.4 g/kg significantly improves outcome
  - Only give once fluid resuscitation is completed as it can cause hypotension in incompletely resuscitated patient
- Alternative osmotic agent is hypertonic saline
  - May have advantage in hypotensive patient since it does not induce diuresis
  - Resuscitation with hypertonic saline demonstrated to result in less hypotension compared with mannitol
    - Has not clearly been shown to result in an improved outcome
- If a surgical lesion identified:
  - Patient immediately taken to operating room for evacuation of lesion

- Invasive monitoring devices inserted either at bedside or in operating room if surgery is required
  - Minimally, ICP monitor, preferably a ventriculostomy drain inserted
  - Other monitoring devices used if available include:
    - $PbtO_2$ monitor
    - $SjvO_2$ catheter
    - Arterial line and a Foley catheter should also be placed
    - Central venous line may be needed, especially if hypotension is present or large doses of mannitol are needed

TREATMENT OF ELEVATED INTRACRANIAL PRESSURE: PRINCIPLES OF CENTRAL NERVOUS SYSTEM RESUSCITATION

General Measures

- Specific factors that may aggravate intracranial hypertension include:
  - Obstruction of venous return (head position, agitation)
  - Respiratory problems (airway obstruction, hypoxia, hypercapnia)
  - Fever
  - Severe hypertension
  - Hyponatremia
  - Anemia
  - Seizures
- Routine management of patient at risk for intracranial hypertension should include measures to prevent these factors.
- Also important to maintain normal brain oxygenation and CPP

Minimize Obstruction to Venous Return

- Elevation of head of bed and keeping head in neutral position to minimize compression of venous return from the brain are standard practice for management of ICP.
  - Elevation of head to 30 degrees results in reduction in ICP without reduction in either CPP or CBF in most patients.
  - **When head elevation is used, both the ICP and blood pressure transducers must be zeroed at the same level (i.e., at the level of the foramen of Monro).**
- In multiple-trauma patients increased intra-abdominal pressure may also impede venous return from the brain, decrease blood pressure (BP), and increase ICP.
  - Abdominal decompression can improve control of ICP when abdominal compartment syndrome is present.

Prevent Fever

- Fever is common during recovery from head injury.
  - Experimentally postinjury fever worsens outcome from fluid percussion injury.
  - Fever is a potent cerebral vasodilator and can raise ICP.
  - Fever can raise cerebral metabolic requirements.
    - Efficient external cooling systems and intravascular cooling devices available to maintain normal body temperature
    - Infectious causes should be investigated appropriately and treated

Prevent Seizures

- Seizures occur in approximately 15% of patients with head injury.
  - Risk related to severity of injury
  - In 4,541 head injury patients, standardized incidence ratio for developing seizures was:
    - 1.5 after mild injuries with no increase over expected number after 5 years
    - 2.9 after moderate injuries
    - 17.0 after severe injuries
  - Patients often sedated and pharmacologically paralyzed to treat intracranial hypertension
    - Clinical monitoring often not helpful
    - Continuous electroencephalogram (EEG) monitoring may be useful for this high-risk group of patients
- Use of anticonvulsants to prevent seizures controversial
  - Seizures dramatically increase cerebral metabolic rate
    - But no clear relationship between occurrence of early seizures and worse neurologic outcome
      - No difference in incidence of seizures with prophylactic phenytoin
      - In a double-blind study of 404 severely head-injured patients randomly receiving phenytoin or placebo for 1 year, phenytoin reduced incidence of seizures during first week but not thereafter

Maintain Brain Oxygenation

- Brain oxygen delivery (DO_2) dependent on oxygen content of blood (CaO_2) and CBF
- Blood O_2 content can be increased by ensuring adequate Hgb concentration and increasing PaO_2
- For the brain, but not other organs, optimal hemoglobin (Hgb) concentration approximates 10 g/dL
  - Lower Hgb concentration reduces oxygen-carrying capacity of blood more than it improves viscosity
  - Higher Hgb concentration increases viscosity and reduces CBF even though it increases oxygen-carrying capacity
- Increasing PaO_2 after hemoglobin is nearly 100% saturated increases CaO_2 minimally
  - By the amount of oxygen dissolved in blood
  - If tissues are ischemic small increases in CaO_2 important
    - PET imaging suggests impaired O_2 diffusion in injured brain tissue
    - May also be mitochondrial dysfunction in injured brain
  - Hyperoxia may improve tissue oxygenation under these conditions
    - There is an increased $PbtO_2$ and decreased extracellular lactate concentration in brain, measured by microdialysis, when patients with very low baseline $PbtO_2$ were placed on 100% oxygen.
    - Reduction in lactate accumulation suggests increased $PbtO_2$ altered ischemic cerebral metabolism favorably.

Maintain Cerebral Perfusion Pressure

- Initial volume resuscitation aimed at achieving euvolemia
  - Once ICP monitor in place, further BP management aimed at maintaining CPP to at least 60 mm Hg
- IV fluid boluses used as initial treatment of low CPP
  - All IV fluids given should be isotonic to avoid worsening cerebral edema

- If fluid resuscitation is insufficient to maintain CPP, treat with pressors
  - Suggestion that norepinephrine results in more predictable BP than dopamine
  - Treating to a CPP >60 mm Hg not shown to improve outcome but does increase acute respiratory distress syndrome risk

First-line Therapies of Intracranial Hypertension

Sedation and Paralysis

- Sedative/analgesic drugs blunt effect of routine nursing care on ICP.
  - Routine paralysis of all patients with severe head injury increases the risk of pulmonary complications and prolongs the intensive care unit stay.
  - However, ICP raised by agitation, posturing, or coughing is prevented by narcotics and nondepolarizing muscle relaxants that do not alter cerebrovascular resistance.
    - Reasonable regimen is morphine and lorazepam for analgesia/sedation
    - Cisatracurium or vecuronium as a muscle relaxant, with dose titrated to twitch response to stimulation (1 to 2 of 4 of a train of four)
  - Neurologic examination cannot be closely monitored while patient is paralyzed.
    - If safe and appropriate, muscle relaxants can be withheld once a day, usually before morning rounds, to obtain a brief neurologic examination.

Osmotic Therapy to Reduce Intracranial Pressure

- One mainstay of treatment of elevated ICP is osmotic therapy with mannitol or hypertonic saline.
  - Treatment can be initiated prior to insertion of ICP monitor if signs and symptoms of herniation are present.
  - Initial dose of mannitol is 1 g/kg
    - Once ICP monitor is inserted, bolus doses can be given to maintain ICP <20 to 25 mm Hg.
    - Bolus dosing of 0.25 mg to 0.5 mg/kg every 2 to 6 hours can be given if serum osmolality <320 mOsm/kg H_2O.
    - Dosing to serum osmolality >320 not demonstrated to improve outcome and increases risk of acute renal failure
- Mannitol reduces ICP through two mechanisms:
  - First is immediate expansion of intravascular volume, resulting in reduced hematocrit and reduced blood viscosity, causing decreased ICP and increased CBF and DO_2
  - Second involves establishment of osmotic gradients between plasma and cells
    - Resulting in decreased cellular volume
    - Long-term treatment with mannitol results in buildup of mannitol within the cells
    - Effect is more marked with continuous infusion of mannitol
- Mannitol more widely studied, but hypertonic saline may be more effective at lowering ICP
  - Studies small and no demonstration of statistical significance in outcome
  - Usual dose form is boluses of 7.5% hypertonic saline

- Other agents include hypertonic saline hetastarch, 7.5% hypertonic saline/6% dextran solution
  - Large randomized controlled studies necessary to define role of hypertonic saline in the treatment of increased ICP

Drainage of Cerebrospinal Fluid

- Placement of ventriculostomy catheter allows drainage of CSF during episodes of increased ICP.
  - Drainage of 3 to 5 mL of CSF can reduce ICP.
  - If CSF is drained continuously, drainage system should not be set lower than 10 cm above the level of foramen of Monro.
    - Approximated by the external auditory canal

Hyperventilation

- Hyperventilation to $PaCO_2$ of 30 to 35 mm Hg can reduce ICP by constricting cerebral blood vessels and reducing cerebral blood volume.
  - Effect of changes in $PaCO_2$ on cerebral vessels mediated by change in pH induced in the extracellular fluid
  - Effects of hyperventilation on ICP are immediate
    - Duration of effect brief because pH of brain, in normal individuals, soon equilibrates to the lower $PaCO_2$ level
- Long-term hyperventilation to $PaCO_2$ of 25 to 30 mm Hg demonstrated to result in worse outcomes after TBI
  - Possibly secondary to reduction in CBF
  - Recommendation is to use hyperventilation only in patients with intracranial hypertension rather than as routine in all head-injured patients
- For patients chronically hyperventilated, abruptly returning $PaCO_2$ to normal can result in a dramatic increase in ICP.
  - This phenomenon occurs after 24 hours of hyperventilation.
  - Associated with vasodilation of cerebral vessels as CSF pH equilibrates at new lower $PaCO_2$ level
  - Hyperventilation should be withdrawn over several days to avoid this increase in ICP.

Additional Treatments for Refractory Intracranial Hypertension

- All treatments outlined below shown in clinical studies to significantly reduce ICP, even when refractory to initial treatments
  - None demonstrated to improve neurologic outcome
  - No data to suggest which of these is most effective or has least morbidity
  - For these reasons, such additional therapies are usually applied selectively
- When refractory intracranial hypertension occurs:
  - Consider whether a delayed intracranial hematoma may have developed
  - Follow-up CT scan may be indicated before these additional treatments
    - Any surgical intracranial hematoma should be evacuated

Pentobarbital Coma

- If CSF drainage and mannitol fail to control elevated ICP, other techniques to be considered.
  - Administration of pentobarbital to achieve burst suppression on EEG

- Routine use of barbiturates in unselected patients not consistently effective in reducing morbidity or mortality after severe head injury
- Nonetheless, a randomized multicenter trial demonstrated barbiturate coma in patients with refractory intracranial hypertension resulted in twofold greater chance of controlling ICP.
- Simple dosing scheme from randomized clinical trial is:
  - Loading dose of 10 mg/kg IV over 30 minutes
  - Followed by 5 mg/kg/hour for 3 hours
  - Followed by maintenance dose of 1 mg/kg/hour
  - Maintenance dose titrated to achieve level of 35 to 50 μg/mL
  - Continuous EEG used to monitor for burst suppression for maximal therapeutic effect
- Significant hypotension may develop during administration of the loading dose
  - Consider placement of pulmonary artery catheter for continuous cardiac monitoring
  - Initial loading dose requires close monitoring of BP
    ○ Hypotension during induction usually responds to fluid bolus
  - Higher doses of pentobarbital can cause myocardial depression and require inotropic or even vasopressor support.
- Goal of treatment is to reduce ICP to < 20 to 25 mm Hg
  - After ICP is controlled for 24 to 48 hours, pentobarbital can be weaned and stopped
    - If ICP increases during reduction of pentobarbital, stop titration and increase dose until ICP controlled
    - Pentobarbital is thought to work through multiple mechanisms
      ○ Alterations in vascular tone
      ○ Decreased cerebral metabolism
      ○ Decreased free radical production
- Pentobarbital coma associated with significant morbidity
  - Hypotension is common and may require concomitant administration of vasopressors.
  - Pentobarbital coma increases risk of pneumonia, pressure ulcers, and paralytic ileus.
- PT characteristics that may indicate a favorable ICP response to barbiturates include:
  - Younger age
  - Diffuse rather than focal brain injury
  - Relatively high level of brain electrical activity
  - High cerebral metabolic rate prior to treatment
  - Preservation of CO_2 reactivity may predict good ICP response to barbiturates

Decompressive Craniectomy

- Kocher initially described in 1901, craniectomy for control of elevated ICP has long history
  - Initially showed improved outcome resulting in increased usage
    - Follow-up studies did not demonstrate same improved outcome and craniectomy became less popular
    - More recently benefits have been seen and is being used for control of elevated ICP
  - Can be considered in patients with elevated ICP uncontrolled by CSF drainage and osmotic therapy
    - If injury primarily involves single hemisphere, a hemicraniectomy can provide adequate decompression.

- Large bone flap should be removed with particular focus on decompressing anterior temporal lobe and visualization of floor of middle fossa.
- Diffuse injury involving both hemispheres may necessitate bifrontal craniectomy, with removal of large bone flap and decompression of both temporal lobes and both frontal lobes.
- Demonstrated to result in significant decrease in ICP
  - Retrospectively suggested to improve outcome
    - Two randomized clinical trials currently under way
    - Craniectomy also useful in treatment of elevated ICP secondary to malignant middle cerebral artery stroke
      ○ Significant reduction in mortality and improved outcome if performed prior to development of symptoms of herniation

Hypothermia

- Hypothermia has several potentially neuroprotective effects, including:
  - Reducing cerebral metabolism and decreasing ICP
  - Randomized, controlled trial in humans did not show a significant improvement in neurologic outcome
    - But ICP was better controlled during hypothermia
  - Routine induction of hypothermia not indicated at present
    - May be effective adjunctive treatment for increased ICP refractory to other medical management

Steroids

- Multiple randomized, controlled studies demonstrated no benefit in treating patients with traumatic brain injury with steroids.
  - Increased risk of death in patients receiving methylprednisolone for 48 hours after injury
  - Steroids not recommended for treatment of head injury
  - Steroids not recommended for treatment of cellular edema accompanying stroke
- Steroids useful in treating vasogenic edema associated with brain tumors or selected infections such as neurocysticercosis
  - Dosing schemes relatively arbitrary with typical dosing scheme for patient with significant symptomatic vasogenic edema from a tumor being dexamethasone, 4 mg IV every 6 hours

Completion of Treatment

- Treatment titrated off once ICP has been controlled below 20 mm Hg for 24 to 48 hours
  - ICP monitors removed if ICP stable below 20 mm Hg for 48 hours after interventions stopped
  - Patients may develop delayed increase in ICP secondary to blossoming of contusions, evolution of a stroke, or development of new mass lesions

OUTCOME WITH INTRACRANIAL HYPERTENSION

- Patients with TBI classified based on initial GCS
  - Patients with mild TBI, GCS of 13 to 15, have minimal chance (3%) of deteriorating into coma and developing elevated ICP

- Patients with moderate TBI, GCS from 9 to 12, have moderate chance (10%–20%) of deteriorating into coma and developing elevated ICP
- Patients with a GCS of 8 or less, severe TBI, have highest chance of developing elevated ICP and also have worst outcome
- Patients with severe TBI more likely to develop increased ICP if they have abnormal head CT or if they meet two of the three criteria of:
  - Age older than 40 years
  - Unilateral or bilateral motor posturing
  - Systolic blood pressure <90 mm Hg
- No study clearly demonstrates that monitoring and treating ICP improves neurologic outcome
  - There are strong associations between intracranial hypertension and poor outcome.
  - Development of refractory intracranial hypertension has a very high mortality rate.
  - In a randomized trial of pentobarbital coma for refractory intracranial hypertension, control of the elevated ICP determined outcome.

- 92% of patients where ICP was controlled survived
- 83% of patients where ICP was not controlled died
- Historically, institution of treatment protocols aimed at controlling elevated ICP significantly improved outcome in TBI.
  - 1977 mortality rate of 50% in comatose patients (GCS <8) in cohort treated without ICP monitoring
  - Significantly lower mortality of 30% in similar patient cohort using ICP monitoring
  - Mortality rates at 30 days for patients with severe TBI slowly declining
    - Mortality of patients in Traumatic Coma Data Bank reduced from 39% in 1984 to 27% in 1996
- Availability of multiple monitoring modalities provided more information on which patients have poor outcomes and provided treatment goals
  - Treatment strategies now aimed at:
    - Maintaining ICP <20 to 25 mm Hg
    - Maintaining CPP >60 mm Hg
    - Maintaining $PbtO_2$ >10 mm Hg
    - Still, TBI associated with significant morbidity and mortality in short and long term

CHAPTER 103 ■ NEUROLOGIC MONITORING

- Neurologic monitoring in intensive care unit (ICU) used:
  - In general sense as part of systems-based approach to assess one of major bodily systems
  - Or with specific intent to guide therapy and/or assess prognosis
  - Imaging studies of central nervous system (CNS) play a central role in assessment by establishing diagnoses and quantifying extent of pathology
- Many interventions in ICU aimed at restoring or maintaining recovery of patient affect results of neurologic monitoring
  - Understanding parameters affecting the state of brain contextually necessary for interpreting results of neurologic monitoring

NEURORADIOLOGIC IMAGING

- Routine imaging studies important in repeated assessment of neurologic status
  - Objective information about structural abnormalities essential for clinical diagnosis
  - Neuroradiologic imaging studies typically are CT or MRI
  - Although not "monitoring" per se, repeated studies or critically timed studies provide clues about time course of pathologic process.
  - Typical imaging workup for various clinical diagnoses presented in Table 103.1
- To maximize utility of imaging study one needs to be aware of strengths and weaknesses of imaging modality

- Questions of contraindications to MRI need to be considered:
  - Metal implants (see www.mrisafety.com)
  - Morbid obesity
  - Claustrophobia
  - Use of contrast agents, require special consideration
- Quality of CT images simply degraded by patient movement
  - MRI images acquired in uncooperative, moving patient may contain "spurious pathology" because of "misregistration" of anatomic structures
- Radiologist needs adequate details of clinical history so imaging protocol can be designed to maximize information
- CT provides a map of degree of radiographic absorption of intracranial structures
  - Test of choice for localizing blood and imaging bone
  - Newer helical CT scanners make image acquisition comparatively fast
    - Allows two- and three-dimensional reconstruction of arterial anatomy during first pass of radiocontrast administration to obtain a CT arteriogram
- MRI provides a map of response of hydrogen nuclei to external magnetic fields
  - More versatile than CT
  - Provides better imaging of posterior fossa contents
  - Considerably more time consuming
  - T1 weighting enhances detection of lipids, methemoglobin (as subacute residua of hemorrhage), and concentrated protein (in a colloid cyst)

TABLE 103.1

TYPICAL IMAGING PROCEDURES FOR NEUROLOGIC DISEASES IN THEIR ACUTE PHASE

Neurologic disease	Initial imaging	Further workup/alternatives
Stroke	CT to rule out hemorrhage	Diffusion- and perfusion-weighted MRI to identify ischemic core and penumbra, respectively
Arteriovenous malformation	CT for hemorrhage	MR angiography or angiography as soon as possible
Intracerebral aneurysm	CT for subarachnoid hemorrhage	CT angiography or angiography to identify aneurysm; TCD for vasospasm
Brain tumor	MRI without and with contrast	
Traumatic brain injury	CT	MRI as indicated later
Multiple sclerosis	MRI without and with contrast	
Meningitis/encephalitis	CT without and with contrast	MRI without and with contrast after initial treatment
Intracranial abscess	CT without and with contrast	MRI without and with contrast even initially, if patient is stable
Granuloma	MRI without and with contrast	

CT, computed tomography; MRI, magnetic resonance imaging; TCD, transcranial Doppler ultrasonography. Modified from Gilman S. Imaging the brain. First of two parts. *N Engl J Med.* 1998;338:812–820.

- Radiofrequency pulse prior to T1 image acquisition suppresses enhancement of lipids ("fat suppression")
  - An example of protocol change affecting resulting image
- T2 weighting enhances detection of unbound water such as in cerebrospinal fluid (CSF) (Fig. 103.1)
  - Radiofrequency pulse prior to T2 image acquisition (fluid attenuation inversion recovery [FLAIR] imaging) suppresses enhancement of CSF and improves edema detection (see Fig. 103.1)
- MRI can also be focused to detect moving elements:
  - MR arteriography or venography
  - CSF flow studies
  - Axoplasmic motion of bulk water imaged with MRI to obtain a diffusion image (apparent diffusion coefficient [ADC] map)
  - Axoplasmic motion stops shortly after brain ischemia
    - Diffusion images provide earliest radiographic evidence for core zone of an ischemic stroke
- Contrast media distribute with blood flow and accentuate areas of increased vascularity as in:
- Inflamed tissue
- Areas of tumor-induced angioneogenesis
- Contrast media also distribute into and highlight brain structures missing blood–brain barrier:
  - As pineal gland or pituitary stalk
  - Brain areas where blood–brain barrier has been disrupted

- Perfusion imaged during bolus administration of contrast medium by MRI or by CT
  - Resulting map of time to peak concentration of contrast medium provides qualitative information on cerebral blood flow (CBF)
  - Qualitative differences in CBF used to identify ischemic penumbra of stroke

CEREBRAL METABOLISM: FLOW–METABOLISM COUPLING

- Cerebral metabolic rate of oxygen ($CMRO_2$) of the brain averages 3.0 to 3.8 mL O_2/minute/100 g
- Only 2% of body weight, human adult brain accounts for:
  - 15% to 20% of resting oxygen consumption
  - 25% to 30% of the glucose consumption of the body
- To meet high demand for oxygen and glucose brain requires perfusion (CBF) of 40 to 60 mL/minute/100 g of brain tissue
- CBF regulated by four primary factors:
  - Metabolic stimuli
  - Chemical stimuli
  - Perfusion pressure
  - Neural stimuli
- In normal brain increased cerebral metabolism rapidly matched by local increases in CBF

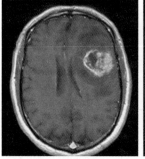
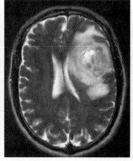
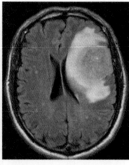

Axial T1 image   Axial T2 image   Axial FLAIR image

FIGURE 103.1. Magnetic resonance images from a patient with a glioblastoma multiforme. The axial, gadolinium-enhanced T1-weighted image demonstrates the enhancing tumor margin with its nonenhancing central necrosis. The axial, T2-weighted image shows water as a bright signal in perifocal edema and the central tumor necrosis, as well as in the cerebrospinal fluid, while the fluid attenuation inversion recovery image highlights only the edema around the tumor and suppresses the cerebrospinal fluid signal and the tumor necrosis. (Images courtesy of Ilona Schmalfuss, MD.)

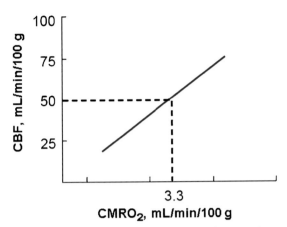

FIGURE 103.2. Flow–metabolism coupling in the central nervous system. As the metabolic needs of the brain—expressed as the cerebral metabolic requirement for oxygen ($CMRO_2$)—increases, cerebral blood flow (CBF) increases in parallel.

- Referred to as regional flow–metabolism coupling or cerebral metabolic autoregulation
- CBF thus linked to brain function and metabolism so that CBF varies in parallel with $CMRO_2$ (Fig. 103.2)
- Two compensatory responses to acute reductions in CBF established:
  ○ Autoregulation
  ○ Increased oxygen extraction
    – Oxygen extraction is able to vary within a narrow range
    – "Misery" perfusion occurs when oxygen extraction is increased in response to increased $CMRO_2$, either when autoregulatory CBF compensation has been exceeded or uncoupling has occurred
    – As cerebral perfusion pressure (CPP) falls, CBF maintained initially by resistance arteriole vasodilation
- Several vasoactive metabolic mediators proposed for cerebral regulation:
  ○ Hydrogen ion
  ○ Potassium
  ○ CO_2
  ○ Adenosine
  ○ Glycolytic intermediates
  ○ Phospholipid metabolites
  ○ Nitric oxide
- Global relationship between CBF and $CMRO_2$ expressed by:
- Fick equation where $DajO_2$ is the arteriojugular difference in oxygen content:

$$CMRO_2 = DajO_2 \times CBF \text{ or } DajO_2 = CMRO_2/CBF$$

- CBF measured within first 6 hours after traumatic brain injury (TBI) was <18 mL/minute/100 g (the threshold for cerebral ischemia) in 33% of patients
  ○ Arterial vasospasm an independent predictor of poor outcome
  ○ Secondary ischemic neurologic damage worsened outcome and was associated with:
    – Systemic factors such as hypotension or hypoxemia
    – Local factors, such as intracranial hypertension
  ○ Disruption of normal homeostatic mechanisms such as autoregulation may also aggravate cerebral ischemia

  ○ Hyperventilation to reduce intracranial pressure (ICP) may be deleterious by decreasing CBF, thus leading to ischemia

Hypothermia

- Cerebral protection by hypothermia attributed to cerebral metabolic suppression
- Temperature coefficient (Q_{10}) is factor by which $CMRO_2$ is decreased by 10°C decrease in temperature
  - Between 37°C and 27°C Q_{10} is 2.23
  - Between 27°C and 17°C, temperature range where electroencephalogram (EEG) activity ceases, Q_{10} doubles to 4.53
  - Below 17°C, the Q_{10} returns to near 2.0
  - Absent EEG activity (during barbiturate coma) Q_{10} remains near 2.0 over entire temperature range
  - With moderate hypothermia (above 27°C) CO_2 reactivity and autoregulation are intact and CBF and $CMRO_2$ remain coupled
    ○ There is a change in coupling of CBF and $CMRO_2$ during deep cerebral hypothermia (below 25°C).
    ○ Nonetheless, metabolic regulation remains the main determinant of CBF even during deep cerebral hypothermia.

Anesthetics

- Except for ketamine, most intravenous (IV) and inhalational anesthetics depress cerebral metabolism with consequent reductions in $CMRO_2$, CBF, and ICP.
- As $CMRO_2$ decreases, CBF is reduced proportionately because of flow–metabolism coupling.
- After administration of propofol and thiopental, coupling usually remains intact and $SjvO_2$ remains unaltered or improves.
- Etomidate can produce rapid reduction in CBF with slower reduction in $CMRO_2$.
  - This mismatching of coupling may induce significant—albeit transient—$SjvO_2$ desaturation.
- Benzodiazepines and opiates have limited intrinsic effects on CBF, $CMRO_2$, and CBF–$CMRO_2$ coupling.
  - They cause decreased CBF and ICP that parallels sedation-induced decrease in $CMRO_2$.
  - Decreased sympathetic tone caused by sedation risks a decrease in mean arterial pressure that may diminish cerebral perfusion.

Arterial Blood Gases: Carbon Dioxide and Oxygen

- CO_2 a potent cerebral vasodilator and a major determinant of CBF
- At normotension, CBF increases almost linearly when $PaCO_2$ increases 25 to 80 mm Hg
- Global CBF varies 2% to 4% for each mm Hg change in $PaCO_2$
- Effects of $PaCO_2$ on cerebral circulation regulated by complex, interrelated system of mediators:

- Initial stimulus of CO_2-induced vasodilation is decreased by brain extracellular pH
- Further mediated by nitric oxide, prostanoids, cyclic nucleotides, potassium channels, and decreased intracellular calcium concentration as final common pathway
- Arteriolar tone an important influence on how $PaCO_2$ affects CBF
  - Moderate hypotension impairs response of cerebral circulation to $PaCO_2$ changes
  - Severe hypotension abolishes it altogether
- $PaCO_2$ modifies pressure autoregulation
  - From hypercapnia to hypocapnia, there is widening of autoregulation plateau
- Moderate changes in PaO_2 do not significantly alter CBF
  - When PaO_2 falls below 50 mm Hg CBF increases so cerebral DO_2 remains constant.
  - Hypoxia acts directly on cerebral tissue to release lactic acid, adenosine, and prostaglandins, which contribute to cerebral vasodilation.
  - Hypoxia acts directly on cerebrovascular smooth muscle to produce hyperpolarization and reduce calcium uptake, enhancing vasodilation.

Pressure Autoregulation

- Refers to ability of brain to maintain total and regional CBF nearly constant despite large changes in systemic arterial blood pressure, independently of flow–metabolism coupling
- Generally expressed as the relationship between CBF and arterial blood pressure when cerebral venous and CSF pressures are low
- Can be more precisely defined using relationship between CBF and CPP that represents difference between systemic MAP and cerebral outflow pressure
  - Because cerebral venous system is compressible and may act as "Starling resistor" or waterfall phenomenon, outflow resistance governed by whichever pressure is higher: ICP or venous outflow pressure (jugular bulb pressure)
  - The cerebral vascular resistance (R) can be expressed as:

$$R = CPP/CBF = (8/\pi) \times h \times (l/r^4)$$

where $(8/\pi)$ is a constant, h is blood viscosity, l is length, and r is radius of vessel
  - Importantly, the radius enters to the fourth power in the equation, making it a most efficient means of controlling vascular resistance.
- In adults under normal conditions, CBF constant between a CPP of roughly 60 and 150 mm Hg
  - Autoregulation curve shifted to the right in hypertensive patients and to the left in neonates
  - At lower limit of autoregulation, cerebral vasodilation maximal
    ○ Below this level, CBF falls passively with CPP
    ○ Beyond upper limit where vasoconstriction is maximal elevated intraluminal pressure may force vessels to dilate, leading to increased CBF and damage to blood–brain barrier.
    ○ Metabolic mediators, such as adenosine, also involved in low-pressure range of autoregulation

Neurogenic Regulation

- Major difference between other systemic circulations and cerebral circulation is relative lack of humoral and autonomic control on normal cerebrovascular tone
  - Maximal stimulation of sympathetic or parasympathetic nerves alters CBF only slightly
  - Is considerable evidence indicating existence of age-related differences in cerebral resistance vessels to neural stimuli
    - Both *in vivo* and *in vitro*, cerebrovascular constrictor responses to noradrenaline or electrical transmural stimuli greater in fetal and neonatal than in adult animals

Other Factors Regulating Cerebral Blood Flow

- CO hardly influences CBF normally, it may significantly influence flow to ischemic regions
- Improving cerebral perfusion by volume loading is indirectly accomplished by improving blood rheology and directly accomplished by increasing systemic arterial pressure, and preventing occult decreases in systemic pressure in hypovolemic patients.
- Blood viscosity a major determinant of vascular resistance
- CBF is inversely related with hematocrit
- Some have claimed viscosity directly participates in cerebral hemodynamic autoregulation, termed *viscosity autoregulation*

CEREBRAL FUNCTION

Clinical Examination

- Cerebral function can be monitored with instrumentation or assessed clinically
  - Each monitor offers only a small window into the state of the CNS
  - Even in combination, current monitors have limitations in spatial and/or temporal resolution
  - A neurologic examination of an alert patient, contrariwise, can comprehensively assess function of CNS
    - Can be repeated as often as needed
    - Requires neither expensive technical equipment nor specialized technologists
  - Clinically the neurologic examination has important limitations
    - First, patient's clinical status or underlying disease may limit amount of information obtainable by a clinical examination
    - Second, results and utility of neurologic examination may be constrained by therapeutic interventions frequently used in ICU
      ○ For example, an intubated patient who is treated with neuromuscular blocking agents
    - Finally, neurologic evaluations performed intermittently by examiners of variable skill, raising problems of reliability
  - Two aspects of examination that are particularly pertinent to ICU environment will be discussed:

TABLE 103.2

GLASGOW COMA SCALE

Category	Grading		Comments
Eye opening	Spontaneous	4	Swelling may interfere with testing.
	To voice	3	
	To pain	2	
	None	1	
Motor response	Follows commands	6	Avoid description of flexion as decorticate
	Localizes pain	5	and extension as decerebrate, because
	Withdraws to pain	4	those terms denote an anatomic
	Flexion to pain	3	location of a lesion.
	Extension to pain	2	
	Flaccid	1	
Verbal response	Oriented	5	Impossible to assess in intubated patients.
	Confused	4	Some centers determine the response by
	Inappropriate	3	inference and designate the final score
	Incomprehensible	2	with the subscript "T."
	None	1	

The GCS score is the sum of the best attainable subscores in the categories of eye opening (E), motor (M), and verbal (V) responses. It ranges from 15 ($E_4 + M_6 + V_5$) to 3 ($E_1 + M_1 + V_1$).

- Assessment of level of consciousness, because of its ties to patient outcome for many different neurologic diseases
- Examination for assessing brain death
  - Because it is a graded assessment of brainstem function
  - Because it illustrates sources of error impacting results of clinical neurologic examination in ICU environment

Level of Consciousness (LOC): Glasgow Coma Scale (GCS)

- LOC typically assessed by GCS
- Numerical scores assigned for best responses in categories of eye opening, motor response, and verbal response (Table 103.2)
- For the GCS association of lower scores with worsened outcome has been shown for:
  - Traumatic brain injury
  - Subarachnoid hemorrhage
  - Brain abscess
  - Survival after cardiac arrest
  - Septic encephalopathy
- GCS has several important limitations even if applied correctly
  - First, information loss inherent in reducing a graded assessment of three responses into a single number
  - Second, mechanical problems, such as swelling and endotracheal intubation, may prevent proper assessment of eye opening and verbal response.
    - In this setting, some assign lowest component score, others try to infer "true" score from related neurologic findings, still others add subscript "T" to indicate intubated patient.
  - Third, sedatives and neuromuscular blocking agents affect GCS score
  - Finally, GCS provides limited information about brainstem function

Determination of Brain Death

- Because clinical determination of brain death requires comprehensive and methodical assessment of patient, steps serve as a guide to neurologic examination of comatose patient (Fig. 103.3)
- Given the gravity of diagnosis of brain death, prerequisite to determination is clinical picture, typically supported by imaging studies, that is consistent with occurrence of brain death
- First step is determination of coma (i.e., lack of responsiveness to external stimuli due to unconsciousness)
- Motor responses *elicited by examination* need differentiation from spontaneous movements *during examination*
  - Latter typically brief, slow movements originating from spinal cord and do not become integrated into decerebrate or decorticate responses
  - Rarely reproducible upon repeat testing
  - Reproducible partial eye opening failing to reveal iris described in response to peripheral painful stimulus in patient fulfilling clinical criteria of brain death
  - Conditions confounding clinical diagnosis of brain death are noted (Table 103.3)
  - In addition to confounding conditions, diagnosis of brain death should be consistent with imaging studies and/or overall clinical picture before formal determination of brain death considered
- Next step in neurologic examination is assessment of brainstem function
  - Typical tests, afferent and efferent pathways, and potentially interfering clinical conditions summarized (Table 103.4)
  - To complete diagnosis of brain death, an apnea test is performed
    - To test response to an acute decrease in pH of CSF due to hypercarbia
      - Hypercarbia induced by disconnecting mechanical ventilation
      - Continued oxygenation is ensured by both preoxygenation and apneic oxygenation
      - Absence of respiratory movements at $PaCO_2$ of 60 mm Hg or after increase in $PaCO_2$ of 20 mm Hg consistent with brain death

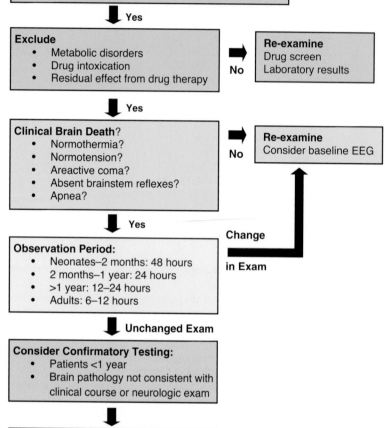

FIGURE 103.3. Algorhythm for the determination of brain death.

- Testing may be complicated by arterial hypotension due to loss of arterial and autonomic tone
  - Such hypotension corroborates diagnosis of brain death but makes hemodynamic stability required for apnea testing difficult to attain
  - Apnea test may trigger movement responses, which reflect residual spinal activity
- Once criteria for brain death are met, either an observation period followed by repeat assessment or a confirmatory test is used to reach a final diagnosis
  - Cerebral angiography is the gold standard among confirmatory tests
  - Contrast media injected into aortic arch and distributes to external carotid circulation, whereas internal carotid and vertebral arteries fill only to level of skull base and atlanto-occipital junction, respectively
  - Similar findings obtained with:
    - Magnetic resonance angiography (MRA)
    - Single photon emission computed tomography 99mTc-HMPAO (SPECT)
    - EEG and transcranial Doppler also frequently used as confirmatory tests

Electrophysiologic Techniques

Diagnostic Electroencephalography: Clinical Utility in the ICU

- Diagnostic EEG studies/EEG monitoring in ICU done primarily for one of three purposes:
- Brain death determination
- Monitoring for evidence of seizure activity or cerebral ischemia
- Determination of drug effect to titrate sedative/analgesic drugs or control ICP
- Criteria for brain death vary from state to state
- Some require a 16- to 32-channel isoelectric EEG on two consecutive recordings at least 24 hours apart to provide corroborating evidence for cessation of brain function.
  - Other factors affecting EEG can produce isoelectric EEG absent brain death.
  - Thus EEG cannot be used as sole evaluation for brain death.
- Drug levels (Table 103.5) decline significantly over 24-hour period.

TABLE 103.3

NEUROLOGIC STATES RESEMBLING BRAIN DEATH

Disease state	Diagnostic aids	Comments
Hypothermia	Core temperature <32°C Osborne waves on ECG Drug screening	May cause central nervous system depression up to clinical brain death
Acute poisoning	Serum concentration measurements	In differentiating from brain death, consider antidote and/or document subtherapeutic drug concentration and/or wait for four elimination half-lives Direct central nervous system depressants may confound confirmatory testing of brain death because of $CMRO_2$–CBF coupling
Metabolic encephalopathy	Laboratory testing Intact lower brainstem function	Imaging studies should document structural central nervous system changes Imaging studies should document structural central nervous system changes
Akinetic mutism	Intact sleep–wake cycle	Imaging study shows frontal or mesencephalic brain lesion
Locked-in syndrome	Clinical course and imaging studies	Central locked-in syndrome: Corticobulbar and corticospinal tracts are interrupted at the level of the base of the pons; vertical eye movements are intact Peripheral locked-in syndrome: Guillain-Barré syndrome, advanced amyotrophic lateral sclerosis, neuromuscular blocking agents, organophosphate poisoning

ECG, electrocardiogram; $CMRO_2$, cerebral metabolic requirement for oxygen; CBF, cerebral blood flow.

- Patients with massive drug overdose or impaired metabolic pathways may show an isoelectric EEG for longer than 24 or 48 hours.
- Other diagnostic testing methods, including other electrophysiologic and nonelectrophysiologic methods, may be helpful.
  - Evoked potentials (see below) are more resistant to drug effects than EEG
  - Frequently used to demonstrate brainstem and cortical function even in face of an isoelectric EEG
  - Additionally, an EEG recorded immediately after cardiac arrest may show isoelectric pattern that subsequently recovers
  - Cortical evoked potentials demonstrated more reliable in assessing neurologic function immediately after ischemic or anoxic insult

- Continuous EEG monitoring or sequential diagnostic EEG studies described for:
- Detection of nonconvulsive seizure (NCS) activity or
- Seizure activity in the pharmacologically paralyzed patient
- Detection of cerebral ischemia
- Processed EEG algorithms developed to facilitate detection of ischemia, epileptiform, and frank seizure activity during continuous EEG monitoring
  - Technology not yet evolved to eliminate need for on-site technologist with monitoring experience
- Continuous EEG monitoring in ICU demonstrated that NCSs much more common than previously thought
  - Reported following:
    - Neurosurgical procedures
    - Subarachnoid hemorrhage

TABLE 103.4

CLINICAL EXAMINATION OF THE BRAINSTEM DURING EVALUATION FOR BRAIN DEATH

Brainstem reflex	Afferent path	Efferent path	Caveats
Pupillary light reaction	II	III	Not confounded by systemic drugs; absence may be caused by **prolonged** administration of neuromuscular blocking agents
Ocular movements (oculocephalic reflex or caloric nystagmus)	VIII	III, VI	Confounded by damage from ototoxic drugs; cervical spine trauma may preclude testing of the oculocephalic reflex; voluntary ocular movements are sometimes the only finding that differentiates a "locked-in" syndrome from brain death
Corneal reflex/pressure on supraorbital nerve	V	VII	
Gag	IX	IX, X	May be difficult to assess in orotracheally intubated patient
Cough	X	X, cervical roots	Best tested by assessing the response to tracheal suctioning

TABLE 103.5

SEDATIVE-HYPNOTIC AND ANALGESIC DRUGS AND THE ELECTROENCEPHALOGRAM (EEG)

Drug		Effect on EEG dominant frequency	Effect on EEG amplitude	Burst suppression
Barbiturates	Low dose	Fast frontal β activity	Slight ↑	Yes, with high doses
	Moderate dose	Frontal α frequency spindles	↑	
	High dose	Diffuse δ → burst suppression → silence	↑↑↑ → 0	
Etomidate	Low dose	Fast frontal β activity	↑	Yes, with high doses
	Moderate dose	Frontal α frequency spindles	↑	
	High dose	Diffuse δ → burst suppression → silence	↑↑ → 0	
Propofol	Low dose	Loss of α, ↑ frontal β	↑	Yes, with high doses
	Moderate dose	Frontal δ, waxing/waning α	↑	
	High dose	Diffuse δ → burst suppression → silence	↑↑ → 0	
Dexmedetomidine		Early appearance of high-amplitude δ frequency that increases with dose, similar to opiates	↑	No
Ketamine	Low dose	Loss of α, ↑ variability	↑↓	No
	Moderate dose	Frontal rhythmic delta	↑	
	High dose	Polymorphic δ, some β	↑↑ (β is low amplitude)	
Benzodiazepines	Low dose	Loss of α, increased frontal β activity	↑	No
	High dose	Frontally dominant δ and θ	↑	
Opiates	Low dose	Loss of β, α slows	↑	No
	Moderate dose	Diffuse θ, some δ	↑	
	High dose	δ, often synchronized	↑↑	

δ, < 3-Hz frequency; θ, 3.5- to 7.5-Hz frequency; α, 8- to 13-Hz frequency; β, > 13-Hz frequency.

- ○ CNS infection
- ○ Head injury
- • Evidence using neuron-specific enolase as a marker of neurologic injury that NCSs may produce neurologic damage
  - ○ Seizure duration and time to diagnosis significantly related to extent of damage and long-term outcome
  - ○ Without continuous EEG monitoring, NCSs cannot be detected
    - – Not consistently and specifically associated with other findings such as hypertension and tachycardia

Processed Electroencephalogram: Monitoring of Sedation

- • EEG to monitor depth of sedation in patients in ICU described extensively:
- • Nearly all techniques utilize processed EEG rather than unprocessed analog signal
- • Generally accomplished using one or two channels of EEG information
  - • Recorded over frontopolar region of cerebral cortex
  - • Location chosen because application of surface recording electrodes easy
    - ○ Most devices designed for this purpose have been validated using frontopolar recording locations
    - ○ Smaller number of channels used based on assumption that drug effect similar in all areas of brain
    - ○ Generally valid except in case of patient with focal brain damage

- ○ None of commercially available devices for monitoring drug effects on the EEG calibrated or validated for monitoring drug effects in patients with abnormal EEG
- ○ Relatively limited information available on use of EEG to monitor drug effects in neurologically damaged patients
- • Most commonly used for titrating sedative drugs
- • Particularly in pharmacologically paralyzed patient
- • Also for titration of barbiturate drugs used to control ICP
- • Devices used to monitor the drug effect utilize either:
- • Unprocessed, raw analog EEG similar to electrocardiogram monitoring in ICU
- • One of three signal processing techniques:
  - ○ Power spectrum analysis
  - ○ Bispectral analysis
  - ○ EEG entropy analysis
- • Bispectral Index (BIS, Aspect Medical Systems, Inc., Natick, MA) monitoring processes EEG signals that are recorded from a self-adhesive electrode strip placed on forehead.
  - ○ Calculates and displays a BIS value
    - – Dimensionless number ranging from 0 to 100 derived from highly processed EEG data that includes:
      - • EEG power
      - • EEG frequency
      - • Bicoherence
    - – Low BIS numbers indicate strong relationships among EEG frequencies and reflect condition consistent with deep hypnotic state (Table 103.6)
    - – Relationship valid despite effects of age and infirmity on sensitivity to sedation

TABLE 103.6

CLINICAL CONDITION EXPECTED WITH BISPECTRAL
INDEX VALUES

100	Awake patient, amnesia unlikely
80	Sedated responsive patient, amnesia prominent unless significant event
70	Heavily sedated or unconscious patient, amnesia probable
60	General anesthesia, unresponsive to verbal stimuli
40	Deep hypnotic state
20	Burst suppression
0	Isoelectric electroencephalogram

- Aspects of imperfect performance of BIS monitor well known
  - BIS can decrease to numbers (20–50) consistent with deep general anesthesia during natural sleep
  - Memory less likely to form at lower BIS values but has been demonstrated even at BIS in range of 40–60, associated with general anesthesia
  - Artifact from electromyogram, electro-oculographic, or pacemaker generators can produce significant but spurious BIS increases (from 50s to 80s)
    - Makes possible overdosing nonrelaxed or paced patients when attempting to maintain a given BIS range
  - Can be driven higher by medications that are CNS stimulants
    - Ketamine
    - Methylphenidate
    - Dexmedetomidine
  - Cannot differentiate deep sedation from cerebral ischemia
    - Both cause loss of higher-frequency EEG waves (α and β slowing and δ and θ wave intrusion)
      - In extreme states, both can produce burst suppression or isoelectric EEG patterns with a low BIS
      - When O_2 delivery decreases below a level sufficient to meet $CMRO_2$, electrical function fails and BIS decreases
        - May partly explain improved ICU outcomes when the BIS is maintained >60

Evoked Potentials (EP)

- Recordings of electrical activity from different parts of the nervous system produced by either sensory or motor stimuli applied to activated portions of sensory and motor systems, respectively

- Except for motor-evoked responses recorded from muscle, EPs much smaller than background EEG or muscle electrical activity
- Responses from repetitive stimuli must be averaged to discern responses from background biologic signals or environmental noise
  - Auditory EPs very small (generally <0.5 μV) and require as many as 1,000 to 2,000 averaged responses to clarify signal
  - Somatosensory EPs larger (0.5–10 μV) and require fewer averages to clarify
- EPs described in terms of:
  - Latency (time [msec] from stimulus application to onset or peak of response)
  - Amplitude (μV)
  - Amplitude more important parameter for ICU studies because voltage mainly related to amount of functional neural tissue generating response
  - Latency related to conduction time from stimulus site to generating site
  - Assumption not always the case since a peripheral or cranial nerve injury may produce a nerve with fibers conducting at many different velocities
- Compared to EEG, EPs much less susceptible to effects of IV sedative-hypnotic drugs and not significantly affected by IV analgesics
- Table 103.7 summarizes different types of evoked potentials monitored in ICU

Peripheral Nerve Stimulation

- Rate of recovery from neuromuscular blocking (NMB) agents depends on:
  - NMB agent chosen
  - Dosing pattern (intermittent or continuous infusion)
  - Numerous patient factors (e.g., pseudocholinesterase deficiency, hepatic or renal dysfunction, induced cytochrome P450 enzyme, organophosphate toxicity, among many others)
- Suitability for extubation following prolonged neuromuscular blockade traditionally relied on functional strength testing
  - Ability to produce a negative inspiratory force
  - Ability to sustain a head lift
  - Incomplete patient cooperation due to sedation or confusion can adversely affect tests
  - Peripheral nerve stimulation (PNS) used for "muscle twitch" testing, or acceleromyography, complements such functional assessments by objectively revealing condition of neuromuscular junction, independent of patient participation

TABLE 103.7

EVOKED POTENTIALS (EPS) IN THE ICU

Type of EPs	Stimulus type and site	Recording sites
Somatosensory	Electrical, peripheral nerve	Peripheral nerve, spinal cord, head
Brainstem auditory	Loud click, ear	Ear, head
Magnetic motor	Magnetic pulse, head	Spinal column, peripheral nerve, muscle
Electrical motor	Electrical, head	Spinal column, peripheral nerve, muscle

TABLE 103.8

PERCENTAGE NEUROMUSCULAR JUNCTION
BLOCKADE WITH NONDEPOLARIZING
NEUROMUSCULAR BLOCKING AGENTS AND
CORRESPONDING TRAIN-OF-FOUR AND CLINICAL
RESPONSES

Response	Blockade (%)
Train-of-four 0/4	95
Train-of-four 1/4	90
Train-of-four 2/4	85
Train-of-four 3/4	80
Train-of-four 4/4	75
Sustained (≥ 5 s) tetanus	50
Sustained (≥ 5 s) head lift	25

- Reliable interpretation of nerve stimulation requires uniform stimulation and placement parameters
  - Conventional PNS delivers current—adjustable up to 80 mA:
    - In a train-of-four (TOF) series at 2 Hz as double-burst stimulation (DBS)
    - As single shocks at 1.0 or 0.1 Hz
    - By tetanic stimuli of 50 or 100 Hz
  - Maximal current settings ensure best chance of delivering suprathreshold stimuli and activation of greatest percentage of motor fibers despite changes of impedance or proximity
    - Occur with electrode separation or desiccation, skin cooling, or peripheral edema
  - TOF and DBS patterns do not require comparison to earlier responses for interpretation
    - Well suited for use in ICU setting where recovery of neuromuscular function may take hours to days and may involve assessments by multiple providers
- Muscle twitch testing measures the force of muscle contractions in response to PNS
  - Ratio of force between last and first stimuli in a series (TOF or DBS) best defines percentage of acetylcholine receptors occupied by *nondepolarizing* NMB agents in the neuromuscular junction
  - Counting loss of twitches in a TOF simpler method for assessing block level (Table 103.8)
  - TOF ratio does not change following administration of *depolarizing* NMB agent such as succinylcholine
    - When depolarizing NMB agents used, force of contraction diminishes equally across all stimuli and disappears altogether with sufficient dose
    - Excessive depolarizing NMB agent dose results in prolonged phase II block
      - TOF responses during a phase II block behave similarly to responses obtained following nondepolarizing NMB agents
- Peripheral nerve stimulator is attached to patient using two pregelled electrocardiogram electrodes; needle electrodes can also be used
  - Electrodes placed closely (without the gels touching) to one another over a site where motor nerve lies relatively superficial to skin

- Antegrade nerve conduction improved if positive lead applied to proximal electrode
- Current path between electrodes should not contain muscle whose movement is monitored
- Separation of electrodes beyond several centimeters increases probability that PNS current may depolarize muscle directly
  - Causing movement unrelated to conduction through neuromuscular junction
  - Misinterpretation of the level of neuromuscular blockade
- Common sites for electrode placement are:
  - Over course of ulnar nerve at medial aspect of the wrist or over ulnar groove at elbow
    - Stimulation of ulnar nerve activates the m. adductor pollicis and twitches thumb
  - Placement of electrodes anterior to tragus will stimulate facial nerve
    - Innervates the m. corrugator supercilii and furrows the eyebrow
  - Stimulation of posterior tibial nerve posterior to the medial malleolus
    - Causes the m. flexor hallucis brevis and great toe to move
- Cold weakens muscle strength even absent NMB agents
  - Making PNS testing valuable in patients recovering from hypothermia
- Patients who have had a stroke will experience up-regulation of acetylcholine receptor density on muscle membrane as affected muscles denervate
  - PNS on affected limb will produce a TOF response exceeding the response seen from same site PNS on normal limb
  - To avoid overdosing or prematurely extubating patient based on TOF testing
    - PNS should be performed on sites unaffected by prior nerve injury
- PNS particularly helpful for monitoring level of relaxation achieved during infusion of NMB agents
  - PNS monitoring helps direct rate of infusion and avoid excessive administration
  - Pharmacokinetic and pharmacodynamic models illustrating TOF response to PNS with succinylcholine and rocuronium NMB infusions are at http://vam.anest.ufl.edu/simulations/simulationportfolio.php

CEREBRAL PERFUSION

- Most common clinical measure aimed at ensuring adequate CBF is to maintain cerebral perfusion pressure (CPP) above lower limit of cerebral autoregulation
- In cases of intracranial disease, relevant pressure opposing adequate perfusion is ICP

Monitoring of Intracranial Pressure

- ICP reflects dynamic interaction of tissues and fluids within a fixed-volume, hard cranial shell of approximately 1,400 mL in an adult
  - Contents divided into:
    - Cerebral parenchyma
    - Arterial and venous blood
    - CSF components

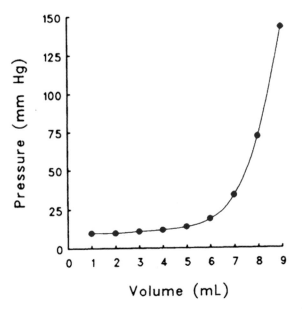

FIGURE 103.4. Pressure–volume relationship of the intracranial vault. Volume in milliliters (abscissa) of water added to a supratentorial extradural balloon in a monkey, 1 mL/hour. Pressure in millimeters of mercury (ordinate). (With permission from Langfitt TW. Increased intracranial pressure. *Clin Neurosurg.* 1969;16:43–71.)

- Cerebral parenchyma accounts for 80% to 90% of contents
  - Includes both intra- and extracellular fluid as well as cellular membranes
- Volume of blood together with CSF makes up the remaining 10% to 20%
- Monro-Kellie doctrine:
  - Any increase in volume of one intracranial component occurs at the expense of another
  - Normal adult ICP is 8 to 15 mm Hg; in babies pressure is 10 to 20 mm Hg
  - Compensation in ICP may be achieved by:
    ○ Changes in volume of CSF
    ○ The slight distention of dura
    ○ Changes in intravascular volume, particularly in the venous channels
    ○ Compression or swelling of brain
  - Rate of change in volume of intracranial contents of importance
    ○ Rapid increase in volume produced by an epidural hematoma may overwhelm compensatory mechanisms and produce a rapid increase in ICP (Fig. 103.4)
    ○ Slowly growing brain tumor may produce a gradual displacement of structures within the cranial vault without a significant increase in ICP
- ICP is not static
- Pressure fluctuations occur with cardiac systole due to distention of the intracranial arteriolar tree and respiration (ICP falling with inspiration and rising with expiration)
- Straining or compression of neck veins can also cause a rise in pressure
- Value in excess of 18 to 20 mm Hg is abnormal and must be treated
- As ICP increases cerebral venous pressure increases in parallel
  - Remaining 2 to 5 mm Hg higher, or else the venous system would collapse

- Because of relationship, CPP satisfactorily estimated as:

$$CPP = MAP - ICP$$

- Cerebral arterial circulation maintains constant CBF for a CPP 60 to 150 mm Hg
- Clinical deterioration in neurologic status widely considered a sign of increased ICP
- Bradycardia, increased pulse pressure, and pupillary dilation are signs of increased ICP
- Five methods most commonly used to monitor ICP are:
  - An intraventricular catheter
    - Considered the gold standard
  - A subarachnoid or subdural bolt
  - A subdural catheter
  - An intraparenchymal fiberoptic filament sensor
  - An extradural fiberoptic sensor
- All ICP monitors are invasive and share a risk of infection of about 5%
- Patients requiring ICP monitoring are generally those:
  - With a closed head injury and a GCS ≤8
  - In whom CT scan shows significant brain distortion
  - With worsening neurologic status
  - In whom there is need to sedate, paralyze, or operate in context of an abnormal brain
  - With postoperative complications
  - Who are unconscious or in shock

Interpretation of Intracranial Pressure Waveforms

- Normal ICP waveform has three characteristic peaks (P1, P2, and P3) of decreasing height correlating with arterial pulse waveform (Fig. 103.5)
- P1 (percussion) wave originates from arterial systole
  - Has sharp peak and constant amplitude
- P2 (tidal) wave more variable and ends on dicrotic notch
  - Elevation of P2 reflects decreased intracranial adaptive capacity and impaired autoregulation
  - However, sustained increases in ICP can occur without P2 elevation
- P3 (dicrotic) wave follows the dicrotic notch and is venous in origin
- Consecutive ICP waveforms observed over time show three distinct patterns observed:
  - A waves, now more commonly referred to as plateau waves, are pathologic (Fig. 103.6)
    - Rapid rise in ICP to 50 to 100 mm Hg, with variable period in which ICP remains elevated ("plateau"), followed by rapid fall to baseline

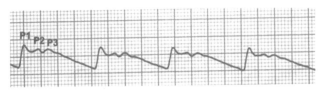

FIGURE 103.5. Intracranial pressure waveform showing the percussion wave (P1), tidal wave (P2), and dicrotic wave (P3). The timing of the peaks corresponds to the arterial pressure waveform. (Image courtesy of Integra Neurosciences, Inc.)

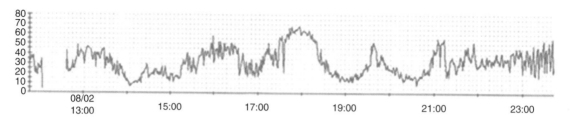

FIGURE 103.6. Lundberg plateau waves. The tracing of the intracranial pressure shows several pathologic increases of intracranial pressure, with plateaus lasting from 20 to 60 minutes. (Image courtesy Integra Neurosciences, Inc.)

- Plateau waves typically last from 5 to 20 minutes
- Generally seen in patients with already elevated ICP
- During a series of plateau waves, both amplitude and duration may increase
  - Leading to "terminal" wave in which ICP may rise to impede CBF
  - "Truncated" or atypical plateau waves not exceeding 50 mm Hg early indicators of neurologic deterioration
- B and C waves are smaller fluctuations in ICP related to respiration and autonomic fluctuations in blood pressure (Traube-Hering-Mayer waves), respectively
  - Of little clinical significance
- Markedly decreased or elevated CPP may lead to ischemia or spontaneous hemorrhage, respectively
- Normal CPP by no means ensures normal CBF
  - Increased cerebrovascular resistance (e.g., because of carotid stenosis, cerebral vasospasm, or microcirculatory compromise) may cause ischemia despite normal CPP
  - Similarly, normal CPP may coexist with abnormally increased CBF in settings such as posttraumatic vasoparalysis or normal perfusion pressure breakthrough after resection of an arteriovenous malformation

Direct Cerebral Blood Flow Measurement

- Ideal clinical method for CBF measurement in patients with intracranial pathology would be:
- Noninvasive, inexpensive bedside procedure
- Continuous or at least frequently repeatable
- Provides good spatial resolution for superficial and deep structures of all vascular territories
  - No currently available method comes close to having characteristics (Table 103.9)
- Direct measurement of CBF possible by determining kinetics of wash-in or wash-out of inert tracer compound
- Widely used measurement uses radioactive isotope of ^{133}Xe per inhalation or IV
- Followed by measurement of radioactivity wash-out, with γ detectors placed over specific areas of brain
  - Method provides spatial resolution of 3 to 4 cm, depending on number of detectors
- In normal brain, flow at different depths may be inferred from the early wash-out
  - Should reflect high-perfusion cortical gray matter and low-perfusion deeper white matter

TABLE 103.9

TECHNIQUES FOR MEASURING CEREBRAL BLOOD FLOW

Category	Technique	Resolution		Invasiveness	Cost
		Temporal	Spatial		
Bedside	Kety-Schmidt	15 min	Hemispheric	Jugular catheter	+
	^{133}Xenon wash-out	3–15 min	3–4 cm	Jugular catheter, radiation	+
	Arteriovenous difference in oxygen content (AVDO$_2$), jugular venous oxygen saturation (SjvO$_2$)	<1 min	Global	Jugular catheter	+
	Double indicator dilution	3 min	Global	Jugular catheter, descending thoracic aortic catheter	+
	Near-infrared spectroscopy	<1 min	Local, bifrontal	No	+
	Thermal clearance probe	<1 min	Local, 1–2 cm	Exposed cortex	+
	Laser Doppler flow probe	<1 min	Local, 1–2 cm	Exposed cortex	+
Tomographic	Positron emission tomography (PET)	4–6 min/section	<1 cm	Radiation from positron emitter	+++++
	Stable Xenon computed tomography (CT)	4–6 min/section	<1 cm	Radiation from CT scan	+++
	Single photon emission tomography (SPECT)	4–6 min/section	<1 cm	Radiation from γ emitter	+++
	Magnetic resonance imaging (MRI)	4–6 min/section	<1 cm	No	+++

- Important disadvantage of technique is lack of sensitivity for focal areas of hypoperfusion
  - Obscured by adjacent areas of adequate flow
    - Phenomenon described as "look-through"
- Methods like SPECT, PET, xenon-enhanced CT or perfusion CT, or MRI provide excellent spatial resolution
- Not available at the bedside
- Some used clinically as confirmatory tests in determination of brain death
  - SPECT and MRA show a "hollow skull phenomenon" and absent intracranial flow, respectively
- Xenon-enhanced CT, which can be combined with standard CT scanning
  - Used to obtain prognostic information and withhold unnecessarily aggressive therapy by assessing severity of decreased CBF during stroke
  - Perfusion imaging allows detection of viable penumbra around areas of ischemia
    - May be restored to normal function if relative ischemia reversed

Transcranial Doppler (TCD)

Theoretical Basis

- Ultrasound waves used to measure velocity of blood flow in basal arteries of brain and extracranial portion of internal carotid artery
  - Waves transmitted through relatively thin temporal bone, orbit, or foramen magnum
  - When they contact moving red blood cells, they are reflected at changed frequency through brain and skull back to detector
  - Change in frequency as blood cells move toward or away from ultrasound transmitter and detector an example of Doppler effect, related to velocity and direction of flow
    - Velocity increases during systole and decreases during diastole
    - Blood in lumen center moves faster than near the vessel wall, producing a spectrum of flow velocities
      - Spectrum resembles shape of waveform produced by intra-arterial pressure transducer
- TCD measurements most commonly made in middle cerebral and internal carotid arteries
  - Also measured in other vessels, including anterior cerebral, anterior communicating, posterior cerebral, posterior communicating, and basilar arteries
  - In approximately 10% of patients, particularly elderly females, technically satisfactory recordings cannot be obtained because of increased skull thickness
  - TCD cannot provide a simple assessment of global or hemispheric CBF
- Beyond question of vessel patency
  - Link between TCD measurements and CBF is indirect and subject to one technical limitation and two principal assumptions inherent in the link
    - Technical limitation is:
      - Accuracy with which the flow velocity can be determined depends on the angle of insonation
      - Variability of repeated measurements can be minimized either by:
        - Using a single examiner
        - Rigidly mounting TCD probe on patient's head with a headset, provided shift in brain structures caused by mass lesion does not displace artery
  - Two principal assumptions that have to be met for TCD-measured blood flow velocity to correspond to CBF are:
    - Flow and flow velocity are directly related only if arterial diameter remains constant
    - Blood flow in basal arteries of brain must be directly related to cortical CBF
  - Assumptions likely represent oversimplification and have not been supported adequately by evidence

Detection of Cerebral Vasospasm

- TCD helpful in identifying vasospasm following aneurysmal subarachnoid hemorrhage
  - As diameter of arterial lumen decreases with vasospasm velocity of blood flowing through the narrowed vessel must increase if flow is to be maintained
    - With absolute flow velocity alone, detection and documentation of severity and duration of vasospasm possible
      - Specificity approaches 100% but with limited sensitivity
- TCD has contributed much to understanding of natural history of vasospasm following aneurysmal subarachnoid hemorrhage (SAH)
  - But most studies predate current therapeutic approach of:
    - Early exclusion of aneurysm
    - Therapy with hypertensive-hypervolemic hemodilution and nimodipine
  - Recent advance in treatment of vasospasm that highlights one limitation of TCD is therapeutic dilation of stenotic arteries
    - TCD flow velocities may remain elevated despite successful dilation as a result of impaired autoregulation in the poststenotic vascular bed.
    - Likewise, TCD cannot assess isolated distal vasospasm.
      - May account for as much as a third of all cases of vasospasm
    - Because of limitations TCD not universally used to assess aneurysmal SAH patients

Assessment of Intracranial Pressure and Confirmation of Brain Death

- TCD-generated waveforms exhibit sequential characteristic changes as ICP increases
- As ICP increases systolic waveform becomes more peaked
- As ICP nears diastolic blood pressure, diastolic flow diminishes and subsequently ceases
- Once ICP exceeds diastolic blood pressure, TCD shows a pattern of to-and-fro movement of blood, indicating imminent intracranial circulatory arrest
  - Change in waveforms used to calculate pulsatility index
    - Relating difference between peak-systolic and end-diastolic velocity either to mean or to systolic velocity
- Such waveform analyses correlate well with ICP but cannot replace ICP monitoring
  - Autoregulation, vasospasm, or proximal arterial stenosis may alter TCD signal independent of ICP
- Clinical brain death demonstrates a characteristic blood flow velocity pattern
  - Short systolic inflow of blood

- Followed by an exit of blood (flow direction reverses) from cranium during diastole
- TCD a validated confirmatory test in diagnosis of brain death
  - Sensitivity exceeds 90%, specificity of 100%
- TCD can ascertain diagnosis in most patients at the bedside
  - Large craniotomy or inadequate bone window may preclude complete examination necessary to confirm brain death

Jugular Venous Oxygen Saturation Monitoring (SjvO$_2$)

- SjvO$_2$ monitoring touted as an indicator of cerebral oxygen homeostasis
  - Changes in SjvO$_2$ from normal range (60%–70%) provide:
    - Indirect information on state of CMRO$_2$
    - Because blood flow normally linked to CMRO$_2$, indirect information on CBF
  - Approximately 50% to 70% of patients with severe head trauma (GCS ≤ 8) will have an episode of desaturation (SjvO$_2$ < 50%)
  - Ischemic threshold widely accepted to be SjvO$_2$ < 50% during early hyperemic conditions following head injury
    - Clinical utility of SjvO$_2$ monitoring remains unsettled
- Complexity of catheter placement, sample collection, and results interpretation may contribute to 20% utilization of SjvO$_2$ monitoring in victims of moderate to severe head injury
  - SjvO$_2$ preferentially measured from flow-dominant internal jugular (IJ) vein
    - Right 60%, left 25%, equal 15%
    - To provide best estimate of *whole* brain CMRO$_2$ conditions
  - Hemispheric dominance established by which side will, in response to unilateral compression of IJ vein, produce greater rise of ICP
    - Alternatively, IJ vein size seen by ultrasound a reasonable estimate of dominance
    - As is relative size of jugular foramina on head CT scan
- Cannulation of the jugular bulb for intermittent or continuous monitoring similar to IJ catheterization for CVL placement
  - However needle, wire, and catheter are advanced in cephalad direction
  - Risk of causing an intracranial vascular injury reduced if wire is not pushed into jugular bulb
  - Catheter advanced slowly until resistance indicates it has reached roof of the bulb
  - Catheter then withdrawn 1 cm so that head movement cannot cause catheter-related vessel injury or thrombosis
    - Recommended not to power-flush or administer infusions through catheter
- Increase in SjvO$_2$ indicates either:
  - Lowered CMRO$_2$ (less extraction) and/or increased or hyperemic CBF
- Decrease in SjvO$_2$ (greater extraction) indicates:
  - Increased CMRO$_2$, hypoxia/anemia, or oligemia
  - Observed changes in SjvO$_2$ might then help guide therapeutic interventions
- Experience validates association of desaturation (SjvO$_2$ <50%) with worsened neurologic outcome

- Mortality reduced 66% when monitoring or managing cerebral extraction of oxygen with SjvO$_2$ in conjunction with CPP than when CPP alone managed
- CMRO$_2$ increased in patients with ICP ≥20 mm Hg and normal to decreased cerebral extraction ("luxury perfusion") of oxygen with hyperventilation therapy
- Elevated ICP associated with normal to increased cerebral extraction of oxygen was treated with mannitol, resulting in improved ICP and cerebral oxygenation
- Profound neurologic deterioration occurs with SjvO$_2$ ≤30%
  - As cerebral circulatory arrest develops, external carotid artery provides blood sampled at jugular bulb
    - SjvO$_2$ then increases
  - In clinical setting where brain death is expected
    - Ratio of mixed venous blood saturation to SjvO$_2$ <1:
      - Highly sensitive (95%), specific (100%), and predictive (92%) for cerebral circulatory arrest
- Limitations with SjvO$_2$ monitoring may explain low utilization
  - Admixture of extracranial blood through collateral venous drainage into superior sagittal, sigmoid, and cavernous sinuses directly into jugular bulb occurs even when catheter correctly placed
  - If samples are drawn faster than 2 mL/minute or catheter tip lies too short of jugular bulb, extracranial blood may further contaminate specimen
    - Spuriously elevate SjvO$_2$
  - "Clean" SjvO$_2$ sample does not distinguish between:
    - Lateralizing differences in flow
    - Metabolism
    - Brain injury
  - Because SjvO$_2$ reflects global average from variety of brain regions
    - Marked regional hypoperfusion may not be reflected by change in SjvO$_2$
  - SjvO$_2$ and brain tissue oxygen pressure (PbtO$_2$), measure of regional ischemia, usually track in same direction
    - But maintaining SjvO$_2$ above conventional thresholds did not reliably protect against occurrence of regional ischemic insults
    - SjvO$_2$ cannot be used alone to:
      - Direct hyperventilation
      - Or to alert clinicians to evolving hypocapnia-induced regional cerebral ischemia
    - "Acceptable" hyperventilation may cause harm clinically undetected by SjvO$_2$
- SjvO$_2$ monitoring most useful as trend monitor in:
  - Patients with diffuse global brain injury
  - When it identifies saturations below ischemic threshold
- Normal-range SjvO$_2$ can represent false-negative measurement
  - Insofar as areas of regional ischemia may be present
- Currently, best technique for guiding therapy to regional area of concern is PbtO$_2$

Near-infrared Spectroscopy (NIRS)

- NIRS utilizes minimal absorption and greater penetration of wavelengths in this portion of electromagnetic spectrum to evaluate changes in CBF and cerebral oxygenation

- Similar to pulse oximetry, NIRS compares differences in absorption of Hgb (670–760 nm) to O_2-Hgb (830 nm)
- NIRS used for noninvasive assessment of brain oxygenation through intact skull by detecting changes in oxyhemoglobin concentrations associated with neural activity
- NIRS offers advantage of continuous, noninvasive monitoring of cerebral cortex
  - Typically done with one sensor each for right and left hemispheres of brain
  - Originally developed for monitoring neonates
    - Penetration in adults significantly less compared to neonates
    - Extracranial changes in blood flow and oxygenation affect absorption values
  - May be as sensitive in detecting progressive cerebral hypoxia as EEG
    - But spatial resolution limited by number of detectors
  - Together with transcranial Doppler evaluation provides useful information in hemodynamic evaluation of carotid artery occlusion
  - Clinical utility in adults remains limited

Brain Oxygenation (PbtO$_2$)/Microdialysis

- In contrast to most other techniques for evaluating brain oxygenation
  - Tissue monitoring/microdialysis offers advantages and disadvantages of monitoring very discrete regions of tissue
  - Continuous PbtO$_2$ monitoring measures oxygen delivery and identifies cerebral hypoxia and ischemia in patients with:
    - Brain injury
    - Aneurysmal SAH
    - Malignant stroke
    - Other patients at risk for secondary brain injury
- 2007 Guidelines for the Management of Severe Head Injury brain tissue oxygenation threshold of <15 mm Hg adopted as level III recommendation
  - Subthreshold levels of PbtO$_2$ associated with increased morbidity and mortality in patients with severe brain injury
    - Increased FiO$_2$ has little effect on PbtO$_2$ in normal tissue
      - In injured brain, PbtO$_2$ increased as long as blood flow is present

- Management strategy in severe TBI includes PbtO$_2$ monitoring and therapy directed at maintaining brain oxygenation >25 mm Hg
  - Multimodal approach results in reduced patient mortality compared to CPP-directed therapy
- In 101 comatose, nonpenetrating head injury patients, whose GCS score was >8
  - Despite aggressive management of both ICP and CPP brain tissue hypoxia frequently occurred
  - Depth and duration of tissue hypoxia associated with unfavorable outcome and death at 6 months after injury
- In patients with severe injury in whom hyperventilation considered
  - Monitoring of brain oxygenation may be considered
  - Significance of local partial pressure of brain tissue oxygen debated
  - However, evidence for inclusion in multimodal monitoring is increasing
- Microdialysis technique can be combined with PbtO$_2$ monitoring using same highly localized probe
  - Microdialysis catheter consists of fluid path surrounded by semipermeable membrane
  - Fluid path perfused with balanced salt solution equilibrating with brain interstitial fluid
    - Fluid returned from path contains brain substances:
      - In proportion to local concentration
      - Specific membrane permeability
      - Perfusate flow rate
      - Concentration of substances of interest can be followed over time
- In research technique used to study the role of excitotoxicity or proteomics of brain ischemia in stroke
  - Monitoring application closest to clinical utility aims to determine state of aerobic glucose utilization by following ratio of metabolic intermediary products such as the pyruvate-to-lactate ratio
  - Ratiometric determinations of chemically similar molecules obviate the need to calibrate the probe based on the permeability of the substance(s) of interest
  - Decrease in pyruvate-to-lactate ratio indicates increase in anaerobic metabolism and/or mitochondrial dysfunction consistent with ischemia

CHAPTER 104 ■ BEHAVIORAL DISTURBANCES IN THE ICU

- Advances in critical care have led to improved survival rates among those admitted to intensive care units (ICUs)
  - In the United States approximately 55,000 patients are treated in ICUs each day.
  - At least 40% of adult ICU patients require mechanical ventilation (MV).

- Patients requiring long-term MV (> 3 days) represent 4% to 10% of critical care admissions and consume 30% to 50% of critical care resources.
- Incidence of neurologic dysfunction or injury has been underestimated, underreported, and only recently studied in critically ill patients

○ Higher severity of initial neurologic dysfunction (lower Glasgow Coma Scale [GCS]) was associated with higher 30-day mortality
○ No change or worsening of severity of GCS from first to third ICU day was also associated with higher 30-day mortality
○ Neurologic morbidities include polyneuropathy, encephalopathy, delirium, and cognitive impairments
• Medical and surgical management of critical illnesses can, and frequently does, result in *de novo* behavioral disturbances, including delirium and cognitive impairments

DELIRIUM: AN ACUTE BEHAVIORAL DISTURBANCE

• A neurobehavioral syndrome characterized by:
• Acute confusion
• Inattention
• Disorganized thinking
• Fluctuating course of mental status changes
• Motoric subtypes of delirium are:
• Hypoactive
• Hyperactive
• Mixed
• *Hypoactive* or "quiet" delirium is characterized by reduced mental and physical activity and inattention
• *Hyperactively* delirious patients are agitated, combative, and at risk for self-extubation, reintubation, pulling out central lines, and falls
• Delirium is a dynamic condition and often fluctuates between the hypoactive or hyperactive.
• In ICU mixed clinical picture is common
• Given multiple possible presentations not uncommon for clinicians to miss diagnosis
○ Delirium underdiagnosed by 80% of physicians
○ Standardized ICU examinations using reliable, sensitive, and specific CAM (Confusion Assessment Method)-ICU allows for accurate detection and analysis of delirium
• Delirium may be most common psychiatric condition experienced by hospitalized elderly
• Affecting between:
• 15% and 20% of hospitalized medical patients
• 25% to 65% of surgical patients
• As many as 80% of ICU patients
• Once considered benign recent evidence links delirium with adverse outcomes:
• Prolonged hospitalization
• Poor surgical recovery
• Increased morbidity and mortality
• Also associated with adverse cognitive outcomes in critically ill patients (see below)
• Delirium is not simply a marker of preexisting subclinical or early dementia.

CHRONIC COGNITIVE IMPAIRMENTS

• Cognitive processes or functions defined as ways of experiencing and thinking about the world and include:
• Intelligence
• Attention

• Learning
• Memory
• Language
• Visual spatial abilities
• Executive function (reasoning, decision making, planning, problem solving, working memory, sequencing, and executive control)
• In ICU survivors, one-third or more will develop chronic cognitive impairment
• Current data suggest cognitive impairments common in survivors of critical illness

NATURE OF COGNITIVE IMPAIRMENTS

• There are 10 cohorts totaling approximately 455 patients assessing long-term cognitive impairments following critical illness
• Evidence suggests that 25% to 78% of ICU survivors experience cognitive impairments
• Among patients with acute respiratory distress syndrome (ARDS), prevalence of cognitive impairments is as high as:
○ 70% to 78% at hospital discharge
○ 45% to 46% at 1 year
○ 47% at 2 years
○ 25% at 6 years
• Cognitive impairments occur in various cognitive domains (Table 104.1)

TABLE 104.1

COGNITIVE IMPAIRMENTS OBSERVED FOLLOWING CRITICAL ILLNESS

Cognitive domains	Specific cognitive impairments
Attention	Divided attention Focused attention Sustained attention
Memory	Explicit or declarative Recall (verbal and nonverbal) Recognition (verbal and nonverbal) Short-term memory
Intelligence	Verbal intelligence Performance intelligence Full-scale (general) intelligence
Language	Verbal fluency
Visual spatial	Apraxia Visuoconstruction
Executive function	Decision making Executive control Impulsivity Perseveration Planning Problem solving Shifting sets Working memory
Mental processing speed	Slow mental processing speed
Motor	Grip strength

- Cognitive impairments in critically ill patients similar to those reported in other populations such as carbon monoxide poisoning and following elective coronary artery bypass graft surgery
- In general, memory the most frequently observed deficit
  - Followed by impaired executive function and attention
  - Memory questionnaire administered to prospective cohort of 87 ARDS survivors found 20% of patients rated memory as poor 18 months after ICU discharge
  - Evaluation of executive function in general ICU survivors at 3 and 9 months found that 35% of patients were impaired
  - Similar findings seen in MV, nondelirious patients who had impaired memory and problem-solving abilities (i.e., executive dysfunction) during ICU treatment, during hospital treatment, and at 2-month follow-up
    - While in ICU, 100% of patients had impaired executive function
    - 67% had impaired memory
    - At 2-month follow-up, 50% had impaired executive function and 31% had impaired memory
- Acute respiratory distress syndrome (ARDS) patients had significantly lower measured IQ compared to their premorbid estimated IQ at hospital discharge
  - Measured IQ returned to premorbid level at 1-year follow-up
  - No additional improvement in IQ at 2 years
  - Does not necessarily suggest comparable recovery in all cognitive domains
    - Data from traumatic and anoxic brain injury literature suggest some cognitive abilities more likely to improve than others

INDICATORS OF COGNITIVE IMPAIRMENTS

- Consistent finding is lack of association between some indicators of illness severity and development of cognitive impairments

- Cognitive impairments not associated with:
  - ICU length of stay (LOS)
  - Acute Physiology and Chronic Health Evaluation II (APACHE II) scores
  - Tidal volume
  - Number of days receiving sedative, narcotic, or paralytic medications
- Impaired executive function measured *during* ICU treatment was associated with ICU and hospital LOS
- Impaired memory measured during ICU and hospital treatment was associated with admission APACHE II scores
- These relationships were not present by 2-month follow-up.
- Age has not been associated with cognitive impairments.
- Most patients in 10 cohorts studied were young or middle-aged adults (mean age, 54 years)

DELIRIUM AND ITS RELATION TO ADVERSE COGNITIVE OUTCOMES

- Studies of association between delirium and adverse cognitive outcomes generally carried out in non-ICU populations
- Data from these investigations likely apply to ICU cohorts
- Important difference between delirium and cognitive impairments is delirium fluctuates but cognitive impairments do not
- Table 104.2 shows comparison of characteristics of delirium, dementia, and cognitive impairments
- Higher incidence of dementia in hospitalized elderly patients with a history of delirium at follow-up evaluation
- Patients 85 years or older, excluding those with dementia, with an episode of delirium during hospitalization were significantly more likely to be diagnosed with dementia at 3-year follow-up compared to patients without delirium
- Over 3-year period, 60% of geriatric medical patients with delirium at hospital admission (after evaluating for dementia at baseline) developed dementia compared to only 18.5% of patients without delirium

TABLE 104.2

COMPARISONS BETWEEN COMPONENTS OF DELIRIUM, DEMENTIA, AND COGNITIVE IMPAIRMENTS

	Delirium	Dementia	Cognitive impairments
Mental status	Marked fluctuation	Chronically impaired—appears stable but deteriorates over time	Normal
Cognitive function	Sudden onset Acute cognitive impairment characterized by disorientation and confusion	Insidious onset Chronic cognitive impairment Often memory is the first observed cognitive impairment Progressive loss of cognitive functions (impaired judgment, executive function, etc.) Progressive decline over time Interferes with daily functioning and work May include changes in personality, mood, and behavior	Sudden onset Chronic cognitive impairment May affect one or multiple cognitive domains, with memory, executive function, and information processing most commonly affected Initially there may be some recovery or improvement of cognitive function Stable over time May interfere with daily functioning and work
Duration	Temporary	Permanent	Permanent

- In critically ill patients, one in three patients with delirium had cognitive impairments at 6-month follow-up
- Patients were not primarily geriatric (mean age of 53 years)
- Findings suggest that presence of delirium may be critical in predicting adverse long-term cognitive outcome

LACK OF RECOGNITION OF COGNITIVE IMPAIRMENTS

- In non-ICU clinical settings, physicians fail to recognize (or assess) cognitive impairment in 35% to 90% of patients
- Cognitive impairments rarely evaluated in critically ill patients
  - May be overlooked in one of every two cases
  - In 42% of ARDS survivors who underwent rehabilitation therapy, most were not evaluated for cognitive impairments, and only 12% of patients were identified as having cognitive impairments by clinical rehabilitation team
- Consequences of cognitive impairments far reaching and may contribute to decreased ability to perform activities of daily living and inability to return to work
  - Two years after hospital discharge:
    - 34% of ARDS survivors returned to full-time work or were full-time students
    - 34% were receiving disability payments started after hospital discharge for ARDS
    - 32% (20 of 62) were not working or were retired

POTENTIAL MECHANISMS OF DELIRIUM AND LONG-TERM COGNITIVE IMPAIRMENTS

- Many physiologic and pharmacologic perturbations affect the central nervous system in critically ill patients
  - Precise mechanisms contributing to delirium and cognitive impairment or both are unknown, various theories proposed, including:
    - Potentially adverse effects of medical illness on cognition
    - Pathologic processes underlying delirium and cognitive impairments
    - The impact of psychoactive medications, including sedatives and analgesics
  - Delirium and cognitive impairments rarely have one causal mechanism
    - They are thought to be multifactorial
    - Pathogeneses likely due to interactions between patient vulnerability and precipitating factors or insults, including critical illness and its treatment

Psychoactive Medications

- Many medications used for sedation or pain control—including those used in ICU setting—known to cause or worsen delirium
  - Association exists between high delirium prevalence rates in surgical and critically ill populations and use of sedatives and narcotics

- Data on impact of anesthetics and sedatives on long-term cognitive functioning conflicting
  - Reports suggest they may have neurotoxic effects, particularly for high-risk groups such as the very old (>75 years) and/or those with a recent history of cognitive impairment
- In some, effects of medications on cognition may be mediated by genetic factors
  - Apolipoprotein E4 (APOE4) allele is one probable genetic factor that may affect individual sensitivity to drug effects
  - Allele a significant risk factor for:
    - Development of certain forms of Alzheimer disease
    - Hippocampal atrophy
    - Worse recovery of neurologic function following traumatic brain injury (TBI)
    - Cognitive decline following cardiopulmonary bypass surgery
    - Delirium
  - More research is needed but appears that certain anticholinergic agents may have particularly adverse effects on cognition when administered to patients possessing the APOE4 allele.
    - Lorazepam increases susceptibility to impaired verbal learning and related cognitive deficits in patients with the APOE4 allele compared to patients without this polymorphism.

DELIRIUM AS A MECHANISM OF COGNITIVE IMPAIRMENTS

- Some researchers have speculated that delirium is a marker of subclinical dementia or cognitive impairment.
  - Which might not otherwise develop for years or decades
  - Data suggest common pathogenic mechanisms might underlie both Alzheimer disease and delirium.
    - Although, from a clinical standpoint, there are similarities and differences

COGNITIVE REHABILITATION

- Cognitive rehabilitation used widely with patients following TBI, stroke, and other neurologic insults
  - Evidence suggests cognitive rehabilitation can be highly effective
  - May be mediated by factors such as cause of brain injury and cognitive domain (i.e., memory, executive functioning, etc.) of focus
    - For example, patients with hypoxic brain injuries may be less responsive to cognitive rehabilitation than those with TBI or stroke

EMOTIONAL DISORDERS

- Psychiatric morbidity following critical illness common and includes depression, anxiety, and posttraumatic stress disorder (PTSD)
  - Unclear whether emotional disorders are a psychological reaction to extraordinary emotional and physiologic stress, sequelae of brain injury sustained due to critical illness and its treatment, or all of the above

- Combination of medications, physiological changes, pain, altered sensory inputs, and an unfamiliar environment may contribute to emotional changes

Posttraumatic Stress Disorder

- Estimates of PTSD prevalence in critically ill cohorts as high as 63%
  - Generally exceed those of other high-risk populations
  - General medical ICU cohorts shown to have both lowest and highest rates of PTSD compared to more specialized populations
    - Reported prevalence rates of PTSD range from 9.7% to 63%
    - Rates of PTSD in specialized populations range from 18.5% to 43%
  - Risk factors for development of PTSD and related symptoms not been systematically studied

- Several probable risk factors have been identified:
  - Delusional memories
  - Younger age
  - Existence of prior mental health history
  - Anxiety
  - Female gender

Depression and Anxiety

- Depression common among medically ill cohorts due both to the specific physical effects of certain illnesses and/or effects of illness on quality of life, independence, employment, and other factors
- Occurs in 25% to over 50% of ARDS survivors
- Regarding anxiety, with the exception of PTSD, less is known
  - Anxiety occurs in 4% to 41% of ARDS survivors
  - Reported in 24% of ARDS survivors at 1 and 2 years
  - Smoking and alcohol abuse may be related to symptoms of depression and anxiety in ARDS survivors

CHAPTER 105 ■ UPPER GASTROINTESTINAL BLEEDING

Acute gastrointestinal (GI) bleeding is a common indication for admission to the intensive care unit (ICU) in the United States, with over 300,000 admissions per year. Most (75%) of these arise from the upper GI tract. Despite advances in critical care medicine, the mortality associated with upper GI bleeding has not changed and remains about 10%, likely due to aging of the population and increasing comorbidities.

EPIDEMIOLOGY

- The annual incidence of hospital admission for upper GI bleeding in the United States is approximately 100 per 100,000.
- Peptic ulcer disease (PUD) is the most common cause of upper GI bleeding, accounting for half of cases (Table 105.1).
- Upper GI bleeding is twice more common in males than females and increases with age.
- Mortality for patients younger than 60 years in the absence of malignancy or organ failure is <1%.
- Patients rarely die from blood loss; rather, death is due to decompensation of other underlying conditions.
- Four major risk factors for PUD are nonsteroidal anti-inflammatory drugs (NSAIDs), *Helicobacter pylori* infection, stress, and gastric acid.
- Duodenal ulcers are more common than gastric ulcers.
- Recent data showed a decline in the proportion of cases caused by PUD—down to 21%—with nonspecific mucosal abnormalities being the most common cause (42%).
- Mallory-Weiss tears account for 5% to 15% of cases, while the proportion of patients bleeding from varices varies widely, depending on the population, from about 5% to 30%.
- Hemorrhagic or erosive gastropathy (usually from NSAIDs or alcohol) and erosive esophagitis often cause mild upper GI bleeding, but major hemorrhage does not usually occur from erosions (Fig. 105.1).
- Esophagogastric varices are also a common cause of upper GI bleeding and usually develop as a consequence of systemic or segmental portal hypertension.
- The outcome of an episode of active variceal hemorrhage depends on the control of active bleeding and the avoidance of complications associated with bleeding and its treatment.

CLINICAL PRESENTATION

- Upper GI bleeding commonly presents with hematemesis and/or melena.
- Hematemesis or coffee-ground emesis indicates an upper GI source of bleeding, which is above the ligament of Treitz, at the junction of the duodenum and jejunum.
- Melena suggests a minimum blood loss of 200 mL. The presence of melena is indicative of blood being present in the digestive tract for at least 12 to 14 hours.
- Although the more proximal the bleeding site in the upper GI tract, the more likely the patient will have melena, a significant percentage of patients with ascending colon sources of bleeding may also present with melena.
- Hematochezia is usually a presentation of lower GI bleeding, but an upper GI source that bleeds rapidly may also present with hematochezia.

TABLE 105.1

ETIOLOGY OF UPPER GASTROINTESTINAL BLEEDING

MUCOSAL (EROSIVE OR ULCERATIVE)
1. Peptic ulcer disease
   a. Idiopathic
   b. Aspirin- or NSAID-induced
   c. Infectious (*Helicobacter pylori*, cytomegalovirus, *Herpes simplex virus*)
2. Stress-related mucosal disease
3. Zollinger-Ellison
4. Esophagitis
   a. Peptic
   b. Infectious (*Candida albicans*, *H. simplex virus*, cytomegalovirus)
   c. Medication-related (aspirin, NSAIDs, alendronate)

VASCULAR
1. Dieulafoy lesion
2. Idiopathic angiomas
3. Osler-Weber-Rendu syndrome
4. Watermelon stomach
5. Radiation-induced telangiectasia
6. Blue rubber bleb nevus syndrome

PORTAL HYPERTENSION
1. Esophageal varices
2. Gastric varices
3. Portal hypertensive gastropathy

TUMORS
1. Benign (leiomyoma, polyp, lipoma)
2. Malignant

TRAUMATIC
1. Mallory-Weiss tear
2. Nasogastric tube (usually while in the intensive care unit)
3. Foreign body ingestion

OTHER
1. Hemobilia
2. Hemosuccus pancreaticus

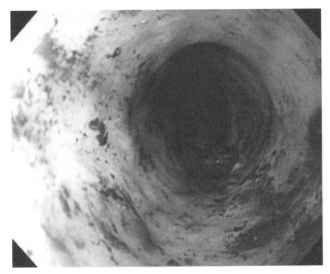

FIGURE 105.1. Severe esophagitis. Endoscopic view of severe esophagitis.

TABLE 105.2

CLINICAL AND LABORATORY DETERMINANTS OF SIGNIFICANT BLOOD LOSS

CLINICAL
1. Resting tachycardia (>100 beats/min or 20 beat increase from baseline if baseline heart rate >100 beats/min)
2. Orthostasis:
   a. Pulse increase >20 beat/min
   b. Systolic BP decrease >20 mm Hg
   c. Diastolic BP decrease >10 mm Hg
3. Hematochezia
4. Failure to clear bright red blood from gastric lavage

LABORATORY
1. High transfusion requirement (more than 1 unit every 8 h)
2. Lactic acidosis
3. Azotemia

BP, blood pressure.

- Patients with upper GI bleeding who have hematochezia usually have hemodynamic instability and rapidly dropping hemoglobin.
- Vomiting, retching, or coughing preceding hematemesis—especially in an alcoholic patient—should increase suspicion for a Mallory-Weiss tear.
- In addition to symptoms, a detailed history should include use of aspirin or other NSAID intake, alcohol consumption, presence of liver disease or variceal bleeding, history of PUD, weight loss, dysphagia, reflux, aortic aneurysm, or abdominal aortic vascular graft.

DIAGNOSTIC EVALUATION

Gastric Lavage

- Nasogastric lavage is important for confirmation of the diagnosis and may be predictive of a high-risk lesion if bright red blood is present in the lavaged.
- A nasogastric tube may also decrease the risk of aspiration in patients with active hematemesis.
- A nonbloody nasogastric aspirate may be seen in up to 16% of patients with upper GI bleeding, usually if bleeding has ceased or if from a duodenal source, particularly if the pylorus is closed.
- The presence of bile in the aspirate is often misleading and does not necessarily rule out a postpyloric source of bleeding in 50% of cases.
- Testing of gastric contents for blood can frequently be misleading because of nasogastric tube-related trauma. In addition, the low pH of gastric contents may interfere with the guaiac test's design for occult blood testing in stool, giving false results.
- An elevated blood urea nitrogen (BUN)-to-creatinine ratio usually indicates an upper GI source as well as major blood loss.
- Patients without renal disease who have a **BUN >25 mg/dL** have lost a minimum of 1 L of blood.

- Persistent azotemia (for more than 24 hours) is an indication of hypovolemia because volume loss contributes quantitatively more than the digestion of blood in raising BUN and is the sole determinant of azotemia 24 hours after cessation of bleeding.

Amount of Blood Loss

- Determination of estimated blood loss is the single most important aspect of care in patients with upper GI bleeding. This estimation helps with the aggressiveness of volume resuscitation and triage to an appropriate level of care (i.e., transfer to ICU).
  - Estimation of blood loss is often incorrect and requires an accurate assessment of vital signs, central venous pressure, hemoglobin and hematocrit, and a degree of clinical experience. Some indicators of clinically significant blood loss are summarized in Table 105.2.
- Most complications associated with blood loss result from the adverse effects of hypovolemia and hemorrhagic shock on organs and are compounded by limited or poor baseline physiologic reserve.
- Initial hematocrit may be misleading due to loss of whole blood, which results in equal loss of plasma and erythrocytes.
- Redistribution of plasma from the extracellular to intravascular space, within 24 to 48 hours of the initial hemorrhage, results in dilution of red cell mass and a fall in hematocrit. The hematocrit fall may occur even more rapidly with volume replacement with crystalloid or nonheme colloid.
- *Acute* responses to blood loss represent a spectrum of changes, including resting tachycardia, orthostasis, peripheral vasoconstriction (cold, clammy skin), and acute end-organ dysfunction (mental status changes, oliguria).
- *Chronic* blood loss is usually associated with stable hemodynamic responses, retention of hypotonic fluid, and an absence of impaired organ function due to compensatory changes in the cardiovascular system.

Diagnostic Workup

- Upper GI endoscopy is the diagnostic modality of choice for further evaluation of upper GI bleeding.
- Endoscopy helps in localization and identification of the bleeding lesion in the upper GI tract and can be therapeutic in establishing hemostasis and preventing recurrent bleeding.
- Upper GI studies with radiocontrast material such as barium are contraindicated in the setting of acute upper GI bleeding due to interference with subsequent endoscopic intervention, angiography, and surgery.
- Angiographic diagnosis of the source of upper GI bleeding is made by extravasation of contrast material. The bleeding must be brisk, with a rate of about **0.5 to 1 mL/minute.** Angiography can be helpful in establishing the diagnosis in 75% of patients; about 85% of bleeding originates from a branch of the left gastric artery.
- Nuclear medicine studies using ^{99m}Tc-pertechnetate-labeled red blood cell scan may also aid in localization of the bleeding site and has the ability to detect bleeding at lower rates (**<0.5 mL/minute**) than contrast angiography.
- Endoscopy is the diagnostic method of choice for esophagogastric varices. In cases where endoscopy is nondiagnostic and gastric variceal bleeding is suspected, studies such as endoscopic ultrasound, portal venography, or computed tomography (CT) angiography can be used.
- Cirrhotic patients with upper GI bleeding should be administered a prophylactic antibiotic—usually a fluoroquinolone—preferably prior to endoscopy.

PREDICTORS OF OUTCOME AND RISK STRATIFICATION

- Three clinical parameters that are independent predictors of death and rebleeding are (1) hemodynamic instability, (2) older age, and (3) presence of comorbidities (Table 105.3).
- Early therapeutic endoscopic intervention plays an important role in achieving hemostasis, reducing the rebleeding rate, and improving morbidity and mortality in high-risk peptic ulcer–related upper GI bleeding.
- On the contrary, early endoscopy increases costs without a change in outcomes in patients with low-risk clinical and endoscopic features.

TABLE 105.3

CLINICAL INDICATORS OF SIGNIFICANT UPPER GI BLEEDING

PATIENT CHARACTERISTICS
Older age (>60 y)
Severe comorbidities (i.e., cardiopulmonary disease)
Onset of hemorrhage after hospitalization

RELATED TO AMOUNT OF BLEEDING
Hematemesis of bright red blood
Hematochezia
Gastric lavage with bright red blood
Hemorrhagic shock
High transfusion requirement

TABLE 105.4

ENDOSCOPIC FINDINGS THAT PREDICT RECURRENT UPPER GI BLEEDING

Endoscopic stigmata of bleeding	Prevalence (%)	Risk of bleeding (%)
Clean ulcer base	35	3–5
Flat spot	10	7–10
Oozing without visible vessel	10	10–20
Adherent clot	10	25–30
Nonbleeding visible vessel	25	50
Active arterial bleeding	10	90

- Risk stratification of patients with upper GI bleeding can be done using clinical and laboratory data and endoscopic findings. Endoscopic risk stratification depends on findings that predict the risk of rebleeding (Table 105.4).

MANAGEMENT

- The initial evaluation of a patient with upper GI bleeding includes the assessment of hemodynamic stability and need for aggressive resuscitation, if necessary.
- Table 105.5 summarizes the general principles of management.

TABLE 105.5

PRINCIPLES OF TREATMENT FOR UPPER GASTROINTESTINAL BLEEDING

GENERAL
1. Close monitoring in the ICU if bleeding is significant
2. Place a large nasogastric tube
3. Large bore IV access
   a. At least two 14- or 16-gauge peripheral IVs
   b. Or a 12 Fr double lumen catheter or a 9 Fr introducer
4. Volume resuscitation with crystalloids to maintain hemodynamic stability
5. Transfuse PRBCs to maintain hemoglobin
   a. >7 g/dL in healthy, young individuals
   b. >10 g/dL in elderly with comorbidities such as ischemic heart disease
6. Correct coagulopathy
7. Consult gastroenterology and surgery if bleeding severe

SPECIFIC (BASED ON THE CAUSE/LESION)
1. Acid suppression
2. Splanchnic vasoconstrictors for variceal bleeding
   a. Octreotide
   b. Vasopressin analogues
3. Antibiotics (fluoroquinolones) for variceal bleeding
4. Upper GI endoscopy
5. Angiography (as indicated)
6. Surgery

ICU, intensive care unit; IV, intravenous; Fr, French; PRBCs, packed red blood cells; GI, gastrointestinal.

Hemodynamic Resuscitation

- The initial management of upper GI bleeding should be directed at restoring blood volume to maintain hemodynamic stability. Hemodynamic stabilization with adequate volume and blood resuscitation also helps to minimize treatment-associated complications.
- Intravenous (IV) access with two large-bore (14- to 16-gauge) catheters should be maintained at all times.
- In cases where peripheral IV catheters cannot be placed, a large-bore central line (9 to 12 French) should be inserted; triple-lumen catheters have one 16- and two 18-gauge ports and are long and should therefore be avoided due to unacceptably high resistance to flow.
- Hypovolemia and hypotension from GI blood loss should be treated promptly with fluid resuscitation using crystalloid and packed red blood cells (PRBCs).
- All patients with hemodynamic instability or a hematocrit drop of more than 6%, a transfusion requirement greater than two units of PRBCs or significant active bleeding as evidenced by continued hematemesis with bright red blood from gastric lavage or hematochezia should be admitted to ICU for close observation and resuscitation.
- High-risk patients, including the elderly or those with severe comorbidities such as ischemic **heart disease** or congestive heart failure, should be transfused to maintain **their hemoglobin >10 g/dL.**
- On the contrary, unnecessary transfusion should be avoided in young, healthy individuals in whom maintenance of hemoglobin >7 g/dL may be sufficient.
- In hemorrhagic shock, close monitoring of end-organ perfusion (coronary, central nervous system, and renal) and preventing ischemic organ injury improves survival.
- In addition to a baseline electrocardiogram (ECG) and telemetry monitoring, urine output should be monitored continuously.
- In patients with massive hemorrhage or variceal bleeding, monitoring of preload via a central venous or pulmonary artery catheter may be useful; less invasive monitoring, including those devices using pulse-wave form variability (LidCO, PICCO, Flow Track) to evaluate preload, may also be useful in these situations.
- Coagulopathy should be corrected as needed to maintain **platelet count >50,000 cells/μL** and **prothrombin time within 2 seconds** of the upper level of normal.
- After replacement of factors and platelets, recombinant activated **factor VII** can rapidly correct severe coagulopathy in hepatic failure.
- Elective intubation should be considered in patients with ongoing hematemesis or altered mental status to facilitate endoscopy and decrease the risk of aspiration. Gastroenterology and, in cases of severe bleeding, surgery consultations should be requested.

Pharmacologic Treatment

Gastric Acid Suppression

- Acid-suppressive therapy with **proton pump inhibitors (PPI)** is an essential adjunct to therapeutic endoscopy for management of patients with PUD-related upper GI bleeding.

- Other acid-suppressing agents, including H$_2$-receptor antagonists (H$_2$RA), have not been shown to reduce the rate of rebleeding or transfusion requirement in PUD.
- High-dose PPI infusion following a bolus injection significantly reduces the rate of rebleeding compared to standard therapy in patients with bleeding from PUD.
- Current recommended doses of IV PPI therapy are lansoprazole, 90- to 120-mg bolus followed by 6 to 9 mg/hour infusion, and pantoprazole, 80 mg bolus followed by 8 mg/hour infusion. The infusion is usually continued for 48 to 72 hours and, if there is no further bleeding, switched to a twice-daily dose.
- The superiority of PPI over H$_2$RAs has been attributed to better maintenance of **gastric pH above 6.0,** which may lead to clot stabilization by prevention of fibrinolysis, and thus rebleeding.

Other Therapies

- Splanchnic vasoconstrictors are important adjunct therapies to variceal hemorrhage. The current agent of choice in the United States is the somatostatin analogue octreotide.
- Somatostatin and its analogues inhibit the release of vasodilator hormones such as glucagon, thereby indirectly causing splanchnic vasoconstriction and decreased portal inflow.
- For octreotide, the recommended dose is a 50-μg IV bolus followed by an infusion of 50 μg/hour for 5 days.
- Additionally, a longer-acting analogue of vasopressin, terlipressin, may also be used. Its efficacy is similar to octreotide and endoscopic sclerotherapy.
- Octreotide may also be considered as an adjunct therapy in the management of nonvariceal bleeding.
- If a vasopressor is needed temporarily for the maintenance of blood pressure, medications that have β_2-adrenergic activity, such as dopamine or albuterol, should be avoided due to potential risk of splanchnic vasodilation.

Endoscopic Treatment

- Identification and hemostasis of the source of upper GI bleeding is critical in the patient's outcome.
- Emergent endoscopy with therapeutic intervention is needed in patients who remain hemodynamically unstable and continue to bleed.
- In cases for which hemodynamic stability can be established quickly with volume resuscitation, endoscopy can be performed within 24 hours.
- The two most commonly used hemostasis techniques in the United States are injection therapy with epinephrine (1:10,000) and contact thermal devices.
- Combination therapy with injection and thermal coagulation are superior to monotherapy in patients with major endoscopic stigmata such as active bleeding or adherent clot.
- Visible vessels should be treated with thermal coagulation, whereas endoscopic intervention is not required for low-risk lesions such as a clean-base ulcer or a flat spot.
- Upper GI endoscopy is associated with potential complications, including aspiration, adverse reactions to conscious sedation, viscus perforation, and increased hemorrhage during therapeutic intervention.

- Contraindications to endoscopy include suspected GI perforation, unstable angina, severe coagulopathy, and severe agitation.
- In patients with recent ischemic cardiac events, the risks of endoscopy may outweigh its benefits, and it should therefore be used judiciously.
- Complications of endoscopic therapy include mucosal ulceration, motility abnormalities, stricture formation, esophageal perforation, and mediastinitis, as well as portal hypertensive gastropathy due to shunting of blood to the gastric mucosa.

Nonvariceal Bleeding

- Early therapeutic endoscopic intervention is important in achieving hemostasis, reducing rebleeding rates, and improving morbidity and mortality in PUD-related upper GI bleeding.
- One-third of patients with active bleeding or a nonbleeding visible vessel require urgent surgery; further bleeding is possible if treated conservatively.
- Patients with recurrent bleeding after endoscopic therapy benefit from repeat endoscopic therapy.
- Treatment of adherent clots is controversial. Double-blind trials of PPI therapy without endoscopic therapy showed extremely low rates of recurrent bleeding. In contrast, two small endoscopic trials showed better results with endoscopic therapy than conservative therapy.
- Bleeding from Mallory-Weiss tear stops spontaneously in 80% to 90% of patients and recurs only in up to 5% of patients. Endoscopic intervention is effective in actively bleeding Mallory-Weiss tears but is not necessary if active bleeding is not present.
- Rarely, surgery may be required to repair the tear. Massive bleeding can be seen if the Mallory-Weiss tear occurs in a patient with portal hypertension.

Variceal Bleeding

- Compared to nonvariceal causes of upper GI bleeding, which stop spontaneously in 90% of cases, variceal bleeding subsides spontaneously in only 50% of patients.
- The development of massive bleeding from gastroesophageal varices is indicative of advanced liver disease.
- Isolated gastric varices can occur due to segmental portal hypertension or as a consequence of obliteration of esophageal varices with endoscopic intervention.
- Active variceal bleeding occurs in about 50% of patients with decompensated cirrhosis, accounting for about one-third of all cirrhosis-related deaths.
- The mortality is very high, ranging between 70% and 80% in patients with continued variceal bleeding or rebleeding; each episode of bleeding is associated with a 30% risk of mortality.
- Variceal hemorrhage can predispose patients to hepatic encephalopathy, hepatorenal syndrome, and systemic infection, all of which increase the mortality in these patients.
- The risk of rebleeding remains high, ranging between 60% and 70%, unless endoscopic intervention is instituted to obliterate the varices.
- The greatest risk of rebleeding is within the first 48 to 72 hours, although it can occur as late as 6 weeks. Table 105.6 summarizes the risk factors for rebleeding from esophageal varices.

TABLE 105.6

RISK FACTORS FOR EARLY (<6 WEEKS) RECURRENT VARICEAL BLEEDING

CLINICAL
Age >60 years
Severity of initial bleed
Severity of chronic liver disease
Presence of ascites
Renal failure

ENDOSCOPIC
Active bleeding during endoscopy
Clot on varices
Red color signs (i.e., cherry red spot)
Increasing size of varices

- Esophageal variceal bleeding is usually amenable to endoscopic therapy via the obliteration of varices by either sclerotherapy or band ligation.
- Endoscopic band ligation is superior to sclerotherapy in initial hemostasis, rate of recurrent bleeding, complications, and mortality.
- **Sclerotherapy** may be indicated in cases where visualization is poor, but is usually followed by band ligation.
- Unlike esophageal varices, endoscopic management of gastric varices is less effective due to deeper localization of varices in the submucosa.
- Injection of cyanoacrylate tissue glue and thrombin are promising therapies in the endoscopic management of gastric varices.
- The transjugular intrahepatic portosystemic shunt (**TIPS**) procedure is done as salvage therapy to artificially create a portosystemic shunt to decompress the portal venous system and, consequently, variceal vasculature. It is recommended in patients with variceal bleeding refractory to pharmacologic and endoscopic therapy, regardless of the severity of cirrhosis.

Angiographic Treatment

- In a few patients with nonvariceal upper GI bleeding, angiographic localization may be necessary, with the option of hemostasis using a vasoconstrictor (i.e., intra-arterial vasopressin) or embolization (i.e., gelatin sponge).
- Embolization carries the risk of bowel ischemia, infarction, and necrosis, which is seen less in the duodenum than in the stomach due to the dual circulation from celiac and superior mesenteric arteries.

Surgery

- Surgical indications for the management of nonvariceal hemorrhage are life-threatening hemorrhage refractory to pharmacologic and endoscopic intervention, failure of medical therapy to resolve or prevent the recurrence of PUD, and related complications such as bleeding.
- The surgical procedure depends on the location of the ulcer and the clinical status of the patient. Mortality from surgical intervention for PUD can be as high as 30%.

TABLE 105.7

RISK FACTORS FOR STRESS ULCER BLEEDING

1. Respiratory failure requiring mechanical ventilation for more than 48 h
2. Coagulopathy
   a. Thrombocytopenia (<50,000 cells/μL)
   b. INR (>1.5)
   c. PTT (greater than two times the upper limit of normal)
3. Other risk factors
   Severe sepsis syndrome
   Shock
   Liver failure
   Renal failure
   Major trauma
   Extensive burns
   Intracranial hypertension

INR, international normalized ratio; PTT, partial thromboplastin time.

- The TIPS procedure has decreased the need for surgical shunt, which is indicated for patients with variceal hemorrhage and preserved hepatic synthetic function.
- Distal esophageal transaction, with or without devascularization, is another surgical option in patients with massive, refractory variceal hemorrhage, but is associated with high mortality.

STRESS-RELATED MUCOSAL DAMAGE

- Splanchnic hypoperfusion plays a pivotal role in the pathogenesis of stress-related mucosal damage. Stress-related mucosa damage (SRMD), also known as stress ulcers, occurs as a consequence of critical illness and is the most common cause of GI bleeding in the ICU. Table 105.7 summarizes the risk factors for bleeding from stress ulcers.
- SRMD occurs within a few hours of critical illness and can present as lesions ranging from subepithelial petechiae to superficial erosions that can progress into true ulcers. These lesions are usually multiple and occur predominantly in the fundus of the stomach, typically sparing the antrum.
- Acute respiratory failure requiring mechanical ventilation for longer than 48 hours and coagulopathy are the two strongest independent risk factors for clinically significant GI bleeding due to SRMD.
- Most SRMD lesions are asymptomatic and clinically insignificant, although some patients may develop clinically evident bleeding, presenting with hematemesis, coffee-ground emesis, melena, and hematochezia.
- Clinically evident bleeding due to SRMD occurs in up to 25% of critically ill patients who do not receive prophylactic therapy, with approximately 20% of these patients having clinically significant bleeding.
- Clinically significant, SRMD-related bleeding is associated with an increased length of ICU stay and morbidity and mortality.

Treatment

- The treatment of stress ulcer bleeding is supportive. Efforts should be focused on reversing the precipitating factors.
- Acid suppression with H$_2$RA or PPIs is routinely used as adjunct therapy, given that luminal acidity is an essential factor in the pathogenesis of SRMD.
- Bleeding from SRMD is usually not amenable to endoscopic intervention because the lesions are diffuse. However, in cases of severe bleeding, endoscopy may be indicated and successful if hemorrhage is from one or several lesions.
- Since the gastric mucosa has a rich collateral blood supply, angiographic treatment—including embolization or intra-arterial vasopressin—may be considered for bleeding refractory to endoscopic therapy.

Prophylaxis

- The incidence of stress ulcer bleeding has been decreasing as a result of more aggressive fluid resuscitation and prophylactic therapy.
- Most deaths in patients with stress ulcer bleeding are not due to GI hemorrhage. Therefore, the contribution of stress ulcer bleeding to overall ICU mortality does not appear to be significant in unselected ICU populations.
- Although gastric acid production is not increased in the most critically ill patients, it is essential in the pathogenesis of SRMD, and thus, therapies targeting gastric acid have been the mainstay of prophylaxis.
- Medications that suppress gastric acid, such as H$_2$RAs and PPIs, prevent SRMD by raising the gastric fluid pH, ideally above 4.0.
- Gastric pH-altering agents, as well as sucralfate, decrease the incidence of clinically significant bleeding by approximately 50%. However, a more recent study showed the superiority of H$_2$RAs over sucralfate in the prevention of SRMD-related bleeding.
- A major concern about using pH-altering medications is an increased risk of ventilator-associated pneumonia due to gastric colonization with the Enterobacteriaceae secondary to increased gastric pH and subsequent retrograde gastro-oropharyngeal contamination.
- Based on available data, the risk of pneumonia attributable to pH-altering drugs can be minimized via the implementation of preventive measures such as maintenance of the semirecumbent position, avoidance of high gastric residuals, and the administration of tube feeds into the small bowel whenever possible.
- Enteral feeding also decreases the risk of clinically evident GI bleeding. The beneficial effects of enteral feeding are probably multifactorial.
- Due to limited data, the use of enteral nutrition as the sole "therapy" for stress ulcer prophylaxis should be discouraged.

CHAPTER 106 ■ APPROACH TO LOWER GASTROINTESTINAL BLEEDING

IMMEDIATE CONCERNS

- Lower gastrointestinal (LGI) bleeding (LGIB) may be the primary cause of admission to the intensive care unit (ICU) or occurs during the course of ICU care for disorders other than LGIB. The initial approach to patients with LGIB, whether occult or acutely overt, is resuscitation to maintain organ perfusion.
- ICU physicians must maintain adequacy of airway and circulation, including ensuring an open airway and adequate intravenous access.
- Thereafter, the severity of bleeding should be graded to determine whether urgent diagnostic and interventional procedures need to be initiated immediately.
- The consequences of LGIB should be prevented or treated, just as would an acute myocardial infarction (AMI) induced by anemia or unstable hemodynamic status. A summary approach to ICU patients is noted in Table 106.1.

Essential Diagnostic Tests and Procedures

- History taking, including previous operative interventions and medications
- Physical examination, including digital examination
- Stool guaiac for anemic patients with suspicious gastrointestinal (GI) blood loss
- Complete blood count
- Endoscopic procedures: sigmoidoscopy, colonoscopy, enteroscopy, and capsule endoscopy
- Barium study
- Radiologic procedures: angiography

TABLE 106.1

SUMMARY OF AN APPROACH TO ICU PATIENTS WITH LOWER GASTROINTESTINAL BLEEDING

1. Immediately assess and stabilize the patient's hemodynamic status
   The ABCs of resuscitation
2. Determine presence of lower gastrointestinal bleeding
   By history, physical examination, and sometimes nasogastric aspiration
3. Arrange appropriate diagnostic and therapeutic interventions to stop any active bleeding
4. Treat any underlying lesions, and monitor and manage the comorbid illness

ICU, intensive care unit.

- Nuclear scintigraphy: technetium-labeled red blood cell scan
- Other examinations for affected organs due to unstable hemodynamics, such as electrocardiogram (ECG) for AMI

Treatment

- Ensure stable hemodynamic status, using fluids and transfusion of blood components.
- Endoscopic therapies include local injection, electrocoagulation, hemoclipping, argon plasma coagulation, and elastic banding according to the nature of the bleeding.
- Radiologic interventions include angiography with intra-arterial vasopressin infusion, embolization, and glue.
- The adverse events caused by treatment modalities, such as perforation caused by endoscopic thermocoagulation or bowel infarction due to angiographic embolization, should be monitored and managed.
- Surgical consultation is warranted for severe LGIB in which the patient cannot be resuscitated or if all available therapeutic modalities fail.

OVERVIEW

- LGIB is defined as a bleeding source distal to the ligament of Treitz, thus involving the small bowel and colon, and accounts for an estimated 20% to 24% of all major GI bleeding.
- The annual incidence of LGIB is approximately 0.03% in the adult population and the annual incidence of hospitalization for LGIB to be 20 to 30 cases per 100,000 persons.
- LGIB is more common in men than women, and the incidence increases with age, with a >200-fold increase from the third to ninth decades of life.
- Patient age is an important factor in the differential diagnosis of GI bleeding. Patients <40 years are more likely to suffer from small bowel tumors, whereas patients >40 years are more prone to bleeding from vascular lesions and neoplasm.
- LGIB is approximately 20% to 33% as common as upper GI bleeding (UGIB) but has a lower mortality rate than does UGIB. Two to 15% of patients with presumed LGIB will have UGIB.
- Patients who develop LGIB while hospitalized for another disease process have a higher risk of death than those admitted with LGIB. Similarly, LGIB patients with comorbid illness have a higher mortality than those without.
- Most deaths are not the direct result of uncontrolled bleeding, but rather exacerbation of an underlying disorder or development of a nosocomial complication.

TABLE 106.2

CAUSES OF LOWER GASTROINTESTINAL BLEEDING

COLONIC SOURCES
- Vascular ectasia
- Diverticulosis
- Ischemic colitis
- Acute hemorrhagic rectal ulcer syndrome
- Neoplasia
- Postpolypectomy
- Inflammatory bowel disease
- Infectious colitis and ulcer
- NSAID-induced colopathy
- Radiation colitis
- Hemorrhoids
- Dieulafoy lesions
- Colon varices
- Aortoenteric fistula

SMALL BOWEL SOURCES
- Vascular ectasia
- Focal active bleeding small bowel tumor:
  - Lymphoma
  - Adenocarcinoma
  - GIST
  - Other tumors
- NSAID-induced enteropathy
- Crohn disease
- Meckel diverticulum
- Vasculitis: SLE, Behçet disease, Schönlein-Henoch purpura
- Infection related ulcer: CMV, and so forth
- Small bowel varices
- Aortoenteric fistula

NSAID, nonsteroidal anti-inflammatory drugs; GIST, gastrointestinal stromal tumor; SLE, systemic lupus erythematosus; CMV, cytomegalovirus.

- LGIB remains a difficult diagnostic and treatment problem for several reasons:
  - Bleeding can originate from any part of the lower GI tract.
  - Blood loss is often intermittent in nature, and it is difficult to identify the source in the absence of active bleeding, especially angiographically.
  - The colon preparation before urgent colonoscopy is, obviously, needed but often incomplete.
  - Recurrent bleeding due to angiodysplasia or diverticula may be seen with LGIB.
  - Unlike UGIB, there are no evidence-based and effective pharmacologic therapies for LGIB.
- Among the many causes of LGIB (Table 106.2), diverticular bleeding, angiodysplasia, colitis, and neoplasm have been reported to be the most frequent.
- In ICU acute hemorrhagic rectal ulcers and ischemic colitis are the most frequent causes of LGIB, followed by colitis, angiodysplasia, and diverticular bleeding (Table 106.3)

Presentation

- LGIB may present in multiple ways, including occult fecal blood; iron deficiency anemia; melena; intermittent scant hematochezia; or acute, massive, and overt bleeding.

TABLE 106.3

CAUSES OF LOWER GASTROINTESTINAL BLEEDING IN SURGICAL, TRAUMA, AND MEDICAL ICUS

Causes	Percent
Acute hemorrhagic rectal ulcer syndrome (AHRUS)	26.7
Ischemic colitis	17.1
Colitis other than ischemia	8.6
Vascular ectasia (angiodysplasia)	6.7
Diverticular bleeding	5.7
Malignancy	5.7
Colonic polyp	3.8
Solitary ulcer	3.8
Hemorrhoid	2.9
Dieulafoy lesions	1.9
Radiation colitis	1.0
Small bowel bleeding	6.7
Undetermined	9.4

ICU, intensive care unit.
From Wang HP. Unpublished data.

- Patients with chronic LGIB may only present with anemia, whereas those with acute LGIB may complain of passing bright red blood per rectum, dark blood with clots, or, less commonly, melena.
- Patients with brown or infrequent stools are unlikely to have brisk bleeding, and those with frequent passage of red or maroon stool may have aggressive ongoing bleeding.
- **Pallor, fatigue, chest pain, palpitations, dyspnea, tachypnea, tachycardia, posture-related dizziness, and syncope** are suggestive of hemodynamic compromise and demand aggressive care.
- The severity of LGIB may be underestimated due to compensatory mechanisms that delay the onset of hypotension. Careful history taking and physical examination are essential to the care of LGIB patients.
- The approach to LGIB patients is initially aimed at immediate assessment and stabilization of the hemodynamic status, followed by identifying the source of bleeding, stopping any active bleeding, treating any underlying lesions, monitoring and managing comorbid illness, and preventing recurrent bleeding.
- Even with the advances in localization studies, approximately 10% of patients still require surgical intervention without having their bleeding source identified.

ANATOMIC CONSIDERATIONS OF LOWER GASTROINTESTINAL BLEEDING (LGIB)

- LGIB is anatomically defined as bleeding located from the ligament of Treitz to the anus, and may include the jejunum, ileum, ileocecal valve, colon (ascending, transverse, descending, sigmoid, rectum), and anus.
- Given the length of lower GI tract (the small bowel averages 6.7 meters), as well as the special anatomic problem for the small bowel, such as its free intraperitoneal location, multiple overlying loops, and active contractility, there are several management issues for LGIB; these include choice of tests

for fecal occult blood, the necessity of nasogastric (NG) tube placement, and the application of endoscopy, radiologic procedures, and ultrasound.

Fecal Occult Blood

- This is the most common form of GI bleeding. In the ICU, patients suspected of having GI blood loss, secondary to findings of persistent anemia, will have a fecal occult blood study as the first investigative step. Although there are numerous types of fecal occult blood tests, the test used determines the location in the GI tract where blood is likely to be detected.

Guaiac-based Tests

- Guaiac-based tests, the classic fecal occult blood study, utilizes hemoglobin's pseudoperoxidase activity. Guaiac turns blue after oxidation by oxidants or peroxidases in the presence of an oxygen donor such as hydrogen peroxide. Because hemoglobin is degraded in the GI tract, guaiac-based tests are more sensitive for detecting bleeding in the lower than upper GI tract.

Immunochemical Fecal Occult Blood Tests

- Immunochemical fecal occult blood tests detect human globin epitopes and are highly sensitive for the detection of stool blood. These tests do not detect upper GI blood because globin molecules are degraded by upper GI tract enzymes.

Heme-porphyrin Test

- The heme-porphyrin test is the most sensitive method of detecting occult blood loss of either the upper or lower GI tract. However, it cannot discriminate between UGIB and LGIB.

Nasogastric Tube Placement

- The necessity of NG tube placement and gastric lavage for acute LGIB to exclude an upper GI source has not been studied prospectively. Routine use of the NG tube to exclude the possibility of an upper GI bleed is controversial and, overall, nasogastric aspiration localizes bleeding accurately only in 66% of attempts. Nonetheless, approximately 2% to 15% of patients presenting with acute severe hematochezia have an upper GI source of bleeding identified on upper GI endoscopy.
  - In the American Society for Gastrointestinal Endoscopy (ASGE) guideline, NG tube placement to rule out an upper GI source of bleeding may be considered if a source is not identified on colonoscopy, particularly if there is a history of upper GI symptoms or anemia.
  - Patients with hemodynamic compromise and hematochezia should have an NG tube placed.
  - The absence of blood in NG aspirate is not sufficient to exclude UGI bleeding—16% of patients with bleeding secondary to a duodenal ulcer have a negative NG tube lavage.

APPROACH TO LOWER GASTROINTESTINAL BLEEDING

Resuscitation

- Approximately 85% of GI bleeding episodes stop spontaneously, whereas the remainder require aggressive resuscitation, diagnostic modalities, and often intense medical and/or surgical management.
- The first management step for a patient presenting with overt LGIB is the ABCs of resuscitation. Resuscitation is imperative to restore euvolemia and prevent complications of blood loss in the cardiac, pulmonary, renal, or neurologic systems.
- Resuscitation takes place in parallel with the initial evaluation of the patient; resuscitation must not be withheld or delayed for diagnostic procedures.
- The patient's respiratory and heart rates, and blood pressure, including orthostatic measurements, should be assessed.
- Attention to the airway is important when the LGIB is caused by an obstructive lesion, which may lead to vomiting with the consequent high risk of aspiration.
- Postural hemodynamic changes, chest pain, palpitations, syncope, pallor, dyspnea, and tachycardia suggest hemodynamic compromise; the severity of bleeding is easy to underestimate due to compensatory mechanisms.
- An **orthostatic decrease** in systolic blood pressure >10 mm Hg or an increase in **heart rate** >10 beats/minute indicates an **acute loss of at least 15%** of blood volume.
- With hemodynamic compromise, two 16-gauge or larger intravenous (IV) catheters should be secured immediately; central venous access can be established in unstable patients.
- Packed red blood cells should be utilized in hemodynamically unstable patients, with the goal of maintaining a hematocrit of approximately 30% in the elderly and in those with heart disease or who are otherwise compromised physiologically and 20% to 25% in younger patients.
- The initial hematocrit may not be the true value, requiring up to **72 hours for equilibration** with the intravascular space.
- The presence of coagulopathy (international normalized ratio [INR] >1.5) or **thrombocytopenia** (<50,000 cells/μL) should be corrected with fresh frozen plasma or platelet transfusions, respectively.
- Oxygen should be administered to keep the SpO_2 between 93% and 95% at a minimum, and vital signs and urine output should be closely monitored. In the elderly or those with a history of cardiac disease, an ECG and cardiac enzyme analysis should be considered.

Determination of Bleeding Site: Noninstrumental

History

- Careful history taking is helpful for determining the level of bleeding from the GI tract and to work out a differential diagnosis of the LGIB.
- Included should be the duration, frequency, and color of the stool; related symptoms of the GI tract such as constipation, fever, or location of pain; medical or surgical history; and history of medications.

- Except for asymptomatic patients with only anemia due to GI bleeding, the *color of the stool* is always queried. Blood that has been in the GI tract for < 5 hours is usually red, whereas blood present for > 20 hours is usually melenic.
- **Massive UGIB** can occasionally masquerade as lower GI bleeding in 10% to 15% of patients presenting with severe hematochezia.
- Upper GI, small bowel bleeding, or slow oozing from the right colon usually produces melena, whereas patients with hematochezia typically have left colonic or rectal lesions.
- If the blood coats the surface of stool, the left colon—especially the rectum and anus—is more likely to be the bleeding source. If the stool is mixed with blood, the source may be in the right colon.
- Blood dripping into the toilet may occur with hemorrhoidal bleeding.
- The duration and frequency of bleeding may help in determining the severity of the problem.
- Related GI tract symptoms may lead to the diagnosis of LGIB. Severe constipation should prompt an investigation for colon cancer or a stercoral ulcer; diarrhea may indicate enterocolitis; and fever or local pain may indicate an inflammation-related bleeding source, such as infectious colitis or inflammatory bowel disease.
- A previous history of colonic polyps, diverticulosis, or colonic tumor should be considered as a possible source of LGIB during the initial evaluation.
- Renal failure is a well-known risk factor for angiodysplasia or arteriovenous malformation (AVM), as is aortic stenosis.
- Note should be made of patients with renal impairment or who are being dialyzed, as these patients may have platelet abnormalities, resulting in a tendency to bleed if a lesion is present.
- Ischemic bowel may be present when severe abdominal pain and bloody stool occur in patients with severe atherosclerotic vascular disease, atrial fibrillation, or hypotension.
- Radiation therapy for prostate or pelvic cancer induces inflammatory changes of the rectum and can produce radiation proctitis, presenting months or even years after the radiation exposure.
- A history of recent colonoscopy with polypectomy indicates postpolypectomy bleeding as the likely source.
- In patients who have undergone aortoiliac reconstructive surgery, the frequency of significant postoperative colonic ischemia ranges between 1% and 7%.
- Medication history is also important. Medications that can damage the GI mucosa or exacerbate bleeding include nonsteroidal anti-inflammatory drugs (NSAIDs), alendronate, potassium chloride, and anticoagulants.
- A family history of colon cancer increases the likelihood of a colorectal neoplasm and generally calls for a complete colonic examination in patients with hematochezia.

Physical Examination

- A thorough physical examination is essential to assess loss of blood volume, a possible bleeding source, and comorbid conditions. The physical examination should also include complete vital signs and heart, lung, and abdominal assessment, as well as an examination of the conjunctiva and skin.
  - Orthostatic vital signs are an important complement to standard monitoring in a patient with severe bleeding but without overt hemodynamic instability.

- Abdominal tenderness on examination may indicate an inflammatory process, such as ischemic colitis or inflammatory bowel disease.
- The rectal examination serves to identify anorectal lesions and confirm the stool color described by the patient. In addition, approximately 40% of rectal carcinomas are palpable during a digital rectal examination.

Laboratory Examination

- Initial laboratory studies should include a complete blood count, serum urea nitrogen, creatinine, coagulation profile (prothrombin time, INR, and partial thromboplastin time), liver tests, blood type and cross-match, and electrolytes.
- The **blood urea nitrogen-to-creatinine ratio** has been used as a noninvasive test to help distinguish UGIB from colonic sources of bleeding; a **ratio of 33 or higher** has a sensitivity of 96% for UGIB.

Determination of the Bleeding Site: Diagnostic Approach

Endoscopic Approach: General

- **Safety of Endoscopic Procedures for Critically Ill Patients.** Colonoscopy remains the procedure of choice for evaluating patients with acute LGIB, and enteroscopy is considered for proximal small bowel bleeding. However, for ICU patients with acquired bleeding and hemodynamic instability, questions remain due to the possibility of severe comorbid illness.
- Colonoscopy complication rates in LGIB of the general population or patients admitted to the ICU primarily for hemorrhage are low and with acceptable diagnostic rate of 67% for ICU patients.
- The complication risk increases in patients with comorbid disease, and in particular, in patients with underlying cardiac disease.
- **Preparation before Endoscopic Procedures.** Good bowel preparation is important for an adequate and sensitive colonoscopy. Studies of urgent colonoscopies performed in an unprepared colon to evaluate for LGIB revealed completion rates as low as 35%.
- In patients with severe diverticular hemorrhage, completion rates may reach up to 100% if aggressive bowel preparation is performed before urgent colonoscopy.
- Bowel preparation regimens may be less effective for LGIB in ICU patients.
- Rapid colon preparation regimens are better suited for those in the ICU or with active LGIB. However, the physician should be aware that hyperosmotic preparations draw plasma water into the bowel lumen to promote evacuation.
- For the critically ill patient with LGIB, there are no data on the "proper timing" of colon preparation. Further, preparation may be incomplete due to poor motility or ileus. Some have suggested that polyethylene glycol electrolyte lavage solution (PEG-ELS) on the day of procedure may be adequate.
- The safety of colon preparation is important for critically ill patients with comorbid illness. PEG-ELS causes no significant change in weight, vital signs, serum electrolytes, or complete blood count and is relatively safe for patients with

electrolyte imbalance, advanced liver disease, poorly compensated congestive heart failure, or renal failure.

- Monobasic and dibasic sodium phosphate (NaP) is a hyperosmotic preparation and may cause alterations in serum electrolytes and extracellular fluid status.

Colonoscopy for Critically Ill Patients

- Advances in endoscopic technology have brought colonoscopy to the forefront of the management of LGIB. However, colonoscopy as the first diagnostic maneuver for brisk LGIB or LGIB with hemodynamic compromise is controversial.
- In hemodynamically unstable patients with ongoing bleeding, angiography in conjunction with surgical consultation may be a more appropriate option.
- Colonoscopy in patients with severe hematochezia is impractical because of inadequate visualization caused by brisk blood loss.
- For acute LGIB colonoscopy can provide a rapid diagnosis and specific therapy if bleeding is found.
- Rapid endoscopic identification of a bleeding source, regardless of whether therapy is administered, may contribute to the clinical management of recurrent bleeding.
- Compared with angiography, urgent colonoscopy has a higher diagnostic yield (80% to 90% vs. 12% to 48%) and a lower complication rate.
- Most patients undergoing radiographic evaluation for LGIB—regardless of findings and interventions—will subsequently require a colonoscopy to establish the cause of bleeding.
- Although most episodes of LGIB will stop spontaneously, 10% to 15% of patients undergoing urgent colonoscopy received endoscopic therapy.
- The lesions most amenable to colonoscopic treatment of LGIB, in most studies, are usually angiodysplasia or diverticulosis.
- In a study of ICU patients with nonprimary LGIB, spontaneous cessation occurred in 53% of patients; 29% achieved hemostasis with endoscopy, but had a higher rate (19%) of recurrent bleeding.

Timing of Colonoscopy

- The use of colonoscopy is controversial for critically ill patients with LGIB. However, evidence suggests that earlier intervention leads to more diagnostic and therapeutic opportunities.
- Urgent colonoscopy after bowel preparation with endoscopic treatment of patients with active diverticular bleeding or stigmata of bleeding has been shown to be highly effective in decreasing the need for surgical intervention.

Sigmoidoscopy or Colonoscopy?

- In studies of the general population with LGIB, diverticular and angiodysplastic bleeding are the most frequent events with bleeding most often occurring in the right colon.
- Flexible sigmoidoscopy can be performed in the initial evaluation of patients with LGIB, but the diagnostic yield of flexible sigmoidoscopy in LGIB is low, ranging from 9% to 58%.
- However, in ICU patients with acquired bleeding, 78% of responsible lesions were in the left colon.
- If the critical situation precludes use of total colonoscopy, sigmoidoscopy as the first maneuver may be acceptable for this patient group.

- If a definite and compatible bleeding source is not identified with flexible sigmoidoscopy, the study should proceed to a full colonoscopy in most patients.

Enteroscopy and Capsule Endoscopy for Critically Ill Patients

- The small bowel is a problematic area to evaluate because of the limitations of standard upper GI endoscopy and colonoscopy. It is estimated that 10% to 25% of LGIB originates in the small bowel.
- Some clinicians have utilized peroral intubation with a standard colonoscope, reaching a point 20- to 60-cm distal to the ligament of Treitz to increase the diagnostic yield of GI bleeding of obscure origin by 17% to 46%.
- Small bowel enteroscopy is currently the best endoscopic investigative modality. Current tools for ruling out small bowel diseases include push-type enteroscopy (PE), double-balloon enteroscopy (DBE), intraoperative enteroscopy, and capsule endoscopy.
- Push-type enteroscopy allows endoscopic evaluation of the proximal 60 cm of the jejunum or 150-cm distal to the pylorus.
- The diagnostic yield of PE is between 38% and 65% of patients in whom upper and lower endoscopy are negative.
- Complications of PE are infrequent, occurring in <1% of cases. Most complications, including bleeding and perforation, are related to the use of an overtube.
- The data on effectiveness and safety of PE for ICU patients are limited.
- Total enteroscopy with DBE can be achieved in 60% to 86% of cases.
- The diagnostic yield of DBE is between 52% and 76%.
- Oral DBE requires no specific preparation other than a 6- to 8-hour fast before the procedure. If a retrograde (anal) approach is undertaken, standard colonic preparation is necessary.
- Complications of DBE are noted in 1.1% to 8.5%, and include aspiration pneumonia, abdominal pain, perforation, and acute pancreatitis.
- The effectiveness and safety of DBE for critically ill patients are unknown.
- Before the advent of capsule endoscopy and DBE, intraoperative endoscopy was the only way to detect and treat lesions beyond the reach of push enteroscopy.
- Diagnostic intraoperative enteroscopy is likely to decrease with introduction of the less invasive capsule endoscopy and DBE; however, it still plays a role in specific clinical situations.
- The yield in detecting bleeding lesions reaches 70% to 100%, making intraoperative endoscopy the most sensitive method of diagnosing small bowel disorders.
- Lesions can be treated endoscopically or marked with a tattoo for surgical resection. The terminal ileum is reached in more than 90% of patients.
- The high sensitivity, however, comes at the cost of extreme invasiveness, making it a procedure of last resort.
- The complication rate is estimated at about 3%, including mucosal tears and bleeding of the mesentery due to traction.
- Capsule endoscopy is a safe and promising diagnostic tool for GI bleeding of unknown origin, focusing especially on the small bowel; it may obviate the need for angiography in some difficult patients.
- Studies comparing capsule endoscopy with other diagnostic procedures, including enteroclysis, PE, computed

tomography (CT) scan, and intraoperative enteroscopy, showed that capsule endoscopy was clearly superior in the diagnosis of occult/obscure/overt small bowel bleeding.

- The overall diagnostic yield rate of capsule endoscopy in patients with GI bleeding ranges from 45% to 66%.
- To increase the diagnostic yield of capsule endoscopy, prokinetic agents, oral bowel preparation (oral sodium phosphate and polyethylene glycol), simethicone, and erythromycin have been recommended.
- Despite the higher diagnostic yield, capsule endoscopy limitations are evident: biopsy specimens cannot be obtained, therapeutic intervention cannot be performed, and localization of some lesions is imprecise.
- The primary risk with capsule endoscopy is capsule entrapment within the GI tract; this occurs in 0.75% to 5% of cases.
- Absolute contraindications to its use include GI obstruction and ileus.
- The use of capsule endoscopy in critically ill patients has been limited and the use of capsule endoscopy for small bowel or obscure bleeding must be made on a case-by-case basis.

Nonendoscopic Approach

Nuclear Medicine

- The two techniques of radionuclide scanning commonly use either ^{99m}Tc-labeled red blood cells or ^{99m}technetium sulfur colloid.
- A ^{99m}Tc-labeled red blood cell scan is the preferred technique, with images that can be detected for up to 12 to 24 hours after injection, whereas the half-life of ^{99m}technetium sulfur colloid is only 2 to 3 minutes.
- This technique can detect bleeding at a rate as low as **0.1 to 0.5 mL/minute** and is thought to be a sensitive diagnostic tool for LGIB.
- The sensitivity of a radionuclide scan for active bleeding has been noted to be >90% and is superior to that of angiography.
- Another role for radionuclide scanning is in the evaluation for Meckel diverticulum, especially in young patients presenting with LGIB with a sensitivity as high as 81% to 90%.
- **Timing the Use of Radionuclide Scanning.** Radionuclide scanning, often performed repeatedly during a hospital course, may be used as the screening test, followed by angiography, small bowel enteroscopy, or surgery to definitively localize and treat the bleeding lesion.
  - Because of its high sensitivity, radionuclide scanning has been utilized as a guide for surgical resection. However, radionuclide scanning is normally not used as a definitive study before surgical therapy.
  - The literature suggests that the localization **accuracy** of radionuclide scanning is quite variable, ranging from **24% to 94%**. Thus, most clinicians use radionuclide scanning as a guide for further diagnostic studies, such as enteroscopy or colonoscopy, rather than for surgical intervention.

Angiography

- Mesenteric angiography is more invasive than technetium-labeled red blood cell scanning, and requires a bleeding rate of at least **0.5 to 1.0 mL/minute** to detect bleeding.
- Angiography is usually undertaken when patients have clinical indicators of severe bleeding (e.g., tachycardia and/or syncope).

- Although colonoscopy is the diagnostic modality of first choice for LGIB, many endoscopists are reluctant to perform colonoscopy in hemodynamically unstable patients with ongoing bleeding and these patients usually undergo radiographic studies.
- Angiography will localize the site of bleeding in 40% to 86% of patients with LGIB.
- Occasionally, the bleeding of colonic lesions, such as vascular abnormalities, can be too massive for colonoscopic visualization, thus precluding the procedure.
- In some centers, a radionuclide scan is requested before mesenteric angiography, because a negative radionuclide scan is unlikely to have a positive angiogram.
- Even if a bleeding site is identified on angiography, localizing the site intraoperatively can be difficult; angiography has a specificity of 100% but a sensitivity of only 30% to 47%.
- Complications include hematoma or bleeding at the catheter site; access site thrombosis; contrast reactions; injury to the target vessels, including dissection and distal embolization; and renal failure. The injured vessels usually involve the SMA, IMA, and celiac artery.
- Angiography also offers therapeutic possibilities via pharmacologic vasoconstriction or selective embolization (transcatheter arterial embolization [TAE]).
- Pharmacologic vasoconstriction is achieved with intra-arterial vasopressin infusion.
- TAE may be a more definitive means of controlling bleeding, but is associated with a risk of **intestinal infarction.** The bowel infarction or colonic necrosis rate from embolization ranges from 10% to 20%.
- Selective embolization initially controls bleeding in up to 100% of patients, but rebleeding rates have been reported to be 15% to 40%.
- Superselective TAE may decrease the incidence of ischemia and rebleeding beyond that of selective embolization. With advances in superselective embolization techniques, clinically significant bowel ischemia has become an uncommon complication.
- The major complication rate was 10% to 20% and included dysrhythmias, pulmonary edema, hypertension, and ischemia.
- Although the efficacies of vasopressin and embolization are reasonably comparable, embolization allows more rapid completion of therapy and a decreased likelihood of systemic complications.
- Embolization should be considered a primary option for LGIB with vasopressin reserved for diffuse lesions or cases in which superselective catheterization is not technically possible.
- **Vasopressin** should not be used in patients with significant coronary artery disease or peripheral vascular disease; mesenteric thrombosis, intestinal infarction, and death have been reported with its use.
- Nitroglycerin reverses the vasopressin-induced coronary vasoconstriction without affecting the therapeutic vasoconstriction of the mesenteric artery.

Computed Tomography Scan and Magnetic Resonance Imaging

- CT scans are not usually considered diagnostic tools for LGIB, except in the context of bleeding bowel tumors. Additionally, there is no current role for the use of magnetic resonance imaging (MRI) in the evaluation of LGIB.

- In the evaluation of colonic vascular lesions, helical CT has a sensitivity of 70% and specificity of 100% compared to colonoscopy and conventional angiography.

Other Modalities

- Data regarding the use of ultrasound for LGIB have been limited. Ultrasound may be considered as a screening tool for LGIB or applied when the bleeding source cannot be identified by other modalities
- Small bowel follow through (SBFT) is of little use in evaluating obscure GI bleeding, with a diagnostic yield that may be as low as 0%.
- Enteroclysis is superior to SBFT for evaluation of the small bowel. However, with the advent of capsule endoscopy, the use of SBFT or enteroclysis for GI bleeding has declined.
- Barium enema cannot detect superficial lesions or confirm a definitive bleeding source of the colon. Furthermore, it may complicate subsequent colonoscopy or angiography and is less useful for critically ill patients with LGIB.

TREATMENT OF LOWER GASTROINTESTINAL BLEEDING

Pharmacologic Therapy

- Unlike pharmacologic therapies for UGIB, there are no medications with a strong evidence base for LGIB.
- The medications for the different causes of LGIB include estrogen/progesterone compounds, octreotide, aminocaproic acid (an antifibrinolytic), and tranexamic acid.
- Estrogen/progesterone compound use is controversial for diffuse ectasias or angiodysplasia refractory to endoscopic therapy and has been noted to be ineffective in recent studies.
- Octreotide at a dose of 0.05 to 1 mg/day may lead to decreased transfusion requirements, but, unfortunately, carefully controlled trials are not available.
- Aminocaproic acid and tranexamic acid may be helpful, but studies with controlled data are not forthcoming.

Endoscopic Procedures

- Endoscopic therapy for LGIB includes injection therapy (epinephrine, saline, or ethanol), heater probe, monopolar

TABLE 106.4

ENDOSCOPIC PROCEDURES FOR BLEEDING

LGIB lesions	Endoscopic procedures
Ulcer	Injection therapy Heater probe Electrocoagulation Hemoclips Band ligation[a] APC[b]
Angiodysplasia	APC Heater probe Electrocoagulation
Diverticulum	Hemoclips APC Injection therapy Heater probe Electrocoagulation
Radiation proctitis	APC Topical formalin
Postpolypectomy bleeding	Hemoclips Band ligation APC Injection therapy Heater probe

LGIB, lower gastrointestinal bleeding.
[a]Especially for Dieulafoy lesions.
[b]APC, argon plasma coagulation. Not recommended for ulcers with big exposed vessels.

and multipolar electrocoagulation, argon plasma coagulation, hemoclips, and band ligation (Table 106.4).
- An alternative treatment for hemorrhagic radiation-induced proctitis, by topical application of formalin, can be performed with or without endoscopy in the operating room.

Radiologic Interventions (See Also Angiography)

- In addition to its diagnostic role, angiography offers therapeutic possibilities via pharmacologic vasoconstriction with vasopressin or selective embolization.
- Comparison between embolization and intra-arterial vasopressin infusion is listed in Table 106.5.

TABLE 106.5

COMPARISON BETWEEN TAE AND INTRA-ARTERIAL VASOPRESSIN INFUSION FOR LGIB

	TAE	Vasopressin infusion
Completion of Tx	Quick	Slow
Definite Tx	Yes	No
Diffuse lesions	Discouraged	Favored
Complications	Bowel infarct	Myocardial ischemia, bowel ischemia, peripheral ischemia, hypertension, arrhythmias, hyponatremia

TAE, transcatheter arterial embolization; LGIB, lower gastrointestinal bleeding; Tx, therapy.

Surgery

- Surgery should be considered in patients in whom a bleeding source has clearly been identified. An emergency procedure is suggested for patients who require more than six units of blood within 24 hours, or a total of 10 units.
- Blind segmental resection is contraindicated, as it is associated with a rebleeding rate of 42% and excessive rates of morbidity and mortality as high as 83% and 57%, respectively.
- If the bleeder cannot be clearly identified, intraoperative enteroscopy may be a management option.
- Recurrent bleeding from colon diverticula occurs in 20% to 40% of patients and is generally considered an indication for surgery.
- Surgery is usually not recommended on the basis of nuclear red blood cell scans alone because of variable accuracy of nuclear red blood cell scans.

LOWER GASTROINTESTINAL BLEEDING AND ACUTE MYOCARDIAL INFARCTION

- Whether LGIB occurs before or after the AMI, selecting an endoscopic procedure is a dilemma.
- The risks versus benefits of endoscopy must be carefully considered in patients with a recent MI because of the potential for cardiopulmonary complications, including myocardial ischemia, hypotension, cardiac arrhythmias, and hypoxia.
- Underlying heart disease, lower blood pressure on arrival in the emergency department, lower hemoglobin level on arrival, and persistent shock before endoscopic examination are all associated with higher risk of MI after emergency endoscopy.
- Establishment of stable hemodynamics and oxygen delivery before emergency endoscopy may reduce the risk of procedure-related MI, especially in patients with known heart disease.
- Colonoscopy in patients with a recent MI is associated with a higher rate of minor, transient cardiovascular complications compared with control patients but is relatively infrequently associated with major complications.
- Colonoscopy may be beneficial after an MI, despite a higher risk in certain circumstances.

Acute Hemorrhagic Rectal Ulcer Syndrome

- Acute hemorrhagic rectal ulcer syndrome (AHRUS) has been reported as one of the most frequent causes of LGIB in the ICU.
- Lesions of AHRUS locate at the lower rectum and account for 26.7% of massive LGIB in the ICU.
- AHRUS characteristically occurs suddenly, with painless, massive, fresh rectal bleeding in elderly, bedridden patients with severe comorbid illness. It is prone to occur in patients with diabetes mellitus who are using anticoagulant or antiplatelet agents.
- Therapies for AHRUS include injection therapy, heater probe, hemoclips, and per anal suturing.
- The prognosis of AHRUS depends on the state of the underlying diseases and achievement of hemostasis.

CHAPTER 107 ■ LIVER FAILURE: ACUTE AND CHRONIC

ACUTE LIVER FAILURE

Definitions and Immediate Concerns

- Acute liver failure (ALF) may be defined as the development of hepatic encephalopathy (HE) and coagulopathy in a patient with no history of previous liver disease, with the onset HE within 26 weeks of jaundice. It should be stressed that ALF is not a disease, but rather a clinical syndrome triggered by numerous etiologic agents.

Overview

- There are three possible outcomes after ALF: spontaneous survival without orthotopic liver transplantation (OLT), OLT, or death.

- In the U.S. Acute Liver Failure Study Group (ALFSG) cohort, one-third of patients died, one-quarter underwent OLT, and the remainder (42%) recovered spontaneously.
- The dismal overall survival of patients with ALF, 25% in the 1970s, has improved to ~65% with the advent of OLT and improvements in intensive care management.

Etiology, Prevalence, and Initial Testing

- In the United States, **acetaminophen** (APAP) accounts for ~45% of cases, half of those due to ingestion of a single large dose with suicidal intent and the other half as "therapeutic misadventures."
- The second most common cause of ALF remains indeterminate even after extensive serologic and historical evaluation (15% of cases).

TABLE 107.1

CAUSE, PREVALENCE, AND EVALUATION OF ACUTE LIVER FAILURE

Cause	Prevalence[a] (%)	Evaluation
APAP	45	History; APAP level
HBV	7	anti-HBc (IgM and total), HBsAg, anti-HBs, HBV DNA, anti-HDV
AIH	5	ANA, ASMA, anti-LKM, immunoglobulins
HAV	4	anti-HAV (IgM and total)
Shock liver	4	Echocardiogram, brain natriuretic peptide
Wilson disease	3	Serum ceruloplasmin and copper; urine copper; slit-lamp eye examination
BCS	2	Doppler ultrasound of liver
Malignancy	1	Contrast-enhanced CT; MRI (preferred)
AFLP/HELLP	1	Pregnancy test
HSV	0.5	Anti-HSV 1/2, HSV DNA
Other	4	Anti-HCV/HCV RNA, anti-CMV/CMV DNA, anti-EBV/EBV DNA, toxicology screen
Indeterminate	14	All of above negative
Idiosyncratic drug	13	History; all of above negative

APAP, acetaminophen; HBV, hepatitis B virus; HDV, hepatitis D virus; AIH, autoimmune hepatitis; ANA, anti-nuclear antibody; ASMA, anti-smooth muscle antibody; anti-LKM, anti-liver kidney microsomal antibody; HAV, hepatitis A virus; BCS, Budd-Chiari syndrome; CT, computed tomography; MRI, magnetic resonance imaging; AFLP/HELLP, acute fatty liver of pregnancy/hemolysis-elevated liver enzymes–low platelet syndrome; HSV, herpes simplex virus; HCV, hepatitis C virus; CMV, cytomegalovirus; EBV, Epstein-Barr virus.
N = approximately 1,000 at the time of publication. (W.M. Lee, personal communication.)
Suggested evaluation of patients with idiosyncratic drug hepatotoxicity and indeterminate ALF should include all of the tests listed, since these are diagnoses of exclusion.
[a]Prevalence of causes are estimates based on the U.S. Acute Liver Failure Study Group Cohort (personal communication).

- Additional causes of ALF are idiosyncratic drug reactions (13%) and acute hepatitis B (7%).
- The remaining causes of ALF are autoimmune hepatitis, acute hepatitis A, hepatic vein thrombosis (Budd-Chiari syndrome), hypotension ("shock liver"), fulminant Wilson disease, malignant infiltration of the liver, and pregnancy-associated ALF (acute fatty liver and HELLP [hemolysis, elevated liver enzymes, and low platelets] syndrome), all constituting fewer than 5% of cases each.
- The initial laboratory and procedural evaluation of patients with ALF to determine cause is indicated in Table 107.1.

Assessment of Prognosis

Outcomes of ALF

- The **cause** of ALF is the single most important prognostic factor.
- The second prognostic factor is the **interval between jaundice and the development of HE;** the shorter the above interval, the higher the likelihood of spontaneous survival.
- In patients with APAP overdose, spontaneous recovery is the rule (63% in the ALFSG cohort).
- Patients with acute hepatitis A, shock liver, and pregnancy-related ALF—assuming prompt delivery of the fetus—also have >50% spontaneous survival. Patients with ALF from all other causes have very poor rates of recovery without OLT.
- Patients with APAP overdose and acute hepatitis A usually have hyperacute progression (jaundice-HE interval within 7 days) and have a relatively good prognosis, whereas most idiosyncratic drug reactions have a more subacute presentation (jaundice-HE interval of more than 28 days) and dismal prognosis without OLT.

Prognostication Schemes

- The most time-honored scheme is the King's College Criteria.
- For patients with APAP-induced ALF, predictors of death included arterial pH <7.30, or azotemia, severe coagulopathy, and high-grade HE (grade 3 or 4).
- In patients with ALF due to other causes, severe coagulopathy or any three of the criteria listed in Table 107.2 also predicted death.

Complications and Treatment

General Management

- ALF commonly causes multiorgan dysfunction, such that management requires close collaboration between intensivists, hepatologists, transplant surgeons, and other specialists.
- Since the progression of complications can be rapid, patients should be transferred to a liver transplant center; in general, higher-volume centers have superior outcomes.
- Sedation should initially be minimized to avoid confusing the effects of drugs with deteriorating mental status.
- Worsening HE is a clear indication for admission to the intensive care unit (ICU); the likelihood of spontaneous survival decreases with a worsening coma grade at admission.

Cause-specific Management

Treatment of Acetaminophen ALF
- The administration of N-acetylcysteine (NAC) has become widely applied to patients with ALF due to APAP.
- Although nomograms to determine whether NAC should be administered are available, the time of ingestion frequently cannot be determined accurately, and ingestions are multiple.
- NAC should be given in cases where the timing, dose ingested, or plasma concentration is in question as the potential benefit outweighs the adverse effects.

TABLE 107.2

SCHEMES FOR PREDICTING POOR PROGNOSIS AND THE NEED FOR ORTHOTOPIC LIVER TRANSPLANTATION IN PATIENTS WITH ACUTE LIVER FAILURE (ALF)

Scheme	Cause of ALF	Criteria for liver transplantation
King's College criteria	APAP	Arterial pH <7.30 *Or* all of the following: 1. PT >100 s 2. Creatinine >3.4 mg/dL 3. Grade 3/4 encephalopathy
	Non-APAP	PT >100 s (INR >6.5) *Or* any 3 of the following: 1. NANB/drug/halothane etiology, 2. Jaundice to encephalopathy >7 d 3. Age <10 or >40 y 4. PT >50 s 5. Bilirubin >17.4 mg/dL
Factor V	Viral	Age <30 y: factor V <20% *Or* Any age: Factor V <30% and grade 3/4 encephalopathy
Factor VIII/V ratio	APAP	Factor VIII/V ratio >30
Liver biopsy	Mixed	Hepatocyte necrosis >70%
Arterial phosphate	APAP	>1.2 mmol/L
Arterial lactate	APAP	>3.5 mmol/L
Arterial ammonia	Mixed	>150–200 μmol/L
APACHE II/III score	APAP	>15
MELD score	Non-APAP	>30

Abbreviations per legend of Table 107.1, as well as: PT, prothrombin time; INR, international normalized ratio; NANB, non-A, non-B viral hepatitis; APACHE, Acute Physiology and Chronic Health Evaluation; MELD, model for end-stage liver disease.
Modified from Sanyal AJ, Stravitz RT. Acute liver failure. In: Boyer TD, Wright T, Manns MP, eds. *Hepatology—A Textbook of Liver Disease.* 5th ed. Philadelphia, PA: Elsevier; 2006:383–415; and Stravitz RT, Kramer AH, Davern T, et al., and the Adult Acute Liver Failure Study Group. Management of acute liver failure: recommendations of the Acute Liver Failure Study Group. *Crit Care Med.* 2007;35:2498–2508.

- Intravenous NAC should be administered when a patient has higher than grade 1 HE or in patients who cannot tolerate oral dosing.
- The administration of NAC, even late after ingestion, appears to confer survival benefit. Thus, dosing should continue until evidence of severe liver injury resolves (international normalized ratio [INR] <1.5 and resolution of HE), rather than by completion of a set number of doses.

Other Cause-specific Treatments

- Specific medications that should be considered in patients with ALF due to other causes are outlined in Table 107.3.
- It should be emphasized that randomized, controlled studies to support these therapies do not exist, and most of these recommendations are made only on the basis of case reports, expert opinion, and a high therapeutic threshold.

Management of Specific Complications of ALF

Neurologic Complications: Pathophysiology

- By definition, patients with ALF develop varying degrees of HE (Table 107.4).

- Worsening mental status may be a consequence of progression to cerebral edema, which is present in 38% to 81% of cases of grade 3 or 4 encephalopathy.
- Patients who develop cerebral herniation have substantially higher serum ammonia levels—usually more than 200 μmol/L—and greater cerebral ammonia uptake. Conversely, herniation rarely occurs when serum ammonia levels remain below 150 μmol/L.
- Ammonia also interferes with cerebral energy metabolism, leading to the accumulation of lactate.
- Increased cerebral blood flow (CBF) remains an important factor in the formation of cerebral edema.
- CBF rises with the accumulation of ammonia and is frequently excessive relative to energy expenditure.
- Although excessive CBF contributes to worsening cerebral edema, patients are also especially vulnerable to ischemia if hypotension occurs. Thus, it is important that cerebral perfusion pressure be carefully controlled and extremes avoided.

Management of HE

- Therapies are aimed at lowering serum ammonia levels in patients with ALF due to the central role of ammonia in the pathogenesis of hepatic encephalopathy.

TABLE 107.3

CAUSE-SPECIFIC THERAPY OF PATIENTS WITH ACUTE LIVER FAILURE

Cause	Therapy
APAP	NAC Oral: 140 mg/kg load, then 70 mg/kg every 4 h
	NAC IV: 150 mg/kg load, then 12.5 mg/kg/h × 4 hr, then 6.25 mg/kg/h
Amanita	Penicillin G: 1 g/kg/d IV & NAC (as in APAP overdose)
HSV	Acyclovir: 30 mg/kg/d IV
AIH	Methylprednisolone 60 mg/d IV
HBV	Lamivudine 100–150 mg/d PO
Wilson disease	? Plasmapheresis, D-penicillamine
AFLP/HELLP	Delivery of fetus

APAP, acetaminophen; NAC, *N*-acetylcysteine; *Amanita* refers to mushroom intoxication; HSV, herpes simplex virus; AIH, autoimmune hepatitis; HBV, hepatitis B virus; AFLP/HELLP, acute fatty liver of pregnancy/hemolysis-elevated liver enzymes–low platelet syndrome.

- Nonabsorbable disaccharides (e.g., lactulose) and oral antibiotics (neomycin, rifaximin, or metronidazole) have not been adequately studied in patients with ALF and appear to have little effect on outcome.
- If lactulose is administered, the dose should be adjusted to achieve no more than three to four bowel movements per day, and care must be taken to avoid excessive abdominal distention, volume depletion, and hypernatremia.
- Oral neomycin is minimally absorbed from the gastrointestinal tract but has been reported to cause acute renal failure and is therefore not recommended.
- A computed tomography (CT) scan of the head should be considered early in the course of ALF to exclude other causes of altered mental status.

Management of Cerebral Edema
- A head CT may be used to detect cerebral edema. However, a normal scan does not rule out clinically important intracranial hypertension.

- Many experts advocate intracranial pressure (ICP) monitor placement in OLT candidates with stage III or IV HE.
- The coagulopathy in patients with ALF increases the bleeding risk of ICP monitor placement, with bleeding complications in up to 20%. Recent series have found lower bleeding rates with the use of recombinant factor VIIa (rFVIIa) shortly before insertion of the device.
- The specific management of cerebral edema in patients with ALF resembles that of other causes of intracranial hypertension, with the important caveat that hyperemia plays an important additional pathogenic role in the former.
- Patients should be cared for in a calm, quiet environment, with limited stimulation. Chest physiotherapy and suctioning should be temporarily minimized.
- The head of the bed should be elevated to at least 30 degrees, as this reduces ICP and decreases the risk of hospital-acquired pneumonia. Additionally, the duration of time that a patient is placed supine or in Trendelenburg position for procedures should be minimized.

TABLE 107.4

HEPATIC ENCEPHALOPATHY GRADES AND RELATIONSHIP TO CEREBRAL EDEMA AND PROGNOSIS IN ACUTE LIVER FAILURE

Stage	Mental status	Cerebral edema	Spontaneous recovery without liver transplantation
I	Euphoria, mild confusion, dysarthria, abnormal sleep rhythm	Rare	52% overall
			87% APAP
			35% drug reaction
II	Accentuation of stage I, lethargy, moderate confusion, incontinence		18% indeterminate cause
			38% other cause
III	Stupor, severe confusion, incoherent speech	40%–80%	33% overall
			50% APAP
IV	Coma or near coma		12% drug reaction
			16% indeterminate cause
			27% other cause

APAP, acetaminophen.
Data modified from Trey C, Davidson C. The management of fulminant hepatic failure. *Prog Liver Dis.* 1970;3:282–298; Gazzard BG, Portmann B, Murray-Lyon IM, et al. Causes of death in fulminant hepatic failure and relationship to quantitative histologic assessment of parenchymal damage. *Q J Med.* 1975;44(176):615–626; and Ostapowicz G, Fontana RJ, Schiodt FV, et al. Results of a prospective study of acute liver failure at 17 tertiary care centers in the United States. *Ann Intern Med.* 2002;137(12):947–954.

- Endotracheal intubation and mechanical ventilation must be implemented in a timely fashion to avoid the potentially injurious effects of hypoxemia and hypercapnia, while also reducing aspiration risk and facilitating management of intracranial hypertension.
- Propofol is preferred over benzodiazepines by some. However, if used over several days, the dose of propofol should be limited to <5 mg/kg/hour to decrease the risk of the potentially fatal propofol infusion syndrome.
- Hyperventilation can be used therapeutically to reduce ICP. Patients with hepatic encephalopathy often spontaneously hyperventilate, with resultant respiratory alkalosis.
- The major concern with using hyperventilation as a means to lower ICP is that vasoconstriction may be severe enough to cause cerebral ischemia.
- If the $PaCO_2$ suddenly normalizes, rebound vasodilatation may occur with consequent elevation in ICP. Thus, sudden changes in $PaCO_2$ should be avoided and arterial blood gases or end-tidal CO_2 should be closely monitored.
- Jugular venous oximetry may be useful to guide therapy, with a high jugular venous oxygen saturation used as evidence that hyperventilation is safe.
- Osmotic agents, including mannitol and hypertonic saline (HTS), lower ICP most effectively in the setting of global cerebral edema with an intact blood–brain barrier.
- A general indication for the administration of mannitol includes persistently (>10 minutes) elevated ICP (>20 mm Hg) after ensuring proper calibration of the ICP monitor.
- A serum osmolality limit of 320 mOsm/L is arbitrary. A more useful surrogate is the osmolar gap, which more reliably predicts the risk of renal failure and should be allowed to normalize (e.g., <15–20) between doses.
- Theoretical advantages of HTS over mannitol include the following: (1) the blood–brain barrier is less permeable to HTS (making it a more effective osmotic agent); (2) it is a volume expander rather than a diuretic; and (3) there is no proven nephrotoxicity.
- Great caution must be taken when HTS is weaned or discontinued to ensure that the serum sodium falls very slowly to avoid precipitating rebound cerebral edema.
- High-dose barbiturates (pentobarbital [3–5 mg/kg intravenous [IV] loading bolus followed by 1–3 mg/kg/hour IV infusion], or thiopental [5–10 mg/kg loading bolus followed by 3–5 mg/kg/hour]) can be used as rescue therapy when other interventions have been maximized but the ICP remains more than 20 mm Hg.
- Electroencephalography (EEG) should be performed to guide dosing, with the goal being to achieve a burst-suppression pattern.
- Corticosteroids are of no value in treating intracranial hypertension in ALF and should not be used for this purpose.
- Fever increases ICP and is an independent predictor of worse outcome in brain-injured patients, such that euthermia should be maintained.
- Temperatures of 32°C to 33°C have been used to control intracranial hypertension in patients with ALF refractory to standard care. Important potential adverse effects of hypothermia in the setting of ALF include interference with coagulation and an increased risk of infection.

Management of Seizures

- Nonconvulsive seizures are a potential cause of worsening cerebral edema and secondary brain injury.

- In general, routinely obtaining an EEG in patients with hepatic encephalopathy, particularly when there is a clinical change in neurologic status, may be useful.
- There is currently insufficient evidence to justify the routine use of prophylactic phenytoin. Sedation with propofol or benzodiazepines is likely to provide more effective antiseizure prophylaxis than phenytoin.

Cardiopulmonary Complications

- Patients with ALF frequently develop **systemic inflammatory response syndrome** (SIRS), regardless of whether or not their course is complicated by infection.
- Hypotension is typical of patients with ALF and can be ascribed to low systemic vascular resistance, the use of sedatives, mechanical ventilation, and relative adrenal insufficiency.
- Lactic acidosis is an important prognostic marker in ALF, but the mechanism is not primarily dysoxia, but rather impaired hepatic clearance and increased splanchnic production.
- Most patients with severe ALF will require an arterial catheter, and various tools are available to optimize volume status and cardiac output.
- The goal mean arterial pressure (MAP) should be individualized to optimize organ perfusion, rather than choosing an arbitrary number, but is generally kept above 60 to 65 mm Hg.
- In patients with relative adrenal insufficiency, treatment with low-dose corticosteroids (e.g., hydrocortisone 50–100 mg IV every 6–8 hours, or 8–10 mg/hour as a continuous IV infusion) reduces vasopressor requirements, although the impact on outcome is uncertain.
- As many as 37% of patients with ALF develop **acute lung injury** (ALI) or acute respiratory distress syndrome (ARDS).
- With established ALI or ARDS, tidal volumes should be limited to 6 mL/kg of predicted body weight, although increases in $PaCO_2$ cannot be tolerated in the setting of cerebral edema and intracranial hypertension.
- Positive end-expiratory pressure settings should be sufficient to achieve adequate oxygenation, while concomitantly ensuring that ICP, blood pressure, and cardiac output are not compromised.

Renal Failure

- Acute renal failure complicates **up to 50%** of cases of ALF and is even more frequent when the cause of ALF is acetaminophen intoxication.
- Hypovolemia, hypotension, and the use of nephrotoxins—including aminoglycosides, nonsteroidal anti-inflammatory drugs, and intravenous contrast—should be minimized.
- Patients with ALF can develop hepatorenal syndrome (HRS) as a consequence of intense renal vasoconstriction.
- The decision to initiate renal replacement therapy (RRT) must consider the magnitude of renal dysfunction, metabolic derangements, and volume overload.
- Continuous renal replacement therapy (CRRT) is preferred over intermittent hemodialysis (IHD) by many clinicians, largely because of more stable volume management and greater time-averaged dialysis dose.
- Transient hypotension is poorly tolerated in patients with cerebral edema; not only does the cerebral perfusion pressure decrease, but cerebral vasodilatation may increase, with further increases in CBF and ICP.

- Excessively rapid correction of metabolic acidosis with bicarbonate-based dialysate may transiently increase cerebrospinal fluid CO_2, reduce central nervous system (CNS) pH, and promote more cerebral vasodilatation.
- Regardless of the mode of RRT, an adequate hemofiltration or dialysis dose should be used, while blood pressure—and preferably ICP—are carefully monitored and maintained.
- With CRRT, regional, rather than systemic, anticoagulation is most often used to improve filter longevity, most often with citrate. Since citrate accumulates with poor hepatic function, ionized calcium levels must be regularly monitored.

Infections

- ALF patients are at high risk of nosocomial infections with both bacterial and fungal pathogens, which occur in almost 40% of these patients.
- Early diagnosis can be difficult since patients often have subtle manifestations of infection but is vital because of the high associated morbidity and mortality.
- Daily surveillance cultures (urine, blood, sputum) and chest radiography should be considered, as they may improve early diagnosis of infection and guide selection of antimicrobial agents.
- Prophylactic antibiotics have not been shown to improve survival and may promote infection with resistant pathogens.
- Empiric broad-spectrum antibiotics (including vancomycin and an antifungal agent, as indicated) should be administered to any patient with ALF who develops significant isolates on surveillance cultures, unexplained progression of HE, or signs of SIRS, as these frequently predict sepsis in patients with ALF.

Coagulopathy

- Despite a deficiency of clotting factors, low fibrinogen, thrombocytopenia, and platelet dysfunction, clinically important spontaneous bleeding is seen in <10% of patients.
- The routine use of blood products to correct these abnormalities is not justified since they are unnecessary, ineffective, and interfere with the prognostic utility of the INR.
- Correction of coagulopathy should be performed in the setting of significant hemorrhage or in anticipation of invasive procedures.
- Vitamin K deficiency has been reported to contribute to the coagulopathy of ALF and should be repleted parenterally (10 mg subcutaneously [SC] or slow [over 30 minutes] IV).
- rFVIIa (40 μg/kg) may be considered in patients with life-threatening bleeding and prior to placement of an ICP monitor or performance of a liver biopsy. However, the risk of thrombosis with rFVIIa is increasingly being documented, even among patients with ALF.
- If fibrinogen levels are low (<100 mg/dL), cryoprecipitate should be given prior to rFVIIa.
- Coagulopathy and mechanical ventilation are well-established indications for gastrointestinal (GI) stress ulcer prophylaxis.
- Mechanical methods of deep venous thrombosis prophylaxis are recommended in place of low-dose unfractionated heparin or low-molecular-weight heparin.

Metabolic Derangements

- ALF is a catabolic state, with increased energy requirements and negative nitrogen balance, which may in turn contribute to immunosuppression.

- Higher-than-usual caloric intake is recommended, with 35 to 40 kcal/kg/day and 0.8 to 1 g/kg/day of protein, preferably provided via the enteral route.
- Reduced hepatic glycogen stores and impaired gluconeogenesis are responsible for the frequent development of hypoglycemia.
- Conversely, hyperglycemia may contribute to increases in ICP and other complications. Thus, blood glucose values must be closely monitored and maintained within the normal range with intravenous short-acting insulin.

Liver Transplantation for ALF

- OLT remains the treatment of last resort for ALF. The decision to list a patient with ALF for OLT requires careful clinical and psychosocial assessment.
- Since OLT candidates with ALF are generally younger and healthier than their counterparts with chronic liver disease, the pretransplant evaluation can usually be abbreviated to include echocardiography, duplex ultrasonography of the liver, and routine pretransplant laboratories (e.g., total anti-cytomegalovirus, human immunodeficiency virus antibody).
- Criteria for listing a patient with ALF for OLT change and current criteria may be found on the United Network for Organ Sharing website (in Policy 3.6). Presently, patients with ALF are given priority to receive a cadaveric organ over all patients with chronic liver disease (status 1).
- Early (3-month) mortality after OLT for ALF is higher than for patients transplanted for all causes of chronic liver disease—about 20% versus 10%, respectively. Thereafter, however, 5- and 10-year survival after OLT for ALF approximates 70% and 65%, respectively.

CHRONIC LIVER FAILURE

Definitions and Immediate Concerns

- Almost all patients with chronic liver failure have underlying cirrhosis, the fibroinflammatory alteration of hepatic architecture that results from numerous chronic insults to the liver. Immediate concerns regarding every patient with chronic liver failure on presentation to the ICU include assessment for possible infection and upper GI bleeding, which precipitate most admissions.

Overview

- Patients with chronic liver disease develop liver failure (decompensation) as a result of portal hypertension and hepatocellular insufficiency.
- Complications of portal hypertension include hemodynamic alterations, functional renal failure, ascites, and GI bleeding, most commonly from variceal hemorrhage.
- Complications of hepatocellular insufficiency include coagulopathy and hepatic encephalopathy, with the latter occurring also as a result of portosystemic shunting.
- ICU use is increasing for patients admitted to the hospital for decompensated cirrhosis (from 18% to 28% of hospitalizations in one major center over 10 years).

Etiology

- The most common cause of end-stage liver disease in the United States is **chronic hepatitis C**, with or without a contribution from alcohol abuse (about 40% of cases).
- Patients with alcoholic cirrhosis and indeterminate (**cryptogenic**) causes occupy the second and third most frequent causes, respectively.
- Other less common causes include chronic hepatitis B, immune-mediated liver diseases (autoimmune hepatitis, primary biliary cirrhosis, primary sclerosing cholangitis), and hereditary liver diseases (hemochromatosis, alpha-1-antitrypsin deficiency).

Assessment of Prognosis in Cirrhotic Patients Admitted to the ICU

- Several prognostic schemes have been assessed (Table 107.5), and those using general organ system assessments, such as the Sequential Organ Failure Assessment (SOFA) score, appear to be more accurate than liver-specific schemes.
- The number of organ systems (cardiovascular, respiratory, hepatic, renal, coagulation, and neurologic) failing 24 hours after ICU admission strongly predicts in-hospital mortality, from 33% in patients with single organ failure to 97% in those with failure of three or more organs.
- In the absence of OLT as a therapeutic option, cirrhotic patients admitted to the ICU have a very poor long-term prognosis, with 69% 1-year mortality and median survival of only 1 month.

Management of Complications of Chronic Liver Failure in the ICU

Evaluation of Abdominal Pain

- The development of abdominal pain in a patient with end-stage liver disease often denotes a life-threatening complication of cirrhosis or portal hypertension (Table 107.6).

- A diagnostic **paracentesis** should be performed immediately in any patient with ascites and abdominal pain to diagnose spontaneous bacterial peritonitis (SBP) or to look for evidence of GI tract perforation into ascites.
- The latter may be distinguished from SBP by its higher total protein and lactate dehydrogenase concentration, the isolation of more than one organism (including anaerobes and *Candida*), lower glucose, and higher white blood cell (WBC) and polymorphonuclear (PMN) leucocyte counts.
- **Hemoperitoneum** from spontaneous rupture of a mesenteric varix or hepatocellular carcinoma may be rapidly detected by diagnostic paracentesis, in which case the patient should be referred for emergent interventional angiography.
- The diagnosis and treatment of intra-abdominal catastrophes in patients with cirrhosis remains challenging. Specifically, complicated gallstone and peptic ulcer disease may present less acutely in patients with cirrhosis, delaying diagnosis; in those requiring surgical intervention, morbidity and mortality remain very high.
- **Acute portal vein thrombosis,** which may complicate cirrhosis and often denotes development of hepatocellular carcinoma (HCC), should be suspected in patients with abdominal pain, GI bleeding, and ileus, and should prompt screening with Doppler ultrasound.
- If the thrombus propagates acutely into the superior mesenteric vein, bowel ischemia and infarction, and death, usually ensue.

Cardiovascular Complications

- The resting hemodynamic state in decompensated cirrhosis consists of systemic hypotension due to systemic and splanchnic arterial dilation. Consequently, patients with decompensated cirrhosis have marked arterial underfilling of systemic vascular beds in the renal arterial and hypothalamic circulations, resulting in the elaboration of compensatory neurohumoral hormones such as renin, vasopressin, and norepinephrine.
- The primary pathogenic mechanism underlying this hyperdynamic state includes release of vasodilatory mediators such as **endothelins** and **nitric oxide** by the portal endothelium.

TABLE 107.5

CALCULATION OF THE SEQUENTIAL ORGAN FAILURE ASSESSMENT (SOFA) SCORE TO PREDICT IN-HOSPITAL MORTALITY IN PATIENTS WITH CIRRHOSIS ADMITTED TO THE ICU

Organ system (criterion)	0 Points	1 Point	2 Points	3 Points	4 Points
Respiratory (PaO_2/FiO_2)	>400	301–400	201–300	101–200 (ventilated)	≤100 (ventilated)
Hemostatic (platelets [$\times 10^3/mm^3$])	>150	101–150	51–100	21–50	≤20
Hepatic (bilirubin [mg/dL])	<1.2	1.2–1.9	2.0–5.9	6.0–11.9	>12.0
Cardiovascular[a] (hypotension)	MAP ≥0 mm Hg	MAP <70 mm Hg	Dopamine ≤5 or dobutamine[a]	Dopamine >5 or epi/norepi ≤0.1	Dopamine >15 or epi/norepi >0.1
Neurologic (Glasgow Coma Score)	15	13–14	10–12	6–9	<6
Renal (creatinine [mg/dL])	<1.2	1.2–1.9	2.0–3.4	3.5–4.9	>5.0

PaO_2/FiO_2, arterial oxygen tension/fractional inspired oxygen; MAP, mean arterial pressure; epi, epinephrine; norepi, norepinephrine.
A SOFA score with a cutoff of 8 points had a sensitivity of 95%, specificity of 88%, overall correctness of 91%, PPV of 87%, and NPV of 96% for predicting in-hospital mortality.
[a]Adrenergic agents in μg/kg/min.
Modified from Wehler M, Kokoska J, Reulbach U, et al. Short-term prognosis in critically ill patients with cirrhosis assessed by prognostic scoring systems. *Hepatology.* 2004;34(2):255–261.

TABLE 107.6

DIFFERENTIAL DIAGNOSIS OF ABDOMINAL PAIN IN PATIENTS WITH CIRRHOSIS

Cause of abdominal pain	Etiologic associations	Clinical presentation
Spontaneous bacterial peritonitis	Low protein ascites	Fever, rebound tenderness, HE, azotemia
Incarcerated hernia (umbilical, inguinal)	Ascites, recanalization of the umbilical vein	Localized pain, bowel obstruction
Cholelithiasis and complications	Pigmented gallstones	Localized pain, jaundice, fever, pancreatitis
Peptic ulcer and complications	Decompensated cirrhosis, *Helicobacter* infection	UGI bleeding, perforated viscous
Hepatocellular carcinoma	Spontaneous rupture	Hemoperitoneum (rare)
Portal/mesenteric venous thrombosis	Hepatocellular carcinoma	Bowel ischemia, GI bleeding, ileus
Rupture of mesenteric varix	Recent large-volume paracentesis	Hemoperitoneum

HE, hepatic encephalopathy; UGI, upper gastrointestinal; GI, gastrointestinal.
In addition to the usual causes of abdominal pain and acute abdomen in the general ICU population, all of the above have been described with higher prevalence in patients with cirrhosis. Appropriate screening tests for the above include diagnostic paracentesis, duplex ultrasonography, contrast-enhanced abdominal computerized tomography (CT), and/or upper endoscopy.

- In addition, patients with decompensated cirrhosis have impaired cardiac contractility in response to stress, in particular, infection or GI bleeding.
- Diagnostic criteria of myocardial failure include blunted inotropic and chronotropic responses to stress, diastolic dysfunction, and prolonged QT interval on electrocardiogram.
- The treatment of **heart failure** in the setting of decompensated cirrhosis remains poorly defined; afterload reduction with angiotensin-converting enzyme inhibitors may precipitate profound hypotension and renal failure, and cardiac glycosides and β-adrenergic agonists have been shown to be relatively ineffective.

Ascites and Renal Complications

- Acute renal failure (ARF) in patients with decompensated cirrhosis is an independent predictor of death in the ICU and frequently denotes the onset of infection.
- The differential diagnosis of ARF in a decompensated cirrhotic includes **prerenal azotemia, hepatorenal syndrome (HRS),** and **acute tubular necrosis (ATN).**
- Analysis of urine sediment and sodium differentiate the above possibilities: the former two diagnoses present with normal urine sediment and low (<10 mEq/L) urine sodium, and the latter with renal tubular cell debris and high urine sodium.
- The distinction of these causes of renal failure remains paramount, since in its late stages, HRS portends a very poor prognosis and is generally irreversible without OLT, in contrast to prerenal azotemia and ATN.
- In practical terms, the diagnosis of HRS is often made after the exclusion of septic shock, intrinsic renal disease, obstructive uropathy, and most important, prerenal azotemia, the latter after a 1.5-L IV fluid (normal saline with or without colloid) challenge (Table 107.7).
- The treatment of **ascites** in the ICU should include judicious administration of diuretics in subjects without marked azotemia (creatinine >2 g/dL), electrolyte abnormalities, or hypotension.

- A combination of furosemide and spironolactone in a ratio of 40 mg and 100 mg has been shown to better effect a diuresis than either agent alone.
- The administration of IV albumin (12.5 g/day) may improve the efficacy of diuretics.
- Large-volume paracentesis should be performed if ascites interferes with ventilation of the patient or if diuretics result in azotemia or electrolyte abnormalities.
- IV colloid administration (albumin 6–8 g for each liter of ascites removed) should accompany paracentesis of $\geq$5 L to prevent **postparacentesis circulatory dysfunction.**
- The insertion of a transjugular intrahepatic portosystemic shunt (TIPS) may be considered in patients who have failed medical therapy.

TABLE 107.7

DIAGNOSTIC CRITERIA OF HEPATORENAL SYNDROME (HRS)

MAJOR CRITERIA
Low GFR (creatinine >2.5 mg/dL; CrCl <20 mL/min)
Absence of shock, infection, nephrotoxins
Absence of improvement after 1.5 L fluid challenge
Absence of intrinsic renal disease
Proteinuria <500 mg/d
Normal renal ultrasound

MINOR CRITERIA
Oliguria (<500 mL/d)
Urine sodium <10 mEq/L
Serum sodium <130 mEq/L

GFR, glomerular filtration rate; CrCl, creatinine clearance.
Adapted from Arroyo V, Gines P, Gerbes AL, et al. Definition and diagnostic criteria of refractory ascites and hepatorenal syndrome in cirrhosis. International Ascites Club. *Hepatology.* 1996;23(1): 164–176.

TABLE 107.8

RELATIVE CONTRAINDICATIONS AND ADVERSE OUTCOMES ASSOCIATED WITH PLACEMENT OF TIPS FOR SALVAGE THERAPY OF ACUTE VARICEAL HEMORRHAGE, REFRACTORY ASCITES, OR REFRACTORY HEPATIC HYDROTHORAX

RELATIVE CONTRAINDICATIONS
Severe liver failure (MELD ≥20; PT >20 s; creatinine
   >2.0 mg/dL; bilirubin >3.0 mg/dL)
Active systemic infection (risk of TIPS infection
   ["endo-TIPSitis"])
Recurrent/severe hepatic encephalopathy
Current hemodynamic instability
Congestive heart failure
Chronic renal failure
Pulmonary hypertension

ADVERSE OUTCOMES
Does not improve long-term patient survival for any
   indication
TIPS-induced hemolytic anemia
Worsening or precipitation of hepatic encephalopathy
TIPS stenosis (>50% at 1 y; lower with covered stents)
Failure of TIPS to prevent recurrence of indication for
   placement (for rescue in variceal bleeding about 5%,
   refractory ascites 15%–60%, hepatic hydrothorax
   30%–40%)

TIPS, transjugular intrahepatic portosystemic shunt; MELD, model for end-stage liver disease; PT, prothrombin time.
The above relative contraindications and adverse outcomes need to be taken in the context of the risk of immediate death as they assume less importance in the setting of rescue therapy for acute variceal bleeding. Data adapted from Laberge JM. Transjugular intrahepatic portosystemic shunt-role in treating intractable variceal bleeding, ascites, and hepatic hydrothorax. *Clin Liver Dis.* 2006;10(3): 583–598; Sanyal AJ. The use and misuse of transjugular intrahepatic portosystemic shunts. *Curr Gastroenterol Rep.* 2000;2(1): 61–71; and Sanyal AJ. Pros and cons of TIPS for refractory ascites. *J Hepatol.* 2005;43(6):924–925.

- In an ICU setting, patients may be too ill to undergo TIPS, and it is important for intensivists to recognize when TIPS placement is inappropriate (Table 107.8).
- The optimal treatment of HRS remains undefined. The ultimate treatment of HRS and the hemodynamic abnormalities of cirrhosis is OLT.
- **Vasoconstrictor therapy** holds promise for reversing HRS by reversing the state of systemic vasodilation. The oral α-adrenergic agonist **midodrine** (5–10 mg orally thrice daily) was found to be effective in one widely cited but preliminary study, when used in combination with octreotide (100 μg SC twice daily).
- **Terlipressin**, an intravenously administered vasopressin analogue with fewer ischemic complications, also reverses systemic vasodilation and has been found to effectively reverse HRS in Europe, but is not yet available in the United States.
- The administration of intravenous colloid, specifically albumin, serves to improve renal vascular perfusion.
- Finally, patients with decompensated cirrhosis should not receive even small therapeutic doses of nonsteroidal anti-inflammatory drugs since these agents exacerbate renal vasoconstriction by inhibiting production of endogenous vasodilatory renal prostaglandins.

- Electrolyte abnormalities frequently accompany ARF in cirrhosis and complicate the treatment of ascites. Hyponatremia and hypomagnesemia result from furosemide administration, and hyponatremia and hyperkalemia result from spironolactone administration.
- Hyponatremia also results from hemodilution in the setting of high vasopressin release from the neurohypophysis and portends a poor prognosis.

Infectious Complications

- Bacterial infections represent the most common cause of admission of cirrhotic patients to the ICU and remain one of the two primary causes of death.
- Risk factors for bacterial infections in hospitalized patients with cirrhosis include ICU admission and GI bleeding.
- Patients with cirrhosis are relatively **immunocompromised** as a result of portal hypertension and immune dysfunction. Portal hypertension results in the formation of a low-protein ascites, which is susceptible to infection because of its low complement concentration and, thus, low opsonic activity.
- **SBP** remains the most common bacterial infection in patients admitted to the ICU, but a shift toward **Gram-positive infections** has occurred. In one major hepatic diseases ICU, 77% of isolates were Gram positive.
- All patients admitted to an ICU with clinical suspicion of sepsis should be empirically given IV antibacterial agents to cover Gram-positive as well as Gram-negative organisms until cultures and sensitivities allow narrowing of the regimen; empiric vancomycin should be considered in patients who have been instrumented.
- The choice of coverage for Gram-negative bacilli should be a third-generation cephalosporin (e.g., cefotaxime [2 g IV every 8 hours] or ceftriaxone [1 g IV every 24 hours]).
- Aminoglycosides should be avoided except in serious infections with a multiply-resistant organism because of the susceptibility of cirrhotic patients to aminoglycoside nephrotoxicity.
- Diagnostic paracentesis should be performed on all cirrhotic patients admitted to the ICU with ascites and renal failure, HE, or any evidence of infection.
- Localizing symptoms and signs of peritonitis—abdominal pain, fever, rebound tenderness—may be absent in up to 30% of patients with this process.
- Blood and ascites should be immediately inoculated into culture bottles at the bedside, which has been shown to increase culture yields. However, **culture yields** may be as low as 40% even with bedside inoculation of a large volume of ascetic fluid (20 mL).
- Culture-negative neutrocytic ascites—that is, with more than **250 PMNs/μL**—should be considered the equivalent of SBP.
- Patients with ascetic fluid PMN count of ≥ 250 cells/μL should receive a third-generation cephalosporin (as above) and IV albumin (1.5 g/kg at diagnosis and 1.0 g/kg 48 hours after diagnosis), which has been shown both to decrease the incidence of HRS after SBP and to improve mortality.
- A similar diagnostic and therapeutic algorithm should be followed for spontaneous bacterial empyema, the infectious equivalent of SBP in patients with hepatic hydrothorax (see below).
- The incidence of **fungal infections** also increases in cirrhotic patients admitted to the ICU. Patients with Child's C cirrhosis have been reported to spontaneously develop invasive

aspergillosis in the ICU. *Candida* species may also infect cirrhotic ascites, with disastrous outcome.

Gastrointestinal Bleeding

- Acute upper gastrointestinal (UGI) bleeding, presenting as hematemesis and/or melena, remains one of the three most common indications for admission of patients with cirrhosis to the ICU.
- Esophageal varices account for most UGI bleeds in patients with cirrhosis, with gastric varices accounting for approximately 5% to 10%, and nonvariceal UGI pathology (gastric or duodenal mucosal lesions) noted in up to 30%.
- Other uncommon causes of UGI bleeding associated with cirrhosis include portal hypertensive gastropathy and gastric antral vascular ectasia, which more often present with occult GI bleeding and anemia.
- Upper endoscopy should be performed in all patients admitted to the ICU with acute UGI bleeding to identify its source as well as administer therapy.
- Patients with cirrhosis who present with acute UGI bleeding should be considered for ICU admission to deliver intensive nursing care and to manage the bleed as well as its complications.
- Despite the trend toward improved survival after variceal hemorrhage in the past two decades, each episode still carries a mortality risk of 10% to 20%, and the risk of rebleeding remains highest during the first few days after the index event.
- General resuscitative measures on admission to the ICU should include correction of hypotension, repletion of blood, and consideration of endotracheal intubation before endoscopy (Table 107.9).
- Factors that should contribute to the decision of whether to intubate a cirrhotic patient with an UGI bleed should include the rate of bleeding, hemodynamic instability, and degree of hepatic encephalopathy.
- Suppression of gastric acid secretion with proton pump inhibitors has been shown to decrease the number, size, and complications from post-band ligation esophageal ulcers.
- Vasopressin, formerly used for lowering portal pressure for this indication, has fallen from favor due to vasospastic adverse effects; although the vasopressin analogue terlipressin has a better safety profile and appears to improve control of acute variceal bleeding.
- The somatostatin analogue octreotide also has a favorable safety profile, and meta-analysis has demonstrated improved rates of sustained bleeding control after acute hemorrhage from esophageal varices.
- Endoscopic therapy after stabilization of the patient remains the definitive treatment for bleeding esophageal varices and controls active bleeding in more than 75% of cases when combined with vasoactive therapy.
- Endoscopic band ligation and sclerotherapy yield similar rates of control of active bleeding, but band ligation results in fewer local complications (esophageal ulcers, recurrent bleeding).
- Recurrent bleeding should prompt a second attempt at endoscopic treatment. In patients with recurrence after a second endoscopic treatment, or in any recurrence with hemodynamic instability, emergent insertion of a TIPS should be considered.
- In such dire situations, the relative contraindications for TIPS placement, outlined in Table 107.8, become less important.
- Patients with acute hemorrhage from fundic gastric varices present a particular therapeutic challenge because the bleeding is more profuse and interventions have been less successful in controlling the acute bleed.
- In the absence of endoscopic and vasoactive control of gastric variceal bleeding, insertion of a large tamponade balloon (Linton tube) can temporize control before insertion of a TIPS.
- Antibiotic prophylaxis after variceal hemorrhage has been shown to decrease the incidence of infection as well as variceal rebleeding, resulting in improved survival.
- Oral or IV fluoroquinolones (norfloxacin 400 mg orally/day or ofloxacin 200 mg IV twice daily) is recommended. Cephalosporins may be used if there is local resistance to fluoroquinolones.

Pulmonary Complications

- Respiratory failure accounts for up to 40% of admissions of cirrhotic patients to the ICU.
- The differential diagnosis of respiratory distress in patients with cirrhosis may be categorized into complications of cirrhosis, pulmonary vascular diseases resulting from portal hypertension, and primary liver diseases with cardiopulmonary manifestations (Table 107.10).
- Complications of cirrhosis include massive ascites and **hepatic hydrothorax** (HH), the accumulation of extracellular fluid with similar protein characteristics as ascites (low-protein, high-albumin gradient as compared to serum) within the pleural space.

TABLE 107.9

SPECIFIC MANAGEMENT OF ACUTE VARICEAL HEMORRHAGE AND ITS COMPLICATIONS

Therapeutic maneuver	Dose/route/indication
Transfusion of RBC	To hemoglobin of 8–9 g/dL
Octreotide	100 μg IV bolus, then 50 μg/h for 5 d
Endoscopy	EVL preferred over EVS
Proton pump inhibitors	Pantoprazole 40 mg IV or PO/d for 9 d
Antibiotic prophylaxis	Norfloxacin 400 mg/d for 7 d, or ceftriaxone 1 g/d for 7 d
TIPS	After two failed therapeutic endoscopies

RBC, red blood cells; IV, intravenous; PO, orally; EVL, esophageal variceal ligation; EVS, endoscopic variceal sclerotherapy; TIPS, transjugular intrahepatic porto-sytemic shunt.

DIFFERENTIAL DIAGNOSIS OF RESPIRATORY
DISTRESS AND HYPOXEMIA IN PATIENTS WITH
CIRRHOSIS

COMPLICATIONS OF CIRRHOSIS
Massive ascites
Hepatic hydrothorax
Muscle wasting
Aspiration pneumonia
**PULMONARY VASCULAR DISORDERS DUE TO
PORTAL HYPERTENSION**
Hepatopulmonary syndrome
Portopulmonary hypertension
**LIVER DISEASES WITH CARDIOPULMONARY
MANIFESTATIONS**
Alpha-1-antitrypsin deficiency (basilar emphysema)
Sarcoidosis (restrictive lung disease, cardiomyopathy)
Hemochromatosis (cardiomyopathy)
Ethanol (cardiomyopathy)

Adapted from Arguedas MR, Fallon MB. Hepatopulmonary
syndrome. *Clin Liver Dis.* 2005;9(4):733–746.

- HH usually occurs in the right pleural space (85%) and may occur in the absence of obvious ascites as a result of negative intrathoracic pressure during inspiration.
- The treatment of HH includes diuretic administration, as for ascites, and therapeutic thoracentesis. Placement of a TIPS in patients with refractory HH may be considered but is not universally effective, and relapse free 1-year survival is only 35%.
- Chest tube placement **and pleurodesis are relatively contraindicated** in refractory HH as they often contaminate the pleural space, precluding OLT.
- An infectious complication of HH, spontaneous bacterial empyema, should be diagnosed and managed similarly to SBP, but has a high mortality.
- **The hepatopulmonary syndrome (HPS)** may be defined as a widened alveolar-arterial oxygen gradient due to intrapulmonary vasodilation in a patient with liver disease. The pathogenesis of HPS remains obscure but likely results from the release of vasoactive mediators from the liver, which increase intrapulmonary **nitric oxide** production.
- In a patient with cirrhosis and resting hypoxemia (PaO_2 <70 mm Hg while breathing a FiO_2 of 0.21), the diagnosis is confirmed by a **contrast echocardiogram.**
- Supplemental oxygen usually bridges patients with HPS to OLT, which improves or reverses the process in 85% of patients.
- Patients with HPS have increased transplant waiting list mortality when compared to patients with normal gas exchange; consequently, patients with HPS and PaO_2 <60 mm Hg on room air are allowed increased priority for OLT in the United States.
- **Portopulmonary hypertension (PPH)** is the development of increased pulmonary vascular resistance due to vasoconstriction and subsequent vascular remodeling in a patient with portal hypertension.
- The diagnosis must be confirmed with right heart catheterization showing **elevated mean pulmonary artery pressure**

DIFFERENTIAL DIAGNOSIS OF ALTERED MENTAL
STATUS IN PATIENTS WITH CIRRHOSIS

HEPATIC ENCEPHALOPATHY
Electrolyte abnormalities
  hyponatremia
  hypokalemia
  hypomagnesemia
Hypoglycemia
Uremia
Intracranial bleeding
  subdural hematoma
  subarachnoid hemorrhage
Alcohol and/or drugs
  intoxication
  withdrawal

(PAP >25 mm Hg), as well as high pulmonary vascular resistance (>240 dynes/second per cm^{-5}) and normal pulmonary capillary wedge pressure.
- The treatment of PPH—indicated when mean PAP is more than 35 mm Hg—has not been well defined; **prostacyclin analogues** (epoprostenol titrated via pulmonary artery [PA] catheter; inhaled iloprost [5 µg six times daily]), **phosphodiesterase inhibitors** (sildenafil, 20 mg orally three times daily), or combination therapy appear to be effective in small case series.
- Unfortunately, the prognosis of patients with PPH is sufficiently poor after OLT that many patients with a mean PAP >35 mm Hg are not offered transplant.

Neurologic Complications

- Changes in mental status frequently accompany admission of patients with cirrhosis to the ICU and should not automatically suggest the presence of HE (Table 107.11).
- HE usually presents as a global decline in cognition and intellect, but focal neurologic deficits and signs of cerebral

PRECIPITATING EVENTS AND MECHANISMS OF
HEPATIC ENCEPHALOPATHY IN PATIENTS WITH
CIRRHOSIS

Event	Mechanism
Excessive protein ingestion	↑ Gut ammonia production
Constipation	
GI bleed	
Portosystemic shunting	↓ Neurotoxin clearance
Fever, infection	(ammonia, endogenous BZD)
Dehydration, azotemia	↓ Renal excretion of ammonium
Hypokalemia	
Sedatives (BZD)	↑ Inhibitory neurotransmission (GABA)

GI, gastrointestinal; BZD, benzodiazepines; GABA, gamma
aminobutyric acid.

TABLE 107.13

INDICATIONS AND CONTRAINDICATIONS FOR LISTING PATIENTS WITH DECOMPENSATED CIRRHOSIS FOR ORTHOTOPIC LIVER TRANSPLANTATION (OLT)

Indications	Contraindications
MELD $\geq$15	Active infection outside the liver
CTP score >7	Advanced cardiopulmonary disease
Hepatopulmonary syndrome (PO$_2$ <60 mm Hg)	Recent or metastatic malignancy
HCC (tumor stage 2)	Uncontrolled HIV infection/AIDS
Hyponatremia (<130 mEq/L)	Cholangiocarcinoma
Ascites refractory to medical therapy[a]	Active substance abuse
Hepatic hydrothorax	Psychosocial issues that would jeopardize
Hepatorenal syndrome	posttransplant compliance

MELD, Model for End-stage Liver Disease; CTP, Child-Turcotte-Pugh; HCC, hepatocellular carcinoma; HIV, human immunodeficiency virus; AIDS, acquired immunodeficiency syndrome.
[a] Refractory ascites may be functionally defined as an inadequate response to, or adverse effects (hyponatremia, hyperkalemia, azotemia) from, maximal medical therapy.

edema—decerebrate posturing and seizures—have also been described rarely.
- After screening for toxic and metabolic derangements, a severely obtunded patient should undergo non–contrast-enhanced head CT to rule out intracranial bleeding.
- High serum ammonia levels may help confirm, but are not necessary to make, the diagnosis.
- Most important, the presentation of a patient with advanced-grade HE should prompt a search for precipitating factors, particularly infection and UGI bleeding (Table 107.12).
- The administration of broad-spectrum antibiotics (e.g., ceftriaxone) should be considered until cultures have returned negative.
- The standard therapy, oral lactulose, must be administered via nasogastric tube in an intubated patient, cannot be given if there is an ileus, and its overzealous administration risks aspiration pneumonia, gaseous distention of the bowel, toxic megacolon, and electrolyte imbalance.
- Rectal lactulose offers an alternative route of administration, but its efficacy over tap water or saline enemas is unknown.
- The "non absorbable" antibiotic neomycin should be avoided, as the absorption of even small quantities from the gut risks renal injury.
- Rifaximin, a rifampin derivative that also decreases gut flora production of neurotoxins, appears to be as effective as lactulose and has a good safety profile.
- The benzodiazepine receptor antagonist flumazenil (1 mg IV) improves HE, but the benefit wanes within 2 hours.

- Extracorporeal albumin dialysis also improves HE in refractory cases and may be considered as a bridge to OLT.

Liver Transplantation for Patients with Chronic Liver Failure in the ICU

- ICUs have been increasingly used to care for patients with decompensated cirrhosis. Therefore, intensivists must have a working understanding of the indications and contraindications for listing cirrhotic patients for OLT (Table 107.13)
- The **model of end-stage liver disease (MELD)** score replaced the Child-Turcotte-Pugh (CTP) score by all OLT centers in the United States.
- The MELD score may be calculated from serum bilirubin, creatinine, and INR (most easily online at UNOS.ORG). Subsequent studies have demonstrated the superiority of the MELD over the CTP system in predicting waiting list mortality.
- A minimal MELD score of **15 points** for activating patients on the liver transplant waiting list has been adopted by most programs based on the observation that a MELD of 15 points predicts a 90-day mortality of about 10% without transplant, the same short-term mortality associated with transplant.
- Many patients in the ICU reach very high MELD scores (e.g., 35–40) with the onset of renal failure and are often removed from the OLT waiting list after developing infection and/or multiorgan system failure.

CHAPTER 108 ■ PANCREATIC DISEASE

OVERVIEW

- Acute pancreatitis has an annual incidence of 5 to 40 per 100,000 with an overall mortality of 1.5 per 100,000.
- The clinical course of acute pancreatitis is often self-limited and results in little, if any, structural alteration of the gland and requires no intervention.
- Approximately one-third of patients, however, develop pancreatic necrosis, which has an associated mortality rate that can be as high as 30%.
- All complications of this disease are potentially lethal and may require aggressive intervention to control or abort the process and to support the patient until the condition is resolved.
- Severe acute pancreatitis often demands an extended stay in the intensive care unit and countless hours of multidisciplinary care.

PATHOPHYSIOLOGY

- Numerous causative factors of acute pancreatitis have been recognized. The most important risk factors for pancreatitis in adults are **gallstones** and excessive **alcohol** use.
- The incidence of gallstone pancreatitis is increased among white women older than the age of 60 years and is highest in patients with gallstones <5 mm in diameter.
- Other causes include metabolic derangements such as hypertriglyceridemia, duct obstruction, medications (i.e., azathioprine, thiazides, and estrogens), and trauma. About 20% of cases remain idiopathic.
- Underlying the pathophysiology of acute pancreatitis is the inappropriate conversion of trypsinogen to trypsin and a lack of prompt elimination of **active trypsin** inside the pancreas.
- Activation of other pancreatic enzymes causes injury to the gland and results in an inflammatory process that is out of proportion to the response of other organs to a similar insult.
- In addition to further direct tissue damage, the inflammatory process may result in the systemic inflammatory response syndrome (SIRS), multiorgan failure, and ultimately, death.

DIAGNOSIS OF THE DISEASE PROCESS

- Even with history, physical examination, laboratory values, radiographic studies, and special procedures, a conclusive diagnosis of acute pancreatitis and its complications is often elusive.
- The recurrence rate of acute pancreatitis has been reported to be as high as 33% and can be even higher in the alcoholic population.

- Disease isolated to the head or tail of the pancreas may result in pain localized to the right or left upper quadrant with diaphragmatic irritation and referred pain to the subcapsular areas.
- The classic presentation of epigastric pain that radiates through to the back may be present in only 50% of patients presenting with acute pancreatitis.
- After the patient develops peritoneal signs, pancreatitis can mimic all other acute abdominal crises, especially those necessitating emergent surgery.

Laboratory Testing

- Serum amylase levels that are more than **three times** the upper limit of normal are almost always caused by acute pancreatitis given the appropriate clinical presentation.
- Serum amylase concentration begins to rise shortly after onset of the disease and it may return to normal levels in 2 to 4 days. Thus, a **normal serum amylase** level does not exclude the disease.
- Up to 19% of patients with an attack of acute pancreatitis had a normal serum amylase level and an abnormal computed tomography scan.
- Acute pancreatitis with normal serum amylase levels has a high proportion of patients with an alcoholic etiology and a longer duration of symptoms before admission.
- Other factors that may contribute to the absence of elevated serum amylase levels include return to normal levels prior to presentation or the inability of an inflamed or chronically diseased pancreas to produce a significant quantity of amylase.
- Pancreatitis secondary to biliary tract disease will often present with some of the highest serum amylase levels.
- An elevated **alanine aminotransferase** level in a patient without alcoholism who has pancreatitis is the single best predictor of biliary pancreatitis; a level more than three times the upper limit of normal has a positive predictive value of 95% for gallstone pancreatitis.
- The clinician must remain aware that an elevated serum amylase is not necessarily diagnostic of acute pancreatitis. The differential diagnosis of hyperamylasemia includes perforated or penetrating gastric ulcer, ruptured ectopic pregnancy, and intestinal obstruction or infarction.
- Measuring urinary amylase, amylase-to-creatinine ratios, and amylase isoenzymes have shown little clinical advantage, with the exception of ruling out macroamylasemias.
- An elevated concentration of serum lipase, however, is quite sensitive for diagnosis of acute pancreatitis secondary to alcohol abuse.
- **Lipase** levels tend to remain **elevated longer** than amylase concentrations. Therefore, an elevated lipase level can be useful information for patients who present later in the course of disease and who may have a normal amylase concentration.

- Serum lipase levels, although thought to be more specific for pancreatic destruction, have little, if any, role in predicting severity of disease.
- Although elevated serum amylase and lipase levels are most widely used for the diagnosis of acute pancreatitis, as stated, they have little, if any, value in predicting the severity of disease.

Radiologic and Diagnostic Studies

- Numerous radiologic findings are suggestive of, but not specific for, pancreatitis. These include dilatation of the first portion of the duodenum (duodenal ileus), dilatation of the first loop of the jejunum (jejunal ileus or sentinel loop), dilatation of the transverse colon or colon cutoff sign (secondary to a transverse colonic ileus), and elevated hemidiaphragm and pleural effusion, especially on the left side (secondary to diaphragmatic irritation and sympathetic pleural effusions).
- Transabdominal pancreatic ultrasonography is not sensitive in the diagnosis of acute pancreatitis, often because of gas in the bowel.
- Transabdominal ultrasound is more sensitive than either computed tomography or magnetic resonance imaging for identifying cholelithiasis and sludge and for detecting dilatation of the biliary ducts, but is insensitive for the detection of distal biliary duct stones.
- Endoscopic ultrasonography may be the most accurate test for diagnosing or ruling out biliary causes of acute pancreatitis and may guide the use of endoscopic retrograde cholangiopancreatography (ERCP).
- It is recommended that patients with severe acute gallstone pancreatitis undergo early ERCP and, if indicated, endoscopic sphincterotomy.
- ERCP is used with endoscopic sphincterotomy to extract impacted gallstones and to drain infected bile in severe acute pancreatitis.
- ERCP can also demonstrate ductal disruptions in traumatic pancreatitis and may also allow identification of pancreas divisum, thought to be a rare cause of acute pancreatitis.
- Although ERCP has recognized risks, including bleeding and either causing or exacerbating pancreatitis, complications are uncommon when performed by experienced endoscopists.
- In patients with abdominal pain of unclear cause, computed tomography can confirm the diagnosis of acute pancreatitis or confirm other causes of abdominal pain.
- In the absence of contraindication, computed tomography with radiocontrast is preferred, as contrast-enhanced computed tomography (CT) remains the gold standard in the diagnosis of pancreatic necrosis.
- When the use of intravenous radiocontrast material is contraindicated, the diagnosis of acute pancreatitis can be inferred from homogenous glandular enlargement and the presence of peripancreatic fluid collections.
- Determination of the extent of pancreatic necrosis correlates with prognosis as mortality increases markedly in patients with **necrosis** involving **more than 30%** of the gland.
- Radiocontrast allows the identification of pancreatic necrosis, which appears as focal or diffuse zones of nonenhanced parenchyma. Areas of necrosis may not be present, however, for 48 to 72 hours after presentation.

- In the clinically stable patient with a contraindication to intravenous contrast, magnetic resonance imaging (MRI) can diagnose and evaluate the extent of pancreatic necrosis. MRI may also identify early duct disruption that is not visible on CT scan.
- There are no imaging techniques that allow precise and reliable identification of infected pancreatic necrosis.
- The appearance of air in the pancreatic parenchyma, caused by gas-producing bacteria, is uncommon in patients with infected pancreatic necrosis; however, when present it usually indicates infection.
- **Fine-needle aspiration,** under CT or ultrasound guidance, with Gram staining and culture of the aspirate is the gold standard for the diagnosis of infected pancreatic necrosis.
- Most series report sensitivity for the prediction of infected necrosis that ranges from 90% to 100% and specificity between 96% and 100%.

CLASSIFICATION

- The most relevant classification to the intensivist determines the degree of severity and progress of an individual episode of pancreatitis. **Ranson's criteria** are well correlated with morbidity, number of days' stay in the ICU, and eventual mortality.
- Admission criteria:
  - Age older than 55 years
  - Blood glucose level >200 mg/dL
  - Leukocyte count >16,000/mm^3
  - Serum lactate dehydrogenase (LDH) level >350 IU/L
  - Serum glutamic-oxaloacetic transaminase (SGOT) >250 Sigma Frankel units
- Criteria to be determined within 48 hours:
  - Serum calcium level <8 mg/dL
  - PaO$_2$ <60 mm Hg, base deficit >4 mEq/L
  - Increase in blood urea nitrogen (BUN) of more than 5 mg/dL
  - Decrease in hematocrit of more than 10 percentage points
  - More than 6 L fluid sequestration
- The presence of fewer than 3 of these 10 criteria within 48 hours of admission correlates with a more benign form and course of disease, with an eventual mortality rate of 3%.
- The presence of three or more of these parameters on admission or within 48 hours usually implies a more severe form of pancreatitis and is associated with high risk of death and major complication.

TREATMENT OF ACUTE PANCREATITIS

- An overall approach to the therapy for acute pancreatitis should include placing the pancreas "at rest," supporting the patient's nutritional and metabolic needs, correcting the acute causes of mortality, detecting complications of disease that require surgical intervention, and preventing and treating delayed causes of mortality.

Gland Suppression

- Suppression of the secretory function of the pancreas has been attempted by elimination of oral fluids, suppression with H$_2$

blockers and antacids, and use of anticholinergics and pro-teolytic enzyme inhibitors. However, controlled randomized studies have not shown significant benefit.

- Recent evidence suggests that **enteral nutrition** is not only feasible but may be desirable in such patients.
- Bacterial translocation from the intestinal tract to the pancreas may have a role in the pathogenesis of infected pancreatic necrosis.
- Lack of enteral feeding may facilitate translocation of bacteria or bacterial products into the circulation. Total parenteral nutrition may, therefore, promote bacterial translocation in patients with pancreatitis.
- Animal studies have shown jejunal feedings result in negligible increases in enzyme, bicarbonate, and volume output from the pancreas. This observation has been confirmed in humans.
- Several studies have shown jejunal feeding to be not only less expensive than total parenteral nutrition but also associated with fewer septic complications and shorter length of stay.
- In addition, enteral nutrition reduces production of proinflammatory mediators that may also have therapeutic potential in such patients.
- Initiating enteral feeding within 48 hours of admission helps to maintain gut function, allowing improved tolerance and fewer problems with ileus and gastric stasis compared with feeding delayed by 4 or 5 days.
- Contrary to the commonly held belief that enteral feedings must be delivered distal to the ligament of Treitz, recent studies suggest that nasogastric feeding is well tolerated and does not appear to exacerbate pancreatitis.
- **Hypocalcemia** can occur in acute pancreatitis, but rarely is there a clinically significant decrease in ionized calcium. If deficits are found, however, calcium and magnesium are easily replaced.

Cardiovascular Collapse, Renal Failure, and Respiratory Insufficiency

- One of the most important determinants of poor outcome in severe acute pancreatitis is the early development and persistence of organ dysfunction.
- The cornerstone of management in early pancreatitis is fluid resuscitation and close monitoring for early manifestations of organ dysfunction.
- In addition to the frequent assessment of vital signs, the intravascular volume status should be monitored by means of physical examination and urinary output.
- Early identification of hypoxemia via either pulse oximetry or arterial blood gas measurement is also paramount.
- **Hypovolemia** occurs as a result of the chemical peritonitis; the associated increased capillary permeability, relative lymphatic obstruction, and partial splanchnic venous obstruction can account for sequestration of up to 40% of the patient's circulatory plasma volume in a few hours. Renal insufficiency may be a result of this massive fluid loss.
- The association of **renal failure** in acute pancreatitis markedly increases the mortality in these patients.
- Whether or not there is a **myocardial depressant factor** associated with severe pancreatitis, inotropic agents may be required to improve cardiac function if cardiac output remains low despite adequate filling pressures.

- The **respiratory insufficiency** associated with severe pancreatitis is complex and is probably a combination of a decrease in functional residual capacity and shunting.
- Respiratory assistance with positive end-expiratory pressure (PEEP) is required until the process resolves and the patient can maintain adequate minute ventilation and oxygenation.
- Patients with severe acute pancreatitis who meet conventional criteria should be admitted to the intensive care unit, as well as those patients who are at high risk of rapid deterioration such as the elderly, patients requiring ongoing volume resuscitation, those with renal failure, respiratory compromise, and evidence of substantial pancreatic necrosis (>30%).
- Morbidly obese patients are at increased risk for developing the severe form of acute pancreatitis. When compared to normal-weight patients, patients with body mass index (BMI) ≥25 kg/m² had an increasing rate and types of complications as the BMI increased.

Therapeutic Peritoneal Lavage

- Despite several early, initially enthusiastic reports, the use of continuous lavage in patients with acute pancreatitis is not supported by the currently available evidence.

Antibiotics

- The natural course of severe acute pancreatitis progresses in two phases. The first 14 days are characterized by the development of the SIRS. The second phase, roughly 2 weeks after the onset of disease, is dominated by sepsis-related complications resulting from infection of pancreatic necrosis.
- In the natural course of the disease, **infection of pancreatic necrosis** occurs in up to 70% of patients and has become the most important risk factor for death from necrotizing pancreatitis.
- The frequency of infected necrosis correlates with the duration of disease. In patients with necrotizing pancreatitis, the proportion of patients with proven infected necrosis at the time of surgery increased from 22% to 24% after the first week to 36% to 55% after the second week and up to 72% after the third week.
- The extent of pancreatic necrosis may also be a risk factor for infection. Patients with more than 50% necrosis of the pancreas have the highest infection rates.
- Among patients with sterile necrotizing pancreatitis, **mortality** rates of 10% to 15% are reported, whereas infected pancreatic necrosis carries with it a mortality rate of up to 50%.
- Multiple investigators have identified **imipenem** as the antibiotic agent of first choice as it can reach higher pancreatic tissue levels and it provides higher bactericidal activity against most of the bacteria present in pancreatic infection compared with other types of antibiotics.
- In a comparison between meropenem and imipenem, there were no significant differences in septic complications, indication for surgery, or mortality, indicating that meropenem is equally effective.
- The combination of quinolones and metronidazole is not an effective antibiotic prophylaxis.

- Longer antibiotic administration in patients with acute necrotizing pancreatitis (> 14 days) is not associated with a reduction in the incidence of septic complications of the disease. However, prolonged imipenem administration in patients with persisting systemic complications tends to reduce mortality in acute necrotizing pancreatitis compared to a 14-day regimen.
- Prophylactic antibiotics may reduce local pancreatic infection rates, episodes of sepsis, and mortality.
- Early versus delayed imipenem–cilastatin in the treatment of acute necrotizing pancreatitis may reduce the need for surgery, the overall number of major organ complications, and the mortality rate.
- The **bacterial spectrum** of infection in acute necrotizing pancreatitis has been described as primarily Gram negative and, in part, anaerobic, with the predominant pathogens including *Escherichia coli*, *Pseudomonas* species, *Enterobacter*, *Bacteroides*, and *Proteus*.
- Early antibiotic treatment of necrotizing pancreatitis results in a dramatic **shift in bacteriology** from Gram-negative to Gram-positive pathogens in those patients who develop infection.
- It is likely that these Gram-positive infections do not originate in the gut, but rather are nosocomial infections acquired via venous catheters, urinary catheters, or endotracheal tubes.
- Antibiotic prophylaxis does not appear to increase the incidence of fungal infections.

SURGICAL MANAGEMENT

- Most episodes of acute pancreatitis are mild and self-limiting, resolving spontaneously within 3 to 5 days. The mortality rate in these patients is <1%, and these patients do not routinely require intensive care or surgical management.
- However, there are several absolute indications for operative intervention in patients with severe acute pancreatitis, including prevention of recurrence and treatment of complications.
- As the conservative management of infected pancreatic necrosis associated with multiple organ failure has a mortality rate of up to 100%, proven infected pancreatic necrosis, as well as septic complications directly resulting from pancreatic infection, are indications for surgical intervention.

Treatment of Biliary Pancreatitis

- Biliary pancreatitis is most often associated with the passage of a small common bile duct stone. Occasionally, a stone may become impacted at the ampulla of Vater. In this case, rapid progressive deterioration of the patient's clinical course may soon follow.
- For patients with severe acute gallstone pancreatitis, urgent biliary drainage and clearance of the common bile duct must be considered.
- There is general agreement that open cholecystectomy with supraduodenal bile duct exploration and insertion of a T tube is an unacceptable emergency procedure in patients with severe gallstone pancreatitis, as both higher morbidity and mortality rates have been shown following early surgery.

- Patients with signs and symptoms consistent with **cholangitis** and patients with severe acute gallstone pancreatitis and obstructive jaundice should undergo **urgent endoscopic retrograde cholangiopancreatography,** and, if choledocholithiasis is confirmed, endoscopic sphincterotomy should be performed.
- In patients with severe acute pancreatitis due to suspected or proven cholelithiasis but without obstructive jaundice, the role of ERCP and endoscopic sphincterotomy is less well defined.
- In severe biliary pancreatitis, emergency ERCP and endoscopic sphincterotomy appears to reduce the overall complication rate and mortality rate. In contrast, ERCP and endoscopic sphincterotomy have no influence on the outcome of mild biliary pancreatitis.
- Recurrence of acute pancreatitis in patients with cholelithiasis has been reported in 29% to 63% of cases if the patient is discharged from the hospital without additional treatment. **Cholecystectomy** and clearance of the common bile duct is indicated in these patients to prevent recurrent biliary pancreatitis.
- In mild gallstone pancreatitis, cholecystectomy should be performed as soon as the patient has recovered from the attack and, preferably, during the same hospital stay.
- In severe gallstone pancreatitis, cholecystectomy should be performed once the inflammatory process has subsided and with sufficient clinical recovery to make the procedure technically easier and safer for the patient.
- If endoscopic sphincterotomy was performed, cholecystectomy should be performed within 6 weeks.
- Cholecystectomy can be performed safely after an episode of gallstone pancreatitis via the laparoscopic approach with a reported conversion to open rate of 0% to 16%.

Vascular Complications

- The systemic vascular effects of acute pancreatitis are probably related to the release of pancreatic proteases, such as trypsin, which locally and distally may activate complement C5a and precipitate the coagulation cascade.
- **Bleeding** from pancreatic pseudocysts and ruptured pseudoaneurysms are the most often fatal complication of pancreatitis, carrying a mortality rate of 25% to 40%.
- Bleeding may present as melena from erosion into the proximal gastrointestinal tract or as hypovolemia and abdominal pain if there is rupture into the peritoneal cavity.
- Most patients with gastrointestinal tract bleeding secondary to acute or chronic pancreatitis are alcoholics, and the cause of the bleeding is usually missed because of more common causes of serious bleeding in this patient population (i.e., peptic ulcer disease, gastritis, varices, Mallory-Weiss tears).
- The development of **aneurysms** is probably related to the severe inflammation and enzymatic autodigestion of the pancreatic and peripancreatic arteries with eventual formation of a pseudoaneurysm. With growth and expansion, the pseudoaneurysms may rupture into pseudocysts, adjacent viscera, the peritoneal cavity, or the pancreatic duct.
- The most common vessel involved in splanchnic pseudoaneurysms related to pancreatitis is the splenic artery, followed by the gastroduodenal and the inferior pancreaticoduodenal,

but such involvement may occur with any of the adjacent splanchnic vessels.

- Patients with chronic pancreatitis may have as high as a 10% incidence of pseudoaneurysms demonstrated on angiographic studies, but bleeding from these rarely occurs unless they are associated with pseudocysts.

- The treatment of **ruptured pseudoaneurysms** requires that the diagnosis be recognized; therefore, the clinician must know of it, must have a high index of suspicion, and must have a well-defined diagnostic and therapeutic plan, including emergency upper endoscopy, selective visceral angiography, ultrasonography, and CT scanning.

- Control can be rendered by either selective arterial infusion of vasopressin or angioembolization with Gelfoam, detachable intravascular balloons, Gianturco coils, or polymerizing adhesives.

- Surgical control is indicated only for immediate life-threatening bleeding or failure of interventional control of bleeding.

- **Hemoductal pancreatitis or hemosuccus pancreatitis** is the complication of pseudoaneurysm rupture into the pancreatic duct and usually encompasses the triad of gastrointestinal bleeding, pancreatitis with epigastric pain, and partial common bile duct obstruction.

- The diagnosis can be confirmed by selective visceral angiography or ERCP. The treatment of this rare complication requires ligation of the pseudoaneurysm and possible pancreatic resection.

- Venous **thrombosis of the portal vein** is a potential complication of acute or chronic pancreatitis. The patient's course is complicated by acute decompensation, hypotension with sequestration in the vascular bed, acidosis, hepatic enzyme elevation, alteration in clotting studies, and venous infarction of the bowel.

- Patients who survive this insult all develop portal hypertension, and some present months to years later with bleeding esophageal varices.

- Selective **splenic venous thrombosis** occurs more frequently, and patients usually present with an increased spleen size, unexplained blood loss, pain in the left upper quadrant and subscapular area, and possibly hypotension and cardiovascular collapse because the subscapular hematoma ruptured into the free peritoneal cavity.

- The treatment is splenectomy with preoperative vascular control by angiographic techniques and balloons.

- During drainage procedures for pancreatic pseudocysts in the presence of associated splenic venous thrombosis, the transgastric approach should be avoided to decrease postoperative bleeding from the rich submucosal plexus of high-pressure veins.

- In the absence of bleeding gastric varices, one may elect to leave the spleen *in situ* even with splenic vein thrombosis, because not all patients develop bleeding from gastric varices.

Pancreatic Pseudocyst

- Peripancreatic fluid collections can occur as a result of acute pancreatitis, chronic pancreatitis, surgery (either pancreatic or other abdominal surgery), trauma, or neoplasia.

- With the exception of a cystic neoplasm, peripancreatic fluid collections form either as a result of a disruption in the pancreatic ductal system with subsequent fluid leakage or the maturation of peripancreatic necrosis.

- The critical clinical distinction between an acute fluid collection and a pseudocyst (or pancreatic abscess) is the lack of a defined wall as defined by the International Symposium on Acute Pancreatitis in 1992.

- Acute fluid collections are common in patients with severe acute pancreatitis, occurring in up to 50% of cases. However, more than half of these lesions regress spontaneously.

- Pseudocyst is defined as a collection of pancreatic juice that arises as a consequence of acute or chronic pancreatitis or pancreatic trauma that is enclosed by a nonepithelialized wall composed of either fibrous or granulation tissue.

- Formation of an acute pseudocyst takes **four or more weeks** from the onset of acute pancreatitis. In contrast, chronic pseudocysts have a well-defined wall but arise in patients with chronic pancreatitis without a preceding episode of acute pancreatitis.

- Pseudocyst formation is a frequent complication of pancreatitis with a reported incidence of 10% to 20% in acute pancreatitis and 20% to 40% in chronic pancreatitis.

- When pus is present, the lesion is more correctly termed a **pancreatic abscess**. The distinction between pancreatic abscess and infected necrosis is critical as the mortality risk for infected necrosis is double that for pancreatic abscess.

- The traditional management of pancreatic pseudocyst is to proceed with a drainage procedure if the pseudocyst persisted **beyond 6 weeks** and/or was **larger than 6 cm.**

- Operative intervention was the mainstay, and the procedure performed was internal drainage via a cyst-enteric anastomosis, primarily cystogastrostomy or cystojejunostomy, depending on the location of the pseudocyst.

  - The traditional method of surgical drainage has been challenged by the introduction of less invasive techniques; percutaneous or endoscopic drainage techniques are comparable to the outcome of surgical drainage techniques in appropriately selected patients.

- Simple aspiration of the cyst has been associated with a recurrence rate of more than 70% and can, therefore, not be regarded as a definitive treatment.

- Continuous catheter drainage has shown better short-term results, with an 84% success rate and an average 7% recurrence rate.

- The prolonged presence of an indwelling catheter for several weeks and frequent fistula formation remain disadvantages of this technique.

- Endoscopic drainage has been increasingly used during the past 10 years, either via a transpapillary route or through the gastrointestinal wall. The short-term results appear to be encouraging.

Biliary Obstruction Due to Pancreatic Inflammation

- Biliary obstruction may be found in as many as 25% of cases presenting with acute pancreatitis, and this obstruction, caused by pancreatic swelling, can be confused with a stone lodged at the ampulla.

- The intrapancreatic portion of the common bile duct becomes involved in the inflammatory process, but this usually resolves over the course of the disease.
- If the biliary obstruction does not resolve, a workup including ultrasonography, **ERCP,** or **transhepatic cholangiography** may be necessary to define the problem and the anatomy so that an appropriate decompressive procedure can be performed.
- If the patient develops cholangitis and becomes septic from infected bile in the obstructed duct, transhepatic cholangiography and drainage may be life-saving to provide decompression without subjecting the patient in septic shock to an emergency operation.

Pancreatic Necrosis, Infected Pancreatic Necrosis, and Abscess

- Little is known of what triggers the release of activated pancreatic enzymes that autodigest the gland and surrounding retroperitoneal tissue and convert acute interstitial or edematous pancreatitis to pancreatic necrosis.
- If venous thrombosis and erosion to the small peripancreatic vessels occur, the combination is hemorrhagic necrotizing pancreatitis.
- Enteric bacterial contamination results in combined abscess and infected necrosis, which carries the highest mortality rate.
- It is rare to see septic complications within the first week of presentation but not unusual after the second week, and they are almost universally present if the patient's course requires therapy for more than 3 weeks.
- Clinical signs of abdominal pain, fever, leukocytosis, associated severe systemic manifestations of hypotension, cardiovascular collapse, pulmonary insufficiency, renal failure, and mental status changes all strongly suggest the onset of this complication.
- The problem is rarely that of making the diagnosis of sepsis, but rather, of differentiating pancreatic necrosis and abscess formation from other sources of systemic sepsis such as pneumonia, urinary tract infection, and intravascular catheter-related infection.
- **Sequential contrast-enhanced computed tomography** is the best tool available for diagnosing and following this disease process. The study is diagnostic of abscess formation if air is seen in the phlegmon.
- Percutaneous **fine-needle aspiration** of the intrapancreatic or peripancreatic fluid collections can be used to confirm bacterial contamination in the absence of air. If necrosis is demonstrated on CT scan, aspirates are sterile, and the patient is not toxic, a conservative approach may be attempted.
- At present there is general agreement that surgery for severe pancreatitis should be deferred as long as the patient continues to respond favorably to conservative management.
- Early operation directed toward debridement of devitalized tissue to prevent septic complications has only led to increased morbidity and incidence of sepsis.
- Optimal surgical timing should occur, at the minimum, 2 to 3 weeks after the onset of pancreatitis to allow a sequestrum to form. The rationale for delaying surgical therapy is to permit proper demarcation of pancreatic and peripancreatic necrosis to occur, limiting the extent of surgery that is needed to facilitate debridement.
- In most studies published over the past decade, indication for surgery was defined by necrosis formation on CT scan and positive fine-needle aspiration. In the unstable patient, CT-guided percutaneous aspiration and drainage of pancreatic abscesses used as a temporizing measure before surgery may improve the patient's overall condition.
- Surgical techniques are still necessary for **debridement and drainage** if percutaneous drainage does not improve the septic course. The goal of surgery in patients with necrotizing pancreatitis is to remove all areas of necrotic tissue, including necrotic pancreatic tissue and any infected necrotic tissue.
- Resective procedures, such as partial or total pancreatectomy that also remove vital pancreatic tissue and healthy organs, are associated with high mortality rates.
- Traditionally, three techniques have been used with comparable results; these include:
  - open necrosectomy with closed continuous lavage of the retroperitoneum
  - open necrosectomy that may or may not be staged with planned relaparotomies followed by delayed primary closure and drainage or with multiple drainage and relaparotomy as required
  - open necrosectomy, often with marsupialization, with open packing and planned relaparotomies.
- The surgical techniques for the treatment of pancreatic necrosis are varied, and the ideal method is still debated. Generally agreed-on principles of surgical management include an organ-preserving approach that involves debridement or necrosectomy, minimization of intraoperative hemorrhage, and maximization of postoperative removal of retroperitoneal debris and exudates.

CHAPTER 109 ■ INFLAMMATORY BOWEL DISEASE AND TOXIC MEGACOLON

FULMINANT COLITIS

- **Ulcerative colitis** is characterized by a diffuse, continuous inflammatory process usually limited to the **superficial mucosa** of the colon. **Crohn disease** entails a more focal, **transmural** inflammation that can affect the colon either alone or accompanied by small bowel involvement. Both have the potential for severe, fulminating, or toxic colitis.
- Since the original classification was published by Truelove and Witts in 1955, severe, acute, ulcerative colitis has been defined by:
  - the presence of six or more bloody bowel movements per day associated with temperature >37.8°C
  - heart rate >90 beats/minute
  - hemoglobin <10.5 g/dL
  - an erythrocyte sedimentation rate (ESR) >30 mm/hour
- The above criteria are indications for hospitalization and intravenous corticosteroid therapy.
- Additionally, the severity of ulcerative colitis can extends beyond the need for hospitalization to *fulminant colitis* and *toxic megacolon,* implying progression of mucosal inflammation into deeper layers of the colon wall.
- These conditions are medical emergencies and require more intense and combined medical and surgical management.
- Patients with **fulminant colitis or toxic megacolon** have evidence of **transmural inflammation,** including more profound tachycardia (heart rate >120 beats/minute), fever (>38°C), hypoactive bowel sounds, hypoalbuminemia, and metabolic alkalosis, accompanied by radiologic and endoscopic evidence of transmural disease and circular muscle paralysis, which precipitates dilatation (Table 109.1).
- Approximately 15% of patients with ulcerative colitis will have a severe flare-up that will require hospitalization. Between 6.3% and 9% will have severe colitis as their initial presentation.
- Mortality from severe colitis is <2%, with a colectomy rate of about 30%.
- The risks of surgery or colectomy with fulminant colitis or toxic megacolon have not been independently assessed, but their prognosis is, most certainly, worse than patients presenting with criteria for severe colitis alone.

Clinical Features

- In contrast to patients with severe colitis, those with **fulminant** colitis are characterized by having more than 10 bowel movements per day, rectal urgency, continuous bleeding, abdominal pain and distention, fevers, weight loss, and dehydration.

- On physical examination, patients present with fever, tachycardia, abdominal tenderness and mild distention, tympany, and decreased bowel sounds.
- Laboratory abnormalities include leukocytosis, anemia (hemoconcentration must be taken into account), hypoalbuminemia, hypokalemia, hyponatremia, and elevated sedimentation rate and C-reactive protein (CRP). The degree of metabolic alkalosis correlates with the severity of colitis.
- A plain abdominal radiograph can determine the extent of ulcerative colitis by the absence of fecal material distal to the margin of disease and the presence of air outlining normal haustrations proximal to the disease margin.
- Radiologic features of fulminant colitis include wall thickening, with islands of edematous mucosa surrounded by deep ulcerations. The presence of **colonic dilatation >5.5 cm** is predictive of the presence of—or evolution to—toxic megacolon.
- A limited proctoscopic examination or flexible sigmoidoscopy with minimal air insufflation may be performed safely to evaluate the mucosa for pseudomembranes or ischemia. Examination generally shows extensive ulceration with friable, bleeding mucosa.
- In rare instances, however, such as with rectal enema therapy or in the setting of Crohn disease, the rectum may be normal.
- In patients whose initial presentation of inflammatory bowel disease is severe colitis, biopsies should be performed to evaluate for Crohn disease and to rule out acute self-limited colitis.
- In those with an exacerbation of known diagnosis, biopsies can help to exclude *Clostridium difficile* or cytomegalovirus.
- More extensive **endoscopic examinations** are **generally contraindicated** due to the risk of perforation or inducing toxic megacolon. However, they have been performed safely in some experienced centers.
- The presence of severe colitis (deep penetrating ulcers) in conjunction with clinical features of severe disease is a poor prognostic sign. Similarly, the presence of extensive and deep ulcerations is a poor prognostic marker in Crohn disease.
- Stool analysis for **ova and parasites,** *C. difficile, Escherichia coli* O157:H7, *Campylobacter, Salmonella,* and *Shigella* should be performed as part of the diagnostic workup.

Management

- Few medical emergencies require as close cooperation between medical and surgical personnel as does fulminant colitis.
- A team approach with early management and continuous assessment by both groups is vital not only to determine whether surgery is indicated but also to support critically ill patients preoperatively and postoperatively.

TABLE 109.1

DETERMINATION OF SEVERITY OF BOWEL DISEASE: CLINICAL/LABORATORY FINDINGS

	Disease severity	
	Severe disease	Fulminant disease
Stools (number/d)	>6	>10
Blood in stool	Frequent	Continuous
Temperature	>37.5°C	>37.5°C
Pulse	>90 bpm	>90 bpm
Hemoglobin	<75% of normal	Transfusion required
Erythrocyte sedimentation rate	<30	>30
Radiographic features	Colon wall edema Thumbprinting	Dilated colon
Clinical examination	Abdominal tenderness	Abdominal distention and tenderness

- Early recognition and institution of therapy by an experienced team can alter the outcome of this life-threatening illness.
- Daily to frequent abdominal radiographs should be performed to follow the progression of the colitis. Additionally, computed tomographic scan may be needed for management in complicated cases.

Medical Treatment

- Resuscitative measures, including vigorous **fluid, electrolyte, and blood** replacement to maintain the serum hematocrit at approximately 30%, are paramount.
- The goal of fluid replacement should be to restore previous losses and continue replenishing those that are ongoing from diarrhea, fever, and third spacing of fluids.
- Despite the fact that bowel rest is an ineffective primary therapy for severe colitis, oral intake of fluids should be discontinued in fulminant colitis or once colonic dilatation is recognized.
- Parenteral **nutritional support** in attempts to correct malnutrition and electrolyte and acid-base balance—including repletion of phosphate, calcium, and magnesium—should be initiated.
- Although severe **hypokalemia** may not be present, total body potassium depletion is common and may be exacerbated by glucocorticoids such that resuscitative measures should include adequate potassium replacement.
- **Aminosalicylates,** a mainstay of maintenance therapy and the treatment of mild to moderate disease, have no role in the treatment of fulminant colitis.
- **Corticosteroids** have long been used in the management of ulcerative colitis as well as in Crohn colitis. Usual doses employed for severe fulminant colitis range from 40 to 80 mg of methylprednisolone (in Europe, often 1 mg/kg) or 400 mg of hydrocortisone provided in divided doses or continuous infusion.
- Prednisone, 25 mg intravenously every 6 hours, and prednisolone sodium phosphate have been used successfully. In the United States, hydrocortisone, 100 mg every 6 hours, and methylprednisolone, 6 to 15 mg every 6 hours, are both available for intravenous administration.
- There is no advantage to doses >60 mg of methylprednisolone daily.

- The use of adrenocorticotropic hormone (ACTH) has not been shown to be superior to corticosteroids and, although it may be preferred in patients not previously exposed to corticosteroids, at a dose of 100 to 150 U/day, its use has become an anachronism.
- The response to corticosteroids in the setting of severe fulminant colitis has remained constant for the past several decades, with approximately 75% of patients responding and less than half failing to achieve remission.
- The most critical assessment in the setting of fulminant colitis is the response to therapy within the first 5 days.
- The presence of hypoalbuminemia, high CRP, short duration of illness, and prior corticosteroid use are predictors of medical failure. In addition, ex-smokers have a worse prognosis.
- Short-term prognosis to corticosteroids in severe disease can be predicted as early as 24 hours. Persistence of more than nine stools per day, an albumin <3 g/dL, or a pulse rate >90 beats/minute was predictive of >60% risk of colectomy.
- Patients with greater than eight stools per day and a CRP >4.5 mg/dL by day 3 had an 85% likelihood of requiring colectomy or cyclosporine therapy.
- Continuation of intravenous (IV) corticosteroids beyond 7 to 10 days does not provide any additional benefits and may increase morbidity and surgical risks.
- **Cyclosporin A,** administered as a continuous IV infusion (2 or 4 mg/kg/day), either alone or in combination with corticosteroids, has been effective in treating severe ulcerative colitis.
- Immediate response rates up to 85% to 92% have been reported and, similar to the experience with the "intensive intravenous corticosteroid" regime, failure to improve—as defined by having eight or more stools per day or persistence of CRP elevation after 3 days of cyclosporine—is predictive of the need for colectomy.
- Forty percent to 50% of patients treated with intravenous cyclosporine experience long-term remission. Improved outcomes are reported for patients who have been transitioned to oral cyclosporine with the addition of **6-MP or azathioprine.**
- Careful daily monitoring for serious side effects of nephrotoxicity, infection, and seizures must be carried out when using cyclosporine.
- Patients who improve, as evidenced by restitution of formed bowel movements with the absence of bleeding and ability to pass flatus without using the toilet, are then transitioned

to oral prednisone at the same daily dose used to achieve the clinical remission.

- Aminosalicylates are added as a maintenance therapy once patients are tolerating oral steroids and a full diet.
- Patients requiring IV cyclosporine are transitioned to oral dosing by doubling the IV dose for twice-daily oral administration (e.g., if the intravenous dose is 100 mg/24 hours, the oral dose would be 100 mg twice daily).
- Patients receiving a combination of corticosteroids and cyclosporine should receive *Pneumocystis* prophylaxis with sulfamethoxazole-trimethoprim three times weekly.
- Patients may be discharged from the hospital when tolerating a low-residue diet with formed stools without blood or rectal urgency; premature discharge is doomed to failure and readmission.
- Most recently, infliximab, a chimeric antitumor necrosis factor (TNF) monoclonal antibody, has been shown to be effective as outpatient therapy for patients with moderate to severe ulcerative colitis. However, the role of infliximab in fulminant ulcerative colitis has been debated; the controversy is likely related to the severity of the disease.

Surgical Management

- Persistence of medical therapy in the setting of fulminant colitis must be balanced against the potential for a surgical "cure" of the disease.
- Indications for surgery in fulminant colitis include clinical deterioration or failure to respond to medical therapy.
- Although the medical management of fulminant colitis and toxic megacolon is similar, the absence of acute colonic dilatation may permit delay of surgical intervention.
- Generally, in the absence of colonic dilatation, medical management may be continued for 5 to 7 days in a further attempt to reverse transmural inflammation, as long as the patient is stable and improving.
- Patients with fulminant colitis who do not begin to respond to the intensive intravenous steroid regimen should be referred to a center experienced in cyclosporin therapy or undergo colectomy.
- The timing of surgical intervention in these less urgent cases requires experienced clinical judgment. Early intervention to reduce mortality must be balanced against the potential for intensive medical management to control the inflammatory process and complications, thereby potentially preventing the psychosocial and medical stigmata of colectomy.
- The type of operation performed for treatment of fulminant colitis depends on the clinical status of the patient and experience of the surgeon.
- A one-stage procedure that cures ulcerative colitis without the need for a second operation is appropriate for older patients or those not desiring restorative ileal pouch–anal anastomosis.
- A limited abdominal colectomy with ileostomy, leaving the rectosigmoid as a mucous fistula or the rectum alone, using a Hartmann procedure has the advantages of limiting the lengthy pelvic dissection in acutely ill patients while allowing for the option of a subsequent restorative, sphincter-saving procedure (ileoanal anastomosis).
- In patients with indeterminate colitis or Crohn disease, preservation of the rectum may provide the opportunity for an eventual ileorectal or ileoanal anastomosis to preserve anal

continence after temporary diversion and pathologic review of the colectomy specimen.

TOXIC MEGACOLON

- Toxic megacolon refers to acute nonobstructive dilatation of the colon, generally as a complication of ulcerative colitis, but it may occur with any severe inflammatory colitis.
- This condition has been described with idiopathic and infectious colitis, including ulcerative colitis, Crohn disease, amebic colitis, pseudomembranous colitis, and other infections (*Shigella, Salmonella,* Chagas disease, and cytomegalovirus [CMV]).
- Toxic megacolon has been reported to complicate 1% to 13% of all ulcerative colitis cases and 2% to 3% of Crohn colitis cases.
- Although mortality in early series was as high as 25%, reaching 50% if colonic perforation occurred, early recognition and management of toxic megacolon has substantially lowered mortality to below 15% generally and, in experienced centers, usually below 2%.
- Factors associated with increased mortality include age older than 40 years, the presence of colonic perforation, and delay of surgery.
- Colonic perforation, whether free or localized, is the greatest risk factor leading to increased morbidity or death.

Predisposing Factors

- The severity of disease activity is the most important predictor of toxic megacolon, which is more common in extensive colitis than in proctitis or proctosigmoiditis.
- Limited right- or left-sided segmental colitis has also been associated with toxic megacolon.
- Toxic megacolon typically occurs early in the course of ulcerative colitis, usually within the first 5 years of disease; 25% to 40% of cases present with the initial attack.
- The onset of toxic megacolon has been temporally linked to diagnostic examinations such as barium enemas or colonoscopy, suggesting that manipulation of the inflamed bowel or vigorous laxative preparation may exacerbate the process, possibly through electrolyte imbalance.
- Certain drug therapies have been implicated in the development of toxic megacolon. Diphenoxylate atropine sulfate (Lomotil), loperamide, and other inhibitors of colonic motility such as opiates and narcotics may contribute to the development of toxic megacolon.
- Electrolyte and pH disturbances are risk factors for toxic megacolon. Severe potassium depletion, secondary to significant diarrhea or corticosteroid therapy, or both, is known to inhibit colonic motility.
- Despite early speculations regarding the role of corticosteroids in inducing toxic megacolon, most no longer accept this idea. Concern remains, however, that corticosteroids may suppress signs of perforation, thereby delaying surgical therapy.
- CMV infection may contribute to fulminant colitis or toxic megacolon. There are no controlled trials regarding the utility of treating CMV and, often, in the absence of systemic manifestations of CMV (e.g., fever, hepatitis), no treatment is necessary.

TABLE 109.2

JALAN'S CRITERIA FOR DIAGNOSIS OF TOXIC MEGACOLON

1. Radiographic evidence of colonic dilatation
2. At least three of the following:
   a. Temperature >38.5°C
   b. Heart rate >120 bpm
   c. White blood cell count >10.5 ($\times10^3$/μL)
   d. Anemia
3. At least one of the following:
   a. Dehydration
   b. Mental status changes
   c. Electrolyte disturbances
   d. Hypotension

Jalan KN, Sircus W, Card WI, et al. An experience of ulcerative colitis. I. Toxic dilation in 55 cases. *Gastroenterology.* 1969;57(1):68–82.

Clinical Features

- Toxic megacolon usually occurs in the background of chronic inflammatory bowel disease.
- Clinical criteria based on signs, symptoms, and diagnostic abnormalities for toxic megacolon are listed in Table 109.2.
- The presentation typically evolves with progressive diarrhea, bloody stools, cramping abdominal pain, and abdominal distention. Impaired consciousness and lethargy may be present and are ominous signs.
- Occasionally, in chronically treated patients, a paradoxical decrease in stool frequency with passage of only bloody discharge or bloody membranes may be an ominous sign. Thereafter, clinical signs of toxemia, including pyrexia (temperature >38.5°C) and tachycardia, develop as abdominal pain and distention become progressive and bowel sounds diminish or cease.
- On physical examination, peritoneal irritation, including rebound tenderness and abdominal guarding, represent transmural inflammation with serosal involvement, even in the absence of free perforation. Conversely, peritoneal signs may be minimal or absent in elderly patients or those receiving high-dose or prolonged corticosteroid therapy.
- In such patients, loss of hepatic dullness may be the first clinical indication of colonic perforation.
- Mental status changes, including confusion, agitation, and apathy, are occasionally noted.
- Leukocytosis, defined as total white blood cell count >10,500 cells/μL, with a left shift, anemia, hypokalemia, and hypoalbuminemia are common laboratory findings.

Diagnosis

- Plain films of the abdomen are usually sufficient radiographic studies, revealing loss of haustration with segmental or total colonic dilatation (see Table 109.2).
- The magnitude of dilatation may not be severe, averaging **8 to 9 cm** (normal is <5–6 cm), although colonic diameter may reach 15 cm before rupture.
- Clinical studies have demonstrated a strong correlation between colonic dilatation and deep ulceration involving the muscle layers.

- Maximal dilatation can occur in any part of the colon. Accompanying mucosal thumbprinting or pneumatosis cystoides coli reflects severe transmural disease.
- Free peritoneal air should serve as an immediate indication for surgery.
- Infrequently, retroperitoneal tracking of air from a colonic perforation may produce subcutaneous emphysema and pneumomediastinum without pneumoperitoneum.
- In patients with severe colitis, small bowel ileus may herald toxic megacolon and is a bad prognostic sign for medical success.
- Discrepancies may exist between physical and radiographic findings. Abdominal distention by physical examination can be minimal despite massive colonic dilatation. Conversely, physical findings may dominate the presentation, and peritoneal signs in the absence of free air or dilatation should not be ignored.

Management

- Just as in fulminant colitis, a coordinated team approach between medical and surgical services to management and monitoring is necessary in patients with toxic megacolon.

Medical Treatment

- The initial treatment is supportive and similar to treatment outlined for fulminant colitis.
- Aggressive resuscitation with **fluids, electrolytes, and blood** is necessary. Blood transfusions should be given to maintain a hematocrit at about 30%.
- Patients with nausea and vomiting or significant abdominal pain should be on complete bowel rest.
- Anticholinergic and narcotic agents should be discontinued immediately. In the presence of small bowel ileus, a nasogastric tube is usually placed, and despite a lack of clear evidence for the placement of long intestinal tubes, they are advocated by some.
- Patient repositioning from front to back or prone knee–elbow position may redistribute colonic air and assist in decompression.
- Rarely, patients with dilatation in the absence of toxic signs or symptoms may benefit from rectal tube decompression.
- **Broad-spectrum antibiotics,** with adequate Gram-negative and anaerobic coverage, are considered standard therapy and should be administered without delay once transmural inflammation or toxic megacolon is suspected.
- Antibiotics should be continued until the patient stabilizes over several days to a week or through the initial postoperative period.
- Whether antibiotics help avert progression of toxic megacolon is not known.
- Generally, most patients with inflammatory bowel disease (IBD) will have been receiving corticosteroids before toxic megacolon developed, in which case they should be continued.
- Similar to therapy for fulminant colitis, augmented doses of corticosteroids should be administered in view of the additional stress of the toxic state. Close monitoring is necessary as there is concern that corticosteroids could mask signs of perforation or peritonitis.

- In cases of toxic megacolon caused by infectious etiologies, corticosteroids should not be used.
- Just as in fulminant colitis, there is no consensus regarding the corticosteroid preparation for treatment in toxic megacolon.

Surgical Management

- After **12 to 24 hours** of intensive medical management, if no improvement or deterioration occurs, surgical intervention is required for toxic megacolon.
- Some physicians actually view early surgical management of toxic megacolon as the conservative approach, noting that delay of operative therapy may promote higher mortality.
- Evidence of colonic perforation is an unequivocal indication for emergent surgery. If physical signs of perforation are absent, 12- to 24-hour radiographic surveillance is necessary.
- Perforation is associated with severe complications, including peritonitis, extreme fluid and electrolyte imbalance, and hemodynamic instability. Early recognition of perforation should lessen morbidity or mortality.
- Other indications for emergent surgery precluding protracted medical management include signs of septic shock, multiorgan dysfunction, and imminent transverse colon rupture (diameter >12 cm).
- Hypoalbuminemia, persistently elevated C-reactive protein or erythrocyte sedimentation rate, small bowel ileus, and deep colonic ulcers are poor prognostic factors for successful medical therapy.
- The surgical management of toxic megacolon must be individualized for each patient. The type of operation is dependent on the clinical condition of the patient and the experience of the surgeon. The types of surgery are outlined in the fulminant colitis section.
- Rarely, "blow-hole" colotomies may be useful in highly selected individuals with poor operative prognoses.

COMPLICATING SCENARIOS IN INFLAMMATORY BOWEL DISEASE

Thrombosis

- Inflammatory bowel disease is associated with an increased risk of **arterial and venous thromboembolism.**
- The prevalence of thromboembolism in IBD patients is as low as 1% to 8% and as high as 39% in a postmortem study.
- The mechanism is unclear, but systemic inflammation is considered a potent prothrombotic stimulus. In addition, coagulation factor abnormalities—factor V Leiden, decreased antithrombin III, protein C and S, increased levels of factors V and VIII, fibrinogen, and plasminogen activator inhibitor—contribute to the hypercoagulable state.
- **Deep vein thrombosis** and pulmonary embolism are the most common presentation of thrombosis in IBD.
- **Portal vein thrombosis** in IBD has 50% mortality and occurs in 9% of patients with deep vein thrombus.
- **Mesenteric vein thrombosis** occurs in about 5% of patients who undergo total colectomy for IBD.
- Approximately 10% of thromboembolisms in IBD manifest as cerebral vascular accidents.

- The treatment of deep vein thrombosis in IBD patients is similar to non-IBD patients. Options include unfractionated heparin, low-molecular-weight heparins, and warfarin for venous thrombosis.
- Those with contraindications to anticoagulation require an inferior vena cava filter to prevent pulmonary embolus. Thrombolytics can be used for large pulmonary emboli.
- Arterial thrombosis treatment in IBD includes surgical thrombectomy or fibrinolysis.

Managing Pregnant Women with Inflammatory Bowel Disease

- A team approach with early management and continuous assessment by the obstetrician, surgeon, and gastroenterologist is vital for the patient.
- The treatment of fulminant colitis and toxic megacolon in the pregnant woman is similar to the nonpregnant patient. However, continued severe illness poses a greater risk to the fetus than the medical or surgical intervention.
- Diagnostic modalities of ultrasound and **magnetic resonance imaging** (MRI) are safe and can be used for detection of abscess or colonic wall thickening and dilation.
- Low-dose radiographs (<5 rads) have minimal risk to fetus.
- Flexible sigmoidoscopy is a valuable tool to assess the severity of disease and anatomic extent of disease. It is considered a safe procedure to perform when indicated. In contrast, full colonoscopy is rarely indicated.
- Polyethylene glycol solution has not been studied in pregnancy; thus, fetal outcomes are unknown. Generally, oral bowel preparations are not recommended and, if a full colonoscopy is necessary, tap water enemas are recommended.
- The indications for surgery—medically refractory severe colitis, obstruction, perforation, and intractable bleeding—are the same as in the nonpregnant IBD patient.
- Surgery for an acute indication in the setting of pregnancy carries a high risk of fetal loss, but case reports of deliveries of healthy infants following colectomy for fulminant colitis are reported.
- There is no evidence that therapeutic abortion improves the outcome of fulminant colitis, so it is not indicated.

Gastrointestinal Bleeding

- Massive gastrointestinal bleeding is an unusual complication in IBD, occurring in 0.9% to 6% of patients.
- The general management is the same as in non-IBD patients. Resuscitation is the first step, followed by diagnostic evaluation—usually with endoscopy—to localize the site of bleeding.
- Colonoscopy can be used to identify the source of bleeding in IBD patients with a reported success rate of 60%.
- Angiography may be used in cases where colonoscopy is not diagnostic.
- Conservative therapy has been advocated, but surgery is indicated when bleeding is not stabilized by transfusions or if recurrent massive bleeding is present.

CHAPTER 110 ■ MESENTERIC ISCHEMIA

- Mesenteric ischemia is a generic term that implies inadequate blood flow to the intestines. It is relevant from a clinical standpoint as two separate disease processes:
  - acute mesenteric ischemia (AMI)
  - chronic mesenteric ischemia (CMI)
- Although the underlying process is similar (i.e., inadequate intestinal blood flow), the clinical presentation, diagnostic concerns, and treatment algorithms are different.
- CMI is almost exclusively related to visceral artery occlusive disease from atherosclerosis and is relevant to intensive care physicians primarily because of the multiple organ dysfunction that occurs after revascularization.
- AMI results from a broad spectrum of underlying conditions including arterial emboli, *in situ* thrombosis in the setting of visceral arterial occlusive disease, mesenteric venous thrombosis, nonocclusive mesenteric ischemia (NOMI), and acute aortic dissections. AMI is relevant to intensivists not only because of the early postoperative concerns, but also because it can occur in critically ill patients with other active problems (e.g., post-coronary artery bypass, acute pancreatitis). A thorough understanding of both clinical entities is essential for all intensive care physicians.

CHRONIC MESENTERIC ISCHEMIA

Pathophysiology

- The underlying pathophysiology of CMI is the inability to achieve postprandial hyperemic intestinal blood flow.
- Intestinal blood flow in the normal fasting state is fairly modest but increases markedly postprandially. In the presence of significant arterial occlusive disease, this postprandial hyperemia is not possible and patients develop ischemic pain similar to angina pectoris, appropriately termed **mesenteric angina.**
- The normal visceral circulation is fairly redundant and has a rich collateral network. The symptoms of mesenteric ischemia usually do not occur unless two of the three visceral vessels (i.e., celiac axis, superior mesenteric artery, inferior mesenteric artery) are significantly diseased.
- However, symptoms may occur with isolated disease in the superior mesenteric artery in the absence of adequate collaterals.
- The majority of visceral artery stenoses are due to atherosclerosis. Other causes, less common, include neurofibromatosis, fibromuscular disease, rheumatoid disorders, aortic dissection, radiation, Buerger disease, and certain drugs.
- The risk factors for visceral artery atherosclerosis are the same as those for the other vascular beds.
- The atherosclerotic process usually involves just the origin of the visceral vessels.

- Patients with occlusive disease in the celiac axis and superior mesenteric artery frequently have renal artery lesions (and vice versa).
- Symptomatic CMI is relatively rare despite the prevalence of visceral artery stenoses. Indeed, a hemodynamically significant visceral artery stenosis (>50% diameter reduction) is noted in up to 27% of patients with peripheral arterial occlusive disease undergoing arteriography and in up to 5 to 10% of unselected patients at autopsy.

Clinical Presentation and Diagnosis

- Most patients with CMI are **cachectic, elderly women** with strong **smoking** histories.
- CMI is more common in women, with a reported ratio of approximately 3:1.
- The mean age of patients undergoing surgery for CMI is 66 years of age. However, CMI may also be found in patients in their fourth and fifth decades of life.
- Abdominal pain is usually the presenting symptom. It initially occurs **postprandially** but may progress to a persistent nature in the latter stages of the disease process.
- Mesenteric angina has no specific characteristics but patients develop a fear of food and avoid eating. The net result is **weight loss** with a mean of 20 to 30 lb in several clinical series.
- Patients may develop nausea or vomiting, constipation, or diarrhea. AMI is a fairly strong cathartic, and motility symptoms rather than pain may be the predominate symptom.
- Patients with CMI frequently have evidence of systemic vascular disease, although there are no characteristic physical findings.
- Although the appearance and clinical presentation of patients with CMI is fairly characteristic, the differential diagnosis of patients with abdominal pain and weight loss is extensive and includes gastrointestinal malignancy first and foremost.
- CMI is usually not considered by most primary care providers, and this is reflected by the fact that the mean duration from presentation to diagnosis exceeds a calendar year and 2.8 diagnostic tests.
- The initial diagnostic workup for patients with abdominal pain and weight loss should include esophagogastroduodenoscopy, colonoscopy, abdominal ultrasound, and an abdominal/pelvic computed tomography (CT) scan.
- Notably, **gastric ulcers** are relatively common in patients with CMI and likely result from ischemia.
- A surprising number of patients are subjected to **cholecystectomy** as part of their workup before the definitive diagnosis of CMI is made.
- **Mesenteric duplex scan** is an excellent *screening* tool for visceral artery stenosis with reported sensitivity and specificity rates of approximately 80%. However, it is technically

challenging, operator dependent, and not available in all centers.

- Various provocative tests have been proposed to unmask clinically significant visceral artery stenoses, although their utility is unclear and they have not achieved widespread use.
- **CT arteriography** has largely replaced catheter-based contrast arteriography as the *diagnostic* study of choice for patients with CMI and is usually sufficient to plan open surgical revascularization.
- CT arteriography is safe, noninvasive, and almost universally available. It is very good for identifying occlusive disease in the superior mesenteric artery and celiac axis.
- CT arteriography is also useful for identifying the presence of collateral vessels between the visceral vessels and/or the internal iliac arteries. Additionally, it is very good for evaluating other intra-abdominal processes.
- The major advantage of contrast arteriography over CT arteriography is that therapeutic interventions can be performed at the time of the diagnostic procedure. However, it is an invasive procedure with a small but finite complication rate.
- A lateral arteriogram is mandatory as part of the examination to accurately assess the origins of the celiac axis and superior mesenteric artery due to their anterior/posterior orientation.
- The significant findings on arteriogram include ostial stenoses of the celiac axis and superior mesenteric artery, the presence of visceral collaterals, and the presence of central aortic atherosclerotic disease.
- A small percentage of patients with CMI may have visceral artery aneurysms, presumably from increased flow through the collateral vessels.
- **Magnetic resonance (MR) arteriography** has been used as a diagnostic study for patients with CMI and offers many of the advantages of CT arteriography. However, it is not as universally available as CT arteriography.
- Furthermore, it is not practical and may be contraindicated for many patients including those in the intensive care unit. Last, MR arteriography tends to overestimate the degree of stenosis in the visceral vessels.

Treatment Strategies

- The natural history of the untreated disease process is death either from inanition or bowel infarction and thus, all patients with CMI require treatment.
- Theoretical treatment options include medical management with total parenteral nutrition or revascularization by either endovascular or open surgical techniques.
- The role of long-term parenteral nutrition is very limited. Additionally, patients with CMI may not be able to metabolize the parenteral nutrition.
- **Endovascular treatment** (angioplasty with or without stenting) has emerged as the initial revascularization option for most patients with CMI but should be viewed as an alternative to the open surgical approach.
- Endovascular treatment has consistently been shown to have a lower mortality rate, a lower complication rate, and shorter hospital length of stay when compared to open surgical revascularization. However, the patency rates for the endovascular approach are lower.

- Decreased patency rates have not been associated with a decrease in survival, and vessel thrombosis and/or recurrent stenosis has not necessarily resulted in AMI.
- The endovascular approach can serve as an excellent bridge to open surgical revascularization for debilitated patients who are poor initial candidates for a major surgical procedure.
- The recent development of lower-profile (i.e., smaller-diameter) angioplasty balloon/stent systems has further extended the applications of the endovascular approach, and reasonable short-term results have been reported for patients with occluded (versus stenotic) vessels.

Endovascular Revascularization

- The preoperative evaluation prior to endovascular treatment is essentially the same for all catheter-based contrast arteriography. Patients with a contrast allergy should be treated with an appropriate steroid preparation.
- Patients with elevated serum creatinine levels (serum creatinine 1.5–2.0 mg/dL) should receive gentle **hydration and acetylcysteine,** although admittedly their benefits are somewhat unsubstantiated.
- A flush aortogram is performed in both the anteroposterior and lateral projections. Since most lesions in the superior mesenteric artery and celiac axis are orificial and located in the proximal 2 cm, selective catheterization is not usually necessary unless a distal lesion is suspected or the extent of the lesion cannot be determined.
- A **>50% diameter reduction of the superior mesenteric artery** is usually considered clinically significant regardless of whether or not the celiac axis is involved. In contrast, the diagnosis of CMI should be questioned in the presence of an isolated celiac axis stenosis.
- Symptomatic stenoses can be treated at the time of the diagnostic arteriogram. The orificial stenoses in the mesenteric vessels are refractory to angioplasty alone, and primary stenting is recommended.
- Balloon angioplasty with selective stenting is reserved for midsegment lesions. Balloon-expandable stents (vs. self-expanding stents) are preferred for the orificial stenoses due to their superior radial forces and controlled deployment mechanism.
- The postoperative care after mesenteric angioplasty/stenting is comparable to that for other peripheral endovascular procedures.

Open Surgical Revascularization

- The preoperative workup for patients undergoing open mesenteric revascularization is comparable to that for other major vascular surgical procedures and includes optimization of all organ systems.
- Multiple algorithms have been developed to reduce the **cardiac risk** for vascular surgical patients undergoing noncardiac procedures, although their utility is unclear given the results of several recent publications.
- Regardless of the specific preoperative cardiac evaluation, all patients should likely be on aspirin, a beta-blocker (if not contraindicated), and a cholesterol-lowering agent (preferably a statin/HMG Co-A reductase inhibitor). A CT or contrast arteriogram is mandatory to both confirm the diagnosis and plan the operative procedure.
- Various open surgical procedures have been reported, although the antegrade aortoceliac/superior mesenteric artery

bypass and the retrograde aortosuperior mesenteric artery bypass are the most common.

- The advantages of the antegrade aortoceliac/superior mesenteric bypass are that both visceral vessels are revascularized and that the supraceliac aorta (the origin of the bypass) is usually free of atherosclerotic occlusive disease. The major disadvantage is the complexity of the procedure.
- In contrast, retrograde aortosuperior mesenteric artery bypass is relatively straightforward, although only a single vessel is revascularized and the graft is prone to kinking given its obligatory retrograde course that traverses both caudal to cephalad and posterior to anterior.
- The optimal choice for a specific patient is contingent on his or her comorbidities with the retrograde bypass generally reserved for patients who will not tolerate the more complex antegrade procedure.
- The immediate postoperative care for patients undergoing revascularization for CMI is frequently complicated by the development of **multiple organ dysfunction** and is distinctly different from that associated with most other abdominal vascular surgical procedures such as aortobifemoral bypass for aortoiliac occlusive disease.
- This propensity to develop multiple organ dysfunction likely accounts for the prolonged intensive care and total hospital length of stays and is one of the leading causes of death in the postoperative period.
- The responsible mechanism for this multiple organ dysfunction is likely the visceral ischemia and **reperfusion phenomenon** inherent to the revascularization. This process has been reported to induce a complex response involving several interrelated inflammatory mediators that have the potential to cause both local and distant organ injury.
- Multiple organ dysfunction syndrome (MODS) occurs after revascularization for both AMI and CMI as demonstrated by marked elevations in serum hepatic transaminases over a 7- to 10-day period, the development of a transient coagulopathy and **thrombocytopenia** below 40,000/μL within 12 to 24 hours, and the development of a significant pulmonary injury.
- The **pulmonary injury** associated with revascularization of AMI or CMI is characterized by an elevated mean shunt fraction and a radiographic picture of the acute respiratory distress syndrome that manifested between 1 to 3 days and persists for 5 to 8 days.
- The optimal management strategy for patients in the early postoperative period after mesenteric revascularization is to support the individual organ systems until the MODS resolves.
- Not all patients develop organ dysfunction, but the incidence is quite high and unpredictable.
- The optimal ventilator management remains unresolved, but it is possible to extubate patients in the early postoperative period when they satisfy the various weaning criteria.
- The thrombocytopenia and coagulopathy are usually managed expectantly with platelet and/or plasma transfusions reserved for severely depressed platelet counts and/or any clinical evidence of bleeding.
- The inherent coagulopathy after mesenteric revascularization does not appear to be responsive to vitamin K.
- Patients should be maintained on total parenteral nutrition throughout the postoperative period until their bowel function returns. This is particularly important given the fact that

most patients are severely compromised from a nutritional standpoint.

- Patients may have a **prolonged ileus** after revascularization and parenteral nutrition is required for some time.
- The bypass should be interrogated prior to discharge to confirm the technical adequacy of the reconstruction.
- Patients with acute changes in their clinical status should also undergo visceral imaging to confirm that their bypass is patent.
- It can be difficult to differentiate MODS from AMI secondary to graft thrombosis. Serum lactate levels may be helpful in this setting.
- All patients who undergo revascularization for CMI require long-term follow-up. Patients are usually seen frequently in the early postoperative period until all their active issues resolve and then every 6 months thereafter with a mesenteric duplex to confirm graft patency.
- Objective assessment of graft patency is critical and significantly better than the return of symptoms that has been used as a surrogate marker. All abnormalities on duplex imaging merit further investigation with additional imaging and/or intervention.
- Diarrhea is a common complaint after revascularization for CMI and can persist for several months. It is more common in patients with preoperative diarrhea and can be so severe that it necessitates total parenteral nutrition.
- The cause of the diarrhea is unclear but may be related to intestinal atrophy, bacterial overgrowth, or disruption of the mesenteric neuroplexus.

Outcome

- The outcome after mesenteric revascularization for CMI is quite good. The perioperative mortality rate after open surgical revascularization is <15%, whereas that for the endovascular treatment is <5%.
- The corresponding complication rates are approximately 30% and 15% for the open and endovascular treatments, respectively.
- The initial technical success rate for the endovascular treatment is ~90%. The objectively documented 5-year patency rates after open revascularization are ~75%; patency rates after endovascular treatment are not as well described, but likely fall short of those reported for the open treatment.
- The 5-year survival after either treatment is ~75%, and most patients return to their presymptoms weight.

ACUTE MESENTERIC ISCHEMIA

- Mesenteric **emboli** and *in situ* **thrombosis** are the most common causes of AMI and account for approximately 50% and 25% of the cases, respectively. Nonocclusive mesenteric ischemia (NOMI, 20%), mesenteric venous thrombosis (5%), and aortic dissections account for the balance.
- Impaired intestinal perfusion leads to mucosal compromise, the release of the intracellular contents, and the influx of substances (including bacteria) from the lumen of the bowel and may lead to the activation of the **systemic inflammatory response.**

- If the impaired perfusion persists, bowel infarction with perforation and peritonitis ensues.
- The immediate clinical concerns for patients with AMI are to reverse the underlying clinical condition and prevent bowel infarction.
- The optimal therapy requires prompt diagnosis and definitive treatment, although this is often difficult given the susceptible patient population and common clinical scenarios.
- The morbidity and mortality associated with AMI are significant. The mortality of patients with AMI and portal/mesenteric venous gas is 86%.

Embolus

Pathophysiology

- Emboli responsible for AMI usually originate from the **heart** and lodge in the superior mesenteric artery. The intracardiac thrombus is related to either atrial fibrillation, an acute myocardial infarction, or a ventricular aneurysm.
- Patients frequently have prior embolic events from the same source, although they are not necessarily limited to the superior mesenteric artery (e.g., common femoral artery bifurcation presenting with acute lower extremity ischemia).
- The extent of bowel ischemia and/or infarction after an embolus to the superior mesenteric artery is contingent on the extent of the collateral circulation, the pattern of the arterial occlusion, and the duration of the ischemia.
- In AMI, the bowel progresses from ischemia to infarction in a time-dependent fashion, although it may remain viable for 6 to 12 hours.
- Acute embolic occlusion of the superior mesenteric usually results in ischemia/infarction of the bowel from the proximal jejunum to the transverse colon. The duodenum and descending colon are usually spared due to separate arterial sources.

Clinical Presentation

- The diagnosis of AMI from an embolus (or other causes of AMI) may be difficult. The differential list of diagnoses includes all the more common causes of acute abdominal pain.
- The diagnosis is confounded by the fact that the patients are often critically ill, and thus, their history and physical examination may not be reliable.
- Diagnosis requires a high index of suspicion and an aggressive approach since delays in diagnosis adversely affect outcome.
- Patients with AMI from an embolus usually present with diffuse abdominal pain. The classic description of the pain secondary to AMI is **pain out of proportion to the physical findings,** although this scenario is not always present.
- Unfortunately, the pain is neither specific nor localized to a particular abdominal quadrant.
- Patients often experience nausea/vomiting and/or diarrhea, but again these are fairly nonspecific complaints.
- Peritoneal signs can be present, but they usually occur late in the process and suggest bowel perforation.
- The hemodynamic status of the patients at the time of presentation ranges from normovolemia to profound hypovolemic shock and is contingent on the status of the bowel and the duration of symptoms.

Laboratory Testing and Diagnostic Studies

- Routine chemistry and hematologic laboratory studies are usually nonspecific and insensitive. Patients frequently have an elevated white blood cell count, a decreased platelet count, an elevated hematocrit, and a mildly elevated amylase level.
- Patients with AMI frequently have either normal plain radiographs or demonstrate nonspecific findings (e.g., ileus) early in the disease process.
- **CT arteriography** is the diagnostic study of choice for patients with AMI secondary to an embolus. Notably, the study is performed using only intravenous contrast since both oral and rectal contrast potentially interfere with the arteriogram itself.
- In patients with AMI secondary to an embolus, a meniscus sign can often be seen in the mid- or distal superior mesenteric artery.
- The images obtained during CT arteriography are also excellent for the nonvascular structures. Significant nonvascular findings of AMI include bowel wall thickening, bowel wall gas, bowel or solid organ infarction, and hepatic or portal venous gas;
- Mesenteric duplex, although an excellent screening test for CMI, is not usually helpful in patients with AMI due to abdominal distention or gas.
- Standard contrast arteriography can be used as an alternative to CT arteriography. Major disadvantages are the obligatory time required to obtain the procedure and the small, but finite, complications associated with the contrast agent and vessel cannulation.
- **Laparoscopy** offers an additional diagnostic modality for patients with AMI. It can be used to assess the viability of the bowel and confirm the diagnosis. Furthermore, it can be performed in the intensive care unit with sedation and, therefore, is feasible for unstable patients with a suspected intra-abdominal process.
- Laparotomy remains the definitive diagnostic test for patients with AMI. However, the diagnostic studies outlined above are usually sufficient.

Treatment Strategies

- Patients should be taken emergently to the operating room for definitive treatment once the diagnosis of AMI from an embolus is made.
- Patients should be systemically **anticoagulated** with heparin to prevent further clot development and started on broad-spectrum **antibiotics** against enteric organisms.
- An extensive preoperative evaluation is unnecessary and may delay urgent and definitive therapy. There is no role for medical management alone in the setting of embolic AMI.
- Patients with AMI are frequently in shock and should be volume resuscitated prior to the induction of anesthesia. This should not delay transfer to the operating room.
- Both midline and transverse abdominal incisions provide adequate exposure to the visceral vessels, and the choice is contingent on surgeon preference.
- A distribution of ischemic/infarcted bowel that extends from the **proximal jejunum to the transverse colon** is consistent with a diagnosis of AMI. Intraoperative interrogation of the visceral vessels with continuous wave Doppler may further substantiate the diagnosis.

- The embolus may be extracted from the superior mesenteric artery using a Fogarty **thromboembolectomy catheter** through various surgical approaches.
- The easiest approach to the superior mesenteric artery is to incise the base of the transverse mesocolon after retracting the transverse colon itself cephalad.
- The arteriotomy in the superior mesenteric artery may be performed either longitudinally or horizontally. Although the longitudinal arteriotomy needs to be closed with a vein patch to prevent narrowing its lumen, it is the preferred approach because it affords greater flexibility in case a bypass procedure is necessary.
- The differentiation between viable and nonviable bowel is difficult. Various complicated modalities have been described but have not been universally adopted. Simple adjuncts include visual inspection for peristalsis, use of continuous wave Doppler to detect arterial signals within the mesentery, and intravenous fluorescein in combination with a Wood lamp.
- Bowel that is ischemic though not frankly necrotic should be revascularized and then reexamined before any final decision about resection. A conservative approach is justified in this setting because many of the borderline areas will remain viable after revascularization.
- Bowel that is obviously dead should be resected, and intestinal anastomoses should be avoided in favor of proximal and distal stomas.
- Approximately **100 to 150 cm** of small bowel is necessary for nutritional absorption.
- A decision to perform a **second-look operation** to reassess the viability of the bowel should be made at the time of the initial procedure. This is routinely performed 24 to 48 hours after the first procedure, a time usually sufficient for the marginal bowel to declare itself.
- A "damage control" operation may be justified in a small subset of unstable patients with AMI. This includes emergent laparotomy, resection of obviously dead bowel, and creation of proximal or distal stomas, leaving the abdomen open and deferring the definitive vascular or gastrointestinal procedure until later.
- Despite its definitive role for patients with CMI, there is likely little role for endovascular therapies in patients with AMI secondary to an embolus. The obligatory time for endovascular treatment, including chemical lysis, is too long given the threatened bowel and the potential to progress from ischemic bowel to infarcted bowel. Furthermore, it does not allow direct assessment of the bowel, and the chemical lysis may cause intestinal bleeding from mucosal sloughing.
- The postoperative course after embolectomy for AMI is similar to that after revascularization for CMI, although the incidence of postoperative complications and multiple organ dysfunction are greater.
- Revascularization may cause an ischemia or reperfusion injury that affects both local and distant organ systems. Accordingly, patients are at risk for developing an abdominal compartment syndrome. Bladder pressures can be measured, and the abdomen closure can be dissembled as necessary.
- Patients should be continued on broad-spectrum antibiotics throughout the early postoperative period. Furthermore, they need to be anticoagulated long term due to the potential for recurrent emboli.

Outcome

- The **mortality rate** for patients with AMI is approximately **70%,** and this rate has changed very little over the past several decades.
- Mortality rates for AMI from mesenteric venous thrombosis (32%) are better than those for arterial problems (54% to 77%) and the mortality rates for mesenteric emboli (54%) are better than those for *in situ* thromboses (77%). Most are due to multiple organ failure.
- Several factors associated with mortality are patient age, time to definitive surgery, shock, acidosis, leukocytosis, cardiac status, and coagulopathy.

In Situ Thrombosis

- Patients with visceral artery occlusive disease may also present with AMI secondary to *in situ* thrombosis.
- The presentation is **superimposed on the symptoms of CMI** in more than 50% of the patients and can usually be differentiated from the other causes of AMI by the history and clinical setting.
- The clinical presentation, diagnostic approach, and immediate postoperative care of patients with AMI secondary to *in situ* thrombosis is similar to that outlined above for embolic AMI, although the operative approach is somewhat different.
- Patients with AMI secondary to *in situ* thrombosis require a **mesenteric bypass.** Although antegrade aortoceliac/superior mesenteric artery bypass is probably the optimal bypass for CMI, retrograde bypass from the infrarenal aorta or common iliac artery is likely the optimal procedure for AMI.
- The main objective is to restore blood flow to the ischemic vascular bed as safely and expeditiously as possible. This usually requires only bypass to the superior mesenteric artery.
- Patients with isolated celiac axis stenosis rarely develop AMI because the **collateral blood flow** to the foregut is so good and the liver may be sustained on portal blood flow alone.
- Prosthetic conduits are relatively contraindicated in the setting of bowel infarction and/or perforation due to the potential for postoperative graft infection. Autogenous conduits with either saphenous or superficial femoral vein are suitable.
- The role of endovascular treatment for patients with AMI secondary to *in situ* thrombosis is likely limited for the reasons noted above for AMI secondary to an embolus.
- An appropriate imaging study (i.e., CT arteriogram, contrast arteriogram) should be obtained in the early postoperative period and the necessary treatment including anticoagulation and revascularization implemented in a timely fashion.

Nonocclusive Mesenteric Ischemia

Pathophysiology

- **Nonocclusive mesenteric ischemia** represents an abnormal or paradoxical mesenteric **vasoconstriction** characterized by the loss of autoregulation. Shock or circulatory stress normally causes mesenteric vasoconstriction in an attempt to maintain cerebral and/or cardiac perfusion. The mesenteric vasoconstriction ordinarily resolves when the underlying circulatory disorders are corrected; persistent vasoconstriction results in NOMI.
- There are multiple potential causes for NOMI, including cardiogenic shock, sepsis, burn injury, trauma, pancreatitis,

digitals, vasopressors, and renal failure. Indeed, almost any underlying condition that can precipitate shock or circulatory stress may precipitate NOMI.

Clinical Presentation and Diagnosis

- Similar to the other causes of AMI, the diagnosis of NOMI requires a high index of suspicion and the proper clinical setting.
- Patients may develop abdominal pain, although the physical examination is frequently unreliable due to the other active medical issues and altered sensorium.
- Laboratory abnormalities are common, including acidosis, leukocytosis, elevated lactate levels, and hyperamylasemia, but these are all relatively nonspecific markers of the underlying shock state.
- Contrast **arteriography** has traditionally been the diagnostic study of choice and is also potentially therapeutic. The significant findings on arteriogram for patients with NOMI include segmental stenosis or narrowing of the superior mesenteric artery in a **string-of-beads** appearance. Furthermore, there is narrowing of the branches of the superior mesenteric artery at their origins, spasm of the mesenteric arcades, and impaired filling of the intramural branches.
- The published experience with CT arteriography in the setting of NOMI is limited, although it likely affords the same advantages as contrast arteriography with fewer risks.

Treatment Strategies

- The initial treatment of patients with NOMI is **nonoperative** and directed at correcting the underlying condition that precipitated the circulatory stress. Specifically, patients should be resuscitated in an attempt to improve their **cardiac output** and systemic perfusion.
- All vasoactive drugs should be stopped (if possible), and patients should be started on broad-spectrum antibiotics directed against enteric organisms. Furthermore, patients should be systemically anticoagulated unless contraindicated.
- Despite these efforts, the characteristic mesenteric vasoconstriction may persist. Continuous intra-arterial papaverine, administered through an infusion catheter placed into the superior mesenteric artery, may reverse the vasoconstriction. A 45-mg test dose of **papaverine** (i.e., short-acting calcium channel blocker) should be given over 15 minutes, and a continuous infusion of 30 to 60 mg/hour should be started if no adverse reactions are encountered.
- **Serial mesenteric arteriograms** should be performed to monitor the response to the papaverine, with the first performed 1 hour after initiating therapy. The intra-arterial infusion may be continued up to 24 hours. It should be noted that the infusion will reverse the mesenteric vasoconstriction only if the underlying hemodynamic instability is corrected.
- Operative treatment of NOMI should be reserved only for the clinical scenario when bowel infarction is suspected.

Mesenteric Venous Thrombosis

Pathophysiology

- Mesenteric venous thrombosis may also result in AMI. However, the associated degree of bowel ischemia is usually less than with arterial occlusion from either an embolus or *in situ* thrombosis.
- Mesenteric venous thrombosis results in **edema in the bowel and mesentery** with significant third-space fluid losses. This may result in bloody ascites and, indeed, a bloody tap at the time of paracentesis may be diagnostic.
- Progression to bowel infarction is contingent on the magnitude of the clot load and its distribution. Clot localized to the portal or superior mesenteric vein does not usually lead to bowel infarction because of the collateral channels, whereas clot in the peripheral mesenteric veins is more likely to do so.
- The natural history of untreated mesenteric venous thrombosis is poor and almost universally progresses from bowel infarction to perforation and death.
- Mesenteric venous thrombosis may result from abnormalities in any of the components of the **Virchow triad** (i.e., stasis, intimal injury, hypercoagulable state). Stasis may result from congestive heart failure or portal hypertension, whereas intimal injury may result from general anesthesia or any number of intra-abdominal infectious processes. A hypercoagulable state is perhaps the strongest of the contributory factors and has been identified in up to 90% of patients with mesenteric venous thrombosis.

Clinical Presentation and Diagnosis

- Patients with mesenteric venous thrombosis usually present with **vague, mild abdominal pain.** The pain is usually insidious in onset and frequently present for some time before the patients seek medical attention. Furthermore, the pain is not usually localized to any specific quadrant.
- Physical examination is notable only for mild, diffuse abdominal pain. Peritoneal signs suggest bowel infarction, but are found only later in the disease process.
- An **abdominal CT** scan is the diagnostic study of choice. The significant findings include bowel edema and thrombus within the mesenteric veins with inflammation of the vessel wall.
- Plain abdominal radiographs may suggest abdominal wall edema and are helpful to rule out other causes of the abdominal pain.
- Standard catheter-based contrast arteriography may be helpful but is inferior to CT. The arteriographic findings that suggest mesenteric venous thrombosis include arterial spasm with a prolonged arterial phase, opacification of the bowel wall, extravasations of the contrast into the bowel lumen, and visualization of the venous thrombus.

Treatment Strategies

- The primary treatment of patients with mesenteric venous thrombosis is **anticoagulation.** Patients should be aggressively anticoagulated with heparin when the diagnosis is made and should be maintained on long-term oral anticoagulation.
- Similar to patients with massive iliofemoral deep venous thrombosis, it may be difficult to achieve effective anticoagulation initially using the standard dosing schedules for heparin, presumably secondary to the clot burden.
- Larger doses of heparin may be required, and the adequacy of heparinization (e.g., partial thromboplastin time) may need to be monitored more frequently.
- Although the required dosage of heparin may be unsettling, the potential clot propagation and its associated complications likely exceed any increased risk from bleeding.

- A **hypercoagulable workup** for the standard hematologic abnormalities should be performed prior to initiation of anticoagulation. However, long-term anticoagulation should be continued even in the absence of an *identifiable* hypercoagulable state since it is likely that many of these patients have some type of hypercoagulable disorder even though it may not be characterized on initial screening.
- Additionally, patients frequently require fluid resuscitation at the time of diagnosis due to the significant third-space losses from the bowel edema.
- Exploratory laparotomy should be reserved for cases in which bowel infarction is suspected. The intraoperative findings include edematous/rubbery bowel, bloody ascites, and thrombus within the mesentery.
- A wide resection of the bowel should be performed in the presence of infarction. Primary enteric anastomosis is probably safe if the margins of resection are free of thrombus within the mesentery. Proximal and distal stomas are advisable if the viability of the bowel at the margins of resection is questionable.
- Patients are at risk for additional or ongoing thrombosis with the most common site being the margins of the resection and/or the anastomosis. Mechanical thrombectomy is not advocated at the time of laparotomy because of the extensive clot burden.
- Endovascular treatment including chemical lysis likely has a limited role for patients with mesenteric venous thrombosis despite several case reports.

Outcome

- The mortality rate (~30%) for mesenteric venous thrombosis is significantly less than for the arterial causes of AMI.
- Death has been associated with portal vein thrombosis, systemic venous thromboembolism, and obesity. The increased mortality rate associated with venous thromboembolism underscores the importance of early, adequate anticoagulation.

Aortic Dissection

- Patients with acute aortic dissection can present with visceral malperfusion and AMI.
- The presence of visceral malperfusion significantly increases the mortality rate. Various endovascular approaches have been used to treat the visceral malperfusion in this setting.
- Endovascular revascularization is probably superior to the open approach provided the patients are candidates from an anatomic and technical standpoint.

COLON ISCHEMIA

- Isolated **colon ischemia** can occur after both open and endovascular aneurysm repair. Furthermore, it can develop as a complication of hemodynamic shock, similar to NOMI.

- Ischemic colitis has been reported to occur in approximately 2% to 13% of open aneurysm repairs. The reported incidence depends on the diagnostic algorithm and modality (routine sigmoidoscopy vs. selective sigmoidoscopy) and is dramatically increased after ruptured aneurysm repair.
- The incidence of colonic ischemia after ruptured aneurysm repair in patients undergoing routine colonoscopy is approximately 25% to 40%.
- The sigmoid colon is affected most frequently, although all the sections of the colon may be involved.
- The ischemia may result from inadequate resuscitation, disruption of collaterals, and/or failure to revascularize a hemodynamically significant inferior mesenteric artery.
- Interestingly, routine reimplantation of the inferior mesenteric artery at the time of aortic reconstruction does not prevent colon ischemia.
- The ischemic colitis associated with endovascular aneurysm repair is more commonly related to atheroembolism rather than acute internal iliac artery occlusion, as might be suspected. The prognosis for ischemic colitis after endovascular aneurysm repair is worse than that for open repair.
- Patients with ischemic colitis usually present with **bloody diarrhea** in contrast to patients with AMI who usually present with abdominal pain.
- In the most common scenario, patients develop bloody diarrhea on the first or second postoperative day after aortic reconstruction. However, the diagnosis should be considered after aortic reconstruction in the absence of bloody diarrhea in patients with thrombocytopenia, multiple-organ dysfunction, increasing abdominal pain/peritonitis, and generalized failure to thrive.
- The diagnosis may be confirmed by endoscopy. Although **sigmoidoscopy** is used most frequently, a complete colonoscopy is likely optimal due to the potential involvement of the other colon segments.
- Treatment depends on the endoscopic findings and clinical setting. The endoscopic findings range from mucosal ischemia to transmural necrosis. Unfortunately, it is often difficult to differentiate diffuse mucosal ischemia from transmural necrosis.
- Patients with mucosal ischemia alone should be treated with bowel rest, broad-spectrum antibiotics, total parenteral nutrition, and serial endoscopic examinations.
- Many of these lesions resolve spontaneously without long-term sequelae, although colonic strictures may develop in a small subset of patients. Patients with **transmural colonic necrosis** should undergo laparotomy with resection of the involved segment, a proximal diverting colostomy, and a distal Hartmann pouch.
- The reported mortality rate in patients with transmural colon necrosis after aortic reconstruction is ~85%.
- Maintaining antegrade flow through the internal iliac vessels, routinely implanting the inferior mesenteric artery, and preserving the colonic collateral circulation may reduce or prevent this adverse outcome.

CHAPTER 111 ■ ACUTE RENAL FAILURE (ARF)

- ARF is a major diagnostic and therapeutic challenge for critical care physicians.
  - *Acute renal failure* describes a syndrome characterized by rapid decrease in the kidney's ability to eliminate waste products.
    - Hours to days
  - Clinically manifested by accumulation of end products of nitrogen metabolism
    - Such as urea and creatinine
  - Other typical clinical manifestations include:
    - Decreased urine output (not always present)
    - Accumulation of nonvolatile acids
    - Increased concentration of potassium and phosphate

DEFINITION AND CLASSIFICATION OF ARF

- Depending on definition of presence
  - ARF reported in 5% to 25% of critically ill patients
  - Consensus definition and classification for ARF developed and validated in hospitalized and critically ill patients
    - Goes by the acronym of *RIFLE*
      - Divides renal dysfunction into the categories of risk, injury, and failure (Fig. 111.1)
      - Likely to be dominant approach to defining ARF in intensive care unit (ICU) for next 5 to 10 years
      - Using this classification incidence of at least some degree of renal dysfunction reported as high as 67%
      - Development of renal dysfunction with a maximum RIFLE category failure has been reported in up to 28% of critically ill patients
        - Associated with an increased risk of in-hospital death by several fold

ASSESSMENT OF RENAL FUNCTION

- Renal function involves:
  - Acid-base balance
  - Water balance
  - Tonicity control
  - Regulation of calcium and phosphate
  - Erythropoiesis
  - Disposal of some cytokines
  - Lactate removal
- In clinical context monitoring of renal function reduced to indirect assessment of glomerular filtration rate (GFR) by measurement of serum creatinine and urea
  - Waste products insensitive markers of GFR
  - Heavily modified by numerous factors such as age, gender, muscle mass, nutritional status, the use of steroids, the presence of gastrointestinal blood, or muscle injury

- Generally start becoming abnormal only when GFR is reduced by more than 50%
  - Thus fail to reflect dynamic changes in GFR
  - Can be grossly modified by aggressive fluid resuscitation
- Use of creatinine clearance via a 2- or 4-hour urine collection or of calculated clearance by means of formulae might increase accuracy of GFR estimation
  - Rarely changes clinical management
- Use of more sophisticated radionuclide-based tests cumbersome in the ICU
  - Useful only for research purposes
- Urine output (UOP) another commonly measured parameter of renal function
  - Often more sensitive to changes in renal hemodynamics than biochemical markers of solute clearance
  - Alone of limited value
    - Patients capable of developing severe ARF while maintaining normal UOP
      - *Nonoliguric ARF*

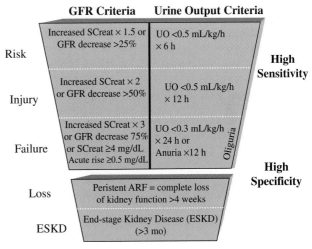

FIGURE 111.1. RIFLE (Risk, Injury, Failure, Loss, End-stage) classification scheme for acute renal failure. The classification system includes separate criteria for creatinine and urine output. The criteria that lead to the worst possible classification should be used. Note that RIFLE-F (F = failure) is present even if the increase in serum creatinine concentration (SCreat) is less than threefold so long as the new SCreat is >4.0 mg/dL (350 μmol/L) in the setting of an acute increase of at least 0.5 mg/dL (44 μmol/L). The designation RIFLE-FC should be used in this case to denote acute-on-chronic disease. Similarly when RIFLE-F classification is reached by urine output criteria only, a designation of RIFLE-FO should be used to denote oliguria. The shape of the figure denotes the fact that more patients (high sensitivity) will be included in the mild category, including some without actually having renal failure (less specificity). In contrast, at the bottom, the criteria are strict and therefore specific, but some patients with renal dysfunction might be missed. GFR, glomerular filtration rate; ARF, acute renal failure; UO, urine output.

– As this has lower mortality rate than oliguric ARF
– UOP is frequently used to differentiate ARF
○ Oliguria defined approximately as UOP <5 mL/kg/day or 0.5 mL/kg/hour
○ RIFLE classification has incorporated oliguria as an important measure for categories of severity of ARF (see Fig. 111.1)

EPIDEMIOLOGY

- Some acute renal injury demonstrated in most ICU patients; manifested by:
  - Albuminuria or loss of small tubular proteins
  - Inability to excrete a water, sodium, or amino acid load
  - Any combination of the above
- Syndrome of ARF occurs in 5% to 8% of all hospitalized patients
  - Incidence greater in ICU patients
    - Occurs in 5% to 25%, depending on definition and specific population studied
    - Incidence and mortality of ARF may be increasing
      ○ May be attributable to major shift from single-organ ARF to the multiorgan dysfunction syndrome typically seen in ICU patients
    - Risk factors for ARF in ICU patients include:
      ○ Older age
      ○ Male gender
      ○ Preexisting comorbid illness
      ○ Diagnosis of sepsis
      ○ Major surgery
      ○ Specifically cardiac surgery
      ○ Cardiogenic shock
      ○ Hypovolemia
      ○ Exposure to nephrotoxic drugs
      ○ Multiorgan dysfunction—specifically concomitant acute circulatory, pulmonary, and hepatic organ dysfunction—commonly associated with ARF

APPROACH TO CLINICAL CLASSIFICATION

- Most practical and useful approach to the etiologic diagnosis of ARF is to divide causes according to probable source of renal injury:

- Prerenal
- Renal (parenchymal)
- Postrenal

Prerenal Failure

- By far the most common in the ICU
- Kidney malfunctions predominantly because of systemic factors that decrease GFR
  - Renal blood flow (RBF) is diminished by:
    - Decreased cardiac output
    - Hypotension
    - Raised intra-abdominal pressure
      ○ Suspected on clinical grounds
      ○ Confirmed by measuring bladder pressure with a urinary catheter
      ○ Pressure > 25 to 30 mm Hg above the pubis prompts consideration of decompression
- If systemic cause of renal failure rapidly removed or corrected
  - Renal function improves and relatively rapidly returns to near normal levels
- If intervention is delayed or unsuccessful, renal injury becomes established
  - Days or weeks then necessary for recovery
- Several tests promoted to help identify development of established ARF
  - Measurement of urinary sodium
  - Fractional excretion of sodium, and other derived indices
  - Accuracy and significance questionable (Fig. 111.2)
    ○ Clinical value of tests in ICU patients receiving vasopressors, massive fluid resuscitation, and loop diuretics is low
    ○ Prerenal ARF and established ARF part of a continuum and that their separation has limited clinical implications
- Principles of management essentially the same:
  - Treatment of cause
  - Promptly resuscitating patient by using invasive hemodynamic monitoring to guide therapy

Parenchymal Renal Failure

- Used to define a syndrome where principal source of damage is within the kidney

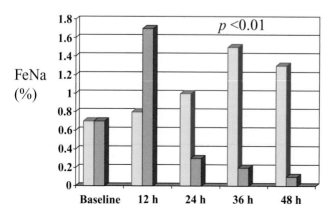

FIGURE 111.2. Histogram showing the effect of experimental sepsis in sheep on the fractional excretion of sodium (FeNa). FeNa decreased in sepsis as would be expected during decreased perfusion. In fact, all experimental animals had a two- to threefold increase in renal blood flow, providing proof of the concept that FeNa cannot be used to infer renal hypoperfusion.

TABLE 111.1

CAUSES OF PARENCHYMAL ARF

Glomerulonephritis
Vasculitis
Renovascular
Interstitial nephritis
Nephrotoxins
Tubular deposition/obstruction
Renal allograft rejection
Trauma

- Typical structural changes seen on microscopy
- Numerous disorders affecting the glomerulus or the tubule responsible (Table 111.1)
  - Nephrotoxins particularly important (Table 111.2)
  - Many cases of drug-induced ARF rapidly improve on removal of offending agent
- More than a third of patients developing ARF in ICU have chronic renal dysfunction, due to:
  - Age-related changes
  - Longstanding hypertension
  - Diabetes mellitus
  - Atheromatous disease of renal vessels
- Chronic renal disease may be manifest by an elevated serum creatinine
  - Not always the case
  - What may seem a relatively trivial insult not fully explaining the onset of ARF in a normal patient is sufficient to unmask lack of renal functional reserve in patient with chronic renal disease

Postrenal Failure

- Obstruction to urine outflow:
  - The most common cause of functional renal impairment in the community
  - Uncommon in the ICU
- Pathogenesis of obstructive ARF involves humoral responses as well as mechanical factors
  - Typical causes of obstructive ARF include:
    - Bladder neck obstruction from an enlarged prostate

TABLE 111.2

DRUGS THAT MAY CAUSE ACUTE RENAL FAILURE IN THE INTENSIVE CARE UNIT

Radiocontrast media
Aminoglycosides
Amphotericin
Nonsteroidal anti-inflammatory drugs
β-Lactam antibiotics (interstitial nephropathy)
Sulphonamides
Acyclovir
Methotrexate
Cisplatin
Cyclosporin A
FK-506 (tacrolimus)
Sirolimus

- Ureteric obstruction from pelvic tumors or retroperitoneal fibrosis
- Papillary necrosis
- Large calculi
- Clinical presentation of obstruction:
  - May be acute or chronic in patients with longstanding renal calculi
  - May not always be associated with oliguria
  - If obstruction is suspected, ultrasonography can be easily performed at the bedside
    - Not all cases of acute obstruction have an abnormal ultrasound.
    - In many cases, obstruction occurs in conjunction with other renal insults:
      ○ Staghorn calculi
      ○ Severe sepsis of renal origin
      ○ Sudden and unexpected development of anuria in an ICU patient suggests obstruction of urinary catheter as the cause.
        – Flushing or changing of catheter should be implemented in this setting

PATHOGENESIS OF SPECIFIC SYNDROMES

Hepatorenal Syndrome (HRS)

- A form of ARF that typically occurs in setting of advanced cirrhosis
  - Can occur with severe liver dysfunction due to alcoholic hepatitis or other forms of acute hepatic failure
- Pathogenesis of HRS is incompletely understood
  - Several potential mechanisms may contribute to HRS, including:
    - Activation of renin-angiotensin system in response to systemic hypotension
    - Activation of sympathetic nervous system in response to systemic hypotension and increased intrahepatic sinusoidal pressure
    - Increased release of arginine vasopressin due to systemic hypotension
    - Reduced hepatic clearance of various vascular mediators such as endothelin, prostaglandins, and endotoxin
- HRS can occur spontaneously in patients with advanced cirrhosis
  - Other precipitants more common
    ○ Sepsis—specifically, spontaneous bacterial peritonitis (SBP)
    ○ Raised intra-abdominal pressure due to tense ascites
    ○ Gastrointestinal bleeding
    ○ Hypovolemia due to paracentesis, diuretics and/or lactulose administration
    ○ Any combination of these factors
  - Other contributing factors for ARF should be routinely ruled out, including:
    ○ Cardiomyopathy due to alcoholism
    ○ Nutritional deficiencies
    ○ Viral infection
    ○ Exposure to nephrotoxins

- Typically, HRS develops in patients with advanced cirrhosis and evidence of portal hypertension with ascites, absent other apparent causes of ARF
  - Generally presents as oligoanuria, with progressive increases in serum creatinine and/or urea, along with bland urinary sediment
  - These patients develop profound sodium and water retention, with evidence of hyponatremia, a urine osmolality higher than that of plasma, and a very low urinary sodium concentration (<10 mmol/L)
- Management is challenging and includes:
  - Systematic identification and treatment of potential reversible precipitants
  - Attenuation of hypovolemia by albumin administration in patients with SBP shown to decrease incidence of ARF
  - Vasopressin derivatives (terlipressin) may improve GFR in this condition
  - Placement of a transjugular intrahepatic, portosystemic stent-shunt (TIPS) associated with modest improvements in kidney function in HRS
    - As well as improvement in outcome
    - Palliative measure for those who are not candidates or awaiting transplant
  - Treatment for reversal of ARF in these patients is to improve hepatic function with therapy for the underlying primary liver disease and/or referral for successful liver transplantation

ARF with Rhabdomyolysis

- Incidence of rhabdomyolysis-induced ARF estimated at 1% in hospitalized patients
  - In critically ill patients, may account for close to 5% to 7% of cases of ARF
- Pathogenesis involves interplay of prerenal, renal, and postrenal factors, including:
  - Concurrent hypovolemia
  - Ischemia
  - Direct tubular toxicity mediated by the heme pigment in myoglobin
  - Intratubular obstruction
- Causes of muscle injury resulting in rhabdomyolysis include:
  - Major trauma
  - Drug overdose such as occurs with narcotics, cocaine, or other stimulants
  - Vascular embolism
  - Prolonged seizures
  - Malignant hyperthermia
  - Neuroleptic malignant syndrome
  - Various infections such as pyomyositis, necrotizing fasciitis, influenza, human immunodeficiency virus (HIV)
  - Severe exertion
  - Alcoholism
  - Result of various agents that can interact to induce major muscle injury, such as the combination of macrolide antibiotics or cyclosporin and statins
- Clinical manifestations of rhabdomyolysis include:
  - Elevated serum creatine kinase
  - Evidence of pigmented granular casts
  - Red-to-brown coloring of the urine

- Patients can also have various electrolyte disorders including:
  - Hyperphosphatemia
  - Hyperkalemia
  - Hypocalcemia
  - Hyperuricemia
- Principles of prevention of ARF include:
  - Identification and elimination of potential causative agents and/or correction of underlying compartment syndromes
  - Prompt and aggressive fluid resuscitation and maintenance of polyuria
    - ≥1.5 to 2 mL/kg ideal or adjusted body weight/hour
      - Usually more than about 300 mL/hour
      - To restore vascular volume and potentially flush obstructing cellular casts
  - Urine alkalinization to a goal of pH >6.5
    - To reduce renal toxicity by myoglobin-induced lipid peroxidation and improve the solubility of myoglobin
  - Mannitol may act as a scavenger of free radicals and reduce cellular toxicity
    - Role of forced diuresis with mannitol controversial

ARF Due to Nephrotoxins

- Alterations in intrarenal hemodynamics is an important initial consequence of many nephrotoxins.
  - Changes to regional renal blood flow may occur through the increased activity of local vasoconstrictors such as angiotensin II, endothelin, adenosine.
  - Also diminished activity of important vasodilators such as nitric oxide and prostaglandins
    - Imbalance can lead to renal vasoconstriction and ischemia
      - Particularly to susceptible regions such as the outer medulla
        - For example, in response to radiocontrast media
    - Imbalance can induce humorally mediated vasoconstriction of afferent arterioles
      - For example, as a result of exposure to nonsteroidal anti-inflammatory drugs and cyclosporine
    - End result of a reduction in regional blood flow is a critical reduction in oxygen delivery, thus predisposing to tubular hypoxia
- Additionally nephrotoxins can directly contribute to impaired tubular metabolism and oxygen usage, for example, after exposure to aminoglycosides.
  - Lead to generation of oxygen-free radical species, including superoxide anions, hydrogen peroxide, hydroxyl radicals, reduced intrinsic antioxidant enzyme activity, intracellular calcium accumulation, mitogen-activated protein kinases, and phospholipase A_2
- Responses to nephrotoxins can induce tubular cell vacuolization, interstitial inflammation, altered cell membrane properties, and disruption of normal tubular adhesion to basement membranes.
  - Failure of these mechanisms contributes to tubular cell apoptosis and necrosis, as well as tubular sloughing into the luminal space, cast formation, and obstruction.
  - Raised intraluminal pressures due to obstruction, altered cellular permeability, and interstitial inflammation can contribute to backup diffusion of fluid and secondary edema formation.

- Radiocontrast media and aminoglycosides are leading agents contributing to nephrotoxin-induced ARF.
  - Radiocontrast media-induced toxicity believed to occur from interplay of alterations in renal hemodynamics due to vasoconstriction, increased intravascular viscosity and erythrocyte aggregation, direct tubular epithelial cell toxicity, and concomitant atheroembolic microshowers in the renovasculature
  - Aminoglycosides are taken up via organic anion transport systems in proximal tubules where they accumulate and generate oxygen-free radical species and increased intracellular calcium, which lead to tubular apoptosis, necrosis, and nonoliguric ARF.

Radiocontrast Nephropathy

- The leading cause of iatrogenic ARF in hospitalized patients
- Results in prolonged hospitalization, higher mortality rates, excessive health care costs, and potentially long-term kidney impairment
- Presents with acute rise in serum creatinine within 24 to 48 hours following injection of radiocontrast media
  - Serum creatinine level generally peaks within 3 to 5 days
  - Returns toward baseline within 7 to 10 days
  - In some patients, kidney function may not return to baseline, and a persistent reduction in function may occur.
- Often associated with preexisting risk factors:
  - Preexisting chronic kidney disease
    - GFR <60 mL/minute/1.73 m^2
  - Diabetes mellitus
  - Use of large quantities of radiocontrast media
- Strategies for prevention include:
  - Early identification of patients at risk and consideration either to delay the investigation or to use an alternative modality until kidney function can be optimized
  - Every effort should be made to correct volume depletion and discontinue potential nephrotoxins.
  - No evidence to support routine use of diuretics, mannitol, or dopamine
  - Periprocedure hydration and use of nonionic iso-osmolar (for example, iodixanol) radiocontrast media can reduce risk
  - Randomized trials and meta-analyses suggest potential benefit with use of N-acetylcysteine

Septic ARF

- Sepsis a leading predisposing factor to ARF in critically ill patients
- Epidemiologic studies estimate 45% to 70% of all ARF encountered in ICU is associated with sepsis
  - Distinction between septic and nonseptic ARF may have particular clinical relevance
  - Considering recent evidence to suggest that septic ARF may be characterized by a unique pathophysiology
  - Classic teaching is:
    - Sepsis brings about hypotension, reducing critical organ blood flow, including to the kidney, causing ischemic injury and ARF
    - Additionally sepsis leads to activation of sympathetic nervous system, stimulating potent vasoconstrictors release

that induce renal vasoconstriction and aggravate kidney ischemia, thus worsening ARF
- Recent data raise serious questions about this ischemic-induced paradigm of septic ARF.
  - A large mammalian model of hyperdynamic sepsis found that RBF was markedly increased above baseline despite significant reductions in kidney excretory function.
  - Small clinical studies of resuscitated patients with septic ARF also show increases in RBF.
  - Implications are that in hyperdynamic sepsis, ARF is hyperemic rather than ischemic, with global RBF considerably increased.
    - Regional cortical and medullary RBF is preserved in sepsis and can be further augmented by infusion of norepinephrine.
- Evolving evidence suggests pathogenesis of septic ARF predominantly involves toxic and immune-mediated mechanisms.
  - Sepsis releases a vast array of proinflammatory and anti-inflammatory mediators such as cytokines, arachidonic acid metabolites, and thrombogenic agents, all of which may participate in the development of ARF.
  - Evidence of renal tubular cell apoptosis in response to inflammatory mediators in endotoxemia
    - May prove to be an important mechanism of septic ARF in critically ill patients
    - Interventions with antiapoptotic properties such as:
      - Intensive insulin therapy
      - Human recombinant activated protein C
      - Selective caspase inhibitors
    - May aid in attenuating renal injury and promote recovery of function

ARF in Association with Major Surgery

- Common complication following major surgery:
- Incidence variable and dependent on prevalence of preexisting comorbid illnesses, preoperative kidney function, and the type and urgency of surgery being performed
- Intraoperative events can negatively affect kidney function, including:
  - Hemodynamic instability (e.g., intravenous or inhaled anaesthetic agents)
  - Hypovolemia due to blood loss or third spacing
  - Details of the operative field (e.g., aortic cross-clamping in major vascular surgery)
  - Increases in intra-abdominal pressure (e.g., laparoscopic insufflation of CO_2)
  - Concomitant sepsis
  - Use of nephrotoxin drugs
- Alone or in combination these contribute to critical reduction in RBF and ischemia, impaired oxygen delivery, and toxin- or inflammatory-mediated injury.
- Postoperative ARF believed partly mediated by proinflammatory mechanisms:
  - Increased endothelial cell adhesion
  - Tubular cell infiltration
  - Generation of reactive oxygen species and proinflammatory cytokines
  - Reperfusion injury

- Cardiac surgery with cardiopulmonary bypass (CPB) commonly induces early postoperative renal injury.
  - Mechanisms of CPB injury incompletely understood
    - Suggestion that CPB is proinflammatory, activating components of the nonspecific immune system
    - Leads to oxidative stress with the generation of oxygen-free radical species and serum lipid peroxidation products
    - CPB shown to deplete serum antioxidative capacity for a prolonged duration after surgery
      - Oxidant stress directly induces renal injury in experimental studies

ARF in Association with Mechanical Ventilation (MV)

- Application of positive pressure MV, particularly with positive end-expiratory pressure (PEEP), can have important physiologic effects on kidney function.
- Clear association between MV and PEEP and alterations in kidney function
- Can occur through several mechanisms including:
  - Alterations in cardiovascular function
  - Alterations in neurohormonal activation
  - Abnormalities in gas exchange
  - Alterations in systemic inflammatory mediators
- Positive pressure during MV increases intrathoracic, intrapleural, and intra-abdominal pressures.
  - During inspiration and for the duration of the respiratory cycle
  - Increased intrathoracic pressure can reduce intrathoracic blood volume, decrease transmural pressure, reduce right ventricular preload, increase right ventricular afterload, exert alterations to pulmonary vascular resistance and volume, and contribute to changes in left ventricular filling and geometry
    - Monitored clinically by changes in mean airway pressure
  - Result may be decreased cardiac output and renal perfusion
- Raised intrathoracic pressure alters transmural pressures and reduces cardiac output and can unload intrathoracic baroreceptors.
  - Initiates a cascade of compensatory neurohormonal events characterized by:
    - Increased systemic and renal sympathetic nervous activity
    - Increased activation of the renin–angiotensin–aldosterone system
    - Increased secretion of vasopressin
    - Reduction in release of atrial natriuretic peptide
  - Culminate in altered renal perfusion and kidney excretory function
    - Renal function may not be, *per se*, impaired with MV
    - Rather may appropriately respond to stimuli by reducing osmolar, sodium, and water clearance
- Acute hypoxemia and/or hypercapnia can act to alter systemic hemodynamics and increase systemic inflammation, both of which may exert negative effects on renal perfusion and function.
  - Particular strategies of MV, specifically in ARDS, contribute to or provoke ventilator-induced lung injury (VILI).
  - Pathophysiology of VILI multifactorial and results from combined effects of:
    - Volutrauma (excessive tidal or end-expiratory volumes)
    - Barotrauma (excessive end-inspiratory peak and plateau pressures)
    - Atelectatic trauma (cyclical opening and closing of alveolar units)
    - Biotrauma (local release of inflammatory mediators from injured lung)
  - Such injurious MV can initiate a cascade of events that increase systemic inflammation and adversely affect kidney function

THE CLINICAL PICTURE

- Most common clinical picture seen in the ICU is a patient who has sustained or is experiencing a major systemic insult, such as trauma, sepsis, myocardial infarction, severe hemorrhage, cardiogenic shock, or major surgery.
- Resuscitation is typically well under way, or surgery may have just been completed.
- Patient may already be anuric or profoundly oliguric, serum creatinine is rising, and a metabolic acidosis is developing; serum potassium and phosphate levels may be rapidly rising.
- Need for mechanical ventilation and vasoactive drugs is common.
- Fluid resuscitation typically undertaken with the guidance of invasive hemodynamic monitoring.
- Vasoactive drugs often used to restore mean arterial pressure (MAP) to acceptable levels
  - Typically >65 to 70 mm Hg
- Patient may improve over time, and urine output may return with or without the assistance of diuretic agents.
- If urine output does not return, renal replacement therapy (RRT) considered
  - If cause of ARF removed and patient is physiologically stable:
    - Slow recovery occurs within 4 to 5 days to as long as 3 or 4 weeks
    - In some cases, urine output can be above normal for several days.
  - If the cause of ARF has not been adequately remedied, patient remains gravely ill, the kidneys do not recover, and death from multiorgan failure may occur.

PREVENTING ARF

- Fundamental principle of ARF prevention is to treat its cause.
- If prerenal factors contribute, these must be identified and hemodynamic resuscitation quickly instituted.

Fluid Resuscitation

- Intravascular volume must be maintained or rapidly restored.
  - Often best done using invasive hemodynamic monitoring
    - Arterial cannula and central venous catheter, pulmonary artery catheter, or pulse contour cardiac output catheter
- Oxygenation must be maintained

- Adequate hemoglobin concentration, usually more than about 7.0 g/dL, must be maintained or immediately restored
- Once intravascular volume restored some patients remain with MAP <70 mm Hg
  - Autoregulation of RBF may be lost
  - Restoration of MAP to near normal levels may increase GFR
  - Such elevations in MAP require addition of vasopressor drugs
- Patients with preexisting hypertension or renovascular disease, MAP of 75 to 80 mm Hg may still be inadequate
  - Vasopressor support in hypotensive sepsis increases renal blood flow and renal medullary blood flow
  - Renal protective role of additional fluid therapy in patient with normal or increased cardiac output and blood pressure is questionable
  - Renal failure may still develop if cardiac output is inadequate.
    - May require various interventions, from the use of inotropic drugs to the application of ventricular assist devices

Fluid Therapy

- The cornerstone in resuscitation of the critically ill patient
  - Primary strategy for preservation of kidney function in the setting of increases in serum creatinine and/or urea and oliguria
  - Evidence has suggested there may be negative consequences to overly aggressive fluid therapy for both renal and nonrenal organ function.
    - No significant difference in incidence of ARF when comparing fluid resuscitation with crystalloid to albumin in critically ill patients
    - Some synthetic colloid therapies, such as hydroxyethyl starches, associated with higher rates of ARF in critically ill patients after resuscitation for severe sepsis
      - Exact mechanism(s) remain uncertain, the hydroxyethyl starches may influence intrarenal hemodynamics or glomerular filtration through alterations in vascular oncotic pressure
  - After apparent optimization of hemodynamics and intravascular volume status achieved
    - Little evidence to support continued aggressive fluid resuscitation to improve kidney function
    - Continued fluid administration and a positive cumulative balance can contribute to notable deteriorations in nonrenal organ function, in particular that of the lungs
    - Restrictive strategy improved lung function, increased ventilator-free days, and reduced ICU length of stay. Moreover, those in the restrictive group had a trend toward a reduced need for RRT

Renal Protective Drugs

Renal Dose or Low-Dose Dopamine

- Evidence of efficacy or safety of dopamine in critically ill patients is lacking
  - Is a tubular diuretic and occasionally increases urine output
  - Incorrectly interpreted as an increase in GFR

- Low-dose dopamine as effective as placebo in the prevention of renal dysfunction

Mannitol

- A biologic rationale exists for the use of mannitol, as is the case for dopamine
  - No controlled human data exist to support its clinical use.
  - Effect of mannitol as a renal protective agent remains questionable

Loop Diuretics

- May protect the loop of Henle from ischemia by decreasing its transport-related workload
  - Animal data are encouraging, as are *ex vivo* experiments
  - No double-blind randomized controlled studies of suitable size to prove that these agents reduce the incidence of renal failure
  - Loop diuretics may decrease the need for RRT in patients developing ARF
    - Achieve this by inducing polyuria
    - Allows for easier control of volume overload, acidosis, and hyperkalemia, the three major triggers for RRT in the ICU
    - Because avoiding dialysis simplifies treatment and reduces the cost of care, loop diuretics are occasionally used in patients with renal dysfunction, especially in the form of continuous infusion

Other Agents

- Other agents such as theophylline, urodilatin, and anaritide, a synthetic atrial natriuretic factor, have also been proposed.
- So far no beneficial effect
- Fenoldopam's role in ARF remains uncertain.
- Similarly, in a single-center study, recombinant human atrial natriuretic factor (rhANF) has been shown to attenuate renal injury in higher-risk patients undergoing cardiac surgery.
  - Large multicenter study of ARF failed to show a benefit

DIAGNOSTIC INVESTIGATIONS

- Etiologic diagnosis of ARF must always be established
  - Such diagnosis may be obvious on clinical grounds; it is best to consider all possibilities and exclude common treatable causes by simple investigations
    - Microscopic examination of the urinary sediment
      - Dysmorphic RBCs or RBC casts virtually diagnostic of active glomerulonephritis or vasculitis
      - Heavy proteinuria suggests some form of glomerular disease
      - White blood cell casts suggests interstitial nephropathy or infection
      - Normal urinalysis can provide important information
        – Suggests ARF is due to a prerenal or obstructive cause
      - Provides evidence of whether a urinary tract infection is present
  - Additional investigations may be necessary to establish diagnosis
    - Evidence of marked anemia in absence of blood loss may suggest acute hemolysis, thrombotic microangiopathy, or paraproteinemia related to malignancy
    - In microangiopathic hemolytic anemia, peripheral blood smear will typically show evidence of hemolysis

– With the presence of schistocytes

– Additional measurement of lactic dehydrogenase, haptoglobin, unconjugated bilirubin, and free hemoglobin are needed

○ If paraproteinemia due to multiple myeloma or lymphoma is suspected:

– Serum and urine protein electrophoresis and serum calcium should be measured

– History of recent cancer diagnosis or chemotherapy should prompt measurement of uric acid for tumor lysis syndrome

• For patients with possible mechanism for muscle injury:

○ Creatine kinase and free myoglobin for possible rhabdomyolysis should be determined

• An elevated anion gap metabolic acidosis with suggestion of a toxic ingestion:

○ Ethylene glycol, methanol, and salicylates should be measured

• Systemic eosinophilia a clue suggesting systemic vasculitis, allergic interstitial nephritis, or atheroembolic disease

• Measurement of specific antibodies—antiglomerular basement membrane (GBM), antineutrophil cytoplasmic antibodies (ANCA), antinuclear antibodies (ANA), anti-DNA, antismooth muscle, and cryoglobulins extremely useful screening tests to support the diagnosis of vasculitis or certain types of collagen vascular diseases or glomerulonephritis

• Imaging by renal ultrasonography a rapid noninvasive investigation principally designed to rule out:

• Obstruction

• Stones

• Cysts

• Masses

• Overt renovascular disease

• Chest radiograph important to assess for pulmonary complications of ARF and if diagnosis of systemic vasculitis is considered

• Occasionally percutaneous renal biopsy necessary to:

• Confirm diagnosis

• Determine severity of renal injury

• Guide therapy

• Estimate potential for renal recovery

• Indicated when thorough noninvasive investigation fails to yield diagnosis, when prerenal and postrenal causes are excluded, and prior to administration of aggressive immunosuppressive therapy

• Can be performed under ultrasound guidance with local anesthetic in critically ill patients undergoing mechanical ventilation without additional risks when compared to standard conditions

MANAGEMENT OF ESTABLISHED ACUTE RENAL FAILURE

• Principles of management of established ARF always include:

• Confirmation of probable cause

• Elimination of potential contributors

• Institution of disease-specific therapy if applicable

• Prevention and management of ARF complications with maintenance of physiologic homeostasis while recovery takes place

• Encephalopathy, pericarditis, myopathy, neuropathy, electrolyte disturbances, or other major electrolyte, fluid, or metabolic derangements are never events in a modern ICU.

• Prevented by several measures, from fluid restriction to the initiation of extracorporeal RRT

• Nutritional support must be started early and must contain adequate calories:

• Around 30 to 35 Kcal/kg/day, as a mixture of carbohydrates and lipids

• Sufficient protein of at least 1 to 2 g/kg/day needed

• No evidence of specific renal nutritional solutions are useful.

• Vitamins and trace elements should be administered at least according to their recommended daily allowance.

• Role of newer immunonutritional solutions controversial

• Enteral route is preferred to the use of parenteral nutrition

• Hyperkalemia

• Serum potassium level of >6 mmol/L

• Must be promptly treated either with:

• Insulin and dextrose administration

• Infusion of bicarbonate if acidosis is present

• Administration of nebulized salbutamol

• All of the above combined

• If "true" serum potassium is >7 mmol/L, or if electrocardiographic signs of hyperkalemia appear:

• Calcium gluconate, 10 mL of 10% solution administered intravenous used

• These measures are temporizing actions while RRT being arranged

• Presence of hyperkalemia a major indication for immediate institution of RRT

• Metabolic acidosis, almost always present, rarely requires treatment *per se*

• Anemia requires correction to maintain Hgb > about 7.0 g/dL

• More aggressive transfusion may be needed based on individual patient assessment

• Drug therapy adjusted to take into account effect of decreased clearances associated with loss of renal function

• Stress ulcer prophylaxis is advisable and should be based on H_2-receptor antagonists or proton pump inhibitors in selected cases.

• Assiduous attention should be paid to the prevention of infection.

• Fluid overload prevented by use of loop diuretics in polyuric patients

• If patient is oliguric only way to avoid fluid overload is to institute RRT at an early stage

• Marked azotemia, defined as:

○ Urea >40 mmol/L (BUN [blood urea nitrogen] of 112 mg/dL)

○ Creatinine level >400 μmol (4.5 mg/dL)

• Undesirable and is treated with RRT, unless recovery is imminent or already under way

○ And return toward normal values is expected within 24 to 48 hours

• Recognized that no randomized trials exist to define the ideal time for intervention with artificial renal support

Recovery and Its Management

• Recovery of renal function after episode of ARF increasingly acknowledged as significant clinical measure of morbidity

TABLE 111.3

INTERVENTIONS THAT MAY POTENTIALLY INFLUENCE RENAL RECOVERY RENAL REPLACEMENT THERAPY (RRT)

Biocompatible membrane
Higher-dose prescription
Modality Continuous Renal Replacement Therapy (CRRT)
Early initiation of RRT
Nutritional support
Intensive insulin therapy
Erythropoietin
Loop diuretics

- Persistent chronic renal impairment, or need for long-term RRT, can negatively influence the health status and quality of life of patients and contribute to considerable annual health care expenditures
- Recovery to independence from RRT occurs in estimated 68% to 85% of critically ill patients by hospital discharge
  - Generally peaks by 90 days
  - Older patients and those with preexisting comorbid illnesses
    - Such as chronic kidney disease or advanced cardiovascular disease
  - Less likely to recover function
  - Those with septic ARF may be more likely to recover function
  - Other potentially modifiable factors linked with improved rates of recovery:
    - Including early and aggressive initiation of RRT when indicated
    - Use of continuous rather than intermittent RRT
    - Early and adequate nutritional support
    - Intensive insulin therapy (Table 111.3)
    - Controversial whether adjuvant erythropoietin and routine use of loop diuretics influence renal prognosis and promote early recovery

PROGNOSIS

- ARF can independently influence both short- and long-term prognoses.

- In hospitalized patients, mortality estimated at 20% among all those developing ARF
  - Rate greatly influenced by severity of renal injury
- Prognosis is worse for critically ill patients and those in whom RRT necessary
  - In-hospital mortality for critically ill patients with ARF estimated at 50% to 60%
    - Depending on case mix, can range between 40% to 80%
  - Better uremic control and more intensive artificial renal support may improve survival
    - Prevent uncontrolled uremia and maintain low urea levels throughout the patient's illness
- Those who survive episode of ARF associated with critical illness:
  - Long-term health status, including health-related quality of life (HRQoL)
  - Functional status
  - Hospital discharge location
  - All important indicators of morbidity
    - These patients frequently describe limitations in daily activities, difficulties with mobility, and high levels of sleep disturbance, fatigue, anxiety, and depression
    - HRQoL is generally good and perceived as acceptable, despite evidence that their quality of life is considerably lower than that of the general population.

FUTURE DEVELOPMENTS

- Consensus definition developed and published that will guide research and translate into improved patient outcome
  - Research needed to explore relationship between survival and subsequent morbidity
    - Specifically recovery of kidney function, HRQoL, and the economic consequences of decisions made during care of critically ill patients with ARF
- Some recent advances made in the prevention of ARF associated with radiocontrast nephropathy with use of N-acetylcysteine
- Although studies with fenoldopam provocative
  - No specific drugs found to help
- Apoptosis shown an important mechanism of renal tubular injury in ARF
  - Therapeutic potential for molecular targets
    - Selective inhibitors of proapoptotic proteins (e.g., capsase inhibitors)
    - May attenuate injury or promote recovery
    - At present, no evidence in humans has emerged

CHAPTER 112 ■ RENAL REPLACEMENT THERAPIES IN THE CRITICALLY ILL PATIENT

ACUTE RENAL FAILURE (ARF) AND THE CRITICALLY ILL PATIENT

- Multinational, multicenter prospective epidemiologic survey of ARF conducted in intensive care unit (ICU) patients who either were treated with renal replacement therapy (RRT) or fulfilled at least one of the predefined criteria for ARF :
  - Predefined ARF criteria were:
    - Oliguria, defined as urine output <200 mL in 12 hours
    - And/or marked azotemia, defined as a blood urea nitrogen level >30 mmol/L
  - Data collected at 54 hospitals in 23 countries
    - Of 29,269 critically ill patients admitted during the 16-month study period
    - 1,738 (5.9%) had ARF during ICU stay
    - Including 1,260 (4.3%) treated with RRT
    - Overall hospital mortality 60.3%
    - Most common contributing factor to ARF was septic shock (47.5%)
      - Approximately 30% of patients had preadmission renal dysfunction
      - 86.2% survivors were independent from dialysis at hospital discharge
      - Independent risk factors for hospital mortality included:
        - Use of vasopressors
        - Mechanical ventilation
        - Septic shock
        - Cardiogenic shock
        - Hepatorenal syndrome
- Crude mortality assessment shows overall hospital outcome of ARF has not changed in past 30 years
  - Despite profound differences indicating much greater illness severity for patients treated in 2005
  - Mortality of ARF has not increased, and perhaps has slightly decreased
- Incidence of ARF requiring extracorporeal support is 11 per 100,000 population per year
  - Annual mortality rate is 7.3 per 100,000 residents
  - Highest rates in males older than 65 years
  - Renal recovery occurs in 78% (68 of 87) of survivors at 1 year
    - Although a great number of patients with severe ARF will die, most survivors will become independent from RRT within a year

INDICATIONS FOR INITIATION AND CESSATION OF RENAL REPLACEMENT THERAPY

General Indications

- Uremic complications of ARF such as pulmonary edema, severe fluid overload, hyperkalemia-induced arrhythmias, and uncontrolled metabolic acidosis have long been described.
- No predefined established indications on when to start RRT
- Medical management attempts to prevent renal dysfunction include the use of diuretics, bicarbonate, fluid restriction, and nutritional restriction to control hyperkalemia.
- When these fail, treatment is escalated to RRT.
- Recently more aggressive blood purification approach advocated and a prevention-based algorithm for initiation of RRT can be used (Table 112.1)
- Once RRT started, there is no scientifically established biochemical or clinical marker that should be targeted by therapy
  - Routine clinical practice is to maintain urea concentration below 30 mg/dL, creatinine below 2.5 mg/dL, and electrolytes within normal values
- Techniques and timing of weaning patients from RRT are poorly described

TABLE 112.1

INDICATIONS FOR STARTING RRT

The presence of one indication *suggests,* two indications *strongly suggest,* three indications *mandate* initiation of RRT.
- Anuria/oliguria (diuresis ≤200 mL in 12 hours)
- Severe metabolic acidosis (pH <7.10)
- Hyperazotemia (BUN ≥80 mg/dL) or creatinine >4 mg/dL
- Hyperkalemia (K^+ ≥6.5 mEq/L)
- Clinical signs of uremic toxicity
- Severe dysnatremia (Na^+ ≤115 or ≥160 mEq/L)
- Hyperthermia (temperature >40°C without response to medical therapy)
- Anasarca or severe fluid overload
- Multiple organ failure with renal dysfunction and/or systemic inflammatory reaction syndrome, sepsis, or septic shock with renal dysfunction

- Following practical clinical concepts
  - Recommended when patient has reached hemodynamic stability, and/or need for vasopressors reduced, and/or severity of illness decreased
    - Intensity of blood purification can be decreased
    - If patient was on a continuous schedule, can be switched to intermittent or semicontinuous modality
    - Process accelerated when urine output and fluid balance become adequate

CONTINUOUS, INTERMITTENT, DIFFUSIVE, CONVECTIVE: AN ONGOING MATTER

RRT Modalities: Description and Nomenclature

- Renal replacement consists of the purification of blood by semipermeable membranes
- A wide range of molecules, from water to urea to low-, middle-, and high-molecular-weight solutes, transported across such membranes by mechanism of ultrafiltration (water), convection, and diffusion (solutes)
- During *diffusion*, movement of solutes depends on tendency to reach same concentration on each side of membrane
  - Practical result is passage of solutes from compartment with highest concentration to compartment with lowest concentration
  - Other components of the semipermeable membrane deeply affect diffusion:
    - Thickness and surface, temperature, and diffusion coefficient
- *Dialysis* a modality of RRT and is predominantly based on the principle of diffusion:
  - A dialytic solution flows through the filter countercurrent to blood flow to maintain the highest solute gradient from inlet to outlet port
- During *convection*, movement of solute across semipermeable membrane takes place in conjunction with significant amounts of *ultrafiltration* (water transfer across the membrane)
  - As solvent (plasma water) is pushed across membrane in response to transmembrane pressure (TMP) by ultrafiltration (UF), solutes are carried with it, as long as the porosity of the membrane allows the molecules to be sieved from blood
- As UF proceeds and plasma water and solutes are filtered from blood, hydrostatic pressure within the filter is lost and oncotic pressure is gained because blood concentrates and hematocrit increase
- Fraction of plasma water removed from blood during UF is called *filtration fraction*
  - Should be kept in 20% to 25% range to prevent excessive hemoconcentration within the filtering membrane and to avoid the critical point at which oncotic pressure is equal to TMP and a condition of filtration/pressure equilibrium is reached
- Finally, replacing plasma water with a substitution solution completes the *hemofiltration* (HF) process and returns purified blood to patient

- Replacement fluid administered after filter, with a process called *postdilution HF*
- Otherwise, solution infused before filter to obtain predilution HF
- Postdilution allows urea clearance equivalent to therapy delivery (i.e., 2,000 mL/hour)
- Predilution, in spite of theoretical reduced solute clearances, prolongs the circuit lifespan, reducing the hemoconcentration and protein caking effects occurring within filter fibers
- Conventional hemofiltration is performed with a highly permeable membrane with a surface area of about 1 m^2, steam sterilized, with a cutoff point of 30 kd

The Concept of RRT Dose

- Conventional view of RRT dose is that it is a measure of quantity of blood purification achieved by means of extracorporeal techniques
- *Operative* view of RRT dose is that it is a measure of quantity of representative marker solute removed from a patient
- Hence, the amount (measure) of delivered dose of RRT can be described by various terms:
- The *efficiency* of RRT is represented by the concept of clearance (K)
- The volume of blood cleared of a given solute over a given time
- K depends on solute molecular size and transport modality (diffusion or convection)
  - As well as circuit operational characteristics (blood flow rate [Qb], dialysate flow rate [Qd], ultrafiltration rate [Qf], and hemodialyzer type and size)
  - K normally used to compare treatment dose during each dialysis session
    - Cannot be used as an absolute dose measure to compare treatments with different time schedules
- The *intensity* of RRT defined by product of clearance times time (Kt)
- Kt more useful than K in comparing various RRTs
- The *efficacy* of RRT represents effective solute removal outcome resulting from administration of a given treatment to a given patient
- Can be described by a fractional clearance of a given solute (Kt/V), where V is the volume of distribution of the marker molecule in the body
- Kt/V an established marker of adequacy of dialysis for small solutes correlating with medium-term (several years) survival in chronic hemodialysis patients
- Urea is typically used as a marker molecule in end-stage kidney disease to guide treatment dose, and a Kt/V$_{UREA}$ of at least 1.2 is currently recommended
- However, Kt/V$_{UREA}$ application to patients with ARF not rigorously validated
  - These aspects particularly evident during intermittent hemodialysis (IHD), less so during sustained low-efficiency daily dialysis (SLEDD), and even less during continuous renal replacement therapy (CRRT)
    - Difference due to fact that, after some days of CRRT, the patient's urea levels approach a real steady state

TABLE 112.2

GUIDELINES FOR RRT PRESCRIPTION

Clinical	Operational	Setting
Fluid balance	Net ultrafiltration	A continuous management of negative balance (100–300 mL/h) is preferred in hemodynamically unstable patients. A complete monitoring (CVC, S-G, arterial line, ECG, pulse oximeter) is recommended.
Adequacy and dose	Clearance/modality	2,000–3,000 mL/hour K (or 35 mL/kg/h) for CRRT; consider first CVVHDF. If IHD is selected, a prescription of every day for 4 h is recommended. Prescribe a Kt/V > 1.2.
Acid-base balance	Solution buffer	Bicarbonate buffered solutions are preferable to lactate buffered solutions in case of lactic acidosis and/or hepatic failure.
Electrolyte	Dialysate/replacement	Consider solutions without K^+ in case of severe hyperkalemia. Accurately manage $MgPO_4$.
Timing	Schedule	Early and intense RRT is suggested.
Protocol	Staff/machine	Well-trained staff should routinely use RRT monitors according to predefined institutional protocols.

CVC, central venous catheter; S-G, Swan-Ganz catheter; ECG, electrocardiogram; CRRT, continuous renal replacement therapy; CVVHDF, continuous venovenous hemodiafiltration; IHD, intermittent hemodialysis.

RRT Prescription

Theoretical Aspects

- Despite uncertainty and shortcomings, the idea that there might be an optimal dose of solute removal continues to have a powerful hold in the literature
- Tables 112.2 and 112.3 provide details that could be followed each time an RRT prescription is indicated

From Continuous to Intermittent: One Treatment Fits All?

- Clearance-based dose quantification methods may not be adequate to compare effectiveness.
- For example, peritoneal dialysis (PD), traditionally providing less urea clearance per week than IHD, has comparable patient outcomes.
- When the critical parameter is metabolic control, an acceptable mean blood urea nitrogen level of 60 mg/dL—easily

TABLE 112.3

EXAMPLE OF A POSSIBLE PRESCRIPTION FOR CONTINUOUS TREATMENT IN A 70-KG PATIENT (V_{UREA}: 42 L) DURING AN IDEAL SESSION OF 24 HOURS (T: 1,440 MINUTES) (NET ULTRAFILTRATION [PATIENT FLUID LOSS] IS CONSIDERED ZERO IN K_{CALC} FOR SIMPLICITY)

	Estimated urea clearance (K_{CALC})	Notes	Value of Q to obtain 35 mL/kg/h	Value of Q to obtain a Kt/V of 1
CVVH postdilution	K_{CALC} = Qrep	Always keep filtration fraction <20% (Qb must be 5 times Qrep)	Qrep: 41 mL/min or 2,450 mL/h	Qrep: 29 mL/min or 1,750 mL/h
CVVH predilution	K_{CALC} = Quf/[1 + (Qrep/Qb)]	Filtration fraction computation changes (keep <20%)	For a Qb of 200 mL/min, Qrep: 53 mL/min or 3,200 mL/h	For a Qb of 200 mL/min, Qrep: 35 mL/min or 2,100 mL/hour
CVVHD	K_{CALC} = Qdo	Keep Qb at least thrice Qdo	Qdo: 41 mL/min or 2,450 mL/h	Qdo: 29 mL/min or 1,750 mL/h
CVVHDF postdilution (50% convective and diffusive K)	K_{CALC} = Qrep + Qdo	Consider notes of both CVVH and CVVHD	Qrep: 20 mL/min + Qdo: 21 mL/min	Qrep: 14 mL/min replacement solution + Qdo: 15 mL/min

CVVH, continuous venovenous hemofiltration; Qrep, replacement solution flow rate; Qb, blood flow rate; Quf, ultrafiltration flow rate (Quf = Qrep + Qnet); CVVHD, continuous venovenous hemodialysis; Qdo, dialysate solution flow rate; CVVHDF, continuous venovenous hemodiafiltration; Qnet, patient's net fluid loss.
Urea volume of distribution V (L): patient's body weight (Kg) × 0.6.
Estimated fractional clearance (Kt/V_{CALC}): K_{CALC} (mL/minute) × prescribed treatment time (minute)/V (mL).
A quantity of 35 mL/kg/hour roughly corresponds to a Kt/V of 1.4. A Kt/V of 1 corresponds to approximately 25 mL/kg/hour.
Filtration fraction calculation (postdilution): Qrep/Qb × 100. Filtration fraction calculation (predilution): Qrep/Qb + Qrep × 100.

obtainable in a 100-kg patient with a 2 L/hour continuous venovenous hemofiltration in a computer-based simulation—has been shown to be very difficult to reach, even by intensive IHD regimens.
- Increased RRT frequency results in decreased ultrafiltration requirements per treatment.
  - Avoidance of volume swings related to rapid ultrafiltration rates may also represent another dimension of dose where comparability is difficult.
- Surviving Sepsis Campaign guidelines for management of severe sepsis and septic shock concluded continuous RRT should be considered equivalent to IHD for the treatment of ARF
  - In 166 critically ill patients with ARF randomized to either CRRT or IHD, the CRRT population, despite randomization, had significantly greater severity of illness scores.
  - In part explains why, despite better control of azotemia and a greater likelihood of achieving the desired fluid balance, CRRT had increased mortality
  - Smaller trial at the Cleveland Clinic failed to find a difference in outcome between one therapy and another
  - Meta-analysis unable to solve debate of continuous versus intermittent treatment
    - Remains uncertain whether the choice of RRT modality (intermittent or continuous) actually matters to patient outcome

TECHNICAL NOTES

RRT Modalities: Description and Nomenclature

- Apart from evidence-based medicine dictates, continuous therapies are used in 80% of ICUs worldwide, whereas intermittent hemodialysis (17%) and peritoneal dialysis (3%) have less common use.
- Accurate ultrafiltration control is now obtained by integrated roller volumetric pumps (blood, replacement dialysate, and effluent) and scales.
  - Monitors display pressure measurements of all crucial segments of the circuit (catheter inlet and outlet, filter inlet and outlet, UF, and dialysate ports)
  - Information is integrated with adequate alarm systems and allows the ICU staff to increase filter efficiency and lengthen circuit patency, with the ability to detect potential sources of clotting, thereby improving patient safety.
  - A complete monitoring of fluid balance also provided by continuous recording of the history of the past 24 hours of treatment
  - When an alarm occurs, a "smart" message on the screen suggests the most appropriate intervention required.
- A complete range of ICU RRT therapeutic modalities includes:
  - Slow continuous ultrafiltration (SCUF)
  - Continuous venovenous hemofiltration (CVVH)
  - Continuous venovenous hemodialysis (CVVHD)
  - Continuous venovenous hemodiafiltration (CVVHDF)
  - Therapeutic plasma exchange (TPE)

Intermittent Hemodialysis
- IHD is a prevalently diffusive treatment in which blood and dialysate are circulated in countercurrent mode, and generally, a low permeability, cellulose-based membrane is used.
- Dialysate must be pyrogen free but not necessarily sterile, since dialysate-blood contact does not occur.
- Ultrafiltration rate is equal to the scheduled weight loss
  - Treatment can typically be performed 4 hours three times a week or daily

Peritoneal Dialysis
- PD is a predominantly diffusive treatment in which blood circulating along the capillaries of the peritoneal membrane is exposed to dialysate.
- Access is obtained by insertion of a peritoneal catheter.
  - Allows abdominal instillation of dialysate
  - Solute and water movement is achieved by means of variable concentration and tonicity gradients generated by the dialysate
  - Treatment can be performed continuously or intermittently

Slow Continuous Ultrafiltration
- SCUF is a technique by which blood is driven through a highly permeable filter via an extracorporeal circuit in venovenous mode.
  - Ultrafiltrate produced during membrane transit is not replaced and corresponds to weight loss.
  - Used only for fluid control in overloaded patients (i.e., congestive heart failure patients who do not respond to diuretic therapy)

Continuous Venovenous Hemofiltration
- CVVH is a technique by which blood is driven through a highly permeable filter via an extracorporeal circuit in venovenous mode.
  - Ultrafiltrate produced during membrane transit is replaced, in part or completely, to achieve blood purification and volume control.
    - Replacement fluid is delivered after the filter, the technique is defined as *postdilution hemofiltration*
    - If delivered before the filter, the technique is defined as *predilution hemofiltration*
    - Replacement fluid can also be delivered both prefilter and postfilter
    - Clearance for all solutes is convective and equals the ultrafiltration rate

Continuous Venovenous Hemodialysis
- CVVHD is a technique by which blood is driven through a low-permeability dialyzer via an extracorporeal circuit in venovenous mode.
  - A countercurrent flow of dialysate is delivered in the dialysate compartment.
  - Ultrafiltrate produced during membrane transit corresponds to the patient's weight loss.
  - Solute clearance is mainly diffusive, and efficiency is limited to small solutes only.

Continuous Venovenous Hemodiafiltration
- CVVHDF is a technique by which blood is driven through a highly permeable dialyzer via an extracorporeal circuit in venovenous mode.

- Countercurrent flow of dialysate is delivered in the dialysate compartment.
- Ultrafiltrate produced during membrane transit is in excess of the patient's desired weight loss.
  - Replacement solution is needed to maintain fluid balance.
- Solute clearance is both convective and diffusive.

Hemoperfusion (HP)

- In HP, blood is circulated on a bed of coated charcoal powder to remove solutes by adsorption.
- Technique is specifically indicated in cases of poisoning or intoxication with agents that can be effectively removed by charcoal
- Treatment may cause platelet and protein depletion

Plasmapheresis (PP)

- PP a treatment that uses specific plasma filters.
- Molecular-weight cutoff of the membrane is much higher than that of hemofilters (100,000 to 1,000,000 kd)
- Plasma as a whole is filtered and blood is reconstituted by the infusion of plasma products such as frozen plasma or albumin.
  - This technique is performed to remove proteins or protein-bound solutes.

High-flux Dialysis (HFD)

- HFD a treatment that uses highly permeable membranes in conjunction with an ultrafiltration control system
- Due to characteristics of membrane, ultrafiltration occurs in proximal part of filter that is counterbalanced by positive pressure applied to dialysate compartment
  - Causes, in the distal part of the filter, a phenomenon called *backfiltration*
    - The convective passage of the dialysate into the blood
    - Diffusion and convection are combined, but due to the use of a pyrogen-free dialysate, replacement is avoided.

High-volume Hemofiltration (HVHF)

- HVHF is a treatment that uses highly permeable membranes and hemofiltration with a high volume setting.

High-permeability Hemofiltration (HPHF)

- HPHF a treatment that uses high-cutoff (60 kd) permeable membranes and hemofiltration
- High treatment flows are not necessary
  - Strict control of bigger molecules, like albumin, is recommended

Anticoagulation

- Need for anticoagulation of CRRT circuit arises from the fact that the contact between blood and the tubing of the circuit and the membrane of the filter induces activation of the coagulation cascade
  - Extracorporeal activation inevitably results in filter or circuit clotting
  - Aims of anticoagulation are as follows:
    - Maintenance of extracorporeal circuit and dialyzer patency
    - Reduction of off-treatment time (downtime) that could have a clinical impact on the overall RRT clearance
    - Reduction of treatment cost by the use of as little material as possible

- Achievement of the above aims with minimal risk for the patient
  - Under no circumstances should the patient be put at risk of bleeding to prolong circuit life.

Circuit Setup Optimization and No Anticoagulation

- Several technical features of the RRT circuit are likely to affect the success of any anticoagulant approach.
  - Vascular access must be of adequate size
  - Tubing kinking should be avoided
  - Blood flow rate should exceed 100 mL/minute
  - Pump flow fluctuations must be prevented (in modern machines this event is mainly due to increased circuit resistances rather than flow rate inaccuracies)
  - Venous bubble trap, where air–blood contact occurs, must be accurately monitored.
- Another component of circuit setup has to be addressed:
  - Plasma filtration fraction should be kept as far as possible below 20%
  - When possible or considered correct, predilutional hemofiltration should be selected
  - Evidence that, when setup is perfectly optimized, anticoagulants are only a relatively minor component of circuit patency
    - Whenever the patient's clinical features present risk factors for bleeding (prolonged clotting times, thrombocytopenia), RRT can be safely performed without use of any anticoagulant

Unfractionated Heparin (UFH)

- UFH a commonly available anticoagulant
- Easy to use
- Antidote available (protamine)
- Heparin doses generally range from 5 to 10 IU/kg/hour
  - In patients with very limited circuit duration, it can also be used in combination with protamine (regional heparinization), with a 1:1 ratio
    - 150 IU of UFH per mg of protamine
    - A strictly monitored activated prothrombin time (aPTT)
    - Problem with UFH is its relatively unpredictable bioavailability, the necessity for antithrombin III (ATIII) level optimization, and the occurrence of heparin-induced thrombocytopenia (HIT)

Low-molecular-weight Heparins (LMWH)

- LMWH a relatively new kind of anticoagulant
  - Prospective studies not yet shown these to be superior to prolong circuit life
  - Molecules appear to have a better bioavailability than UFH and a lower incidence of HIT with a 10% increased cost

Prostacyclin

- Prostacyclin (PGI_2) a potentially useful drug for RRT anticoagulation
- The most potent inhibitor of platelet aggregation with the shortest half-life
- PGI_2 infused at a dose of 4 to 8 ng/kg/hour, with or without adjunct of low dose of UFH
- Hypotension may be induced by higher doses of PGI_2
- High cost and harmful side effects might limit the use of this agent to patients with short circuit duration

TABLE 112.4

TABLE 112.4

ANTICOAGULATION STRATEGIES

Drug	PRO	CON
No anticoagulation	High risk of bleeding in patients	Relatively shorter circuit life span
Unfractionated heparin	Routine	HIT
Low-molecular-weight heparin	Routine (alternative to UH)	HIT
Prostacyclin	Very short circuit life span	Hypotension
Citrate	Routine/very short circuit life span	Hypocalcemia
Danaparoid	HIT	Insufficient data available
Argatroban	HIT	Insufficient data available
Irudine	HIT	Insufficient data available
Nafamostat mesilate	HIT	Insufficient data available
Heparin-coated circuits	Routine	Insufficient data available

HIT, heparin-induced thrombocytopenia; UH, unfractionated heparin.

Citrate

- Citrate provides a form of regional anticoagulation
  - Depends on the ability of citrate to chelate calcium, which prevents clot formation
    - A calcium-free sodium citrate containing replacement solution and/or dialysate solution is prepared and administered at the appropriate rate to achieve the desired aPTT (60 to 90 seconds)
    - Calcium chloride is then administered to replace chelated/dialyzed calcium and maintain normocalcemia
    - Effective in maintaining excellent filter patency and compares favorably with heparin
    - Avoids the risk for HIT and does not lead to systemic anticoagulation
  - Relative drawbacks of this anticoagulation management strategy include:
    - Risk for hypocalcemia and metabolic alkalosis
    - Use of cumbersome replacement/dialysate fluid preparation

Other Strategies

- Alternatives to the techniques presented above are listed in Table 112.4 for completeness.

Vascular Access

- The fundamental role played by vascular access must be emphasized
  - Circuit failure more often due to inadequate vascular access than insufficient anticoagulation
  - Optimal dialysis catheter can save patient from inappropriate increases of anticoagulation dose
  - Venovenous RRT relies on use of temporary double-lumen catheter
    - Such catheters inserted in a central vein and available in different brands, shapes, and sizes
    - Site of insertion of double-lumen catheters implies several considerations (clinician expertise, body habitus of the patient, the presence of other intravenous catheters)
    - Femoral vein is generally the first choice of vascular access
    - Internal jugular or subclavian accesses often associated with inadequate performance
      - Inguinal puncture is safer and easier to perform in coagulopathic critically ill patients
      - Valid alternative may be achieved by cannulation of the right internal jugular vein with tip of catheter reaching right atrium
      - Circuit blood flow rates with this approach can reach 300 mL/minute
      - Catheter sizes for adult patients range from 12 to 14 French and length from 16 to 25 cm
        - The bigger and shorter the catheter, the higher the performance
        - When femoral vein is selected, a 20-cm-long catheter has its tip positioned close to the inferior vena cava, allowing optimal flows within the circuit
        - When an inadequate blood flow or a catheter malfunction is suspected, venous and arterial lumens should be flushed with saline.
          - With goal of testing resistance to injection and aspiration
          - Limb clotting of the line versus kinking due to the patient's position must be distinguished
          - In the first case, a switching of arterial and venous limb can be attempted
          - Maneuver increases circuit recirculation, but clinical consequences are negligible
          - In the second case, a heparin or urokinase lock can be tried for a few hours
          - Another approach is a catheter (guidewire) exchange

THE ROLE OF RENAL REPLACEMENT THERAPIES IN DIFFERENT SETTINGS

Sepsis and Multiple Organ Dysfunction Syndrome

- Interest in the past 10 years concerning extracorporeal blood purification therapies (EBPT) as adjuvants in the complex therapy of sepsis and multiple organ dysfunction syndrome (MODS)
  - RRT was first and still is most used and effective type of EBPT

- Evidence is growing about its ability to maintain homeostatic balance in critically ill patients—specifically, septic patients with MODS
- Beyond correcting specific uremic toxins
  - RRT seems to restore other physiologic homeostatic mechanisms (*renal dose* of CRRT)
  - At *overdoses*, it may play a role in blood purification from water-soluble cytokines produced during systemic inflammatory and septic states (*sepsis dose*)
  - Concept leads to speculation that higher-volume hemofiltration may be beneficial in septic patients beyond the removal of classic markers
    - If a UF rate of 1,400 to 2,400 mL/hour for a 70-kg man (equivalent to 20 to 35 mL/kg/hour) can be considered *traditional dose*
    - Then increasing effluent production to more than 45 mL/kg/hour can be considered as high-volume CVVH
    - One of the main challenges of HVHF is the technical limit of currently available machines (UF ranges from 4 L/hour to 9 or 10 L/hour)
      - Sessions are often intermittent or interrupted by traditional CVVH after 2 to 8 hours
  - The first reports of application of HVHF to the treatment of septic shock in humans with MODS have appeared recently.
  - Beneficial effect on macrophage function with restoration of the ability to produce tumor necrosis factor-α (TNF-α) in response to endotoxin exposure, showing the potential of EBPT for immunomodulation at a cellular and humoral level in sepsis
  - Prospective cohort analysis in 306 patients who received HVHF at a mean UF rate of 4 L/hour found an improvement in cardiac index (CI), blood pressure (BP), and stroke volume (SV) in hypodynamic patients, and an increase in systemic venous resistance (SVR) with a decrease in dopamine dose in those who were hyperdynamic.
  - Evaluation of the effects of short-term, high-volume hemofiltration (STHVH), lasting 4 hours with 9 L/hour hemofiltration flow and followed by conventional CVVH in 20 patients affected by intractable cardiocirculatory failure resulting from severe septic shock
    - Eleven patients ("responders") attained all therapeutic end points (increase in CI; increase in mixed venous saturation; increase in arterial pH; reduction in epinephrine dose)
    - Rate of survival to 28 days in this group was markedly higher (9 of 11) than among nonresponders (0 of 9)
  - Hemodynamics, serum cytokines, and complement concentration measured in 11 patients with septic shock and MODS
  - Patients randomly assigned to HVHF (8 hours at 6 L/hour) or to standard CVVH
  - Decrease in vasopressor requirement significantly higher in HVHF group
  - In the HVHF group, the concentration of the measured soluble mediators in the ultrafiltrate was negligible, indicating a greater role in filter adsorption of studied mediators.
  - All of these data support the hypothesis that HVHF techniques are safe and feasible and show that adequate blood purification can restore and maintain cardiac and circulatory function as well as metabolic and gas exchange parameters.

- Large randomized trials are still lacking, and these types of therapies are still far from becoming routine.
- A more complex evolution of EBPT, combining the need for high-sieving coefficients of larger molecules and continuous therapy, led to a technique called *coupled plasma filtration adsorption* (CPFA).
  - Technique separates plasma from blood using a plasma filter
  - Plasma then passed through a synthetic resin cartridge and returned to the blood
  - A second blood filter is used to remove excess fluid and low-molecular-weight toxins
    - The resin was chosen based on its adsorption capacity for important inflammatory mediators, low levels of extractable toxins, and good pressure flow performance.
    - In a randomized clinical trial, the adsorbent removed almost 100% of TNF-α and interleukin-β (IL-β), allowing a significant reduction of vasopressor dosage when compared to CVVH alone.

Congestive Heart Failure (CHF)

- Fluid overload may occur in patients with CHF
  - When diuretics fail, fluid removal becomes uncontrolled, and other therapeutic options must be undertaken
- Extracorporeal ultrafiltration a possible solution
  - Acute isolated schedules of ultrafiltration may be too aggressive and could result in severe hemodynamic instability
  - Continuous extracorporeal techniques applied in such patients
  - Excellent hemodynamic stability, a good cardiovascular response
    - Often, diuresis restoration the most common effects encountered
- One specific comment must be made concerning difference between CVVH and other techniques, including dialysis and use of diuretics.
  - In all pharmacologic and dialytic techniques, removal of sodium and water cannot be dissociated.
    - Diuretic effect is based on a remarkable natriuresis.
    - Ultrafiltration during dialysis may result in hypotonicity or hypertonicity, depending on interference with diffusion and removal of other molecules such as urea and other electrolytes.
    - In such circumstances, water removal is linked to other solutes in proportions that are dependent on the technique used.
    - In SCUF, the mechanism of ultrafiltration produces a fluid that is substantially similar to plasma water except for a minimal interference due to Donnan effects.
      - Ultrafiltration is basically iso-osmotic and isonatremic.
      - Water and sodium removal cannot be dissociated, with sodium elimination linked to the sodium–plasma water concentration
    - In CVVH and hemofiltration in general, the ultrafiltrate composition is definitely similar to plasma water.
      - Sodium balance can be significantly affected by sodium concentration in replacement solution.
      - Sodium removal can be dissociated from water removal.
      - This effect cannot be achieved with any other technique.

Contrast-induced Nephropathy

- Radiocontrast-induced nephropathy (RCIN) causes acute kidney injury and increases mortality
- Systematic review of published trials to determine whether periprocedural extracorporeal blood purification prevents RCIN:
  - Incidence of RCIN, defined as an increase in serum creatinine concentration (>0.5 mg/dL [>44 mmol/L]), was 35.2% in the standard medical therapy group and 27.8% in extracorporeal blood purification group
  - Extracorporeal blood purification did not decrease the incidence of RCIN significantly as compared with standard medical therapy (risk ratio, 0.97; 95% confidence interval, 0.44–2.14)
  - Periprocedural hemodialysis did not decrease the incidence of RCIN

RRT for Children

- Important differences in RRT indications, methods, and prescription between children and adult patients; nevertheless, the technique is essentially the same
- Main indication is correction of water overload
  - Different from adult setting, where solute control may play a key role
  - Shown that restoring adequate water content in small children is the main independent variable for outcome prediction

- This concept is much more important in critically ill, smaller children, in whom a relatively larger amount of fluid must be administered to deliver an adequate amount of drug infusion, parenteral/enteral nutrition, blood derivates, and so on.
- Corrections of acid-base imbalance and electrolyte disorders strong indications for RRT in children
- Catheter size ranges from:
  - 6.5 French (10 cm long) for patients weighing <10 kg
  - 8 French (15 cm long) for patients weighing 11 to 15 kg
- Blood priming may be indicated if more than 8 mL/kg of patient's blood volume necessary to fill a RRT circuit
- Full anticoagulation must always be maintained to avoid excessive blood loss in case of circuit clotting.
- Predilution hemofiltration is generally the preferred modality and is delivered in a continuous fashion.
- Fluid balance requires strict monitoring and highest accuracy due to the risk of excessive patient dehydration.
- Prescription of RRT clearance should be titrated based on the patient body surface area, an approach that will usually lead to relatively higher doses for small children with respect to adult patients when considered per kilogram.
- Critically ill children weighing below 10 kg and neonates with ARF are often treated with peritoneal dialysis (PD).
- An important exception to this general approach is the case of children with ARF during an extracorporeal membrane oxygenation treatment (ECMO).
  - In this case, the RRT circuit is placed in parallel to the ECMO circuit, and it is possible to let a significant blood flow run into the filter even in the smallest patients.

CHAPTER 113 ■ ENDOCRINOPATHY IN THE INTENSIVE CARE UNIT

- During critical illness, the stressors are multiple and include emotional and physical stress such as trauma or infection, and various therapeutic or diagnostic interventions such as surgery, arterial or venous catheterization, laryngeal intubation and mechanical ventilation, and drugs. In response, the host adapts to counteract prolonged stress while maintaining the ability to adjust to unpredictable surges of stress. The integrity and flexibility of host response to these stressors is essential to survive critical illness.

- It is now recognized that the "stress system" has two main components: the corticotropin-releasing hormone (CRH)/vasopressin neurons of the hypothalamus and the locus ceruleus noradrenaline/autonomic neurons of the brainstem. This chapter summarizes recent knowledge on how immune molecules signal the brain to generate both neurologic and hormonal responses aimed at downgrading the immune system when the inflammatory response is no longer needed. Abbreviations used in this chapter are presented in Table 113.1.

TABLE 113.1

ABBREVIATIONS

ACTH	adrenocorticotropic hormone
ADH	antidiuretic hormone
CRH	corticotropin-releasing hormone
FSH	follicle-stimulating hormone
GABA	gamma-aminobutyric acid
GH	growth hormone
GHRH	GH-releasing hormone
GHRP	GH-releasing peptide
GLUT	glucose transporter isoform 4
GNRH	gonadotropin-releasing hormone
HMGB	high mobility group box
IGF	Insulin-like growth factor
IL	interleukin
iNOS	inducible nitric oxide synthase
IRR	insulin receptor-related receptor
LH	luteinizing hormone
LHRH	LH-releasing hormone
LTH	luteotrophic hormone
MIF	macrophage migration inhibitory factor
NO	nitric oxide
NTIS	nonthyroidal illness syndrome
PRL	prolactin
T_3	tri-iodothyronine
T_4	serum thyroxine
Th1	helper T cell 1
Th2	helper T cell 2
TNF	tumor necrosis factor
TRH	thyrotropin-releasing hormone
TSH	thyroid-stimulating hormone

PHYSIOLOGY OF THE ENDOCRINE RESPONSE

- Two pathways are used by the organism for interorgan communication—the central nervous system and the endocrine system.
- The central nervous system and its peripheral arms allow rapid communication between different tissues.
- The endocrine system is made of several organs or tissues distributed throughout the body. Nevertheless, all endocrine tissues are directly linked to the pituitary and the hypothalamus.
- In vertebrates, the endocrine organs include anterior and posterior pituitary, ovary and testis, adrenal cortex and medulla, thyroids and parathyroids, islets of Langerhans in the pancreas, and various parts of the intestinal mucosa. The pineal and thymus can also be considered endocrine organs.
- Many other organs have some endocrine properties. The kidney secretes renin and the heart secretes natriuretic factors.
- Hormones are divided into steroids (cholesterol-derived proteins), peptides, and amines.
- The main known **hormones** are listed in Table 113.2.

General Organization of the Endocrine System

- The **pituitary gland** (**hypophysis**) is a pivotal endocrine organ. It is connected to the central nervous system by the pituitary stalk and is divided into two parts: the anterior pituitary and the posterior pituitary, which is developed from the brain.
- The **anterior pituitary** is made up of the *pars distalis*, which is richly vascular and has three cell types (chromophobe and two types of chromophil cells), the *pars intermedia*, which is the least vascular part and contains only a few cells, and the *pars tuberalis*.
- The anterior pituitary produces seven hormones: gonadotropic hormones (follicle-stimulating hormones (FSH), luteinizing hormone (LH) and luteotropic hormone (LTH), thyrotropic (thyroid-stimulating) hormone (TSH), adrenocorticotropic hormone (ACTH), growth hormone (GH), and prolactin (PRL).
- The **posterior pituitary** has three parts: the median eminence, infundibular stem, and infundibular process or neural lobe. Its tissues consist of unmyelinated fibers, fusiform cells, neurons, and mast cells.
- The posterior pituitary produces mainly vasopressin, also called the antidiuretic hormone (ADH).

TABLE 113.2

LIST OF HORMONES

Hormones	Organ	Carrier in bloodstream	Target tissues	Main actions
Insulin	Pancreas: β cells of the islets of Langerhans	Free	Liver, muscle, fat	Decreases blood glucose level Decreases gluconeogenesis, proteinolysis, lipolysis Increases fatty acid and glycogen synthesis
Glucagon	Pancreas: α cells of the islets of Langerhans	Free	Liver	Increases blood glucose level by increasing glycogenolysis and gluconeogenesis
Somatostatin	Hypothalamus cells and cells of pancreas, intestine, stomach	Free	Pancreas	Suppresses gastrointestinal hormone secretion Inhibits insulin and glucagon secretion Inhibits GH and TSH release
Thrombopoietin	Liver, kidney, striated muscle, stromal cells of the bone marrow	Free	Bone marrow	Regulates the differentiation of megakaryocytes and platelets
Angiotensinogen	Liver	Free	Plasma	Releases aldosterone Causes vasoconstriction
Insulin growth factor	Liver	IGF-binding proteins	Muscle, cartilage, bone, liver, kidney, nerves, skin, and lungs	Regulates cell proliferation and apoptosis
Tri-iodothyronine (T_3) Thyroxine (T_4) Calcitonin	Thyroid	Thyroxine-binding globulin (TBG 70%) Thyroxine-binding prealbumin (TBPA 10%–15%) Albumin (15%–20%) Free	Whole body Intestines, bone, kidney, central nervous system	Increases metabolic rate Promotes growth Metabolic effects: stimulates carbohydrate metabolism, fat metabolism; decreases cholesterol, phospholipid, and triglyceride plasma levels Prohormone for the active T_3 Reduces blood calcium levels Regulates vitamin D and bone mineral metabolism Controls satiety
Adrenocorticotropin hormone (ACTH)	Anterior pituitary	Free	Adrenal cortex	Produces glucocorticoids and mineral corticoids
Luteinizing hormone (LH)		Free	In females, granulosa cells and theca cells In males, Leydig cells of the testis	Reproduction: In females, triggers ovulation and maintains luteal function during the first 2 weeks of menstruation. In males, increases testosterone production
Follicle-stimulating hormone (FSH)		Free	In females, graafian cells In males, Sertoli cells of the testes	Reproduction: In females, initiates follicular growth In males, enhances androgen-binding protein and acts in the spermatogenesis

(*continued*)

TABLE 113.2

CONTINUED

Hormones	Organ	Carrier in bloodstream	Target tissues	Main actions
Growth hormone (GH)		Free	Liver, chondrocytes, and whole body	Anabolic hormone: promotes lipolysis, increases protein synthesis, reduces liver uptake of glucose Enables height growth in childhood Increases calcium retention and increases bone mineralization Stimulates the immune system
Prolactin		Free	Mammary glands	Stimulates lactation
Oxytocin	Posterior pituitary	Free	Brain, mammary gland, myometrium, endometrium, kidney, heart	Peripheral actions: Letdown reflex in lactating Uterine contraction Reduces diureses and stimulates sodium excretion Embryonal development of heart Brain actions: Sexual arousal Social behavior Maternal behavior Increases trust and reduces fear
Antidiuretic hormone (ADH)		Free	Vessels, liver, pituitary gland, kidney, brain	Peripheral actions: V1a: vasoconstriction, gluconeogenesis, platelet aggregation and release of factor VIII and von Willebrand factor V1b: ACTH secretion V2: water reabsorption in the collecting ducts Brain actions: Memory formation Response to stress
Cortisol	Adrenal cortex	Corticosteroid-binding globulin (CBG 90%) Albumin Free (about 4%)	Liver, vessels, immune system, hippocampus	Metabolic properties: Enhances hepatic gluconeogenesis and glycogenolysis Induces peripheral insulin resistance Induces free-fatty acid and amino-acid release Cardiovascular properties: Maintains vascular tone Maintains endothelial and vascular permeability Anti-inflammatory and immunosuppressive actions
Aldosterone		Free	Collecting ducts of the kidney	Reabsorption of sodium and excretion of potassium H^+ secretion
Estrogen	Ovary, placenta	Free	Uterus, coagulation system, liver, gastrointestinal tract	Promotes development of female secondary sex characteristics Regulates the menstrual cycle Causes thickening of the endometrium Promotes lipid metabolism, protein synthesis, fluid balance

(continued)

TABLE 113.2

CONTINUED

Hormones	Organ	Carrier in bloodstream	Target tissues	Main actions
Progesterone		Free	Endometrium, vaginal epithelium, brain, smooth muscle, immune system, thyroid, skeleton	Reproduction Neurosteroid: involved in myelinization, synaptic function
Testosterone	Testes of males and ovaries of females	Sex hormone binding globulin (SHBG)	In males,	Anabolic effects: Growth of muscle mass Increases bone density and maturation Virilizing effects: Maturation of sex organs Development of male secondary sex characteristics
Parathormone	Parathyroid	Free	Skeleton, gastrointestinal tract, kidney	Increases blood calcium concentration in three ways: Enhances calcium release from the bone Enhances calcium reabsorption from renal tubules Enhances calcium absorption in the intestine
Human chorionic gonadotropin (HCG)	Placenta	Free	Uterus	Maintains the corpus luteum and progesterone production during pregnancy
Atrial natriuretic peptide (ANP)	Atrial myocytes of the heart	Free	Kidney, vessels, adrenal, adipose tissue	Reduces blood volume, central venous pressure, cardiac output, arterial blood pressure
Brain natriuretic peptide (BNP)	Cardiac ventricles			Increases renal sodium secretion and excretion Increases lipolysis
Melatonin	Pineal gland, retina, gastrointestinal tract	Free	Brain	Circadian rhythms Antioxidant Immune system: increases T-cell response
Renin	Kidney	Free	Plasma	Activates the renin–angiotensin–aldosterone system by cleaving angiotensinogen to angiotensin 1
Calcitriol	Kidney	Free	Intestinal epithelium	Increases calcium absorption from the gastrointestinal tract

- The anterior pituitary exerts control of most endocrine organs, and insufficiency of the anterior pituitary results in atrophy of ovary or testis, adrenal cortex, and thyroid.
- The thyroid and adrenal cortex have no specific target organ, and the hormones they secrete act broadly to contribute to homeostasis.
- The gonads also produce hormones that act on tissues in general and on specific target organs (urogenital apparatus).
- The adrenal medulla secretes adrenalin and noradrenalin, which are released during stressed states enhancing the sympathetic system in a "fight or flight" response.

Physiologic Control of the Endocrine System

- There is no single mechanism for the regulation of hormone activity. However, two main mechanisms of endocrine activity regulation occur though (1) feedback loops, and (2) interaction with the central nervous system.
- Feedback mechanisms allow circulating hormones from the target organs as well as from the anterior pituitary to down- or up-regulate the release of hypothalamic molecules.

- The feedback loop also involves the central nervous structures such as the hippocampus, which contains the highest concentration of glucocorticoid receptors in the central nervous system.
- This self-balancing system stabilizes the endocrine activity under resting conditions but is insufficient in case of enhanced endocrine activity. In the latter case, neurologic control is the key regulator of the endocrine activity, and the hypothalamus plays a key role in the regulation of these hormones.
- The hypothalamus is directly connected to the posterior pituitary and the adrenal medulla. Additionally, it influences the anterior pituitary by releasing in synchronous pulses stimulatory or inhibitory hormones in the hypophyseal portal vessels of the pituitary stalk.
- Complex interactions between distinct feedback loops can occur through interconnections between distinct functional regions within the hypothalamus.
- The effect of CRH on ACTH release by the pituitary is permissive, and vasopressin acts in synergy with CRH. In addition, there are tight interconnections between projections of CRH-synthesizing neurons from the parvocellular nuclei to the brainstem, and reciprocally noradrenergic projections originating from the locus coeruleus and ending in the parvocellular reticular nuclei. Thereby, noradrenaline, CRH, and vasopressin can stimulate one another.
- CRH, vasopressin, and noradrenaline are under the stimulatory control of the serotoninergic, cholinergic, and histaminergic systems, and are inhibited by gamma-aminobutyric acid, benzodiazepine, and opioids.

POTENTIAL MECHANISMS OF REGULATION OF THE ENDOCRINE ACTIVITY DURING CRITICAL ILLNESS

The Stressors

- Critical illness is a condition involving multiple stressors of both emotional and physical types.
- Physical stressors can be classified into disease related (e.g., infection, burns, trauma) and intervention related (e.g., surgery, invasive diagnostic or therapeutic procedures, drugs).
- The unpredictable nature, duration, and intensity of the stressors renders the host response more problematic.

Mechanisms of Neuroendocrine Activation in Acute Inflammation

Signals Sent to the Hypothalamic–Pituitary Axis

- Acute inflammatory response to insults such as lipopolysaccharide (LPS) include the release of a number of mediators such as tumor necrosis factor alpha (TNF-α), interleukin (IL)-1, IL-6, IL-8, nitric oxide (NO), and the late mediators, macrophage migration-inhibiting factors (MIF), and high mobility group box-1 (HMGB-1).
- These mediators reach the hypophyseal portal capillaries in the median eminence via the anterior hypophyseal arteries. Cytokines can diffuse into the pituitary as these areas are free of the blood–brain barrier and be carried to the hypothalamus and the brain areas lacking a blood–brain barrier. Addition-

ally, active transport of cytokines can provide a pathway to nuclei inside the blood–brain barrier.
- In addition to the blood-borne cytokines, glial cells can produce a number of cytokines, such as IL-1, IL-2, and IL-6. Similarly, LPS challenge induces IL-6 expression in the anterior pituitary in animals.
- In humans, sepsis induces hypothalamic expression of TNF and IL-1β within the parvocellular and supraoptic nuclei.
- The induction of IL-1β and inducible nitric oxide synthase (iNOS) occurs in the meninges, areas lacking a blood–brain barrier, and also in the parvocellular nuclei and the arcuate nucleus, which contain the hypothalamic-releasing and -inhibiting hormones.
- LPS can also be carried by the cerebrospinal fluid to the third ventricle where it crosses the ependyma or acts on projections from parvocellular neurons. Thus, it is likely that delayed overexpression of NO through iNOS activation prolongs the synthesis of hypothalamic hormones induced by LPS.
- In addition, cytokines, via activation of GABAergic (gamma-aminobutyric-acid-releasing) neurons, block NO-induced LH-releasing hormone (LHRH) but not FSH release, inhibit GH-releasing hormone (GHRH) release, and stimulate somatostatin and prolactin release. The regulatory action of NO is mediated by the combined activation of guanylate cyclase, cyclo-oxygenase, and lipoxygenase.
- Cytokines can also directly act on the anterior pituitary, particularly to stimulate ACTH synthesis and release.
- A second pathway of activation of the hypothalamic–pituitary axis is the neural route. Various afferent neurons of the peripheral system sense the threat at the inflammatory sites and stimulate the noradrenergic system and the hypothalamus.
- Stimulation of vagal afferent fibers by LPS results in activation of the locus coeruleus where neurons have projections that synapse on cholinergic interneurons in the parvocellular nucleus.
- It has been shown that CRH is released on acetylcholine stimulation of muscarinic receptors, and that this effect is prevented by nonspecific NO antagonists.
- NO diffuses in the parvocellular cells and induces the generation of both cyclo-oxygenase and lipoxygenase, which in turn stimulate CRH synthesis.

PATTERNS OF ENDOCRINE ACTIVITY DURING CRITICAL ILLNESS

- Infection, LPS challenge, major surgery, trauma, or burns elicit very similar patterns of pituitary hormone secretion. Plasma ACTH and prolactin increase within a few minutes following the insult and are associated with a rapid inhibition of LH and TSH but not FSH. Growth hormone secretion is also stimulated in humans but inhibited in rats.

Hypothalamic–Pituitary–Adrenal Axis

- Acute stress is associated with an immediate increase in the amplitude of hypothalamic hormones, mainly CRH and vasopressin, resulting in increases in amplitude and frequency of ACTH and cortisol pulses and the loss of the circadian rhythm.

- To achieve this enhanced and accelerated release of hormones, the host recruits additional secretagogues of CRH, vasopressin, and ACTH, mainly magnocellular vasopressin and angiotensin II.
- In addition, catecholamines, neuropeptides Y, and to a lesser extent CRH released from the adrenal medulla, as well as direct autonomic neural input to the adrenal cortex, stimulate glucocorticoid secretion.
- The common feature is characterized by high circulating levels of ACTH and cortisol, which remain in plateau as long as the stressful condition is maintained. However, in critical illness, circulating levels of cortisol reflect not only cortisol release, but also cortisol clearance from plasma.
- In critically ill patients, cortisol levels may vary from <5 μg/dL to >100 μg/dL and do not reflect the hypothalamic–pituitary–adrenal (HPA) axis function.

Vasopressin

- Circulating vasopressin levels are regulated through various stimuli including changes in blood volume or blood pressure, plasma osmolality, cytokines, and other neuromediators.
- Acute illness may be associated with inappropriately high circulating levels of vasopressin resulting in water retention and hyponatremia.
- In sepsis, vasopressin levels in plasma seem to follow a biphasic response with initially high concentrations, probably related to the release from posterior pituitary stores on strong baroreflex activation, followed by a decline in 72 hours with relative vasopressin insufficiency occurring in about one-third of cases.
- The delayed decrease in vasopressin levels in plasma is not related to altered hormone clearance from plasma and may result from NO overexpression in the parvocellular nuclei.

The Hypothalamic–Pituitary–Thyroid Axis

- Low T_3-T_4 syndrome has been described for more than 20 years in fasting conditions and in a wide variety of diseases (e.g., sepsis, surgery, myocardial infarction, transplantation, heart, renal and hepatic failure, cancers, malnutrition, inflammatory diseases) and is also called euthyroid sick syndrome or nonthyroidal illness syndrome (NTIS).
- In the early phase following an acute stress, there is a decrease in serum tri-iodothyronine (T_3) level, an increase in rT_3 level. Then serum thyroxine (T_4) levels decrease within 24 to 48 hours, and TSH levels remain within normal range without a circadian rhythm.
- Underlying mechanisms include the following:
  - Decrease in conversion of T_4 and T_3 in extrathyroid tissues due to inhibition of the hepatic 5'-monodeiodination;
  - The lack of substrates due to the presence of transport protein inhibitors preventing T_4 fixation on the protein;
  - Dysfunction of the thyrotrophic negative feedback on the hypothalamic–pituitary axis;
  - Cytokines (IL-1, IL-6, TNF-α, interferon-gamma [IFN-γ]) inhibiting the thyrotrophic centers and/or affecting the expression of thyroid hormone nuclear receptors;
  - The presence of other inhibitory substances such as dopamine.

- Prolonged critical illness is associated with centrally induced hypothyroidism as suggested by restoration of T_3 and T_4 pulses by exogenous thyrotropin-releasing hormone (TRH) infusion.

Growth Hormone

- The acute phase of critical illness is characterized by high GH levels with attenuated oscillatory activity associated with low levels of insulin-like growth factor-1 (IGF-1).
- This pattern is interpreted as a state of resistance to GH that is mainly related to decreased expression of GH receptors.
- This GH resistance seems to be beneficial: the direct lipolysis and anti-insulin effects may be enhanced, liberating metabolic substrates such as free fatty acids and glucose to vital organs, while costly metabolism mediated by IGF-1 is postponed.
- When critical illness–related stress is sustained, the pattern of GH secretion shows less pulsatile fraction and elevated nonpulsatile fraction. It correlates with the low circulating levels of peripheral effectors such as IGF-1.
- However, contrary to the acute phase of critical illness, this reduced secretion of IGF-1 does not reflect resistance to GH, but rather, suggests a hypothalamic origin as confirmed by the restoration of the pulsatile GH secretion pattern by infusion of GH secretagogues.

Adrenal Medulla Hormones

- It is well known that under resting conditions very small amounts of adrenaline and noradrenaline are released from the adrenal medulla (i.e., <50 ng/kg/minute in the dog). Therefore, absence of the adrenal medulla is well tolerated under resting conditions.
- However, exposure to stressors like fright, pain, anesthesia, exercise, cold, or endotoxin cause within seconds an increase in circulating adrenaline and noradrenaline concentrations by 2 to 3 logs. This response is absent if the adrenal medulla is removed.
- The release of catecholamines into the circulation accounts for the tachycardia, pupillary dilation, pilar erection, and spitting observed in the stressed animals.
- Adrenaline is stored in the adrenal medulla in vesicles. Noradrenaline is present in the subcellular granules of the sympathetic nervous endings.
- Catecholamines have a very short half-life (10 to 20 seconds for adrenaline) and are metabolized through captation, enzymatic inactivation (methylation in liver or kidney; oxidative deamination by monoamine oxydase), or renal excretion.
- The regulation of catecholamine secretion involves hormonal and nervous factors and negative feedback through calcium channels.
- The hormonal regulation depends on cortisol, which is necessary for the enzymatic degradation of catecholamine synthesis. This interaction relies on nerve transmission, paracrine effect, and the local vascular system.
- The neurogenic regulation involves the cholinergic preganglionic parasympathetic nervous system through the splanchnic nerves.
- Like cortisol, catecholamine levels in plasma can remain elevated as long as the stress is maintained, even up to a few months after recovery.

- Obtaining circulating plasma levels of adrenaline and noradrenaline is useless to assess the appropriateness of the catecholamine response to critical illness.

Insulin

- Insulin is involved in glucose metabolism through (1) mobilization of the store of glucose transport molecules in target cells such as muscle and fat tissue, (2) activation of hepatic glucokinase gene transcription, and (3) activation of glycogen synthetase and inhibition of glycogen phosphorylase.
- Other actions of insulin include growth stimulation, cellular differentiation, intracellular traffic, increased lipogenesis, glycogenesis, and protein synthesis. Insulin also modulates leptin and other adipokine release from fat cells.
- Insulin binds a ubiquitous membrane receptor belonging to the tyrosine kinase family, the IGF-1 and insulin receptor–related (IRR) receptor.
- Insulin levels in plasma are rapidly increased following an acute stress as a result of both increased secretion and tissue resistance.
- Insulin suppresses and antagonizes the effects of TNF, macrophage migration inhibitory factor (MIF), and superoxide anions and decreases the synthesis of the acute phase reactants.

CLINICAL CONSEQUENCES OF ENDOCRINE ACTIVITY DURING CRITICAL ILLNESS

- The immediate activation for the endocrine system, mainly the sympathoadrenal hormones, results in alertness, insomnia, hyperactivity, pupillary dilation, pilar erection, sweating, salivary secretion, tachycardia, rise in blood pressure with vasodilation of skeletal muscle and coronary arteries, bronchiolar dilation, skin vasoconstriction, mobilization of glucose from liver with hyperglycemia, increased oxygen capacity of the blood via spleen constriction and mobilization of red blood cells, and shortening of coagulation time.
- However, in the intensive care unit where flight is not possible, fighting is the only option, and the appropriateness of the neuroendocrine activity to the intensity and duration of the stress determines host survival and recovery (Table 113.3).
- The clinical consequences of the stress system activation include behavioral changes and cardiovascular, metabolic, and immune adaptations.

Behavioral Changes

- In animals, infections are associated with anorexia and body weight loss, hypersomnia, psychomotor retardation, fatigue, and impaired cognitive abilities. Similar behavioral changes are consistently reported in humans after cytokine or LPS challenge.
- The so-called depression due to a general medical condition is likely mediated through release of peripheral and brain cytokines.
- When glucocorticoids and catecholamine responses are insufficient, critically ill patients will develop brain dysfunction that can result to coma.

Cardiovascular Changes

- The cardiovascular adaptation is mainly driven by the sympathoadrenal hormones, even though thyroid hormones and

TABLE 113.3

CLINICAL CONSEQUENCES OF ENDOCRINE ACTIVITY DURING CRITICAL ILLNESS

	Appropriate response to stress	Inappropriate response to stress
Behavioral changes	Alertness, hyperactivity Insomnia, depression	Psychomotor retardation Hypersomnia Impaired cognitive abilities Anorexia and body weight loss
Cardiovascular changes	Tachycardia Rise in blood pressure Dilation of skeletal blood vessels and coronary arteries Skin vasoconstriction	Vasodilatory shock Multiple organ dysfunction
Metabolic changes	Mobilization of glucose from liver Hyperglycemia Mobilization of red blood cells Shortening coagulation time	Generation of free radicals and peroxynitrites Mitochondrial dysfunction Acquisition of superinfection Damage to central and peripheral nervous system Catabolism of muscle protein
Immune changes	Leukocytes accumulating into the inflammatory focus Activation of immune and immune accessory cells Generation of cytokines, neuropeptides, and lipid mediators of inflammation	Change the Th1/Th2 balance toward excess Th2 cells Release of proinflammatory mediators Apoptosis of T lymphocytes, eosinophils, epithelial cells Immune suppression

vasopressin contribute to cardiac adaptation, blood volume, and vasomotor tone regulation.

- Corticosteroids exert important actions on the various elements of the cardiovascular system, including the capillaries, the arterioles, and the myocardium.
- Corticosteroids enhanced vessel responsiveness to various vasoactive agents, particularly catecholamines.
- The underlying mechanisms are not fully understood and may involve direct mobilization of intracellular calcium, enzymatic metabolism of adrenaline, increased binding affinity of adrenaline for its receptor, or facilitation of the intracellular signalization that follows the coupling of adrenaline to its receptor.
- Corticosteroids also have catecholamine-independent effects on the heart and the vessels, and by retaining salt and water help maintain an appropriate blood volume.
- When the hypothalamic—pituitary–adrenal axis or the noradrenergic responses are inappropriate, critically ill patients will develop cardiovascular dysfunction.
- It has been shown that **septic shock patients with adrenal insufficiency,** as defined by an increase in cortisol of 9 μg/dL or less to ACTH challenge, have more pronounced hypotension than those with presumed normal function and are more likely to develop refractory shock. Adrenal failure also resulted in a more prolonged cardiovascular dysfunction and death in the septic patients.
- Adrenal insufficiency can develop in other critical illnesses, particularly in chronically ventilated patients where an association with weaning failure has been observed.
- Adrenal insufficiency is at best diagnosed in critically ill patients by either low baseline cortisol levels (of 10 μg/dL or less) or cortisol increment after 250 μg of corticotropin (ACTH) of 9 μg/dL or less.
- Failure of the noradrenergic system will also result in cardiovascular dysfunction during critical illness.
- A decrease in the pulsatile activity of the HPA axis and the noradrenergic system results in regularity within the circulatory and respiratory functions, enabling the patient to adjust to stressful conditions, losing the interorgan communications that result in multiple organ dysfunction and death.
- Finally, inappropriately low vasopressin levels contribute to the vasodilatory shock associated with many critical illnesses.

Metabolic Changes

- The net result from the activation of the endocrine system is hyperglycemia. The rise in blood glucose follows the activation of the so-called counter-regulatory hormones (glucocorticoids, adrenaline, and glucagon) and results in mobilization of glucose mainly from the liver.
- Subsequently, tissues that are insulin dependent cannot uptake glucose, which is then available for insulin-independent tissues like the brain or inflammatory cells.
- The main reason for critical illness–associated insulin resistance is impairment in glucose transporter isoform-4 (GLUT-4) metabolism. Proinflammatory cytokines such as TNF result in the generation of intracellular ceramides that block the transcription of the gene coding for GLUT-4, preventing the translocation of GLUT-4 to the cell's membrane and entry of glucose into the cells.

- Hyperglycemia has been shown to increase mortality in critical illness. The mechanism underlying glucose toxicity for the cells is still unknown and may include an overloading of the insulin-independent cells such as neurons.
- Excess in the catabolic hormones (cortisol, adrenaline, and glucagon) will also elicit an imbalance between muscle protein breakdown rate and the rate of muscle protein synthesis, resulting in a net catabolism of muscle protein, which may contribute to critical illness–induced muscle weakness and affect long-term prognosis.

Immune Changes

- The changes in the immune function are mainly related to the sympathoadrenal hormones, even though insulin and vasopressin can also influence immunity.
- Glucocorticoids suppress most, if not all, T-cell–derived cytokines and change the T-helper (Th)1/Th2 balance toward excess Th2 cells.
- Glucocorticoids up-regulate lymphocyte-derived IL-10 but do not effect IL-10 synthesis. They also inhibit the synthesis of many other inflammatory mediators such as cyclo-oxygenase and iNOS and down-regulate cell surfaces markers such as endotoxin receptor and adhesion molecules.
- Glucocorticoids enhance the occurrence of apoptosis of thymocytes, mature T lymphocytes, eosinophils, epithelial cells, and precursors of dermal/interstitial dendritic cells, but delay apoptosis of neutrophils.
- Catecholamines also drive a Th2 shift in both antigen-presenting cells and Th1 cells. In LPS-stimulated human blood cultures, noradrenaline and adrenaline inhibit IL-12 synthesis and enhance IL-10 release, an effect that is mediated via beta-adrenergic receptors.
- While the stress hormones glucocorticoids and catecholamines induce systemically a shift of the Th1/Th2 balance in favor of Th2 cells, catecholamines also promote locally at the level of inflamed tissues the synthesis of proinflammatory mediators.
- In addition, at the inflammatory sites, tight cross talk between cytokines and the cortisone/cortisol shuttle, with TNF and IL-1 converting cortisone to cortisol and IL-4 and IL-13 inactivating cortisol into cortisone, helps balance the proinflammatory and anti-inflammatory responses.
- When critical illness is associated with an impaired HPA axis, the Th1/Th2 shift favors the release of proinflammatory mediators in the circulation and in body tissues, allowing cytokine-induced cell deaths either through ischemic or apoptotic mechanisms.

MANIPULATION OF ENDOCRINE ACTIVITY DURING CRITICAL ILLNESS

- The use of exogenous hormones in critical illness has become a standard of care (Table 113.4).
- Although there are no randomized controlled trials of adrenaline, noradrenaline, or dopamine versus a placebo or no treatment, these drugs are routinely administered in critically ill patients with cardiovascular dysfunction.

TABLE 113.4

MANIPULATION OF ENDOCRINE ACTIVITY DURING
CRITICAL ILLNESS

Endocrine intervention	Main effects
Vasopressin	Increases systemic vascular resistance and mean arterial pressure Improves cardiac performance Improves renal function
Corticosteroids	Improves systemic hemodynamics and hastens shock recovery Improves organ dysfunction and mortality
Insulin	Improves morbidity and mortality in both surgical and medical patients
Thyroid hormones	Improves hemodynamics No evidence of survival benefit
Growth hormone	High doses associated with increased morbidity and mortality
Coadministration of GHRP-2, TRH, and GNRH	Beneficial metabolic effects?

Refer to Table 113.1 for abbreviations.

- Although it is clear that exogenous administration of catecholamines or vasopressin can restore hemodynamic stability in critical illness, whether manipulating these hormones helps survival remains uncertain.

- The use of corticosteroids in patients with septic shock has been controversial for several decades and continues to be controversial.
- The effects of corticosteroid administration have been studied, particularly in patients with severe infections. There is enough evidence in the literature supporting the benefit of corticosteroids on hemodynamic and systemic inflammation.
- It is well recognized that a short course of high-dose glucocorticoids should be avoided. In contrast, combined administration of low doses of glucocorticoid and mineralocorticoid improved survival in septic shock patients with demonstrable failure of the HPA axis.
- The updated Surviving Sepsis campaign has given the following recommendation: "We suggest intravenous hydrocortisone be given only to adult septic shock patients after blood pressure is identified to be poorly responsive to fluid resuscitation and vasopressor therapy."
- Additional recommendations are as follows: fludrocortisone is optional when hydrocortisone is used, and steroid therapy should not be guided by the corticotropin test results.
- In critically ill patients who failed to wean from the ventilator because of adrenal insufficiency, hydrocortisone replacement significantly improved outcome.
- Although there is conflicting evidence, intensive treatment with insulin may significantly improve morbidity and mortality in both surgical and medical patients.
- Thyroid hormone replacement in various critical illnesses, including in patients with cardiac disease, sepsis, acute respiratory distress syndrome, or with burn and trauma patients, was associated with some hemodynamic improvement. However, there is also evidence for side effects–related increased risk of death.
- Growth hormone therapy in critically ill patients is associated with increased mortality.

CHAPTER 114 ■ DISORDERED GLUCOSE METABOLISM

- Disordered glucose metabolism is a significant medical problem in patients in the outpatient, emergency room, ward, and intensive care settings. Diabetes mellitus (DM), the most important group of medical conditions resulting from disordered glucose metabolism, results in significant short-term and chronic morbidity and is increasing in prevalence around the globe.
- In the United States alone, nearly 6% of the population (18.2 million people) are estimated to have this disease. In addition to the many associated chronic health conditions developed by patients with DM, there are several acute and life-threatening conditions that also develop in these patients. Hyperglycemic emergencies, such as diabetic ketoacidosis

(DKA) and hyperosmotic hyperglycemic nonketotic syndrome (HHS), are important causes of morbidity and mortality in patients with DM who are admitted to the intensive care unit.

DIABETIC KETOACIDOSIS

- DKA remains a serious and potentially fatal complication of DM. Overall mortality from DKA is <5%; however, mortality increases substantially with extremes of age, the presence of coma, or the development of hypotension.

- DKA is the initial presentation of DM in up to 30% of patients overall, with approximately 40% of children and 17% of adults presenting in DKA without prior diagnosis of DM.
- While most patients presenting with DKA have type 1 DM, those with type 2 DM can also develop DKA during times of significant physiologic stress.

Pathophysiology

- Normal glucose metabolism is typically tightly regulated to maintain a serum glucose concentration between **70 and 115 mg/dL** (about 3.9–6.4 mm/L) by carefully balancing glucose production in the liver and glucose utilization in peripheral tissues.
- Insulin is mainly responsible for this tight glucose control by stimulating hepatic glucose uptake and storage (glycogen synthesis) and suppressing hepatic gluconeogenesis and glycogenolysis.
- In DKA, either relative or absolute insulin deficiency combined with increased counter-regulatory hormones (CRHs)—glucagon, catecholamines, cortisol, and growth hormone—promotes metabolic pathways opposite to insulin in both hepatic and peripheral tissues.
- Most patients with **type 1 DM** who develop DKA have an absolute or near-absolute insulin deficiency, whereas most patients with **type 2 DM** have either normal or elevated insulin levels.
- These changes are typically the result of a **precipitating event** in patients with severely imbalanced DM (Table 114.1). Infection accounts for 30% to 50% of precipitating causes of DKA, with urinary tract and pulmonary infections making up the vast majority.
- Myocardial infarction, cerebrovascular accident, pulmonary embolism, pancreatitis, trauma, alcohol abuse, and drugs that affect carbohydrate metabolism can also precipitate DKA.
- DKA is also associated with **ketosis,** an additional product of worsening glucose homeostatic decompensation, which occurs as a result of increased lipolysis from increased action of hormone-sensitive lipase.
- Hormone-sensitive lipase is highly up-regulated during periods of insulin deficiency and elevations in CRHs. Hepatic oxidation of free fatty acids induced by hormone-sensitive lipase produces **ketone bodies,** mainly β-hydroxybutyrate (β-OHB) and acetoacetic acid, strong acids that present a large hydrogen ion load to the body.
- The normal buffering systems are rapidly overwhelmed by the ongoing hydrogen load, and an **anion gap acidosis** develops.
- Hyperglycemia and ketonemia produce a hypertonic intravascular environment, resulting in an intracellular water shift into the intravascular and interstitial compartments. The ensuing **cellular dehydration** is accompanied by electrolyte shifts as well.
- When the renal glucose reabsorption rate is exceeded, an osmotic diuresis of water and electrolytes occurs. Sodium, potassium, magnesium, calcium, chloride, and phosphate are all lost during this osmotic diuresis. Commonly, water and electrolyte deficits are compounded by poor oral intake and protracted vomiting.
- The effects of hypovolemia are responsible for the clinical picture as the depletion of the intravascular space produces

TABLE 114.1

PRECIPITATING FACTORS IN DIABETIC KETOACIDOSIS AND HYPEROSMOLAR HYPERGLYCEMIC NONKETOTIC SYNDROME

INFECTION
- Urinary tract infection
- Pneumonia
- Dental infection
- Cellulitis

COEXISTING CONDITIONS
- Acute myocardial infarction
- Cerebral vascular accident
- Pancreatitis
- Pulmonary embolism
- Hyperthermia
- Hypothermia
- Renal failure/dialysis
- Severe thermal injury
- Thyrotoxicosis
- Cushing syndrome
- Mesenteric thrombosis

MEDICATIONS
- Calcium-channel blockers
- β-Blockers
- Chlorpromazine
- Cimetidine
- Diazoxide
- Diuretics
- Ethacrynic acid
- Phenytoin
- Steroids
- Total parenteral nutrition

SUBSTANCE ABUSE
- Alcohol
- Cocaine

UNDIAGNOSED DIABETES MELLITUS

the life-threatening signs and symptoms. The body's response is a further increase in CRH, and the cycle is perpetuated.

Presentation and Diagnosis

- The presentation and diagnosis of DKA is typically straightforward and relies on a thorough patient history, focused physical examination, and appropriate laboratory analysis.
- Patients typically report a history of poor glucose control and symptoms associated with hyperglycemia, such as polyuria, polydipsia, weight loss, and lethargy that may progress over the course of days to weeks.
- **Nausea, vomiting, and abdominal pain** are also common presenting complaints and frequently signify the progression from symptomatic hyperglycemia to overt DKA.
- Physical examination may reveal evidence of dehydration—for example, tachycardia, hypotension, prolonged capillary refill time, poor skin turgor, dry mucous membranes, and weight loss.
- Additionally, **Kussmaul respirations** (very deep, gasping breaths taken in response to severe metabolic acidosis), an acetone or fruity breath odor, depressed mental status, and even focal neurologic deficits or coma may also be seen.

TABLE 114.2

DIAGNOSTIC CRITERIA FOR DIABETIC KETOACIDOSIS (DKA) AND
HYPEROSMOLAR HYPERGLYCEMIC NONKETOTIC SYNDROME (HHS)

Parameter	Normal range	DKA	HHS
Plasma glucose (mmol/L)	<6.7	>13.9	>33
Arterial pH	7.35–7.45	<7.30	>7.30
Serum bicarbonate (mmol/L)	22–28	<15	>15
Anion gap	>10	>12	<12
Serum osmolality (mOsm/kg)	Variable	Variable	>320
Serum ketones	Negative	Moderate to high	None
Urine ketones	Negative	Moderate to high	None

Adapted from Kitabchi AE, Umpierrez GE, Murphy MB, et al. Management of hyperglycemic crises in
patients with diabetes. *Diabetes Care.* 2001;24:131–153; and Chiasson JL, Aris-Jilwan N, Belanger R, et al.
Diagnosis and treatment of diabetic ketoacidosis and the hyperglycemic hyperosmolar state. *CMAJ.*
2003;168:859–866.

- **Laboratory analysis** is usually confirmatory of DKA in these patients (Table 114.2). A complete blood count, blood glucose, serum electrolytes, serum osmolality, blood urea nitrogen, serum creatinine, arterial or venous blood gas, serum ketones, and urinalysis should be ordered in patients with suspected DKA.
- Caution should be exercised when using the **serum sodium levels** in patients with DKA, as the reported laboratory value can be artificially low, normal, or elevated, depending on the spurious effects of glucose and triglycerides in these patients and the relative loss of water compared to sodium.
- In the presence of hyperglycemia, serum sodium measurement can be corrected by adding **1.6 mg/dL** to the measured serum sodium for **each 100 mg/dL increase** of glucose above normal.
- Appropriate cultures should be requested if infectious triggers of DKA are suspected.
- Other tests, such as serum lactate, β-human chorionic gonadotropin (β-HCG), electrocardiography, chest radiography, and computed tomography may be indicated, depending on the clinical scenario.
- A plasma anion gap–associated metabolic acidosis, due to the high ketone concentration, is typically seen in laboratory analysis of patients with DKA. However, in up to 11% of patients, a nongap hyperchloremic metabolic acidosis may occur instead.
- Other causes of anion gap–associated metabolic acidosis, which must be excluded during DKA evaluation, include alcoholic ketoacidosis, starvation ketoacidosis, and lactic acidosis, as well as methanol, ethylene glycol, paraldehyde, and salicylate ingestion.
- Ketonemia and ketonuria can both be assessed semiquantitatively with the nitroprusside reaction test. This test estimates the relative levels of acetoacetate and acetone in the blood, but does not detect the presence of β-OHB, potentially underestimating the degree of ketosis.
- Because the ratio of β-OHB to acetoacetate may increase from 1:1 to as much as 5:1 during the development of DKA, β-OHB may represent the predominant ketone during illness. Of note, β-OHB monitoring may significantly improve the diagnostic specificity in DKA patients with euglycemia or only mild hyperglycemia—as with prolonged vomiting, starvation, pregnancy, hepatic insufficiency, or following insulin administration—where blood glucose levels can be misleading.

Management

- Management of DKA includes the phases of initial resuscitation, correction of hyperglycemia and resolution of ketosis, and treatment of any precipitating causes.
- As with all resuscitations, evaluation and treatment of airway and breathing dysfunction should be done first. DKA can cause loss of protective airway reflexes, hypoxia, and hyperventilation.
- If the patient's **Glasgow Coma Scale is 8 or less,** or in situations that require sedation and transport away from the acute care environment for further evaluation, tracheal intubation may be necessary to ensure adequate **airway protection** and ventilation.
- Because these patients have a high incidence of **gastroparesis,** the placement of a decompressive gastric tube may also be warranted in the presence of an altered level of consciousness, and elevation of the head of bed to between 30 and 40 degrees may serve to prevent passive regurgitation.
- Mechanical ventilation, if utilized, should be set to maintain respiratory compensation of the accompanying severe metabolic acidosis initially and adjusted appropriately as the acidosis corrects.
- Following airway and respiratory care, initial therapy should be directed at restoring adequate **blood volume and organ perfusion** with intravascular volume resuscitation.
- In addition to correcting the hemodynamic insults associated with severe hypovolemia, appropriate volume administration can also decrease CRH levels and plasma glucose concentration.
- The goal during this phase is to replace the fluid deficit over the first 24 hours, half of which should be replaced in the first 6 to 8 hours. Typically 1 to 2 L of isotonic saline in the first 1 to 2 hours is sufficient for initial resuscitation; however, in more severe cases the resuscitation may require larger volumes, and some prefer to add colloids.
- The following clinical estimations of volume deficit using orthostatic blood pressure and heart rate may also be used

to guide initial fluid replacement, although these criteria may be less reliable in patients with neuropathy and/or impaired cardiovascular reflexes:

- An **increase in pulse** without change in blood pressure with orthostatic position change indicates approximately a **10% decrease** in extracellular volume (i.e., 2 L).
- A **decrease in blood pressure** (> 15/10 mm Hg) with position change indicates approximately a **15% to 20% decrease** in extracellular volume (i.e., 3–4 L).
- Supine hypotension indicates a decrease of > 20% in extracellular fluid volume (i.e., > 4 L).

- Invasive monitoring should be provided as necessary; patients with mild to moderate DKA may require only noninvasive blood pressure monitoring, continuous electrocardiography, pulse oximetry, and a urinary catheter, whereas patients with the most severe disease states and comorbidities may, in addition, require arterial and central venous catheterization.
- Additionally, patients with oliguria or hypotension refractory to initial rehydration, mental obtundation, sepsis, respiratory insufficiency, pregnancy, or significant comorbidities or precipitating events, such as myocardial infarction or decompensated congestive heart failure, should be managed in a critical care environment.
- After the initial resuscitation phase, both the rate of infusion and type of intravenous fluid must be adjusted. Current recommendations are to decrease the infusion rate to 250 mL/hour or to **4 to 14 mL/kg/hour,** depending on the patient's hydration status and goal replacement volume.
- Depending on the patient's corrected serum sodium, isotonic saline is continued or changed to hypotonic saline. If the patient's corrected serum sodium is low, 0.9% saline solution should be continued as the replacement fluid.
- Once plasma glucose levels reach 250 mg/dL, either 5% or 10% dextrose solution should be added to the replacement fluids to maintain serum glucose levels between 150 and 200 mg/dL, to allow the insulin infusion to continue until ketosis is reversed, and to prevent the too rapid correction of serum glucose levels.
- Concomitant with aggressive fluid resuscitation, insulin therapy to decrease glucose production and increase glucose utilization with subsequent improvements in ketosis, acidosis, and hyperglycemia should be instituted.
- Most experts recommend **low-dose insulin infusion** over intermittent intravenous or subcutaneous administration, as the former is more physiologic and more therapeutically reliable and decreases the risk of hypoglycemia and hypokalemia.
- Continuous insulin infusion is the preferred route of insulin in all but the mildest cases of DKA.
- For continuous insulin infusion, many experts recommend an **initial bolus** of regular insulin of 0.1 to 0.15 U/kg followed by an infusion at 0.05 to 0.1 U/kg/hour, with a goal of decreasing plasma glucose levels by **no more than 50 to 75 mg/dL/hour.**
- If the plasma glucose level does not respond appropriately in the first few hours, and if the intravascular volume status is adequate, the infusion rate may be doubled every hour until a constant decline in plasma glucose level is achieved.
- In addition to serum glucose and bicarbonate levels, the American Diabetic Association recommends evaluation of β-OHB levels as the preferred method of monitoring DKA, which may become the preferred method for rapid diagnosis.

- Typically, **β-OHB concentrations** are <1 mmol/L; however, in patients with DKA, plasma β-OHB concentration can be elevated to concentrations in excess of 4 to 12 mmol/L (mean 7 mmol/L). Adequate DKA treatment should prompt a decrease in β-OHB concentration by approximately 1 mmol/L/hour, and should return to baseline (< 1 mmol/L).
- Despite massive potassium losses (3–5 mEq/kg) in patients presenting with DKA, the serum potassium concentration may be normal due to intravascular volume contraction and intracellular electrolyte shifts. The addition of potassium to the fluids, once adequate renal function is ensured, can help prevent hypokalemia during DKA treatment.
- In patients with significant hemodynamic compromise or severe hypokalemia (i.e., with a serum potassium level <3.3 mEq/L), insulin should be temporarily withheld as resuscitation occurs, because the reduction in plasma glucose levels and acidosis can cause significant intracellular fluid and potassium shifts that may worsen cardiovascular function to the point of collapse.
- Severe hypokalemia may occur with resuscitation and insulin therapy and potentially cause life-threatening cardiac dysrhythmias and respiratory muscle weakness. **Potassium replacement** should begin once the serum potassium concentration falls **below 5.5 mEq/L,** assuming adequate urine output, using the following guidelines:
  - If the serum potassium is 4 to 5 mEq/L, 20 to 30 mEq of potassium should be added to each liter of intravenous fluid.
  - If the serum potassium is 3 to 4 mEq/L, 30 to 40 mEq of potassium should be added to each liter of intravenous fluid.
  - If the serum potassium is <3 mEq/L, 40 to 60 mEq of potassium should be added to each liter of intravenous fluid.
- In addition to potassium, other electrolytes such as **magnesium, phosphate, and calcium** are also depleted in patients with DKA. Inadequate serum concentrations of these electrolytes may cause respiratory depression, cardiac dysfunction, and alteration of tissue oxygenation that can be avoided by aggressive monitoring and appropriate replacement.
- Measurement of these electrolytes should be done at presentation to identify significant abnormalities in order to facilitate appropriate correction as early as clinically indicated. And they should be repeated as necessary, depending on the clinical scenario.
- Of note, hypocalcemia may become problematic in the face of overaggressive phosphate replacement.
- Adequate treatment of DKA—intravascular volume repletion with reversal of hyperglycemia and ketosis—is generally associated with improvements in both physiologic and laboratory parameters. Criteria for resolution of DKA include plasma **glucose < 200 mg/dL, serum bicarbonate concentration ≥ 18 mEq/L, venous pH > 7.3, anion gap < 12 mEq/L,** and, recently, β-OHB < 1 mmol/L.
- After resolution of the DKA episode, when the patient is able to tolerate enteral nutrition, a multidose subcutaneous insulin regimen that includes a combination of short- and intermediate- or long-acting insulin should be instituted.
- To allow for sufficient insulin plasma levels, intravenous insulin should be continued for 1 to 2 hours following the first dose of subcutaneous insulin.
- Following these acute phase, it is essential to also provide chronic therapy to prevent repeated episodes and secondary sequelae of diabetes mellitus.

COMPLICATIONS OF DIABETIC KETOACIDOSIS AND HYPEROSMOLAR HYPERGLYCEMIC NONKETOTIC SYNDROME TREATMENT

- Hyperglycemia
- Hypoglycemia
- Electrolyte disturbances (hypokalemia, hyperkalemia)
- Hyperchloremic metabolic acidosis
- Cerebral edema
- Intravascular volume overload
- Hypoxemia
- Noncardiogenic pulmonary edema
- Acute respiratory distress syndrome
- Rhabdomyolysis
- Thromboembolism
- Pancreatitis

Complications

- Common **complications** encountered during DKA treatment include hypoglycemia and hyperglycemia, various electrolyte disturbances, lactic acidosis, intravascular volume overload, cerebral edema, acute respiratory distress syndrome, coagulopathy, rhabdomyolysis, and thromboembolism (Table 114.3).
- **Hypoglycemia** and hyperglycemia are common complications of DKA treatment. While intensive intravenous insulin therapy decreases blood glucose levels, reverses ketone body formation, and improves insulin sensitivity, it also places the patient at significant risk for hypoglycemia and its associated serious complications, including significant cognitive dysfunction, coma, and death.
- The incidence of serious hypoglycemic episodes associated with DKA treatment can be substantially decreased with the institution of low-dose insulin protocols, the addition of **dextrose-containing solutions** to intravenous fluid management when the blood glucose concentration reaches **250 to 300 mg/dL**, and the institution of frequent blood glucose monitoring with frequent insulin infusion rate titration.
- Additionally, hyperglycemia—with the potential for DKA to recur—can be seen following the resolution of DKA, due in large part to abrupt termination of the intravenous insulin infusion without adequate overlap of nonintravenous therapies, including subcutaneous insulin.
- Hypokalemia may be responsible for associated dysrhythmias, skeletal muscle weakness, and ileus. Treatment of the acidemic state with bicarbonate and inadequate potassium replacement predisposes patients to hypokalemia.
- Cerebral edema is a rare, but devastating, complication of DKA therapy. It occurs more commonly in pediatric populations and may be seen in up to 1% of the patients treated for DKA. The exact reason for the development of cerebral edema during DKA treatment remains unproven; however, it is felt to be related to an overly **rapid correction** of the hyperosmolar state. For this reason, current recommendations state that the change in serum osmolality resultant from therapy should not exceed 3 mOsm/kg/hour, and, in patients with concomitant cardiac and renal compromise, serum osmolality should be monitored frequently.

- With worsening cerebral edema, intracranial pressure may significantly increase—occasionally to the point of brainstem herniation with associated respiratory arrest and cardiovascular derangements. For this reason, careful monitoring should be done during DKA treatment for signs of cerebral edema and brainstem herniation such as the acute onset of headache, changes in the level of consciousness, the development of papilledema, or the onset of seizures.
- Sodium and water deficits are slowly corrected, and rapid decreases in blood glucose levels are avoided. Treatment of this condition is largely supportive and may be improved with the use of mannitol as an osmotic diuretic to decrease the amount of cerebral edema.
- Acute respiratory distress syndrome is also a rare but potentially fatal complication that may occur at any time during the process of DKA. The disorder may be linked to the underlying cause of DKA as a source of infection or the treatment phase with associated fluid resuscitation, fluid shifts, and changing osmotic gradients.

HYPEROSMOLAR HYPERGLYCEMIC NONKETOTIC SYNDROME

- HHS is a medical emergency that develops in response to one of many **precipitating conditions** (see Table 114.1) in patients with type 2 DM.
- Among adults in the United States, the incidence of HHS is approximately 17.5 cases per 100,000 persons per year and results in significant morbidity and mortality. The mortality rate from HHS is related directly to patient age, considering that mortality is, for example, <10% in patients younger than 75 years of age compared to 35% in patients older than 84 years of age.
- In approximately 20% of patients presenting with HHS, this diagnosis is their initial presentation with type 2 diabetes. Additionally, the diagnosis is usually made after significant delay and is made more complex because HHS can coexist with DKA in approximately 30% of patients.

Pathophysiology

- The basic pathophysiologic abnormality in HHS is a **relative insulin deficiency** caused by both an increase in peripheral insulin resistance and an increase in blood levels of the counter-regulatory hormones glucagon, cortisol, and growth hormone.
- Various catecholamines increase hepatic and renal glucose production and further worsen peripheral tissue glucose utilization.
- Together, the above defects cause an insidious but dramatic rise in serum glucose concentration, typically over days to weeks.
- With increasing serum glucose concentration, an **osmotic gradient** develops between the intravascular and extravascular compartment. Because water moves from the extravascular compartment down this osmotic gradient, both intracellular dehydration and a transiently increased intravascular volume with relative serum hyponatremia can occur.
- As the serum glucose concentration continues to rise, osmotic diuresis causes profound decreases in intravascular volume,

coupled with losses of vital electrolytes such as sodium, potassium, phosphate, and magnesium.

- This **large intravascular volume loss** can result in life-threatening end-organ hypoperfusion and nonketotic metabolic acidosis.
- Compared to DKA, ketones are minimally produced in patients with HHS likely due to the ability of the pancreas to secrete insulin. The amount of insulin, while not sufficient to prevent hyperglycemia in these patients, does prevent fatty acid lipolysis and the formation of ketone bodies and development of ketoacidosis.

Presentation and Diagnosis

- Because patients with HHS typically fail to develop ketoacidosis, the time from onset to diagnosis and treatment can be significantly longer than in patients with DKA. The clinical diagnosis of these patients, therefore, requires a high index of clinical suspicion.
- Patients with suspected HHS may initially exhibit nausea/vomiting, visual disturbances, muscle weakness, and leg cramps. Left untreated, these patients eventually develop confusion, lethargy, hemiparesis, seizures, and coma.
- Physical examination may reveal both signs of profound dehydration—such as decreased skin turgor and dry mucous membranes—as well as abdominal distension from gastroparesis.
- Initial laboratory evaluation in patients with suspected HHS should include serum glucose, ketones, electrolytes, and creatinine concentration; serum measured and calculated osmolality; urinalysis; and appropriate empiric bacterial and fungal cultures (see Table 114.2).
- Because these patients can have significantly elevated serum glucose concentrations—as ≥1,000 mg/dL—the serum osmolality can be quite high and seems to correlate with neurologic symptoms.

Management

- The treatment goals for HHS include aggressive intravascular fluid replacement, insulin administration to correct hyperglycemia, appropriate electrolyte replacement, and, if indicated, respiratory system support. Ultimately, effective patient education and long-term patient support are also important.
- First, treatment of the triggering disorder should be started.
- HHS treatment is typically undertaken in two phases. The first is the acute—emergency—phase and consists of rapid **restoration of circulatory volume and electrolyte deficits** with concomitant insulin administration to correct serum hyperglycemia, hyperosmolality, and metabolic acidosis.
- The second phase is a transitional phase centered on changing insulin replacement to appropriate chronic diabetes therapy (i.e., subcutaneous or oral hypoglycemic regimen), as well as patient education and support.
- In patients with HHS, the total body water deficit can be as high as 100 to 200 mL/kg in adults; thus, fluid replacement is the mainstay therapy for intravascular collapse and poor organ perfusion.

- Initially, 0.9% saline solution should be infused at **15 to 20 mL/kg total body weight per hour** to restore extracellular fluid volume deficit. Normal saline infusion should continue until blood pressure and end-organ perfusion have been normalized. The intravenous solution should then be changed to 0.45% saline solution at a reduced rate to restore the intracellular fluid deficit.
- The overall fluid resuscitation goal should be replacement of one-half of the estimated fluid deficit over the first 8 hours, and the other half of the estimated fluid deficit over the next 16 hours. Care should be taken to ensure that the serum osmolality does **not decrease more than 3 mOsm/kg/hour** to reduce the risk of acute cerebral edema.
- The cornerstone of therapy for HHS is intravenous insulin given to restore normal peripheral glucose uptake, suppress lipolysis, and decrease hepatic gluconeogenesis.
- **Insulin** should be initially given as an intravenous **bolus of 0.15 units/kg**, followed by a continuous infusion of **0.1 unit/kg/hour** with a goal glucose decrease of 50 to 75 mg/dL/hour. While the patient is receiving intravenous insulin, the glucose should be **monitored every 1 to 2 hours** via either capillary or serum samples.
- Once the serum glucose decreases to 250 mg/dL, dextrose should be added to the intravenous fluid administration and the insulin infusion should be decreased to 0.05 to 0.1 U/kg/hour.
- Complications of insulin therapy include hypoglycemia, hypokalemia (insulin infusion should not begin with serum potassium <3.5 mEq/dL), and hypophosphatemia.
- Electrolyte replacement is also an important component to the management of HHS. **Hypokalemia** can develop during HHS due to intracellular shift of potassium ions from the extracellular compartment and losses due to the osmotic diuresis. For this reason, electrocardiographic monitoring should be utilized during this phase of therapy, and aggressive potassium replacement—with up to 40 mEq/hour—may be necessary.
- **Hypophosphatemia** may also develop secondary to the ongoing osmotic diuresis. Replacement of phosphate during HHS treatment seems prudent; however, several prospective randomized studies have failed to show a definitive benefit to phosphate replacement in the absence of decreased cardiac or respiratory function and anemia.

Complications

- In addition to the electrolyte abnormalities discussed above, complications from HHS include pancreatitis, rhabdomyolysis, thromboembolism, hyperchloremic metabolic acidosis, cerebral edema, acute gastric dilatation, and acute respiratory distress syndrome (see Table 114.3).
- Patients with HHS are at increased risk for **thromboembolism,** and thus, subcutaneous heparin administration may be warranted to prevent thromboembolic complications.
- Complications of HHS treatment include intravascular volume overload and acute cerebral edema from overaggressive intravenous fluid administration. Intravascular volume overload is seen as hypoxemic respiratory failure—often with pulmonary edema—and lower extremity pitting edema.
- **Acute cerebral edema** is manifested by headache, lethargy, and depressed levels of consciousness that can rapidly progress to brainstem herniation. Treatment of this

TABLE 114.4

RELATION BETWEEN INTENSIVE INSULIN THERAPY AND OUTCOME IN CRITICALLY ILL PATIENTS

Study	DIGAMI	Leuven I	Portland	Stamford	Leuven II
Patient population	Acute MI ($N = 620$)	Surgical ($N = 1,548$)	CABG ($N = 3,554$)	Medical ICU ($N = 1,600$)	Medical ICU ($N = 767$)
Diabetes	100%	13%	100%	17%	15%
Decrease in mortality rate	30%	34%	53%	29%	18%
Reason for reduced mortality rate	N/K	Sepsis	HF, VT, VF	N/K	Multiple
Hypoglycemia (%) (glucose level, mmol/L)[a]	17 (<3.0)	5.2 (<2.2)	0.8 (<3.3)	1.3 (<3.3)	25 (<2.2)
Mean glucose (mmol/L):					
Intensive treatment	9.2	5.7	9.8	7.3	5.8
Conventional treatment	12.0	8.5	11.8	8.4	8.6

CABG, coronary artery bypass graft; HF, heart failure; ICU, intensive care unit; MI, myocardial infarction; VF, ventricular fibrillation; VT, ventricular tachycardia; N/K, unknown.[a]1 glucose mmol/L = 18 mg/dL.

potentially devastating complication consists of administering an osmotic diuretic such as mannitol and supportive care.

GLYCEMIC CONTROL AND INSULIN THERAPY IN THE INTENSIVE CARE UNIT

- Over the past decade, multiple published studies (Table 114.4) suggested that intensified glycemic control of intensive care unit (ICU) patients by using intravenous insulin infusion results in improved outcomes, including decreased mortality rate. Although these observations led to dramatic changes in the management of ICU blood glucose control in both Europe and North America, concerns have been raised about the optimal range of glycemic control for ICU patients and the clinical implication of the increased risk of iatrogenic hypoglycemia.
- Although there were significant differences in design, blood sugar target, and patient population among all studies listed in Table 114.4, the results were, for the most part, fairly similar. Intensive therapy with intravenous insulin produced a consistent decrease in mortality rate in a variety of patient populations.
- In contrast, two recent multicenter randomized control trials (RCTs) of intensive insulin therapy—one focused on patients with severe sepsis (VISEP) and the second on medical and surgical ICU patients—failed to demonstrate improvement in mortality.
- The benefit of intensive insulin therapy may be a result of decreased infection rates with improving glycemic control.
- A higher rate of hypoglycemia was observed in the intensive insulin groups. This finding is particularly important for ICU patients who are commonly sedated and mechanically ventilated since aggressive lowering of serum glucose levels may

carry the risk of hypoglycemia, which is potentially more difficult to detect.
- In the case of sepsis, the most current Surviving Sepsis Campaign (Table 114.5) provides recommendations for glycemic control in the ICU.
- Until the full results of the ongoing studies become available, intensive insulin therapy to *all ICU patients* remains unsupported, and should be viewed with a healthy degree of scientific skepticism.

TABLE 114.5

THE SURVIVING SEPSIS CAMPAIGN 2008 CONSENSUS RECOMMENDATION ON GLUCOSE CONTROL DURING SEVERE SEPSIS

1. Following initial stabilization, intensive care unit patients with severe sepsis and hyperglycemia to receive intravenous insulin therapy to reduce blood glucose levels (grade 1B)
2. Validated protocol to be used for insulin dose adjustments and targeting glucose levels to the <150 mg/dL range (grade 2C)
3. All patients receiving intravenous insulin to receive a glucose calorie source in addition to monitoring blood glucose values every 1–2 h until glucose values and insulin infusion rates are stable, then every 4 h thereafter (grade 1C)
4. Caution taken if using point-of-care testing for capillary blood glucose as it may overestimate arterial blood or plasma glucose values (grade 1B)

Adapted from Dellinger P, Levy MM, Jean M, et al. Surviving Sepsis Campaign: international guidelines for management of severe sepsis and septic shock: 2008. *Crit Care Med.* 2008;36(1):296–327.

CHAPTER 115 ■ THE ADRENAL GLAND IN CRITICAL ILLNESS

- The most important adrenal problem affecting the intensivist is impaired production of adrenal steroids. Individuals with impaired capacity to produce adrenal steroids can become critically ill with illnesses that are otherwise trivial and are unlikely to improve in the absence of steroid replacement. Critically ill patients may also develop adrenal insufficiency in the course of an intensive care unit (ICU) admission secondary to the effects of the underlying disease, or its treatment, on either the pituitary or adrenal gland.
- Furthermore, it has been suggested that conditions such as septic shock and acute respiratory distress syndrome (ARDS) might frequently be associated with a relative deficiency of adrenal steroids and, thus, patients with these conditions might benefit from steroid treatment, even in the absence of preexisting adrenal disease.

STRESS POINTS

- The most important hormones synthesized by the adrenal gland are cortisol (the main glucocorticoid) and aldosterone (the main mineralocorticoid). **Cortisol** production is regulated by adrenocorticotropin hormone (ACTH) secretion, whereas **aldosterone** secretion is primarily regulated by the renin–angiotensin system.
- Corticosteroid insufficiency (hypoadrenalism) is the most important clinical problem involving the adrenal gland in the ICU setting. It can occur as a result of diseases that directly affect the adrenal gland (primary adrenal insufficiency) or those that impair ACTH production from the pituitary (secondary adrenal insufficiency). Corticosteroid insufficiency can be difficult to recognize since its clinical features are similar to those of other severe illnesses, and some features are masked by ICU interventions. Unrecognized, corticosteroid insufficiency is associated with a high mortality. The **clinical findings** associated with adrenal insufficiency are shown in Table 115.1.
- The diagnosis of adrenal insufficiency is difficult in critically ill patients due to the insensitivity of clinical features and the dramatic and variable changes that occur normally in the **hypothalamic–pituitary–adrenal (HPA) axis** during severe illness. The interpretation of biochemical tests is difficult and will depend on the clinical context. Where there is uncertainty, empiric glucocorticoid replacement is indicated.
- When the possibility of adrenal insufficiency during critical illness has been raised, definitive testing to determine whether it is present, persistent, and its nature (e.g., pituitary vs. Adrenal) will be needed, but only when the patient's condition has improved so as to safely allow the studies.

ESSENTIAL DIAGNOSTIC TESTS AND PROCEDURES

- The symptoms, physical signs, and laboratory findings traditionally associated with hypoadrenalism are not sufficiently sensitive to be reliable in making the diagnosis of adrenal insufficiency. Rather, these may suggest the need for biochemical testing.
- The diagnosis will usually be made on either a random serum **cortisol level,** the level of cortisol achieved after a **short ACTH test,** or (in the specific situation of septic shock) a poor **increment** in cortisol across a short ACTH test (Figs. 115.1 and 115.2).

PHYSIOLOGY OF THE ADRENAL GLAND

- The adrenal cortex is the site of synthesis of adrenal corticosteroids, whereas the medulla synthesizes catecholamines.

TABLE 115.1

CLINICAL FINDINGS IN ADRENAL INSUFFICIENCY

SYMPTOMS
Weakness/fatigue
Anorexia
Nausea, vomiting, abdominal pain
Salt craving[a]
Postural dizziness
Myalgias/arthralgias

SIGNS
Weight loss
Hyperpigmentation[a]
Hypotension
Vitiligo[a]

CLINICAL FINDINGS
Hyponatremia
Hyperkalemia[a]
Hypoglycemia
Uremia
Anemia
Eosinophilia
Vasopressor insensitivity
Systemic inflammatory response in absence of infection

[a]Features usually present in primary adrenal insufficiency but not secondary adrenal insufficiency.

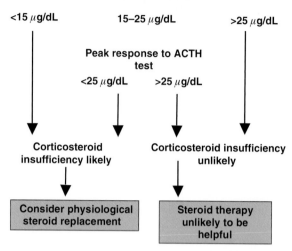

FIGURE 115.1. The combination of basal values and peak responses to ACTH tests is intended to avoid missing corticosteroid insufficiency of either central or adrenal origin.

- The cortex is structurally and functionally divided into layers (zones) that secrete mineralocorticoids, glucocorticoids, and adrenal androgens.

Adrenal Hormones

- The main hormones synthesized by the adrenal cortex are aldosterone (the main mineralocorticoid), cortisol (the main glucocorticoid), and dehydroepiandrosterone (the main adrenal androgen).
- **Aldosterone,** in conjunction with cortisol, regulates salt and water balance. The main action is to **increase sodium resorption** within the distal nephron; it also regulates sodium excretion from the skin (in sweat), the pancreas, and the colon.
- Cortisol action affects almost all tissues in the body and is important in maintaining homeostasis under resting and stress conditions. Cortisol in the circulation is **heavily bound** to serum proteins—**corticosteroid-binding globulin** (CBG) and **albumin**—such that only a small fraction is available in a tissue in free form.
- Adrenal androgens are the most abundantly produced adrenal steroids, but their clinical significance is minor compared to the other adrenal steroids, and they are not routinely substituted in patients with adrenal insufficiency.
- Adrenaline is the main catecholamine secreted from the adrenal medulla. Although this hormone may modify some aspects of the stress response, the relative normality of individuals who have had both adrenal medullas removed suggests that this action is of limited importance in most situations.

Regulation of Adrenal Hormone Synthesis

- Cortisol is synthesized in response to ACTH, which is released from the anterior pituitary.

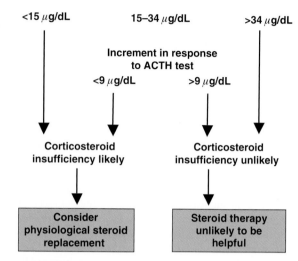

FIGURE 115.2. An adequate basal response is required to rule out central causes of corticosteroid insufficiency, whereas an adequate increment has been reported to be needed to exclude relative adrenal insufficiency. The use of an incremental response outside of the setting of septic shock is not recommended. (Adapted from Cooper MS, Stewart PM. Corticosteroid insufficiency in acutely ill patients. *N Engl J Med.* 2003;348:727–734.)

- **ACTH** release is controlled by hypothalamic **corticotrophin-releasing hormone** (CRH) secretion. Central activation of the HPA axis occurs with all physiologic stressors and also entrains the diurnal rhythm of cortisol secretion.
- ACTH has an important trophic action on the adrenal cortex, and continued ACTH secretion is essential to maintain the structural integrity of the cortex and the capacity to generate cortisol.
- Impairment of ACTH secretion leads to a prolonged reduction in the capacity of the adrenal to respond to exogenous ACTH.
- During severe illness, factors such as hypotension, pain, anxiety, and endotoxin substantially increase ACTH and cortisol secretion. The level of CBG also decreases rapidly due to a combination of reduced synthesis and increased breakdown. These combined effects lead to increased **free cortisol levels** and increase cortisol levels within target tissues.
- Aldosterone synthesis is under control of **both ACTH and angiotensin II** (AngII) with the rate-limiting step regulated by AngII.
- The activity of the renin–angiotensin system is thus the most important factor in regulating aldosterone synthesis.

Glucocorticoid Action

Metabolic Effects

- Glucocorticoids strongly influence most of the metabolic pathways involved in energy homeostasis. The effects ensure that **glucose is readily available** as a fuel.
- Glucocorticoids induce enzymes responsible for hepatic gluconeogenesis and antagonize the anabolic actions of insulin on glycogen deposition.

- Glucocorticoids also increase the production of fuels for gluconeogenesis by stimulating muscle amino acid generation and adipose tissue fatty acid synthesis.
- Prolonged glucocorticoid stimulation may result in adverse outcomes. Increased gluconeogenesis increases the risk of glucose intolerance and hyperglycemia. Continued breakdown of protein leads to myopathy, skin thinning, easy bruising, and poor wound healing. Increased peripheral lipolysis leads to loss of fat on limbs but accumulation of central fat.

Cardiovascular Effects

- Glucocorticoids have important effects on salt and water balance, which are likely to be an important part of the stress response protecting against hemorrhage or sepsis.
- Glucocorticoids contribute to renal **sodium reabsorption,** even though the dominant regulatory pathway is via aldosterone, and also have a major impact on the capacity to excrete water through the kidneys.
- A deficiency of glucocorticoids can result in excessive water retention and **hyponatremia.**
- In the absence of glucocorticoids, the vasculature can become **insensitive** to the pressor effects of **catecholamines.**

Immunologic Effects

- Glucocorticoids impact the development, migration, and survival of leukocytes, reduce the synthesis of proinflammatory cytokines by immune cells, and block tissue production of eicosanoids such as prostaglandins and leukotrienes.
- While excessive glucocorticoid action can lead to immunosuppression, glucocorticoid deficiency states are also associated with impaired resistance to microbial infection.

Other Effects

- Glucocorticoids can alter bone metabolism, leading to osteoporosis and fractures.
- Glucocorticoids may also induce a range of neuropsychiatric symptoms ranging from sleep disturbance to frank psychosis.

CORTICOSTEROID INSUFFICIENCY

- Corticosteroid insufficiency can occur with diseases or interventions that involve the adrenal gland directly (**primary adrenal insufficiency**) or occur from impaired ACTH production due to hypothalamic or pituitary disease (**secondary adrenal insufficiency**).

Causes of Corticosteroid Insufficiency

- Worldwide, the most common cause of permanent hypoadrenalism is tuberculous adrenalitis.
- In the general population, adrenal insufficiency is most frequently encountered in patients who have developed hypoadrenalism secondary to recent oral glucocorticoid usage.
- During critical illness, reversible adrenal insufficiency may develop secondary to many factors, including the use of anesthetic agents and antibiotics, central nervous system (CNS) disease, and adrenal insults that may comprise hemorrhage, infection, and hypoperfusion (see Table 115.1).

- Increased proinflammatory cytokine production during sepsis can also induce systemic glucocorticoid resistance such that normal adrenal responses may be insufficient to control systemic inflammation.
- Secondary hypoadrenalism due to recent exogenous glucocorticoid therapy may suppress the HPA axis, with consequent adrenal atrophy that may last for months after cessation of glucocorticoid treatment.
- Adrenal atrophy and subsequent deficiency depends on both the dose and duration of treatment but should be anticipated in any patient taking (or having recently stopped) more than 30 mg hydrocortisone per day or equivalent for more than 3 weeks.
- In such subjects, hypoadrenalism may be precipitated by failure to give adequate glucocorticoid replacement for intercurrent stress.

Clinical Presentation

- The clinical presentation of adrenal insufficiency differs greatly between the endocrine outpatient setting and the ICU. In critically ill patients, **classical features may be masked.**
- In the outpatient setting, clinical features depend on the rate of onset and severity of adrenal deficiency. The onset may be insidious, with presenting symptoms such as weakness, weight loss, nausea, abdominal pain, arthralgia, and postural syncope, and the diagnosis being made only with the development of an acute crisis during an intercurrent illness.
- Skin pigmentation usually differentiates primary from secondary hypoadrenalism, reflecting the persistently high circulating ACTH concentrations in the former condition. In autoimmune Addison disease, there may be associated vitiligo.
- In secondary adrenal insufficiency due to hypopituitarism, the presentation may relate to symptom complexes due to deficiency of hormones other than ACTH, notably leutenizing hormone (LH)/follicle-stimulating hormone (FSH)—presenting with infertility, oligomenorrhea/amenorrhea, and/or poor libido—and thyroid-stimulating hormone (TSH)—presenting with weight gain and cold intolerance.
- Rarely, presentation may be more acute in patients with pituitary apoplexy.
- In critically ill patients, these features may be masked, and the only signs may be **hemodynamic instability** despite adequate fluid resuscitation, usually with a **hyperdynamic circulation** and decreased systemic vascular resistance, or ongoing evidence of inflammation without an obvious source or response to empiric treatment.
- Acute adrenal insufficiency (Addisonian crisis) is a medical emergency manifesting as hypotension and circulatory failure.

Laboratory Findings

- In established primary hypoadrenalism, hyponatremia is present in 90% of cases and hyperkalemia in 65%.
- **Hyperkalemia** occurs due to aldosterone deficiency and is therefore usually absent in secondary hypoadrenalism.
- **Hyponatremia** may be depletional in Addisonian crisis, but elevated vasopressin levels can cause dilutional hyponatremia in secondary adrenal insufficiency.

- Usually, free thyroxine concentrations are low or normal, but **TSH** values are frequently elevated. This is a direct effect of glucocorticoid deficiency and reverses with glucocorticoid replacement. Thyroxine levels may also be low in secondary hypoadrenalism. Thyroid hormone administration without glucocorticoids in these situations can precipitate adrenal insufficiency and should be avoided.
- **Eosinophilia** may be seen and can occasionally alert the astute clinician to the diagnosis.

Biochemical Diagnosis

- The biochemical diagnosis of hypoadrenalism can be straightforward in an outpatient setting but is often much more difficult in the critical care unit.
- Clinical suspicion of hypoadrenalism should be confirmed biochemically and, in the outpatient setting, the gold standard stimulation test is the **insulin tolerance test** (ITT).
- In the critical care unit setting, the ITT is problematic as it cannot be performed in patients with ischemic heart disease, epilepsy, or severe cortisol deficiency (a 0900 hr or early morning cortisol <7 μg/dL).
- The cortisol response to hypoglycemia obtained during the ITT can be reliably predicted by the ACTH stimulation test—a safer, quicker, and less expensive study.
- The **ACTH stimulation test** (Table 115.2) involves intramuscular (IM) or intravenous (IV) administration of 250 μg tetracosactrin. In critically ill patients, the IV route is preferred.
- In critically ill patients, plasma cortisol levels are measured at 0 and 30 minutes and an additional sample 60 minutes after baseline is often used, with the peak value defined as the higher of the 30- and 60-minute values.
- The peak value is unaffected by the time of day, but the basal value varies with the diurnal rhythm.
- The use of the 60-minute sample is not standard practice when basing decisions on peak levels but is reasonable when an increment is being used (e.g., septic shock).

- The ACTH test should not be used after a recent pituitary insult (surgery, apoplexy), as it may take 2 to 3 weeks for the adrenal cortex to readjust to the reduced level of ACTH secretion.
- The test can be performed in patients who have recently commenced corticosteroid replacement therapy with dexamethasone, as it does not cross-react in the cortisol assay.
- In a critically ill patient, the testing regimen is more complex and more difficult. The use of the short ACTH is controversial in critical illness but remains the test that is most useful to intensivists.
- In patients with suspected primary adrenal insufficiency, the **peak value** obtained during an ACTH test should be at least 20 μg/dL, but in patients with hypotension or sepsis, it would be reasonable to expect values to exceed 25 μg/dL.
- In patients found to have abnormal responses to the 250-μg study, further tests may be required to determine the cause, for example, studies for adrenal autoantibodies, abdominal imaging for primary adrenal failure, and/or pituitary magnetic resonance imaging and other anterior pituitary function tests for secondary adrenal failure.
- Clinical improvement with hydrocortisone replacement is good evidence for adrenal insufficiency when the diagnosis is uncertain.
- A general scheme for investigating adrenal insufficiency in critical illness, combining basal and stimulated tests, is given in Figure 115.1.
- In vasopressor-dependent septic shock, the **incremental response** (<9 μg/dL) post-ACTH administration is associated with increased mortality.

Management

- In addition to measurement of plasma electrolytes and blood glucose, samples for ACTH and cortisol should be taken before initiating corticosteroid therapy.
- If the patient is not critically ill, an ACTH stimulation test can be performed. In critically ill patients, intravenous

---

TABLE 115.2

ACTH STIMULATION TEST

Short Adrenocorticotropin Hormone (ACTH) Stimulation Test
Procedure. Serum samples are obtained just before and 30 (and/or 60) minutes after an IV injection of 250 μg of tetracosactrin (Synacthen, Cosyntropin, 1-24 ACTH).

INTERPRETATION

Unstressed patient:	Peak cortisol value <20 μg/dL suggests AI
During critical illness:	Peak cortisol <20 μg/dL suggests AI (patients without sepsis or hypotension)
	Peak cortisol <25 μg/dL suggests AI (patients with sepsis or hypotension)
	Cortisol increment <9 μg/dL indicates relative AI (of use *only* in vasopressor-dependent septic shock)

Comments. The diagnosis of adrenal insufficiency (AI) in the intensive care unit usually depends on the short ACTH stimulation test, but its interpretation is difficult and depends on clinical context. Peak cortisol values of either 20 or 25 μg/dL have been proposed and should be used depending on the severity of the illness. In septic shock, the use of the increment has been proposed for diagnosing relative adrenal insufficiency and may identify patients likely to benefit from glucocorticoid replacement; however, it should *not* be used outside this setting without evidence. The test does not differentiate between primary and secondary hypoadrenalism and is unreliable in recent-onset secondary AI.

TABLE 115.3

RELATIVE POTENCY OF GLUCOCORTICOIDS AND
APPROXIMATE DOSE EQUIVALENTS WHEN USED
FOR GLUCOCORTICOID REPLACEMENT

	Relative glucocorticoid potency[a]	Replacement dose (mg)
Hydrocortisone[b]	1	30[d]
Cortisone[b,c]	0.8	37.5
Prednisolone	4.5	5–7.5
Prednisone[c]	4.5	5–7.5
Methylprednisolone	5	4
Dexamethasone	35	0.75

[a]Relative glucocorticoid potency varies with the parameter studied so
is only approximate and refers predominantly to glucocorticoid
replacement in Addison disease.
[b]Physiologic glucocorticoids that are preferred for replacement
purposes.
[c]These steroids are inactive prodrugs so are used only via the oral
route.
[d]This is the standard initial replacement dose in patients with possible
adrenal insufficiency but can often be reduced to 15–20 mg when
needed long term.

hydrocortisone should be given in a dose of 100 mg every
6 hours either as a bolus dose or a continuous infusion.
- Clinical improvement, especially in blood pressure, should be
evident within 6 hours if the diagnosis is correct.
- After 24 hours, the hydrocortisone dose can be reduced, usually to 50 mg every 6 hours and subsequently, if possible,
to oral hydrocortisone, 40 mg in the morning and 20 mg at
6:00 p.m. This can then be rapidly reduced to standard replacement doses of 20 mg on wakening and 10 mg at 6:00 p.m.
- Although synthetic glucocorticoids have been used in adrenal
replacement—their relative potencies and dose equivalents
are given in Table 115.3—they have no advantage over hydrocortisone.
- Mineralocorticoid replacement is not required during high-
dose hydrocortisone therapy, but patients with adrenal disease will also require fludrocortisone when daily hydrocortisone dose drops below 50 mg/day.
- In septic shock, the recommended replacement is 50 mg of
hydrocortisone every 6 hours.

ADRENAL HORMONE EXCESS (CUSHING SYNDROME)

- States of endogenous corticosteroid excess are rare. Cushing
disease is due to an ACTH-secreting pituitary adenoma and
has an incidence of approximately 1 per 1 million of population.
- Endogenous *Cushing syndrome* is otherwise from a cortisol-
secreting adrenal adenoma or ectopic ACTH secretion, often
from a benign or malignant pulmonary tumor.
- The diagnosis of Cushing disease/syndrome and the determination of the site of the lesion are difficult to make, involving
dynamic suppression tests, imaging, and venous sampling.
- Much more common is iatrogenic Cushing syndrome caused
by therapeutic glucocorticoids. Patients with this disorder are
likely to have the classic features of Cushing syndrome—
namely, central obesity, myopathy, skin fragility, glucose
intolerance, osteoporosis, and hypertension.
- The main clinical issue in this situation is to ensure that a
physiologic replacement dose of steroid is maintained during
intercurrent stress.
- In any patient on long-term oral steroid doses above 5 to
7.5 mg prednisolone or its equivalent, intravenous steroid
replacement should be administered if the patient is unable to
continue the oral dose, since it is likely that he or she will have
a variable degree of adrenal atrophy secondary to prolonged
ACTH suppression.

OTHER ADRENAL DISEASES

Hyperaldosteronism

- Primary hyperaldosteronism was previously thought to be
uncommon, but is increasingly recognized as a major cause
of hypertension.
- This form of mineralocorticoid-mediated hypertension is
associated with **hypokalemia and a raised aldosterone-to-
renin ratio.**
- The use of this ratio has increased the number of diagnoses
of primary hyperaldosteronism, mainly due to an increased
incidence of bilateral adrenal hyperplasia.
- Treatment is with surgery or with long-term **spironolactone.**

CHAPTER 116 ■ PHEOCHROMOCYTOMA

IMMEDIATE CONCERNS

Major Problems

- Pheochromocytoma is a rare catecholamine-secreting tumor
with a wide spectrum of presentations ranging from minimal
symptoms to sudden death. Although early diagnosis can lead
to a curative treatment course, outcomes are often fatal when
the condition is unrecognized. Critical care physicians should

be familiar with pheochromocytoma crisis, as it is a medical
emergency requiring the highest level of specialty care.

Stress Points

- The diagnosis of pheochromocytoma should be considered
in any patient who presents with **severe hypertension** or
the classic symptoms of episodic **headache, palpitations,** and
diaphoresis.

- Furthermore, pheochromocytoma should be included in the differential diagnosis in any patient with an **unexplained cardiovascular event,** including congestive heart failure, myocardial infarction, or stroke.
- Fractionated **plasma metanephrines** or **24-hour urine metanephrines** are the initial laboratory studies to rule out pheochromocytoma.
- *α*-**Blockade** with phenoxybenzamine should be started as soon as the biochemical diagnosis of pheochromocytoma is established.
- After adequate *α*-blockade is established, *β*-**blockers** can be used as an adjuvant means of controlling tachycardia.
- Pheochromocytoma crisis is a medical emergency requiring immediate *α*-blockade and invasive hemodynamic monitoring; additional pharmacologic agents, such as *β*-blockers, calcium channel blockers, and intravenous nitrates, are often needed to control heart rate and blood pressure.
- The only curative therapy for pheochromocytoma is surgical resection; however, this should be attempted only on an elective basis after several weeks of adrenergic blockade.

PATHOPHYSIOLOGY

- Intermittent and unregulated catecholamine release is the hallmark pathophysiologic feature of pheochromocytoma.
- The morbidity of pheochromocytoma is primarily related to the cardiovascular impact of unregulated systemic catecholamine excess.
- Pheochromocytomas originate from chromaffin cells and, by definition, are located in the adrenal medulla.
- Approximately 90% of pheochromocytomas are histologically benign.
- There are three sequential products synthesized in the adrenal medulla from the precursor L-tyrosine—dopamine (DA), norepinephrine (NE), and epinephrine (EPI).
- The rate-limiting step in catecholamine synthesis is the production of the precursor peptide L-DOPA. By decarboxylation, L-DOPA is converted to DA, which is then converted to NE by *β*-hydroxylase. Ultimately, NE is converted to EPI by phenylethanolamine-N-methyltransferase (PNMT).
- Although NE is the predominant catecholamine secreted by most pheochromocytomas, there are reports of rare tumors that secrete DA, adrenocorticotropic hormone, vasoactive intestinal peptide, and calcitonin gene–related peptide.
- Because PNMT is found only in the adrenal medulla and the organ of Zuckerkandl, EPI-secreting tumors are typically located in these two locations.

EPIDEMIOLOGY OF PHEOCHROMOCYTOMA

- Pheochromocytoma is a rare tumor with an incidence ranging from 0.1% to 0.25% in large autopsy studies.
- The prevalence in hypertensive patients is in the range of 0.1% to 1%.
- Pheochromocytoma can occur sporadically or in association with several familial syndromes. Approximately 84% of cases are estimated to be sporadic.
- Up to 24% of nonsyndromic pheochromocytoma patients have specific germ line mutations, including RET (**MEN-2**),

VHL (**von Hippel-Lindau**), and succinate dehydrogenase subunit D (SDHD) and B (SDHB).
- Approximately 40% of MEN-2 patients develop pheochromocytoma. Because of the relatively high incidence, patients with the RET proto-oncogene mutation should be routinely screened for elevation in serum or urine metanephrines.
- Bilateral and multicentric tumors are more common in MEN-2 patients, while extra-adrenal and malignant lesions are uncommon.
- VHL disease is inherited in an autosomal dominant fashion and is characterized by retinal hemangiomatosis, pancreatic tumors, cerebellar hemangioblastoma, kidney lesions, and epididymal cystadenoma.
- Pheochromocytoma can be found in up to 20% of people with VHL disease. As in MEN-2, bilateral disease is more common than in sporadic cases.
- SDHB and SDHD are susceptibility genes for pheochromocytoma associated with extra-adrenal lesions. Whereas SDHD mutation carriers are more likely to have multifocal extra-adrenal pheochromocytomas, SDHB mutation carriers are more likely to develop malignancy and may be associated with kidney and thyroid cancer.
- Other rare familial disorders that are associated with pheochromocytoma include von Recklinghausen disease and Carney syndrome.

CLINICAL PRESENTATION

Signs and Symptoms

- Symptoms are highly variable but classic symptoms include episodic headache, palpitations, diaphoresis, and visual blurring.
- Other complaints may include tremors, anxiety, dizziness, nausea, diarrhea, abdominal discomfort, Raynaud phenomenon, and weight loss.
- **Hypertension** is the most common feature and occurs in up to 90% of patients. Less commonly, some present with diastolic hypertension and postural hypotension, in the absence of antihypertensive therapy.
- Patients may be normotensive between episodes of catecholamine excess, and **postural tachycardia and hypotension** is another commonly seen feature of pheochromocytoma.
- Conversely, some patients can be normotensive for many years and only suffer a hypertensive crisis after being stressed.
- Up to 23% of all "incidentalomas" are discovered during abdominal imaging in trauma patients, further underscoring the significance of this tumor in the critical care setting.
- On specific questioning, many of these patients with incidentalomas report symptoms referable to the hyperadrenergic state.
- Moreover, among patients with a known history of another malignancy, up to a fourth of radiologically discovered adrenal tumors are pheochromocytomas and not metastatic disease.

ESSENTIAL DIAGNOSTIC TESTS

Biochemical Identification

- The biochemical diagnosis of pheochromocytoma is dependent on the detection of the metabolic products of the catecholamines. Monoamine oxidase catalyzes the conversion of catecholamines into **vanillylmandelic acid** and **homovanillic acid.** Furthermore, carboxyl-O-methyl transferase converts NE, EPI, and DA to **normetanephrine, metanephrine,** and **methoxytyramine,** respectively.

- Because functional pheochromocytomas release catecholamines heterogeneously and intermittently, spot checks of NE, EPI, or DA are often within a normal range and cannot reliably exclude the diagnosis of pheochromocytoma.
- Conversely, free metanephrines are continuously elevated in patients with functional pheochromocytomas. Total metanephrine measurement is less sensitive than determining the fractionated amount of normetanephrine, metanephrine, and methoxytyramine.
- **Fractionated plasma metanephrine** measurement is more sensitive than 24-hour urinary total metanephrines and catecholamines but is less specific.
- In the critically ill patient with clinical characteristics that are highly suspicious for pheochromocytoma, measurement of fractionated plasma metanephrines is the most appropriate test. Conversely, when low-risk patients are screened, 24-hour urinary studies will yield the lowest proportion of false-positive results.
- Certain medications and radiographic contrast agents can interfere with the laboratory results and should be withheld before the draw. The list of medications that can affect the biochemical testing for pheochromocytoma is long and includes: **acetaminophen, β-blockers, vasodilators, α-blockers, stimulants, antipsychotics, antidepressants, and calcium channel blockers.**
- Provocative tests with agents such as histamine, glucagon, and naloxone are no longer recommended, as they can be dangerous and are ineffective in patients with normal urinary studies.

Tumor Localization

- Tumor localization will not likely change the therapeutic plan for patients in the intensive care unit. However, localization studies are important for surgical planning and can confirm the diagnosis.
- Ultrasound is particularly useful in critically ill patients, as it can be done at the bedside without exposing them to nephrotoxic contrast agents or ionizing radiation. Although ultrasound can accurately rule out a large adrenal lesion, it is also highly user dependent.
- **Magnetic resonance imaging** (MRI) can identify pheochromocytoma lesions and delineate the anatomy important for surgical planning. Pheochromocytomas have a characteristic high-intensity signal on **T2-weighted images.**
- **Computed tomography** (CT) **scanning** from the chest to pelvis is recommended to evaluate for extra-adrenal lesions. Drawbacks to consider include (1) the possibility of exacerbating a pheochromocytoma crisis from contrast injection; (2) the exposure to ionizing radiation, which may be important in some obstetric or pediatric patients; and (3) the obscuring artifacts that can occur from implanted devices and surgical clips.
- **Meta-[^{131}]iodobenzylguanidine (MIBG)** is particularly useful in patients at risk for multiple or extra-adrenal tumors, such as in young children, and in patients with a family history

or familial syndrome associated with pheochromocytoma. MIBG is less sensitive than CT or MRI.

Workup of Incidental Lesions

- The finding of an adrenal "incidentaloma" should prompt the biochemical workup described above, as well as the measurement of plasma aldosterone, renin activity, and 24-hour urine cortisol. These studies will rule out aldosteronoma and Cushing syndrome.
- Although many clinicians continue to perform fine-needle aspiration biopsy and selective venous sampling for patients with adrenal tumors, these interventional studies may precipitate a pheochromocytoma crisis and are relatively contraindicated.
- All functioning adrenal lesions, including pheochromocytoma, should be resected electively.

MANAGEMENT

Treatment of Nonemergent Pheochromocytoma

- Pheochromocytoma is a potential cause of cardiovascular emergencies such as heart failure, myocardial infarction, and stroke. When pheochromocytoma is the cause of these events, appropriate therapy to control the hyperadrenergic state can often reverse or minimize disability.
- Although surgical intervention remains the only curative therapy for pheochromocytoma, the tumor should be resected only after appropriate preoperative steps are undertaken.
- Preoperative preparation for elective resection includes α-blockade to control hypertension, prevent cardiac arrhythmias, and allow adequate volume resuscitation before resection.
- Effective preoperative preparation and α-blockade reduces operative mortality. Even in the normotensive patient, complete α-blockade will prevent hemodynamic instability caused by operative stress and tumor manipulation during elective resection.
- **Phenoxybenzamine** is an ideal α-blocker for preoperative patients because it has a relatively long half-life. The starting dose is 10 mg every 12 hours and should be titrated upward, as tolerated. Dose escalation can be halted when the patient has postural hypotension.
- **β-Blockers** are sometimes needed to control heart rate and should be given only after adequate α-blockade, to avoid severe hypertension from unopposed α-stimulation.
- **Metyrosine,** an inhibitor of tyrosine hydroxylase, reduces catecholamine production and can be added to the preoperative regimen.
- Narcotics should generally be avoided, as they may stimulate **histamine release,** which may in turn trigger a crisis.

Managing the Postoperative Patient

- Perioperative complications are either related to inadequate adrenergic blockade, lack of appropriate intravascular volume expansion, or to a technical problem. Surgical complications include bleeding, infection, and damage to nearby structures, such as the spleen or renal vessels.

- Most pheochromocytomas smaller than 6 cm can be resected using the laparoscopic technique. Larger tumors may require laparotomy or thoracoabdominal access for safe resection.

- Despite preoperative α-blockade, many patients have either arrhythmias or some form of hemodynamic instability during adrenalectomy. Some compensatory hypotension often results after tumor extirpation. Typically, this drop in blood pressure is minimized when blood volume is restored appropriately and when α-blockade is adequate preoperatively.

- Although many patients are hyperglycemic due to chronic catecholamine excess before resection, they may be profoundly **hypoglycemic** in the early postoperative period. Intravenous glucose and frequent blood sugar checks are required in many of these patients.

- Essential hypertension may persist after resection. Disease may recur from the contralateral adrenal gland or metastases years after surgery. Reoperative resection is the treatment of choice when complete extirpation is feasible.

- Palliative debulking is often desirable in patients with disease that cannot be completely resected, as it can improve symptoms and the effectiveness of medical therapy.

- An uncommon surgical complication of adrenalectomy is renovascular hypertension, a result of injury to, or thrombosis of, the renal artery or vein.

Treatment of Pheochromocytoma Crisis

- Pheochromocytoma crisis is uncommon but requires prompt diagnosis and emergent medical intervention. The clinical presentation of pheochromocytoma crisis includes (1) multisystem **organ failure;** (2) **fever,** often exceeding 40°C; (3) **encephalopathy;** and (4) **hemodynamic instability.**

- A common error is the **misdiagnosis of sepsis** in patients whose condition continues to decline despite empiric antibiotic therapy.

- Episodes of pheochromocytoma crisis are typically precipitated by traumatic stress, which is often iatrogenic.

- Patients in pheochromocytoma crisis should be transferred urgently to an **intensive care unit** or to the highest level of care available.

- **Phentolamine,** an intravenous α-blocker, should be given in 2-mg boluses. **Phenoxybenzamine** and **prazosin** can be used but can be more difficult to titrate.

- β-Blockade, without α-blockade, can precipitate hemodynamic instability. However, after initial α-blockade is started, β-blockade can effectively control heart rate and blood pressure. **Labetalol,** which has both α- and β-blocker effects, can be given intravenously during crisis situations.

- **Nitrates,** such as **sodium nitroprusside** and nitroglycerine, result in prompt venodilation, which can decrease cardiac preload and cause an immediate decline in blood pressure. Side effects from sodium nitroprusside include cyanide accumulation after long-term use. These agents should be used as adjuvant therapies after α-adrenergic blockade is achieved.

- Monitoring should include real-time arterial pressure and measurement of urinary output with a bladder catheter. Central venous monitoring is not essential, and placement should not delay pharmacologic treatment. Central venous catheters are useful for monitoring volume status, and many pharmacologic agents require central venous delivery.

- Emergent adrenalectomy should be avoided in patients with pheochromocytoma crisis. After the patient is stabilized and α-blockade instituted, planning should begin for elective adrenalectomy with curative intent. This can be performed during the same admission after preoperative planning, including the completion of localization studies and at least 2 weeks of α-blockade.

Pregnancy and Pheochromocytoma

- The stress of pregnancy and labor can prompt pheochromocytoma crisis and elicit symptoms in patients with unrecognized pheochromocytoma.

- On rare occasions, symptoms are minimal during gestation and manifest only after delivery.

- Obstetric outcomes are exceptionally poor when maternal pheochromocytoma is unrecognized; fetal and maternal mortality rates exceed 50% in such cases. However, others have reported favorable results when the diagnosis is established and the mother is adequately treated antenatally.

- In obstetric patients, maternal hypertension is often **erroneously attributed to pre-eclampsia or eclampsia.** Because of the grave consequences related to this missed diagnosis, pheochromocytoma should be considered in any hypertensive gravid woman.

- The localization of pheochromocytoma lesions in pregnant women should avoid fetal exposure to ionizing radiation. **Ultrasound** and **MRI** are safe, but CT and MIBG scanning result in some fetal exposure to radiation.

- Both α- and β-blockade can be given safely to the obstetric patient. The timing of surgical resection should be carefully planned.

- Emergent adrenalectomy is not required and should be delayed until delivery, which should be accomplished by cesarean section, or thereafter.

- If the diagnosis is made early in the gestational period and medical therapy is poorly tolerated, the second trimester is the ideal time period for elective laparoscopic resection. Surgery in the first trimester is associated with fetal loss, and resection in the third trimester can be technically challenging because of the larger uterus and can cause premature labor.

CHAPTER 117 ■ THYROID DISEASE IN THE INTENSIVE CARE UNIT

THYROID FUNCTION TESTS

- The purpose of this section is to provide an overview of the most commonly ordered labs. A later section will delineate how to interpret these values in the critically ill patient.

Serum Thyroid-Stimulating Hormone/ Free Thyroxine

- Measurement of serum thyroid-stimulating hormone (**TSH**) and free thyroxine (**FT$_4$**) is sufficient to diagnose most thyroid disorders.
- The ultrasensitive TSH test is recommended. Currently, the most widely accepted range of **0.45 to 4.12 mIU/L** is based on values from the NHANES III (National Health and Nutrition Examination Survey) database.

Total T$_4$ Measurement

- Total T$_4$ (TT$_4$) includes both bound and free thyroxine. Therefore, conditions or medications that affect serum levels of thyroid-binding globulin (TBG) will also affect the total T$_4$ value.
- The use of FT$_4$ value can eliminate this shortcoming. If FT$_4$ is not available, this level can be estimated by looking at the FT$_4$ index, FTI.

Serum Tri-iodothyronine (T$_3$)

- Serum tri-iodothyronine (T$_3$) may be measured in the free and bound fractions, although it is generally recommended that the **total T$_3$** be used, as only a minute fraction of T$_3$ is free.

- T$_3$ levels should be measured in patients suspected of having **hyperthyroidism**, as some patients may have excess secretion of only T$_3$ early in the course of thyrotoxicosis.
- Measurement of this hormone is not helpful in hypothyroidism as the elevated TSH stimulates preferential formation of T$_3$ to typically maintain the level in the normal range.

T$_3$ Resin Uptake

- T$_3$ resin uptake (T^{3}RU) is an indirect, inverse test to estimate the number of **unoccupied serum protein-binding sites.**
- T^{3}RU (the binding of ^{125}I-T$_3$ to an adsorbent) is increased if the number of unoccupied binding sites on TBG is decreased. This may be due to either low TBG levels such as in nephrotic syndrome or chronic liver disease, or increased thyroid hormone levels as in hyperthyroidism.
- In contrast, the T$_3$RU is low if the number of unoccupied binding sites is increased. Low thyroid hormone concentrations (hypothyroidism or high TBG concentrations), estrogen therapy, or pregnancy may lead to a low T$_3$RU.

Reverse T$_3$

- Reverse T$_3$ (rT$_3$) differs from T$_3$ in that the iodine is missing from the inner ring instead of the outer ring of T$_4$. It is largely bound to proteins in the serum.
- Its half-life in the serum is quite short, and furthermore, the biologic function of rT$_3$ is not completely understood in humans.
- The clinical utility of measuring these levels is chiefly in the setting of **sick euthyroidism.**
- Table 117.1 details the interpretation of thyroid function tests.

TABLE 117.1

INTERPRETATION OF THYROID FUNCTION TESTS

	TSH	Free T$_4$	Total T$_3$	T$_3$U	rT$_3$
Hypothyroidism					
Primary	High	Low	Normal	Low	Low/normal
Secondary	Low/normal	Low	Normal	Low	Low/normal
Hyperthyroidism	Low	High/normal	High	High	Low/normal
Sick euthyroid	Low/normal	Low/normal	Low	High	High

TSH, thyroid-stimulating hormone; T$_4$, thyroxine; T$_3$, tri-iodothyronine; T$_3$U, T$_3$ resin uptake; rT$_3$, reverse T$_3$.

DRUGS AND THYROID FUNCTION

- The vast majority of the effects of pharmacologic agents on thyroid hormone homeostasis may be divided into four categories:
  - Agents that alter the synthesis or secretion of thyroid hormones
  - Agents that alter hormone concentration by changing serum levels of binding proteins or by competing for their binding sites
  - Agents that modify the cellular uptake and metabolism of thyroid hormones
  - Agents that interfere with thyroid hormone action at the tissue level
- Typically these effects on thyroid hormone metabolism are transient, but they may complicate the interpretation of the thyroid function tests.
- Commonly used compounds that interfere with thyroid function and their mechanisms of action are listed in Table 117.2.

Thyrotoxicosis

Clinical Presentation

- In the intensive care unit (ICU), patients with thyrotoxicosis may have an atypical presentation, with tachyarrhythmias or central nervous system disturbance as the primary sign.
- It is important to consider thyroid dysfunction in the differential diagnosis of such patients, since treatment with

TABLE 117.3

SIGNS AND SYMPTOMS OF THYROTOXICOSIS

Symptoms	Signs
Anxiety	Goiter
Hyperdefecation	Lid lag/lid retraction
Sweating/heat intolerance	Proximal muscle weakness
Palpitations	Tremor
Weight loss	Tachycardia/arrhythmias
Weakness	Hyperreflexia
Increased appetite	Thyroid bruit
Scant/absent menses	Dermopathy

β-blockers and antithyroid medications can rapidly improve the clinical course.
- Table 117.3 lists the symptoms and signs that may be seen in a patient with thyrotoxicosis.

Cardiovascular Manifestations

- Sinus **tachycardia** and **atrial fibrillation** are the most commonly seen cardiovascular disorders in hyperthyroidism. Since atrial fibrillation may be the only indication of thyrotoxicosis, it is important to screen such patients with a TSH and FT_4.
- Congestive **heart failure** typically occurs only in patients with underlying heart disease, but may also manifest as a result of chronic tachycardia-induced cardiomyopathy.

TABLE 117.2

COMMONLY USED DRUGS THAT AFFECT THYROID FUNCTION

Drug	Mode of action	Thyroid function abnormality
Amiodarone	Inhibits cellular hormone uptake	Hyperthyroidism
	Alters hormone secretion	Hypothyroidism
	Alters intracellular metabolism	
Lithium	Reduced hormone secretion (acute)	Hypothyroidism (acute)
	Autoantibody immune response (chronic)	Hyperthyroidism (chronic)
Dopamine	Reduced hormone secretion	Reduced TSH, T_4
Cholestyramine		
Ferrous sulfate		
Charcoal		
Sucralfate	Reduced absorption from gut	Elevated TSH, reduced T_4
Propranolol	Altered hormone synthesis	Reduced T_4-to-T_3 conversion
Phenobarbital	Alters intracellular metabolism	Reduced total T_4
Sodium ipodate		
Iopanoic acid	Reduced hormone secretion	Reduced T_4-to-T_3 conversion
	Altered hormone synthesis	
Glucocorticoids	Reduced TSH secretion	Reduced total T_4
	Altered hormone synthesis	Reduced T_4-to-T_3 conversion
Heparin	Inhibits T_4 binding to TBG	Transient increase in fT_4
Lasix	Inhibits T_4 binding to TBG	Reduced total T_3, total T_4
Salicylates	Inhibits T_4 binding to TBG	Reduced total T_3, total T_4
		Increased free T_3, free T_4
Carbamazepine	Alters intracellular metabolism	Reduced total T_4
Radiographic contrast agents	Alters hormone secretion	Increased free T_4
		Decreased free T_3
Cytokines	Autoantibody immune response	Transient hypothyroidism or hyperthyroidism

TSH, thyroid-stimulating hormone; T_4, thyroxine; T_3, tri-iodothyronine; TBG, thyroid-binding globulin.

- Physical examination findings in a thyrotoxic patient include widened pulse pressure, hyperdynamic precordium, tachycardia, and systolic ejection murmur.
- The typical electrocardiographic changes seen in thyrotoxicosis are sinus tachycardia and atrial fibrillation. Patients may also present with complete heart block, and cases have been reported that showed reversal with treatment of the underlying thyroid disorder.

Pulmonary Manifestations

- Dyspnea on exertion is a common presenting symptom of patients with hyperthyroidism. **Respiratory muscle strength** is significantly reduced in thyrotoxicosis and improves with reduction of thyroid hormone levels.
- Several studies have also shown that thyrotoxicosis is a risk factor for the development of **pulmonary hypertension.**
- Pulmonary emboli may be seen in patients with atrial fibrillation who are not on anticoagulation therapy.
- Pulmonary edema has been described in uncontrolled thyrotoxic patients.

Laboratory Findings

- The laboratory findings in hyperthyroidism are the combination of a low TSH and a high FT_4 (see Table 117.1).
- If the FT_4 is normal and TSH suppressed in a patient suspected of having thyrotoxicosis, it is important to check the T_3 level, as this may be elevated in early Graves disease or in T_3-secreting toxic adenomas.
- In the event that the patient presents with an elevated T_4 or T_3 and a detectable or "normal" TSH, the clinician should consider the effects of **nonthyroidal illness** or drugs (see Table 117.2) on thyroid function testing.
- Rarely, the patient may have a TSH-secreting pituitary tumor or thyroid hormone resistance.
- Consultation with an endocrinologist may be warranted if the patient has unusual thyroid function tests that cannot be readily corroborated with the entire clinical picture.

Etiology

- The two most common causes of thyrotoxicosis in the outpatient setting are **Graves disease** and **toxic multinodular goiter.**
- Young women are more likely to present with the classic stigmata of Graves disease: thyroid bruit, ophthalmopathy, and diffuse goiter.
- Elderly patients tend to have a solitary or multiple nodules that become autonomously functioning and lead to hypersecretion of thyroid hormone.
- In the ICU it is important to consider other causes of hyperthyroidism. **Factitious** thyrotoxicosis is rare but should be considered in a patient with a history of taking herbal supplements or over-the-counter weight loss medications.
- Surreptitious use of thyroid hormone may be diagnosed by measurement of serum **thyroglobulin levels.** If low, this would indicate that the patient is self-medicating. Typically, the thyroglobulin levels are high in patients with true thyroid disorders.
- Patients with a history of Graves disease, multinodular goiter, or even subclinical hyperthyroidism may develop frank thyrotoxicosis several days after the administration of iodinated contrast media. However, patients with normal thyroid function are, in general, not at risk of this complication.

Treatment

- The treatment of thyrotoxicosis is based on the underlying pathophysiology. Patients with Graves disease, toxic multinodular goiter, or toxic adenoma should be started on a **thionamide**, such as methimazole (MMI) or propylthiouracil (PTU).
- The dosage of antithyroid medication should be tailored to the degree of thyrotoxicosis; hence, consultation with an endocrinologist is advisable.
- Patients with peripheral manifestations of hyperthyroidism may also benefit from the addition of a β-adrenergic antagonist drug. **Propranolol** is the drug most commonly used in the United States.
- Patients who have overdosed on thyroid hormone or are taking a supplement with thyroid hormone extract should be counseled regarding the complications of taking thyroid hormone supplements in excess, and the offending agent should be discontinued.
- If the patient requires treatment, β-adrenergic antagonists and bile acid sequestrants may be used.

Thyroid Storm

- Thyroid storm is a rare but life-threatening syndrome of exaggerated clinical manifestations of thyrotoxicosis. The clinical picture is one of decompensation of one or more **organ systems.**
- It is a medical emergency typically caused by exacerbation of hyperthyroidism following a precipitating event or illness; Table 117.4 lists the precipitants of thyroid storm.
- There are no universally accepted criteria for its diagnosis, and consequently, the incidence is unknown. However, four main features noted in thyroid storm are tachycardia, fever, central nervous system (CNS) disturbances, and gastrointestinal symptoms.
- The CNS symptoms vary from marked hyperirritability and anxiety to confusion and coma.
- Laboratory testing is unreliable in distinguishing patients with thyrotoxicosis and thyroid storm; thus the diagnosis of thyroid storm is primarily a clinical one.

TABLE 117.4

PRECIPITANTS OF THYROID STORM

Infection
Parturition
Nonthyroid surgery
Radioactive iodine therapy
Postthyroidectomy
Vigorous palpation of the thyroid
Iodine therapy/radiographic contrast agents
Diabetic ketoacidosis
Hypoglycemia
Withdrawal of antithyroid drug therapy
Myocardial infarction
Cerebrovascular accident
Pulmonary embolus
Trauma
Medications
Thyroxine
Haldol
Pseudoephedrine

TABLE 117.5

SUMMARY OF TREATMENT FOR THYROID STORM

Medication	Dose and route of administration	Action
Propranolol	0.5–1 mg IV over 10 min, then 1–3 mg IV as needed 80–120 mg PO every 6 h	β-Adrenergic blockade and inhibition of T_4-to-T_3 conversion
Thionamides PTU	200–400 mg PO/NG/PR every 4 h	Inhibit hormone synthesis and block conversion of T_4 to T_3
Methimazole	20 mg PO/NG every 4 h	Inhibits hormone synthesis
Iodine[a] SSKI Lugol solution	5 drops POo/NG every 6 h 10 drops PO/NG every 8 h	Blocks release of thyroid hormone
Iodinated contrast agents[a] Sodium ipodate or iopanoic acid	0.5 g PO/NG every 12 h	Blocks release of thyroid hormone and conversion of T_4 to T_3
Glucocorticoids Hydrocortisone Dexamethasone	200 mg IV load, then 100 mg IV every 8 h 2 mg PO/NG/IV every 6 h	Stress-dose steroids and blocks conversion of T_4 to T_3
Lithium	300 mg PO/NG every 6 h titrate to lithium level of 1 mEq/L	Inhibits hormone synthesis
Cholestyramine	4 g PO/NG every 6 h	Lowers serum T_3 and T_4

IV, intravenously; PO, orally; PTU, propylthiouracil; NG, nasogastrically; SSKI, saturated solution of potassium iodide.
[a]Either iodine or iodinated contrast agents should be used, but not both. Administration of iodine should be preceded by PTU by 2–3 hours to avoid enhancement of thyroid hormone synthesis.

- Mortality rates range from 20% to 100%, so prompt, multifaceted therapy is essential.

Management

- The treatment of thyroid storm takes a four-pronged approach (Table 117.5).
  - First, an antithyroid drug must be given to reduce thyroid hormone production and peripheral conversion of T_4 to T_3.
  - Second, supportive care must be administered against the systemic disturbances of fever, hypovolemia, and cardiovascular compromise.
  - Third, the peripheral actions of thyroid hormone should be blocked.
  - Finally, any precipitating factors should be addressed.
- A thionamide is given to block synthesis of T_3 and T_4. **PTU is** the favored agent because it also inhibits peripheral conversion of T_4 to T_3. By reducing T_3 concentrations in the serum, it is postulated that the manifestations of thyrotoxicosis are more rapidly improved with PTU than with MMI.
- Neither of these drugs is available parenterally, so administration is typically by mouth or nasogastric (NG) tube. In patients with altered mental status, or in whom an NG cannot be placed, rectal administration of PTU has been reported to be used successfully in a few patients.
- It is conventional to use high doses of antithyroid drugs, such as 200 to 400 mg PTU every 4 hours or 20 mg MMI every 4 hours.
- Thionamides do not inhibit the release of preformed T_3 and T_4 from the thyroid. Inorganic iodide, however, can accomplish this goal. It may be administered orally as **Lugol solution**

(10 drops every 8 hours) or as saturated solution of potassium iodide (SSKI, 5 drops every 6 hours).
- Oral radiographic contrast agents, sodium ipodate or iopanoic acid, may be substituted for iodine. These drugs block the release of preformed thyroid hormone from the gland and inhibit the extrathyroidal conversion of T_4 to T_3.
- It is critical to administer **thionamide therapy about an hour before the iodide** or contrast agent is given, because the sudden influx of iodide into the thyroid can lead to increased thyroid hormone production and thereby prolong the thyrotoxicosis.
- When the iodide or contrast agent is given after the antithyroid drug, serum T_3 and T_4 levels are substantially reduced in 2 to 3 days and may reach the normal range in 5 to 7 days.
- If the patient has an allergy to iodide or cannot tolerate thionamides, lithium may be substituted to inhibit T_3 and T_4 synthesis. It may be given initially at a dose of 300 mg every 6 hours and titrated to maintain serum lithium concentrations around 1 mEq/L.
- Fever is preferentially treated with acetaminophen. **Salicylates should not be used** as they inhibit T_3 and T_4 binding to serum proteins and thereby increase serum free T_3 and T_4 levels.
- The patient's fluid losses should be appropriately replaced, bearing in mind the insensible losses from high fever and, if present, diarrhea.
- Hypercalcemia, if present, will usually be reversed by adequate hydration.
- High-dose **glucocorticoids** have been given historically for empiric treatment of relative adrenal insufficiency. Such

TABLE 117.6

FEATURES OF AMIODARONE-INDUCED THYROTOXICOSIS

	Iodine-induced thyrotoxicosis (type I)	Destructive thyrotoxicosis (type II)
Underlying thyroid abnormality	Yes	No
Goiter	Diffuse or multinodular usually present	Occasionally small, firm goiter
RAIU	Low/normal/high	Low
Serum IL-6 concentrations	Slightly elevated	Markedly elevated
Pathogenic mechanism	Excessive thyroid hormone synthesis	Excessive hormone release (destructive thyroiditis)
Treatment	Thionamides and $KClO_4$	Glucocorticoids
Subsequent hypothyroidism	Unlikely	Possible
Color flow Doppler sonography	Normal or increased blood flow	Decreased blood flow

RAIU, radioactive iodine uptake; IL-6, interleukin-6; $KClO_4$, potassium perchlorate.

treatment also has the added benefit of inhibition of peripheral conversion of T_4 to T_3.

- In patients with Graves disease, glucocorticoids also directly inhibit secretion of thyroid hormone. A loading dose of hydrocortisone 200 mg may be given initially followed by 100 mg every 8 hours; this therapy can be tapered rapidly after 2 to 3 days.
- Dexamethasone or methylprednisolone at equivalent doses may be substituted for hydrocortisone if preferred.
- β-Adrenergic antagonist drugs can provide rapid amelioration of many of the symptoms of thyroid storm and should be dispensed immediately.
- In the thyrotoxic state, drug clearance is increased and higher-than-usual doses are necessary to achieve the desired effect. If rapid β-blockade is necessary to reduce heart rate, or if the patient's mental status precludes oral drugs, intravenous (IV) administration is preferred.
- In extreme cases, it may be beneficial to use a method to remove T_3 and T_4 from the patient's serum. The simplest approach is to administer oral **cholestyramine**. This drug binds the hormones in the gastrointestinal tract, interrupting the enterohepatic circulation. Plasmapheresis has also been used successfully to lower T_3 and T_4 levels.
- Patients treated with the above regimen usually recover in 12 to 24 hours if the syndrome is recognized and treated in a timely fashion.
- Long-term treatment of hyperthyroidism is required if the patient has Graves disease or toxic multinodular goiter. In patients with Graves disease, it may be preferable to treat with thionamides, as there is a chance of remission of the autoimmune condition. However, others advocate total thyroidectomy in cases that progress to thyroid storm.
- Radioiodine ablation is not an option for several months because the inorganic iodide used in treatment of the thyroid storm saturates the gland and precludes further uptake of iodide.

Drug-Induced Alterations in Thyroid Function

Amiodarone

- Amiodarone is a lipophilic drug that contains 75 mg iodine per 200-mg tablet.

- The drug has a half-life of several months, and, during that time, it releases approximately 9 mg of inorganic iodine per day.
- In euthyroid patients, chronic administration of the drug results in increased serum TT_4, FT_4, and rT_3 levels; lower T_3 concentrations; and normal TSH.
- Most patients remain euthyroid while on amiodarone despite the hormonal derangements that may be seen; on the other hand, about **14% to 18%** of patients develop either **hypothyroidism or hyperthyroidism** while on amiodarone.
- On discontinuation of the amiodarone, most patients return to euthyroidism, although it may take several months because of the prolonged half-life of the drug.
- Hypothyroidism is more commonly encountered in iodine-replete areas, such as the United States. Treatment is aimed at normalization of the TSH with levothyroxine replacement while the amiodarone therapy is continued.
- In iodine-deficient regions, it is more common to see hyperthyroidism as a result of amiodarone therapy. There are two mechanisms (Table 117.6) of amiodarone-induced thyrotoxicosis (AIT).
  - Type I AIT occurs in glands with an underlying abnormality. Areas of autonomy, such as a toxic nodule or autoimmune disease in the thyroid, produce increased levels of hormone in response to the excess iodine released from the amiodarone.
  - Type II AIT develops as a result of a direct cytotoxic effect of amiodarone on the thyrocyte.
- Treatment of type I AIT is difficult because most patients do not respond to thionamides, as these drugs have decreased efficacy in states of iodine excess. If possible, it is important to discontinue the amiodarone.
- Use of potassium perchlorate ($KClO_4$) blocks further iodine entry into the thyrocyte and may enhance the efficacy of thionamides.
- It is important to note that both thionamides and $KClO_4$ may cause agranulocytosis, so serial monitoring of blood counts is advisable.
- The treatment of type II AIT is primarily with glucocorticoids and by discontinuation of the amiodarone, although in some cases it is reasonable to continue the antiarrhythmic medication. In patients in whom chronic therapy with amiodarone is essential, thyroidectomy is a potential option for treatment of AIT.
- Radioiodine ablation is not an option given the low iodine uptake as a result of the iodine excess from the amiodarone.

CONTRAST MEDIA AND THYROID FUNCTION

- Another potential source of excess iodine is radiographic contrast media. The oral cholecystographic agents, iopanoic acid and sodium ipodate, may be used short term in thyrotoxic patients for their side effect of decreasing peripheral conversion of T_4 to T_3 and blocking hormone secretion from the thyroid. Used over a longer period of time, however, such agents will only exacerbate the underlying hyperthyroidism.
- Many other agents are available that have variable effects on the thyroid gland. Typically, patients with no underlying thyroid disease will not be affected by the use of these agents, but patients with Graves disease, multinodular goiter, or the elderly are at risk to develop **thyrotoxicosis** after their use.
- The lipid-soluble agents used for myelography, bronchography, and uterosalpingography are cleared slowly and release inorganic iodine for months to years.
- Newer water-soluble preparations used in arteriography and computed tomography are cleared from the plasma more quickly, but the iodine they release during these procedures can still affect thyroid function.
- The degree of thyroid dysfunction can range from mild transient subclinical hyperthyroidism to thyroid storm. Most patients experience only transient thyrotoxicosis, and the syndrome resolves when the excess iodine is cleared. If treatment is required, thionamides and β-adrenergic blockade may be used until the thyrotoxicosis resolves.

THYROTOXIC PERIODIC PARALYSIS

- Thyrotoxic periodic paralysis (TPP) is a complication of hyperthyroidism characterized by localized or generalized attacks of weakness or flaccid paralysis and hypokalemia.
- Although it has been reported in Western countries and in women, it is more common in Asian men, where the incidence is 1.9% in thyrotoxic patients.
- The clinical presentation is identical to familial hypokalemic periodic paralysis, but the pathophysiology is distinct. Although the mechanism of the syndrome is not clearly defined, hypokalemia alone is not enough to elicit the paralysis.

Clinical Presentation

- The clinical presentation is one of flaccid weakness that is symmetrical; lower extremities are generally affected more than the upper extremities.
- Breathing may be impaired if the patient has a more generalized weakness.
- The onset of the attacks is usually sudden and may be preceded by cramping.
- Ingestion of alcohol or carbohydrates and strenuous physical exercise commonly precipitate the episodes of weakness.
- Patients have decreased or absent deep-tendon reflexes. The symptoms may last from a few hours to several days.

Treatment

- Treatment is aimed at correction of the hyperthyroidism. If hypokalemia is present, replacement should be given.

- Some patients are given a potassium-sparing diuretic in addition to the potassium supplementation until euthyroidism is achieved. β-Adrenergic antagonists also decrease the frequency of attacks in these patients.

Preoperative Management

- Adequate preparation for surgery in thyrotoxic patients is critical to the successful outcome of the procedure. Surgery in a hyperthyroid patient can precipitate thyroid storm, with high morbidity and mortality if preoperative care is inadequate.
- The type of treatment will depend on the amount of time before the surgery. Elective procedures should be postponed until the T_3 and T_4 levels are normalized with thionamides and β-adrenergic blockade. This can usually be achieved within approximately 2 weeks.
- TSH may not normalize for months, and this value should not be used as the criteria to assess the thyroid status.
- Urgent or emergent procedures may be safely done after initiation of PTU and a β-adrenergic antagonist. Inorganic iodide should also be administered to block release of thyroid hormone and decrease peripheral conversion of T_4 to T_3.
- Finally, a glucocorticoid should also be used if the patient is suspected of having concomitant adrenal insufficiency, or additional inhibition of T_4 to T_3 conversion is needed.

HYPOTHYROIDISM

- Hypothyroidism is a common clinical problem, affecting approximately 4.6% of the population in the United States.
- Hypothyroidism is most often caused by autoimmune thyroiditis, also known as *Hashimoto thyroiditis*. Other common causes of hypothyroidism are noted in Table 117.7.
- Nonthyroidal illness, surgery, or diagnostic testing can lead to metabolic decompensation in patients with undiagnosed or untreated hypothyroidism.
- Untreated hypothyroidism may slow the metabolism of certain drugs, thereby increasing the risk of problematic side effects.

TABLE 117.7

CAUSES OF HYPOTHYROIDISM

Autoimmune, Hashimoto thyroiditis
Postthyroidectomy
Postradiation
^{131}I treatment
External beam radiation
Iodine deficiency
Drugs
Lithium
Iodine-containing drugs (amiodarone, radiocontrast agents)
Secondary hypothyroidism
Pituitary tumor, irradiation, empty sella syndrome, infiltrative disorders
Hypothalamic disease
Transient disorders
Silent, subacute thyroiditis

TABLE 117.8

CLINICAL MANIFESTATIONS OF HYPOTHYROIDISM

Symptoms	Signs
Fatigue and weakness	Delayed relaxation of tendon reflexes
Cold intolerance	Bradycardia
Weight gain	Hypoventilation
Constipation	Diastolic hypertension
Dyspnea on exertion	Reduced pulse pressure
Depression	Pericardial and pleural effusions
Menorrhagia	Generalized and periorbital edema
Myalgia	Macroglossia
Dry skin and hair	Loss of eyebrows

- The clinical manifestations of hypothyroidism are manifold. Most of the symptoms are nonspecific, which can lead to a delay in the diagnosis.
- In elderly patients, the diagnosis may be missed because the patient may be asymptomatic or the signs attributed to aging.
- Patients in the ICU may present with severe CNS disturbances, cardiovascular derangements, hyponatremia, or respiratory failure.
- Table 117.8 notes the signs and symptoms of hypothyroidism.

Cardiovascular Manifestations

- The symptoms of cardiovascular dysfunction are much less pronounced in patients with hypothyroidism compared to their thyrotoxic counterparts.
- Cardiovascular hemodynamics are affected by hypothyroidism in several ways. In particular, patients have **decreased cardiac output,** mediated by reduced contractility and heart rate.
- These patients also have increased systemic vascular resistance, predisposing them to hypertension.
- Diastolic filling and compliance are reduced, leading to diastolic dysfunction. Elevation of diastolic pressure, out of proportion to systolic pressure, may lead to a decreased pulse pressure.
- Although congestive heart failure can occur with hypothyroidism, it is rare for hypothyroidism to be the sole causative agent. Typically, patients have underlying cardiac disease that is exacerbated by hypothyroidism.
- Pericardial effusion associated with hypothyroidism may also compromise cardiac function.
- Angina may also worsen in patients with hypothyroidism.
- Patients without preexisting cardiac dysfunction typically do not manifest symptoms and signs of congestive heart failure or coronary artery syndrome unless the hypothyroidism is profound.

Pulmonary Manifestations

- **Dyspnea on exertion** is a common presenting complaint in patients with hypothyroidism, in part due to the impaired cardiac function and reduced pulmonary function. Respiratory muscle weakness also appears to play a role in this dyspnea.

- There is a reduction in central pulmonary drive in response to hypoxia and hypercapnia, leading to hypoventilation.
- Upper airway obstruction may occur as a result of goiter (see below: Acute Airway Obstruction). Additionally, sleep apnea may occur as a result of macroglossia.
- Finally, a restrictive pattern of disease may be seen in the presence of a pulmonary effusion.

Gastrointestinal Manifestations

- **Peristalsis** is slowed in patients with hypothyroidism. Most patients have normal bowel motility, but a small proportion with hypothyroidism requires laxative use.
- Patients may report vague abdominal pain and distention. Rarely, severe cases may present with ileus.
- Severely hypothyroid patients may also have **malabsorption.** The mechanism of this abnormal absorption is not clearly defined; theories include myxedematous infiltration of the mucosa, associated autoimmunity, and decreased intestinal motility.

Metabolic Manifestations

- Hypothyroidism may lead to decreased free water clearance and subsequent **hyponatremia.** The magnitude of sodium derangement is directly related to the severity of hypothyroidism.
- Hyperlipidemia is more commonly seen than hyponatremia. Lipid clearance is decreased in patients with hypothyroidism, resulting in elevated levels of free fatty acids, low-density lipoprotein (LDL), and total cholesterol.
- Treatment of the hypothyroidism results in improvement of the lipid panel.

Treatment

- Thyroid hormone is preferentially replaced with T_4. In adults, the starting dose of T_4 is typically 1.7 μg/kg/day (based on ideal body weight). Elderly patients or those with coronary disease should be started at lower doses and titrated based on TSH levels every 6 weeks.

Complications

Myxedema Coma

- Myxedema coma is a rare but life-threatening complication of hypothyroidism. It may occur after severe longstanding hypothyroidism or after an acute precipitating event such as surgery or infection. It is more likely to occur in elderly women during the winter months.
- Any of the usual causes of hypothyroidism (see Table 117.6) may induce myxedema coma. Prompt recognition and treatment are essential, even before laboratory results are available.
- Mortality rates are improving due to early diagnosis and treatment, but mortality remains at 30% to 40%. Patients with cardiac complications and the elderly are at greatest risk.

Clinical Presentation

- Most patients with myxedema coma have had symptoms of hypothyroidism for many months. There is a gradual onset of lethargy, progressing to stupor, which is precipitated by cold exposure, infection, or medications. Other precipitating events are stroke, congestive heart failure, trauma, or gastrointestinal bleeding.
- The patient is typically an obese elderly woman with yellow discoloration of the skin. The principal features of myxedema are hypothermia, bradycardia, and decreased mental status or coma.
- Patients also characteristically have a **decreased respiratory rate** as a result of reduced hypoxic ventilatory drive. The resultant hypercarbia can exacerbate the altered mental status.
- **Hypothermia** is present in nearly all patients with myxedema coma. Temperature may be quite low (<80°F, [20°C]); values below 90°F (32°C) predict a poorer prognosis.
- The severity of hypothermia may go unrecognized if the proper thermometer is not used; many thermometers may not be able to measure below 93°F (34°C).
- The diagnosis of myxedema coma should be considered in any unconscious patient with infection who does not have a fever. Warming should be gradual, using ordinary hospital blankets. Electric heating blankets should not be used, as they may cause peripheral vasodilation and subsequent hypotension.
- The cardiovascular abnormalities seen in myxedema coma are similar to those associated with severe hypothyroidism. Patients can present with **bradycardia, reduced cardiac output,** and decreased cardiac contractility, which may lead to hypotension.
- Signs of congestive heart failure may be found. In patients with diminished heart sounds, low-voltage electrocardiogram, or cardiomegaly on chest radiograph, an investigation for pericardial effusion should be performed.
- This profound level of hypothyroidism may lead to impaired free water excretion. As a result, over half of patients can have **hyponatremia.**
- Patients should be managed by free water restriction; the condition will improve with thyroid hormone replacement.
- Bladder atony may occur, so patients should be monitored for residual volumes postvoiding.
- Hypoglycemia is a common feature that is the result of the hypothyroidism or concomitant adrenal insufficiency.

Diagnosis

- The diagnosis of myxedema coma is initially made based on historical and clinical clues. It is important to investigate other causes of altered mental status, such as cerebrovascular accident and infection.
- Serum should be obtained for measurement of TSH, free T_4, and cortisol.
- If the clinical picture is consistent with myxedema coma, treatment should be initiated before laboratory confirmation of the diagnosis.

Treatment

- Because of the high mortality rate of this endocrine emergency, patients with myxedema coma should be treated aggressively.
- Patients should be presumed to have adrenal insufficiency and treated with **stress-dose steroids** (hydrocortisone, 100 mg IV every 8 hours) until laboratory data exclude the diagnosis.

- The administration of levothyroxine prior to glucocorticoids in such patients can provoke an adrenal crisis.
- The optimal replacement strategy for levothyroxine is unknown because of the rarity of the condition. Clinical judgment must be used to weigh the risk of rapid administration of thyroid hormone—with the possibility of precipitation of myocardial infarction—against the risk of not replacing the thyroid hormone fast enough in light of the high mortality of undertreated myxedema coma.
- It is preferable to administer both T_3 and T_4 intravenously to patients with myxedema because of the possibility of impaired gastrointestinal absorption.
- Supportive care should be directed to the coexisting medical conditions. Hyponatremia can usually be managed with free water restriction, but 3% saline may be given in extreme circumstances.
- Hypotension will usually improve with initiation of levothyroxine. Refractory hypotension should be treated with vasopressor agents until the thyroid hormone has had time to act.
- Patients may require mechanical ventilation because of respiratory muscle weakness, depressed mental status, or decreased hypoxic ventilatory drive.
- Finally, it is important to address the underlying medical illness that precipitated the myxedema coma.

Preoperative Management of Hypothyroidism

- Patients with mild to moderate hypothyroidism may proceed to surgery, as no convincing evidence exists to show that there is an adverse effect on outcomes; if the procedure is elective, it is optimal to begin replacement with thyroid hormone and delay the surgery until the patient is euthyroid.
- The exception to this rule is a patient with coronary artery disease awaiting bypass or stenting. Such patients should have their **coronary vasculature addressed first,** and then have their thyroid hormone replaced postoperatively.
- Evidence suggests that replacement of thyroid hormone before restoring coronary blood flow could tax an already ischemic myocardium.
- A patient with severe hypothyroidism—for example, very low levels of thyroid hormone, or myxedema coma, or clinical symptoms of chronic thyroid hormone deficiency such as altered mentation, pericardial effusion, or heart failure—who requires urgent surgery should be given a loading dose of intravenous T_4 and possibly T_3.
- In addition, stress-dose glucocorticoids should be given if adrenal or pituitary function is uncertain, as replacement of thyroxine in a patient with adrenal insufficiency can precipitate adrenal crisis.

THYROID FUNCTION IN NONTHYROIDAL ILLNESS

- Aberrations in thyroid function during illness occur along a continuum, with wider deviations from the mean as the patient becomes more severely ill. Several names have been ascribed to the condition, including euthyroid sick syndrome, low T_3 syndrome, low T_4 syndrome, and nonthyroidal illness.

- Interpretation of thyroid function tests in critically ill patients is complex. For this reason, thyroid function should not be measured in this setting unless a thyroid disorder is strongly suspected.
- When it is deemed appropriate to evaluate the hypothalamic–pituitary–thyroid axis, the clinician should check a TSH, total T_4, free T_4, and total T_3.
- The most commonly seen change in thyroid hormone function tests in hospitalized patients is a low serum T_3 concentration. Most T_3 in the serum is produced by deiodination of T_4 to T_3 in the peripheral tissues.
- Many commonly used medications in the ICU may also decrease the peripheral conversion of T_4 to T_3, further lowering the circulating T_3 levels.
- Glucocorticoids and β-adrenergic antagonists are the most common offending agents. In addition, free fatty acids inhibit the deiodinase activity.
- Cytokines have also been shown to have a role in the development of the sick euthyroid syndrome by their role in decreasing the conversion of T_4 to T_3.
- Concomitant with the decline in T_3 levels is a rise in rT_3 (reverse T_3) in nonthyroidal illness. Fasting may produce this clinical picture within 24 to 36 hours and is reversed as quickly with refeeding.
- This pattern of low T_3/high rT_3 is found in many patients with various acute and chronic illnesses such as infection, surgery, cancer, cardiovascular diseases, pulmonary processes, burns, or trauma.
- The metabolic rate of formation of rT_3 is unchanged in the setting of illness. The increase in this value is, instead, a reflection of the attenuated rates of clearance of rT_3.
- The complicating factor with measuring the rT_3 levels in patients suspected of having nonthyroidal illness is that it may take up to a week to process the test in the laboratory.
- T_4 levels may also be reduced in up to 20% of hospitalized patients and 50% of critically ill patients. These low T_4 levels are correlated with a higher mortality rate.
- The reduction in T_4 can, in part, be attributed to decreased concentrations of one of the three thyroid hormone–binding proteins: TBG, transthyretin, and albumin.
- Serum TSH levels are typically normal in most patients with nonthyroidal illness, although during the recovery phase of the illness, thyrotropin concentrations may rise.
- In more critically ill patients, the TSH may simultaneously fall with the decline in T_4 levels. Such findings have led some to suggest that some patients may have an acquired transient central hypothyroidism during the nonthyroidal illness.
- Thyroid hormone replacement has not been shown to improve outcomes in critically ill patients. Medications may also alter TSH levels (see Table 117.2). Dopamine infusions are frequently associated with a reduction in serum thyrotropin concentration.
- When measuring TSH levels in the ICU, it is important to use a high-sensitivity assay with a lower detection limit of at least 0.01 mU/L. The vast majority of hospitalized patients with low, but detectable, TSH by this assay have sick euthyroid syndrome.
- In contrast, patients with undetectable thyrotropin are more likely to be hyperthyroid.
- Finally, those patients with high TSH (up to 20 mU/L) are likely recovering from a nonthyroidal illness and should be reassessed 6 weeks after the hospitalization.

Acute Airway Obstruction and Goiter

- Acute airway obstruction is a life-threatening complication of an enlarged thyroid gland.
- Fortunately quite rare, but important to consider, is anaplastic **thyroid cancer.** Patients with this disease may present with considerable growth of the thyroid within a few weeks.
- Thyroid **lymphoma** can also show a rapid growth pattern but will quickly respond to appropriate chemotherapy and/or radiation therapy.
- **Riedel thyroiditis,** also rare, with a prevalence of 0.06% to 0.3%, may present with a rapidly enlarging, hard neck mass that must be differentiated from thyroid cancer or lymphoma. The fibrous tissue may invade soft tissue and muscle and lead to tracheal compression.
- The more common scenario is a patient who presents with a nodule that rapidly increases in size over several minutes to hours. In these cases, the patient has underlying nodular disease that has encroached on a nearby blood vessel and **bled into a cystic compartment** of the nodule. Typically, patients have regression of such a nodule over the ensuing weeks.
- The clinical presentation of a compressive goiter is varied. Patients may present with complaints of a pressure sensation in the neck, particularly with movement of the head. Difficulty swallowing and vocal cord paralysis also may be encountered.
- The **Pemberton sign,** facial flushing and jugular venous distention on raising the arms over the head, is an indication of obstruction of venous outflow from the head.
- Many patients with a goiter have a mild degree of airway obstruction when screened with pulmonary function tests.
- It is critical to recognize that a patient presenting with new-onset wheezing or stridor may have a substernal goiter.
- The management of acute airway compromise is primarily surgical. If airway collapse is imminent, it is critical to protect the airway with intubation.
- The type of surgery necessary depends on the size of the goiter and whether there is an associated malignancy. Radioiodine treatment can take months to years to shrink the goiter.

Postthyroidectomy Hypocalcemia

Hypoparathyroidism

- The most common cause of hypoparathyroidism is surgery on the neck, with resultant removal of, or injury to, the parathyroid glands. This is typically seen after cancer surgery, total thyroidectomy, or parathyroidectomy.
- It is most often a transient condition with symptoms occurring 1 to 2 days postoperatively. Symptoms may vary from subtle perioral numbness and tingling to profound fatigue to tetany.
- Table 117.9 lists the symptoms and signs that may be seen in patients with hypocalcemia.
- Risk of hypocalcemia is dependent on the extent of surgery, localization and preservation of the parathyroids, and skill of the surgeon. Incidence rates of postoperative, transient hypocalcemia range from 1.6% up to >50%, but most of these patients will regain parathyroid function over the ensuing months.
- The risk of permanent hypoparathyroidism is variable, between 0% and 10%. During nonparathyroid neck surgery,

TABLE 117.9

SYMPTOMS AND SIGNS OF ACUTE HYPOCALCEMIA

Symptoms	Signs
Perioral numbness and tingling	Chvostek sign
Tingling paresthesias in distal extremities	Trousseau sign
Muscle cramps	Hypotension
Hyperreflexia	Bradycardia
Carpopedal spasm	Prolonged QT interval
Seizures	Arrhythmias

it is critical for the surgeon to recognize a compromised parathyroid gland and autotransplant the gland into the adjacent neck muscle to ensure the gland will regain function.

Treatment

- Treatment is aimed at normalization of the serum calcium. Many surgeons begin thrice-daily prophylactic oral calcium supplementation the night of the surgery.
- If the patient develops progressive symptoms, tetany, or seizures, the use of IV **calcium gluconate** is warranted. In life-threatening situations, 10 mL of calcium gluconate may be administered intravenously over a 5- to 10-minute period and repeated as necessary.

- In less acute situations, a continuous calcium infusion may be used by mixing 10 ampules of calcium gluconate in 500 mL of 5% dextrose in water. The infusion rate may vary between 0.3 mg/kg/hour to 2 mg/kg/hour, depending on the clinical setting.
- The goal of therapy is to reverse hypocalcemic symptoms and restore calcium levels to the low-normal range.

Hungry Bone Syndrome

- Hungry bone syndrome (HBS) is a well-recognized complication of surgical correction of severe hyperparathyroidism.
- Patients with very high levels of parathyroid hormone (PTH) may develop significant hypocalcemia after surgical removal of the offending parathyroid adenoma(s). The mechanism of this metabolic derangement is rapid skeletal mineralization.
- Less commonly seen is HBS after thyroidectomy for thyrotoxicosis. Patients with hyperthyroidism may develop secondary osteoporosis and resultant hypercalcemia from the increased bone resorption. After surgical removal of the thyroid gland, patients have a reversal of the thyrotoxic osteodystrophy and, instead, have a net flux of calcium and phosphorous deposition into bone.
- In extreme thyrotoxicosis, the patient may develop hypocalcemia. This condition typically resolves within a few days to weeks with treatment of the hypocalcemia.

CHAPTER 118 ■ COAGULATION DISORDERS IN THE INTENSIVE CARE UNIT

- Coagulopathic conditions frequently encountered in the intensive care unit (ICU) arbitrarily divided (Table 118.1):
  - Those associated with serious bleeding or a high probability of bleeding
  - Thrombotic syndromes or conditions associated with higher probability of thrombosis
  - Systemic diseases associated with acquired selective coagulation factor deficiencies
    - A few conditions associated with abnormal coagulation screening tests that represent laboratory phenomena not associated with increased bleeding risk

OVERVIEW OF COAGULATION

- For years teaching was that process of blood clotting divided into the intrinsic, extrinsic, and common pathways (Fig. 118.1)

TABLE 118.1

OVERVIEW OF COAGULATION DISORDERS SEEN IN THE ICU

Conditions Associated with Serious Bleeding or a High Probability of Bleeding
Disseminated intravascular coagulation (DIC)
Liver disease/hepatic insufficiency
Vitamin K deficiency/depletion
Massive transfusion syndrome
Anticoagulant overdose (heparin, warfarin)
Thrombocytopenia (drug-induced, immunologic)
Acquired platelet defects (drug-induced, uremia)

Thrombotic Clinical Syndromes
Thrombotic thrombocytopenia purpura/hemolytic uremic syndrome
Deep venous thrombosis
Pulmonary embolism
Coronary thrombosis/acute myocardial infarction

Laboratory Abnormalities Not Associated with Clinical Bleeding
Lupus anticoagulant
Reactive hyperfibrinogenemia

Other Selected Clinical Syndromes
Hemophilia (A and B)
Specific factor deficiencies associated with specific diseases
Amyloidosis, factor X; Gaucher, factor IX; nephrotic syndrome, factor IX, antithrombin III
Cyanotic congenital heart disease (polycythemia, qualitative platelet defect)
Depressed clotting factor levels (newborns)

- Students come away with thought that clotting occurs as result of orderly sequential process
- Obscures fact that once initiated, clot production and clot destruction (fibrinolysis) occur simultaneously
  - Minimizes role that platelets and the endothelium play in overall process
- Previously thought that intrinsic pathway, beginning with activation of factor XII (fXII) to activated factor XII (fXIIa) in contact with some biologic or foreign surface, was physiologically most important in initiation of clot formation
  - Now know that the activation of fX to fXa through action of fVIIa/tissue factor (TF) complex paramount
  - Also evident that various elements of clotting cascade frequently act in concert
    - Use of term *tenase* to describe the action of fVIIa/TF complex along with the fIXa/fVIIIa complex on activation of factor X to Xa
    - Use of term *prothrombinase* to describe factor Xa/Va complex, which cleaves prothrombin (factor II) to form thrombin (factor IIa)
    - There is cross talk between two arms of the clotting cascade, with fVIIa being able to enhance the activation of fIX (to fIXa) and fXI (to fXIa), further pointing out the central role that fVIIa and TF play *in vivo* (Fig. 118.2)
      - There are various positive feedback loops principally involving thrombin that enhance the upstream activation of clotting process
- TF for activation of coagulation present in subendothelial matrix
  - Found circulating freely in plasma as soluble TF and contained on cellular elements such as monocytes
  - Clotting does not occur in free-flowing blood but rather on surfaces
  - Platelets, endothelial cells, subendothelial matrix, and biologic polymers, for example, catheters, grafts, stents, and so on, provide these surfaces for clot formation
- Platelets initiate clot formation through formation of platelet plug
  - More significantly bring specialized proteins that regulate clotting response, for example, fVIII, inhibitors of fibrinolysis, and so on, to area of bleeding
  - Provide surface for colocalization of clotting factors for efficient clot formation (Fig. 118.3)
  - Do not ordinarily adhere to vascular endothelium unless mechanically disrupted (e.g., cut) or activated by inflammation
    - Then platelets bind to endothelial cells or subendothelial matrix via a von Willebrand factor (vWf)-dependent mechanism
    - Once adherent platelets become activated and secrete various molecules, that further enhances platelet

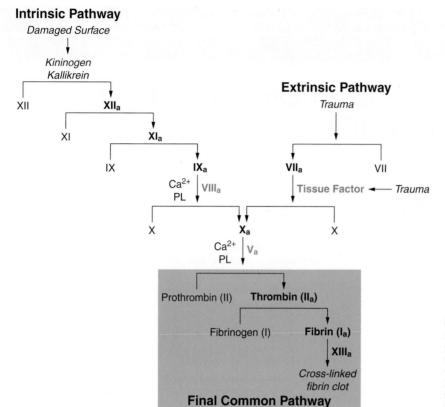

FIGURE 118.1. Coagulation is initiated either through the intrinsic pathway by activation of factor XII by the generation of high-molecular-weight kininogen and kallikrein, or through activation of the extrinsic pathway by tissue factor. Roman numerals indicate zymogen clotting factors; "a" indicates activated forms of the clotting factors.

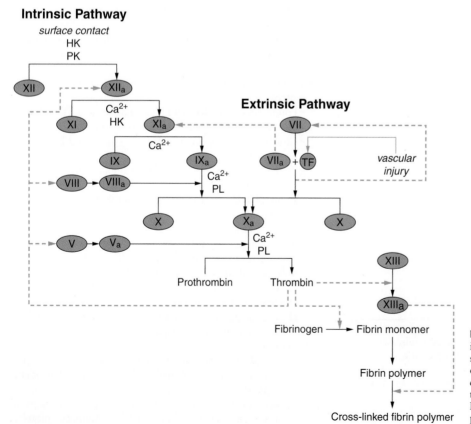

FIGURE 118.2. Modified clotting cascade indicating cross talk between the intrinsic and extrinsic pathways by the action of VIIa/tissue factor (TF) enhancing the conversion of factor XI to activated factor XI (XIa) (*dotted lines*). Ca²⁺, calcium; HK, high-molecular-weight kininogen; PK, prekallikrein; PL, phospholipids.

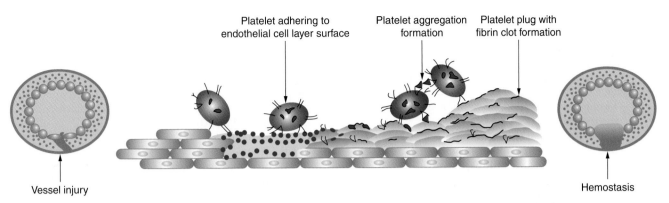

FIGURE 118.3. The role of platelets in mediating primary hemostasis at sites of vascular injury. Platelets are initially activated and express specific adhesion receptors on their surface, followed by adhesion to activated endothelial cells and exposed subendothelial components (e.g., collagen, von Willebrand factor). Subsequent platelet aggregation occurs with the development of a primary platelet plug. Coagulation occurs on the developing platelet plug with the creation of a fibrin clot.

adherence and aggregation, vascular contraction, clot formation, and wound healing
- Endothelium a specialized organ that plays central role in regulation of clot formation (i.e., hemostasis) by presenting a nonthrombogenic surface to flowing blood and by enhancing clot formation when disrupted by trauma or injured by infection or inflammation (Fig. 118.4)
  - Normal endothelium produces inhibitors of blood coagulation and platelet activation, and modulates vascular tone and permeability
  - Endothelial cells synthesize and secrete components of subendothelial extracellular matrix, including adhesive glycoproteins, collagen, fibronectin, and vWf
  - When disrupted, bleeding occurs
  - When *injured*, endothelium often becomes *pro*thrombotic rather than *anti*thrombotic, and unwanted clot formation may occur

INTERACTION OF COAGULATION AND INFLAMMATION

- Many inflammatory cytokines have been identified as promoters of a procoagulant milieu
  - Interconnection of TF and tumor necrosis factor-α (TNF-α) may potentially be most important of these
- During sepsis, TF expression is up-regulated in activated monocytes and endothelial cells as a response to endotoxin
  - Consequence being both secretion of proinflammatory cytokines, interleukin-6 (IL-6), and TNF-α from activated mononuclear cells, and the activation of coagulation
  - Results in increased thrombin production, which plays a central role in coagulation and inflammation through the induction of procoagulant, anticoagulant, inflammatory, and mitogenic responses

Protein C Pathway

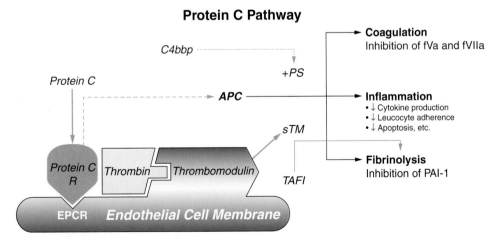

FIGURE 118.4. The interaction of the protein C system with the endothelium: thrombin bound to thrombomodulin (TM) modifies protein C bound to the endothelial protein C receptor (EPCR) on the cell surface to generate activated protein C (APC). APC acts as a natural anticoagulant by inactivating activated factors V (fVa) and VIII (fVIIa), modulates inflammation by down-regulating the synthesis of proinflammatory cytokines, leukocyte adherence, and apoptosis and enhances fibrinolysis by inhibiting thrombin-activatable fibrinolysis inhibitor (TAFI) and plasminogen activator inhibitor type-1 (PAI-1). sTM, soluble thrombomodulin; sEPCR, soluble endothelial protein C receptor; PS, protein S; C4bbp, C$_{4b}$ binding protein; PAI-1, plasminogen activator inhibitor type 1.

○ Thrombin results in activation, aggregation, and lysis of leukocytes and platelets, and activation of endothelial cells, with resultant increase in proinflammatory cytokines IL-6 and TNF-α expression

○ Net result of thrombin generation is to produce a proinflammatory and procoagulant state

  – Leading to formation of fibrin and microvascular thrombosis

  – These proinflammatory effects of thrombin are counterbalanced by the anti-inflammatory effects of activated protein C (see Fig. 118.4)

• Second important point of connection of coagulation and inflammation is through protein C (PC) system

  • Anticoagulant effects of activated protein C (aPC) and its cofactor, protein S, well known; only recently have anti-inflammatory roles of these proteins been appreciated

  • Experimentally, aPC increases secretion of anti-inflammatory cytokines, reduces leukocyte migration and adhesion, and protects endothelial cells from injury

  • Balance between anticoagulant and anti-inflammatory roles of aPC may be mediated by relative distribution of free and complement factor C_{4b}-bound protein S

  • *In vitro,* aPC inhibits TNF-α elaboration from monocytes and blocks leukocyte adhesion to selectins, as well as having an influence on apoptosis

  • Protein C pathway is engaged when thrombin binds to thrombomodulin on surface of endothelial cell

  • Binding of PC to the endothelial cell protein C receptor (EPCR) augments protein C activation by thrombin-TM complex more than 10-fold *in vivo*

  • EPCR is shed from the endothelium through the action of inflammatory mediators and thrombin, thereby downregulating aPC generation in sepsis and inflammation

• Third important link between inflammation and coagulation occurs at level of fibrinolysis and also involves PC system

  • aPC capable of neutralizing fibrinolysis inhibitors, *plasminogen activator inhibitor type-1* (PAI-1) and *thrombin activatable fibrinolysis inhibitor* (TAFI)

  • Consequently, depressed levels of aPC promote clot formation by reducing *inactivation* of procoagulant molecule-activated factors V and VIII (fVa, fVIIIa), leading to increased generation of thrombin and fibrin clots and by limiting fibrinolytic response needed to degrade clots

  • TAFI (also known as carboxypeptidase R) also shown to inactivate inflammatory peptides, such as complement factors C3a and C5a, which play role in contact activation of coagulation

  • Polymorphisms of promoter region of the PAI-1 gene that lead to differences in PAI-1 production have been demonstrated to affect prognosis in meningococcal sepsis and multiple trauma

AN APPROACH TO THE PATIENT WITH AN ACTUAL OR SUSPECTED COAGULATION DISORDER

Clinical History

• Diagnostic assessment begins at the bedside

  • Specific questions regarding bleeding should investigate occurrence of any of following:

  • Spontaneous, easy, or disproportionately severe bruising

  • Intramuscular hematoma formation (either spontaneous or related to trauma)

  • Spontaneous or trauma-induced hemarthrosis

  • Spontaneous mucous membrane bleeding

  • Prior problems with bleeding related to surgery (including dental extractions, tonsillectomy, and circumcision)

  • The need for transfusions in the past

  • Menstrual history

  • Current medications

    ○ Innumerable aspirin-containing medications available, all of which can potentially interfere with platelet-mediated primary hemostasis

• Prior history of significant thrombosis, deep vein thrombosis (DVT), pulmonary embolus, or stroke, suggests possibility that hypercoagulable condition may be present

• Occurrence of thrombotic events, particularly early cardiovascular events such as myocardial infarction, in young adult relatives should cause consideration of:

  • Deficiencies of antithrombin-III, protein C, or protein S

  • Presence of factor V Leiden R506Q mutation, prothrombin G20210A (or the newly described A19911G) polymorphism or mutation

  • C677T mutation or polymorphism of the MTHFR (methylenetetrahydrofolate reductase) gene

  • Vasculitis associated with autoimmune disorder such as systemic lupus erythematosus (SLE) must always be considered in evaluation of an individual with unexplained pathologic clot

Physical Examination

• Generalized bleeding in critically ill ICU patients presents a special problem

  • Often associated with severe underlying multiple organ system dysfunction

    • Correction of coagulopathy usually requires improvement in patient's overall clinical status

  • Supportive evidence or physical findings of other concurrent organ system dysfunction, such as oliguria or anuria, respiratory failure, or hypotension, often are readily apparent

  • Bleeding in critically ill patients is often caused by sepsis-related disseminated intravascular coagulation (DIC)

  • Must also consider coagulopathy of severe liver dysfunction, undiagnosed hemophilia, or, in elderly or debilitated, vitamin K deficiency in differential diagnosis

  • Physical examination of patient with bleeding disorder should answer basic questions:

    • Is process localized or diffuse?

    • Is it related to an anatomic or surgical lesion?

    • Is there mucosal bleeding?

    • Are there signs of either arterial or venous thrombosis?

  • During the course of the examination, attention paid to presence of specific physical findings:

    • Enlarged spleen coupled with thrombocytopenia suggests that splenic sequestration may be a contributor to the observed thrombocytopenia

    • Evidence of liver disease, such as portal hypertension and ascites, points to decreased factor synthesis as a possible cause of a prolonged prothrombin time (PT) or activated partial prothrombin time (aPTT)

- If lymphadenopathy, splenomegaly, or other findings suggestive of disseminated malignancy detected, acute or chronic DIC should be suspected as the cause of prolonged coagulation times, hypofibrinogenemia, and/or thrombocytopenia
- Purpura that are palpable suggest capillary leak from vasculitis
  - Purpura associated with thrombocytopenia or qualitative platelet defects generally not elevated and cannot be distinguished by touch
- Venous and arterial telangiectasia may be seen in von Willebrand disease and liver disease, respectively
  - Selective pressure centrally applied to arterial telangiectasia, whole lesion fades
  - Venous telangiectasia requires confluent pressure across entire lesion, as with a glass slide, for blanching to occur

Diagnostic Laboratory Evaluation

- Importance of correct specimen collection for hemostatic evaluation must be emphasized
- In ICU, common for laboratory samples to be drawn through an indwelling arterial or central venous cannula
- Heparin-containing solution commonly present
  - In cannula flush medium to transduce a waveform
  - As a component of intravenous infusion
- Depending on heparin concentration

- Fibrin degradation products (FDPs) can be falsely elevated
- Fibrinogen can be falsely low
- PT, aPTT, and thrombin time (TT) can be spuriously prolonged
- Minimum of 20 mL of blood in adolescents and adults, and 10 mL of blood in younger children, should therefore be withdrawn through the cannula and either discarded or used for other purposes before obtaining a specimen for laboratory hemostasis analysis
- Should minimize any influence of heparin on results
  - May not be reasonable to withdraw this volume of blood, and a peripheral venipuncture may be necessary
  - aPTT sensitive to presence of small amounts of heparin
    - Unexpected prolonged aPTT obtained through a heparinized catheter should raise suspicion of sample contamination
    - TT will also be prolonged but will normalize if heparin neutralized (e.g., with toluidine blue or HEPA sorb)
- Most suspected bleeding disorders confirmed using routine tests (Table 118.2):
- Evaluation of peripheral blood smear, including an estimate of the platelet count and platelet and red blood cell (RBC) morphologic features
- Measurement of PT, aPTT, and TT
- Assays for fibrinogen or presence of fibrin degradation products or the d-dimer fragment of polymerized fibrin
  - Latter test more specific for fibrinolytic fragment produced when polymerized fibrin monomer, produced

TABLE 118.2

HEMORRHAGIC SYNDROMES AND ASSOCIATED LABORATORY FINDINGS

Clinical syndrome	Screening tests	Supportive tests
DIC	Prolonged PT, aPTT, TT; decreased fibrinogen, platelets; microangiopathy	(+) FDPs, d-dimer; decreased factors V, VIII, and II (late)
Massive transfusion	Prolonged PT, aPTT; decreased fibrinogen, platelets ± Prolonged TT	All factors decreased; (−) FDPs, d-dimer (unless DIC develops); (+) transfusion history
Anticoagulant overdose		
Heparin	Prolonged aPTT, TT; ±prolonged PT	Toluidine blue/protamine corrects TT; Reptilase time normal
Warfarin (same as vitamin K deficiency)	Prolonged PT; ± prolonged aPTT (severe); normal TT, fibrinogen, platelets	Vitamin K-dependent factors decreased; factors V, VIII normal
Liver disease		
Early	Prolonged PT	Decreased factor VII
Late	Prolonged PT, aPTT; decreased fibrinogen (terminal liver failure); normal platelet count (if splenomegaly absent)	Decreased factors II, V, VII, IX, and X; decreased plasminogen; ± FDPs unless DIC develops
Primary fibrinolysis	Prolonged PT, aPTT, TT; decreased fibrinogen and ± platelets decreased	(+) FDPs, (−) d-dimer; short euglobulin clot lysis time
TTP	Thrombocytopenia, microangiopathy with mild anemia; PT, aPTT, fibrinogen generally WNL/mildly abnormal	ADAMTS13 deficiency/inhibitor, unusually large vWf multimers between episodes; mild increase in FDPs or d-dimer
HUS	Microangiopathic hemolytic anemia, ± thrombocytopenia; PT, aPTT generally WNL	Renal insufficiency; FDPs and d-dimer generally (−)

DIC, disseminated intravascular coagulation; PT, prothrombin time; aPTT, activated partial thromboplastin time; TT, thrombin time; FDPs, fibrin degradation products; TTP, thrombotic thrombocytopenic purpura; WNL, within normal limits; vWf, von Willebrand factor; HUS, hemolytic uremic syndrome.

through the action of thrombin on fibrinogen, cleaved by proteolytic enzyme, plasmin
  • D-dimer assay positive only if fibrinogen cleaved to fibrin by action of thrombin

Evaluation of Thrombosis

• Patients presenting with thrombotic event generally don't display abnormalities of usual clotting studies
  • Hyperfibrinogenemia and persistent elevations of fVIII associated with increased risk of thrombosis
  • Both elevated by acute inflammation
    • Finding of elevations of these clotting factors is generally not helpful in the evaluation of a thrombotic event in an acutely ill individual
  • Several inherited or acquired abnormalities that increase risk for thrombosis identified:
    • Prior to initiation of anticoagulation, plasma levels of protein C (antigen and activity), protein S (antigen and activity), total and free, and antithrombin III (antigen and activity) should be obtained
    • Polymerase chain reaction (PCR) analysis for mutations in factor V (factor V Leiden; [Arg]R506Q[Gln]), prothrombin ([Gly]G20210A[Ala], and [Ala]A19911G[Gly]) and MTHFR ([Cys]C677T[Thr]) genes should be performed
    • Baseline serum homocysteine obtained as thrombosis risk of MTHFR mutation related to elevations of homocysteine caused by alterations in the metabolism of folic acid rather than the mutation *per se*
  • Acquired thrombotic risk factors include:
    ○ Presence of lupus anticoagulants, antiphospholipid, and anticardiolipin antibodies
    ○ In adult populations, approximately 40% of patients with thrombosis will not display known thrombophilic risk factors
    ○ Intensivist must look for confounding clinical conditions:
      – Severe dehydration with marked hemoconcentration

CONDITIONS ASSOCIATED WITH SERIOUS BLEEDING OR A HIGH PROBABILITY OF BLEEDING

Disseminated Intravascular Coagulation

Pathogenesis

• Often occurring in conjunction with more serious, life-threatening disorders, one of most serious hemostatic abnormalities seen in ICU
• Clinical syndrome results from activation of blood coagulation
• Then leads to excessive thrombin generation
• Final result of this process is the widespread formation of fibrin thrombi in the microcirculation, with resultant consumption of certain clotting factors and platelets
• Consumption generally results in development of significant bleeding due to rate of consumption outpacing rate at which clotting factors and platelets are produced (Table 118.3)

TABLE 118.3

UNDERLYING DISEASES ASSOCIATED WITH DIC

- Sepsis
- Liver disease
- Shock
- Penetrating brain injury
- Necrotizing pneumonitis
- Tissue necrosis/crush injury
- Intravascular hemolysis
- Acute promyelocytic leukemia
- Thermal injury
- Freshwater drowning
- Fat embolism syndrome

- Retained placenta
- Hypertonic saline abortion
- Amniotic fluid embolus
- Retention of a dead fetus
- Eclampsia
- Localized endothelial injury (aortic aneurysm, giant hemangiomata, angiography)
- Disseminated malignancy (prostate, pancreatic)

Clinical Presentation and Diagnosis

• Suspicion that DIC is present usually stems from one of two situations:
  • Unexplained generalized oozing or bleeding
  • Unexplained abnormal laboratory parameters of hemostasis
• Usually occurs in context of suggestive clinical scenario or associated disease (see Table 118.3)
• Infection and multiple trauma most common underlying conditions associated with development of DIC
• A list of laboratory studies in DIC is found in Table 118.4
• In addition to liver disease, several other conditions have presentations similar to DIC and must be considered in differential diagnosis:
• Massive transfusion
• Primary fibrinolysis
• Thrombotic thrombocytopenic purpura/hemolytic uremic syndrome
• Heparin therapy
• Dysfibrinogenemia

Management

• Primary treatment for DIC is correction of underlying problem that led to its development
  • Specific therapy for DIC should not be undertaken unless:
    • Patient has significant bleeding or organ dysfunction secondary to DIC

TABLE 118.4

LABORATORY TESTS FOR THE DIAGNOSIS OF DIC

Test	Discriminator value
Platelet count	<80–100,000 cells/μL or a decrease of >50% from baseline
Fibrinogen	<100 mg/dL or a decrease of >50% from baseline
PT	>3 s prolongation above ULN
FDPs	>80 mg/dL
d-Dimer	Moderate increase

PT, prothrombin time; FDPs, fibrin degradation products; ULN, upper limit of normal.

- Significant thrombosis has occurred
- If treatment of underlying disorder—for example, acute promyelocytic leukemia—is likely to increase the severity of DIC
- Supportive therapy for DIC includes use of several component blood products
  - Packed RBCs are given according to guidelines in face of active bleeding
  - Fresh whole blood, <24 to 48 hours old, may be given to replete both volume and oxygen-carrying capacity
  - Additional potential benefit of providing coagulation proteins, including fibrinogen, and platelets
  - Cryoprecipitate contains higher concentration of fibrinogen than whole blood or fresh frozen plasma (FFP)
  - FFP of limited value for treatment of significant hypofibrinogenemia
    - May effectively replete other coagulation factors consumed with DIC such as protein C
    - Large volumes of FFP needed
  - Use of cryoprecipitate or FFP in treatment of DIC has been debated
    - Concern that products provide further substrate for ongoing DIC
    - Clinical (autopsy) studies failed to confirm this concern
- Goal of blood component therapy to produce clinical stability
  - Serum fibrinogen level <75 to 50 mg/dL, repletion with cryoprecipitate to raise plasma levels to 100 mg/dL or higher is goal
    - Starting dose is one bag of cryoprecipitate for every 10 kg body weight every 8 to 12 hours
    - Recheck fibrinogen level after infusion to document fibrinogen level
    - Amount and timing of next infusion adjusted according to results
  - Platelet transfusions when thrombocytopenia contributes to bleeding
    - Fibrin/fibrinogen fragments produced in DIC have potential to impair platelet function by inhibiting fibrinogen binding to platelets
    - May be clinically significant at the concentration of FDPs achieved with DIC
    - Platelet transfusions to maintain platelet counts up to 40,000 to 80,000 cells/μL
  - Pharmacologic therapy for DIC has two primary aims:
    - To "turn off" ongoing coagulation so that repletion of coagulation factors may begin
    - To impede thrombus formation and ensuing ischemic injury
  - Two new recombinant blood products have some usefulness
    - Recombinant-activated protein C
      - Results in 6% reduction in sepsis mortality in adults and possibly a reduction in the incidence of DIC
      - Recombinant-activated factor VII (rhfVIIa)
        - Potent agent for control of bleeding from several medical and surgical causes, including DIC and other consumptive coagulopathies
    - Other anticoagulant molecules such as heparin and antithrombin III and thrombolytic agents studied as therapy for DIC and sepsis

Liver Disease and Hepatic Insufficiency

Abnormal Hemostasis in Liver Disease
- Common cause of abnormal hemostasis in ICU patients
  - Abnormal coagulation studies or overt bleeding occurs in 15% of patients with clinical or laboratory evidence of hepatic dysfunction
  - Common cause of a prolonged PT or aPTT, often without any clinical sequelae
- Hemostatic defect associated with liver disease multifactorial
  - Synthesis of several plasma coagulation proteins impaired
    - Include factors II, V, VII, IX, and X
  - Fibrinogen synthesis usually maintained at levels that prevent bleeding until terminal liver failure supervenes
    - Function of fibrinogen synthesized by diseased liver may not be normal
      - Increased sialic acid content in structure
      - May result in a diminished ability to form clots (i.e., a dysfibrinogen)
  - Factor XIII activity often decreased in hepatocellular disease
    - Clinical significance of decrease in factor XIII uncertain
    - Levels as low as 3% provide normal fibrin clot stabilization
  - Although apparently synthesized by liver, factor VIII (i.e., factor VIII coagulant protein [VIII:C], antihemophilic factor A [AHF]) synthesis seems independent of state of hepatic function
    - Factor VIII levels may be increased in some types of liver disease
    - Plasma protein C and antithrombin III levels are low in hepatic insufficiency
  - Patients with liver disease, particularly cirrhosis, have increased fibrinolytic activity
    - Mechanism for heightened fibrinolytic state not clear
    - Related to increased amounts of plasminogen activator noted in these patients
  - Thrombocytopenia present to variable degree in patients with hepatic dysfunction
    - Usually ascribed to splenic sequestration
    - Rarely profound and generally does not produce clinically significant bleeding
      - *In vitro* platelet aggregation may be affected
    - Increased plasma concentrations of FDPs possible cause of qualitative platelet abnormalities
    - Thrombocytopenia in conjunction with other coagulation or hemostatic defects secondary to liver disease may result in difficult to manage bleeding
  - Patients with hepatocellular disease may exhibit decreased synthesis of:
    - Vitamin K-dependent anticoagulant proteins
    - Protein C and protein S
    - Antithrombin-III
  - Decreased levels of these natural anticoagulants may increase risk of thrombosis
    - Neither PT, aPTT, nor TT affected by levels of any of these naturally occurring anticoagulants

Presentation
- Factor VII activity levels usually first to decrease due to its short half-life—4 to 6 hours—and increased turnover
  - Results in prolonged PT

- Prolonged thrombin time in setting of liver disease may indicate:
  - Presence of dysfibrinogenemia as result of altered hepatic fibrinogen synthesis
  - An acquired defect in fibrin polymerization (e.g., increased FDPs)
- As severity of liver disease increases, aPTT also may be affected
  - Reflecting more severely impaired synthetic function
  - Plasma concentrations of vitamin K-dependent coagulation proteins decrease, as does factor V, which is not vitamin K dependent
  - Plasma levels of fibrinogen generally maintained until disease approaches end stage
    - Synthetic hypofibrinogenemia of liver disease not accompanied by marked increase in either FDPs or d-dimers
  - Fibrinolysis may complicate clinical management
    - Differentiating between concomitant DIC and fibrinolysis attributable to liver disease alone may be difficult
    - D-dimer assay result should be negative in the patient with liver disease and elevated FDPs, but no active bleeding

Management

- If patient is not actively bleeding, with certain provisos, no specific therapy is required.
  - With prolonged PT, postoperative or preoperative patient, correction of PT may be attempted
  - FFP provides most immediate source of specific coagulation factors (i.e., factor VII)
    - Usually corrects isolated mild PT prolongation
  - Cryoprecipitate required if fibrinogen levels <50 to 100 mg/dL or if documentation of significant dysfibrinogenemia
- Vitamin K deficiency relatively common in patient population
  - Correction of PT in vitamin K-responsive critically ill patients typically requires longer than 12 to 24 hours
  - Patients with significant hepatic impairment may manifest partial response or may not respond
  - Immediate use of FFP is therefore appropriate when rapid correction is necessary.
- Recombinant human-activated factor VII (rhfVIIa) infusions shown to control bleeding in severe liver disease
  - Does not necessarily result in reduced mortality
- When synthetic capability of liver more profoundly impaired and aPTT prolonged
  - Greater volumes of FFP or more specific therapy needed
  - Use of factor IX concentrates (prothrombin complex concentrates) or rhfVIIa has been advocated
    - Particularly if bleeding present; however, use remains controversial
    - Products produced from plasma pooled from multiple donors carry a significant risk of both hepatitis B and C
    - May provoke DIC and actually worsen hemostasis
    - Use of prothrombin complex concentrates or rhfVIIa reserved for patients with poorly controlled bleeding unresponsive to other therapeutic modalities such as infusion of FFP
- Comprehensive therapeutic approach needed in patient with active bleeding as result of liver disease
  - Initially, FFP, 10 to 15 mL/kg body weight, given every 6 to 8 hours until bleeding slows significantly
    - Then continued at maintenance levels as dictated by clinical status and coagulation studies

- Recombinant human-activated factor VII or prothrombin complex concentrates used in patients unresponsive to FFP infusions
- Cryoprecipitate infused for fibrinogen levels <50 to 100 mg/dL
- Platelet transfusions required if platelet count <40,000 to 80,000 cells/μL
- Vitamin K empirically administered on presumption that part of synthetic defect results from a lack of cofactor
- Anticipate poor response to vitamin K in presence of severe liver disease
- Transfusions of packed red blood cells (PRBCs) given as deemed appropriate by the clinician

Vitamin K Deficiency

- Most common cause of prolonged PT in ICU is vitamin K deficiency
- Necessary for the gamma-carboxylation of factors II, VII, IX, and X
- Without which factors cannot bind calcium and are not efficiently converted into activated forms
- Factor VII has shortest half-life of these coagulation proteins
- PT is the most sensitive early indicator of vitamin K deficiency
- Differential diagnosis of isolated prolongation of PT, with or without bleeding, includes:
  - Vitamin K deficiency
  - Liver disease
  - Clinical presentation of these patients quite similar
    - Distinction sometimes made only on basis of response (or lack thereof) to empirical vitamin K therapy
  - Warfarin administration (overt or covert) should be excluded
    - Newer, long-acting vitamin K antagonist rodenticides (so-called *super-warfarin*) produce profound, prolonged, vitamin K-resistant reduction in vitamin K-dependent clotting factors
    - May produce an isolated prolongation of PT initially
    - Treatment of poisoning with these agents requires aggressive prolonged use of vitamin K and, in bleeding patient infusions of FFP or rhfVIIa
    - Confirmation of warfarin exposure as cause of prolonged PT possible by toxicologic methods
    - Laboratory findings of an isolated vitamin K deficiency
      ○ Prolonged PT, include a normal fibrinogen level, platelet count, and factor V level
      ○ Factor V not a vitamin K-dependent protein
        - Should therefore be normal except in cases of DIC (consumption) or severe liver disease (decreased production)
        - Prolongation of aPTT from vitamin K deficiency, warfarin therapy, or from liver disease a relatively late event
          - Occurs initially as result of factor IX depletion

Management

- Management of vitamin K deficiency consists primarily of its repletion
- Usually by intravenous (IV) or subcutaneous routes in critically ill patients

- Should not await development of bleeding or oozing
- Should be administered when PT abnormality detected and vitamin K deficiency thought responsible
- Adequate blood pressure (BP) and subcutaneous perfusion needed to ensure reliable absorption
- Possibility of anaphylactoid reactions with IV use of vitamin K of concern
  ○ Risk markedly reduced when drug given as infusion over 30 to 45 minutes in small volume of fluid
    – Anaphylaxis still reported with this mode of infusion
- Usual dose of vitamin K in adults is 10 to 15 mg IV or subcutaneously
  ○ 1 to 5 mg in young children
  ○ Up to 10 mg in larger children
- PT should correct within 12 to 24 hours after this dose
- Serial dosing of critically ill patients often used and PT may require up to 72 hours to normalize
  - If PT does not correct within 72 hours after three daily doses of vitamin K, intrinsic liver disease suspected
  - Further administration of vitamin K is of no additional benefit in this setting
- When patient actively bleeding:
- Not sufficient to only provide vitamin K
- FFP used in this setting
- To restore hemostasis to acceptable level, 30% to 50% of normal factor activity
- 10 to 20 mL/kg body weight of FFP is typically required
- Similar approach is used in patients previously given warfarin
- rhfVIIa used with success to reverse bleeding noted in vitamin K deficiency and in warfarin overdose

Massive Transfusion Syndrome

- Transfusion of large quantities of blood can result in multifactorial hemostatic defect
  - Related to washout of plasma coagulation proteins and platelets
  - Exacerbated by development of DIC with consequent:
    - Factor consumption
    - Hypothermia
    - Acidosis
    - Rarely, by citrate toxicity or hypocalcemia
- Washout syndrome results from transfusion of large amounts of stored blood products devoid of clotting factors and platelets
  - Develops exclusively in patients receiving large volumes of PRBCs
    - Trauma victims
    - Patients with massive gastrointestinal hemorrhage or hepatectomy
    - Those undergoing cardiopulmonary bypass
  - Without also receiving FFP and platelets
    - Factors V and VII have short shelf half-lives
      ○ Often deficient in blood banked longer than 48 hours
      ○ Qualitative platelet defect noted in whole blood within hours of storage
        – Especially if acid–citrate–dextrose solution used
      ○ Transfusion of large quantities of stored whole blood may produce limited improvement of bleeding, resulting from decreased clotting factors and platelets.

- Development of washout coagulopathy directly dependent on volume of blood transfused relative to patient's blood volume
  - Generally residual plasma clotting activity after one blood volume exchange falls to 18% to 37% of normal
  - After two–blood volume exchange, residual activity is only 3% to 14%
  - After three–blood volume exchange, <5% of normal clotting function remains
- DIC may develop in many clinical settings
- Including some associated with major hemorrhage or massive transfusion
- In presence of hypotension associated with hypovolemia or hemorrhagic shock
- Major trauma especially with release of tissue factors into plasma
- Exsanguinating hemorrhage
  - May require blood replacement faster than type-and-crossmatch of each unit can be performed
  - Donor–recipient incompatibility, even when mismatch is minor blood group systems, can lead to DIC
- Human error resulting in major incompatibility produces severe hemolysis and may be lethal
- Microaggregates of blood cells formed within stored blood products can cause DIC
  - Smaller pore effective filtering systems for blood product administration has essentially eliminated this as a source of problems
- Patient bleeding as consequence of massive transfusion or washout presents with:
- Diffuse oozing and bleeding from all surgical wounds and puncture sites
- Laboratory abnormalities include:
  - Prolonged PT, aPTT, and TT
  - Fibrinogen levels and platelet counts are typically decreased
  - FDPs not usually increased unless concurrent DIC present (see Table 118.2)
- Likelihood clinico-laboratory picture resultant from massive transfusion estimated from:
  - Amount of bleeding that has occurred
  - Blood volume administered relative to patient's blood volume
    ○ Number of blood volume exchanges given
    ○ The more PRBCs transfused relative to patient's blood volume
      – Greater the chance of coagulopathy development due to massive transfusion

Management

- Therapeutic approach to patients developing coagulopathy from massive transfusion is supportive
- Platelets and FFP given to replete components of coagulation typically lacking
  - Platelet administration may help stem bleeding from anatomic wounds
  - Severe bleeding associated with thrombocytopenia alone uncommon unless:
    ○ Counts fall below 20,000 to 30,000 cells/μL of blood
    ○ Nonetheless, patients may benefit from platelet transfusion at counts as high as 80,000 to 100,000 cells/μL

- FFP preferred over cryoprecipitate
  - More complete coagulation protein composition
  - Cryoprecipitate specifically given when fibrinogen depletion a major contributor to bleeding
- Prospective identification of those at risk of coagulopathy from massive transfusion critical:
  - Magnitude of insult and anticipated need for blood are large:
    - Both platelets and FFP given before coagulopathy develops
  - In most patients (weight $\geq$30 to 40 kg or body surface area [BSA] $\geq$1.0 m^2):
    - 4 units of platelets (0.5 unit of apheresis-collected platelets) and 1 unit of FFP
    - Given for each 5 units of whole blood or PRBC transfused
  - Should prevent washout and attendant bleeding
- If patient continues to bleed despite what should be adequate therapy for massive transfusion syndrome, other causes should be considered
  - Anatomic bleeding and possibility of DIC should be investigated
  - Therapy here may include rhfVIIa infusion

Anticoagulant Overdose

- Anticoagulant therapy usual in ICU
- Possibility of administration error exists
- Poorly standardized and can lead to overdose

Heparin

- A repeating polymer of two disaccharide glycosaminoglycans
  - Commercially prepared from either porcine intestinal mucosa or bovine lung
  - Currently found in two forms:
    - Unfractionated heparin (UH)
    - Low-molecular-weight heparin (LMWH)
- They have different mechanisms of action and associated precautions
  - UH
    - Has immediate effect on coagulation
    - Mediated primarily through interaction with antithrombin III
  - Resulting heparin–antithrombin III (AT-III) complex possesses greater affinity for thrombin than does AT-III alone
    - Inactivates thrombin
    - Damping-down clot formation
  - Additionally has direct inhibition of activated factor X (fXa)
    - This anticoagulant effect of UH relatively minor
      - Consequently, achieving therapeutic aPTT with UH very difficult in face of low levels of AT-III
  - Degree of anticoagulation produced by heparin monitored by prolongation of aPTT
  - LMWH
    - Produced by controlled enzymatic cleavage of heparin polymers
    - Produces anticoagulation almost exclusively through inhibition of fXa
    - Produces more stable degree of anticoagulation
    - Due to longer half-life (3 to 5 hours) and biologic activity (24 hours), allows for intermittent bolus therapy every 12 or 24 hours
    - Does not produce consistent prolongation of aPTT

- Requires assay of anti-Xa activity for monitoring, if desired
- Heparin hepatically metabolized by "heparinase" enzyme in dose-dependent fashion
  - Excess heparin renally excreted
  - As rate of heparin administration is increased
    - Half-life of drug prolonged due to increased percentage excreted by kidney
    - 10-unit/kg bolus of heparin infused IV, average half-life is 1 hour
    - If bolus increased to 400 or 800 units/kg half-life prolonged to 2.5 and 5 hours, respectively
    - Nonlinear response results in greater drug effects on coagulation with smaller dosage increments
      - Increases in heparin infusion rate in response to inadequate prolongation of aPTT results in point when further small infusion increments result in greater prolongation of aPTT
  - Risk of pathologic bleeding associated with heparin increases when aPTT is:
    - 1.5 to 2.5 times the patient's baseline aPTT
    - Corresponds to plasma heparin concentration of 0.2 to 0.4 units/mL
    - Administration of heparin as continuous infusion rather than intermittent bolus dose less likely to be associated with bleeding
- **Management:** Serious bleeding associated with heparin overdose rapidly reversed by protamine sulfate
  - Protamine binds ionically with heparin to form complex lacking anticoagulant activity
  - 1 mg of protamine neutralizes approximately 100 units of heparin
    - Dose of protamine needed is calculated from number of units of active heparin remaining in patient's system
    - Estimated from original heparin dose and typical half-life for infusion rate
    - aPTT used to gauge residual effects of heparin
    - Protamine itself potentially has anticoagulant effects
      - Drug given by slow IV push over 8 to 10 minutes
      - Single dose should not exceed 1mg/kg, with 50-mg maximum dose
      - Dose may be repeated
        - No more than 2 mg/kg, to a 100-mg maximum dose, given as cumulative dose without rechecking coagulation parameters
      - Dose of protamine always be monitored by coagulation studies
  - Significant side effects most commonly seen in overly rapid drug administration
    - Hypotension
    - Anaphylactoid-like reactions
  - LMWH not consistently neutralized by protamine
    - Invasive procedures should not be performed within 24 hours of administration
  - Bleeding following LMWH therapy treated effectively with rhfVIIa

Warfarin

- Warfarin and vitamin K structurally similar in respective 4-hydroxycoumarin nucleus and naphthoquinone ring
- Mechanism of action of warfarin through competitive binding at the vitamin K receptor site:

- Postribosomal γ-carboxylation of vitamin K-dependent coagulation proteins occurs:
  - Factors II, VII, IX, and X
  - Modification necessary to produce calcium-binding site on molecule
    - Allows for efficient activation of zymogen clotting factor into enzymatically active form
- When warfarin present in sufficient plasma concentrations, there is depletion of active forms of vitamin K-dependent factors
- PT/international normalized ratio (INR) calculated from PT, an accurate indicator of effects of warfarin when use continued beyond 2 or 3 days
  - Factor VII has half-life of 4 to 6 hours and active form rapidly depleted after one or two doses of warfarin
  - Remainder of vitamin K-dependent factors take up to a week to become depleted
  - PT becomes prolonged and INR elevated with factor VII depletion alone
    - Does not reflect overall state of anticoagulation until equilibrium period of several days has passed
      - Over this time, other vitamin K-dependent factors depleted
  - In severe cases of warfarin overdose, aPTT becomes prolonged
    - Resultant from depletion of active forms of factors II, IX, and X
- Several drugs and pathophysiologic conditions associated with potentiation of warfarin's effects on coagulation (Table 118.5)
  - Aspirin has no direct effect on warfarin metabolism
    - So profoundly influences qualitative platelet function that is considered potentiator of warfarin's anticoagulant effects
    - Same true for clofibrate
  - Conditions of acute and chronic hepatic dysfunction can alter warfarin metabolism and vitamin K-mediated γ-carboxylation

TABLE 118.5

DRUGS THAT POTENTIATE THE ANTICOAGULANT EFFECTS OF WARFARIN

Antibiotics
Broad-spectrum antibiotics (especially cephalosporins)
Griseofulvin (oral)
Metronidazole
Sulfinpyrazone
Trimethoprim-sulfamethoxazole

Anti-inflammatory Drugs
Steroids (anabolic, in particular)
Acetylated salicylates
Phenylbutazone (oxyphenbutazone)
Sulfonamides

Other Drugs
Cimetidine
Clofibrate
Disulfiram
Phenytoin
Thyroxine (both D- and L-isomers)
Tolbutamide

- Clinical syndrome termed warfarin (Coumadin) necrosis noted during initial stages of anticoagulation with vitamin K antagonist
  - Characterized clinically by development of skin and subcutaneous necrosis
    - Particularly in areas of subcutaneous fat
  - Pathologically by thrombosis of small blood vessels in fat and subcutaneous tissues
  - Syndrome caused by rapid depletion of vitamin K-dependent anticoagulant protein C
    - Prior to achieving depletion of procoagulant proteins
    - Occurs predominantly in individuals heterozygous for protein C deficiency
    - Anticoagulation requires decrease in procoagulant protein levels to about 20% to 25%
      - Prothrombotic milieu created with protein C levels of 40% or less
        - Individuals heterozygous for protein C deficiency
          - With baseline protein C levels of 50% to 60% of normal
          - May develop prothrombotic environment during first few days of warfarin therapy
  - Risk of developing warfarin necrosis greater when initial dose of warfarin >10 to 15 mg administered
  - Development of syndrome avoided if heparin and warfarin therapy are overlapped until "Coumadinization" complete and if large loading doses of warfarin are avoided
- **Management:** When overanticoagulation with warfarin presents with bleeding
  - Immediate reversal usually mandated
  - Treatment of choice is FFP
    - Provides prompt restoration of deficient vitamin K-dependent coagulation proteins, along with restoration of hemostatic function
    - 10 to 15 mL/kg FFP sufficient to produce significant correction of PT
      - Repeat infusions of FFP may be needed to effect continued correction
      - Due to the short half-life of fVII
  - Vitamin K may be administered in less acute situations
  - For severe bleeding or bleeding not controlled by FFP infusions
    - rhfVIIa used successfully

Platelet Disorders

- Platelets necessary for efficient clot formation
  - Produce physical barrier at site of vascular injury, the so-called *platelet plug*
  - Also serve to focus clotting process at point of bleeding
    - Delivering vasoconstrictors, clotting factors, and surface on which clot development occurs
    - Quantitative and qualitative platelet disorders a common cause of clinical ICU bleeding (Table 118.6)

Quantitative Platelet Disorders

- Decreased number of circulating platelets reflects:
  - Increased peripheral destruction or sequestration
  - Decreased marrow production
  - Combination of these factors

TABLE 118.6

PLATELET DISORDERS SEEN IN THE ICU

Quantitative	Qualitative
Increased Destruction	**Drugs**
Immune	**Anti-inflammatory agents**
Idiopathic thrombocytopenic purpura	Aspirin (irreversible)
Systemic lupus erythematosus	Nonsteroidal anti-inflammatory agents
Acquired immunodeficiency syndrome	Corticosteroids
Drugs (gold salts, heparin, sulfonamides, quinidine, quinine)	**Antibiotics**
Sepsis	Penicillins (e.g., ampicillin, carbenicillin, ticarcillin, penicillin-G)
Nonimmune	Cephalosporins (e.g., cephalothin)
Thrombotic thrombocytopenic purpura/hemolytic uremic	Nitrofurantoin
syndrome	Chloroquine, hydroxychloroquine
Mechanical destruction (e.g., cardiopulmonary bypass,	**Phosphodiesterase inhibitors**
hyperthermia)	Dipyridamole
Consumption (i.e., DIC)	Methylxanthines (e.g., theophylline)
Decreased Production	**Other drugs**
Marrow suppression	Antihistamines
Chemotherapy	Alpha-blockers (e.g., phentolamine)
Viral illness (e.g., cytomegalovirus, Epstein-Barr virus, herpes	Beta-blockers (e.g., propranolol)
simplex, parvovirus)	Dextran
Drugs (thiazides, ethanol, cimetidine)	Ethanol
	Furosemide
Marrow replacement	Heparin
Tumor	Local anesthetics (e.g., lidocaine)
Myelofibrosis	Phenothiazines
	Tricyclic antidepressants
Other conditions	Nitrates (e.g., sodium nitroprusside, nitroglycerin)
Splenic sequestration	**Metabolic Causes**
Dilution (see Massive Transfusion Syndrome)	Uremia
	Stored whole blood
	Disseminated intravascular coagulation (i.e., FDP-mediated
	inhibition)
	Hypothyroidism

DIC, disseminated intravascular coagulation; FDP, fibrin degradation product.

- Examples of increased peripheral destruction include:
  - Immune-mediated processes (both autoimmune and drug-induced)
  - Abnormal consumption (as in DIC)
  - Mechanical destruction (e.g., cardiopulmonary bypass, hyperthermia)
  - Autoimmune processes such as idiopathic thrombocytopenic purpura (ITP), SLE, acquired immunodeficiency syndrome (AIDS), lymphocytic leukemia, or lymphoma
    - Result in increased peripheral destruction and splenic sequestration
  - Drug-induced, immune-mediated platelet destruction a cause of thrombocytopenia frequently considered in thrombocytopenic ICU patient
    - Usually reversible with withdrawal of offending drug
    - Exact mechanism related to binding of drug to platelet membrane
      - Subsequent binding to platelet, platelet–drug complex, or both, of a specific antibody
      - Resulting platelet–drug–antibody complexes cleared by RES

  - Drugs in the ICU commonly associated include:
    - Quinidine and quinine
    - Heparin
    - Gold salts
    - Various penicillin and cephalosporin antibiotics
    - Sulfonamide antibiotics
    - Anticonvulsant valproic acid (Depakote, Depakene) (in part, is immunologic in nature)
- Various drugs associated with nonimmune mechanism of thrombocytopenia by bone marrow suppression:
  - Most cancer chemotherapeutic agents
  - Thiazide diuretics
  - Cimetidine
  - Ethanol
  - Several of the cephalosporin and penicillin antibiotics
  - Generalized infection, bacterial sepsis, and many viral illnesses
  - Gaucher disease
- Consumption of platelets also can cause thrombocytopenia
  - Mechanical destruction occurs during cardiopulmonary bypass

- ○ Not uncommon to note a 50% drop in platelet count postbypass
    - ○ Platelet counts may decrease for 48 to 72 hours after bypass before recovering
  - • May also be destroyed by high body temperatures
    - ○ Severe hyperthermic syndromes
  - • Consumed during microvascular coagulation in DIC

Qualitative Platelet Disorders

- Drugs frequently used in ICU have the potential to impair platelet function
  - • The sicker the patient, the greater the likelihood of exposure to one of these drugs (see Table 118.6)
  - • Terminating offending drugs usually results in restoration of normal function
    - • Aspirin the notable exception
      - ○ It irreversibly inhibits platelet cyclo-oxygenase
      - ○ Resulting in defect lasting for duration of platelet lifespan, 8 to 9 days
      - ○ Effect is profound: single 325-mg aspirin results in qualitative platelet defect remaining in 50% of circulating platelets 5 days after ingestion
      - ○ Prefer to avoid aspirin ingestion for at least 7 days prior to an elective invasive procedure
    - • Nonsteroidal anti-inflammatory drugs (NSAIDs) such as ibuprofen or naproxen sodium inhibit platelet cyclo-oxygenase
      - ○ Effects are reversible
      - ○ Normal platelet function usually restored within 24 hours of last dose
      - ○ Degree of platelet inhibition produced by NSAIDs is not clinically significant
        - – Patients can receive these drugs for analgesia and fever control
        - – Reasonable to minimize use of NSAIDs in bleeding, severely thrombocytopenic patient
    - • Clopidogrel (Plavix) or dipyridamole (Persantine) produce platelet inhibition that remains evident for several days after discontinuing drug
    - • β-lactam antibiotics sterically hinder binding of platelet aggregation agonist adenosine diphosphate (ADP) to specific platelet receptor, resulting in impaired platelet aggregation
      - ○ Reversed on removal of the drug
- In ICU one must also always consider possibility that patient with bleeding suggestive of a platelet defect may have an inherited disorder of platelet function
  - • Rare but encountered from time to time and include:
    - • Glanzmann thrombasthenia (abnormal platelet GP IIb/IIIa)
    - • Bernard-Soulier syndrome (abnormal GP Ib/IX)
    - • Wiskott-Aldrich syndrome, platelet storage pool deficiency (abnormal platelet dense bodies)
    - • Gray platelet disorder (abnormal platelet granules)
- **Management:** Unnecessary medications *always* discontinued when platelet function impaired
  - • Never acceptable to leave nonessential agent on patient's medication list because it is benign
  - • More controversial issue is deciding whether platelet transfusions warranted
    - • Relationship of thrombocytopenia to clinical bleeding is relative

- ○ Massive transfusion syndrome and DIC may respond to empirical platelet transfusion at counts as high as 80,000 to 100,000 platelets/μL
- ○ Although bleeding with platelet count of 80,000 cells/μL (or greater) unlikely to be a result of thrombocytopenia
- ○ With cancer chemotherapy and bone marrow aplasia
  - – Therapy not required until counts <10,000 to 20,000 cells/μL
  - – rhfVIIa used to reverse hemostatic defect caused by aspirin or clopidogrel
- ○ Administration of platelets limits both morbidity and mortality
  - – Finding generalized to all patients with platelet counts in this range
  - – Appropriateness of this approach unclear
  - – Major concern is development of alloimmunization
  - – Potentially negating future benefit from platelet transfusion in time of need
  - – Patients with acute leukemia have self-limited marrow aplasia resulting from chemotherapy
    - • Need for platelet transfusion is limited
  - – Patients with aplastic anemia have ongoing need for platelet transfusion
    - • Risk of alloimmunization high
  - – Autoimmune disorders associated with increased peripheral platelet destruction, disorders of splenic sequestration, and drug-related thrombocytopenia unlikely to benefit from platelet transfusion
    - • Exception related to planned invasive procedure associated with increased risk of bleeding
    - • Transfusions in presence of type II HIT contraindicated

Uremia

- Commonly seen in ICU and associated with increased risk of bleeding
- Shown to cause reversible impairment of platelet function
- "Toxin" responsible for defect not well defined
- Some studies have demonstrated an impairment of platelet–vessel wall interactions and suggest defects in vWf
- Degree of platelet impairment related to severity of uremia for given patient
- Thrombotic events are also increased with uremia
  - • Appear to be multifactorial in cause but reflect increased renal loss of antithrombin III and protein S in nephrotic-range proteinuria
- Therapeutic approaches may modulate the qualitative platelet defect
  - • Dialysis
  - • Cryoprecipitate
  - • 1-deamino-8-D-arginine vasopressin (DDAVP) 0.3 μg/kg, maximum dose 21 mg
  - • Conjugated estrogens (10 mg/day in adults)
- Benefit derived by treatment with cryoprecipitate or DDAVP related to increase in plasma concentration of large multimeric forms of vWf
  - • Greatly improving platelet adhesion
- Duration of action of these agents is limited
  - • Reaching their zenith between 2 and 6 hours
  - • Additional doses of DDAVP during same 24-hour period may result in a diminished response to the drug (tachyphylaxis) with little or no further benefit

- ○ May require 48 to 72 hours before again responding to this agent
- Mechanism of action of conjugated estrogens not known
  - Effect of estrogen more protracted and does not diminish with repeat dosing
  - Benefit is not noted for 3 to 5 days after starting therapy

THROMBOTIC SYNDROMES

- Often the cause of admission to an ICU
  - Particularly if acute coronary syndromes included in this category
  - Noncardiac thrombotic syndromes encountered in ICU include:
    - DVT (specifically in association with a central venous catheter)
    - Heparin-induced thrombocytopenia
    - Pulmonary embolism syndrome
    - Thrombotic thrombocytopenic purpura (TTP) or hemolytic uremic syndrome (HUS)
    - Thrombotic DIC
    - Stroke
    - Central nervous system (CNS) venous sinus thrombosis
      - ○ Most commonly in infants and elderly associated with dehydration
- Many conditions, particularly venous thromboembolic events, develop while patient in ICU
  - May be preventable
  - Assess risk of DVT and risks of thromboprophylaxis in all patients and institute appropriate therapy on a case-by-case basis
  - Postoperative patients and those immobilized for long periods of time are at risk
    - Candidates for some sort of thromboprophylaxis
  - Approximately 10% of ICU patients will develop DVT while in ICU
    - *Despite* receiving thromboprophylaxis
    - Up to 15% of these experience symptomatic pulmonary embolism (PE)
    - Not all patients at same risk
    - Not all respond to prophylactic measures equally

Management

- Initial management approach for patient with documented or highly suspected thrombotic event:
  - Anticoagulation with either UH or LMWH
  - Efficacy of either appears equivalent
    - Some studies suggest incidence of severe bleeding less with LMWH
    - LMWH may produce a more stable level of anticoagulation
      - ○ May result in fewer laboratory tests and dose adjustments
    - Choice of which agent to use is at discretion of intensivist
  - If repeated invasive procedures anticipated UH may be preferred agent
    - Owing to shorter half-life
    - Most patients started on UH with bolus dose of 50 units/kg

- Followed by a continuous infusion of 10 units/kg/hour
  - ○ Doses may be reduced for elderly or frail patient
- Once initiated adjust to keep aPTT 1.5 to 2.5 times baseline
  - ○ Corresponds to plasma heparin concentration of 0.2 to 0.4 units/mL
- Dosing of LMWH weight related
- Dose of warfarin titrated to maintain INR of the PT between 1.5 and 4.0

SELECTED DISORDERS

Systemic Diseases Associated with Factor Deficiencies

- Amyloidosis, Gaucher disease, and nephrotic syndrome occasionally seen in ICU
  - Each may have one or more associated factor deficiencies
    - Amyloidosis or Gaucher disease develop factor IX deficiency
    - Factor X deficiency also associated with amyloidosis
    - Deficiencies generally result from absorption of specific clotting factor onto abnormal proteins present with each disorder
  - In nephrotic syndrome, factor IX deficiency may develop
    - ○ Originally thought proteinuria responsible for development of factor IX deficiency
      - – May not be the case
    - ○ Deficiency typically remits with corticosteroid therapy
    - ○ Antithrombin III deficiency seen along with nephrotic syndrome and may lead to thrombosis
      - – Loss of antithrombin III **DOES** appear related to proteinuria

Laboratory Disorders Not Associated with Bleeding: Lupus Anticoagulants

- Lupus anticoagulant received much attention as potential cause of bleeding
  - By virtue of name and associated laboratory abnormalities
  - As isolated hemostatic defect thrombosis more likely a problem
    - 25% incidence rate
    - Bleeding in one series occurred in only 1 of 219 patients
- PT and aPTT assays depend on interaction of various coagulation factors with either lipoprotein or phospholipid to activate coagulation efficiently
  - Lupus anticoagulant is an antiphospholipid antibody directed against phospholipids or lipoproteins
    - Produces prolongation of the PT, aPTT, or measured recalcification time of platelet-rich plasma
    - Prolongation of aPTT more common than prolongation of PT
      - ○ Although isolated prolongation of PT seen
    - 25% of patients with active SLE and lupus anticoagulant also have associated:
      - ○ Thrombocytopenia or hypoprothrombinemia
      - ○ Therefore at risk for bleeding
        - – In contrast to those patients with lupus anticoagulant alone

- Lupus anticoagulant originally described in patients with SLE
- Not limited to this class of diseases
- Lupus anticoagulants or anticardiolipin antibodies, or both demonstrated in:
  - Large percentages of patients with human immunodeficiency virus (HIV) infection
  - Hemophilia A
  - Both HIV and hemophilia A
  - Also observed chronic and acute inflammatory disorders
- Thrombotic events in patients who exhibit lupus anticoagulant may occur independent of underlying disorder and be directly related to lupus anticoagulant itself
  - Likelihood of thrombosis associated with lupus anticoagulant appears greatest when:
    - Lupus anticoagulant has specificity for:
      - β_2-glycoprotein I or
      - Phosphatidylserine
  - Some forms of disorder, such as associated with pregnancy, respond to anti-inflammatory drugs such as aspirin or prednisone
  - Thrombosis equally likely to be venous or arterial
  - Venous thrombosis more common in extremities
  - Arterial thrombosis more common in CNS
  - Placental infarcts frequently seen in placental specimens in patients with repeated fetal wastage
  - Stroke, myocardial infarction (MI), and PE are well described in patients with the lupus anticoagulant

Reactive Hyperfibrinogenemia

- Defined as plasma fibrinogen concentration >800 mg/dL
  - In clinical laboratory, fibrinogen measured using functional assay
    - Time to fibrin clot formation is end point in presence of excess thrombin
    - Time to clotting proportional to amount of fibrinogen present in sample
    - When excessive amounts of fibrinogen present, clotting is incomplete
      - Fibrin fragments formed inhibit further fibrin clot formation
- Other hematologic parameters, the aPTT, PT, and TT, consequently prolonged
  - Suggesting potential, although artifactual, risk for bleeding
  - Can be evaluated by diluting plasma to normal fibrinogen concentration using saline or defibrinated plasma
  - Clotting studies will now be normal
  - Bleeding not seen unless fibrinogen also is dysfibrinogen
    - Even in these patients bleeding remains uncommon problem
    - In patients with dysfibrinogenemia:
      - Clotting studies fail to correct when saline or defibrinated plasma dilutions undertaken
      - Distinguishes from patients with reactive hyperfibrinogenemia

CHAPTER 119 ■ ANTITHROMBOTICS AND THROMBOLYTIC THERAPY

- Venous (VTE) and arterial (ATE) thromboembolism major causes of morbidity and mortality
  - Arterial thromboembolism commonly implicated in:
    - Myocardial infarctions
    - Stroke
    - Limb ischemia
    - Responsible for more deaths yearly than next seven leading causes combined
  - Venous thrombosis may lead to:
    - Pulmonary embolism
    - Right heart dysfunction
    - Venous insufficiency
    - Postthrombotic syndrome
    - Incidence of intensive care unit (ICU) patients developing VTE ranges from 5% to 33%
      - Estimated 2 million cases of VTE yearly in United States alone
      - Annual estimated mortality of about 60,000 from pulmonary embolism

  - Ability to rapidly diagnose and initiate effective therapy paramount

ANTIPLATELET AGENTS

- Platelets play key role in inflammatory and thrombotic cascade
  - Integral in pathogenesis of arterial thrombosis
  - Particularly in regions of high fluid shear stress:
    - Coronary, cerebrovascular, peripheral circulations
  - Aggregation leading to disruption of blood flow can have devastating outcomes

Aspirin (ASA)

- ASA most widely used antiplatelet drug in the world
  - Used as antipyretic agent since the mid-1800s
  - Antiplatelet effect recognized only about 50 years ago

- Activated platelets cleave phospholipids to generate arachidonic acid
  - Converted to thromboxane-A2 through a series of reactions
    - Mediated by cyclo-oxygenase-1 (COX-1) and thromboxane-A2 synthase
    - Three isoforms of COX enzyme
      - COX-1 being the major type
      - COX-3 being a variant of COX-1
      - COX-2 the inducible form present in cells at site of inflammation
- ASA an irreversible inhibitor of COX-1 and COX-3 at low concentrations
  - Rapid onset of action, approximately 30 minutes
  - Exerts its effect by acetylating serine 529 site of platelet COX-1 enzyme
    - Anucleate platelets unable to synthesize new enzyme
    - Single daily ASA dose sufficient to inhibit function for platelet lifespan
    - Restoration of normal aggregation on cessation of ASA therapy results from newly released, nonacetylated platelets replacing ASA-treated ones
  - ASA dose required to inhibit platelet function relatively low
    - Antithrombotic effect of ASA saturates at doses of approximately 100 mg
- Efficacy of ASA in acute coronary syndrome established
  - For acute myocardial infarction (MI) ASA alone reduced mortality to similar extent as streptokinase alone
    - No additive benefit when using both agents
  - Meta-analysis found ASA reduced risk of MI, stroke, or death from 13.3% to 8.0% in patients with unstable angina
    - Greatest risk reduction occurred with dose of 75 to 150 mg/day
    - Higher doses such as 325 mg/day conferred no added benefit
- Risk reduction of ischemic strokes in atrial fibrillation associated with oral vitamin K-inhibiting anticoagulant therapy is greater than that provided by ASA

Aspirin Resistance

- ASA efficacy in inhibition of platelet function differs between patients
  - Cardiovascular events occur preferentially in patients with low responses to ASA therapy
    - Low response is referred to as *aspirin resistance*
    - Prevalence varies between 5% and 60%, depending on laboratory studies used
  - ASA-resistant patients noted to have a 24% risk of death, MI, or stroke
    - Compared with a 10% risk for ASA sensitive patients
  - Two aspects of resistance: biochemical and clinical
    - Biochemical resistance refers to ASA inability to initiate platelet inhibition
    - Clinical resistance indicates an increased risk of cardiovascular events in patients receiving ASA treatment
    - Platelet receptor polymorphism is thought to be responsible for resistance
- Risk of hemorrhage, especially from the gastrointestinal tract, a major concern when doses higher than 325 mg/day used
  - Local effect of ASA on gastric mucosa more prevalent with higher doses
    - Patients with vascular malformations or mucosal lesions may bleed at lower doses

- Risk of cerebral hemorrhage in patients with prior stroke or uncontrolled hypertension
  - In event of hemorrhage discontinue ASA and measure bleeding time
  - If needed, treat with fresh platelet transfusion
- For elective surgical procedures ASA stopped 5 days before surgery
- ASA not recommended for VTE prophylaxis
  - Other forms of standard VTE prophylaxis preferred
    - Subcutaneous heparin
    - Pneumatic compression devices

Clopidogrel

- Clopidogrel a member of the thienopyridine family
  - A potent platelet inhibitor
  - Irreversibly binds to low-affinity adenosine diphosphate (ADP) receptors
  - Rapidly absorbed and metabolized by hepatic cytochrome P-450 enzyme system
    - Active metabolite selectively and irreversibly inhibits ADP-induced platelet aggregation
    - Metabolite also impairs activation of glycoprotein (GP) IIb/IIIa complex
    - Prevents fibrinogen binding to platelets
  - Platelets exposed to drug affected for remainder of their lifespan
- Dose-dependent platelet inhibition can be seen within 2 hours after a single oral dose
  - Maximum effect, patients given loading dose of 300 to 600 mg
    - Followed by 75 mg/day
  - Repeated doses of 75 mg/day (no load)
    - Maximum platelet inhibition can be achieved within 3 to 7 days
- When steady state achieved, platelet aggregation inhibited by 40% to 60%
  - Prolongation of bleeding time independent of age, renal impairment, or gender
  - Platelet aggregation and bleeding time return to baseline about 5 days after discontinuation
- Clopidogrel more effective than ASA in reducing atherosclerotic events by 8.7%
  - Peripheral vascular disease
  - Myocardial infarction
  - Stroke
- Efficacy and safety of clopidogrel evaluated in acute coronary syndrome patients
  - Shows 20% relative risk reduction in composite triple end points:
    - Nonfatal myocardial infarction
    - Death
    - Stroke
- Clopidogrel, like ticlopidine, prolongs bleeding time
  - Incidence of neutropenia reported at 0.1%
  - Rare case reports of clopidogrel-associated thrombotic thrombocytopenic purpura
  - Incidence of gastrointestinal bleeding is less when compared to ASA
  - Incidence of bleeding is higher among patients taking clopidogrel, requiring urgent surgical procedures

- Clopidogrel effect can be reversed by transfusion of fresh platelets

Ticlopidine

- An older thienopyridine compound
- Inhibits platelet aggregation irreversibly
- Interferes with ADP-induced binding of fibrinogen to platelet receptors
- Fallen out of favor because of two major side effects: neutropenia and thrombotic-thrombocytopenic purpura
  - Rare case reports of severe bone marrow toxicity limit ticlopidine use to patients intolerant or unresponsive to ASA

Cilostazol

- A newer platelet aggregation inhibitor with vasodilatory activity
- Causes platelet inhibition by inhibiting phosphodiesterase (PDE) type III activity
- Has greater vasodilatory effect on femoral arteries than on vertebral, carotid, or superior mesenteric arteries
- Approved U.S. Food and Drug Administration for reduction of symptoms related to intermittent claudication in severe peripheral vascular disease

Glycoprotein IIb/IIIa Antagonists

Abciximab

- The most successful GPIIb/IIIa antagonist
- A human-murine Fab chimeric monoclonal antibody (Ab) fragment to GPIIb/IIIa binding site
- Large protein with rapid and prolonged response
- Causes bleeding time to remain elevated for 12 hours after injection
- Used in combination with ASA and heparin in patients with unresponsive unstable angina or undergoing percutaneous coronary intervention
  - Delivers 60% relative risk reduction in triple end points: myocardial infarction, emergent revascularization, or cardiovascular deaths
- Major complications—reported as frequently as 10.5%—of agent include:
  - Intracranial bleeding
  - Decrease in hemoglobin of more than 15%,
  - High incidence of thrombocytopenia
    - May be spurious in 4% of cases due to platelet clumping
    - True and severe thrombocytopenia may also develop, resulting in profound bleeding
  - In the event of profuse bleeding, platelet transfusions required to normalize platelet count
  - Desmopressin has been shown to normalize the bleeding time

Eptifibatide

- A disintegrin derived from the southeastern pygmy rattlesnake
  - Rapidly bound and rapidly reversed

- Normalization of the bleeding time within 1 to 4 hours
- More effective in milder forms of acute coronary syndromes

Tirofiban

- A small nonpeptide compound derived from tyrosine
  - Interacts with arginine—glycine–aspartic acid fibrinogen receptor
  - Used in unstable angina with mixed results

Dipyridamole

- A phosphodiesterase inhibitor, reversibly inhibiting platelet aggregation
  - Increases cyclic adenosine monophosphate and cyclic guanosine monophosphate levels through inhibition of phosphodiesterases
  - Potentiates the effect of nitric oxide
  - Used adjunctively with ASA to reduce stroke events in patients younger than 70 years of age

ANTITHROMBOTIC THERAPY

Unfractionated Heparin (UH)

- UH a naturally occurring acidic glycosaminoglycan whose anticoagulant effect originates from its pentasaccharide sequence
  - Sequence binds to antithrombin
  - Causes conformational change at arginine reactive site
  - Potentiates effect of antithrombin, causing enhanced effect on inhibition of coagulation enzymes, in particular thrombin (factor IIa) and factor Xa
  - Heparin also inhibits activation of factors V and VIII by thrombin
- Increase in inhibition of enzymes in presence of UH up to 2,000 times faster than in its absence
  - Due to the variable size and structure of heparin about one-third of dose demonstrates therapeutic anticoagulant activity
  - Different-sized molecules cleared at different rates by kidney
    - Larger ones cleared more rapidly
    - Necessitates need for monitoring with activated partial thromboplastin time (aPTT)
- Obtained from bovine lung or porcine intestine, available as a sodium or calcium salt
  - Unit of heparin measured in animals in a biologic assay
  - Unit measurement variable by as much as 50% on a weight basis
  - UH prescribed for patients on a unit basis per kilogram
- UH clearance involves a combination of rapid, saturable, and slower first-order mechanisms
  - Saturable phase of UH clearance via binding to receptors on endothelial cells and macrophages, where it becomes depolymerized
  - Slower-phase first-order saturable mechanism is renal
  - At therapeutic doses cleared predominantly through the rapid, saturable dose-dependent mechanism
    - Anticoagulant effects are nonlinear
    - Intensity and duration of effect rising disproportionately to increasing dose

TABLE 119.1

WEIGHT-BASED HEPARIN DOSING NOMOGRAM

aPTT, s[b]	Dose change, U/kg/h	Additional action	Next aPTT, h
<35 (<1.2 × mean normal)	+4	Rebolus with 80 IU/kg	6
35–45 (1.2–1.5 × mean normal)	+2	Rebolus with 40 IU/kg	6
46–70[a] (1.5–2.3 × mean normal)	0	0	6[c]
71–90 (2.3–3.0 × mean normal)	−2	0	6
>90 (>3 × mean normal)	−3	Stop infusion 1 h	6

aPTT, activated prothrombin time; s, seconds.
Initial dosing: Loading 80 IU/kg; maintenance infusion: 18 IU/kg/hour (aPTT in 6 hours)
[a]Therapeutic range in seconds should correspond to a plasma heparin level of 0.2–0.4 IU/mL by protamine sulfate or 0.3–0.6 IU/mL by amidolytic assay. When aPTT is checked at 6 hours or longer, steady-state kinetics can be assumed.
[b]Heparin, 25,000 IU in 250 mL D$_5$W. Infuse at rate dictated by body weight.
[c]During the first 24 hours, repeat aPTT every 6 hours. Thereafter, monitor aPTT once every morning unless it is outside the therapeutic range.
From Hyers TM, Agnelli G, Hull RD, et al. Antithrombotic therapy for venous thromboembolic disease. *Chest.* 2001;119(Suppl):179S, with permission.

Uses of Unfractionated Heparin

- UH indicated for prophylaxis of VTE, treatment of deep vein thrombosis (DVT) and pulmonary embolism (PE), and for early treatment of acute coronary syndromes
- **Prevention of Thromboembolism:** UH at fixed low dose of 5,000 units, subcutaneously every 8 to 12 hours, results in a 60% to 70% relative risk reduction for DVT and fatal PE
  - In high-risk surgical and acutely ill medical patients low-molecular-weight heparin (LMWH) becoming standard for prevention of thrombosis
  - In patient unable to tolerate any type of anticoagulation, compression stockings useful as mechanical means for preventing DVT
    - Intermittently squeezing patient's calves
    - Leads to increased blood flow through venous system
    - May also stimulate fibrinolysis by stimulating vascular endothelium
- **VTE and PE:** Therapy aimed at preventing extension of clot with further embolization and recurrence
- Most efficient and safe method for initiating intravenous (IV) UH therapy is using weight-adjusted nomograms
  - In first days of treatment, there is weak association between supratherapeutic aPTT and bleeding
  - This in *marked contrast* to significant relationship between subtherapeutic aPTT and VTE recurrence in first 24 hours
  - Must maintain therapeutic range when heparin anticoagulation therapy is initiated
    - Best achieved with monitoring of plasma aPTT
- The weight-based method results in a significant decrease in the time required to reach therapeutic levels
  - 97% of patients dosed using weight-based nomogram achieve therapeutic levels within 24 hours of initiation as opposed to 77% in standard dosing group (Tables 119.1 and 119.2)

TABLE 119.2

GUIDELINES FOR ANTICOAGULATION USING UNFRACTIONATED HEPARIN

Indication	Guidelines
VTE suspected	- Obtain baseline aPTT, PT, CBC - Check for contraindication to heparin therapy - Order imaging study, consider giving heparin 5,000 IU IV
VTE confirmed	- Rebolus with heparin 80 IU/kg IV and start maintenance infusion at 18 U/kg (see text and Table 119.1) - Check aPTT at 6 hours to keep aPTT in a range that corresponds to a therapeutic blood heparin level (see text and Table 119.1) - Check a platelet count between days 3 to 5 - Start warfarin therapy on day 1 at 5 mg and adjust subsequent daily dose according to INR - Stop heparin therapy after at least 4 to 5 d of combined therapy when INR is >2.0 - Anticoagulate with warfarin for at least 3 mo at an INR of 2.5; range: 2.0–3.0 (see Table 119.4)

aPTT, activated prothrombin time; PT, prothrombin time; CBC, complete blood count; IV, intravenously; INR, international normalized ratio.
For subcutaneous treatment with unfractionated heparin, give 250 IU/kg subcutaneously every 12 hours to obtain a therapeutic aPTT at 6–8 hours.
From Hyers TM, Agnelli G, Hull RD, et al. Antithrombotic therapy for venous thromboembolic disease. *Chest.* 2001;119(Suppl):180S, with permission.

- Therapy initiated with IV loading dose of 80 units/kg
  - Followed by 18 units/kg/hour
  - Doses adjusted using a standard nomogram to reach and maintain aPTT corresponding to therapeutic heparin levels of 1.5 to 2.5 times baseline
  - Alternatively, therapeutic heparin anticoagulation determined by achieving a plasma anti-factor Xa level of 0.35 to 0.7 units/mL
- UH anticoagulation continued for up to 5 days so adequate anticoagulation achieved
  - aPTT monitored every 6 hours until therapeutic range achieved
    - Once daily thereafter
- Preferably on day 1 patient transition begun to long-term oral warfarin (5 mg)
  - Anticoagulation effect of warfarin monitored by international normalized ratio (INR) to achieve a therapeutic range of two to three times normal level for a first thrombotic episode
  - Warfarin considered at therapeutic level if INR of 2 to 3 maintained for 2 consecutive days
- Warfarin interacts with many commonly used ICU drugs and metabolism may be affected by hepatic and renal impairment
  - May lead to erratic variation in anticoagulant effect of warfarin and exposes patient to increased risks of bleeding and thrombotic complications
- Minimum recommended duration of warfarin therapy is 3 months
  - Longer treatment beneficial
    - Now recommended warfarin therapy be continued for at least 6 to 12 months after an acute thromboembolic episode arising from an idiopathic DVT
    - With recurrent events or those who have permanent or long-term risk factors, indefinite therapy recommended
- **Acute Coronary Syndromes:** American College of Cardiology/American Heart Association updated guidelines for management of patients with acute myocardial infarction demonstrate clear benefit of LMWH over UH when it came to a lower event rate and relative risk reduction
- Guidelines recommend using LMWH due to:
  - Greater inhibition of factor Xa
  - Ability to administer the drug subcutaneously
  - High bioavailability
  - Other benefits include potential to prevent thrombin generation and inhibit thrombin, the lack of need to monitor coagulation, and the lower incidence of heparin-associated thrombocytopenia

Monitoring UH

- Most widely used test for evaluating the adequacy of UH anticoagulation is aPTT
  - Global coagulation test not always a reliable indicator of plasma heparin levels and/or the antithrombotic activity of heparin
  - aPTT can be impacted by various acute phase reactant plasma proteins, including factor VIII
  - aPTT can be influenced by coagulation timer and reagents used to perform test
  - If unable to measure plasma heparin levels directly:
    - Standardize therapeutic range of the aPTT to correspond to plasma levels of 0.3 to 0.7 IU/mL anti–factor Xa activity by an amidolytic assay

Complications of Anticoagulation Therapy

Heparin Resistance

- Patients considered heparin resistant if daily requirement exceeds 35,000 units per 24 hours
- At least 25% of patients with VTE heparin resistant
- May be associated with antithrombin deficiency, increased heparin clearance, increases in heparin-binding proteins, and increases in factor VIII, fibrinogen, and platelet factor 4
- Aprotinin and nitroglycerin reported to cause drug-induced resistance
  - Association with nitroglycerin controversial
- Factor VIII and fibrinogen elevated in response to acute illness or pregnancy
  - Elevation of factor VIII alters response of aPTT to heparin without decreasing the antithrombotic effect
    - Anticoagulant effect measured by plasma aPTT and antithrombotic effect measured by anti-factor Xa activity become dissociated
- For patients considered heparin resistant:
  - Dose of heparin adjusted to maintain the anti-factor Xa heparin levels between 0.35 and 0.7 mIU/mL
- In patients with VTE and manifesting heparin resistance:
  - Monitoring aPTT *versus* anti-factor Xa activity showed no difference in clinical outcomes, the anti-factor Xa heparin levels group required significantly less heparin with no differences in bleeding

Hemorrhagic Complications

- Incidence of major hemorrhagic complications, such as intracranial or retroperitoneal hemorrhage, hemorrhage requiring a transfusion, or hemorrhage directly related to death, from therapeutic anticoagulation is <5%
  - Risk increases with age, total dose of heparin per 24 hours, premorbid condition of patient, concomitant use of ASA, GPIIb/IIIa antagonists, or thrombolytic therapy
  - IV heparin infusion produces less marked bleeding complications than subcutaneously administered
    - May be due to lower total dose of heparin via IV route
- Anticoagulant effect of UH neutralized rapidly by IV protamine
  - A cationic protein derived from fish sperm
  - Strongly binds to anionic heparin compound in ratio of approximately 100 units of UH/mg of protamine
    - For example, 50 mg of protamine required to neutralize 5,000 units of IV heparin
    - When heparin infused, only drug given over prior 2 hours included in calculation
    - If heparin infusion discontinued for more than 30 minutes but less than 2 hours, use one-half of calculated protamine dose
    - If infusion discontinued for more than 2 hours use one-quarter of calculated protamine dose
    - Avoid giving 50 mg of protamine at one time
      - If given by infusion, it should not exceed 5 mg/minute to reduce incidence of adverse reactions
      - Heparin neutralization can be confirmed by a fall in the aPTT
  - Risks of severe adverse reactions to protamine:
    - Such as hypotension and bradycardia
- Reduced with slow administration of drug over >3 minutes

- Some begin protamine infusion following a 3 to 5 mg test dose over 1 minute
- Allergic reactions including anaphylaxis associated with:
  - Previous exposure to protamine-containing insulin (NPH-insulin)
  - Fish hypersensitivity
  - Vasectomy
  - Patients at risk for antiprotamine antibodies pretreated with corticosteroid and antihistamine medications

Heparin-associated (Induced) Thrombocytopenia (HIT)

- HIT an antibody-mediated adverse reaction to the administration of UH and/or LMWH
- May lead to both arterial and venous thrombosis
- Diagnosis is made on clinical and serologic findings
- HIT antibody formation, accompanied by otherwise unexplained fall in platelet count by >50% from baseline and/or skin lesions at injection sites are the manifestations of HIT
- Incidence of HIT is <1% when heparin is given for <7 days
  - Thereafter, when given to patients with extended need for anticoagulation
    - Incidence may rise to as much as 10% to 20% for mild form (type 1) of HIT
      - To more than 5% for type 2, the more severe manifestation
  - Risk of developing HIT increased by use of heparin flush, prophylactic treatments, and increasing doses of heparin
- HIT may occur more rapidly if patient has had recent exposure, within 100 days, to heparin
  - Can also develop after >9 to 30 days following cessation of therapy
    - Often goes undetected
  - Precipitous fall in platelet count from baseline platelet count usually seen with the type 1 syndrome
    - 50% to 75% of these patients go on to develop more ominous type 2 syndrome
    - Manifests with development of arterial or, more commonly, venous thrombotic complications
- Patients who develop HIT generate large amounts of thrombin
- *In vivo,* platelet activation results from binding of heparin platelet factor-4/immunoglobulin-G (PF4-IgG) immune complexes to platelet factor IIa receptors
- Increased levels of thrombin demonstrated by elevated levels of thrombin–antithrombin complexes
  - Serve as an *in vivo* marker of thrombin generation
  - Much higher than what is seen in control patients with DVT
  - Diagnosis confirmed with platelet function testing or identification in blood of the antibody to heparin-platelet factor 4 complex
    - Using enzyme-linked immunosorbent assay
- Once the determination of HIT is made patients at risk of thrombosis if no anticoagulation given
  - Alternative antithrombotic agents are detailed in Tables 119.3 and 119.4

Low-molecular-weight Heparin

- Prepared from UH by controlled depolymerization of parent drug into short segments

- Molecular weight of LMWH ranges from 1,000 to 10,000
- About 20% of LMWH chains contain pentasaccharide sequences needed for antithrombin binding

Mechanism of Action

- LMWH chains too short to bridge thrombin to antithrombin
  - Binds to antithrombin
  - Brings about conformational changes, leading to inhibition of factor Xa
  - Ratio of inhibition of thrombin to factor Xa varies from 1:2 to 1:4 for different preparations of LMWH
- LMWH increasingly used for treatment of VTE disease in non-ICU patients
  - Administered as subcutaneous (SC) injection once or twice daily and IV when rapid effect needed
  - As safe and effective as IV/SC UH
  - Shorter LMWH chains bind less avidly to endothelial cells, macrophages, and heparin-binding proteins and have better bioavailability
  - Accumulate *in vivo,* leading to longer half-life
    - More predictable renal clearance
    - Greater ability to inactivate factor Xa
      - Compared to inactivation of thrombin
      - Consequently negligible effect on aPTT
- Clearance of LMWH dose independent
  - Accomplished almost exclusively kidneys
    - Drug can accumulate in renal insufficiency
  - Cost effective because of reduced need for monitoring
  - Several advantages of LMWH over the UH (Table 119.5)
  - Disadvantages of LMWH, may be more pertinent to the ICU, include:
    - Absence of established dose for obese patients
    - Impaired clearance in patients with renal failure
      - Can be overcome by monitoring anti–factor-Xa levels
      - Adjusting subsequent doses
      - Based on anti–factor-Xa levels, LMWH has plasma half-life of 4 hours
        - Therapeutic levels range from 0.5 to 1.2 U/mL
        - When measured 3 to 4 hours after drug administration
      - No rapid/complete antagonist to anticoagulant effect of LMWH (Table 119.6)

Dosing

- Most commonly prescribed LMWHs are:
  - Enoxaparin
  - Dalteparin
  - Newer agents like tinzaparin
- *Enoxaparin* primarily metabolized in liver by desulfation and/or depolymerization
  - To lower-molecular-weight species with reduced biologic potency
  - Renal clearance of active fragments represents about 10% of administered dose
  - Total renal excretion of active/nonactive fragments about 40% of dose
- **DVT Prophylaxis following Abdominal Surgery in Patients at Risk for Thromboembolic Complications:** Patients at risk include those who are:
- Older than 40 years of age
- Obese
- Undergoing surgery under general anesthesia lasting longer than 30 minutes

TABLE 119.3

ALTERNATIVES TO HEPARIN FOR THE TREATMENT OF HEPARIN-INDUCED THROMBOCYTOPENIA (HIT)[a]

Agent	Clearance	Therapeutic dose	Monitoring	Adverse effects
Direct thrombin inhibitors Lepirudin (Refludan, Berlex)[b]	Renal	IV, 0.4 mg/kg of body weight (up to 110 kg); IV bolus[c] followed by 0.15 mg/kg/hr (up to 110 kg) (maximal initial bolus, 44 mg; maximal initial infusion, 16.5 mg/hr)	Measure aPTT 2 hr after therapy started and after each dose adjustment; therapeutic range, 1.5 to 2.5 times the baseline value (optimal aPTT, <65 sec[d]); check baseline PT before switching therapy to warfarin[e]	Bleeding with therapeutic dose in 17.6% of patients; antilepirudin antibodies develop in 30% of patients
Argatroban (Novastan, GlaxoSmithKline)[b]	Hepatic	2 μg/kg/min continuous infusion (maximal infusion, 10 μg/kg/min)	Measure aPTT 2 hr after initiation of therapy and after each dose adjustment; therapeutic range, 1.5 to 3 times the baseline value (not to exceed 100 sec); switching to warfarin complicated by baseline prolongation of the PT[f]	Bleeding with therapeutic dose in 6 to 7% of patients
Bivalirudin (Angiomax, The Medicines Company)[g]	Enzymatic (80%) and renal (20%)	For PCI, 0.75 mg/kg IV bolus followed by 1.75 mg/kg/hr for remainder of procedure; infusion may be continued for 4 hr after the procedure or administered as low-dose infusion (0.2 mg/kg/hr) for an additional 20 hr	Measure ACT 5 min after completing IV bolus	Bleeding with dose used in PCI in 2.4% of patients
Anti-factor Xa therapy Danaparoid (Orgaran, Diosynth)[b]	Renal	IV, 2,250 U bolus followed by 400 U/hr for 4 hr, then 300 U/hr for 4 hr, then 150 to 200 U/hr	Not required, but if needed, maintain anti-factor Xa level, 0.5 to 0.8 U/mL	Bleeding with therapeutic dose in 8.1% of patients; cross-reactivity with PF4-heparin antibodies in 3.2% of patients

aPTT, activated partial thromboplastin time; PT, prothrombin time.
[a]Except where indicated, the guidelines for dosing and monitoring are from the manufacturers of the drugs. Guidelines for therapeutic dosing are for intravenous (IV) infusion, except for bivalirudin, which is used in patients undergoing percutaneous coronary intervention (PCI). The guidelines of the American College of Chest Physicians recommend overlap use of direct thrombin inhibitor therapy and warfarin therapy for more than 5 days, whereas the Hemostasis and Thrombosis Task Force of the British Committee for Standards in Haemotology recommend overlap use of direct thrombin inhibitor therapy and warfarin therapy until the international normalized ratio (INR) is at a therapeutic level for at least 48 hours.
[b]These drugs have been approved in the United States for the treatment of heparin-induced thrombocytopenia.
[c]Bolus therapy is not advised in older patients or patients with renal insufficiency.
[d]This value is the maximal aPTT recommended by Lubenow et al.
[e]Therapeutic lepirudin may prolong the baseline PT slightly, but it generally does not interfere with conversion from lepirudin to warfarin therapy. If the PT is prolonged by more than a few seconds, further evaluation should be undertaken before initiating warfarin.
[f]Combined anticoagulant therapy with argatroban and warfarin produces an INR response that is significantly greater than that obtained with warfarin alone. To change therapy from argatroban to warfarin for outpatient anticoagulant therapy, the INR should be monitored daily, and when the INR is greater than 4, the argatroban infusion should be withheld and the INR rechecked to determine whether it is therapeutic. An alternative strategy would be to use a chromogenic factor X assay to monitor warfarin therapy while the patient is also receiving argatroban.
[g]This drug has been approved in the United States for the treatment of patients undergoing percutaneous coronary intervention (PCI) who have heparin-induced thrombocytopenia or a history of heparin-induced thrombocytopenia.
[h]This drug is not available in the United States.
From Arepally GM, Ortel TL. Heparin-induced thrombocytopenia. *N Engl J Med*. 2006;355:809, with permission.

- Have additional risk factors such as malignancy or history of DVT or PE
- Recommended dose of enoxaparin for this indication 40 mg SC daily
  - Beginning 2 hours preoperatively
- **Treatment of DVT with or without PE:** In patients with acute DVT with PE or acute DVT without PE who are not candidates for outpatient treatment
  - Recommended dose of enoxaparin is 1 mg/kg every 12 hours SC
- **Unstable Angina and Non-Q Wave MI:** Recommended dose of enoxaparin is 1 mg/kg SC every 12 hours in conjunction with oral ASA (100–325 mg daily)
- Based on currently available data on efficacy and safety of LMWHs
  - Enoxaparin the only LMWH consistently demonstrating short- and long-term improvements in major ischemic outcomes compared with UH
- **Hip or Knee Replacement Surgery:** Recommended dose of enoxaparin is 30 mg SC every 12 hours

TABLE 119.4

GUIDELINES FOR TRANSITION TO ORAL ANTICOAGULANT IN A PATIENT WITH HEPARIN-ASSOCIATED OR INDUCED THROMBOCYTOPENIA (HIT)

Step	Description
1	Stop heparin or LMWH therapy
2	Ensure adequate levels of anticoagulation with a DTI or alternative anticoagulant
3	Avoid interruptions during treatment with a DTI or alternative anticoagulant
4	Wait until the platelet count has "cooled" or is near normal before beginning therapy with an oral anticoagulant
5	Initiate modest doses of an oral anticoagulant (2.5–5 mg warfarin)
6	Avoid overshooting the target INR[a]
7	Avoid using warfarin (or equivalent) as monotherapy

LMWH, low-molecular-weight heparin; DTI, direct thrombin inhibitor; INR, international normalized ratio.

[a]Recognize that cotherapy with a direct thrombin inhibitor prolongs the INR for a longer time than warfarin therapy alone.

From Bartholomew J. Transition to oral anticoagulants in patient with heparin-induced thrombocytopenia. *Chest.* 2005;127:32s, with permission.

- If hemostasis established initial dose given 12 to 24 hours after surgery
- Hip replacement surgery, 40 mg SC daily, given initially 12 (±3) hours **prior** to surgery may be considered
  - Enoxaparin prophylaxis 40 mg SC daily recommended for 3 weeks
  - Usual duration of administration is 7 to 10 days
- **Restricted Mobility:** Medical patients at risk for thromboembolic complications
  - Recommended dose of enoxaparin 40 mg SC daily
- **Mechanical Prosthetic Heart Valves:** Use of enoxaparin not adequately studied for thromboprophylaxis or long-term use in patients with mechanical prosthetic valves
- Isolated cases of prosthetic valve thrombosis reported in patients who have received enoxaparin for thromboprophylaxis
  - Some were pregnant women in whom thrombosis led to maternal and fetal deaths
- Pregnant women with mechanical prosthetic valves may be at higher risk for thromboembolism
- *Dalteparin* consists of small heparin molecules ranging from 2,000 to 9,000 Da
- Administered SC, has better availability and longer half-life than UH
- Similar mechanism as enoxaparin, selectively inhibiting factor Xa
  - Inhibitory activity is 2.7:1 compared to 1:1 for UH
  - Inhibition of factor Xa prevents formation of fibrin clots
- Elimination of drug occurs via renal route and is dose independent
  - Plasma half-life of 3 to 5 hours
- Does not significantly affect platelet activity, prothrombin time (PT), or aPTT
- Superior to warfarin in preventing DVT following total hip replacement surgery

TABLE 119.5

ADVANTAGES OF LOW-MOLECULAR-WEIGHT HEPARIN OVER UNFRACTIONATED HEPARIN

Advantage	Consequence
Better bioavailability and longer half-life	Can be given subcutaneously once or twice after subcutaneous injection daily for both prophylaxis and treatment
Dose-independent clearance	Simplified dosing
Predictable anticoagulant response	Coagulation monitoring is unnecessary in most patients
Lower risk of heparin-induced thrombocytopenia	Safer than heparin for short- or long-term administration
Lower risk of osteoporosis	Safer than heparin for extended administration

From Weitz JI. Anticoagulants and fibrinolytic drugs. In: *Hematology: Basic Principles and Practice.* 4th ed. Orlando, FL: Churchill Livingstone; 2005:2254, with permission.

TABLE 119.6

DOSAGE REGIMENS FOR PATIENTS WITH SEVERE RENAL IMPAIRMENT

Indication	Dosage regimen
Prophylaxis in abdominal surgery	30 mg administered SC once daily
Prophylaxis in hip or knee replacement surgery	30 mg administered SC once daily
Prophylaxis in medical patients during acute illness	30 mg administered SC once daily
Prophylaxis of ischemic complications of unstable angina and non-Q wave myocardial infarction when concurrently administered with aspirin	1 mg/kg administered SC once daily
Inpatient treatment of acute deep vein thrombosis with or without pulmonary embolism when administered in conjunction with warfarin sodium	1 mg/kg administered SC once daily
Outpatient treatment of acute deep vein thrombosis without pulmonary embolism when administered in conjunction with warfarin sodium	1 mg/kg administered SC once daily

SC, subcutaneously.

- Dalteparin decreases risk of death or acute myocardial infarction (AMI) by 36% as compared to ASA alone
- Dalteparin found as effective as IV UH in preventing death or AMI in acute phase following unstable angina or non-Q wave MI
- *Tinzaparin* is a relatively new drug with a similar mechanism of action and pharmacokinetic profile as enoxaparin and dalteparin.
  - Approved for treatment of symptomatic DVT

Complications

- **Bleeding:** Major complication of LMWHs is bleeding
  - Is as frequent as with UH
  - Of course, more common in patients receiving antiplatelet/antifibrinolytic therapy in addition to LMWH
  - Recent surgery, coagulopathy, or trauma increases risk of bleeding
  - Protamine sulfate can be used as antidote
    - Incompletely neutralizes anticoagulant activity by binding to longer chains of LMWH
      - These are responsible for antithrombin activity
      - Short chains, which inhibit factor Xa activity, don't bind to protamine
        - Only partially reverses effect of LMWH
- **Thrombocytopenia:** LMWH binds less avidly to platelets
  - Causes less release of PF4 and has reduced affinity for PF4
  - Less likely to trigger formation of antibodies
    - Incidence of HIT is lower compared to UH
    - Ab already formed in established HIT can cross-react with LMWH
      - Lead to thrombosis or other complications of disorder
      - LMWHs should not be used as substitute for UH in HIT patients

Warfarin (Coumadin)

- The most frequently prescribed oral anticoagulant
  - Fourth most prescribed cardiovascular agent
  - Overall, one of the most commonly prescribed drugs in United States
- Well absorbed in gut
  - Transported in plasma bound to albumin
- An antagonist of vitamin K

- Vitamin K required for posttranslational modification of:
  - Factors II, VII, IX, and X
  - As well as naturally occurring endogenous anticoagulant proteins C and S
- These factors biologically inactive without carboxylation of selected glutamic acid residues
  - Requires reduced vitamin K as cofactor
- Antagonism of vitamin K or vitamin deficiency reduces rate at which these factors are produced
  - Creating state of anticoagulation
- Therapeutic doses reduces production of functional vitamin K-dependent factors 30% to 50%
  - Concomitant reduction in carboxylation of secreted clotting factors yields 10% to 40% decrease in biologic activity of clotting factors
- Thus, coagulation system becomes functionally deficient
- PT the primary assay used in monitoring warfarin therapy
  - Changes noted in first few days of therapy primarily due to reduction in factors VII and IX
    - Have shortest half-lives, 6 and 24 hours, respectively
- PTs performed with different thromboplastins not always directly comparable
  - INR adopted using thromboplastins with international sensitivity index values near 1.0
- Warfarin used in lower extremity DVT patients to prevent extension and reduce risk of PE
  - Patients with PE treated with warfarin to prevent further thromboemboli
- Warfarin is used in patients with atrial fibrillation and artificial heart valves to reduce risk of embolic strokes
- Helpful in preventing blood clot formation in certain orthopedic surgeries:
  - Knee or hip replacements
- Helps prevent thrombotic stenosis of coronary artery stents (Table 119.7)
- Most common complication of warfarin therapy is bleeding
  - Occurs in 6% to 39% of patients annually
  - Incidence related to intensity of anticoagulation
    - Need for intense anticoagulation has evolved and been reduced over past 20 years
      - Incidence of bleeding decreased significantly
      - Moderate bleeding (elevated INR) treated by adjusting down dose
      - Severe bleeding can be treated with fresh frozen plasma

TABLE 119.7

THERAPEUTIC GOALS AND DURATION OF WARFARIN ANTICOAGULATION

Indication	INR	Duration
Prophylaxis of venous thrombosis for high-risk surgery	2–3	Clinical judgment
Treatment of venous thrombosis		
First episode	2–3	3–6 mo[a]
High risk of recurrent thrombosis	2–3	Lifelong
Thrombosis associated with antiphospholipid antibody	3–4	Lifelong
Treatment of pulmonary embolism		
First episode	2–3	3–6 mo
High risk of recurrent embolism	2–3	Lifelong
Prevention of systemic embolism		
Tissue heart valves	2–3	3 mo
Acute myocardial infarction (to prevent systemic embolism)[b]	2–3	Clinical judgment
Valvular heart disease (after thrombotic event or dilated left)	2–3	Lifelong
Atrial fibrillation		
Chronic or intermittent	2–3	Lifelong
Cardioversion	2–3	3 wk before and 4 wk after atrial fibrillation if normal sinus rhythm is maintained
Prosthetic heart valves		
Aortic position		
Mechanical	2.5–3.5[c]	Lifelong
Bioprosthetic	2–3	Clinical judgment (3 mo optional)
Mitral position		
Mechanical	2.5–3.5[c]	Lifelong
Bioprosthetic	2–3	3 mo

INR, international normalized ratio.

[a]All recommendations are subject to modification by individual characteristics. First event with reversible or time limited risk factors (surgery, trauma, immobilization, estrogen use). Hyers TM, Agnelli G, Hull RD, et al. Antithrombotic therapy for venous thromboembolic disease. *Chest.* 2001;119(Suppl):176s–193s.

[b]If oral anticoagulant therapy is elected to prevent recurrent myocardial infarction, an INR of 2.5–3.5 is recommended.

[c]Depending on the type of prosthetic valve and valve position (mitral), some patients may benefit from INR in upper therapeutic range. From Horton JD, Bushwick BM. Warfarin therapy: evolving strategies in anticoagulation. *Am Fam Physician.* 1999;59(4):636, with permission.

Alternative Therapies

Thrombin Inhibitors

- Heparin, LMWH, and warfarin used for treatment of venous and arterial thromboemboli
- These drugs have drawbacks
- Biophysical limitations of heparin include inability of heparin or antithrombin complex to inhibit factor Xa within the prothrombinase complex and thrombin bound to fibrin, clotting enzymes that are important triggers of thrombin growth
- Direct thrombin inhibitors (DTIs) have advantageous properties over indirect thrombin inhibitors (ITIs) (heparins, including LMWH)
- Thrombin is a trypsin-like serine protease that converts fibrinogen to fibrin
- Inhibited either directly or indirectly
  - ITIs act by catalyzing reaction of antithrombin and/or heparin cofactor II
  - Thrombin substrate specificity due to surface binding sites (i.e., exosite 1)
  - DTIs directly bind thrombin (at exosite 1 or other active site of thrombin)

  - ○ Block this procoagulant from reacting further
  - ○ More advantageous than ITIs, such as heparin
    - – Don't bind plasma proteins
    - – Produce more predictable response
    - – DTIs do not bind PF4
      - • Anticoagulant activity unaffected by large quantities of PF4 released in surrounding region of platelet-rich thrombi
    - – DTIs inactivate fibrin-bound and fluid-phase thrombin
- Three parenteral DTIs approved for limited use in United States and Canada:
  - Hirudin and argatroban approved for treatment of patients diagnosed with heparin-associated thrombocytopenia
  - Bivalirudin approved as alternative therapy for heparin-sensitive patients undergoing percutaneous coronary interventions
- **Hirudin:** A 65 amino acid polypeptide originally isolated from salivary glands of medicinal leech
  - Now available via recombinant DNA technology
  - Recombinant form exhibits 10-fold reduced affinity for thrombin compared to native form
  - Directly inhibits thrombin in bivalent manner
    - • Globular amino-terminal domain interacts with thrombin active site

- Anionic carboxy-terminal tail binds to exosite 1 on thrombin
  - The substrate recognition site
- Hirudin/thrombin complex essentially irreversible
- May create problem if significant bleeding occurs
  - No specific antidote
- Recombinant hirudins, for example, desirudin and lepirudin
  - Have leucine substituted for isoleucine at N-terminal end of molecule
  - Lepirudin (Refludan) approved in North America for treatment of heparin-induced thrombocytopenia subtypes 1 and 2
- Plasma half-life of hirudin approximately 60 minutes following IV injection
  - 120 minutes following SC administration
- Cleared via kidneys
  - Should be used with caution, if at all, in patients with renal insufficiency
- Anticoagulant activity measured using aPTT
  - Dose adjustment made to maintain aPTT within therapeutic range ratio of 1.5 to 2.0
    - Approximately 4 hours after drug initiation
    - Correlation between plasma hirudin levels and aPTT nonlinear
    - Ecarin clotting time more preferable monitor of anticoagulation
    - Dose adjustments needed in those with renal impairment
    - Rarely nonneutralizing hirudin antibodies prolonging anticoagulant effect due to delayed hirudin-antibody complex clearance may develop
- Successfully used and licensed for treatment of arterial or venous thrombosis complicating HIT
  - Also used in patients with HIT undergoing cardiopulmonary bypass
  - Shown superior to heparin or LMWHs for DVT prophylaxis in patients undergoing elective hip arthroplasty
    - Does not increase bleeding risk in this high-risk setting
- Used extensively in patients with acute coronary syndromes and for VTE prophylaxis
  - Narrow therapeutic index and high risk of bleeding
  - Must be used with extreme caution and not approved for this use
- **Bivalirudin:** A 20 amino acid synthetic polypeptide analogue of hirudin
  - The amino terminal D-Phe-Pro-Arg-Pro sequence, which binds to the active site of thrombin, is connected via four Gly residues to a carboxyl-terminal dodecapeptide that interacts with exosite 1 on thrombin
  - Differs from hirudin in that once bound to thrombin, Arg-Pro bond on amino terminal extension of bivalirudin is cleaved
    - Converting bivalirudin to lower-affinity thrombin inhibitor
    - Producing transient inhibition of active site of thrombin
    - Allowing recovery of thrombin activity
  - Shorter half-life of bivalirudin, 25 minutes after IV injection
  - Only about 20% renally excreted
  - Safer alternative to hirudin
- Patients with a high risk of developing HIT
  - Bivalirudin typically administered as weight-adjusted (1 mg/kg) bolus dose given prior to percutaneous coronary interventions

- Followed by 4-hour infusion (0.2–0.5 mg/kg/hour)
- Dose adjusted according to renal function
  - Plasma clearance of in patients with moderate or severe renal impairment reduced by approximately 20%
- Suggests infusion reduction by 20% in patients with moderate to severe renal impairment
- Anticoagulant effect monitored by activated clotting time (ACT)
- Additional bolus given if ACT <350 seconds
- **Argatroban:** A synthetic L-arginine derivative competitive inhibitor of thrombin
  - Binds noncovalently to active site of thrombin to form reversible complex
  - Plasma half-life is 45 minutes
  - Monitored using aPTT
    - Dose adjusted to maintain therapeutic aPTT ratio of 1.5 to 3.0
    - Therapy can prolong INR more than other DTIs
      - May complicate overlap therapy with vitamin K antagonists
  - Metabolized in liver and is used with caution in patients with hepatic dysfunction
  - Considered drug of choice for patients with severe renal impairment
  - Approved for use in patients with:
    - Documented HIT
    - For anticoagulation in HIT patients undergoing percutaneous coronary intervention
- **Melagatran/Ximelagatran:** Melagatran a dipeptide mimetic of region of fibrinopeptide A that interacts with active site of thrombin
  - Drug has poor oral bioavailability and must be given SC
  - **Ximelagatran** an uncharged lipophilic prodrug
    - Exhibits about 20% bioavailability after oral administration
    - Once absorbed, ximelagatran rapidly transformed to melagatran
      - Has half-life of approximately 4 to 5 hours
  - Primary route of excretion for melagatran is kidneys
    - Approximately 80% eliminated renally
    - Dose adjustments needed in elderly and those patients with renal impairment
    - No adverse food or drug interaction to influence absorption of ximelagatran
      - Produces predictable anticoagulant effect
  - Need for routine monitoring usually unnecessary
  - Ximelagatran under evaluation for thromboprophylaxis in orthopedic patients and for treatment of VTE and atrial fibrillation

Factor Xa Inhibitors

- Factor Xa the rate-limiting step in thrombin generation
  - Situated at beginning of common coagulation pathway
  - Where both intrinsic and extrinsic pathways converge
- Drugs blocking factor Xa considered either indirect or direct inhibitors
  - Indirect factor Xa inhibitors act by binding to and activating antithrombin
    - Which then inhibits free factor Xa
  - Direct factor Xa inhibitors bind to and inhibit factor Xa without antithrombin

TABLE 119.8

PROPERTIES OF LOW-MOLECULAR-WEIGHT HEPARIN, FONDAPARINUX, AND IDRAPARINUX

Property	LMWH	Fondaparinux	Idraparinux
Source	Porcine mucosal heparin	Chemical synthesis	Chemical synthesis
Molecular weight (daltons)	Mean 5,000	1,728	1,727
SC bioavailability	~90%	100%	100%
Target(s)	Multiple: FXa > FIIa >FIXa, FXIa, FXIIa	FXa only	FXa only
Binding to proteins other than target	Yes	No	No
Anti-Xa:anti-IIa	2–5:1	Anti-Xa only	Anti-Xa only
TFPI release from endothelium	Yes	No	No
Clearance	Renal primarily	Renal	Renal
Half-life (SC route)	3–4 h	17–21 h	80–130 h
Effects of protamine	Partial neutralization	No effect	No effect
Potential for HIT	Low	Very low	Very low

LMWH, low-molecular-weight heparin; SC, subcutaneous; FXa, factor Xa; FIIa, factor IIa; FIXa, factor IXa; FXIa, factor XIa; FXIIa, factor XIIa; TFPI, tissue factor pathway inhibitor; HIT, heparin-induced thrombocytopenia.
From Weitz JI, Middledorp S, Geerts W, et al. Thrombophilia and new anticoagulant drugs. *Hematology.* 2004;1:429, with permission.

- **Indirect Factor Xa Inhibitors:** *Fondaparinux* and *idraparinux* two new parenteral indirect factor Xa inhibitors
  - Synthetic analogues of antithrombin-binding pentasaccharide sequence found in heparin and LMWH
  - Drugs are modified to increase affinity for antithrombin
    - As compared to heparin and LMWH
    - Chain length of molecules too short to bridge thrombin to antithrombin
      - Act by catalyzing factor Xa inhibition by antithrombin
      - Properties are different from those of LMWH (Table 119.8)
  - Potential benefits of fondaparinux over LMWH:
    - Synthetically produced
    - Has longer half-life
    - Does not bind to plasma proteins other than antithrombin
    - Does not bind to PF4 to form heparin/PF4 complexes
      - Serve as antigenic target for antibodies causing HIT
      - May be safer to use in these patients
    - Fondaparinux extensively studied and as effective as antithrombotic agent for prevention and treatment of both venous and arterial disorders
      - Currently approved as thromboprophylaxis:
        - Following orthopedic procedures
        - As initial treatment for VTE
        - Investigated as antithrombotic agent in cardiac disease
- Idraparinux a chemically modified analogue of fondaparinux
  - Binds to antithrombin with such high affinity that half-life approximates that of antithrombin
  - Requires SC dosing weekly
  - Under evaluation for:
    - Treatment of VTE
    - Long-term prevention of stroke in chronic atrial fibrillation patients
  - May be useful in patients intolerant of vitamin K-antagonist medications
  - Possible drawback to use of drug is long half-life and lack of antidote
    - Healthy volunteers had anticoagulant effect reversed by hrfVIIa

- **Direct Factor Xa Inhibitors:** Several synthetic direct factor Xa inhibitors undergoing clinical trials
  - Inhibit both free and activated platelet-bound factor Xa trapped within thrombus as part of prothrombinase complex
  - Property may offer advantage over LMWH and indirect factor Xa inhibitor agents
  - Appear to inhibit thrombus formation while allowing time for sufficient thrombin to be generated to activate platelets
    - May be associated with a lower incidence of major bleeding

Thrombolytic Therapy

- Fibrinolytic system aids in dissolution of intravascular clots via fibrin digesting plasmin
  - Inactive plasminogen converted to plasmin by cleavage of single peptide bond
  - Plasmin a nonspecific protease
    - Acts by digesting fibrin clots as well as other proteins
- Thrombolytic drugs act as plasminogen-activating agents
  - Catalyze conversion of endogenous plasminogen to plasmin
  - Dissolve fibrin deposits and pathologic thrombi at sites of vascular injury
    - May be associated with significant hemorrhage
    - When thrombolytic therapy initiated, massive fibrinolysis may occur
    - Potentially overwhelming body's inhibitory controls
- Use of thrombolytic therapy in treatment of DVT and PE highly individual specific
  - Early use of thrombolytic therapy in setting of DVT may decrease subsequent pain, swelling, and loss of venous valves
    - Reportedly reduces incidence of postphlebitic syndrome
    - Guidelines do not recommend thrombolysis for treatment of DVT unless limb ischemia and limb loss imminent
  - In treatment of PE
    - Thrombolytic therapy followed by heparin more efficacious in thromboembolus dissolution compared to heparin alone

– In acute (first 24 hours) setting
– Lead to more rapid resolution of lung scan abnormalities and hemodynamic improvements
– Benefit over longer term questionable
- Thrombolytic therapy standard treatment for patients presenting with:
  ○ Acute ST-segment elevation MI and new-onset left bundle branch block
  ○ Ischemic stroke, cerebral vein and sinus thrombosis, thrombosed mechanical valves, and thrombosed arteriovenous shunts and catheters
- Agents have evolved from non–fibrin-selective first generation agents to more fibrin-selective third generation agents
- There are still limitations with currently available agents
- *First-generation thrombolytic agents*
- Not fibrin specific and convert circulating plasminogen to plasmin
- Constant equilibrium between circulating plasminogen and plasminogen in thrombus
- Eventual depletion of plasminogen, reducing clot lysis
- Associated with increased risk of allergic reaction
- Have comparatively short half-lives
- *Streptokinase*
  ○ Single-chain polypeptide, molecular weight of 47 to 50.2 Kd, produced by group C β-hemolytic streptococci
  ○ Works by binding with circulating plasminogen to form activator complex, converting plasminogen to plasmin
    – 1:1 complex has increased catalytic activity compared to plasmin
    – Leads to stimulation of locally bound streptokinase–plasmin and streptokinase–plasminogen complexes
      * Results in acceleration in plasminogen activation and clot dissolution
    – Streptokinase increases levels of activated protein C
  ○ Half-life of streptokinase–plasminogen complex is 23 minutes
    – Lytic effect ranging from 82 to 184 minutes
    – No metabolites of streptokinase
    – Eliminated by the liver
  ○ Adverse reactions include allergic reactions, rarely anaphylaxis, and bleeding
    – Hypotension not related to bleeding or anaphylaxis seen during infusion in 1% to 10% of patients
    – Decreasing infusion and close monitoring recommended
  ○ For PE
    – Recommended dose 1 million IU infusion over 24 hours
  ○ For AMI
    – Adult dose is 1.5 million IU in 50 mL D$_5$W IV over 5 minutes
- *Urokinase*
  ○ A two-chain serine protease containing 41 amino acid residues
  ○ Isolated from human urine and fetal kidney cell cultures
  ○ Single-chain precursor
    – Precursor converted to active two-chain urokinase plasminogen activator through limited hydrolysis by plasmin and kallikrein

– Active form increases efficacy of plasmin activation
  * Enhances further conversion
○ Has a 15- to 20-minute half-life and metabolized in liver
  – Produces less sustained fibrinolysis
  – Potential disadvantages of significant bleeding
○ For PE regimen is administration of 4,400 IU/kg load
  – Followed by infusion of 4,400 IU/kg for 12 to 24 hours
○ For AMI less well studied than other agents
  – Most common regimen is 2 million U as IV load
  – Followed by 1 million U over the next 60 minutes
- *Second-generation thrombolytics* fibrin selective
- Developed with intention to limit or avoid systemic thrombolysis
- Present agents may cause mild to moderate depletion in levels of circulation fibrinogen and plasminogen
- *Tissue-type plasminogen activator* (TPA, Alteplase)
  ○ Glycoprotein of 527 amino acids
  ○ First recombinant tissue-type plasminogen activator (rtPA)
  ○ Enzyme responsible for most of body's natural physiologic responses to clear and reduce excessive thrombus propagation
  ○ TPA binds fibrin with a greater affinity than streptokinase, converting plasminogen to plasmin once bound to fibrin clot surface
    – Hence term "clot selective"
  ○ TPA rapidly cleared from plasma, primarily by liver
    – Initial half-life of <5 minutes
    – Heparin usually administered with TPA due to short half-life to avoid reocclusion
  ○ Not antigenic and almost never associated with allergic reactions
  ○ For AMI, drug given as accelerated infusion (over 1.5 hours) or long infusion (>3 hours)
    – Must be given in 1 mg/mL concentration in sterile water
    – Accelerated infusion of rtPA 15 mg IV, followed by 0.75 mg/kg, up to 50 mg IV over 60 minutes
      * Maximum total dose of 100 mg
    – The >3-hour infusion begins as 10-mg IV load over 2 minutes, followed by a 50-mg infusion over first hour, and by a 20-mg/kg infusion over next 2 hours
  ○ For acute ischemic stroke with time of symptom onset of <3 hours
    – Dose of TPA 0.9 mg/kg, to maximum of 90 mg IV over 60 minutes
    – 10% of total dose administered as IV bolus over 1 minute
  ○ For thrombolysis of PE
    – 100 mg TPA as continuous infusion over 2 hours
      * Initial 15-mg IV load
      * Followed by 85 mg over 2 hours
      * Heparin improves clinical course in stable patients with acute submassive PE when receiving TPA
      * Beneficial to administer alteplase with heparin
- *Third-generation thrombolytics* based on modifications of TPA structure
- May give agent longer half-lives, increased resistance to plasma protease inhibitors, and/or cause more selective binding to fibrin

TABLE 119.9

CHARACTERISTICS OF U.S. FOOD AND DRUG ADMINISTRATION–APPROVED THROMBOLYTIC AGENTS

	Streptokinase	Anistreplase	Alteplase	Reteplase	Tenecteplase
Molecular weight (Da)	47,000	131,000	70,000	39,000	70,000
Half-life (minutes)	23	100	<5	13–16	20–24
Dose/time	1.5 MU × 30–60 min	30 mg × 5 min	100 mg × 90 min	10 + 10 U × 30 min	0.5 mg/kg × 5–10 s
Bolus administration	No	Yes	No	Yes	Yes
Metabolism	Hepatic	Hepatic	Hepatic	—	—
Allergic reactions	1%–4%		<0.2%	No	<1%
Hypotension	Yes	Yes	No	No	No
Early heparin[a]	?Yes	?Yes	Yes	Yes	Yes
Fibrin selective	No	No	Yes	Yes	Yes
Systemic fibrinogen	Marked	Marked	Mild	Moderate	—
Fibrinogen breakdown	4+		1–2+	Unknown	4–15
Plasminogen binding	Indirect	Indirect	Direct	Direct	Direct
TIMI 3 flow (%)	32	43	54	60	66
≈90-minutes patency (%)	50	65	75	80	75
Intracerebral hemorrhage (%)	0.5	0.6	0.8	0.9	
Mortality rates (%)	7.3	10.5	7.2	7.5	

TIMI 3, thrombolysis in myocardial infarction flow 3 (normal)
[a]The need for concomitant heparin has been formally tested with only streptokinase and alteplase.
From Khan IJ, Gowda RM. Clinical perspectives and therapeutics of thrombolysis. *Int J Cardiol.* 2003;91:117, with permission.

- *Reteplase* (rtPA), a synthetic, nonglycosylated deletion-mutant form of TPA containing 355 of 527 amino acids of native TPA
  - Produced in *Escherichia coli* via recombinant technology
  - Binds fibrin five times less avidly than native TPA
    - Allowing drug to diffuse through clot rather than binding to it
    - In high concentrations allows plasminogen at clot to be converted into plasmin
      - Results in faster clot resolution compared to alteplase
  - More rapidly cleared from plasma
    - Somewhat extended half-life, 11 to 19 minutes, than alteplase
    - Primarily renal and some hepatic clearance
  - Not antigenic and is rarely associated with allergic reactions
  - NOT given with heparin due to physical incompatibility
  - For AMI adult dose of reteplase two IV loads of 10 U
    - Each given over 2 minutes
    - Second load given 30 minutes following first
  - Approved only for use in AMI
    - Reteplase has wide off-label use in acute DVT and PE
    - Dosing schedule same as for AMI
- *Tenecteplase* a genetically engineered mutation of TPA with similar mechanism of action to alteplase
  - Produced recombinantly with Chinese hamster ovary cells
    - A 527 amino acid glycoprotein
    - Has decreased plasma clearance
    - 15- to 19-minute half-life
    - Reduced sensitivity to plasminogen activator inhibitor
    - Greater fibrin specificity
      - May lead to decreased hemorrhagic complications
  - Administered a 30- to 50-mg IV bolus over 5 seconds
    - Dose calculated based on patient's weight as follows:
      - 0.5 mg/kg
    - Currently under investigation for ischemic stroke
- Thrombolytic agents differ in:
  - Ability to lyse clots
  - Fibrin selectivity
  - Ability to activate thrombosis and platelet aggregation
  - Clinical effectiveness of same agent can be altered by:
    - Dose
    - Route of administration
    - Concomitant use of adjunctive agents
  - All thrombolytic agents administered via IV route in dosing regimens designed to achieve >90% activation of the fibrinolytic system (Table 119.9)

CHAPTER 120 ■ TRANSFUSION THERAPY: WHEN TO USE IT AND HOW TO MINIMIZE IT

- Routine, safe administration of blood products required several important scientific advances
  - Discovery of A, B, and O blood types by Landsteiner in 1900
  - The AB blood type by Decastello and Sturli in 1902
  - The first blood bank established in 1932 in a Leningrad hospital
  - The first blood bank in the United States established by Fantus in 1937 at Cook County Hospital in Chicago
  - 1940s techniques of cross-matching, anticoagulation, and storage of blood, and establishment of blood banks made routine blood transfusion a reality
  - Introduction of plastic storage containers in 1950 and the introduction of refrigerated centrifugation instruments in 1953 made component therapy possible

BLOOD PRODUCT COLLECTION AND ADMINISTRATION

- Approximately 14 million units of RBCs (packed RBCs [PRBCs] and whole blood), 9,875,000 units of platelets, and 4 million units of plasma are transfused annually in United States
  - Represents 11.8% increase since 1999 and 56% increase since 1980
  - Use of other components, especially platelets, has also increased
  - Only about 5% of eligible donors ever donate blood
  - Transfusion rates in the United States for 2001 estimated at 48.75 units of RBC transfusion per 1,000 population
    - Compared to 44.93 units of RBC transfusion per 1,000 population in England
    - 28 units of RBC transfusion per 1,000 population in Australia
    - 54.8 units of RBC transfusion per 1,000 population in Denmark
- Anemia in critical illness is common
  - 25% to 37% of patients receive at least one blood transfusion during intensive care unit (ICU) stay
  - 85% of patients with ICU length of stay over 1 week received at least one transfusion
    - Blood transfusion not associated with acute blood loss in >66% of cases
    - Phlebotomy and decreased production of blood cells implicated as significant contributors to ICU anemia
    - Many studies estimated daily blood loss from phlebotomy at least 40 mL/day

  - Practitioners should carefully consider need for frequent blood draws in ICU

Collection and Preparation of Blood Products

- Blood is collected from donors and separated into individual components
  - PRBCs, plasma, platelets, and proteins
  - Collected into plastic bags containing a citrate solution that binds calcium, preventing coagulation
    - Citrate phosphate dextrose (CPD)
    - Citrate phosphate double dextrose (CP2D)
    - Citrate phosphate dextrose adenine (CPDA-1)
  - Solutions now available that extend the shelf life of PRBCs, and contain dextrose, adenine, sodium chloride, and phosphate (AS-3) or mannitol (AS-1 and AS-5)
  - After collection, each unit gently centrifuged to pack RBCs
    - Leaving approximately 70% of platelets suspended in plasma
      - Platelet-rich plasma removed and centrifuged to sediment the platelets
      - All but a small amount of the resulting supernatant plasma is removed and rapidly frozen
      - Platelets are then resuspended, yielding a platelet concentrate
    - When frozen plasma is stored at <18°C, referred to as fresh frozen plasma (FFP)
      - If frozen plasma allowed to thaw at 4°C, precipitate that remains can be collected to yield cryoprecipitate
      - Albumin and other proteins extracted from remaining plasma
  - Another option for collection of blood leukocytes, platelets, or plasma is automated cell separators (apheresis)
    - Blood is withdrawn from donor and separated by centrifuge
    - Desired component removed
    - Remaining blood returned to donor
    - Allows blood banks to offer products such as single-donor platelet packs
      - Administration of a single-donor unit of platelets exposes recipient to only one person's antigens
      - Equivalent dose of pooled platelet transfusion ("six pack" or "ten pack") exposes patient to six or ten sets of antigens, respectively
        - Making subsequent platelet transfusion less effective
        - Additionally bacterial contamination less likely with single-donor apheresis platelets

Storage Lesion

- Storage or refrigeration creates progressive changes in PRBCs, *storage lesion,* and include:
  - Increase in concentration of potassium, phosphate, and ammonia
  - Decrease in pH
  - Altered affinity of hemoglobin for oxygen
  - Changes in RBC deformability
  - Hemolysis
  - Development of microaggregates
  - Release of vasoactive substances
  - Denaturation of proteins
  - Lifespan of RBCs becomes shorter the longer cells are stored
    - Associated with decreased intracellular 2,3-diphospho-glycerate (2,3-DPG) and adenosine triphosphate (ATP)
- Large volumes of cold blood contributes to development of hypothermia
  - A clinically significant effects of storage on subsequent transfusion
  - Except for hypothermia, many of these changes reversed shortly after transfusion
  - In some cases, cause metabolic effects different from predicted based on *ex vivo* observations
  - Critical not to empirically treat theoretically anticipated effects of blood transfusions using "cookbook" approaches (such as giving one ampule of bicarbonate and one ampule of calcium with every "*x*" units of blood)

Administration of Blood Products

- Progressive abandonment of "10/30" transfusion "trigger" for red cell transfusion in favor of lower triggers
  - Even more appropriately, transfusion practice based on patient physiology
  - 10/30 transfusion trigger likely resulted from recommendation in 1942 that it was "wise" to maintain hemoglobin levels "between 8 and 10 grams per cubic centimeter" for patients who were poor surgical risks by giving a preoperative transfusion
    - No data were available to support this recommendation
    - Stood relatively unchallenged for about 50 years
  - Expanding body of literature suggests arbitrary transfusion for a set transfusion trigger (e.g., the "10/30 rule") ill-advised
    - Purported cardiac risks with anemia overemphasized

Whole Blood

- Few widely accepted indications for whole blood in modern transfusion practice
  - Storage of whole blood precludes extraction of components
  - From systems perspective, is highly inefficient
  - Experience with use of whole blood by the U.S. military has rejuvenated use
    - Experience, especially with fresh whole blood having potentially beneficial effects on coagulopathy and hypothermia, may result in modification of civilian practices in future

Red Blood Cells

- PRBCs the most commonly utilized blood product
  - Providing oxygen-carrying capacity in cases of acute or chronic blood loss
  - Longest storage life currently allowed by U.S. Food and Drug Administration (FDA) is 42 days
  - Longer storage times result in fewer than 75% of RBCs remaining viable in circulation 24 hours after transfusion
  - Platelets degenerate at refrigerator temperatures
    - Refrigerated PRBCs contain essentially no functioning platelets
  - Levels of factors V and VIII decrease significantly at 1°C to 6°C
    - Levels of other factors remain essentially unchanged
- PRBCs provide oxygen-carrying capacity and maintain oxygen delivery provided:
  - Intravascular volume and cardiac function are adequate
  - Decision to transfuse, and amount of PRBCs transfused, depend on clinical situation
    - Hematocrit (Hct) 30% (or hemoglobin [Hgb] of 10 g/dL) as transfusion trigger no longer acceptable
    - One or more units of PRBC transfused with no predetermined number of units applicable
    - Each PRBC unit typically raises Hct 2% to 3% in 70-kg adult
      - Varies depending on the donor, the recipient's fluid status, the method of storage, and its duration
- With blood loss, O_2 delivery maintained through a series of complex interactions and compensatory mechanisms, including:
  - Increased cardiac output
  - Increased extraction ratio
  - Rightward shift of oxyhemoglobin curve
  - Expansion of volume
- Many anemic patients tolerate Hgb of 7 to 8 g/dL or less
  - Demonstrated in chronic renal failure and Jehovah's Witnesses
  - Cardiac output does not increase significantly until Hgb below about 7 g/dL
  - Young healthy patients tolerate acute anemia to Hgb 7 g/dL or less through increases in CO, provided they have a normal intravascular volume and high arterial oxygen saturation
- Multicenter, randomized controlled study of transfusion in 838 patients in ICU
  - Liberal transfusion strategy (transfusion for Hgb <10 g/dL) compared with a restrictive strategy (transfusion for Hgb <7 g/dL)
  - Restrictive strategy at least as effective as liberal strategy
    - Possible exception of patients with acute myocardial infarction (MI) and unstable angina
- Suggested guidelines for RBC transfusion are listed in Table 120.1

Leukocyte-reduced Red Blood Cells

- Transfusion of PRBCs has been associated with immunosuppression
  - Effect thought to be related to exposure to leukocytes
  - Use of leukocyte-reduced components proposed to minimize immunosuppression

TABLE 120.1

GUIDELINES FOR TRANSFUSION OF PACKED RED BLOOD CELLS

- Ongoing bleeding with hemodynamic instability unresponsive (or incompletely responsive) to infusion of 2,000 to 3,000 mL crystalloid
- Hemoglobin <7 g/dL

- Majority of PRBC and platelet transfusions in United States are leukocyte reduced
- Efficacy of these preparations remains controversial, and data are lacking
- Recommendations for transfusion of leukocyte-reduced blood components are listed in Table 120.2

Platelets

- Platelet transfusions indicated for patients at significant risk of bleeding
- Because of quantitative or qualitative platelet deficits
- A unit of platelets prepared from individual (or "random") donors or by apheresis
  - A single donor provides equivalent of 6 to 10 single "random" donor units
  - In selected cases human leukocyte antigen (HLA)-matched platelets can be obtained by apheresis from HLA-matched donors
  - Platelet count 1 hour posttransfusion of 1 unit of platelets increases by 5,000 to 10,000 platelets/μL
    - Less pronounced responses expected with:
      - Repeated transfusion and development of alloimmunization
      - In presence of fever, sepsis, or splenomegaly
      - If alloimmunization thought to be cause of a poor response, platelets from an HLA-matched donor may be needed
- Prophylactic transfusion of platelets should be considered inappropriate:
  - Absent microvascular bleeding
  - With a low platelet count in a patient undergoing a surgical procedure

TABLE 120.2

INDICATIONS FOR TRANSFUSION OF LEUKOCYTE-REDUCED BLOOD COMPONENTS

- To decrease the incidence of subsequent refractoriness to platelet transfusion caused by human leukocyte antigen (HLA) alloimmunization in patients requiring long-term platelet support
- To provide blood components with reduced risk for cytomegalovirus transmission
- To prevent future febrile nonhemolytic transfusion reactions (FNHTRs) in patients who have had a documented FNHTR
- To decrease the incidence of HLA alloimmunization in nonhepatic solid-organ transplant candidates

Data from Ratko TA, Cummings JP, Oberman HA, et al. Evidence-based recommendations for the use of WBC-reduced cellular blood components. *Transfusion.* 2001;41:1310–1319.

TABLE 120.3

INDICATIONS FOR TRANSFUSION OF PLATELETS

- Disseminated intravascular coagulation: 20,000–50,000 platelets/μL
- Major surgery in leukemia: 50,000 platelets/μL
- Thrombocytopenia with massive transfusion: 50,000 platelets/μL
- Invasive procedures in cirrhosis: 50,000 platelets/μL
- Cardiopulmonary bypass: 50,000–60,000 platelets/μL
- Liver biopsy: 50,000–100,000 platelets/μL
- Neurosurgical procedures: 100,000 platelets/μL

Data from Rebulla P. Platelet transfusion trigger in difficult patients. *Transfus Clin Biol.* 2002;9:249–254.

- A platelet count that has fallen below 10,000 platelets/μL, in most medical patients
- Disease state-specific triggers for platelet transfusion are noted in Table 120.3
- Hypothermia depresses platelet function
  - Platelet transfusion generally ineffective with depressed temperatures
  - Restoration of normal temperature returns platelet function to normal
    - Ameliorates microvascular bleeding

Plasma

- A source of clotting factors in patients with coagulopathy and documented factor deficiency
  - May occur with liver dysfunction, congenital absence of factors, and transfusion of factor-deficient blood products, or after the use of warfarin
  - One unit of plasma contains near-normal levels of all factors including:
    - About 400 mg of fibrinogen
    - Generally increases factor levels by about 3%
  - Adequate clotting usually achieved with factor levels >30%
    - Higher levels advisable in patients undergoing operative or invasive procedures
    - Prothrombin time (PT) and activated partial thromboplastin time (aPTT) used to assess patients for plasma transfusion
      - Also to follow the efficacy of administered plasma
    - Recent experience suggests that use of thromboelastography (TEG) may provide advantages over the PT as a guide for the treatment of coagulopathy
  - Plasma can be frozen and stored for up to 1 year
- Should not be given routinely or prophylactically by "cookbook" formula after RBC transfusion or "prophylactically" after cardiac bypass or other procedures
  - Plasma should not be used as a volume expander
    - Crystalloids are cheaper, safer, and at least as effective
    - Broadly accepted guidelines plasma transfusion are noted in Table 120.4

Cryoprecipitate

- Indications for use of cryoprecipitate include (Table 120.5):
  - Factor deficiency (hemophilia A)
  - von Willebrand disease
  - Hypofibrinogenemia

TABLE 120.4

INDICATIONS FOR TRANSFUSION OF PLASMA

- International normalized ratio (INR) >1.5 with an anticipated invasive procedure or surgery
- Massive hemorrhage (over one blood volume) with an INR >1.5
- Treatment of thrombotic thrombocytopenia purpura
- Inherited coagulopathies where a specific factor concentrate is not available
- Emergent reversal of anticoagulant therapy

Data from Toy P, Popovsky MA, Abraham E, et al., and the National Heart, Lung and Blood Institute Working Group on TRALI. Transfusion-related acute lung injury: definition and review. *Crit Care Med.* 2005;33:721–726.

- Some patients with uremic bleeding may benefit from cryoprecipitate transfusion
- Usually administered as a transfusion of 10 single units. Each 5 to 15 mL unit contains over 80 units of factor VIII and about 200 mg of fibrinogen
  - Relatively high concentrations allow use of smaller volume of cryoprecipitate than would be required if plasma were used

Risks of Blood Transfusion

- Blood transfusion is potentially life-saving, but significant risks still involved
  - Risks range from (Table 120.6):
    - Minor febrile transfusion reactions
    - To transmission of viral infection
    - To potentially fatal transfusion of incompatible blood
  - Blood banks in United States conduct over 10 tests or checks on donated units of blood in addition to screening interview
    - 9 are for infectious diseases
    - Donor screening and introduction of effective tests for hepatitis and human immunodeficiency virus (HIV) have dramatically reduced the risks of transmission
  - Recent data reveal leading causes of fatalities after blood transfusion are:
    - Administrative error leading to transfusion of ABO-incompatible blood
    - Bacterial contamination
    - Transfusion-related acute lung injury (TRALI)
    - Infectious risks of transfusion far outweighed by noninfectious risks
    - TRALI the leading cause of transfusion-related mortality in 2003

TABLE 120.5

INDICATIONS FOR TRANSFUSION OF CRYOPRECIPITATE

- Hemophilia A
- von Willebrand disease
- Hypofibrinogemia
- Uremic bleeding
- As substitute for plasma if lower volume is desired

TABLE 120.6

RISKS OF BLOOD TRANSFUSION

- Transfusion-related acute lung injury
- Bacterial contamination of blood products
- Administrative error leading to transfusion of ABO-incompatible blood
- Viral infection transmission
  Hepatitis B
  Hepatitis C
  Human immunodeficiency virus 1 and 2
  Human T-cell leukemia virus 1 and 2
  Epstein-Barr virus
  Cytomegalovirus
  Parvovirus B19
  Human herpesvirus 8
  Transfusion-transmitted virus
  Mad cow disease (bovine spongiform encephalopathy)
  West Nile virus
- Bacterial/protozoal infection transmission
  Syphilis
  Malaria
  Babesia microti
  Trypanosoma cruzi
  Yersinia enterocolitica
  Serratia marcescens
  Staphylococcus aureus
  Staphylococcus epidermidis
  Klebsiella pneumoniae
  Trypanosoma cruzi
- Transfusion reactions
  Acute
  Delayed
- Immunosuppression

- Average of 11.7 deaths from bacterial sepsis per year in United States reported to FDA from 2001 to 2003
  - Decreased to 7.5 deaths per year in 2004 and 2005
    - Partly due to 2004 mandating of bacterial screening of platelets
- Transfusion of blood to the wrong person a serious threat
  - Review of a 10-year experience in New York State risk of an ABO-incompatible transfusion estimated at 1 in 38,000 units of PRBC
    - Risk of a fatal reaction 1 in 1.8 million transfusions
    - Rate of ABO-incompatible transfusion of 1 in 12,000 units of PRBC transfused reported from hemovigilance program in Quebec
- Given risks and benefits of blood transfusion
  - Informed consent for transfusion of components crucial in nonemergent situations
  - Summary of rates of more common or more concerning risks is in Table 120.7
    - Data useful for discussions with patients and families

Transfusion Reactions

- Given Classification of American Association of Blood Banks for transfusion reactions shown in Table 120.8

Transfusion-related Acute Lung Injury

- Acute onset of pulmonary edema associated with transfusion and leading to death first described in 1951 by Barnard

TABLE 120.7

INFORMATION FOR PATIENTS: COMMONLY ASKED QUESTIONS ABOUT BLOOD TRANSFUSION

Complication	Risk from blood product transfusion	Comments
Febrile nonhemolytic transfusion reactions	Occurs in 0.5%–38% of all transfusions	Usually mild fever only More common with platelet transfusions
Severe acute hemolytic reaction	Fatal in 1 of 600,000 transfusions	Stop transfusion immediately and initiate supportive measures
Delayed hemolytic reaction	1 in 260,000 transfusions	Suspect when unexplained fever, fall in hematocrit, or jaundice occur
Bacterial contamination	1 in 15,000 platelet transfusions	Among leading causes of transfusion-related fatalities
Cytomegalovirus	Of concern in low-birth-weight infants and immunocompromised patients (e.g., transplant)	Between 50% and 85% of adults in the United States are carriers
Hepatitis B virus	<1 in 137,000	25% of carriers have active hepatitis and may progress to cirrhosis
Hepatitis C virus	<1 in 1 million	Most infected persons asymptomatic, but 80% become chronic
Human immunodeficiency virus	<1 in 1.9 million	Potentially fatal
Human T-cell leukemia virus 1 and 2	Very small	Rarely found in U.S. blood donors
West Nile virus	Very small when donors are properly screened	80% of those infected remain asymptomatic, 20% develop mild symptoms, and 1 in 150–200 infected people develop severe disease that may be fatal
Transfusion-related lung injury	1 in 5,000 units (estimated)	5%–10% fatal

Source: American Association of Blood Banks. www.aabb.org/content/About_Blood/Facts_About_Blood_and_Blood_Banking/fabloodtrans.htm.

- TRALI currently leading cause of death after transfusion
- Estimated rate of 1 in 5,000 units transfused, although higher rates have been reported
- TRALI likely underappreciated and underdiagnosed
- Other more commonly recognized conditions (acute lung injury and acute respiratory distress syndrome [ARDS] often associated with blood transfusion
- Makes diagnosis of TRALI more difficult

TABLE 120.8

TRANSFUSION REACTIONS: AMERICAN ASSOCIATION OF BLOOD BANKS CLASSIFICATION

Type	Clinical features	Comments
Immunologic		
Hemolytic	Chills, fever, hypotension, renal failure, back pain, hemoglobinuria	Caused by red blood cell mismatch
Fever and/or chills, nonhemolytic	Temperature elevation >1°C, chills and/or rigors, headache, vomiting	
Urticarial	Pruritus, urticaria, flushing	
Anaphylactic	Hypotension, urticaria, bronchospasm, respiratory distress, wheezing, local edema, anxiety	Varies from isolated urticaria to fatal anaphylaxis
Transfusion-associated acute lung injury	Hypoxemia, respiratory failure, hypotension, fever	Leading cause of transfusion-associated mortality
Nonimmunologic		
Hypotension (associated with angiotensin-converting enzyme inhibition)	Flushing, hypotension	
Circulatory overload	Dyspnea, orthopnea, cough, tachycardia, hypertension, headache	
Nonimmune hemolysis	Hemoglobinuria	Caused by physical destruction of blood (heating, freezing, etc.)
Air embolus	Sudden dyspnea, cyanosis, chest pain, cough, hypotension, cardiac arrhythmia	
Hypocalcemia	Paresthesia, tetany, arrhythmia	
Hypothermia	Cardiac arrhythmia	
Transfusion-associated sepsis	Bacterial contamination of transfused blood	Consider in patients with fever >40°C and/or cardiovascular collapse

- Mortality rate associated with TRALI ranges 5% to 10%
  - All patients receiving blood products should be monitored, including SpO_2
- TRALI occurs with transfusion of all blood components
  - Especially with platelets and plasma
- Clinical syndrome characterized by:
  - Acute onset of dyspnea, hypotension, hypoxemia, fever, and noncardiogenic pulmonary edema
  - Symptoms appear within 6 hours of transfusion
    ○ Most often within 30 minutes
  - Diagnosis of TRALI made by exclusion
    ○ TRALI causes increased pulmonary microvascular permeability with increased protein levels in edema fluid
    ○ Two theories:
      – First hypothesis suggests leukocyte antibodies from donor unit activate recipient leukocytes in pulmonary circulation, leading to increased microvascular permeability and noncardiogenic pulmonary edema
        - Blood donations from multiparous women have been implicated
      – Second hypothesis assumes an initial predisposing event that primes the patient's neutrophils and sequesters them in lung
        - Biologically active lipids and cytokines in donor unit then further prime and activate recipient's neutrophils
          - Resultant microvascular permeability and noncardiogenic pulmonary edema
- Treatment of TRALI supportive and consists of appropriate hemodynamic and ventilatory support
  - Once TRALI suspected transfusion terminated immediately and blood bank notified
  - Donor unit can be tested for anti-HLA and/or antigranulocyte antibodies

Bacterial Contamination

- Most frequent cause of transfusion-transmitted infectious disease
  - After hemolytic reactions and TRALI bacterial contamination the most frequently reported cause of transfusion-related fatalities to the FDA
  - Agents most often implicated in PRBC bacteremia were:
    - *Serratia* and *Yersinia*
  - For platelets:
    - *S. aureus*, *Escherichia coli*, *Enterobacter*, and *Serratia* species more frequently identified
- Fever, chills, hypotension, tachycardia, and shock after transfusion should raise suspicion of bacterial contamination
  - Blood cultures of patient AND unit should be obtained
  - Platelets are stored at 20°C to 24°C and are good bacterial growth medium
  - Platelets are now screened for bacterial contamination in the United States

Hepatitis

- Transmission of hepatitis agents among most serious risks of blood transfusion
  - Past estimates of posttransfusion hepatitis were approximately 10%
  - Current data suggest infectious risk of hepatitis is <0.01% per unit transfused
    - Pooled nucleic acid amplification testing (NAT) used to test for HIV and hepatitis C virus (HCV)

- Involves pooling of 16 to 24 individual blood samples and using polymerase chain reaction (PCR) or other amplification techniques to test for HIV and HCV nucleic sequences
- All blood screened for hepatitis B virus (HBV), with tests for HB_SAg and anti-HB_C
  - Also screened for HCV with anti-HCV testing
  - Risk of transfusion-associated HBV infection approximately 1 in 30,000 to 1 in 250,000 per unit
  - With pooled NAT tests for HCV the window period has decreased
    ○ The risk of HCV transmission now as low as 1 in 1 million
    ○ No new case of transfusion-associated HCV detected by Centers for Disease Control and Prevention Sentinel Counties Viral Hepatitis Surveillance System since 1994 in United States
  - Approximately half of blood recipients who contract HBV infection develop symptoms
    ○ Much smaller percentage requires hospitalization
  - Approximately half of patients contracting posttransfusion HCV infection develop chronic form of disease
    ○ Many patients eventually develop significant liver dysfunction, including cirrhosis

Human Immunodeficiency Virus

- Risk of HIV transmission from blood transfusion decreased dramatically since early 1980s
- Despite increasing incidence of HIV infection in general population
- Window period from initial infection to development of antibody to the virus poses problem with ability to detect all seropositive donors
- With pooled NAT window period for detection of HIV reduced by 30% to 50%
  - Risk of HIV transmission estimated to be as low as 1 in 2 million units

Human T-cell Leukemia Virus

- Blood carries risk of transmission of human T-cell leukemia virus (HTLV) 1 and 2 infection
- Transmission of virus especially to immunocompromised patients may cause illnesses such as T-cell leukemia, spastic paraparesis, and myelopathy
- Prompted routine screening of donors in United States since 1989
- Risk of HTLV 1 and 2 transmission is estimated to be 1 in 641,000 units

Herpesviruses

- Cytomegalovirus (CMV) infection is endemic, so routine screening is not performed in the United States
- 20% of blood donors infected with CMV by 20 years of age
- Approximately 70% infected by 70 years of age
- Infection carried in white blood cells
- Most patients who encounter problems with CMV are immunocompromised
  - Especially transplant recipients on immunosuppressive drugs
  - Such patients require transfusion with CMV-reduced-risk–leukocyte-reduced or seronegative blood products to avoid transmission of viral infection

- Human herpesvirus 8 causes Kaposi sarcoma and lymphoma in patients with acquired immunodeficiency syndrome (AIDS) and other immunosuppressed states

Graft versus Host Reaction

- Blood transfusion exposes recipient to many cells and proteins from donor
  - When immunologically competent lymphocytes introduced into immunocompromised patient
    - Graft versus host reaction can occur
    - Functional donor lymphocytes attack recipient tissues
      - Notably bone marrow, causing aplasia
    - Patients present with fever, rash, nausea, vomiting, diarrhea, liver function test abnormalities, and depressed cell counts
    - Complication fatal in as many as 90% of cases
    - Prevalence of complication in United States not known but thought to be rare
    - Rare cases also reported from familial directed donations and with HLA-matched platelets
      - γ-Irradiation of blood products eliminates this risk

Immunomodulation

- Allogeneic blood transfusion may alter immune response and susceptibility to infection, tumor recurrence, and reactivation of latent viruses
  - Known since 1974 that transfusion of PRBCs depresses immune response in patients undergoing renal transplantation
  - Unclear to what extent immunosuppressive effects exist in other recipients
  - Contradictory evidence exists concerning increased infections in patients given allogeneic blood transfusions
    - Controversy exists regarding exact relationship of blood transfusions to increased recurrence of tumor and poor prognosis
    - Early studies on colorectal cancer showed decreased survival and increased tumor recurrence in heavily transfused patients
    - Blood transfusion may represent a covariable
      - Very ill patients and those undergoing more difficult procedures for more extensive disease more likely to receive blood transfusion

- In light of immunomodulating effects of allogeneic blood transfusion:
  - Leukocyte-depleted transfusions suggested as alternative
  - Reasonable to adopt a policy of blood conservation in perioperative period in absence of clear indications and acute symptoms
  - Leukocyte reduction of blood products thought to decrease risk of immunomodulation

Decision Making in Blood Transfusion

Blood Transfusion in Hemorrhagic Shock

- Goal of resuscitation from shock is prompt restoration of adequate tissue and end-organ perfusion and oxygen transport
- American College of Surgeons Committee on Trauma developed a classification of hemorrhagic shock that permits useful guidelines for resuscitation (Table 120.9)
  - Crystalloid infused at 3:1 ratio for every unit of RBCs administered, and therapy is monitored primarily by hemodynamic response
  - Resuscitation proceeds with use of blood products, depending on patient's response
  - Colloid solutions offer no advantages over crystalloids for resuscitation in critically ill patients
  - Crystalloid solutions considered solutions of choice because:
    - They are less expensive
    - Need not be cross-matched
    - Do not transmit disease
    - Probably result in less fluid accumulation in lung
    - No data indicate using colloid rather than crystalloid solutions prevents pulmonary edema
      - Updated review of randomized controlled trials of albumin resuscitation yielded no suggestion of reduction in mortality when the colloid was used in hypovolemia or in critically ill patients with burns and hypoalbuminemia
- Several crystalloid solutions available for resuscitation
- Isotonic solutions used to avoid free water overload
- Lactated Ringer (LR) solution recommended as initial therapy
- Metabolic alkalosis common after successful resuscitation with this solution and blood products

TABLE 120.9

CLASSES OF HEMORRHAGIC SHOCK

Class of hemorrhage	Blood volume loss	Characteristics	Treatment
I	15% (750 mL)	Vital signs essentially normal	No resuscitation generally needed
II	15%–30% (750–1,500 mL)	Tachycardia, decreased pulse pressure, anxiety, pallor, diaphoresis, acidosis	Crystalloid resuscitation needed; blood transfusion given if no response to fluids (or if response is transient)
III	30%–40% (1,500–2,000 mL)	Hypotension, tachycardia, decreased mental status, oliguria	Blood transfusion generally needed, with crystalloids in 3:1 ratio
IV	>40% (>2,000 mL)	Severe tachycardia and hypotension, lethargy	Massive resuscitation with fluids and blood products needed

Adapted from the American College of Surgeons, Advanced Trauma Life Support.

- Due to lactate in LR solution and citrate in banked blood
- Both converted to bicarbonate in liver
- LR solution contains calcium and if mixed with blood product blood may clot in bag
- Normal (0.9%) saline solution (SS) an acceptable alternative to LR solution
  - Large volumes can produce hyperchloremic metabolic acidosis
  - May complicate use of base deficit in resuscitation
  - 0.9% SS compatible with all blood products
    - Use is sometimes preferred if transfusion a possibility
- Decision to transfuse blood highly dependent on acuity of blood loss
  - Patients with acute, massive hemorrhage, trauma or gastrointestinal bleeding, show signs of hemodynamic instability early in presentation
  - Diagnosis of hemorrhagic shock and decision to administer blood transfusion not based solely on hypotension, tachycardia, or anemia
    - Hypotension does not occur until >30% of blood volume lost
      - Particularly so in children who maintain blood pressure despite severe blood loss
      - Elderly patients on β-blocking agents may not manifest significant tachycardia
      - Hgb levels obtained early in course of hemorrhagic shock do not reflect severity of blood loss
        - Not been enough time for fluid shifts to occur
      - Blood transfusion based on comprehensive assessment of patient, including vital signs and estimation of amount of blood loss
        - As well as clinical and laboratory evaluation of end-organ perfusion
- Acute, massive hemorrhage managed initially with aggressive crystalloid replacement
  - After 2,000 to 3,000 mL of crystalloid solution
  - Blood transfusion initiated in patients who continue to manifest unstable vital signs
    - Should occur concomitantly with expeditious surgical control of bleeding sites
    - Cross-matched blood given as soon as available
    - If needed:
      - Type O negative blood given to women of childbearing age
      - Type O positive blood given to men of all ages and women older than 50 years until cross-matched blood available
    - Correction of coagulopathy and hypothermia paramount
      - "Damage control" surgical approach
        - Aimed at rapid control of bleeding while delaying less urgent procedures utilized
        - Helps reduce transfusion requirements
        - Allows patient to recover more quickly from shock

Blood Transfusion in the Normovolemic Patient

- Anemic patients with normal blood volume are generally hemodynamically intact
  - Concerns regarding diminished oxygen-carrying capacity of blood may persist in some patients
  - For years standard of care dictated that Hct level of 30% should be maintained

- Rationale included faster recovery and prevention of myocardial ischemia
  - Especially in patients with coronary artery disease
- Recent data indicate lower Hct levels well tolerated
  - Even in patients at risk for myocardial ischemia
  - Has resulted in lowering the trigger level for transfusion
- Many reports demonstrating blood transfusion an independent risk factor for:
  - Worse outcome, including increased mortality, especially in trauma patients
  - Maintaining Hgb at or above 10 g/dL in euvolemic critically ill patients compared to 7 g/dL was not associated with improvement in overall mortality
    - Mortality was significantly lower with conservative strategy (Hgb 7 g/dL) among patients less acutely ill and those younger than 55 years of age
    - In patients with unstable angina and acute MI, maintaining Hgb at or above 10 g/dL remains standard of care
      - Although there are conflicting data on that subject
  - Medicare discharge records showed elderly patients with acute MI had lower mortality if Hct was 30% or higher
  - Another review suggested a higher hematocrit on admission to ICU after coronary artery bypass grafting was associated with higher rate of MI
  - Reports advocating Hct level of 30% in septic patients
    - Reports do not establish blood transfusion to Hct of 30% an independent factor contributing to improved outcome
  - General trend is that of increasingly restrictive strategy of blood transfusion

MINIMIZING TRANSFUSIONS IN THE INTENSIVE CARE UNIT

Immediate Concerns

- Comprehensive strategy of blood conservation should be followed
- Need to correct anemia should be assessed
- Sources of ongoing blood loss controlled
- Measures to enhance erythropoiesis should be entertained

Minimizing Unnecessary Blood Loss

- Significant blood can be lost with repeated phlebotomy in the ICU
- Particularly significant in children
- Routine serial "blood draws" should be avoided
- Obtaining laboratory results only when clinically indicated should be followed
- Microsampling techniques, including bedside point-of-care testing, limit amount of blood lost with each draw
- Estimated daily blood loss from phlebotomy at least 40 mL/day
  - Practitioners should carefully consider need for frequent phlebotomy in ICU

Optimization of Red Cell Production

Iron

- Essential for properly functioning Hgb
  - Site of attachment of oxygen molecule
  - Other oxygen-carrying proteins, myoglobin and cytochrome *a-a*3, depend on iron
  - Many enzymes in Kreb cycle contain iron in functional groups
  - In critically ill patient, iron deficiency anemia multifactorial:
    - Poor gastrointestinal absorption
    - Nutrient antagonism
    - Concomitant copper and vitamin A deficiencies
  - Patients with systemic inflammatory response syndrome (SIRS) have circulating cytokines, impairing release of iron stored in reticuloendothelial system
    - Creates situation where total body iron levels are normal
    - But iron not available for incorporation into RBC precursors (functional iron deficiency anemia)
  - Not known whether iron supplementation in critically ill anemic patients beneficial
    - Iron deficiency could be functional, not an absolute reduction in total body iron
    - Iron supplementation implicated with increased risk and severity of infection, since free iron acts as a chelator of free radicals
      - Currently no clear indication to administer supplemental iron to critically ill patients who are anemic

Erythropoietin

- A circulating glycoprotein secreted primarily by kidneys in response to hypoxia
  - Principal action to stimulate production and release of RBCs from bone marrow
  - Commercially available using recombinant DNA technology
  - Approved for use in anemic patients with end-stage renal disease
    - Indications extended to include anemic patients with chronic renal insufficiency, cancer, and AIDS
    - Indications still being expanded
    - Patients undergoing elective surgical procedures typically associated with severe blood loss may benefit from preoperative erythropoietin therapy.
      - Combined with autologous blood transfusion
    - Potential therapeutic value of erythropoietin in anemia of critical illness an area of intense research
      - Erythropoiesis in critically ill patients suppressed for variety of reasons
        - Including renal and hepatic failure
        - Circulating cytokines in SIRS suppress erythropoiesis both by blunting response to and inhibiting production of erythropoietin
        - Erythropoietin formation in patients with multiple organ dysfunction was inadequate to stimulate reticulocytosis in relative erythropoietin deficit
        - High doses of recombinant human erythropoietin therapy stimulated erythropoietic system
          - Evidenced by higher rate of reticulocytosis
          - No increase in Hct or reduction in PRBC transfusion

- Corwin in two randomized controlled trials demonstrated a reduction of up to 19% in PRBC units transfused and a greater increase in Hct in group treated with erythropoietin
  - No differences in morbidity or mortality between two groups
- Georgopoulos showed similar results
  - Additional finding that effects of erythropoietin therapy are dose dependent
- More recently less favorable results
  - Use of erythropoietin alfa did not reduce incidence of PRBC transfusion among critically ill patients
    - Treatment with agent associated with increase in incidence of thrombotic events
  - Second study concluded use of target hemoglobin level of 13.5 g/dL in chronic kidney disease was associated with:
    - Increased risk of complications
    - No improvement in quality of life
- Several reports demonstrated adverse outcomes in cancer patients
  - Adverse effects potentially attributable to erythropoietin therapy include:
    - Hypertension
    - Thrombotic complications
    - Cardiovascular events
    - Tumor progression
    - Increased risk of death
  - FDA issued alert to provide new safety information for erythropoiesis-stimulating agents (ESAs)
    - Alert based on analyses of studies on cancer and orthopedic surgery patients
      - Found to have a higher chance of serious and life-threatening effects and/or death with the use of ESAs
      - FDA recommends using lowest dose possible to achieve a Hgb that
        - Avoids need for transfusion
        - And withholding dose of ESA if Hgb level exceeds 12 g/dL
          - Or rises by 1 g/dL in any 2-week period

Autotransfusion

- Blood lost during surgical procedures can be:
  - Retrieved, spun, washed, and filtered
    - Recovered RBCs then reinfused back into patient
  - Blood from drains such as thoracostomy tubes can be retrieved
    - Collected in containers with citrate solutions to prevent clotting and reinfused
  - Relative contraindications include:
    - Contamination of blood with bacteria, malignant cells, or amniotic or ascitic fluids
- Other strategies of blood conservation include:
  - Preoperative autologous donation and acute normovolemic hemodilution

Hemoglobin-based Oxygen Carriers

- Current investigation focused on hemoglobin-based oxygen carriers (HBOCs)

- Hemoglobin obtained from three sources:
  - Human blood from discarded units of PRBCs
  - Animal blood
  - Recombinant DNA technology

Structure and Function of Normal Human Hemoglobin

- Hgb a large molecule made up of four polypeptide chains:
- Two α- and two β-chains
- Molecular weight of 64,450
- Each chain is conjugated with heme moiety
  - Iron-containing porphyrin derivative to which O_2 attaches, forming oxyhemoglobin
  - When fully saturated each Hgb molecule has four O_2 molecules attached
    - Iron has to be in ferrous state (Fe^{2+}) for oxygen to attach
    - When blood is exposed to various drugs and other oxidizing agents
      - Ferrous iron converted to ferric iron (Fe^{3+})
      - Forming methemoglobin (met-Hgb)
        - Cannot bind oxygen
        - Enzyme within red cells, met-Hgb reductase, converts met-Hb back to Hgb
- Affinity of Hgb for O_2 increases exponentially as more oxygen molecules attach
  - Hence sigmoid nature of oxygen–Hgb dissociation curve
  - Factors that decrease the affinity of Hgb to oxygen (i.e., making off-loading of oxygen easier) include:
    - Acidosis and 2,3-DPG

Characteristics of Cell-free Hemoglobin

- **Dissociation:** When free in plasma, the Hgb tetramer dissociates into two $\alpha\beta$-dimers
  - Filtered through renal glomeruli and can precipitate in renal tubules
  - Causing obstruction
  - Further compounded by decreased renal blood flow that results from the vasoconstrictive effect of Hgb
- Technologies developed to produce large stable Hgb polymers by cross-linking Hgb molecules
  - Most commonly used cross-linking reagent is glutaraldehyde
    - Results in formation of polymers of varying sizes that do not filter through glomeruli
  - Another strategy to stabilize Hgb was intramolecular cross-linking
    - Cross-link was between α-chains of same molecule so that neither polymerization nor subunit dissociation occurred
      - Product was abandoned due to intense vasoconstrictive features
- **Viscosity:** Lower viscosity of Hgb solutions initially thought advantageous
  - Provided less systemic vascular resistance
  - Deeper insight into physiology of vascular endothelium revealed that reduced shear stresses on blood vessel wall were associated with decreased secretion of relaxing factors such as prostacyclin and endothelin
    - With net vasoconstrictive effect
  - Resulting decrease in blood flow antagonizes oxygen delivery function of Hgb

- **Vasoactivity:** Most HBOCs have systemic pressor effect, some have same effect on pulmonary circulation
  - Two other pressor mechanisms described:
    - Binding of nitric oxide
    - Stimulation of catecholamine release
  - Effects associated with decreased cardiac output
- **Affinity for Oxygen:** Once released from RBC, Hgb loses its 2,3-DPG
  - Affinity for oxygen increases
  - Causes leftward shift of the oxygen–Hgb dissociation curve
  - Impairing off-loading of oxygen
  - Strategies to decrease the affinity of Hgb for oxygen include:
    - Pyridoxalation
    - Use of bovine Hgb
    - Not clear whether decreasing affinity of Hgb for oxygen is beneficial
      - Higher levels of oxygen at tissue level may trigger autoregulatory response by blood vessel wall
        - With decreased secretion of relaxing factors, resulting in vasoconstriction and decreased flow
- **Oxidation:** Deprived of met-Hgb reductase in red cells, free Hgb at higher risk of being oxidized into met-Hgb
  - Antioxidants such as glutathione available in plasma to serve this function
  - Levels of met-Hgb in patients receiving HBOCs not physiologically significant
- **Effects on the Inflammatory Response:** HBOCs lack ability to stimulate neutrophils and incite inflammatory response with attendant systemic manifestations of multiple organ dysfunction

Clinical Trials of Hemoglobin-Based Oxygen Carriers

- Most widely studied HBOC in clinical practice is human polymerized Hgb product (PolyHeme, Northfield Laboratories, Evanston, IL)
- First randomized trial in acute trauma and emergency surgery published in 1998 showing that PolyHeme maintained total hemoglobin *in lieu* of RBCs despite marked fall in RBC Hgb
  - Reduced use of blood transfusion
  - Study concluded that PolyHeme appears to be a clinically useful blood substitute
  - Phase III trial involving 720 patients from 32 level I trauma centers recently completed
    - Trial randomized trauma patients with evidence of hemorrhagic shock at scene to either normal saline or PolyHeme
    - Treatment started in field and continued for up to 12 hours after injury
    - Primary end point was survival at 30 days
    - Preliminary results showed no statistically significant difference in survival
      - PolyHeme may be useful when blood is needed but not available

REFUSAL OF BLOOD TRANSFUSION

- Critically ill patients with transfusion preferences present a challenging management problem

- Jehovah's Witnesses' refusal of blood and blood products part of religious beliefs
  - Genesis 9:4–5, Leviticus 17:10–12
- Honoring these beliefs requires modification of medical management strategies
- Care of these patients requires early identification of transfusion preferences
- All patients admitted to critical care setting should have treatment preferences (including blood transfusion) discussed with them or legal representative as soon as possible
- Transfusion may be emergent in some situations but in most circumstances should be able to discuss the risks, benefits, and potential complications of transfusion of various blood products with patient or representative
- Discussion with patient and family members includes detailed explanation of each product
  - Origin and technical aspects of products may affect acceptance
  - In case of Jehovah's Witnesses, or other groups with religious preferences, assistance from church representative or elder may be helpful to family and physician
- Survival at lower levels of Hgb (>3 g/dL) reported
  - Mortality exceeds 50% when Hgb below 3 g/dL
  - Implementation of blood conservation strategies, hormonal stimulation, and use of RBC substitutes as available are options in the management of these patients
  - Use of high-dose erythropoietin (40,000 units subcutaneously every other day) and supplemental iron provide accelerated erythropoiesis under extreme circumstances

TABLE 120.10

MANAGEMENT STRATEGIES FOR JEHOVAH'S WITNESSES WITH SEVERE ANEMIA

- **Blood conservation**
  No routine blood draws
  Consequential blood tests only
  Use of capillary tubes for arterial blood gas analysis
  Pediatric-size tubes for other tests
  Decisive surgical interventions in cases of bleeding
  Intraoperative and peri-procedure blood conservation
- **Hemostasis**
- **Autologous transfusion (cell salvage device)**
- **Normovolemic hemodilution**
- **Maximization of oxygen delivery**
  Maintain high oxygen saturation
  Minimize oxygen demand
- **Sedation**
- **Mechanical ventilation**
- **Neuromuscular blockade**
- **Allow permissive hypercapnia/metabolic acidosis**
- **Hormonal stimulation**
  High-dose recombinant erythropoietin
  Iron supplementation
- **Red cell substitutes (as they become available)**

- Table 120.10 lists potential strategies useful in management of Jehovah's Witnesses and others requesting blood transfusion not be administered
- Some of these strategies are considered for all patients in critical care setting to minimize the need for transfusion

CHAPTER 121 ■ HEMATOLOGIC CONDITIONS IN THE ICU

HEMATOPOIESIS

Cellular Components

- Hematopoiesis a polyclonal process responsible for production and maintenance of blood and immune cells
  - Large numbers of blood and immune cells traced to pool of hematopoietic stem cells (HSCs) from which these clones originated
  - Two hallmarks of an HSC:
    - It can renew itself
    - It can produce cells that give rise to all the different types of blood cells
  - These cells also can mobilize out of bone marrow into circulating blood and can undergo programmed cell death

- Called *apoptosis*—process by which detrimental or unneeded cells undergo programmed self-destruction to maintain homeostasis
- Most primitive stem cell in bone marrow responsible for:
  - Production of all lymphoid (T, B, and natural killer lymphocytes), myeloid (granulocytes, monocytes), erythroid, and megakaryocytic (platelets) cell lineages
  - While maintaining sufficient numbers of pluripotent stem cells to sustain hematopoiesis throughout adult life
  - These cells found in small population of cells characterized by the surface expression of CD34 molecule and by lack of markers of differentiation
- In course of producing mature, circulating blood cell
  - Original single hematopoietic stem cell undergoes between 17 and 19.5 divisions

- Providing net output between approximately 170,000 and 720,000 blood cells
- Wide array of environmental factors regulate quantity and behavior of stem cells including:
  - Cytokines and chemokines
  - Extracellular matrix components
  - Hematopoietic and nonhematopoietic cells such as natural killer (NK) cells, T cells, macrophages, fibroblasts, osteoblasts, adipocytes, and perhaps even neurons

Humoral Mediators

- Production of specific type of differentiated blood cell from stem cell thought to occur randomly
  - Cytokines promote proliferation and survival of certain types of cells
    - But do not affect which cell type is produced from stem cell
  - As progenitors differentiate phenotype-specific receptors evolve so that only certain cytokines affect these new and more mature cells
  - Others maintain stem cell self-renewal and expansion
- Cytokines made and secreted mainly by helper T lymphocytes and macrophages and other stroma cells such as fibroblasts and endothelial cells
  - Some cytokines have been synthesized and are U.S. Food and Drug Administration–approved for clinical use:
    - Erythropoietin (epoetin alfa, or long-acting darbepoetin alfa) for erythrocyte production
    - Granulocyte colony-stimulating factor (G-CSF, filgrastim or long-acting pegfilgrastim), and granulocyte–macrophage colony-stimulating factor (GM-CSF, sargramostim) for neutrophil production
    - Stem cell harvest for transplantation and interleukin-11 (IL-11; oprelvekin) for stimulation of megakaryocytes and production of platelets
  - *Cytokine*, a general term, more specific terms include:
    - *Lymphokine*, for cytokines made by lymphocytes
    - *Monokine*, for cytokines made by monocytes
    - *Chemokine*, for cytokines with chemotactic activities
    - *Interleukin*, cytokine made by one leukocyte and acting on other leukocytes
  - Cytokines act on target cells by binding specific membrane receptors through which they mediate their effect on inflammation, immunity, and hematopoiesis
  - Responses to cytokines include:
    - Increasing or decreasing expression of membrane proteins—including cytokine receptors, proliferation, and secretion of effector molecules
    - Cytokines in clinical use today mainly interferon-α and interferon-γ
- Cytokines important in critical care medicine, especially those proinflammatory cytokines released by monocytes or macrophages in response to infectious and noninfectious inflammation
  - Release results in whole body inflammation such as that seen in SIRS
  - These patients also undergo an anti-inflammatory phase
    - Includes release of cytokines with opposing—anti-inflammatory—biologic effects or naturally occurring cytokine antagonists, such as interleukin-1 receptor

antagonist and tumor necrosis factor-α soluble receptors p55 and p75

DECREASED BLOOD COUNTS

Anemias

- Hemoglobin concentration <12 g/dL
  - Present in 95% of patients in the intensive care unit (ICU)
  - About one-third of those having upon admission concentration of <10 g/dL
  - In the assessment attention paid to:
    - Time of onset
    - Patient's ethnic origin
    - Concurrent illness
    - Procedures patient has undergone
    - Drugs patient is receiving
    - History of transfusions
- One approach to classify anemia into two major categories:
  - Anemia resulting from underproduction
  - Anemia due to increased destruction of red blood cells (RBCs) (Table 121.1)
- Obtain diagnostic tests prior to transfusions, including:
  - Complete blood count

TABLE 121.1

ANEMIA CLASSIFICATION

Anemias Secondary to Marrow Underproduction
- **Decreased erythropoietin production**
  Renal disease
  Endocrine deficiency
  Starvation
- **Inadequate response to erythropoietin**
  Iron deficiency
  B_{12} deficiency
  Folic acid deficiency
  Anemia of chronic disease
  Marrow infiltration
  Sideroblastic anemia
  Myelodysplastic syndrome
- **Marrow failure**
  Congenital dyserythropoietic anemia
  Aplastic anemia
  Pure red cell aplasia
  Toxic marrow damage

Anemias Secondary to Increased Destruction
- **Acquired**
  Immune-mediated hemolytic anemia
  Paroxysmal nocturnal hemoglobinuria
  Hemolytic anemia due to red cell fragmentation (TTP, DIC)
  Hemolytic anemia due to chemical or physical agents
  Infections
  Acquired hemoglobinopathies (methemoglobinemia)
- **Hereditary**
  Congenital hemoglobinopathies (sickle cell disease)
  Enzyme deficiency (G6PD, pyruvate kinase)
  Red cell membrane defects (spherocytosis, elliptocytosis)

TTP, thrombotic thrombocytopenic purpura; DIC, disseminated intravascular coagulation.

- Including hematocrit, hemoglobin, mean corpuscular volume (MCV) and hemoglobin (MCH)
- Reticulocyte count
- Stained blood smear
- Additionally serum bilirubin and lactic acid dehydrogenase useful to determine presence of hemolysis
- If immune hemolysis is suspected:
  - Direct Coombs test should be ordered
  - Indirect Coombs test done routinely with cross-match request to blood bank
- If hemoglobinopathy suspected:
  - Hemoglobin electrophoresis obtained before transfusion
- Does patient require transfusion with packed RBC (PRBCs)?
  - Hemoglobin (Hgb) of 10 g/dL/hematocrit (Hct) of 30% thought desirable
    - Especially those undergoing surgery and/or with critical illness
    - The main reason for high transfusion rates in ICU patients
    - Replaced by a more physiologic approach
      - Patient's intravascular volume and tissue oxygen needs considered
  - Restrictive transfusion policy:
    - Hgb maintained between 7 and 9 g/dL effective
      - Yields decreased death rates compared to liberal strategy
      - Young traumatized patients Hgb allowed to drift to 5 g/dL
        - As long as no signs of DO$_2$ deficit such as elevated lactate levels, an unacceptable heart rate, or other symptoms
      - These patients most often started on recombinant erythropoietin and have iron stores repleted to keep from undergoing transfusion
  - Patients with acute myocardial infarction or unstable angina and some cancer patients may benefit from higher Hgb level
  - Patients with Hgb ≥10 g/dL unlikely to benefit from blood transfusion

Anemia in Critical Illness

- Anemia with Hgb ≤8.5 g/dL the most frequent type in the ICU
  - More than 50% of these patients receive RBC transfusions during ICU stay
  - As do more than 85% of patients with ICU length of stay >7 days
  - Studies showed that number of RBC transfusions independently associated with longer ICU stay and increase in mortality
    - Vast majority of critically ill patients have anemia on admission to ICU
    - Most common indication for RBC transfusion in ICU was treatment of anemia
    - Transfusion trigger in all studies Hgb about 8.5 g/dL
    - RBC transfusions increased in patients with prolonged ICU length of stay and increased age
- Possible mechanisms involved in anemia of acute critically ill patients include:
  - Blunted erythropoietin (EPO) response to anemia

- Blood concentrations of EPO inappropriately low in these patients
- Suppression of erythropoiesis by proinflammatory cytokines
- Possible blood loss from frequent phlebotomies
- Blood loss from gastrointestinal bleeding as a result of gastric tubes, stress-induced mucosal ulcerations, acute renal failure, and frequent coagulation problems in ICU patients
- Shares characteristics with anemia of chronic inflammation such as high ferritin concentrations and low-to-normal transferrin saturation with functional iron deficiency
- Appears inflammatory cytokine IL-6 induces production of hepcidin
  - Iron-regulatory hormone may be responsible for hypoferremia and suppressed erythropoiesis
- Approach to treatment of this type of anemia includes:
- Measures to reduce blood loss
- Restrictive blood transfusion policy
- Possibly the use of recombinant human EPO (rh-EPO)
  - Subcutaneous administration of rh-EPO at 40,000 units weekly
  - Starting between days 3 and 7 of ICU stay
  - Resulted in significant reduction in RBC transfusions and a higher hemoglobin level
- Iron is locked up in the phagocytic system and unavailable
  - Administration of intravenous (IV) iron, together with rh-EPO, may result in an enhanced rh-EPO effect
  - Only about 10% of oral iron bioavailable, so not appropriate in ICU patients
  - Have been anaphylactoid reactions reported with iron dextran
    - Iron gluconate the preferred formulation
      - Dose is 125 mg diluted in 100 mL saline over 1-hour infusion
      - To a total cumulative dose of 1,000 mg

Autoimmune Hemolytic Anemia (AIHA)

- A patient critically ill from AIHA presents with:
- Signs and symptoms of normovolemic anemia
- Unless massive hemolysis associated with hypotension, significant hemoglobinuria, and acute renal failure
- Variable levels of jaundice may be present in nonmassive AIHA
- Initial laboratory data may show:
  - Elevated reticulocyte index (>2) identifying mechanism of anemia as hemolytic
  - Elevated indirect bilirubinemia and lactate dehydrogenase
  - Blood smear shows increased numbers of diffusely basophilic red cells
    - Reflecting increased reticulocytes
  - Variable numbers of microspherocytes and fragmented cells, indicative of hemolysis
  - Urine may be discolored red, brown, or black if sufficient intravascular hemolysis to produce hemoglobinuria
  - Positive result on direct antiglobulin (Coombs) test
    - Indicates immunoglobulin or complement is on surface of circulating RBCs
    - Identifies immune etiology of hemolysis
    - Absent recent transfusion, the diagnosis of AIHA is confirmed

○ Information may become available when blood bank attempts to cross-match patient's blood for transfusion
- Important to determine, by history and appropriate laboratory studies:
  - Whether hemolysis related to drug patient is taking
  - Whether caused by warm-reacting (usually immunoglobulin [Ig] G) or cold-reacting (usually IgM) antibodies (Ab)
  - Mechanisms whereby drugs produce immune hemolysis not absolutely clear
    - Evidence suggests alteration of RBC surface antigens by drug and production of antibodies that lead to hemolysis
    - Underlying diseases associated with AIHA include:
      ○ Infections, such as infectious mononucleosis and pneumonia caused by *Mycoplasma pneumonia*
      ○ Collagen vascular diseases, especially systemic lupus erythematosus
      ○ Lymphoproliferative disorders such as chronic lymphocytic leukemia
- Mainstay of treatment of AIHA caused by warm-reacting antibodies is corticosteroids:
  - Usually given in dosages equivalent to 60 to 80 mg/day of prednisone
  - In nonresponders splenectomy, high-dose intravenous gamma globulin, rituximab chimeric anti-CD20 antibody, alemtuzumab humanized anti-CD52 antibody, or treatment with other immunosuppressive drugs may be useful
- Steroids usually ineffective in AIHA caused by cold-reactive antibodies (cold agglutinin disease), but responses observed using larger doses
  - Patients with cold agglutinins may have symptoms related to impaired blood flow in acral parts where blood temperature low enough to permit agglutination of RBCs by antibodies
  - Warming usually prevents or alleviates such symptoms
  - Rarely, plasmapheresis needed to reduce concentration of offending IgM Ab
  - If drug-induced immune hemolysis, discontinuation usually the only treatment needed
- When transfusion considered
  - May be impossible to find compatible RBCs by usual cross-matching procedures
  - Transfused cells may be subject to rapid antibody-mediated destruction
  - Patient must not be allowed to die because of undue caution regarding transfusion of incompatible RBCs
    - Key to optimal care is close communication between the intensivist and blood bank physician
    - When transfused, patient must be observed closely for signs of accelerated hemolysis, such as visible hemoglobin in the plasma or urine
  - Certain special considerations for transfusion of patients with cold-reacting Ab:
    - Administered blood should be warmed to body temperature
    - Transfusion of plasma, which contains complement, should be avoided because hemolysis is complement mediated and may be limited by depletion of complement *in vivo*
    - In massive hemolysis, therapeutic efforts directed at maintenance of blood pressure, renal blood flow, and urinary output
    - IV fluids and diuretics such as furosemide used to maintain a urine flow of 100 mL/hour

Hemolytic Anemia from G6PD Deficiency

- RBC glucose-6-phosphate dehydrogenase (G6PD) deficiency an X-linked recessive disorder
  - Affects various population groups around the world
  - In United States African Americans most often affected
    - Gene frequency of about 11%
    - Have G6PD A–variant of the enzyme and a mild to moderate deficiency
  - Study by U.S. Army found 2.5% of males and 1.6% of females were deficient
    - Highest rates of G6PD deficiency in:
      ○ African American males (12.2%) and females (4.1%)
      ○ Asian males (4.3%)
  - RBC G6PD levels in affected men are 8% to 20% of normal
  - Clinically significant hemolysis occurs when RBCs subjected to oxidative metabolic challenge
    - May occur with exposure to certain drugs or with certain illnesses
    - Drugs include some sulfonamides, nitrofurantoins, and antimalarials such as primaquine
    - Illnesses most likely to trigger hemolysis are acute infections
      ○ Infectious hepatitis, in particular, associated with severe hemolytic episodes in G6PD-deficient patients
  - Hemolysis, sudden and massive, usually apparent 1 to 3 days after inciting stress
    - Hemoglobinemia and hemoglobinuria may occur
    - Blood smear shows polychromatophilia within a few days, reflecting developing reticulocytosis
    - Early in course of hemolytic episode Heinz bodies may be identified
      ○ Precipitates of oxidatively denatured hemoglobin
      ○ Useful diagnostic clue should be sought if G6PD deficiency is suspected
      ○ Absence of Heinz bodies does not exclude diagnosis
  - RBC enzyme deficiency readily detected by laboratory assay when patient is in stable state, more difficult during hemolytic episode
    - Because the enzyme deficiency greatest in oldest red cells
    - These are the first destroyed in hemolytic episode
      ○ As replaced by newly produced young cells, overall RBC enzyme level may rise to the normal range
      ○ Tends to ameliorate the hemolysis with time
  - If diagnosis suspected, potentially offending drugs should be stopped
    - Supportive care usually all that is necessary
    - Deficiency an X-linked trait, female heterozygotes may have hemolytic episodes

Hemolytic Anemia from Red Cell Injury in the Circulation

- Fragmentation and destruction of RBC in circulation may result from increased shear stresses caused by turbulent blood flow
- Two major categories of disease in which this hemolysis occurs are:
  - Malfunctioning intravascular prosthetic devices: heart valves, vascular grafts, and shunts
  - Disorders affecting blood vessels that result in microangiopathic hemolytic disease, such as disseminated intravascular coagulation or thrombotic microangiopathy (TMA)

○ Encompasses spectrum of thrombotic thrombocytopenic purpura (TTP) and hemolytic uremic syndrome
- Hemolysis is intravascular, hemoglobinemia and hemoglobinuria may be present
  - Characteristically blood smear shows RBC fragmentation producing micropoikilocytes (schistocytes)
  - TMA patients also have thrombocytopenia, fever, and possibly neurologic and renal involvement
- Specific treatment directed at underlying disorder
- Supportive measures include:
  - Blood transfusion and hydration to ensure good urine flow
  - Badly malfunctioning prosthesis, such as an artificial heart valve, may require replacement
  - Treatment of TMA with plasma administration, either infusion or plasmapheresis, the only effective therapy

Sickle Cell Anemia

- Sickle cell Hgb (Hgb S) the result of a single nucleotide mutation in the sixth codon of the β globin gene (β^s)
  - Heterozygous inheritance does not usually cause disease or symptoms–sickle trait
  - Homozygous inheritance or compound heterozygous inheritance with another β globin gene results in disease (Table 121.2)
- Clinical symptoms of sickle cell disease (SCD) affect multiple organs and may vary widely among patients
  - Chief among clinical features are episodes of severe pain (crises)

- In chest, back, abdomen, or extremities
- Acute chest syndrome, frequent and sometimes fatal complication
  ○ Affects more than 40% of all patients with SCD
  ○ Can lead to:
    – Acute and chronic respiratory insufficiency,
    – Including pulmonary hypertension
  ○ Cardinal features are fever, pleuritic chest pain, referred abdominal pain, cough, lung infiltrates, and hypoxia
- Other complications of SCD include:
  ○ Recurrent strokes in young adults
  ○ Parvovirus B19-induced aplastic crisis
  ○ Hyperbilirubinemia from cholestatic syndrome or cholecystitis
  ○ Liver disease
  ○ Splenic infarctions
  ○ Autosplenectomy with increased risk of fulminant septicemia caused by encapsulated organisms such as *Streptococcus pneumoniae* and *Haemophilus influenzae*
  ○ Hematuria
  ○ Priapism
  ○ Bone infarctions with the risk of avascular necrosis, osteomyelitis, and other musculoskeletal manifestations
  ○ Leg ulcers
  ○ Spontaneous abortions
- Many patients survive into fifth and sixth decades in industrialized countries
- Goals of SCD treatment are:
  - To relieve symptoms of complications

TABLE 121.2

CLINICAL AND HEMATOLOGIC FINDINGS IN THE COMMON VARIANTS OF SICKLE CELL DISEASE AFTER THE AGE OF 5 YEARS

| Disease group | Clinical severity | Hemoglobin electrophoresis | | | Hematologic values | | | | |
		S (%)	F (%)	A₂ (%)	A (%)	Hb g/dL	Retic (%)	MCV (fl)	RBC morphology
SS	Usually marked	>90	<10	<3.5	0	6–11	5–20	>80	Sickle cells, NRBC, normochromia, anisocytosis, poikilocytosis, target cells, Howell-Jolly bodies
Sβ° Thal	Marked to moderate	>80	<20	>3.5	0	6–10	5–20	<80	Sickle cells, NRBC, hypochromia, microcytosis, anisocytosis, poikilocytosis, target cells
Sβ^+ Thal	Mild to moderate	>60	<20	>3.5	10–30	9–12	5–10	<75	No sickle cells, hypochromia, microcytosis, anisocytosis, poikilocytosis, target cells
SC	Mild to moderate	50	<5	[a]	0	10–15	5–10	75–95	"Fat" sickle cells, anisocytosis, poikilocytosis, target cells
S HPFH	Asymptomatic	<70	>30	<2.5	0	12–14	1–2	<80	No sickle cells, anisocytosis, poikilocytosis, rare target cells

MCV, mean corpuscular volume; RBC, red blood cell; NRBC, nucleated red blood cells; Hb, hemoglobin; S, Hb S; F, Hb F; A2, Hb A2; A, Hb A.
[a]50 percent Hb C.
Hematologic values are approximate. There is tremendous variability between disease groups and between individual patients of the same group, particularly regarding clinical severity.
For findings in younger children, see Brown AK, Sleeper LA, Miller ST, et al. Reference values and hematological changes from birth to five years in patients with sickle cell disease. *Arch Pediatr Adolesc.* 1994;48:796–804.
Adapted from NIH Publication No. 96–2117.

- To prevent complications using new treatments targeting disease mechanisms
- Treatment of painful crisis is supportive
  - Dehydration, acidosis, infection, and hypoxemia promote red cell sickling and should be prevented or corrected
  - Adequate relief of pain usually requires parenteral administration of opioid analgesics at frequent fixed intervals
    - Analgesics should be used without worrying about addiction or side effects of opiates
    - Patients can be given oral analgesics to take at home
  - Oxygen is often administered in sickle cell crisis; benefits uncertain
  - Antibiotics covering major pulmonary pathogens should be administered in acute chest syndrome
  - Transfusions of blood:
    - No clear evidence transfusion therapy shortens simple painful crisis; thus not a treatment for uncomplicated painful crisis
    - Urgent transfusions are needed when:
      - There is severe sudden drop in hemoglobin, especially in children in whom splenic sequestration or aplastic crises present in this manner
      - Severe acute chest syndrome with hypoxia
      - Chronic RBC transfusions shown to prevent strokes in patients with SCD
        - Optimal duration of transfusion is unknown
      - Risks of transfusions must be weighed against the benefits
        - Alloimmunization
        - Infections
        - Iron overload
      - For patients undergoing general anesthesia, preoperative transfusion to hematocrit above 30% reduced postoperative complications
      - Leukocyte-depleted RBC phenotypically matched for antigens most frequently associated with immune response are preferred
      - Exchange transfusion most rapid method to reduce Hgb S concentration to <30% in urgent situations
        - Such as stroke and severe acute chest syndrome, and in patients with striking cholestatic syndrome and signs of liver failure
- Preventive treatments should include:
  - Early vaccinations against *S. pneumoniae* and *H. influenzae*
  - Prophylactic penicillin in children until age of 5 years
  - Folic acid (1 mg daily) to prevent megaloblastic erythropoiesis
  - Hydroxyurea treatment to prevent complications
    - Shown to reduce pain episodes, acute chest syndrome, blood transfusions, and hospitalizations
    - Improvements noted correlate to increases in Hgb F levels and a decrease in granulocytes, monocytes, and reticulocytes
    - Reserved for SCD patients with severe complications

Specific Clinical Problems of SCD

- If abdominal symptoms present possibilities of cholecystitis and complications of cholelithiasis must be considered
- Rarely, bone marrow infarction may be extensive, producing syndrome of fat embolism

- Manifested by severe bone pain, fever, neurologic abnormalities, and respiratory distress
- May be fatal
- Treatment by exchange transfusion can be life saving
- May be a cause of some cases of acute chest syndrome
- Hematuria occurs as complication SCD, including sickle cell trait, and may be severe
  - Usually results from sickling and vaso-occlusion in the renal medulla, but other causes unrelated to SCD must be excluded
- Treatment with hydration and, perhaps, urinary alkalinization often sufficient for this self-limited complication
- Priapism, a frequent and painful complication of SCD
  - Arises from vaso-occlusion that produces congestion and sickling in corpora cavernosa
    - May resolve spontaneously, and initial conservative treatment with analgesics, hydration, and alkalinization is appropriate
    - Exchange transfusion and various surgical procedures successful in terminating priapism

Aplastic Crisis in Hemolytic Anemia

- Sudden intensification of anemia in hemolytic disease resulting from a precipitous reduction in rate of RBC production
- May occur in course of any hemolytic disease but most commonly reported in congenital hemolytic disorders:
  - Hereditary spherocytosis
  - Sickle cell anemia
- Most common in children but also occurs in adults
- Patients characteristically have:
  - Fever
  - Anorexia
  - Nausea and vomiting
  - Abdominal pain and headache common
- Anemia usually severe and may be life-threatening
  - Mild leukopenia and thrombocytopenia often present
  - Aplastic nature of anemia demonstrated by extremely low reticulocyte count and marked reduction in erythroid precursors in bone marrow
    - Episode self-limited, and recovery usually begins by 2 weeks
    - In recovery phase a return of vigorous erythropoiesis
      - Often outpouring of nucleated RBC and reticulocytes
      - Frequently accompanied by leukocytosis and immature white blood cells (WBCs)
  - Convincing evidence that parvovirus B19 the cause of most aplastic crises
- Prompt recognition of syndrome important because of suddenness and severity of anemia
- Low reticulocyte count in patient with hemolytic disease usually main clue to diagnosis
- Treatment is via RBC transfusion
- Volume given sufficient to alleviate signs and symptoms of inadequate tissue DO_2

LEUKOPENIAS

- Refers to total WBC count of <4,000 cells/μL
  - Granulocytopenia/neutropenia refers to circulating granulocyte count below 1,500 cells/μL

- Clinical importance of granulocytopenia relates to increased risk of bacterial infection
- If the absolute neutrophil count ≤500 cells/μL bacterial infection the rule
- Agranulocytosis implies severe neutropenia or a complete absence of granulocytes
- Three patient groups most pertinent to critical care situations:
  - Patients with neutropenia from primary bone marrow diseases or cytotoxic treatment
  - Patients in whom neutropenia exists alone or in combination with other cytopenias as an aplastic process
  - Patients with neutropenia or agranulocytosis caused by immunologic mechanisms

Primary Bone Marrow (BM) Diseases and Cytotoxic Treatment

- Largest and most frequent entity that causes neutropenia
  - BM diseases such as leukemias, myelodysplastic syndrome, and marrow fibrosis frequently present with neutropenia
  - Chemotherapy-induced neutropenia common complication of treatment of cancer
  - Risk of life-threatening infections increases with:
    - Increased severity of neutropenia and its duration
    - Increasing patient age
    - Coexistence of other severe illnesses
- These patients end up in the ICU due to a rapid onset of septic shock
- Neutropenic fever an indication for hospitalization and institution of IV wide-spectrum antibiotics
  - Before antibiotics, cultures of blood, sputum, and urine obtained
  - Other sites cultured as indicated in individual patients
  - Patients should have chest radiographs taken
  - Common effects of bacterial infections
    - Purulent sputum in pneumonia
    - Pyuria in urinary tract infection
    - Abscess formation
    - Usually absent because of lack of granulocytes
- Choice of antibiotic regimen should take into account findings in individual patient that suggest specific site of infection and any knowledge of patterns of infection in a given institution
  - If cultures are positive antibiotic treatment should be adjusted accordingly
  - If cultures are negative empirical therapy continued if patient remains neutropenic and until counts recover
  - If fever continues and patient's condition deteriorates with persistent neutropenia:
    - Appropriate to prescribe empirical antifungal agent, such as amphotericin B
    - Patients screened by obtaining a computed tomography (CT) scan of sinuses, chest, abdomen, and pelvis for possible foci of invasive fungal infections
    - Galactomannan antigen test for aspergillus should be done routinely on blood and sputum (usually bronchoalveolar lavage) of immunosuppressed patients with neutropenia
    - If patients have a central venous line (CVL), fungal and bacterial blood cultures obtained

- Removal of CVL considered if blood cultures are positive
- Routine therapeutic use of colony-stimulating factors (G-CSF, GM-CSF) not recommended by American Society of Clinical Oncology (ASCO)
  - Should be considered in patients at high risk for infection-related complications or who have prognostic factors that are predictive of poor clinical outcomes, including:
    - Expected prolonged (>10 days) and profound (<0.1 × 10^3 cells/μL) neutropenia
    - Age older than 65 years
    - Uncontrolled primary disease, pneumonia, hypotension, multiorgan dysfunction, invasive fungal infection, or being hospitalized at the time of development of the fever
    - CSFs recommended for primary and secondary prophylaxis used to prevent chemotherapy-induced neutropenia
    - Respiratory status deterioration or acute respiratory distress syndrome can develop during neutropenia recovery with or without the use of G-CSF
    - Could be related to release of inflammatory cytokines by resident alveolar neutrophils and macrophages
    - Mortality as high as 62% in these patients
      - Immediate evaluation by bronchoscopy to rule out infection and early use of high-dose steroids could be critical for their survival

Bone Marrow Aplasia

- Neutropenia part of pancytopenia commonly present in aplastic anemia
  - Etiologies:
    - Autoimmune basis
    - Drug or chemical exposure may be suspected
    - No tests are available to prove an association in individual cases
      - Benzene and derivatives potentially toxic to bone marrow
      - Other chemicals, dichlorodiphenyltrichloroethane (DDT), other insecticides, suspect
      - Toluene exposure in glue sniffers may be associated
      - Many medications linked with aplastic anemia
        - Occurs as idiosyncratic reaction in small percentage of patients exposed to drug:
          - Chloramphenicol
          - Phenylbutazone
          - Indomethacin
          - Diphenylhydantoin
          - Sulfonamides
          - Gold preparations
      - In 50% of cases of aplastic anemia, no cause found or suspected
- Principles of treating infectious complications resulting from neutropenia in aplastic states the same as those outlined earlier for neutropenia in malignant diseases
  - Allogeneic bone marrow transplantation in suitable patients
  - Immunosuppressive therapy including antithymocyte globulin
  - Other supportive care measures
    - Antibiotic prophylaxis
    - Colony-stimulating factors

Immune and Drug-Related Granulocytopenia

- Neutropenia in adults often occurs as:
  - Isolated finding
  - In association with autoimmune disease:
    - Rheumatoid arthritis
    - Systemic lupus erythematosus
    - Other similar conditions
- Evaluation includes:
  - Peripheral blood smear to seek out large granular lymphocytes (LGL)
  - Measurement of antinuclear antibodies, rheumatoid factor, and other autoantibodies
  - Possibly bone marrow examination
- Chronic neutropenia, idiopathic or autoimmune, usually does not require treatment
- Patients with absolute neutrophil count <500 cells/μL prone to develop recurrent fevers and infections
  - Antibiotics and G-CSF may improve neutrophil count during infection
  - Patients with LGL syndrome may not respond well to G-CSF
    - May require immunosuppressive therapy, such as methotrexate or cyclosporine, alone or with G-CSF
- Chronic neutropenia in association with rheumatoid arthritis, or Felty syndrome
  - Usually seen in severe cases with elevated rheumatoid factor
  - Patients who have recurrent fevers and infection require treatment similar to patients with LGL syndrome
  - Splenectomy should be considered in refractory cases
- Drug-induced agranulocytosis a serious medical problem
  - Occurs in 1% to 3% of patients treated with certain medications
  - Characteristic clinical syndrome includes:
    - High fever
    - Chills
    - Severe sore throat (agranulocytic angina) caused by bacterial infection
  - Oral and pharyngeal ulcers, necrotizing tonsillitis, pharyngeal abscesses, and bacteremia may occur
  - Blood demonstrates virtual absence of granulocytes
    - Bone marrow may show absence of all granulocyte precursors or only the mature cells
    - May superficially resemble acute leukemia, or state of maturation arrest
  - Serial blood counts recommended for patients on some drugs:
    - Phenothiazines
    - Clozapine
    - Sulfasalazine
    - Antithyroid drugs
  - Management includes prompt withdrawal of all potentially offending drugs and use of broad-spectrum antibiotics
  - Bone marrow examination not usually indicated
  - Time to recovery may be proportional to severity but usually within about a week after withdrawal of the offending drug

THROMBOCYTOPENIAS

- Thrombocytopenia a common laboratory abnormality in ICU patients associated with adverse outcomes
  - Defined as platelet count <150 $\times$ 10^3 cells/μL
  - Incidence reported to be 23% to 41.3%, with mortality rates up to 54%
  - Incidence of more severe thrombocytopenia lower, about 10% to 17%
    - Associated with greater mortality
    - Defined as fewer than 50 $\times$ 10^3 cells/μL
- Systematic evaluation of thrombocytopenia essential to identification and management of causes (Table 121.3)
  - Sepsis the most common cause
    - Accounts for >48% of thrombocytopenia cases in ICU
    - More than 25% of ICU patients have more than one cause
  - Drug-induced thrombocytopenia a diagnostic challenge
  - Many medications can cause thrombocytopenia
    - Critically ill patients often receive multiple drugs
    - Heparin is the most common cause of drug-induced thrombocytopenia due to immune mechanisms
  - Steps in diagnosis of true thrombocytopenia:
    - Mechanism
      - Increased destruction
      - Decreased production
      - Sequestration
    - Presence of large platelets on blood smear or by mean platelet volume (MPV) suggests active thrombopoiesis
    - Examination of bone marrow for megakaryocytes often necessary to distinguish between increased destruction (presence of megakaryocytes) and decreased production (absence of megakaryocytes)
    - Splenomegaly raises possibility of sequestration
    - Other laboratory tests not necessary to evaluate thrombocytopenia itself
    - Also the possibility of platelet clumping induced by:
      - Commonly used anticoagulant EDTA (ethylenediaminetetraacetic acid)
      - Platelet cold agglutinins
      - Partial clotting of blood sample
      - Platelet satellitosis, a disorder in which platelets cluster around white blood cells
    - When pseudothrombocytopenia is suspected, examining the peripheral blood smear and close communication with the laboratory necessary
- Treatment of thrombocytopenia depends on cause

TABLE 121.3

POTENTIAL CAUSES OF THROMBOCYTOPENIA

Sepsis, infections
Disseminated intravascular coagulation
Perioperative and postresuscitation hemodilution
Immune thrombocytopenias
Drug-induced thrombocytopenias
Liver disease/hypersplenism
Massive transfusion
Primary marrow disorder
Antiphospholipid antibody syndrome/lupus anticoagulant
Intravascular devices

- General principles of platelet transfusion are outlined:
  - Thrombocytopenia caused by destruction or sequestration of patient's own platelets means transfused platelets subject to same fate
    - Platelet transfusions most often are of little benefit
    - Reserved for treatment of severe bleeding
  - Thrombocytopenia caused by decreased platelet production
    - Hematologic malignancies
    - Recovery from stem cell transplantation
  - Serious hemorrhage prevented by regular transfusion of platelets
    - Generally acceptable to use prophylactic transfusion to keep platelet count >10,000 to 20,000 cells/μL
    - Transfusion of one random donor platelet unit per 10 kg of recipient weight, or single-donor unit from apheresis usually used to achieve that goal
    - Effectiveness of platelet transfusions diminished in febrile, infected patients who may require larger and more frequent transfusions
    - Actively bleeding patients require more frequent transfusion and a higher target of platelet count, usually above 50,000 cells/μL
      - Chronically transfused patients become refractory to transfusions from random donors because of alloimmunization
      - Single-donor platelets limit exposure to foreign antigens and may delay immunization
      - Platelets obtained from family members by platelet apheresis used in patients at risk for bleeding and refractory to random-donor platelets

Thrombocytopenia with Infection

- Mild and transient thrombocytopenia occurs with many systemic infections
  - Mechanism may be a combination of suppressed bone marrow production, increased destruction, and increased splenic sequestration
  - In bacteremia, platelets consumed because of disseminated intravascular coagulation (DIC)
  - In viral infection, platelet production may be suppressed
  - Thrombocytopenia common with human immunodeficiency virus (HIV) infection, mainly due to decreased production, although sometimes autoimmune mechanism involved
    - Thrombotic thrombocytopenic purpura (TTP) or thrombotic microangiopathy (TMA) associated with HIV as well with streptococcal and *Escherichia coli*
    - Treating underlying infection usually adequate to correct thrombocytopenia

Drug-Induced Thrombocytopenia

- Presents diagnostic challenge because many medications cause thrombocytopenia, and patients in ICU often on multiple medications
  - Most common reported drugs with probable or definite relation to thrombocytopenia were:

- Quinidine, quinine, rifampin, and trimethoprim-sulfamethoxazole
- Many other drugs can cause thrombocytopenia:
  - Heparin (see below)
  - Intravenous antibiotics
  - Anticonvulsants
  - Diuretics
  - Platelet glycoprotein (GP) IIb/IIIa antagonists used in acute coronary syndrome
- Underlying mechanism of drug-induced thrombocytopenia usually immune
  - At least three different types of antibodies appear to play a role:
    - Hapten-dependent antibodies
    - Drug-induced platelet-reactive autoantibodies
    - Drug-dependent antibodies
  - Targets for drug-dependent antibodies GP on cell membrane of platelets, such as GP Ib/IX and GP IIb/IIIa
  - Diagnosis of drug-induced thrombocytopenia supported by recovery to a normal platelet count within 5 to 7 days
- Treatment may require only withdrawal of the offending drug
  - Prednisone given if diagnosis of ITP cannot be ruled out
  - Patients with severe thrombocytopenia caused by GP IIb/IIIa antagonists may require platelet transfusions because they are typically also receiving heparin and aspirin for acute coronary syndrome
  - Platelet serology tests available but may not be available in time frame that allows information to be used in decision-making process

Heparin-Induced Thrombocytopenia (HIT)

- HIT an anticoagulant-induced prothrombotic disorder caused by platelet activation of heparin-dependent antibodies of IgG class
  - Diagnosis of HIT considered when platelet count, between days 5 and 14 from start of heparin therapy falls:
    - To <150 × 10^3 cells/μL
    - More than 50% decrease from baseline platelet count
    - High index of suspicion key in making diagnosis
  - Thrombocytopenia usually moderate and resolves within a few days of discontinuing heparin
  - HIT without thrombosis:
    - Called isolated HIT
  - *HIT thrombotic syndrome* (HITTS) denotes HIT complicated with thrombosis
  - Mortality rate associated with HIT ranges between 10% and 20%
- HIT an immune-mediated hypersensitivity reaction to platelet factor 4 (PF4)/heparin complex
- PF4 a heparin-binding protein found naturally in platelet α granules
  - Undergoes conformational changes once bound to heparin
- Anti-PF4/heparin antibodies produced by many patients taking heparin
  - Only a few develop thrombocytopenia
- Anti-PF4/heparin antibodies transient and usually undetectable within median of 50 to 85 days
  - If heparin is readministered to patient with high levels of HIT antibodies, abrupt thrombocytopenia can occur.
    - Likely will be more than 100 days after the last exposure to heparin

- Seroconversion found by enzyme-linked immunosorbent assay (ELISA) in up to 15% of patients on heparin
  - Does not constitute a diagnosis of HIT
- Patients more likely to develop HIT are:
  - Surgical patients
  - Individuals exposed to higher doses of heparin for longer time
  - Patients receiving unfractionated heparin (UFH), as opposed to low-molecular-weight heparin (LMWH)
- Small minority of ICU patients with thrombocytopenia receiving UFH have HIT
  - PF4/heparin-reactive antibodies more likely to be detected by ELISA assay than serotonin release assay (SRA)
    - Suggests *over* diagnosis, due to a high false-positive rate by ELISA, of HIT
  - Thrombotic sequelae of HIT carry significant morbidity and may be lethal:
    - Deep venous thrombosis (DVT) most common
      - Lower extremity predominates
    - Pulmonary embolism
    - Skin necrosis
    - Limb ischemia
    - Thrombotic stroke
    - Myocardial infarction
- All strategies should be used to prevent HIT in ICU patients
  - Elimination of heparin locks for CVLs and hemodialysis catheters
  - Hemodialysis without heparin is safe and effective
- To reduce risk of life-threatening thromboembolic events, once diagnosis of HIT recognized heparin promptly substituted with:
  - Direct thrombin inhibitor, such as argatroban or lepirudin
  - Heparinoid danaparoid (not available in United States)
  - Warfarin temporarily reduces synthesis of protein C and S, causing a hypercoagulable state, so is never be used alone in initial treatment of HIT
    - Use should be postponed until substantial platelet recovery has occurred
    - Consultation with a hematologist should be considered
  - Argatroban dose is 2 μg/kg/minute IV infusion and dilution of 1 mg/mL
    - Dose adjustment needed for hepatic impairment (25% of the dose)
    - Aim of a 1.5 to 3 times prolongation of activated partial thromboplastin time (aPTT) compared to baseline
  - Lepirudin treatment consists of a bolus 0.4 mg/kg (maximum of 44 mg)
    - Given over 10 to 15 seconds
    - Followed by continuous infusion at 0.15 mg/kg/hour
    - Goal of a 1.5 to 3 times prolongation of aPTT over baseline
    - Dose should be modified if creatinine is >1.5 mg/dL or clearance is <60 mL/minute
    - If given with warfarin, discontinue lepirudin when international normalized ratio (INR) of 2.0 obtained
- Approach to patients with suspected or confirmed HIT includes the following:
  - Discontinuation of all heparin
  - Administration of nonheparin anticoagulation, such as argatroban or lepirudin
  - Testing for anti-PF4/heparin antibodies, followed, if positive, by SRA

- Avoiding prophylactic platelet transfusions
- Allowing platelet recovery before starting warfarin
- Assessing for lower extremity DVT
- Patients with previous HIT who are antibody negative and require cardiac surgery should receive UFH in preference to other anticoagulants
- Preoperative and postoperative anticoagulation handled with anticoagulant other than UFH or LMWH
- Patients with recent or active HIT should have surgery delayed until antibody is negative
  - Otherwise, alternative anticoagulant should be used

Idiopathic Thrombocytopenic Purpura

- Idiopathic thrombocytopenic purpura (ITP):
- Also known as immune thrombocytopenic purpura
- Categorized as acute, chronic, or refractory
- Common cause of thrombocytopenia in both adults and children
- Usually in differential diagnosis of thrombocytopenia diagnosis of ITP made only after exclusion of other causes of thrombocytopenia
- When history, physical examination, and blood count with peripheral smear consistent with ITP, and other causes not suggested, few diagnostic tests necessary
  - Bone marrow examination important to rule out other primary marrow diseases
    - Myelodysplastic syndrome or lymphoproliferative disorders
    - In ITP, marrow shows increased number of megakaryocytes with immature forms and normal erythroid and myeloid lineages
  - Test for HIV important in patients with risk factors
  - Tests for platelet Abs not helpful because of limited specificity and sensitivity
  - TTP may occur as one of autoimmune complications of collagen vascular diseases such as systemic lupus erythematosus, or lymphoproliferative diseases such as chronic lymphocytic leukemia
    - May even be the presenting manifestation of these disorders
- Many forms of treatment have demonstrated effectiveness in ITP
  - Platelet transfusions used only in case of severe, life-threatening hemorrhage
  - Initial therapy usually with corticosteroids
    - Dosage equivalent to 1 mg/kg/day of prednisone
  - If platelet count does not rise substantially within 2 to 3 weeks
    - Splenectomy usually the next step
      - Produces prolonged remissions in two-thirds of cases
      - Partial remission in 15% of patients
      - May be necessary in patients who responded to steroids but cannot be weaned from drug without recurrence
  - The 10% to 20% of patients who don't respond to splenectomy may benefit from:
    - Vincristine or immunosuppressive agents such as cyclophosphamide
  - Anabolic steroid, danazol, given for several months, effective in some cases of ITP
  - Large doses of IVIG may increase platelet count in ITP

○ Perhaps through blockage of reticuloendothelial sites of platelet destruction
○ Therapy costly and short duration
 – Usually 2 to 3 weeks
• Anti-D therapy effective only in Rh(D)+ patients
 ○ Not effective in splenectomized patients
• Rituximab, a chimeric anti-CD20 monoclonal antibody shown to be effective in chronic ITP
 ○ Goal in treating chronic or refractory ITP to maintain a safe platelet count
  – Defined as >10,000 to 20,000 cells/μL
  – And minimize morbidity and mortality associated with treatment
• When ITP occurs during pregnancy additional concern that IgG autoantibody may cross placenta and produce thrombocytopenia in fetus and newborn
 • Lowest platelet count usually seen several days after birth
 • Current practice is to use standard obstetric management of pregnancy and delivery
 • ITP should be differentiated from gestational thrombocytopenia
  • Occurs in about 5% of normal women with uncomplicated pregnancies
  • Most important clue to differentiating is a history of previous thrombocytopenia when woman was not pregnant
  • More severe thrombocytopenia occurring before third trimester more likely to be ITP

Thrombotic Thrombocytopenic Purpura

• TTP and its closely related disorders may be catastrophic and rapidly fatal:
 • Hemolytic-uremic syndrome (HUS)
 • Thrombotic microangiopathy (TMA)
 • Peripartum HELLP (hemolysis, elevated liver enzymes, and low platelets) syndrome
• TTP a pentad of abnormalities:
 • Thrombocytopenia from increased platelet destruction
 • Microangiopathic hemolytic anemia (MHA)
  • Caused by mechanical damage to RBCs as a result of the vascular lesions
 • Neurologic abnormalities
 • Renal abnormalities
 • Fever
• Thrombocytopenia and MHA sufficient to begin plasmapheresis
• Clinical presentation variable, but thrombocytopenia and hemolytic anemia often severe
• Wide variety of fluctuating neurologic abnormalities may be present, including:
 • Seizures
 • Altered consciousness
 • Delirium
 • Paresis
• Renal abnormalities may include:
 • Uremia
 • Hematuria
 • Proteinuria
• Reasons for fever are unclear
• Typical presentation for young children:

• Prodrome of bloody diarrhea caused by the Shiga toxin-producing enterohemorrhagic strain of *E. coli*
• Laboratory findings in TTP those related to the above features:
• Thrombocytopenia
• Hemolytic anemia with red cell fragmentation
• Renal dysfunction
• Elevation of serum lactic acid dehydrogenase from intravascular hemolysis, and perhaps also damage to other tissues, is an index of activity of the disease
• Coagulation tests usually normal
• Basic pathogenic mechanism behind these syndromes most likely vascular endothelial cells
 • Role for ultralarge von Willebrand factor (vWf) multimers identified
  • Linked to endothelial damage and occurrence of disseminated platelet thrombi
  • Specific metalloprotease (ADAMTS13) that rapidly cleaves multimers identified
  • Deficiency of metalloprotease activity associated with many TTP cases
• Plasma exchange has dramatically changed TTP-HUS prognosis and outcome
 • Plasma infusion less effective in adults
 • Could be adequate in congenital TTP caused by ADAMTS13 deficiency
 • Duration of plasma exchange is unpredictable
  • Up to several months, may be required in patients with repeated relapses
 • Efficacy of additional treatments such as prednisone, platelet aggregation inhibitors, and splenectomy unknown

Alcoholism-Associated Thrombocytopenia

• Platelet counts <100,000 cells/μL present in >25% of critically ill alcoholic patients
 • Many possible causes for thrombocytopenia in such patients
  • Hypersplenism
  • Folic acid deficiency
  • Reversible severe thrombocytopenia may be direct effect of alcohol ingestion in some patients
 • Studies of mechanism have demonstrated:
  • Decreased effective platelet production
  • Shortened platelet survival
  • Abnormalities of platelet function have been noted
 • Recovery begins 2 to 3 days after cessation of alcohol ingestion
  • Maximum platelet counts reached in 1 to 3 weeks
  • Often an overshoot to abnormally high platelet counts
  • Then return to baseline levels
 • Therapy consists of having patient discontinue alcohol ingestion and providing appropriate supportive measures

Thrombocytopenia Associated with Bone Marrow Disorders

• Severe thrombocytopenia from impaired platelet production a frequent concomitant of bone marrow disorders
 • Aplastic anemia
 • Leukemia

- Other malignancies metastatic to the bone marrow
- Cytotoxic chemotherapy
- Treatment is directed at the underlying disease

INCREASED BLOOD COUNTS

Erythrocytosis

- An abnormally increased red cell mass
  - May require critical care due to:
    - Complications of blood hyperviscosity
    - Hemorrhagic or thromboembolic complications
  - Initial clue to presence of erythrocytosis usually high value for Hgb/Hct
    - May be present without true erythrocytosis if plasma volume contracted
    - Red cell mass (RCM) usually increased when hematocrit above 60% in a man or 57% in a woman
- True erythrocytosis results from one of two general mechanisms:
  - Polycythemia vera (PV), a clonal abnormality of bone marrow stem cells resulting in autonomous overproduction of RBCs and often of granulocytes and platelets
  - Secondary erythrocytosis, resulting from excess erythropoietin production in response to:
    - Hypoxemia
    - Abnormalities of oxygen release from hemoglobin
    - Autonomous hormone production (e.g., by renal or other tumors)
  - When RCM expanded and hematocrit increased
    - Blood viscosity is increased
    - Diminished blood flow, stasis, thrombosis, and tissue hypoxia may ensue
    - Hemorrhagic tendency also increased, particularly in PV
      - Elevated platelet counts and abnormalities of function may be present

Polycythemia Vera

- Diagnosis of PV shown in Table 121.4
  - Detection by polymerase chain reaction (PCR) of Janus kinase 2 (JAK2) tyrosine kinase in up to 97% of patients with PV increases sensitivity/specificity of early diagnosis
    - JAK2 V617F point mutation makes hematopoietic progenitors hypersensitive to the different growth factors, resulting in proliferation of all lineages
  - Uncontrolled PV risks primarily hyperviscosity and thromboembolic or hemorrhagic events
  - Patients at highest risk those:
    - Whose disease has shown particularly active cell proliferation, requiring extensive therapy
    - With a prior history of complications
    - The elderly
    - Level of Hct or platelet count not a reliable predictor
  - Symptoms resulting from decreased cerebral flow:
    - Headache
    - Dizziness
    - Changes in vision the most common manifestations of hyperviscosity

TABLE 121.4

PROPOSED MODIFIED CRITERIA FOR THE DIAGNOSIS OF POLYCYTHEMIA VERA (PV)

A1: Raised red cell mass
25% above mean normal predicted value, or a hematocrit value >60% in males or 56% in females
A2: Absence of causes of secondary erythrocytosis
A3: Palpable splenomegaly
A4: Clonality marker (i.e., acquired abnormal marrow karyotype)
B1: Thrombocytosis
Platelet count >400 × 10³ cells/μL
B2: Neutrophil leukocytosis
Neutrophil count >10 × 10³ cells/μL, or >12.5 × 10³ cells/μL in smokers
B3: Splenomegaly demonstrated on isotope or ultrasound scanning
B4: Characteristic BFU-E growth or reduced serum erythropoietin
A1 + A2 + A3 or A4 establishes PV
A1 + A2 + two of B establishes PV

BFU-E, erythroid burst-forming units.
Adapted from Pearson TC, Messinezy M, Westwood N, et al. A polycythemia vera updated: diagnosis, pathobiology, and treatment. *Hematol Am Soc Hematol Educ Program.* 2000;51.

- Hemorrhage or thrombosis can affect almost any body part
  - Peptic ulcer disease with bleeding common
  - Thromboses may be arterial or venous
- Fatigue, plethora, pruritus particularly with hot bath, excessive sweating, paresthesias (erythromelalgia), fullness in the left upper abdomen (splenomegaly), and shortness of breath PV manifestations
- Surgery poses enormous risk in patient with uncontrolled PV
  - High incidence of thrombotic or hemorrhagic complications
  - Uncontrolled PV patients may present as medical emergencies requiring ICU care and urgent therapy
    - Mainstay of such therapy is phlebotomy to reduce Hct to <45%
    - May be done as rapidly as 1 unit RBC every other day in young adults
    - Electrolyte solutions administered with phlebotomy to avoid circulatory instability
    - Elderly patients may tolerate phlebotomy less well
      - Removal of volumes of 200 to 300 mL at less frequent intervals may be necessary
    - Clinical observations of increased thrombosis with aggressive phlebotomy
      - Simultaneous use of cytotoxic chemotherapy is recommended as part of the initial therapy of patients older than 60 years and in younger patients with thrombotic risk factors or a history of thrombosis
      - Hydroxyurea used for this purpose
        - Initial dose of 15 to 30 mg/kg/day
        - Long-term treatment with hydroxyurea may be linked with increased risk of transformation to acute leukemia
        - Emergency plateletpheresis may also be considered in such emergencies to lower an elevated platelet count

○ Other treatment options include:
  – Low-dose aspirin (81 mg/day)
  – Interferon-α
  – Anagrelide
- Patients with PV should avoid practices and habits that augment hypercoagulability:
  - Smoking
  - Use of oral contraceptives
  - Hormone replacement therapy
  - Aggressive antithrombotic prophylaxis given postoperatively in addition to maintaining normal hematocrit and platelet counts

Secondary Erythrocytosis or Polycythemia

- Diagnosis of secondary erythrocytosis is made in patient with:
- Increased RCM in whom the criteria for PV not met
- These patients either have:
  - Physiologically appropriate increased RCM (i.e., secondary to tissue hypoxemia)
  - Inappropriately increased RCM (i.e., secondary to increased erythropoietin production)
- Additional studies needed to differentiate diverse causes of polycythemia
- Indications for phlebotomy in secondary erythrocytosis less clear than in PV
  - Best current advice to individualize therapy to maximize patient's exercise tolerance and overall sense of well-being

Thrombocytosis

- Literature dealing with thrombocytosis in ICU patients very scant
  - Presence of thrombocytosis predicts a favorable outcome in ICU patients
  - Blunted rise in platelet count may be associated with worse outcome
  - Classified according to origin into primary (clonal) and secondary (reactive) forms
    - Primary, a persistent elevation of platelet count due to clonal thrombopoiesis
      ○ Occurs in myeloproliferative disorders including essential thrombocythemia (ET), PV, myelodysplastic syndrome, chronic myelogenous leukemia, and myelofibrosis
    - Secondary, due to various conditions, some of them short-lived, such as acute bleeding, infection, trauma or other tissue injury, and surgery
      ○ Other causes, such as malignancy, postsplenectomy, chronic infection, iron deficiency, or chronic inflammatory disease may persist for a longer time
  - Multiple studies conducted on adult and pediatric hospitalized patients with an elevated platelet count ($>500 \times 10^3$ cells/μL)
    - Most patients have secondary thrombocytosis
      ○ Higher platelet count and increased thromboembolic complications are significantly associated with primary thrombocytosis
      ○ Even when using $\geq 1,000 \times 10^3$ cells/μL as the basis for defining extreme thrombocytosis

○ 82% of 231 patients analyzed were found to have an elevated platelet count due to reactive (secondary) thrombocytosis
  – Risk of bleeding and/or thrombosis:
    • 56% in primary thrombocytosis
    • 4% in secondary type
    • Unless additional risk factors present, secondary thrombocytosis not associated with increased risk of thromboembolic events
- Treatment for primary thrombocytosis, such as ET, based on risks for thrombosis or bleeding in presence of vasomotor symptoms
- Patients at increased risk should receive platelet-lowering agents such as hydroxyurea, anagrelide, or interferon-α (IFN-α)
  - Age older than 60 years
  - History of thromboembolism
  - Platelet count $>1,500,000$ cells/μL
- Low-dose aspirin can be used for relief of vasomotor symptoms
  - If no relief, platelet-lowering agents should be added
  - Hydroxyurea the recommended drug in patients ≥ 60 years of age
  - IFN-α is the cytoreductive agent of choice for childbearing women
- Aim to lower the platelet count to $<400,000$ cells/μL
- Arterial or venous thrombosis treated with heparin, possibly, thrombolysis
- Plateletpheresis may be indicated in both types of events
- Low-dose aspirin may be useful in arterial thrombosis
- In hemorrhage, it is appropriate to stop antiplatelet agents and transfuse platelets if bleeding persists
- Some patients with uncontrolled thrombocytosis ($>1,500,000$ cells/μL) have an acquired defect of vWf
  - Contributes to risk of bleeding
  - DDAVP, cryoprecipitate, or factor VIII concentrate may be indicated

Leukocytosis

- Can be due to primary bone marrow disorders or secondary disorders in response to acute infection or inflammation
- Secondary leukocytosis is physiologic and transient, resolving after treating the underlying cause
  - *Leukemoid reaction* refers to a persistent leukocytosis of more than 50,000 cells/μL with shift to left
    ○ Major causes for such a reaction include severe infections, severe hemorrhage, acute hemolysis, hypersensitivity, and malignancies (paraneoplastic syndrome)
- Due to a primary bone marrow disorder with uncontrolled clonal growth of immature cells can result in an emergency situation known as hyperleukocytosis syndrome
  - Occurs in leukemic states when the WBC count is high
  - Signs and symptoms are most commonly related to the central nervous system, eyes, and lungs and include:
    ○ Stupor
    ○ Altered mentation
    ○ Dizziness
    ○ Visual blurring
    ○ Retinal abnormalities

○ Dyspnea
○ Tachypnea
○ Hypoxia
- Intracranial and pulmonary infarction or hemorrhage and sudden death may occur
- Priapism and peripheral vascular insufficiency linked with syndrome
- Pathogenesis incompletely understood, but autopsies have shown WBC aggregates, microthrombi, and microvascular invasion (leukostatic tumors)
- Syndrome occurs more commonly in acute (AML) and chronic myelogenous leukemia (CML) than in acute lymphoblastic leukemia
  ○ Rarely in chronic lymphocytic leukemia
- Level of WBC count syndrome appears is variable
  ○ Depending on maturity and size of WBCs present and degree of coexisting anemia
  ○ WBC count >100,000 cells/μL in AML or accelerated phase of CML usually an alarming sign and indication for prompt treatment
  ○ Signs or symptoms attributable to the hyperleukocytosis syndrome:
    – Leukophoresis indicated, rapidly/safely decrease WBC count
    – Chemotherapy initiated
      • Treatment with allopurinol and IV hydration with urine alkalinization started in anticipation of hyperuricemia
      • Hydroxyurea (6 g by mouth) frequently used initially to produce rapid leukemic cell kill

OTHER HEMATOLOGIC DISORDERS

Plasma Cell Dyscrasias

- Presenting symptoms for these malignant disorders may include:
- Severe infection
- Spinal cord compression
- Hyperviscosity syndrome
- Total serum protein abnormally high on routine chemistry blood test
  - Subsequent evaluation will reveal monoclonal gammopathy:
    ○ IgM in Waldenstrom macroglobulinemia
    ○ IgG/IgA in multiple myeloma

- Hyperviscosity syndrome rare and less frequent when IgG or IgA, respectively, are abnormal proteins
- Most common manifestations of the hyperviscosity syndrome are:
  ○ Neurologic, including headache, visual disturbances, hearing loss, vertigo, altered consciousness (ranging from stupor to coma), paresis, seizures, and peripheral neuropathy
  ○ Bleeding tendency may exist because of associated thrombocytopenia or interference by abnormal protein with function of platelets or plasma coagulation factors
- Most rapidly effective form of therapy for hyperviscosity from serum protein abnormalities is plasmapheresis
  ○ Hydration and specific therapy for underlying disease should start

STEM CELL TRANSPLANTATION (SCT)

- After allogeneic SCT a large proportion admitted to ICU
- Usually admitted with respiratory distress requiring mechanical ventilation, multiorgan failure, or septic shock
- Have the highest mortality among cancer patients admitted to ICU
- Because of generally poor outcome, especially for patients requiring mechanical ventilation, utility of such support questioned
- Generally accepted that patients admitted to ICU during engraftment period be fully supported because of better outcome
- Patients may have *engraftment syndrome*, can result in cytokine-induced capillary leak syndrome with multiorgan failure or alveolar hemorrhage
  - Early high-dose steroids dramatically reverse downhill course
  - Patients should also undergo bronchoscopy to rule out infection while receiving steroid therapy
- Early intervention and transfer to ICU in septic shock results in improved outcome
- After autologous SCT patients usually have better survival in ICU than after allogeneic SCT
- Even those requiring mechanical ventilation
- Admission to surgical ICU less frequent for patients after SCT, most frequent reasons include:
- Intestinal perforation
- Intracranial bleeding

CHAPTER 122 ■ ONCOLOGIC EMERGENCIES

- Cancer the second leading cause of death in United States, surpassed only by heart disease
  - Approximately 1 million new cases of squamous and basal skin cancers, and 1,445,000 new cases of all other cancers (excluding carcinoma *in situ*, with the exception of *in situ* bladder carcinoma) diagnosed yearly
  - 5-year relative survival rate of 66% calculated for all cancers diagnosed between period of 1996 and 2002
    - Compared to 51% between 1975 and 1977

HYPERCALCEMIA

- The most common of paraneoplastic syndromes
- Develops in 10% to 30% of all patients with malignancy at some time during disease
  - Breast cancer, lung cancer, and multiple myeloma most common associated malignancies
  - Presence in patient with cancer portends an extremely poor prognosis
    - Particularly when elevated parathyroid hormone-related protein (PTHrP) levels detected
    - About 50% of cancer patients with hypercalcemia die within 30 days

Pathophysiology

- Results from increased bone resorption
  - Subsequent release of calcium from bone into extracellular fluid
  - Classification based on mechanism by which elevated calcium generated; four recognized types:
    - Humoral hypercalcemia of malignancy (HHM)
    - Local osteolytic hypercalcemia
    - Tumor production of the active form of vitamin D
    - Ectopic parathyroid hormone (PTH) secretion

Humoral Hypercalcemia of Malignancy

- Most common cause of cancer-induced hypercalcemia (CIH)
  - Seen in 80% of cases
  - Mechanism mediated by PTHrP
  - Secreted into systemic circulation by malignant tumors
    - Most frequently squamous cell carcinoma, renal cell carcinoma, ovarian and endometrial carcinomas, human T-cell lymphoma/leukemia virus (HTLV)-associated lymphomas, and breast carcinoma
  - Normally PTHrP expressed in nonneoplastic adult and fetal tissues
    - Involved in cell growth and differentiation
    - Not systemically secreted in significantly detectable levels

- Due to structural homology with parathyroid hormone at amino terminal end, humoral PTHrP binds to PTH receptors in bone and kidney
  - With increased bone resorption, distal tubular calcium resorption

Local Osteolytic Hypercalcemia

- Seen in about 20% of cases of malignant hypercalcemia
  - Occurs when tumor cells in bone metastases induce osteoclastic bone resorption
    - By secreting cytokines such as tumor necrosis factor (TNF), interleukin-1 (IL-1), IL-6, macrophage inflammatory protein, and lymphotoxin
      - Stimulate local macrophages within tumor to differentiate into osteoclasts
  - Seen frequently in breast cancer, non–small cell lung cancer, and multiple myeloma

Tumor Production of the Active Form of 1,25-dehydroxyvitamin D

- Occurs in <1% of cases
- Seen in some lymphomas
- Hypercalcemia mediated by:
  - Enhancement of osteoclastic bone resorption
  - Intestinal resorption of calcium

Ectopic Parathyroid Hormone Secretion

- Final mechanism of hypercalcemia of malignancy is ectopic PTH secretion
- Adequately described in only eight patients

Differential Diagnosis

- Malignancies and primary hyperparathyroidism account for about 90% of hypercalcemia cases
  - May coexist in critically ill cancer patient
  - In hospitalized patients, neoplastic disease most common cause in >65% of cases
  - Renal failure, thyrotoxicosis, granulomatous diseases (sarcoid, tuberculosis), adrenal insufficiency, immobilization, vitamin A or D intoxication, milk alkali syndrome, familial hypocalciuric hypercalcemia, and medications (thiazide diuretics, lithium, estrogens, and tamoxifen) included in the differential diagnosis of hypercalcemia

Clinical Presentation

- Multiple symptoms of hypercalcemia (Table 122.1)
  - Nonspecific and often attributed to coexisting chronic or terminal illness

---

TABLE 122.1

CLINICAL MANIFESTATIONS IN HYPERCALCEMIA

NEUROLOGIC
Drowsiness, weakness, lethargy
Stupor, coma
Psychosis
Visual and speech impairment
Focal neurologic deficits

GASTROINTESTINAL
Anorexia
Nausea, vomiting
Constipation
Abdominal pain
Peptic ulcer disease
Pancreatitis

RENAL
Nephrogenic diabetes insipidus
Acute renal failure

CARDIAC
PR interval prolongation
QRS complex widening
QT interval shortening
T wave changes
Bradyarrhythmias
Bundle branch block
Atrioventricular nodal block
Cardiac arrest

BONE
Pain
Pathologic fractures

Data from Stewart AF. Hypercalcemia associated with cancer. *N Engl J Med.* 2005;352:373; Halfdanarson TR, Hogan WJ, Moynihan TJ. Oncological emergencies: diagnosis and treatment. *Mayo Clin Proc.* 2006;81(6):835; Hypercalcemia. *CancerMail from the National Cancer Institute.* http://cancerweb.ncl.ac.uk; Germano T. The parathyroid gland and calcium-related emergencies. *Top Emerg Med.* 2001;23(4):51; Bushinsky DA, Monk RD. Calcium. *Lancet.* 1998;352:306; Cogan MG, Covey GM, Arieff AL, et al. Central nervous system manifestations of hyperparathyroidism. *Am J Med.* 1978;65:963; 2005 American Heart Association Guidelines for Cardiopulmonary Resuscitation and Emergency Cardiovascular Care. *Circulation.* 2005;112(24 Suppl):IV1–121; and Berensen JR. Treatment of hypercalcemia with bisphosphonates. *Semin Oncol.* 2002:29(6 Suppl 21):12.

- Symptoms generally correlate with absolute concentration and rapidity in rise of serum calcium
  - Neurologic symptoms mild at lower levels or when hypercalcemia developed slowly
    - Mild drowsiness or fatigue may progress to weakness, lethargy, stupor, and eventually coma in hypercalcemic crisis or in acutely rising hypercalcemia
    - Psychotic behavior, visual and speech abnormalities, hypotonia, and occasionally localizing signs on examination, often attributed to metastatic disease, may be exhibited
      - May resolve with therapy that lowers serum calcium
    - In older patients, neurologic dysfunction more pronounced at lower concentrations of serum calcium
  - Gastrointestinal symptoms related to smooth muscle hypotonicity and include anorexia, nausea, vomiting, constipation, and abdominal pain
    - Infrequently may present as peptic ulcer disease and pancreatitis
  - Renal manifestations due to impairment of renal water-concentrating ability
    - Antidiuretic hormone (ADH) secretion inhibited by hypercalcemia
    - Dehydration decreases glomerular filtration rate (GFR) and renal excretion of excess calcium
    - With expansion of extracellular volume (ECV), compensatory proximal tubular resorption of sodium and calcium occurs
      - Leads to paradoxical increase in serum calcium
      - Frank renal failure may ensue
        - Particularly in patient with multiple myeloma
    - Hypercalcemia of malignancy rarely associated with nephrolithiasis and nephrocalcinosis
      - Hypercalciuria must be chronic for these to occur
  - Cardiovascular symptoms of hypercalcemia marked by:
    - Increased myocardial contractility and irritability
    - Electrocardiogram (ECG) changes include:
      - PR-interval prolongation
      - QRS-complex widening
      - QT-interval shortening
      - T-wave changes
    - At increasing serum calcium levels patients may experience bradyarrhythmias and bundle branch block
      - With progression to atrioventricular (AV) nodal block and cardiac arrest at serum concentrations of 18 mg/dL
  - Bone symptoms of hypercalcemia include:
    - Pathologic fractures and pain
    - Due to osteolytic metastases or humorally mediated bone resorption

---

Diagnosis

- Calcium present in ECF in three fractions:
  - 50% is ionized free fraction
  - 40% is protein bound (primarily to albumin) and is not renally filtered
  - 10% complexed to anions
- Hypercalcemia diagnosed by measuring ionized calcium level
  - Biologically active level correlating with signs and symptoms of hypercalcemia
  - Except in presence of hypoalbuminemia ionized calcium inferred from total plasma calcium
  - In cancer patients, hypoalbuminemia common
    - Total plasma calcium must be corrected to reflect the calcium level measured as if albumin were in normal range
    - For each 1 g/dL decrease in serum albumin, there is a 0.8 mg/dL decrease in serum calcium
    - Calculation inaccurate with calcium-binding immunoglobulins (multiple myeloma)
      - Warrants measurement of ionized calcium level
        - Total serum calcium significantly overestimates ionized fraction
        - Ionized calcium concentrations increase with acidosis and decrease with alkalosis
          - Changes small and not clinically significant
- Once diagnosis of hypercalcemia confirmed by obtaining corrected calcium levels

- Measurement of intact PTH level necessary:
  - Suppressed in hypercalcemia of malignancy
  - Elevated in primary hyperparathyroidism
  - PTH lowers serum phosphate and increases serum Cl– concentrations
    - Low serum Cl– (<100 mEq/L) suggests hypercalcemia of malignancy
    - Elevation of serum Cl– caused by hyperchloremic acidosis resulting from PTH-induced renal bicarbonate loss
    - Ectopic hyperparathyroidism rare cause of malignant hypercalcemia
      - Elevations in PTH levels more likely indicate concomitant primary hyperparathyroidism
  - Determination of serum PTHrP concentration not routine
    - Useful in identifying mechanism of hypercalcemia
      - Low in patients with primary hyperparathyroidism
      - High in patients with either HHM alone or concomitant primary hyperparathyroidism and malignant hypercalcemia
      - Used in evaluating response to bisphosphonate therapy
        - Patients with PTHrP levels >12 pmol/L less responsive to pamidronate
        - More likely to develop recurrent hypercalcemia within 14 days

Treatment

- **Only effective long-term therapy of malignancy-associated hypercalcemia reduction in tumor burden** (Table 122.2)
- Antihypercalcemic therapy a temporizing measure
  - **Does not affect survival**
- Hypercalcemia classified based on serum calcium levels into:
  - Mild hypercalcemia (10.5–11.9 mg/dL)
  - Moderate hypercalcemia (12.0–13.9 mg/dL)
  - Severe hypercalcemia (14.0 mg/dL or greater)
  - Treatment strategy dependent on:
    - Magnitude of hypercalcemia
    - Severity of symptoms
    - Cause of hypercalcemia
- Severe hypercalcemia requires emergent, aggressive treatment regardless of symptoms
- Interventions in mild to moderate hypercalcemia contingent on severity of symptoms
  - Prior to initiating therapy assess for correctable factors contributing to hypercalcemia
    - Exogenous sources of calcium
    - Thiazide diuretics, vitamins A and D, calcitriol, lithium, and estrogens or antiestrogens used as therapy for breast carcinoma

---

TABLE 122.2

TREATMENT OF HYPERCALCEMIA OF MALIGNANCY

Definitive Treatment
Antitumor therapy to reduce tumor burden

Initial Treatment
Removal of exogenous calcium sources:
Intravenous fluids, parenteral nutrition, oral calcium supplements, thiazide diuretics, vitamins A and D, calcitriol, lithium, estrogens, antiestrogens
Weight-bearing ambulation
Phosphate repletion
Fluids and diuresis
Saline hydration

Loop diuretics	Judicious use in euvolemic or hypervolemic patients; now less favorable because of hypokalemia, hypomagnesemia, volume depletion

Pharmacologic Treatment
Bisphosphonate therapy
Principal agents in hypercalcemic treatment

Zoledronate	15-min infusion
Pamidronate	2-h infusion
	Bisphosphonate adverse effects: acute and chronic renal failure, fever arthralgias, ocular inflammation, electrolyte imbalance, osteonecrosis of the jaw

Other agents

Calcitonin	Useful in congestive heart failure or renal failure
Glucocorticoids	Used in lymphomas with elevated levels of 1,25-vitamin D
Mithramycin	Use limited by adverse effects: thrombocytopenia, anemia, leukopenia, renal failure
Gallium nitrate	Use limited by 5-day continuous infusion, nephrotoxicity

Dialysis
For patients with renal failure or congestive heart failure

Data from Stewart AF. Hypercalcemia associated with cancer. *N Engl J Med.* 2005;352:373; Halfdanarson TR, Hogan WJ, Moynihan TJ. Oncological emergencies: diagnosis and treatment. *Mayo Clin Proc.* 2006;81(6):835; Hypercalcemia. *CancerMail from the National Cancer Institute.* http://cancerweb.ncl.ac.uk; Germano T. The parathyroid gland and calcium-related emergencies. *Topics in Emerg Med.* 2001;23(4):51; Bushinsky DA, Monk RD. Calcium. *Lancet.* 1998;352:306; Cheng C, Chou C, Lin S. An unrecognized cause of recurrent hypercalcemia: immobilization. *South Med J.* 2006;99(4):371; Body JJ. Hypercalcemia of malignancy. *Semin Nephrol.* 2004;24:48; Berenson JR, Lipton A. Bisphosphonates in the treatment of malignant bone disease. *Annu Rev Med.* 1999;50:237; and Tanveyanon T, Stiff PJ. Management of the adverse effects associated with intravenous bisphosphonates. *Ann Oncol.* 2006;(17):897.

○ Immobilization well-established cause of hypercalcemia
  – Weight-bearing ambulation recommended whenever possible
○ In the presence of hypophosphatemia, hypercalcemia more difficult to treat
  – Observed in cancer patients for multiple reasons including:
    • Poor nutrition
    • Saline diuresis
    • PTHrP effects
    • Use of antacids and loop diuretics
    • Hypercalcemia itself
  – Oral/nasogastric tube phosphate supplementation administered to keep the calcium-phosphate product between 30 and 40
    • Intravenous (IV) phosphorous may precipitate hypocalcemia, seizures, and acute renal failure
    • Reserved for patient in whom oral/nasogastric tube administration cannot be performed

Fluids and Diuretics

• Initial intervention administration of isotonic saline at a rate of 200 to 500 mL/hour
  • Based on degree of hypovolemia and renal and cardiovascular dysfunction
  • Once fluid deficit replaced
    • Rate decreased to 100 to 200 mL/hour
    • In patients without cardiac or renal impairment
  • Reduces serum calcium level by:
    • Increasing glomerular filtration rate
    • Increasing calcium delivery to proximal tubule
      ○ Urinary calcium excretion augmented by calciuric effects of saline
  • Loop diuretics inhibit calcium reabsorption at loop of Henle, increasing calciuresis
    • Judiciously used after euvolemia achieved in hypovolemic patients or in patients presenting with volume overload
    • Complications include hypokalemia, hypomagnesemia, and volume depletion

Bisphosphonate Therapy

• Inhibit osteoclastic bone resorption
  • The principal agents in management of hypercalcemia of malignancy
• Compared to saline and diuretics alone, and other antiresorptive agents including calcitonin
  • Bisphosphonates superior treating hypercalcemia of malignancy
  • Only 1% to 2% of oral bisphosphonates absorbed
  • Drugs administered IV
• Pamidronate and zoledronate most commonly used bisphosphonates for treatment of hypercalcemia of malignancy
  • Clodronate and ibandronate available in Europe and elsewhere
• Patients respond to bisphosphonate therapy within 2 to 4 days
  • Nadir in serum calcium occurring within 4 to 7 days
  • Normocalcemia may persist for 2 to 4 weeks
• Zoledronate 850 times more potent than pamidronate and is more efficacious

• Pooled analysis of two randomized controlled trials
  ○ Single 4-mg dose of zoledronic acid to 90-mg dose of pamidronate
  ○ Serum calcium concentrations normalized within 10 days
    – In 88% versus 70% of patients, respectively
  ○ Duration of response was 32 days versus 18 days, respectively
• Zoledronate administered over shorter interval of 15 minutes
  ○ Advantageous in outpatient setting
  ○ Pamidronate requires a 2-hour infusion
• Both zoledronate and pamidronate associated with acute and chronic renal failure
  • More adverse events reported with zoledronate
  • Dose reduction of zoledronate recommended in patients with creatinine clearance between 30 and 60 mL/minute
  • No change in dose or infusion rate of pamidronate in patients with serum creatinine of <3 mg/dL
• Other complications of bisphosphonates include:
  • Acute systemic inflammatory reactions such as fever and arthralgias
  • Ocular inflammation
  • Electrolyte imbalance
  • Osteonecrosis of the jaw

Other Agents

• Calcitonin a well-tolerated synthetic polypeptide analogue of salmon calcitonin
  • Reduces serum calcium levels by inhibiting bone resorption
  • Administered subcutaneously or intramuscularly, produces rapid, transient decrease in serum calcium in 12 to 24 hours
  • Useful in patients with congestive heart failure (CHF) or renal failure where saline, diuresis, and bisphosphonates contraindicated
  • Tachyphylaxis may occur with continued use
• Glucocorticoids effective in decreasing serum calcium in hypercalcemia of malignancy associated with some lymphomas, particularly Hodgkin lymphoma
  • Elevated 1,25-vitamin D present in Hodgkin lymphoma
  • Glucocorticoids
    • Increase renal calcium excretion
    • Block vitamin D–mediated calcium absorption in gastrointestinal (GI) tract
    • Have limited utility in acute setting because reduction in serum calcium may not be observed for 1 to 2 weeks
• Mithramycin, an inhibitor of osteoclast RNA synthesis
  • Formerly first-line hypocalcemic agent
  • Has serious adverse effects including:
    • Thrombocytopenia
    • Anemia
    • Leukopenia
    • Renal failure
• Gallium nitrate
  • Disadvantage of requiring continuous IV infusion over 5 days
  • Potential nephrotoxicity
• Dialysis may be used to treat patients with hypercalcemia complicated by renal failure or CHF

ACUTE TUMOR LYSIS SYNDROME (ATLS)

Definition

- ATLS occurs as a consequence of rapid and massive destruction of tumor cells, resulting in
  - Release of intracellular metabolites into circulation
    - In quantities sufficient to exceed renal excretory capacity
  - The four biochemical disturbances generated by this process that characterize the syndrome are life threatening:
    - Hyperkalemia
    - Hyperphosphatemia
    - Hypocalcemia
    - Hyperuricemia
- ATLS is most frequently observed after administration of cytotoxic chemotherapy in patients with high-grade hematologic malignancies:
  - Burkitt's lymphoma
  - Acute lymphocytic leukemia (ALL)
  - Incidence of clinically significant ATLS in non-Hodgkin lymphoma and ALL:
    - Reported as 6% and 5.2%, respectively
  - Metabolic derangements in patients may develop within hours to days after chemotherapy
- Other malignancies in which ATLS has been described include:
  - Chronic leukemia
  - Low-grade lymphoma
  - Rarely, multiple solid tumors such as:
    - Metastatic breast carcinoma
    - Lung carcinoma
    - Seminoma
    - Thymoma
    - Medulloblastoma
    - Ovarian carcinoma
    - Rhabdomyosarcoma
    - Melanoma
    - Vulvar carcinoma
    - Merkel cell carcinoma
  - Syndrome can also occur after:
    - Radiation therapy
    - Immunotherapy (rituximab and interferon)
    - Endocrine therapy (corticosteroids and tamoxifen)
- Spontaneous tumor lysis syndrome (STLS) a rare entity that develops primarily in Burkitt lymphoma and leukemia absent any treatment
  - Increased purine metabolism from high tumor cell turnover rates leads to hyperuricemia and consequent uric acid nephropathy
  - Prompt recognition of STLS essential because it is associated with poor outcomes and high mortality rates
- Predisposing factors for developing ATLS include:
  - Large tumor burdens
  - Bulky lymphadenopathy
  - Extensive bone marrow involvement
  - Rapid tumor cell proliferation
  - Leukocytosis ($>50 \times 10^3$ cells/μL)
  - Elevated lactate dehydrogenase (LDH) ($>1,500$ IU)
  - High tumor chemosensitivity
- Pretreatment hyperuricemia, renal dysfunction, and hypovolemia, and treatment with nephrotoxic agents confer increased risk of ATLS

Pathophysiology

- Rapid dissolution of cells with aggressive cytotoxic therapy results in:
- Increase in plasma uric acid, potassium, and phosphorus levels
  - Hyperphosphatemia results in precipitation secondary hypocalcemia
  - Hyperkalemia occurs 6 to 72 hours after administration of chemotherapy
    - Associated manifestations include:
      - Lethargy
      - Nausea and vomiting
      - Diarrhea
      - Muscle weakness
      - Paresthesias
      - ECG abnormalities such as peaked T waves, PR-interval prolongation, and QRS-complex widening
      - Ventricular arrhythmias may lead to sudden death
  - Hyperphosphatemia is seen 24 to 48 hours following chemotherapy
    - Malignant cells have up to four times more phosphorous than nonneoplastic cells
    - As plasma phosphorous increases with cell lysis:
      - The normal renal mechanism that excretes excess phosphate and prevents distal tubular reabsorption becomes overwhelmed
        - Leading to hyperphosphatemia
    - Signs and symptoms of acute hyperphosphatemia are manifestations of secondary hypocalcemia, and range from:
      - No symptoms to anorexia, vomiting, confusion, neuromuscular irritability, tetany, carpopedal spasm, seizures, dysrhythmias, and cardiac arrest
  - Secondary hypocalcemia seen with hyperphosphatemia because:
    - Calcium phosphate precipitates when product exceeds 60, into:
      - Renal interstitium and tubules, resulting in nephrocalcinosis
    - Hypocalcemia persists after correction of hyperphosphatemia
      - Inappropriately low plasma calcitriol level present
      - Causes rise in serum PTH
        - Increases phosphate resorption in proximal tubule
        - Leads to nephrocalcinosis, acute renal failure
  - Hyperuricemia occurs 48 to 72 hours after chemotherapy
    - Patients may exhibit nonspecific symptoms such as:
      - Nausea, vomiting, anorexia, and lethargy
    - Acute renal failure with associated oliguria, edema, hypertension, and altered sensorium seen in untreated patients
    - Uric acid generated from hepatic purine metabolism
      - Adenosine and guanosine nucleotides degraded to hypoxanthine and xanthine, respectively
      - Xanthine oxidase converts these to uric acid

– Rapidly proliferating neoplastic cells have high turnover rates:
  • With accelerated purine catabolism from DNA and RNA degradation
  • Cells contain large amounts of purine nucleotides
  • With cytotoxic therapy, there is rapid rise in plasma uric acid
  • Uric acid excreted by kidneys through processes of:
    • GFR
    • Partial proximal tubular reabsorption
    • Distal tubular secretion
    • Clearance of uric acid independently proportional to:
      □ Intravascular volume status
      □ Urinary flow rate
      □ May be significantly reduced in presence of dehydration or tubular obstruction from acute nephrocalcinosis or uric acid nephropathy
– Uric acid nephropathy develops when:
  • Urate deposit in renal tubules and collecting ducts because of acidic conditions
  • Urinary pKa of uric acid is 5.4
  • Luminal pH of distal tubules and collecting ducts is 5.0
    • Resulting in poor solubility of uric acid in acidic urine
    • Poor solubility, coupled with the marked hyperuricosuria present in ATLS, leads to:
      □ Uric acid precipitation
      □ Intraluminal obstruction
      □ Oliguria
      □ Acute renal failure
• Acute renal failure (ARF) in ATLS may also be mediated by:
  • Renal calculi from phosphate and uric acid precipitation
  • Ischemic acute tubular necrosis caused by renal hypoperfusion
  • Drug toxicity, sepsis, and tumor-associated obstructive uropathy or renal parenchymal infiltration may exacerbate ATLS-induced ARF

Classification

• No widely accepted definition of ATLS currently exists
  • First classification of ATLS into laboratory TLS and clinical TLS
  • Modified/further developed classification system into the Cairo-Bishop definition:
    • Uses laboratory and clinical data and grading scale to assess severity of ATLS
      ○ Laboratory TLS (LTLS) defined as <u>two or more</u> of following metabolic abnormalities occurring 3 days before or 7 days after chemotherapy:
      – Uric acid 8 mg/dL or greater
      – Potassium 6 mEq/L or greater
      – Phosphorous 6.5 mg/dL or greater
      – A 25% increase in baseline levels of these metabolites
      – Calcium 7 mg/dL or less
        • Or 25% decrease from baseline level
      ○ Clinical tumor lysis syndrome is defined as LTLS in addition to one or more of the following findings:

– Increased serum creatinine (1.5 times the upper limit of normal
– Cardiac arrhythmia/sudden death
– Seizure
• The grading of ATLS from 0 through 5 is determined by:
  • Presence or absence of LTLS
  • Degree of serum creatinine elevation
  • Presence and severity of the cardiac arrhythmia and seizure

Prevention and Treatment

• Early recognition of patients at high risk for ATLS an essential component of management strategy so appropriate prophylactic interventions can be instituted

Fluids and Alkalinization

• Except in patients at risk for CHF
  • Aggressive IV hydration with isotonic or hypotonic saline the single most important intervention for both prevention and treatment of ATLS
  • Cytotoxic therapy should be delayed if possible to administer appropriate hydration
  • IV hydration should commence 2 days before and for 2 to 3 days after chemotherapy
  • At rate of 3,000 mL/m^2/day or two to four times daily fluid maintenance
  • To achieve urine output of $\geq$100 mL/m^2/hour
  • IV fluid increases intravascular volume, renal blood flow, GFR, and urine output (UOP):
    ○ Results in correction of electrolyte derangements by ECF dilution
    ○ Prevents phosphate and uric acid precipitation by increasing urinary excretion
• Volume expansion alone may be insufficient to maintain adequate UOP
  • Necessitating administration of diuretics
  • Once euvolemia achieved, and no signs of acute obstructive uropathy present
    ○ Furosemide, 0.5 to 1 mg/kg
    ○ 2 to 4 mg/kg for severe oliguria or anuria
    ○ May induce or improve UOP
  • Effectiveness of furosemide diminished with uric acid precipitation in renal tubules
    ○ Here, mannitol 0.5 mg/kg may be administered
• Alkalinization of urine to pH 7.0 or greater remains controversial
  • Practice based on biochemical properties of uric acid
  • 13 times more soluble at pH 7.0 than at pH 5.0
    ○ Maximal solubility attained at pH 7.5
    ○ Urine alkalinization (pH $\geq$6.5) enhances renal excretion of uric acid
  • Calcium phosphate precipitation increases with systemic alkalinization
    ○ Exacerbating nephrocalcinosis
  • Hypoxanthine and xanthine solubility substantially reduced
    ○ Leading to xanthine nephropathy with concurrent allopurinol therapy

Management of Hyperuricemia

- Allopurinol reduces risk of ATLS when administered 2 to 3 days prior to chemotherapy
- Inhibits production of uric acid
- Allopurinol a synthetic structural analogue of hypoxanthine and competitive inhibitor of xanthine oxidase
  - In presence of allopurinol, xanthine oxidase cannot catalyze conversion of hypoxanthine to xanthine and xanthine to uric acid
- Allopurinol
  - Administered orally at 300 to 800 mg daily
    - 10 mg/kg/day, or up to 400 mg/m²/day
    - In one to three divided doses
    - Titrated to uric acid level
  - IV allopurinol approved 1999; administered in doses of 200 to 400 mg/m²/day
    - To a maximum 600 mg/day in patients unable to tolerate orally
  - Dose adjustment of allopurinol required for reduced creatinine clearance
  - Several limitations with allopurinol therapy:
    - Reduction in serum uric acid level not seen before 48 to 72 hours after initiating drug
      ○ Agent inhibits uric acid synthesis but does not affect pretreatment concentration
      ○ Inhibition of xanthine oxidase by allopurinol leads to increased plasma levels of xanthine and hypoxanthine, which may precipitate in renal tubules
      ○ 3% of patients develop hypersensitivity reactions
        – Including Stevens-Johnson syndrome
      ○ Interacts with drugs, including cyclosporine and azathioprine
- Another agent that lowers uric acid concentration is urate oxidase
  - Converts uric acid to allantoin
  - Five to 10 times more soluble in urine than uric acid
  - Urate oxidase not expressed in human beings resultant from nonsense mutation in coding region during hominoid evolution
  - Recombinant urate oxidase, rasburicase, developed due to 4.5% of hypersensitivity reactions in nonrecombinant form
  - Rasburicase approved in 2002 for use in pediatric patients at risk for ATLS
    - Injectable dose of 0.15 to 0.20 mg/kg normalizes uric acid levels within 4 hours of administration in children and adults
    - May be repeated daily for a total of 5 days
    - Chemotherapy should be initiated 4 to 24 hours after first dose
    - Rasburicase does not generate increased xanthine and hypoxanthine levels
      ○ Thereby minimizing risk of uric acid nephropathy
    - Rasburicase contraindicated in patients with G6PD deficiency
    - Bronchospasm and anaphylaxis rarely occur with rasburicase therapy
    - Insufficient evidence that rasburicase reduces incidence of dialysis in ATLS
      ○ 5-day course of therapy is approximately 2,000 to 3,000 times more expensive than a 5-day course of oral allopurinol

– Cost-effectiveness must be considered in treatment plan

Correction of Electrolyte Abnormalities

- Because of potential for life-threatening dysrhythmias, prompt recognition imperative
  - Laboratory monitoring every 4 to 6 hours in first 24 hours of chemotherapy in patients at high risk for ATLS
  - Every 6 to 8 hours thereafter
  - Baseline ECG obtained to assess for cardiac effects
- Hyperkalemia
  - Treated with calcium gluconate to stabilize the cardiac membrane
  - IV insulin/dextrose and inhaled β_2 agonists to facilitate intracellular shift of K+
  - Sodium bicarbonate shifts K+ intracellularly by improving the metabolic acidosis
    - May result in inappropriate volume expansion
  - K+ binding resins
    - Sodium polystyrene sulfate, increase K+ elimination in GI tract
    - Have delayed hypokalemic effect
  - Diuretics administered to reduce serum K+ in patients without renal failure
    - When acute renal failure occurs, dialysis may be required emergently
- Asymptomatic hypocalcemia should be left untreated
  - To preclude calcium phosphate precipitation
  - Symptomatic hypocalcemia managed with IV calcium gluconate
  - Hyperphosphatemia treated with oral phosphate binders
    - Aluminum hydroxide or aluminum carbonate
    - Usually concurrently correct the hypocalcemia

Dialysis

- Indicated in patients with marked elevations in serum uric acid, phosphate, and potassium
  - That do not respond to aggressive treatment
  - In patients with ARF with volume overload, severe uremia, or acidosis
  - Hemodialysis used in ATLS
    - Superior to peritoneal dialysis in clearance of both uric acid and phosphorous

OBSTRUCTIVE SYNDROMES

Superior Vena Cava Syndrome (SVCS)

Definition

- SVCS describes set of signs and symptoms associated with obstruction of SVC
  - May be caused by extrinsic compression, vascular invasion, or intraluminal thrombosis of vein
  - SVC a thin-walled, compliant, low-pressure middle mediastinal vessel
    - Easily vulnerable to disease processes in adjacent right lung, paratracheal and perihilar lymph nodes, main stem bronchi, esophagus, and thoracic spinal cord
  - Percentage of cases attributable to cancer varies from 78% to 90% to 97%

○ Recent retrospective study reported malignancy the cause of SVCS in 60% of patients
  – Bronchogenic carcinoma 85% to 90% of malignancies in which SVCS presents
  – SVCS develops in 2% to 10% of lung malignancies
  – Risk of SVCS higher in small cell lung cancer
    • Incidence of 6.6% to 12%
    • Because it involves the central mediastinal structures
  – Because of anatomic location of SVC
    • Right-sided lung cancers cause SVCS four times as often as left-sided lung cancers
    • Other neoplasms include:
      • Malignant lymphomas
      • Hodgkin lymphoma often involves mediastinum but rarely causes SVCS
      • Primary germ cell cancers, thymoma, mesothelioma, metastatic disease (primarily breast carcinoma) constitute a small proportion of SVCS cases
• Increasing proportion of benign causes related to presence of IV devices
  ○ Central venous catheters
  ○ Pacemaker wires
• Other benign causes of SVCS include:
  ○ Fibrosing mediastinitis from prior irradiation or histoplasmosis
  ○ Aortic dissection
  ○ Complications of surgery, such as aortic dissection repair

Clinical Presentation

• SVCS may be initial presentation of bronchogenic carcinoma and lymphoma
  • May arise in patients with previously documented malignancy
• Severity of signs/symptoms depends on extent, location, and onset rapidity of SVC occlusion
  • In general, obstruction within or below azygos vein results in more dramatic symptoms
    • Azygos venous capacity increases from 11% to 35% to augment head/neck drainage
    • Impedance of flow from obstruction precludes this auxiliary function
    • With slowly developing SVCS
      ○ Collateral vessels in chest wall and upper extremities are recruited as a diversion for existing SVC engorgement
      ○ SVCS here of insidious onset, as in fibrosing mediastinitis
• Most commonly reported symptom in SVCS:
  • Dyspnea
  • Followed by head and facial swelling
• Other cardiopulmonary symptoms include:
  • Cough, orthopnea, and chest pain
• Associated signs are:
  • Neck and arm vein distention
  • Plethora or cyanosis of the head and neck
  • Venous collateralization in the arms and upper chest wall
  • Chronic pleural effusions
• More extensive airway or vascular obstruction predicted when positional maneuvers such as lying supine or leaning forward exacerbate respiratory or cardiac symptoms
  • Respiratory insufficiency in supine position worsens as weight of mediastinal structures impinges on tracheobronchial tree

• In the substantially compromised patient with SVCS, cardiopulmonary arrest may ensue with sedative administration or general anesthesia
• Other head and neck signs and symptoms:
  • Conjunctival and periorbital edema, nasal congestion
  • Dysphagia and hoarseness due to laryngeal nerve compression
  • Proptosis, glossal edema, stridor secondary to laryngeal edema
  • Tracheal obstruction
• Central nervous system (CNS) manifestations include:
  • Mild headaches, dizziness, and lethargy with progression to syncope
    ○ In rapidly developing or complete SVC obstruction
  • Seizures or coma
    ○ From cerebral edema and increased intracranial pressure
• Bleeding complications such as epistaxis, hemoptysis, and GI hemorrhage from esophageal varices (in longstanding SVC) may occur

Diagnostic Investigations

• **Imaging:** Once clinical diagnosis of SVC syndrome is suspected, confirmation obtained using both radiologic and nuclide techniques
  • Chest x-ray (CXR) shows:
    • Widening of superior mediastinum in approximately 60% of patients
    • Pleural effusions, most frequently right-sided, in up to 25% of patients
    • Normal chest radiograph does not exclude diagnosis
  • Contrast-enhanced helical computed tomography (CT) accurately delineates site, extent, and cause of occlusion
    • As well as any associated thrombus and collateral vessel development
    • Radiologic diagnosis of SVCS made by demonstrating both decreased or absent venous opacification below level of obstruction and prominent collateral vessel opacification
  • Magnetic resonance imaging (MRI) an alternative imaging method in patients with iodinated contrast allergy or without adequate venous access for contrast administration
    • Offers no distinct advantage over CT
  • Venography most useful when planning bypass or stenting procedures
    • Superior to CT in identifying site and extent of obstruction and in mapping collateral circulation
    • Does not elucidate underlying cause of SVCS unless SVC thrombosis alone is the causative factor
  • Radionuclide ^{99m}technetium venography a less invasive alternative to standard venography
    • Lacks image resolution of the latter
  • Although not well established, helical CT phlebography
    • Involves simultaneous bilateral antecubital vein injection with IV contrast
    • Produces both detailed CT images of the mediastinum and CT venogram that correlates well with digital venography
    • Flow artifact (inhomogeneous contrast opacification) created by physiologic mixing of contrast-opacified and nonopacified blood may mimic intraluminal filling defects in patent vessels
    • Remains the major limitation of technique

- **Histologic Diagnosis:** Sputum cytology, thoracentesis, percutaneous needle biopsy, bronchoscopy, mediastinoscopy, or thoracotomy all methods used to obtain pathologic specimens
  - Diagnostic yields are as follows:
    - Bronchoscopy, 50% to 70%
    - Transthoracic needle aspiration biopsy, 75%
    - Mediastinoscopy or mediastinotomy, >90%
  - Well established that absent tracheal obstruction or severe laryngeal or cerebral edema, SVCS itself results in no life-threatening complications
    - Forgoing pathologic diagnosis unjustified, except in severe airway obstruction or cerebral edema
    - Identification of underlying condition guides appropriate treatment of SVCS in both benign and malignant disease

Treatment

- Primary goals of treatment are symptom relief and eradication or palliation of underlying malignancy
- Initial symptomatic management involves bed rest, head elevation to reduce venous pressure, and supplemental oxygen administration
  - Diuretics and sodium restriction anecdotally may decrease edema
  - Glucocorticoids to minimize inflammatory responses to tumor or radiotherapy (XRT) controversial
    - Steroids are mainstay of treatment in non-Hodgkin lymphoma (NHL)
- **Endovascular Stenting:** If above ineffectual in controlling symptoms, percutaneously placed endovascular stent can be inserted with or without balloon angioplasty
  - Relief of symptoms occurs immediately after stent placement in 80% to 95% of patients
    - Morbidity increases with stent insertion if thrombolytics administered
    - Recurrence of SVCS occurs in 10% to 30% of patients after primary therapy with chemotherapy and/or radiation
      - Here, stent placement may be used for palliation
- **Thrombolysis:** With increased use of intravascular devices, thrombus accounts for larger proportion of the benign causes of SVCS
  - SVCS attributable to thrombosis of central venous line and catheter preservation desired
    - Thrombolytic therapy given within 5 days of symptom onset associated with an 88% success rate versus 25% after 5 days
- **Radiotherapy and Chemotherapy:** Treatment modality selected individualized to type of malignancy, stage, and performance status of each patient
- Primary management of solid tumors and non–small cell lung cancer (NSCLC) involves XRT
  - NSCLC associated with SVCS carries a poor prognosis
  - 1-year survival 17%
  - In review of 1,635 patients median survival of 5 months
  - Treatment of choice in NSCLC is XRT and possible stent insertion
    - Within 72 hours of XRT, patients have relief of symptoms
    - Within 2 weeks, 70% to 90% of patients are symptom free
- Chemotherapy prolongs survival and improves quality of life in patients with small cell lung cancer (SCLC)

- Addition of thoracic irradiation may reduce recurrence risk of SVCS
- SVCS relieved in 77% of patients receiving chemotherapy and/or radiation
  - Relapse in 17% of patients
- Lymphoma and germ cell tumors usually treated with chemotherapy based on histologic type, grade, and stage of disease
  - Hodgkin lymphoma, chemotherapy followed by XRT to areas of bulky disease may be indicated
  - NHL, XRT alone may be used in early-stage disease, and chemotherapy is treatment for higher-stage tumors
  - Whether to irradiate areas of bulky disease in NHL after chemotherapeutic remission unclear
    - With residual tumor or progression of disease after chemotherapy, radiotherapy is administered
- **Surgery:** Surgical bypass of obstruction with vein grafts or prosthetic grafts may be appropriate in benign SVCS
  - In patients with malignancy, surgical intervention, when no further treatment options are possible is palliative measure with poor long-term survival

ACUTE AIRWAY OBSTRUCTION

Oropharyngeal and Tracheal Obstruction

- Sudden upper airway obstruction (UAO) of the larynx, pharynx, or extrathoracic trachea is uncommon with cancers of the head and neck
  - Tumors of larynx, pharynx, base of tongue, and thyroid are primarily slow growing
  - Obvious signs and symptoms of airway compromise usually evident prior to development of acute obstruction
  - Tracheal masses, which take years to be discovered, first become symptomatic when the airway lumen is narrowed by 75%
  - Mechanisms of UAO include:
    - Direct tracheal invasion
    - Extrinsic tracheal compression
- Direct tracheal invasion seen with:
  - Locally advanced oropharyngeal tumors, laryngeal neoplasms associated with bulky or supraglottic lesions, and rarely, thyroid cancer and primary tracheal tumors
  - Tracheal impingement in lung cancer occurs with tracheal ingrowth of primary tumor
    - Originating in a main stem bronchus or from enlarging paratracheal or subcarinal lymph nodes
  - Bilateral vocal cord paralysis with recurrent laryngeal nerve paralysis associated with lung malignancies
  - Extrathoracic malignancies may metastasize to mediastinal and endobronchial lymph nodes, causing airway obstruction
    - Renal cell carcinoma, sarcomas, breast cancer, and colon cancer most commonly involved
    - Melanoma may arise as a primary tracheal tumor
      - More often is a metastatic lesion
- Tracheal compression
  - Usually attributable to benign disease
  - A secondary mechanism of UAO in neoplastic disease

- Often the initial presentation of mediastinal tumors and extensive lymphoma

Clinical Presentation

- Patients present with dysphagia, hoarseness, intractable cough, hemoptysis, dyspnea, or stridor
  - Important goals during physical examination are:
    - To determine whether impending airway obstruction present
    - To localize site of lesion
  - Once stridor apparent, airway caliber has narrowed to approximately 6 mm
    - Without intervention, complete UAO imminent
    - Inspiratory stridor implies an extrathoracic lesion at the level of the glottis or above
    - Expiratory stridor suggests an intrathoracic lesion
    - Biphasic stridor may be indicative of a subglottic or tracheal mass
    - Voice alteration, such as muffling and hoarseness, accompanies subglottic lesions and unilateral vocal cord paralysis, respectively

Diagnostic Investigations

- CXR may identify an obstructive neck mass and consequent tracheal deviation
  - Flexible oropharyngeal or nasopharyngeal endoscopy performed to assess airway
  - Once the airway stabilized, high-resolution CT of head and neck obtained
    - Provides comprehensive evaluation of sites of narrowing and size and extent of tumor in relation to adjacent structures
    - Spirometry demonstrates a plateau in inspiratory limb of flow-volume loop if there is a fixed obstructive lesion in extrathoracic trachea

Treatment

- Initial management includes head elevation and administration of cool humidified oxygen
  - Inhalation of helium–oxygen mixture reduces the work of breathing
  - Airway obstruction in patients with bulky oropharyngeal, laryngeal, or thyroid carcinomas will require emergent or elective tracheostomy.
    - Endotracheal intubation not recommended as it may exacerbate existing airway edema and hemorrhage.
- For intraluminal tracheal lesions, bronchoscopy with interventions such as laser therapy, brachytherapy, photodynamic therapy, or stenting may be performed to rapidly alleviate symptoms.
  - Stents also useful in palliating symptomatic extrinsic compression
  - Endotracheal intubation or stenting used to maintain airway when there is extrinsic compression from lymphoma or other highly radiosensitive or chemosensitive tumors with anticipation of rapid reduction of tumor mass
- Surgical resection indicated for primary airway tumors and for lung cancers without mediastinal lymph node involvement
  - In lung and thyroid cancers directly invading trachea, surgery may be curative

- Metastatic disease to the trachea requires palliative treatment

Intrathoracic Obstruction

- Intrathoracic airway obstruction may be present with intrinsic primary endobronchial tumors:
  - Bronchogenic carcinoma and carcinoid
  - With metastatic tumors or their associated lymphadenopathy (lung, renal, breast, thyroid, and colon cancers, and sarcoma or melanoma)
  - With bulky disease causing airway compression
- Symptoms often progress slowly over time
  - Patients complain of dyspnea, wheezing, or chest discomfort
  - Leading to misdiagnosis of asthma or bronchitis prior to development of fulminant airway obstruction
  - Postobstructive pneumonia a finding on initial presentation
  - With impending obstruction, patients may exhibit:
    - Hypertension, tachycardia, tachypnea, and significant pulsus paradoxus
    - Poor air movement, use of accessory muscles, and mental status changes, indicators of severe obstruction
    - Progressive symptoms may result in negative pressure pulmonary edema and anoxic brain injury
- Chest examination may reveal a prolonged expiratory time and wheezing
  - Respiratory symptoms unilateral with lesions below the carina
  - The CXR shows asymmetric lung fields, particularly on end expiration
- Stable patients should have a flow–volume loop performed
  - Intrathoracic, mobile tracheal lesion above the carina will demonstrate airway compression during expiratory phase
    - Producing flattening of expiratory limb of flow–volume loop
  - Whereas a plateau in both inspiratory and expiratory limbs will be observed with fixed obstructive lesions
- Chest CT defines tumor extent and location
  - Rigid bronchoscopy usually necessary to evaluate airway in impending obstruction
  - When obstruction severe, flexible bronchoscopy hazardous
    - Does not permit ventilatory support
    - Bronchoscope may obstruct the already narrowed airway lumen
- Treatment proceeds with general measures:
  - Oxygen or helium/oxygen supplementation, and possibly, steroids
  - If endotracheal intubation required, must recognize potential for hemodynamic compromise associated with asymmetric obstruction and significant increases in airway pressure distal to obstruction
  - Bronchoscopy with various interventions, including debridement, dilation, endotracheal stent placement, laser ablation, photodynamic therapy, and placement of brachytherapy catheters, may relieve symptoms.
  - External beam radiotherapy may also play a role.
  - In lung cancer, tracheal and carinal resection indicated in patients without mediastinal lymph node involvement for a potential cure

NEUROLOGIC SYNDROMES

Spinal Cord Compression

Etiology and Pathophysiology

- Malignant spinal cord compression (MSCC) a profoundly debilitating, but usually nonfatal, manifestation of metastatic cancer
  - Occurs in 5% to 10% of cancer patients
  - Term *malignant spinal cord compression* refers to epidural, intramedullary, and leptomeningeal disease
  - Focus of this section is on epidural spinal cord compression (ESCC)
    - Literature primarily discusses this population
- Any malignancy capable of metastatic spread may give rise to MSCC
  - Prostate, breast, and lung cancers most commonly involved
  - Each accounting for 15% to 20% of cases
  - In combination, 60% of cases
- Cumulative incidence of MSCC is specific to tumor type
  - Highest rates occurring in multiple myeloma (8%), prostate cancer (7%), and nasopharyngeal cancer (6.5%)
  - Other tumors include:
    ○ NHL and renal cell carcinoma, each representing 5% to 10% of cases
    ○ GI cancers, sarcoma, melanoma, thyroid cancer, and unknown primary carcinoma
    ○ Enlarging meningiomas, nerve sheath tumors, and leptomeningeal metastases may also compress the spinal cord
- Nonmalignant causes of MSCC in cancer patients are:
  - Epidural abscesses in presence of immune compromise
  - Hematoma with bleeding diatheses
- MSCC has proclivity for thoracic spine
  - Estimated to occur in this location in approximately 60% to 66% of cases
  - 20% of cases involve lumbar spine
    - Prostate and colorectal carcinomas
  - Cervical spine is uncommon, 7% to 10% of cases
- MSCC the initial manifestation of malignancy in 20% of patients
  - Carcinomas of the lung and unknown primary, multiple myeloma, and NHL accounted for 78% of patients with MSCC presenting with malignancy
  - Compared to 26% in patients with previously established malignancy
- Mechanisms by which MSCC occurs include:
  - Vertebral body invasion by tumor with possible vertebral collapse causing encroachment on anterior spinal cord (85%)
  - Direct extension into intervertebral space by paraspinal lymphoma, sarcoma, or lung cancer (10% to 15%)
  - Epidural or intramedullary space invasion (<5%)
- Mechanism of injury to the spinal cord mediated by white matter vasogenic edema and axonal swelling that result from cord compression
  - Venous hypertension, decreased spinal cord blood flow, and cord infarction ensue
    - Resulting in ischemic hypoxic neuronal injury
- Vascular endothelial growth factor (VEGF) generated in association with spinal cord hypoxia
  - Dexamethasone may down-regulate VEGF expression
  - Resulting in the beneficial actions of steroids in MSCC

Clinical Presentation

- Pain the primary presenting symptom in MSCC, occurring in 83% to 95% of patients
  - Characterized as localized, radicular, or referred
  - Seen for a median of 8 weeks prior to diagnosis
  - Focal bony pain is typically localized, dull or aching, and constant
  - Direct tenderness of involved vertebral body seen with periosteal destruction
    - With time, radicular pain occurs in dermatome of affected nerve root
    - Is severe, deep, and lancinating
    - Radicular symptoms occur most often in lumbosacral spine
      ○ May be unilateral or bilateral
      ○ The latter more frequent with thoracic spine involvement
  - Referred pain does not radiate, but appears in a region distal to the area of pathology
    - Sacroiliac pain may result from L1 compression
  - Pain of MSCC typified by worsening with recumbency
    - Secondary to distention of epidural venous plexus
    - Coughing, sneezing, or Valsalva maneuvers also exacerbate pain
    - Straight-leg raising identifies a lumbosacral radiculopathy
    - Neck flexion reproduces symptoms of thoracic radiculopathy
- Motor weakness present in 60% to 85% of patients on diagnosis of MSCC
  - Only one-third of patients complain of lower extremity weakness on initial presentation
    - Two-thirds are not ambulatory at time of diagnosis
  - Motor deficits at level of conus medullaris or above have a symmetric distribution
    - Paresis usually seen in extensors of upper extremities
    - Or flexors of the lower extremities, depending on location of lesion in spine
    - Upper motor neuron signs such as spasticity, hyperreflexia, and Babinski responses, may be present
    - Cervical lesions may lead to quadriplegia and respiratory collapse
- Sensory deficits, varying degrees of paresthesias, less common than motor deficits
  - Found in 40% to 90% of patients
  - Level of hypesthesia on examination occurs 1 to 5 levels below anatomic level of cord compression
  - Sensation of electric shock radiating through spine and extremities with neck flexion–*Lhermitte sign*–seen infrequently with cervical or thoracic neoplasms
  - Perineal paresthesias occur with cauda equina lesions
    - Gait ataxia may follow sensory loss impairment
    - In absence of sensory findings, impairment of spinocerebellar tract is considered
- Bowel and bladder dysfunction reflect autonomic dysfunction
  - A late manifestation of MSCC
  - Patients report urinary hesitancy and frequency
  - Both incontinence of urine, from poor sphincter tone or overflow of urine, and urinary retention may ensue

- At diagnosis, 50% of patients incontinent or catheter dependent
- Patients may also exhibit erectile dysfunction and impotence
- Constipation and incontinence of stool with diminished sphincter tone may be present
- Narcotics widely used in cancer patients
  - Are capable of precipitating urinary retention and constipation
  - Spinal lesions must be excluded before narcotic use is implicated

Diagnostic Investigation

- Imaging study of choice in evaluating MSCC is MRI
  - Noninvasive and provides high resolution of the tissues, including bony metastases and intramedullary pathology
  - MRI has sensitivity, specificity, and overall accuracy of 93%, 97%, and 95%, respectively
    - In detecting MSCC in patients with known malignancies, excluding primary CNS tumors
    - When entire spine is imaged beyond area of clinically determined cord compression
      - Multiple epidural metastases (MEMs) found in 30% of patients
      - Presence of MEMs may alter treatment strategy
      - Using whole-spine MRI in all patients undergoing imaging may be needed
      - Relative paucity of cervical spine metastases
        - If clinical presentation does not suggest cervical disease
        - May be acceptable to image thoracolumbar spine alone
- Myelography with or without CT myelogram a more invasive tool than MRI
  - Used in imaging MSCC when MRI contraindicated
  - CT alone does not adequately define soft tissues and spinal cord
  - Plain radiographs and radionuclide testing have low sensitivity and specificity for MSCC
    - Plain films detect vertebral metastases at site of known cord compression only 80% of the time
    - Many metastases missed
      - The ability to visualize lesions requires that 30% to 40% of bone be eroded
      - Bone scintigraphy the most cost-effective and sensitive technique in imaging vertebral metastases

Treatment

- Goals of therapy are pain control and preservation of neurologic function
  - To improve quality of life
  - Narcotic and corticosteroids administration, XRT, and surgery may all be used
- **Corticosteroids:** 81% of patients receiving corticosteroids and XRT versus 63% of those receiving XRT alone remained ambulatory
  - At 6 months percentages were 59% and 33% in the two groups, respectively
  - Less well-established data regarding use of high-dose dexamethasone regimens
    - Although higher doses (100-mg vs. 10-mg boluses) may have greater clinical efficacy in improving posttreatment ambulation
    - Associated with higher proportion of adverse effects
  - Typical regimens include a 10-mg bolus

- Followed by 16 mg divided four times daily
- Tapered over 2 weeks
- High-dose regimens (100-mg bolus)
  - Then 96 mg divided four times daily
  - Tapered over 2 weeks reserved for patients with paresis or paraplegia
- Ambulatory asymptomatic patients undergoing XRT may have corticosteroids withheld
- **Surgery and Radiation:** Direct decompressive surgery followed by XRT superior to XRT alone for patients with MSCC
  - 84% of surgery group versus 57% of XRT group were ambulatory after therapy
  - Those in surgery group were ambulatory for 122 days compared to 13 days in XRT group after treatment
  - Of patients unable to ambulate on entering study:
  - 62% of those receiving surgery and radiation versus 19% receiving XRT alone regained ability to ambulate
  - XRT alone should be used only for patients who are not surgical candidates
    - Radiotherapy useful in preserving neurologic function in subclinical MSCC
    - Most tumors causing MSCC are not chemosensitive

Prognosis

- Median survival in MSCC patients receiving XRT is 3 to 6 months
  - Patients who initially present with paralysis or become paralyzed after treatment
    - Have shorter life expectancy than those who are ambulatory
    - Ambulatory function on diagnosis of MSCC the most important predictor of outcome of ambulatory function after XRT
      - Underscores need for education of both clinician and patient to enable prompt recognition of MSCC
      - Delay in diagnosis attributed to patient's failure to identify symptoms AND diagnostic delays by the generalist and hospital practitioner
        - Leading to deterioration in motor or bladder function

CARDIAC TAMPONADE

- Primary neoplasms of myocardium and pericardium are uncommon
- Metastatic disease to pericardial space is frequently seen
- Primary pericardial tumors
  - Mesothelioma represents largest proportion
  - 40 times less common than metastatic disease
- Secondary malignancies include most frequently:
  - Lung
  - Breast and ovarian carcinomas
  - Melanoma
  - Lymphoma and leukemia
- Malignancy a primary cause of pericardial effusion in the United States
  - Pericardial tamponade resulting from malignant pericardial effusion (MPCE) represents at least 50% of reported cases of pericardial fluid collection requiring intervention
  - Autopsy series report MPCE seen in 2% to 22% of cancer patients

○ These effusions are clinically quiescent, remaining unrecognized

○ In some patients, MPCE the initial presentation of cancer
  – It signifies dismal prognosis, with most patients dying within 1 year

○ Pericardial effusions in some cancer patients due to comorbid conditions
  – Radiation-induced pericarditis
  – Infection
  – Uremia
  – Myocardial infarction
  – Congestive heart failure
  – Pneumonia

Pathophysiology

• Mechanisms by which malignant disease generates MPCEs include:
• Direct invasion of the pericardium or myocardium
• Disruption of lymphatic flow from lymph node metastases or from prior radiotherapy to chest or mediastinum
• Tumors that invade the pericardium directly or hematogenously, most often:
  • Lung cancer
  • Followed by lymphoma and breast cancer
• With either of aforementioned mechanisms
• Pericardial fluid accumulates
• Inhibits passive diastolic filling of normally low-pressure right heart structures
  • Producing jugular and abdominal venous hypertension
  • As pericardial effusion expands, the heart is further compressed
    ○ Leading to reduced diastolic compliance, decreased diastolic filling, and decreased stroke volume, cardiac output, and blood pressure
    ○ Right atrial and right ventricular collapse ensues
    ○ Resulting in frank tamponade, which, untreated, will lead to shock
• *Pericardial reserve volume* is about 10 to 20 mL
  • Defined as volume that will just distend the pericardium
  • As pericardial effusion enlarges, capacity for stretch is exceeded
    ○ When fluid accumulates rapidly pericardium cannot stretch rapidly enough to accommodate added volume, and heart becomes compressed
    ○ Acute tamponade may occur with as little as 50 mL of fluid
    ○ When effusions develop chronically pericardium is able to compensate by stretching slowly over time
      – Phenomenon of stretch relaxation
      – In cancer patients, MPCE develops slowly
        • 2 L of pericardial fluid may be present before critical symptoms occur

Clinical Presentation

• Patients may be asymptomatic with small pericardial effusions
  • Symptoms correlate with compressive effect of effusion on surrounding structures

• Including lung, trachea, and esophagus
• Symptoms include dyspnea, cough, chest pain, hoarseness, hiccups, and dysphagia
  ○ Patients may report feeling of uneasiness
• Most commonly reported physical sign is distension of jugular veins
  ○ Classic finding of the Beck's triad of hypotension, increased jugular venous pressure, and quiet heart sounds may be present in addition to the Kussmaul sign
    – Paradoxical jugular venous distention and increased jugular venous pressure on inspiration
  ○ Sinus tachycardia, hepatomegaly, and peripheral edema may be apparent
  ○ On cardiac examination, dullness beyond apical impulse and rales noted
    – In patients with inflammatory effusions pericardial rub often heard
    – Narrow pulse pressure frequently noted
    – Pulsus paradoxus observed in 77% of patients with acute tamponade
      • Decrease in systolic blood pressure >10 mm Hg
  ○ When low-output shock results from failure of compensatory mechanisms to maintain cardiac output
    – Patient exhibits cold, clammy skin, cyanosis, oliguria, and altered mental status

Diagnostic Investigations

• CXR shows water bottle–shaped heart
  • With widening of cardiac silhouette and, occasionally, pericardial calcifications
  • Pleural effusions present in one-third of cases
• ECG may demonstrate low-voltage QRS or nonspecific ST-T wave changes
  • Electrical alternans in the P wave and QRS complex rare noted in 0% to 10% of patients
    • Every other QRS complex has a lower voltage and/or reversed polarity
• Echocardiogram precisely localizes pericardial fluid
  • Discerns quality of effusion (homogeneous vs. heterogeneous)
  • Determines whether loculations or bulky tumor are present
  • Assesses right and left ventricular function
  • Ascertains whether right atrial and right ventricular diastolic collapse present
  • On echocardiography, heart may swing in pendular fashion within pericardial fluid
• Right heart catheterization the definitive standard for further defining pericardial effusion
  • Classically equalization of diastolic pressures across all cardiac chambers

Treatment

• Cardiac tamponade a class I indication for performing pericardiocentesis
  • Initial emergent intervention in malignant cardiac tamponade is to drain the effusion
    • Usually in conjunction with echocardiographic guidance

- Fluid sent for chemical analysis, microbiology, and cytology
- Effusion removed successfully in 97% of patients
- In absence of tamponade, systemic chemotherapy is administered as baseline treatment
  - Precluding recurrences in 67% of cases
  - Effective in controlling malignant effusions when tumors are chemosensitive
    - As in lymphoma, leukemia, and breast cancer
    - XRT highly effective (93%) in controlling malignant pericardial effusions in patients with lymphoma and leukemia
      ○ Radiation myocarditis or pericarditis a complication of radiotherapy
  - Pericardiocentesis is performed in MPCE for symptomatic relief and to establish a cause
    ○ Fluid reaccumulates within 48 hours of initial pericardiocentesis
    ○ Intrapericardial sclerosing or cytostatic agents according to tumor type
      – Administered to prevent recurrence
      – Mechanism of action of sclerosing agents effect symphysis of visceral and parietal pericardia
      – Surgical approach to MPCE management:
        • Subxiphoid pericardiotomy for a pericardial window
        • Performed using local anesthesia
        • Has low recurrence rate
        • Tissue can be obtained for pathologic review
        • Small risk of myocardial laceration, pneumothorax, and mortality with procedure
      – 12% recurrence at 1 year and 4% reoperation rate for subxiphoid pericardiotomy
      – Pleuropericardiotomy and pericardiectomy have higher morbidity and mortality rates
        • Require general anesthesia
        • Rarely used in MPCE management
      – Percutaneous balloon pericardiotomy may become procedure of choice in future
        • Requires only local anesthesia
        • Facilitates passage of pericardial fluid into left pleural or peritoneal spaces
          • Have greater resorptive capacity
        • Major side effect is asymptomatic pleural effusion in most patients
        • Appears to be safe and effective technique in patients with large MPCEs and recurrent tamponade (90% to 97%)
        • Reaccumulation rates 0% to 6%
    ○ Reaccumulation rates for other therapies administered after initial pericardiocentesis performed are:
      – Radiotherapy, 33%
      – Systemic chemotherapy, 30%
      – Sclerotherapy with tetracycline, 15% to 30%
      – Mechanical therapies, including indwelling pericardial catheter placement, balloon pericardiotomy, and thoracotomy with pericardiostomy, 0% to 15%
  - Even if no reaccumulation of fluid
    ○ Cardiac function may remain impaired in presence of epicardial tumor infiltration
    ○ Diastolic dysfunction occurs due to constrictive effect of diseased epicardium surrounding heart
    ○ Effusive-constrictive pericarditis results in combination of tamponade and cardiac restriction

– Considered in differential diagnosis when patient develops hemodynamic collapse a few days after pericardiocentesis
– Pericardiectomy useful in alleviating constrictive component
– Mortality extremely high

Prognosis

- Survival after development of MPCE extremely poor
  - Pericardial lesions contribute to or directly cause death in 86% of untreated patients with symptomatic MPCE
    - In a 275 patient series with MPCE
      ○ Median survival was 135 days
      ○ Chance of surviving the first year was 26%
      ○ Findings of male gender, lung cancer, positive fluid cytology for malignant cells, and clinical presentation of cardiac tamponade or hemodynamic collapse independently associated with poor survival
  - Another series concluded that poor prognosis was associated with positive fluid cytology
    ○ Median survival was 7.3 weeks versus 29.7 weeks in positive cytology and negative cytology groups, respectively
    ○ MPCE and abnormal cytology found to be independent predictors of death
    ○ These prognostic factors used to make practical and realistic treatment decisions

GASTROINTESTINAL EMERGENCIES

Neutropenic Enterocolitis (NE)

- NE is also known as necrotizing enteropathy, ileocecal syndrome, or typhlitis
- First described in adult patients with leukemia and lymphoma over 40 years ago
- Typhlitis recognized in 1970 as equivalent entity involving the cecum in children undergoing induction therapy for acute leukemia
- A life-threatening inflammatory syndrome in immunocompromised patient involving the terminal ileum, ascending colon, and cecum
- Disease affects both small and large bowel *neutropenic enterocolitis* most commonly used
- Cardinal features defining the syndrome are:
  - Fever, abdominal pain, and bowel wall thickening in patient with neutropenia
  - *Neutropenia* defined as neutrophil count of either:
    ○ <500 neutrophils/μL
    ○ Or <1,000 neutrophils/μL with expected precipitous decline to <500 neutrophils/μL
  - Disease may progress to bowel ulceration, necrosis, and perforation, and ultimately, sepsis and death
- NE occurs primarily in patients following aggressive cytotoxic therapy for:
- Acute leukemia and other hematologic malignancies such as lymphoma, chronic leukemia, multiple myeloma
- Rarely in solid tumors, such as colon, breast, testicular, lung, and pancreatic cancers

- Administration of drugs toxic to bowel mucosa can result in NE, such as:
  - Cytosine arabinoside
  - Cytarabine
  - Cisplatin
  - Fluorouracil
  - Vincristine
  - Doxorubicin
  - 5-fluorouracil
  - Thioguanine
  - Mercaptopurine
- NE rare in solid tumors
  - Case reports identifying syndrome in breast cancer patients receiving taxanes
  - Case reports of acute leukemia patients presenting with NE in absence of chemotherapy
    - Indicating that drug toxicity a predisposing factor not a prerequisite in the disease pathogenesis
- Other immunocompromised patients in whom NE occurs include:
  - Aplastic anemia
  - Cyclic neutropenia
  - Agranulocytosis
  - Felty syndrome
  - Thalassemia minor
  - Systemic lupus erythematosus
  - Human immunodeficiency virus (HIV) disease
  - Patients receiving immunosuppressive therapy for bone marrow/renal transplantation also at risk
- Incidence of NE in adults varies widely, ranging from 0.8% to 26%
  - Pooled incidence rate for adults hospitalized for treatment of hematologic malignancies and solid tumors and for aplastic anemia was 5.3%
  - In acute leukemia group receiving myelosuppressive therapy, with exclusion of transplant patients, it was 5.6%
  - Extrapolating from these findings, neutropenia rather than acute leukemia the primary risk factor for NE
  - Elsewhere, 88 (6%) of 1,450 consecutive patients treated for leukemia had clinical manifestations of NE
  - While incidence low, the high mortality rate associated with NE underscores its designation as an oncologic emergency
    - Initially mortality rates ranged from 50% to 100%
    - The above systematic review noted an observed rate of 50% or higher
    - Other published figures ranging between 40% and 50%

Pathogenesis

- NE has a predilection for the terminal ileum, cecum, and appendix
  - An explanatory factor is overall decreased blood supply to colon
  - Inherent to cecum is decreased vascularity and increased distensibility compared to other colonic segments
    - Progressive cecal distention may cause increasing intraluminal pressure and exacerbation of submucosal edema
  - Pathogenesis of NE is multifactorial and remains unclear
    - Drug-induced cytotoxic mucosal injury initiates the process

- Limiting cellular proliferation and generating glandular epithelial atypia and necrosis (cytosine arabinoside)
- Producing myenteric plexus degeneration (vincristine)
- Subsequently, mucosal barrier integrity is breached
  - Cells cannot rapidly regenerate to repair the damaged surface
- Bacterial translocation occurs, resulting in microbial infection and sepsis
- Marked neutropenia impairs host defense and promotes further microbial invasion
  - Bowel flora becomes altered
- Blood cultures are often positive for:
  - *Clostridium septicum, C. difficile*
  - *Escherichia coli*
  - *Pseudomonas*
  - *Klebsiella*
  - *Enterobacter*
  - *Staphylococcus*
  - Candidiasis, primarily *Candida albicans*, which colonizes mucosal surfaces, the most common fungal infection in neutropenic patients
    - Associated with high morbidity and mortality
    - These microbial infections lead to inflammation and edema
- With sustained profound neutropenia
  - Bacterial invasion is unconstrained
  - Results in transmural necrosis, hemorrhage, ulceration, and perforation
  - In addition to drug-induced mucosal injury, infiltration of mucosa with leukemic and lymphoproliferative cells and mucosal ischemia from sepsis-related hypotension may also participate in initiating and perpetuating mucosal injury

Symptoms

- Onset of NE is 7 to 10 days after treatment, when neutropenia is evident
  - Clinical presentation includes:
    - Fever, occurring in 90% of all hospitalized neutropenic patients at any time
    - Nausea and vomiting
    - Abdominal pain
    - Watery or bloody diarrhea
  - Physical examination may show:
    - Stomatitis with diffuse mucositis
    - Abdominal tenderness
    - Abdominal distention
    - Peritoneal signs suggestive of bowel perforation
    - In 60% to 80% of patients
      - Right lower quadrant tenderness is elicited
      - Palpation of a right lower quadrant mass usually indicates a thickened, dilated, fluid-filled cecum

Differential Diagnosis

- NE included in differential diagnosis whenever a neutropenic patient presents with fever and abdominal pain, particularly right lower quadrant pain
- Other entities that may mimic NE are:

- Pseudomembranous colitis
- Acute appendicitis
- Acute cholecystitis
- Acute pancreatitis
- Diverticulitis
- Ischemic colitis
- Ogilvie syndrome (colonic pseudo-obstruction)
- Chemotherapy-induced abdominal pain
- Ileus secondary to vincristine toxicity
- GI bleeding may occur in 35% of typhlitis cases
  - Hemorrhage should suggest NE rather than appendicitis

Diagnostic Investigation

- On laboratory analysis, in addition to neutropenia, thrombocytopenia often seen
  - Blood cultures positive in 50% to 82% of cases for bowel organisms
  - Stool studies notable for absence of *C. difficile* toxin A
- Plain abdominal radiographs usually normal or nonspecific
  - Findings may include:
    - Decreased right lower quadrant gas with dilated small bowel loops and air fluid levels consistent with distal bowel obstruction
    - Free intraperitoneal air after perforation
    - Pneumatosis coli
    - Localized or diffuse "thumb-printing" characteristic of mucosal edema
- Sonography assists in confirming diagnosis of NE
  - Excluding other differential diagnoses by detecting bowel wall thickening
  - Ultrasound useful in following clinical course of disease
  - Sonographic manifestations of NE include:
    - Rounded mass with dense central echoes and a wider hyperechoic periphery
    - Pseudopolypoid changes of the cecal mucosa
    - Pericolic fluid collections
    - Patients with sonographically detected bowel wall thickness >10 mm had significantly higher mortality rate (60%) than did those with bowel wall thickness ≤10 mm (4.2%)
- CT a more accurate modality for assessing cecal wall thickening and evaluating the extent of the colitis
  - Has utility in differentiating NE from appendicitis, appendiceal abscess, or pseudomembranous colitis
  - CT findings include:
    - Diffuse submucosal thickening and edema of the terminal ileum and ascending colon
    - Mural hemorrhage
    - Pericolic fluid collections
    - Abscess formation
    - Pneumatosis coli
    - Intraperitoneal free air
- False-negative rates in identifying NE for CT, ultrasound, and plain radiographs are 15%, 23%, and 48%, respectively
- Barium enema unsafe because it may result in bowel perforation in presence of severely damaged, necrotic bowel
- Endoscopic evaluation generally avoided because it involves a high risk of perforation
  - In addition to hemorrhagic and infectious complications
  - May precipitate fulminant mural necrosis

- Colonoscopy has been performed in a few patients and shows irregular nodular mucosa, ulcerations, hemorrhagic friability, and a masslike lesion resembling carcinoma

Histopathology

- With difficulty of obtaining biopsy specimens, a tissue diagnosis is not required to confirm NE

Management

- Prospective trials or case control studies evaluating therapeutic interventions in NE lacking
- Management strategy remains controversial regarding decision to proceed with early surgical intervention versus conservative approach
  - Conservative management involves:
    - Bowel rest
    - IV fluid and blood product resuscitation
    - Broad-spectrum antibiotics, granulocyte colony-stimulating factor (G-CSF)
    - Parenteral nutrition
    - Use of omeprazole and gastric decompression not advocated
    - Antidiarrheal and narcotic agents should be avoided
      - Perpetuate ileus and promote bacterial overgrowth
- Chemotherapy-induced NE may recur with future treatment
    - Further chemotherapy withheld until NE has completely resolved
    - Bowel decontamination helpful before subsequent chemotherapy
- Selection of broad-spectrum antibiotics incorporates:
    - Infectious Diseases Society of America 2002 recommendations for febrile neutropenia
    - 2003 ISDA guidelines for complicated intra-abdominal infections
    - Without prompt antibiotic therapy, neutropenic patients with Gram-negative bacteremia have 40% mortality rate
      - Antibiotic(s) of choice in NE must have activity against both Gram-negative and anaerobic organisms
      - Options include:
        - Monotherapy
          - Carbapenem or piperacillin—tazobactam
        - Duotherapy
          - Antipseudomonal β-lactam plus aminoglycoside
          - Cefepime or ceftazidime plus metronidazole
        - Antifungal therapy with amphotericin B therapy
          - Considered for empiric therapy
          - In profoundly neutropenic patients with fevers beyond 5 days
            - Despite appropriately dosed antibiotics
- G-CSF:
    - Increases cell division in myeloid precursor cells
    - Decreases bone marrow transit time
    - Modulates activity and function of developing and mature neutrophils
- G-CSF recommended in febrile neutropenic patients with:
    - High risk for infection-associated complications

○ Poor prognostic factors, such as:
– Profound neutropenia (<100 cells/μL)
– Sepsis
– Pneumonia
– Hypotension
– Invasive fungal infection
– Uncontrolled primary disease
• NE undisputedly meets these criteria
• G-CSF administration in chemotherapy-related febrile neutropenia:
○ Reduces hospitalization time and time to neutrophil recovery
○ May have impact on infection-related mortality
– Warrants further study
• Clinical improvement in NE patients usually seen:
○ After normalization of neutrophil count with discontinuation of chemotherapy
– Symptoms start as white blood cell (WBC) count declines after chemotherapy
– Recovery begins after the nadir when WBC is increasing
• No standard recommendations regarding surgical intervention in NE
○ Most patients unlikely to be surgical candidates
○ Surgery with laparotomy alone for patients with perforation and ileus
○ Patients who fail to improve or worsen (bowel perforation, peritonitis) after 2 or 3 days of conservative therapy warrant consideration for surgery
○ Surgery recommended for severe complications:
– Abscess, necrotic bowel, and obstruction
○ Definitive indications for surgery include:
– Intraperitoneal free air/perforation
– Generalized peritonitis
– Persistent bleeding in spite of correction of coagulopathy
○ Important considerations influencing decision to surgically intervene:
– Patient's prognosis and comorbidities
– Postoperative morbidity/mortality greater with coexistent disease
– If surgery warranted, the procedure of choice is colectomy with ileostomy and mucous fistula
• Primary anastomosis used in few patients
• Extent of mucosal necrosis may be underestimated by the appearance of the serosa
• Ensure complete resection of edematous bowel
• Even in absence of necrosis and inflammation, to preclude fatal outcome

TOXICITY OF CHEMOTHERAPY

• Most antineoplastic agents therapeutic actions target rapidly proliferating malignant cells
• Agents interrupt fundamental cellular processes such as DNA, RNA, and protein synthesis
• Not completely specific to malignant cells and will also act on normal tissues
• Causing multiple toxicities
• Rapidly regenerating cells, hematopoietic, GI mucosa, spermatogonia, and hair follicles may suffer transient toxicity

Pulmonary Toxicities

• Pulmonary toxicity–both acute and chronic–increasingly seen
• Chemotherapy-induced lung disease (CLD) describes:
• Lung injury with multiple etiologic agents
• Varying pathophysiologic mechanisms, including
○ Direct lung toxicity
○ Immunologic response
○ Increased capillary permeability
• Corresponding clinical presentations are:
○ Interstitial pneumonitis/fibrosis
○ Hypersensitivity syndrome
○ Capillary leak syndrome
• Each may result in fulminant respiratory failure
• Symptoms can appear immediately or months after termination of therapy

Antitumor Antibiotics

• **Bleomycin:** An antitumor antibiotic used in treatment of lymphoma, germ cell tumors, cervical carcinoma, and head and neck squamous cell carcinoma
• Absence of bleomycin hydrolase in skin and lungs prevents deactivation of drug, accounting for selective toxicity
• Bleomycin interstitial pneumonitis the most ominous toxicity
• Associated with 3% mortality rate
• Occurring in 0% to 46% of patients receiving bleomycin-containing regimens
○ Either during treatment or up to 6 months after discontinuation
• Toxicity mediated by mechanism of direct lung injury via generation of cytokines and free radicals
○ Sequelae are endothelial damage, inflammatory cell infiltration, fibroblast activation, and fibrosis
• Conflicting evidence whether perioperative FiO_2 >0.24 causes synergistic toxicity with bleomycin through production of free radicals
• **Mitomycin C:** Antibiotic used in treating solid tumors, primarily breast and lung carcinomas
• Mechanism of injury alkylation of endothelial cell DNA, precluding cell division
• Associated with development of an interstitial pneumonitis/fibrosis
○ Usually 3 to 12 months after therapy
○ With 3% to 14% incidence
○ Mortality as high as 14% to 50%
• Risk factors include:
○ Oxygen exposure
○ Prior irradiation
○ Other cytotoxic drug administration, such as:
– Bleomycin
– Cisplatin
– Vinca alkaloids
– Cyclophosphamide
– Doxorubicin
○ Drug withdrawal, steroids, and avoidance of supplemental oxygen may be helpful
• Mitomycin–vinca alkaloid syndrome a unique entity
• Occurs with 6% incidence after vinca alkaloid administered to patients receiving combination therapy with mitomycin and vinblastine
○ Not with vinca alkaloid alone

- Severe hypoxemia ensues with development of interstitial infiltrates on CXR
- Most patients show acute improvement within 24 hours with:
  - Oxygen
  - Diuretics
  - Occasionally, mechanical ventilation
- Chronic lung damage occurs in 60% of patients

Alkylating Agents

- **Carmustine (BCNU):** A nitrosourea used in management of CNS tumors and in induction therapy for bone marrow transplant (BMT)
- Cytoxicity mediated by alkylation of guanine in DNA
- Carmustine causes dose-dependent pulmonary fibrosis
  - Carries highest incidence of fibrosis among nitrosoureas
  - Mortality rate ranges from 24% to 90%
  - In 1% and 30% of patients receiving high- and low-dose carmustine, respectively, early-onset fibrosis and alveolitis occurs
  - In up to 40% of patients undergoing induction for BMT, pulmonary fibrosis develops within 2 years
    - Late fibrosis observed up to 17 years after exposure
    - Concomitant radiotherapy, chronic obstructive pulmonary disease, and pneumoconioses increase risk of carmustine toxicity
      - 60% of patients will respond dramatically to steroids

Microtubule-Targeting Agents

- **Taxanes:** Paclitaxel inhibits microtubule disassembly
- Has activity against solid tumors such as non–small cell lung carcinoma, breast carcinoma, and ovarian carcinoma
- Prepared in Cremophor, a castor oil-based solution
  - A type I hypersensitivity reaction, characterized by urticaria, bronchospasm, angioedema, and hypotension, occurs within 2 to 10 minutes of infusion of paclitaxel with a 3% to 10% incidence
  - Attributable to Cremophor vehicle rather than paclitaxel itself
  - Premedication with steroids and H_1 and H_2 blockers can curtail reaction

Antimetabolites

- **Cytosine Arabinoside:** Ara-C is a substituted nucleoside antimetabolite that disrupts DNA replication
- Used in therapy of leukemia and NHL
- One toxicity is abrupt onset of endothelial inflammation and capillary leak syndrome
  - Causing noncardiogenic pulmonary edema, acute dyspnea, and a diffuse interstitial and alveolar pattern
  - Management supportive and includes oxygen, diuretics, and mechanical ventilation when needed
- **Gemcitabine:** A pyrimidine analogue, structurally similar to ara-C
- Has activity against tumors of the pancreas, lung (NSCLC), breast, and ovaries
- Incidence of lung toxicity <1% to 1.4%
- Proposed mechanism of injury involves pulmonary endothelial cell damage resulting in capillary leak syndrome
- Symptoms of gemcitabine pulmonary toxicity range from:
  - Mild dyspnea to a fatal acute respiratory distress syndrome (ARDS)

- Increasing age, pulmonary neoplasm, and prior radiotherapy may be contributing risk factors
- Patients respond rapidly to corticosteroids, but fatalities do occur

Differentiation Agents

- **All-*trans*-Retinoic Acid:** ATRA is a differentiation agent used for the treatment of acute promyelocytic leukemia (APL)
- It is associated with retinoic acid syndrome
  - Develops in 20% to 50% of APL patients receiving ATRA
  - Median of 7 days (range 0–35 days) after induction therapy
  - Clinical presentation includes fluid retention, weight gain, fever, and musculoskeletal pain, with progression to respiratory distress, pulmonary infiltrates, pleural and pericardial effusions, renal insufficiency, skin infiltrates, hypotension, and death
  - Corticosteroids highly effective when syndrome commences
    - Have limited utility once pulmonary symptoms apparent
    - Mechanism of pulmonary toxicity of ATRA is capillary leak syndrome

Monoclonal Antibodies

- **Trastuzumab:** A humanized monoclonal antibody targeting epidermal growth factor type 2 (HER2) receptor
- In approximately 25% of breast cancers HER2 receptor overexpressed
  - Associated with a poor prognosis
  - Analysis of 25,000 patients identified bronchospasm as only manifestation of pulmonary toxicity
    - Nine cases (0.04%) were fatal
    - Most serious reactions commenced within 2 hours of infusion
    - Most fatalities were observed in patients with poor performance status and severe underlying pulmonary disease
- **Bevacizumab:** Recombinant humanized monoclonal antibody directed against VEGF
- Inhibits binding of VEGF to receptors impairing angiogenesis
- Approved for first-line treatment of advanced colorectal cancer in combination therapy
- **Alemtuzumab:** Monoclonal antibody to lymphocyte and monocyte CD52 antigen
- Salvage therapy for chronic lymphocytic leukemia
- In 16 patients with B-cell chronic lymphocytic leukemia, associated pulmonary toxicity in one patient was severe bronchospasm, responding to corticosteroids

Cardiac Toxicities

Antitumor Antibiotics

- **Anthracyclines:** Red-pigmented antibiotics (rhodomycins), which include doxorubicin, daunorubicin, idarubicin, and epirubicin
- Active against broad spectrum of tumors, such as breast and esophageal carcinomas, Hodgkin and non-Hodgkin lymphomas, osteosarcomas, Kaposi sarcoma, and soft-tissue sarcomas

- Three mechanisms that lead to oxidative stress contribute to cardiac toxicity:
  - Mitochondrial dysfunction and consequent adenosine triphosphate depletion
  - Free radical lipid peroxidation by iron–doxorubicin complexes
  - Glutathione peroxidase depletion
  - Histopathology demonstrates myofibril dropout, vacuolization of myocardial cells, and necrosis
  - Acute cardiotoxicities include nonspecific ST-T wave changes, supraventricular tachycardia (SVT), ventricular arrhythmias, myopericarditis, cardiomyopathy, and sudden death
    - Cardiomyopathy is dose dependent
      ○ Classified as subacute and late
        – Subacute cardiomyopathy presents within 8 months of therapy, with a peak onset of 3 months
        – Late cardiomyopathy is observed after 5 or more years
    - Continual decline in left ventricular function results in CHF
  - Liposomal doxorubicin may reduce cardiotoxicity
  - Dexrazoxane, an iron chelator with cardioprotective properties substantially reduces toxicity
  - Toxic effects compounded by other therapies:
    - Trastuzumab, cyclophosphamide, dactinomycin, mithramycin, mitomycin, etoposide, melphalan vincristine, bleomycin, dacarbazine, and taxanes
- **Mitoxantrone:** Agent has structural similarity to anthracyclines
  - Used in metastatic breast cancer, acute myeloid leukemia, and NHL
  - Cardiac injury, like the anthracyclines, may involve iron chelation complexes
  - Arrhythmias and dose-dependent heart failure are toxicities
  - Incidence of moderate to severe decrease in left ventricular ejection fraction (LVEF) and of CHF is 13% and 2.6%, respectively, with cumulative dose ≤ 140 mg/m^2
    - Doses below 110 mg/m^2 decrease incidence of heart failure
    - Incidence increases with doses >160 mg/m^2
- **Mitomycin C:** In addition to lung toxicity, mitomycin is cardiotoxic
  - Results in increased incidence of cardiac failure with cumulative doses >30 mg/m^2
  - Additive cardiotoxicity occurs when used in conjunction with anthracyclines
    - Superoxide free radicals may mediate toxicity

Alkylating Agents

- **Cyclophosphamide:** A nitrogen mustard alkylating agent effective in treating leukemia, lymphoma, multiple myeloma, mycosis fungoides, neuroblastoma, and ovarian cancer
  - Acute cardiotoxicity may develop with doses of 120 to 170 mg/kg given over 1 to 7 days in preparation for bone marrow transplantation
    - ECG may reveal decreased QRS amplitude, nonspecific T-wave abnormalities, poor R-wave progression, SVT and VT, and second-degree atrioventricular block
    - Acute fulminant CHF may occur in up to 28% treated with high-dose cyclophosphamide
      ○ CHF usually short lived and reversible
  - Drug is metabolized to its active form in the liver by the cytochrome P-450
    - More rapid metabolism amplifies the risk of CHF

- Another cardiotoxicity is hemorrhagic myocarditis
  - Putatively mediated by endothelial capillary injury
  - Results in pericardial effusion, tamponade, and death
  - Most effusions are treatable with corticosteroids and analgesics
- When purine analogue pentostatin used in bone marrow conditioning regimens in combination with cyclophosphamide
  - An increased incidence of fatal cardiac toxicity that includes myocardial infarction, CHF, and arrhythmias
- Possible additive effect of cyclophosphamide and anthracycline-induced cardiomyopathy, but data are conflicting
- **Iphosphamide:** An alkylating agent, with similar properties to cyclophosphamide
  - Used to treat lymphoma, leukemia, and testicular and bladder tumors
  - Arrhythmias and transient, reversible, dose-dependent CHF may be seen
- **Cisplatin:** Cross-links interstrand DNA
  - Used in treating cancers of the testes, bladder, ovaries, and other tumors
  - Bradycardia, SVT, acute ischemia, myocardial infarction (MI), and ischemic cardiomyopathy observed
  - Acute chest pain and palpitations associated with cisplatin infusion
  - Late complications occur 10 to 20 years after therapy
  - Hypomagnesemia and hypokalemia generated by cisplatin-induced tubular defects may exacerbate arrhythmias

Microtubule-Targeting Agents

- **Vinca Alkaloids:** Vinca alkaloids include vincristine and vinblastine
  - Used for management of hematologic malignancies and solid tumors
  - Vinorelbine, a semisynthetic derivative used in NSCLC therapy
  - Exert toxicity by inhibiting microtubule assembly
    - All possess vasoconstrictive properties
    - Hypertension, vasospastic myocardial ischemia, and myocardial infarction seen
    - Vinorelbine toxicity is more common in women than men
- **Taxanes:** Hypertension and cardiac arrhythmias, most commonly transient asymptomatic bradycardia observed with paclitaxel
  - Incidence of more significant bradyarrhythmias—Mobitz type I and II heart block and complete heart block—was 0.1%
  - Rarely see atrial and ventricular tachycardias, myocardial ischemia, and MI
    - Often in patients with underlying cardiac disease or electrolyte derangements
  - Docetaxel may lead to the potentiation of anthracycline cardiomyopathy

Antimetabolites

- **5-Fluoruracil and Capecitabine:** 5-FU a synthetic pyrimidine antimetabolite used in regimens for managing multiple solid tumors including gastrointestinal, breast, ovarian, and head and neck malignancies
  - Myocardial ischemia, possibly triggered by coronary vasospasm, well-known cardiac toxicity occurring with increased frequency in combination with cisplatin

- Silent ischemic ECG changes identified during 24 hours of observation in up to 68% of patients receiving a continuous 5-FU infusion
- Other cardiac manifestations include chest pain, angina, atrial and ventricular arrhythmias, MI, persistent ventricular dysfunction, sudden death, and cardiogenic shock requiring inotropic support
- Preexisting cardiac morbidity significantly increases risk of cardiotoxicity
  - Compared to no prior cardiac disease (15.1% vs. 1.5%)
- Given potential for severe cardiotoxicity, infusions terminated when chest pain occurs
- Oral equivalent of infused 5-FU is capecitabine
- Exhibits a similar cardiotoxicity profile to 5-FU

Topoisomerase Inhibitors

- **Etoposide:** A topoisomerase II inhibitor used primarily for treatment of refractory testicular tumors and small cell lung carcinoma
  - Hypotension the most common side effect
  - MI and vasospastic angina may also occur
  - Prior chemotherapy or mediastinal irradiation may increase MI risk after etoposide therapy

Biologic Response Modifiers (BRM)

- **Interferons:** Glycoprotein BRM classified according to their respective derivations:
  - Interferon-*alfa* (leukocytes)
  - Interferon-*beta* (fibroblasts)
  - Interferon-*gamma* (lymphocytes)
    - Used to treat various tumors including renal cell carcinoma, metastatic melanoma, multiple myeloma, Kaposi sarcoma, and some leukemias and lymphomas
    - Cardiovascular toxicities include hypertension or hypotension, ischemia in patients with coronary artery disease (CAD), MI, arrhythmias (20% incidence), sudden death, and cardiomyopathy characterized by resolution with termination of the infusion
- **Interleukin-2 (IL-2):** A glycoprotein BRM derived from helper T-lymphocytes
  - Approved for treatment of metastatic renal cell cancer
  - Most patients develop capillary leak syndrome and hypotension associated with decreased peripheral vascular resistance necessitating vasopressors
    - In 423 treatment courses with IL-2, 65% of patients required pressor support
    - In patients with CAD, direct myocardial toxicity precipitates ischemia, MI, arrhythmias, and death
    - IL-2 may also predispose to ventricular and supraventricular arrhythmias
      - Seen in 14% to 21% of patients

Differentiation Agents

- **All-*trans*-Retinoic Acid:** (See also Pulmonary Toxicities.) Pericardial effusions, cardiac tamponade, myocardial ischemia, fatal infarction, and thrombosis
- **Arsenic Trioxide:** A differentiation agent effective in treating relapsed acute promyelocytic leukemia
  - Like all-*trans*-retinoic acid, may cause the retinoic acid syndrome
  - Prolongation of QT interval is another complication seen in up to 63% of patients

- Leading to torsades de pointes and sudden death
- Degree of QT prolongation higher in presence of hypokalemia
  - Careful monitoring of electrolytes and maintaining levels in high normal range is prudent

Monoclonal Antibodies

- **Trastuzumab:** (See also Pulmonary Toxicities.) An increased risk of cardiotoxicity associated with trastuzumab
  - Highest in patients receiving concurrent:
    - Anthracycline plus cyclophosphamide (27%)
    - Concomitant trastuzumab and paclitaxel (13%)
    - Trastuzumab alone (3%–7%)
  - Mechanism of cardiac toxicity not well understood
    - Cardiac erbB2 essential for myocyte function
    - Trastuzumab targets both HER2 and erbB2 receptors
    - Early symptom following initial treatment may be an asymptomatic decline in LVEF
      - With late progression to dilated cardiomyopathy
    - Risk factors for cardiovascular toxicity include older age, cumulative doxorubicin dosage 400 mg/m^2 or greater, and concurrent anthracycline and trastuzumab administration, rather than temporally separated dosing
- **Rituximab:** The CD20 antigen, present on normal and malignant B cells, the target of the chimeric murine/human monoclonal antibody rituximab
  - Used to treat leukemias and lymphomas, as well as benign diseases
  - Cardiac toxicity involves dysrhythmias and angina in <1% of infusions
    - Most adverse effects infusion related, usually occurring within 2 hours of first infusion
    - Acute infusion-related deaths reported in 0.04% to 0.07% of cases
    - Clinical presentation in these patients includes hypoxia, pulmonary infiltrates, ARDS, MI, ventricular fibrillation, and cardiogenic shock
    - Hypersensitivity reactions, including hypotension, angioedema, hypoxia, or bronchospasm, occur in up to 10% of cases
    - Management is supportive, using IV fluids, antihistamines, acetaminophen, bronchodilators, and vasopressors
- **Cetuximab:** Agent is human/mouse chimeric monoclonal antibody designed to target human epidermal growth factor receptor
  - Used alone or in combination therapy with irinotecan to treat metastatic colorectal cancer
  - Life-threatening infusion reactions occur in 3% of patients with:
    - Bronchospasm, urticaria, and hypotension
  - Interstitial pneumonitis with noncardiogenic pulmonary edema a rare toxicity
- **Bevacizumab:** (See also Pulmonary Toxicities.) Associated with CHF, hypertension, and arterial thromboembolism
  - With monotherapy, 2% of patients developed moderate to life-threatening (grades 2 to 4) left ventricular dysfunction
  - CHF developed in 14% of patients concurrently receiving anthracyclines, and in 4% of patients previously receiving anthracyclines or left chest wall irradiation
  - Clinical trials documented hypertension in 5% of patients, with reports of hypertensive crisis, hypertensive encephalopathy, and subarachnoid hemorrhage

- U.S. Food and Drug Administration warning to health care providers announcing demonstrated increased risk of arterial thromboembolic events, which include cerebrovascular accident, transient ischemic attack, MI, and angina
- Risk of fatal arterial thrombotic events doubled to 5% in patients receiving intravenous 5-FU and bevacizumab

Hematologic Toxicities

Thalidomide

- A sedative-hypnotic with anti-inflammatory properties
- Used in multiple myeloma patients to treat advanced and chemotherapy-refractory disease
- Mechanism of action is unclear
  - Immune modulation, antiangiogenesis, and tumor necrosis factor-α may play role
- Increased risk of venous thromboembolism (VTE) associated with agent
  - Occurs at a mean of 2 months of therapy
  - Lower extremity deep vein thrombosis (DVT) the most frequent thrombotic complication
  - Approximately 50% of patients will develop pulmonary embolism (PE)
  - Mechanism of thalidomide-induced DVT not well defined
    - Thalidomide may exert direct effect on endothelial cells injured by other chemotherapy agents such as doxorubicin
    - VTE rates with thalidomide monotherapy, thalidomide–dexamethasone, thalidomide–doxorubicin, and thalidomide–dexamethasone–doxorubicin
      – Were <5%, 9%, 12%, and 22%, respectively
      – This suggests role for VTE prophylaxis

Hormones

- **Estramustine:** Estramustine phosphate has hormonal properties because it contains nor-nitrogen mustard linked to 17 beta-estradiol.
  - Used in treatment of prostate cancer
  - Up to 10% of patients receiving estramustine have:
    - VTE and PE
    - Myocardial and cerebrovascular ischemia
- **Tamoxifen and Aromatase Inhibitors:** Tamoxifen and the aromatase inhibitors—anastrozole, letrozole, and exemestane—adjuvant therapy for early-stage estrogen receptor–positive breast carcinoma
  - Increased risk of VTE with tamoxifen
    - Incidence of VTE in general population is 0.12% per year and 0.09% per year in women
    - In women with early-stage breast cancer and no adjuvant treatment, compared to those receiving tamoxifen
      - Incidence increases to 0.4% over 5 years and 1.4% to 1.7% over 5 years, respectively
      - Incidence escalates to 10.8% over 5 years in same population of women
        – Receiving concurrent tamoxifen and chemotherapy
  - Aromatase inhibitors (AI) generally associated with lower risk of VTE than tamoxifen
    - At 5 years incidence of VTE with anastrazole 1.6% versus 2.4% with tamoxifen

Gastrointestinal Toxicities

Bevacizumab

- Associated with both bowel perforation and GI hemorrhage
  - In patients with metastatic colon cancer receiving irinotecan, fluorouracil, and leucovorin (IFL) plus bevacizumab, or IFL alone
    - GI perforation observed in six patients (1.5%) treated with IFL plus bevacizumab with one fatality compared to none in IFL group
  - More recent phase II trial adding bevacizumab to bolus 5-FU and leucovorin
    - Bowel perforation in 2% of cases
    - In advanced refractory colorectal cancer, severe to life-threatening GI hemorrhage (grades 3 and 4) seen in 3.8% patients

Genitourinary Toxicities

Cyclophosphamide and Ifosfamide

- Cyclophosphamide and ifosfamide induce early (within 72 hours of administration) hemorrhagic cystitis via their metabolite, acrolein
- Causes denudation of bladder mucosa and bleeding
- Early hemorrhagic cystitis was observed in over 40% of bone marrow transplants
  - Rate dramatically declined to 5% with aggressive hydration regimens and administration of the thiol mesna
  - Mesna a type of thiol that inactivates acrolein in bladder after being converted to active form in kidney
    - Must be administered prior to cyclophosphamide infusion and continued after infusion terminated consequent to its shorter half-life
- Cases of hemorrhagic cystitis progressing to intractable or profuse bleeding
  - Bladder irrigation and cystoscopy with clot extraction and fulguration may be necessary to achieve hemostasis
  - Cystectomy, vascular ligation, or hyperbaric therapy required in recalcitrant cases
- Late occurring hemorrhagic cystitis starts 72 hours after administration of preparatory regimens in bone marrow transplantation
  - Risk factors including viral infections, busulfan use, pelvic irradiation, older age at transplantation, allogenic transplantation, and graft versus host disease

Mitomycin C

- One life-threatening manifestation of mitomycin is thrombotic thrombocytopenic purpura-hemolytic uremic syndrome (TTP-HUS)
  - A distinct multiorgan disorder distinguished by:
    - Thrombocytopenia
    - Microangiopathic hemolytic anemia (MAHA)
    - Tissue ischemia
  - Precipitated by platelet agglutination in the arterial microvasculature
  - Classic pentad no longer required to make the diagnosis
    - Fever, thrombocytopenia, MAHA, renal failure, neurologic dysfunction

- New definition encompasses a broad spectrum of conditions in which unexplained thrombocytopenia and MAHA are present
- Of chemotherapeutic agents associated with TTP-HUS, mitomycin the most common
  - Bleomycin, cisplatin, and gemcitabine also causes of syndrome
- Pathogenic mechanism of mitomycin C–induced TTP-HUS may involve:
  - Chemotherapy-induced endothelial cell injury
  - Circulating immune complexes against tumor-related antigens
- In some cancer patients difficult to attribute TTP-HUS to mitomycin
  - Because malignancy-induced TTP-HUS clinically indistinguishable from mitomycin-induced disease

- TTP-HUS typically seen 4 to 8 weeks following final dose of mitomycin
  - Usually present with dyspnea from noncardiogenic pulmonary edema
    - May progress to ARDS and may mimic mitomycin lung toxicity
  - Renal failure generally present
  - Neurologic symptoms infrequent
- Patients with mitomycin-induced TTP-HUS do not respond to plasmapheresis
  - Immunoadsorption of plasma over a staphylococcal protein A column to remove immune complexes may be effective
  - Prognosis of mitomycin-induced TTP-HUS is poor
    - Most patients succumb to pulmonary or renal failure or to underlying malignancy within 4 months

APPENDIX A: FLUIDS AND ELECTROLYTES

TABLE A.1

INTRAVENOUS FLUIDS

Solution			Na	Cl	K	Ca	Mg	Acetate	Gluconate	Albumin	Lactate	Dextrose
Units	mOsm/L	pH	mmol/L			mg/dL				g/L		
5% Dextrose (D$_5$W)	250–253	5	—	—	—	—	—	—	—	—	—	50
0.45% NaCl (½ NS)	155	5–5.6	77	77	—	—	—	—	—	—	—	—
0.9% NaCl (NS)	308	5.7	154	154	—	—	—	—	—	—	—	—
0.45% NaCl + D$_5$W (D$_5$ ½ NS)	406	4–4.4	77	77	—	—	—	—	—	—	—	50
0.9% NaCl + D$_5$W (D$_5$NS)	561	4–4.4	154	154	—	—	—	—	—	—	—	50
Ringer solution	309	6	147	156	4	4–4.5	—	—	—	—	—	—
Lactated Ringer (LR)	275	6.7	130	109	4	3	—	—	—	—	28	—
5% Dextrose + lactated Ringer (D$_5$LR)	525–530	4.7–5	130	109	4	3	—	—	—	—	28	50
Plasma protein fractions 5%	294	6.7–7.3	130–160	90	0–5	—	0–3	0–27	0–23	0–12.5	—	—
3% NaCl	1,026	5.8	513	513	—	—	—	—	—	—	—	—
5% NaCl	1,710	5–6	855	855	—	—	—	—	—	—	—	—
Mannitol 5%	275	6										
Mannitol 1.0%	550	6										
Mannitol 15%	825	6										
Mannitol 20%	7.100	6										
Mannitol 25%	1,375	6										
Fresh frozen plasma	31.0–33.0		7.68	76	3.2	3.2	8.2	—	—	—	—	—
Dextran–40 in NS	310	5–5.5	154	154	—	—	—	—	—	—	—	—
Dextran–70 in D$_5$W	287	3.5–7										50
5% Albumin	300	6.9	145	145						50		
25% Albumin		6.9	145	145						250		
Hydroxyethyl starch 6% (Hetastarch)	310	5.5	1.54	154								

Na, sodium; Cl, chloride; K, potassium; Ca, calcium; Mg, magnesium; D$_5$W, 5% dextrose in water; NaCl, sodium chloride; NS, normal saline.

OSMOLALITY

Calculated serum osmolality

$$= 2[Na^+] + \frac{[glucose]}{18}$$

$$+ \frac{[BUN]}{2.8} + \frac{[mannitol]}{18} + \frac{[EtOH]}{4.6} + \frac{[ethylene\ glycol]}{6.2}$$

$$+ \frac{[methanol]}{3.2}$$

[Normal 275–290 mmol/kg]

Osmolar gap =

Measured serum osmolality − Calculated serum osmolality

[0–5 mOsm/kg]

Sodium (Na$^+$)

Pseudohyponatremia with hyperglycemia

Each 100-mg/dL increase in serum glucose (above 100 mg/dL) decreases Na$^+$ by 1.6 mmol/L

Free water deficit in hypernatremia

$$= (0.6)(body\ weight\ in\ kg)\left(\frac{[Na^+]}{140} - 1\right)$$

Free water excess in hyponatremia

$$= (0.6)(body\ weight\ in\ kg)\left(1 - \frac{[Na^+]}{140}\right)$$

POTASSIUM (K$^+$)

[K$^+$] increases 0.6 mmol/L for each 0.1-unit decrease in pH

APPENDIX B: ACID-BASE

TABLE B.1

ANTICIPATED CHANGES IN SIMPLE DISTURBANCES

Primary disorder	Primary	Secondary	Compensation	Limit	Net effect
Metabolic acidosis	↓ [HCO$_3$]	↓ PaCO$_2$	Δ PaCO$_2$ = 1.0–1.4 × δ [HCO$_3$]	10 mm Hg	↑ [H$^+$](↓ pH)
Metabolic alkalosis	↑ [HCO$_3$]	↑ PaCO$_2$	Δ PaCO$_2$ = 0.5–1.0 × δ [HCO$_3$]	55 mm Hg No hypoxia	↓ [H$^+$](↑ pH)
Respiratory acidosis	↑ PaCO$_2$	↑ [HCO$_3$]	Acute: Δ [H$^+$] 0.75 δ PaCO$_2$ Δ [HCO$_3$] = 1 mmol/L ↑ /10 mm Hg ↑ PaCO$_2$ Δ [HCO$_3$] = 0.1 × δ PaCO$_2$ Chronic: Δ [HCO$_3$] = 0.35 × PaCO$_2$ Δ [HCO$_3$] = mmol/L ↑ /10 mm Hg ↑ PaCO$_2$	30 mmol/L HCO$_3$ 45 mmol/L HCO$_3$	↑ [H$^+$](↓ pH)
Respiratory alkalosis	↓ PaCO$_2$	↓ [HCO$_3$]	Acute: Δ [HCO$_3$] = 0.2 × δ PaCO$_2$ Δ [HCO$_3$] = 1 mmol/L ↓ /10 mm Hg ↓ PaCO$_2$ Δ [H$^+$] 0.75 δ PaCO$_2$ Chronic: Δ [HCO$_3$] = 0.5 × δ PaCO$_2$ Δ [HCO$_3$] = 2–5 mmol/L ↓ /10 mm Hg ↓ PaCO$_2$	18 mmol/L 12–15 mmol/L	↓ [H$^+$](↑ pH)

CAUSES OF SIMPLE ACID-BASE DISTURBANCES

A. Metabolic acidosis
  1. Increased anion gap (usually decreased chloride)
    a. Acidosis
      1. Alcoholic ketoacidosis
      2. Diabetic ketoacidosis
      3. Starvation ketoacidosis
      4. Ethylene glycol ingestion
      5. Paraldehyde
      6. Methanol ingestion
      7. Lactic acidosis
      8. Uremic acidosis
      9. Hyperosmolar nonketotic coma
    b. Nonacidosis
      1. Hypokalemia
      2. Hypocalcemia
      3. Hypomagnesemia
      4. Hyperalbuminemia
      5. Nitrate usage
      6. Penicillin/carbenicillin
      7. Pseudohypernatremia
      8. Pseudohypochloremia
      9. False decrease in serum HCO$_3^-$

2. Normal anion gap (usually increased chloride)
   a. Acidosis
      1. Carbonic anhydrase inhibitors
      2. Ureterosigmoidostomy
      3. Ileostomy
      4. Diarrhea
      5. Pancreatic fistula
      6. Parenteral nutrition
      7. Ingestion of NH_4Cl
      8. Ingestion of HCl or other acid
      9. Renal tubular acidosis
      10. Dilutional acidosis
      11. Following respiratory alkalosis
      12. Cholestyramine
      13. Normal saline infusions
   b. Nonacidosis
      1. Hyperkalemia
      2. Hypocalcemia
      3. Hypomagnesemia
      4. Hypoalbuminemia
      5. IgG
      6. Lithium
      7. Pseudohyponatremia
      8. Pseudohyperchloremia
      9. False increase in serum HCO_3^-

B. Metabolic alkalosis
   1. Loss of H^+
      a. Gastrointestinal loss
         1. Vomiting, nasogastric suction
         2. Antacids
         3. Chloride-depleting diarrhea
      b. Renal loss
         1. Diuretics
         2. Excess mineralocorticoid
         3. Postchronic hypercapnia
         4. Decreased chloride intake

      5. High-dose penicillins
      6. Hypercalcemia
   c. Intracellular H^+ shift
      1. Hypokalemia
      2. Refeeding
   2. HCO_3^- retention
      a. Massive transfusions
      b. $NaHCO_3$ therapy
      c. Milk-alkali syndrome
   3. Volume contraction
      a. Diuretics
      b. Gastrointestinal losses in patients with achlorhydria
      c. Sweat losses in cystic fibrosis

C. Respiratory acidosis
   1. Central nervous system (CNS) depression
   2. Chronic obstructive lung disease
   3. Severe asthma
   4. Pneumothorax
   5. Abdominal distention
   6. Pulmonary edema
   7. Mechanical underventilation
   8. Idiopathic hypoventilation
   9. Neuromuscular disease

D. Respiratory alkalosis
   1. Salicylate toxicity
   2. Hepatic failure
   3. Psychogenic hyperventilation
   4. Pulmonary edema
   5. Asthma
   6. Systemic inflammatory response syndrome
   7. Restrictive lung disease
   8. Primary CNS disease
   9. Mechanical overventilation
   10. Hypoxemia

APPENDIX C: FORMULAS

CEREBRAL/NEUROLOGIC FORMULAS

Intracranial pressure (ICP)
   [<20 cm H_2O, <15 mm Hg]

   Cerebral perfusion pressure (CPP) = MAP − ICP

[70–100 mm Hg]

Cerebral vascular resistance (CVR)
   [1.5–2.1 mm Hg/100 g/min/mL]

   Cerebral blood flow (CBF) = CPP/CVR

[75 mL/100 g gray matter/min]
[45 mL/100 g white matter/min]

Jugular bulb saturation ($S_{jv}O_2$)
   [55%–70%]

Cerebral metabolic rate ($CMRO_2$) = (CBF) ($CaO_2 - C_{jv}O_2$)

[3–3.5 mL/100 g/min]

$$\text{Cerebral oxygen extraction} = \frac{CMO_2}{(CBF)(CaO_2)} = \frac{CaO_2 - C_{jv}O_2}{CaO_2}$$

HEMODYNAMIC FORMULAS

Pulse pressure = systolic BP − diastolic BP

$$\text{Mean arterial pressure (MAP)} = \frac{SBP + 2(DBP)}{3}$$

[70–105 mm Hg]

Central venous pressure (CVP)
   [0–8 mm Hg]

Mean pulmonary artery pressure ($\overline{PA}$)
   [10–20 mm Hg]

Pulmonary artery occlusion pressure (PAOP)
   [4–12 mm Hg]

Cardiac output (CO) = Stroke volume (SV) × Heart rate (HR)

[4–8 L/min]

$$\text{Cardiac index (CI)} = \frac{CO}{BSA}$$

[2.5–4.0 L/min/m^2]

Pulmonary vascular resistance (PVR) $= \dfrac{(\overline{PA} - PAOP)80}{CO}$

[150–250 dyne/s/cm^{-5}]

Pulmonary vascular resistance index (PVRI) $= \dfrac{(\overline{PA} - PAOP)80}{CI}$

[100–240 dyne/s/cm^{-5}/m^2]

Systemic vascular resistance (SVR) $= \dfrac{(MAP - CVP)80}{CO}$

[800–1,200 dyne/s/cm^{-5}]

Systemic vascular resistance index (SVRI) $= \dfrac{(MAP - CVP)80}{CI}$

[1,300–2,900 dyne/s/cm^{-5}/m^2]

Stroke volume index (SVI) $= \dfrac{CI}{HR}$

[40 ± 7 mL/beat/m^2]

Right ventricular stroke work index (RVSWI)

$= SVI(\overline{PA} - CVP)(0.0136)$

[6–10 g · meter/m^2 per beat]

Left ventricular stroke work index (LVSWI)

$= SVI(MAP - PAOP)(0.0136)$

[43–56 g · meter/m^2 per beat]

Arterial O_2 content (CaO_2) = O_2 combined with hemoglobin + O_2 dissolved in the plasma

[1 g Hb binds 1.36 mL O_2]

$= (1.36)(Hb)(SaO_2) + 0.0031(PaO_2)$

[20 mL O_2/dL]

Mixed venous O_2 saturation ($S\overline{v}O_2$)
[75%]

Mixed venous O_2 content ($C\overline{v}O_2$) $= (1.36)(Hb)(S\overline{v}O_2)$

$+ 0.0031(PvO_2)$

[15 mL O_2/dL]

O_2 delivery ($\dot{D}O_2$) = CO × CaO_2 × 10

[600–1,000 mL O_2/min]

Oxygen delivery indexed (DO_2I) = CI × CaO_2 × 10

[500–600 mL/min/m^2]

O_2 consumption ($\dot{V}O_2$) = CI($CaO_2 - C\overline{v}O_2$)

[110–150 mL/min/m^2]

O_2 extraction ratio $= \dfrac{(CaO_2 - C\overline{v}O_2)}{CaO_2}$

[25%]

RESPIRATORY FORMULAS

Oxygenation

Fraction of inspired O_2 (FIO_2)
[0.21–1.0]

Respiratory quotient (R) = VCO_2 expired/VO_2 inspired

[Normal: 0.8]
Barometric pressure (PB)
[760 mm Hg at sea level]
Partial pressure of H_2O (PH_2O)
[47 mm Hg at 37°C]

Partial pressure of inspired O_2 (PIO_2) = FIO_2 (PB − PH_2O)

[150 mm Hg at sea level]

Partial pressure of alveolar O_2 (PAO_2) (alveolar gas equation)

$$PAO_2 = FIO_2 (PB - PH_2O) - \dfrac{PaCO_2}{R}$$
$$= (FIO_2 × 713) - (PaCO_2/0.8) \text{ (at sea level)}$$
$$= 150 - (PaCO_2/0.8) \text{ (at sea level on room air)}$$

[Range: 100 mm Hg on room air; 673 mm Hg on 100% O_2]
Partial pressure of arterial O_2 (PaO_2)
[70–100 mm Hg]
Increased: hyperventilation, increased FIO_2, contaminated sample
Decreased: hypoventilation, decreased FIO_2, $\dot{V}/\dot{Q}$ mismatch, intrapulmonary or anatomic R → L shunt, diffusion abnormalities

Alveolar–arterial O_2 gradient (P(A − a)O_2) = PAO_2 − PaO_2

[3–16 mm Hg on room air; 25–65 mm Hg on 100% O_2]

Ventilation

Partial pressure of arterial CO_2 ($PaCO_2$)
[46 mm Hg]
Partial pressure of alveolar (expired) CO_2 ($P\overline{E}CO_2$)
Dead-space ventilation (VD): Portion of VT that does not participate in gas exchange

VD = anatomic dead space + physiologic dead space

[150 mL]
Engelhoff modification of the Bohr formula for dead space

$$\dfrac{VD}{VT} = \dfrac{PaCO_2 - PECO_2}{PaCO_2}$$

Minute ventilation (VE) = respiratory rate × VT

Pulmonary capillary blood O_2 content (CcO_2)

$= 1.36 (Hb)(SaO_2)(FIO_2) + 0.003 (PBH_2O - PaCO_2)(FIO_2)$

Shunt fraction ($\dot{Q}s/\dot{Q}t$) $= \dfrac{CcO_2 - CaO_2}{CcO_2 - CvO_2}$

Lung Volumes

Tidal volume (VT): Volume inspired/expired with each breath
   [500 mL; 6–7 mL/kg lean body weight]
Inspiratory reserve volume (IRV): Maximal inspired volume end-tidal inspiration
   [25% of vital capacity (VC)]
Inspiratory capacity (IC): Maximal volume inspired from resting expiratory level

$$IC = IRV + VT$$

   [1–2.4 L]
Expiratory reserve volume (ERV): Maximal expired volume from end-tidal inspiration
   [25% of vital capacity (VC)]
Residual volume (RV): Volume remaining in lungs after maximal expiration
   [1–2.4 L]
Functional residual capacity (FRC): Volume remaining in lungs at end-tidal expiration

$$FRC = ERV + RV$$

   [1.8–3.4 L]
Vital capacity (VC): Maximal volume expelled by forceful effort after maximal inspiration

$$VC = IRV + ERV + VT$$

   [3–5 L; 50–60 mL/kg lean body weight in females; 70 mL/kg lean body weight in males]
Total lung capacity (TLC): Volume in lungs at end of maximal inspiration

$$TLC = VC + RV$$

   [4–6 L]

Lung Mechanics

Plateau pressure (Pplat)
Peak inspiratory pressure (PIP)
Positive end-expiratory pressure (PEEP)

Compliance = change in volume/change in pressure

$$Static\ compliance\ (Cst) = \frac{VT}{Pplat - PEEP}$$

   [70–160 mL/cm H_2O (paralyzed/anesthetized and supine)]

$$Dynamic\ compliance\ (Cdyn) = \frac{VT}{PIP - PEEP}$$

   [50–80 mL/cm H_2O (paralyzed/anesthetized and supine)]

RENAL FORMULAS

$$Creatinine\ clearance\ (Cl_{Creat}) = \frac{(U_{Creat})(urine\ volume)}{P_{Creat}}$$

Fractional excretion of sodium (FeNa$^+$)

$$= \frac{urine\ [Na^+]}{plasma\ [Na^+]} \times \frac{plasma\ [creatinine]}{urine\ [creatinine]} \times 100$$

Free water clearance

$$= urine\ vol - \frac{urine\ osmolality}{plasma\ osmolality} \times urine\ vol$$

TABLE C.1

DAILY RENAL EXCRETION OF CATIONS AND ANIONS IN NORMALS

Electrolyte	Urinary excretion (mmol/d)
CATIONS	
Na	127 ± 6
K	49 ± 2
Ca	4 ± 1
Mg	11 ± 1
NH_4	28 ± 2
Total	**219 ± 3**
ANIONS	
Cl	135 ± 5
SO_4	34 ± 1
PO_4	20 ± 1
Organic anions	29 ± 1
Total	**221 ± 6**

Na, sodium; K, potassium; Ca, calcium; Mg, magnesium; NH_4, ammonia; Cl, chloride; SO_4, sulfate; H_2PO_4, phosphate.
From Goldstein MB, Bear R, Richardson RMA, et al. The urine anion gap: a clinically useful index of ammonium excretion. *Am J Med Sci.* 1986;292:198, with permission.

TABLE C.2

USE OF URINE ELECTROLYTES

Diagnostic problem	Urinary value	Primary diagnostic possibilities
Volume depletion	Na = 0–10 mmol/L	Extrarenal sodium loss
	Na >10 mmol/L	Renal salt wasting or adrenal insufficiency
Acute oliguria	Na = 0–10 mmol/L	Prerenal azotemia
	Na >30 mmol/L	Acute tubular necrosis
Hyponatremia	Na = 0–10 mmol/L	Severe volume depletion, edematous
	Na >dietary intake	Inappropriate antidiuretic hormone secretion; adrenal insufficiency
Hypokalemia	K = 0–10 mmol/L	Extrarenal K loss
	K >10 mmol/L	Renal K loss
Metabolic alkalosis	Cl = 0–10 mmol/L	Cl-responsive alkalosis
	Cl = dietary intake	Cl-resistant alkalosis

Na, sodium; K, potassium; Cl, chloride.

TABLE C.3

INTERPRETATION OF URINE ELECTROLYTES

Electrolyte	Normal response	Patient response	Potential pitfalls
Na^+	Reflects diet and ECF volume; <10 mmol if ECF vol contracted	>20 mmol in ECF vol contraction suggests renal tubular damage	Diuretic use No reabsorbed anions Recent vomiting, drugs
Cl^-	Reflects diet and ECF volume; <10 mmol if ECF vol contracted	>20 mmol with ECF vol contraction suggests renal damage	Diuretic Diarrhea
K^+	Reflects diet, plasma [K], aldosterone action	If hypokalemia and urine [K] >20 mM or rate of K excretion >30 mmol/d then K excretion too high	K-sparing diuretics Low urine [Na] Water diuresis
pH	Depends on acid-base status Useful for bicarbonaturia	Useful once low NH_4^+ excretion confirmed to define cause of low NH_4^+	Unreliable for urine NH_4^+ Urinary tract infection
HCO_3^-	Depends on diet and acid-base status; >10 mM indicates HCO_3^- load 0 in acidemia	High urine HCO_3^- with chronic metabolic alkalosis indicates vomiting or HCO_3^- input High urine HCO_3 with acidemia in pRTA	Urinary tract infection Carbonic anhydrase inhibitors
(Na^+, K^+, Cl^-)	Depends on diet and acid-base status	Na + K > Cl = low urine NH_4^+ Cl > Na + K = high urine NH_4^+	Ketonuria Drug anions Alkaline urine

Na^+, sodium; Cl, chloride; K^+, potassium; HCO_3^-, carbonate; NH_4, ammonia; ECF, extracellular fluid; pRTA, partial renal tubular acidosis; vol, volume.
From Halperin ML, Goldstein MB. *Fluid, Electrolyte and Acid-Base Emergencies*. Philadelphia: WB Saunders; 1988, with permission.

TOXICOLOGY FORMULAS

Serum methanol concentration [MeOH] in mg/dL
$$= 3.2(Osm_s - (2 \times [Na^+]) - ([BUN]/2.8) - ([glucose]/18) - ([ETOH]/4.6) - 10)$$

Ethylene glycol concentration $= 6.2(Osm_s - (2 \times [Na^+]) - ([BUN]/2.8) - ([glucose]/18) - ([EtOH]/4.6) - 10)$

INFECTIOUS DISEASES FORMULAS

Antibiotic kinetics:
The *volume of distribution* (V_D) of an antimicrobial is calculated as:

$$V_D = \frac{A}{C_p}$$

where A = total amount of antibiotic in the body and C_p = antibiotic plasma concentration.

Repetitive dosing of antibiotics depends on the principle of *minimal plasma concentrations* (C_{min}):

$$C_{min} = \frac{D}{(V_D)(2^n - 1)}$$

where D = dose and n = dosing interval expressed in half-lives.

The *plasma concentration at steady state* (C_{ss}) of an antimicrobial can be estimated utilizing the following formula:

$$C_{ss} = \frac{\text{Dose per half-life}}{(0.693)(V_D)}$$

Antibiotic adjustments:
Renal dysfunction in critically ill patients is common. In those patients receiving aminoglycosides, dosage modification is required according to the *aminoglycoside clearance*:

$$\text{Aminoglycoside clearance} = (C_{cr})(0.6) + 10$$

where C_{cr} = creatinine clearance in mL/minute.

In order to estimate the *creatinine clearance*, the *Cockcrof and Gault formula* is utilized:

$$C_{cr} \text{ (mL/min)} = \frac{(140 - \text{age}) \times \text{weight}}{Cr \times 72}$$

where Cr = serum creatinine in mg/dL. Another modification to this formula is the *Spyker and Guerrant method*:

$$C_{cr} \text{ (mL/min)} = \frac{(140 - \text{age}) \times (1.03 - 0.053 \times Cr)}{Cr}$$

APPENDIX D: PHARMACOLOGY

DRUG FORMULAS

Drug clearance $= V_d \times K_{el}$

Drug half-life $(T_{1/2}) = 0.693/K_{el}$

Drug elimination constant $(K_{el}) = \dfrac{\ln([peak]/[trough])}{{}^t peak - {}^t trough}$

Drug loading dose $= V_d \times [target\ peak]$

Drug dosing interval
$= (-1/K_{el}) \times \ln([desired\ trough]/[desired\ peak])$
$+ infusion\ time\ (h)$

TABLE D.1

DRUG DOSAGE ADJUSTMENTS IN RENAL FAILURE

	Dose adjustment	GFR (mL/min)			Removed by	
		>50	10–50	<10	Hemodialysis	Peritoneal dialysis
Aminoglycosides						
Gentamicin	D	60–90	30–70	20–30	Yes	Yes
	I	8–12	12	24		
Tobramycin	D	60–90	30–70	20–30	Yes	Yes
	I	8–12	12	24		
Antifungals						
Amphotericin B	I	24	24	24–36	No	No
Flucytosine	I	6	12–24	24–48	Yes	Yes
Antituberculous						
Ethambutol	I	24	24–36	48	Yes	Yes
Isoniazid	D	100	100	66–75	Yes	Yes
Rifampin	I	None	None	None	No	No
Antivirals						
Acyclovir	I	8	24	48	Yes	—
Amantadine	I	12–24	48–72	168	No	No
Cephalosporins						
Cefamandole	I	6	6–8	8	Yes	—
Cefazolin	I	6	12	24–48	Yes	—
Cefotaxime	I	6–8	8–12	12–24	Yes	—
Cefoxitin	I	8	8–12	24–48	Yes	—
Cephalothin	I	6	6	8–12	Yes	Yes
Chloramphenicol	D	None	None	None	Yes	No
Clindamycin	D	None	None	None	No	No
Erythromycin	D	None	None	None	No	No
Metronidazole	I	8	8–12	12–24	Yes	No
Nitrofurantoin	D	100	Avoid	Avoid	Yes	—
Penicillins						
Amoxicillin	I	6	6–12	12–16	Yes	No
Ampicillin	I	6	6–12	12–16	Yes	No
Carbenicillin	I	8–12	12–24	24–48	Yes	Yes
Dicloxacillin	D	None	None	None	No	—
Nafcillin	D	None	None	None	No	—
PCN G	I	6–8	8–12	12–16	Yes	No
Piperacillin	I	4–6	6–8	8	Yes	—
Ticarcillin	I	8–12	12–24	24–28	Yes	Yes
Sulfas/trimethoprim						
Sulfamethoxazole	I	12	18	24	Yes	No
Trimethoprim	I	12	18	24	Yes	No
Tetracyclines						
Doxycycline	I	12	12–18	18–24	No	No
Minocycline	D	None	None	None	No	No
Vancomycin	I	24–72	72–240	240	No	No

(continued)

TABLE D.1

CONTINUED

	Dose adjustment	GFR (mL/min)			Removed by	
		>50	10–50	<10	Hemodialysis	Peritoneal dialysis
Antihypertensives						
Atenolol	D	None	50	25	Yes	—
Captopril	D	None	None	50	Yes	—
Clonidine	D	None	None	50–75	No	—
Hydralazine	D	8	8	12–24	No	No
Methyldopa	I	6	9–18	12–24	Yes	Yes
Metoprolol	D	None	None	None	Yes	—
Minoxidil	D	None	None	None	Yes	
Nadolol	D	None	50	25	Yes	—
Nitroprusside	D	None	None	None	Yes	—
Prazosin	D	None	None	None	No	No
Propranolol	D	None	None	None	No	—
Antiarrhythmics						
Bretylium	D	None	25–50	Avoid	?	—
Disopyramide	I	None	12–24	24–40	Yes	—
Lidocaine	D	None	None	None	No	—
Procainamide	I	4	6–12	8–24	Yes	—
Quinidine	I	None	None	None	Yes	Yes
Calcium blockers						
Diltiazem	D	None	None	None	—	—
Nifedipine	D	None	None	None	—	—
Verapamil	D	None	None	None	No	—
Digoxin	D	100	25–75	10–25	No	No
	I	24	36	48		
H$_2$ blockers						
Cimetidine	D	800/d	600/d	400/d	No	No
Ranitidine	D	None	150/d	150/d	No	—
Nizatidine	D	None	150/d	150 qod	—	—
Famotidine	D	None	None	20/d or (40 qod)	—	—

GFR, glomerular filtration rate; PCN G, penicillin G; D, dosage reduction method of dosage adjustment; I, interval extension method of dosage adjustment; qod, every other day; H$_2$, histamine.
From Bennett WM, Aronoff GR, Golper TA, et al. *Drug Prescribing in Renal Failure*. Philadelphia: American College of Physicians; 1987, with permission.

APPENDIX E: DERMATOMES

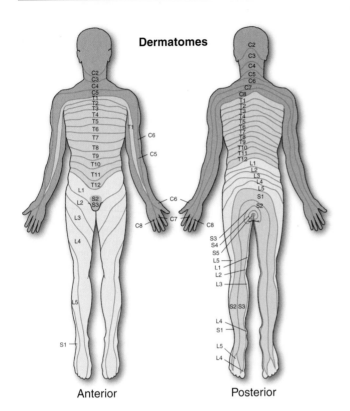

FIGURE E.1.

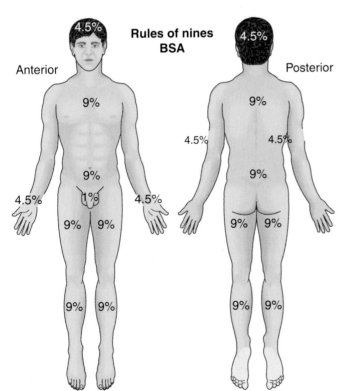

FIGURE E.2. BURNS: To estimate the extent of burn, the *rule of nines* for body surface area (BSA) is commonly used: Children: arms 9% each; legs 9% each; head 13%; trunk 18% anterior, 18% posterior; genitalia 1%. Lund and Browder chart for estimation of burn extent. (From Artz CP and Yarbrough DR III. Burns: including cold, chemical, and electric injuries. In: Sabiston CC Jr, ed. *Textbook of Surgery: The Biological Basis of Modern Surgical Practice,* 11th ed. Philadelphia: WB Saunders; 1977, with permission.

APPENDIX F: ORGAN INJURY SCALING, TRAUMA SCORING SYSTEMS

TRAUMA SCORING SYSTEMS

TABLE F.1

ABBREVIATED INJURY SCORE (AIS)

Score	Injury[a]
1	Minor
2	Moderate
3	Serious
4	Severe
5	Critical
6	Unsurvivable

[a]Injuries are ranked on a scale of 1 to 6, with 1 being minor, 5 severe, and 6 an unsurvivable injury. This represents the "threat to life" associated with an injury and is not meant to represent a comprehensive measure of severity.
From Copes WS, Sacco WJ, Champion HR, et al. Progress in characterizing anatomic injury. In *Proceedings of the 33rd Annual Meeting of the Association for the Advancement of Automotive Medicine, Baltimore,* with permission.

TABLE F.2

GLASGOW COMA SCORE (GCS)[a]

Score[b]	Best eye response (E)
1	No eye opening
2	Eye opening to pain
3	Eye opening to verbal command
4	Eyes open spontaneously
Score[b]	**Best Verbal Response (V)**
1	No verbal response
2	Incomprehensible sounds
3	Inappropriate words
4	Confused
5	Orientated
Score[b]	**Best Motor Response (M)**
1	No motor response
2	Extension to pain
3	Flexion to pain
4	Withdrawal from pain
5	Localizing pain
6	Obeys commands

[a]Note that the phrase "GCS of 11" is essentially meaningless, and it is important to break the figure down into its components, such as E3V3M5 = GCS 11.
[b]A coma score of 13 or higher correlates with a mild brain injury, 9–12 is a moderate injury, and 8 or less a severe brain injury.
From Teasdale G, Jennett B. Assessment of coma and impaired consciousness. *Lancet.* 1974;ii:81–83, with permission.

TABLE F.3

REVISED TRAUMA SCORE (RTS)[a]

Glasgow coma score (GCS)[b]	Systolic blood pressure (SBP)	Respiratory rate (RR)	Coded value
13–15	>89	10–29	4
9–12	76–89	>29	3
6–8	50–75	6–9	2
4–5	1–49	1–5	1
3	0	0	0

[a]The coded form of the RTS is calculated as follows: RTS = 0.9368 GCS + 0.7326 SBP + 0.2908 RR. Values for the RTS are in the range 0 to 7.8408. The RTS is heavily weighted toward the GCS to compensate for major head injury without multisystem injury or major physiologic changes. A threshold of RTS <4 has been proposed to identify those patients who should be treated in a trauma center, although this value may be somewhat low.
From Champion HR, Sacco JW, Copes WS. A revision of the trauma score. *J Trauma.* 1989;29:623–629, with permission.

TABLE F.4

INJURY SEVERITY SCORE (ISS)[a]

Region	Injury description	Abbreviated injury score (AIS[b])	Square top three
Head and neck	Cerebral contusion	3	9
Face	No injury	0	
Chest	Flail chest	4	16
Abdomen	Minor contusion of liver	2	25
	Complex rupture of spleen	5	
Extremity	Fractured femur	3	
External	No injury	0	
	Injury severity score:		50

[a]The ISS takes values from 0 to 75. If an injury is assigned an AIS[b] of 6 (unsurvivable injury), the ISS is automatically assigned to 75. The ISS is virtually the only anatomic scoring system in use and correlates linearly with mortality, morbidity, hospital stay, and other measures of severity.
From Baker SP, O'Neill B, Haddon W, et al. The injury severity score: a method for describing patients with multiple injuries and evaluating emergency care. *J Trauma.* 1974;14:187–196.

APPENDIX G: SEDATION SCORES

TABLE G.1

RAMSAY SCALE

Level	Characteristics[a]
1	Patient awake, anxious, agitated, or restless
2	Patient awake, cooperative, orientated, and tranquil
3	Patient drowsy, with response to commands
4	Patient asleep, brisk response to glabella tap or loud auditory
5	Patient asleep, sluggish response to stimulus
6	Patient has no response to firm nailbed pressure or other noxious stimuli

From Ramsay MAE, Savege TM, Simpson BRJ, et al. Controlled sedation with alphaxalone/alphadolone. *BMJ.* 1974;ii:656–659, with permission.

TABLE G.2

RICHMOND AGITATION-SEDATION SCALE (RASS)

Score	Term	Description
+4	Combative	Overtly combative or violent; immediate danger to staff
+3	Very agitated	Pulls on or removes tube(s) or catheter(s) or has aggressive behavior toward staff
+2	Agitated	Frequent nonpurposeful movement or patient–ventilator dyssynchrony
+1	Restless	Anxious or apprehensive but movements not aggressive or vigorous
0	Alert and calm	
−1	Drowsy	Not fully alert, but has sustained (>10 seconds) awakening, with eye contact, to voice
−2	Light sedation	Briefly (<10 seconds) awakens with eye contact to voice
−3	Moderate sedation	Any movement (but no eye contact) to voice
−4	Deep sedation	No response to voice, but any movement to physical stimulation
−5	Unarousable	No response to voice or physical stimulation

From Sessler CN, Gosnell MS, Grap MJ, et al. The Richmond agitation-sedation scale: validity and reliability in adult intensive care unit patients. *Am J Respir Crit Care Med.* 2002;166:1338–1344, with permission.

APPENDIX H: SEVERITY SCORING SYSTEMS

TABLE H.1

ACUTE PHYSIOLOGIC AND CHRONIC HEALTH EVALUATION (APACHE II)

A: Acute physiological score (APS; 12 variables)

Physiologic variable	High abnormal range				0	Low abnormal range			
	+4	+3	+2	+1		+1	+2	+3	+4
Temperature rectal (°C)	≥41	39–40.9		38.5–38.9	36–38.4	34–35.9	32–33.9	30–31.9	≤29.0
Mean arterial pressure (mm Hg)	≥160	130–159	110–129		70–109		50–69		≤49
Heart rate—ventricular response	≥180	140–179	110–139		70–109		55–69	40–54	≤39
Respiratory rate—nonventilated or ventilated	≥50	35–49		25–34	12–24	10–11	6–9		≤5
Oxygen: A-a DO$_2$ or PaO$_2$ (mm Hg)									
a. FiO$_2$ ≥0.5 record A-a DO$_2$	≥500	350–499	200–349		≤200				
b. FiO$_2$ <0.5 record only PaO$_2$					PO$_2$ >70	PO$_2$ 61–70		PO$_2$ 55–60	PO$_2$ <55
Arterial pH	≥7.7	7.6–7.69		7.5–7.59	7.33–7.49		7.25–7.32	7.15–7.24	<7.15
Serum HCO$_3$—only if no ABGs	≥52	41–51.9		32–40.9	23–31.9		18–21.9	15–17.9	<15
Serum sodium (mmol/L)	≥180	160–179	155–159	150–154	130–149		120–129	111–119	≤110
Serum potassium (mmol/L)	≥7	6–6.9		5.5–5.9	3.5–5.4	3–3.4	2.5–2.9		<2.5
Serum creatinine (μmol/L)	≥350	200–340	150–190		60–140		<60		
Hematocrit (%)	≥60		50–50.9	46–49.9	30–45.9		20–29.9		<20
White blood cell count (×1,000/mm^3)	≥40		20–39.9	15–19.9	3–14.9		1–2.9		<1
Glasgow coma score (GCS) Score = 15 minus actual GCS									

B: Age points

Age (years)	Points
≤44	0
45–54	2
55–64	3
65–74	5
≥75	6

C: Chronic health points

History	Points for elective surgery	Points for emergency surgery
Liver: Biopsy-proven cirrhosis and documented portal hypertension or prior episodes of hepatic failure	2	5
Cardiovascular: NYHA Class IV	2	5
Respiratory: e.g., severe COPD, hypercapnia, home O$_2$, pulmonary hypertension	2	5
Immunocompromised	2	5
Renal: Chronic dialysis	2	5

Apache II score

A: APS	
B: Age points score	
C: Chronic health points score	
Sum of A + B + C	
Total:	

ABG, arterial blood gas; NYHA, New York Heart Association; COPD, chronic obstructive pulmonary disease.
From Knaus WA, Draper EA, Wagner DP, et al. APACHE II: a severity of disease classification system. Crit Care Med. 1985;13:818–829, with permission.

TABLE H.2

SIMPLIFIED ACUTE PHYSIOLOGY (SAPS II) (SCORE)

Variable	26	13	12	11	9	7	6	5	4	3	2	1	0	1	2	3	4	6	7	8	9	10	12	15	16	17	18
Age in years						40–59							<40										60–69	70–74	75–79		≥80
Heart rate (beat/min)				<40		≥160			120–159		40–69		70–119														
Systolic blood pressure (mm Hg)		<70						70–99			≥200		100–199														
Body temperature (°C)													<39°C			≥39°C											
PaO₂/FiO₂ (mm Hg) only if VENT or CPAP				<100	100–199		≥200																				
Urinary output (L/d)				<0.500					0.500–0.999				≥1.000														
Blood urea (mmol/L) (g/L)							10.0–29.9 / 0.60–1.79						<10.0 / <0.60									≥30.0 / ≥1.80					
WBC count (10³/mL)			<1.0							≥20.0			1.0–19.9														
Serum K⁺ (mEq/L)										<3.0	≥5.0		3.0–4.9														
Serum Na⁺ (mEq/L)								<125					125–144	≥145													
Serum HCO₃ (mEq/L)							<15			15–19			≥20														
Bilirubin (if jaundice μmol/L) (mg/L)													<68.4 / <40.0				68.4–102.4 / 40.0–59.9				≥102.5 / ≥60.0						
Glasgow coma score (points)	<6	6–8				9–10		11–13					14–15														
Chronic diseases																					Met. Cancer	Hem. Mal				AIDS	
Type of admission													Elective surgery					Medical		Surgery emergency							

VENT, ventilator; CPAP, continuous positive airway pressure; WBC, white blood cell; Met Cancer, metastatic carcinoma; Met, metastatic; hem mal, hematologic malignancy; AIDS, acquired immunodeficiency syndrome.

The SAPS II score registers the worst value of selected variables, within the first 24 hours after admission.

From Le Gall JR, Lemeshow S, Saulnier F, et al. A new simplified acute physiology score (SAPS II) based on a European/North American multicenter study. *JAMA.* 1993;270:2957–2963, with permission.

TABLE H.3

SEQUENTIAL ORGAN FAILURE ASSESSMENT (SOFA) SCORE

Organ system		Score 0	Score 1	Score 2	Score 3	Score 4
Respiration	Lowest PaO$_2$/FiO$_2$ (mm Hg) or (Kpa) Respiratory support (yes/no)	>400 >53.33	≤400 40–53.33	≤300 26.67–40	≤200 13.33–26.67 and yes	≤100 ≤13.33 and yes
Coagulation	Lowest platelet (10^3/mm^3)	>150	≤150	≤100	≤50	≤20
Hepatic	Highest bilirubin (mg/dL) or (μmol/L)	<1.2 <20	1.2–1.9 20–32	2.0–5.9 33–101	6.0–11.9 102–204	≥12 >204
Circulatory	Lowest mean arterial pressure (mmHg)	>70	<70			
	Highest dopamine dose (μg/kg/min)			≤5	>5	>15
	Highest epinephrine dose (μg/kg/min)				≤0.1	>0.1
	Highest norepinephrine dose (μg/kg/min)				≤0.1	>0.1
	Dobutamine (yes/no)			Any dose[a]		
Neurologic	(GCS, see Table H-2)	15	13–14	10–12	6–9	<6
Renal	Highest creatinine level (mg/dL) or (μmol/L) Total urine output (mL/24 h)	<1.2 <110	1.2–1.9 110–170	2.0–3.4 171–299	3.0–4.9 300–440 <500	≥5.0 >440 <200

GCS, Glasgow Coma Score.
SOFA total (Σ **6 items**). The SOFA score assesses the function of 6 different organ systems: respiratory (partial arterial oxygen pressure (PaO$_2$)/fraction of inspired oxygen [FiO$_2$]), cardiovascular (blood pressure, vasoactive drugs), renal (creatine and diuresis), hepatic (bilirubin), neurological (Glasgow Coma Score), and hematological (platelet count).
From Vincent JL, Moreno R, Takala J, et al. The SOFA (Sepsis-related Organ Failure Assessment) score to describe organ dysfunction/failure. On behalf of the Working Group on sepsis-related problems of the European Society of Intensive Care Medicine. *Intensive Care Med.* 1996;22:707–710, with permission.

TABLE H.4

MULTIPLE ORGAN DYSFUNCTION SCORE (MODS)

Variables	Points				
	0	1	2	3	4
PaO$_2$/FiO$_2$	<300	226–300	151–225	76–150	≤75
Creatinine serum	≤100	101–200	201–350	351–500	≥500
Bilirubin	≤20	21–60	61–120	121–240	>240
Heart rate	≤10	10.1–15	15.1–20	20.1–30	>30
Platelet count	>120	81–120	51–80	21–50	≤20
Glasgow coma score	15	13–14	10–12	7–9	≤6

From Marshall JC, Cook DJ, Christou NV, et al. Multiple organ dysfunction score: a reliable descriptor of a complex clinical outcome. *Crit Care Med.* 1995;23:1638–1652, with permission.

TABLE I.1

AMINOPENICILLINS

Drug	Drug class	Adults (usual dose[a])	Spectrum of activity, indications, and active against most strains of	Actions, interactions, and others	Route, reduce dose, and contraindications
Ampicillin	Aminopenicillin	Usual dose: IV: 2.0 g IV q4h; PO: 500 mg q6h	*Streptococcus pneumoniae*; *Staphylococcus aureus* (penicillinase and nonpenicillinase producing); *Haemophilus influenzae*, and group A β-hemolytic *Streptococci*. Bacterial meningitis caused by *Escherichia coli*, group B *Streptococci*, and other gram-negative bacteria (*Listeria monocytogenes*, *Neisseria meningitidis*). Endocarditis caused by susceptible gram-positive organisms including *Streptococcus sp.*, penicillin G–susceptible *Staphylococci*, and *Enterococci*. Endocarditis due to enterococcal strains usually respond to intravenous therapy. Gram-negative sepsis caused by *E. coli*, *Proteus mirabilis*, and *Salmonella sp.* Gastrointestinal infections caused by *Salmonella typhosa* (typhoid fever), other *Salmonella sp.*, and *Shigella sp.* Urinary tract infections caused by *E. coli* and *Proteus mirabilis*	Allopurinol (increased frequency of rash); Warfarin (increased INR)	Primary mode of elimination: Renal. Reduce dose in moderate to severe renal impairment
Amoxicillin	Aminopenicillin	Usual dose: IV: 500 mg–1 g tds (higher doses: 2 g 4 hourly in endocarditis); PO: 1 g q8h	• *Streptococcus pneumoniae* • *Haemophilus influenzae* (except COPD patients) • β-Hemolytic *Streptococci* • *Streptococcus pyogenes* do not produce β-lactamase • *Enterococcus faecalis*	Bactericide; Some gram-negative activity	• Primary mode of elimination: Renal • Reasonable oral absorption (oral preparation) • Reduce dose in moderate to severe renal impairment
Amoxicillin/clavulanate	Aminopenicillin/β-lactam inhibitor combination	Usual dose: 500/125 mg (PO) q8h or 875/125 mg (PO) q12h for severe infections or respiratory tract infections	Aerobic gram-positive microorganisms; *Streptococcus pneumoniae* (including isolates with penicillin MICs ≤2 μg/mL). Aerobic gram-negative microorganisms; *Haemophilus influenzae* (including β-lactamase–producing isolates); *Moraxella catarrhalis* (including β-lactamase–producing isolates). The following *in vitro* data are available, but their clinical significance is unknown. Aerobic gram-positive microorganisms; *Staphylococcus aureus* (including β-lactamase–producing isolates). NOTE: *Staphylococci* that are resistant to methicillin/oxacillin must be considered resistant to amoxicillin/clavulanic acid. *S. pyogenes*		• Primary mode of elimination: Renal • Reduce dose in moderate to severe renal impairment • 875/125 mg formulation should not be used in patients with CrCl <30 mL/min

(continued)

TABLE I.1

CONTINUED

Drug	Drug class	Adults (usual dose[a])	Actions, interactions, and others	Spectrum of activity, indications, and active against most strains of	Route, reduce dose, and contraindications
Ampicillin/ sulbactam	Aminopenicillin/β-lactam inhibitor combination	Usual dose: IV: 1.5–3.0 g q6h Remember: Na$^+$ content = 4.2 mEq/g Total dose of sulbactam should not exceed 4 g/day	Bactericide Broad-spectrum antibiotic and a β-lactamase inhibitor For mild or moderate infection, 1.5 g IV q6h Pseudoresistance with E. coli/ Klebsiella (in vitro)	**Gram-negative bacteria** Haemophilus influenzae (β-lactamase and non–β-lactamase producing); Moraxella (Branhamella) catarrhalis (β-lactamase and non–β-lactamase producing); Escherichia coli (β-lactamase and non–β-lactamase producing); Klebsiella spp. (all known strains are β-lactamase producing); Proteus mirabilis (β-lactamase and non–β-lactamase producing); Proteus vulgaris; Providencia rettgeri; Providencia stuartii; Morganella morganii; Neisseria gonorrhoeae (β-lactamase and non–β-lactamase producing). **Anaerobes** Clostridium sp.; Peptococcus sp.; Peptostreptococcus sp.; Bacteroides sp., including B. fragilis	• Primary mode of elimination: Renal and hepatic • Ampicillin and sulbactam for injection may be administered by either the IV or the IM routes • In patients with impairment of renal function, the elimination kinetics of ampicillin and sulbactam are similarly affected

INR, international normalized ratio; COPD, chronic obstructive pulmonary disease; MIC, minimum inhibitory concentration; CrCl, creatinine clearance.
Cunha BA. *Antibiotic Essentials*, 5th ed. Royal Oak, MI: Physicians Press; 2006.
From http://www.drugs.com (drug information online). Revised from November 2006.

TABLE I.2

ANTIPSEUDOMONAL PENICILLINS

Drug	Drug class	Adults (usual dose[a])	Actions, interactions, and others	Spectrum of activity, indications, and active against most strains of	Route, reduce dose, and contraindications
Piperacillin	Antipseudomonal penicillin	Usual dose: IV: 34 g q48h	Drug interaction with aminoglycosides in renal failure	**Prophylaxis:** Piperacillin is indicated for prophylactic use in surgery including intra-abdominal (gastrointestinal and biliary) procedures, vaginal hysterectomy, abdominal hysterectomy, and cesarean section. Piperacillin should only be used to treat or prevent infections that are proven or strongly suspected to be caused by susceptible bacteria. **Indications and use** Intra-abdominal infections including hepatobiliary and surgical infections caused by *E. coli, Pseudomonas aeruginosa, Enterococci, Clostridium* spp., anaerobic cocci, or *Bacteroides* spp., including *B. fragilis.* Urinary tract infections caused by *E. coli, Klebsiella* spp., *P. aeruginosa, Proteus* spp. including *P. mirabilis,* or *Enterococci* Gynecologic infections including endometritis, pelvic inflammatory disease, pelvic cellulitis caused by *Bacteroides* spp. including *B. fragilis,* anaerobic cocci, *Neisseria gonorrhoeae,* or *Enterococci* (*E. faecalis*) Septicemia including bacteremia caused by *E. coli, Klebsiella* spp., *Enterobacter* spp., *Serratia* spp., *P. mirabilis, S. pneumoniae, Enterococci, P. aeruginosa, Bacteroides* spp., or anaerobic cocci. Lower respiratory tract infections caused by *E. coli, Klebsiella* spp., *Enterobacter* spp., *P. aeruginosa, Serratia* spp., *H. influenzae, Bacteroides* spp., or anaerobic cocci. Skin and skin structure infections caused by *E. coli, Klebsiella* spp., *Serratia* spp., *Acinetobacter* spp., *Enterobacter* spp., *P. aeruginosa, Morganella morganii, Providencia rettgeri, Proteus vulgaris, P. mirabilis, Bacteroides* spp. including *B. fragilis,* anaerobic cocci, or *Enterococci* Bone and joint infections caused by *P. aeruginosa, Enterococci, Bacteroides* spp., or anaerobic cocci	• Primary mode of elimination: Renal • Reduce dose in moderate to severe renal impairment
Piperacillin/ tazobactam	Antipseudomonal penicillin	Usual dose: IV: 4.5 g q8h Pneumonia nosocomial, use 4.5 g (IV) q6h	Drug interaction with aminoglycosides and vecuronium	Indicated for nosocomial pneumonia (moderate to severe) caused by piperacillin-resistant, β-lactamase–producing strains of *Staphylococcus aureus* and by piperacillin/tazobactam-susceptible *Acinetobacter baumannii, Haemophilus influenzae, Klebsiella pneumoniae,* and *Pseudomonas aeruginosa* (nosocomial pneumonia caused by *P. aeruginosa* should be treated in combination with an aminoglycoside) Community-acquired pneumonia (moderate severity only) caused by piperacillin-resistant, β-lactamase–producing strains of *H. influenzae* Appendicitis (complicated by rupture or abscess) and peritonitis caused by piperacillin-resistant, β-lactamase–producing strains of *Escherichia coli* or the following members of the *Bacteroides fragilis* group: *B. fragilis, B. ovatus, B. thetaiotaomicron,* or *B. vulgatus*	• Mode of elimination: 20% in bile, 80% unchanged in urine • Reduce dose in moderate to severe renal impairment

(continued)

TABLE I.2

CONTINUED

Drug	Drug class	Adults (usual dose^a)	Actions, interactions, and others	Spectrum of activity, indications, and active against most strains of	Route, reduce dose, and contraindications
				Uncomplicated and complicated skin and skin structure infections, including cellulitis, cutaneous abscesses, and ischemic/diabetic foot infections caused by piperacillin-resistant, β-lactamase–producing strains of *S. aureus* Infections caused by piperacillin-susceptible organisms for which piperacillin has been shown to be effective are also amenable to piperacillin tazobactam content. Postpartum endometritis or pelvic inflammatory disease caused by piperacillin-resistant, β-lactamase–producing strains of *E. coli*	
Ticarcillin disodium	Antipseudomonal penicillin	Usual dose: IV: 3 g q6h	Drug interaction with aminoglycosides in renal failure	Ticarcillin is a semisynthetic antibiotic with a broad spectrum of bactericidal activity against many gram-positive and gram-negative aerobic and anaerobic bacteria. Ticarcillin is, however, susceptible to degradation by β-lactamases, and therefore, the spectrum of activity does not normally include organisms that produce these enzymes.	• Primary mode of elimination: Renal • Reduce dose in moderate to severe renal impairment
Ticarcillin/ clavulanate	Ticarcillin disodium (Antipseudomonal penicillin) + β-lactamase inhibitor clavulanate potassium (the potassium salt of clavulanic acid), for intravenous administration	Usual dose: IV: 3.1 g q4–6h (3.1 g vial containing 3 g ticarcillin and 100 mg clavulanic acid) Moderate infections 200 mg/kg/d in divided doses every 6 h Severe infections 300 mg/kg/d in divided doses every 4 h For patients weighing <60 kg, the recommended dosage is 200–300 mg/kg/d, based on ticarcillin content, given in divided doses every 4–6 hours.	Drug interaction with aminoglycosides in renal failure	Ticarcillin is a semisynthetic antibiotic with a broad spectrum of bactericidal activity against many gram-positive and gram-negative aerobic and anaerobic bacteria. Ticarcillin is, however, susceptible to degradation by β-lactamases, and therefore, the spectrum of activity does not normally include organisms that produce these enzymes. **Gram-positive aerobes** *Staphylococcus aureus; Staphylococcus epidermidis* **Gram-negative aerobes** *Citrobacter* sp.; *Enterobacter* sp., including *E. cloacae; Escherichia coli; Haemophilus influenzae; Klebsiella* sp. including *K. pneumoniae; Pseudomonas* sp. including *P. aeruginosa; Serratia marcescens* **Anaerobic bacteria** *Bacteroides fragilis* group; *Prevotella* (formerly *Bacteroides*) *melaninogenicus* **Gram-positive aerobes** *Staphylococcus saprophyticus; Streptococcus agalactiae* (group B); *Streptococcus bovis; Streptococcus pneumoniae* (penicillin-susceptible strains only); *Streptococcus pyogenes; Viridans* group streptococci **Gram-negative aerobes** *Acinetobacter baumannii; Acinetobacter calcoaceticus; Acinetobacter haemolyticus; Acinetobacter lwoffi; Moraxella catarrhalis; Morganella morganii; Neisseria gonorrhoeae; Pasteurella multocida; Proteus mirabilis; Proteus penneri; Proteus vulgaris; Providencia rettgeri; Providencia stuartii; Stenotrophomonas maltophilia* **Anaerobic bacteria** *Clostridium* sp. including *C. perfringens, C. difficile, C. sporogenes, C. ramosum,* and *C. bifermentans; Eubacterium* sp.; *Fusobacterium* sp. including *F. nucleatum* and *F. necrophorum; Peptostreptococcus* sp.; *Veillonella* sp.	• Primary mode of elimination: Renal • Reduce dose in moderate to severe renal impairment

Cunha BA. *Antibiotic Essentials*, 5th ed. Royal Oak, MI: Physicians Press; 2006.
From http://www.drugs.com (drug information online). Revised from November 2006.

TABLE I.3

CARBAPENEMS

Drug	Drug class	Adults (usual dose[a])	Actions, interactions, and others	Spectrum of activity, indications, and active against most strains of	Route, reduce dose, and contraindications
Ertapenem	Carbapenem	Usual dose: IV/IM: 1 g q24h	Not a substrate/inhibitor of cytochrome P450 enzymes Probenecid (decrease clearance of ertapenem)	**Aerobic and facultative gram-positive microorganisms** *Staphylococcus aureus* (methicillin-susceptible isolates only); *Streptococcus agalactiae; Streptococcus pneumoniae* (penicillin susceptible isolates only); *Streptococcus pyogenes* Note: Methicillin-resistant *Staphylococci* and *Enterococcus* spp. are resistant to ertapenem. **Aerobic and facultative gram-positive microorganisms** *Escherichia coli; Haemophilus influenzae* (β-lactamase negative isolates only); *Klebsiella pneumoniae; Moraxella catarrhalis; Proteus mirabilis* **Anaerobic microorganisms** *Bacteroides fragilis; Bacteroides distasonis; Bacteroides ovatus; Bacteroides thetaiotaomicron; Bacteroides uniformis; Clostridium clostridiiforme; Eubacterium lentum; Peptostreptococcus* sp.; *Porphyromonas asaccharolytica; Prevotella bivia*	Primary mode of elimination: Renal Reduce dose in moderate to severe renal impairment.
Imipenem/ cilastatin	Carbapenem	Usual dose: IV: 1,000 mg q6h (4 g) only in severe life-threatening infections (mainly in some Pseudomonas species) no more than 50 mg/kg/24h IV: 250 mg q6h in mild infections IV: 500 mg q8h (1.5 g) or q6h (2.0 g) in moderate infections Total dose of sodium 37.5 mg (1.6 mEq) by 500 mg Imipenem	The bactericidal activity of imipenem results from the inhibition of cell wall synthesis	**Conditions:** Bacterial septicemia. Lower respiratory tract infections. Urinary tract infections (complicated and uncomplicated). Nosocomial pneumonia, peritonitis, sepsis. Gynecologic infections. Bone and joint infections. Skin and skin structure infections. Endocarditis. Polymicrobic infections. **Gram-positive aerobes** *Enterococcus faecalis* (formerly *S. faecalis*) (NOTE: Imipenem is inactive *in vitro* against *Enterococcus faecium* [formerly *S. faecium*]); *Staphylococcus aureus* including penicillinase-producing strains; *Staphylococcus epidermidis* including penicillinase-producing strains; *Streptococcus agalactiae* (group B streptococci); *Streptococcus pneumoniae; Streptococcus pyogenes* **Gram-negative aerobes** *Acinetobacter* spp.; *Citrobacter* spp.; *Enterobacter* spp.; *Escherichia coli; Gardnerella vaginalis; Haemophilus influenzae; Haemophilus parainfluenzae Klebsiella* spp.; *Morganella morganii; Proteus vulgaris; Providencia rettgeri; Pseudomonas aeruginosa* (NOTE: Imipenem is inactive *in vitro* against *Xanthomonas* [*Pseudomonas*] *maltophilia* and some strains of *P. cepacia*); *Serratia* spp., including. *S. marcescens*	Central nervous system adverse experiences such as confusional states, myoclonic activity, and seizures have been reported during treatment with imipenem. Reduce dose in moderate to severe renal impairment. For patients on hemodialysis, imipenem is recommended only when the benefit outweighs the potential risk of seizures.

(*continued*)

TABLE I.3

CONTINUED

Drug	Drug class	Adults (usual dose[a])	Actions, interactions, and others	Spectrum of activity, indications, and active against most strains of	Route, reduce dose, and contraindications
				Gram-positive anaerobes *Bifidobacterium* spp.; *Clostridium* spp.; *Eubacterium* spp.; *Peptococcus* spp.; *Peptostreptococcus* spp.; *Propionibacterium* spp. **Gram-negative anaerobes** *Bacteroides* spp., including *B. fragilis*; *Fusobacterium* spp. **Gram-positive aerobes** *Bacillus* spp.; *Listeria monocytogenes*; *Nocardia* spp.; *Staphylococcus saprophyticus*; group C streptococci; group G streptococci; *Viridans* group streptococci **Gram-negative aerobes** *Aeromonas hydrophila*; *Alcaligenes* spp.; *Capnocytophaga* spp.; *Haemophilus ducreyi*; *Neisseria gonorrhoeae* including penicillinase-producing strains *Pasteurella* spp.; *Providencia stuartii*. **Gram-negative anaerobes** *Prevotella bivia*; *Prevotella disiens*; *Prevotella melaninogenica*; *Veillonella* spp. *In vitro* tests show imipenem to act synergistically with aminoglycoside antibiotics against some isolates of *Pseudomonas aeruginosa*.	
Meropenem	Carbapenem	Usual dose: IV: 500 mg q8h Usual dose: IV: 1 g q8h Usual dose: IV: 2 g q8h	Pneumonia, urinary tract infection, gynecologic infections, skin and skin structure infections Nosocomial pneumonia, peritonitis, neutropenic patients, sepsis Meningitis and cystic fibrosis	Meropenem is a broad-spectrum carbapenem antibiotic. It is active against gram-positive and gram-negative bacteria. Meropenem has significant stability to hydrolysis by β-lactamases of most categories, both penicillinases and cephalosporinases produced by gram-positive and gram-negative bacteria. Meropenem should not be used to treat methicillin-resistant *Staphylococcus aureus* (MRSA). *In vitro* tests show meropenem to act synergistically with aminoglycoside antibiotics against some isolates of *Pseudomonas aeruginosa*.	Reduce dose in moderate to severe renal impairment.

Cunha BA. *Antibiotic Essentials*, 5th ed. Royal Oak, MI: Physicians Press; 2006.
From http://www.drugs.com (drug information online). Revised from November 2006.

TABLE I.4

MONOBACTAMS

Drug	Drug class	Adults (usual dose[a])	Actions, interactions, and others	Spectrum of activity, indications, and active against most strains of	Route, reduce dose, and contraindications
Aztreonam	Monobactam It was originally isolated from *Chromobacterium violaceum*.	Usual dose: IV: 1–2 g q8h Usual dose: IV: 2 g q6h	• Synthetic bactericidal antibiotic • Synthetic bactericidal antibiotic • Meningeal dose	Aerobic gram-negative microorganisms: *Citrobacter* spp., including *C. freundii; Enterobacter* spp., including *E. cloacae; Escherichia coli; Haemophilus influenzae* (including ampicillin-resistant and other penicillinase-producing strains); *Klebsiella, Proteus,* and *Serratia* species.	Reduce dose in moderate to severe renal impairment.

Cunha BA. *Antibiotic Essentials,* 5th ed. Royal Oak, MI: Physicians Press; 2006.
From http://www.drugs.com (drug information online). Revised from November 2006.

TABLE I.5

CEPHALOSPORINS (PARENTERAL)

Drug	Drug class	Adults (usual dose[a])	Actions, interactions, and others	Spectrum of activity, indications, and active against most strains of	Route, reduce dose, and contraindications
Cefazolin	First-generation cephalosporin	Usual dose: IV: 1 g q8h Remember: Na+ content = 46 mg per g cefazolin	*In vitro* tests demonstrate that the bactericidal action of cephalosporins results from inhibition of cell wall synthesis **Drug interactions** None	*Staphylococcus aureus* (including penicillinase-producing strains); *Staphylococcus epidermidis;* methicillin-resistant staphylococci are uniformly resistant to cefazolin. Group A β-hemolytic *Streptococci* and other strains of streptococci (many strains of enterococci are resistant) *Streptococcus pneumoniae; Escherichia coli; Proteus mirabilis; Klebsiella* sp.; *Enterobacter aerogenes; Haemophilus influenzae*	Reduce dose in moderate to severe renal impairment.
Cefuroxime	Second-generation IV/oral cephalosporin	Usual dose: IV: 1.5 g q8h PO: 500 mg q12h Remember: Na+ content = 2.4 mEq/g	Cefuroxime has *in vitro* activity against a wide range of gram-positive and gram-negative organisms, and it is highly stable in the presence of β-lactamases of certain gram-negative bacteria. The bactericidal action of cefuroxime results from inhibition of cell wall synthesis.	**Aerobes, gram-positive** *Staphylococcus aureus; Staphylococcus epidermidis; Streptococcus pneumoniae; Streptococcus pyogenes* (and other streptococci) NOTE: Most strains of enterococci (e.g., *Enterococcus faecalis* [formerly *Streptococcus faecalis*]), are resistant to cefuroxime. Methicillin-resistant staphylococci and *Listeria monocytogenes* are resistant to cefuroxime. **Aerobes, gram-negative** *Citrobacter* spp.; *Enterobacter* spp.; *Escherichia coli; Haemophilus influenzae* (including ampicillin-resistant strains); *Haemophilus parainfluenzae; Klebsiella* spp. (including *Klebsiella pneumoniae*); *Moraxella (Branhamella) catarrhalis* (including ampicillin- and cephalothin-resistant strains); *Morganella morganii* (formerly *Proteus morganii*); *Neisseria gonorrhoeae* (including penicillinase- and non-penicillinase-producing strains); *Neisseria meningitidis; Proteus mirabilis; Providencia rettgeri* (formerly *Proteus rettgeri*); *Salmonella* spp.; *Shigella* spp.	Reduce dose in moderate to severe renal impairment. Do not use for meningitis prophylaxis.
Cefotaxime	Third-generation cephalosporin	Usual dose: 2 g IV q6h	Administer by IV injection or infusion or by deep IM injection.	Lower respiratory tract infections, including pneumonia, caused by *Streptococcus pneumoniae* (formerly *Diplococcus pneumoniae*), *Streptococcus pyogenes[b]* (group A streptococci) and other streptococci (excluding enterococci, e.g., *Enterococcus faecalis*), *Staphylococcus aureus* (penicillinase and nonpenicillinase producing), *Escherichia coli, Klebsiella* sp., *Haemophilus influenzae* (including ampicillin-resistant strains), *Haemophilus parainfluenzae, Proteus mirabilis, Serratia marcescens,[b] Enterobacter* sp., indolepositive *Proteus* and *Pseudomonas* sp. (including *P. aeruginosa*).	Reduce dose in moderate to severe renal impairment.

Genitourinary infections

Urinary tract infections caused by *Enterococcus* sp., *Staphylococcus epidermidis, Staphylococcus aureus*[b] (penicillinase and nonpenicillinase producing), *Citrobacter* sp., *Enterobacter* sp., *Escherichia coli, Klebsiella* sp., *Proteus mirabilis, Proteus vulgaris,*[b] *Providencia stuartii, Morganella morganii,*[b] *Providencia rettgeri,*[b] *Serratia marcescens,* and *Pseudomonas* sp. (including *P. aeruginosa*). Also, uncomplicated gonorrhea (cervical/urethral and rectal) caused by *Neisseria gonorrhoeae,* including penicillinase-producing strains.

Gynecologic infections, including pelvic inflammatory disease, endometritis, and pelvic cellulitis caused by *Staphylococcus epidermidis, Streptococcus* sp., *Enterococcus* sp., *Enterobacter* sp.,[b] *Klebsiella* sp.,[b] *Escherichia coli, Proteus mirabilis, Bacteroides* sp. (including *Bacteroides fragilis*[b]), *Clostridium* sp., and anaerobic cocci (including *Peptostreptococcus* sp. and *Peptococcus* sp.) and *Fusobacterium* sp. (including *F. nucleatum*[b])

Bacteremia/septicemia caused by *Escherichia coli, Klebsiella* sp., *Serratia marcescens, Staphylococcus aureus,* and *Streptococcus* sp. (including *S. pneumoniae*)

Skin and skin structure infections caused by *Staphylococcus aureus* (penicillinase and nonpenicillinase producing), *Staphylococcus epidermidis, Streptococcus pyogenes* (group A streptococci) and other streptococci, *Enterococcus* sp., *Acinetobacter* sp.,[b] *Escherichia coli, Citrobacter* sp. (including *C. freundii*[b]), *Enterobacter* sp.,[b] *Klebsiella* sp., *Proteus mirabilis, Proteus vulgaris,*[b] *Morganella morganii, Providencia rettgeri,*[b] *Pseudomonas* sp., *Serratia marcescens, Bacteroides* sp., and anaerobic cocci (including *Peptostreptococcus*[b] sp. and *Peptococcus* sp.)

Intra-abdominal infections including peritonitis caused by *Streptococcus* sp.,[b] *Escherichia coli, Klebsiella* sp., *Bacteroides* sp., and anaerobic cocci (including *Peptostreptococcus*[b] sp. and *Peptococcus*[b] sp.) *Proteus mirabilis,*[b] and *Clostridium* sp.[b]

Bone and/or joint infections caused by *Staphylococcus aureus* (penicillinase- and nonpenicillinase-producing strains), *Streptococcus* sp. (including *S. pyogenes*[b]), *Pseudomonas* sp. (including *P. aeruginosa*[b]), and *Proteus mirabilis*[b]

(*continued*)

TABLE I.5

CONTINUED

Drug	Drug class	Adults (usual dose[a])	Actions, interactions, and others	Spectrum of activity, indications, and active against most strains of	Route, reduce dose, and contraindications
				Central nervous system infections (e.g., meningitis and ventriculitis), caused by *Neisseria meningitidis*, *Haemophilus influenzae*, *Streptococcus pneumoniae*, *Klebsiella pneumoniae*,[b] and *Escherichia coli*[b]	
Ceftazidime	Third-generation cephalosporin	Usual dose: 2 g IV q8h	Ceftazidime is bactericidal in action, exerting its effect by inhibition of enzymes responsible for cell wall synthesis.	Lower respiratory tract infections, including pneumonia, caused by *Pseudomonas aeruginosa* and other *Pseudomonas* spp.; *Haemophilus influenzae*, including ampicillin-resistant strains; *Klebsiella* spp.; *Enterobacter* spp.; *Proteus mirabilis*; *Escherichia coli*; *Serratia* spp.; *Citrobacter* spp.; *Streptococcus pneumoniae*; and *Staphylococcus aureus* (methicillin-susceptible strains).	Reduce dose in moderate to severe renal impairment.
				Skin and skin structure infections caused by *Pseudomonas aeruginosa*; *Klebsiella* spp.; *Escherichia coli*; *Proteus* spp., including *Proteus mirabilis* and indole-positive *Proteus*; *Enterobacter* spp.; *Serratia* spp.; *Staphylococcus aureus* (methicillin-susceptible strains); and *Streptococcus pyogenes* (group A β-hemolytic streptococci).	
				Urinary tract infections, both complicated and uncomplicated, caused by *Pseudomonas aeruginosa*; *Enterobacter* spp.; *Proteus* spp., including *Proteus mirabilis* and indole-positive *Proteus*; *Klebsiella* spp.; and *Escherichia coli*	
				Bacterial septicemia caused by *Pseudomonas aeruginosa*, *Klebsiella* spp., *Haemophilus influenzae*, *Escherichia coli*, *Serratia* spp., *Streptococcus pneumoniae*, and *Staphylococcus aureus* (methicillin-susceptible strains)	
				Bone and joint infections caused by *Pseudomonas aeruginosa*, *Klebsiella* spp., *Enterobacter* spp., and *Staphylococcus aureus* (methicillin-susceptible strains)	
				Gynecologic infections, including endometritis, pelvic cellulitis, and other infections of the female genital tract caused by *Escherichia coli*	
				Intra-abdominal infections, including peritonitis caused by *Escherichia coli*, *Klebsiella* spp., and *Staphylococcus aureus* (methicillin-susceptible strains) and polymicrobial infections caused by aerobic and anaerobic organisms and *Bacteroides* spp. (many strains of *Bacteroides fragilis* are resistant)	

| Cefepime | Fourth-generation cephalosporin | Usual dose: 1–2 g IV q12h For proven serious systemic *P. aeruginosa* infections, febrile neutropenia, or cystic fibrosis: 2 g (IV) q8h (max dose) Meningeal dose: 2 g (IV) q8h (max dose) | Local intolerances to IV or IM administration of cefepime were not statistically different from those of ceftazidime administration | *In vitro*, activity against **gram-positive organisms** including *Streptococcus agalactiae*, *Streptococcus pneumoniae*, *Streptococcus pyogenes*, and penicillin-susceptible *Staphylococcus aureus* **The broad range of gram-negative organisms sensitive to include** family Enterobacteriaceae, *Klebsiella pneumoniae*, *Haemophilus influenza*, *Neisseria meningitidis*, *Neisseria gonorrhoeae*, and *Pseudomonas aeruginosa* **Central nervous system infections, including meningitis, caused by** *Haemophilus influenzae* and *Neisseria meningitidis*. Ceftazidime has also been used successfully in a limited number of cases of meningitis due to *Pseudomonas aeruginosa* and *Streptococcus pneumoniae*. | Reduce dose in moderate to severe renal impairment |

[b]Usual dose, assumes normal renal/hepatic function.
Cunha BA. *Antibiotic Essentials*, 5th ed. Royal Oak, MI: Physicians Press; 2006.
From http://www.drugs.com (drug information online). Revised from November 2006.

TABLE 1.6

GLYCOPEPTIDES

Drug	Drug class	Adults (usual dose[a])	Actions, interactions, and others	Spectrum of activity, indications, and active against most strains of	Route, reduce dose, and contraindications
Vancomycin	Glycopeptide	The initial dose should be no <15 mg/kg, even in patients with mild to moderate renal insufficiency Usual dose IV: 1 g q12h	The bactericidal action of vancomycin results primarily from inhibition of cell wall biosynthesis. In addition, vancomycin alters bacterial cell membrane permeability and RNA synthesis. Concomitant administration of vancomycin and anesthetic agents has been associated with erythema and histaminelike flushing and anaphylactoid reactions.	Indicated for the treatment of serious or severe infections caused by susceptible strains of methicillin-resistant (β-lactam–resistant) staphylococci. It is indicated for penicillin-allergic patients; for patients who cannot receive or who have failed to respond to other drugs, including the penicillins or cephalosporins; and for infections caused by vancomycin-susceptible organisms that are resistant to other antimicrobial drugs. Also indicated for initial therapy when methicillin-resistant staphylococci are suspected, but after susceptibility data are available, therapy should be adjusted accordingly. Effective in the treatment of staphylococcal endocarditis. Its effectiveness has been documented in other infections due to staphylococci, including septicemia, bone infections, lower respiratory tract infections, and skin and skin structure infections. Effective alone or in combination with an aminoglycoside for endocarditis caused by *S. viridans* or *S. bovis.* For endocarditis caused by enterococci (e.g., *E. faecalis*), vancomycin hydrochloride has been reported to be effective only in combination with an aminoglycoside. Effective for the treatment of diphtheroid endocarditis Has been used successfully in combination with rifampin, an aminoglycoside, or both, in early-onset prosthetic valve endocarditis caused by *S. epidermidis* or diphtheroids The parenteral form of vancomycin may be administered orally for treatment of antibiotic-associated pseudomembranous colitis produced by *C. difficile* and for staphylococcal enterocolitis	Dosage adjustment must be made in patients with impaired renal function. Vancomycin dosage schedules should be adjusted in elderly patients Dosage table for vancomycin (adapted from Moellering et al.)[b] Creatine Clearance/ Dose mL/min—mg/24 h 100—1,545 90—1,390 80—1,235 70—1,080 60—925 50—770 40—620 30—465 20—310 10—155

Cunha BA. *Antibiotic Essentials*, 5th ed. Royal Oak, MI: Physicians Press; 2006.
From http://www.drugs.com (drug information online). Revised from November 2006.

TABLE I.7

CHLORAMPHENICOL, CLINDAMYCIN, ERYTHROMYCIN GROUP, KETOLIDES

Drug	Drug class	Adults (usual dose[a])	Actions, interactions, and others	Spectrum of activity, indications, and active against most strains of	Route, reduce dose, and contraindications
Chloramphenicol	Chloramphenicol sodium succinate	Chloramphenicol sodium succinate is intended for intravenous use only. It has been demonstrated to be ineffective when given intramuscularly. 0.25–1 g IV q6h (max. of 4 g/d) Administration of 50 mg/kg/d in divided doses will produce blood levels of the magnitude to which the majority of susceptible microorganisms will respond.	The most serious adverse effect of chloramphenicol is bone marrow depression. Serious and fatal blood dyscrasias (aplastic anemia, hypoplastic anemia, thrombocytopenia, and granulocytopenia) are known to occur after the administration of chloramphenicol.	Chloramphenicol must be used only in those serious infections for which less potentially dangerous drugs are ineffective or contraindicated: 1. Acute infections caused by *Salmonella typhi* 2. Serious infections caused by susceptible strains: • *Salmonella* sp. • *H. influenzae*, especially meningeal infections • *Rickettsia* • Lymphogranuloma-psittacosis group • Various gram-negative bacteria causing bacteremia, meningitis, or other serious gram-negative infections • Other susceptible organisms that have been demonstrated to be resistant to all other appropriate antimicrobial agents 3. Cystic fibrosis regimens	Total urinary excretion of chloramphenicol in these studies ranged from a low of 68% to a high of 99% over a 3-d period. From 8% to 12% of the antibiotic excreted is in the form of free chloramphenicol
Clindamycin	Clindamycin phosphate	IV or IM: 600–900 mg q8h PO: 0.15–0.45 g q6h	Pseudomembranous colitis has been reported with nearly all antibacterial agents, including clindamycin, and may range in severity from mild to life threatening.	Aerobic gram-positive cocci, including: *Staphylococcus aureus* (penicillinase- and nonpenicillinase-producing strains); *Staphylococcus epidermidis* (penicillinase- and nonpenicillinase-producing strains); *Streptococci* (except *Enterococcus faecalis*); *Pneumococci* Anaerobic gram-negative bacilli, including *Bacteroides* sp. (including *Bacteroides fragilis* group and *Bacteroides melaninogenicus* group) and *Fusobacterium* species Anaerobic gram-positive non–spore-forming bacilli, including *Propionibacterium*, *Eubacterium*, and *Actinomyces* sp. Anaerobic and microaerophilic gram-positive cocci, including *Peptococcus* sp., *Peptostreptococcus* sp., *Microaerophilic streptococci*, and *Clostridia*	The elimination half-life of clindamycin is increased slightly in patients with markedly reduced renal or hepatic function. Hemodialysis and peritoneal dialysis are not effective in removing clindamycin from the serum.

(*continued*)

TABLE 1.7

CONTINUED

Drug	Drug class	Adults (usual dose[a])	Actions, interactions, and others	Spectrum of activity, indications, and active against most strains of	Route, reduce dose, and contraindications
Clarithromycin	Semisynthetic macrolide antibiotic	Usual dose: PO: 0.5 g q12h	**Drug Interactions:** Patients who are receiving single doses of clarithromycin and theophylline or carbamazepine may be associated with an increase of serum theophylline and carbamazepine concentrations.	**Aerobic gram-positive microorganisms** *Staphylococcus aureus; Streptococcus pneumoniae; Streptococcus pyogenes* **Aerobic gram-negative microorganisms** *Haemophilus influenzae; Haemophilus parainfluenzae; Moraxella catarrhalis* **Other microorganisms** *Mycoplasma pneumoniae; Chlamydia pneumoniae* **Mycobacteria** *Mycobacterium avium* complex consisting of *Mycobacterium avium* and *Mycobacterium intracellulare* β-Lactamase production should have no effect on clarithromycin activity. Most strains of methicillin-resistant and oxacillin-resistant staphylococci are resistant to clarithromycin. **Helicobacter** *Helicobacter pylori*	Contraindications: Any of the following drugs: cisapride, pimozide, astemizole, terfenadine, and ergotamine or dihydroergotamine. If clarithromycin is coadministered with cisapride, pimozide, astemizole, or terfenadine resulting in cardiac arrhythmias (QT prolongation, ventricular tachycardia, ventricular fibrillation, and torsades de pointes), this is most likely due to inhibition of metabolism of these drugs.
Linezolid	Oxazolidinone	Usual dose: PO or IV dose: 600 mg q12h all indications except 400 mg q12h for uncomplicated skin infections	**Reversible myelosuppression** including anemia, leukopenia, pancytopenia, and thrombocytopenia has been reported in patients. In cases where the outcome is known, when linezolid was discontinued, the affected hematologic parameters have risen toward pretreatment levels. **Lactic acidosis** has been reported with the use of linezolid. Spontaneous reports of **serotonin syndrome** associated with the coadministration of linezolid and serotonergic agents, including antidepressants **Peripheral and optic neuropathy** have been reported in patients treated with linezolid	**Aerobic and facultative gram-positive microorganisms** *Enterococcus faecium* (vancomycin-resistant strains only); *Staphylococcus aureus* (including methicillin-resistant strains); *Streptococcus agalactiae; Streptococcus pneumoniae* (including multidrug-resistant isolates); *Streptococcus pyogenes* **Aerobic and facultative gram-positive microorganisms** *Enterococcus faecalis* (including vancomycin-resistant strains); *Enterococcus faecium* (vancomycin-susceptible strains); *Staphylococcus epidermidis* (including methicillin-resistant strains); *Staphylococcus haemolyticus; Viridans* group streptococci **Aerobic and facultative gram-negative microorganisms** *Pasteurella multocida*	Linezolid is primarily metabolized by oxidation of the morpholine ring, which results in two inactive ring-opened carboxylic acid metabolites: The aminoethoxyacetic acid metabolite (A) and the hydroxyethyl glycine metabolite (B). Nonrenal clearance accounts for approximately 65% of the total clearance of linezolid. Under steady-state conditions, approximately 30% of the dose appears in the urine as linezolid, 40% as metabolite B, and 10% as metabolite A.

Cunha BA. *Antibiotic Essentials*, 5th ed. Royal Oak, MI: Physicians Press; 2006.
From http://www.drugs.com (drug information online). Revised from November 2006.

TABLE 1.8

TETRACYCLINES

Drug	Drug class	Adults (usual dose[a])	Actions, interactions, and others	Spectrum of activity, indications, and active against most strains of	Route, reduce dose, and contraindications
Doxycycline	Derived from oxytetracycline	Usual dose: PO: 0.1 g q12h IV: 0.1 g q12h	The tetracyclines are primarily bacteriostatic and are thought to exert their antimicrobial effect by the inhibition of protein synthesis.	Wide range of gram-positive and gram-negative microorganisms **Aerobic gram-positive microorganisms** *Bacillus anthracis; Listeria monocytogenes; Staphylococcus aureus* **Aerobic gram-negative microorganisms** *Bartonella bacilliformis; Brucella sp.; Calymmatobacterium granulomatis; Campylobacter fetus; Francisella tularensis; Haemophilus ducreyi; Haemophilus influenzae; Neisseria gonorrhoeae; Vibrio cholerae; Yersinia pestis.* **Anaerobic microorganisms** *Actinomyces israelii; Fusobacterium fusiforme; Clostridium sp.* **Other microorganisms** *Borrelia recurrentis; Chlamydia psittaci; Chlamydia trachomatis; Mycoplasma pneumoniae; Rickettsiae; Treponema pallidum; Treponema pertenue*	Can be used in patients with renal failure Hemodialysis does not alter serum half-life.
Oxytetracycline	Tetracycline	Usual dose: PO: 0.25–0.5 g q6h IV: 0.5–1.0 g q12h	Primarily bacteriostatic	Wide range of gram-positive and gram-negative microorganisms, similar to other tetracyclines	Contraindicated in pregnancy, hepatotoxicity in mother, transplacental to fetus. Intravenous dosage over 2.0 g/d may be associated with fatal hepatotoxicity

Cunha BA. *Antibiotic Essentials*, 5th ed. Royal Oak, MI: Physicians Press; 2006.
From http://www.drugs.com (drug information online). Revised from November 2006.

TABLE 1.9

FLUOROQUINOLONES

Drug	Drug class	Adults (usual dose[a])	Actions, interactions, and others	Spectrum of activity, indications, and active against most strains of	Route, reduce dose, and contraindications
Ciprofloxacin	Fluoroquinolone	Usual dose: IV: 400 mg q8–12h (infusion over a period of 60 min) PO: 500–750 mg q12h	Inhibition of bacterial topoisomerase IV and DNA gyrase (both of which are type II topoisomerases), enzymes required for DNA replication, transcription, repair, and recombination **Drug interactions** with theophylline, caffeine, warfarin phenytoin, sulfonylurea glyburide, metronidazole, probenecid, piperacillin sodium, and cyclosporine	**Aerobic gram-positive microorganisms** *Enterococcus faecalis* (many strains are only moderately susceptible); *Staphylococcus aureus* (methicillin-susceptible strains only); *Staphylococcus epidermidis* (methicillin-susceptible strains only); *Staphylococcus saprophyticus; Staphylococcus pneumoniae* (penicillin-susceptible strains); *Staphylococcus pyogenes* **Aerobic gram-negative microorganism** *Citrobacter (diversus, freundii); Enterobacter cloacae; Escherichia coli; Haemophilus (influenzae, parainfluenzae); Klebsiella pneumoniae; Moraxella catarrhalis; Morganella morganii; Proteus (mirabilis, vulgaris); Providencia (rettgeri, stuartii); Pseudomonas aeruginosa; Serratia marcescens.* Also ciprofloxacin has been shown to be active against *Bacillus anthracis* both *in vitro* and by use of serum levels as a surrogate marker.	Contraindications: Concomitant administration with tizanidine Patients with impaired renal function: Creatinine clearance (mL/min): • >30 (see usual dose) • 5–29 (200–400 mg q18–24h)

| Levofloxacin | Fluoroquinolone | Usual dose: 250–750 mg qd PO or IV | Inhibition of bacterial topoisomerase IV and DNA gyrase (both of which are type II topoisomerases), enzymes required for DNA replication, transcription, repair, and recombination **Drug interactions** with theophylline, caffeine, warfarin, phenytoin, sulfonylurea glyburide, metronidazole, probenecid, piperacillin sodium, and cyclosporine | **Acute bacterial sinusitis** due to *Streptococcus pneumoniae, Haemophilus influenzae,* or *Moraxella catarrhalis*
Acute bacterial exacerbation of chronic bronchitis due to *Staphylococcus aureus, Streptococcus pneumoniae, Haemophilus influenzae, Haemophilus parainfluenzae,* or *Moraxella catarrhalis.*
Nosocomial pneumonia due to methicillin-susceptible *Staphylococcus aureus, Pseudomonas aeruginosa, Serratia marcescens, Escherichia coli, Klebsiella pneumoniae, Haemophilus influenzae,* or *Streptococcus pneumoniae.* Adjunctive therapy should be used as clinically indicated. Where *Pseudomonas aeruginosa* is a documented or presumptive pathogen, combination therapy with an antipseudomonal β-lactam is recommended.
Community-acquired pneumonia due to *Staphylococcus aureus, Streptococcus pneumoniae* (including multidrug-resistant strains [MDRSP]),[a] *Haemophilus influenzae, Haemophilus parainfluenzae, Klebsiella pneumoniae, Moraxella catarrhalis, Chlamydia pneumoniae, Legionella pneumophila,* or *Mycoplasma pneumoniae*
Complicated skin and skin structure infections due to methicillin-susceptible *Staphylococcus aureus, Enterococcus faecalis, Streptococcus pyogenes,* or *Proteus mirabilis.*
Uncomplicated skin and skin structure infections (mild to moderate) including abscesses, cellulites, furuncles, impetigo, pyoderma, and wound infections, due to *Staphylococcus aureus* or *Streptococcus pyogenes*
Chronic bacterial prostatitis due to *Escherichia coli, Enterococcus faecalis,* or *Staphylococcus epidermidis*
Complicated urinary tract infections (mild to moderate) due to *Enterococcus faecalis, Enterobacter cloacae, Escherichia coli, Klebsiella pneumoniae, Proteus mirabilis,* or *Pseudomonas aeruginosa*
Acute pyelonephritis (mild to moderate) caused by *Escherichia coli*
Uncomplicated urinary tract infections (mild to moderate) due to *Escherichia coli, Klebsiella pneumoniae,* or *Staphylococcus saprophyticus* | Clearance of levofloxacin is substantially reduced and plasma elimination half-life is substantially prolonged in patients with impaired renal function (creatinine clearance <50 mL/min), requiring dosage adjustment in such patients to avoid accumulation. Neither hemodialysis nor continuous ambulatory peritoneal dialysis (CAPD) is effective in removal of levofloxacin from the body, indicating that supplemental doses of levofloxacin are not required following hemodialysis or CAPD.
Adverse reactions:
Opiate screen false positives; photosensitivity; QTc interval prolongation and tendinopathy |
| Moxifloxacin | Fluoroquinolone | Usual dose: 400 mg PO or IV qd | The bactericidal action of moxifloxacin results from the interference with topoisomerase II and IV. | **Community-acquired pneumonia** (CAP), including CAP caused by multidrug-resistant *Streptococcus pneumoniae*[b]
Complicated skin and skin structure infections, including diabetic foot infections
Complicated intra-abdominal infections, including polymicrobial infections such as abscesses | Similar to other fluoroquinolones |

[a]MDRSP (multidrug-resistant *Streptococcus pneumoniae*) are strains resistant to two or more of the following antibiotics: Penicillin (minimum inhibitory concentration [MIC] = 2 μg/mL), second-generation cephalosporins (e.g., cefuroxime), macrolides, tetracyclines, and trimethoprim/sulfamethoxazole).
[b]Multidrug-resistant *S. pneumoniae* includes isolates previously known as PRSP (penicillin-resistant *S. pneumoniae*), and are strains resistant to two or more of the following antibiotics: Penicillin (MIC ≥2 mg/mL), second-generation cephalosporins (e.g., cefuroxime), macrolides, tetracyclines, and trimethoprim/sulfamethoxazole.
Cunha BA. *Antibiotic Essentials,* 5th ed. Royal Oak, MI: Physicians Press; 2006.
From http://www.drugs.com (drug information online). Revised from November 2006.

TABLE 1.10

POLYMYXINS

Drug	Drug class	Adults (usual dose[a])	Actions, interactions, and others	Spectrum of activity, indications, and active against most strains of	Route, reduce dose, and contraindications
Polymyxin B	Phospholipid cell membrane-altering antibiotic	0.75–1.25 mg/kg (IV) q12 h (1 mg = 10,000 units)	Colistin is polycationic and has both hydrophilic and lipophilic moieties. These interact with the bacterial cytoplasmic membrane, changing its permeability. This effect is bactericidal. The main toxicities described with intravenous treatment are nephrotoxicity and neurotoxicity. At a dose of 160 mg colistimethate IV q8h, very little nephrotoxicity is seen. (Conway SP, Etherington C, Munday J, et al. Safety and tolerability of bolus intravenous colistin in acute respiratory exacerbation in adults with cystic fibrosis. *Ann Pharmacother* 2000;34:1238–1242.)	Colistin is effective against gram-negative bacilli, except *Proteus* and *Burkholderia cepacia*, and is used as a polypeptide antibiotic. Multidrug-resistant *Acinetobacter baumannii*, even in *Acinetobacter baumannii* meningitis with intrathecal polymyxin E Mycobacterium aurum was susceptible to the antibiotic colistin (polymyxin E), which had an MIC of 5 μg/mL and an apparent bactericidal effect at concentrations above 50 μg/mL. Cited from David HL, Rastogi N. Antibacterial action of colistin (polymyxin E) against *Mycobacterium aurum*. *Antimicrob Agents Chemother.* 1985;27(5):701–707	Usage in pregnancy: The safety of this drug in human pregnancy has not been established.
Polymyxin E	Colistin (Polymyxin E) is a polymyxin antibiotic produced by certain strains of *Bacillus polymyxa* var. *colistinus*. There are 2 forms of colistin available commercially: colistin sulfate and colistimethate sodium (colistin methanesulfonate sodium, colistin sulfomethate sodium).	Colomycin 1,000,000 units is 80 mg colistimethate Coly-Mycin M 150 mg "colistin base" is 360 mg colistimethate or 4,500,000 units	Polymyxins bind to the cell membrane and alters its structure making it more permeable. The resulting water uptake leads to cell death. They are cationic, basic proteins that act like detergents. Intereactions: Anphoctericin B, amikacin, gentamicin, tobramycin, vancomycin. Adeverse effects: Renal failure (tubular necrosis). Neurotoxicity associated with very prolongued or high serum levels; neuromuscular blockade with renal failure and or neuromuscular disorders	Bactericidal for gram-negative; little to no effect on gram-positive since cell wall is too thick to permit access to membrane	Colistin sulfate and colistimethate sodium are eliminated from the body by different routes.

Cunha BA. *Antibiotic Essentials*, 5th ed. Royal Oak, MI: Physicians Press; 2006.
From http://www.drugs.com (drug information online). Revised from November 2006.

TABLE I.11

AMINOGLYCOSIDES

Drug	Drug class	Adults (usual dose[a])	Actions, interactions, and others	Spectrum of activity, indications, and active against most strains of	Route, reduce dose, and contraindications
Gentamicin	Aminoglycoside antibiotic, derived from *Micromonospora purpurea*, an actinomycete	**Usual dose:** Gentamicin sulfate 3 mg/kg/d q8h In patients with life-threatening infections: 5 mg/kg/d q24h (preferred over q8h dosing) Intravenous use only for gentamicin sulfate in 0.9% sodium chloride.	Bactericidal antibiotic that acts by inhibiting normal protein synthesis in susceptible microorganisms. **Drug interactions:** Amphotericin B, cephalothin, cyclosporine, enflurane, methoxyflurane, polymyxin B, radiographic contrast, vancomycin (increase nephrotoxicity), cisplatinum, etc. (see specifications of the product)	*Escherichia coli; Proteus* sp. (indole-positive and indole-negative); *Pseudomonas aeruginosa*; species of *Klebsiella-Enterobacter-Serratia* group; *Citrobacter* sp.; and *Staphylococcus* sp. (including penicillin and methicillin-resistant strains) · Gentamicin is also active *in vitro* against species of *Salmonella* and *Shigella*.	To adjust the doses for patients with renal impairment **Adverse reactions:** Nephrotoxicity: Adverse renal effects have been reported. They occur more frequently in patients with a history of renal impairment and in patients treated for longer periods or with larger dosages than recommended. Others such as neurotoxicity (serious adverse effects on both vestibular and auditory branches of the eighth nerve), peripheral neuropathy, or encephalopathy, including numbness, skin tingling, muscle twitching, convulsions, and a myasthenia gravis-like syndrome, have been reported. (See specifications of the product.)
Amikacin	Semisynthetic aminoglycoside antibiotic, derived from kanamycin	**Usual dose:** Amikacin sulfate IV: 15 mg/kg or 1 g q24h (preferred to q12h dosing)	**Drug interactions:** See gentamicin sulfate.	**Gram negative** Amikacin is active *in vitro* against *Pseudomonas* sp., *Escherichia coli, Proteus* sp. (indole-positive and indole-negative), *Providencia* sp., *Klebsiella-Enterobacter-Serratia* sp., *Acinetobacter* (formerly Mima-Herellea) sp., and *Citrobacter freundii* When strains of the above organisms are found to be resistant to other aminoglycosides, including gentamicin, tobramycin, and kanamycin, many are susceptible to amikacin *in vitro*. **Gram positive** Amikacin is active *in vitro* against penicillinase and nonpenicillinase-producing *Staphylococcus* sp. including methicillin-resistant strains. However, aminoglycosides in general have a low order of activity against other gram-positive organisms.	See gentamicin sulfate.
Tobramycin	Aminoglycoside antibiotic, derived from the actinomycete *Streptomyces tenebrarius*	**Usual dose:** Tobramycin sulfate: IV: 5 mg/kg q24h or 240 mg q24h (preferred over q8h dosing). The dosage should be reduced to 3 mg/kg/d as soon as clinically indicated.	Tobramycin acts by inhibiting synthesis of protein in bacterial cells. **Drug interactions:** See gentamicin sulfate.	**Gram-positive aerobes** *Staphylococcus aureus* **Gram-negative aerobes** *Citrobacter* sp., *Enterobacter* sp., *Escherichia coli, Klebsiella* sp., *Morganella morganii, Pseudomonas aeruginosa, Proteus mirabilis, Proteus vulgaris, Providencia* sp., *Serratia* sp. Aminoglycosides have a low order of activity against most gram-positive organisms, including *Streptococcus pyogenes, Streptococcus pneumoniae,* and *Enterococci*	See gentamicin sulfate.

Cunha BA. *Antibiotic Essentials*, 5th ed. Royal Oak, MI: Physicians Press; 2006.
From http://www.drugs.com (drug information online). Revised from November 2006.

TABLE I.12

MISCELLANEOUS

Drug	Drug class	Adults (usual dose[a])	Actions, interactions, and others	Spectrum of activity, indications, and active against most strains of	Route, reduce dose, and contraindications
Metronidazole	Nitroimidazole antiparasitic/ antibiotic	Usual dose: IV: 1 g q/24h PO: 500 mg q12h	Metronidazole is a synthetic antibacterial compound. **Drug interactions:** Warfarin and other oral coumarin anticoagulants, phenytoin or phenobarbital, cimetidine, and disulfiram	**Anaerobic gram-negative bacilli,** including *Bacteroides* sp., including the *Bacteroides fragilis* group (*B. fragilis, B. distasonis, B. ovatus, B. thetaiotaomicron, B. vulgatus*); *Fusobacterium* sp. **Anaerobic gram-positive bacilli,** including *Clostridium* sp. and susceptible strains of *Eubacterium* **Anaerobic gram-positive cocci,** including *Peptococcus* sp.; *Peptostreptococcus* sp.	Primary mode of elimination: Hepatic
Trimethoprim (TMP)/sulfame-thoxazole (SMX) or cotrimoxazole	Synthetic folate antagonist/ sulfonamide	Usual dose: IV or PO: 2.5–5 mg/kg q6h	Sulfamethoxazole is bacteriostatic and trimethoprim is bactericidal **Drug interactions:** Warfarin (monitoring carefully); phenytoin (folate deficiencies when is used concomitantly); thiazides increased incidence of thrombocytopenia with purpura in elderly patients; cyclosporine (nephrotoxicity reversible); digoxin; indomethacin; pyrimethamine; tricyclic antidepressants; amantadine; methotrexate; and oral hypoglycemic agents	Primary agent in the treatment of *Pneumocystis carinii pneumonia* (PCP), an opportunistic infection in patients with HIV/AIDS, and as secondary prophylaxis of PCP in patients who have already had at least one episode of PCP. Also is indicated for the treatment of chronic bronchitis, enterocolitis caused by strains of *Shigella* (*flexneri* and *sonnei*), acute otitis media in children, traveler's diarrhea caused by enterotoxigenic *Escherichia coli* and *Shigella* sp., and bacterial urinary tract infections	SMX-TMP is metabolized in the liver. Urinary concentrations of both active drugs are decreased in patients with impaired renal function. Only small amounts of trimethoprim are excreted in feces via biliary elimination. Trimethoprim and active sulfamethoxazole are moderately removed by hemodialysis.

Cunha BA. *Antibiotic Essentials*, 5th ed. Royal Oak, MI: Physicians Press; 2006.
From http://www.drugs.com (drug information online). Revised from November 2006.

TABLE I.13

ANTIFUNGALS

Drug	Drug class	Adults (usual dose[a])	Actions, interactions, and others	Spectrum of activity, indications, and active against most strains of	Route, reduce dose, and contraindications
Amphotericin B	Antifungal Polyene macrolide antibiotic produced by soil bacteria *Strepto-myces nodosus*	Usual dose: IV: 0.5–0.8 mg/kg q24h	Amphotericin B is the gold standard for the treatment of serious and invasive systemic mycosis as well as for Kala-Azar. **Drug interactions:** Avoid concomitant administration of nephrotoxic drugs and bone marrow suppressants.	Amphotericin B has useful activity against candidiasis, cryptococcosis, histoplasmosis, blastomycosis, paracoccidioidomycosis, coccidioidomycosis, aspergillosis, extracutaneous sporotrichosis, zygomycosis (mucormycosis), penicilliosis (*Penicilliosis marneffei*) pseudallescheriasis, hyalohyphomycosis (including infection due to *Acremonium, Fusarium, Penicillium*, etc.) and phaeohyphomycosis (including infection due to *Alternaria, Bipolaris, Cladosporium, Cladophialophora, Curvularia, Exophiala, Exserohilum, Fonsecaea, Phialophora, Wangiella*, etc.). Empirical antifungal therapy is useful to granulocytopenic patients with persistent or recurrent fever.[a]	Primary mode of elimination: Metabolized The most common cause for withdrawal of or failure to continue amphotericin B therapy is its severe renal toxicity in nearly half of all the patients. The second problem, which is a major one, is the nephrotoxicity of amphotericin B.
Liposomal amphotericin B	Antifungal Polyene macrolide antibiotic True liposomal preparation of ampho-tericin B in which lipid complex of liposomes is constituted of lecithin and cholesterol	Usual dose: IV: 3–6 mg/kg q24h	Is the most effective and affordable drug for treatment of both systemic mycosis and **Kala-Azar.** **Drug interactions:** As with conventional amphotericin B, avoid concomitant administration of nephrotoxic drugs and bone marrow suppressants, only and in patients with hypokalemia.	Amphotericin B shows a high order of *in vitro* activity against many species of fungi *viz. Histoplasma capsulatum, Cryptococcus immitis, Candida* sp., *Blastomyces dermatitidis, Rhodotorula, Cryptococcus neoformans, Sporothrix schenckii, Mucor* sp., *Aspergillus fumigatus, Malassezia furfur, Trichosporon beigelii, Saccharomyces cerevisiae, Scedosporium* sp., *Paecilomyces* sp., *Penicillium* sp., *Fusarium* sp., *Bipolaris* sp., *Exophiala* sp., *Cladophialophora* sp., *Absidia* sp., *Apophysomyces* sp., *Cunninghamella* sp., *Rhizomucor* sp., *Rhizopus* sp., *and Saksenaea* sp. These fungi are inhibited by concentrations of amphotericin B ranging from 0.03 to 1 μg/mL *in vitro.* Amphotericin B also has activity against species of *Leishmania* and is found to be effective in the treatment of Kala-Azar.	Primary mode of elimination: Metabolized

[a]Walsh TJ, Lee J, Lecciones J. Empiric therapy with amphotericin B in febrile granulocytopenic patients. *Rev Infect Dis.* 1991;13:496–503.

(*continued*)

TABLE I.13

CONTINUED

Drug	Drug class	Adults (usual dose[a])	Actions, interactions, and others	Spectrum of activity, indications, and active against most strains of	Route, reduce dose, and contraindications
Fluconazole	Triazole antifungal agent	**Usual dose:** 400 mg (IV/PO) × 1 dose, then 200 mg (IV/PO) q24h Usual dose for candidemia: 400 mg (IV/PO) q24h after loading dose of 800 mg (IV/PO) Meningeal dose: 400 mg (IV/PO) q24h	Fluconazole is a highly selective inhibitor of fungal cytochrome P450 sterol C-14 α-demethylation. **Drug interactions:** Oral contraceptives, cimetidine, antacid, hydrochlorothiazide, rifampin, warfarin, phenytoin, cyclosporine, zidovudine, theophylline, terfenadine, oral hypoglycemic agents, tolbutamide, glipizide, glyburide, rifabutin, tacrolimus, cisapride, midazolam, azithromycin (not significant)	**Prophylaxis** Fluconazole is also indicated to decrease the incidence of candidiasis in patients undergoing bone marrow transplantation who receive cytotoxic chemotherapy and/or radiation therapy. Fluconazole exhibits *in vitro* activity against *Cryptococcus neoformans* and *Candida* spp. Fungistatic activity has also been demonstrated in normal and immunocompromised animal models for systemic and intracranial fungal infections due to *Cryptococcus neoformans* and for systemic infections due to *Candida albicans*. **Fluconazole is indicated for the treatment of:** 1. Vaginal candidiasis (vaginal yeast infections due to *Candida*) 2. Oropharyngeal and esophageal candidiasis. In open noncomparative studies of relatively small numbers of patients, fluconazole was also effective for the treatment of *Candida* urinary tract infections, peritonitis, and systemic *Candida* infections including candidemia, disseminated candidiasis, and pneumonia. 3. Cryptococcal meningitis	**Primary mode of elimination:** Renal **Contraindications:** Terfenadine and cisapride Fluconazole has been associated with rare cases of serious hepatic toxicity.
Voriconazole	Triazole antifungal agent	**Usual dose:** **IV dosing:** Loading dose of 6 mg/kg (IV) q12h × 1 day, then maintenance dose of 4 mg/kg (IV) q12h. It is possible to switch to weight-based PO maintenance IV dose. **PO dosing:** 1. If weight ≥40 kg: Loading dose of 400 mg (PO) q12h × 1 day, then maintenance dose of 200 mg (PO) q12h. If response is inadequate, increase dose to 300 mg (PO) q12h. 2. If weight <40 kg: Loading dose of 200 mg (PO) × 1 day, then maintenance dose of 100 mg (PO) q12h. If response is inadequate, increase dose to 150 mg (PO) q12h. In patients with chronic and/or non life-threatening infections, loading dose may be given PO.	**Mode of action** of voriconazole is the inhibition of fungal cytochrome P450-mediated 14 α-lanosterol demethylation, an essential step in fungal ergosterol biosynthesis. **Drug interactions:** Benzodiazepines, vinca alkaloids, carbamazepine, ergo alkaloids, rifampin, rifabutin, sirolimus, long-acting barbiturates (see contraindications), cyclosporine, omeprazole, tacrolimus, phenytoin, warfarin, statins, dihydropyridine, calcium channel blockers (low arterial pressure), sulfonylureas (hypoglycemia). Potential hepatotoxicity risk	**Invasive aspergillosis** Indicated for the primary treatment of acute invasive aspergillosis (*Aspergillus* spp.) Also with *Fusarium* spp. and *Scedosporium* spp. **Other disease-causing agents** Voriconazole was shown to be effective against both *Scedosporium apiospermum* and *Fusarium* spp. For *Scedosporium apiospermum*, a successful response to Vfend was reported in 15 of 24 subjects (63%). In those with *Fusarium* spp., 9 of 21 (43%) were successfully treated with voriconazole.	**Primary mode of elimination:** Hepatic **Contraindications:** Long-acting barbiturates

Itraconazole	Antifungal agent	**Itraconazole exhibits *in vitro* activity against** *Blastomyces dermatitidis, Histoplasma capsulatum, Histoplasma duboisii, Aspergillus flavus, Aspergillus fumigatus, Candida albicans,* and *Cryptococcus neoformans.* **Itraconazole also exhibits varying *in vitro* activity against** *Sporothrix schenckii, Trichophyton species, Candida krusei,* and other *Candida* species. Fungistatic activity has been demonstrated against disseminated fungal infections caused by *Blastomyces dermatitidis, Histoplasma duboisii, Aspergillus fumigatus, Coccidioides immitis, Cryptococcus neoformans, Paracoccidioides brasiliensis, Sporothrix schenckii, Trichophyton rubrum,* and *Trichophyton mentagrophytes.*	Usual dose: 200 mg (IV/PO) q24h 200 mg capsule/solution (PO) q24h. Begin itraconazole for acute/severe infections with a loading regimen of 200 mg (IV) q12h × 2 days (4 doses), then give 200 mg (IV or PO) q24h maintenance dose. Each IV dose should be infused over 60 minutes. **Drug interactions:** Coadministration of cisapride, pimozide, quinidine, *dofetilide,* or levacetylmethadol (levomethadyl) with itraconazole.

Primary mode of elimination: Hepatic; metabolized predominantly by the cytochrome P450 3A4 isoenzyme system (CYP3A4) Patients with impaired hepatic function should be carefully monitored when taking itraconazole.
If signs or symptoms of congestive heart failure appear during administration of itraconazole, monitor carefully and consider other treatment alternatives.
Contraindications: Cisapride, oral midazolam, pimozide, quinidine, dofetilide, triazolam, and levacetylmethadol (levomethadyl) are contraindicated with itraconazole.

Caspofungin	Echinocandin antifungal	Caspofungin is active against all species of *Candida.* It is extremely active against all species except *Candida parapsilosis, Candida guilliermondii,* and *Candida lusitaniae,* against which it is moderately active. Caspofungin is also very active against all *Aspergillus* sp. It does not kill *Aspergillus* completely in test tubes. There is a very limited amount of activity against *Coccidioides immitis, Blastomyces dermatitidis, Scedosporium* sp., *Paecilomyces varioti,* and *Histoplasma capsulata* but it is likely that the activity is not sufficient for clinical use.	Usual dose: 70 mg (IV) × 1 dose, then 50 mg (IV) q24h In patients weighing more than 80 kg it is recommended that 70 mg/d is given rather than 50 mg/d. Patients with moderate liver insufficiency should receive a dose of 35 mg/d.

Caspofungin is not an inhibitor and is a poor substrate for cytochrome people P450 enzymes.
Drug interactions: Cyclosporine, tacrolimus, carbamazepine, rifampin, dexamethasone, efavirenz, nelfinavir, nevirapine, phenytoin

Primary mode of elimination: Hepatic

From Cunha BA. *Antibiotic Essentials*, 5th ed. Royal Oak, MI: Physicians Press; 2006, with permission.
From http://www.drugs.com (drug information online). Revised from November 2006.

Note: Page numbers followed by *f* indicate figures; page numbers followed by *t* indicate tables.